Contents in Brief

T0156199

Each update, each change has been made in hopes of providing a premier text to guide the nursing student in their quest for a quality education toward the entry into what I believe to be one of the most satisfying career choices. With each topic I have read and each page written I am in awe of nursing and all it encompasses. None of this would have been possible without the unwavering support of my family, friends, and colleagues.

To my husband Anthony and my daughter Jaelyn Elizabeth, whose love and cheers have encouraged me in this process, I appreciate your support and understanding of the long hours and hard work needed to bring this book to publication. I love you both.

To my writing partner, Kelly Gosnell, words cannot express my respect for your hard work and dedication to our dream to produce a work we are infinitely proud of. You have been a source of strength and friendship in this endeavor. I look forward to many future chapters of writing adventures. Finally to the Elsevier team, I thank you for the continued belief in this title and the partnership striving to produce it.

Kim Cooper

To my husband Ed and my daughters Katelyn and Kinsey, I thank you for your love, patience, and understanding during the time it took to complete this endeavor starting with the seventh edition. Your acceptance of the demands on my time made it all possible. In the last edition I expressed my gratitude to the newest family members, Jared and Miles. Since that time, we have added three new family members to the life of a nursing textbook author. Taj, Ivory, and Owen have now become a part of our textbook! I appreciate all you have done to support and brighten the road along the way.

To all my wonderful family, friends, and colleagues, your constant support and belief in me while completing this project mean more to me than I can express.

To my writing partner, Kim Cooper, without you getting me into the crazy world of ancillary writing years ago, I would not have had the opportunity to tackle this fantastic opportunity of nursing textbook authorship with you. It has been, and hopefully will continue to be, an awesome ride.

Kelly Gosnell

A tailored education experience —

Sherpath book-organized collections

ELSEVIER

Sherpath book-organized collections offer:

Objective-based, digital lessons, mapped chapter-by-chapter to the textbook, that make it easy to find applicable digital assignment content.

Adaptive quizzing with personalized questions that correlate directly to textbook content.

Teaching materials that align to the text and are organized by chapter for quick and easy access to invaluable class activities and resources.

Elsevier ebooks that provide convenient access to textbook content, even offline.

Sherpath is the digital teaching and learning technology designed specifically for healthcare education.

Foundations of Nursing

EDITION
9

Foundations of Nursing

Kim Cooper, RN, MSN
Associate Professor and Dean
School of Nursing
Ivy Tech Community College
Terre Haute, Indiana
President, Indiana State Board of Nursing

Kelly Gosnell, RN, MSN
Associate Professor and Department Chair
School of Nursing
Ivy Tech Community College
Terre Haute, Indiana

ELSEVIER

Elsevier
3251 Riverport Lane
St. Louis, Missouri 63043

FOUNDATIONS OF NURSING, NINTH EDITION   ISBN: 978-0-323-81203-0

Notice

Practitioners and researchers must always rely on their own experience and knowledge in evaluating and using any information, methods, compounds or experiments described herein. Because of rapid advances in the medical sciences, in particular, independent verification of diagnoses and drug dosages should be made. To the fullest extent of the law, no responsibility is assumed by Elsevier, authors, editors or contributors for any injury and/or damage to persons or property as a matter of products liability, negligence or otherwise, or from any use or operation of any methods, products, instructions, or ideas contained in the material herein.

Previous editions copyrighted 2019, 2015, 2011, 2006, 2003, 1999, 1995, and 1991.

Library of Congress Control Number: 2021945622

Senior Content Strategist: Brandi Graham
Senior Content Development Specialist: Laura Goodrich
Publishing Services Manager: Julie Eddy
Senior Project Manager: Cindy Thoms
Senior Book Designer: Renee Duenow

Printed in the United States of America

Last digit is the print number: 9   8   7   6   5   4   3   2   1

Working together
to grow libraries in
developing countries

www.elsevier.com • www.bookaid.org

Acknowledgments

The ninth edition has undergone revisions geared to prepare the nursing student for NCLEX® Next Generation. The questions at the end of each chapter show increasing rigor and include increased numbers of alternative format styled questions. Chapters have case studies that challenge the student to critically process information.

Chapter 6 focuses on health disparities between populations. The responsibilities facing the LPN/LVN concerning transcultural nursing and the importance of cultural competence is highlighted. The rights and needs of individuals with disabilities is discussed.

The Covid-19 pandemic has shaken the healthcare industry to its core. Chapter 7, Asepsis and Infection Control, contains updates about not only the coronavirus but other common pathogens commonly encountered by the LPN/LVN.

Chapters 14 and 15 reflect updated procedure descriptions. New devices and practice expectations are featured.

In Chapter 20 alternative and complementary therapies are reviewed. The updates to the chapter focuses on the growing choices available to patients and families. The timely information will allow the LPN/LVN student to consider the impact on their own future practice.

Key family definitions and compositions are updated in Chapter 24. As society works to increase recognition and acceptance of expanded family structures the LPN/LVN requires the information presented.

Americans are aging. The baby boomers are approaching retirement and the onset of those health concerns that often begin in middle and late adulthood. The stressors of caring for those individuals is discussed in Chapter 38. As LPN/LVNs often seek employment in longterm or assistive care settings this chapter will outline the populations impacted most.

The nurturing of the youth is a focus for nursing. Chapter 30 with its focus on health promotion for children outlines potential barriers to health care for children. In addition, areas of growing concern to today's youth including obesity, media exposure, and the use of alternative smoking devices are investigated.

At the same time, this edition has maintained the strong foundation that it has had since very the first edition. Special thanks to our photographer, Katelyn Gosnell Richey, for her hard work in adding over 100 new photographs between *Foundations of Nursing* and *Adult Health Nursing;* to our many family, friends, and colleagues for volunteering to be our models; and to Ivy Tech Community College, Terre Haute, Indiana, for their willingness to share their facility setting for many of the updated photographs.

The work on the ninth edition kicked off under the direction of Nancy O'Brien, Content Strategist. She was a returning team member from the eighth edition. Shortly after work began she transitioned to a much deserved retirement.

Laura Goodrich, Senior Development Specialist, and Cindy Thoms, Senior Project Manager. Their unwavering support and continued belief in our vision were invaluable in the completion of the works.

The role of the practical nurse is to be a key member of the health care team. The United States Department of Labor forecasts that between 2020 and 2030 the need for LPN/LVNs will grow nearly 10%. More than 60,000 job openings will be present annually for the LPN/LVN. The education of these dedicated men and women is needed to prepare them for entry to practice. Those contributors, reviewers, and dedicated colleagues have shared invaluable expertise in this journey in bringing this work to life, and we are forever indebted.

Contributors and Reviewers

CONTRIBUTORS

Terra Ripple Baughman, MSN Nursing
Assistant Professor of Nursing
Nursing
Ivy Tech Community College of Indiana
Wabash Valley Region, Indiana

Tracy Blanc, RN, MSN
Associate Professor
Nursing
Ivy Tech Community College of Indiana
Terre Haute Indiana

Emily Cannon, DNP, RN
Assistant Professor
School of Nursing
Indiana State University
Terre Haute, Indiana

Ashley Carter, DNP, RN, CNE
Assistant Professor of Nursing
College of Nursing and Health Professions
University of Southern Indiana
Evansville, Indiana

Charlotte Connerton, EdD, RN, CNE
Assistant Professor
Nursing
University of Southern Indiana
Evansville, Indiana

Michele Gonser, RN, MSN
Director of Quality Improvement
Nursing
Ivy Tech Community College
Fort Wayne, Indiana

Traci Michelle McNeil, RN, BSN, MSN
Associate Professor
School of Nursing
Ivy Tech Community College
Terre Haute, Indiana

Catherine S. Moe, BSN, MS, EdD
Associate Professor-Dean (Retired)
Nursing
Lakeview College of Nursing
Danville, Illinois
Visiting Faculty
Nursing
University of Illinois
Champaign, Illinois
Assistant Professor
Nursing
Lakeview College of Nursing
Charleston, Illinois

Amy Pierce, MSN, RN
Instructor of Nursing
College of Nursing and Health Professions
University of Southern Indiana
Evansville, Indiana
Registered Nurse
Deaconess Comprehensive Pain Management Center
Deaconess Health Systems
Newburgh, Indiana

REVIEWERS

Amanda Churchman, RN, MSN
PN Program Director
Red River Technology Center
Duncan, Oklahoma

Heather L. Clark, DNP, RN
Practical Nursing Program Director
Penn State University
Center Valley, Pennsylvania

Linda Cline, RN, MSN/Ed
Practical Nursing Program Director
Assistant Professor
Southwest Virginia Community College
Cedar Bluff, Virginia

Odelia Garcia, MS, MSN, BSN, RN
Vocational Nursing Instructor
Texas State Technical College – Harlingen
Harlingen, Texas

Alice M. Hupp, BS, RN
Lead Instructor
North Central Texas College
Gainesville, Texas

Lorraine Kelley, BSHA, RN
Faculty
Pensacola State College
Pensacola, Florida

Molly M. Showalter, MSN Ed, RN
Interim Director Vocational Nursing Program
Texas Southmost College
Brownsville, Texas

Elaine Kay Strouss, MSN, BSN, RN
Dean of the School of Health Sciences
Community College of Beaver County
Monaca, Pennsylvania

LPN/LVN Advisory Board

Nancy Bohnarczyk, MA
Adjunct Instructor
College of Mount St. Vincent
New York, New York

Nicola Contreras, BN, RN
Faculty
Galen College
San Antonio, Texas

Dolores Cotton, MSN, RN
Practical Nursing Coordinator
Meridian Technology Center
Stillwater, Oklahoma

Patricia Donovan, MSN, RN
Director of Practical Nursing and Curriculum Chair
Porter and Chester Institute
Rocky Hill, Connecticut

Nancy Haughton, MSN, RN
Practical Nursing Program Faculty
Chester County Intermediate Unit
Downingtown, Pennsylvania

Dawn Johnson, DNP, RN, Ed
Practical Nurse Educator
Reno, Nevada

Mary E. Johnson, RN, MSN
Director of Nursing
Dorsey Schools
Roseville, Michigan

Bonnie Kehm, PhD, RN
Faculty Program Director
Excelsior College
Albany, New York

Tawnya S. Lawson, MS, RN
Dean, Practical Nursing Program
Hondros College
Westerville, Ohio

Kristin Madigan, MS, RN
Nursing Faculty
Pine Technical and Community College
Pine City, Minnesota

Hana Malik, DNP, FNP-BC
Academic Director
Illinois College of Nursing
Lombard, Illinois

Mary Lee Pollard, PhD, RN, CNE
Dean, School of Nursing
Excelsior College
Albany, New York

Barbara Ratliff, MSN, RN
Nursing Program Chair
Cincinnati State Great Oaks School of Practical
    Nursing
Cincinnati, Ohio

Mary Ruiz-Nuve, RN, MSN
Director of Practical Nursing Program
St. Louis College of Health Careers
St. Louis, Missouri

Renee Sheehan, RN, MSN/Ed
Director of Nursing, Vocational Nursing
Nursing Assistant Programs
Summit College
Colton, California

Fleur de Liza S. Tobias-Cuyco, BSc, CPhT
Dean, Director of Student Affairs, and Instructor
Preferred College of Nursing
Los Angeles, California

To the Instructor

The ninth edition of *Foundations of Nursing* was developed to educate the practical/vocational nursing student in the fundamentals of nursing required to care competently and safely for a wide variety of patients in various settings. As the level of knowledge and responsibility increases for LPN/LVNs in all health care settings from acute to community-based care, it is essential that a text such as *Foundations of Nursing* be available to educate the student for the growing demands of this profession.

This full-color companion text to *Adult Health Nursing* provides the knowledge base necessary for the expanding role of the LPN/LVN while remaining accessible, clearly written, user-friendly, and portable. This new edition was revised to incorporate the most current and clinically relevant information available on the following topics:

- Historical, legal, and ethical aspects of nursing
- Communication
- Physical assessment
- Nursing process and critical thinking
- Documentation
- Cultural and ethical considerations in nursing interventions
- Growth and development across the life span
- Death and dying
- Safety
- Medical-surgical asepsis
- Pain management, comfort, rest, and sleep
- Complementary and alternative therapies
- Basic nutrition and nutritional therapy
- Fluids and electrolytes
- Mathematics review and medication administration
- Emergency first aid nursing, including terrorism and bioterrorism interventions
- Maternal, neonatal, and pediatric care
- Gerontologic nursing and care of the older adult
- Mental health and community health
- Role of the LPN/LVN and leadership

Finally, it is our belief that nursing will always be both an art and a science. This philosophy is reflected throughout the text.

ORGANIZATION AND STANDARD FEATURES

The organization of the eighth edition continues to follow the strengths of the previous edition, based on positive comments from educators and students. The basic nursing skills are provided throughout the text. Two new chapters have been added to provide the student with greater focus on individual concepts. Oxygenation concepts are now found in Chapter 14, and elimination concepts are housed in Chapter 15. Some additional changes include moving eye, ear, and vaginal irrigations to the medication chapter; nasogastric feedings to the nutrition chapter; and heat and cold therapy has moved to the newly named Hygiene and Care of the Patient's Environment chapter. Medical-surgical nursing—with an overview of anatomy and physiology and a separate chapter on care of the surgical patient—are available in the companion text, *Adult Health Nursing*.

TABLE OF CONTENTS

The text is divided into 7 units with 41 chapters. Chapters have been reorganized for easy, logical association of content. Updates have been made to ensure that students have access to the most current information. To match a growing emphasis on holistic care, there are significant updates to alternative and complementary therapy information presented. The legal, ethical, and professional aspects of nursing practice have been updated. Revision to health care and nursing practice have been made to provide students with an updated viewpoint.

CHAPTER ORGANIZATION

Disorders chapters typically are organized in the following format for more effective learning:
- Etiology and Pathophysiology
- Clinical Manifestations
- Assessment (with subjective and objective data)
- Diagnostic Tests
- Medical Management
- Nursing Interventions (including relevant medications)
- Nursing Diagnoses
- Patient Teaching
- Prognosis

NURSING PROCESS

The nursing process as applied to specific disorders is integrated throughout. A special nursing process summary section appears at the end of appropriate chapters, enabling the reader to see more clearly its application to the chapter content as a whole. For this text the authors have replaced nursing diagnoses with a patient problem list to better describe health problems the patient experiences. These statements provide a problem-centered approach to nursing care. We have emphasized the role of the LPN/LVN in the nursing process as follows:

- The LPN/LVN will participate in planning care for the patient based on the patient's needs.
- The LPN/LVN will review the patient's plan of care and recommend revisions as needed.
- The LPN/LVN will follow defined prioritization for patient care.
- The LPN/LVN will use clinical pathways, care maps, or care plans to guide and review patient care.

REFERENCES AND SUGGESTED READINGS

References and Suggested Readings are grouped by chapter and listed at the end of the book for easy access. *Additional Resources* such as websites and agencies are included where applicable.

In the appendixes, *Common Abbreviations* are listed along with The Joint Commission's *Lists of Dangerous Abbreviations, Acronyms, and Symbols* to promote safety in clinical practice in such areas as avoiding dosage errors, and *Laboratory Reference Values* provide quick access to important information. *Answers to the Review Questions* for the NCLEX® Examination are provided in Appendix C.

LPN THREADS

The ninth edition of *Foundations of Nursing* shares some features and design elements with other Elsevier LPN/LVN textbooks. The purpose of these *LPN Threads* is to make it easier for students and instructors to use the variety of books required by the relatively brief and demanding LPN/LVN curriculum. *LPN Threads* include the following:

- Efforts are continually made to keep the *reading level* of our LPN texts around 10th grade to increase the consistency among chapters and ensure the text is easy to understand.
- *Full-color design, cover, photos,* and *illustrations* are visually appealing and pedagogically useful.
- *Objectives* (numbered) begin each chapter. Chapter objectives provide a framework for content and are especially important in providing the structure for the TEACH Lesson Plans for the textbook.
- *Key Terms* with phonetic pronunciations and page number references are listed at the beginning of each chapter. Key terms appear in color in the chapter and are defined briefly, with full definitions in the *Glossary.* Simple phonetic pronunciations accompany difficult medical, nursing, or scientific terms or other words that may be difficult for students to pronounce.
- A wide variety of *special features* related to critical thinking, clinical practice, care of the older adult, health promotion, safety, patient teaching, complementary and alternative therapies, communication,

home health care, delegation and assignment, and more. Refer to the To the Student section of this introduction on page xiv for descriptions of each of these features.

- *Critical Thinking Questions* with each Nursing Care Plan give students opportunities to practice critical thinking and clinical decision-making skills with realistic patient scenarios. Answers are provided in the Instructor Resources section on the Evolve website.
- *Key Points,* located at the end of chapters, follow the chapter objectives and serve as a useful chapter review.
- A full suite of *Instructor Resources* including TEACH Lesson Plans and Lecture Outlines, PowerPoint Lecture Slides, Test Bank, and Image Collection. Each of these teaching resources is described in detail below.
- In addition to consistent content, design, and support resources, these textbooks benefit from the advice and input of the *Elsevier LPN/LVN Advisory Board.*

TEACHING AND LEARNING PACKAGE

FOR STUDENTS

- An *Evolve website* provides free student resources, including additional review questions for the NCLEX Examination for every chapter, calculators, and animations and video clips.
- The *Study Guide for Foundations of Nursing* is designed to promote learning, understanding, and application of the content in the textbook. Each chapter ties specific activities to specific objectives rather than simply listing objectives and activities separately. Activities include hundreds of labeling, matching, and fill-in-the-blank questions, each with textbook page references; critical thinking questions with clinical scenarios; and multiple-choice and alternate-format questions for NCLEX review. The complete answer key is provided to instructors in the Instructor Resources section of the Evolve website. *Sold separately.*
- *Virtual Clinical Excursions* is an interactive workbook/online package that guides the student through a multifloor virtual hospital in a hands-on clinical learning experience. Students can assess and analyze information, diagnose, set priorities, and implement and evaluate care. NCLEX-style review questions provide immediate testing of clinical knowledge. *Sold separately.*

FOR INSTRUCTORS

The comprehensive *Evolve Resources With TEACH Instructor Resource* provides a rich array of teaching tools and includes the following:

- *TEACH Lesson Plans With Lecture Outlines,* based on the textbook learning objectives, provide ready-to-use lesson plans that tie together all the text and ancillary components provided for *Foundations of Nursing.*

- A collection of more than 200 *PowerPoint Lecture Slides* are specific to the text.
- A *Test Bank,* delivered in ExamView, provides approximately 1500 multiple-choice and alternate-format NCLEX-style questions. Each question includes the correct answer, rationale, topic, objective, cognitive level, step of the nursing process, and

NCLEX category of patient needs, as well as corresponding textbook page references.

- An *Image Collection* contains nearly 500 images from the textbook. Images are suitable for incorporation into classroom lectures, PowerPoint presentations, or distance-learning applications.
- *Answer Keys* are provided for the Critical Thinking Questions in Nursing Care Plans and for the activities in the Study Guide.

To the Student

Designed with you in mind, *Foundations of Nursing* presents fundamental nursing concepts in a visually appealing and easy-to-use format. Here are some of the numerous special features that will help you understand and apply the material.

READING AND REVIEW TOOLS

Objectives introduce the chapter topics, *Key Terms* are listed with page number references, and difficult medical, nursing, or scientific terms are accompanied by simple phonetic pronunciations. Key terms are in color where they are briefly defined in the text, and complete definitions are provided in the Glossary.

Each chapter ends with a *Get Ready for the NCLEX® Examination!* section. *Key Points* follow the chapter objectives and serve as a chapter review. An extensive set of *Review Questions for the NCLEX® Examination* provides immediate opportunity for testing your understanding of the chapter content. *Answers* are located in Appendix C in the back of the book.

ADDITIONAL LEARNING RESOURCES

The online *Evolve Resources* at http://evolve.elsevier.com/Cooper/foundations give you access to even more Review Questions for the NCLEX Examination, animations, and much more.

CHAPTER FEATURES

Skills are presented in a logical step-by-step format with accompanying full-color illustrations. Clearly defined *nursing actions* followed by *rationales* in italicized type show you how and why skills are performed. Each skill includes icons that serve as a reminder to perform the basic steps applicable to *all* nursing interventions:

 Check orders.

 Gather necessary equipment and supplies.

 Introduce yourself.

 Check patient's identification.

 Provide privacy.

 Explain the procedure/intervention.

 Perform hand hygiene.

 Don gloves (if applicable).

Nursing Care Plans, developed around specific case studies, include patient problem statements in place of nursing diagnoses. These patient problem statements better describe health problems the patient experiences. These statements provide a problem-centered approach to nursing care. An emphasis is placed on patient goals and outcomes and questions to promote *critical thinking*. These sample care plans are valuable tools that can be used as a guideline in the clinical setting. The critical thinking aspect empowers you to develop sound clinical decision-making skills.

Patient problem statements and interventions are screened and set apart in the text in a clear, easy-to-understand format to help you learn to participate in the development of a nursing care plan.

Evidence-Based Practice boxes summarize the latest research findings and highlight how they apply to LPN/LVN practice.

Medication tables developed for specific disorders provide quick access to action, dosage, side effects, and nursing considerations for commonly used medications.

Safety Alert! boxes emphasize the importance of maintaining safety in patient and resident care to protect patients, residents, family, health care providers, and the public from accidents and the spread of disease.

Health Promotion boxes emphasize a healthy lifestyle, preventive behaviors, and screening tests to assist in the prevention of accidents and disease.

Patient Teaching boxes appear frequently in the text to help develop awareness of the vital role of patient/family teaching in health care today.

Coordinated Care boxes throughout the text promote comprehensive patient care with other members of the health care team, focusing on prioritization, assignment, supervision, collaboration, and leadership topics.

Complementary and Alternative Therapies boxes in nearly every chapter give a breakdown of specific non-traditional therapies, along with precautions and possible side effects.

Cultural Considerations boxes explore broad cultural beliefs and how to address the needs of a culturally diverse patient and resident population when planning nursing care.

Communication boxes focus on communication strategies with real-life examples of nurse-patient dialogue.

Life Span Considerations for the Older Adult boxes bring a gerontologic perspective to nursing care, focusing on the nursing interventions unique to the older adult patient or resident.

Home Care Considerations boxes discuss the issues facing patients and caregivers in the home setting.

Contents

32 Care of the Child With a Physical and Mental or Cognitive Disorder, 994

33 Health Promotion and Care of the Older Adult, 1080

UNIT V FUNDAMENTALS OF MENTAL HEALTH NURSING, 1122

34 Concepts of Mental Health, 1122

APPENDIXES

Foundations of Nursing

The Evolution of Nursing

1

Objectives

1. Describe the evolution of nursing and nursing education from early civilization to the 20th century.
2. Identify the major leaders of nursing history in America.
3. Discuss the significant changes in nursing in the 21st century.
4. Discuss societal influences on nursing.
5. Identify the major organizations in nursing.
6. Define the three purposes of the National Association for Practical Nurse Education and Service (NAPNES) and the National Federation of Licensed Practical Nurses (NFLPN).
7. Identify the components of the health care system.
8. Describe the complex factors involved in the delivery of patient care.
9. Identify the participants in the health care system.
10. Define practical and vocational nursing.
11. Describe the purpose, role, and responsibilities of the practical and the vocational nurse.

Key Terms

accreditation (ŭ-CRĔD-ĭ-TĀ-shŭn, p. 11)
approved program (p. 11)
articulation (ăr-tĭc-ū-LĀ-shŭn, p. 11)
certification (sĕr-tĭ-fĭ-KĀ-shŭn, p. 14)
health (p. 18)
health care system (p. 13)
holistic (hŏ-LĬS-tĭk, p. 14)

holistic health care (p. 13)
illness (p. 1)
licensure (LĪ-sĭn-shŭr, p. 5)
patient (p. 18)
pesthouses (p. 2)
portfolio (p. 11)
wellness (p. 13)

Nursing is one of today's most exciting and challenging careers. Each nurse receives a formal education in an institution with a set curriculum that has been approved by each state's board of nursing. Degrees and certificates are awarded by the school. Licensure is conferred by the individual state. On completion of the nursing program, individuals are eligible to request permission to sit for the National Council Licensing Examination (NCLEX®). The nursing profession has not always had such an organized body of knowledge or a regulated process for licensure. To best understand the position of today's nursing profession and nursing education, a look back at the history of nursing is warranted.

HISTORY OF NURSING AND NURSING EDUCATION

The word *nursing* can be traced back to the Latin word *nutrire*, which means "to nourish, feed, foster and support." Each of these terms reflects elements of the underlying role of the nurse. Throughout the ages, the perception and the roles of nursing has evolved as the profession has grown and changed. Many influences have led to changes in nursing and nursing education: the methods our society uses to care for the sick, the relationship of people to their environment, the search for knowledge and truth through education, increasing recognition of the values of preventative care, and technological advances. Nursing evolves as society and health care needs and policies change. The field responds and adapts to these changes, meeting new challenges as they arise.

CARE OF THE SICK DURING EARLY CIVILIZATION

The concepts of health, wellness, and illness and their relationships with one another and with nursing have evolved throughout history. Illness (an abnormal process in which aspects of the social, emotional, or intellectual condition and function of a person are diminished or impaired) was considered to be an indicator of how one stood with God; it was understood as a direct outcome of divine disfavor. Primitive people believed that a person became sick when an evil spirit entered the body and that the presence of a good spirit kept disease away.

Medicine men performed witchcraft and rituals to induce the bad spirits to leave the body of the ailing person. Some of their methods involved the use of frightening masks, noises, incantations, vile odors, charms, spells, and even sacrifices. They used purgatives (laxatives) and emetics, application of hot and cold substances, cautery, cupping (the use of suction on the skin to promote blood flow), and massage directly on the body or the affected part. Although others assisted the medicine men in treating illnesses, few were women. The role of women in health care was focused on helping other women during childbirth.

NURSING EDUCATION IN THE 19TH CENTURY

The hospitals of the early 19th century were very different from those of today. Hospitals, or **pesthouses** as they were called, were dirty, overcrowded facilities filled with patients. The scope of care delivered was limited. The providers of care typically were untrained. Hygienic practices were poor. These factors resulted in high infection and mortality rates. Hospitals of this era were places to contract diseases rather than be cured of them. Societal interest in care of the sick and disabled was limited. Training programs for health care providers were scarce, which led to recruitment of care providers with questionable qualifications. Women of "proper upbringing" did not work outside of the home. The ranks of workers loosely referred to as nurses were filled with women who drank heavily, engaged in prostitution, or were inmates in jails and prisons. Although religious orders did train and educate a small number of nurses, they were unable to meet the health care needs of communities.

Under the guidance of Theodor Fliedner, a German pastor in Kaiserswerth, Germany, the Lutheran Order of Deaconesses established the first school of nursing in the mid-1800s. The reputation of the school soon spread throughout Europe. It reached a young woman in England, Florence Nightingale, whose interest in nursing spurred her to overcome the opposition of her family, her friends, and the social class to which she belonged.

Florence Nightingale (1820 to 1910)

Florence Nightingale (Fig. 1.1), a strong-minded, intelligent, and determined young woman, joined the Kaiserswerth program in 1851 at age 31 years and became the superintendent of a charity hospital for ill governesses in 1853. The quality of patient care improved, but the governing board of the hospital was

Fig. 1.1 Florence Nightingale, the first nursing theorist. (From the Dolan Collection, *Nursing Times* photograph.)

not always pleased with the changes and innovations she made and the guidance she gave her uneducated nurses.

In the following year, concerned by the news of the number of casualties and deaths among soldiers in the Crimean War and the atrocious conditions suffered by the wounded, Nightingale sent the secretary of war, a long-time friend, a letter offering her services. Ironically, it crossed with his request for her to lead a group of nurses to Scutari, Turkey, to care for the wounded. Within a week of receiving the secretary's letter, she and 38 other nurses were on their way.

With use of the principles she learned at Kaiserswerth, Nightingale began to provide care to the wounded soldiers. Her nursing skills, dedication, and leadership turned the tide at the Barrack Hospital. Sanitary conditions, nonexistent before her arrival, were established. The hospital units were cleaned, and clothes were washed regularly. The mortality rate dropped significantly. The changes did not end with the physical environment of the hospital. Through Nightingale's patience, dedication, and empathic treatment of the soldiers, a psychological change took place as well. The soldiers grew to respect her and looked forward to her presence on the wards. They looked for her smile and took strength from her personality. When she made her rounds late at night through the rows of the injured and sick, she carried a lamp to light her way. Soon she was known as the "Lady with the Lamp." The small lamp became her trademark and continues to be the symbol of the nursing profession around the world (Fig. 1.2).

The standards of nursing care Nightingale established gained the respect of the medical community and led to improved care for the sick and a much-improved

Fig. 1.2 The Nightingale lamp. (Courtesy the College and Association of Registered Nurses of Alberta Museum and Archives P-650.)

Fig. 1.3 Nursing students in an early training program. (Courtesy the National Library of Medicine.)

image of nursing in general. She is credited as the first nursing theorist. The need for educated and trained nurses had become painfully evident, and the time was right for a shift in the approach to nursing education (Ellis, 2008).

Nursing From Occupation to Profession

Prior to Nightingale's time, nursing was largely unregulated. The decision of which actions were best were primarily "trial and error." She realized the importance of developing nursing theories and the promotion of standardized education. In 1860, Florence Nightingale began the reformation of nursing from occupation to profession by establishing the nursing school at Saint Thomas Hospital in London. With a reputation as a progressive medical facility, it was the ideal place to promote the new standards of nursing in which she so strongly believed.

The nursing program operated separately from the hospital. It was financially independent to ensure that the major emphasis of its activity was placed squarely on the education of nursing students (Fig. 1.3). Students had to pass strict procedures for admission, and a residence was provided for them. The nurses' training lasted 1 year and included formal instruction and practical experience. Complete records were kept on each student's progress. This practice was known as the "Nightingale Plan," which became the model for nursing education in the 20th century. After the students graduated, records were also kept on their places of employment. The "register" that resulted was the beginning of a movement to exercise control over the nursing graduate and to establish a standard for the practicing nurse.

Students admitted into the nursing program at Saint Thomas had to provide excellent character references, show a strong commitment to a career in nursing, and demonstrate that they were intellectually capable of passing the course of study before them. The new "Nightingale nurses" improved patient care by such measures as good hygiene and sanitation, patient observation, accurate record keeping, nutritional improvements, and the introduction and use of new medical equipment. The demand for their services was overwhelming.

DEVELOPMENT OF NURSING EDUCATION IN THE UNITED STATES

At the same time Florence Nightingale was active in Europe, circumstances in the United States were creating similar patient care problems. The American Revolution and the Civil War involved severe casualties, disease, infected wounds, and archaic medical care. As in the Crimean War, nurses were scarce, and those who were available were poorly trained to handle the horrors of war.

In 1849, Pastor Theodore Fliedner of Germany, who had established Nightingale's alma mater, traveled to the United States with four of his highly trained nurse deaconesses. He was instrumental in the establishment of the first Protestant hospital on American shores. Located in Pittsburgh, it was called the Pittsburgh Infirmary and is still in existence under the name Passavant Hospital. While Fliedner was busy with the hospital, his deaconesses began the first formal education of nurses in the United States.

As hospitals in the large cities grew to meet the demands for health care, a shortage of nurses developed. Most early nursing programs were supported by these large hospitals. In 1869, the American Medical Association recommended that every large hospital should establish and support its own school of nursing to meet the need for patient care. Schools of nursing would be established by the turn of the century, all modeled after the Nightingale Plan.

In May 1873, the Bellevue Hospital School of Nursing in New York was established as the foremost proponent of the Nightingale Plan in the United States. In October of that same year, the Connecticut Training School opened in New Haven. In November, the Boston Training School began operating at the Massachusetts General Hospital.

Isabel Hampton Robb (Fig. 1.4) and Lavinia Dock organized the American Society of Superintendents of Training Schools of Nursing in 1893. The primary goal of these dedicated women was to set educational standards for nurses. The organization became the first of its kind for nursing. The structure of the organization was modeled after that of the American Medical Association. See Table 1.1 for a list of American nursing leaders.

CHANGES IN NURSING DURING THE 20TH CENTURY

Like the superintendents who operated at the national level, the graduates of the training schools also attempted to establish standards. They established the alumnae association for the actual practice of nursing at the local level.

LICENSING

At the beginning of the 20th century, more than 400 schools of nursing were in existence in the United

Fig. 1.4 Isabel Hampton Robb. (Courtesy the National Library of Medicine.)

Table 1.1	Leaders in the Development of Nursing in America
NURSE	**CONTRIBUTION TO NURSING**
Dorothea Dix (1802–1887)	Pioneer crusader for elevation of standards of care for the mentally ill. Superintendent of Female Nurses of the Union Army.
Clara Barton (1821–1912)	Developed the American Red Cross in 1881.
Mary Ann Ball (1817–1901)	One of the greatest nurse heroines of the Civil War. Championed the rights and comforts of the soldiers; organized diet kitchens, laundries, ambulance service; and supervised the nursing staff.
Linda Richards (1841–1930)	First trained nurse in America. Responsible for the development of the first nursing and hospital records. Credited with the development of our present-day documentation system.
Isabel Hampton Robb (1859–1910)	Organized the first graded system of theory and practice in the schools of nursing. One of the founders of the *American Journal of Nursing*.
Lavinia Dock (1858–1956)	Responsible, with Robb, for the organization of the American Society of Superintendents of Training Schools, which evolved into the National League for Nursing Education.
Mary Eliza Mahoney (1845–1926)	Graduated from the New England Hospital for Women and Children in 1879, becoming the first African American professional nurse. Worked for acceptance of African Americans in the nursing profession.
Lillian D. Wald (1867–1940)	Responsible for the development of public health nursing in the United States through the founding of the Henry Street Settlement in New York City.
Mary Adelaide Nutting (1858–1948)	A leader in nursing education. Developed curriculum concepts and guidelines for student nurses. Assisted in the development of the International Council of Nurses.
Mary Breckenridge (1881–1965)	Pioneer in nurse-midwifery. Established the Frontier Nursing Service to deliver obstetric care to mothers in the hills of Kentucky; these nurses traveled on horseback to reach the mothers.

States, with variations in the curricula and program lengths and differences between the competencies of program graduates. In 1903, North Carolina, New Jersey, New York, and Virginia became the first states to mandate licensure (the granting of permission by the overseeing authority to engage in practice or activity that would otherwise be illegal) as a criterion for entry to professional practice. The nursing organizations recognized the need to amend their purpose and redirect their focus. As part of the reorganization that followed, in 1911, the American Society of Superintendents of Training Schools became the National League for Nursing Education (NLNE, n.d.). In the years that followed the organization developed and released their first nursing curriculum plan.

WORLD WAR I

In 1917, the United States' entry into World War I brought an increased demand for nurses. The newly formed Army and Navy Nurse Corps sought nurses who certifiably demonstrated "good moral character and professional qualifications." The available supply of nurses could not meet the demand, so once again, untrained women volunteered their services. Nursing leaders, concerned that these untrained personnel would be caring without adequate training for wounded and ailing soldiers, moved quickly to establish the Army School of Nursing. At the height of their service, more than 20,000 women are estimated to have served in the Nurse Corps (U.S. Army Heritage Center Foundation, n.d.).

After the war, most of the women who had served as military nurses returned to their homes and their previous jobs and careers. The image of professional nurses still posed a problem for most women, and few had the desire to remain in nursing as civilians. Furthermore, they were disenchanted because nurses' training still focused heavily on "service to the patient" rather than on a comprehensive professional education, which was far removed from what the Nightingale Plan had proposed for aspiring nurses.

WORLD WAR II

Twenty-five years later, World War II escalated the demand for trained nurses once again. The number of patient casualties and level of acuity skyrocketed. Early in the war, the Cadet Nurse Corps was established to provide an abbreviated training program designed to meet the needs of the war effort. In addition, federally subsidized programs in nursing were developed and implemented to offer women and, for the first time, men an education and a career in nursing while serving their country in the war.

After the war, many of the nurses trained by these programs remained in military service. Prestige, pay, and the opportunity for advancement were much greater in military service than for civilian nurses. In the major hospitals, particularly in urban areas, civilian nurses received low pay and worked long shifts in atrocious conditions. These conditions were hardly likely to attract those who became nurses as a result of the war and who, ironically, enjoyed a certain lifestyle that war provided. The aftereffects of World War I, the Great Depression, and World War II led to an increased nursing shortage.

State boards of nursing, which had licensure responsibility, came under increasing pressure to mandate requirements for nurses. State-administered licensing examinations no longer seemed adequate for the country's needs. The parochial state examinations were in no way standardized and allowed people with a wide spectrum of competence to enter nursing. National norms of competence were sorely needed.

Contemporary Nursing

The focus of health care from care of the sick to an ever-expanding profit-driven industry resulted in a change in its culture and characteristics. Growth and diversity of services became the major emphases as the industry became increasingly lucrative. Contemporary nursing was born as the demand for nurses increased at a rate greater than could be met. This demand was accompanied by a growth in specialized inpatient services and an intensive growth in community-based services such as occupational and home health nursing. The number of advanced practice nursing roles, including nurse anesthetists, nurse practitioners, and midwives, has surged in recent decades.

The future of nursing as a profession has remained a source of deliberation. In 1903, Isabel Hampton Robb and Adelaide Nutting published a position paper recommending the baccalaureate degree level as the minimum acceptable preparation for entry into the profession. The associate degree was recommended as the minimum for technical nursing practice. Decades later, in 1965, the American Nurses Association (ANA) took a position recommending that nursing education take place in institutions of learning within the general system of education, much as Robb and Nutting had proposed.

Since that time there has been a change in the settings for nursing education. Although many early nursing programs were managed by hospitals, in the mid-1960s, hospitals began moving away from operating schools of nursing. Today, registered nursing and licensed practical nursing programs are conducted primarily in technical schools, colleges, and universities. Licensed practical nurse (LPN) and licensed vocational nurse (LVN) programs may also be administered by high schools in some parts of the country. The shift toward colleges and universities provides the student nurse a broader educational base with an emphasis on not only skill development but also the integration of nursing theory and related general education courses (Box 1.1). In 2010, the Institute of Medicine (IOM) released a publication entitled *The Future of Nursing:*

Box 1.1   The Patient Care Partnership: Understanding Expectations, Rights, and Responsibilities

When you need hospital care, your doctor and the nurses and other professionals at our hospital are committed to working with you and your family to meet your health care needs. Our dedicated doctors and staff serve the community in all its ethnic, religious, and economic diversity. Our goal is for you and your family to have the same care and attention we would want for our families and ourselves.

The sections below explain some of the basics of how you can expect to be treated during your hospital stay. They also cover what we will need from you to care for you better. If you have questions at any time, please ask them. Unasked or unanswered questions can add to the stress of being in the hospital. Your comfort and confidence in your care are very important to us.

WHAT TO EXPECT DURING YOUR HOSPITAL STAY

- **High-quality hospital care.** Our first priority is to provide you the care you need, when you need it, with skill, compassion, and respect. Tell your caregivers if you have concerns about your care or if you have pain. You have the right to know the identity of doctors, nurses, and others involved in your care, and when they are students, residents, or other trainees.
- **A clean and safe environment.** Our hospital works hard to keep you safe. We use special policies and procedures to avoid mistakes in your care and keep you free from abuse or neglect. If anything unexpected or significant occurs during your hospital stay, you will be told what happened, and any resulting changes in your care will be discussed with you.
- **Involvement in your care.** You and your doctor often make decisions about your care before you go to the hospital. Other times, especially in emergencies, those decisions are made during your hospital stay. When decision making takes place, it should include the following:
  1. Discussing your medical condition and information about medically appropriate treatment choices. To make informed decisions with your doctor, you need to understand the following:
     - The benefits and risks of each treatment.
     - Whether your treatment is experimental or part of a research study.
     - What you can reasonably expect from your treatment and any long-term effects it might have on your quality of life.
     - What you and your family will need to do after you leave the hospital.
     - The financial consequences of using uncovered services or out-of-network providers.

     Please tell your caregivers if you need more information about treatment choices.
  2. *Discussing your treatment plan.* When you enter the hospital, you sign a general consent to treatment. In some cases, such as surgery or experimental treatment, you may be asked to confirm in writing that you understand what is planned and agree to it. This process protects your right to consent to or refuse a treatment. Your doctor will explain the medical consequences of refusing recommended treatment.

It also protects your right to decide if you want to participate in a research study.
  3. *Getting information from you.* Your caregivers need complete and correct information about your health and coverage so that they can make good decisions about your care. That includes the following:
     - Past illnesses, surgeries, or hospital stays.
     - Past allergic reactions.
     - Any medications or dietary supplements (e.g., vitamins and herbs) that you are taking.
     - Any network or admission requirements under your health plan.
  4. *Understanding your health care goals and values.* You may have health care goals and values or spiritual beliefs that are important to your well-being. They will be taken into account as much as possible throughout your hospital stay. Make sure your doctor, your family, and your care team know your wishes.
  5. *Understanding who should make decisions when you cannot.* If you have signed a health care power of attorney that states who should speak for you if you become unable to make health care decisions for yourself, or a "living will" or "advance directive" that states your wishes about end-of-life care, give copies to your doctor, your family, and your care team. If you or your family need help making difficult decisions, counselors, chaplains, and others are available to help.
  6. *Protection of your privacy.* We respect the confidentiality of your relationship with your doctor and other caregivers, and the sensitive information about your health and health care that are part of that relationship. State and federal laws and hospital operating policies protect the privacy of your medical information. You will receive a Notice of Privacy Practices that describes the ways that we use, disclose, and safeguard patient information and that explains how you can obtain a copy of information from our records about your care.
  7. *Preparing you and your family for when you leave the hospital.* Your doctor works with hospital staff and professionals in your community. You and your family also play an important role in your care. The success of your treatment often depends on your efforts to follow medication, diet, and therapy plans. Your family may need to help care for you at home. You can expect us to help you identify sources of follow-up care and to let you know if our hospital has a financial interest in any referrals. As long as you agree that we can share information about your care with them, we will coordinate our activities with your caregivers outside the hospital. You can also expect to receive information and, where possible, training about the self-care you will need when you go home.
  8. *Help with your bill and filing insurance claims.* Our staff will file claims for you with health care insurers or other programs such as Medicare and Medicaid.

Box 1.1   The Patient Care Partnership: Understanding Expectations, Rights, and Responsibilities—cont'd

They will also help your doctor with needed documentation. Hospital bills and insurance coverage are often confusing. If you have questions about your bill, contact our business office. If you need help understanding your insurance coverage or health plan, start with your insurance company or health benefits manager. If you do not have health coverage, we will try to help you and your family find financial help or make other arrangements. We need your help with collecting needed information and other requirements to obtain coverage or assistance.

While you are here, you will receive more detailed notices about some of the rights you have as a hospital patient and how to exercise them. We are always interested in improving. If you have questions, comments, or concerns, please contact: _____.

From American Hospital Association: *The patient care partnership: understanding expectations, rights, and responsibilities,* Chicago, 2003, AHA. Reprinted with permission from the American Hospital Association.

Focus on Nursing Education. The purpose of the document was to present identified challenges to health care and the nursing profession. The report identified as a weakness the limited number of nurses who have a baccalaureate degree education. The IOM has taken the position of promoting the need for changes in the nursing workforce, with a goal for 80% of working nurses to be prepared with a baccalaureate degree. In recognition of the pathways taken by some nurses to begin as unlicensed assistive personnel (UAP) with movement to LPN or LVNs and eventually on to registered, it emphasizes the need for smoother transitions to higher degrees by nurses. In the years since the highly discussed IOM report, nursing has seen an increase in baccalaureate nurses. This group represented only 49% of nurses, and when reevaluated in 2017, baccalaureate-prepared nurses had increased to 56% (Stringer, 2019).

The National League for Nurses (NLN) released a position paper in 2014 recognizing the LPN/LVN as a valued member of the professional nursing team. The NLN voiced the need for LPN/LVNs to have continued support for their entry into practice. The education of the LPN/LVN should contain experiences of acute- and long-term settings. Colleges and universities have been challenged further to develop programming geared to promote smooth transitions into increasingly advanced levels of education upon the LPN/LVN's return to school. Growing the practical and vocational nursing curricula to incorporate roles and content characteristic of associate of science and baccalaureate level education was discouraged (NLN Board of Governors, 2014). Currently, there are LPN/LVN education programs around the country. The majority of these programs (45%) are located in the southern portion of the United States.

Challenges in Nursing Education

Nursing education has come an incredible distance since the days of Florence Nightingale. Expectations of the profession have expanded beyond the management of the activities of daily living and medication administration. Nurses are responsible for providing care to increasingly complex health conditions and managing complicated treatment modalities. Educating nurses who are able to meet the challenges of the health care environment can be difficult for nursing schools. Identified concerns include issues related to health care reform, defining the scope of practice, high-stakes testing, diversity, academic progression, and faculty shortages.

Nursing Caps, Uniforms, and Pins

Originally, nurses wore the practical white, pleated cap and the apron of the maidservant, which signified respectability, cleanliness, and servitude. As the nursing profession gained recognition, nurses' caps became less utilitarian and more symbolic, a badge of office and achievement.

Since World War II, the nurse's cap has lost much of its significance. The "capping ceremony," a ritual in which junior nurses receive their first cap, has disappeared. The movement of nurses away from wearing the traditional nursing cap can be attributed to several reasons. The cap began its gradual decline in popularity around the same time as a movement toward a more informal uniform made the cap a dated piece of apparel. Nurses often reported that the cap interfered with the care being provided because it caught on equipment in the patient care area. Some nurses even reported hair loss from the constant friction of the hat. The movement of men into the profession, for whom there was no cap, was accompanied by discontent. Washing and starching the hat was a chore, and there were growing concerns about the caps harboring bacteria (Medscape Today News, n.d.) (Fig. 1.5).

The nursing uniform is another area that has seen and will continue to see change. Decades ago, nursing uniforms consisted of plain white dresses or skirts and later pant suit options. Controversy exists within the medical profession about the need for nursing uniforms. Many nurses do not approve of mandatory dress codes. They argue that other health care professionals do not depend on uniforms for their authority (Fig. 1.6).

A professional appearance is nonetheless important. Patients feel more comfortable and confident when they can easily find and distinguish nurses from other staff members. Agencies typically have dress codes in place. Some mandate the style of uniform; others assign certain colors to different health care groups. Facilities require staff members to wear nametags and identification badges and dress to promote professionalism. As a result of technological advances and the need for security, some facilities use fingerprint scans for access into the record-keeping and medication administration systems.

Pinning ceremonies began as a means to demonstrate successful program completion by nursing students. The practice of awarding a pin at the time of graduation dates back to the later 1800s in England (Early, 2015). In the United States the first nursing pins were awarded in New York's Bellevue Hospital in 1880. This first pin had a symbolic design. The center displayed a crane, which demonstrated vigilance.

Fig. 1.5 Nursing caps in history. (Courtesy Ona Wilcox College of Nursing Records, Archives & Special Collections at the Thomas J. Dodd Research Center, University of Connecticut Libraries.)

There were bands of color around the outer portion of the pin. A blue band signaled constancy and a red band illustrated mercy and a relief of suffering. Most schools of nursing continue to award a nursing pin to the graduate nurse. Pinning does not bestow credentials such as degree completion or state licensure but is considered a rite of passage by many in the profession. Many pins bear the Nightingale lamp as a common component, along with an emblem of the school of nursing.

SIGNIFICANT CHANGES IN NURSING FOR THE 21ST CENTURY

Nursing practice is affected by various societal factors, along with developments that are more internal to the field. Demographics of the population, women's health care issues, men in nursing, rising numbers of people with fewer socioeconomic advantages seeking health care, and bioterrorism threats are a few of the societal factors that influence nursing today.

DEMOGRAPHIC CHANGES

Because the demographics of the population are changing, nursing education and practice must also change and adapt. Life expectancy of the population is increasing, and growing numbers of older adults are seeking health care for chronic illnesses.

WOMEN'S HEALTH CARE ISSUES

The biological gender differences impacting women are increasingly becoming a health care focus. "Women's health research is the study of health across a woman's lifespan in order to preserve wellness and to prevent, diagnose, and treat disease. It

Fig. 1.6 (A) Nursing uniforms in the early years. (B) Nursing uniforms today. (A, Copyright the Royal Columbian Hospital, New Westminster, BC)

includes all health conditions for which women and men experience differences in risk, presentation, and treatment response, as well as health issues specific to women, such as pregnancy and menopause." Disease pathology, progression, and treatment can differ for women (Society for Women's Health Research, 2020). Every decade the US Department of Health and Human Services presents a series of national health objectives in a series entitled "Healthy People." The 2020 series has identified 42 heath focused objectives. Women and girls are the focus in 16 of these (CDC, 2020).

Nursing is responding in two ways to women's health care issues and the women's movement. Nurses, most of whom are women, are increasingly asserting their equal rights as humans, employees, and health care professionals. Encouraged by the women's movement, they have sought greater autonomy and responsibility in providing care. In addition, the women's movement has helped women to become more aware of their own unique needs. Nurses have learned to encourage female patients to seek more responsibility for and control over their bodies, health, and lives in general.

MEN IN NURSING

Men have had a role in nursing throughout its history. However, in more modern times the number of men in nursing has decreased. The influences of war promoted the profession for women rather than men. Some critics also associate Florence Nightingale with the decreasing number of men in nursing. She recommended that "gentlewomen" replace workers who were unskilled. This verbiage promoted the idea that nursing was more "woman's work." Fortunately, the past few decades have shown increases in the number of men in nursing. Presently, fewer than 10% of nurses identify as male (AACN, 2019). The majority of men in nursing are registered nurses (RNs).

To combat the shortage of men in nursing, education and professional settings have programs to attract and recruit men to the profession. Studies are showing that drawing men to the profession is not where the challenge ends. The attrition rate for men in nursing education is higher than that of women. Men are also more likely than their female counterparts to leave the profession once licensed. Reports indicate that challenges related to feelings of social isolation, stereotypes about men who choose nursing, nursing instructors' inability to incorporate masculine styles of caring into the curriculum, and a lack of male role models in the profession may be to blame.

MINORITY NURSES

The faces of patients needing care represent a diverse demographic. To best provide culturally responsive care the nursing profession will need to further work in an effort to present a demographic that is more consistent with the country's population. National Council State Boards of Nursing (NCSBN) perform a workforce study every 2 years. During the study, the racial composition of the nursing profession is assessed: 19% of RNs self-identified as minorities. LPN/LVNs displayed a higher level of diversity with 29% (NCSBN, 2017). Diversity is not limited to race or ethnicity. Age should also be a consideration. The average age of the LPN/LVN workforce in 2017 was 52 years. This is reflective of an aging group, because this is 1 year older than the 2015 survey.

The promotion of diversity in nursing must begin with nursing faculty and students. The percentage of minority representation in nursing faculty is less than other nursing career areas, with less than 20% of nursing educators identifying as non-White (NLN, 2017). Looking at the working nurses in the country and the educators, it is clear that efforts to recruit and retain diverse students is needed.

HUMAN RIGHTS

Nursing advocates for the rights of all individuals. Beyond this basic requirement, the profession has promoted the rights of specific segments of the population through the creation of bills of rights. Such bills address the rights of hospitalized patients, those who are dying, older adults, and pregnant women. These bills of rights address the need to respect all patients as individuals and ensure quality care for all.

MEDICALLY UNDERSERVED

Soaring rates of unemployment, homelessness, undocumented workers, and poverty, combined with the enormous rise in health care costs, have led to an increased number of individuals in the United States who are unable to afford health care. These groups, when combined, represent a sizable population of those who are potentially unable to obtain health insurance or pay outright for health care.

An estimated 18% of the US gross domestic product (GDP) is spent on health care (CMS, 2020). The average spending on health care in the United States was just more than $10,500 per person (CDC, 2019). Health care spending in the United States is significantly greater than in other industrialized nations. Germany is the next in line, spending less than $6000 per person per year (McCarthy, 2019). The rate of uninsured further complicates discussions related to heath care spending. In 2018, the rate of uninsured in the United States was 8.5%, or 27.5 million people (US Census Bureau, 2019). There are regional differences noted with the percentages of uninsured. Several southern states show higher rates than others. Overall the Northeast has lower rates of uninsured. Limited access to health care is another concern that hinders individuals with mental health disorders and those who live in rural areas. Initiatives to provide increased services in rural and community-based clinics offer assistance to these populations. Nursing engagement in health promotion activities to prevent and manage illness and chronic conditions is one such solution.

Frequently, nurses who work in these settings have a higher degree of training and function as advanced practice nurses, so they have the capability to provide direct health care. This area of nursing is expanding rapidly as more nurses seek to work with this underserved population.

NURSING SHORTAGE

The United States continues to face a nursing shortage. The nation is expected to need an increase of 9% LPN/LVNs between 2019 and 2029 (Bureau of Labor Statistics, 2021). This increase will require more than 65,000 more LPN/LVNs. Despite strategies to reduce the shortfall of nurses, the supply is not expected to meet the growing demand. The nursing workforce is aging. In the coming decade, many nurses who currently are working are expected to retire.

The nursing shortage is not related to a single cause but is tied to a series of interrelated factors. The aging workforce is problematic. The majority of nurses are in the middle phase of their careers, and, although not ready to retire now, they will be leaving the workforce in the coming years. Nursing faculty shortages limit the abilities of programs of nursing to expand to meet the demands. Nursing, once considered a prime career choice for women, now faces competition as women look at other promising career options (American Association of Colleges of Nursing, 2012). Schools of nursing also are facing a shortage of qualified educators, which further hinders growth of the profession.

DEVELOPMENT OF PRACTICAL AND VOCATIONAL NURSING

ATTENDANT NURSES

The first school for training practical nurses opened in Brooklyn, New York, in 1892 under the auspices of the Young Women's Christian Association (YWCA). The Ballard School, as it was known, gave a course that lasted approximately 3 months and trained its students to care for invalids, children, the chronically ill, and the elderly. The main emphasis was on home care and included cooking, nutrition, basic science, and basic nursing procedures. Graduates of this program were referred to as attendant nurses.

Two other programs were patterned after the Ballard School. In 1907, the Thompson Practical Nursing School opened in Brattleboro, Vermont (still in operation and accredited by the NLN), and in 1918, the Household Nursing Association School of Attendant Nursing (later changed to the Shepard-Gill School of Practical Nursing) opened in Boston. Hospital experience was not a part of the training in the early programs. The focus was on home nursing care and light housekeeping duties.

PRACTICAL NURSING PROGRAMS

Practical nursing programs developed slowly during the first half of the 20th century, with only 36 schools opening. The practical nursing schools before 1940 had few controls, little educational planning, and minimal supervision. Between 1948 and 1954, a sharp increase in the formation of practical and vocational nursing programs was attributed to the increased demand for nursing services in World War II and the postwar years and the excellent bedside nursing care demonstrated by the practical nurse. These programs varied in administrative design. Some were affiliated with hospitals or chronic care institutions, whereas others aligned themselves with private agencies or private schools. Students in these programs provided nursing services while they were obtaining their education and training. Technical and vocational education emphasized apprentice training. Federal funds allocated for training practical and vocational nurses helped recruit men and women.

FUTURE OF THE LICENSED PRACTICAL NURSE AND LICENSED VOCATIONAL NURSE

There are an estimated 825,000 LPN/LVNs in the United States (The Henry J. Kaiser Family Foundation, 2017). Their practice settings are vast. Although they once were a visible member of the health care team in acute care facilities, currently only an estimated 25% are working in hospital settings. The position of the LPN/LVN has been in many areas of the country removed or sharply limited in acute care settings. With a looming nursing shortage, there is a need for the LPN/LVN to be a key member of the team addressing this nationwide concern.

ORGANIZATIONAL INFLUENCE

As practical nursing programs continued to grow in number, the need to establish standards of curricula became increasingly evident. The Association of Practical Nurse Schools was founded in 1941 and was dedicated exclusively to practical nursing. Its membership was multidisciplinary and included LPNs, RNs, physicians, hospital and nursing home administrators, students, and public figures. Together they planned the first standard curriculum for practical nursing. By 1942, they saw the need to change the name to the National Association of Practical Nurse Education (NAPNE). They broadened their focus to include education and practice and established an accrediting service for schools of practical and vocational nursing in 1945. The association changed its name once more in 1959 to the National Association for Practical Nurse Education and Service (NAPNES). NAPNES remains a guiding force in the development of practical nursing education.

In 1949, the National Federation of Licensed Practical Nurses (NFLPN) was founded by Lillian Kuster. Limited to LPNs and LVNs, this association is the official membership organization for the LPN/LVN. Working together, NAPNES and NFLPN set standards for practical and vocational nursing practice, promote and protect the interests of LPN/LVNs, and educate and inform the general public about practical and vocational nursing.

In 1961, the NLN broadened its scope of service because of the growth of practical and vocational nursing programs. The NLN established the Department of Practical Nursing Programs and developed an accreditation service for these programs, which is now called the Council of Practical Nursing Programs.

For 20 years, the NLN and the NAPNES provided accreditation services. Nursing programs had the option of seeking accreditation from either organization. However, in recent years, NAPNES has discontinued this service.

PROGRAM CREDENTIALING

Accreditation of a program differs from program approval. Approval is required for a program to open and operate. An approved program is one that satisfies the minimum standards set by the state agency responsible for overseeing educational programs: for example, it meets the needs of the student, has adequate course content and qualified faculty, is of sufficient length, has adequate facilities, and provides clinical experience. To protect the welfare of the public, the state requires programs to demonstrate all these elements for graduates to be eligible for licensure. Accreditation is a higher standard that signifies that the accrediting organization has judged that a program has met its preestablished criteria. The administrators of the program seeking accreditation submit voluntarily to the accreditation process; they do so because of the recognition of quality it confers. The accreditation process provides an intensive review of the programs structure, curriculum, and outcomes. Often the standards established by professional organizations that give accreditation are far higher than those established by the state. Although graduates of nonaccredited programs can take the licensure examination required in most states, accreditation is extremely important when programs seek federal funding. Graduates from nonaccredited programs may face challenges when attempting to transfer completed course work to another institution for further education.

CONTEMPORARY PRACTICAL AND VOCATIONAL NURSING EDUCATION

Practical nursing programs are offered by various organizations, including high schools, trade or technical schools, hospitals, junior and community colleges, colleges and universities, and private education agencies.

Programs are required to meet the minimum state standards. The length of the programs is usually 12 to 18 months, with a focus on nursing skills and theory that is correlated with clinical practice.

Educational programs in nursing offer various creative approaches to the education of student LPN/LVNs. The combination of practical and vocational nurse education with associate degree programs in 2-year colleges is available. At the successful completion of the first academic year and of the requirements for the practical nursing portion of the program, the student can either exit and take the licensure examination for practical or vocational nursing or continue for another year and earn an associate degree in nursing, becoming eligible to take the licensure examination for registered nursing. Many other programs offer other combinations of education and degrees throughout the United States. Most states have some type of articulation plan.

Articulation allows nursing programs to plan their curricula collaboratively; the purpose is to lessen duplication of learning experiences and support a process of progressive buildup. Thus one program becomes the foundation for another program. An LPN/LVN may receive as much as 50% credit toward the associate degree; the associate degree–prepared RN may receive as much as 50% credit toward the bachelor of science in nursing (BSN) degree. This process is sometimes referred to as a 1-plus-1 program or a 2-plus-2 program, respectively. Articulation acknowledges the student's existing knowledge base and permits the student to continue her or his advancement in education without repeating previous course work.

CAREER ADVANCEMENT

The career ladder is a model that some institutions use to allow for professional advancement. A career ladder recognizes the clinical expertise of the nurse and provides a mechanism for financial compensation. Each institution clearly lists and defines its criteria for advancement on the ladder. Items generally include adherence to facility policies, completion of mandatory education programs, and demonstration of leadership and clinical skills. Nurses make application for consideration of the career ladder by submitting a portfolio illustrating their accomplishments. A portfolio is an organized account of an individual's education and professional accomplishments.

FACTORS THAT INFLUENCED PRACTICAL AND VOCATIONAL NURSING

Before 1860, nursing care in the United States was provided generally by people who were self-taught and who gained what knowledge they could through experience. Registration, licensing, and title differentiation were unclear or nonexistent. Duties and responsibilities were not defined clearly. The term *nurse* was used only in the broadest sense as "a person who takes care of the sick."

NEED FOR TRAINED CAREGIVERS

Practical nursing in the United States evolved from the need for caregivers who could be trained and ready for service in a short time. The cost of the services provided by these caregivers was expected to be reasonable and easily affordable by the patient. There was also the need to provide a vocation for the many unskilled women who were migrating to the larger cities to seek better opportunities. Women generally were not skilled or trained for jobs other than manual labor.

WORLD WAR I

World War I increased the need for trained nurses abroad, and in the United States, the Spanish influenza epidemic strained the resources of the nursing community. The Smith-Hughes Act was passed in 1917 to provide vocational and public education. Federal funding then provided the means for vocational-based practical and vocational nursing programs throughout the country. Even with these resources, the demand for nurses caused by the war and the epidemic could not be met.

SELF-TAUGHT PRACTICAL NURSE

By 1940, thousands of self-taught "practical nurses" were working to meet the needs of the country. They lacked the education and experience obtainable only under supervision in an established program. Few states had minimum standards for the practice of practical and vocational nurses. There was no agreement on the duties, the role, and the responsibilities of practical and vocational nurses, and they were known by many job descriptions and titles. The absence of standards and licensing created difficulties and safety concerns.

The state of New York was the first to have mandatory licensure laws. A state pool of test questions was adopted in 1945 by the State Boards of Nursing Examiners in 25 states (Smith, 2009). By 1950, all states had joined the momentum and required testing and licensure for entry into practice.

DUTIES OF LICENSED PRACTICAL NURSES AND LICENSED VOCATIONAL NURSES

In 1944, the US Department of Vocational Education commissioned an intensive study of practical and vocational nursing tasks. The outcome of this study differentiated the tasks performed by the LPN/LVN in relation to those tasks performed by the RN. As a result of this study, individual state boards of nursing began to specify the duties and responsibilities that could be accomplished by each group of nurses.

POSITION PAPER OF THE AMERICAN NURSES ASSOCIATION

In 1965, the American Nurses Association's *First Position on Education for Nursing* was released. The document outlined recommendations for the educational levels for the nurse to enter practice. It recommended a 2-year technical education be provided in vocational and community college settings. Graduates of these programs would earn an associate of science degree. The professional nurse would earn a baccalaureate degree. The paper did not specifically discuss the LPN/LVN. Practical and vocational nurses nonetheless have proved their worth. Under the supervision of an RN or a physician, they provide excellent bedside nursing skills in many areas of service. The 1965 position paper of the ANA was another influence that brought about a change in attitude toward practical and vocational nursing.

LICENSURE FOR PRACTICAL AND VOCATIONAL NURSING

Licensing laws have been passed to protect the public from unqualified practitioners in most fields and professions. In the mid-1950s, states moved toward mandatory licensure for nurses. The laws passed were managed by state agencies such as the state boards of nursing. The state's nurse practice acts provide specific information about the scope of practice for the differing nursing levels. On completion of a nursing program, the graduate is eligible to take the National Council Licensing Examination for Practical Nursing (NCLEX-PN). Once the examination is completed successfully, licensure is awarded by the state of application.

LAWS THAT MONITOR THE LICENSED PRACTICAL NURSE AND THE LICENSED VOCATIONAL NURSE

Licensing for practical and vocational nurses in the United States began in 1914, when the state legislature in Mississippi passed the first laws pertaining to that group. This licensing followed the passage of laws on licensing for RNs. The passage of such laws governing practical and vocational nursing in other states did not rapidly follow. After the outbreak of World War II and the opening of a large number of practical and vocational nurses training programs, all the states were forced to pass legislation concerning their licensure. By 1955, all states had passed laws in this area in consonance (agreement) with the standards set by NAPNE. The State Board Test Pool of the NLN Education Committee established a testing mechanism for all states and administered the examination several times a year throughout the country. Graduates of a state-approved practical or vocational nursing education program were eligible to sit for the examination; if they passed, they became LPNs, or LVNs as they are called in Texas and California. Each state set its own required passing score on the examination.

Graduates of an approved LPN/LVN education program are eligible to apply to take the licensure examination. This application must be approved by the

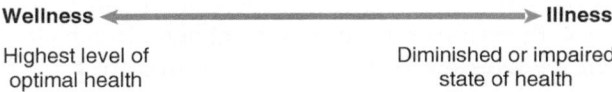

Fig. 1.7 Health care continuum.

individual's state board of nursing. On completion of the computerized examination with a "pass" score (numerical scores are no longer given), the graduate is issued a license to practice as an LPN or an LVN.

HEALTH CARE DELIVERY SYSTEMS

LPN/LVNs practice within the health care delivery system as a whole. To achieve their greatest potential, nurses must be aware of the complexity of this system and the vital role that nursing plays in its functioning.

HEALTH CARE SYSTEM DEFINED

The health care system consists of a network of agencies, facilities, and providers involved with health care in a specified geographic area. Many categories of health care professionals operate within this system, including the LPN/LVN. This health care environment includes the patient, the patient's family, the community in which the system operates, technology, governmental and regulatory agencies, the medical profession, third-party participants (e.g., insurance companies), and many other forces that affect the patient's care. The major goal of the system is to achieve optimal levels of health care for a defined population. The means of achieving this goal is provision of adequate and appropriate health care services. The LPN/LVN is an integral member of the team of health care professionals who provide these services within the scope of practice as defined by the state's nurse practice act.

WELLNESS-ILLNESS CONTINUUM

The range of a person's total health is described along the *wellness-illness continuum.* One's position on this continuum is ever changing and is influenced by the individual's physical condition, mental condition, and social well-being. At one end of the spectrum is wellness (a dynamic state of health in which an individual progresses toward a higher level of functioning, achieving an optimal balance between internal and external environment). Wellness represents the highest level of optimal health. Illness, at the opposite end of the spectrum, represents a diminished or impaired state of health (Fig. 1.7).

A balance of all aspects of life is the key to maintaining one's health. Factors that affect the level of wellness include age, gender, family relationships, emotional stressors, ethnic and cultural influences, and economic status. Consideration of the interrelationships among these variables is paramount when the nurse is planning and providing care. An all-inclusive approach to

Fig. 1.8 Maslow's hierarchy. (Data from Maslow A: *Motivation and personality*, ed 2, New York, 1970, Harper & Row.)

health care is known as holistic health care (a system of comprehensive or total patient care that considers the physical, emotional, social, economic, and spiritual needs of a person).

MASLOW'S MODEL OF HEALTH AND ILLNESS

Several models of the wellness-illness continuum have been developed. These models enable the nurse to understand the patient's individual level of wellness and position on the continuum. The most common model was developed in the 1940s by Abraham Maslow. He believed that an individual's behavior is formed by the individual's attempts to meet essential human needs, which he identified as physiologic, safety and security, love and belongingness, and esteem and self-actualization. Maslow placed these needs into a conceptual hierarchy, or pyramid, that ranks them according to how basic each one is. A person has to meet needs at the base of the pyramid before advancing to the needs higher on the pyramid. Those needs placed higher on the pyramid are not requirements for life but rather enhance it. Remember that each patient may view or prioritize individual needs according to his or her own value system (Fig. 1.8).

HEALTH PROMOTION AND ILLNESS PREVENTION

From the earliest recorded civilizations to the 20th century, the primary focus of health care was on the care of the sick. The current focus has broadened to include an emphasis on an awareness of the causes of disease and the prevention of its spread through the use of health promotion activities.

In contrast to their origins as dirty, unsanitary, and ill-kept institutions where unsuspecting patients acquired diseases, hospitals have become clean, increasingly safe locations where patients and their families are cared for with limited fear that they will be exposed to additional illness and medical problems. The US Department of Public Health works to help in the identification of disease types and related risk factors. These statistics identify problem areas for researchers and health care providers, who then direct their efforts at developing treatment for the illness, isolating its cause, and establishing methods to decrease its spread. The determination of cause-and-effect relationships provides a starting point for the development and implementation of health promotion initiatives.

Today three levels of health promotion are recognized. Their purpose is to promote health through maintaining wellness, preventing disease-related complications, and reducing the infirmity associated with disease states. *Primary prevention* seeks to avoid disease states through wellness activities and preemptive screening programs such as mammograms, colonoscopies, and glucose screening. *Secondary prevention* recognizes the presence of disease but seeks to reduce the impact of the condition by encouraging behaviors to promote health. An example of this type of prevention is dietary teaching to a patient with diabetes with the intention to reduce episodes of hyperglycemia. The management of care activities for those with serious health problems who seek to improve the quality of life and reduce further loss of function are captured by *tertiary prevention*.

CONTINUITY OF CARE

The patient is the focus of the health care system. However, many factors in our holistic health care system determine what actually happens in the care of each patient. The number of health care providers and health care agencies involved in the care and treatment of a single patient is extensive. Increased specialization by health care providers and health care institutions, reimbursement procedures by third-party payers (e.g., insurance companies), cumbersome federal regulatory organizations, and state health care regulatory agencies affect the consumer (the patient) and the type and quality of care provided.

One of the greatest challenges for the consumer of medical care is artful navigation of the health care delivery system. The consumer faces challenges to maintain autonomy and obtain continuity of care. Patients who already are weakened by the stressors of actual or potential medical conditions can become frightened as they attempt to understand the medical care and related choices available to them.

DELIVERY OF PATIENT CARE

The care of patients is a humanistic enterprise. It involves not only treating disease and injury but also preventing disease, restoring optimal wellness through rehabilitation, caring for the chronically ill, and educating patients and families. To identify the individual needs of the patient and to plan a systematic approach to meet those needs, nurses participate in developing an individualized care plan with use of the nursing process (see Chapter 5). The purpose of the care plan is to meet the expressed needs of the patient. Its development involves the patient and all health care providers who, through a coordinated and cooperative effort, work toward meeting the patient's total needs in a holistic, caring manner.

PARTICIPANTS IN THE HEALTH CARE SYSTEM
Professional Health Care Specialists
The patient is the central focus of activities performed by more than 200 types of health care providers identified in the health care system in the United States. Many professions require certification or licensure of their members. Within many disciplines are subspecialties of individuals who have advanced training and licensure.

Registered Nurses
The RN is a direct health care provider who is licensed after completion of one of three types of nursing education programs: a 4-year baccalaureate degree program, a 2-year associate degree program, or a 3-year diploma program. RNs practice in a variety of settings inside and outside of the care facility. The RN's duties and tasks vary according to educational background and the state's nurse practice act. Educational and career opportunities exist for the RN beyond initial licensure. Nurses with master's degrees or doctorates represent a small but growing segment of the profession. These individuals often are termed advanced practice nurses. Their roles are expanded and may involve educator, administrator, and prescriptive authority.

Licensed Practical and Licensed Vocational Nurses
The LPN/LVN practices under the supervision of the RN or the physician. Working together, the LPN/LVN and the RN are the direct patient caregivers in most institutions. The role of the LPN/LVN is based on the scope of practice outlined in each state's nurse practice act (see Chapter 40 for more information on nurse practice acts).

Other Caregivers
Other caregivers also are required to be registered or licensed and to have the specialized education and training dictated by their professional organizations. Holistic care requires that professionals from differing areas come together to provide comprehensive care. When a patient's condition dictates, referral to other care providers may be indicated. For example, social workers are trained to counsel patients who have social, emotional, or environmental problems. Physical therapists use precise methods of massage, exercise, and hydrotherapy to help restore physical function of the body. Dietitians are trained to determine the foods that meet the nutritional requirements of the patient. Respiratory therapists assist the patient by

administering oxygen, monitoring and maintaining ventilators, drawing blood for blood gas analysis, and performing other pulmonary function tests.

Technologists, Medical Technicians, and Paraprofessionals

Diagnostic personnel work in the laboratory and radiology departments. Their roles involve assisting the medical professional staff in testing for disease states and injury. The term *technologist* refers to those who have a baccalaureate degree, whereas the term *technician* refers to those who have had training and have earned an associate degree or certificate. Paraprofessionals are educated to assist the professional in providing care for patients. UAP are educated in basic nursing techniques and perform under the supervision of the RN. The unit secretary prepares and maintains patient records, orders supplies, schedules tests, and performs receptionist duties on the care unit.

These are only a sampling of the health care participants in the health care system. Each participant has a valuable contribution to make toward ensuring the safety and well-being of the patient.

ECONOMIC FACTORS THAT AFFECT HEALTH AND ILLNESS

Rising Health Care Costs

Health care costs have reached a critical height. A large portion of the country's financial resources are committed to health care–related costs. Several factors have been highlighted as playing a role in the increase in costs, including an aging population, increased use of advanced technologies, rising cost of private health care insurance, the rising cost of medical malpractice insurance, and a struggling economy.

Increasing number of aging Americans. As the baby boomer generation nears the age of retirement, their health problems increase; this onset of chronic diseases in a large segment of the population strains the health care system. Diseases associated with aging include heart disease, diabetes, and osteoporosis. As the US population ages, an increasing number of older adults need nursing home care, which is costly and has limited coverage under traditional insurance plans.

Advances in technology. Advances in technology have led to better diagnosis and treatment of illness, but such progress carries a large price. Research and the development of technology cost millions of dollars, a price that is passed on to the patient in the cost of the individual tests or treatments. Technological advances have resulted in concerns for patient privacy as electronic piracy has become an increasing threat. Safeguards for the electronic health records add to the costs for health care.

Health care insurance. Private health care insurance initially was developed to defray some or all of the cost of health care. It made health care more affordable, but it also raised the demand for it. As more individuals sought care, the price of health care services and insurance costs spiraled. This trend continues at an alarming and seemingly uncontrollable speed. The underinsured and uninsured populations face hardship when health care is needed. Determination of who receives care and who does not is becoming an ethical issue at all levels of the health care delivery system. The uninsured often find themselves limiting preventative or routine care activities. They may seek care only when in a crisis situation or unduly tax the health care system by using emergency care services for mild or routine health needs.

Malpractice insurance. Nurses and doctors carry medical malpractice insurance to protect themselves in the event a malpractice claim is filed against them. As malpractice claims have increased in frequency and amount, the premiums for this insurance have also risen. In response, physicians sometimes resort to practicing "defensive medicine." That is, they become overly cautious out of fear of a claim, ordering costly tests and procedures not because they are medically necessary but to protect themselves. These behaviors have resulted in higher medical costs for the patient.

These issues are alarming for health care providers. Nurses can help keep costs to a minimum by using materials and time economically and providing knowledgeable efficient care.

CHANGES IN DELIVERY SYSTEM

Hospitals throughout the United States are changing delivery systems to make care more cost effective. Case management and cross-training are two commonly encountered methods for modifying the systems used to deliver care.

Case management nursing revolves around the use of clinical pathways, which map out expectations of the hospitalization according to a designated time frame. The RN functions as a case manager, coordinating and planning the care of a group of patients, or caseload. An LPN/LVN works with the RN to assist the patient in attaining desired outcomes of care. Case management nursing has been proven to reduce the length of stay for the patient, which in turn reduces the overall cost of the patient's health care.

Cross-training allows employers to maximize the use of available staff. Workers are trained to perform duties that cross traditional role boundaries. Cross-training may involve combining the roles of differing categories of workers or expanding the responsibilities of staff members to cover multiple care units. Two groups of workers that frequently cross-trained to expand their roles are clerical support staff and UAP. This training enables a single worker to perform UAP-related tasks (e.g., ambulating patients and taking vital signs) as well as clerical support duties (e.g., transcribing orders and ordering unit supplies). Another type of cross-training involves linking patient care units, frequently identified as sister units. Common sister units are maternal child care and women's health, and the nursing staff are trained to work in both areas. Individuals receive training to perform duties that vary according to the needs at a given time. This training can be as narrowly defined as medical training to care for surgical patients or as broadly defined as housekeeping personnel training to give basic morning care to patients. The scope of cross-training usually is defined by the individual institution, and the purpose is to reduce the number or cost of employees without compromising the quality of patient care.

Other trends that affect the economics of health care include the development of multisystem health care chains or networks that may include several hospitals, clinics, nursing homes, and pharmacies. These systems share expenses and generally achieve an overall reduction in operating expenses. Health maintenance organizations (HMOs) or group health care practices provide health care to members for a fixed prepaid rate. This service includes medical care, nursing care, diagnostic tests, hospitalization, and various inpatient and outpatient treatments. This service has shown a high quality of low-cost health care.

SOCIAL AND ENVIRONMENTAL FACTORS THAT AFFECT HEALTH AND ILLNESS

Social and environmental factors do not necessarily cause illness, but they do influence the development or progression of an illness. Financial hardship, lifestyle choices, and social pressures all influence an individual's willingness or ability to actively maintain health or prevent illness. In addition, personal behavior choices such as smoking, drug abuse, alcoholism, and obesity affect an individual's health and wellness. The individual's mental state has an influence on patient outcomes. Emotions associated with fear, loss of identity, and loss of control commonly are experienced during illness. An imbalance in body functions can affect one's physical condition and ultimately the position along the wellness-illness continuum. Although there is often a tendency to separate social factors from physical factors, remember that the two areas affect each other reciprocally.

Each patient possesses a unique personality, background, lifestyle, and level of education. Early recognition of the effect of environmental factors on a patient and prompt intervention by family, health care providers, or the patients can decrease or minimize any negative impact.

HEALTH PROMOTION

Most people in the United States believe that everyone has a right to health care, regardless of race, color, creed, or economic status. This health care includes the treatment of disease and health promotion and preventive medicine. In many cases, treatment of illness is less of a concern than its prevention. The acute awareness of preventive medicine has resulted in the present emphasis on education about issues such as smoking, heart disease, drug and alcohol abuse, weight control, and mental health and wellness promotion activities.

During illness or after a change in health status, people often feel they are not in control of their health, but they typically do trust in the health care system. The presumption is that care will be highly satisfactory and lead to a cure. Health care providers are expected to provide service in a knowledgeable, safe, and expeditious manner and to work in a cooperative manner for their benefit. Patients also expect the cost of care to be reasonable and, most importantly, paid by somebody else (an insurance company or the government).

Patients' Rights

In 1972, the American Hospital Association (AHA) issued the *Patient's Bill of Rights* in an effort to ensure the patient's fundamental rights for treatment with dignity and compassion were protected. The trailblazing document was revised again in the 1990s and finally was replaced in 2003 when the AHA adopted the *Patient Care Partnership* (Box 1.2). According to the terms of this document, patients are assured that they can expect high-quality hospital care, a clean and safe environment, involvement in their care and the decision-making process, protection of privacy, help when leaving the hospital, and help with billing concerns (AHA, 2003). Nursing home patients' rights also are protected. The *Resident's Bill of Rights* is a document developed to provide clarity to the needs and rights of the individual who resides in a long-term care environment. It is the responsibility of the facility staff to provide copies of these rights and to explain them to the residents (Centers for Medicare and Medicaid Services, n.d.).

Health Care Providers' Rights

The delivery of health care must be a process of mutual exchange between patients and health care providers. Patients expect their rights to be respected, but health care workers have expectations as well. Health care professionals expect that patients will do the following to actively participate in their care as much as possible: take an active role in the planning process, understand the care and the treatment given, ask questions, follow the treatment plan prescribed, act responsibly with respect to their own conditions, and give health care workers the same respect to which patients are entitled.

INTERDISCIPLINARY APPROACH TO HEALTH CARE

The primary goal of the health care team is the optimal physical, mental, and social well-being of the

Box 1.2 **Nursing Conditions in the Past**

The following job description was given to floor nurses by a hospital in 1887.

In addition to caring for your 50 patients, each nurse will follow these regulations:

- Daily sweep and mop the floors of your ward, dust the patient's furniture and windowsills. Maintain an even temperature in your ward by bringing in a scuttle of coal for the day's business.
- Light is important to observe the patient's condition. Therefore, each day, fill kerosene lamps, clean chimneys, and trim wicks. Wash the windows once a week.
- The nurse's notes are important in aiding the physician's work. Make your pens carefully; you may whittle nibs to your individual taste.
- Each nurse on day duty will report every day at 7 a.m. and leave at 8 p.m., except on the Sabbath, on which day you will be off from 12 noon to 2 p.m.
- Graduate nurses in good standing with the director of nurses will be given an evening off each week for courting purposes or two evenings a week if you go regularly to church.
- Each nurse should lay aside from each payday a goodly sum of her earnings for her benefits during her declining years so that she will not become a burden. For example, if you earn $30 a month, you should set aside $15.
- Any nurse who smokes, uses liquor in any form, gets her hair done at a beauty shop, or frequents dance halls will give the director of nurses good reason to suspect her worth, intentions, and integrity.
- The nurse who performs her labors and serves her patients and doctors without fault for 5 years will be given an increase of 5 cents a day, providing there are no hospital debts outstanding.

It is interesting to compare current practical and vocational nursing tasks with those that were expected in 1887. Practical and vocational nursing has indeed come a long way.

From Hill SS, Howlett HA: *Success in practical/vocational nursing: from student to leader*, ed 7, St. Louis, 2013, Saunders.

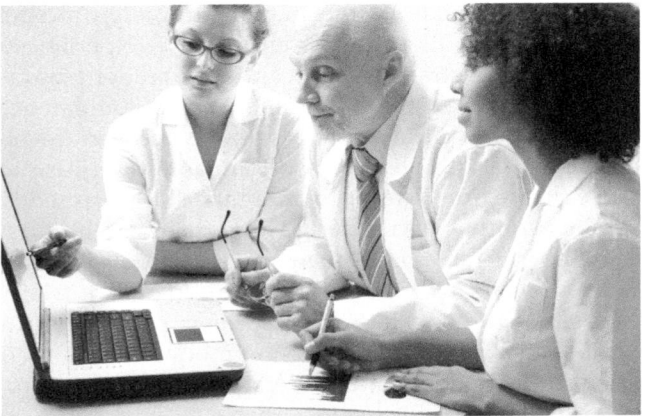

Fig. 1.9 Nurse collaborating with other members of the interdisciplinary team. (Copyright 1999–2012 Thinkstock. All rights reserved.)

Care Plan

The care plan is a document that outlines the individual needs of the patient and the approach of the health care team to meet these needs. It is developed in cooperation with the patient and, in some cases, the patient's family. It further identifies who will assist in treating the patient. The plan of care is a "living document" that is updated as the patient's condition warrants. The goal of the document is to guide and direct the activities surrounding the patient's care, ensure continuity and consistency of care, and eliminate duplication of services. (See Chapter 5 for further discussion of use of the nursing care plan in the nursing process.)

Communication

Good communication is essential for the exchange of information among the members of the health care team. Communication is the prerequisite for meeting the needs of the patient or, if necessary, making appropriate changes to do so. (See Chapter 4 for further discussion of communication.)

Documentation

Documentation in any form is the permanent record of the patient's progress and treatment. It constitutes the formal and legal record of care received by the patient and the patient's response to that care (Fig. 1.10). The information recorded during the entire course of treatment serves many purposes. It provides a progress record of treatment so that all the involved health care members are aware of what treatment the patient is receiving. It also provides a chronicle of events, which becomes a valued piece of the patient's health history that may be referenced for future health care needs. (See Chapter 3 for further discussion of documentation.)

NURSING CARE MODELS

Since the time of Florence Nightingale, nursing and health care technology have continued to change

patient. This goal is achieved by promoting and restoring health within the wellness-illness continuum. Health care personnel, when working to meet the needs of the patient, must work together as a health care team. Following this interdisciplinary approach to treatment prevents the fragmentation of patient care. Just as the plan of care for patients is developed in a holistic manner, so is the actual delivery of health care. All health care providers must remember that the central focus of all their activity is the patient.

Each member of the team is responsible for coordinating activity with every other member of the team by developing a comprehensive care plan, effectively communicating, and keeping accurate records (Fig. 1.9).

to meet the needs of the patient. Initially, nursing education was like an apprenticeship. Experienced nurses demonstrated skills, and the student nurse practiced these skills until technical competence was achieved. Little emphasis was placed on development of a knowledge base to enable the nurse to solve future problems or to adapt the skills learned to various complex situations. Through research, nursing theorists have developed several models to assist with problem solving and organization of care. Many schools of nursing loosely base their curriculum or philosophy on a specific nursing model to help their students learn about and understand the nursing process (see Chapter 5).

Fig. 1.10 Nurse documenting patient care at a computer. (Copyright 1999–2012 Thinkstock. All rights reserved.)

As early as the 1970s, nursing leaders identified the following four major concepts that were the basis for all nursing models of care:

- *Nursing:* Encompasses the roles and actions of the nurse
- **Patient:** The individual who receives the care
- **Health:** The area along the wellness-illness continuum that the patient occupies
- *Environment:* The setting for the nurse-patient interaction

Several leading nurse theorists have developed nursing models of care, and their work is ongoing. Table 1.2 shows six leading nursing theories that incorporate those basic concepts.

CONTEMPORARY PRACTICAL AND VOCATIONAL NURSING CARE

As stated earlier, the existence of the LPN/LVN in the health care delivery system is not new. What is new is the expansion of the LPN/LVN's role and responsibilities from bathing patients and doing light housekeeping to performing skilled tasks needed to provide health care to people along the wellness-illness continuum.

The ongoing evolution of the role is influenced by various state nurse practice acts, individual changes within the health care agencies, the availability of health care workers, and the needs of patients. LPN/LVNs are finding careers in hospitals, clinics, outpatient agencies, home health agencies, long-term care facilities, insurance companies, physician offices, and the military services.

Table 1.2 Leading Theories

THEORIST	NURSING OBJECTIVE	SETTING
Nightingale (1860)	To facilitate "the body's reparative processes" by arranging the patient's environment.	Patient's environment is arranged; includes appropriate noise control, nutrition, hygiene, lighting, comfort, socialization, and hope.
Orem (1971)	To care for and help patient attain total self-care.	This is self-care deficit theory. Nursing care becomes necessary when patient is unable to fulfill biologic, psychological, developmental, or social needs.
Leininger (1978)	To provide care consistent with nursing's emerging science and knowledge, with caring as the central focus.	In this transcultural care theory, caring is the central and unifying domain for nursing knowledge and practice.
Roy (1979)	To identify types of demands placed on patient, assess adaptation to demands, and help patients adapt.	This adaptation model is based on the physiologic, psychological, sociologic, and dependence-independence adaptive modes.
Parse (1981)	To focus on humans as unitary living beings and humanity's qualitative participation with the health experience (nursing as science and art).	Humans continually interact with environment and participate in maintenance of health. Health is a continual open process rather than a state of well-being or absence of disease.
Benner and Wrubel (1989)	To focus on patient's needs for caring as a means of coping with stressors of illness.	Caring is central to the essence of nursing. Caring creates the possibilities for coping and enables possibilities for connecting with and concern for others.

PRACTICAL AND VOCATIONAL NURSING DEFINED

Practical and vocational nursing is defined as the activity of providing specific services to patients under the direct supervision of an RN or a licensed physician. The services are provided in a structured setting surrounding the caring for the sick, the rehabilitation of the sick and injured, and the prevention of sickness and injury.

The nurse has a unique function: to assist individuals, sick or well, in the performance of those activities that contribute to health, to their recovery, or to a peaceful death—activities that patients would perform unaided if they had the necessary strength, will, or knowledge—and, if feasible, to do this in such a way as to help patients gain independence as rapidly as possible. The practical or vocational nurse is educated to be a responsible member of a health care team, performing basic therapeutic, rehabilitative, and preventive care to assigned patients. Currently, there are more than 700,000 LPN/LVNs working in the United States (Bureau of Labor Statistics, 2021).

The practice of discharging patients from acute care facilities for continued recuperation in extended care units and nursing homes, places of employment for LPN/LVNs, is evident in the increasing number of patients who need more complex care. Every 2 years, the National Council of State Boards of Nursing performs a job analysis. This analysis helps to determine the content areas for the NCLEX-PN. The findings of the latest job analysis indicate that newly licensed LPN/LVNs are continuing to provide care in all types of settings, with the majority continuing to be employed in long-term care settings. No statistically significant changes have occurred in work settings since the last job analysis.

OBJECTIVES AND CHARACTERISTICS OF PRACTICAL AND VOCATIONAL NURSING EDUCATION

The objectives for practical and vocational nursing education are the following:
- To acquire the specialized knowledge and skills needed to meet the health care needs of patients in a variety of settings
- To participate in the intradisciplinary health care team.
- To be a graduate of a state-approved practical or vocational nursing program
- To apply for state licensure, sit for, and pass the NCLEX-PN examination

To accomplish these objectives, students must assume responsibility for their own education, intensive study, and dedication to duty. Organization of time effectively helps accomplish these objectives and ultimately ensures the patient of safe and competent care.

Distinguishing characteristics, roles, and responsibilities for the LPN/LVN are shown in Box 1.3.

ROLES AND RESPONSIBILITIES

NAPNES (2007) issued the following statement of responsibilities required for practice as an LPN/LVN:
- Demonstrate professional behaviors of accountability and professionalism according to the legal and ethical standards for a competent licensed practical/vocational nurse.
- Effectively communicate with patients, significant support person(s), and members of the interdisciplinary health care team incorporating interpersonal and therapeutic communication skills.
- Collect holistic assessment data from multiple sources, communicate the data to appropriate health care providers, and evaluate patient responses to interventions.
- Collaborate with the RN or other members of the health care team to organize and incorporate assessment data to plan/revise patient care and actions based on established nursing diagnoses, nursing protocols, and assessment and evaluation data.
- Demonstrate a caring and empathic approach to the safe, therapeutic, and individualized care of each patient.
- Implement patient care, at the direction of an RN, a licensed physician, or a dentist through performance of nursing interventions or directing aspects of care, as appropriate, to UAP.

LPN/LVNs are required to be aware of the content of the nurse practice act of the state in which they are employed. The role of the LPN/LVN is found in this law, and the law differs from state to state.

A major criterion in differentiating between the roles of the RN and the LPN/LVN is the level of

---

Box 1.3	Characteristics, Roles, and Responsibilities of the Practical or Vocational Nurse

- Is a responsible and accountable member of the health care team
- Maintains a current license
- Practices within the scope of the state's nurse practice act
- Practices under the supervision of the registered nurse, or physician, or designated healthcare provider
- Supervises other practical and vocational nurses and unlicensed assistive personnel
- Participates in continuing education activities
- Contributes to and follows the nursing process to meet patients' needs
- Promotes and maintains health, prevents disease, and encourages and assists in rehabilitation
- Maintains a professional appearance
- Subscribes to recognized ethical practices
- Participates in activities of professional organizations
- Assists in developing the role of the licensed practical nurse and licensed vocational nurse of tomorrow

independence for the practice activities. The LPN/LVN never functions independently. LPN/LVNs provide care in basic and complex situations under the general supervision of an RN or physician. They are responsible for functioning safely and are accountable for their actions.

LPN/LVNs function interdependently when they offer input to the RN about the effectiveness of care or offer suggestions to improve the patient's care. Because LPN/LVNs provide actual care at the bedside in acute care situations, the data collected during the giving of care are valuable in determining whether progress is being made toward meeting patient goals.

Practical and vocational nursing is an exciting, challenging career that provides an opportunity to care for others while receiving personal satisfaction. The focus is on bedside and personal care of patients in a variety of settings. Performance in a responsible and accountable manner calls for knowledge, skill, and expertise.

Get Ready for the NCLEX® examination!

Key Points

- The evolution of nursing was influenced greatly by the way care was given to the sick and injured.
- The influence of Florence Nightingale on nursing practice and nursing education was highly significant in the 19th century.
- Nursing practice and education in the United States were influenced significantly by the activities of Florence Nightingale.
- The Association of Practical Nurse Schools was organized in Chicago in 1941 to address the needs of practical nursing education. Its name was changed in 1942 to the National Association of Practical Nurse Education (NAPNE).
- NAPNE changed its name again in 1959 to the National Association for Practical Nurse Education and Service (NAPNES).
- In 1949 the National Federation of Licensed Practical Nurses (NFLPN) was founded by Lillian Kuster.
- Mandatory licensure laws were established for practical and vocational nursing education and practice.
- The wellness-illness continuum is a range that comprises the entirety of a person's health.
- Prevention of illness and injury and continuity of patient care are integral components of holistic health care.
- The practical or vocational nurse is one of many of the large groups of health care workers who provide health care services.
- The practical and vocational nursing community functions in accordance with several states' nurse practice acts.
- Roles and responsibilities of the nurse are varied and complex and evolve with new technologies and research advances.
- Ongoing education is valued, expected, and required for continued licensure.

Additional Learning Resources

SG Go to your Study Guide for additional learning activities to help you master this chapter content.

Be sure to visit the Evolve site at http://evolve.elsevier.com/Cooper/foundations/ for additional online resources.

Review Questions for the NCLEX® Examination

1. **A prospective nursing student questions what program accreditation means. What should be included in the information provided?**
   1. Accreditation is a voluntary review by a given organization to determine whether the program meets that organization's preestablished criteria.
   2. An accredited program is one that meets the minimal standards set by the respective state agencies responsible for overseeing educational programs.
   3. Program accreditation is necessary before the graduate is eligible to take the National Council Licensing Examination for Practical Nursing (NCLEX-PN).
   4. Nursing program accreditation is a federally funded health care program that educates practical nurse students.

2. **The nursing student is discussing the impact of preventative medicine. Which change has resulted from this focus?**
   1. Anxiety over diagnostic workups such as colonoscopies or gynecologic examinations
   2. The number of admissions for inpatient services
   3. The length of a hospitalization stay
   4. Knowledge and services to promote health and prevent illness (wellness-illness continuum)

3. **Growth and advancement of the nursing profession in the 21st century can be attributed to:**
   1. growth of cities.
   2. better education of nurses.
   3. teachings of Christianity.
   4. improved conditions for women.

4. **Nursing education programs may seek voluntary accreditation by which agency?**
   1. American Nurses Association
   2. International Council of Nurses
   3. Congress for Nursing Practice
   4. National League for Nursing

5. When developing a definition of "health," a person should consider that health is:

   1. a condition of physical, mental, and social well-being and absence of disease.
   2. the ability to pursue activities of daily living.
   3. a function of the physiologic state.
   4. a static condition; the absence of pathology.

6. Which philosophy is described as comprehensive or total patient care that considers the physical, emotional, social, economic, and spiritual needs of the person; the person's response to the illness; and the impact of the illness on the person's ability to meet self-care needs?

   1. The wellness-illness continuum
   2. The Patient Care Partnership
   3. Holistic nursing
   4. The health care delivery system

7. The student nurse reviewing the history of nursing knows that the "Lady with the Lamp" is:

   1. Clara Barton.
   2. Florence Nightingale.
   3. Phoebe.
   4. Lavinia Dock.

8. The American Society of Superintendents of Training Schools of Nursing was established in 1894. What was the major goal of the organization?

   1. To promote development of new schools of nursing
   2. To train nursing leaders
   3. To set educational standards for nurses
   4. To develop standards for licensure

9. Nurses correctly recognize what as the key determinant of their scope of practice?

   1. The nursing process
   2. The agency's policies
   3. The Hippocratic Oath
   4. The nurse practice act

10. Nursing theorists are helpful in enabling the nursing profession to problem solve and establish standards. Who is largely recognized as the first nursing theorist?

    1. Phoebe
    2. Clara Barton
    3. Florence Nightingale
    4. Sister Calista Roy

11. The most commonly used model that assists in the understanding of the patient's place on the wellness-illness continuum is that of:

    1. Abraham Maslow.
    2. Dorothea Dix.
    3. Clara Barton.
    4. Theodore Fliedner.

12. Which person was the first nurse to train in America?

    1. Lavinia Dock
    2. Linda Richards
    3. Clara Barton
    4. Mary Breckenridge

13. Which was the first school dedicated to the training of the practical nurse in the United States?

    1. The Ballard School
    2. The Young Women's Christian Association (YWCA)
    3. The Thompson Practical Nursing School
    4. The Shepard-Gill School

14. What is health?

    1. The absence of illness
    2. A state of complete physical, mental, and social well-being
    3. A condition between disease and good health
    4. The opposite of disease

15. Which statement about men in nursing is the most correct description?

    1. Men were not permitted to serve in the military.
    2. The prominence of men in nursing increased during the Civil War.
    3. The number of men in the profession is decreasing.
    4. Men are regaining their historical position in the profession as nurses.

16. The nurse is reviewing the planned health promotion activities for a local community center. Which primary prevention activities may be included? *(Select all that apply.)*

    1. Screening for complications of diabetes
    2. Dietary teaching focused on prevention of obesity
    3. Support group development for the victims of partner violence
    4. Weight loss programs for patients with diabetes
    5. Exercise programs for teens
    6. PSA levels following prostate cancer treatment
    7. Mammograms starting at the age of 40 years
    8. Education for patients with celiac disease on how to best control their symptoms

17. Which factors affect male students' success in nursing programs? *(Select all that apply.)*

    1. Men have more difficulty studying for examinations.
    2. Men may feel isolated in the nursing program.
    3. Many men have difficulty showing their feelings of care and empathy.
    4. There are limited role models for men in nursing.
    5. Instructor attitudes may not embrace male students.

Legal and Ethical Aspects of Nursing

http://evolve.elsevier.com/Cooper/foundations/

Objectives

1. Summarize the structure and function of the legal system.
2. Compare and contrast nursing negligence and malpractice.
3. Discuss the legal relationship that exists between the nurse and the patient.
4. Explain the importance of maintaining standards of care.
5. Give examples of ways the nursing profession is regulated.
6. Give examples of legal issues in health care.
7. Discuss federal regulations of the Health Insurance Portability and Accountability Act of 1996 (HIPAA) privacy rule and its impact on the health care system.
8. Give examples of ways the licensed practical/vocational nurse can avoid being involved in a lawsuit.
9. Differentiate between a legal duty and an ethical duty.
10. Explain advance directives.
11. Summarize how culture affects an individual's beliefs, morals, and values.
12. Identify how values affect decision making.
13. Distinguish between ethical and unethical behavior.
14. Explain the meaning of a code of ethics.
15. Explain the nurse's role in reporting unethical behavior.
16. Give examples of ethical issues common in health care.

Key Terms

accountability (ăk-kŏwnt-ă-BĬL-ĕ-tē, p. 25)
advocate (ĂD-vō-kăt, p. 25)
deposition (dĕ-pō-SĬ-shŭn, p. 24)
doctrine of informed consent (p. 27)
ethical dilemmas (ĔTH-ĭ-kăl, p. 35)
ethics (ĔTH-ĭks, p. 32)
euthanasia (ūth-ĕn-Ā-zhă, p. 31)
laws (p. 23)
liability (lĭ-ă-BĬL-ĕ-tē, p. 25)

liable (LĪ-ă-bl, p. 24)
malpractice (p. 24)
nonmaleficence (nŏn-mă-LĔF-ĭ-sĕns, p. 36)
respondent (add pronunciation p. 24)
standards of care (p. 26)
value clarification (p. 35)
values (p. 34)
verdict (p. 24)

Today's health care system is dynamic and complex. It has undergone significant changes over the decades. Health care providers are guided by established laws, rules, regulations, and ethical principles. The rising cost of health care and growing consumer awareness have had an impact on the practice of nursing and the distribution and use of available health care resources. Additional challenges are presented by the rapid advances in technology and communication. Practice opportunities and settings for the licensed practical/vocational nurse (LPN/LVN) are changing with the focus on managed care, community health, and home health care.

Nursing practice of the LPN/LVN is guided by a combination of legal principles, established laws, moral standards, and ethical principles. Nurses must understand the legal standards and ethical principles that affect practice. Each state has laws that govern the scope and practice of nursing that are referred to as nurse practice acts. The law sets an obligatory minimum standard in any given situation. Ethical principles, which evolve out of society and culture, frequently impose an even higher duty. These legal standards and ethical principles serve as a support for all members of the health care system and help protect the rights of all members of society.

LEGAL ASPECTS OF NURSING

The legal relationship that exists between the nurse, patient, and family is influenced by the existing laws, rules, and regulations that govern nursing practice. Acting outside the established scope of practice or failing to meet the established standard of care has the potential to result in injury to the patient and give rise to legal liability and the potential loss or sanction of the

Box 2.1	Characteristics of Criminal and Civil Law

CRIMINAL
- Conduct at issue is offensive to society *in general.*
- Conduct at issue is detrimental to society *as a whole.*
- The law involves *public* offenses (such as robbery, murder, assault).
- The law's purpose is to *punish* for the crime and deter and *prevent* further crimes.

CIVIL
- Conduct at issue violates a *person's* rights.
- Conduct at issue is detrimental to that *individual.*
- The law involves an offense that is against an *individual.*
- The law's purpose is to *make the aggrieved person whole again,* to restore the person to where he or she was.

Box 2.2	Busta v Columbus Hospital Corporation (1996)

While he was a postoperative patient at Columbus Hospital in Great Falls, Mr. Busta died from injuries sustained in a fall from his third-floor window; apparently, he had tried to climb down on an improvised rope. At trial, the nurse assigned to care for Mr. Busta testified that during her last evening visit with him, he had experienced an episode of tachycardia and hypertension. He had also behaved atypically, desiring isolation and refusing all nursing care and his prescribed medication, known to have adverse effects, including confusion, anxiety, and psychosis. The nurse did not report the symptoms and the change in behavior to the physician. She also testified that when she observed the patient at midnight, he appeared to be sleeping; she did not reassess his vital signs.

Mr. Busta's surgeon testified that, because of the mind-altering adverse effects of the patient's medication, he would have reassessed his patient if he had been notified of the changing signs and symptoms. Expert testimony opined that the nurse was negligent in failing to adequately monitor Mr. Busta on the evening and night before he died and in failing to report the constellation of signs and symptoms to the surgeon and that the hospital was negligent in failing to maintain a safe environment (evidence presented at trial showed that the hospital had not acted on a directive from The Joint Commission [TJC] to restrict the opening of windows in patients' rooms).

The jury found that the negligence of Columbus Hospital combined with the patient's contributory negligence caused the patient's injuries and death; the jury apportioned 70% of the liability to the hospital and 30% to Mr. Busta. The jury found that Mr. Busta and his estate were damaged in the amount of $5000 and his heirs $800,000. On the basis of the jury's apportioned liability, the district court entered a judgment in favor of Mr. Busta's estate in the amount of $3500 and in favor of his heirs $560,000.

From Croke E: Nurses, negligence and malpractice, *Am J Nurs* 103(9):59–60, 2003.

nursing license. Nurses must be aware of their scope of nursing practice and the standards of care that constitute professional duties.

Many legal issues are related to health care, and health care–related litigation that involves nurses is common. Today's patients are more educated, are more aware of their rights, and have higher expectations regarding the care they receive than patients from previous generations. To practice safely, the nurse must have a familiarity with common legal issues in nursing. Reviews of nursing errors often find a series of preventable failures in performance.

OVERVIEW OF THE LEGAL SYSTEM

The legal system is a complex set of rules and regulations that has developed in response to the needs of society. **Laws** prescribe proper behavior in society; they sanction acceptable behavior and prohibit unacceptable behavior. Nurses must have a basic understanding of the legal system, which mandates and protects. The law assigns fundamental legal duties and provides protection for all members of the health care system.

The two primary categories of law are criminal and civil (Box 2.1). Matters related to criminal law are those that involve the needs of the public. Cases that concern matters of criminal law are charged by agents that represent either the federal or the state government. Civil cases are between individuals. The charges involved in a civil matter are brought by an individual or agency. Some degree of overlap may exist with the cases. For example, a criminal matter may result in individuals filing a civil lawsuit. The penalties that result from the cases also differ. Criminal cases are resolved with a finding of guilt or innocence. The penalty may involve fines, incarceration, or a combination of the two. Civil matters conclude with a determination of accountability or innocence. Monetary settlements are assigned based on the type of liability assessed. Civil law and criminal law are established in one of two ways: (1) federal, state, and local governments develop *statutory law;* and (2) *common law,* or case law, evolves in response to specific legal questions that come before the court and usually follows *precedent* (previous rulings on an issue).

Negligence

The terms *negligence* and *malpractice* often are used interchangeably. However, this is incorrect. There are distinct differences between them. *Negligence* refers to the absence of due care. It is more of a general action that often can be attributed to being careless. Nurses and unlicensed assistive personnel may be charged with negligence. Professional-level accountability and judgment are not required elements to establish negligence. Negligence refers to the failure to act in a manner demonstrating the care and knowledge any prudent individual would use. Examples of negligence may include medication errors, patient falls, use/misuse of restraints, and equipment injuries. An example of negligence can be found in Box 2.2.

Malpractice

Malpractice refers to professional negligence. Nursing responsibilities include actions taken and those omitted. The concept of malpractice must contain four key elements. Each of the elements must be present for liability to be established.

1. *Duty* refers the established relationship between the patient and the nurse.
2. *Breach* of duty is failure to perform the duty in a reasonable, prudent manner.
3. *Harm* has occurred; this does not have to be physical injury.
4. The breach of duty was the *proximate cause* of the harm; the occurrence of harm depended directly on the occurrence of the breach.

If the court finds that malpractice has occurred, the nurse is subject to legal punishment or restitution as the court determines. The best way to avoid being charged with malpractice is to practice within the rules and regulations, the standards of care, and the employing agency's policies and procedures. The nurse-patient relationship is also very important; strive to maintain a positive relationship. A poor nurse-patient relationship has been identified as a leading factor in whether a patient seeks legal action.

There are four options for establishing the levels of responsibility. The individual may be personally responsible for the act of negligence or malpractice committed. A manager or supervisor may be implicated if there was inappropriate supervision or delegation by another member of the health care team. The employer may be found responsible for the employee's actions if there are deficits in education or inappropriate credentials for the role. The employer is also responsible for ensuring the staff members have the needed supplies and equipment (Missouri Department of Health & Human Services, n.d.).

OVERVIEW OF THE LEGAL PROCESS

Civil litigation involves the legal exchange between individuals as opposed to legal concerns that involve a criminal matter, which would involve the state or federal government bringing charges. Most legal suits in health care involve civil litigation. The process for filing a claim begins when an individual believes that a breach of duty has taken place and resulted in pain, suffering, or injury. At that time, the plaintiff (the complaining party) typically seeks legal representation. In some states, a prelitigation panel may meet to ascertain the validity of the suit being proposed. If this process results in a finding that litigation in this case has a legal basis, the plaintiff writes a statement called a *complaint* and files it in the appropriate court. The complaint names the *defendant* or **respondent** (the person alleged to be **liable** [legally responsible]), states the facts involved in the case, defines the legal issues the case raises, and outlines the *damages* (compensation that the plaintiff is seeking). The defendant/respondent (the

person accused of the offense) is served a *summons* (a court order that notifies the defendant of the legal action), which constitutes the necessary legal notice, and the defendant usually hires an attorney to represent him or her in the lawsuit. The defendant is asked to provide a response to the charges. This response is either an admission of guilt or a denial of allegations listed in the complaint.

Discovery is the next step in the process. Discovery allows both sides of the case to review documents and interview witnesses. The witnesses may be the defendant being named in the suit or individuals who have facts about the case. Witnesses are required to undergo questioning by the attorneys. This process is referred to as the **deposition**. Witnesses are under oath. The statements made are recorded. This transcript becomes a part of the evidence.

Other tools also serve the process of discovery. The *interrogatory* is a written question that one party sends to the other party, to which an answer is legally required. A *Request for Production of Documents and Things* is a formal request by the agents filing the charges for all items that are deemed to be related to the case at hand. In a health care–related case, these items may include policies and procedures, standards of care, medical records, assignment sheets, personnel files, equipment maintenance records, birth certificates, marriage certificates, medical bills, and other documents pertinent to the issues at hand. A fourth discovery technique is the admission of facts. This tool requests the party to admit or deny certain statements to streamline the factual presentation of the case.

Once the evidence has been presented, the court renders a **verdict** (decision) based on the facts of the case, the evidence and testimony presented, the credibility of the witnesses, and the laws that pertain to the issue. Either party has the right, in case of disagreement with the outcome of the lawsuit, to file an *appeal* (request a review of the decision) asking that a higher court review the decision. The outcome of litigation is never certain.

In a criminal trial, the question is whether the defendant is answerable for a crime against the people (because criminal law concerns crimes against society rather than individuals). At trial, the people's attorney and the defendant's attorney present their cases. The judge or the jury (if a jury trial) then *deliberate* (consider and decide) the guilt or innocence of the defendant. If the judge or jury reaches a verdict of *not guilty,* the defendant is cleared of the charges. If the verdict is *guilty,* the judge passes a *sentence* (penalty) based on the severity of the offense, the defendant's past criminal record, and applicable laws. The defendant who receives a guilty verdict may appeal if there has been an error either: (1) in the process in which the conviction was obtained or (2) by the court during the proceedings. Box 2.3 presents some common legal terminology.

| Box 2.3 | Common Legal Terminology |

Abandonment of care	Wrongful termination of providing patient care
Assault	An intentional threat to cause bodily harm to another; does not have to include actual bodily contact
Battery	Unlawful touching of another person without informed consent
Competency	A legal presumption that a person who has reached the age of majority can make decisions for herself or himself unless proved otherwise (if she or he has been legally declared incompetent)
Defamation	Spoken or written statements made maliciously and intentionally that may injure the subject's reputation
Harm	Injury to a person or the person's property that gives rise to a basis for a legal action against the person who caused the damage
Libel	A malicious or untrue writing about another person that is brought to the attention of others
Malpractice	Failure to meet a legal duty, thus causing harm to another
Negligence	The commission (doing) of an act or the omission (not doing) of an act that a reasonably prudent person would have performed in a similar situation, thus causing harm to another person
Slander	Malicious or untrue spoken words about another person that are brought to the attention of others
Tort	A type of civil law that involves wrongs against a person or property; torts include negligence, assault, battery, defamation, fraud, false imprisonment, and invasion of privacy

LEGAL RELATIONSHIPS

Legal liability for alleged harm may be held solely or shared between multiple parties. The patient or family may choose to pursue charges against the facility, nursing personnel, medical staff, or ancillary departments. Each may be charged separately or in a group. In the past, nurses did not hold legal liability for alleged harm suffered by a patient while receiving medical care, but the physician and/or the hospital did. As nurses gained recognition for their expertise and gained more autonomy, dissatisfied patients (and their attorneys) began to look at nurses as potential defendants and to seek to hold nurses accountable under the law. **Accountability** (being responsible for one's own actions) is a concept that gives rise to a legal duty, and thus **liability** (legal responsibility), in nursing.

Indeed, the nurse is not immune from liability in the practice of nursing. An analysis of statistics shows sharp increases in the amount of litigation against nurses by patients. A variety of reasons explain the increases (Boxes 2.4 and 2.5). Nurses are facing increased responsibilities in the health care arena. Technological advances require more knowledge and competence. Staffing shortages and budgetary constraints also may play a role. High levels of patient acuity and an emphasis on early discharge may result in the need for more comprehensive referrals and improved discharge teaching. Flaws in either may result in litigation. Finally, insurance experts believe that some responsibility may rest with the large payout to litigants. Legal findings against nurses can be categorized. The practice setting most commonly involved litigation is labor and delivery (35%) followed by surgery (28%) and emergency department (32%). The most common area resulting

| Box 2.4 | Preventable Omissions in Nursing |

Nursing errors can be tied to seven largely preventable omissions. These involve failures to:
1. Collaborate with other health care team members
2. Clarify interdisciplinary orders
3. Ask for and offer assistance
4. Utilize evidence-based performance
5. Communicate information to patients and families
6. Limit overtime
7. Adequately staff patient care units with appropriately credentialed staff

Source: Nursing Made Incredibly Easy. How to avoid the top seven nursing errors. Deamont, Ann MSN, RN, VHA-CM. March/April 2013 Volume 11, Issue 2, pages 8–10. Retrieved from http://journals.lww.com/nursingmadeincredibleyeasy/Fulltext/2013/03000/How_to_avoid_the_top_seven_nursing_errors.4.aspxhttp://journals.lww.com/nursingmadeincrediblyeasy/Fulltext/2013/03000/How_to_avoid_the_top_seven_nursing_errors.4.aspx.

in the legal action is communication. This can refer to failure to report patient condition changes, medication errors, and interventions (failure to perform or unsafe performance) (Miller and Zois, 2020).

When a nurse accepts a patient care assignment, the nurse-patient relationship is initiated. This relationship, beyond its more personal human component, has a legal basis: the duty to provide professional care. A failure to provide care to the expected level of expertise gives rise to legal liability (see the discussion on standards of care in the next section). In the nurse-patient relationship, the nurse accepts the role of advocate for the patient. An **advocate** is one who defends or pleads a cause or issue on behalf of another. A nurse advocate has a legal and ethical obligation to safeguard the patient's interests.

Box 2.5   Common Breaches of the Standard of Care

PRACTICE
Failure to:

- Use proper judgment
- Properly assess
- Properly administer medication
- Protect patients from burns
- Properly maintain the airway
- Restock crash cart
- Honor advance directives
- Take an accurate and thorough history
- Provide a safe environment
- Properly administer injections
- Go through hierarchy to get the care needed
- Detect that the patient has an allergy
- Protect the patient from abuse
- Prevent abuse, neglect, or injury by other patients
- Obtain physician orders—practicing outside the scope of nursing practice by writing orders
- Practice safely (by using drugs or alcohol while working)
- Protect and prevent falls

MONITORING

- Properly monitor
- Recognize and report signs and symptoms of patient's deteriorating condition
- Properly use monitoring equipment
- Protect against injuries from monitoring equipment
- Detect or prevent decubitus ulcers
- Monitor and detect polypharmacy effects on patient
- Detect signs and symptoms of a medical condition in a timely and proper fashion
- Detect signs and symptoms of drug toxicity
- Properly use restraints

COMMUNICATION

- Document in a timely and proper fashion
- Notify physician of laboratory values in a timely and proper fashion
- Report child or elder abuse
- Notify physician of a change in status
- Communicate with other health care personnel about advance directives
- Properly give discharge instructions
- Document patient's status or condition in a timely and proper fashion
- Document communications between health care providers in a timely and proper fashion
- Document the need for restraints in a timely and proper fashion
- Properly document (precharting)

A landmark case that addressed nursing liability was *Darling v Charleston Community Memorial Hospital.* In this case, an 18-year-old man fractured his leg and had a cast applied in the hospital. He was admitted to a room, and the nurses caring for the patient noticed that the toes on his casted leg were edematous and discolored. The patient reported decreased feeling in his toes to the nursing staff. Over the next few days, gangrene developed, and the man's leg had to be amputated.

The Illinois Supreme Court heard the case and held that the nurses were liable, along with the physician, because the nursing staff had failed to adhere to the standards of care. This case established a precedent that almost every state has adopted.

REGULATION OF PRACTICE

Standards of care define acts whose performance is required, permitted, or prohibited. These standards of care derive from federal and state laws, rules, and regulations and codes that govern other professional agencies and organizations such as the American Nurses Association (ANA) and the Canadian Nurses Association (CNA). These organizations regularly evaluate existing standards and revise them as needed. Standards of care coupled with the *scope of nursing practice* give direction to the practicing nurse. They define the obligations of the nurse, including those activities that are obligatory and those that are prohibited. Failure to adhere to these standards gives rise to legal liability. Ignorance of the requirements and limitations does not absolve liability.

Nursing liability falls into several areas: practice, monitoring, and communication. Box 2.5 shows common breaches of the standards of care. The legal test is the comparison with the hypothetical actions under similar circumstances of a reasonably *prudent* (careful, wise) nurse of similar education and experience. The standards of care follow those laws of the individual state. In reality, application of the standards is not always easy. Nursing shortages in some states have led to a need for individual nurses to take on increased responsibilities and work more hours. Personnel cutbacks often leave units short-staffed, and nurses feel pressure to take on expanded duties; this increases their risk for liability considerably. In addition, special challenges face entry-level licensed nurses when they enter the workforce. Orientation programs often fail to adequately cover all the skills needed to be a competent practitioner. It is the nurse's responsibility to seek additional instruction and supervision when faced with an unfamiliar practice or procedure. Remember that it is not possible for the nurse to meet every patient's needs.

The laws that formally define and limit the scope of nursing practice are called *nurse practice acts.* All state, provincial, and territorial legislatures in the United States and Canada have adopted nurse practice acts, although the specifics they contain often vary. It is the nurse's responsibility to know the nurse practice act that is in effect for the geographic region. A free copy of the state's nurse practice act can be obtained by writing to the board of nursing in a given state or accessing its website.

In addition to the boundaries made by the state's nurse practice act, the employing institution often places limitations on practice. The institution has the right to establish policies and procedures for nursing

Box **2.6**   Evidence of Nursing Standards

- Accreditation criteria of The Joint Commission (formerly the Joint Commission on Accreditation of Healthcare Organizations [JCAHO])
- Agency policy and procedure manuals
- American Nurses Association Code for Nurses (2001)
- American Nurses Association Standards of Practice (1995)
- Customs and usual community practices
- Education, continuing education, staff development, and orientation
- Experience
- Expert nurse witness, other experts, and peers
- Nursing literature, textbooks, and journals
- Nursing specialty standards of care and certification
- Other accreditation standards depending on the practice setting (e.g., National League for Nursing, National Association of Home Care)
- Practice protocols, contracts, practice agreements, employment agreements, and personnel or employee manuals
- State and federal licensing laws and regulations that govern health care agencies: state, professional, and occupational legislation and regulations
- State nurse practice acts and regulations

activities within the confines of the state's nurse practice act. When a question comes before the court regarding whether the standard of care was met in a particular situation, the court uses a variety of resources to answer the question (Box 2.6).

LEGAL ISSUES

Many legal issues affect the LPN/LVN and influence the level of care delivered to the patient. Statutory and common law play important roles in defining the rights and responsibilities of the patient and the nursing professionals. The patient has a right to expect the nurse to act in the patient's best interest by providing care that meets and is consistent with the established legal standards and principles.

Patients' Rights

Patients have expectations regarding the health care services they receive. In 1972, the American Hospital Association (AHA) developed the Patient's Bill of Rights. Since its inception, the Patient's Bill of Rights has undergone revisions; the modified version of 2003 is called The Patient Care Partnership: Understanding Expectations, Rights, and Responsibilities (see Box 1.1). The AHA encourages health care institutions to adapt the template bill of rights to their particular environments. This involves considering the cultural, religious, linguistic, and educational backgrounds of the population the institution serves. In 1980, the Mental Health Patient's Bill of Rights and the Pregnant Patient's Bill of Rights were adopted into law. The goal of the AHA is to promote the public's understanding of

their rights and responsibilities as consumers of health care. Failure of the nurse to embrace the outlined rights of the patient can promote breaches in the relationship between the nurse and the patient.

The Joint Commission is an independent accrediting agency responsible for accrediting and certifying more than 19,000 facilities in the United States. The Joint Commission has developed a brochure titled *Know Your Rights,* which is a statement on the rights and responsibilities of patients. The Patient Self-Determination Act (included in the Omnibus Budget Reconciliation Act of 1990, U.S. Code vol. 42, sec. 1395 cc[a][1]) regulates any institution that receives federal funding. The Patient Self-Determination Act requires that institutions maintain written policies and procedures regarding advance directives (including the use of life support if the patient is incapacitated), the right to accept or refuse treatment, and the right to participate fully in health care–related decisions.

The Health Insurance Portability and Accountability Act (HIPPA) was passed into legislation in 1996. In the years that followed there were modifications. Then agencies and facilities had until 2003 to become compliant with the mandates. Health care providers who maintain and transmit health care information must provide reasonable and appropriate administrative, technical, and physical safeguards on a patient's health information. The law sets rules and limits on who has permission to look at and receive health information and assigns penalties for wrongful disclosure of individually identifiable health information. All health care providers must be knowledgeable about the HIPAA standards and protect the privacy rights of patients and residents (www.hhs.gov/ocr/hipaa).

Health care institutions are obligated to uphold the patient's rights to (1) access to health care without any prejudice, (2) treatment with respect and dignity at all times, (3) privacy and confidentiality, (4) personal safety, and (5) complete information about one's own condition and treatment.

Patients' responsibilities to the health care institution include (1) providing accurate information about themselves, (2) giving information regarding their known conditions, and (3) participating in decision-making regarding treatment and care.

Informed Consent

The Patient Care Partnership establishes the patient's right to make decisions regarding his or her health care. The doctrine of informed consent refers to full disclosure of the facts the patient needs to make an intelligent (informed) decision before any invasive treatment or procedure is performed (Fig. 2.1). The patient has the right to accept or reject the proposed care but only after understanding fully what is being proposed—that is, the benefits of the treatment, the risks involved, any alternative treatments, and the consequences of refusing the treatment or procedure. The

AUTHORIZATION FOR AND CONSENT TO OPERATION. ADMINISTRATION OF ANESTHETICS, SPECIAL DIAGNOSTIC OR THERAPEUTIC PROCEDURES AND THE RENDERING OF OTHER MEDICAL SERVICES

Patient ___Jaelyn Horrall_____ Date ___January 9, 2021___ Time ___0800_____

1. **Operation or Procedure and Alternatives**
   a. I hereby authorize Dr. _____Kelly Cooper_____ and whomever she may designate as her assistants to perform the following procedure and/or alternative procedure necessary to treat my condition: (state nature of procedure(s) to be performed).

   _____Right total hip replacement_____

   _____OK for blood transfusion_____

   (LIST PROCEDURE(S))

   b. I understand the reason for the procedure is: __to replace my right hip joint and the head of my right hip bone. OK to receive__

   __blood transfusion_____

   _____

   c. For the purpose of advancing medical education and care, I consent to the admittance of observers to the operating room.
   d. It has been explained to me that conditions may arise during this procedure whereby a different procedure or an additional procedure may need to be performed and I authorize my physician and her assistants to do what they feel is needed and necessary.
   e. I understand that no guarantee or assurance has been made as to the results of the procedure and that it may not cure the condition.
   f. I consent to the examination and disposal by hospital authorities of any tissues or body parts that may be removed.

2. **Risks:** This authorization is given with the understanding that any operation or procedure involves some risks and hazards. The more common risks include: infection, bleeding, nerve injury, blood clots, heart attack, allergic reactions, and pneumonia. These risks can be serious and possibly fatal. Specific risks for this procedure and alternative methods of care have been explained to me by my physician.

3. **Anesthesia:** The administration of anesthesia also involves risks, most importantly a rare risk of reaction to medications causing severe injury or death. I consent to the use of such anesthetics as may be considered necessary by the person responsible for these services.

4. **Photography:** I consent to the photographing of operations to be performed, including appropriate portions of my body for medical, scientific, or educational purposes, providing my identity is not revealed by the pictures or by the descriptive texts accompanying them.

5. **Patient's Consent:** I have read and fully understand this consent form, and I understand I should not sign this form if all items, including all my questions, have not been explained or answered to my satisfaction or if I do not understand any of the terms or words contained in this consent form.

   IF YOU HAVE ANY QUESTIONS AS TO THE RISKS OR HAZARDS OF THE PROPOSED SURGERY OR TREATMENT, OR ANY QUESTIONS CONCERNING THE PROPOSED SURGERY OR TREATMENT ASK YOUR SURGEON NOW! **BEFORE SIGNING THIS CONSENT FORM.**

   DO NOT SIGN UNLESS YOU HAVE READ AND THOROUGHLY UNDERSTAND THIS FORM!

6. I certify that I have read and fully understand the above consent after adequate explanations were made to me, and after all blanks were filled in or crossed out before I signed.

   Kim Richey
   _____
   (Witness to Signature only)

   Betty Berg RN
   _____
   (Second Witness Signature if needed)
   (i.e., Telephone Consent)

   Signed ____*Jaelyn Horrall*_____
   _____
   (Patient, Parent, or Legal Guardian's Signature)

   _____
   (Doctor Signature)

   AUTHORIZATION AND CONSENT

   Kell-Russell Memorial Hospital
   12 West Industrial Blvd.
   Terre Haute, IN 47805
   (800) 555-0000

   NS-81 (Rev. 2/01)

   LABEL

   4532

Fig. 2.1 Sample consent form for a special procedure.

explanation of the procedure must be in nontechnical terms and in a language the patient can understand. Failure to secure informed consent may result in civil liability for battery. *Civil battery* (also called technical battery) is the unlawful touching of a person; an intent to harm is not necessary. Consent must be given freely. Coercion negates the spirit of informed consent. Patients who seek treatment sign forms to indicate acceptance of care interventions. Additional consent for treatment may be needed for further invasive actions. Patients may withdraw or limit consent at any time. Consent may be communicated in a variety of ways. Patients may imply consent by their actions. Patients may verbalize their acceptance of treatment interventions. Invasive procedures may require a written consent document to be completed.

Consent must be provided by the appropriate person. To provide consent, the patient must be at least 18 years of age. Minors under the age of 18 years may consent for treatment if they meet certain criteria, including the following:

- Marriage
- Court-approved emancipation
- Living apart from parents or guardians for at least 60 days and independent of parental support
- Service in the armed forces

In some situations, a minor may consent for care, including treatment for sexually transmitted infections, drug and alcohol abuse, sexual assault, and family planning.

There also must be competence to consent for care. Competence requires that the patient be of sound mind to accept the treatment. In addition, consent cannot be obtained from one who is impaired or under the influence of alcohol or drugs. If the patient is deemed incompetent to provide consent, a legal process exists for the determination of the individual legally eligible to provide the consent. In many cases, consent is provided by the spouse. In the absence of the spouse, this role may be passed to another legally identified individual.

It is the duty of the physician or nurse practitioner who is performing the procedure or treatment to provide the needed information to the patient. The nurse often has the responsibility to witness the patient signing the consent. In this case, the nurse's responsibility is limited to the actual witnessing of the signature, not provision of information. The nurse does not discuss with the patient the elements of disclosure that the physician or the nurse practitioner are required to make. Involvement in providing this type of information to the patient potentially places the nurse in a position of liability. Answers to any unanswered questions that the patient has about the procedure are the responsibility of the health care provider who will perform the procedure.

Certain situations may require consent for treatment to be obtained over the telephone. Health care facilities have policies that govern telephonic consent. This type

---

Box 2.7 HIPAA Patient Identifiers

1. Names
2. Geographic locations smaller than a state—includes zip code, city, county, precinct
3. Dates—includes admission date, discharge date, date of death, and all ages over 89
4. Phone numbers
5. Fax numbers
6. Electronic mail addresses
7. Social security numbers
8. Medical record number
9. Health plan beneficiary
10. Account numbers
11. Certificate/license numbers
12. Vehicle identifiers
13. Device identifiers and serial numbers
14. URLs
15. Internet protocol (IP) addresses
16. Biometric identifiers, including fingerprints and voice prints
17. Full face photographic images
18. Any other unique identifying number, characteristic, or code

Modified from HIPAA PHI: List of 18 Identifiers and Definitions. UC Berkeley Human Research Protection Program.
HIPAA, Health Insurance Portability and Accountability Act of 1996.

---

of consent traditionally is needed in management of emergency procedures.

Confidentiality

Nurses have a duty to protect information about a patient regardless of how the information is kept. Information should be accessed only on a need-to-know basis. For example, on a patient care unit only those health care personnel directly involved in an individual's care should be able to access that patient's information. Failure to maintain patient confidentiality risks legal liability, and civil and criminal filings may result. Employers consider violations of confidentiality an offense that justifies termination. The responsibility of maintaining confidentiality is not limited to the work shift. All matters committed to the nurse's keeping are to be held in confidence. Securing the materials that contain confidential information is a responsibility of the nurse. These materials include not only the physical chart forms but the technological resources as well. When accessing computerized patient files, the nurse must ensure the appropriate log-out information is entered to prevent others from viewing the records. Written notes and chart forms must be stored in restricted areas. Information that can be used to identify a patient is considered protected health information (PHI) (Box 2.7). These identifiers extend well beyond the patient's name and include admission and discharge dates; social security number; photographs; addresses and phone numbers; and date of birth. The age of patients who are 89 years of age or older also is considered an identifier and PHI. Conversations discussing

Box 2.8	**Common Myths About the Use of Social Media for the Health Care Professional**

1. Posted communication is private between the individual posting it and the initial intended recipient.
2. Content is deleted easily from a social media site.
3. If transmitted information is shared with a few people and the patient does not find out, it is acceptable.
4. If names are not used in posted communication, the patient's privacy is protected and violations are avoided.

patients and their personal information should be held in private conference rooms. Discussions away from the patient care areas, such as the elevator or cafeteria, are problematic and should be avoided.

Social Media

Social media refers to online platforms to exchange and share information, viewpoints, and experiences. The information provided may include images or video. The advance of social media has had an impact on health care. Smartphones and handheld devices are common. There are benefits to social media for the nursing profession. Educational resources are readily available on social media. These may be for minimal or no cost. Support from within the profession can be achieved through social media pages. The availability of social media allows connectivity that transcends physical locations and time.

Nurses have banded together and utilized their political powers using social media. Facebook is the largest social networking site with more than 1 billion users. It contains countless nursing groups. These groups have been formed in response to political concerns, to offer support to colleagues, and in response to the Covid-19 pandemic.

Students and licensed nurses are encouraged to use restraint in their social media activities. Information posted, even if deleted, can be detrimental. Nurses and students need to be aware of the social media policies of their institutions. An assessment of an applicant's social media activities may be included in the consideration for employment.

The ready access to these sites and personal electronic devices has resulted in a serious situation. Most health care facilities have policies about the use and accessibility of smartphones and handheld devices in the care environment. Violations relating to the use of social media most often result when nurses violate or blur the boundaries between themselves and their patient (Box 2.8). Simply taking a picture or uploading information about patients, families, or the facility can be tempting. Nurses who violate social media policies established by their employers can be disciplined up to and including termination. The nursing board may choose to take sanctions against the license. Discipline can range from fines and changes in the status of the license to other sanctions.

In a case that caught national attention, an established emergency department nurse photographed scenes from an empty emergency trauma room that was in disarray from the recent treatment of a victim who had been hit by a New York subway train. She titled the photo #Man vs 6 Train. After 7 years on the job, she was terminated. Some violations may not involve what many would consider a violation by divulging personal information, but instead may be considered poor judgment. A nurse was terminated from her place of employment after posting on Facebook at the same time that she was providing patient care (Stokowski, 2011).

Social media violations are not limited to patient care delivery or to privacy issues. Discussing the care facility in a disparaging manner can be viewed negatively by employers. Making comments about sensitive subjects such as staffing or airing concerns or opinions about management may result in a sanction by the agency.

In response to growing concerns the ANA and National Council State Boards of Nursing (NCSBN) worked together in 2011 to release a position paper discussing social media (ANA and NCSBN, 2011). They outlined the benefits of social media and warned nurses of pitfalls that can result from inappropriate use of such forums. In addition, they have made posters, pamphlets, and videos available to nurses and students at http://www.ncsbn.org/NCSBN_SocialMedia.pdf.

Medical Records

Laws govern the collection, maintenance, and disclosure of information in medical records. Each health care institution also has policies and procedures regarding patient medical records. Medical records are not public documents, and the information they contain must be kept secure. Any breach in the confidentiality of information kept in a patient's medical record risks legal liability.

In a lawsuit, both parties are permitted to use the patient's medical record to argue facts of the case. Entries made in the chart often show whether the standards of care were met in each situation. It is essential that the employing institution's policies and procedures regarding the patient's medical record be followed. All entries in the medical record must be permanent, accurate, complete, and legible. Two current trends potentially affect patient confidentiality. Many smaller health care organizations are merging to form large corporations to save resources while continuing to provide services. Also, computer-based health care records are becoming common. Together, these two trends have the potential to increase drastically the number of people with access to confidential patient information. Those implementing these trends are required to take federal HIPAA privacy standards into consideration and prevent unauthorized disclosure of medical records and patient information.

Invasion of Privacy

The legal concept of invasion of privacy involves a person's right to be left alone and remain anonymous if he or she chooses. Consent for treatment does not waive the right to privacy. Privacy-related concerns may include the physical exposure or disclosure of patient information to others. When providing care, health care professionals must protect the patient from unnecessary exposure with the use of drapes and remember to close the door or use available signage to restrict admission to rooms during procedures as needed. Handle calls and inquiries concerning the patient with care. Providing information to callers can result in a breach in confidentiality. Refer calls to the charge nurse or available family members. Nurses frequently take notes during change-of-shift report. Monitor these notes closely during the shift. Destroy report sheets and communication tools at the end of the shift before leaving the worksite. Use of any patient information (name, photograph, specific facts regarding an illness, and so on) without authorization is a violation of the patient's legal rights. Safeguard the patient's right to privacy at all times.

Reporting Abuse

There are exceptions to the right to privacy. The law stipulates that the health care professional is required to report certain information to the appropriate authorities. The report should be given to a supervisor or directly to the police, according to agency policy. When acting in good faith to report mandated information (e.g., certain communicable diseases or gunshot wounds), the health care professional is protected from liability.

To respond to the growing problem of child abuse, the federal Child Abuse Prevention Treatment Act of 1973 made the reporting of child abuse *mandatory*. Health care professionals are mandated reporters. Failure to report suspected cases to the appropriate authorities may result in fines or imprisonment. Facilities have procedures in place to assist the nurse when making reports. Withholding medical treatment to an infant born with serious life-threatening handicaps is a form of child abuse. Congress enacted the Child Abuse Amendments in 1984 to protect the rights of these handicapped newborns to proper treatment and care. These regulations make any institution that receives federal funds legally responsible to investigate the withholding of medical treatment to an infant. In general, withholding of lifesaving treatment and care is a form of passive euthanasia (letting a person die) and medical neglect. This act carries the risk of professional neglect (medical malpractice) charges.

Spousal and elder abuse also may be a hidden problem within a family. Populations at increased risk include women and older adults (see the Lifespan Considerations box). Most states have responded to the issue of spousal and elder abuse by enacting laws to protect victims. Fines, restraining orders that prohibit contact by the abusing person, and even imprisonment are some of the ways often attempted to protect the victims of abuse. Abuse is an underreported crime. Only a portion of abuse cases are ever reported. It is the responsibility of the nurse to know the signs of abuse and the procedures for reporting suspected cases.

 Lifespan Considerations
Older Adults

Elder Adults

Factors that put older adults at risk for physical, emotional, or financial abuse include the following:
- Declining physical health
- Declining mental ability
- Decreased strength and mobility
- Loss of independence
- Isolation
- Loss of loved ones, friends, and relatives

These factors often make the older adult feel helpless and frightened. Impaired communication, decreased hearing acuity, and anxiety make assessment of an older adult more difficult. Nonetheless, be sure to watch for the signs of abuse.

Workplace violence is another form of abuse that occurs at times in the health care setting. This form of violence includes verbal abuse, emotional abuse, sexual harassment, physical assault, and threatening behavior. Health care institutions are currently implementing policies and procedures to promote a safe work environment, and education is an important component of this. Strategies to provide adequate supervision, employ security personnel, monitor work areas, and facilitate reporting of incidents represent efforts to decrease the incidence of workplace violence.

HOW TO AVOID A LAWSUIT

The best way to avoid a lawsuit is to provide compassionate, competent nursing care. The nurse–patient relationship should be based on trust and respect. Open and honest communication is the key to building a therapeutic relationship and often helps resolve patient dissatisfaction before the patient resorts to legal action (Fig. 2.2). Following the standards of care and the policies and procedures of the facility and adhering to the scope of practice for the LPN/LVN reduce the likelihood of lawsuit. Remaining current on practice developments and taking advantage of continuing education opportunities help to ensure competence.

Nurses may be in settings outside of the worksite in which an individual is injured and needs assistance. Concerns may result about the responsibility of the nurse and the decision to offer assistance to a victim. Nurses are not required to offer assistance when they are acting as a "private citizen." If the nurse chooses to offer help, liability may be limited under Good

Fig. 2.2 A patient–nurse relationship built on trust and open communication is the best way to prevent a lawsuit.

Samaritan laws. These statutes have been developed to provide immunity from liability in certain circumstances. The goal of this protection (except in cases of gross negligence) is to encourage assistance in emergencies that occur outside of a medical facility. State and provincial laws vary, so it is important to know the Good Samaritan laws that apply.

Proper documentation in the medical record is another important factor in assessment of liability. The medical record is examined thoroughly in the event of a lawsuit, and its use is permitted to demonstrate in court the level of care that was provided to the patient. An important legal presumption to remember is, "Care was not given if it was not charted." Simply stating care was provided does not provide legal protection. Omissions in charting provide a great boost to the team bringing the lawsuit.

INSURANCE

Obtaining insurance is an important part of being a professional, providing protection of personal assets or garnishment of wages. The determination about carrying insurance is personal, but nurses must evaluate their personal level of vulnerability when making a decision.

Professional Liability Insurance

Employers carry insurance for their facilities. This coverage provides insurance to the employees. Still, many nurses choose to purchase individual coverage. Many experts support the decision to have professional liability insurance. A careful review of policy options before purchase is important to ensure that the terms of the policy meet the needs of the individual nurse. The two types of policies are as follows:

- *Claims-made policy:* This type of policy provides protection when the claim for nursing or negligence is made while the policy is in force (during the policy period or during extended coverage).
- *Occurrence-basis policy:* This type of policy protects against claims made about events that occurred during the policy period or extended coverage period.

A *"tail" agreement* offers extended coverage for periods when a nurse is exposed to professional liabilities but no longer has a claims-made policy.

Disciplinary Defense Insurance

Disciplinary defense insurance or license protection insurance provides the following if a nurse is brought before the LPN/LVN board of nursing for disciplinary actions and problems with the license:

- A qualified nurse attorney or attorney to represent the nurse
- Wage loss reimbursement
- Travel, food, lodging reimbursement
- Legal fees paid or reimbursement for payment

DISCIPLINARY PROCESS

If a nurse receives a letter from the board of nursing alleging breaches of the standards of care or infractions of patient safety practices, it is best to seek legal representation. Every state has a variation of the disciplinary process. The process plays on various levels, such as investigation of the allegations, meeting with investigators, hearings with the board, and appeals through the court system. Licensure issues fall under administrative law (Box 2.9).

Potential Sanctions Against a Nursing License

Any of the following may result from investigation of a claim by the state board of nursing regarding licensure issues or disciplinary actions:

- Dismissed charge
- Investigations agreement
- Letter of reprimand, formal or informal
- Probation with stipulations (e.g., education, practice environment limitations, fines, monitoring fees, worksite monitors, and evaluation by psychiatrist, psychologist, or drug addiction specialists)
- Mandated diversion program for drug-related or alcohol-related charges or mental condition
- Suspension with stipulations
- Revocation of license

ETHICAL ASPECTS OF NURSING

The science of ethics studies the relationships between actions and moral values and how these affect society. The word **ethics** refers to values that influence a person's behavior and the individual's feelings and beliefs about what is right or wrong. Nursing ethics involve moral values and principles that affect personal and professional conduct. As previously mentioned, the LPN/LVN has the responsibility to practice within the legal and ethical boundaries of nursing practice. Nursing ethics propose the duties and obligations of nurses to their patients, other health care professionals, the profession, and society.

Box 2.9	Common Grounds for Licensure Proceedings

- Aiding and abetting a criminal
- Aiding and abetting someone in violating the nurse practice act
- Attempting to sell or selling, or falsely obtaining or providing, a nursing diploma or license to practice as a registered nurse
- Being convicted of a crime or offense that shows the inability of a nurse to practice without due regard for the safety and health of patients or clients
- Being found to be legally insane or mentally incompetent by the courts
- Being guilty of moral turpitude
- Committing Medicare/Medicaid fraud
- Diverting or stealing narcotics
- Documentation errors
- Entering a plea of guilty or *nolo contendere* to a criminal charge regardless of the disposition of the proceeding (e.g., expungement)
- Failure to exercise technical competence
- Failure to maintain confidentiality of patient information
- Failure to practice nursing according to the legal standards of nursing practice
- Failure to properly cooperate with the state board of nursing
- Failure to properly delegate or assign nursing care, treatment, or duties
- Failure to properly notify appropriate person when leaving or refusing an assignment
- Failure to report health care providers who are practicing in an illegal, unethical, or incompetent manner
- Failure to report previous criminal actions
- Failure to report to the state board of nursing status as a carrier of HIV or hepatitis B when participating in or performing exposure-prone procedures
- Failure to use good nursing judgment
- Falsifying information on a renewal or application
- Falsifying records
- Having a license in nursing or in another health care profession that has been revoked, suspended, probated, denied, or restricted
- Having a mental or physical impairment that interferes with nursing skills, abilities, judgment, or a combination of these
- Misappropriating patient, facility, or individual items
- Patient abuse
- Performing duties when competency has not been attained, maintained, or achieved
- Practicing outside the scope of the nurse practice act
- Practicing without a valid license
- Sexual misconduct
- Using, when on duty, alcohol, illegal drugs, or drugs that impair nursing judgment
- Violating rules or orders adopted by the state board of nursing
- Violating state or federal law relating to nursing practice
- Violating state or federal narcotics or controlled substance laws

ADVANCE DIRECTIVES

Advance directives are signed and witnessed documents that provide specific instructions for health care if a person is unable to make these decisions personally at the time they are needed.

The two basic types of advance directives are living wills and durable powers of attorney for health care. Many patients have instituted one or both.

The Patient Self-Determination Act (PSDA; 1991) requires health care institutions to provide written information to patients concerning the patient's rights under state law to make decisions, including the right to refuse treatment and formulate advance directives (Levin, 1990). It is especially important to understand patients' cultural beliefs and values when explaining advance directives. Regulatory mandates to benefit the public are based on the dominant value in American society of self-determination, which may conflict with a patient's cultural heritage.

Under the act, whether the patient has signed an advance directive must be documented in the patient's record. The hospital also is required to ensure that state law is followed. The institution must provide education for the staff and the public concerning living wills and durable powers of attorney. For either type of advance directive to be enforceable, the patient must be legally incompetent or lack capacity to make decisions regarding health care treatment. The termination of legal competency is made by a judge, and the determination of decisional capacity usually is made by the physician and the family. Therefore the advance directive is implemented within the context of the health care team and the health care institution. Be familiar with the institution's policies involving the act.

A *living will* is a written document that directs treatment in accordance with a patient's wishes in the event of a terminal illness or condition (Fig. 2.3). Living wills are often difficult to interpret and are not clinically specific in unforeseen circumstances. Each state has its own requirements for executing living wills. Generally, the presence of two witnesses is required when the patient signs the document; neither may be a relative or physician. If health care workers follow the directions of the living will, they are immune from liability.

A *durable power of attorney* for health care designates an agent, surrogate, or proxy to make health care decisions on the patient's behalf based on the patient's wishes.

In addition to federal statutes, the ethical doctrine of autonomy ensures the patient the right to refuse medical treatment. This right was upheld in the *Bouvia v Superior Court* case in 1986. That case allowed the discontinuation of the patient's tube feedings per the patient's prior request. The courts also have upheld the right of a legally competent patient to refuse medical treatment based on religious beliefs. Jehovah's Witnesses, for example, accept medical treatment but

---

LIVING WILL DECLARATION OF

_____

If I should lapse into a persistent vegetative state or have an incurable and irreversible condition that, without the administration of life-sustaining treatment, will, in the opinion of my attending physician, cause my death within a relatively short time and I am no longer able to make decisions regarding my medical treatment, I direct my attending physician, pursuant to the Rights of the Terminally Ill Act, to withhold or withdraw life-sustaining treatment that is not necessary for my comfort or to alleviate pain.

Declarant Signature

Signed this _____ day of _____, 20 _____

Social Security Number: _____ Date of Birth: _____

Address: _____ Signature: _____

City/State: _____

The declarant voluntarily signed this writing in my presence.

Signature of witness: _____ Printed name/Date: _____

Signature of witness: _____ Printed name/Date: _____

-OR-
NOTARY

The declarant voluntarily signed this document in my presence.

STATE OF NEBRASKA   )
) SS.
COUNTY OF_____   )   Notary Public

Fig. 2.3 Example of a living will.

---

refuse blood transfusions. In the absence of a truly compelling reason otherwise, the right to make such choices is protected. The US Supreme Court stated in the _Cruzan v Director, Missouri Department of Health_ case in 1990, "We assume that the United States Constitution would grant a competent person a constitutionally protected right to refuse lifesaving hydration and nutrition" (Cornell University Law School, 1990). In cases that involve the patient's right to refuse or withdraw medical treatment, the courts balance the patient's interest with the state's interest in protecting life, preserving medical ethics, preventing suicide, and protecting innocent third parties. Children generally are considered innocent third parties. Although the courts do not force adults to undergo treatment that is refused for religious reasons, they do grant an order that allows hospitals and physicians to treat children of Christian Scientists or Jehovah's Witnesses who have denied consent for treatment of their minor children.

When patients are legally incompetent and are unable to make health care decisions, the court intervenes. Balancing the state's interest with that of the patient, the court attempts to deliver a judgment that represents what the patient would have chosen if competent. The Supreme Court held in the Cruzan case

that states had the right to require "clear and convincing evidence" of a legally incompetent patient's prior wishes when making determinations to discontinue life-sustaining treatment. In that case, nutrition and hydration were recognized as life-sustaining medical treatment that could be withdrawn.

Every state now requires "clear and convincing" evidence of the patient's choice, but individual states differ as to what standard satisfies the requirement. In the absence of evidence indicating the patient's prior choice, most states allow treatment to be stopped based on other factors, including the best interest of the patient balanced with the state's interest (Box 2.10).

DEVELOPMENT OF ETHICAL PRINCIPLES

Values are personal beliefs about the worth of an object, an idea, a custom, or an attitude. Values vary among people and cultures; they develop over time and undergo change in response to changing circumstances and necessity. Each individual adopts a value system that governs what is deemed right or wrong (or good and bad) and influences behaviors in a given situation.

Values influence everyday decisions. Each person has many values and at times has to choose between competing or conflicting values. Some values are more

Box **2.10**   The Living Will and Durable Power of Attorney

- People who receive extraordinary measures to prolong life are often unconscious or mentally incompetent by the time these measures are put into effect. Therefore, only by deciding ahead of time what kind of care you want and communicating these decisions to others can you ensure that you receive the extent of care that you want. This can be done through such documents as a living will and a medical durable power of attorney. If your state has adopted legislation for either or both documents, you should use the legally approved wording.
- Address the living will and send copies of it to your family physician, your attorney, and close family members. It specifies that if the time comes when you can no longer take part in decisions for your own future, this statement will stand as an expression of your wishes and directions while you are still of sound mind.
- You may, for example, direct that if a situation should arise in which there is no reasonable expectation of recovery from extreme physical or mental disability, you be allowed to die and not be kept alive by medications, artificial means, or "heroic measures." You may also, of course, use a living will to request such measures to keep you alive as long as possible. You may request pain-relieving medication, even though it may shorten your life. You may spell out specific provisions regarding, for example, cardiac resuscitation, mechanical respiration, antibiotics, tube feeding, and permission to offer your organs as transplants to other people.
- Some "living will" legislation applies only to terminally ill patients, not to patients who are incapacitated by illness or injury but may live many years in severe pain, who are in a coma, or who are in some other greatly disabled

state. Thus, it is advisable to draw up a durable power of attorney, an instrument that appoints another person (a health care surrogate) to make decisions in the event of your incompetence. Some states have enacted statutes expressly for decisions about health care, known as a "medical durable power of attorney." In these states, filling out a form is all that is required; you do not have to consult an attorney.
- Depending on the statute, the agent you appoint (someone you trust and have confidence in) may give, withdraw, or withhold consent to specific medical or surgical measures; hire and fire medical personnel; gain access to your medical records; go to court to carry out your wishes; spend or withhold funds for treatment; and interpret your living will.

REMEMBER

- Both documents must be signed and dated before two witnesses who are not blood relatives and to whom you are not leaving property.
- For the durable power of attorney, you must have your signature notarized. If you choose more than one proxy for decision-making on your behalf (a good idea in case your first choice is not available), give an order of priority (1, 2, 3).
- Give a copy to your physician to keep in your medical file, and be sure that the physician agrees with your wishes.
- Give copies to close relatives, friends, or both.
- Tell these people about your intentions now.
- Look over your living will once a year. Redate it and initial the new date to make it clear that your wishes are unchanged.

---

important than others, and the choices made are based on the priority placed on each value. A person's values are learned through experience, observation, and reasoning. Some values are consciously chosen; others are adopted unconsciously. Society has a strong influence on children's behaviors and values retained and learned. Acceptable behavior is rewarded, and unacceptable behavior is punished. The development of an individual value system occurs with maturity and largely reflects culture (see the Cultural Considerations box).

 Cultural Considerations

Culture and Ethics

People of different cultural backgrounds often define health and illness in different ways. Culture is learned as the individual grows up and is influenced (usually subconsciously) by the surrounding environment. The nurse must be aware of cultural differences and should avoid: (1) transferring personal expectations to patients; (2) making generalizations based on personal views; (3) assuming patients can understand what is being said just because they speak English; and (4) treating each patient the same. To meet patients' needs, respect for their cultural heritage is vital.

Nurses must reflect on and assess their own values. **Value clarification** is the process of self-evaluation that helps gain insight into personal values. To clarify values, do the following: (1) select the belief or behavior and consciously examine it; (2) decide its value; and (3) incorporate the value into everyday responses and behaviors. These steps exercise freedom of choice and determine which values are most important. Nurses are in a unique position of having the ability to assist in value clarification as well, by encouraging the patient to express feelings and thoughts related to a situation, without contributing personal opinions. Patients need to act on their own values, not those of the nurse. Sometimes the patient may be referred to a clergy member or other professional who can help deal with ethical issues. Most health care institutions have an ethics committee to help resolve ethical questions that arise and to act as an advising body for issues encountered.

Ethical dilemmas are situations that do not have a clear right or wrong answer (Box 2.11). They are complex, confusing, and often frustrating situations that call for careful rational analysis. First, the problem must be identified as an ethical one. This means that

Box 2.11 Ethical Dilemmas

WHAT WOULD YOU DO?

The following are scenarios with an ethical dilemma. What would you do or say in each one?

1. You see a nursing assistant stealing the patient's ring. She says she needs money to pay her house note or the bank will foreclose. What should you do?
2. The patient has a do-not-resuscitate order and a living will. He has not designated a health care proxy or representative. The patient goes into arrest, and the daughter who has not seen her dad in 10 years yells, "Do something, or I will sue you if he dies!" Whose wishes should you follow?
3. You know your friend at work is diverting drugs. You have confronted her, but she says it is not for her but for a friend. What should you do?
4. You suspect elder abuse by a family member of one of your relatives. What should you do?
5. You made a mistake, and your charge nurse tells you to just rewrite the nurse's notes to protect the unit and the hospital. What should you do?

the question presented cannot be answered by applying external laws, rules, policies, and procedures. Many situations present a combination of legal and ethical questions. It is important to sort out the questions and seek guidance as needed. The next step is complete assessment of the situation, with as much information as possible gathered to aid in the decision-making process. Before a decision is finalized, any ethical principles that may apply to the situation should be considered. Ethical principles are general, but they provide a framework for decision making.

ETHICAL PRINCIPLES IN NURSING PRACTICE

Several ethical principles are important for a health care professional to consider when confronted with an ethical question. The first, most fundamental principle is *respect for people.* This principle leads us to view all human life as sacred, with each individual having inherent worth. To the nurse, this principle means that no one person is more important than another; each patient has the same worth and is always entitled to respect. *Autonomy* is another ethical principle; it refers to freedom of personal choice, a right to be independent and make decisions freely. Frequently the patient may ask the nurse for opinions or assistance in making decisions. The nurse does not have the authority to make decisions for the patient. *Beneficence* means doing good or acting for someone's good; this principle is of primary importance to nurses. The nurse has an ethical duty to protect life and promote the wellbeing of all patients. Another ethical principle is **nonmaleficence,** which means to do no harm. It is paramount to nursing practice to act in the patient's best interest and an ethical and legal duty to do nothing that has a harmful effect on the patient. Finally, there is the principle of *justice,* or the concept of what is fair. In the context of

nursing, justice means that all patients have the same right to nursing interventions.

It is a great challenge to the nurse to balance these ethical principles when they seem in conflict. Rarely are options clear or black and white. Decisions often come down to choosing what seems more right and less wrong, more good and less bad.

CODES OF ETHICS

As members of society and of the health care community, nurses use personal and professional ethical principles to govern professional practice. Professional organizations have developed codes of ethics for the nursing profession that serve as a way to regulate the nurses' actions and give guidelines for ethical behavior. By helping health care practitioners become more competent, trustworthy, and accountable, such codes of ethics help safeguard society. The National Federation of Licensed Practical Nurses (NFLPN) has developed a code for LPN/LVNs. This code specifies what is expected: (1) to know and function within the scope of practice for a licensed LPN/LVN; (2) to maintain patient confidences; (3) to provide health care without discrimination; (4) to maintain a high standard of professional and personal behavior; and (5) to take an active role in the development of the LPN/LVN profession. The ANA and the CNA also have developed codes of ethics that specify the ethical duties required of the nursing professional.

REPORTING UNETHICAL BEHAVIOR

Nurses have a duty to report behavior witnessed that does not meet the established standards. Unethical behavior involves failing to perform the duties of a competent, caring nurse. Making a decision to report unethical behaviors can be stressful. When making a decision about reporting unethical behaviors, the nurse must consider key issues, including asking if the behavior or practice (NCSBN, n.d.):

- Puts the patient or facility at risk
- Demonstrates incompetence
- Involves the use of alcohol or drugs
- Is related to a physical or mental condition
- Violates a nursing statute

When reporting unethical behavior, always follow the proper chain of command and explain the facts as clearly as possible. Any documentation of the incident must be objective and accurately state what occurred, when and where it occurred, and any other pertinent facts. The state's board of nursing can provide direction to the complainant. Reporting a coworker is never an easy task. However, always remember that a nurse's first duty is to the patient and his or her health, safety, and wellbeing.

ETHICAL ISSUES

Ethical issues are difficult for the nurse, as for everyone, because there is often no absolutely right nor absolutely wrong answer to the question. Like many other issues in health care, ethical issues change as society changes. Some of the current ethical issues in nursing include practitioner-assisted suicide (PAS), the right to refuse treatment, the nurse's right to refuse to provide care, and genetic research.

Practitioner-Assisted Suicide

Health care professionals and patient advocacy groups on both sides of the issue are debating the ethics of PAS. Also called physician-assisted suicide, this is a form of active euthanasia in which a health care provider takes an active role in ending a patient's life. Two cases, *Vacco v Quill* and *Washington v Glucksberg,* were brought before the US Supreme Court regarding the legality of state bans on assisted suicide. The Supreme Court ruled in 1997 that there is no constitutional right to assisted suicide. This ruling allows each state to decide whether to legalize or ban assisted suicides. The ANA has taken a firm stand on the issue of PAS: PAS is not consistent with the philosophy of nursing. ANA's specific objections to PAS are based on the principle of nonmaleficence, to do no harm, and beneficence, the duty to protect life.

In 1944, the ANA adopted a position statement concerning PAS. The ANA wrote that such an act is in violation of the *Code of Ethics for Nurses* and the ethical tradition of the profession. Nurses have an obligation to provide compassionate end-of-life care that includes providing comfort and pain relief. However, proponents of PAS cite the ethical principles of the right to autonomy and the right to self-determination in support of their position.

Right to Refuse Treatment

In the context of health care, competent adults have the right to refuse treatment. This right derives from their right to determine what is done, or not done, to them. Medicine's technical capacity to sustain life and postpone death further complicates this complex issue. It is the right of the patient to accept or refuse a treatment, even if the refusal has the potential to or is certain to result in death. To exercise the right to refuse treatment, many patients prepare advance directives. Living wills, one kind of advance directive, become effective when patients are incapacitated and are not able to make their own wishes known; these documents specify which lifesaving treatments are acceptable and which are not. Some patients choose to designate a *health care proxy* (assign durable power of attorney) to make decisions regarding medical treatment if the patient becomes unable to make them. The proxy is another person who will speak for the patient and make decisions regarding the patient's care. The proxy is obligated to act on the patient's behalf according to the patient's expressed wishes. State laws vary on the legalities of the various forms of advance directives, and nurses need to know the applicable laws in their state.

Do-Not-Resuscitate Orders

The patient usually is not involved directly at the time a *do-not-resuscitate (DNR) order* is written. Although many people make their wishes regarding DNR status known in an advance directive, at this stage the patient usually is incapacitated with little hope for recovery. The physician, after consultation with the patient's family, writes the DNR order in the medical record. The physician is responsible for following the applicable policies and procedures for writing DNR orders. When a DNR order is written in the chart, the nurse has the duty to follow the order.

Refusal to Treat

Refusal to treat is an issue that arises when a patient's care requires a nurse to do something that conflicts with his or her personal moral beliefs. A typical example of this dilemma involves assisting in or caring for a woman having an abortion. There is a legal right to abortion, but this does not establish whether abortion is morally right or wrong. If the nurse has a strong moral or religious belief regarding abortion, these concerns must be communicated with the appropriate supervisor. Do not abandon the patient; instead, ask for another assignment. Remember that the right to disqualify oneself from assisting with an abortion does not extend to the complete ability to avoid caring for the patient after the abortion. Disagreement with care decisions made by patients does not allow the nurse to refuse to care for them.

Patient diagnoses and lifestyles do not allow the nurse the legal right to refuse to care for a person. Examples include an infectious disease, such as HIV, or sexual orientation. The rationale is that the need for standard precautions (infection control measures) applies to every patient, and therefore the nurse is at no greater risk for infection from one patient than from another. The ethical principle of respect for all people without discrimination underlies this issue. The patient has the right to receive care, and the nurse has the responsibility to provide nursing interventions.

CONCLUSION

There are no easy, quick answers to legal or ethical issues. The nurse has the charge of working to manage difficult situations effectively. Today's health care system is facing many challenges, as is the profession of nursing. The health care system will continue to undergo changes in response to the enormous problem of containing health care costs while improving quality of care. The nursing profession will be called on to adjust and adapt to these changes. The legal system also is undergoing changes. Members of the legal community and the health care system have to work together to ensure that the legal and ethical rights of all individuals are considered and protected.

Get Ready for the NCLEX® Examination!

Key Points

- Laws regulate the practice of the licensed practical/vocational nurse (LPN/LVN).
- The Patient Care Partnership and other legislative directives outline what the patient can expect from the health care system.
- LPN/LVNs are legally and ethically obligated to know the scope of practice and the standards of care that apply in the state or province where they are licensed.
- Every patient has the right to receive care that meets the established standards of care.
- Malpractice (professional negligence) is when the health care professional fails to meet the standard of care.
- Prevention is the best defense against a lawsuit. A competent, caring nurse who follows the standards of care is less likely to be sued.
- Values systems have developed over the history of civilization.
- Ethical decisions regarding health care are influenced by a person's culture, beliefs, attitudes, and values.
- A code of ethics and ethical principles helps guide the practice of nursing.
- On April 14, 2003, the Health Insurance Portability and Accountability Act of 1996 (HIPAA) for regulating patient privacy standards took effect; these federal regulations have had an impact on the field of health care.

Additional Learning Resources

SG Go to your Study Guide for additional learning activities to help you master this chapter content.

Be sure to visit the Evolve site at http://evolve.elsevier.com/Cooper/foundations/ for additional online resources.

Review Questions for the NCLEX® Examination

1. The newly licensed practical/vocational nurse (LPN/LVN) has reviewed the nurse practice act (NPA) of the state of licensure. What is the purpose of this documentation?
   1. Determine the quality of nursing care
   2. Enforce the standards of nursing practice
   3. Define the scope of nursing practice
   4. Set the nurse's educational requirements

2. The nurse working in a nursing home correctly recognizes that duties include patient advocacy. Which role is considered a primary duty of patient advocacy?
   1. To complete all nursing responsibilities on time
   2. To maintain the patient's right to privacy
   3. To safeguard the well-being of every patient
   4. To act as the patient's legal representative

3. The health care provider's order read "assist the patient with walking." The nurse allowed the patient to walk alone. The patient fell, fracturing the humerus. Which verdict is the most likely occurrence?

   1. The nurse will be found guilty of malpractice.
   2. The nurse will be guilty of negligence.
   3. The nurse will be charged with technical battery.
   4. The nurse will not be found liable for any harm.

4. The patient refused to take the medication his doctor ordered for relief of pain. The LPN/LVN knows this is a patient right established by:
   1. the principle of beneficence.
   2. the doctrine of negligence.
   3. specific nurse practice acts.
   4. the Patient Self-Determination Act.

5. The LPN/LVN knows that one of the best defenses against a lawsuit is for a nurse to:
   1. work only in a large hospital or nursing home.
   2. provide for every patient's needs as quickly as possible.
   3. promote a positive nurse–patient relationship.
   4. carry individual professional liability insurance.

6. The nurse believes that all patients should be treated as individuals. The ethical principle that this belief reflects is:
   1. autonomy.
   2. beneficence.
   3. nonmaleficence.
   4. respect for people.

7. LPN/LVNs have a code of professional and personal ethics to follow. The purpose of a code of ethics is to:
   1. establish penalties for any unethical behavior.
   2. promote trustworthy, accountable LPN/LVNs.
   3. make certain that all nurses are competent and always honest.
   4. give the nurse guidelines for ethical decision making.

8. The patient admitted for surgery has a lump in her breast. The patient's daughter asks the LPN/LVN if her mother should have the surgery. Which issue must be considered before responding?
   1. Confidentiality and invasion of privacy
   2. Informed consent, beneficence, and respect
   3. Respect for people and personal autonomy
   4. Nonmaleficence, justice, and liability

9. The nurse's first job as an LPN/LVN is on a unit that cares for terminally ill children. What action should be taken by the nurse before helping families cope with their children's illnesses?
   1. Study the nurse practice act to find rules relating to the medical care of terminally ill children
   2. Spend time performing value clarification to aid in identifying her feelings about this new role
   3. Evaluate her own personal mores and customs that may affect the practice of nursing in general
   4. Review the state and federal laws that prescribe how a child may be treated when near death

10. The LPN/LVN is reviewing the patient's medical record. The nurse notes the presence of an advance directive. The nurse recognizes that the purpose of this documentation is to:

1. help every person exercise the right to die with dignity.
2. encourage a person to determine how he or she will die.
3. allow a patient to exercise the right of autonomy.
4. provide a means to prevent medical maltreatment.

11. The nurse knows that all patients have the right to nursing interventions regardless of their race, religion, or gender. The ethical principle that best describes this concept is:

   1. nonmaleficence.
   2. justice.
   3. autonomy.
   4. beneficence.

12. An alert adult patient has refused an intramuscular injection. The nurse waits until the patient is asleep and gives the injection anyway. The nurse could be charged with:

   1. civil battery.
   2. malicious homicide.
   3. criminal assault.
   4. invasion of privacy.

13. The nurse loves photography and brings his camera to work at the nursing home. He takes a picture of one of his coworkers walking a patient. What best describes the actions taken by the nurse?

   1. He violated the patient's right to privacy.
   2. He failed to get proper medical clearance.
   3. He performed an act of nursing malpractice.
   4. He legally obtained a realistic picture.

14. The nurse gets a report, puts his patient assignment notebook in his pocket, and goes on break. His notebook has very specific information about his patients and is missing from his pocket when he returns to the unit. The book is found later on the floor in the cafeteria by a visitor and is returned to the information desk. The nurse:

   1. may have breached the Patient Self-Determination Act.
   2. is guilty of criminal misconduct.
   3. could be fired for malpractice.
   4. has violated the Health Insurance Portability and Accountability Act of 1996 (HIPAA).

15. The newly licensed nurse is assigned a patient who needs catheterization. The nurse has not performed the procedure before. What would be the best action for the nurse?

   1. Contact the nursing supervisor and explain that the procedure will need to be done by another nurse.
   2. Review the agency procedure for catheterization in the unit's resource area and see the assistance of another experienced nurse for help during the procedure.

3. Immediately advise the charge nurse that someone else will need to assume care of this patient.
4. Promptly notify the staff development office that an instructor needs to do this procedure.

16. A nurse who has recently been promoted to unit manager questions her immediate supervisor if there is any potential liability for her as a result of the actions of her nursing staff member. What information included in the supervisor's response would be appropriate? *(Select all that apply.)*

   1. "An individual nurse is solely responsible for their actions."
   2. "As long as you are working in good faith, you cannot be found liable."
   3. "As a supervisor, there is some liability if measures are not followed to ensure staff understand how to utilize the care equipment."
   4. "A supervisor is required to assess the performance of their staff to ensure competency."
   5. "Employer liability is limited to cases in which a death occurs."
   6. "The nurse is very seldom held liable in any court cases so you don't have anything to worry about."
   7. "You are completely covered with liability insurance by the facility so no personal complaints can be lodged against you."

17. Social media use can have positive benefits including which outcomes? *(Select all that apply.)*

   1. Networking between professionals
   2. Reduction in the amount of lateral violence between staff members
   3. Provides readily available education opportunities
   4. Access to mentoring answer
   5. Use of social media is an inexpensive answer

18. A nurse reported that she posted on a social media site about her clinical experiences. The nurse reports she did not use the patient's name. Which information should be given to the nurse? *(Select all that apply.)*

   1. "Names are the only identifiers that are of concern when considering patient privacy."
   2. "Any patient information that can aid in the identification of the patient's identity can be problematic and a violation."
   3. "As long as the information is erased, there is not a problem."
   4. "Any distribution of information regarding the patient or clinical assignment is a violation of confidentiality."
   5. "Personal e-mails are lesser violations than posting on large websites."

3 Documentation

Objectives

1. List the five purposes for patient records.
2. Describe the electronic health record (EHR) and the personal health record (PHR).
3. Determine when the use of Situation, Background, Assessment, and Recommendation is beneficial.
4. State important legal aspects of chart ownership, access, confidentiality, and patient care documentation.
5. Describe differences between traditional and problem-oriented medical records.
6. Describe the basic guidelines for and the mechanics of charting.
7. Describe the differences in documenting care with activities of daily living and physical assessment forms, narrative, SOAPE, and focus formats.
8. Discuss documentation and clinical (critical) pathways.
9. Discuss home health care documentation.
10. Discuss long-term health care documentation.
11. Discuss issues related to computerization in documentation.

Key Terms

auditors (p. 41)
chart (health care record) (p. 40)
charting (p. 40)
charting by exception (p. 48)
computers on wheels (p. 42)
database (DĂ-tă-bās, p. 42)
diagnosis-related groups (p. 41)
documenting (p. 40)
electronic health record (p. 40)
electronic medical record (p. 40)
informatics (p. 43)
ISBAR (p. 43)
Kardex (or Rand) (p. 48)
narrative charting (p. 45)
nomenclature (NŌ-měn-klā-chŭr, p. 43)

nursing care plan (p. 48)
nursing notes (p. 42)
patient portal (p. 43)
peer review (p. 41)
personal health record (p. 43)
point-of-care (p. 42)
problem list (p. 46)
problem-oriented medical record (p. 46)
quality assurance, assessment, and improvement (p. 41)
recording (p. 40)
SOAPE (SŌP, p. 46)
SOAPIER (SŌP-ē-ŭr, p. 46)
traditional (block) chart (p. 45)

The chart (health care record) has never been more important in the health care system than it is today; it is a legal record that is used to meet the many demands of the health, accreditation, medical insurance, and legal systems.

The process of adding information to the chart is called charting, recording, or documenting. Documenting involves recording the interventions carried out to meet the patient's needs. In the charting of interventions, documenting the type of intervention, the time care was rendered, and the signature and title of the person providing care is essential. Anything written or printed that is a record or proof of activities will play a role in this process. Although many details are necessary to remember when documenting in the chart, the process is not difficult but is often time consuming. Good documentation reflects the nursing process. Documentation is an integral part of the implementation phase of the nursing process (see Chapter 5) and is necessary for the evaluation of patient care and for reimbursement for the cost of care provided. In the past, all documenting in the patient's health records involved written documentation. Today a majority of facilities use some form of electronic health record (EHR), also sometimes referred to as electronic medical record (EMR). EHRs are used in various settings, including hospitals, long-term care settings, health care provider's offices, clinics, and home care agencies.

The licensed practical/vocational nurse (LPN/LVN) must understand how to use medical records

Table 3.1 Essential Elements of Documentation

NURSING PROCESS	OBSERVATION SOURCES	WHERE TO DOCUMENT
ASSESSMENT		

Physiologic status
  Functional status
  Knowledge
  Psychosocial well-being
  Family
  Safety
	Patient and family interview
	History and physical examination
	Laboratory and radiology results
	Medication records
	Environment
		Discharge and transfer forms
		Progress notes
		Flow sheets

Diagnosis	Nursing judgment	Patient care plan Critical pathways Protocols Progress notes Patient problem lists Admission sheets
OUTCOMES IDENTIFICATION/PLANNING		

Outcome definition
  Defining care priorities
  Defining intervention strategy
  Activation of care plan
	Patient care plan
	Critical pathways
	Projected length of stay
	Standards of care
	Admission assessment data
	Staff reports
		Patient care plan
		Critical pathways
		Protocols
		Progress notes
		Patient problem lists

Implementation	Progress notes Patient rounds Direct patient care	Progress notes Critical pathways Protocols
Evaluation	Patient and family interview Physical assessment Staff reports Progress notes Diagnostic test results Flow sheets	Patient care plan Critical pathways Progress notes Protocols Patient problem lists

effectively and efficiently. This chapter addresses the purposes for health records, the common types of records, the basic guidelines and rules for documentation, and legal concerns. Knowledge of these guidelines and the ability to chart completely, accurately, and legibly (when using written records) are requirements for licensure and employment as a nurse. See Table 3.1 and Chapter 5 for information on the nursing process and documentation.

PURPOSES OF PATIENT RECORDS

The five basic purposes for accurate and complete patient records are (1) documented communication; (2) permanent record for accountability; (3) legal record of care; (4) teaching; and (5) research and data collection.

The patient's chart provides a concise, accurate, and permanent record of past and current medical and nursing problems, plans for care, care given, and the patient's responses to various treatments. The record facilitates accurate communication and continuity of care among all members of the health care team. Recorded information is not as easily lost or altered as the spoken word. Proper charting covers all areas of patient needs and concerns: physical, emotional, psychological, social, and spiritual.

This permanent record sometimes is used by various government and other agencies to evaluate the institution's patient care, to justify cost reimbursement for care provided, and to establish or review accreditation. Current regulations require chart audits (review of specific chart components for completion and appropriateness) by officially appointed auditors (people appointed to examine patient charts and health records to assess quality of care). Auditors check to see whether all ordered care was charted as given and whether responses to specific care plan items and treatments are noted. Institutions have medical and peer review systems (an appraisal by professional coworkers of equal status). Peer review appraises the manner in which an individual nurse conducts practice, education, or research. Institutions also have specific procedures to provide for quality assurance, assessment, and improvement, which is an audit in health care that evaluates services provided and the results achieved compared with accepted standards. Accurate and legible records are the only means institutions have to prove that they are providing care to meet patient needs and established standards.

Cost reimbursement rates by the government plans (Medicare, Medicaid) are based on the prospective payment system of diagnosis-related groups (DRGs; a system that classifies patients by age, diagnosis, surgical procedure, and other information with 25 major diagnostic categories and hundreds of different subcategories to predict the use of hospital resources, including length of stay, resulting in a fixed payment amount) (CMS, 2019). Many private insurance companies now use similar illness categories when setting hospital payment rates. Institutions are reimbursed by insurance companies or government programs only for documented patient care. The payers carefully review various items in patient medical records, including the **nursing notes** (the form on the patient's chart on which nurses record their observations, the care given, and the patient's responses), when deciding whether the necessary and ordered care is being given or was given.

The patient chart or health record is a legal document; when necessary and appropriate, it is used in court proceedings. Although the physician or institution owns the original record, lawyers and courts are able to gain access to it. Therefore it is important to chart in a very detailed manner to protect those involved in patient care.

Patient health records also are used for teaching. Students in the health care professions learn more quickly and easily if examples of good charting are shared. Individuals also learn from their mistakes and the mistakes of others. It is important for students to remember that the patient's information is to be held confidential.

Patient records that involve research and data collection have many uses in the health field. For example, the government periodically publishes data on certain diseases and the effectiveness of new treatments. In addition, the pressure to contain or limit health care costs has made data regarding the usual length of hospitalization and the cost of treatment for specific illnesses or surgeries important for governmental and other health insurance providers.

ELECTRONIC HEALTH RECORD

In many health care settings, the EHR facilitates delivery of patient care and supports the data analysis necessary for coordinating patient care. EHRs contain information that is identical to that found in traditional records but eliminate repetitive entries and allow more freedom of access to the **database** (Fig. 3.1). In general, EHRs increase efficiency, consistency, and accuracy and decrease costs. Legibility is a further benefit of these systems.

The scope of the use of EHR for documentation in health care agencies varies depending on the agency. In addition to documentation of nursing care and interventions, most health care agencies have incorporated information systems for management of admissions, billing, and the communication of orders for diet, pharmacy, and diagnostic tests. A benefit of the EHR is the ability for all health care providers to view a patient's

Fig. 3.1 Nurses use computers for documentation.

records, encouraging increased continuity of care. In addition, agency-wide computer information systems are more efficient because information entered in the system can be transferred automatically to other areas. In regard to nursing documentation, systems often include options for generating individualized care plans, automated Kardex forms, acuity levels, and medication administration records (MARs). Although the terms EMR and EHR often are used interchangeably, a key difference between the EHR and the EMR is that the EHR allows the exchange of patient data not only within a facility but also from one facility to another. The EMR typically is set up to exchange patient data within a facility (Office of the National Coordinator for Health Information Technology, 2011).

EHR systems vary in the way they are accessed, depending on the facility. Some systems permit computer input only at the nurses' station; some facilities have bedside systems, also referred to as **point-of-care** (POC) systems; and others use handheld systems that look similar to a cell phone. POC systems are sometimes housed on wheeled carts referred to as **computers on wheels,** or COWs. Nurses should be sure that patients and their family members are aware that the handheld systems are an EHR device in order to prevent the patient or family member from perceiving the staff to be on their personal cell phones during their shift. Charting at the bedside saves time and allows current information to be immediately available to all who need it. Some systems automatically retrieve and record information from electronic devices (e.g., vital signs) and simultaneously enter the data in all relevant locations in the record, which cuts down on duplication of effort. In addition, some systems prompt for certain data to be entered, which results in more accurate and complete record keeping.

Electronic charting procedures vary by agency. Data often are recorded in flow-sheet format for easy storage and retrieval. Some agencies incorporate the use of free-text narratives in addition to standardized phrases to allow specific and individualized documentation. The standard phrases indicate information such as patient health problems, interventions, and outcomes classification systems. Assessment data, for instance, are entered by selecting from a list of preformulated choices, which means that the accuracy and pertinence of the data entered depend on the nurse's familiarity with the language the system uses to name the patient problems, the lists of data for assessment, and anything else that is entered by picking from a list.

Naming conventions, or nomenclature (a classified system of technical or scientific names and terminology), must be considered when choosing computer-based documentation. The field of medical or nursing informatics (the study of information processing) is evolving constantly, which requires that software programs be updated on a regular basis to stay current with changes in terminology. In addition, considerable time must be invested in training personnel in charting procedures and the terminology the system uses and in conducting ongoing refresher training. Newly hired personnel need to learn a new system even if they already have had considerable experience in the field.

In addition to the EHR, the personal health record (PHR) is an extension of the EHR that allows patients to input their information into an electronic database. One benefit of a PHR system is for those patients who see health care providers who are not part of the same organization and EHR system. In this case the patient inputs information from these providers into one system so all health information is stored in one place. Points of contention for the PHR are how the information is going to be stored, and the PHR must be updated by the patient themselves manually and in a timely manner to be kept current (Mayo Clinic Staff, 2020).

Patient portals (an Online system through a healthcare facility that provides a patient with access to their own health information, correspondence with providers, logging of appointments, etc.) are another method of tracking health information. Most health care systems have patient portals in which patients have electronic access to their health information. Patient portals contain information such as lab, radiology, and other test results as well as the patient's current medication lists. In addition, most patient portals allow patients to send messages to their health care provider. The patient portal differs from a PHR in that the patient cannot add their own health information to a patient portal. It should be noted that lab and diagnostic results will not be visible to the patient until their provider has viewed and released the information for the patient to see. This usually occurs in approximately 24 to 72 hours after results are available.

ISBAR

ISBAR (identification, situation, background, assessment, and recommendation) is a method of communication among health care workers and a part of documentation of communication that has occurred among health care staff. ISBAR is considered a safety measure

---

Box 3.1   ISBARR

I Introduction: "Hello Dr. Reads, this is Nurse Schwenk from Kell-Russell Memorial Hospital."

S *Situation:* "I am calling you about Mr. Walter's predischarge laboratory results."

B *Background:* "All his laboratory results are within normal range, except for his serum potassium level. It is 3.1."

A *Assessment:* "When I was speaking with him about his home medications, he said he has not been taking his potassium supplement for about 2 weeks. He says he forgot to refill the potassium but has continued taking his Lasix."

R *Recommendation:* "Could we give him a new prescription for potassium and include this information on his discharge instructions?"

R *Read back:* "Let me read that order back to you to make sure I understood you correctly. 'Prescription for K-tab, 10 mEq, p.o. B.I.D. and include on discharge instructions.'"

---

in preventing errors from poor communication during interactions between health care personnel, the communication between nurses that occurs from one shift to the next, or when a nurse phones a health care provider with information about a patient. SBAR is recognized by The Joint Commission as one method of meeting National Patient Safety Goals (TJC, 2017; TJC, 2020). When ISBAR occurs between a nurse and a health care provider over the telephone and an order is received from the health care provider, a facility often mandates using an additional "R" in the communication exchange. The additional "R" (ISBARR) represents "read back." This occurs when the nurse reads back the order to the health care provider to ensure what the nurse heard was accurate. See Box 3.1 for an example of the use of ISBARR.

BASIC GUIDELINES FOR DOCUMENTATION

The quality and accuracy of the nursing notes are extremely important. They have a decisive impact on the success or failure of communication. Sometimes the nursing notes clearly and concisely convey the intended message; sometimes, in contrast, they cause confusion and errors in communication and patient care. Correct choice of words and spelling; grammar and punctuation; and good penmanship and other writing skills (with non–computer-based systems) are critical. The LPN/LVN must ensure the information recorded in the chart is clear, concise, complete, and accurate.

The registered nurse (RN) has primary responsibility for each patient's initial admission nursing history, physical assessment, and development of the care plan based on the patient health care problem identified. Contributions by all team members during this initial process as well as during later updating sessions are important.

The forms used to provide documentation of patient care vary based on each health care institution's policy. Each facility uses a combination of graphics, care flow sheets, and narrative or SOAPE notes (see description

Box 3.2 Basic Rules for Documentation

- All documents should have the correct patient name, identification number, date of birth, date, and time if appropriate.
- Avoid use of generalized empty phrases such as "status unchanged" or "had good day."
- Be objective in charting: only what you hear, see, feel, smell.
- Be timely, specific, accurate, and complete.
- Chart after care is provided, not before.
- Chart all ordered care as given or explain the deviation (e.g., nothing by mouth [NPO] for laboratory, off unit, refused).
- Chart as soon and as often as necessary.
- Chart facts; avoid judgmental terms and placing blame.
- Chart only your own care, observations, and teaching; never chart for anyone else.
- Describe each item as you see it: for example, "white metal ring with clear stone" (rather than "diamond ring"). Do not speculate, guess, or assume.
- Document only what you observe, not opinions. Never use charting to accuse someone else.
- Fill all spaces; leave no empty lines. Chart consecutively. Go line by line. Do not indent left margin.
- Follow each institution's policies and procedures for charting.
- Follow rules of grammar and punctuation.
- If a charting error is made, identify the error according to facility policy and make the correct entry.
- If you question an order, record that clarification was sought. For example, do not record "physician made error," but chart "Dr. Bradley was called to clarify order for _____."
- Note patient response to treatments and response to analgesics or other special medications.
- Sign each block of charting or entry as directed by the agency policy.
- Use direct quotes when appropriate.
- Use only approved abbreviations and medical terms.
- Use only hard-pointed, permanent black ink pens; no erasures or correcting fluids are allowed on charts for written patient records.
- When a patient leaves a unit (e.g., to go to x-ray, laboratory, or office), chart the time and the method of transportation on departure and return.
- When making a late entry, note it as a late entry and then proceed with your notation: for example, "Late entry _____," or as dictated by the facility policy.
- Write legibly (for written documentation).

in later material) to document observations, care, and responses. The LPN/LVN should be sure that nursing notes correlate with the medical orders, Kardex information, and nursing care plan.

CHARTING RULES

See Box 3.2 for generally accepted documentation rules that provide consistency in documentation between health care providers and facilities. These rules also meet the standards expected by the individuals and the agencies that use the charts. Some of the rules apply to handwritten documentation. With a computerized documentation system, as is used with an EHR or EMR, the LPN/LVN should follow the guidelines for that particular system.

LEGAL BASIS OF DOCUMENTATION

Accurate documentation is one of the best defenses in the event of legal claims associated with nursing care (see Chapter 2). To limit nursing liability, the nursing documentation must indicate clearly that individualized, goal-directed nursing care was provided to a patient based on the nursing assessment. The record has to describe exactly what happened to a patient. This is best achieved when the chart is updated immediately after providing care. Although nursing care may have been excellent, if the care was not documented, a court of law will consider that care was not provided. It is the nurse's responsibility to indicate all assessments, interventions, patient responses, instructions, and referrals in the medical record.

Inappropriate documentation may lead to nursing malpractice. Some examples of inappropriate documentation include not charting the correct time that events occurred or that an event occurred at all, failing to record verbal orders, charting nursing care in advance, and documenting incorrect data. Table 3.2 lists some legal guidelines for documentation to be kept in mind. Again, some of the rules apply to handwritten documentation. With a computerized documentation system, follow the guidelines for that particular system.

COMMON MEDICAL ABBREVIATIONS AND TERMINOLOGY

Use standard medical abbreviations and terminology for effective documentation. Avoid using abbreviations or terms that are not standard or in question. Use of the complete word is always better if unsure of the proper abbreviation. Many abbreviations that once were accepted are now found on "abbreviations to avoid" lists because of the probability of error if these terms are used. Most facilities have a published list of generally accepted medical abbreviations and the terms approved for use in charting. The use of abbreviations when charting can be confusing if a facility's approved abbreviations are not followed. For example, is "BS" breath sounds, bowel sounds, or blood sugar? In addition, abbreviations used for communication outside of the health care facility, such as cell and smartphone texting abbreviations, must never be used in patient records. (See Appendix A for a list of commonly used abbreviations and The Joint Commission's list of abbreviations to avoid.)

METHODS OF RECORDING

The documentation system selected by a health care facility optimally reflects the philosophy of the facility and the way nursing care is implemented.

Table 3.2   Legal Guidelines for Documentation

GUIDELINES	RATIONALE	CORRECTIVE ACTION
Do not erase, apply correction fluid, or scratch out errors made while recording when using handwritten records.	Charting becomes illegible. It may appear as though there was an attempt to hide information or deface the record.	Draw a single line through error, and follow agency policy for identifying errors. Then record note correctly.
Do not document retaliatory or critical comments about patient or care by other health care professionals.	Statements can be used as evidence for unprofessional behavior or poor quality of care.	Enter only objective descriptions of patient's behavior; record patient comments as quotations.
Correct all errors promptly.	Errors in recording often lead to errors in treatment.	Avoid rushing to complete charting; be sure information is accurate.
Record all facts.	Record is required to be accurate and reliable.	Be certain entry is factual; do not speculate or guess.
Do not leave blank spaces in nursing notes when using handwritten records.	It is possible for another person to insert additional or incorrect information in the space.	Chart consecutively, line by line; if space is left, draw line horizontally through it and sign at the end.
Record all entries legibly and in black ink when using handwritten records.	Illegible entries are open to misinterpretation, which causes errors and lawsuits. Ink is not subject to erasure; black ink is more legible when records are photocopied.	Never erase entries or use correction fluid, and never use pencil.
If an order was questioned, record that clarification was sought.	Seeking clarification is the correct action to take because the nurse is just as liable for prosecution as the health care provider is if an order was carried out that is known to be improper. It is not professional to criticize another professional in the notes (see previous entry).	Do not record "physician made error." Instead, chart that "Dr. Smith was called to clarify order for analgesic."
Chart only for yourself.	You are accountable for information you enter into chart.	Never chart for someone else. (EXCEPTION: If caregiver has left unit for day and calls you with information that has to be documented, include the name of the source of information in the entry and include that information was provided via telephone.)
Avoid using generalized, empty phrases, such as "status unchanged" or "had good day."	Specific information about patient's condition or case is sometimes accidentally deleted or overlooked if information is too generalized.	Use complete, concise descriptions of care.
Begin each entry with time of entry, and end with your signature and title as specified by facility policy.	This guideline ensures that correct sequence of events is recorded; signature documents who is accountable for care delivered.	Do not wait until end of shift to record important changes that occurred several hours earlier; be sure to sign each entry.
Keep computer passwords for documentation confidential.	Maintains security and confidentiality.	Once logged into the computer, do not leave the terminal unattended.

Professionally executed charting is legal proof of care given and communicates the patient's status and progress. The nursing process shapes the approach to providing care, and in turn, effective documentation of the care the nurse provides reflects the nursing process.

TRADITIONAL CHART

The traditional (block) chart is divided into sections or blocks. Emphasis is placed on specific sections (or sheets for noncomputerized charts) of information. Typical sections are the following: admission information, physician's orders, progress notes, history and physical examination data, nurse's admission information, care plan and nursing notes, graphics, and laboratory and x-ray examination reports. The order, the content, and the number of the sections vary among institutions. Nurses use flow sheets, graphics, and narrative charting (recording of patient care in descriptive form) (Fig. 3.2) to chart observations, care, and responses. Narrative charting is used for computerized and noncomputerized nurse's notes. Narrative charting includes the data (subjective, objective, or both) about the basic patient need or problem, whether anyone has been contacted or consulted, care and treatments provided (implementation), and the patient's response to treatment (evaluation). Information obtained from the nurse's assessment of the patient is clustered (see Chapter 5) and organized in a head-to-toe manner. This type of charting is documented in an abbreviated story form instead of in the outline style of the problem-oriented medical record format described in the following section.

PROBLEM-ORIENTED MEDICAL RECORD

The problem-oriented medical record (POMR) is organized according to the scientific problem-solving system or method. The principal sections are database,

Nurse's Notes: 0800 Alert and oriented x 3, pt. is conversing with nurse. B/P 132/84, P 88 and regular, R 20 and unlabored, T 98.7. Reports 2/10 pain is tolerable to right anterior chest wall incision, states "PCA is controlling my pain well." Hand grip and arm strength strong to right, weak on the left. Push pull strength to lower extremities strong to right and weak to left. PERRL. Oral mucosa pink, moist, and intact. Apical pulse auscultated for 1 min at 88bpm, strong and regular rhythm, lungs clear anterior and posterior in all fields. O_2 sat. 95% with O_2 @2L via N/C. Using incentive spirometer every hour with 10 breaths reaching a maximum of 1300 mL. Abdomen soft and non-distended with bowel sounds x 4 quads. No edema to extremities, skin turgor immediate return, capillary refill less than 3 seconds. Dressing to chest wall incision dry and intact, due to be changed today. Jackson-Pratt has 75 mL of serosanguinous fluid. IV D5 ½ NS infusing into right forearm with no signs of infiltration, PCA

Fig. 3.2 Example of narrative charting.

problem list, care plan, and progress notes. The accumulated data, or **database**, from the history, the physical examination, and the diagnostic tests are used to identify and prioritize the health problems on the master medical and other problem lists.

This **problem list** (Fig. 3.3) of active, inactive, potential, and resolved problems serves as the index for chart documentation. Together, representatives of all the disciplines involved with the patient's care develop a care plan with identified patient problems (Fig. 3.4). All health care providers—physicians, nurses, social workers, and therapists—chart on the same progress notes with forms such as narrative notes, flow sheets, and discharge summaries to document patient progress. This is done to facilitate and enhance communication between care providers.

SOAPIER (SOAPE documentation) (Box 3.3) is an acronym for seven different aspects of charting. For notes on specific patient problems, only the necessary parts needed for completeness are used.

S *Subjective* information is what the patient states or feels; only the patient can provide this information.

O *Objective* information is what the nurse can measure or factually describe.

A *Assessment* refers to an analysis or potential diagnosis of the cause of the patient's problem or need.

P *Plan* is the general statement of the plan of care to be given or action to be taken.

I *Intervention* or implementation is the specific care given or action taken.

E *Evaluation* is an appraisal of the response and effectiveness of the plan.

R *Revision* includes the changes that may be made to the original plan of care.

SOAPE is the briefer adaptation of the charting format for the POMR. In this more compact form, the care given or action taken (intervention [I]) is included in the notations under planning. The needed plan revisions (R) are noted in the evaluation section after the evaluation of the response to treatment is recorded. Fig. 3.5 shows the SOAPE charting forms in the progress notes that commonly are used in the patient's medical record.

MASTER PROBLEM LIST				
Date	**Problem**	**Resolved**	**Reviewed**	**Reactivate**
7/4/22	#1 Insufficient knowledge R/T preoperative and postoperative procedures.	7/6/22		
7/5/22	#2 Recent onset of pain R/T incision.	7/6/22		
7/5/22	#3 Inability to regulate body temperature 2° due to bladder infection.			
		Addressograph 000-123, DOB 11/1/1954 Serbane, Donna M. - Room 348A Female - 63 Dr. Janeston		

Fig. 3.3 Master problem list.

Kell-Russell Memorial Hospital

000-123, DOB 11/1/1954
Serbane, Donna M. - Room 348A
Female - 63
Dr. Janeston

PATIENT CARE PLAN

Admitting Diagnosis:	Cholelithiasis	Operation: Cholecystectomy	Surgery Date: 7/4/22
Additional Diagnosis:	UTI	Surgeon: Dr. Janeston	Adm. Date: 7/3/22 Dism. Date:

Patient Problem Statement with Goal	Start Date	Nursing Interventions	Date D/Cd	Init	Reassessment	Date D/Cd	Init
#3 Inability to regulate body temperature r/t infection	7/4/22	Vital signs q̄ 4 and PRN		MH			
in bladder AEB (as		Encourage fluids as tolerated					
evidenced by)		I & O, provide high calorie in					
T 101.2, urine		between meal snacks. Assess comfort					
becoming cloudy,		Medicate for temperature > 102° (0)					
report of burning on		q̄ 4 PRN					
urination. Goal: #1							
Temp will remain							
within normal limits							
within 48 hours of							
starting ordered							
antibiotic; #2 Urine							
will begin turning							
clear with no burning							
within 48 hours of							
starting ordered							
antibiotic							

INITIALS AND SIGNATURE *M.H., Michaela Heldeman, RN* _____ _____

Fig. 3.4 Patient care plan.

Box 3.3   SOAPE and SOAPIER Documentation Formats

Subjective	**S**ubjective
Objective	**O**bjective
Assessment	**A**ssessment
Plan	**P**lan
Evaluation	**I**ntervention
	Evaluation
	Revision

FOCUS CHARTING FORMAT

In the *focus charting format* (Box 3.4), which was developed by nurses, a modified list of patient problems statements is used as an index for nursing documentation. Note the similarity of this list to the problem list used for the POMR. Focus charting can be used with traditional and POMR charting.

Focus charting uses the nursing process and the more positive concept of the patient's needs rather than medical diagnoses and problems. The focus is sometimes a current patient concern or behavior and sometimes a significant change in patient status or behavior or a significant event in the patient's therapy. A focus is not a medical diagnosis.

DARE is the acronym for four different aspects of charting using the focus format (see Box 3.4). Data *(D)* are subjective and objective and are equivalent to the assessment step of the nursing process. Action *(A)* is a combination of planning and implementation. Response *(R)* of the patient is the same as evaluation of effectiveness. Some facilities include education or patient teaching *(E)*. The nurse does not need to use all the DARE steps each time notes are documented on a particular focus (Fig. 3.6).

CHARTING BY EXCEPTION

Some facilities require the narrative notes for each shift to include a minimum of three entries and a flow sheet on which the nurse charts care given. Behind this policy is the legally derived charting concept that if the care was not documented, it is considered that care was not provided. All care must be charted, but this is a time-consuming, detailed, and defensive method.

Last name: Serbane		First name: Donna M.	Attending Physician Dr. Janeston	Room No. 348A	Hosp No. 000-123, DOB 11/1/1954
Date	**Notes Should Be Signed by Physician**				
7-5-22	0930 Problem #1 Inability to regulate body temperature				
	(Patient problem: elevated body temperature)				
	[S] Feels hot & flushed. Has burning on urination and heavy feeling over bladder area. c/o "some discomfort" in lt. flank				
	[O] Temperature 101^2 (0) elevated from 99^8 @ 0730 AM. Skin warm, flushed, dry. Urinating in 100-200 mL am'ts. Urine dark,				
	amber and cloudy. Foley Cath. dc'd 7/4 @ 2200. Lungs clear.				
	[A] Possible bladder infection secondary to Foley catheter.				
	[P] Notify Dr. Janeston of temperature elevation, dysuria and back discomfort. Assess for other signs of infection. To x-ray				
	for chest evaluation. Begin oral antibiotics after catheterization and urine specimen to laboratory for C & S per Dr. Janeston				
	orders. Encourage increased oral fluids.				
	[E] Urine to laboratory, x-ray of chest ordered, chest and breath sounds clear. Nonproductive cough. Drank 500 mL of water this				
	shift. 2230 urine less concentrated.				

Fig. 3.5 SOAPE charting progress notes.

To alleviate this problem, many facilities now have a policy called **charting by exception** (CBE). The nurse charts complete physical assessments, observations, vital signs, intravenous (IV) site and rate, and other pertinent data at the beginning of each shift. During the shift, the only notes the nurse makes are for additional treatments done or planned treatments withheld, changes in patient condition, and new concerns. Notations are made reflecting progress or revisions for all active patient problems on the nursing care plan.

With the CBE method of documentation, the nurse uses more detailed flow sheets, which enhances the focus on existing concerns. One format that may be used is the problem, intervention, and evaluation (PIE) format. It is a problem-solving approach, so PIE is similar to the SOAPE format; the main difference is that SOAPE charting originated from the medical model, whereas PIE charting arose from the nursing process. The SOAPE method of documentation also is oriented to the problems, interventions, and evaluations involved in nursing care. It was designed to provide an ongoing plan of nursing care with daily documentation. The care and assessment flow sheets consist of standardized assessment criteria and interventions. With this method, the nurse assesses all areas and compares the results with normal standards. The PIE format may be written in several ways, so the nurse should use the format dictated by the agency's policy. At each shift, the nurse evaluates each patient problem at least once, and if the problem remains unresolved, the nurse ensures it is addressed continually until resolution is reached. After the patient problem is resolved, it no longer is covered by the daily documentation.

Sometimes the nurse uses a variation of the PIE format that includes assessment (A) data before the PIE (APIE). These assessment data include subjective (S) and objective (O) data. This assists the nurse to follow the steps of the nursing process (Fig. 3.7).

RECORD-KEEPING FORMS AND EXAMPLES

Different facilities use a variety of forms to make medical record documentation easy and quick, yet comprehensive. Many forms help eliminate the need to duplicate data repeatedly in the nursing notes. The forms present several types of information in a format more accessible than compilation of all progress notes. Most of the forms are self-explanatory regarding the type of information required from the nurse (Fig. 3.8). It is unnecessary to chart a narrative note each time a medication is given (see Chapter 17) or a bath (see Chapter 9) or measurement of vital signs (see Chapter 12).

The nursing **Kardex (or Rand)** system is used by some facilities to consolidate patient orders and care needs in a centralized, concise way. The cumulative care file or Rand is kept at the nursing station for quick reference or is part of the EHR or EMR. Forms vary among institutions based on information required for care (Fig. 3.9).

The **nursing care plan** (which outlines the proposed nursing care based on the nursing assessment and the identified patient problems to provide continuity of care) is developed to meet the nursing care needs of a patient. Many facilities use standardized care plans for certain conditions or surgeries; however, individualization of the plan of care based on each patient's own needs or circumstances is also important. This kind of plan, developed by nurses for nurses, is based on

EXAMPLE OF FOCUS CHARTING

Date	Time	Focus	Data, Actions, Patient Response, and Education
7/5/22	0820	Hypotension	D BP in left arm 90/60, patient's skin diaphoretic, patient responds to name A Placed patient in Trendelenburg position, increased IV fluid rate to 100 mL/hr per protocol, called Dr. Janeston. R Patient remains responsive, BP in left arm 94/68 3 min after increasing fluid *S Wilson, RN*
7/5/22	1620	Pain	D Twisting in bed, grimacing with movement, states "has sharp lower back pain" A Administered morphine sulfate 10 mg IV in RVL R Verbalized relief within 15 min, lying quietly. E Instructed patient to move slowly when getting out of bed and to call for assistance *T. Newson, RN*

Fig. 3.6 Focus charting nurse's notes.

Date	Time	Progress notes
7/6/22	0900	A - Assessment: (s) states -"sharp shooting pain in epigastric region" Patient reports 7/10 on pain scale (o) guarding abdomen and refuses lunch tray. States "I am nauseated."
	0915	P - Problem: Pain related to unknown cause
	0920	I - Intervention: Demerol 100 mg given IM in R ventral gluteal region
	1000	E - Evaluation: States "the pain is gone." *C. Sommers, LPN*

Fig. 3.7 APIE (assessment, problem, intervention, and evaluation) documentation.

nursing assessment and identified patient problems. Standardized nursing care plans include the pertinent patient problems, goals, and plans for care and specific actions for care implementation and evaluation.

Incident Reports

An *incident report* (form used to document any event not consistent with the routine operation of a health care unit or the routine care of a patient, Fig. 3.10) is sometimes necessary in response to an unplanned occurrence within a health care facility. For example, if a nurse neglects to give a medication or treatment or gives an incorrect dose of a drug, an incident report must be filed. Either of these events has the potential to cause injury. Incident reports also are filled out for any unusual event in a hospital (e.g., injuries to a patient, visitor, hospital personnel). Many staff members are reluctant to fill out these forms, but this information helps the facility risk manager and unit managers to track occurrences of incidents. One of the benefits of tracking particular incidents is to prevent future problems through education and other corrective measures.

When filling out an incident report, give only objective, observed information. Do not admit liability or give unnecessary details. Include in the incident report care given to the patient in response to the incident and the name of the health care provider notified. When charting the incident in the patient's nursing notes, do not mention the incident report, because doing so makes it easier for an attorney to request that document for a court case (Table 3.3).

Twenty-Four–Hour Patient Care Records and Acuity Charting Forms

The nursing records may be consolidated into a system that accommodates a 24-hour period. A 24-hour record-keeping system helps eliminate unnecessary record-keeping forms. It is easier to obtain accurate assessment information and documentation of activities of daily living with 24-hour notations. In addition, 24-hour patient care records often use flow sheets and checklists to enhance efficiency further.

Twenty-four–hour patient care records provide the foundation for an acuity charting system. *Acuity charting* uses a score that rates each patient by severity of illness. With documentation and analysis of nursing interventions, an overall level of acuity for each patient is determined. For example, perhaps an acuity system rates patients from 1 to 5 (1 is high, 5 is low). A patient returning from surgery with multisystem problems is an acuity level 1. On the same continuum, another patient awaiting discharge after a successful recovery from surgery is an acuity level 5. One benefit is the ability to determine efficient staffing patterns according to the acuity levels of the patients on a particular nursing unit. The patient-to-staff ratios depend on a composite gathering of data in regard to the 24-hour interventions necessary for implementing care.

Discharge Summary Forms

Much emphasis is placed on preparing a patient for a timely discharge from a health care institution. Ideally, discharge planning begins at admission, and in some cases, even before admission, as is necessary with same-day surgery admissions and childbirth. Nurses continue discharge planning as the patient's condition changes. Patients and family should be involved in the discharge planning process.

PHYSICAL ASSESSMENT (HEAD TO TOE)
TIME OF ASSESSMENT: _____

	NOTES:
1. NEUROLOGIC: Level of consciousness	
Confused	
Oriented x 1. person 2. place 3. time 4. purpose	
PERRLA—Babinski: Positive or Negative	
Hand strength: Strong or Weak	
Leg movement: Strong or Weak	
2. INTEGUMENTARY	
Condition: Moist or Dry	
Temperature:	
Turgor	
Tenting	
Incision	
Location:	
Without erythema	
Exudate:	
Sutures/staples intact	
Sutures/staples not intact	
Open wound	
Hemovac: Color Amt	
Davol: Color Amt	
Jackson-Pratt: Color Amt	
Penrose: Color Amt	
Wound vac: Color Amt	
Dressing	
Clean & dry	
Needs changed	
3. CARDIOVASCULAR	
Apical pulse rate:	
Capillary refill <3 sec: Yes or No	
Pedal pulses (1-4+): L & R	
Pedal edema (1-4+): L & R	
Nonpitting edema	
IV	
Solution	
Peripheral	
Central line	
Rate:	
Site & condition:	
4. RESPIRATORY	
Anteriorly	
Posteriorly	
O$_2$ Saturation level: %	
Crackle	
Wheezes: Sonorous or Sibilant	
Pleural friction rub	

Fig. 3.8 Nursing care record.

Dyspnea Tachypnea Orthopnea	
O_2 Therapy: type:	
Rate: Liters per:	
Incentive spirometer	
Inspiratory capacity: mL	
Chest tube to H_2O seal _____ cm	
Chest tube to H_2O seal and wall suction _____ mm Hg	
Color and amount _____ mm Hg	
5. GASTROINTESTINAL	
Appetite _____ Type of diet _____	
Dentures: Yes or No	
Oral fluid intake:	
Bowel sounds *4:	
Active Hyper Hypo Absent	
Distention Tympanic Tenderness	
Flatulence	
BM #: Color: Consistency:	
Stoma pink & viable: Yes or No	
N/G	
Amt: mL	
Color of drainage	
Peg tube _____	
Site condition _____ Flush _____ Feeding _____	
Gastrostomy tube _____	
Site condition _____ Flush _____ Feeding _____	
Jejunostomy _____	
Site condition _____ Flush _____ Feeding _____	
6. URINARY	
Output amount: _____ hours of output _____	
Color:	
Odor:	
Catheter	
Type: Foley Ureterostomy	
Suprapubic Nephrostomy	
Urostomy	
CBI credit:	
True urine:	
7. MOBILITY	
Activity level:	
Bed rest. chair. up with assistance. walker.	
crutches. cane	
Up ad lib: Yes or No	
Gait: Unsteady or Steady	
Level of tolerance:	
Traction: Kind: Weight:	

Fig. 3.8, cont'd

Continued

8. REPRODUCTIVE	
Prostate problems: Yes or No	
Hysterectomy: Yes or No	
Breast—monthly breast self-exam: Yes or No	
Mastectomy:	
____ Rt ____ Left ____ Appearance	
Vaginal drainage: Yes or No	
9. SENSORY	
Hard of hearing: Yes or No	
Hearing aid: Yes or No	
Glasses	
Contacts	

VITALS	VITALS	ADLs
TIME TAKEN: hr	TIME TAKEN: hr	BED BATH-TIME:
Temp:	Temp:	Supplies needed: 1 linen bag
Pulse:	Pulse:	2-3 towels
Respirations:	Respirations:	2-3 washcloths
Blood pressure:	Blood pressure:	4-5 disposable washcloths
How taken:	How taken:	Soap, shampoo, deodorant, comb
Level of pain:	Level of pain:	1disposable garbage bag
NOTES:	NOTES:	Cotton swabs
		Orange stick/nail file
		Lip conditioner
		Toothbrush, toothettes, toothpaste
		Denture supplies
CHECK:	CHECK:	Other supplies need by pt:
Water filled & cool	Water filled & cool	
Bed straightened	Bed straightened	
Patient comfortable?	Patient comfortable?	LINEN CHANGE OF BED:
Patient requests:	Patient requests:	1 linen bag (if not doing @ bedtime)
		1 contour sheet
		1 flat sheet
		1 pull sheet
		Pillow case(s) - How many pillows?
		1 blanket
		1 bedspread
		Add'l supplies needed for pt:
___ ALL INFO CHARTED	___ ALL INFO CHARTED	___ ALL INFO CHARTED

Fig. 3.8, cont'd

A discharge summary form provides important information that pertains to the patient's continued health care after discharge. A discharge summary always should be provided to the patient or the family (or both) so that there is written documentation of instructions given to the patient and so that the patient can refer to those instructions after being discharged. Discharge summary forms (see Fig. 11.5) make the summary concise and instructive. Often the form includes a copy that is given to the patient, a family member, or a home health care nurse and a copy that is kept with the patient records. Home health care agencies or extended nursing care facilities also benefit from receiving information on these summary forms and use it to provide better continuity of care.

DOCUMENTATION AND CLINICAL (CRITICAL) PATHWAYS

Documentation tools that integrate the standards of care of multiple disciplines have been developed to meet the needs of managed care. Managed care is a

Date Activities	Date Elimination	Date Supportive	Date Wounds	Date Hygiene	Date	Diet
7/5 Bed rest 7/6 BRP ___ Dangle ___ Chair ___ w/Chair ___ Crutched ___ Walker ___ Ad. Lib. ___ Turn 7/7 Up with Assistance	7/5 Catheter dc'd 7/6 ___ Commode ___ Adult Diaper ___ Colostomy Old/New ___ Ileostomy Old/New ___ Hematest ___ Save Stools ___ Strain all Urine ___ Urostomy 7/5 Intake/Output ___ Ileo Conduit ___ Enema/Flush PRN ___ CBI	___ Cradle/Footboard ___ Overhead Frame ___ TED Hose ___ Telemetry #___ ___ NG Tube ___ Tracheotomy ___ Traction ___ Oxygen ___ Siderails ___ Restraints ___ Egg Crate 7/5 IV's/Int. lock ___ Isolation ___ PCA Pump ___ Oral Suction ___ K-Pad	___ Packing ___ Hemo drain ___ Drain 7/5 Incision ___ Suction ___ Solcotrans 7/5 T-Tube ___ Chest Tube	7/6 Bed Bath 7/7 Assist ___ Self Bath ___ Shower/Tub ___ Sitz ___ Towel Bath ___ Oral ___ Hair ___ Skin/Decubitus	7/6	Clear liquids

Snacks	Beverages
	B Hot tea
	D Hot tea
	S Hot tea

Food Allergies: milk

LABORATORY and RADIOLOGY

7/5 Chest x-ray ECG CBC

7/7 Chest x-ray UA/C&S

DATE	TREATMENTS	DISC.
	DAILY WEIGHT SCALE	
7/5	Incentive spirometer every hour while awake.	
7/5	Vital signs q 4 hr.	
7/5	Turn, cough, and deep breath q 2 hr.	
7/5	Reinforce dressings PRN.	
7/6	Chg. abdominal dressings PRN.	
7/6	Record T-tube drainage.	

CONTACT (next of kin)
W.L. Spaur – husband
534-3974
Chaplain/Minister
G Timmons

BLUE DOT:

RECENT/PRESENT SURGERY:
Open Cholecystectomy   7/5/18

ADDITIONAL DIAGNOSIS:
UTI 7/7

Room:	Date of Birth (DOB):	Name:	Sex:	S (M) W.D.	Religion	Diagnosis:	Attending Physician:	Consulting Physician:
348A	11/1/1954	Serbane, Donna M.	Fe		Prot	Cholelithiasis & Cholecystitis	D. Janeston, MD	J.W. Richtey, MD

Fig. 3.9 Nursing Kardex (or Rand) card.

systematic approach to care that provides a framework for the coordination of medical and nursing interventions.

These documentation tools are called *clinical (critical) pathways.* Clinical (critical) pathways allow staff from all disciplines to develop standardized, integrated care plans for a projected length of stay for patients of a specific case type. The case types that have clinical (critical) pathways are usually those that occur in high volume and are predictable. A clinical (critical) pathway for a total hip repair may recommend on a day-to-day basis the level of activity, pain control therapy, advancement in diet, and educational topics necessary for a patient's recovery.

The exact contents and format of these clinical (critical) pathways vary among institutions. The contents include a care plan, interventions specific for each day of hospitalization, and a documentation tool. The clinical (critical) pathway replaces other nursing forms such as the nursing care plan.

The LPN/LVN and other team members use the pathways to monitor a patient's progress and as a documentation tool. CBE is frequently the method used with pathways. Staff members document only when anticipated interventions are not provided as projected.

Many agencies use military time, a 24-hour system that uses digit numbers to indicate morning, afternoon, and evening times regardless of which method of documentation is used (Fig. 3.11).

HOME HEALTH CARE DOCUMENTATION

The home health care industry continues to grow in our society for a number of reasons. Limitations in coverage within the acute care setting are a major cause for the growth, as is the desire patients have to be cared for in their home rather than in a health care facility.

Documentation in the home health care system has different implications than in other areas of nursing. The primary difference is the nature of the home setting, which dictates that a narrower scope of people (e.g., patient, family, direct health care provider) witness the majority of care. Home health care requires that the entire health care team work closely together. The documentation of care must be accurate and complete so that all members of the team are able to ascertain what care is rendered in the home. In addition,

KELL-RUSSELL MEMORIAL HOSPITAL

Report of Medication, Patient (Visitor)
Safety Variance

To be completed by the person most closely
involved or the person discovering the
incident/occurrence.

PATIENT NAME: *Longe, John*   AGE: *70*   SEX: *male*

ADDRESS: *59 W Bass Ave*

TYPE OF PATIENT: _____ Inpatient _____ Outpatient _____ Emergency
(check one) _____ *X* _____ Visitor _____ Employee

Date and time of variance: *07/07/2021*

Exact location of variance: *Room 3001*

Description of variance: *Visitor found lying on floor at foot of patient's bed. "I got light headed when I saw all of the tubes and machines on my dad."*

What was the nature of the injury to the patient (visitor) etc.: *no injuries noted*

Equipment or supplies involved: *none*

ID # & Present Location: *3001*

Why did variance occur? *Visitor states "I got light headed when I saw all of the tubes and machines on my dad. I didn't get hurt because my brother caught me and eased me down to the floor." Visitor refuses to see a physician.*

Physician notified? _____ yes _____ no *X* when? _____

Signature *Sandra Suey, RN*   Physician: *Dr. Janeston*

Witness *Mary Pinkton, RN*

If the incident is related to patient care, this sheet must remain on inpatient medical record for 24 hours, after which it shall be taken to the Risk Management Department.

CONFIDENTIAL - NOT PART OF THE MEDICAL RECORD

Fig. 3.10 Incident report.

Table 3.3   Examples of Incident Report Entries

PROPER ENTRY	INCORRECT ENTRY
1900 Resident found on floor in a sitting position beside table in activity room. Complete assessment performed. Vital signs stable; 1-cm abrasion on anterior left forearm noted. No complaints by resident. Abrasion recorded on skin assessment record. Notified Dr. Reads per phone. Orders received to perform neurologic assessment every 2 hours for 24 hours and place on fall risk protocol.	1900 Resident found on floor in activity room. Apparently missed chair when trying to move chair and sit down. Minor abrasion on left arm. Dr. Reads notified and orders received.
0800 Administered hydrochlorothiazide 25 mg p.o. Hydrochlorothiazide 12.5 mg ordered. Vital signs measured and remain stable. Dr. Reads notified. Order received to continue monitoring vital signs every hour × 4 hours. If stable, monitor every 4 hours for 24 hours.	0800 Administered 25 mg hydrochlorothiazide by mistake. Patient had no complaints and states he "feels fine." Notified Dr. Reads and orders received.
1700 Felt sharp pain in lower back, 8/10, after assisting patient from bed to chair. Gait belt used to assist in patient transfer. Notified employee health department.	1700 Injured back while helping patient transfer from bed to chair. Notified employee health department.

© Elsevier

Fig. 3.11 Military time clock.

the documentation provides the quality control and the justification for reimbursement from Medicare, Medicaid, or private insurance companies. Nurses have to document all their services for payment (e.g., direct skilled care, patient instructions, skilled observations, evaluation visits). The nurse is the pivotal person in the documentation of the delivery of home health care.

Home health care documentation has several components that the nurse must consider. Medicare, Medicaid, and private insurance typically have similar requirements in regard to documentation. The patient's eligibility for home care must be assessed thoroughly and documented. The nurse must document in detail any procedures, treatments, or medications administered and response to these interventions. Another important aspect of health care documentation is noting any patient education and demonstration of learning. Home health documentation also must reflect coordination of services by all members of the health care team and evidence of compliance with regulations (CMS, n.d.). Home health care is discussed in more detail in Chapter 37.

LONG-TERM HEALTH CARE DOCUMENTATION

An ever-increasing number of older adults need care in long-term health care facilities. Because many individuals live in this setting for the rest of their lives, they are referred to as residents rather than as patients. The acuity of residents' conditions, and the number of their disabilities, continues to escalate commensurate with their age. Nursing personnel often face challenges much different from those in the acute care setting.

These differences establish a significantly different basis for nursing documentation.

Outside agencies are instrumental in determining the standards and policies for documentation in long-term health care. For example, the Omnibus Budget Reconciliation Act (OBRA) of 1987 instituted significant Medicare and Medicaid requirements for long-term care provision and documentation. Among the requirements of OBRA are minimum data sets (MDS) and regulated standards for resident assessments, individualized care plans, and qualifications for health care providers (RNs and LPN/LVNs). In addition, the department of health in each state governs the frequency of the required nursing entries in the records of residents in long-term care facilities. Long-term care documentation supports a multidisciplinary approach in the assessment (referred to as the MDS) and the planning process (referred to as resident assessment protocols) of the residents. Often long-term care agencies also have skilled care units where patients or residents stay when, in response to mandates for shorter hospital stays, they need increased levels of care and are not able to return directly to their usual residence after a hospital admission. Multidisciplinary communication among such health care providers as nurses, unlicensed assistive personnel (UAP), social workers, physical therapists, and dietitians is essential in the regulated documentation process. The fiscal management of long-term care hinges on the justification of nursing care as demonstrated in sound documentation of the services rendered. Additional documentation information in long-term care is discussed in Chapter 38.

SPECIAL ISSUES IN DOCUMENTATION

RECORD OWNERSHIP AND ACCESS

The original health care record or chart is the property of the institution or the health care provider. On admission to the health care facility, the patient usually is asked to sign a form granting permission for appropriate people, such as insurance carriers, to have access to the record as necessary. Patients may not have immediate access to their full records, depending on the agency policy. Lawyers, with the patient's written permission, are given access to the patient's medical records. Courts have the legal right to obtain records for review and use in the case of a lawsuit.

Patients have gained access rights to their records in most states, but only if they follow the established policy of each facility. A written request for chart access may be required, and institutions can specify a period that allows the physician and the facility to review the record and give a response. Sometimes the institution requires that a staff member or physician be present while the individual looks through the chart to answer questions and to protect the integrity of the record. Patients also may ask for a copy of their medical records. The use of patient portals has helped immensely in giving access to much of a patient's record. While it doesn't allow viewing of the primary provider's anecdotal notes or nurse's notes, as previously mentioned the patient portal does allow for viewing of items such as lab and diagnostic test results.

CONFIDENTIALITY

Health care personnel are required to respect the confidentiality of the patient's record. The Patient Care Partnership (patients, when admitted to a facility, receive this information regarding their rights and responsibilities) and the law guarantee that medical information is kept private, unless the information is needed in providing care or the patient gives permission for others to see it (American Hospital Association, n.d.). The Health Insurance Portability and Accountability Act (HIPAA), an act of Congress passed in 1996, affords certain protections to persons covered by health care plans, including continuity of coverage when changing jobs, standards for electronic health care transactions, and primary safeguards for the privacy of individually identifiable patient information (see Chapter 2).

Ethical codes of practice also emphasize the LPN/LVN's obligation to preserve patient privacy by holding patient information in highest confidentiality. Health care personnel may not read a record, or allow others to do so, without a clinical reason, and personnel must hold the information regarding the patient in confidence. Furthermore, trust is necessary for good nurse-patient relationships, and breaking confidences is a way to lose patient trust. Breaking laws concerning patient confidentiality often leads to job termination, lawsuits, or both (see Chapter 2).

Student nurses are reminded that no information is to leave the clinical site and that any documents that have patient identifying information must be closely guarded at all times within the facility. Any printouts or notes with patient identifiers that have been used by the student must be shredded before leaving the clinical agency. In addition, the student must be vigilant in keeping documents in a safe place when in the clinical agency; documents with patient identifiers never should be left anywhere unattended, such as on bedside tables in the patient's room, at the nurses' station, or on conference room tables. Any information that the student does need for course assignment purposes regarding assigned patients should have no identification information on the documents. Identification information is not limited to the patient's name, age, or identification number. Any unique information about the patient, such as medical diagnosis or past medical history, is considered a patient identifier.

ELECTRONIC DOCUMENTATION SAFEGUARDS

Charting with an electronic system is an efficient method of documentation, but the security of the system must be considered when considering legal and

---

Box 3.5   Guidelines for Safe Computer Documentation

- Do not share with another caregiver the password that you use to enter and sign off computer files. (NOTE: A good system requires frequent changes in personal passwords to prevent unauthorized people from accessing and tampering with records. Some facilities use fingerprint scanners instead of passwords.)
- After logging on, never leave the computer terminal unattended without first logging off.
- Follow the correct protocol for correcting errors. To correct an error after storage, follow the facility policy for identifying documentation errors, then add the correct information and date and initial the entry. If you record information in the wrong chart, follow facility policy for identifying this error.
- Make sure that stored records have backup files, an important safety check. If you inadvertently delete part of the permanent records, type an explanation into the computer file with the date, the time, and your initials and submit an explanation in writing to your manager.
- Do not leave information about a patient displayed on a monitor where others have the opportunity to see it.
- Follow the agency's confidentiality procedures for documentation.
- Printouts of computerized records also have to be protected. Shredding of printouts and keeping a log that accounts for every copy (whether electronic or printed) of a computerized file that you have generated from the system are ways to keep waste and creation of duplicate records to a minimum and protect the confidentiality of patients.

---

ethical issues. Confidentiality, access to information, and inappropriate alterations in patient records are areas of concern. Networks typically are protected by a firewall from illegitimate outside access. Some computer systems permit online access from remote sites, but this further complicates the task of keeping the system secure. To protect the patient's rights and keep the patient's record confidential, anyone who enters data into or consults a computerized record has to log on to the system with a secure password. The institution may require the user to change passwords at certain time frames, such as every 90 days, to maintain security. Because the password is assigned only to individual health care personnel, any data entered are credited automatically to whoever signed in; thus personnel must never share the password with anyone. Be sure to log off the system before leaving the terminal to ensure that information about a patient does not remain on the monitor display for others to view.

It is also necessary to protect computer-generated printouts and prevent the indiscriminate duplication or distribution of information about patients. Most facilities that use computer charting incorporate a system for logging and tracking computer printouts (Box 3.5) and have protocols for shredding the copies that are made.

USE OF FAX MACHINES

Fax machines send written documents over telephone lines to transmit data quickly between health care facilities, such as health care provider's offices, hospitals, long-term care facilities, and laboratories. HIPAA rules allow for a patient's medical records and information to be faxed. Information can be transmitted from health care providers to health care facilities and vice versa. For example, laboratory results can be sent via fax, email, or phone to a health care provider, or a health care provider may fax medical information to another professional for consultation. Various safeguards must be in place to maintain patient confidentiality and privacy. Some facilities require that the sender verify the fax number with the recipient. Similarly, a facility may preprogram frequently faxed numbers into the system to prevent incorrect dialing of the intended number. Although fax machines are still used, they are being used less by facilities that have an EHR system in place.

Get Ready for the NCLEX® Examination!

Key Points

- Documentation is part of the implementation phase of the nursing process and is used in evaluation.
- Only approved abbreviations and medical terms should be used when charting in a patient's record. Knowledge of the common abbreviations and terms is required.
- The five purposes for patient records are (1) a means of communication to facilitate continuity of care; (2) a permanent record for accountability purposes (audits, accreditation, and cost reimbursement); (3) a legal record; (4) usage in teaching; and (5) usage for research and data collection.
- Many facilities have an electronic health record (EHR) or electronic medical record (EMR) system in place to facilitate documentation and coordination of patient care.
- ISBAR (*i*ntroduction, *s*ituation, *b*ackground, *a*ssessment, and *r*ecommendation) aids in communication during "hand-off" or "handover" interactions with other health care personnel.
- Two common types of medical records or charts are the traditional (block) chart and the problem-oriented medical record (POMR).
- The POMR uses a master patient problem list as an index to the chart. These listed problems are usually medical diagnoses.
- SOAPIER is one format for charting in the POMR. The letters stand for subjective *(S)*, objective *(0)*, assessment *(A)*, plan *(P)*, implementation *(I)*, evaluation *(E)*, and revision *(R)*.
- Two other common formats for charting nursing notes are narrative and focus. Focus charting includes data *(D)*, action *(A)*, response and evaluation *(R)*, and education and patient teaching *(E)*.
- Charting must be legible (with handwritten documentation), clear, concise, accurate, and complete. These guidelines serve as a national standard for licensed nurses.
- The specific institution or unit often has specific forms and charting formats; in addition, the general guidelines and rules for charting should be followed.
- Medical records are legal documents. The health care provider or institution owns the original record.
- Lawyers, courts, and patients are able to gain access to the record by following specified access procedures.

- The contents of a health record are confidential information protected by the law and the Patient Care Partnership.
- The nursing Kardex or Rand is a card-filing system used in some facilities by nurses to condense all the orders and other care information needed quickly for each patient. It is updated frequently.
- Computerized information systems provide information about a patient in an organized and easily accessible fashion.
- Clinical pathways allow staff from all disciplines to develop integrated care plans for a projected length of stay for patients of a specific case type.
- Many agencies use military time. This system uses four-digit numbers to indicate morning, afternoon, and evening times.
- A 24-hour record-keeping system helps eliminate unnecessary record-keeping forms.
- The acuity level determined by analyzing what nursing care is necessary allows patients to be rated in comparison with one another. Staffing patterns then can be determined by examining the acuity levels for the patients on a particular nursing unit.
- Fax machines are used to send written documents over telephone lines to transmit data quickly between hospitals and other facilities, such as health care provider offices.

Additional Learning Resources

SG Go to your Study Guide for additional learning activities to help you master this chapter content.

Be sure to visit the Evolve site at http://evolve.elsevier.com/Cooper/foundations/ for additional online resources.

Review Questions for the NCLEX® Examination

1. The nursing preceptor is preparing to speak with the new licensed practical/vocational nurse (LPN/LVN) regarding documentation. Which statement by the preceptor is correct?

    1. "It is important to use only approved medical terms and abbreviations when documenting in the electronic health record (EHR)."

2. "Our facility discourages nurses from using complete words when documenting because it takes up too much space in the chart."

3. "To prevent errors, our facility does not allow the use of abbreviations for documentation."

4. "The physician uses more abbreviations when writing orders than the nurse uses when documenting."

2. The patient asks the LPN/LVN if he can take his chart with him on discharge from the hospital. Which response by the nurse is most accurate?

1. "The chart has confidential information in it and cannot be taken out of the facility."

2. "The chart belongs to you, so I will check to see whether this is permissible."

3. "We need to complete the proper forms for you to take your chart with you."

4. "The chart is the property of the hospital, but if you need copies of your records, we can arrange that for you."

3. When reviewing information regarding the problem-oriented medical record (POMR), the LPN/LVN correctly identifies which guideline?

1. The problem list has only active and resolved problems.

2. Only the physician charts on the progress notes.

3. The charting format is SOAPE or SOAPIER.

4. Focus charting format is used with this type of record.

4. The LPN/LVN is using the SOAPE method to chart for a patient on the orthopedic unit who had a total hip replacement 2 days ago. When documenting the *S* portion, which entry demonstrates correct documentation? *Select all that apply*

1. Patient's vital signs are stable.

2. Patient reports left hip pain 8/10.

3. Patient's wife was present during patient teaching.

4. Patient ambulated 20 ft unassisted with steady gait.

5. Patient reports a feeling of nausea after eating.

6. Patient asked when they will be discharged.

7. Patient's abdomen is distended upon palpation.

8. Patient reports a feeling of numbness below the incision site.

9. Patient's incision is well approximated.

10. Patient's daughter visits every day during her lunch break.

5. The student nurse is correct when identifying which concept regarding documentation as being correct?

1. Chart as soon and as often as necessary.

2. Remember to chart only basic care information.

3. Leave blank lines for others if asked.

4. Chart facts with use of judgmental terms if needed.

6. Understanding that health care personnel must respect the confidentiality of patient records, which action by the nurse is appropriate?

1. Looking at a friend's chart to see the diagnosis

2. Stating that only the Patient Care Partnership advocates confidentiality

3. Reading charts only for a professional reason

4. Sharing information from a chart to protect a friend

7. Following orientation to the facility's computer system, which statement by the new nurse is most accurate?

1. "I can save on charting time once I am comfortable using this system."

2. "The computer system is not that efficient."

3. "Documentation can be done only on a shared terminal at the desk."

4. "Most computerized systems lack security measures to protect confidentiality."

8. The nurse demonstrates knowledge of correctly completing an incident report with which action?

1. Documenting in the chart that the incident report has been filed

2. Having all parties involved sign the report

3. Asking the supervising nurse to complete the incident report

4. Documenting facts regarding the incident

9. Which statement is correct about formats for documentation? *Select all that apply*

1. Focus charting is a goal-oriented system.

2. Clinical pathways are the most commonly used format now.

3. Charting by exception documents those conditions, interventions, or outcomes outside the norm.

4. Standardized care plans are not cost effective.

5. EHR systems allow for patient data to be shared for collaboration of care.

10. Which statement is a recommended guideline for charting?

1. Documentation should be lengthy and detailed.

2. Content that suggests a risk situation should be included.

3. One should skip lines between charting entries.

4. The patient's name and identification number should be on all documents.

11. Which statement is a safe principle of computerized charting?

1. It is acceptable to chart in advance of care being given.

2. Each unit or department has its own password.

3. There is no room for mistakes in computerized charting.

4. Do not leave patient information displayed on the monitor.

12. The student nurse is reviewing the chart of a 3-year-old patient who was admitted to the hospital with the diagnosis of RSV. The assessment data includes:

- Temperature 102.6°F (38.9°C)
- Oxygen saturation 89% on 2L O_2 via nasal/cannula
- Heart rate 112 bpm
- Complains of chest hurting
- Respirations 40 and labored
- Substernal retractions noted with breathing
- States, "I'm not hungry."
- Frequent coughing noted
- Moans, "I don't feel good."

Choose the *most likely* options for the information missing from the statements below by selecting from the list of options provided.

The student nurse is aware that the assessment data "Respirations 40 and labored" is an example of _____ data. If looking for subjective data in the assessment the student nurse chooses _____ as a good example.

OPTIONS
Subjective
Irrelevant
Moans, "I don't feel good."
Frequent coughing noted
Objective
Oxygen saturation 89% on 2L O_2 via nasal/cannula

13. What is the primary purpose of Title II of the Health Insurance Portability and Accountability Act (HIPAA)?

    1. Ensure proper documentation in patient's medical records
    2. Maintain privacy and confidentiality of patient's health information
    3. Regulate the availability and range of group insurance plans
    4. Limit restrictions on insurance coverage based on preexisting conditions

14. Which statement is correct about abbreviations? *Select all that apply*

    1. The nurse should be aware of any abbreviations on the "do not use" list.
    2. Creating abbreviations saves time for the reader.
    3. Abbreviating drug names and dosages helps reduce medication errors.
    4. When in doubt, the nurse should use the complete word and not the abbreviation.
    5. The nurse should include medical abbreviations on discharge instructions.

15. The nurse documents in the patient record, "0830 patient appears to be in severe pain and refuses to ambulate. Blood pressure and pulse are elevated, physician notified, and analgesic administered as ordered with adequate relief. J. Doe RN." Which statement about the documentation is most accurate?

    1. The documentation is inadequate because the pain is not described on a scale of 1 to 10.
    2. The documentation is good because it shows immediate responsiveness to the problem.

3. The documentation is acceptable because it includes assessment, intervention, and evaluation.
4. The documentation is unacceptable because it is vague, nondescriptive data without supportive data.

16. The nurse works in a facility that uses narrative charting for nurse's notes. Identify which documentation is an example of narrative charting. *(Select all that apply.)*

    1. "Patient alert and oriented ×3, PERRLA, hand grips strong and equal."
    2. "S—The patient complains of pain in the lower back, 6 out of 10."
    3. "Patient ambulated 60 ft in the hall, unassisted with steady gait. Currently resting in chair with no complaints."
    4. "Problem #1—Elevated blood glucose. Plan—Measure patient's blood glucose with finger stick method before meals and at bedtime."
    5. "Patient asking for pain medication for incisional pain 7/10. Hydrocodone 10–325, 2 tablets administered by mouth while patient was eating lunch. Patient resting in bed with side rails up × 2, and call light in reach."

17. In most states, patients can gain access to their medical records by which means?

    1. Asking the nursing staff to allow them to view each entry in the record
    2. Submitting a written request to the facility to view the record
    3. Requesting the state board of health to allow access to the record
    4. Asking the staff for copies of their records

18. The charge nurse in a long-term care facility has been asked by the facility administrator to be sure that the staff documents in a way that will help ensure appropriate reimbursement for services provided. The charge nurse should instruct the staff to chart using what system as a guide?

    1. Minimum data sets (MDS)
    2. Charting by exception (CBE)
    3. DARE (*d*ata, *a*ction, *r*esponse, *e*ducation)
    4. Problem-oriented medical record (POMR)

19. An elderly patient with pneumonia is in an acute care hospital. Medicare will pay for 4 days of care in the facility. What prospective payment system is responsible for determining this reimbursement?

    1. Evaluation of nursing documentation
    2. Submission of appropriate physician progress notes
    3. Clinical (critical) pathways
    4. Diagnosis-related groups (DRGs)

4 Communication

Objectives

1. Recognize that communication is inherent in every nurse–patient interaction.
2. Discuss the concepts of verbal and nonverbal communication.
3. Discuss the impact of nonverbal communication.
4. Recognize assertive communication as the most appropriate communication style.
5. Use various therapeutic communication techniques.
6. Identify various factors that have the potential to affect communication.
7. Discuss potential barriers to communication.
8. Recognize trust as the foundation for all effective interaction.
9. Apply the nursing process to patients experiencing difficulty with verbally communicating.
10. Apply therapeutic communication techniques to patients with special communication needs.

Key Terms

active listening (p. 65)
aggressive communication (p. 63)
altered cognition (p. 73)
assertive communication (p. 63)
assertiveness (p. 63)
clarifying (p. 69)
closed posture (p. 62)
closed question (p. 62)
communication (kŏ-MYŪ-nĭ-KĀ-shŭn, p. 60)
connotative meaning (kŏn-nō-TĀ-tĭv, p. 61)
denotative meaning (dĭ-nō-TĀ-tĭv, p. 61)
expressive aphasia (ă-FĀ-zhă, p. 76)
focusing (p. 69)
gestures (p. 62)
jargon (JĂR-gŏn, p. 61)
minimal encouragement (p. 66)
nontherapeutic communication (nŏn-thĕr-ă-PYŪ-tĭk, p. 64)

nonverbal communication (p. 63)
one-way communication (p. 61)
open posture (p. 62)
open-ended question (p. 69)
paraphrasing (p. 69)
passive listening (p. 65)
posture (p. 62)
receiver, (p. 60)
receptive aphasia (p. 76)
reflecting (p. 69)
restating (p. 69)
sender, (p. 60)
therapeutic communication (p. 64)
two-way communication (p. 61)
unassertive communication (p. 63)
verbal communication (p. 61)

Communication is one of the most important aspects of care in nursing. Some form of communication occurs each time an interaction takes place. Interactions occur between two parties, such as the nurse and the patient or the nurse and a family member, a physician, or a coworker, or other combinations. Remember that the message intended is not always the message received. The licensed practical/licensed vocational nurse (LPN/LVN) should always strive to communicate effectively and minimize miscommunication. This chapter explores various aspects of communication.

Communication can be described simply as the exchange of information. The way in which information is exchanged may vary greatly. Communication takes verbal and nonverbal forms and conveys a variety of messages (e.g., information, emotions, humor, acceptance, rejection). Many variables influence the effect of the message.

OVERVIEW OF COMMUNICATION

For communication to occur, a sender and a receiver of a message are necessary. The **sender** is the one who conveys the message, whereas the **receiver** is the person or people to whom the message is conveyed. The individual who receives the message is sometimes the intended receiver and sometimes an unintended receiver. Consider the following scenario:

The night nurse, reporting to the day nurse outside Ms. B.'s room: "Ms. B. was on her call light all night. She's a real complainer!"

Ms. B overhears the exchange.

The day nurse is the intended receiver, or the one with whom the night nurse means to communicate regarding Ms. B.'s behavior. Because Ms. B. also hears the statement, she becomes an unintended receiver. Consider the possible effect of this message on the relationship between Ms. B. and the night nurse. Negative consequences for the relationship between Ms. B. and the day nurse are another possible outcome, if Ms. B. believes that the day nurse shares the night nurse's view of her.

Communication can be one-way or two-way, and which type of communication actually occurs depends partly on the roles of the people in the interaction. One-way communication is highly structured; the sender is in control and expects and gets little response from the receiver. A lecture to a large audience is an example of one-way communication. One-way communication is of limited use in the nurse–patient relationship. Two-way communication requires that the sender and the receiver participate in the interaction. It allows for exchange between the nurse and the patient, and its purpose is to meet the needs of the nurse and the patient and to establish a trusting relationship. It is important to always strive to seek and accept the patient's input and feedback rather than simply talk to the patient.

VERBAL COMMUNICATION

Verbal communication involves the use of spoken or written words or symbols. It may seem that there is little room for misunderstanding or misinterpretation of the intended message as long as the receiver understands the words and symbols being used. Frequently this is not the case. Sometimes words have very different meanings, or connotations, for different people. The connotative meaning of a word is subjective and reflects the individual's perception or interpretation. There is a potential for miscommunication that lies in such subjective variation. Take, for example, the word *stable*. If the family members are informed that their loved one's condition is stable, they perhaps may understand that for the moment, the patient's condition is not deteriorating. On the other hand, they may hear a different message, not the one that was intended: the patient is doing well and is out of danger.

Denotative meaning refers to the commonly accepted definition of a particular word. For example, the word *telephone* means the same thing to anyone who is familiar with the English language. The key word here is *familiar.* No guarantee exists that both parties know the word or assign the same definition to it. Consider the situation in which the nurse asks the patient when he last voided or had a stool. Although these terms and phrasing are familiar to health care professionals, the patient may have no idea that the nurse is asking when he last urinated or had a bowel movement. This is an example of the nurse using hospital jargon. Jargon is commonplace "language" or terminology unique to people in a particular work setting, such as a hospital, or to a specific type of work, such as nursing. It is as though the nurse and the patient have different dictionaries for what is thought to be a shared language. The nurse must be cautious of the terminology used when communicating with patients.

NONVERBAL COMMUNICATION

Messages transmitted without the use of words (either oral or written) constitute nonverbal communication. Nonverbal cues include tone and rate of voice, volume of speech, eye contact, physical appearance, and use of touch (Table 4.1). Some degree of nonverbal communication usually accompanies verbal communication.

Voice

Aspects of the voice affect nonverbal messages, including tone, volume, and the rate of speech. Characteristics of people's voices vary depending on their emotions, familiarity with a situation, confidence, and geographic and cultural influences. Meaning cannot be interpreted accurately on the basis of tone, rate, and volume alone. For example, a high-pitched, loud voice and rapid speech may indicate that an individual is frightened, but people also speak that way out of excitement or enthusiasm. In fact, some people always tend to use this speech pattern, and thus no conclusions are appropriate at all. The nurse should consider the voice characteristics in the context of the situation as a whole so that interpretation of the message is accurate.

Eye Contact

Eye contact is responsible for much communication and miscommunication. Generally, eye contact communicates an intention to interact. However, the nature of the interaction and the results of eye contact are not necessarily always positive. Extended eye contact sometimes implies aggression and arouses anxiety. On the other hand, the person who maintains eye contact for 2 to 6 seconds during an interaction helps involve the other person in what is said without being threatening or intimidating. An absence of eye contact communicates many things: shyness, lack of confidence, disinterest, embarrassment, or hurt, or in contrast, deference and respect. Sensitivity to eye contact of each communication partner helps with perceiving what actually is occurring in an interaction. Culture significantly affects how people interpret eye contact. Most Americans view eye contact in a positive manner, whereas some cultures may view eye contact differently. Some people of certain cultures may view eye contact as impolite, aggressive, or improper. It is important for the nurse to assess the situation and determine how eye contact is interpreted by their patient.

Physical Appearance

The physical appearance of the participants in an interaction has the potential to greatly influence the perceptions they form of each other. Physical appearance

Table **4.1**   **Nonverbal Cues**

ATTRIBUTE OR BEHAVIOR EXHIBITED BY SENDER (CUE)	COMPONENTS	POSSIBLE INTERPRETATION OR PERCEPTION BY RECEIVER
Voice	Tone, volume, pitch, rate of speech	Fear, excitement, enthusiasm, stress, anger, comfort, concern, confidence, calm
Eye contact	Extended (longer than 6 s)	Aggression, intimidation, disrespect
	Brief but direct (2–6 s)	Interest, respect, caring
	Absent or fleeting	Shyness, lack of confidence, low self-esteem, disinterest, anxiety, fear, uneasiness, hurriedness, or deference or respect (culture-specific)
Physical appearance	Size, color of skin, dress, grooming, body carriage, age, gender	Professional or nonprofessional, trust or distrust, respect or disrespect, comfort or intimidation, interest or disinterest, competence or incompetence
Gestures	Distinct movements of hands, head, body	Emphasis, clarification, pleasure, helpfulness, anger, threat, disrespect
Posture	*Open:* Relaxed stance, facing receiver, uncrossed arms and legs, slight shift toward receiver, direct eye contact, smile	Warmth, acceptance, caring
	Closed: Formal, distant stance; arms and possibly legs tightly crossed	Disinterest, coldness, nonacceptance, authority, control, intimidation, condescension

includes attributes of size, color of skin, dress, grooming, posture, and facial expression. Although often these attributes have absolutely nothing to do with any messages the sender intends to convey, they can have a major impact on the receiver's interpretation. Consider, for example, the patient with a personal bias against individuals with numerous tattoos or body piercings. Although the tattoos and piercings have no impact on the competency of the nurse, the patient with a bias against these may have difficulty establishing a trusting and therapeutic relationship with a nurse who has tattoos or piercings.

A professional appearance conveys self-respect and competence. How the nurse chooses to dress while on duty sends a strong message to the patient. The LPN/LVN who chooses to wear wrinkled uniforms or soiled shoes may risk sending the message that the patient is not worth the time it would take for the nurse to look professional. This may lead the patient to view the nurse as uncaring or incompetent.

Many health care facilities have adopted specific dress codes to convey professionalism in the workplace. Scrubs of one design or color often are worn by specific personnel as a means of communicating to the patient the role of that professional. In some facilities, the nurse may wear one color of scrubs, and the unlicensed assistive personnel (UAP) may wear another. Jewelry and hair also may be addressed in dress codes within health care facilities for safety purposes.

Gestures. **Gestures** are movements people use to emphasize the idea they are attempting to communicate.

Gestures also play a useful role in clarifying. A patient is often better able to express where pain is on the body by pointing to a particular area than trying to describe it in words. However, many gestures affect communication negatively. For example, a nurse who frequently looks at a watch while interviewing a patient conveys disinterest in what the patient is saying or that the nurse has a limited amount of time to spend with the patient. Also, gestures often have different meanings from individual to individual and from culture to culture. It is essential to be constantly aware of gestures the participants use during interactions and to consider the implication of gestures used.

Posture. The way that an individual sits, stands, and moves is called **posture**. Posture has the potential to convey warmth and acceptance or distance and disinterest. An **open posture** conveys a willingness to communicate with another person. This posture is typically demonstrated with the speaker facing the receiver, often leaning toward them slightly with arms unfolded. **Closed posture** does not convey a willingness to communicate. It is commonly demonstrated with arms folded and not relaxed, no eye contact, and facing away from the person. Closed posture does not encourage a good interaction between the nurse and patient. A person often interprets closed posture as disinterest, coldness, and even nonacceptance. Standing at the bedside looking down at the patient in the bed places the nurse in a position of authority and control. The patient is likely to experience this as intimidating and condescending. Whenever possible, the nurse should be at the same level as the patient during conversations; this is especially important with pediatric

Fig. 4.1 Whenever possible, place yourself level with the patient.

patients. Sitting at the bedside in a relaxed and open posture is one example (Fig. 4.1).

Consistency of Verbal and Nonverbal Communication

No definitive studies prove what percentage of communication is verbal or nonverbal; however, most people and communication experts believe that nonverbal communication is often more accurate and makes up the largest percentage of our communication. Nonverbal communication is very powerful. If nonverbal cues are inconsistent or incongruent with the verbal message, the nonverbal message is most likely the one received. At the very least, this incongruence frequently is the cause of misinterpretation and misunderstanding. The following scenario is an example of incongruence between what the nurse is stating and what she is demonstrating.

Nurse M. has been having a very busy morning. While trying to get Ms. D. ready to go to surgery, Nurse M. has been interrupted several times by staff members asking for help or advice. Now Mr. R., a patient also assigned to Nurse M., has put on his call light. As she enters Mr. R.'s room in an obvious hurry, Mr. R. states, "I'm very sorry to bother you, but could you refill my water pitcher?" Nurse M. grabs the pitcher from the bedside stand and takes it to the sink, while muttering through tight lips, "It's no bother, Mr. R. I'm happy to do it!"

The words Nurse M. used are appropriate. However, Nurse M.'s nonverbal cues are "speaking" much louder than her words, and Mr. R. is sure to pick up on her anger and frustration from her posture, tone of voice, and facial expression. How is it possible for him to really believe that he has not been a bother and that Nurse M. is "happy" to help him?

STYLES OF COMMUNICATION

The manner, or style, in which a message is communicated greatly affects the mood and the overall outcome of an interaction. Every time an interaction

Box **4.1**	Assertive Communication for Nurses

Communicating assertively means:
- Being able to express your needs while being aware of others' needs
- Being confident in communicating directly and honestly
- Feeling comfortable and in control of anxiety, tenseness, shyness, or fear
- Honoring the fact that you and the other person have rights

An assertive nurse:
- Appears self-confident and composed
- Ensures that verbal and nonverbal communication is congruent
- Is unapologetic
- Maintains eye contact
- Speaks firmly and with a positive attitude
- Speaks genuinely, without sarcasm
- Takes initiative to guide situations
- Uses clear, concise speech

Modified from Balzer Riley J: Communication in nursing, ed 8, St. Louis, 2021, Mosby.

occurs between a nurse and a patient the tone is set for the nurse–patient relationship. The style of communication the nurse demonstrates is often what makes the difference between a positive or negative interaction.

ASSERTIVE COMMUNICATION

Assertiveness is one's ability to confidently and comfortably express thoughts and feelings while still respecting the legitimate rights of the patient. An assertive communication style is interaction that considers the feelings and needs of the patient yet honors the nurse's rights as an individual (Box 4.1). It makes interactions more even and has positive benefits for all involved (Balzer Riley, 2021).

AGGRESSIVE COMMUNICATION

Aggressive communication occurs when an individual interacts with another in an overpowering and forceful manner to meet one's own personal needs at the expense of the other. Aggressive communication is destructive and nontherapeutic. In the situation just described, Nurse M. responds to Mr. R. in an aggressive manner. Neither party benefits from such an interaction. After the fact, Nurse M. most likely feels guilty and disrespectful for having responded to Mr. R. in this harsh manner, and Mr. R. undoubtedly feels humiliated and unworthy.

UNASSERTIVE COMMUNICATION

Another choice for Nurse M., although not a favorable one, would have been to respond unambiguously to Mr. R. but in an unassertive communication style. In this style, the nurse agrees to do what the patient requests, even though doing so creates additional problems for the nurse. Use of this style sacrifices one's legitimate personal rights to the needs of the patient, and there is a price to pay: resentment.

Imagine that Nurse M. had responded like this to Mr. R.'s request to have his water pitcher refilled:

Well, I'm really busy right now, but … well, I guess I can do it if I hurry. I just don't know how I'm ever going to get my other patient ready for surgery in time. Here, give me your pitcher.

This interaction is much like the previous one, although more open. The problem with this interaction is that no one really benefits from the interaction. Mr. R. now has fresh water but probably feels like he has imposed on the nurse unduly. Perhaps he even feels angry, thinking that his needs are not as important as those of another patient. Nurse M. now is even further behind than before and is likely to feel resentment toward Mr. R. and as guilty or ashamed as before for giving Mr. R. the impression he is a "bother."

The most effective way for Nurse M. to address the situation is with an assertive communication style. Perhaps the interaction sounds like this:

Well, Mr. R., if you don't mind waiting about 10 minutes, I will be glad to fill your water pitcher with fresh ice and water. If you need it filled before that, I can ask one of the nursing assistants to fill it for you now.

With assertive communication, the needs of Nurse M. and Mr. R. can be met, with neither of them feeling unworthy, belittled, resentful, or guilty.

ESTABLISHING A THERAPEUTIC RELATIONSHIP

A therapeutic nurse–patient interaction is one in which the nurse demonstrates caring, sincerity, empathy, and trustworthiness. If the patient senses that the nurse is not being genuine in conveying these feelings, a therapeutic, trusting relationship does not develop. If the nurse appears hurried or detached from the interaction, a message is sent that the patient is not as important as the other things on the nurse's mind, which very likely leaves the patient feeling frustrated and diminished in self-worth.

Ensure that the *patient* is the focus of each interaction, not the equipment or the task. On entering a patient's room, look at and address the patient before assessing or adjusting any equipment. In addition, be diligent in following through with commitments. If you have promised to assist the patient with a bath in 15 minutes, then this commitment should be fulfilled. If this is not going to be possible, explain this to the patient and establish another mutually agreeable plan for completing the bath. Failure to follow through on commitments undermines the relationship and erodes trust.

Trust is essential to effective nurse–patient interaction. Much of the information that the patient shares with the nurse is personal and often highly sensitive. The patient must be able to trust the nurse to treat the information confidentially and share it only with those individuals who need it to provide safe and competent care for the patient. Although confidentiality is critical to maintain, certain limits exist. The nurse is obligated to report a patient's statement of intent to do self-harm or to harm others. This obligation should be made clear to all patients.

Be careful to maintain professional boundaries in nurse–patient relationships. Sharing of personal information, such as address and phone number, is not advisable. Doing so often leads to situations that the nurse is not prepared to handle.

COMMUNICATION TECHNIQUES

Communication in nursing has the potential to be therapeutic or nontherapeutic. **Therapeutic communication** is the ideal. It consists of an exchange of information that facilitates the formation of a positive nurse–patient relationship and actively involves the patient in all areas of care. In contrast, **nontherapeutic communication** usually blocks the development of a trusting and therapeutic relationship.

Specific communication techniques are used to facilitate the development of therapeutic interaction. Some techniques are verbal, and others are nonverbal. Individual nurses are more or less comfortable with the various techniques, and the LPN/LVN should choose a communication technique that fits the nurse's style and the patient's, and a given situation. The use of therapeutic communication techniques does not guarantee that therapeutic communication will occur. Therapeutic communication requires the nurse to have an awareness of the patient's feelings and the ability to respond to the patient's needs through the use of verbal and nonverbal communication skills (see the Coordinated Care box).

 Coordinated Care

Supervision

Communication Skills

- Nurses who have many years of education and experience continue to develop and improve effective communication skills, particularly cross-cultural communication.
- New and inexperienced unlicensed assistive personnel (UAP) often need guidance to make their communication skills more effective.
- It is a responsibility of the nurse to monitor how effective the UAP are when communicating with patients and ancillary personnel from other departments such as x-ray, laboratory, and dietary departments.
- Two methods to help UAP become better communicators are role modeling effective communication techniques and in-service education programs.

NONVERBAL THERAPEUTIC COMMUNICATION TECHNIQUES

Listening

Listening is an acquired skill that is vital to the nurse-patient relationship. Nurses who have mastered this skill are quiet while the patient is speaking, pay attention to not only the verbal but also the nonverbal communication of the patient, and truly focus on what the patient is saying. One of the most effective methods of therapeutic communication, listening also can be one of the most difficult to master (Table 4.2). It often feels awkward and uncomfortable at first. This nonverbal communication technique is a behavior that conveys interest and caring toward the patient. It is not always the result that counts the most: it is possible to *hear* without *listening*.

Listening is sometimes active and sometimes passive. Active listening requires full attention to what the patient is saying. The nurse hears the message, interprets its meaning, and gives the patient feedback, indicating understanding of the message. The patient has an opportunity to validate that the message was received or not received as intended.

In passive listening, listening to the speaker is indicated either nonverbally through eye contact and nodding, or verbally through encouraging phrases such as "Uh-huh" and "I see" (Balzer Riley, 2021). Although it is not possible for the patient to be sure that the nurse has received or understood the message accurately, passive listening lets the patient know that the nurse is interested and being attentive to what is being said by the patient. The nurse's level of confidence affects the ability to listen attentively. Novice nurses often are "thinking ahead" to the most appropriate response to the patient and, by so doing, miss what the patient really is trying to communicate. As experience and confidence are attained, the LPN/LVN gains the capacity to give full attention to the patient's message, thus allowing for more appropriate intervention.

Silence

Maintaining silence is an extremely effective, yet sometimes difficult, therapeutic communication technique. In American society, silence often feels awkward, which leads to the desire to interrupt silence by making conversation. This impulse does not always allow the people involved in an interaction time to organize their thoughts sufficiently to communicate their needs or response. A person commonly needs several seconds after hearing a verbal message to interpret what has been stated and to formulate the most appropriate response. Unfortunately, the receiver often does not get this amount of time before a response is necessary. In many cases, the sender becomes uncomfortable with the silence and begins speaking again before the receiver has had an opportunity to formulate a response.

The ability to use silence effectively requires skill and timing. Prolonged silence is often difficult to maintain but is vital to an interaction. Silence conveys support, compassion, and caring. Holding the patient's hand or placing one's hand on the shoulder of a patient or loved one when combined with silence conveys caring and concern. An example of effective use of silence is when a patient dies. The nurse can communicate support and compassion by remaining with the family after relaying the news to them. Allowing family members time to express their feelings while remaining silent and using therapeutic touch communicates that the nurse cares about the family without trying to talk away the situation.

In some cases, it is helpful for nurses to let patients know that they do not have to speak and to convey that they are willing to just sit and wait until patients feel ready to respond. However, the nurse's nonverbal cues must be congruent with this willingness to wait. Actions such as fidgeting, writing, and looking at one's watch communicate the opposite message. Therapeutic silence requires practice to master the skill in a way that it becomes easy and natural.

Table **4.2** Therapeutic Communication Techniques: Nonverbal	
NONVERBAL TECHNIQUES	**BENEFITS**
Active listening	Conveys interest and caring; gives patient full attention; allows feedback to verify understanding of the message
Maintaining silence (often used in conjunction with touch)	Allows time to organize thoughts and formulate an appropriate response; often conveys respect, understanding, caring, and support; allows observation of patient's nonverbal responses
Minimal encouragement by nodding occasionally and maintaining eye contact (usually also involves brief verbal comments; e.g., "Yes, go on" or "Then what happened?")	Communicates to the patient that the nurse is interested and wants to hear more
Touch	Often conveys warmth, caring, comfort, support, and understanding
Conveying acceptance (usually also involves a verbal component)	Demonstrates acceptance of patient's rights to current beliefs and practices without condoning them; nonjudgmental, therefore encourages honesty and openness on the part of the patient; provides an opportunity to bring about change in health behaviors while still maintaining the patient's personal integrity

Touch

Touch is another form of nonverbal communication that is inherent in the practice of nursing. Nearly every nursing intervention for the purpose of providing physical care calls for touch. When a nurse provides nursing care, touch is often highly personal or intimate (e.g., giving a bed bath, assisting a patient on or off a bedpan, inserting a urinary catheter). Because of the intimate nature of touch in the nursing context, it must be used with great discretion to fit into sociocultural norms and guidelines. Some nurses are uncomfortable with touch because of a fear of its seeming inappropriate or being misinterpreted. When the nurse is comfortable with physical contact with a patient, touch has the potential for conveying warmth, caring, support, and understanding (Fig. 4.2). For the nurse to convey warmth, the nature of touch must be sincere and genuine. However, if the nurse is not comfortable with touch, or the nurse touches the patient in a manner that communicates hesitancy or reluctance, a very strong negative message, such as rejection, is sent to the patient.

Interpretation of touch depends on several factors, such as the duration and intensity of the contact; the body part touched; the culture, gender, and age of the patient and the nurse; the environment; and the stage of development of the relationship. Depending on the patient's culture, holding the hand of a patient who does not speak English during a difficult procedure may be more effective and comforting than efforts to communicate verbally. A small child who is frightened by the hospital environment often responds better to being cuddled than to a verbal explanation of what is taking place. Older adult patients frequently reach out to touch the person caring for them. Many patients who are sad find a warm embrace to be very comforting. A back rub

Fig. 4.2 Touch has the potential to communicate caring and comfort.

for the patient who is in pain often promotes relaxation and eases the pain. However, because of sociocultural differences, the nurse must always be alert to and aware of the possible variations in interpretation of touch. When used appropriately, touch has powerful potential as a communication technique.

VERBAL THERAPEUTIC COMMUNICATION TECHNIQUES

Conveying Acceptance

Many issues in the nurse–patient relationship are highly personal. Some patients are hesitant to give the nurse complete information, particularly as it relates to values, beliefs, lifestyles, and practices. Often this reluctance has to do with a fear of disapproval from the nurse in regard to the patient's values, beliefs, or practices, or even rejection of the individual as a person.

The nurse's acceptance and willingness to listen and respond to what a patient is saying without passing judgment on the patient is key to the development of a therapeutic nurse–patient relationship. It is likely that, given variances in sociocultural influences (e.g., economic status, religion, upbringing, cultural background, and age), a patient's values, beliefs, and practices will differ from that of the nurse. The nurse must be cognizant of conveying disapproval or communicating disapproval nonverbally through gestures or facial expressions.

Minimal encouragement is a subtle therapeutic technique that communicates to the patient that the nurse is interested and wants to hear more. It indicates acceptance of the patient as a person. It usually involves nonverbal cues, such as maintaining appropriate eye contact, nodding occasionally, and verbal comments such as "Yes, go on" to encourage the patient to continue.

The nurse may be confronted with a patient whose practices are harmful to a healthy lifestyle. Acceptance of the patient and the lifestyle is not synonymous with approving of the lifestyle choices. The challenge for the nurse is to facilitate changes in the patient's health behaviors while helping the patient to maintain personal integrity. Keep in mind that the nurse and the patient have the right to their own beliefs. The nurse can demonstrate acceptance of the patient's right to his or her present beliefs and practices without condoning them. The next step is to communicate a healthier alternative to the present behavior and assist patients in initiating the new behavior if they choose to make these practices a part of their life.

Questioning: Closed

Much of the information gathered by the nurse about a patient comes from questioning the patient directly. The type of information sought determines what type of questioning is most appropriate (Table 4.3). A closed question is focused and seeks a particular answer. For example, when interviewing a newly admitted patient with diabetes, the nurse asks, "What is your insulin

Table 4.3   Therapeutic Communication Techniques: Verbal

VERBAL TECHNIQUES	BENEFITS	EXAMPLES
CLOSED QUESTIONING		
Focused and seeks a particular answer; usually requires and elicits only a "yes" or "no" or one-word to two-word answer	Provides a very specific answer to a very specific question	"How old are you?" "How many children do you have?" "Have you had a tetanus shot in the past 5 years?"
OPEN-ENDED QUESTIONING		
Does not require a specific answer and cannot be answered by "yes," "no," or a one-word response; usually begins with words such as "how," "what," "can you tell me about," "in what way"	Allows the patient to elaborate freely; useful in assessing feelings; elicits the patient's thoughts without influencing the response	"How do you feel about having surgery tomorrow?" "What concerns do you have about going home?" "How are these symptoms different from the last time you were ill?"
RESTATING		
Repeating to the patient what the nurse believes to be the main point that the patient is trying to communicate; tone of voice rises slightly at the end of the phrase as if asking a question	Lets the patient know whether the nurse heard what was said; encourages the patient to offer additional information	*Patient:* "I'm not sure how I will manage the housework when I get home. My husband will expect me to do the cooking and cleaning just like always, and I don't think I'll be able to do it so soon after my surgery." *Nurse:* "Your husband will expect you to do the cooking and cleaning when you get home?" *Patient:* "Yes. I don't think he understands how difficult this surgery has been for me, and how weak and tired I feel."
PARAPHRASING		
Restatement of the patient's message in the nurse's own words	Verifies that the nurse's interpretation of the message is correct	*Patient:* "I wish I was having a general anesthetic instead of a spinal. My neighbor had a relative who had a spinal anesthetic and never walked again." *Nurse:* "You are concerned that you might have complications from the spinal anesthetic?" *Patient:* "I sure am." *Nurse:* "I can have the anesthesiologist come talk to you some more about the risks and benefits of a spinal anesthetic. Would that be helpful?" *Patient:* "Oh, yes. Would you do that, please?"
CLARIFYING		
Seeks to understand the patient's message by asking for more information or for elaboration on a point; expressed as a question or statement followed by a restatement or paraphrasing of part of the patient's message	Allows the patient to verify that the message received is accurate; particularly useful when the message is ambiguous or not easily understood	*Nurse:* "How are you getting along with the new blood pressure medication?" *Patient:* "Well, the doctor told me to take one every day, but they are so darned expensive, I've only been taking them every other day. It seems to be working out okay." *Nurse:* "Let me make sure I understand this correctly. The cost of the medication is keeping you from being able to take it each day?" *Patient:* "Yes, I just can't afford it on my fixed income."

Continued

Table 4.3 Therapeutic Communication Techniques: Verbal—cont'd

VERBAL TECHNIQUES	BENEFITS	EXAMPLES
FOCUSING		
The nurse encourages the patient to select one topic over another as the primary focus of discussion	Allows the nurse to gather more specific information when the patient's message is too vague; focuses on specific data	*Patient:* "Don't let them give me any morphine. The last time they gave me that I almost died!" *Nurse:* "Will you please tell me, as accurately as you can, what you experienced the last time you were given morphine?"
REFLECTING		
Assists the patient to reflect on feelings and thoughts rather than seeking answers and advice from another	Promotes independent decision making; allows the patient to see that her or his ideas and thoughts are important	*Patient:* "Sometimes I think my family is falling apart. All we ever do is fight and argue. My kids don't take responsibility for themselves, much less help out around the house. This makes my husband furious, and we all end up in a shouting match with everyone feeling miserable. What should I do? Sometimes I just feel like walking out." *Nurse:* "What do you think you should do?" *Patient:* "I don't know. I would like for us to go to counseling, but I'm afraid my husband won't hear of it." *Nurse:* "Have you discussed this with him?" *Patient:* "No. I suppose that is where I need to start."
STATING OBSERVATIONS		
The nurse makes observations of the patient during an interaction and communicates these observations back to the patient	Allows for clarification of the intended message when verbal cues do not match nonverbal cues; allows for more accurate interpretation of patient concerns	(Ms. C. denies having any concerns about her upcoming hysterectomy. However, the nurse notes that Ms. C.'s posture and facial expression are tense, her eye contact is brief and darting, and she is fidgeting about in bed. The nurse shares these observations with Ms. C.) *Nurse:* "Ms. C., you seem to understand the information about your surgery that we have discussed, but you still seem to be quite tense and anxious. Can you tell me what is bothering you?" *Patient:* "Well, it's just that my husband and I always wanted to have one more child and now that will never happen. It all seems so final."
OFFERING INFORMATION		
The nurse provides the patient with relevant data and asks for feedback to determine the patient's level of understanding	Useful for patient teaching; promotes informed decision making	Preoperative teaching Diabetes education Discharge instruction
SUMMARIZING		
Concise review of main ideas from a discussion	Focuses on key issues and allows for additional information that was perhaps omitted; particularly useful when interaction has been lengthy or has covered several topics	"We've covered a lot of information in the past few minutes. The main things to keep in mind are _____." (Review the primary topics covered in the interaction.)

dosage in the morning?" A specific question with a specific answer, it is typical of closed questions, which generally require only one or two words in response. This direct type of questioning is useful if this is the type of information desired. However, if the LPN/LVN wants the patient to give more details on a subject, an open-ended question is a more effective communication technique.

Questioning: Open-Ended

Open-ended questions do not require a specific response and allow the patient to elaborate freely on a subject when replying. This type of question is useful in assessing the patient's feelings. Consider the different responses possible for a patient who is asked the following questions:

Closed: "Mr. A., are you worried about your scheduled surgery?"

Open-ended: "How you are feeling about having surgery tomorrow, Mr. A.?"

The closed question requires only a yes or no answer and probably elicits a very short response. The open-ended question invites Mr. A. to elaborate in whatever direction he chooses with regard to his feelings about having surgery. Given the opportunity to explore his feelings, Mr. A. may reveal information about other aspects of his life or questions and concerns he may have regarding his upcoming surgery. Open-ended questions also convey the message that the nurse is interested in the patient as an individual, not just in obtaining information.

Restating

When using the technique of restating, the nurse repeats to the patient what is believed to be the main point that the patient is trying to convey. It is another way of letting the patient know that the nurse is listening. Simply by repeating the central theme of the patient's comments, the nurse encourages the patient to provide more information. If the nurse also slightly raises the tone of his or her voice at the end of the restatement, the patient probably will take this as a signal that the nurse is interested in hearing more information.

Restating often feels awkward to the nurse who is not experienced in using this technique. Avoid overuse of this technique, because this sounds as though you are "parroting" what the patient is saying. Parroting can sound like a planned response and often is annoying to the patient. When used selectively, restating is a valuable technique to encourage the patient to offer helpful information.

Paraphrasing

Although paraphrasing bears some similarity to restating, it differs in intent. Paraphrasing is the restatement of the patient's message in the nurse's own words in an attempt to verify that the nurse has interpreted the patient's message correctly.

Clarifying

Clarifying takes restating and paraphrasing a step further and is useful when the patient's message is incomplete or confusing or does not go deeply enough into the area being explored. When clarifying, the LPN/LVN suggests to the patient some of his or her own ideas about what the patient is trying to communicate in a manner that asks the patient to verify that the nurse's understanding of the message is accurate. Clarifying prevents misinterpretation of the patient's comments.

Focusing

The technique of focusing also is used when more specific information is needed to understand the patient's message accurately. The patient may be providing the nurse with important information, but if the message is too vague or strays from the topic being discussed, it is difficult for the nurse to identify the actual message.

Reflecting

Reflecting is like restating, but it involves feelings and thoughts more than facts. This therapeutic technique is used to assist patients to explore their own feelings, often about a choice that lies before them, rather than seeking answers or advice from someone else, such as the nurse. The nurse allows for the expression of the patient's feelings but, rather than offering advice, reflects the thoughts back to the patient. This empowers the patient to verbalize a possible solution and at the same time places the patient in a position of control and promotes self-esteem and autonomy.

Reflecting allows patients to see that their ideas and thoughts are important and have worth. Patients gain confidence in their own decision making instead of feeling the need to rely on others for decision making.

Stating Observations

While interacting with a patient, the nurse also is observing the patient. Communicating the nurse's observations to the patient is called *stating observations* and is often useful in validating the accuracy of observations. This technique can be especially helpful when the patient's verbal message does not seem to match the nonverbal behaviors witnessed by the nurse. With description of the patient's observed behavior, feedback is provided, and the patient is invited to verify that the message received was the one the patient intended to send. Clarification of the confusion between verbal and nonverbal cues allows the nurse to address the patient's concerns more effectively.

Offering Information

Much of the communicating that the nurse does takes the form of *offering information*. Preparing a patient for what to expect before, during, and after an invasive diagnostic procedure is one example of how the nurse uses this communication technique. Discharge teaching to prepare the patient for self-care at home is another example. The nurse should use the patient's feedback to determine whether the information given has been understood. Offering information is not the same as giving advice. Giving advice takes decision making away from the patient and puts the nurse-patient relationship at risk.

Summarizing

Summarizing means providing a review of the main points covered in an interaction. This technique is used most often after a lengthy interaction or one that has covered several issues (e.g., at the end of a patient teaching session). It helps the patient to separate the essential information from the "nice to know" information and gives a sense of closure to the session.

Use of Humor

The power of humor during interactions with patients should not be underestimated as an effective communication tool. Yoshikawa and Ohmaki (2019) found that laughter therapy reduces systolic blood pressure, heart rate, and raises serum serotonin levels. Study participants also reported less pain. From a psychological standpoint the study showed less depression and anxiety feelings as a result of laughter, as well as increased desire for social interaction (Fig. 4.3).

Humor can help put the nurse and the patient at ease. However, it is important for the nurse to know when humor is appropriate and when it is inappropriate. It is never appropriate to laugh *at* a patient; it is only appropriate to laugh *with* a patient. The timing and context of humor are also important. In some serious situations, humor is not appropriate, such as when a patient has just received a serious diagnosis or when a patient is trying to convey thoughts or feelings. In general, get to know the patient before using humor. Correct perception of the patient and situation allows you to take cues from the patient or the patient's significant others to predict how the patient

Fig. 4.3 Help reduce stress and support a therapeutic relationship by sharing a joke or laughing with patients.

may respond to humor. In some situations, remember to be especially cautious with the use of humor (e.g., when the patient is from a different culture or background or is confused or cognitively impaired). Another pitfall to watch out for is use of humor to avoid confronting or dealing with issues. Rather than allowing yourself or the patient to resort to humor to mask fears and other difficult emotions, try to find a more appropriate technique that helps the patient communicate effectively. Humor is certainly effective and therapeutic in some situations, but it becomes a hindrance, and potentially destructive, if it is the only tool used by the nurse.

FACTORS THAT AFFECT COMMUNICATION

POSTURING AND POSITIONING

Where and how the nurse sits or stands conveys a message to the patient. Standing at the bedside while the patient lies in the bed sends the message that the LPN/LVN has power and the patient does not. The crossing of arms over the chest may convey a lack of openness to the patient. Assuming a position of total relaxation, such as leaning back into the chair, possibly even slouching, sends a message of disinterest.

The most therapeutic posture and positioning is the same position and level as the patient, or as close to it as feasible. For example, if the patient is lying in bed, the nurse should sit on a chair at the bedside facing the patient during a conversation. In addition, the head of the bed should be elevated, unless contraindicated, so that the patient is at the same level as the nurse. Sitting in a comfortable position and leaning slightly forward toward the patient convey a message of interest and openness.

SPACE AND TERRITORIALITY

Generally, Western cultures recognize four zones of personal space. From the face to about 18 inches away is the *intimate space*. Because of the nature of many nursing interventions, the LPN/LVN must enter the patient's personal space. Bathing, inserting urethral catheters, and changing dressings are just a few examples. Entering this space can cause uneasiness for the nurse and the patient. Approaching these interventions in a professional manner can help alleviate much of the uneasiness felt by the nurse and patient (Fig. 4.4). The *personal space* comprises the area from 18 inches to 4 feet away from a person. Sitting and talking with a patient is an example of an interaction in the personal space. This area tends to be a comfortable space for most people during an interaction such as that between a nurse and patient. The *social space* is 4 to 12 ft from a person. An example of a social space is a nurse conducting a diabetes class for a group of patients. Beyond 12 ft to approximately 25 ft from a person is considered *public space* (Krauss Whitbourne, 2012) Factors such as the patient's culture, individual

Fig. 4.4 Much of the nursing care provided to a patient occurs in the intimate space.

preferences, and the situation determine the level of comfort with the various types of space. The nurse should be especially aware of the patient's nonverbal communication when interacting with the patient in these zones of personal space.

ENVIRONMENT

The general environment surrounding an interaction often has a significant impact on the interaction's effectiveness. A therapeutic interaction between the nurse and the patient is extremely difficult if a lot of commotion is occurring in the room. Key elements for a successful interaction are a calm, relaxed atmosphere and privacy. Ideally, the initial interaction should take place in a private room with the door closed. However, this degree of privacy is not always possible. If the patient has a roommate, taking the patient to a private conference room is sometimes a good option, depending on the status of the patient and the nature of the interaction. At the very least, the privacy curtain should be pulled between the two patients during interaction with a patient.

LEVEL OF TRUST

A trusting relationship is essential to an effective nurse-patient interaction. Without trust, interaction does not progress past superficial social interaction. The nurse first must gain the patient's trust before expecting to have a meaningful or therapeutic interaction. One way for the LPN/LVN to build trust is by demonstrating confidence and competence. A trusting relationship is often difficult to establish with a patient who has had

negative encounters with other health care providers. The LPN/LVN should be sensitive to the patient's previous experiences and demonstrate a sincere effort to make the current situation a positive experience for the patient.

LANGUAGE BARRIERS

In today's culturally diverse society, care of a patient who speaks a different language is not unusual. Language barriers can pose a major threat to effective communication and development of a therapeutic nurse–patient relationship. Some larger hospitals or hospitals where the community has a very diverse population often have a translator on staff or one who is easily accessible. If the LPN/LVN is employed in a health care facility that does not have a translator available, the nurse should use all available means (e.g., social services) to find one. If an interpreter cannot be located, the nurse may rely on the patient's family members or friends to assist with communication if they speak the same language as the nurse. The nurse should be very cautious that misinterpretation does not occur with use of family members as interpreters and should avoid use of younger children as the interpreter. Keeping messages simple and avoiding the use of medical terminology can help in preventing misinterpretations. Use of gestures and pictures also may be helpful in communicating with the patient. The LPN/LVN also must comply with Health Insurance Portability and Accountability Act of 1996 (HIPAA) regulations and guidelines when using a family member or friend as an interpreter.

Some health care institutions may have resources such as translation dictionaries in the languages most common to its geographic location available, or the nurse may use an online resource (Boxes 4.2 and 4.3). Use these resources with caution. There is a high risk of mispronouncing words or using incorrect words, and doing so can convey unintended or inaccurate messages. Consider information concerning barriers in language and communication that may exist between subcultures of a group, including the use of slang terms.

CULTURE

Nursing is concerned with holistic care of the patient. Culture is a significant component of a patient's psychosocial well-being. The nurse must attempt to seek specific information regarding cultural practices and beliefs of the patients being cared for, especially when the patient is from a culture different from that of the nurse. The effect of culture on communication is immense, and a complete discussion is beyond the scope of this chapter. Julia Balzer Riley (2021) offers useful guidelines when relating to patients of different cultures (see the Cultural Considerations box). For more complete information, refer to Chapter 6.

Cultural Considerations

Communicating With Patients of Different Cultures From Your Own

DOMINANT LANGUAGE AND DIALECTS
- Identify the dominant language of the group.
- Identify dialects that have the potential to interfere with communication.
- Explore contextual speech patterns of the group. What is the usual volume and tone of speech?

CULTURAL COMMUNICATION PATTERNS
- Explore the willingness of individuals to share thoughts, feelings, and ideas.
- Explore the practice and meaning of touch in the given society: within the family, among friends, with strangers, with members of the same gender, with members of the opposite gender, and with health care providers.
- Identify typical personal spatial and distancing characteristics during one-to-one communication. Explore how distancing changes with friends compared with strangers.
- Explore the use of eye contact within the group. Does avoidance of eye contact have special meaning? How does eye contact vary among family, friends, and strangers? Do eye contact practices change when communication occurs between members of different socioeconomic groups?
- Explore the meaning of various facial expressions. Do specific facial expressions have special meanings? Do people tend to smile a lot? How are emotions displayed or not displayed in facial expressions?
- Are there acceptable ways of standing and greeting outsiders?

ATTITUDES TOWARD TIME
- Explore attitudes in the group toward time. Are individuals oriented primarily to the past, present, or future? How do individuals see the context of past, present, and future?
- Identify differences in the interpretation of social time versus clock time.
- Explore how time factors are interpreted by the group. Are individuals expected to be punctual in arrival to jobs, appointments, and social engagements?

FORMAT FOR NAMES
- Explore the format for personal names.
- How does the individual expect to be greeted by strangers and health care practitioners?

From Balzer Riley J: Communication in nursing, ed 9, St. Louis, 2021, Mosby.

AGE AND GENDER

The effects of *age* and *gender* on communication are influenced strongly by cultural or societal beliefs and attitudes. A significant age difference between the nurse and the patient does, in some cases, raise a barrier to communication. Nurses who have had limited interaction with children may find it difficult to communicate effectively with children in the health care setting. Teenagers also may present a unique challenge when

---

Box 4.2   Guidelines for Communicating With Patients Who Are Partially Fluent in English

- Ask for feedback. Provide the patient with paper and pencil.
- Assess the patient's nonverbal and verbal communication.
- Avoid using medical terms.
- Remain at eye level with the patient. Assess whether the patient is comfortable with eye contact.
- Remember that patients usually understand more than they can express. They need time to process the discussion and to determine what they want to respond.
- Remember that stress interferes with the patient's ability to think and speak in English.
- Speak slowly and never loudly (unless the patient has a hearing impairment).
- Use pictures when possible.

Modified from Balzer Riley J: Communication in nursing, ed 8, St. Louis, 2021, Mosby.

Box 4.3   Guidelines for Communicating With Non–English-Speaking Patients

If an interpreter is available:
- Address questions to the patient, not the interpreter.
- Avoid using children and relatives as interpreters.
- Be aware that more time will be needed for interactions to allow for translation and interpretation.
- Give the patient and interpreter time alone together.
- Select same-age and same-gender interpreters if possible.
- Use dialect-specific interpreters, not translators.

If an interpreter is *not* available:
- Be aware of the patient's nonverbal communication. This helps in determining if the translation is accurate of the patient's feelings.
- Determine whether there is a third language that you and the patient speak. In many cultures, it is common for patients to speak several languages.
- Pantomime simple words and actions to help the patient understand the desired message.
- Talk with your facility's administration about the importance of using trained medical interpreters when caring for the non–English-speaking patient.
- Until medical interpreters are available, use formal and informal networking to locate a suitable interpreter.
- Use a translator.
- Use picture boards.

Modified from Balzer Riley J: Communication in nursing, ed 8, St. Louis, 2021, Mosby.

communicating with nurses. Their vocabulary and expressions are often unique to their age group and include the use of slang terms. At the other end of the spectrum, the nurse may encounter an older adult who does not have confidence in a very young nurse or has some physiologic or cognitive impairment that hampers effective communication. Communication is most effective if the nurse tries to understand as much about patients across the lifespan as possible and selects the most appropriate communication techniques for a variety of circumstances.

When communicating with older adults who may have communication barriers because of hearing loss or cognitive barriers, consider ways to improve communication. Speaking directly to patients by getting their attention and facing them enhances the interaction. If the patient wears a hearing aid, be sure it is in place and in working order. Eliminate background noise when speaking with the patient and do not shout at the patient. Also give the patient time to process what has been said and allow ample time for the patient to respond. Last, do not talk to the patient as a child, or in a simplified and slow manner, with terms of endearment such as "honey" or "sweetie," commonly referred to as "elder speak."

Male and female patterns of communication often are related closely to cultural, familial, and lifestyle patterns developed over a lifetime. The beliefs, values, and attitudes that an individual or a society in general holds regarding male or female status and expectations are likely to affect how messages are sent and received (Balzer Riley, 2021).

PHYSIOLOGIC FACTORS

Many physiologic factors may interfere with the patient being able to communicate effectively. *Pain* is a common example. While a patient is experiencing pain, all available energy is focused on coping with the pain; it is difficult, if not impossible, for the patient to communicate about anything except the pain. The LPN/LVN first should address the patient's pain before trying to communicate with the patient, especially before performing any patient teaching.

Altered cognition is another physiologic factor that frequently hinders effective communication. If the patient lacks the cognitive ability to receive, process, and send information, communication is disrupted. Several factors have the potential to affect a patient's cognitive ability. A cerebrovascular accident (stroke), sedative effects of medication, dementia, and developmental delays are examples of such factors.

Careful assessment of a patient's level of cognitive function is important when beginning any interaction. The nurse should assist with keeping the patient's sensory abilities operating at their maximum potential. For example, if the patient wears glasses or a hearing aid, the nurse should ensure these assistive devices are in place to help the patient process information accurately. If there is decreased ability to comprehend, the environment should be kept quiet during communicating. Box 4.4 lists strategies for communicating with patients who are cognitively impaired.

Box 4.4   **Communicating With Patients Who Are Cognitively Impaired**

- Do not rush patients to respond to questions. Allow the patient time to think before they respond.
- Avoid asking more than one question at a time.
- Actively listen to the patient when they are speaking.
- Be sure the patient is focusing on you when speaking to them.
- If necessary, use a communication board or cards to help the patient express themself.
- Ensure that distractions are limited when speaking to the patient.
- Use short sentences that convey important points.

Box 4.5   **Communicating With Patients Who Have Hearing Impairment**

- Be sure to get the patient's attention when entering the room before you begin speaking.
- Ensure the patient is wearing hearing aids and/or glasses if he or she has them.
- Ensure the patient can see your lips because many lip-read.
- Face the patient.
- If the patient hears better from one ear, stand nearer to that ear when speaking.
- Reduce environmental noise, such as the television or radio.
- Rephrase comments rather than repeating if the patient continues to have difficulty understanding.
- Speak at a normal volume rather than shouting.
- Try to lower the tone of your voice. Hard-of-hearing individuals usually have difficulty with high-pitched sounds and voices.
- Use sign language or provide a sign language interpreter if needed.

Impaired hearing is another common physiologic factor that impedes communication. Hearing impairment may lead to misinterpretation of messages and frustration for the sender and the receiver. The LPN/LVN should be sure that all efforts are made to ensure that effective communication is not sacrificed because of a patient's impaired hearing. See Box 4.5 for strategies for communicating with the patient with a hearing impairment.

PSYCHOSOCIAL FACTORS

A multitude of factors place patients under stress. The patient may be frightened, in pain, deprived of sleep, nauseated, or experiencing a host of other unpleasant circumstances. Stress can lead to problems with communication between the patient and the nurse. While experiencing increased stress, the patient may respond with anger, impatience, or even withdrawal. Realize that these behaviors are not directed at you personally but are coping mechanisms used by the patient.

When the patient is experiencing stress, especially extreme stress, you may need to modify communication methods. Keep information simple, basic, and concrete and offer only essential information. Let the patient direct the conversation. Being supportive of the patient aids in keeping the lines of communication open and effective.

An illness often is accompanied by some degree of *grieving* as a result of actual or perceived loss. This loss can take many possible forms, including role or lifestyle change, physical change, altered function, terminal prognosis, and anticipated or actual loss of a loved one.

Nurses often feel uncomfortable interacting with a grieving patient for fear of not knowing what to say or saying the wrong thing. Because of this uneasiness, nurses may sometimes say nothing or avoid the subject entirely. The challenge for the LPN/LVN in dealing with patients and their loved ones who are grieving is to attempt communication with them despite any feelings of personal inadequacy. A silent presence is often all that is necessary. The grieving process may be facilitated by using therapeutic touch, displaying warm and caring behaviors, listening, and using open-ended statements to assist those who are grieving to understand their own feelings and behaviors.

BLOCKS TO COMMUNICATION

Just as therapeutic techniques enhance the quality of an interaction, barriers to communication block its effectiveness. The list of possible responses that block communication is extensive. The most common are presented in Table 4.4.

Table 4.4 Responses That Block Communication

CATEGORY OF RESPONSE	EXPLANATION OF CATEGORIES	EXAMPLES	OUTCOME
False reassurance	Using falsely comforting phrases in an attempt to offer reassurance	"It will be okay." "Don't worry. Everything will be just fine." "You'll be fine."	You promise something that will not occur or is unrealistic
Giving advice or personal opinions	Making a decision for a patient; offering personal opinions; telling a patient what to do with phrases such as "should do," "ought to"	"If I were you I would …" "I think you should …" "Why don't you …"	Takes decision making away from the patient; impairs decision making; creates doubt; encourages blaming the nurse if decision has unwanted outcome
False assumptions	Making an assumption without validation; jumping to conclusions	"It seems like you don't care to learn about your diagnosis." "Your husband isn't very supportive." "You aren't really trying."	Easily leads to a wrong conclusion; often viewed as accusatory or argumentative
Approval or disapproval	Trying to impose the nurse's own attitudes, values, beliefs, and moral standards on a patient about what is right and wrong	"I don't agree with your decision to not try this treatment option!" "Having cosmetic surgery seems like a waste of money." "You shouldn't even think that." "He really is a good doctor."	Easily leads the patient to doubt personal values; creates feelings of guilt and resentment; causes friction between you and the patient
Automatic responses	Stereotyped or superficial comments that do not focus on what the patient is feeling or trying to say	"You can't win them all." "Isn't that nice?" "I don't make the rules; I just follow them." "The doctor knows best."	Tends to belittle the individual's feelings and minimize the importance of the message; communicates the message that you are not taking the patient's concerns seriously
Defensiveness	Responding negatively to criticism; often in response to feelings of anger or hurt on your part; usually involves making excuses	"I'm doing the best I can." "We are never short-staffed." "You must have misunderstood what I said."	Implies that the patient has no right to an opinion; results in ignoring or minimizing the patient's concerns; displays defensive behavior

Table 4.4 Responses That Block Communication—cont'd

CATEGORY OF RESPONSE	EXPLANATION OF CATEGORIES	EXAMPLES	OUTCOME
Arguing	Challenging or arguing against the patient's statements or perceptions	"How can you say you didn't sleep all night? You were sleeping every time I came into your room." "How could your pain level be so high? You were just talking and laughing with your visitor."	Denies that the patient's perceptions are real and valid; implies that the patient is not being truthful, is misinformed, or uneducated
Asking for explanations	Asks the patient to explain her or his actions, beliefs, or feelings with "why" questions	"Why aren't you following the directions your primary care provider gave you?" "Why do you feel that way?" "Why didn't you go to the doctor sooner?"	Frequently viewed by the patient as accusatory; puts patient on the defensive; risks causing resentment, insecurity, and mistrust of the nurse
Changing the subject	Inappropriately focusing the discussion on something other than the patient's concern	"We'll worry about that later. It's time for you to go to physical therapy." "Let's talk about something happier. Talking about your cancer diagnosis is making you too sad."	Rude and shows lack of empathy; blocks further communication, and sometimes makes patient feel uncomfortable about expressing feelings; interrupts thoughts, and often inhibits the sharing of important information

Modified from Potter PA, Perry AG: *Fundamentals of nursing,* ed 9, St. Louis, 2016, Mosby; Arnold E, Boggs KU: *Interpersonal relationships: Professional communication skills for nurses,* ed 7, Philadelphia, 2016, Saunders.

❖ NURSING PROCESS

When a patient experiences difficulty with verbally communicating, the care plan is geared toward assisting the patient with communicating by other means. With input from the patient, significant others, and members of the intraprofessional health care team, the nurse determines which methods of communication will best work for each individual patient.

◆ ASSESSMENT

Any of the factors that affect communication discussed previously in this chapter potentially are related to difficulty with verbally communicating. Factors that indicate difficulty with verbally communicating include the patient's inability to produce words (either by complete aphasia or expressive aphasia), lack of nonverbal communication, struggle with speech pattern, and being disoriented to person, place, or time.

◆ PATIENT PROBLEM

If one or more of certain patient factors are present, the patient problem of *Compromised Verbal Communication* may be indicated. For example, a patient with an endotracheal tube in place to relieve respiratory distress that occurred after a traumatic chest injury will have this patient problem. The presence of the endotracheal tube renders him unable to speak. The loss of speech hampers his abilities to express his needs and supports the identification of the patient problem of difficulty with verbally communicating.

◆ SETTING PATIENT GOALS AND PLANNING

The goal for any patient experiencing difficulty with verbally communicating is that the patient will be able to communicate effectively with others in the environment by sending and receiving clear, concise, and understandable messages. The patient goals must be specific and realistic for the patient and address the patient's needs and concerns. In general, the desired patient goals include:

- The patient will use effective communication techniques.
- The patient will use alternative methods to communicate.
- The patient's verbal communication will match nonverbal communication.

◆ IMPLEMENTATION

Nursing interventions appropriate to the patient difficulty with verbally communicating depend on the type of communication problem that exists and the factors contributing to the problem. Thus nursing interventions may vary greatly from one patient to another. See Box 4.6 for examples of helpful nursing interventions related to specific types of difficulty with communication.

| Box 4.6 | Nursing Interventions for Patients Experiencing Difficulty Verbally Communicating |

1. Determine language spoken; obtain language dictionary or interpreter if possible and accepted by the patient.
2. Listen carefully. Validate verbal and nonverbal expression, particularly when dealing with pain.
3. Anticipate patient's needs until effective communication is possible.
4. Use simple communication; speak in a well-modulated voice, smile, and show concern for the patient.
5. Maintain eye contact at patient's level if culturally appropriate.
6. Use touch as appropriate and if culturally appropriate. Holding a patient's hand or stroking the arm is a simple, unobtrusive way of showing empathy and concern.
7. Spend time with the patient, allow time for responses, and make the call light readily available.
8. Explain all health care procedures.
9. Determine the patient's literacy status.
10. Obtain communication equipment such as electronic devices, paper and pen, letter boards, picture boards, and magic slates as indicated.
11. With an individualized approach, establish an alternative method of communication, such as writing or pointing to letters, words, phrases, picture cards, or simple drawings of basic needs.
12. If there is a comprehension deficit, keep environment quiet when communicating and get the patient's attention before attempting to communicate (e.g., touch patient's shoulder, call patient's name).
13. Give praise for progress noted. Ignore mistakes and watch for frustration or fatigue.
14. Never raise your voice or shout at a patient.
15. Be persistent in deciphering what the patient is saying, and do not pretend to understand when the message is unclear.

Modified from Ackley BJ, Ladwig GB: Nursing diagnosis handbook: An evidence-based guide to planning care, ed 12, St. Louis, 2020, Mosby.

◆ EVALUATION

The nurse evaluates the effectiveness of communication based on the patient's ability to meet the established goals. A good way to accomplish this is by observing the patient's response to an interaction and considering what kind of message is received from the patient's verbal and nonverbal communication. Does the patient appear to have received the message, and is the patient satisfied with it? If the patient goals have been achieved but the impairment is ongoing, continue with the current plan of care. If the impairment no longer exists, on the other hand, consider the patient problem to be resolved. If the goals have not been met, reexamine the phases of the nursing process to determine what revisions are necessary.

COMMUNICATION IN SPECIAL SITUATIONS

The communication techniques discussed thus far are generally applicable to any type of nurse–patient interaction. Some patients have unique communication needs. Three examples of such situations follow.

PATIENTS WITH VENTILATOR DEPENDENCE

Patients who receive mechanical ventilation via endotracheal tube or tracheostomy experience an inability to speak because the trachea is obstructed by the tube. Patients often find this inability to speak devastating, and it often disrupts their sense of well-being and control. When the patient is unable to produce sound, it is essential to identify and implement *alternative methods of communication*.

To determine which communication method is most appropriate, the nurse should carefully assess the patient's ability (e.g., cognitive level, literacy, visual acuity, consciousness level, primary language, gross motor skills, and fine motor skills) to use a particular alternative. One valuable tool is a *communication board*. Depending on the patient's literacy, a communication board includes the alphabet, commonly used phrases, pictures, or a combination of all three. If able to point, the patient points to pictures or phrases on the board to communicate a need or thought. If the desired picture or phrase is not on the board, the patient points to the letters that spell out the message. This method is not feasible for the patient who does not read or cannot see well enough to select from the board.

If the patient is unable to move well enough to point, alternative selection methods are necessary. Possibilities include setting up a "signal" system, such as one eye blink for "yes" and two blinks for "no." The receiver (e.g., the nurse or a family member) systematically points to items or letters on the board, and the patient "signals" when the correct item is selected. This is a slow and rather cumbersome process for communicating and requires patience of the patient and the receiver of the message. In many cases, it is also very tiring for the patient. Nevertheless, it has the potential to be a helpful tool when no other means of communicating is available or feasible. Box 4.7 lists additional alternative methods of communication to use with the patient who is unable to speak.

PATIENTS WITH APHASIA

Aphasia is a deficient or absent language function that results from ischemic insult to the brain, such as stroke (cerebrovascular accident), brain trauma, or anoxia. Some patients experience **expressive aphasia**, in which they are unable to *send* the desired verbal message; and some suffer **receptive aphasia**, or an inability to recognize or interpret the verbal message being *received*. Communication methods recommended for the patient with aphasia are summarized in Box 4.8.

Box 4.7	Alternative Methods of Communicating With Patients Who Are Unable to Speak

- *Clock face communicator:* Messages placed at intervals around the clock face; clock hand scans the messages, and the patient presses a button to stop the hand on the desired message.
- *Computer-assisted communication:* Patient uses keyboard to type messages.
- *Eye blinks:* Predetermined system in which the number of times a patient blinks in response to a question indicates yes or no answer.
- *Lip-reading:* Patient mouths words to be interpreted by the receiver.
- *Magnetic boards with plastic letters:* Patient moves letters around on board to spell words or phrases.
- *Paper and pencil or magic slate:* Patient writes messages to communicate needs.
- *Picture board:* Patient points to pictures on a board or poster of typical patient needs.
- *Sign language:* Hand and finger signals used to indicate letters; used throughout the world for hearing-impaired patients.
- *Word or picture cards:* 3 × 5 cards with words or pictures on them; patient picks appropriate card or sorts cards into short phrases or sentences.

Box 4.8	Communicating With Patients With Aphasia

- Avoid patronizing and childish phrases.
- Collaborate with a speech pathologist.
- Do not shout or speak loudly (hearing loss is not the problem).
- Encourage patients to speak as much as possible when they are able and ready, not to provide just yes or no answers.
- Give the patient time to understand; be calm and patient; do not pressure or tire the patient.
- If the patient has expressive aphasia, ask questions that require simple yes or no answers or blinking of the eyes. Offer pictures or a communication board to which the patient can point.
- If the patient has problems with comprehension, use simple, short questions and facial gestures to give additional clues.
- Listen to the patient, and wait for the patient to communicate.
- Speak of things familiar and of interest to the patient.
- Use communication aids (see Box 4.7).

Modified from Potter PA, Perry AG: Fundamentals of nursing, ed 10, St. Louis, 2021, Mosby.

UNRESPONSIVE PATIENTS

It is not certain whether, or how much, the unresponsive patient is able to hear or interpret verbal stimuli. Some patients, after regaining consciousness, have reported hearing actual statements that were made in the room while the patient was still in an unconscious state. Because of this, anyone interacting with the unresponsive patient must assume that all sound and verbal stimuli may be heard by the patient. Caution people nearby about making negative or anxiety-producing statements. Encourage health care providers and family and friends to speak to the unresponsive individual as if he or she were awake. This sometimes feels awkward, and family members and friends often need support and encouragement to talk with the patient as they would have before the illness or accident. Talking about daily activities and reading books, cards, and newspapers is beneficial. Also, always explain to the patient any procedure or activity that involves the patient. Remember not to have conversations with other health care providers about topics that do not place the patient at the center of the discussion or that may cause stress or anxiety if the patient were to hear it.

CONCLUSION

No interaction takes place that does not involve communication. Every time the LPN/LVN interacts with a patient, there is opportunity for a positive or negative outcome. By becoming familiar with therapeutic communication techniques and practicing them to become proficient in their use, the nurse can promote a helping relationship with the patient. By also being aware of factors that affect communication and of blocks to communication, the LPN/LVN succeeds in preventing interactions that may negatively affect the patient's self-esteem and sense of worth.

Get Ready for the NCLEX® Examination!

Key Points

- All interactions result in the occurrence of some form of communication.
- Communication is verbal and nonverbal.
- Nonverbal communication is very powerful.
- The manner, or style, in which a message is communicated greatly influences the mood and the overall outcome of an interaction.
- Communication in nursing should be therapeutic.
- Trust is essential to effective nurse–patient interaction.
- Active listening is one of the most effective methods of therapeutic communication.
- Touch is a form of nonverbal communication that is inherent to the practice of nursing.
- Humor is potentially a powerful tool in promoting the well-being of an individual.
- Numerous factors affect communication.
- Impaired verbal communication requires alternative methods for communicating effectively.

Additional Learning Resources

SG Go to your Study Guide for additional learning activities to help you master this chapter content.

Be sure to visit the Evolve site at http://evolve.elsevier.com/Cooper/foundations/ for additional online resources.

Review Questions for the NCLEX® Examination

1. The patient is fearful concerning his upcoming surgery. Which statement by the nurse is most therapeutic?
   1. "Sometimes anxiety is not easy to deal with. Can you tell me what is bothering you the most about your upcoming surgery?"
   2. "Don't worry. Everyone has some anxiety about having surgery."
   3. "Just try to think about the positive results from the surgery. You'll recover quickly."
   4. "I had surgery once, and it still scares me to think about it, so I know how you feel."

2. During an admission interview, the patient refers several times to "all the problems I had last time I was in the hospital." What is the most appropriate communication technique for the nurse to use in this situation?
   1. Reflection
   2. Paraphrasing
   3. Minimal encouragement
   4. Focusing

3. The patient states, "I'm so nervous about being hospitalized." Which statement is the nurse's best response to get the patient to elaborate?
   1. "It's normal to be nervous, but we'll take good care of you."
   2. "You're feeling especially nervous?"
   3. "How many times have you been hospitalized?"
   4. "Nurses will be here all the time to check on you."

4. The nurse is talking with the patient about her husband's death 2 years ago. Tears form in the patient's eyes, and she stops talking. What is the most appropriate therapeutic response by the nurse?
   1. Change the subject to something less difficult for the patient.
   2. Remain silent and hold the patient's hand.
   3. Leave the room to provide privacy.
   4. Pretend not to notice the tears and continue the conversation.

5. Which question is an example of clarification? (*Select all that apply.*)
   1. "You will take your medicine now, won't you?"
   2. "Does this headache have anything in common with your previous headaches?"
   3. "In other words, you feel that your stomach aches are associated with stress at work?"
   4. "What do you mean by that?"
   5. "Do I understand you correctly that you are saying that you don't understand why the doctor prescribed this medication for you?"

6. A newly admitted patient speaks almost no English. The patient has a fever of 102.6 and is suspected of having a urinary tract infection. The nurse needs to obtain from the patient a urine specimen for culture and sensitivity. An interpreter is not readily available. What is the best nursing action to assist in obtaining the specimen?
   1. Speak very slowly and distinctly.
   2. Show the patient the equipment and illustrations of the process.
   3. Obtain a physician's order to catheterize the patient to collect the specimen.
   4. Delay the collection of the specimen until an interpreter can be found.

7. Abdominal surgery has revealed that the patient, a young mother, has advanced metastatic colon cancer. While the nurse is changing her dressing, the patient begins to cry and states, "If I had just gone to the doctor sooner, my kids wouldn't have to grow up without a mother." **For each response by the nurse use an X to identify if the response is therapeutic (promotes communication) or non-therapeutic (blocks communication).**

Assessment Finding	Therapeutic	Non-Therapeutic
"It's natural to blame yourself in a situation like this."		
"Is there someone that will be able to care for the children?"		
"Don't give up. The chemotherapy and radiation therapy may prove to be effective."		

"I hear you saying that you feel that if you had been diagnosed earlier, the outcome may have been different?"

"Thinking negative like that is not going to help anyone."

"Tell me more about how you are feeling."

8. During his admission interview, an older patient states, "I can't hear you very well." After determining that the patient does not have a hearing aid, which action assists with communicating with this patient? (*Select all that apply.*)

   1. Speak in a higher-pitched voice.
   2. Speak loudly into his "good" ear.
   3. Exaggerate lip movement while speaking.
   4. Face the patient and speak slowly and distinctly.
   5. Be sure to get the patient's attention before speaking.

9. Which statement by the student nurse is an example of assertive communication? (*Select all that apply.*)

   1. "It's time for your morning care. Do you prefer to use the shower chair, or do you think you are strong enough to stand during your shower today?"
   2. "I'd like you to take your shower now, but if you'd rather do it later, I guess that would be okay."
   3. "It would be best if we completed your morning care now, but since you want to wait until tonight, I'll ask my instructor if that would be okay."
   4. "I'm sure you'll feel better after you have your morning care. Will you please take your shower now?"
   5. "Since you will be going to physical therapy soon, it's important we get your morning care completed. Do you want to take a sponge bath or a shower?"

10. The patient has a long history of smoking and has just been diagnosed with lung cancer. He states to the nurse, "There's no point in trying to stop smoking now. I might as well enjoy the time I have left." Which is the best response by the nurse?

    1. "You're probably right. It won't do much good to stop smoking now."
    2. "You feel that there is no reason to stop smoking now?"
    3. "It's never too late to stop smoking."
    4. "I know it's hard, but if you stop smoking now, your condition might improve."

11. The patient tells the nurse that he is frightened about having cancer. Which response by the nurse is most effective in getting the patient to vent his concerns?

    1. "Fear is a common reaction to having cancer."
    2. "Tell me more about being frightened by having cancer."
    3. "Have you told your wife you are afraid?"
    4. "Would you like me to call the chaplain to visit with you?"

12. The nurse is admitting a patient with long-standing type 1 diabetes. The nurse knows that a closed question will best ascertain the number of units of insulin the patient usually takes. **Choose the *most likely* options for the information missing from the statements below by selecting from the list of options provided.** What is the number of _____ of _____ that you take in order to keep your _____ under control?

OPTIONS
Elevated
Cholesterol
Units
Blood glucose
Blood pressure
Insulin
Grams
Weight
Bilirubin

13. The patient is being seen in the clinic for a follow-up visit after fracturing her ankle. The nurse notes that she is not using her crutches correctly. Which statement by the nurse is most appropriate?

    1. "You are not using your crutches correctly."
    2. "Let me show you some ways to make crutch walking easier for you."
    3. "Who taught you to use your crutches like that?"
    4. "Do your crutches seem to fit you properly?"

14. Which method is most appropriate for communicating with an alert patient on a ventilator with an endotracheal tube in place?

    1. Open-ended questions
    2. Communication board
    3. Reflection
    4. Restatement

15. The patient is in a coma after a motor vehicle accident. Which statement regarding communication with the patient is most appropriate? (*Select all that apply.*)

    1. Speak to the patient as if he can hear what is being said.
    2. Avoid verbal stimulation because of its potential to trigger excitability.
    3. Encourage family members to limit visitation to no more than 5 minutes per hour.
    4. Leave the television on continuously to stimulate the patient.
    5. Encourage family members to read a book or newspaper to the patient.

16. Which statement about communication is most accurate?

    1. Use of therapeutic communication techniques guarantees that a therapeutic interaction takes place.
    2. Some form of communication takes place each time there is an interaction between individuals.
    3. The intended receiver is always the person receiving the communication.

4. Verbal communication is more effective than nonverbal communication.

17. Which communication technique is considered appropriate in all interactions?

1. Listening
2. Clarifying
3. Touch
4. Eye contact

18. The nurse is providing discharge instructions to a patient. Which action provides the most accurate assessment of understanding by the patient?

1. Asking the patient whether he understands the instructions
2. Repeating the instructions a second time
3. Providing the patient with written instructions
4. Asking the patient to repeat the instructions

19. Which nurse–patient interaction usually occurs in the "personal zone" of space surrounding the patient? (*Select all that apply*.)

1. Urethral catheterization
2. Complete bed bath
3. Discharge instructions
4. Injection administration
5. Admission interview

20. Which approach is most appropriate for effective communication with a patient with cognitive impairment?

1. Repeating a phrase until the patient indicates understanding
2. Asking friends and family to step out of the room to decrease distraction
3. Using simple sentences and avoiding detailed explanations
4. Directing communication to significant others rather than the patient

Nursing Process and Critical Thinking

Objectives

1. Explain the use of each of the six phases of the nursing process.
2. List the elements of each of the six phases of the nursing process.
3. Describe the establishment of the database.
4. Discuss the components of a patient problem statement.
5. Differentiate between types of health problems.
6. Describe the development of patient-centered goals.
7. Discuss the creation of nursing orders.
8. Explain the evaluation of a nursing care plan.
9. Demonstrate the nursing process by preparing a nursing care plan.
10. Explain North American Nursing Diagnosis Association International (NANDA-I), *Nursing Interventions Classification (NIC)*, and *Nursing Outcomes Classification (NOC)*.
11. Describe the use of clinical pathways in managed care.
12. Discuss critical thinking in nursing.
13. Define evidence-based practice.

Key Terms

assessment (p. 81)
biographic data (bī-ō-GRĂF-ĭk DĂ-tă, p. 83)
case management (kās MĂN-ĭj-mĕnt, p. 92)
clinical pathway (CLĬN-ĭ-căl PĂTH-wā, p. 92)
collaborative problems (kŏ-LĂB-ŭr-ă-tĭv PRŎB-lĕmz, p. 86)
cue (kyū, p. 83)
database (p. 83)
defining characteristics (dē-FĪN-ĭng kăr-ăk-tŭr-ĬS-tĭks, p. 85)
diagnose (dī-ăg-NŌS, p. 84)
evaluation (ē-văl-yū-Ā-shŭn, p. 90)
goal (p. 86)
implementation (ĭm-plĕ-mĕn-TĀ-shŭn, p. 90)

managed care (p. 92)
medical diagnosis (MĔD-ĭ-kăl dī-ăg-NŌ-sĭs, p. 86)
NANDA-I (p. 84)
nursing diagnosis/patient problem statement (p. 84)
nursing interventions (p. 88)
nursing process (p. 81)
nursing-sensitive patient outcomes (p. 91)
objective data (ŏb-JĔK-tĭv DĂ-tă, p. 83)
outcome (goal) (p. 91)
planning (p. 87)
potential patient problem statement (p. 85)
standardized language (p. 91)
subjective data (sŭb-JĔK-tĭv DĂ-tă, p. 83)
variance (VĂR-ē-ăns, p. 92)

According to the American Nurses Association (ANA), the current definition of nursing states, "Nursing is the protection, promotion, and optimization of health and abilities, prevention of illness and injury, facilitation of healing, alleviation of suffering through the diagnosis and treatment of human response, and advocacy in the care of individuals, families, groups, communities, and populations" (ANA, n.d.a). This broad definition seeks to illustrate nursing's growth as a profession. The nursing process serves as the organizational framework for the practice of nursing.

The nursing process is a systematic method by which nurses plan and provide care for patients. This involves a problem-solving approach that enables the nurse to identify patient problems and potential problems. Once these problems are identified, the nurse is then able to plan, deliver, and evaluate nursing care

in an orderly, scientific manner. The nursing process consists of the following six dynamic and interrelated phases: assessment, diagnosis, outcomes identification, planning, implementation, and evaluation (Fig. 5.1). Box 5.1 describes how the nursing process is carried out by the registered nurse (RN) and licensed practical/vocational nurse (LPN/LVN). The LPN/LVN has a significant role in the nursing process, which is discussed subsequently in the chapter.

ASSESSMENT DATA

The ANA defines assessment as "a systematic, dynamic way to collect and analyze data about a client, the first step in delivering nursing care. Assessment includes not only physiological data, but also psychological, sociocultural, spiritual, economic, and life-style

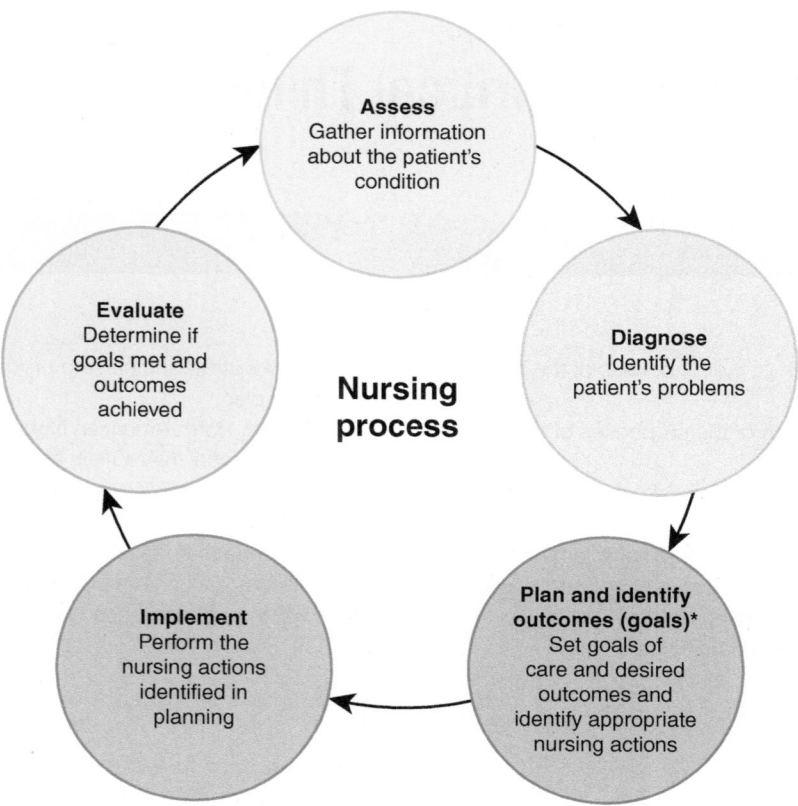

Fig. 5.1 Relationships among the steps of the nursing process. *Note: Combined American Nurses Association (ANA) standards 3 and 4.

Box 5.1	Implementation of the Nursing Process by the Registered Nurse (RN) and Licensed Practical/Vocational Nurse (LPN/LVN)

Assessment: The RN is responsible for the initial assessment of the patient; the LPN/LVN assists the RN with ongoing assessments.

Diagnosis: The RN is responsible for identifying the appropriate nursing diagnosis (patient problem) for the patient with the assistance of the LPN/LVN.

Outcomes Identification: The RN develops individualized goals or expected outcomes directly associated with the nursing diagnoses. The LPN/LVN also can assist the RN with identifying these outcomes.

Planning: The RN, with assistance from the LPN/LVN, plans interventions that will help meet the patient's desired goals/expected outcomes.

Implementation: The RN and LPN/LVN implement the proposed plan.

Evaluation: The RN and LPN/LVN perform ongoing assessments, allowing the RN to determine whether proposed goals/outcomes have been met.

factors as well" (ANA, n.d.b). Information is gathered by the nurse to identify the condition of the patient's health. The nurse performs a patient assessment on initial contact with the patient, with the remaining phases of the nursing process dependent on the accuracy and completeness of this initial data collection. Either a complete assessment or a focused assessment is performed, depending on the patient's status and the type of facility. The LPN/LVN assists the RN by performing ongoing complete and focused assessments of patients, depending on the facility and scope of practice within a state.

A complete assessment involves a review and physical examination of all body systems (e.g., musculoskeletal, respiratory, gastrointestinal) (see Chapter 13). This type of assessment also includes cognitive, psychosocial, emotional, cultural, and spiritual components and is appropriate for a patient with a stable condition who is not in acute distress. Information about functional abilities, lifestyle, and developmental concerns is also important.

A focused assessment is advisable when the patient is critically ill, disoriented, or unable to respond. A focused assessment is used to gather information about a specific health problem. For example, if the patient reports abdominal distention, lack of appetite, and straining to have a bowel movement, one possible patient problem statement might be *Infrequent or difficult bowel elimination.* To further investigate the situation, the nurse may ask additional questions about the intake of foods high in fiber, fluid intake, and amount of exercise.

Focused assessments also are performed continually throughout nurse–patient contact. The nurse

Table 5.1   Comparison of Subjective and Objective Data

SUBJECTIVE DATA	OBJECTIVE DATA
"I feel nauseated."	50 mL dark green–tinged vomitus
"My chest hurts."	Blood pressure, 100/60 mm Hg; pulse, 100/min; respirations, 32/min; patient holds fist over sternum
"I'm nervous."	Wringing hands, pacing in the hall; pulse, 112/min; respirations, 28/min
"I'm tired."	Dark circles under eyes, yawning, naps during the day
"My foot hurts."	1-cm × 2-cm open lesion on the left heel

who monitors intake and output, skin turgor, and oral mucous membranes is performing a focused assessment for inadequate fluid volume. Assessments made to determine progress toward the achievement of desired outcomes (outcomes, or goals, are something that a person strives to achieve) are also focused assessments.

TYPES OF DATA

In an assessment, the nurse gathers subjective and objective data. A cue is a piece or pieces of data that often indicate that an actual or potential problem has occurred or will occur. Subjective data are information that is provided by the patient. Statements about nausea and descriptions of pain, fatigue, and anxiety are examples of subjective data. Other terms for subjective data are *symptoms* and *subjective cues*. Subjective data are hidden until shared by the patient.

Objective data are observable and measurable signs. For example, the LPN/LVN is able to observe capillary refill, measure a patient's blood pressure, and observe and measure edema. Other terms for objective data are *signs* and *objective cues*. Table 5.1 shows a comparison of subjective and objective data.

SOURCES OF DATA

Data are obtained from primary or secondary sources. The primary source of data is the patient. In most instances, the patient is considered the most accurate reporter. The alert and oriented patient is able to provide information about past illnesses and surgeries as well as present symptoms and lifestyle.

When the patient is unable to supply adequate information because of deterioration of mental status, age, or seriousness of illness, the nurse turns to secondary sources. Secondary sources include family members, significant others, medical records, diagnostic procedures, and previous nursing progress notes. Members of the patient's support system often are able to furnish information about the patient's past health status, current illness, allergies, and current medications.

Health team professionals are also helpful secondary sources. Health care providers, nurses, dietitians, respiratory and physical therapists, and others frequently provide data about the patient. The nurse should review nursing literature to determine what information may be needed. Nursing textbooks are a good resource for information about etiology (cause), pathophysiology, clinical manifestations, assessment, diagnostic tests, medical management, nursing interventions, patient teaching needs, and prognosis. This important information then guides further data collection.

METHODS OF DATA COLLECTION

Two basic methods are used to collect data. In the first method, the nurse conducts an interview, the nursing health history, to obtain information about the patient's health history. The nurse commonly assesses several common components in the course of the interview. Biographic data provide information about the facts or events in a person's life. Additional information collected includes the reason the patient is seeking health care, a history of the present illness, the health history, and the family history. Because the environment in which the patient lives and works often plays a part in the patient's health status, an environmental history is important to obtain. A psychosocial history yields information about a combination of psychological and social factors. When gathering information about the function of each body system, the nurse follows the nursing health history with a review of systems.

The second method of data collection is the physical examination. The physical examination often is guided by subjective data provided by the patient. For example, the nurse should follow up with a thorough assessment of any body part or system for which the patient has reported symptoms or concerns. A head-to-toe format provides a systematic approach that helps avoid the omission of important data (see Chapter 13).

A completed nursing health history and a physical examination allow the nurse to establish a database (a large store or bank of information) for the patient. Analysis of the database leads to the identification of nursing diagnoses. In addition, the database makes information available for the health care provider who assists in the medical management of the patient and all health care personnel who are involved in the patient's care.

DATA CLUSTERING

Data obtained from the health history, physical examination, and related diagnostic procedures are analyzed in the development of a plan of care. Data clustering is one method of data organization. The clustering of related data helps to identify patterns that assist with the identification of patient's health problems. Some schools of nursing or health care facilities use the term *defining characteristics* as a synonym for data clustering.

Table 5.2	Determination of Significant Cues		
PATIENT VALUES	**NORM**[a]		**CONCLUSION**
42-year-old man with blood pressure 165/92 mm Hg	<120/80 mm Hg		High blood pressure
18-year-old patient with respirations of 32/min	16/min–22/min		Tachypnea
Small-frame woman with the weight of 178 lb, height 5'1"	105–118 lb		Weight above the accepted normal standard
22-month-old child not walking	12 months		Walking delayed
Male adult patient with hemoglobin of 8 g/dL	14–18 g/dL		Below normal limits
Female adult patient with hemoglobin of 12 g/dL	12–16 g/dL		Within normal limits
25-year-old patient with a pulse of 120 beats/min	60–100 beats/min		Tachycardia
Newborn patient with a pulse of 132 beats/min	130–150 beats/min		Within normal limits
Adult patient with thrombocyte count of 20,000/mm²	150,000/mm²–400,000/mm²		Thrombocytopenia

[a]Conclusion is based on the appropriate norm for the age and gender of the patient.

DIAGNOSIS

To **diagnose** is to identify the type and cause of a health condition. Only the physician or other medically qualified health care provider such as a nurse practitioner can provide a medical diagnosis. The LPN/LVN and the RN observe and collect data. Once the initial assessment has been completed, the data require analysis. In most situations, the RN is responsible for analyzing and interpreting data to identify health problems that the nurse can treat, referred to as the nursing diagnosis or patient problem statement (Table 5.2). The RN often collaborates with the LPN/LVN when determining the nursing diagnosis.

NURSING DIAGNOSIS/PATIENT PROBLEM STATEMENT

A **nursing diagnosis/patient problem statement** is a type of health problem that can be identified by the nurse. In 1990, the North American Nursing Diagnosis Association (NANDA) was created; in 2002, NANDA became NANDA International **(NANDA-I)** to reflect nursing diagnosis terminology used around the world. NANDA-I approves the official definition for a nursing diagnosis. In 2013, NANDA-I updated the definition of a nursing diagnosis as "a clinical judgment concerning a human response to health conditions/life processes, or a vulnerability for that response, by an individual, family, group or community. A nursing diagnosis provides the basis for selection of nursing interventions to achieve outcomes for which the nurse has accountability" (NANDA-I, 2018). The assessment and development of nursing diagnoses or patient problem statements are the responsibility of the RN. These are the foundational elements for the patient care plan. The RN is permitted legally to identify and prescribe the primary interventions to treat or prevent problems that are identified as nursing diagnoses or patient problems. Nurses must be aware of this important point. If the nurse is not able to prescribe the primary treatment, the problem is *not* a nursing diagnosis or a patient problem statement. As a member of the health care team, the LPN/LVN actively participates in patient care planning. This role includes collaboration with the RN to update the care plan and to implement prescribed nursing interventions.

Components of a Patient Problem Statement

The nursing community views the NANDA-I nursing diagnosis designations as being RN focused. In this text, *patient problem statements* are used to guide the development of a nursing care plan. This terminology allows for active participation in the care planning process by the LPN/LVN and other members of the intraprofessional health care team. When identifying patient problems, consider the following factors: the patient's presenting signs and symptoms; contributing, etiologic (causative), and related factors; and defining characteristics.

Patient problem statement. Patient problems may be actual or potential. The nursing assessment determines how to classify the problem. If the patient's condition is expected to change, add the phrase "potential for" before the patient problem statement. For example, it is reasonable to expect that a patient being prepared for surgery will experience pain, alteration in mobility, or the need for education. Therefore, a patient problem statement would be *Potential for Discomfort.* This problem is identified based on a pattern of related cues or data that support the patient problem statement. A list of the most commonly seen patient problem statements to be used throughout *Foundations of Nursing and Adult Health Nursing* may be found on the back inside cover.

Adjectives add meaning to the patient problem statement by describing or modifying the statement. Examples of adjectives include *inability, insufficient, impaired,* and *willingness.* The patient problem statement given in the nursing care plans and nursing process sections of this text include the appropriate adjectives. Similarly, if assessment findings of the identified patient problem characterize it to be a potential problem, *Potential for* is placed in front of the patient problem statement. Examples include *Inability to Clear Airway* or *Potential for Inability to Clear Airway*.

Definition. Chronic conditions are things that are always present or consistently recur. These conditions commonly last 3 months or longer. Acute problems are typically rapid in onset and are limited in the duration of time. Acute problems can become chronic if the condition is not resolved. For this text, the patient problems that are acute will be labeled as either *acute* or *recent*. Chronic patient problems will be labeled as either *chronic* or *prolonged*. The definition presents a clear, precise description of the patient problem statement. This description helps identify the difference between similar patient problems. An example of an acute patient problem related to a recent injury is *Recent Onset of Pain*. A patient with a debilitating illness whose pain is present on some level for more than 3 months would have the patient problem *Prolonged Pain*.

Contributing, etiologic, and related factors and risk factors. Contributing, etiologic, and related factors are conditions that often are involved in the development of a problem. The factors may become the focus for nursing interventions. These authors will refer to a contributing factor as a "related to." Contributing, etiologic, and related factors are written as the "related to" in actual patient problem statements. A patient who has limited mobility and refuses to get out of bed would have the patient problem statement *Potential for Pressure Injury, related to lack of mobility, and refusal to get out of bed.*

Defining characteristics. **Defining characteristics** are the clinical cues, signs, and symptoms that furnish evidence that the problem exists. The cues, signs, and symptoms identified in the patient's assessment are prefaced with "as evidenced by" in the patient problem statement. Examples are presented in the following discussion of the writing of patient problem statements. If utilizing NANDA-I nursing diagnoses, the defining characteristics for each nursing diagnosis title or label are listed in nursing diagnosis handbooks.

Data Clustering

Data obtained from the health history, physical examination, psychosocial history, and related diagnostic procedures are analyzed in the development of a plan of care. Data clustering is one method of data organization. The clustering of related data helps to identify patterns that assist with the identification of the patient problem statement. Some schools of nursing or health care facilities use the term *defining characteristics* as a synonym for data clustering. Examples of data clustering and the related patient problem include the following:

- Urine loss associated with physical exertion, such as lifting a heavy object, and urine loss associated with increased abdominal pressure, such as with

pregnancy, are cues for the patient problem *Inability to Control Urination Due to Physical Stress.*
- Abnormal blood pressure, increased heart rate response to activity, exertional dyspnea, and verbal report of fatigue or weakness are cues for the patient problem *Inability to Tolerate Activity.*

Actual patient problem statement. An actual patient problem statement identifies health-related problems that exist and are discovered during the nursing assessment. These health problems can be treated by the nurse, which is how they differ from a medical diagnosis. In an educational setting, the actual patient problem statement usually is represented by a three-part statement. In a clinical setting, only the first two parts of the statement typically are used. The three parts are written in the following order: (1) the patient problem statement; (2) the contributing, etiologic, or related factor(s); and (3) the specific cues, signs, and symptoms from the patient's assessment that support the patient problem statement. Connecting phrases are used to join the three parts of the statement. "Related to" (r/t) links the first and second parts of the statement. "As evidenced by" (AEB) joins the second and third parts of the patient problem statement. Note the bold italicized connecting words of an actual patient problem statement in the following example.
- Infrequent or Difficult Bowel Elimination, **related to** insufficient fluid intake **as evidenced by** increased abdominal pressure, no bowel movement for 5 days, and straining with defecation.

Potential patient problems. Potential patient problem statements are health-related problems that the nurse deems as having a strong possibility of occurring. The nursing assessment indicates that risk factors are present that are known to contribute to the development of the problem. **Potential patient problems** are written as two-part statements: (1) the patient problem statement with the adjective "potential" in front of it, and (2) the risk factor(s). As in an actual patient problem statement, the two parts are connected by the words "related to." An example of a potential patient problem statement is as follows:
- Potential for Compromised Skin Integrity, **related to** physical immobilization

Note that no third part (as evidenced by) is seen in this statement. If signs or symptoms were found, an actual problem would exist.

Health promotion patient problem statements. A health promotion patient problem statement refers to the willingness of the patient, caregiver, or significant others to participate in activities that will aid in keeping the patient well. Health promotion problem statements are identified with the adjective *"willingness."* An example of a health promotion patient problem statement is *Willingness to Learn Breastfeeding, related to delivery of infant AEB mother's interest in meeting with the lactation consultant.*

OTHER TYPES OF HEALTH PROBLEMS

Collaborative problems and medical diagnoses must be distinguished from patient problem statements. These two types of problems are defined and discussed separately.

Collaborative Problems

Collaborative problems are health-related problems that the nurse anticipates based on the condition or diagnosis of a patient. Both health care provider–prescribed and nursing-prescribed interventions (discussed subsequently in this chapter) are used in the management of collaborative problems (Carpenito, 2021). An example of a collaborative problem is the care of a patient with hypertension who is taking a new medication for the condition. The potential for hypotension is considered a collaborative problem because prevention uses physician-prescribed interventions (e.g., adjustment of the hypertensive medications as needed) and nursing-prescribed interventions (e.g., monitoring of the patient's blood pressure, assistance when the patient goes from a sitting to standing position). If the prevention or treatment of the problem is primarily the nurse's responsibility, the problem is identified as a patient problem statement. *Potential for Infection* for the new postoperative surgical case is a potential complication that is a nursing responsibility.

Medical Diagnosis

A medical diagnosis is the identification of a disease or condition with the evaluation of physical signs, symptoms, patient interviews, laboratory tests, diagnostic procedures, review of medical records, and patient history. The health care provider is licensed to make and treat medical diagnoses. Examples of medical diagnoses are congestive heart failure, pneumonia, diabetes mellitus, and hepatitis B.

Differentiation of Medical and Patient Problems

Students often have difficulty with the distinction between a medical and a patient problem statement. Health care providers, including physicians and advanced practice nurses, diagnose diseases or disorders such as those listed previously. These diseases or disorders are the results of changes in the structure or the function of an organ or body system. Diagnostic studies such as x-ray examinations and laboratory studies help with identifying medical diagnoses. Although the patient is often able to recover from a medically diagnosed condition, the diagnosis does not change. The patient who recovers from a heart attack (myocardial infarction) has a history of a myocardial infarction. The patient who was diagnosed with diabetes is likely to still have diabetes.

In the case of a patient problem statement, the situation is different. Patient problem statements address *human responses* to health problems and life processes. The nurse addresses the patient's concerns about the medical problem. If a patient is diagnosed with cancer, the nurse has the opportunity to address the patient's responses to the diagnosis; responses to the disease may include anxiousness, fear of the disease or treatment, grief, inability to tolerate activity, and nausea associated with treatment. These problems often change as the LPN/LVN carries out interventions. The nurse may assist the patient who is concerned about dying with grief resolution or perhaps teach the patient coping strategies. A patient problem statement may change or resolve as care is provided or the condition changes. The medical diagnosis of cancer may not go away; however, the goal for the patient may be the ability to resolve feelings of fear regarding the diagnosis, prognosis, and treatment through nursing interventions addressed in the care plan.

GOAL IDENTIFICATION

The nurse, in collaboration with the patient, develops expected outcomes for the established patient problem. The goal statement indicates the degree of wellness desired, expected, or possible for the patient to achieve and contains a patient goal statement. The ANA uses the term *outcome identification*, but alternative terms for this statement are a patient goal, a patient-centered goal, an objective, a behavioral objective, or a patient outcome. The authors of this text have chosen to use the term patient goal statement. A patient goal statement provides a description of the specific, measurable behavior (outcome criteria) that the patient will be able to exhibit in a given time frame after the interventions. The nurse must avoid writing a goal statement that is centered on nursing interventions because this indicates what the nurse is meant to do rather than what the patient is to do.

Desired patient goal statements serve two functions. First, they guide the selection of nursing interventions. Nursing interventions are selected to promote the achievement of the desired outcome. Second, the goal statement establishes the measuring standard that is used to evaluate the effectiveness of the nursing interventions. Therefore, the goal statement has to provide specific details that can be used as the benchmark to judge progress or the solution of the problem.

A well-written patient-centered goal statement does the following:
- Uses the word *patient* or a part of the patient as the subject of the statement
- Uses a measurable verb
- Is specific for the patient and the patient's problem
- Does not interfere with the medical plan of care
- Is realistic for the patient and the patient's problem
- Includes a time frame for patient reevaluation

Because the subject of the patient goal statement is meant to be the patient or a part of the patient, the goal statement should begin with the words, "The patient will" or "The patient's … will."

Measurable verbs indicate the precise behavior that the nurse anticipates hearing or seeing. *Define, describe, list, walk, demonstrate,* and *verbalize* are examples of measurable verbs.

The properly written patient goal statement is specific to the patient and the patient's health problem. A patient who is in traction because of a bone fracture has mobility restrictions. A goal statement indicating that all joints will be moved through a full range of motion is not safe for this patient's problem.

The patient goal statement also must be realistic for the patient and the patient's health problem. Although some 88-year-old patients are joggers, the expectation that an 88-year-old patient will learn to jog is probably not reasonable.

A time frame is written into the patient goal statement to provide a deadline for evaluation of the patient's progress. Nursing experience assists the nurse in accurately predicting realistic time frames.

Patient goal statements indicate a reversal of the patient problem statement, as shown in the following example:

PATIENT PROBLEM STATEMENT	GOAL STATEMENT
Compromised Skin Integrity, related to prolonged immobility as evidenced by (AEB) 2-cm–diameter excoriated area on coccyx	Patient will have intact skin within 3 wk. (NOTE: Intact skin is a reversal of the impaired skin.)

Patient goal statements can be written in two ways. The previous example illustrates the simple reversal of the problem statement in a concise fashion. A second approach is to list the desired behavior in broader terms and then list exact criteria or standards; this also may be referred to as a long-term and short-term goal. In the following list, the first example is the long-term goal, and the second and third examples are short-term goals:

- The patient will use her walker to ambulate at all times rather than using her wheelchair within the next 2 months. (Long-term goal)
- The patient will participate in range-of-motion exercises on her lower extremities bilaterally two times a day. (Short-term goal)
- The patient will ambulate 20 feet every day with the assistance of her walker, increasing distance ambulated by 5 feet daily. (Short-term goal)

PLANNING

During the **planning** phase of the nursing process, priorities of care are established and nursing interventions are chosen to best address the patient problem statement. This information typically is communicated through the care plan so that all health care personnel directly involved in the care of the patient can follow the same plan, resulting in continuity of care. The nurse must work with the patient and significant others in choosing appropriate interventions and in considering evidence-based practice guidelines. The plan of care should comprise standardized languages or recognized terminology to document and effectively communicate the plan.

PRIORITY SETTING

The nurse in today's busy health care facility is caring for many patients with complex problems and is challenged daily to use time and effort wisely. Priorities must be established to provide care for each patient.

Once patient problem statements have been identified, the RN must prioritize the patient problem statements according to the patient's current health status. The framework most often used to guide the prioritization is Maslow's hierarchy of needs. This structure is based on the principle that lower-level needs must be met before higher-level needs can be satisfied. The physiologic needs are more vital than the safety and security needs, and the safety and security needs are more critical than the love and belonging needs. Review Maslow's hierarchy in Fig. 1.8. Life-threatening and health-threatening problems are ranked before other types of problems. Actual problems often are ranked before potential problems, unless the potential problems, if they were to develop, are life threatening. For example, *Potential for Inability to Clear Airway* may be prioritized higher than an actual problem of *Inability to Control Urination* due to urgency. With the use of Maslow's hierarchy, the nurse can determine whether the actual or *potential* patient problem statement has the highest priority. The nurse also must take into consideration the patient's thoughts and feelings regarding the prioritization of problems. If patients are not active participants in the plan of care, they are not likely to be driven to work toward meeting the agreed-upon goals.

Time factors and severity of illness are important considerations in determining which problems to initially address. The patient who is admitted to the emergency department with a possible heart attack (myocardial infarction) is not ready at that time to contemplate dietary instructions to reach a goal of reducing cholesterol.

Priorities change as the patient progresses through time in a health care facility. As some problems are resolved, the approach to other problems comes into focus. Consider the following scenario and how the concerns of nursing change during one patient's hospital stay.

A 28-year-old woman admitted for an abdominal hysterectomy may have the preoperative patient problem of *Fearfulness. Recent Onset of Pain* is an important patient problem in the first few days after surgery. As the pain is controlled, *Deficient Nutrition* and *Potential for Infrequent or Difficult Bowel Elimination* are managed.

When the patient approaches discharge, teaching about wound care and activity restrictions becomes the focus for patient problems. Because of the loss of reproductive ability, self-esteem problems have to be confirmed or ruled out as possible patient problems for this patient. Note how the patient's problems changed, but the medical procedure did not.

SELECTING NURSING INTERVENTIONS

Nursing interventions are those activities that promote the achievement of the desired patient goal. Interventions include activities that the nurse selects, in partnership with the patient, to resolve a patient problem, monitor for the development of a potential problem, or carry out physician orders. Nursing interventions are classified as physician prescribed or nurse prescribed.

Physician-prescribed interventions are those actions ordered by a physician for a nurse or other health care professional to perform. Remember that physician orders are not orders for nurses but are prescriptive instructions for patients (Carpenito, 2021). Although the physician has given the order, nursing judgment must still be used. The LPN/LVN must follow orders when administering medications, performing wound care, and ordering diagnostic tests. Assessing, teaching, and validating the safety of physician orders are important nursing responsibilities. In this text, the term "health care provider" has been used to encompass those health care professionals who have prescriptive authority, such as physicians, advanced practice nurses, and physician assistants. The term "physician-prescribed interventions" applies to these individuals.

Nurse-prescribed interventions are any actions that a nurse is legally able to order or begin independently. Nurses write interventions for themselves or other nursing staff (Carpenito, 2021). Examples of independent nursing interventions are providing a back massage, turning a patient every 2 hours, and monitoring for complications. When determining appropriate nursing interventions, the nurse should consider the contributing, etiologic, and related factors; risk factors; the patient-centered goal; and the patient problem itself. Nursing interventions are focused on any or all of these areas.

Nursing interventions often are aimed at reducing or eliminating the causative factor. For example, for the patient problem statement *Anxiousness, related to lack of knowledge about hospital procedures,* an appropriate nursing intervention is to teach the patient about typical routines and procedures. Providing information addresses any knowledge deficit, which helps to reduce the fear of the unknown, thereby reducing anxiety.

The patient goal also is considered when selecting nursing interventions. For example, when the patient goal statement says, "The patient will plan a week's menu for an 1800-calorie diabetic diet within 1 week," the interventions are selected to increase the patient's knowledge about planning for a diabetic diet.

The patient problem statement also may direct the interventions. If the patient's problem is *Recent Onset of Pain,* interventions to relieve acute pain are selected.

A variety of sources list nursing interventions. Nursing textbooks, periodicals, and care planning books are helpful sources of information. The *Nursing Interventions Classification (NIC)* may be another helpful source for nursing interventions and activities. (The *NIC* is discussed subsequently in this chapter.) Nursing colleagues and previous experience in nursing care are also good sources of ideas for interventions, as are patient suggestions regarding care. In addition, nursing conferences held to plan patient care often provide an environment for the development of creative approaches to patient care.

WRITING NURSING INTERVENTIONS

Because nursing interventions offered in textbooks and care planning resources are often broad, general statements that indicate an activity to be performed, these nursing interventions must be converted to more specific instructional statements when writing a care plan for an actual patient. Suggested interventions for constipation may include increase dietary bulk, increase activity, and encourage fluids.

This information is helpful because it prescribes a direction for care, but the information provided is lacking in specific details. The nurse must determine specific information regarding interventions so that any person following the direction of the care plan can carry out interventions without question. For care planning purposes, the nurse must be able to change the guiding general statement about the nursing intervention to a more specific statement. Nursing interventions have to be written to reduce the likelihood of misinterpretation. Details are provided to convey the intended meaning. Written nursing interventions should include the subject (the nurse is assumed unless stated otherwise), action verb, and qualifying details. Consider the following interventions:

- Ambulate the patient three times a day at 0900, 1400, and 1900.
- Ambulate the patient 30 feet three times a day at 0900, 1400, and 1900.

The correctly written nursing intervention is the second one because it contains the subject (the nurse is assumed), the action verb (ambulate), and the qualifying details (30 feet three times a day). This intervention is specific and easily interpreted by any health care professional following the care plan.

A properly written nursing intervention is specific for the problem, realistic for the patient, compatible with the medical plan of care, and based on scientific, evidenced-based principles. The following examples illustrate an appropriate conversion of general nursing interventions into specific nursing interventions:

- Add four servings of fruits and vegetables of the patient's choice to the daily menu, one extra serving per meal, and one snack.

- Turn the patient every 2 hours with the assistance of two personnel and the lift sheet.
- Offer water and juices up to 2000 mL/day according to the following schedule: 7 to 3 shift, 1200 mL; 3 to 11 shift, 600 mL; 11 to 7 shift, 200 mL.

COMMUNICATING THE NURSING CARE PLAN

After completing the initial assessment, analyzing the data, writing the patient problem statement, selecting goals, and selecting appropriate nursing interventions (which are then made more specific with written nursing interventions), the nurse has the responsibility to communicate the detailed plan of care for the patient. The written nursing care plan is the tangible product of the nursing process (Table 5.3). (Refer to Chapter 3 for additional information on charting and documentation.)

Because the nursing staff constantly changes (nurses work different shifts and have days off), written guidelines are important for the continuity of patient care. Continuity increases patient trust in the nursing staff and promotes outcome achievement.

Nursing care plans may be written specifically for a patient, or the nurse may use a standardized care plan for a patient. The nurse must individualize each care plan to the patient, even with the use of standardized care plans. Individually prepared care plans are the most time-consuming but often provide care that is best matched to the specific patient's needs and situation. An individualized plan of care takes into consideration pertinent patient characteristics such as age, culture, and medical diagnosis.

Table 5.3 Nursing Care Plan Form

PATIENT PROBLEM STATEMENT	NURSING ORDER	SCIENTIFIC PRINCIPLE	EVALUATION
Patient 1 *Recent Onset of Pain, r/t tissue trauma from broken fibula and tibia, AEB grimaces, reports right leg pain at 8/10, and has elevated blood pressure 140/100 mm Hg.* DESIRED PATIENT GOAL: Patient will demonstrate an improved comfort level as evidenced by relaxed facial expression, statements of pain relief, and return of vital signs to the patient's normal range within 30 min of nursing interventions.	1. Assess verbal and nonverbal indications of pain. 2. Monitor blood pressure and pulse for an increase over baseline value q 4 h. 3. Elevate the right leg on two pillows at all times except meals. 4. Offer back rub and position change when statements of pain are made.	1. Fractures cause swelling and pressure on nerves. Patient pain report establishes the need for intervention. 2. Pain increases heart rate and blood pressure. 3. Gravity helps reduce edema, which reduces pain. 4. Sensory nerve impulses from the skin "close the gate" and prevent pain transmission.	Goal achieved. D = States pain in lower right leg 8/10. Blood pressure 140/100 mm Hg. A = Right leg elevated on two pillows. Back rub given for 10 min. R = States pain improved to 2/10. Blood pressure 132/88 mm Hg; no facial grimacing.
Patient 2 *Potential for Compromised Skin Integrity, r/t pressure on bony prominences, impaired circulation, and physical immobilization.* DESIRED PATIENT GOAL: Short-term goal: Patient will remain free of any skin impairments, such as reddened areas, by 10/28/2018. Long-term goal: Patient will have no skin breakdown with q 2 h turning during the duration of stay in the facility.	1. Monitor skin condition for skin color and texture changes q 2 h with turning. 2. Identify areas that are more at risk for skin impairment, such as bony prominences (e.g., elbows, heels, and sacral area). 3. Use lotions or moisturizers to prevent dry skin with a.m. care and PRN. 4. Change patient's position at least q 2 h	1. Early identification of any skin impairment can prevent breakdown. 2. Identifying problem areas makes knowing where to look and how often to look for skin impairment a more effective process. 3. Dry skin can lead to cracks in the skin and infection. 4. Changing position in immobile residents prevents pressure ulcers from forming.	Goal achieved. D = Patient has no areas of skin impairment. A = Patient's position changed q 2 h and lotion applied in a.m. and PRN. R = Voices no reports of discomfort regarding skin condition.

CRITICAL THINKING QUESTIONS

1. The patient experiencing pain (patient 1) asks why he has an elevated blood pressure. How should the nurse respond?
2. What interventions can the nurse initiate to prevent this patient's pain from reaching an 8/10 level in the future?
3. What nutritional measures can the nurse include in the plan of care for the patient who is at risk for impaired skin integrity (patient 2)?

A, Action; *AEB,* as evidenced by; *D,* data; *PRN,* as needed; *q 2 h,* every 2 hours; *R,* response/evaluation; *r/t,* related to.

Standardized nursing care plans are appropriate for patient populations with routine, expected care requirements. Women who have had a vaginal delivery or a cesarean delivery are ideal patient populations for standardized care plans. Many standardized care plans include blank spaces that the nurse fills in to individualize to some degree.

Linear Care Plans Versus Concept Maps

Among nursing faculty, a range of different expectations often exists for the care planning process. Formats for the written nursing care plan vary from school to school. Components that are common in an educational setting are NANDA-I diagnostic labels, patient-centered goals and desired patient outcomes, and nursing interventions and orders.

Nursing faculty may require students to submit the care plan in a four-column or five-column format that is referred to as a *linear style*. With this system, rationale is often necessary to explain why the intervention is needed or how the intervention will work. This encourages the student to use critical thinking skills and evidence-based practice for supporting the nursing interventions chosen.

Other nursing faculty may prefer the care plan to be represented as a concept map. Concept maps typically use different shapes, and sometimes colors that are connected with lines when there is a relationship between one or more items. A concept map is especially beneficial for visual learners. With concept mapping, the student may put the patient problem statement into a rectangular shape in the middle of the page; interventions are in circles that branch off from the nursing diagnosis, and outcomes are placed into a triangle. The student should follow the specific guidelines of the nursing program for topics to be included on a concept map and its organization.

IMPLEMENTATION

During the implementation phase of the nursing process, the nurse and other members of the team put the established plan into action to promote goal achievement. This is the fifth phase of the nursing process. With evidence-based interventions, the nurse should ensure that the plan is implemented in a timely and safe manner.

In emergency situations, the nursing process as a means of problem-solving is accelerated. The nurse proceeds directly from assessment of the problem to intervention. If a patient has gone into cardiac or respiratory arrest, the nurse initiates cardiopulmonary resuscitation immediately.

Nursing interventions include nurse-prescribed and physician-prescribed activities. (See the discussion of selecting nursing interventions in the previous "Planning" section in this chapter.) Implementation refers to actions that carry out the planned interventions established in the care plan. Implementation includes actions such as patient teaching, medication administration, monitoring the patient's condition through assessment, delegating care to appropriate personnel, and providing ordered treatments.

EVIDENCE-BASED PRACTICE

Nursing research is the basis for evidence-based practice (EBP). Nursing research was cultivated in the 1950s, leading to the development of nursing theories in the 1960s and 1970s. In the 1990s, nursing theories were researched and further tested to expand the field of nursing and EBP. Nursing research today continues to solidify theories and practice and introduce new theories. Other disciplines such as sociology, psychology, biology, and physics are incorporated into nursing theory.

The ANA Scope and Standards of Practice (2015) defines EBP as: "a scholarly and systematic problem-solving paradigm that results in the delivery of high-quality health care. In order to make the best clinical decisions using EBP, external evidence from research is blended with internal evidence (i.e., practice-generated data), clinical expertise, and healthcare consumer values and preferences to achieve the best outcomes for individuals, groups, populations, and healthcare systems." Evidenced-based practice gives meaning and provides rationale to nursing actions. EBP provides accountability for the actions we as nurses implement on a daily basis.

EVALUATION

Evaluation is a determination made about the extent to which the established goals have been achieved. The nurse takes several steps to complete the evaluation phase. (1) Review the patient-centered goals or desired patient outcomes that were established previously. These goal statements present standards and criteria that are observable and measurable. (2) Reassess the patient to gather data that indicate the patient's actual response to the nursing interventions. (3) Compare the actual outcome with the desired outcome and make a critical judgment about whether the patient-centered goal or desired patient outcome was achieved.

This critical judgment leads the nurse to make one of three conclusions or decisions: the goal was achieved, the goal was not achieved, or the goal was partially achieved. Evaluation of the desired patient goal is illustrated in the following statement:

PATIENT GOAL STATEMENT	EVALUATION AND DOCUMENTATION
1. The patient will demonstrate self-administration of insulin with sterile technique and selection of correct site by 10/21/2020.	1. 10/21/2020: Patient goal achieved. Patient correctly administered regular insulin into the upper thigh with a sterile technique.
2. Patient's left hip ulcer will measure 1 cm (W) × 2.5 cm (L) in 3 wk (10/28/2020).	2. 10/28/2020: Patient goal partially achieved. Patient's left hip ulcer measures 0.3 cm (W) × 0.5 cm (L).

The plan of care generally undergoes changes during this phase of the nursing process. The nurse makes modifications according to whether the goal has been achieved, partially achieved, or not achieved. When a problem has been resolved, it is removed from the nursing care plan.

When the goal has been achieved partially or not achieved, further analysis is needed. At this point, the nurse should review all phases of the nursing process. The following are examples of questions the nurse should consider to ensure the accuracy of the nursing process:

- Was the assessment complete and accurate?
- Was the problem identified correctly?
- Was the desired patient goal realistic and specific?
- Were the interventions realistic, and did all personnel implement them consistently?
- Did new problems develop?
- Was adequate time allowed?

Once the nurse has determined the answers to these questions, the nursing care plan can be modified accordingly.

STANDARDIZED LANGUAGES: NANDA-I, *NIC*, AND *NOC*

Effective communication in the health care setting is vital to provide consistent quality care for patients. Nurses work in a variety of settings, and patients may be cared for in a variety of settings, sometimes with transfer from one facility to another. The use of a standardized language (terms that have the same definition and meaning regardless of who uses them) fosters communication regarding aspects of patient care.

NANDA-I, *Nursing Interventions Classification (NIC),* and *Nursing Outcomes Classification (NOC)* provide standardized nursing diagnoses (patient problem statements), nursing interventions, and nursing-sensitive patient outcomes (goals). These classification systems further provide research-based information regarding nursing treatments and judgments. NANDA-I, *NIC,* and terminology are used internationally in all patient settings, including acute care hospitals, long-term care facilities, outpatient and ambulatory settings, rehabilitation facilities, and home care. These systems aid in supporting clinical decisions, provide EBP used in plans of care and in supporting effective staffing, student learning, and staff education. NANDA-I, *NOC,* and *NIC* (NNN) comprise the components of a care plan by identification of the nursing diagnosis, nursing outcome(s), and nursing interventions. In this text, the authors illustrate this process as follows:

PATIENT PROBLEM	GOAL STATEMENT	NURSING INTERVENTION
Inefficient Oxygenation	Arterial blood gases within normal limits	Ensure use of incentive spirometer 10 breaths every hour

NURSING INTERVENTIONS CLASSIFICATION

This standardized language, developed at the University of Iowa, encourages enhanced communication between nurses regarding nursing interventions. The current edition of *Nursing Interventions Classification (NIC)* lists more than 500 interventions and 13,000 activities. Each *NIC* intervention has a label, a definition for that label, a list of activities that can be used for that intervention, and background information. The label and definition should not be altered when they are used, but the activities must be individualized to the patient's needs. The title given to nursing interventions is concise. Examples of nursing interventions are *Airway management; Analgesic administration; Teaching: prescribed diet;* and *Therapeutic play.* Some *NIC* interventions are called *indirect interventions* because they occur away from the bedside but on behalf of the patient. Examples of indirect care interventions are *emergency cart checking, shift report, staff development,* and *supply management* (Butcher et al., 2019).

The list of activities is a helpful guide for beginning nurses. The following example shows a *NIC* intervention and lists 3 of the 36 possible activities for the intervention (Butcher et al., 2019). NOTE: The definition is given and the indicated number that can be retrieved with computer systems. These numbers "run in the background" and are not for memorization.

NIC intervention: 6540

Infection control: Minimizing the acquisition and transmission of infectious agents

Activities:
- Isolate individuals exposed to communicable disease.
- Wash hands before and after each patient-care activity.
- Ensure appropriate wound care technique.

NURSING OUTCOMES CLASSIFICATION

Nursing Outcomes Classification (NOC), which measures the effects of nursing care, is the effort of a group of researchers working at the University of Iowa. These researchers have developed a standardized system with an organized structure to name and measure nursing-sensitive patient outcomes. Identification of outcomes that are responsive to nursing care is important work for nursing, especially in connection with efforts to contain costs and establish best practices (Moorhead et al., 2018). There are currently 385 outcomes with accompanying definitions, measurement standards, indicators, and references (Moorhead et al., 2018).

The *NOC* outcomes use brief phrases to describe the result of nursing care. Indicators are given as subheadings for each outcome. These indicators use a measurement scale to evaluate the degree of outcome attainment. The outcome statement and indicator can be described with selected keywords from a patient goal statement ("The patient will demonstrate beginning *grief resolution* as evidenced by the ability to *verbalize reality of loss* after nursing interventions"). NOTE:

The coded nature of the outcome and indicators that are used to enhance entry and retrieval of information from a computer database.

Grief resolution (outcome 1304). Verbalizes reality of loss (indicator 130403). The scale used for this indicator measures from "never demonstrated" to "consistently demonstrated" (1 to 5 scale) (Moorhead et al., 2018).

These measurement scales can be used to establish a baseline assessment and then the scale can be applied again during the evaluation phase. Some facilities use these indicators to plan for patient discharge. For example, if the patient does not achieve a 4 or 5 on a scale, then a referral is sometimes necessary.

ROLE OF THE LICENSED PRACTICAL/VOCATIONAL NURSE

The LPN/LVN plays a vital role in the collaborative care of the patient. The role of the LPN/LVN in the nursing process may vary from state to state and with different institutions. All practical and vocational student nurses should be knowledgeable regarding their own state's practice. In many states, the RN is responsible for the coordination of care, initiation of the nursing care plan, and evaluation of patient outcomes with the assistance of the LPN/LVN. The LPN/LVN is frequently responsible for providing direct bedside nursing care. This direct care position allows the LPN/LVN to closely observe, prioritize, intervene, and evaluate the care provided to and for the patient. See Box 5.2 for a summary of the role of the LPN/LVN in the nursing process.

MANAGED CARE AND CLINICAL PATHWAYS

To practice in the changing world of health care today, nurses are called on to go beyond performing technical skills and providing direct patient care. Responsibilities include working with outcomes, cost, resources, and other members of the health care team. One way of addressing cost containment issues is through managed care. Managed care refers to health care systems that have control over primary health care services and attempt to trim down health care costs by reducing unnecessary or overlapping services; an emphasis is placed on health promotion, education, and preventive medicine. Case management is one-way managed care achieved in a health care setting. Case management encompasses planning, coordination of care, and patient advocacy in providing quality, cost-effective outcomes for the patient. The case management system of care allows for continuity in care because one person coordinates the plan of care for an individual patient within the health care setting, including discharge planning.

Case management usually depends on the use of clinical pathways. A clinical pathway is a multidisciplinary plan that incorporates EBP guidelines for high-risk, high-volume, high-cost types of cases while

Box 5.2	Role of the Licensed Practical/Vocational Nurse in the Nursing Process

ASSESSMENT
- Observe and report significant cues to the nurse in charge or to the health care provider.

DIAGNOSIS
- Assist with the determination of accurate patient problem statements.
- Gather further data to confirm or eliminate problems.

GOAL IDENTIFICATION AND PLANNING
- Assist with setting priorities.
- Suggest interventions.
- Assist with the development of realistic patient-centered goals and desired patient outcomes.

IMPLEMENTATION
- Assist with the establishment of priorities.
- Carry out health care provider and planned nursing interventions.
- Evaluate the effectiveness of nursing activities.

EVALUATION
- Assist with reevaluation of the patient's health state after nursing interventions.
- Suggest alternative nursing interventions when necessary.

providing for optimal patient outcomes and maximizing clinical efficiency. Synonyms for clinical pathways are critical pathways, multidisciplinary action plans, action plans, and care maps. The clinical pathway guides care with the coordination of actions from all disciplines in a health care facility, such as nursing, respiratory therapy, medicine, pharmacy, social services, dietary therapy, occupational therapy, speech therapy, and physical therapy, to develop the plan of care. Clinical pathways, like any method of planning care for a patient, are aimed at providing continuity of care, efficiency in the care provided, and reducing facility costs. Clinical pathways are generally standardized documents, so it is important for the nurse to be sure to individualize them to the patient's needs. If a patient does not achieve the projected outcome, it is considered a variance. A variance must be evaluated to determine why the patient did not meet the outcome. Possible reasons an outcome was not achieved include the patient's condition changed, interventions were not performed or were not effective, or a new problem developed. Variance analysis then is used to promote continuous quality improvement. Repetition of variances often leads the health care team to revise a clinical pathway.

Whether the health care facility uses the traditional care plan, clinical pathways, or another system for organizing care, the goal remains the same: efficient care with positive patient outcomes. In addition, the nurse and all health care professionals must be cognizant of cost containment when providing care.

CRITICAL THINKING

"Thinking with a purpose" describes the term *critical thinking*. Critical thinkers question information, conclusions, and points of view and look beneath the surface. They are logical and fair in their thinking. The skills related to critical thinking are applied to reading, listening, and writing across all subjects. Critical thinking is a complex process, and no single simple definition explains all aspects of critical thinking. Each author who writes about critical thinking has his or her own definition. Papathanasiou (2014) defines critical thinking for nursing as "the mental process of actively and skillfully perception, analysis, synthesis and evaluation of collected information through observation, experience and communication that leads to a decision for action."

Critical thinking is essential to providing quality nursing care for patients in various situations. One of the first skills a nursing student learns is to take a temperature. The student nurse must choose among obtaining tympanic (ear), oral, rectal, skin, temporal, or axillary measurements. Critical thinking enables the nurse to use the nursing process in choosing the appropriate method. One consideration is the need for accuracy in the results. Also, certain medical or surgical problems may interfere with the accuracy of the reading. If a patient has an ear infection, the results of a tympanic reading may not be accurate. The nurse avoids a rectal thermometer when the patient is recovering from hemorrhoid surgery. If the patient is likely to have a seizure, an oral thermometer is contraindicated because the patient may bite down on the device. The condition of the site to be used also should be taken into consideration. Heavy perspiration often interferes with axillary temperature readings; oral temperature is affected by the ingestion of hot or cold beverages. All of these variables are taken into consideration by the student nurse who uses critical thinking skills in the decision-making process.

It is crucial for nurses to not only be able to *perform skills* (the "doing" of nursing) but also *think about* what they are doing. Nurses use a knowledge base to make decisions, generate new ideas, and solve problems. Nursing students add to their knowledge base by studying facts, principles, EBP guidelines, and theories. Knowledge of psychology, anatomy, physiology, pharmacology, and other related course work helps the student to gain the scientific knowledge base to think critically.

Nurses also must reflect on situations or care given to determine what was effective and what was not effective. Critical thinkers are able to analyze this information and adjust care accordingly, if necessary. Critical thinkers are also able to explore the relationships between concepts and ideas and apply these concepts to unique patient care situations.

To help determine the difference between thinking and critical thinking, consider the following nonclinical situations:

- *Situation 1:* On the day before classes begin, the student is anxious about getting started and is unsure of her chances of success. She is thinking, "I hope I don't get lost. I hope the teachers are nice. I wonder if I will be able to pass the tests. Will I succeed?" On the day classes begin, she drives to school, finds a parking space, and enters the building to locate her classroom.
- *Situation 2:* On the day before classes begin, the student is anxious about getting started and is unsure of her chances of success. She is thinking, "I will drive to the school so that I can judge how much time to allow for travel. I want to go early and locate my classroom today so that I will have an easier time tomorrow. Maybe I can get some course materials early so that I can organize my notebook."

Both of these situations involve individuals who are thinking. The student in situation 1 is experiencing a mental activity, but it is aimless and without purpose. The student in situation 2 has recognized the need to gain control and get organized. This student is beginning to think critically and with a purpose, which is to decrease the anxiety associated with her first day of class.

The following clinical situations provide examples of some aspects of critical thinking at the bedside.

- *Situation 1:* The nurse was caring for a patient with chronic obstructive pulmonary disease and peripheral vascular disease. During the assessment, the nurse used a pulse oximeter on the patient's finger to measure the patient's oxygen saturation level. The measurement yielded an oxygen saturation of 87%. The assessment revealed clear lung sounds, no difficulty with respirations or reports of shortness of breath, capillary refill less than 2 seconds, and extremities cool to the touch. The nurse demonstrates critical thinking skills by realizing that the assessment does not match the oxygen saturation measurement and decides to recheck the oxygen saturation level with the earlobe probe because the patient's hands were cool to the touch. The oxygen saturation level with the earlobe probe was 93%, which matched the assessment findings. With the use of critical thinking skills, the nurse was able to make comparisons between the assessment findings and the oxygen saturation level and problem solve by determining how to address the situation.
- *Situation 2:* A patient with diabetes was admitted to the hospital for a bladder infection. At the change of shift, the oncoming nurse entered the room to perform an assessment. The nurse noted that the patient was unresponsive. The nurse demonstrates critical thinking skills by realizing the patient is most likely experiencing one of two problems: hypoglycemia or hyperglycemia. The nurse first performed a quick "ABC" assessment and determined that the patient's airway was open, the patient was breathing, and the patient's heart was circulating blood. Then, because the patient was admitted with an infection, the nurse

suspected that the patient was experiencing a rise in blood glucose levels, or hyperglycemia. He obtained a finger-stick blood glucose reading of 346. The nurse also noted that the patient's skin was warm, dry, and flushed. The patient's respirations were deep, and her breath smelled "fruity." The nurse quickly called the physician to report these findings and anticipated receiving orders to give the patient more insulin. Critical thinking skills enabled the nurse to deal with this patient's situation appropriately.

Anticipating questions, asking an expert, and asking *why* are examples of other strategies to improve critical thinking. The more experience the student nurse or nurse gains, the better their critical thinking skills become. Hearing others think aloud also may help the student learn how other people reason. The student should take advantage of every learning opportunity and realize that every experience, mistake, and encounter is a potential learning opportunity.

Get Ready for the NCLEX® Examination!

Key Points

- The nursing process consists of six interconnected phases: assessment, diagnosis, outcome identification, planning, implementation, and evaluation. In this text, diagnosis is frequently referred to as *patient problem statement*, and outcome identification is frequently referred to as *patient goal*.
- A complete and valid assessment influences the remaining phases of the nursing process.
- The patient is the primary source of data; all others are secondary sources.
- The nurse prescribes the primary interventions to treat a nursing diagnosis or patient problem statement.
- The nurse uses assessment data to develop the nursing diagnosis (patient problem statement).
- The nurse projects end results that are measurable, desirable, and observable during outcome identification or patient goal.
- The nurse develops an individualized plan of care that considers pertinent patient characteristics such as age, culture, medical diagnosis, and mutual interest.
- Nursing interventions are planned activities to promote outcome (patient goal) achievement.
- Evaluation is an ongoing component of each phase of the nursing process.
- During evaluation, the actual patient outcome (goal) is compared with the desired patient outcome (goal), and a judgment is made about outcome (goal) achievement.
- The plan of care is changed according to evaluation and the resulting identification of needs.
- NANDA-I, *NIC*, and *NOC* continue to develop standardized nursing languages to aid communication and research.
- The LPN/LVN has a significant role in the nursing process.
- Managed care and case management systems have emerged in response to rising health care costs.
- A clinical pathway is a multidisciplinary plan that schedules clinical interventions over an anticipated time frame for specific types of patient health problems.
- Critical thinking involves thinking with a purpose and using reasoning with decision-making.
- EBP provides the latest guidelines for patient care based on best practices provided by research.

Additional Learning Resources

SG Go to your Study Guide for additional learning activities to help you master this chapter content.

Be sure to visit the Evolve site at http://evolve.elsevier.com/Cooper/foundations/ for additional online resources.

Review Questions for the NCLEX® Examination

1. The student nurse correctly identifies which as a medical diagnosis? *(Select all that apply.)*

   1. Acute pain
   2. Pneumonia
   3. Inability to tolerate activity
   4. Inability to clear airway
   5. Neuropathy, secondary to type 2 diabetes mellitus

2. A patient is admitted to a hospital for coronary artery bypass graft surgery. His wound continues to drain, and when he is discharged, home health nurses will visit to continue to care for him. Who is most likely responsible for coordinating the patient's discharge plans?

   1. RN team leader
   2. Social worker
   3. Case manager
   4. Physician

3. Which patient problem statement includes all appropriate components of an actual patient problem statement? *(Select all that apply.)*

   1. *Inefficient Oxygenation*
   2. *Potential Complication: Gastric Bleeding, related to gastric ulcer*
   3. *Fearfulness, related to separation from support system as evidenced by statements of being scared, pallor, and increased respirations*
   4. *Potential for Falling, related to confusion as evidenced by calling nurse by name of aunt*
   5. *Anxiousness, related to upcoming surgery as evidenced by the patient stating, "I am very worried that something is going to go wrong."*

4. *Prolonged Infrequent or Difficulty With Bowel Elimination, related to the effects of analgesic medications on the bowel as evidenced by statements of straining to have a bowel movement and no bowel movement in 5 days is an example of which type of patient problem statement?*

   1. An actual patient problem statement
   2. A potential patient problem statement
   3. A wellness patient problem statement
   4. A patient problem statement

5. Based on Maslow's hierarchy of needs, which patient problem statement label has the highest priority?

   1. *Potential for Aspiration Into Airway*
   2. *Insufficient Knowledge*
   3. *Recent Onset of Pain*
   4. *Inability to Control Urination Due to Physical Stress*

6. Which patient goal statement is best stated and contains necessary criteria? *(Select all that apply.)*

   1. The patient will identify the types of foods to include in a high-fiber diet.
   2. The nurse will teach the patient about constipation prevention.
   3. The nurse will increase total fluids during hospitalization.
   4. The patient will have a soft, formed bowel movement on the third day after surgery.
   5. The patient will ambulate 50 feet three times per day, with the assistance of 1, starting on postoperative day 1.

7. The patient is admitted to the hospital with an upper respiratory infection. The nurse writes the following problem statement: *Potential for Inadequate Fluid Volume, related to refusal to drink fluids, secondary to a sore throat.* Which is the best patient goal statement for the patient?

   1. The nurse will offer 2000 mL of fluids per day during hospitalization.
   2. The patient will experience a less of a sore throat in 8 hours.
   3. The nurse will maintain an intravenous infusion of fluids for the ordered length of time.
   4. The patient will maintain adequate hydration as evidenced by moist mucous membranes, elastic skin turgor, and voiding of clear dilute urine.

8. A woman who has had four children comes to the clinic. She tells the nurse that when she laughs or coughs, she loses control of some urine. Which nursing intervention is properly written in the care plan?

   1. The nurse will teach the patient Kegel exercises.
   2. The patient will perform Kegel exercises 10 times a day with four to six repetitions each time.
   3. The nurse will teach the patient how to perform Kegel exercises 10 times a day with four to six repetitions each time.
   4. The patient will not experience stress incontinence after 2 months of performing Kegel exercises 10 times per day.

9. A 14-year-old patient is admitted to the emergency department with a possible medical diagnosis of acute appendicitis. Who should the nurse interview first when performing the assessment?

   1. The patient's parents
   2. The patient
   3. The physician
   4. The admissions nurse

10. Which statement by the student nurse best demonstrates knowledge of the nursing process when describing defining characteristics?

   1. "Defining characteristics are a description of the patient problem."
   2. "Defining characteristics tell how the nursing diagnosis was determined."
   3. "Defining characteristics are a cluster of clinical cues."
   4. "Defining characteristics are factors such as signs and symptoms that support the nursing diagnosis."

11. Which phrases are most appropriate to use to connect the parts of a patient problem statement?

   1. "Related to" and "due to"
   2. "Due to" and "as evidenced by"
   3. "Related to" and "as evidenced by"
   4. "Due to" and "as evidenced by"

12. What occurs during the last phase of the nursing process?

   1. The nurse gathers data to use in planning care.
   2. The nurse selects nursing interventions to achieve the desired outcomes.
   3. The nurse compares the desired outcome with the actual outcome.
   4. The nurse prioritizes nursing interventions.

13. Which statement best describes a patient problem statement?

   1. Statement of the patient's needs according to Maslow's hierarchy
   2. Description of the patient's disease process
   3. Listing of the required nursing interventions
   4. A patient's health-related problem that can be treated by the nurse.

14. The patient is experiencing severe respiratory distress that is related to his chronic obstructive pulmonary disease. The patient is alert and oriented and is capable of answering questions. Which source of information is most accurate when performing a nursing history during the admission assessment?

   1. The patient
   2. The patient's wife
   3. The physician
   4. The medical record

15. The student nurse is correct in identifying which statement as objective data? *(Select all that apply.)*

   1. "When I walk to the mailbox, I get very short of breath."
   2. "My legs ache when I climb stairs."
   3. 4-cm Transverse abdominal incision.
   4. Report of pain 6 on a scale of 0 to 10.
   5. B/P 178/90.

16. A newborn was born 4 weeks premature and weighs 5 pounds, 3 ounces. Based on the prematurity of this infant the nurse has identified the problem statement *Potential for Inability to Regulate Body Temperature.* What is the most accurate patient goal for this patient problem statement?

   Choose the *most likely* options for the information missing from the statements below by selecting from the list of options provided.

   The parents _____ that they will keep their infant's _____ between 97.5 and 98.6 degrees _____ by _____ the infant's temperature as listed in the discharge instructions.

OPTIONS
Demonstrate
Blood glucose
Fahrenheit
State
Measuring
Temperature
Celsius
Indicate
List

17. While giving a bath, the nurse notes skin breakdown on a patient's coccyx. What part of the patient problem statement is this observation?

1. The patient problem statement
2. The etiologic or related factor
3. The patient goal
4. The defining characteristic

18. Which example includes all appropriate components of a *potential* patient problem statement? *(Select all that apply.)*

1. *Potential for Inability to Tolerate Activity*
2. *Potential for Aspiration Into Airway, related to difficulty swallowing*
3. *Potential Complication: Hemorrhage*
4. *Potential for Inability to Clear Airway, related to accumulation of mucus in trachea*
5. *Potential for Compromised Skin Integrity, related to immobility as evidenced by 2-cm abrasion*

Cultural and Ethnic Considerations

6

Objectives

1. Identify the importance of transcultural nursing.
2. Explain what health disparities are and what nurses can do to improve health care in these populations.
3. Explain how personal cultural beliefs and practices affect nurse-patient and nurse-nurse relationships.
4. Identify and discuss cultural variables that potentially influence health behaviors.
5. Explain how cultural data can be used to help develop therapeutic relationships with the patient.
6. Discuss cultural and religious influences as they relate to the older adult.
7. Discuss the use of the nursing process in the care of culturally diverse patients.

Key Terms

ableism (p. 102)
biomedical health belief system (Table 6.2, p. 106)
cultural bias (p. 98)
cultural competence (KŬL-chŭr-ăl KŎM-pĕ-tĕns, p. 98)
culture (p. 98)
deaf culture (p. 105)
ethnicity (ĕth-NĬS-ĭ-tē, p. 100)
folk medicine (p. 107)

health disparities (p.97)
holistic health belief system (Table 6.2, p. 108)
race (p. 100)
society (p. 97)
stereotype (STĔR-ē-ō-tīp, p. 98)
subculture (p. 98)
transcultural nursing (p. 99)
unconscious bias (p. 98)

The United States has been described as a "melting pot" of people from many different countries. This description implies that people are blended so completely together that everyone shares the same values, beliefs, health practices, communication styles, and religion. A better description is to say the country is like a pot of vegetable soup—many different, but distinct, pieces are combined to form a rich assortment. This assortment makes up our **society** (a nation, community, or broad group of people who establish particular aims, beliefs, or standards of living and conduct). In addition, the "soup recipe" is no longer what it had been in the past; as a result, our societal "flavor" is changing.

US Census projections anticipate a decrease in the percentage of the population identifying as the majority, designated as "white only," over the next 40 years. Before the 2000 US Census, respondents had no way to select more than one race. Because of this, the comparison to previous years is not completely accurate. However, the prediction of a decreasing "white only" population is supported by recent data that shows increases in the percentage of minority children under the age of 5. In fact, more than half the population under the age of 1 are a racial minority. The racial composition of the United States will continue to be influenced by immigration as well as family size and multiple race identification. More people are identifying as biracial, Hispanic, and Black (US Census Bureau, 2012).

Despite the changes in the general composition of our country, racial and ethnic differences continue to be risk factors for health problems that extend beyond expected genetic and biological differences. **Health disparities** are preventable, negative health outcomes that disproportionately affect socially and economically disadvantaged populations. As the racial composition changes to include more Hispanic, Black, and biracial individuals, there will also be a greater need to address the health disparities that affect those populations.

Certainly, racial and ethnic groups are not the only groups at risk of lesser health outcomes. Many cultures and subcultures have also increased health risks that can, and should, be addressed with specific interventions aimed at improving health. The nurse's goal is to provide the best care possible. Learning about cultural variations can be a starting point for providing culturally competent care. It is easy to see that the practices that were considered culturally acceptable even a few years ago are not the same as today. To establish a trusting relationship with a patient, the nurse must be receptive to the patient's preferred language and cultural practices and understand that they may change over time.

CULTURE DEFINED

Culture is a set of learned values, beliefs, customs, and practices that are shared by a group and are passed from one generation to another. Because of the influx of diverse cultures, the United States is multicultural and multilingual. Some immigrants have come from areas of the world devastated by wars, natural disasters, famine, and poverty. Sometimes they have had little preparation or time to learn English or American culture before arriving.

Often separate subcultures exist within a given group. A **subculture** shares many characteristics with the primary culture but has characteristic patterns of behavior and ideals that distinguish it from the rest of a cultural group. Even among Americans who have lived here for several generations, these subcultures exist. For example, a person who grew up in the mountains of Appalachia has very different cultural practices than a person from New York City. Understanding of these variables and acceptance of each person as an individual are the first steps in giving holistic care to patients.

Although cultures often differ considerably from one another, they share certain basic characteristics. Box 6.1 identifies four common characteristics of all cultures.

All members of a culture do not exhibit the same behaviors. These variations within a cultural group occur because of individual differences. Examples of these differences are as follows:

- Age
- Amount and type of interaction between younger and older generations
- Degree to which values in current country are adopted
- Dialect or language spoken

Box **6.1**	Common Characteristics of Cultures

Culture is learned, beginning at birth, through language and socialization. Behaviors, values, attitudes, and beliefs are learned within the cultural family system.

Culture tends to be dynamic and ever changing. Language, traditions, and norms of customs may act as stabilizers for a culture.

Members of the same cultural group may share patterns that are present in every culture. These include communication, means of economic and physical survival, transportation systems, family systems, social customs and mores, and religious systems. (Mores are accepted traditional customs, moral attitudes, or manners of a particular social group.)

Culture is an adaptation to specific factors or conditions in a specific location, such as the availability of natural resources. When people are removed from that location, their customs continue even though they are no longer called for in the new setting.

- Gender identity and roles
- Geographic location of country of origin or current residence
- Religion
- Socioeconomic background

CULTURAL COMPETENCE AND TRANSCULTURAL NURSING

People look at the world from their own cultural viewpoint and tend to prefer people who have similar experiences to their own. **Unconscious bias**, or implicit bias, is an unintentional bias that occurs from one's cultural **stereotypes** (an idea or image of a person or culture that is not easily changed). In healthcare, unconscious bias contributes to health inequities (Marcelin, 2019). People often believe that the beliefs and practices of their particular culture are best. This belief is called **cultural bias**. Unconscious bias is an inherent decision-making shortcut that nearly all people possess as a part of brain efficiency. Even though this unconscious bias is a nearly universal human condition, some research suggests that people are very aware of many of their biases and view them as part of their "core values.." (Chamorro-Premuzic, 2020) To meet the needs of patients, the nurse must become aware of their biases and recognize the value and impact of their patients' core values. Nurses need to work toward greater understanding, rather than impose their own perspective on others. It is often easier to identify the faults and biases of others, than it is to identify our own. When the nurse identifies systemic biases, the nurse can advocate for patients by working to address them directly or through service on committees.

The diversity that we see in the United States is not always reflected in the demographics of the people who provide healthcare to our diverse population. Increasing the diversity of health care providers has been shown to improve health care delivery. The improvement in healthcare is most notable in patients that are typically more at risk of negative health outcomes. Unconscious bias does not just affect the ways that nurses interact with patients. It appears to impact the hiring practices of employers. The percentage of health care workers that identify as Black, Hispanic, LGBT, and persons with disabilities are underrepresented when compared to the general population (Marcelin, 2019). Evidence suggests this contributes to health disparities. Learning about cultural differences that exist improves working relationships between members of the health care team. In much the same way that this kind of openness helps in caring for patients, it helps in understanding and accepting differences among nurses and their colleagues.

In the care of patients from many different cultures, the nurse must develop **cultural competence**: the awareness of one's own cultural beliefs and practices and their relation to those of others, which may be different. One way to identify these beliefs and practices is through a self-assessment. This self-assessment is important. Personal beliefs and practices influence, and sometimes put some limitations on, the ability to care for those from other cultures. Understanding personal beliefs enables one to respond to those from different cultures with openness, understanding, and acceptance of cultural differences.

The nurse needs to accept that it is not possible to act the same with all patients and still give effective, individualized, holistic care. Rather than ignore the differences, the nurse should include questions about cultural practices during the nursing process. This information is critical and is important in developing a plan of care to meet patient needs. Box 6.2 gives some guidelines for cultural information that can be gathered in the patient assessment.

Because of the many variations in cultural and subcultural practices, culturally appropriate nursing care is a challenge. Understanding these variables and integrating an understanding into all aspects of nursing care is referred to as **transcultural nursing**. The nurse should strive to achieve a high level of transcultural nursing in day-to-day practices.

It is important to understand that people from different cultures have a variety of practices related to healthcare, treatment methods, and responses to illness and death (see the Evidence-Based Practice box). In many cases, these differences extend to practices related to childbirth and the ways people of different age groups are cared for (see the Lifespan Considerations for Older Adults box). In addition, cultural beliefs frequently affect diet and nutrition. Remember to assess areas that potentially are influenced by cultural factors.

Box 6.2 Cultural Assessment for Health Care

NURSING DATA COLLECTION (OBTAINED THROUGH INTERVIEW OR OBSERVATION)
- What language is used? If the patient does not commonly use English, how well does the patient understand English? Whom does the patient depend on to translate information?
- What cultural practices have the potential to interfere with receiving health care?
- Differences in health care beliefs
- Difficulty with care being performed by members of the opposite sex
- Modesty and privacy concerns
- Personal space practices
- Use of folk medicines or treatments
- What dietary practices have the potential to interfere with treatment for this illness?

INTERVIEW QUESTIONS
- Who will make decisions about your treatment?
- Who is the person in your family who must be involved with health care decisions?
- Will members of your community be asked to help with making decisions about your care?
- Can you describe what is wrong?
- What do you think has caused your problem (illness, condition)?
- Why do you think this has happened at this time?
- Why did it happen to you?
- Why did it affect your (body part)?
- How long have you had this problem?
- Why did you come for help now?
- What do you think will help to clear up your problem?
- Who else do you think can help you?
- Have you gone to this person for help?
- What did the person do?
- Did this treatment help?
- What results do you hope to get from your care?
- How will your illness affect your family?

Modified from Potter PA, Perry AG, Stockert P, et al: *Fundamentals of nursing*, ed 9, St. Louis, 2017, Mosby.

Evidence-Based Practice

Cultural Beliefs and Rituals Regarding Death

EVIDENCE SUMMARY

Although culture and religion are important to people who are dying, and to their families, practices regarding the death of a loved one vary among cultures and religions. Focus groups were used in this research study to find similarities and differences among cultural and religious beliefs, ceremonies, and rituals about death. Many cultures and religions use beliefs for praying, talking, and remembering loved ones. Rituals often accompany ceremonies and are used to delay death, ward off evil, ensure that the dying person is remembered, and help the family cope with the death. All participants in the study indicated that respect and protection of the dying person's soul were important. Many practices that surround death are influenced by religion and culture. Hispanic and Latino rituals often are influenced heavily by Catholicism. African American and Caribbean participants identified the importance of faith, hope, and prayer and similarities were found between Hindu and Buddhist beliefs about funeral arrangements, afterlife, family customs, and Karma.

APPLICATION TO NURSING PRACTICE
- Be aware of religious and cultural preferences when helping patients and families prepare for death.
- Ask families about the rituals and ceremonies they use to help them cope with the death of a loved one.
- Allow patients and families the ability to participate in planning which rituals will be done at the patient's bedside.
- Be sensitive to cultural perceptions regarding organ donation, viewing the body, and preparing for burial.

REFERENCE
Lobar SL, Youngblut JM, Brooten D: Cross-cultural beliefs, ceremonies, and rituals surrounding death of a loved one, *Pediatr Nurs* 32(1):44–50, 2006.

From Potter PA, Perry AG, Stockert P, et al: *Fundamentals of nursing: concepts, process, and practice*, ed 9, St. Louis, 2017, Mosby.

Lifespan Considerations

Older Adults

Cultural Background

- Cultural background has an impact on family dynamics and plays an important role in determining the role and the status of the older person.
- Older adults form a unique cultural group based on shared historical experiences. Often fewer differences are found between two older individuals of diverse cultural backgrounds than between two people of the same culture but from different age groups because of shifts in value systems that occurred over time.
- Some older adults are less tolerant of other cultures as a result of influences or experiences early in their lives, which raises the possibility of misunderstandings and distrust when the caregiver is of a cultural group different from the older person.
- Older people experiencing disturbed cognitive function from Alzheimer's disease or other conditions sometimes speak without regard for the cultural sensitivity of others and thus make hurtful comments to caregivers and other people.
- Older adults may value home remedies and cultural practices regarding health care and sometimes resist the attempts of caregivers to change even their harmful practices. Practices that are not harmful are left alone out of respect for their wishes.

RACE AND ETHNICITY

There are various reasons why a given individual demonstrates a given cultural practice. Perhaps the person is from a foreign country or a region of the United States where that practice is common. Perhaps the person's practice is related to race (a group of people who share biological physical characteristics) and hereditary factors. Ethnicity refers to a group of people who share a common social and cultural heritage based on shared traditions, national origin, and physical and biological characteristics. They often share social practices such as language, religion, dress, music, and food. Factors related to culture, race, and ethnicity often overlap, and many people combine a variety of practices related to several of these factors. It is important to understand that not everyone in a cultural, racial, or ethnic group has identical practices and that each person should be treated in an individual, holistic manner.

ETHNIC AND RACIAL GROUPS IN THE UNITED STATES

The United States is home to people from many cultures. Do not make assumptions about a patient's beliefs or practices based on the person's name, skin color, or language. Assumptions commonly are made about the predominant cultures and subcultures in our country based on one's own family or community. A larger view of our society is necessary for a better understanding of our country.

Changes in the nation's demographic are illustrated in Table 6.1. Significant decreases are noted in the white population accompanied by increases in most other racial groups. The largest increase has occurred in the Hispanic population, which rose from 12.5% to 16.3% of the population between 2000 and 2010. Predictions for the future indicate that this trend will continue and that the minority cultures will, in combination, make up a majority of the US population by the middle of this century (US Census Bureau, Census 2010).

One significant aspect of this diversity is the language used to communicate. New immigrants from these diverse cultures may not speak English or may have a limited grasp of the language. Often the younger members of the family are the ones who help the adults communicate with others outside of the cultural community. Adults frequently bring a young child

Table 6.1 **Changes in Racially Designated and Hispanic Populations, 2000–2010**

| | 2000 | | 2010 | | |
RACE	NUMBER	PERCENTAGE OF TOTAL POPULATION	NUMBER	PERCENTAGE OF TOTAL POPULATION	PERCENT CHANGE
Total population	281,421,906	100.0%	308,745,538	100.0%	+9.7%
White	211,460,626	75.1%	223,553,265	72.4%	−5.7%
Black or African American	34,658,190	12.3%	38,929,319	12.6%	+12.3%
American Indian or Alaska Native	2,475,956	0.9%	2,932,248	0.9%	+18.4%
Asian	10,242,998	3.6%	14,674,252	4.8%	+43.3%
Native Hawaiian and other Pacific Islander	398,835	0.1%	540,013	0.2%	+35.4%
Some other race	15,359,073	5.5%	19,107,368	6.2%	+24.4%
Two or more races	6,826,228	2.4%	9,009,073	2.9%	+32%
Hispanic or Latino (of any race)	35,305,818	12.5%	50,477,594	16.3%	+3.8%

From US Bureau of the Census: Table DP-1: General population and housing characteristics, 2010; US Bureau of the Census: Profile of general population and housing characteristics, 2010. Retrieved from http://factfinder2.census.gov.

along as a translator when shopping or seeking health care. A professional translator is preferable as opposed to a friend or family member to prevent bias, inaccuracy, or compromises in confidentiality. Adults who are asked about personal health issues may be reluctant to answer these questions if answers are translated through their children or grandchildren.

GENDER IDENTITY AND SEXUAL ORIENTATION

Patients that identify as LGBT, sometimes referred to as LGBTQ+, are a part of a community which includes lesbian, gay, bisexual, transgender, queer/questioning, as well as a variety of other gender identities and sexual orientations outside of gender conforming heterosexual relationships. Sexual orientation is not about sexual activity but about the attraction felt toward others. Similarly, gender identity is about the internal sense of self as being male, female, neither male nor female, or being both male and female. Gender identity is not about the clothes one wears, if they choose to have romantic relationships with men or women, or if they ultimately wish to have surgery to modify their outward sexual appearance. It is an internal experience that is a part of that person's identity.

Sexual health and matters affected by sexual health are personal topics. The nurse should perform the history with a goal to obtain necessary information without engaging in irrelevant questions out of personal curiosity. The dignity and privacy of the patient needs to be maintained to the greatest extent possible, just as the nurse would when caring for a non-LGBT patient. The patient's gender identity may be documented as a "trans woman" or a "trans female" to identify a patient that identifies as a woman but was born with male genitalia. The appropriate abbreviation is "M2F" or "MTF" to designate male to female. A "trans man" or "trans male" was born with female genitalia but identifies as male. "F2M" or "FTM" designates the trans man. The trans patient should be addressed with their preferred pronouns, which may be she/her, he/him, or they/them regardless of outward appearance. If the gender identity is in question, it is appropriate to clarify by asking if they have preferred pronouns.

The LGBT community faces many challenges in health care as well as violations of their basic civil and human rights. Social stigma and discrimination contribute to increased victimization and violence. People in the LGBT subculture remain a part of larger cultures, communities, and families that may or may not support their needs. LGBT individuals have an increased risk of substance abuse, mental health problems, and suicide. The use of proper pronouns and respectfully addressing sexual orientation, are measures that can increase access and encourage appropriate use of health care. Additionally, acceptance of LGBT individuals improves their mental health and safety (*Healthy People 2020,* 2020).

INDIVIDUALS WITH DISABILITIES

People with disabilities have barriers to health care and tend to have poorer outcomes. The Centers for Disease Control and Prevention (CDC) defines a disability as "any condition of the body or mind (impairment) that makes it more difficult for the person with the condition to do certain activities (activity limitation) and interact with the world around them (participation restrictions)" (CDC, 2020). The CDC reports that 26% of adults in the United States have some form of disability. The most common disabilities are those of mobility and cognition. People with disabilities have less access to health care and more modifiable risk factors for disease and disease severity. To put it simply, they are not making it to their doctors to learn about behaviors that could improve their health. The rates of obesity, smoking, heart disease, and diabetes are higher in people who have disabilities than in people without disabilities. These missed opportunities for teaching are likely contributing to worsening health. Barriers to health care access include transportation difficulties, financial concerns, and communication challenges (CDC, 2020).

Some disabilities are present at birth and some are acquired. Like the LGBT subculture, people who have the shared experience of having a disability can find their way into a subculture that is not necessarily a part of the family heritage and may be very unfamiliar at first. Disability culture is not a single culture and it is not defined just by the presence of a disability. The experience of a person that has experienced a stroke in adulthood is very different from a person who has had cerebral palsy since birth. Even if both had similar physical limitations the experience of acquiring a disability later in life is different than the experience of the person who has always had the disability. The person who has had the stroke is learning new skills and may be adapting their environment to accommodate the physical limitations. They may have a goal of recovering their previous level of functioning. Adapting to the changes would be a psychological challenge as well as a physical one. The person who has had cerebral palsy likely already has many skills to work around the limitations. Through previous experience, they choose businesses that are designed to meet the needs of all customers, not just the able-bodied ones (Fig. 6.1). The home environment already meets their needs. The psychological state, coping, and adaptation to the environment for these two people would be very different from each other. Both of these individuals may be a part of disability culture, but the person who has adapted to their condition and recognizes the biases toward people with disabilities is more likely to be a part of the culture.

The experience of being disabled is varied. Disability culture recognizes the individuality of each person and their experience. While the experience of having a disability is very different, they often experience similar

Fig. 6.1 Adaptive gym setting. (©iStock.com/FatCamera.)

types of ableism. **Ableism** is discrimination and prejudice toward people with disabilities where the person is defined by their disabilities and preference is given to people without disabilities. A common example of ableism in health care is when the conversation and health questions are directed at someone other than the patient who happens to have a disability. Nurses and other health care providers often direct the questions to the person accompanying the patient and may not even recognize it. There is no logical reason for addressing questions to the guest not in a wheelchair, the one that has both legs, or the sighted friend. It is likely an unconscious bias.

Even in patients that have a cognitive disability, the conversation should be directed to them. When interacting with patients with severe cognitive disability, the patient should be encouraged to voice their concerns and health care preferences. They may or may not have the ability to make their own health care choices. Sometimes the experience of being hospitalized and in a new environment is overwhelming. If a patient with intellectual or developmental disability enters the health care system alone, they may request an advocate. Patients with cognitive difficulties that also find it difficult to communicate may have difficulty making the request. If they do not make the request for an advocate, the nurse may ask if there is an advocate they would like contacted. This can be especially helpful for a patient with autism, a disability that affects communication. Ultimately, the patient should be given as much decision-making authority as possible. The nurse and healthcare team should work with the thought of "presumed competence." The patient is presumed competent unless there is a reason to doubt competence.

Ableism is demonstrated in other types of improper communication. Some patients need assistance or additional time to answer questions. Ask what type of communication is preferred. If a person needs an ASL interpreter, a communication board, or more time to answer their own questions, this should be accommodated. It is acceptable to touch or wave to get the attention of a patient with hearing loss. Patients with severe hearing impairments tend communicate directly and be physically expressive. Communication with the patient should reflect the communication you use with other adults in the room. "Ma'am", "Sir", "Mr.", "Miss.", or "Mrs." are most appropriate unless you have been asked to address them otherwise. People with all types of disabilities also have sexual identities and preferences so you may need to clarify pronouns before using gender specific language.

When people think of disabilities, they often think of visible disabilities. Invisible disabilities include the fatigue and pain experienced with medical conditions and their treatments, learning disorders, and other neurological disorders. It also includes visible disorders that affect the individual but may not have reached the level of severity that it is apparent to most people. With a person with a visible disability, it is usually assumed that they are less capable. Whereas the person with an invisible disability is often expected to do more than they can do or are denied the supports they need to accomplish the task.

Disability etiquette often comes down to treating the person with a disability with respect and not making assumptions. Sometimes mistakes are made. When you make a mistake, apologize and continue giving your best care. People with disabilities are not much different than people without disabilities and most people appreciate a sincere apology. People with disabilities want you to remember that they are people first. In fact, people first language is the way they want to be addressed. "A person with blindness" is more respectful than saying "a blind person." The person who uses a wheelchair is empowered by the mobility it provides. They are not "wheelchair bound." Rather, they utilize a wheelchair for mobility. It is important to recognize appropriate and derogatory terminology. The disability community has several terms that have gone out of favor. This includes the medical terminology of "mental retardation" which is now called a cognitive or intellectual disability. Dwarfism is a diagnosis that may be identified in some little people or people of short stature. The term "dwarf" may or may not be acceptable to the individual of short stature. Not all little people have dwarfism as the reason for short stature. In Spanish, the expectations are similar. Disability does not define the person. As an example, the person with autism would say they have autism (tiene autismo), rather than saying they are autistic (son autistas).

In disability culture, the disability is often seen as a human condition that does not need to be fixed. It needs to be accommodated. Disabilities are largely defined by what the person cannot do that most people can do. The CDC's definitions of disabilities exemplifies this view by defining disabilities by what the person cannot do (CDC, 2020). Making our environment accessible to more people allows them to do more. If you are unsure if a patient needs assistance, ask if they need help. We all need help sometimes. Even if a person is not your patient, if you suspect that a person needs help, you can offer to help. Just do not assume they need help, or worse, give "help" without being asked.

Part of disability etiquette is the respect extended to the person's assistive equipment. Examples of assistive equipment include a talking board, prosthetics, a smart phone, braces, and a simple notebook and pen. Recognize that the patient's assistive equipment is their personal property. Damage or loss of the property can cause the person to lose independence until it is replaced. The replacement of items may be quite expensive and time consuming. The patient's assistive devices are a part of their personal space and should be treated as an extension of the person. Do not touch any device without getting permission from the patient first. This includes wheelchairs. Nurses are very accustomed to transporting hospitalized patients in wheelchairs. If an individual utilizes a wheelchair normally, the nurse should treat the wheelchair as an extension of the person. Ask permission before pushing the chair and do not lean or rest on the chair at any time. When possible, sit at eye level with your patient (United Cerebral Palsy, 2018). To learn more about disability etiquette for specific conditions, visit United Cerebral Palsy's website at ucp.org.

CULTURALLY RELATED ASSESSMENTS

To care for a patient from a different culture, the nurse should assess the patient's beliefs. Patients cannot be expected to accept care and health teaching if they do not believe that the practices will help them to recover.

Brief examples of specific beliefs and practices of some cultures are presented later in this chapter. Stereotyping an individual according to common cultural practices should be avoided. The individual may or may not accept all of the practices within a culture or subculture.

When the nurse assesses a patient, several areas should be explored: communication, space, time, social organization, religious beliefs, health practices, and biological variations.

VERBAL COMMUNICATION

The most apparent communication variation is the language spoken. Whether the nurse and the patient can understand each other must be determined. When patients do not understand what is being said, they sometimes say "yes" or nod their head nonetheless, giving the mistaken impression of agreeing with the nurse. Many people do this to avoid embarrassment or to be polite. The nurse must not assume that the patient or the family understands.

Sometimes the patient understands some English, or the nurse speaks some of the patient's language. If patients have a poor grasp of English, they may tire quickly when trying to understand what is being said. In addition, medical terminology potentiates an even greater risk without a medical interpreter in the native language of the client. Questions and directions should be kept brief and simple. It is better to provide more information later than to give long explanations. Sometimes, the patient's ability to read written English is better than his or her speaking ability. In such cases, the patient benefits from written explanations accompanied by pictures when possible.

The preferred approach is the use of a professional interpreter. Many health care facilities have employees on call to translate when a language barrier exists. Availability of a translator may require that the nurse work with a family member who is able to translate. Note that this intervention affects confidentiality surrounding the patient's care. The patient must understand essential information such as why care is being given and why medications are ordered. The nurse's responsibility is to make every effort to provide this information to the patient. Use of effective communication techniques is beneficial as the nurse cares for patients from different cultures (Box 6.3).

Even among English-speaking people, different cultural groups assign different meanings to the same words. For example, a person from the United Kingdom may say he is going to take the "lift." An American may not understand that this refers to an elevator. Within the United States, the variety of regional accents further complicates communication. People from different areas of the country (e.g., people from the north and the south) often struggle to understand each other because of the different accents or regional expressions they use. Some cultural or regional groups speak very rapidly, which adds to the difficulty of understanding. In addition, people from Spain use many words with different meaning than that of Spanish people from Central America.

Other cultural patterns also play a role in communication. In some cultural groups, many family members commonly accompany a person to the health care setting. Large groups of family members tend to make communication difficult. They sometimes all try to assist by answering at once. Or perhaps, when in the presence of strangers, a person from another group only answers direct questions and thus appears rude or uncommunicative. Unfortunately, the appearance of rudeness is a common by-product of a cross-cultural mismatch in communication. Sometimes a person speaks more loudly to emphasize a point out of the mistaken belief that this helps the listener understand better. In fact, it often has the opposite effect of the one desired. Members of some cultures interpret the raised voice as rudeness or aggression and shut out the sound altogether.

| Box 6.3 | Strategies for Communication With Patients From Different Cultures |

- Take a little extra time to establish a level of comfort between you and the patient.
- Ask questions in an unhurried and calm manner. Rephrase a question and ask it again if the answer seems inconsistent with other information the patient has provided.
- Observe the cultural differences in communication and honor those differences. Use eye contact, touch, and seating arrangements that are comfortable for the patient.
- Ask patients about the meaning of health and illness and their understanding of treatments and planned care. Investigate how the illness is likely to affect their life, relationships, and self-concept. Find out what patients consider to be the cause of their illness. Ask how patients prefer to manage their illness.
- To establish a therapeutic relationship, listen to the patients' perceptions of their needs, and respect the patients' perspectives.
- Listen actively and attentively; try not to anticipate the patient's response.
- Talk to patients in an unhurried manner that considers social and cultural amenities.
- Give patients time to answer.
- Use validation techniques to verify that the patient understands. Remember that smiles and head nodding may indicate that the patient is trying to please the nurse, not necessarily that the nurse is understood.
- Sexual concerns may be difficult for patients to discuss. Having a nurse of the same gender may facilitate communication.
- Use alternative methods of communication, such as a foreign language phrase book, an interpreter, gestures, or pictures, for patients who do not speak English.
- Learn key phrases in languages that are commonly spoken in your community.

From Harkreader H, Hogan MA, Thobaben M: *Fundamentals of nursing: caring and clinical judgment,* ed 4, Philadelphia, 2007, Saunders.

Consider, in contrast, the use of silence. Silence indicates many things to many cultures: a lack of understanding, stubbornness, apprehension, discomfort, agreement, disagreement, respect, or disdain. In some cultures, the presence of silence may result in feelings of discomfort and anxiety. It is not uncommon for people to make attempts to fill periods of silence with conversation. Among American Indian, Chinese, and Japanese cultures, silence sometimes is used to allow the listener to consider what the speaker has said before continuing. Members of other cultures, such as Russians, the French, and the Spanish, tend to become silent to indicate consensus between parties. In Asian cultures, people often use silence as a sign of respect, especially to elders (see the Cultural Considerations box). In contrast, people from other cultures, such as those of Mexican descent, may use silence when they disagree with a person of authority.

🌐 Cultural Considerations

Culturally Sensitive Communication

- It should be noted that any reference to cultural practices among a specific culture are commonalities. Individuals within a culture may or may not possess the same practices, beliefs, or values.
- Ask all patients how they like to be addressed. If in doubt, address them formally.
- Determine the patient's preferences for touch. For example, Americans often greet each other with a firm handshake. Many Native Americans, however, see this as a sign of aggression. Touch outside of marriage sometimes is forbidden in older adults from the Middle East.
- Investigate the patient's preferences for silence. Generally, Eastern cultures value silence, whereas Western cultures are uncomfortable with silence.
- Be aware of the patient's beliefs about eye contact during conversation. Direct eye contact in European American cultures is a sign of honesty and truthfulness. Older Native Americans may avoid eye contact. Asian adults sometimes avoid eye contact with authority figures because this is considered disrespectful, and direct eye contact between the sexes in Middle Eastern cultures sometimes is forbidden except between spouses.

From Potter PA, Perry AG, Stockert P, et al: *Fundamentals of nursing,* ed 9, St. Louis, 2017, Mosby; Meiner SE: *Gerontologic nursing,* ed 4, St. Louis, 2010, Mosby.

NONVERBAL COMMUNICATION

Nonverbal communication is usually expressed through body language. Some groups are more comfortable than others with touching or maintaining eye contact. Touch is particularly culturally or regionally related. In parts of the United States, many people consider even casual touching inappropriate. In other regions, casual touch and embracing between acquaintances is the norm. Recent immigrants from England and Germany may be less likely to touch each other in public or allow casual touching by strangers. Spanish, French, Italian, Jewish, and South American individuals are likely to be much more comfortable about touching each other and being touched.

Eye contact also has significant cultural interpretations. Many people in the United States regard maintaining eye contact as an indication of openness, interest in others, attentiveness, and honesty. Lack of eye contact thus is interpreted as a sign of shyness, humility, guilt, embarrassment, rudeness, thoughtlessness, or dishonesty. Other cultures have various other reasons for not maintaining eye contact. Some Asian cultures and American Indians relate eye contact to impoliteness or an invasion of privacy. Certain East Indian cultures avoid eye contact with people of lower or higher socioeconomic classes. Among some Appalachian people, maintaining eye contact indicates hostility or aggressiveness.

Body language and gestures often are related culturally. In the United States, certain gestures generally are understood by most people who have lived in the United States for an extended period of time. However, some commonly used gestures have the potential to offend someone from another culture. For example, a "thumbs up" hand gesture conveys acceptance or a "good job" in the United States. To someone from another culture this may mean something else that may not have a positive connotation. Traditionally, Italian people use a great deal of hand gestures when communicating.

Assessing the communication variables of a patient from another culture is important. First, an assessment of cultural factors is performed; then the nurse has to respond appropriately. Every effort should be made to communicate with others at their personal level of comfort to establish good rapport. If the patient is from a culture that avoids eye contact, try to look away when talking with the patient. If touch is unacceptable among casual acquaintances, avoid patting the shoulder or touching a hand when talking with the patient. The nurse should be sensitive to any difficulty a patient is having with the more intimate touching that inevitably accompanies many nursing interventions.

Violations of cultural beliefs and practices by the nurse are likely to interfere with establishing a therapeutic relationship with the patient and the patient's family. Do not expect to completely adjust individual personal cultural practices but try to understand and accept the differences among practices in various cultures. Do not judge the patient's behavior according to personal practices.

AMERICAN SIGN LANGUAGE

American Sign Language (ASL) is the primary language spoken by many Americans who are deaf. The language incorporates both verbal and nonverbal aspects of communication. Individuals that use ASL use hand positions and movements as well as facial expressions and expressive movements to complete the meaning beyond the words. For many people, ASL holds greater meaning than the language spoken. It is a key component of a subculture known as "Deaf culture." Deaf culture is more than communicating with ASL and it is more than hearing loss. People immersed in Deaf culture, have often attended schools where classes are taught in ASL and have an ASL speaking community. Within this culture, being deaf is not seen as a disability, nor is it something that needs "fixed." The nurse needs to keep in mind that people with deafness or significant hearing loss may or may not be a part of Deaf culture and may or may not view hearing loss as a disability. Regardless, a person with ASL as the primary language may need an interpreter, just like other non-native English speakers. Members of American Deaf culture may have different social expectations, communication style, and beliefs than those of Americans not a part of this subculture.

SPACE

Cultural interpretation of space varies and is an important element of assessment. Cultures assign different comfort areas and meanings to personal space. In the United States, people are often more comfortable when given a larger amount of personal space than what is common in many other countries. Closer contact is reserved for more intimate relationships. Members of some cultures are accustomed to more close contact, which may be interpreted as an invasion of one's space in other cultures. A nurse who is receptive to the patient's interpretation of a comfortable space may find it easier to establish a therapeutic relationship. Occasionally, the need for personal space also is manifest in a desire to use a certain space. For example, perhaps a resident in a nursing home always wishes to sit in a particular chair or in a specific part of the room. Another resident chooses to sit at the same table for each meal. A change in any of these arrangements may cause either of these residents to become upset.

TIME

The measurement of time and the rhythms of people's activities and interactions often have different meanings in various cultures. These different meanings have the potential to create some problems in the care of patients from other cultures. Traditional nursing practice emphasizes that medications and treatments are provided on a rigid schedule. The United States and many Northern European cultures generally give a high priority to being on time for appointments, and people typically expect everyone to follow this pattern. Japanese American culture also places emphasis on promptness and the adherence to fixed schedules, especially when meeting with a person who is regarded highly. People in many cultures believe that other concerns regarding time are more important. In Eastern cultures, including Chinese, East Indian Hindu, Filipino, and Korean, schedules and time are much more flexible concepts. Some Asians spend a lot of time getting to know someone and view abrupt endings to a conversation as rude. Mexican Americans may be late for an appointment because they focus more on a current activity and are less concerned about a previously planned meeting. According to Giger (2017), this concept, known as "elasticity," implies that future activities are possible to recover but not present ones. If these cultural differences are not understood, the nurse may feel angry when a patient is late for an appointment, fails to come at all, or does not follow therapeutic schedules. Similarly, health care providers should strive to plan for and communicate realistic wait times for procedures and appointments. In lower-income areas, patients may rely more heavily on public transportation or family and friends to get to appointments. In communities where patients have less control over transportation, patients may have a more relaxed outlook about schedules. In areas with fewer transportation barriers, appointments may be seen as more rigid. Long wait times may be seen as a lack of respect for the patient's time.

Perception of time or time orientation also varies among cultures. Many people in the United States tend to be future oriented. Present actions are taken based on a future outcome. An example is a person who takes medication to treat hypertension to prevent illness. Among members of other cultures, notably African American or Black, Hispanic, and American Indian, individuals tend to be more present-oriented. Sometimes, like people described previously who prolong a current encounter rather than rushing off to be on time for another one, a present-oriented person chooses to satisfy a current, more urgent need rather than prepare for a less immediate one that is in the future. A pregnant woman, for instance, may miss her own health care provider's appointments to take care of her family; if her older child needs a ride to school, the mother skips the appointment and drives the child. A patient with this belief system is often difficult to encourage to follow through on treatment for a chronic illness. Such a patient perhaps views the cost of a medication for hypertension to prevent future problems as an optional expense. Paying the rent or buying food for the family is a current need that takes precedence.

SOCIAL ORGANIZATION

Cultural behavior is socially acquired, not genetically inherited. How nurses react to members of other cultures reflects an internalized response that is part of their own culture. Often, we are not aware of the strong impact these patterns of cultural behavior have each day in our lives. We may behave in a hostile manner toward a person of a particular ethnic group or a person with a different skin color merely because of a culture-related belief. It is important to recognize these biases and to deal with them rationally. Understanding other cultures and that one culture is not superior over another helps to overcome prejudices that have nothing to do with an individual.

Self-concept is also influenced by culture and cultural identity. Individuals view themselves as part of a particular social group. They describe themselves in terms such as "African American" or "Black," "Hispanic," "German American," "Irish Catholic," or "Texan." Clearly, these descriptions vary greatly. What is important is to understand how the person sees herself or himself. A good cultural assessment takes this self-description into account.

The varying social structures within a culture also have an impact on how individuals and families function. Some cultures are patriarchal, and the men (often the oldest) make most of the decisions. In a culture that is matriarchal, the women usually make the decisions about health care, provide the care, and discipline the children. The structure of the family is important

to determine in a health care setting. For example, a family in a patriarchal society sometimes delays any decision making regarding health care for one of the family members until the oldest man in the family is consulted. Another family, in a matriarchal society, expects the women to give care to a family member in the hospital.

The description of family may differ among cultures. Some family structures are based on biological relationships. Others are based on meeting basic needs for family by forming a group among unrelated individuals. Knowledge of the family structure assists the nurse to better understand the patient. A common mistake is to assume that every family is a traditional nuclear family. In fact, this family structure is becoming increasingly rare. Knowing who the patient depends on for comfort and decision making and how the patient describes the family or support system is more important.

RELIGIOUS BELIEFS AND HEALTH CARE

Religious beliefs frequently are entwined with cultural beliefs. Some cultures expect all members to adhere to a particular religion. In these societies, religious and cultural beliefs are difficult to separate. In the United States, wide variations are found in religious practices. In addition, as people from varying cultures intermarry, religious practices also become more varied.

Data for religious affiliations are not collected by the US Bureau of the Census, making an accurate way to determine the numbers of followers of the various religions in the United States difficult. Despite the inability to quantify the religious preferences in the country, nursing care clearly is affected by patients' religious beliefs and practices. The nurse must be aware of and open to the wide range of such beliefs to ensure that care provided is sensitive to the needs of individual patients.

Assessment of family and social organization becomes increasingly more complicated as our society brings together more and more diverse cultures. It is not unusual for a family to be bicultural or biracial or to follow two different faith practices. Be constantly on guard against making assumptions about patients based on appearance, language, ethnic origin, names, or religious practices. Assessment of the individual and family on their own terms helps the nurse to understand each person.

HEALTH PRACTICES

For many years, the belief popular in the United States was that modern biomedical health care was the best and only way to treat diseases. The **biomedical health belief system** remains the primary method of preventing and treating diseases in the United States. The biomedical model is characterized by a scientific, mechanical belief that does not include spiritual beliefs and separates the issues of the mind from those of the body. https://geriatrics.stanford.edu/culturemed/overview/knowledge_fund/belief_systems.html Today many health care providers still find it difficult to believe that any alternative therapies are as effective as the biomedical methods that they have seen used for many years. In recent years, a variety of alternative health services such as folk remedies, holistic therapies, and spiritual interventions have aroused attention in the traditional medical community. Scientific research is being done in these areas to determine the effectiveness of these methods. Some are now accepted more readily and sometimes are used concurrently with biomedical methods (see Chapter 20).

Several factors are driving this change in thinking about health care. Some of the long-established methods have become less effective, notably antibiotics used to treat infections. A number of complementary therapies and folk remedies have been shown effective in treatment of certain diseases. More health care providers with varied backgrounds and beliefs about health and illness now practice in the United States. Increasing mobility and use of electronic media have resulted in more sharing of information, which has promoted diversity. Movement of cultural groups to new areas provides exposure of new information and methods of managing health issues (Fig. 6.2). Some health care practices among cultures are benign and ineffective, and others are therapeutic and useful. The concern lies with those that can pose danger to health and wellness. It is important to allow patients to follow practices that are in accordance with their cultural identity and personal beliefs when they are receiving health care in the traditional health care system, without allowing the effectiveness of either approach to be compromised. The characteristics of four basic concepts of health beliefs are described in Table 6.2. For many

Fig. 6.2 While providing information in a home care setting, a nurse compares traditional and Western remedies. Culture influences how people perceive health, illness, and pain. The nurse must take cultural variations into account to effectively communicate with patients and their families.

years, Western cultures have used almost universally the biomedical method of treating illness and maintaining health. **Folk medicine** are the traditional healing practices that are passed down within a culture. Folk medicine often includes herbs, foods, rituals, and spiritual practices. There is no single system of folk remedies and the folk remedies of one culture can differ greatly from the next. It often includes native healers who may incorporate religious practices and magic (Fig. 6.3).

Do not assume that patients born in the United States accept the biomedical view of health care. Individuals in many subcultures of the United States practice folk medicine. These people sometimes avoid seeking care from health care providers or practice folk medicine while also receiving traditional care. The Appalachian people have many traditions that have been passed down for common ailments. Like folk medicine practiced in other parts of the world, foods, herbs, and rituals are part of the remedies. The Appalachian folk medicine practices are not unlike other folk medicine in that some of the remedies are safe and effective, some are not dangerous but also not effective, and some are unsafe practices (Medicinal Remedies From Appalachia, 2012)

As our medical system becomes more open to considering a variety of alternative health care systems, the nurse is expected to understand the relationships between different views. Assessing the health practices of patients is an important part of achieving this understanding. If individual beliefs are discussed openly, the patient probably will be more willing to tell the nurse about using other health care methods in addition to those directed by the health care provider. Be aware that this information must be shared with the doctor to prevent conflicts among treatments.

BIOLOGICAL VARIATIONS

Cultural groups are identified in a variety of ways. In some instances, the members share strong biological characteristics. This is especially true if the cultural group is made up primarily of individuals from a particular race or geographic region. When assessing these individuals, include these characteristics. Some of the obvious ones are body structure, skin color, and hair color and texture. For example, the nurse probably expects a cultural group from the Scandinavian region to have many people with blond hair and blue eyes. Asians are likely to have straight, coarse, dark hair. More important to health care practice is a family history of diseases that are common within the ethnic group. Some diseases, such as sickle cell anemia, are found more frequently among those of African ancestry. Other diseases, such as diabetes, asthma, or heart disease, tend to be more prevalent among certain cultural groups. Even with consideration of diet, diabetes occurs more frequently among American Indians.

Table 6.2   Health Belief Systems

BELIEF SYSTEM	CHARACTERISTICS
Biomedical health belief system	Life is regulated by biomedical and physical processes. Life processes can be manipulated by humans with mechanical interventions. Health is the absence of disease or signs and symptoms of disease. Disease is an alteration of the structure and function of the body. Disease has a specific cause, onset, course, and treatment. It is caused by trauma, pathogens, chemical imbalances, or failure of body parts. Treatment focuses on the use of physical and chemical interventions.
Folk health belief system	This commonly is referred to as "third-world" beliefs and practices. It often is called strange or weird by nurses and other health professionals who are unfamiliar with folk medicine beliefs. In most instances, these practices do not seem "strange or weird" once health care providers become acquainted with them. This system classifies illnesses or diseases as natural or unnatural. According to this belief system, natural events have to do with the world as God made it and as God intended it to be. Thus there is a certain amount of predictability for daily life. Unnatural events imply the exact opposite because they upset the harmony of nature. Thus unnatural events are those events that interrupt the plan intended by God and at their very worst represent the forces of evil and the machinations of the devil. They have no predictability and are beyond the control of ordinary mortals. Treatment is done by carrying out rituals or repentance or giving in to the supernatural force's wishes.
Holistic health belief system	Religious experiences are based on cultural beliefs and may include such things as blessings from spiritual leaders, apparitions of dead relatives, and even miracle cures. Healing powers also may be ascribed to animate or inanimate objects. Religion dictates social, moral, and dietary practices designed to assist an individual in maintaining a healthy balance and in playing a vital role in illness prevention (e.g., burning of candles, rituals of redemption, and prayer). Baptism may be seen as a ritual of cleansing and dedication and prevention of evil. Anointing the sick may be seen as preparation for death and also may be performed as the hope of a miracle. Circumcision also is viewed as a religious practice. Treatment is designed to restore balance with physical, social, and metaphysical worlds. It may extend beyond treating the person to treating the environment to decrease pollution or prevent hunger, homelessness, etc.
Alternative or complementary belief system	Today many Americans use one or more nonmedical forms of therapy to treat an illness. Acupuncture, aromatic therapy, meditation, therapeutic touch, and a variety of other techniques provide feasible alternative therapies (see Chapter 20). Alternative therapies address the whole patient by viewing symptoms as the tip of the iceberg and as the body's means for communicating to the mind that something must be changed, removed, or added to one's life. The mind and body are seen as a whole unit.

Data from Giger JM: *Transcultural nursing: assessment and intervention,* ed 7, St. Louis, 2017, Elsevier.

Another important health consideration is the effect of culturally determined dietary practices. Many traditional foods are high in saturated fats, sodium, and sugar. If these foods are eaten frequently, they have the potential to affect patients' health and the health of their family members. In some cases, members of some cultural groups have dietary deficiencies caused by low intake of protein, complex carbohydrates, and fresh fruits and vegetables. When assessing the patient, include questions to determine whether the patient follows cultural dietary practices or eats a more general diet. Several diverse cultural groups (Chinese, Korean, Mexican, Puerto Rican, and Vietnamese) have beliefs that diseases and foods are classified as either "hot" or "cold." The diet is adjusted according to the perceived balance, and thus diseases are treated with the proper foods. This practice sometimes leads to a failure to meet basic nutritional needs and to dietary problems (see Chapter 19).

NURSING PROCESS AND CULTURAL FACTORS

When caring for patients, the nurse typically uses the nursing process to develop a plan of care. With use of the information gathered in an assessment, cultural behaviors can be determined and included in a plan of care accordingly.

North American Nursing Diagnosis Association–International (NANDA-I) nursing diagnoses and similar patient problem statements may be difficult to appropriately apply to culturally diverse patients. People from other cultures often do not share the biomedical health belief system on which these diagnoses or problems are based. Classifying patient problems and needs according to a rigid standard is unrealistic. Unfortunately, a patient's behavior may be labeled as abnormal when it is actually normal in the person's own cultural context. The difficulties go even further, however. The goal of the nursing diagnosis or patient

Fig. 6.3 Within the Mexican American folk medicine system, the *curandero* is the folk healer. (From Harkreader H, Hogan MA: *Fundamentals of nursing: caring and clinical judgment*, ed 3, Philadelphia, 2007, Saunders.)

problem system is to help change patient behavior; however, doing so by imposing biomedically based health care beliefs and practices without regard to cultural identity violates the basic tenets of nursing's patient-centered approach.

Certain nursing diagnoses or problem statements are particularly difficult to tailor to particular patients. It is necessary to be cautious with using nursing diagnoses or patient problem statements such as *Insufficient Knowledge, Compromised Verbal Communication, Impaired Health Maintenance,* and *Noncooperation.*

To provide care and lessen the limitations of the NANDA-I nursing diagnoses or patient problem statements, patient behavior should be evaluated from the perspective of the individual's culture. The nurse, the health care system, or both may be required to change to accommodate, maintain, or reinforce the patient's health beliefs and practices. Perhaps the nurse will do this by reprioritizing nursing goals and changing procedures. A compromise is important between individual health beliefs and practices and those of the patient. The patient and family or support system are unlikely to accept any of the health teaching or treatments the nurse attempts to provide if their own beliefs are not recognized. A mutually acceptable alliance with the patient is imperative. Equally important is a mutual respect between the patient and nurse. If the patient defers health care decisions to clergy, a family member, or a significant other, it is also important for the nurse to recognize and communicate respectfully with that person, if possible, under the guidelines of the Health Insurance Portability and Accountability Act (HIPAA). If the nurse or health care team does not recognize this relationship and respect the dynamics, then compliance is in jeopardy in the event of a conflict. Remember that the ultimate goal is to assist the patient to achieve optimal health. One implication of this is that the nurse may need to adjust many of the accepted nursing interventions to accommodate patients and their cultures.

Because of a patient's cultural background, the nurse sometimes must modify how an assessment is performed or care is provided or must adapt the usual routines of the institution to the patient's needs. For instance, consideration should be given when accommodating cultural practices among Muslim patients. The nurse should allow Muslim women to keep the head, arms, and legs covered as much as possible. In addition, every attempt should be made to assign female staff members to care for Muslim women. Because Muslims pray several times each day, care should be scheduled around these times to allow the patient privacy and the necessary leisure to pray. The nurse should be ready to consider similar accommodations to meet the needs of patients in other culturally dependent, special circumstances.

CULTURAL PRACTICES OF SPECIFIC GROUPS

Hispanics make up a large percentage of the population in the United States and account for as much as 50% of the population in some counties. Subcultures also exist within the Hispanic culture, and Hispanics' origins vary as well. According to the 2010 US Census Bureau report, the largest Mexican populations are found in areas of California, Texas, Illinois, and Arizona. Puerto Ricans are concentrated in New York, Florida, Illinois, and Pennsylvania. About two-thirds of all Cubans in the United States live in Florida (US Census Bureau, Census 2010). Although these groups share some common beliefs, they each have distinct practices. The place of origin is important to determine when caring for a Hispanic patient.

Numerous tribes of American Indians live throughout various regions of the United States (US Census Bureau, Census 2010). Nursing care of this population is complicated by the fact that each nation or tribe of American Indians has its own language, religion, and belief system. Practices differ significantly among groups and among members of the same tribe. When the term "American Indian" is used, it is intended to refer to tribes residing within the continental United States. The nurse should respect how a person wishes to be identified. Patients may prefer to be identified based on their specific tribe or they may prefer another term such as Indigenous People, Native Americans, American "Indians, Native People, or First Nations". Preferred terms used in the United States may be offensive in Canada; https://www.infoplease.com/history/native-american-heritage/american-indian-versus-native-american

A complete picture of all cultural practices and beliefs for groups living in the United States is impossible in the context of this chapter. Table 6.3 gives examples

Table 6.3 **Cultural Beliefs and Practices***

MEXICAN AMERICANS	AFRICAN AMERICANS	CHINESE AMERICANS	MUSLIM AMERICANS	AMERICAN INDIANS
Predominant Health Belief System				
Sometimes accept biomedical, but belief system is often heavily mixed with folk practices.	Highly diverse. Many adhere to biomedical system. Others, particularly from rural areas, more closely follow folk health beliefs. Often the two belief systems are practiced concurrently. Prayer is important.	Holistic belief system is primary influence. Accept biomedical interventions for serious illness, but possibly continue to practice traditional methods to reestablish natural balance.	Holistic. Essential to preserve modesty and privacy. Obligatory to keep body parts covered as much as possible. Use same-sex health care providers if at all possible. Always examine a female patient in presence of another female. Patient may wish to have doctor consult with Imam (religious leader) when planning care.	Historically, American Indians have been guided by sacred myths and legends that describe the tribes' evolution from inception to the present time. Supernatural beings portrayed in these stories symbolize the culture in which religion and healing practices are blended. Values and beliefs intrinsic to culture and religion form the day-to-day living experiences. Traditional American Indian concepts focus on the need for the individual to be in harmony with the surrounding environment and with the family. Health and religion cannot be separated within the American Indian culture.
Language				
Spanish, often mixed with English. Children often are better able to speak English and sometimes translate for adults. Some adults never learn English.	English is understood and used when speaking with those outside of cultural group. Black English dialect sometimes is used when speaking with family and friends. Words commonly used in this dialect sometimes are intermixed with standard English when speaking with those in outside community.	Sometimes continue to speak native language even after many years in United States. It is possible to view this as honoring ancestors and native country. Learning to speak English is often difficult because there is little common basis for pronunciation, written characters, or word order.	Varies with country of origin. New immigrants often need family member or community leader to help with translations.	American Indian language has been shown to be derived from the languages used by the people in northwestern Canada. It is also similar to the language spoken by some people living in Alaska, some on the northern coast of the Pacific Ocean, and some in northern California. The language involves tonal speech in which the pitch is of great importance. Every vowel and consonant are fully sounded, regardless of how many times they are doubled or tripled within a word. Vowels are often interchanged, creating several variations and meanings of a word. Even today, many American Indians still speak the native language and are fluent in English, but some do not speak English and need the assistance of an interpreter.

Table 6.3	Cultural Beliefs and Practices—cont'd

MEXICAN AMERICANS	AFRICAN AMERICANS	CHINESE AMERICANS	MUSLIM AMERICANS	AMERICAN INDIANS
Communication				
Sustained direct eye contact is considered rude, immodest, or dangerous. Women and children are susceptible to *mal ojo* (evil eye) and so avoid eye contact. Touch is used often. Touch has potential to neutralize mal ojo. Closeness and physical contact are valued in familiar situations. Modesty is highly valued, so it is possible that men and women will be embarrassed when exposure of body is necessary.	Personal space comfort area tends to be close. Eye contact is sometimes uncomfortable, especially among older generation.	Maintaining eye contact often is considered ill-mannered and disrespectful. Uncomfortable when face to face. Prefer to sit side-to-side or at right angles to carry on conversation. Touching is not usual during conversation; it is regarded as disrespectful or impolite. Touch possibly acceptable among same-sex acquaintances, but touching in public between opposite sexes is not acceptable.	Women do not usually shake hands with men. Women prefer to keep head, arms, and legs covered. Allow Imam to visit. Allow privacy to pray. Identify Muslim patients on chart and bracelet. Post signs to alert male staff members to avoid room with female Muslim patient.	Until recently, the Navajo language was unwritten. In World War II, a special branch of the US Marine Corps was developed for Navajos who served as Navajo code talkers. It has been estimated that this highly esteemed group saved millions of lives because the enemy was unable to understand the Navajo language or infiltrate the code. Instead of shaking hands, people of this culture extend a hand and lightly touch the hand of the person they are greeting. Initially these people are silent and reserved, but once they become familiar, warm behavior usually is demonstrated. When introducing themselves by name, they give honor to ancestors by stating the clan and the location of their home area. They avoid eye contact, which is considered a sign of disrespect.
Family Roles				
Families sometimes expect to help care for patient. Male family members usually are consulted before health care decisions are made. Only a wife is permitted to give care to husband at home if genitalia are touched.	Women are primary decision makers in family and are frequently head of the household. Extended family plays important role. Even when not related by blood, close ties exist. May refer to these people as "Aunt," "Uncle," "Grandmother," and include them in family decisions.	Loyalty and devotion to family is more important than individual feelings. Taking care of family members brings honor to family. Older children have authority over younger children in family. Decision making is organized in this way, and younger siblings must show respect and deference or it shames the family.	Decision-making unit is the family, not the individual. Husband is consulted in any decisions about family. Imam often included in health-related decisions.	This culture is extremely family oriented, but "family" has a much broader meaning than just father, mother, and children. The biological family is the center of social organizations and includes all members of the extended family. They are traditionally a matriarchal society. Thus, when a couple marries, the husband makes his home with his wife's relatives and his family becomes one of several units that live in a group of adjacent hogans or other type of dwelling.

Continued

Table 6.3   Cultural Beliefs and Practices—cont'd

MEXICAN AMERICANS	AFRICAN AMERICANS	CHINESE AMERICANS	MUSLIM AMERICANS	AMERICAN INDIANS
				Usually, a male family member who is looked on as having the greatest amount of prestige rises as leader for the extended family and provides necessary direction. However, in settling issues, all sides are listened to and the entire group determines the outcome. To be without relatives is to be really poor.

Birth Rites

The husband may not be present during birth. Female family members sometimes request to be present during labor and delivery.	Many folk customs potentially influence birth. Mother often supported through birth process by female family members. Breast-feeding initiation after birth in this population is less at 69% compared with rates of white infants at 89% (Beauregard, et. al., 2019).	Fathers generally are not present in labor and delivery areas. Some mothers prefer acupuncture for birth rather than Western pain-control methods. Traditionally, mother does not see child for 12–24 h.	Men are not present during labor and delivery. Some husbands wish to be present during the birth process. Women seek a female physician. Pregnant women are exempt from fasting during Ramadan, the sacred ninth month during which Muslims fast from food and drink from dawn to dusk.	The tradition of massaging the newborn baby as a bonding experience between the mother and baby is still practiced. Assistance with ceremonies, particularly those associated with birth, is shared and has great importance. After delivery, the umbilical cord is taken from the newborn, dried, and buried near an object or place that symbolizes what the parents want for the child's future. The infant death rate remains disproportionately high for American Indians.

Death Rites

Small children are shielded from the dying and death scene. Families take turns staying around the clock with the dying person. Grief sometimes is expressed with hyperkinetic or seizure type of behavior that serves to release emotions.	Extended family is very supportive during final illness. Family members generally take turns staying with dying person. Some fear touching the body or being present when a person has died.	Often have aversion to death and anything concerning death. Donation of body parts is encouraged. Eldest son is responsible for all arrangements for the deceased. White, yellow, or black clothing is worn as sign of mourning.	Life is unique and precious; any intervention to hasten death is forbidden. Autopsy is acceptable with medical and legal need. It is important to allow family and Imam to follow Islamic practices to prepare body for funeral. Organ donations are permitted.	Assistance with ceremonies, particularly those associated with death, is a shared responsibility and has great importance. People of this culture have a taboo against touching a dead person or any article associated with the deceased individual. Taboos associated with death in a hogan include the need to seal the entry and warn others to stay away; frequently the need to abandon or burn the hogan is observed.

Table 6.3   Cultural Beliefs and Practices—cont'd

MEXICAN AMERICANS	AFRICAN AMERICANS	CHINESE AMERICANS	MUSLIM AMERICANS	AMERICAN INDIANS
Dietary Practices				
Lactose intolerance is sometimes present. Eggs, rice, corn, and beans are good sources of protein. Meats include beef, pork, poultry, and goat. Diet is high in fat because frying is common method of cooking. Fruits and vegetables that are native are included in diet. Sometimes there is an inadequacy in calcium, iron, vitamin A, folic acid, and vitamin C.	High incidence of lactose intolerance, so intake of milk and milk products is low. Many celebrations and rites revolve around food and feasting on traditional dishes (soul food). Traditional dishes such as collard greens, other leafy and yellow vegetables, legumes, beans, rice, and potatoes are high in nutritive value. Overall, the diet tends to be low in fiber, calcium, and potassium and high in fat. Dietary restrictions sometimes related to religious practices.	Diet is low in fat and sugar. Fat intake is limited because of cooking methods. Fish, pork, and poultry, and nuts, dried beans, and tofu, are protein sources. Milk products are avoided because of lactose intolerance. Salt intake sometimes high as a result of eating preserved foods and seasoning with soy sauce. Rice is eaten with almost every meal.	Fasting during daylight hours during Ramadan. Medical condition often exempts person from fasting. Allow family to provide meals if allowed with treatment. Alcohol and drugs are forbidden. Ensure that no pork products are included in foods.	Lack of food and food storage sometimes contributes to nutritional deficiencies. Lactose intolerance is extremely prevalent, affecting 79% of the American Indian population. One hypothesis suggests that some have a predisposition for diabetes that is seemingly triggered by changes in dietary practices and increasing obesity. Contemporary American Indian diet combines food indigenous to the areas with modern processed foods. Food practices are also influenced by tribal beliefs, practices, geographic area, and local availability of selected food. Foods preferred by many include meat and blue cornmeal. Milk is not a preferred food. The fat intake is primarily of saturated fats, and fiber intake is low. Commodity foods are supplied by the US Department of Agriculture's food distribution program.

*It should be noted that any reference to cultural practices among a specific culture are commonalities. Individuals within a culture may or may not possess the same practices, beliefs, or values.

of common cultural practices of prevalent minority groups. Always keep in mind the strong influence culture has on patients, colleagues, and the nurse. An awareness of the community in which the nurse practices is especially important. If the nurse resides in an area that is populated heavily by a culture that is unlike his or her own, it is the nurse's responsibility to learn as much as possible about the people and the culture.

Get Ready for the NCLEX® Examination!

Key Points

- Transcultural nursing is practiced when the nurse consistently attempts to apply knowledge about culture to all aspects of care.
- To achieve cultural competence, the nurse needs an understanding of individual cultural beliefs and practices and an ability to perceive the health care setting from the patient's point of view. This understanding helps the nurse to be more open and sensitive to the patient's cultural values.
- The impact of culture on behaviors, attitudes, and values depends on individual factors and varies among members of a specific cultural group.
- Beliefs and practices vary among and within cultures.
- Unconscious bias can interfere with development of cultural competence. It is essential to be open to other cultures and value their beliefs and to recognize that your own cultural beliefs are not necessarily superior to those of others.
- A preconceived idea that all members of a particular group possess the same attributes is known as stereotyping.
- Ethnic and racial stereotyping can lead to assumptions about an individual that are often inaccurate.
- Recognition of different health belief systems assists the nurse to develop a plan of care that incorporates varying beliefs.
- Nursing diagnoses and patient problems are based on the biomedical health belief system and may have limitations when used to develop a plan of care for culturally diverse patients with different health beliefs.
- Increased knowledge about cultural groups is imperative as transcultural nursing continues to be important in health care.

Additional Learning Resources

SG Go to your Study Guide for additional learning activities to help you master this chapter content.

Be sure to visit the Evolve site at http://evolve.elsevier.com/Cooper/foundations/ for additional online resources.

Review Questions for the NCLEX® Examination

1. The nurse works in a community with many Mexican American families. What is the best method for the nurse to learn about the Mexican American culture?

   1. Eat at Mexican American restaurants in the area.
   2. Schedule a home visit with a Mexican American family.
   3. Conduct a library study or Internet search of information on the culture.
   4. Observe cultural behaviors in a movie theater in the area.

2. The patient is admitted to the hospital with reports of diffuse symptoms such as nausea, vomiting, weight loss, headaches, insomnia, and chest pain, which she describes by saying, "My heart aches." Which intervention is appropriate for this patient, whose cultural beliefs may differ from the nurse's beliefs about physical illness?

   1. Adhere to the philosophy, "I treat all my patients the same."
   2. Encourage the patient to describe her symptoms using only English.
   3. Contact an adviser who is familiar with the cultural beliefs of the patient.
   4. Allow the patient to continue taking herbal preparations while she is hospitalized.

3. A Muslim patient visiting the health care provider's office was told she had to remove her clothes and put on an examination gown. The patient said she preferred to remain in her own clothes. Why should the nurse allow the patient to remain in her clothes?

   1. The patient is embarrassed.
   2. Her beliefs may require her to keep as much of her body covered as possible during the examination.
   3. The patient is being uncooperative.
   4. The patient cannot disrobe in front of another female.

4. The patient explains to the nurse that he became ill because the natural balance in his body was upset when he moved into a new apartment. He has been taking herbs and rearranging objects to change the environment. The patient is most demonstrating what health belief system?

   1. Biomedical
   2. Folk
   3. Holistic
   4. A combination of all three

5. A patient, who speaks a language different from the nurse's, asks that her daughter remain with her while the nurse performs a history and physical examination. What action by the nurse is most appropriate?

   1. Ask the daughter to leave to maintain privacy for the patient.
   2. Explain to the patient that family members are not allowed to stay in the examining room because of infection control.
   3. Consider that the daughter may be there to serve as an interpreter for her mother.
   4. Ignore the daughter while performing the history and physical examination.

6. The student nurse tells her instructor that she does not understand why a Chinese American family is not grieving for their dying father. What behaviors are being demonstrated by the student nurse?

   1. Subculture orientation
   2. Stereotyping
   3. Cultural bias
   4. Culturally racist

7. A male nurse is assigned to care for a female patient. The patient's husband tells the nurse that he cannot care for his wife due to religious reasons. Which statement best describes the patient's spouse's position?

   1. The couple are prejudiced against the nurse's race.
   2. The patient's religion requires that women should be assigned to care for her.
   3. The nurse is not the same religion as the patient and therefore cannot care for the patient.
   4. The couple does not speak English.

8. The nurse is planning to do a cultural assessment of an elderly Chinese American patient. What position of the nurse is most therapeutic?

   1. The nurse sits facing the patient.
   2. The nurse touches the patient frequently to convey concern.
   3. The nurse positions the chair so that the nurse sits at a right angle to the patient.
   4. The nurse maintains good eye contact while asking questions.

9. A female nurse who is African American is assigned to care for a new 86-year-old resident in a long-term care facility. When she enters his room, he makes several racially offensive remarks. What is an appropriate response?

   1. The nurse should refuse to give care to the patient.
   2. The nurse should understand that he is possibly less tolerant of other races because of his own cultural experiences or he perhaps has disturbed cognitive functions.
   3. The nurse should become angry and retaliate by making racial statements directed at the patient.
   4. The nurse should tell her supervisor that she will not take care of any other white patients.

10. Upon entering a patient's room the nurse realizes that the patient is praying. What action by the nurse is most appropriate?

    1. The nurse should stay in the room and wait until the patient is finished with his prayers.
    2. The nurse should quietly leave the room and give the patient privacy to pray.
    3. The nurse should interrupt the patient and tell him it is time for his care to be given.
    4. The nurse should tell the patient that he cannot pray while he is in the hospital.

11. A Mexican American is pregnant with her second child. When the nurse is reviewing her diet, the patient states that she never drinks milk. What culturally related factor may explain this?

    1. The patient does not like the taste of milk.
    2. Milk is forbidden in her cultural diet.
    3. Lactose intolerance occurs often among Mexican Americans.
    4. The patient cannot afford to buy milk.

12. An elderly patient has been diagnosed with type 2 diabetes and hypertension. The student nurse tells the patient that her vegetables should be steamed and served plain. The patient responds, "I always cook my green beans with ham and salt and pepper. How can I eat them plain?" Which response by the nurse is most culturally sensitive?

    1. "I'm sorry, but you will just have to change your method of cooking."
    2. "I guess you will just have to give up eating green beans."
    3. "You must follow the health care provider's order if you want to get better."
    4. "Could you try cooking the beans with half as much ham and not add salt?"

13. When caring for a patient who speaks a foreign language, the patient problem statement *Compromised Verbal Communication* would be inappropriate for what reason?

    1. An inability to understand each other is the problem, not impaired verbal communication.
    2. The patient is using a different health belief system that interferes with communication.
    3. The patient is perhaps following acceptable communication guidelines within his or her culture.
    4. The patient has deficient knowledge, not impaired verbal communication.

14. What term describes a nurse who is aware of her or his own cultural beliefs and the beliefs and practices of other cultures and who has the ability to interact effectively with people from other cultures?

    1. Stereotyping
    2. Ethnocentric
    3. Culturally aware
    4. Culturally competent

15. Before implementation of any newly prescribed procedure, the nurse notices that the family of an older adult patient always consults the eldest son. What is the social organization of this family? *(Select all that apply.)*

    1. Hispanic in origin
    2. Patriarchal
    3. Male dominated
    4. Traditional nuclear
    5. Matriarchal

16. The nurse caring for a Chinese American woman after an appendectomy can anticipate which intervention?

    1. Maintaining eye contact with education
    2. Sitting side by side to communicate
    3. Touching the patient frequently to comfort
    4. Providing a same-gender caregiver
    5. Allowing the patient to keep head, arms, and legs covered

17. _____ means the nurse is aware of his or her own cultural beliefs and practices and how they relate to those of others.

18. A woman, 43, is brought to the ED by three friends after suffering an apparent GTC seizure during a birthday dinner at a local restaurant. The woman is in a wheelchair with visible muscle rigidity and spasticity. She reports postictal headache and sleepiness, but no apparent confusion or vision changes. There is no sign of fever, infection, or head injury. BP is 90/50 mm Hg; pulse: 60 BPM; respirations: 14 breaths per minute. The nurse asks one of the client's friends about the wheelchair, and after hesitating a moment, the friend says, "Sheryl has cerebral palsy." The client herself begins to explain that this is the first time she has ever had a seizure. The nurse nods and gently breaks eye contact with her and tries again to address her questions to the friend.

Highlight the *most likely* options to complete the statement below.

This nurse's assessment actions are **best described as** ____1_____. Another member of the treatment team should intervene and ____2_____ in order to ____3_____.

OPTIONS FOR 1	OPTIONS FOR 2	OPTIONS FOR 3
Health disparity	Give other friends a chance to speak instead of favoring one individual	Demonstrate transcultural nursing sensitivity
Cultural bias	Pause assessment to wait for a speech therapist advocate before proceeding	Gently sidestep the problem of this client's inability to speak clearly
Ableism	Halt assessment and invite collaboration from a learning disabilities expert	Practice "presumed competence"
Stereotyping	Address the next question directly to the client	Complete an ED assessment more efficiently

Asepsis and Infection Control

7

http://evolve.elsevier.com/Cooper/foundations/

Objectives

1. Explain the difference between medical and surgical asepsis.
2. Explain how each element of the chain of infection contributes to infection.
3. List five major classifications of pathogens.
4. Identify the body's normal defenses against infections.
5. Discuss nursing interventions used to interrupt the chain of infection.
6. Describe the signs and symptoms of a localized infection and those of a systemic infection.
7. Discuss the events in the inflammatory response.
8. Discuss standard precautions.
9. Demonstrate the proper procedure for hand hygiene.
10. Demonstrate technique for gowning and gloving.
11. Identify principles of surgical asepsis.
12. Describe the accepted techniques of preparation for disinfection and sterilization.
13. Discuss patient teaching for infection prevention and control as an element of health promotion.
14. Discuss infection prevention and control measures in the home.

Key Terms

antiseptic (ăn-tĭ-SĔP-tĭk, p. 118)
asepsis (ā-SĔP-sĭs, p. 118)
carrier (KĂR-ē-ŭr, p. 122)
Centers for Disease Control and Prevention (CDC) (SĔN-těrz fŏr dĭ-ZEZ kŏn-trol ănd prē-VĔN-shŭn, p. 128)
contamination (kŏn-tăm-ĭ-NĀ-shŭn, p. 117)
disinfection (dĭs-ĭn-FĔK-shŭn, p. 118)
endogenous (ĕn-DŎJ-ĕn-ŭs, p. 127)
exogenous (ĕks-ŎJ-ĕn-ŭs, p. 127)
fomite (FŌ-mīt, p. 117)
health care–associated infection (hĕlth kăr ā-SŌ-sē-ā-tĭd ĭn-FĔK-shŭn, p. 116)
host (HŌST, p. 127)

infection prevention and control (ĭn-FĔK-shŭn prē-VĔN-shŭn, p. 118)
medical asepsis (MĔD-ĭ-kăl ā-SĔP-sĭs, p. 118)
microorganisms (mī-krō-ŌR-găn-ĭz-ĕmz, p. 117)
reservoir (RĔZ-ŭr-vwăhr, p. 122)
spore spōr, p. 119)
standard precautions (STĂN-dŭrd prē-KĂW-shŭnz, p. 128)
sterilization (stĕr-ĭ-lĭ-ZĀ-shŭn, p. 153)
surgical asepsis (SŬR-jĭ-kăl ā-SĔP-sĭs, p. 118)
vector (VĔK-tŭr, p. 122)
vehicle (VĒ-ĭ-kĕl, p. 122)
virulent (VĪR-ū-lĕnt, p. 127)

With the discovery that microorganisms cause infection came the realization that illness or disease caused by infection is prevented by inhibiting or stopping the growth and reproduction of microorganisms. The aseptic technique is a method developed by Joseph Lister (1827–1912) to reduce morbidity and mortality from infection. Lister is known as the father of the aseptic technique, although many researchers have contributed to its development.

In today's health care environment, nurses and other health care workers must practice effective infection prevention and control measures to protect patients and themselves. In addition to protecting patients, nurses and health care workers must be aware of the risk involved with drug-resistant microorganisms and occupational exposure to infectious material. Diligent attention to infection prevention reduces the incidence of patient deaths, disabilities, and extended health care days of admission. Health care delivery costs are reduced when infection prevention is implemented at all facilities. Most importantly, patient lives are in danger when infections are not prevented.

ASEPSIS

The increase of transmissible infections, not only in health care facilities but also in the home, is an issue of great societal concern. Microorganisms (tiny, usually microscopic entities capable of carrying on living processes) are naturally present on and in the human body and in the environment. Many of these microorganisms are harmless (nonpathogenic) and in most individuals do not produce disease. Some are even helpful. If an individual is highly susceptible to infection, nonpathogenic microorganisms can be dangerous. There are a variety of reasons a patient may be more susceptible to infection, including treatments for diseases such as cancer (chemotherapy and radiation), autoimmune diseases (immune suppressants), and asthma and chronic obstructive pulmonary disease (corticosteroids). Additionally, certain diseases make patients more susceptible to infection. For example, the high glucose seen in some patients with diabetes encourages bacterial growth. Additionally, the lack of sleep, poor nutrition, and open areas on the skin put the patient at a higher risk for infection.

Any patient who enters a health care facility has a greater risk of an infection because of reduced immunologic function. Increased stressors to the patient's immune system are the presenting illness, exposure to disease-causing microorganisms, and portals created by invasive procedures. In addition, health care facilities are conducive to the spread of these microorganisms because of the many ill carriers within their walls. The nurse's knowledge about infection and the application of infection prevention and control principles help protect patients from infection. With each patient care activity, the nurse should ensure that infection prevention and control are routine.

Infection prevention and control involve the implementation of policies and procedures in hospitals and other health care facilities to minimize the spread of health care-associated or community-acquired infections to patients and other staff members. During patient care, the nurse may be exposed to pathogenic microorganisms. The nurse is a chief player in the prevention of the spread of infection, which is accomplished with learning and continued observation of routine and specialized practices of cleanliness and disinfection. These techniques aid in accomplishing **asepsis** (the absence of pathogenic microorganisms). Asepsis is divided into the following two categories:

1. **Medical asepsis** consists of techniques that inhibit the growth and transmission of pathogenic microorganisms. Medical asepsis is also known as the *clean technique* and is used in many daily activities, such as hand hygiene and changing patient bed linens.
2. **Surgical asepsis** consists of techniques designed to destroy all microorganisms and their spores (the reproductive cell of some microorganisms, such as fungi or protozoa). Surgical asepsis is known as the sterile technique and is used in specialized areas, such as the operating room, or during invasive procedures, such as urinary catheter insertion, wound care, and injections.

INFECTION

For an infection to develop, a specific cycle or chain of events must occur. The following six elements are necessary for infection and are referred to as the chain of infection (Fig. 7.1):

1. *Infectious agent*: A pathogen
2. *Reservoir*: Where the pathogen can grow

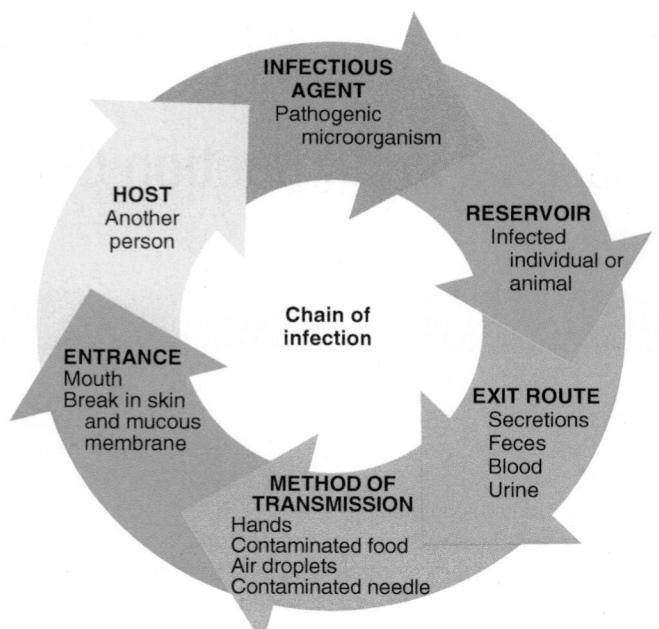

Fig. 7.1 The chain of infection.

3. *Portal of exit (exit route)*: Exit route from the reservoir
4. *Mode (method) of transmission*: Method or vehicle of transportation, such as exudate, feces, air droplets, hands, and needles
5. *Portal of entry (entrance)*: Entrance through the skin, mucous lining, or mouth
6. Host: Another person or animal that is susceptible to the pathogen

For prevention of the transmission of an infection, the cycle must be interrupted. Medical asepsis is an effective way to disrupt the chain of infection. This practice helps to inhibit (to stop or slow a process) the growth and reduce the number of microorganisms.

INFECTIOUS AGENT

Pathogenic microorganisms are infectious agents. Pathogens can be bacteria, viruses, yeasts, fungi, and protozoa. All these microorganisms need food for growth and a suitable environment in which to live. Unwashed hands, wound drainage, soiled linen, and decaying teeth provide ideal areas for pathogenic growth. The microorganism strength, number of microorganisms present, effectiveness of a person's immune system, and length of exposure to the microorganisms determine the ability to produce disease. The role of the nurse is to provide a safe environment by working to prevent the transmission of infection.

Health care workers have several ways to help their patients remain free of infection. Proper disinfection (the use of a chemical that can be applied to objects to destroy microorganisms), appropriate use of an antiseptic (a substance that tends to inhibit the growth and reproduction of microorganisms and may be used on humans) and use of surgical asepsis when indicated are important ways to help reduce the presence of microorganisms.

Fig. 7.2 (A) Aerobic bacteria. (B) Anaerobic bacteria. (Courtesy the Centers for Disease Control and Prevention. A, Bill Schwartz; B, Dr. Richard L. Levin, Greater Southeast Community Hospital, Washington, DC.)

Bacteria

Bacteria have many different characteristics. In addition to their three basic shapes (round, oblong, and spiral), there are many variations. Some are elongated or have pointed ends, and some are flattened on one side. Some are shaped like commas, and others appear square. Spirilla are often tightly coiled, like a corkscrew. During cell division, some bacteria remain together to form pairs, whereas others form long chains. Diagnostic testing focuses on the unique characteristics for identifying specific types of bacteria.

Bacteria also can be differentiated by their chemical compositions, the nutrients that they need to grow, and the waste products the bacteria form. *Aerobic* bacteria grow only in the presence of oxygen, whereas *anaerobic* bacteria grow only in the absence of oxygen (Fig. 7.2A and B). Some bacteria are capable of movement. Motility is possible because of fine, hairlike projections—flagella—that extend from the bacterial cell. These projections move in a wavelike fashion to propel the cell. Some bacteria have only one flagellum attached to one end of the cell, and others have many flagella surrounding the cell. Locomotion of the spirochete is achieved with a wiggling motion that involves the entire cell body.

Some bacteria form a specialized structure called a spore. The spore is a round body that is formed by the bacterium when conditions are unfavorable for growth of the bacterium. The spore enlarges until it is as large as the bacterial cell and is surrounded by a capsule.

Eventually, the portion of the cell that surrounds the spore disintegrates. The spore remains dormant until environmental conditions become favorable for growth. Then, the spore germinates and begins reproducing. Characteristically, spores have a high degree of resistance to heat and disinfectants.

Some bacteria can form capsules around the cell wall. These mucilaginous (of a thick, sticky, slimy substance) envelopes form when the bacterial environment is hostile. The formation of the capsule is a defense mechanism to help protect the bacteria. Capsule formation also contributes to the development of multidrug resistance. When capsules are present, antibiotic therapy is sometimes ineffective because the capsule prevents the drug from reaching the bacteria within the capsule and destroying it.

Identification of the specific organism is vital to the development of the appropriate plan of treatment. Antimicrobial therapies provide a system of attack that is individualized to specific microorganisms. Specially trained laboratory personnel perform this identification. In some instances, they examine a specimen before staining it, but this method is usually less satisfactory. Most bacteria are not visible without a special staining process, in which a dye is applied to a specially prepared glass slide that contains a small amount of the material to be examined. Identification of most bacteria is possible with this simple process; however, other bacteria necessitate additional staining.

Depending on whether a color can be removed with a solvent or the color is retained after the use of the solvent, the organism is identified as gram positive or gram negative. Special staining techniques are required for bacteria that have flagella, spores, or capsules.

If a bacterial infection is suspected, it is important to identify the type of bacteria and the antibiotics that the bacteria is sensitive to. In order to determine the type of bacteria, the nurse collects specimens of body fluids and secretions (culture) suspected of containing pathogenic organisms in sterile containers and sends them to the laboratory for testing. Laboratory personnel transfer the specimen to a special culture medium that promotes growth. They then study the culture and identify the pathogens.

To determine the antimicrobial (antibiotic) that will best inhibit the pathogen's (bacteria's) growth, the laboratory personnel will test the bacteria against several antibiotics and note the results. This is known as sensitivity. The report details which antibiotics the bacteria is both sensitive to (inhibits growth) and which the bacteria is resistant to (will not inhibit growth). The results of the sensitivity tests assist the practitioner in determining which antimicrobial (antibiotic) medication will effectively inhibit the pathogens' growth. The practitioner then orders appropriate antimicrobial agents based on these tests, which typically take 48 to 72 hours to complete. Different organisms require different antibiotics to be destroyed effectively. Often, the practitioner will prescribe an antibiotic they believe will be the correct antibiotic (based on experience, type of infection, location, and type of antibiotic) when the patient is initially evaluated. This antibiotic is continued as prescribed unless the culture and sensitivity (C&S) result indicates a different antibiotic would be more beneficial to the patient. Because the C&S results are not available for up to 3 days, it is imperative the nurse communicate to the patient quickly if another antibiotic is prescribed. The nurse should explain the change to the patient in a way that assures the patient that the first prescribed antibiotic was not erroneously prescribed. The patient may think the practitioner made a mistake in prescribing the original antibiotic and that a medical error or a lapse in judgment has occurred. The nurse would explain that the practitioner made a 'best guess' on the appropriate antibiotic pending the results of the C&S, and now that the lab results have been received, a more effective antibiotic has been prescribed. The nurse would also include details about the need to discontinue the first antibiotic based on the provider's orders. When the nurse reviews the C&S results, the nurse would then assure the patient has been prescribed an antibiotic noted as "sensitive" to the organism identified in the culture. If the bacteria is "resistive" to the antibiotic, the nurse would alert the provider and expect a change in antibiotic to one the bacteria is "sensitive" to. Bacterial infections are transmitted from person to person by direct contact, by inhalation, and by indirect contact with articles contaminated with the pathogen. Some also are transmitted through the ingestion of contaminated food and drink (Fig. 7.3).

The *Streptococcus* bacterium is responsible for more diseases than any other organism, but methicillin-resistant *Staphylococcus aureus* (MRSA) has been proven responsible for several serious and sometimes fatal infections. Patients with immunocompromised conditions who are admitted to health care facilities have an increased risk of exposure to strains of MRSA that are multidrug resistant and therefore more difficult to treat.

Rocky Mountain spotted fever has been found in almost every area of the United States, and its prevalence continues to increase. It is transmitted to humans through the bite of an infected tick. Several varieties of ticks carry the disease. The ticks live on many kinds of animals found in rural and wooded areas. They are also able to live on common house pets, such as cats and dogs. People who work in areas where ticks are known to be abundant are more likely to become infected. The tick attaches itself to the skin, and the longer it remains attached, the more likely the person is to become infected. Great care must be taken not to crush or squeeze the tick on removal from the skin.

The spore-forming bacterium *Bacillus anthracis* causes the acute infectious disease of anthrax. Anthrax infection occurs in three forms:
* Cutaneous (skin) (Fig. 7.4)
* Gastrointestinal
* Inhalation

Anthrax occurs more commonly in animals, but it also can infect humans. It is seen more often in agricultural regions of South and Central America, southern and eastern Europe, Asia, Africa, the Caribbean, and the Middle East, where it is found in animals. It rarely infects domesticated animals in the United States.

B. anthracis spores can live in the soil for many years. Casual contact from person to person does not spread anthrax. In cases of intentional exposure (e.g., during a biologic terrorism event), the most likely routes of infection are inhalation of the spores and spore contact with skin. *B. anthracis* is considered by the Centers for Disease Control and Prevention (CDC, 2020) to be one of the most likely agents that may be used during a biologic terrorism event (see Chapter 10).

Anthrax infection is diagnosed when *B. anthracis* is detected in blood, skin lesions, or respiratory secretions by means of a laboratory culture or measurement of specific antibodies in the blood of infected people.

Treatment of all forms of anthrax (inhalational, gastrointestinal, and cutaneous) consists of antibiotics such as Doxycycline and penicillin G procaine (US FDA, 2017). A vaccine is available for preventing

Fig. 7.3 Some common disease-producing bacteria. (A) Streptococci. (B) Staphylococci. (C) Diplococci. (D) Bacilli. (E) Spirilla. (Courtesy the Centers for Disease Control and Prevention. A, Dr. Gilda Jones; B, Dr. Richard Facklam; C, Dr. Norman Jacobs; D, Dr. Roger Feldman.)

Fig. 7.4 Cutaneous anthrax infection. (Courtesy of the Centers for Disease Control and Prevention.)

anthrax infection. Vaccination is recommended for those at high risk of exposure (US FDA, 2018). If left untreated, anthrax can be fatal with a mortality rate of 20% for cutaneous and 80% for inhalation anthrax (US FDA, 2018).

Viruses

Viruses are the smallest known agents to cause disease. They are not complete cells but are composed of either RNA or DNA. They consist of a protein coat around a nucleic acid core and depend on the metabolic processes of the cell they enter. Before 1900, scientists discovered that certain agents, unlike bacteria, can pass through a laboratory filter. In addition, they were unable to observe these tiny bodies with the ordinary microscope. In 1898, Martinus W. Beijerinck called these small bodies *viruses,* and they became known as filterable viruses.

For years, scientists knew little about viruses, even though they were able to observe their effect on humans and animals. In 1941, the electron microscope became available. With this advancement, the science of virology was born, and a whole new era in the study of human disease was opened. In addition, the development of other tools and techniques has resulted in rapid advances in the study of viruses: the use of certain dyes that become luminous when exposed to ultraviolet light (fluorescent microscopy), tissue culture methods, ultracentrifuge, cytochemistry, and the development of other technical laboratory aids.

Viruses gain entrance to the body through various portals such as the respiratory tract, gastrointestinal tract, and broken skin. Sometimes, a virus can infect a susceptible host through a mosquito bite or during a needlestick with a contaminated needle. Viruses are selective in the type of body cells they attack, but once they have found cells for which they have an affinity, they enter the cell and reproduce rapidly. As they multiply, they interrupt the cell activities and use the cell material to produce new virus material.

Antibiotics are not effective against viruses. This is often misunderstood by the patient, who will expect a prescribed antibiotic for the diagnosis of a viral infection. When a patient is diagnosed with a viral infection, the nurse should offer education about why the practitioner is not prescribing an antibiotic while acknowledging the symptoms the patient is experiencing. When diagnosed with a viral infection such as influenza or a cold, the nurse should offer input on suggested remedies that will ease the symptoms the patient reports, such as over-the-counter medications, fluids, rest, use of a humidifier, warm or cool compresses, antipyretics, analgesics, or nasal rinses. The nurse should recommend only those treatments approved by the practitioner based on the type of viral infection.

Viral infections are usually self-limiting. They run a given course, and recovery usually occurs. One exception is acquired immunodeficiency syndrome (AIDS). Without adequate treatment with specific types of medication, the human immunodeficiency virus (HIV) reproduces, and the immune system continues to be stressed to the point at which it can no longer fight off even the most common infection; the patient then receives the diagnosis of AIDS.

Other viral diseases have the capacity to cause death if complications occur or if they attack individuals with extremely weak or debilitated conditions. One recent example of this type of virus is the Coronavirus (COVID-19) which became prevalent in late 2019 and early 2020. People who are at either end of the age spectrum are also at increased risk for complications. For a select few viruses, such as influenza, antiviral medications are considered as a treatment (CDC, 2019). The nurse should be educated on the methods of transmission, common symptoms, and recommended treatments for viruses in order to protect themselves and the patients they care for daily. Viruses are classified in various ways, either according to the diseases they cause or by the characteristics of a specific group. In the latter classification system, each subgroup often has many types or strains (Table 7.1).

In early 2020, the news of a viral infection, known as the Coronavirus (COVID-19) made headlines globally and indeed continues to be a topic of much research. Declared as a pandemic in March 2020 by the World Health Organization (WHO) and as a national health emergency in the same month, this virus has changed many aspects of our health care system. For the first time in decades, the average lay person without health care training learned about the various types of masks, face coverings, eye protection, and hand washing. Masks and social distancing of 6 feet or more were recommended by health officials to prevent the spread of the virus. Many states enacted orders for masks to be worn by every individual while in all public settings. At the time of updating this textbook edition, more than 8 million people have been infected with COVID-19, and more than 200,000 people have died from the virus in the United States (CDC 2020).

Suddenly, the health care system was burdened with the task of rationing supplies, personal protective equipment (PPE), and various other resources. The CDC continued to issue pandemic guidelines that may be different than the guidelines commonly used in everyday practice. These guidelines are specific to the viral threat and the constant flow of information that comes from research. The situation was and is very fluid, and both those working in health care and those who are not trained health care workers must be diligent in both educating themselves and understanding the changes. For the purpose of testing, the student would be accurate to follow the typical guidelines of mask use and contact precautions that were and continue to be in place before the Coronavirus pandemic. For example, the care of a patient with tuberculosis (TB) patient has not changed. The equipment needed for the room of a patient in airborne precautions continues to be the same before and after the Coronavirus pandemic. In early 2021 vaccines for Covid-19 received emergency approval. Many healthcare facilities started requiring that their employees be vaccinated in the late summer and early fall of 2021.

At the same time, while learning, remembering, and practicing the traditional guidelines, the student must maintain an overview of the changing guidelines during, and perhaps after, the pandemic. These guidelines are especially important to the student completing clinicals in facilities, and it is also important for the student to understand the broader scope of diseases present both before and after Coronavirus.

Fungi

Fungal (mycotic) infections are among the most common diseases found in humans. Fungi are among the most plentiful forms of life. They belong to the plant kingdom, and although many of them are harmless, some are responsible for infections. Fungus types that many people are familiar with include the fuzzy black, green, or white growth on stale bread. Mycotic infections are diseases caused by yeasts and molds. Some are superficial and involve the skin and the mucous membranes. Most frequently, the infections involve the external layers of the skin, the hair, and the nails.

Fungi also may invade the deeper tissues of the body. These types of infections may produce no signs or symptoms; however, some become serious and potentially fatal, especially in a patient with severe immunocompromise. Coccidioidomycosis (valley fever) and histoplasmosis (a systemic fungal respiratory disease) are examples of systemic fungal infections.

Protozoa

Protozoa are single-celled animals; in some form, they exist everywhere in nature. Some of the parasitic forms of protozoa are found in the intestinal tract, the genitourinary tract, the respiratory tract, and the circulatory system of humans and other animals. Protozoa are responsible for malaria, amebic dysentery, and African sleeping sickness (see Table 7.1).

RESERVOIR

To thrive, organisms need a proper atmosphere. Characteristics of an environment that supports organism growth include an available food source, oxygen, water, light, and desirable temperatures and levels of acidity or alkalinity. Any natural habitat of a microorganism that promotes growth and reproduction is a reservoir. Many areas of the body typically host a variety of microorganisms, but the presence of these microorganisms does not always cause illness. Reservoirs include humans, animals, and environmental sources. Within the health care environment, infection may breed and thrive in soiled dressings and medical equipment, including stethoscopes, bedside tables, and overbed tables.

A carrier, or vector, is a person or animal that does not become ill but harbors and spreads an organism, causing disease in others.

The nurse must be aware of the potential risk presented within the health care environment. Ensuring cleaning between patient use, prompt changing of soiled materials, and proper disposal of contaminated materials are critical (Box 7.1).

PORTAL OF EXIT

A microorganism does not have the capacity to cause disease in another host without finding a point of escape from the reservoir. Examples of exit routes in humans are any body fluids produced from the patient, such as those from the gastrointestinal, respiratory, and genitourinary systems or from an open area on the patient's body.

With hand hygiene, the nurse can help prevent the spread of microorganisms. Also, the nurse should teach the patient to cover the nose and mouth when coughing or sneezing.

MODE OF TRANSMISSION

A contaminated vehicle is the means by which microorganisms are carried about and transported to the next host once they have left the reservoir. Contamination means a condition of being soiled, stained, touched by, or otherwise exposed to harmful agents (i.e., the entry of infectious materials into a previously clean or sterile environment), making an object potentially unsafe for use. If the vehicle is a living carrier, it is called a vector. If the vehicle is an inanimate (nonliving) object, it is called a fomite. Some examples of fomites found in health care facilities are computers (many people touch the computer throughout the day), medical records and charts, stethoscopes, thermometers, bandage scissors, used tissues, drinking glasses, needles, and soiled dressings.

Transmission via this kind of common contact with a fomite or vector is known as the indirect method of transmission. Transmission through direct contact is also possible, such as when the nurse uses a poor hand hygiene technique and then touches a patient while providing care such as assessing, bathing, or repositioning the client or during medication administration.

Air currents can carry microorganisms. To help reduce the number of microorganisms in the air, do not shake the linens when making a bed. Use of a dampened or treated cloth when dusting can help prevent the circulation of dust particles.

The floor is one of the dirtiest areas in any building. Do not use anything that has been dropped on the floor. Linens that have been dropped on the floor should be treated as soiled and placed in the appropriate container to be sent for laundering. Supplies (such as dressings) should be discarded. During care, it may be necessary to squat to provide care such as emptying an indwelling urinary catheter or assisting in bathing the patient's legs and feet. During such situations, squat in a way to avoid the knees touching the floor. Feet and furniture are the only items that belong on the floor.

Table 7.1   Common Pathogens, Reservoirs, and Infections or Diseases

ORGANISM	PRIMARY RESERVOIR	INFECTION OR DISEASE
Bacteria		
Staphylococcus aureus	Skin, hair, anterior nares	Wound infection, pneumonia, food poisoning
β-Hemolytic group A streptococci	Oropharynx, skin, perineal care	Strep throat, rheumatic fever, scarlet fever, impetigo
β-Hemolytic group B streptococci	Adult genitals	Urinary tract infection, wound infection, neonatal sepsis
Escherichia coli	Colon	Enteritis
E. coli serotype O157:H7	Colon—food and water	Hemolytic-uremic syndrome (HUS)
Neisseria gonorrhoeae	Genitourinary tract, rectum, mouth, eye	Gonorrhea, pelvic inflammatory disease, conjunctivitis
Staphylococcus epidermidis	Skin	IV line infection, bacteremia, endocarditis
Tubercle bacillus (*Mycobacterium tuberculosis*)	Lungs	Tuberculosis infection Tuberculosis disease
Bacillus anthracis	Infected animals or their products; bioterrorist release	Cutaneous anthrax Inhalation anthrax Gastrointestinal anthrax
Rickettsia rickettsii	Wood tick	Rocky Mountain spotted fever
Viruses		
Herpes simplex virus I and II	Lesions of the mouth, skin, adult genitals	Cold sores, sexually transmitted infections
Hepatitis A and E	Food or water, feces	Hepatitis A and E
Hepatitis B, C, D, and G	Blood, body fluids, and excretions	Hepatitis B
Human immunodeficiency virus (HIV)	Blood, semen, vaginal secretions, breast milk	HIV-positive status, HIV infection
Varicella zoster virus	Vesicle fluid, respiratory tract infections	HIV disease Varicella (chickenpox) primary infection, herpes zoster (shingles) reactivation
Fungi		
Pneumocystis jiroveci (carinii)	Intestinal tract, genitourinary tract, respiratory tract, and circulatory system of humans and animals	Pneumonia referred to as an opportunistic infection in acquired immunodeficiency syndrome (AIDS)
Candida albicans	Mouth, skin, colon, genital tract	Thrush, dermatitis, sexually transmitted diseases
Cryptococcus species	Bird feces	Pneumonia-like illness, meningoencephalitis
Protozoa		
Plasmodium falciparum	Mosquito	Malaria
Entamoeba histolytica	Intestinal tract (specifically the large intestine)	Diarrhea, colitis

IV, Intravenous.

Because so many factors can promote the spread of infection to a patient, all health care workers who provide direct care (physical therapists, physicians, nurses) and those who perform diagnostic and support services (laboratory technicians, respiratory therapists, dietary workers) must follow infection prevention and control practices to prevent or minimize the spread of infection.

PORTAL OF ENTRY

Once the microorganism has exited the reservoir and has been transmitted to a susceptible host, it must find a way to enter the host. When the host's defense mechanisms are reduced (see the section "Host"), the microorganism has a greater chance to gain entry to the host and produce infection. If the patient's skin is punctured with a contaminated needle, microorganisms can enter the bloodstream. If the nurse is not careful when changing a wound dressing, contamination of the new dressing or the wound could occur and could introduce possibly pathogenic microorganisms into the open wound and cause an infection.

Many of the entrance and exit routes microorganisms take are the same, and methods used to prevent

Box 7.1   Measures to Reduce Reservoirs of Infection

BATHING
- Use soap and water to remove drainage, dried secretions, excess perspiration, or sediment from disinfectants.

DRESSING CHANGES
- Change wet or soiled dressings.

CONTAMINATED ARTICLES
- Place used tissues, soiled dressings, and soiled linen in moisture-resistant bags for proper disposal. Place dressings that can be poured, dripped, or squeezed in biohazard bags.

CONTAMINATED NEEDLES AND SHARPS
- Place syringes, uncapped hypodermic needles, and sharps such as scalpels in moisture-resistant, puncture-proof containers (often called "sharps containers"). Keep these in patients' rooms or treatment areas so that carrying exposed, contaminated equipment any distance is not necessary.
- Do not recap needles or attempt to break them.

BEDSIDE UNIT
- Keep table surfaces clean and dry.

BOTTLED SOLUTIONS
- Do not leave bottled solutions open for prolonged periods.
- Keep solutions tightly capped.
- Date bottles when opened.
- Use only as directed by the manufacturer.

SURGICAL WOUNDS
- Maintain the patency of drainage tubes and collection bags to prevent the accumulation of serous fluid under the skin surface.

DRAINAGE BOTTLES AND BAGS
- Empty and dispose of drainage suction canisters according to agency policy.
- Empty all drainage systems on each shift unless otherwise ordered by a physician.[a]
- Never raise a drainage system (e.g., urinary drainage bag) above the level of the site being drained unless it is clamped off.

[a]Closed, water-sealed chest drainage system receptacles are never emptied, only replaced if necessary, per hospital protocol.

Box 7.2   Factors That Affect Immunologic Defense Mechanisms

- Chemotherapy
- Diagnostic procedures
- Disease processes
- Environmental factors
- Fatigue
- Hereditary factors
- Increasing age and extreme youth
- Lifestyle
- Medical therapy
- Nutritional status
- Occupation
- Radiation
- Stress
- Trauma
- Travel history

of sharp instruments, often referred to as "sharps containers." Needles should never be recapped.

An indwelling urinary catheter or another type of drainage equipment often provides an entrance for microorganisms. Ensure that tubes remain connected and intact. Take care when turning, positioning, or transferring a patient to prevent any tubes from becoming tangled or pulling apart. Care should be taken to clean the tubing according to agency policy. For example, indwelling urinary catheters should be cleaned with soap and water or cleaned 6 inches from the patient outward with chlorhexidine (CHG) per policy (AHRQ, 2013). Patients with invasive medical devices such as infusion ports and those being cared for in an intensive care unit are bathed with chlorhexidine gluconate (CHG), typically using prepackaged CHG-infused disposable cloths (John Hopkins Medicine, 2020).

In the care of open areas of the skin or mucous membranes, specific techniques can be used to prevent the entrance of microorganisms. Wear gloves when handling soiled dressings and place the dressings in the appropriate type of waste container for disposal per facility policy.

HOST

A **host** is an organism in which another organism is nourished and harbored.

Susceptibility to an infection is defined by the amount of resistance that the host can exhibit against the pathogen. Microorganisms are constantly in contact with people, but an infection does not develop unless a person is susceptible to the microorganism's strength and numbers. As the pathogen's strength and numbers increase, the person becomes more susceptible. Factors that affect a person's immunologic defense mechanisms are described in Box 7.2.

Immunizations have proven effective in reducing susceptibility to some types of infectious diseases.

or control both processes are also similar. The skin is the first line of defense of the body. It should be kept intact, lubricated, and clean. Observe the patient's skin closely for any open areas and treat them accordingly (see Chapter 9).

Accidental needlesticks are a potential hazard for all personnel who work in a health care facility. Any injury caused by a sharp piece of possibly dirty equipment (such as a used needle or scalpel) should be reported immediately so that procedures can be initiated to help prevent the development of specific types of infections (such as hepatitis B and HIV). Available and appropriate waste containers are essential for the safe disposal

Table 7.2   Normal Defense Mechanisms Against Infection

DEFENSE MECHANISMS	ACTION	FACTORS THAT MAY ALTER DISEASE
Skin		
Intact multilayered surface (body's first line of defense against infection)	Provides a barrier to microorganisms	Cuts, abrasions, puncture wounds, areas of maceration
Shedding of the outer layer of skin cells	Removes organisms that adhere to skin's outer layers	Failure to bathe regularly
Sebum	Contains fatty acid that kills some bacteria	Excessive bathing
Mouth		
Intact multilayered mucosa	Provides a mechanical barrier to microorganisms	Lacerations, trauma, extracted teeth
Saliva	Washes away particles that contain microorganisms Contains microbial inhibitors (e.g., lysozyme)	Poor oral hygiene, dehydration
Eye tearing and blinking	Provides mechanisms to reduce entry (blinking) or to assist in washing away (tearing) particles that contain pathogens, thus reducing the number (dose) of organisms	Injury, exposure—splash or splatter of blood or other potentially infectious material into the eye
Respiratory Tract		
Cilia lining upper airway coated by mucus	Trap inhaled microbes and sweep them outward in mucus to be expectorated or swallowed Engulf and destroy microorganisms that reach lungs' alveoli	Smoking, high concentration of oxygen and carbon dioxide, decreased humidity, cold air
Urinary Tract		
Flushing action of urine flow	Washes away microorganisms on the lining of the bladder and urethra	Obstruction to normal flow by urinary catheter placement, obstruction from growth or tumor, delayed micturition Introduction of a urinary catheter, continual movement of the catheter in the urethra
Gastrointestinal Tract		
Acidity of gastric secretions	Chemically destroys microorganisms incapable of surviving low pH	Use of antacids
Rapid peristalsis in the small intestine	Prevents retention of bacterial contents	Delayed motility resulting from impaction of fecal contents in a large bowel or mechanical obstruction by masses
Vagina		
At puberty, normal flora cause vaginal secretions to achieve low pH	Inhibit the growth of many microorganisms	Antibiotics, excessive douching, and oral contraceptives disrupting normal flora

These are given before a person has been exposed to a disease (to provide protection before contact) or after exposure (if the person's history indicates possible contact with an infectious microorganism). Table 7.2 lists the normal defense mechanisms against infection.

Health care facility policies may mandate that workers be current with immunizations. Many facilities also recommend preventive medications and vaccines. As role models, nurses should provide teaching and encouragement to their patients concerning the benefits of these practices.

INFECTIOUS PROCESS

When the nurse understands the chain of infection, the nurse gains the ability to intervene to prevent infections from developing. When the patient acquires an infection, the nurse can observe certain signs and symptoms and take appropriate actions to prevent its spread. Infections follow a progressive course (Box 7.3). The severity of the patient's illness depends on the extent of the infection, virulence (disease-causing power) of the microorganisms, and susceptibility of the host.

If the infection is *localized* (e.g., a superficial wound infection), proper care helps control its spread and

Box 7.3	Stages of an Infectious Process (Localized or Systemic)

INCUBATION PERIOD

Interval between the entrance of the pathogen into the body and the appearance of first symptoms (e.g., chickenpox, 1–3 weeks; common cold, 1–2 days; influenza, 1–3 days; mumps, 12–26 days). The host may be infectious during this period.

PRODROMAL STAGE

The interval from the onset of nonspecific signs and symptoms (malaise, low-grade fever, fatigue) to more specific symptoms; during this time, microorganisms grow and multiply, and the patient is more capable of spreading the disease to others. For example, the herpes simplex begins with itching and tingling at the site during the prodromal stage before the lesion appears.

ACUTE STAGE

The interval when the patient manifests signs and symptoms specific to the type of infection (e.g., common cold manifested by sore throat, sinus congestion, rhinitis; mumps manifested by earache, high fever, and parotid and salivary gland swelling). This is often the period in which the individual is most contagious.

CONVALESCENCE

Interval when acute symptoms of infection disappear; the length of recovery depends on the severity of infection and patient's general state of health, and recovery takes from several days to months.

Fig. 7.5 Localized skin infection. (Courtesy the Centers for Disease Control and Prevention/Bruno Coignard, MD; Jeff Hageman, MHS.)

minimizes the illness (Fig. 7.5). The patient usually experiences localized symptoms such as pain and tenderness at the wound site. An infection that affects the entire body instead of just a single organ or part is *systemic* and has the potential to be fatal.

The course of an infection influences the level of nursing care that must be provided. The nurse is responsible for the administration of prescribed antimicrobial agents (antibiotics, antivirals, or antifungals). Monitoring patients to assess their response to the therapies includes the objective nursing assessment and vital signs, laboratory studies (e.g., white blood cell levels and albumin values), and subjective reports from the patient. Supportive therapy includes providing adequate nutrition and rest to bolster the body's defense against the infectious process. The complexity of care further depends on the body systems affected by the infection.

Regardless of whether the infection is localized or systemic, the nurse plays a critical role in minimizing its spread. For example, the organism that causes a simple wound infection often spreads to involve an incisional wound site if the nurse uses improper technique during the dressing change. If nurses have a break in their own skin, they may acquire infections from patients if the technique for controlling infection transmission is inadequate.

INFLAMMATORY RESPONSE

Inflammation is the body's response to injury or infection at the cellular level. Inflammation is a protective vascular reaction that delivers fluid, blood products, and nutrients to interstitial tissues in the area of an injury. The process neutralizes and eliminates pathogens or necrotic (dead) tissues and establishes a means of repairing body cells and tissues. Signs of inflammation frequently include edema (swelling), rubor (redness), heat, pain or tenderness, and loss of function in the affected body part. When inflammation becomes systemic, other signs and symptoms develop, including fever, leukocytosis (increased white blood cell count), malaise (generalized discomfort), anorexia, nausea, vomiting, and lymph node enlargement.

The inflammatory response is triggered by physical agents, chemical agents, or microorganisms. Mechanical trauma, temperature extremes, and radiation are examples of physical agents. Chemical agents include external and internal irritants, such as harsh poisons or gastric acid. Microorganisms trigger this response as well, as previously discussed. The inflammatory response sometimes occurs in the absence of an infectious process.

HEALTH CARE–ASSOCIATED INFECTIONS

Approximately 1 in every 31 hospitalized patients have at least one **health care–associated infection** (HAI) (CDC, 2020). These infections previously were referred to as nosocomial infections and include infections patients get when undergoing medical treatment in a health care facility. Much attention has been given to the prevention of HAIs, including monitoring and surveillance by the CDC (2019) and The Joint Commission's National Patient Safety Goal standards. The National Patient Safety Goal 7 focuses on increased compliance with hand hygiene as a preliminary way to decrease the number of HAI in health care settings (TJC, 2020). Nurses will be involved in monitoring and preventing HAIs, such as central line–associated bloodstream infections (CLABSIs), catheter-associated urinary tract infections (CAUTIs), surgical site infections (SSIs), and ventilator-associated pneumonia (VAP) (CDC, 2015). These infections pose a far-reaching and serious problem. Hospitals harbor microorganisms that are often highly **virulent** (exceedingly pathogenic), making them more likely places for infection. The hospitalized patient's immune system is probably already weakened from disease or invasive procedures, making the patient more susceptible to pathogens. HAIs not only necessitate longer hospital (or any health care facility) stays for the patient and increase costs for the patient and the hospital but also can result in disability and death.

An **exogenous** (growing outside the body) infection is caused by microorganisms from another person (e.g., an infection transmitted to the patient by a health care worker). An **endogenous** (growing within the body) infection is caused by the patient's own normal microorganisms, which become altered and overgrow or are transferred from one body site to another (e.g., microorganisms in fecal material are transferred to skin by hands and infect a wound).

HAIs are most commonly transmitted via direct contact between health care workers and patients or from patient to patient. For this reason, a strong emphasis must be placed on the prevention of transmission with measures such as hand hygiene and environmental cleaning.

The nurse is responsible for providing the patient with a clean and safe environment. The nurse must be conscientious and thorough while performing clean and aseptic procedures to reduce the transmission of infection. To decrease the occurrence or duration of HAIs, many facilities have an infection prevention and control department, which investigates and establishes policies to ensure that all personnel maintain aseptic techniques while performing a procedure on a patient. These procedures include clean technique, which is used in all areas, and sterile technique, which is used in invasive procedures.

HAIs significantly increase health care costs. Extended lengths of stay in health care facilities increase disability, and prolonged recovery times add to the expenses the patient has to bear, and to those of the health care facility and any funding bodies (e.g., health insurance companies, Medicare, and Medicaid). The Centers for Medicare and Medicaid Services (CMMS) require hospitals to collect and report data regarding the incidence of HAIs to receive funding. This position encourages facilities to focus on activities that prevent HAIs to avoid financial penalties.

INFECTION PREVENTION AND CONTROL TEAM

Infection prevention and control is a valuable discipline in the health care arena. The Occupational Safety and Health Administration (OSHA), hospital accrediting agencies, and hospital administration place a strong emphasis on infection prevention and control. Administratively, infection control nurses and other members of the infection prevention and control team function within the hospital via the infection prevention and control committee.

INFECTION CONTROL NURSE

Many facilities employ nurses or other professionals who are specially trained in infection prevention and control. They are responsible for advising hospital personnel on the development and implementation of safe patient care delivery practices and for monitoring infection within the health care agency. The duties of an infection control nurse are as follows:

- Assessing microorganism sensitivity to antibiotics presently in use and communicating with medical staff regarding current sensitivity and resistance patterns.
- Compiling data and analyzing the results regarding the epidemiology of HAIs (or health care–acquired infections).
- Conferring with various hospital departments and other resources to investigate unusual events or clusters of infection.
- Consulting with occupational health departments concerning recommendations to prevent and control the spread of infection among health care personnel, such as testing for tuberculosis.
- Educating patients and families in the prevention and control of infection.
- Identifying infection control problems associated with medical or patient equipment.
- Notifying the local public health department of incidences of specific reportable communicable diseases.
- Providing staff education on infection prevention and control.
- Reviewing and revising infection prevention and control policies and procedures to ensure they are in compliance with local, state, and federal regulations and with hospital accrediting agencies.
- Reviewing patient medical records and laboratory reports and recommending appropriate transmission-based isolation procedures.
- Screening patient records for community-acquired infections (those that are acquired outside of the health care setting). These infections often are distinguished from HAIs by the type of organisms that affect patients who are recovering from a disease or injury.

| Box 7.4 | Vaccination and Follow-Up Care for Health Care Workers |

HEPATITIS B

1. Federal law requires that health care employers make available at no cost the hepatitis B vaccine and vaccination series to all employees who have occupational exposure. If an employee declines the vaccine, the employee is required to sign a declination form. Evaluation and follow-up care are available to all employees who have been exposed.
2. A blood test (titer) is offered in some facilities 1–2 months after completion of the three-dose vaccine series (check the health care facility or agency policy).
3. After exposure, no treatment is needed if a positive blood titer is on file. If no positive titer is on file, it is mandatory to follow the CDC guidelines.

HEPATITIS C

1. The employee is offered a baseline blood test to test for the presence of the disease within 48 h.
2. Additional testing is conducted to monitor for the disease approximately 3 weeks after exposure (check the health care facility or agency policy). If the source patient is identified and tests positive for hepatitis C (HCV), the employee may receive a baseline test (CDC, 2017).
3. If the results are positive, the employee is started on treatment. (No prophylactic treatment exists for HCV after exposure.)
4. Early treatment for infection has the potential to prevent chronic infections.

HUMAN IMMUNODEFICIENCY VIRUS

1. If the patient tests positive for HIV infection, a viral load study is performed to determine the amount of the virus present in the blood.
2. If the exposure meets the CDC criteria for HIV prophylactic treatment, or postexposure prophylaxis (PEP), it optimally is started as soon as possible.
3. If PEP medication regimens are warranted, they are continued for 4 weeks following exposure.
4. It is recommended that PEP medication regimens contain three or more suggested antiretroviral drugs.
5. Expert consultation should be provided to any health care worker that experiences occupational exposure. Consultation should begin within 72 h after exposure.
6. Follow-up postexposure testing should occur at 6 weeks, 12 weeks, and 6 months. All medical evaluations and procedures, including the vaccine and vaccination series and evaluation after exposure (prophylaxis), are made available at no cost to at-risk employees. A confidential written medical evaluation is available to employees who have experienced exposure incidents.
7. If newer fourth-generation antiretroviral drugs are available, treatment may end at the 4-month postexposure time rather than 6 months postexposure.

From Centers for Disease Control and Prevention (CDC): Updated US Public Health Service Guidelines for the management of occupational exposures to HIV and recommendations for postexposure prophylaxis, 2015. Retrieved from https://npin.cdc.gov/publication/updated-us-public-health-service-guidelines-management-occupational-exposures-human

An infection control nurse is a valuable resource in the prevention and control of HAIs.

OCCUPATIONAL HEALTH SERVICE

The occupational health service plays an important role in the prevention or the control of an infection in a health care setting by taking measures to protect the health care worker and patients from certain infections. Federal law requires that health care employers make available the hepatitis B vaccine and vaccination series to all employees who have the risk for occupational exposure.

When any needle stick occurs, the health care worker must report it immediately. Hepatitis B, or serum hepatitis, is the most commonly transmitted infection from contaminated needles. Health care agencies require workers who have had a needlestick to complete an injury report and seek appropriate treatment (Box 7.4).

Many facilities mandate that all workers and students obtain titers as proof of immunity against varicella, measles, mumps, and rubella. Titers are laboratory tests that measure the amount of an antibody in the bloodstream. If the amount of the antibody is not high enough, the health care agency often requires personnel to receive a vaccination or be revaccinated to prevent the disease.

STANDARD PRECAUTIONS

With the understanding that exposure to bloodborne pathogens (e.g., hepatitis B virus, HIV) can produce illness and infection came the realization that specific precautions can be used to help prevent infections.

The **Centers for Disease Control and Prevention (CDC)**, part of the US Department of Health and Human Services, provides facilities and services for investigation, prevention, and control of the disease. The nurse should utilize appropriate forms of protective measures and equipment to avoid becoming infected. Actions such as handwashing, use of appropriate PPE, avoiding the recapping of used needles, wearing gloves during contact with blood or other body fluids, maintaining a routine of changing out of work clothing and shoes after contact with potentially infected surfaces.

Accurate identification of all patients infected with bloodborne pathogens is difficult. In the past, the CDC recommended that health care workers use "universal blood and body fluid precautions," or "universal precautions," and body substance isolation when caring for all patients. These two sets of precautions have now been incorporated into one standard set of guidelines, called **standard precautions** (Box 7.5).

Box 7.5 | Standard Precautions

HAND HYGIENE

- Hand hygiene is considered of utmost importance when practicing standard precautions. Hands are to be washed before patient care and after touching blood, body fluids, secretions, excretions, and contaminated items, regardless of whether gloves are worn. Perform hand hygiene immediately after gloves are removed, between patient contacts, and when otherwise indicated to prevent the transfer of microorganisms to other patients or environments. Washing hands may be necessary between tasks and procedures on the same patient to prevent cross-contamination of different body sites.
- Use approved soaps and alcohol-based hand sanitizers and lotions.

GLOVES

- Wear clean gloves when the potential for touching blood, body fluids, secretions, excretions, and contaminated items exists. Put on clean gloves just before touching mucous membranes and nonintact skin. Change gloves between tasks and procedures on the same patient after contact with material that possibly contains a high concentration of microorganisms. Remove gloves promptly after use, before touching noncontaminated items and environmental surfaces. Perform hand hygiene immediately after removing gloves to prevent the transfer of microorganisms to other patients or the environment.

MASK, EYE PROTECTION, FACE SHIELD

- Wear a mask and eye protection or a face shield to protect the mucous membranes of the eyes, nose, and mouth during procedures and patient care activities that are likely to generate splashes or sprays of blood, body fluids, secretions, and excretions.

GOWN

- Wear a fluid-resistant gown (a clean, unsterile gown is adequate) to protect skin and prevent soiling of clothing during procedures and patient care activities that are likely to generate splashes or sprays of blood, body fluids, secretions, or excretions or cause soiling of clothing. Select a gown that is appropriate for the activity and amount of fluid likely to be encountered. Remove the soiled gown as promptly as possible and perform hand hygiene to prevent the transfer of microorganisms to other patients or environments.

MISCELLANEOUS GUIDELINES

- Place used sharps, such as needles or scalpels, in a designated sharps disposal container.
- Do not purposefully bend, break, or recap needles.
- Place disposable wastes and articles contaminated with blood or large amounts of body fluids in a biowaste container for a trash pickup.
- Clean up spills of blood or body fluids per facility protocol (i.e., blood spill kit).
- Place all soiled linen in a laundry bag. Do not overfill the bag, to prevent contamination of the environment.
- For patients with diarrhea, strongly recommend soap and water for hand hygiene in place of alcohol-based hand cleansers because the spores of *Clostridium difficile* are not killed by alcohol (CDC, 2019).
- For patients who are coughing, wear a face mask if within 3 feet of the patient and teach the patient about respiratory hygiene.
- Use mouthpieces, resuscitator bags, or other ventilation devices if resuscitation is needed.
- Health care workers: If you have exudative (draining) lesions, refrain from all direct patient care and from handling patient care equipment until the wound is healed.
- Handle laboratory specimens from all patients as if they are infectious (refer to agency manual).
- Use private rooms for patients with communicable diseases subject to airborne transmission or patients who soil their environment uncontrollably with body substances. For certain diseases (e.g., meningococcal meningitis), personnel and family entering the patient's room are to wear masks. This is true for the first 24 h until antibiotics have been started, then is no longer required per the CDC. Roommates who are immune to the patient's disease or who currently are infected with the same disease are permitted to share rooms (institutional policy may vary on this specific procedure).

From Guideline for Isolation Precautions: Preventing Transmission of Infectious Agents in Healthcare Settings (2007)

The increased incidence of TB has led to heightened stress, along with these precautions, on wearing the particulate respirator mask (Fig. 7.6) to protect against airborne pathogens.

The CDC guidelines for transmission-based precautions in health care settings are the second tier of infection prevention to be used along with standard precautions (CDC, 2016). Transmission-based precautions are used when a patient has a known or suspected infection and specific methods of isolation are used to prevent the patient's infection from causing infection in other patients, visitors, and health care staff, including nurses. Specifics on types of transmission-based precautions are discussed later in the chapter. The goal of these guidelines is to interrupt the chain of infection and reduce the transmission of bloodborne pathogens and other potentially infectious materials. The guidelines apply to (1) blood; (2) all body fluids, secretions, and excretions except sweat, regardless of whether they contain visible blood; (3) nonintact skin; and (4) mucous membranes. Standard precautions are designed to reduce the risk of transmission of microorganisms from recognized and unrecognized sources of infections.

These precautions promote hand hygiene and the use of gloves, masks, eye protection, and gowns when appropriate for patient contact.

Fig. 7.6 Nurse wearing a particulate respirator mask.

HAND HYGIENE

Hand hygiene is the single most important and basic preventive technique that health care workers can use to interrupt the infectious process. Box 7.6 indicates when the initiation of hand hygiene is essential.

Performing hand hygiene (Skill 7.1) provides the necessary protection before the nurse cares for a patient. For effective cleansing of hands soiled with dirt or organic matter, or if the nurse has handled a contaminated item, soap or detergents that contain antiseptic and water are required. The standard is to wash for at least 15 to 20 seconds with facility-approved soap, running hands under water (CDC, 2020). Box 7.7 contains an overview of the CDC hand hygiene guidelines, and Box 7.8 addresses the use of alcohol-based waterless antiseptics for hand hygiene. All forms of HAIs can result from improper hand hygiene and the use of contaminated equipment.

Increased use of artificial fingernails has prompted several research studies. A variety of regulatory agencies, including the CDC, The Joint Commission, and the Association of Perioperative Registered Nurses (AORN), have adopted position statements concerning their use. Only natural nails should be worn in the health care setting; these should be no longer than 1/4 inch long. The use of artificial and acrylic nails should be avoided because of their potential status as carriers of harmful microorganisms, including pin worm. Artificial nails may harbor microorganisms even after the wearer has completed hand hygiene (CDC, 2020). When tools used for the care of fingernails are shared among residents or patients, they should be sanitized before and after use on each patient.

In addition to hand hygiene, other actions can be taken to reduce the chance of transmitting microorganisms. Teach patients and visitors about appropriate times for hand hygiene (see the Patient Teaching box on infection prevention and control). Provide patients with their own set of personal care articles, such as a bedpan, urinal, bath basin, water pitcher, and drinking glass, to prevent cross-contamination. Because microorganisms are also transmitted by indirect contact with contaminated equipment and soiled linen, place these articles in special waste containers or laundry bags. Keep these items should be kept away from your uniform. The risk of transmitting HAIs or infectious diseases among patients is high when standard precautions are not followed. Health care workers need to stay informed about patients who have a known source of infection and communicate the information with other health care workers as appropriate. By following recommendations for infection prevention and control practices, health care workers experience more protection from exposure and reduce the patient's risk for acquiring an HAI.

Skill 7.1 Performing Hand Hygiene With Soap and Water

CHECK GATHER HELLO ID PRIVACY EXPLAIN WASH GLOVES

NURSING ACTION (RATIONALE)

1. Inspect hands, observing for visible soiling, breaks, or cuts in the skin and cuticles. (*Poor personal hygiene and an open area of the skin provide areas in which microorganisms are able to grow.*)
2. Determine the amount of contaminant on hands. (*Determines the type of hand hygiene needed.*)
3. Assess areas around the skin that are contaminated. (*Prevents contamination of hands during and after hand hygiene procedure.*)
4. Adjust the water to the appropriate temperature and force. (*Water that is too hot can chap skin, and too much force causes splashing and may spread microorganisms to other areas, especially your clothing.*)
5. Wet hands and wrists under the running water, always keeping hands lower than elbows. (*Hands are the most contaminated part of the upper extremities; water should flow from the wrists [least contaminated area] over the hands and then down the drain.*)
6. Lather hands with liquid soap (about 1 teaspoon). (*Soap lather emulsifies fat and aids in cleansing.*)
7. Wash hands thoroughly with a firm, circular motion and friction on the back of hands, palms, and wrists. Wash each finger individually, paying special attention to areas between fingers and knuckles by interlacing fingers and thumbs and moving hands back and forth, causing friction. (*Helps to loosen soil and microorganisms, both resident [normally present] and transient [acquired from contamination].*)

8. Wash for at least 20 s (CDC, 2015a). (*The greater the contamination, the more need for longer washing.*)

9. Rinse wrists and hands completely, again keeping hands lower than elbows. (*Water should run from cleaner area [the wrists] over the hands and then down the drain, rinsing the dirt and microorganisms away.*)

10. Dry hands thoroughly with paper towels. Start by patting at fingertips, then hands, and then wrists and forearms.
11. If it is necessary to turn off faucets manually, use a dry paper towel. (*Keeps clean hands from touching contaminated handles.*)
12. Use hospital-approved hand lotion if desired.
13. Inspect hands and nails for cleanliness. (*Ensures cleanliness of hands and nails.*)
14. If hands are not visibly soiled, use an alcohol-based waterless antiseptic for routine decontamination of hands in all clinical situations, unless you are caring for a patient with Clostridium difficile or Candida infection. These spores are unaffected by alcohol, so soap and water must be used in these instances (see Box 7.8).

Continued

Skill 7.1 Performing Hand Hygiene With Soap and Water—cont'd

15. Provide patient teaching (see the Patient Teaching box on infection prevention and control).

16. Explain to the patient the importance of hand hygiene. (*Helps the patient understand*

that hand hygiene slows down the spread of infection.)

17. If contamination occurs, it is necessary to reassess the technique.

From Centers for Disease Control and Prevention (CDC): Handwashing: clean hands save lives: Show me the science–how to wash your hands, 2015. Retrieved from https://www.cdc.gov/handwashing/show-me-the-science-handwashing.html.

Box 7.7 Overview of CDC Hand Hygiene Guidelines

The Centers for Disease Control and Prevention (CDC) makes recommendations for hand hygiene in health care settings. Hand hygiene is a term that applies to hand washing, use of an antiseptic hand sanitizer, and surgical hand antisepsis. Evidence suggests that hand antisepsis, the cleansing of hands with an antiseptic hand sanitizer, is more effective in reducing HAIs than is plain hand washing.

FOLLOW THESE GUIDELINES IN THE CARE OF ALL PATIENTS

- Continue practice of washing hands with either facility-approved soap or antimicrobial soap and water whenever hands are visibly soiled.
- Use an alcohol-based hand sanitizer to routinely decontaminate the hands in the following clinical situations: (NOTE: If alcohol-based hand sanitizers are not available, the only alternative is hand washing; see Skill 7.1, step 14.)
  - Before and after patient contact.
  - Before donning sterile gloves when inserting central intravascular catheters.
  - Before performing nonsurgical invasive procedures (e.g., urinary catheter insertion, nasotracheal suctioning).
  - After contact with body fluids or excretions, mucous membranes, nonintact skin, and wound dressings.
  - If moving from a contaminated body site (rectal area or mouth) to a clean body site (surgical wound, urinary meatus) during patient care.
  - After contact with inanimate objects (including medical equipment) in the immediate vicinity of the patient.
  - After removing gloves.
  - Before eating and after using a restroom, wash hands with facility-approved soap and water.
- Antimicrobial-impregnated wipes (i.e., towelettes) are not a substitute for using an alcohol-based hand sanitizer or antimicrobial soap.
- If exposure to *Bacillus anthracis* is suspected or proven, wash hands with facility-approved soap and water.

The physical action of washing and rinsing hands is recommended because alcohols, chlorhexidine, iodophors, and other antiseptic agents have poor activity against spores.

FOLLOW THESE GUIDELINES FOR SURGICAL HAND ANTISEPSIS (SEE SKILL 7.6)

- Surgical hand antisepsis reduces the resident microbial count on the hands to a minimum.
- The CDC recommends using an antimicrobial soap to scrub hands and forearms for the length of time recommended by the manufacturer. Refer to agency policy for time required.
- When using an alcohol-based surgical hand-scrub product with persistent activity, follow the manufacturer's instructions. Before applying the alcohol solution, prewash hands and forearms with a non-antimicrobial soap and dry hands and forearms completely. After application of the alcohol-based product as recommended, allow hands and forearms to dry thoroughly before donning sterile gloves.

GENERAL RECOMMENDATIONS FOR HAND HYGIENE

- Use facility-approved hand lotions or creams to minimize the occurrence of irritant contact dermatitis associated with hand antisepsis or hand washing.
- Do not wear artificial fingernails or nail polish when having direct contact with patients at high risk (e.g., those in intensive care units or operating rooms).
- Keep natural nail tips less than 1/4 inch long.
- Wear gloves when contact with blood or other potentially infectious materials, mucous membranes, and nonintact skin could occur.
- Remove gloves after caring for a patient. Do not wear the same pair of gloves for the care of more than one patient, and do not wash gloves between uses with different patients.
- Change gloves during patient care if moving from a contaminated body site to a clean body site.

HAIs, Health care-associated infections.

Modified from Boyce JM, Pittet D; Healthcare Infection Control Practices Advisory Committee; Society for Healthcare Epidemiology of America; Association for Professionals in Infection Control Infectious Diseases Society of America Hand Hygiene Task Force: Guideline for hand hygiene in health-care settings: Recommendations of the Healthcare Infection Control Practices Advisory Committee and the HICPAC/SHEA/APIC/IDSA Hand Hygiene Task Force. *Infect Control Hosp Epidemiol*. 23(12 Suppl):S3–S40, 2002.

| Box 7.8 | Using an Alcohol-Based Waterless Antiseptic for Routine Hand Hygiene |

The Centers for Disease Control and Prevention (CDC) recommends the use of alcohol-based waterless antiseptics to improve hand hygiene practices, protect health care workers' hands, and reduce transmission of pathogens to patients and personnel in health care settings. Alcohols have excellent germicidal activity and are more effective than either plain soap or antimicrobial soap and water. Emollients are added to alcohol-based antiseptics to prevent drying of the skin.

If hands are not visibly soiled, use an alcohol-based waterless antiseptic for routine decontamination of hands in most clinical situations.

1. Apply an ample amount of product to the palm of one hand. *(Enough product is needed to thoroughly cover the hands.)*
2. Rub hands together, covering all surfaces of hands and fingers with antiseptic.

3. Rub hands together for several seconds until the alcohol is dry. Allow hands to dry before applying gloves. If an adequate volume is used, 15–25 s are needed for hands to dry. *(Drying ensures full antiseptic effect.)*
4. If hands are dry or chapped, a small amount of facility-approved lotion or barrier cream can be applied. *(Use the hospital-provided container of lotion because other lotions possibly interfere with antimicrobial action or disintegrate gloves.)*

NOTE: Alcohol-based waterless antiseptics are not recommended if caring for a patient with *Clostridium difficile* (*C. diff*) diarrhea or *Candida* species infections. The spores are unaffected by the alcohol in the hand sanitizer.

NOTE: Because of the risk of alcohol poising with ingestion of large amounts, alcohol-based waterless antiseptics should be kept out of reach of children who may swallow them.

Data from Boyce JM, Pittet D; Healthcare Infection Control Practices Advisory Committee; Society for Healthcare Epidemiology of America; Association for Professionals in Infection Control Infectious Diseases Society of America Hand Hygiene Task Force: Guideline for hand hygiene in health-care settings: Recommendations of the Healthcare Infection Control Practices Advisory Committee and the HICPAC/SHEA/APIC/IDSA Hand Hygiene Task Force. *Infect Control Hosp Epidemiol.* 23(12 Suppl):S3–S40, 2002.

Patient Teaching

Infection Prevention and Control

- Teach the patient about the infection process, especially how an infection is transmitted, and stress the importance of interrupting the process. Use a simple diagram to illustrate this (see Fig. 7.1). Teaching caregivers is extremely important as well.
- Use an example for each step that is familiar to the patient.
- Provide a simple explanation of clean and contaminated items.
- Although hand hygiene is a basic hygiene technique, emphasize when and how the procedure should be performed to be effective in preventing infection. Demonstrate hand hygiene within sight of the patient whenever possible.
- Instruct the patient about the signs and symptoms of infection.
- Teach the applications of aseptic principles to self-care activities, such as wound care and medication administration.
- When isolation apparel (such as mask, gown, or gloves) is to be used, demonstrate the procedures for the patient and visitors.
- Instruct the patient to place contaminated dressings and other disposable items that contain infectious body fluids in a leak-resistant bag. At home, needles should be placed in bleach bottles with the cap taped or glued on or placed in a sharps container and taken to a local hospital for disposal.

Always allow a question-and-answer session for the patient (some patients need special assistance in understanding the precautions).

Patient Teaching

Gloving Technique

- Ensure that the patient understands the rationale for the use of gloves.
- Some patients need special assistance in understanding the precautions.
- Demonstrate to the patient how to don gloves.

- Wear gloves only once, and change gloves if they are damaged or torn, or when patient care has been completed.
- If you have not completed the patient's care but have come into contact with infectious material, change the gloves before continuing the patient's care.
- Because of the risk of perforating the gloves during use, perform hand hygiene after removing the gloves (Skill 7.2).

Family members need to understand the importance of the use of gloves. Explain that gloves become contaminated if they touch infected material or a contaminated object (see the Patient Teaching box on gloving technique).

Latex Allergy

Latex allergy causes an individual to have a reaction to certain proteins found in natural rubber latex, a product manufactured from a milky fluid derived from the rubber tree found in Africa and Southeast Asia. The latex proteins can enter the body through the skin and mucous membranes, intravascularly, and by inhalation. Suspect the presence of a latex allergy and obtain an evaluation by a physician when anyone has the development of red, watery, itchy eyes; sinus or nasal congestion; tachycardia; or hypotension after exposure to latex. Anaphylaxis is a potentially life-threatening

GLOVING

Nurses and other health care personnel should don gloves if any possibility exists of contact with infectious material with their hands. The WHO gives the following advice regarding gloves:

Skill 7.2　Gloving

CHECK　GATHER　HELLO　ID　PRIVACY　EXPLAIN　WASH　GLOVES

NURSING ACTION (RATIONALE)

Donning Gloves

1. Remove gloves from the dispenser. (*Keeps gloves handy and ready for use.*)
2. Inspect gloves for perforations. (*Prevents pathogenic microorganisms from entering through the perforations in the gloves.*)
3. Don gloves when ready to begin patient care. Wearing gloves with a gown does not necessitate any special technique for putting them on; wear them pulled over cuffs of the gown. (*Ensures full coverage of your wrists.*)
4. Change gloves after direct handling of infectious material such as wound drainage. (*Prevents cross-contamination.*)
5. Do not touch side rails, tables, or bed stands with contaminated gloves. (*Prevents spread of microorganisms throughout the environment.*)

Removing Gloves

6. Remove the first glove by grasping the outer surface at the palm with the other gloved hand and pulling the glove inside out and off. Place this glove in the hand that is still gloved. (*Prevents you from touching your own skin with a contaminated glove.*)

7. Remove the second glove by placing a finger under the cuff and turning the glove inside out and over the other glove. Drop gloves into a waste container. (*Prevents you from touching a contaminated glove; wraps contamination inside gloves to help protect others.*)

8. Perform hand hygiene. (*Helps prevent cross-contamination.*)
9. Provide patient teaching (see the Patient Teaching box on gloving technique).
10. If contamination occurs, it is necessary to reassess the technique.

condition that can develop when someone is exposed to latex and has a severe latex allergy.

Some medical products contain latex. Synthetic versions of many products are available. Even though an individual product is "latex free," an environment is "latex safe" only when all items of latex that have the potential to come in contact with the allergic individual are removed (Box 7.9).

GOWNING

The nurse should don a gown when preparing to provide care for a patient in isolation to help protect the nurse's clothing from becoming soiled and to avoid transmitting the infection. The gown also provides

---

Box 7.9　Preventing Latex Allergy

The American Nurses Association (ANA) provides the following suggestions for nurses to avoid becoming allergic to latex:

1. Whenever possible, wear powder-free gloves (they are lower in protein allergens).
2. Wear gloves that are appropriate for the task (e.g., avoid use for cleaning).
3. Wash with a pH-balanced soap immediately after removing gloves.
4. Apply only non–oil-based hand care products (oil-based products break down latex).
5. If a reaction or dermatitis occurs, report to employee health or seek medical treatment immediately.

protection against unknown infectious microorganisms. Recommendations are that the nurse discards the gown when leaving the patient's room rather than reuse it. This aids in preventing the spread of pathogens to other patients or personnel. This procedure also applies to visitors.

Another rationale for the use of a gown is the protection of a patient whose immune system is inadequate. In this situation, health care workers and visitors wear a gown to prevent the transfer of microorganisms from themselves to the patient.

There are several types of isolation. Some necessitate the wearing of a gown, whereas others do not. Donning of an isolation gown is indicated in the care of patients with diseases characterized by heavy drainage or exudate, infectious and acute diarrhea, other gastrointestinal disorders, respiratory disorders, skin wounds or burns, and urinary disorders.

Isolation gowns open at the back and have ties at the neck and the waist to keep the gown securely closed, protecting the back and the front of the nurse's uniform. The gown must be long enough to cover the uniform and, for added protection, have long sleeves with cuffs.

To don gowns correctly, follow the procedure listed in Skill 7.3.

MASK AND PROTECTIVE EYEWEAR

When a mask is applied correctly, it fits snugly below the health care worker's chin and securely over the nose and mouth; the top edge fits below eyeglasses, if worn (this prevents fogging of glasses). Masks are available with eye shields to cover the wearer's eyes (or glasses). Goggles are another way to protect the eyes (see Fig. 7.6). Nurses should change their masks at least every 20 to 30 minutes and/or when they become moist. Nurses should not reuse their masks or allow them to dangle around their necks and then reuse them (Skill 7.4). Masks and protective eyewear guard members of the health care team in the following ways:

- They protect the wearer from inhaling microorganisms that travel on airborne droplets for short distances or that remain suspended in the air for longer periods and from splashing if it should occur. Masks also prevent the mucous membranes of the nose and mouth from coming into contact with contaminants.
- They prevent the patient from inhaling pathogens if resistance is reduced or if a patient with an airborne respiratory infection is being transported to another care area.
- Eyewear shields protect the membranes and conjunctiva of the eye.

DISPOSING OF CONTAMINATED EQUIPMENT

Health care facilities generate immense quantities of contaminated materials, some of which are disposable and some of which are reusable. It is essential to design and implement an effective mechanism to handle this material within the facility. The process for the disposal of contaminated materials is reviewed by the infection control nurse and the infection prevention and control committee. Some facilities manage the waste onsite, and other facilities rely on waste haulers to remove the waste. A major risk to health care workers and facility personnel is in the improper disposal of sharps (needles, scalpels), which often are contaminated by blood or bodily fluid. When left in linens, these sharp items have the potential to injure workers cleaning patient care areas. For prevention of this problem, all patient care areas in which sharps are ever used must be provided with puncture-proof containers into which health care workers place used disposable sharp items.

HANDLING LINEN

The CDC recommends the following guidelines for handling linen:

- Place soiled linen in a laundry bag in the patient's room.
- Treat all linen as though it were infectious.

Note that double bagging (placing a plastic bag that contains contaminated linen into another clean plastic bag) is no longer recommended as a universal practice unless a cloth bag is being placed in a plastic bag. In most cases, a single bag is adequate if it is possible to place the contaminated articles in the bag without contamination of the outside of the bag.

ISOLATION TECHNIQUE

The CDC issued isolation guidelines, in addition to standard precautions, that contain two tiers of approach (CDC, 2019). The first tier contains precautions designed for health care workers to use when caring for all patients in health care facilities regardless of their diagnosis or presumed infectiousness. This first tier is called *standard precautions*.

The second tier condenses the disease-specific approach to isolation into transmission categories: airborne, droplet, and contact precautions. These precautions are designed to be used in the care of patients with a specific type of confirmed or suspected infection (Box 7.10 and Figs. 7.7 to 7.9).

The type of isolation techniques followed for a given patient depends on how transmissible the pathogen in question is. The nurse should follow some basic principles regardless of which technique is used:

- Perform thorough hand hygiene before and after caring for a patient.
- Have an adequate understanding of the disease process and the method of transmission of the infectious microorganism to help determine which protective barriers to use.
- Dispose of contaminated equipment and articles in a safe and effective manner to prevent the transmission of pathogens to other individuals.

Skill 7.3   Gowning for Isolation

 CHECK GATHER HELLO ID PRIVACY EXPLAIN WASH GLOVES

NURSING ACTION *(RATIONALE)*

1. Push up long sleeves, if you have them. (*Ensures that the uniform sleeve is under the gown sleeve for protection.*)
2. Perform hand hygiene. (*Reduces spread of microorganisms.*)
3. Don gown and tie it securely at neck and waist. (*Provides protective covering of the entire uniform.*)

4. Remove gown after providing necessary patient care. (*Has protected the nurse.*)

5. Discard soiled gown appropriately. (*Prevents contamination.*)

Skill 7.3 Gowning for Isolation—cont'd

6. Perform hand hygiene. (*Prevents spread of microorganisms.*)
7. Record use of gown in isolation procedure if required by the health care agency. (*Provides proof that appropriate procedure was followed.*) Some agencies charge a daily rate for isolation precautions. This is noted on a daily basis in the patient's record. Therefore, repeated notations throughout the 24 h are not necessary.
8. Provide patient teaching (see the Patient Teaching box on infection prevention and control).
9. If contamination occurs, it is necessary to reassess the technique.

Skill 7.4 Donning a Mask

NURSING ACTION (RATIONALE)

The nurse should perform the following steps when donning a mask:

1. Remove mask from the container. (*Mask is readily available for use.*)
2. Don mask when ready to begin patient care by covering your nose, mouth, and eyes (or glasses) with the device. Wear a mask with a protective eye shield when there is a risk of splashing. Secure the mask in place with an elastic band or by tying the strings behind your head. (*Provides protection from microorganisms.*)

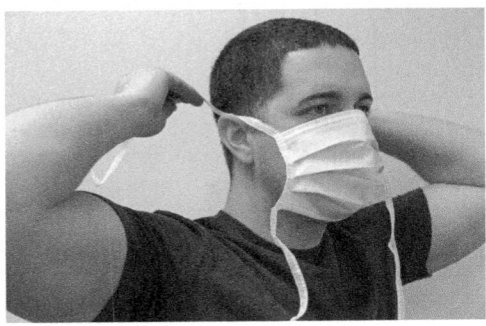

3. Wear a mask until it becomes moist, but no longer than 20–30 min. (*Moisture renders a mask ineffective.*)

4. Remove mask by untying the strings or moving the elastic. Be certain not to touch a contaminated area (*Prevents your contact with a contaminated mask*).

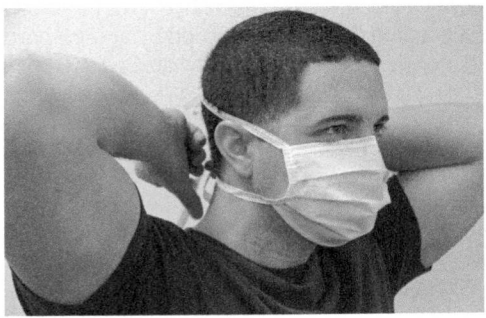

5. Dispose of the soiled mask in an appropriate container. (*Protects other health care workers.*)
6. Wash hands thoroughly. (*Removes microorganisms.*)
7. Record use of a mask during patient care (some agencies require documentation of specific barriers used). (*Provides proof of wearing a mask for protection of patient and nurse.*)
8. Provide patient teaching (see the Patient Teaching box on infection prevention and control).
9. If contamination occurs, it is necessary to reassess the technique.

• If the patient is to be transported to other areas in the agency (away from the isolation room), take necessary measures to protect those who potentially will be exposed. The patient should be transported in accordance with hospital protocol.

Environmental barriers keep pathogens in a confined area. Examples of such barriers are placing a patient in a private or isolation room, closing the patient's door, and wearing PPE (e.g., gown, mask, goggles, gloves).

The patient with an infectious disease should be placed in a private or isolation room equipped with the appropriate hand hygiene and toilet facilities. Private rooms used for airborne illness isolation have negative-pressure airflow that prevents infectious particulates from flowing out of the closed environment. Special rooms with positive-pressure airflow also are used for patients with immunocompromised conditions, such as transplant recipients or patients who are receiving certain kinds of chemotherapy. In this case, a reduced

Box **7.10** Types of Precautions and Patients Who Require Those Precautions

STANDARD PRECAUTIONS (TIER 1)

Use standard precautions for the care of all patients. This general mandate is necessary because whether the patient is colonized or infected with certain pathogenic microorganisms is sometimes not known. Barrier precautions reduce the need to handle sharps.

TRANSMISSION PRECAUTIONS (TIER 2)
Airborne Precautions (See Fig. 7.7)

In addition to standard precautions, use airborne precautions for patients known or suspected to have serious illnesses transmitted by airborne droplet nuclei. Examples of such illnesses include the following:

- Measles
- Varicella zoster virus (including disseminated zoster), responsible for chickenpox and shingles
- Tuberculosis and Covid-19
    - Airborne precautions should be practiced for all patients with known or suspected TB or Covid-19. (Suspected TB is defined by agency policy and generally means any patient with a positive acid-fast bacillus [AFB] smear, a cavitated lesion seen on a chest x-ray, or identification as high risk with a screening tool; suspected Covid-19 is defined by agency policy and generally means any patient with Covid-19 symptoms and/or chest x-ray indicative of Covid-19 pneumonia)
    - Isolation is mandatory in a single-patient room designated as negative-pressure airflow and having at least 6–12 air exchanges per hour. It is necessary to vent room air to the outside and to ensure that the door is closed (before and after entering the room) to maintain negative pressure.
    - It is mandatory that health care workers wear an N-95 or higher particulate respirator mask or a powered air-purifying respirator (PAPR) when entering an AFB isolation room (check agency's policy for the type of mask).
    - It is mandatory for health care workers to undergo a fit test before using a respirator for the first time. This ensures that the type and the size of the respirator are appropriate for the individual.
    - It is mandatory for health care workers to fit-check the respirator's fit before each use.
    - Respirators are permitted to be reused and stored according to manufacturer recommendations and agency policy.
- Fit-test: Procedure to determine the adequate fit of respirator, usually with qualitative and Covid-19 measure (wearers are exposed to a concentrated saccharin solution and asked if they can detect taste while wearing a respirator. Also asked about the ability to smell substances).

DROPLET PRECAUTIONS (SEE FIG. 7.8)

In addition to standard precautions, use droplet precautions for patients known or suspected to have serious illness transmitted by large particle droplets. Examples of such illnesses include the following:

- Invasive *Haemophilus influenzae,* including meningitis, pneumonia, epiglottitis, and sepsis
- Invasive *Neisseria meningitidis* disease, including meningitis, pneumonia, and sepsis

Examples of other serious bacterial respiratory infections spread by droplet transmission include the following:
- Diphtheria (pharyngeal)
- Mycoplasma pneumonia
- Pertussis
- Pneumonic plague
- Streptococcal pharyngitis, pneumonia, and scarlet fever in infants and young children

Examples of serious viral infections spread by droplet transmission include the following:
- Adenovirus
- Influenza
- Mumps
- Parvovirus B19
- Rubella

CONTACT PRECAUTIONS (SEE FIG. 7.9)

In addition to standard precautions, use contact precautions for patients known or suspected to have serious illnesses easily transmitted by direct patient contact or by contact with items in the patient's environment. Examples of such illnesses include the following:

- Gastrointestinal, respiratory, skin, or wound infections or colonization with multidrug-resistant bacteria judged by the infection prevention and control committee, and current state, regional, and national recommendations, to be of special clinical and epidemiologic significance
- Enteric infections with a low infectious dose or prolonged environmental survival, including the following:
    a. *Clostridium difficile*
    b. Diapered or incontinent patients with the following:
        1. Escherichia coli O157:H7
        2. Shigella
        3. Hepatitis A
        4. Rotavirus
- Respiratory syncytial virus, parainfluenza virus, and enteroviral infections in infants and young children
- Skin infections that are highly contagious or that tend to occur on dry skin, including the following:
    a. Diphtheria (cutaneous)
    b. Herpes simplex virus (neonatal or mucocutaneous)
    c. Impetigo
    d. Major (noncontaminated) abscesses, cellulitis, or decubitus ulcers
    e. Pediculosis
    f. Scabies
    g. Staphylococcal furunculosis in infants and young children
    h. Methicillin-resistant *Staphylococcus aureus* (MRSA)
    i. Vancomycin-resistant enterococci (VRE)
    j. Extended-spectrum beta-lactamase (ESBL); this enzyme attaches to the cell wall of *E. coli* and some *Klebsiella* organisms, which in turn makes the organisms multidrug resistant
    k. Varicella zoster virus (disseminated or in the immunocompromised host)
    l. Viral or hemorrhagic conjunctivitis
    m. Viral hemorrhagic infections (Ebola, Lassa, Marburg)

PATIENTS WITH IMMUNOCOMPROMISED CONDITIONS

Patients with immunocompromised conditions vary in their susceptibility to health care–associated infections depending

| Box 7.10 | Types of Precautions and Patients Who Require Those Precautions—cont'd |

on the severity and the duration of immunosuppression. They are generally at increased risk for bacterial, fungal, parasitic, and viral infections from endogenous and exogenous sources. In general, the use of standard precautions for all patients and transmission-based isolation precautions for specified patients reduces the acquisition by these patients of institutionally acquired organisms from other patients and environments. Patients with leukopenia sometimes require protective measures in addition to standard precautions. These precautions are typically called neutropenic precautions. In such instances, the physician or infection control nurse instructs nursing staff about the necessary protective measures (e.g., masks, private room). They place an isolation sign on the door that lists the additional protective measures that staff and visitors are required to follow for the safety of the patient.

MONITORING OF ISOLATION

Transmission-based isolation practices are monitored on an ongoing basis by the infection control nurse.

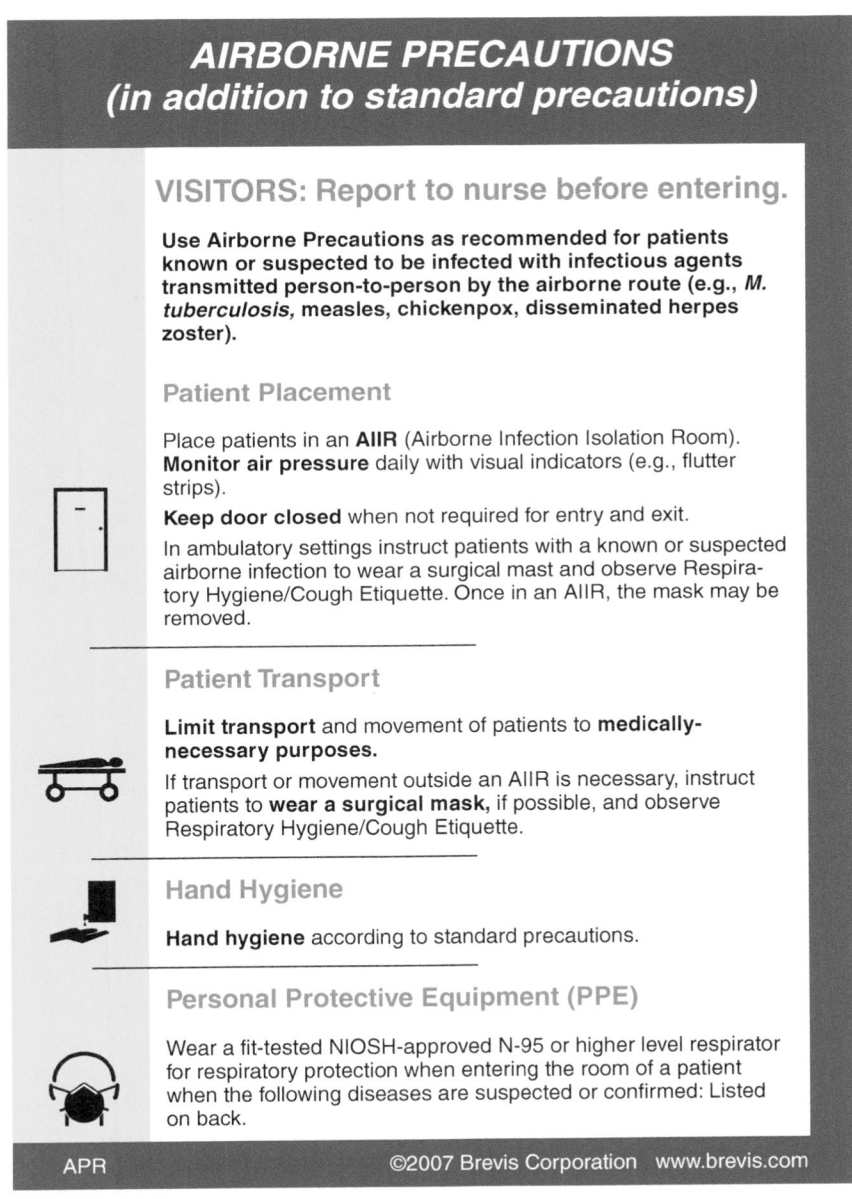

Fig. 7.7 Airborne precautions. (Copyright 1997–2007 Brevis Corporation. Courtesy Brevis Corporation, Salt Lake City, Utah.)

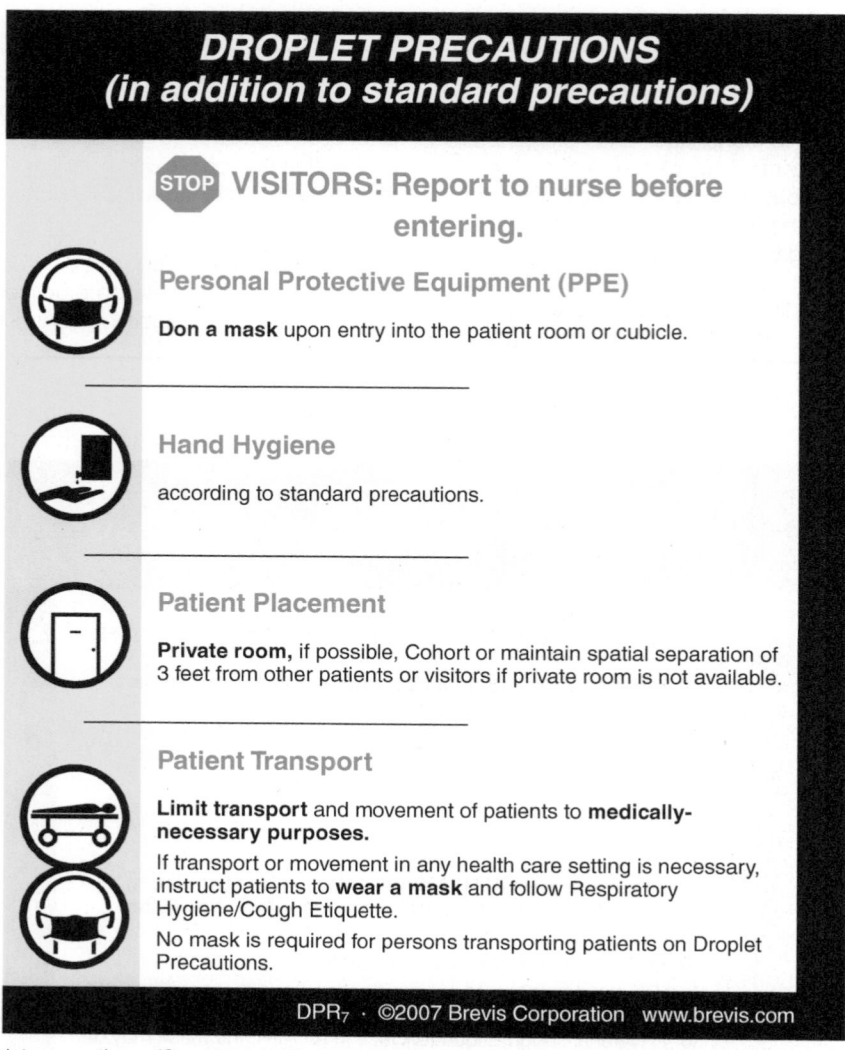

DROPLET PRECAUTIONS
(in addition to standard precautions)

STOP VISITORS: Report to nurse before entering.

Personal Protective Equipment (PPE)

Don a mask upon entry into the patient room or cubicle.

Hand Hygiene

according to standard precautions.

Patient Placement

Private room, if possible, Cohort or maintain spatial separation of 3 feet from other patients or visitors if private room is not available.

Patient Transport

Limit transport and movement of patients to **medically-necessary purposes.**

If transport or movement in any health care setting is necessary, instruct patients to **wear a mask** and follow Respiratory Hygiene/Cough Etiquette.

No mask is required for persons transporting patients on Droplet Precautions.

DPR₇ · ©2007 Brevis Corporation   www.brevis.com

Fig. 7.8 Droplet precautions. (Copyright 1997–2007 Brevis Corporation. Courtesy Brevis Corporation, Salt Lake City, Utah.)

number of microorganisms are able to enter the room. All articles that come into contact with the patient are contaminated, and these items should be handled appropriately to help reduce the transmission of microorganisms. Dedicated equipment for assessment of vital signs remains in the room if possible. Otherwise, it is mandatory for the health care worker to disinfect the equipment when it must be removed from the room to use on another patient.

The psychological or emotional deprivation that may result from the use of these transmission-based isolation precautions must be considered in the care of the patient. The patient is forced into solitude and deprived of normal social contacts. If possible, spend extra time with the patient to reduce feelings of isolation. Keep the room clean and pleasant. Provide instruction about the rationale for the precautions to the patient and family members. Teach the family and visitors how to apply and dispose of any PPE that they may need to wear and ensure that the procedure is followed (Skill 7.5).

PULMONARY TUBERCULOSIS PRECAUTIONS

Pulmonary TB infections continue to concern health care workers. Some strains of these bacteria are multi-drug resistant, making treatment of the infection very difficult. The best way to prevent the transmission of pulmonary TB is to quickly identify, isolate, and treat patients with TB. The nurse should suspect a patient has pulmonary TB if the patient has respiratory symptoms that last longer than 2 weeks. Other suspicious symptoms include fatigue, unexplained weight loss, dyspnea, fever, night sweats, and hemoptysis (a cough that can be productive of blood). Good assessment skills hasten the possibility of a diagnosis, which is essential because the risk of exposure is greatest before a diagnosis is made and isolation precautions are implemented. Isolation for patients with known or suspected TB includes a negative-pressure isolation room (see Box 7.10). Such rooms have negative pressure in relation to surrounding areas in the facility so that room air is vented directly to the outside or through special high-efficiency particulate air (HEPA) filters if

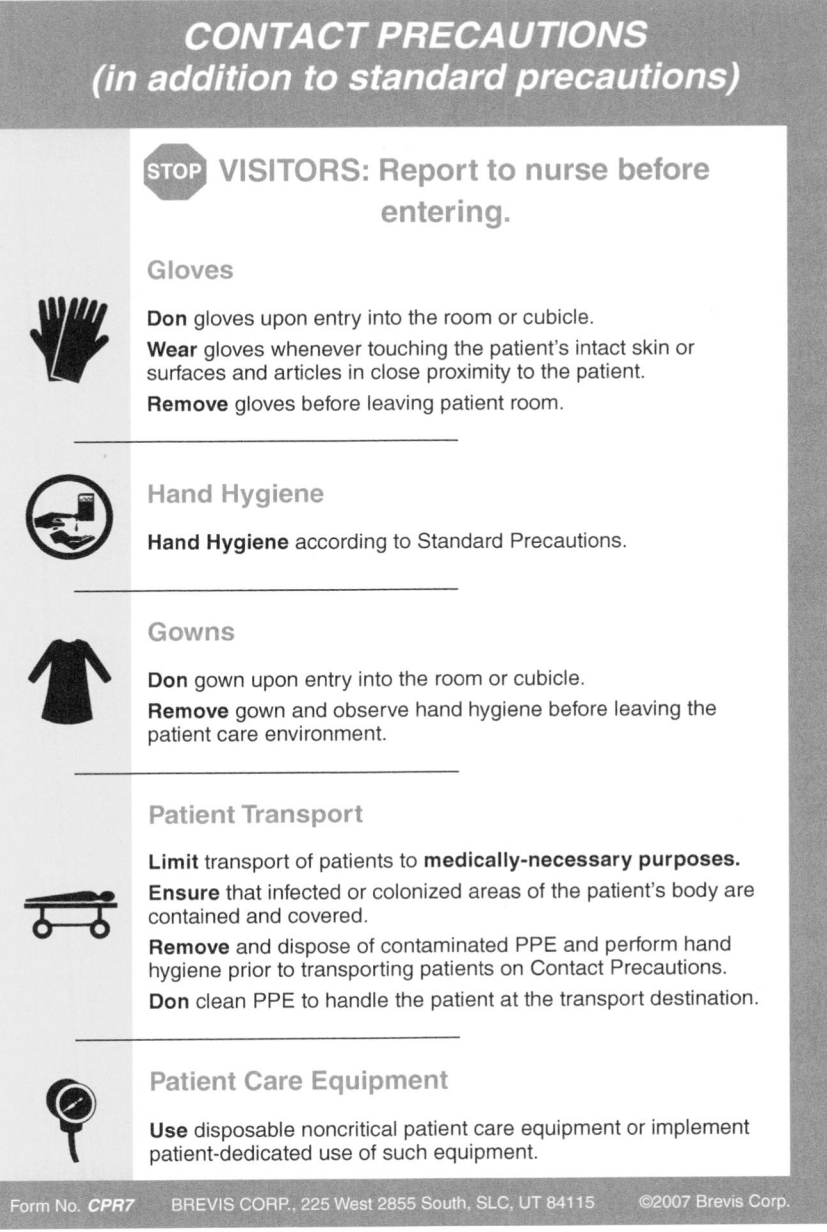

Fig. 7.9 Contact precautions. (Copyright 1997–2007 Brevis Corporation. Courtesy Brevis Corporation, Salt Lake City, Utah.)

recirculation is unavoidable. High-risk procedures on patients with suspected or confirmed infectious TB must be performed in negative-pressure rooms. Some negative air pressure rooms have an anteroom, a small room outside the negative air flow room equipped with isolation equipment, a sink, and an area to dispose of contaminated PPE. If an anteroom is not used, the equipment is kept in the hallway, at the entrance of the patient's room.

OSHA and CDC guidelines require health care workers who care for patients with known or suspected TB to wear an N-95 (or higher) respirator or mask (CDC, 2019). The respirators have the capacity to filter particles smaller than 5 μm with a filter efficiency of 95% or higher. The masks of health care employees who work with TB cases must undergo a fit-test to obtain a face-seal leakage of 10% or less. To ensure correct fit and efficiency, workers who experience a significant weight loss or weight gain should repeat the fitting process. Under National Institute for Occupational Safety and Health (NIOSH) criteria, the minimally acceptable level of respiratory protection for TB is the N-95 respirator (see Skill 7.5). Training in the wearing and storage of the respirator is required for hospital staff. OSHA also requires employers to provide training concerning the transmission of TB, especially in areas where the risk of exposure is high, such as areas where bronchoscopies are performed. Other requirements include annual TB skin testing for health care workers and appropriate follow-up when a previously negative skin test becomes positive.

Skill 7.5   Isolation (Transmission-Based) Precautions

NURSING ACTION (RATIONALE)

1. Determine the causative microorganism and the patient's immune system status. (*Determines virulence of the causative pathogen and how well the patient's immune system is working.*)
2. Recognize the mode of transmission and how the microorganism may exit the body. (*Determines the category or type of isolation to use.*)
3. Follow agency policy for the specific type of transmission-based precautions used. (*Increases awareness of isolation categories available in the agency.*)
4. Ensure that the environment has the equipment and supplies for the type of isolation:
   a. Private or isolation room with ante-room. (*Reduces spread of pathogens.*)
   b. Adequate hand hygiene facilities. (*All workers and visitors are to perform hand hygiene before entering and leaving the area.*)
   c. Containers for trash, soiled linen, and sharp instruments (such as needles). (*Ensures safe disposal of contaminated articles.*)
5. Provide an explanation of isolation precautions to the patient, family, and visitors. (*Relieves apprehension and promotes cooperation of those involved.*)
6. Post a sign on the door of the patient's room or wall outside the room stating the type of protective measures in use for patient care. (*Informs personnel, patient, family, and visitors entering the room of precautions to be followed and encourages cooperation.*)
7. Be certain to supply the room with lined containers designated for soiled linens and for trash. (*Prevents transmission of pathogens from seepage through the container.*)
8. Assess vital signs with designated equipment if possible, administer medications, administer hygiene, and collect specimens (Table 7.3). (*Administers patient care.*)

9. Report any changes in the patient's health status to the primary health care provider or supervisor. (*Ensures continuity of care and helps determine patient progress.*)
10. Record assessments and performance of transmission-based precautions. (*Provides proof of appropriate patient care.*) Document per agency policy.
11. Determine the patient's understanding of activities in the room. (*Increases patient's comfort and feeling of well-being.*)
12. Provide patient teaching (see the Patient Teaching box on infection prevention and control).
13. Additional techniques for acid-fast bacillus (AFB) isolation (*airborne precautions*):
    a. Before entering the room, don an N-95 respirator mask for which you have undergone a fit-test. (*Reduces transmission of airborne droplet nuclei.*)
    b. Educate patient, family, and other visitors about how AFB is transmitted. (*Improves the ability of the patient to participate in care. TB cannot be transmitted through contact with clothing, bedding, food, or eating utensils.*)
    c. Explain to the patient that TB is transmitted by inhalation of droplets that remain suspended in the air when the patient coughs, sneezes, or speaks (CDC, 2006). Offer an opportunity for questions. (*Improves the ability of the patient to participate in care.*)
    d. Instruct patient to cover their mouth with tissue when coughing, educate patient about when to perform hand hygiene, and educate about the importance of wearing a regular disposable surgical mask while out of the room. (*Reduces spread of droplet nuclei.*)
    e. Record assessments and performance of patient care. (*Promotes continuity of care.*)

Another option for health care workers who work around patients with known or suspected airborne infections such as TB is called a powered air-purifying respirator (PAPR). A PAPR may be selected instead of an N-95 respirator if an N-95 respirator does not fit adequately. Facial hair and facial deformities may interfere with the face seal of an N-95. A PAPR also may be worn if an N-95 respirator is unavailable.

SURGICAL ASEPSIS

Surgical asepsis, or sterile technique, requires that the nurse use different precautions from those of medical asepsis. *Surgical asepsis* is the complete removal of all microorganisms, including spores, from an object. The slightest break in technique, when working with a sterile field or with sterile equipment, results in contamination. The nurse must practice surgical asepsis during

Table 7.3 Specimen Collection Techniques for the Patient in Isolation

AMOUNT NEEDED[a]	COLLECTION DEVICE[a]	SPECIMEN COLLECTION AND TRANSFER
Wound (Culture) Specimen		
As much as possible (after cleaning the surface of the skin or wound bed to remove flora or debris)	Sterile cotton-tipped swab or syringe	Clean site with sterile water or saline solution before wound specimen collection. Don gloves and place a clean test tube or culturette tube on a clean paper towel. After swabbing the center of the wound site, grasp a collection tube by holding it with a paper towel. Carefully insert a swab without touching the outside of the tube. After removing gloves, washing hands, and securing the tube's top, transfer the labeled tube into a bag for transport to the laboratory. Document that procedure was performed.
Blood (Culture) Specimen		
This specimen usually is obtained by the laboratory technician 10 mL per culture bottle, from two different venipuncture sites (volume may differ based on collection containers and age of patient)	Syringes, needles, and culture media bottles	Don gloves and perform venipuncture per hospital protocol at two different sites to decrease the likelihood of both specimens being contaminated by skin flora. Inject 10 mL of blood into each bottle. Remove gloves and wash hands. Secure tops of bottles, label specimens, complete requisition, and send to the laboratory. Document that procedure was performed.
Stool (Culture) Specimen		
Small amount, approximately size of a walnut	Clean specimen cup with seal top (not necessary to be sterile) and sterile tongue blade	Don gloves and place a cup on a clean paper towel in the patient's bathroom. With a tongue blade, collect the needed amount of feces from the bedpan, not the toilet. Transfer feces to specimen cup without touching cup's outside surface; cover with lid provided. Remove gloves, wash hands, and place a seal on the cup. Repeat hand washing. Transfer specimen cup into a clean bag for transport to the laboratory after ensuring cup is correctly labeled. Document procedure was performed.
Urine (Culture) Specimen		
5–15 mL for adults	Syringe and sterile cup	Don gloves and place cup or tube on a clean towel in patient's bathroom. Use an alcohol swab pad, syringe, and needle to collect specimens if the patient has an indwelling urinary catheter. (All indwelling urinary catheters are equipped with needleless ports, which must be cleaned per manufacturer guidelines; alcohol swabs are not sufficient.) Otherwise, have the patient follow a procedure to obtain a clean-voided specimen (see Chapter 23). Transfer urine into a sterile container by injecting urine from a syringe or pouring it from the container. Secure top of the labeled container, remove gloves, and wash hands. Transfer labeled specimen into clean bag for transport to the laboratory, after ensuring the container is labeled correctly. Document procedure was completed.

[a]Agency policies may differ on the type of container. Ensure that all specimen containers used have the biohazard symbol on the outside and the amount of specimen required and are bagged for transport to a laboratory.
From Pagana KD, Pagana TJ: *Mosby's diagnostic and laboratory test reference*, ed 14, St. Louis, 2019, Mosby.

the period of care to keep microorganisms away from the area.

Although surgical asepsis is practiced in the operating room, the labor and delivery area, and major diagnostic or procedure areas, the nurse also uses surgical aseptic techniques at the patient's bedside. This includes, for example, when the nurse inserts intravenous (IV) lines, gives injections, inserts urinary catheters, suctions the patient's lower airway, and applies sterile dressings. In an operating room, the nurse follows a series of steps to maintain sterile techniques, including donning a mask, protective eyewear, and a cap; performing surgical hand hygiene; and donning a sterile gown and gloves. In contrast, when changing a dressing at a patient's bedside, the nurse often only performs hand hygiene, dons sterile gloves, and maintains a sterile area during the procedure. In the event of inserting IV lines and administering injections, the nurse does not use sterile gloves, but instead uses sterile equipment and avoids contamination of the sterile equipment, including not talking unnecessarily over the sterile equipment or touching the sterile items with the nurses "clean" exam gloves.

Box 7.11   Principles of Sterile Technique

1. *A sterile object remains sterile only when touched exclusively by other sterile objects.* (This principle guides your placement of sterile objects and how you handle them.)
   a. Sterile touching sterile remains sterile; for example, wear sterile gloves and use sterile forceps to handle objects on a sterile field.
   b. Sterile touching clean becomes contaminated; for example, if the tip of a syringe or other sterile object touches the surface of a clean disposable glove, the object is contaminated.
   c. Sterile touching contaminated becomes contaminated; for example, when you touch a sterile object with an ungloved hand, the object is contaminated.
   d. Sterile touching questionable is contaminated; for example, when you find a tear or break in the covering of a sterile object, discard the object regardless of whether it appears untouched or not.
2. *Place only sterile objects on a sterile field.* Properly sterilize all items before use. It is essential to keep the package or container holding a sterile object intact and dry. A package that is torn, punctured, wet, or open is unsterile.
3. *A sterile field out of the range of vision or an object held below a person's waist is contaminated.* Never turn your back on a sterile field or leave it unattended. Contamination can occur accidentally from a dangling piece of clothing, falling hair, or an unknowing patient touching a sterile object. Consider any object below waist level contaminated because you are not able to keep it in constant view. Keep sterile objects in front of you with your hands as close together as possible.
4. *A sterile object or field becomes contaminated by prolonged exposure to air.* Avoid activities that potentially create air currents, such as excessive movements or rearranging linen after a sterile object or field becomes exposed. When opening sterile packages, keep to a minimum the number of people walking into the area. Microorganisms also travel by droplets through the air. Be sure no one talks, laughs, sneezes, or coughs over a sterile field or when gathering and using sterile equipment. Never perform sterile procedures if you have a cold or other respiratory ailment unless you are wearing a specialized mask. Microorganisms have the potential to travel through the air and fall on sterile items or fields if you reach over the work area. When opening sterile packages, hold the item or piece of equipment as close

as possible to the sterile field without touching the sterile surface. Do not continue to rearrange the sterile items on the sterile field to help reduce the contamination that can occur by microorganisms traveling through the air.

5. *When a sterile surface comes in contact with a wet, contaminated surface, the sterile object or field becomes contaminated.* Moisture seeping through a sterile package's protective covering permits microorganisms to travel to the sterile object. When stored sterile packages become wet, discard the objects immediately or send the equipment for resterilization. When working with a sterile field or tray, you sometimes have to pour sterile solutions. Any spill is a possible source of contamination unless the object or field rests on a sterile surface impervious to moisture. For example, urinary catheterization trays contain sterile supplies that rest in a sterile, plastic container. Any sterile solution spilled within the container does not contaminate the catheter or other objects. In contrast, if you place a piece of sterile gauze in its wrapper on a patient's bedside table and the table surface is wet, consider the gauze to be contaminated.
6. *Fluid flows in the direction of gravity.* A sterile object becomes contaminated if gravity causes a contaminated liquid to flow over the object's surface. To prevent contamination during a surgical hand scrub, raise and hold your hands above your elbows. This allows water to flow downward without contaminating your hands and fingers. The principle of water flow by gravity is also the reason for drying in a sequence from fingers to elbows, with hands held up, after the scrub (see Skill 7.6).
7. *Consider the edges of a sterile field or container to be contaminated.* Frequently, you place sterile objects on a sterile towel or drape. Because the edge of the drape touches an unsterile surface, such as a table or bed linen, a 1-in (2.5-cm) border around the drape must be considered contaminated. The edges of sterile containers become exposed to air after they are open and thus are contaminated. After you remove a sterile needle from its protective cap or after removing a forceps from a container, do not allow the objects to touch the container's edge. The lip of an opened bottle of solution also becomes contaminated after it is exposed to air. When pouring a sterile liquid, first pour a small amount of solution and discard it. The solution thus washes away microorganisms on the bottle lip. Then, pour a second time on the same side to fill a container with the desired amount of solution.

Because surgical asepsis requires exact techniques, the nurse needs the patient's cooperation. For this reason, the nurse should prepare the patient before any procedure. Some patients may fear moving or touching objects during a sterile procedure, whereas other patients may try to assist. The nurse should explain how a procedure is to be performed and instruct the patient how to avoid contaminating sterile items, including the following measures:

- The patient should try not to make sudden movements of body parts covered by sterile drapes.

- The patient should refrain from touching sterile supplies, drapes, and the nurse's gloves and gown.
- The patient should avoid coughing, sneezing, or talking over a sterile area.

PRINCIPLES OF STERILE TECHNIQUE

When beginning a surgically aseptic procedure, follow the principles listed in Box 7.11 to ensure maintenance of surgical asepsis. Failure to follow each principle conscientiously endangers patients by placing them at risk for infection.

Assemble all the equipment necessary for a sterile procedure before the procedure begins. By doing so, avoid the need to leave a sterile area unattended to locate missing equipment or supplies. Have a few extra supplies available in case something accidentally becomes contaminated. If an object becomes contaminated during the procedure, it should be discarded immediately per facility policy.

SURGICAL HAND SCRUB

In the operating room setting, effective hand washing or the use of appropriate surgical hand rub to achieve surgical hand hygiene is imperative. To reduce patients' risk of postoperative infection, the nurses and other surgical personnel use an antimicrobial solution for hand hygiene as an integral part of the presurgical scrubbing procedure. Although sterilizing the skin is not possible, the number of microorganisms can be reduced greatly by chemical, physical, and mechanical means.

The surgical hand scrub (Skill 7.6) is the traditional method for surgical asepsis. With the use of an antimicrobial agent and sterile brushes, the surgical hand scrub removes debris and transient microorganisms from the nails, hands, and forearms. This technique also reduces the resident microbial count to a minimum and inhibits the rapid or rebound growth of microorganisms. According to the CDC (2020), use of an alcohol-based surgical hand rub, following a prewash of the hands, is also acceptable as long it has met US Food and Drug Administration requirements to be used for this purpose. Both hand antiseptic methods currently are used in operating room settings. Skill 7.6 addresses both techniques. Surgical personnel wear surgical attire (i.e., scrubs) in the operating room to reduce the chance for contamination from themselves to patients and vice versa. Fingernails should be short, clean, and natural. Do not wear artificial nails. Artificial nails harbor microorganisms (CDC, 2020). Remove all rings, watches, and bracelets before the surgical scrub and while assisting with procedures that require surgical asepsis.

The AORN (2013) has a revised set of policies and procedures; in addition, refer to agency policy on surgical hand hygiene (refer to *Adult Health Nursing*, Chapter 2).

MANAGING STERILE PACKAGES

Sterile items such as syringes, gauze dressings, and catheters are packaged in paper or plastic containers that are impervious to (unable to be penetrated by) microorganisms if the items remain dry and intact. Paper packages are permeable to steam and thus allow for steam autoclaving. A disadvantage of paper wrappers is that they tear or puncture relatively easily. Sterile items should be placed in clean enclosed storage cabinets and never kept in the same room as dirty equipment.

Sterile supplies have dated labels or chemical tapes that indicate the date when the sterilization expires. The tapes change color during the sterilization process. Failure of the tapes to change color means the item is not sterile. Never use or allow the use of a sterile item or piece of equipment after the expiration date. Some agencies use the "event-related" contamination rule. If the integrity of the sterile package is questionable (i.e., wet, torn, discolored), the item is discarded or resterilized per policy. If the nurse finds moisture present after a sterile tray is opened, the item is either discarded or returned to the institution's supply area for resterilization.

Before opening a sterile item, perform thorough hand hygiene. Assemble the supplies at the work area, such as the bedside table or in the treatment room before packages are opened. A bedside table or countertop provides a large, clean working area for the opening of items. Ensure that the work area is above your waist level. Sterile supplies should not be opened in a space where a dirty object may fall on or come into contact with them.

Sterile packaged items can be opened without contamination of the contents even when you are not wearing sterile gloves. Commercially packaged items usually are designed so that you only have to tear away or separate the paper or plastic cover from the rest of the tray or kit. Hold the item in one hand while pulling the wrapper with the other (Fig. 7.10). Be careful after opening to keep the inner contents sterile before use. When opening items packed in linen and some commercially prepackaged items, use the steps described in Box 7.12 and illustrated in Figs. 7.10 and 7.11.

PREPARING A STERILE FIELD

Performing sterile procedures requires a sterile work area that provides room for handling and placing sterile items. A sterile field is an area that is free of microorganisms and has been prepared to receive sterile items. The nurse should prepare the field by using the inner surface of a sterile wrapper as the work surface or by using a sterile drape (Skill 7.7).

Sometimes, nurses choose to wear sterile gloves while preparing items on the field. The nurse is then able to touch the entire drape, but an assistant must open and pass sterile items to the nurse unless the nurse applies new sterile gloves to prevent contamination of the sterile items. The nurse should not allow the gloves to touch the outside wrapping of the package that contains the sterile items.

POURING STERILE SOLUTIONS

The nurse may be required to pour sterile solutions into sterile containers. A bottle that contains a sterile solution is sterile on the inside and contaminated on the outside. The bottle's neck is also contaminated, but the inside of the bottle cap is sterile. After opening a cap or lid, hold it in the hand or place it, sterile side

Skill 7.6   Surgical Hand Hygiene

CHECK   GATHER   HELLO   ID   PRIVACY   EXPLAIN   WASH   GLOVES

NURSING ACTION *(RATIONALE)*

1. Inspect hands for the presence of abrasions, cuts, or open lesions. (*These conditions increase the likelihood of more microorganisms residing on skin surfaces.*)

2. Apply surgical shoe covers, cap or hood, face mask, and protective eyewear. (*Mask prevents escape into the air of microorganisms that can contaminate hands. Other protective wear prevents exposure to blood and body fluid splashes during the procedure.*)

3. Perform surgical hand hygiene (traditional method):

   a. Turn on water using knee or foot controls and adjust to a comfortable temperature.

   b. Wet hands and arms under running lukewarm water and lather with detergent to 5 cm (2 inches) above elbows. (Keep hands above elbows at all times.) (*Hands become the cleanest part of the upper extremity. Keeping hands elevated allows water to flow from least to most contaminated areas because water runs by gravity from the fingertips to the elbows. Washing a wide area reduces the risk of contaminating the gown that you will don later.*)

   c. Rinse hands and arms thoroughly under running water. **Remember to keep hands above elbows.** (*Rinsing removes transient microorganisms from fingers, hands, and forearms.*)

   d. Under running water, clean under nails of both hands with a nail pick. Discard after use. (*Removes dirt and organic material that harbor large numbers of microorganisms.*)

   (1) Wet a clean sponge and apply antimicrobial detergent. Scrub nails of one hand with 15 strokes. Holding sponge perpendicular to hand, scrub palm, each side of thumb and fingers, and posterior side of each hand with 10 strokes.

   (2) Mentally divide your arm into thirds, and scrub each third 10 times. The entire scrub should last 5–10 min. Rinse the sponge and repeat the sequence for the other arm. It is permitted to substitute with a two-sponge method. Check agency policy. (*Friction loosens resident bacteria that adhere to skin surfaces. Ensures coverage of all surfaces. Scrubbing is performed from the cleanest area [hands] to a marginal area [upper arms.]*)

   e. Discard sponge and rinse hands and arms thoroughly. Turn off water with foot or knee control and back into room entrance with hands elevated in front of and away from the body. (*After it has touched skin, consider the sponge contaminated. Rinsing removes resident bacteria. Prevents accidental contamination.*)

Skill 7.6   Surgical Hand Hygiene—cont'd

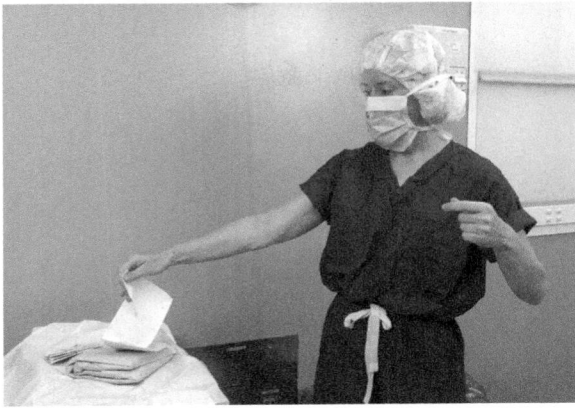

(1) Walk up to the sterile tray and lean forward slightly to pick up a sterile towel.

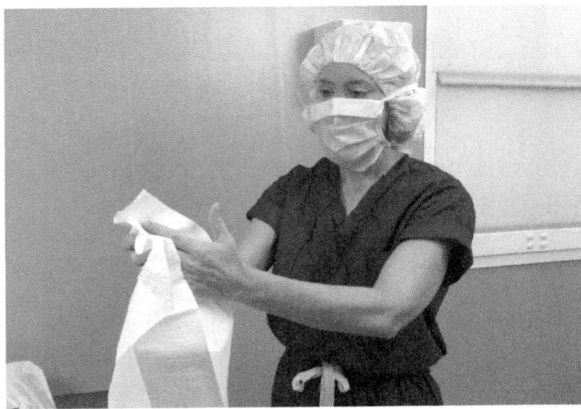

(2) Dry one hand thoroughly, moving in sequence from fingers to elbow. Dry in a rotating motion. Dry from the cleanest to the least clean area. *(Drying prevents chapping and facilitates donning of gloves. Leaning forward prevents accidental contact of arms with scrub attire.)*

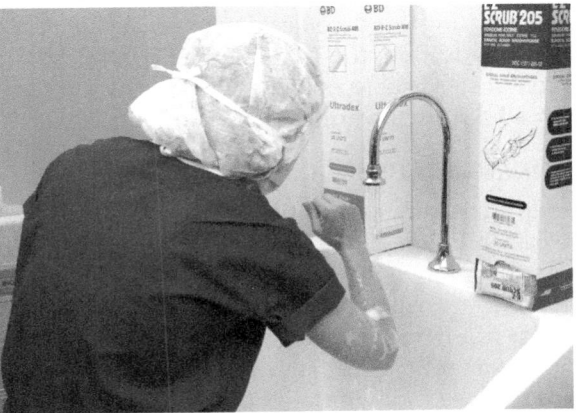

f. Repeat the drying method for the other hand by carefully reversing the towel or using a new sterile towel. *(Prevents accidental contamination.)*

g. Discard towel. *(Prevents accidental contamination.)*

5. Proceed with sterile gowning.

4. Alternate method of surgical hand hygiene using an alcohol-based antiseptic:

a. Wash hands with soap and water for 15–30 s to remove soil. *(Removes dirt and organic material that harbor large numbers of microorganisms.)*

b. Under running water, clean under nails of both hands with a nail pick. Discard after use and dry hands with a paper towel. *(Removes dirt and organic material that harbor large numbers of microorganisms.)*

c. Apply enough alcohol-based waterless antiseptic to one palm to cover both hands thoroughly. Spread the antiseptic over all surfaces of the hands and the fingernails. Follow product instructions for length of time to rub over hand surfaces. Allow to air dry. *(Ensures coverage of all surfaces. Air drying ensures complete antisepsis.)*

d. Repeat the process and allow hands to air dry before applying sterile gloves.

Figures from Potter PA, Perry AG: *Fundamentals of nursing: concepts, process, and practice,* ed 9, St. Louis, 2016, Elsevier.

Fig. 7.10 When opening a commercially packaged sterile item, tear the wrapper away from your body.

Fig. 7.11 Placement of items on a sterile field.

Box 7.12   Opening Sterile Packages

1. Perform hand hygiene.
2. Place the item flat in the center of the work surface.
3. Remove the tape or seal that indicates the sterilization date.
4. Grasp the outer surface of the tip of the outermost flap.
5. Open the outer flap away from your body, keeping your arm outstretched and away from the sterile field.
6. Grasp the outside surface of the first side flap.
7. Open the side flap, allowing it to lie flat on the table surface. Keep your arm to the side and not over the sterile surface. Do not allow flaps to spring back over the sterile contents.
8. Grasp the outside surface of the second side flap and allow it to lie flat on the table surface.
9. Grasp the outer surface of the last and innermost flap.
10. Stand away from the sterile package and pull the flap back, allowing it to fall flat on the surface.
11. Use the inner surface of the package cover (except for the 1-in border around the edges) as a sterile field to handle this or additional sterile items (see Fig. 7.10). Grasp the 1-in border to maneuver the entire field on the table surface.
12. When opening a small sterile item, hold it in your hand so that you can pass it to a person wearing sterile gloves or transfer it to a sterile field. Hold the package in your nondominant hand while you open the top flap and pull it away from you. With your dominant hand, carefully open the side and top flaps away from the enclosed sterile item in the same order as in the previous steps (see Fig. 7.9).

(inside) up, on a clean surface. Thus, you can see the inside of the lid as it rests on the table surface. Never allow a bottle's cap or lid to rest sterile side down on a sterile surface because the cap's outer edge is unsterile and will contaminate the surface. Likewise, the placement of a sterile cap down on an unsterile surface increases the chances of the inside of the cap becoming contaminated.

Hold the bottle with its label in the palm of the hand to prevent the solution from wetting the label. If the solution wets the label, it may cause it to fade or smear and reduce its legibility. Keep the edge of the bottle from touching the edge or the inside of the receiving container, which is unsterile. Pour the solution slowly to avoid splashing the underlying drape or field. Never hold the bottle so high above the recipient container that even slow pouring causes splashing. Hold the bottle over the outside of the edge of the sterile field (Fig. 7.12).

DONNING A STERILE GOWN

A nurse must don a sterile gown (Skill 7.8) before working in the operating room and before assisting with certain sterile procedures or working in special treatment areas. The sterile gown decreases the risk of contaminating sterile objects when the nurse handles them. In addition, the sterile gown prevents contamination of sterile objects or sterile fields by microorganisms shed from the nurse's skin (Potter et al., 2019).

DONNING STERILE GLOVES

Sterile gloves are an additional barrier used to prevent the transmission of microorganisms. The two methods of donning gloves are open (Skill 7.9) and closed (Fig. 7.13). Nurses who work in general nursing divisions use open gloving before procedures such as dressing changes or urinary catheter insertions. Nurses should use the closed gloving method when donning a sterile gown before procedures in the operating room and special treatment areas.

When donning sterile gloves, select the proper glove size. The glove must be snug enough for you to

Skill 7.7   Preparing a Sterile Field

NURSING ACTION *(RATIONALE)*

1. Prepare a sterile field just before the planned procedure. *(Prevents exposure of sterile field and supplies to air contamination.)* Be sure to use supplies immediately.
2. Select a clean work surface that is above waist level. *(Consider sterile objects held below waist contaminated.)*
3. Assemble necessary equipment. *(Preparing equipment in advance prevents breaks in technique.)*
   - Sterile drape
   - Assorted sterile supplies
4. Check dates, labels, and condition of the package for sterility of equipment. *(Consider equipment stored beyond expiration date, or a package that is damaged, unsterile.)*
5. Wash hands thoroughly. *(Prevents spread of microorganisms.)*
6. Place package containing sterile drape on the work surface and open. *(Ensures sterility of packaged drape.)*

7. With fingertips of one hand, pick up the folded top edge of the sterile drape. *(Up to the 1-inch border around drape is unsterile and permitted to be touched.)*
8. Gently lift the drape up from its outer cover and let it unfold by itself without touching any object. Discard the outer cover with your other hand. *(If a sterile object touches any unsterile object, it becomes contaminated.)*
9. With the other hand, grasp the adjacent corner of the drape and hold the entire edge straight up and away from your body. Now, properly place the drape while using two hands and be sure to keep the drape away from unsterile surfaces. *(Prevents contamination.)*
   a. Holding the drape, first position the bottom half over the intended work surface. *(Prevents from reaching over the sterile field.)*
   b. Allow the top half of the drape to be placed over the work surface last. *(Creates a flat, sterile work surface.)*
10. Perform the procedure using a sterile technique. *(Prevents contamination.)*

Fig. 7.12 Place receptacle into which you pour fluids near the edge of the sterile table to prevent the need for reaching over the sterile field to pour.

pick up things easily and yet not so tightly stretched that it tears easily.

Closed Gloving

Closed gloving is practiced when the nurse also needs to wear a sterile gown. With closed gloving, contamination of the sterile gown is prevented. The wearer of a sterile gown and sterile gloves can safely handle sterile materials and instruments during surgery or other types of sterile procedures.

CLEANING, DISINFECTION, AND STERILIZATION

Microorganisms are present on items in the home and public areas, including health care agencies. By following a basic clean or aseptic technique, the nurse can help interrupt the spread of infection. Antiseptics are a means to inhibit the growth of microorganisms, although killing them this way is not possible. Antiseptics also are referred to as *bacteriostatic* solutions. *Bacterio-* means "microorganism," and *static* means "referring to that which cannot move or grow." Use of antiseptics (e.g., alcohol or CHG) on human tissue is acceptable and often is performed before sterile procedures such as surgery and during wound care. Antiseptics can be used for mouth care and when performing hand hygiene.

CLEANING

Cleaning is the removal of foreign materials, such as soil and organic material, from objects. Generally, cleaning involves the use of water and mechanical action with or without detergents.

When an object comes in contact with potentially infectious material, the object is contaminated. If the object is disposable, it is discarded per facility policy. Reusable objects must be cleaned thoroughly and then either disinfected or sterilized before reuse, per facility policy.

Skill 7.8   Donning a Sterile Gown

NURSING ACTION *(RATIONALE)*

The nurse should perform the following steps when applying a sterile gown:

1. Don surgical cap, shoe covers, protective eyewear, and mask and then perform surgical hand hygiene. (*Prevents contamination of the surgical field and protects the nurse from blood and body fluid exposure.*)

2. Ask the circulating nurse to open the sterile gown package and the sterile glove package. (*Prevents contamination of the hands after the surgical hand wash because the outer wraps are not sterile.*)

3. Don the gown.
   a. If available, the scrub nurse assists by pulling the gown over your extended hands and arms. If no assistance from a scrub nurse is available:
      (1) Pick up the gown touching only the inner surface below the neck. (*Touching the outer, sterile surface causes the gown to become contaminated because the hands are not yet gloved and thus unsterile.*)
      (2) Maintain constant control of the folded layers of the gown. (*Prevents the gown from brushing against unsterile surfaces.*)
      (3) While holding the gown at arm's length, allow the gown to unfold from top to bottom. Be sure that the gown does not touch the floor. (*Prevents contamination.*)

(4) While holding the inside of the gown near the shoulders and below the neckband, slide hands and arms into the sleeves with your fingers stopping at the end of the cuffs. (*The fingers remain inside the sleeves to don the sterile gloves by means of closed gloving.*)

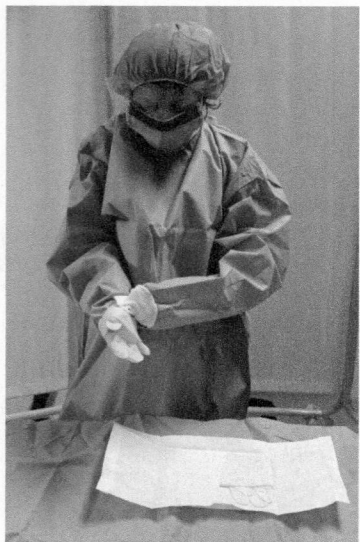

(5) Ask another staff member to grasp the cord that is attached to the ties of the gown to draw the ties around to the back with the gown overlapping itself. The staff member should now tie the gown, avoiding touching any part of the gown except the ties. (*Do not allow the front or the sides of the gown to be touched by the staff member because these areas are sterile.*)

CHECK GATHER HELLO ID PRIVACY EXPLAIN WASH GLOVES

NURSING ACTION (RATIONALE)

1. Have a package of properly sized sterile gloves at the treatment area. (*Facilitates procedure.*)
2. Perform thorough hand hygiene. (*Removes bacteria from skin surfaces.*)
3. Remove outer glove package wrapper by carefully separating and peeling apart sides. (*Prevents inner glove package from accidentally opening and touching contaminated objects.*)

4. Grasping the inner side of the package, lay the package on a clean flat surface just above waist level. Open package, keeping gloves on wrapper's inside surface. (*Inner surface of the glove package is sterile. Sterile objects held below the waist are considered contaminated.*)

5. Identify right and left gloves. Each glove has a cuff approximately 2-in (5-cm) deep. (*Proper identification of gloves prevents contamination by improper fit.*)

6. Glove dominant hand first. With the thumb and first two fingers of the nondominant hand, grasp the edge of the cuff of the glove for the dominant hand. Touch only the glove's inside surface. (*Gloving of dominant hand first improves dexterity. Touching the inside surface is permitted because the inner edge of the cuff will lie against skin. If the glove's outer surface touches a hand or wrist, it is contaminated.*)

7. Carefully pull the glove over the dominant hand, leaving the cuff; be sure the cuff does not roll up the wrist. Be sure the thumb and fingers are in proper spaces. (*If the glove's outer surface touches a hand or wrist, it is contaminated.*)

Continued

8. With a gloved dominant hand, slip fingers underneath the second glove's cuff in such a fashion that the cuff will protect the gloved fingers. *(Sterile touching sterile prevents glove contamination.)*

9. Carefully pull the second glove over the nondominant hand. Do not allow fingers and thumb of the gloved dominant hand to touch any part of the exposed nondominant hand. Keep the thumb of the dominant hand abducted back. *(Contact of gloved hand with exposed hand results in contamination.)*

10. After the second glove is on, interlock hands. *Be sure to touch only sterile sides.* The cuffs usually fall down after application. *(Ensures smooth fit over fingers.)*

GLOVE REMOVAL AND DISPOSAL

11. Grasp the outside of one cuff with the other gloved hand; avoid touching the wrist. *(Minimizes contamination of underlying skin.)*

12. Pull the glove off, turning it inside out. Discard in a receptacle. *(The outside of the glove does not touch the skin surface.)*

13. Take fingers of the bare hand and tuck inside the remaining glove cuff. Peel glove off, inside out. Discard in a receptacle. *(Reduces spread of microorganisms.)*

Fig. 7.13 Closed gloving. (A) Open glove package. (B) Grasp back of dominant hand's glove cuff with nondominant hand and stretch over the end of dominant hand's sleeve. (C) Glove nondominant hand in the same manner. (D) Use the gloved dominant hand to pull on the glove, keeping the nondominant hand inside the sleeve until it emerges into the glove.

When cleaning equipment that is soiled by organic material such as blood, fecal matter, mucus, or pus, put on a mask and protective eyewear or goggles (or a face shield), a fluid-resistant gown, and waterproof gloves. These barriers provide protection from infectious organisms (as discussed previously). A stiff-bristled brush and detergent or soap are necessary for cleaning.

Perform the following steps when cleaning equipment:

1. Rinse a contaminated object or article with cold running water to remove organic material. Hot water causes the protein in organic material to coagulate and stick to objects, making removal difficult.
2. After rinsing, wash the object with soap and warm water. Soap or detergent reduces the surface tension of water and emulsifies dirt and remaining material. Rinse the object thoroughly to remove the emulsified dirt.
3. Use a brush to remove dirt or material present in the equipment's grooves or seams. Friction dislodges contaminated material for easy removal. Open any hinged items for cleaning.
4. Rinse the object in warm water.
5. Dry the object and prepare it for disinfection or sterilization if indicated by the intended use of the item.
6. The brush, gloves, and sink in which the equipment is cleaned are considered contaminated and must be cleaned and dried per facility policy.

DISINFECTION

Disinfection is used to destroy microorganisms. However, it does not destroy spores. The solutions used during disinfection are called *disinfectants,* or possibly *bactericidal solutions* (the suffix *-cidal* is derived from a Latin word meaning "to kill"). These solutions are too strong to use on human skin and are appropriate to use on inanimate objects. If a disinfectant solution comes in contact with human tissue, the tissue may feel "slippery." This is the first step of tissue breakdown. When using a disinfectant, use clean gloves to protect the skin (Skill 7.10).

STERILIZATION

Sterilization refers to methods used to kill all microorganisms, including spores. The two types of sterilization methods are physical and chemical (Box 7.13).

Most health agencies have a central supply department that disinfects and sterilizes reusable equipment and supplies. Although most supplies used today for patient care are disposable, some supplies and equipment still require the use of disinfection and sterilization. The patient and family members should be taught the principles of cleansing and disinfecting in the home environment (see the Patient Teaching box on disinfection and sterilization).

There are two accepted methods of disinfection and sterilization (see Box 7.13). One is a physical process that uses heat or radiation; the second process uses chemicals. Both methods destroy microorganisms. The method used depends on the following factors: (1) the type of microorganisms present (spore-forming bacteria are resistant to destruction); (2) how many microorganisms may be present (it takes longer to kill a large number); and (3) the type of item that must be disinfected and sterilized (some materials are so sensitive that heat or certain chemicals destroy them). Other determinants of the sterilization method used are (1) the intended use for the article (e.g.,

Skill 7.10   Preparing for Disinfection and Sterilization

NURSING ACTION (RATIONALE)

1. Prepare equipment and supplies. (*Ensures organization of procedure.*)
   - Disinfectant to use for cleansing. (*Aids in the appropriate care of equipment and reusable supplies.*)
   - Method of sterilization. (*Ensures that appropriate method is used.*)
   - Gloves. (*Protects you from contamination.*)
   - Running water. (*Aids in cleansing and rinsing of articles.*)
   - Scrub brush. (*Aids in cleaning grooves.*)
   - Cloth wrapper. (*Provides the means for wrapping articles that require sterilization.*)
2. Don gloves. (*Protects you from contamination.*)

3. Rinse the article under cool running water. (*Emulsifies or softens soil for removal.*)
4. Wash the article with detergent. (*Emulsifies or softens dirt for easy removal.*)
5. Use the scrub brush to remove material in grooves. (*Friction loosens material in corners and grooves.*)
6. Dry the article thoroughly. (*Prevents the growth of microorganisms.*)
7. Prepare the article for sterilization by wrapping it in a cloth wrapper. (*Promotes appropriate sterilization of the article.*)
8. Clean the work area and put it in order. (*Prevents the spread of microorganisms.*)
9. Perform patient teaching (see the Patient Teaching box on disinfection and sterilization in the home).

Box 7.13   Methods of Disinfection and Sterilization

PHYSICAL METHOD

1. Steam under pressure, or moist heat, is the most practical and dependable method for the destruction of all microorganisms. This process is called sterilization. Examples of sterilization equipment are the autoclave, which is used in hospitals and other agencies, and the pressure cooker, which is used in a home environment.
2. Boiling water is the best method for home use and is the least expensive. However, this technique does not destroy bacterial spores and some viruses. The article must be boiled for a minimum of 15–20 min for disinfection.
3. Radiation is used to sterilize pharmaceutical goods, foods, and heat-sensitive items. It is extremely effective on articles that are difficult to sterilize with other methods.
4. Dry heat is a method used for disinfecting articles that are destroyed by moisture. Health agencies seldom use this method, but in the home, an article can be disinfected by being placed in the oven for 2 h at 320°F (160°C) or for 45 min at 350°F (176.7°C).

CHEMICAL PROCESS

1. Gas (ethylene oxide) is used for sterilization. It destroys spores formed by bacteria.
2. Chemical solutions often are used to disinfect instruments because they are effective in destroying microorganisms. One way to store clinical thermometers is in a chemical solution, and some articles are soaked in a solution to prepare them for another, more definitive method of disinfection or sterilization.

---

surgery requires that all organisms be destroyed, whereas medical asepsis consists of techniques that inhibit the growth and transmission of pathogenic microorganisms) and (2) the methods of sterilization available.

Liquid and gaseous chemicals are used to sterilize and disinfect equipment. Examples may include iodine, alcohol, dialdehyde, and chlorine bleach compounds. Chlorine bleach is useful for household disinfection and disinfection of water, but it must never be mixed with ammonia because of the resulting emission of toxic fumes. Chlorine bleach has a tendency to corrode some metals. Iodine is a good bactericidal agent (i.e., it kills bacteria but not spores). Iodine leaves behind stains and is not used as widely as it was previously.

PATIENT TEACHING FOR INFECTION PREVENTION AND CONTROL

Patients and families often have to learn to use infection prevention and control practices at home. The aseptic technique becomes almost second nature to the nurse, who practices it daily. However, the patient is less aware of the factors that promote the spread of infection and of the ways to prevent its transmission. The nurse should educate patients about the nature of infection and the techniques to use in planning or controlling its spread (see the Lifespan Considerations for Older Adults and Cultural Considerations boxes regarding infection control).

Lifespan Considerations
Older Adults

Infection Prevention and Control

- The older adult experiences an alteration in the integrity of the oral mucosa. Promote careful oral hygiene and emphasize the importance of routine dental care.
- The older adult experiences a decrease in the production of digestive acid. Teach the older patient to wash hands carefully before food preparation, to cook foods adequately, and to refrigerate unused portions promptly.
- The dermal and epidermal skin layers of the older adult become thinner, and elasticity is decreased. Turn the bedridden patient frequently, and carefully observe the skin for impairment.
- The older adult may experience urethral stricture, neurogenic bladder, and prostatic enlargement (in males). In the older patient with an indwelling urinary catheter, assess for adequate drainage and maintain the cleanliness of the urethra and the perineal area.
- Older adults experience a decrease in rib cage movement during inspiration. When caring for older adults after surgery, elevate the head of the bed (if indicated) and encourage the patient to cough and breathe deeply and to get out of bed as soon as possible to prevent postoperative complications such as pneumonia.

Cultural Considerations

Infection Prevention and Control

- Cultural heritage affects all dimensions of health. The patient's cultural background must be considered when educating a patient about infection prevention and control measures.
- The way that culture influences behaviors, attitudes, and values depends on many factors and is often not the same for every member of a cultural group.
- Clean water may be a difficult commodity for some of the populations who live in remote areas of the Arctic region. In some villages near the ocean, drinking water is brought in as ice from several miles upriver. In this process, the chunks of ice destined for human consumption often are handled by many people and must be melted, boiled, and cooled.
- Some cultures have a traditional belief that disease is caused by contact with contaminated agents such as blood, corpses, and skin diseases.
- The germ theory can be confusing to individuals with animistic beliefs (a belief in the existence of spirits and demons). They may believe that the supernatural or spirit world causes disease.
- Some religions have customs that promote good hygiene or have been proven medically sound practices, such as washing the hands on awakening from sleep, after elimination of body wastes, after hair cutting, after touching vermin (insects and small animals), after being close to a dead body, and before eating or drinking.
- In some cultures, people may trust faith healers and be less likely to take preventive health measures.

INFECTION PREVENTION AND CONTROL FOR HOME AND HOSPICE SETTINGS

Patients commonly are discharged from acute care to their homes more quickly than in the past. Thus, they often require care from home health personnel. An infection that develops within 30 days after discharge, such as a wound infection at an operative site, may be an outcome of hospitalization, and the acute care facility's infection control department must receive a report. As more patients elect to die at home, care for the dying makes similar care and reporting measures necessary more often. The epidemiologic (pertaining to the study of the occurrence, distribution, and causes of disease in humankind) basis of infections that develop in homes sometimes is related to the diseases that affect a community. The patient developing influenza, an enteric infection, or a streptococcal pharyngitis as it passes through the community is an example of diseases that an epidemiologist my track.

As home care and hospice programs continue to expand, questions emerge about infection prevention and control in these settings. The reliability of hospital infection rates depends directly on the accurate identification of the source of infection. Such accuracy tends to be problematic when rapid hospital discharges leave the source of an infection unclear. Hospitalized patients need to receive education and instruction at discharge about reporting the occurrence of any signs and symptoms of infection such as pain, erythema (redness), edema (swelling), drainage or exudate, and fever to the appropriate acute care personnel after discharge (see the Health Promotion box).

❖ NURSING PROCESS

The role of the LPN/LVN in the nursing process as stated is that the nurse:
- Participates in planning care for patients based on patient needs.
- Reviews patient's plan of care and recommends revisions as needed.
- Reviews and follows defined prioritization for patient care.
- Uses clinical pathways, care maps, or care plans to guide and review patient care.

◆ ASSESSMENT

By evaluating signs and symptoms revealed during assessment, the nurse can determine whether a patient's clinical condition indicates a risk for infection. Early recognition of infection helps the nurse identify a patient problem and thus establish an appropriate treatment plan. In addition, the nurse should consider how well the patient is dealing with the disease and whether any resources could benefit the patient. It is important to include the patients: how does the infection affect them?

Health Promotion

Prevention of Infection in the Home Setting

The basic principles of hygiene are bathing; not sharing personal articles such as combs, toothbrushes, razors, and washcloths; and covering the mouth when coughing and sneezing. These practices are important to help prevent the spread of infection in the home setting. Patient education about the risk of spreading microorganisms responsible for hospital-acquired infections to family or friends is important, especially when family members are assisting at home in changing dressings or managing hygiene for patients with incontinence.

The licensed practical/vocational nurse (LPN/LVN) helps educate patients and family members about the following activities:

- *Hand hygiene.* Wash hands after using the bathroom, after contact with any secretions, before inserting contact lenses, before eating, and before and after patient care. Use water, soap, and friction for at least 20 seconds, and dry hands thoroughly. Use of an alcohol-based hand sanitizer can be used if soap and water are not available and hands are not visibly soiled. It is recommended that the product contain at least 60% alcohol.
- *Food preparation.* Ensure the patient has the resources needed to maintain basic food safety such as indoor plumbing with hot and cold water and power for a refrigerator (electricity or gas). Do not allow any person with an infectious gastrointestinal disease to prepare food until symptoms resolve. Do not thaw and then refreeze foods. Be sure cooked foods are stored immediately in clean containers in the refrigerator. Wash hands before food preparation. Do not allow raw meat items to come in contact with other food items because of a risk of spreading disease. Using a dishwasher or washing dishes in hot soapy water decreases the risk of contamination (CDC, 2017).
- *Tube feedings.* Prepare enough formula for only 8 hours (commercially prepared) or 4 hours (home prepared). Contaminated enteral feeding may cause infections in patients (e.g., *Salmonella* or staphylococcal infections). The feeding bag and tubing should be cleansed or replaced per manufacturer recommendations.
- *Linens.* Wash linens that are contaminated with blood or body fluids separately in hot, soapy water with 1 cup of bleach per load, and dry them in a dryer on the hot cycle.
- *Waste containers.* Keep waste containers available in the patient contact area for the disposal of dressings, diapers, tissues, and other disposable items. Place a sturdy bag inside the waste container to prevent spilling and leakage. Flush body fluids such as urine, vomitus, feces, and blood down the toilet.
- *Body fluid spills.* Clean up any accidental body fluid spill as soon as possible, while wearing gloves. To disinfect, spray a solution of 1 cup of bleach diluted with 10 cups of water over the spill, and clean up with paper towels. Then, place the paper towels in the plastic-lined waste container.

Prompt assessment of laboratory data will provide information about potential infections. Laboratory values such as increased white blood cell count or a positive blood culture often indicate infection. In the assessment of laboratory data, the nurse should consider the age of the patient. For example, in the older adult, smaller amounts of bacteria such as *Salmonella* have the potential to cause gastrointestinal infections because of the decrease in bactericidal gastric acids and deterioration of the mucosal layer of the stomach.

Sometimes positive laboratory results indicate the need to use transmission-based isolation precautions. In this case, the nurse should consult the infection control nurse or refer to the facility's infection prevention and control policy manual.

◆ PATIENT PROBLEMS

The selection of patient problems is based on data collected during the assessment. Possible patient problems for patients susceptible to or affected by an infection include the following:

- Compromised Tissue Integrity
- Potential for Infection (Nursing Care Plan 7.1)
- Social Seclusion

◆ EXPECTED OUTCOMES AND PLANNING

The plan of care focuses on achieving specific goals and outcomes related to the patient problems chosen. Interventions are determined with the aid of the patient, the family, the physician, and other members of the health care team. These goals and outcomes possibly include the following:

Goal 1: Transmission of an infectious organism is prevented.

Outcome: Patient does not experience the onset of HAI.

Goal 2: Progress of infection is controlled or decreased.

Outcome: Inflammation or signs and symptoms over an involved site decrease in 5 days.

◆ IMPLEMENTATION

The nurse's role is to prevent the onset and spread of infection and promote healing. By recognizing and assessing a patient's risk factors and implementing appropriate measures, the nurse has the capacity to help reduce the risk of transmitting infections. Use good hand hygiene techniques, properly use sterile supplies, and wear appropriate PPE, as indicated.

◆ EVALUATION

The success of the nurse who practices infection prevention and control techniques is measured according to the extent to which the goals are achieved for reducing or preventing infection. Evaluation is by nature ongoing because a patient's condition can change at any time. The nurse is then in a position to decide to continue nursing interventions, revise them as necessary,

🤝 Nursing Care Plan 7.1   The Patient With an Infection

This care plan has been created for the patient who is at risk for infection. Mr. R. is a 68-year-old man in the nursing unit for 8-hour postoperative care after a bowel resection. He has intravenous fluids infusing and a urethral catheter in place.

PATIENT PROBLEM

Potential for infection related to the presence of abdominal incision, intravenous devices, age, presence of an indwelling catheter

Patient Goals and Expected Outcomes	Nursing Interventions	Evaluation
Patient remains free of the signs and symptoms of infection as evidenced by normal vital signs and absence of purulent drainage from abdominal incision, tubes, and catheter	Assess for the presence or existence of risk factors, such as abdominal incision, indwelling catheter, and venous or arterial devices. Monitor white blood count (WBC). Monitor the following for signs and symptoms of infection: • Erythema (redness) • Edema (swelling) • Increased pain • Purulent exudates (drainage) at incision, exit sites of IV, in-dwelling urinary catheter • Elevated temperature • Color of respiratory secretions • Appearance of urineAssess nutritional status. Perform asepsis for wound care, catheter care, and IV access management. Maintain hand hygiene before patient contact and between procedures with the patient. Encourage diet and fluid intake (contact dietitian as necessary). Encourage coughing and deep breathing; consider use of incentive spirometer. Teach patient and family how to perform hand hygiene correctly.	Patient demonstrates an understanding of necessary precautions to prevent infection. Patient remains free of infection.

CRITICAL THINKING QUESTIONS

1. Mr. R. has a peripheral IV infusing and reports discomfort at the site of insertion. What should the nurse do?
2. Mr. K. has a urinary catheter connected to continuous drainage. He reports burning at the site of insertion, and the nurse notes dark, concentrated urine in the tubing. What should the nurse do next?
3. The nurse notes on the sheet of laboratory results for the patient that his WBC count is $2800/mm^3$. Why is this a concern, and what is recommended as a precautionary measure?

---

or determine that the problem has been resolved. This is accomplished by referring to the goals and outcomes identified when planning care.

Goal 1: Transmission of infectious organisms is controlled.

Evaluative measures: Assess patient's temperature; observe wound sites for erythema, edema, tenderness, or exudate.

Goal 2: Progression of infection is controlled or decreased.

Evaluative measures: Inspect the size of the inflamed area over consecutive intervals; gently palpate the involved site to note a reduction in tenderness.

See the Coordinated Care box for infection prevention and control procedures.

Coordinated Care

Delegation

Infection Prevention and Control

Hand hygiene or antisepsis involves a set of basic procedures that all caregivers are obliged to perform correctly. If you observe other caregivers or family caregivers cleanse their hands incorrectly, reinforce the importance of the correct technique and procedural steps.

Observe the Consistency and Thoroughness of Staff in Washing or Disinfecting Hands

Application of disposable gloves is a basic procedure that should be performed correctly by unlicensed assistive personnel (UAP). If you observe UAP failing to use gloves when necessary, reinforce the importance of the procedure.

Clarify for the Unlicensed Assistive Personnel the Type of Isolation Precautions to Use (see Figs. 7.7 to 7.9)

Basic care procedures (e.g., bathing and feeding) that are performed for patients in transmission-based isolation can be delegated to UAP. The nurse is responsible for assessing whether it is more effective to provide direct care or delegate care activities, depending on the patient's clinical status. Procedures such as medication administration and care of IV lines require the application of critical thinking knowledge unique to the nurse.

Clarify for Unlicensed Assistive Personnel Special Precautions in Use of a Fitted Respirator Mask

Basic care procedures (e.g., bathing, feeding) that are performed under airborne infection isolation (see Skill 7.5) can be delegated to UAP. The nurse is responsible for assessing whether it is more effective to provide direct care or delegate care activities, depending on the patient's clinical status. Procedures such as medication administration and care of IV lines require critical thinking and knowledge application unique to the nurse.

Get Ready for the NCLEX® Examination!

Key Points

- The mucous membranes of the respiratory, gastrointestinal, and genitourinary tracts provide primary defense against pathogenic microorganisms, as does intact skin.
- An infection has the potential to develop as long as the six elements that compose the infectious chain are uninterrupted.
- A microorganism's virulence depends on its ability to resist attack by the body's normal defenses.
- Age, poor nutrition, stress, inherited conditions, chronic disease, and treatments or conditions that compromise the immune system increase susceptibility to infection.
- The signs of local inflammation and infection are similar, but the inflammatory response can occur in the absence of an infectious process.
- Surgical asepsis requires more stringent techniques than medical asepsis and is directed toward eliminating all microorganisms and their spores.
- Contamination of a sterile object or field occurs when it comes into contact with a wet surface that contains microorganisms or when it is exposed to airborne microorganisms.
- The CDC recommends that health care workers consider all patients as infectious and that health care workers use standard precautions to reduce the risk of exposure to blood and body fluids.
- Following aseptic principles is the key to a nurse's success in preventing patients from acquiring infection.
- Some types of equipment (e.g., sphygmomanometer or blood pressure cuff) are designated best for use in a patient who has been placed in transmission-based precautions. The item should be disinfected per hospital policy before use on other patients or discarded if it is disposable.
- Lack of proper hand hygiene is the main cause of the spread of infections.
- An infection control nurse monitors the incidence of infections within an institution and provides educational and consultative services to maintain aseptic practices to staff, patients, and their caregivers.
- Isolation transmission-based precautions are used to prevent personnel and patients from acquiring infections and prevent the transmission of microorganisms to other people.
- Wearing gloves, gowns, and masks in combination with eye protection devices such as goggles or glasses with solid side shields is mandatory when contact with blood or potentially infectious material is possible or whenever splashing or spraying of blood or potentially infectious material is possible.
- The restricted environment subjects a patient in transmission-based isolation to psychological and emotional deprivation.
- Standard precautions are used to prevent the spread of organisms present in blood, all other body fluids, nonintact skin, and mucous membranes.
- Standard precautions are used with all patients because it is often unknown which patients have an infection. This includes the use of barrier protection when appropriate.
- If the skin is broken or if the nurse performs an invasive procedure into a body cavity normally free of microorganisms, surgical aseptic practices are followed.

- The major sites for health care–associated infections include the urinary and respiratory tracts, the bloodstream, and surgical or traumatic wounds.
- Nurses must be role models and keep up to date with their own immunizations and teach patients to do so.
- Proper cleansing requires the mechanical removal of all foreign materials from an object or area.
- Cultural influences play a major role in patient education and follow-up care.

Additional Learning Resources

SG Go to your Study Guide for additional learning activities to help you master this chapter content.

Be sure to visit the Evolve site at http://evolve.elsevier.com/Cooper/foundations/ for additional online resources.

Review Questions for the NCLEX® Examination

1. A young adult patient is admitted to a medical unit with the diagnosis of hepatitis A and placed in contact precautions. What is the primary goal of this action?

   1. To prevent transmission of infectious microorganisms
   2. To control the environment of the patient during hospitalization
   3. To protect the patient from infectious microorganisms
   4. To protect only the family from the transmission of the disease

2. The nurse is working in a clinical medical area with a census of 15. Each patient has a different illness. When planning care, the nurse recognizes which is the most important action to provide protection to each patient from health care–associated infections?

   1. Wearing a gown
   2. Placing each patient in isolation
   3. Hand hygiene
   4. Wearing gloves

3. The nurse is caring for the patient in isolation and plans to wear latex gloves. Which is an important consideration?

   1. Assess the patient and the patient's record for potential latex allergy.
   2. Vinyl gloves provide higher barrier protection than latex.
   3. The cost of latex gloves is significantly higher than that of synthetic gloves.
   4. Latex gloves are so reliable as barriers that hand hygiene is not required.

4. The nurse is speaking with a patient about the need to prevent infection. The nurse recognizes the patient understands proper hand hygiene when the patient makes what statement?

   1. "The water I wash my hands with should be as hot as I can tolerate to kill all of the germs on my skin."
   2. "If there isn't time to completely wash my hands, it will be all right to rinse them quickly in warm water."
   3. "After washing my hands with soap for at least 20 seconds, I will rinse them thoroughly under running water."
   4. "I will put soap into a basin of warm water, lather my hands for 15 seconds, and then rinse them in the basin."

5. The nursing instructor is discussing the chain of infection with a group of student nurses. What is the most important information about identifying the chain of infection for the health care provider?

   1. Understanding of the chain of infection allows for tests to be performed to assess resistance to communicable diseases.
   2. Recognition of the chain of infection provides information about which patients will most benefit from isolation precautions.
   3. The need for antibiotic therapy can be determined by assessing the chain of infection.
   4. Points at which the infection can be stopped or prevented can be located by identifying the chain of infection.

6. A patient in isolation is experiencing signs of social deprivation. Which intervention by the nurse is appropriate?

   1. Allow visitors to remove masks while in the patient's room.
   2. Leave the door of the negative-pressure room open slightly.
   3. Remind the patient that the isolation is for his or her own benefit.
   4. Set specific times when the nurse will return to the patient's room.

7. A middle-aged client is admitted to the hospital with cellulitis of the right foot. Three days later, the patient develops bacterial pneumonia. How would the patient's bacterial pneumonia be classified?

   1. Acute primary
   2. Health care–associated
   3. Interstitial
   4. Mycoplasmic

8. The student is reviewing the sterile technique. When using the technique, the student nurse remembers to hold sterile objects in which location?

   1. Close to shoulder level
   2. Just below waist level
   3. Over the patient's bed
   4. Above waist level

9. The nurse is planning care for several patients undergoing procedures. For which procedure will the nurse gather supplies to implement surgical asepsis? *(Select all that apply.)*

   1. Inserting an IV line
   2. Performing perineal care
   3. Performing oral care
   4. Obtaining a sputum specimen
   5. Inserting an indwelling catheter

10. The nurse is performing a surgical hand scrub. During a surgical hand scrub, how are the hands to be held?

    1. Above the elbows
    2. With the fingers pointing downward
    3. Whichever way is convenient
    4. Just below the waist

11. To practice strict surgical asepsis, the nurse:

    1. adheres to principles of sterile technique.
    2. performs routine environmental cleaning.
    3. disinfects surfaces that come into contact with body fluids.
    4. maintains proper hand hygiene before and after patient care.

12. The student nurse is preparing to don sterile gloves. What action by the student indicates an understanding of the needed procedure?

   1. Touch only the inside surface of the first glove while pulling it onto the hand.
   2. Place the fingers of the dominant hand into the outside cuff of the first glove.
   3. Let the cuff of the glove roll up over the hand as it is being pulled onto the hand.
   4. Begin the procedure by pulling the first glove upward and over the nondominant hand.

13. The nurse has completed a sterile procedure and is preparing to remove the soiled gloves. Place the steps in the correct order:

   1. Grasp the outer surface of the glove.
   2. Place the glove in the hand that is still gloved.
   3. Peel the second glove off, turn inside out, and discard.
   4. Take fingers of bare hand and tuck inside remaining glove cuff.

14. To remove the gloves, what action is required of the nurse?

   1. Pull each finger from each of the gloves first, then roll the glove back over the hand.
   2. Remove the glove from the nondominant hand by reaching inside the glove and pulling it off.
   3. Remove one glove, then use the bare fingers to push the remaining glove off from inside the cuff.
   4. Hold both gloved hands under running water and roll the gloves down to keep microorganisms contained.

15. Which is a principle of surgical asepsis?

   1. Any sterilized item is considered unsterile once it is allowed to fall below knee height.
   2. Sterile fields and sterilized items are no longer sterile if they contact a clean surface.
   3. A person not wearing sterile garments can come no closer to a sterile field than 3 feet.
   4. The front and back of a sterile gown being worn are considered sterile from shoulders to knees.

16. A patient isolated for pulmonary tuberculosis is expressing anger at the nurse. What action by the nurse is most appropriate? *(Select all that apply.)*

   1. Provide a dark, quiet room to calm the patient.
   2. Explain isolation procedures and provide meaningful stimulation.
   3. Reduce the level of precautions to keep the patient from becoming angry.
   4. Limit family and other caregiver visits to reduce the risk of spreading the infection.
   5. Talk with the patient about how they are feeling.

17. The nurse is assisting the physician with irrigation of a draining abdominal wound by preparing the sterile tray. To maintain sterility of the tray, which action by the nurse is correct?

   1. Use sterile forceps while reaching across it to move the contents around.
   2. Wear clean gloves to open and touch the contents of the tray.
   3. Allow the open tray to stand unattended for 20 minutes, then cover it with a towel.
   4. Put on sterile gloves before handling the contents of the tray.

18. The nurse is presenting an educational program on the CDC's hand hygiene recommendations for implementation in a hospital. Which statement by the nurse demonstrates an understanding of the CDC's recommendation? *(Select all that apply.)*

   1. Health care providers will always wear gloves when providing patient care.
   2. Disinfecting hands after glove removal is not necessary according to the guidelines.
   3. Alcohol-based hand cleaner is effective on hands that are not visibly soiled with blood and body fluids.
   4. It is necessary to remove waterless alcohol-based hand cleaner with paper towels to remove pathogens from hands.
   5. The nurse should use water and soap to wash hands after caring for a patient diagnosed with *Clostridium difficile*.

19. The nurse is preparing to open the outer sterile wrap of an indwelling catheter tray. Which flap of the wrap (in which direction) should be opened first?

   1. The flap that opens away from the nurse
   2. The flap that opens to the left
   3. The flap that opens to the right
   4. The flap that opens toward the nurse

20. The patient asks the nurse how his skin will be sterilized before his surgery. What is the best response by the nurse?

   1. "We will use alcohol to sterilize your skin."
   2. "It is not possible to sterilize skin, but we will use an antimicrobial solution to eliminate most microorganisms."
   3. "There are a series of steps used in sterilizing your skin to prevent you from getting an infection."
   4. "We will use Betadine solution to sterilize your skin."

21. A man, 63, has been brought by a friend to the ED after 4 days of profuse diarrhea. He reports frequent watery stools up to 12 times per day, severe abdominal pain, and nausea. Blood pressure is 120/90, pulse 100 BPM. He exhibits a low-grade fever (102°F). Labs show blood and pus in the stool. He is diagnosed with *Clostridium difficile* (*C. diff*) and is started on vancomycin while being stabilized in the ED. Two floors up in ICU, the RN asks the LPN to prepare this client's room for him.

Identify the nursing actions below as 1—indicated (appropriate or necessary), 2—indicated contraindicated (could be harmful), or 3—non-essential (not necessary) for the client's care at this time. *Only one selection can be made for each nursing action.*

NURSING ACTION	INDICATED	CONTRAINDICATED	NON-ESSENTIAL
a. Reserve a room designated as negative-pressure airflow with at least 6–12 air exchanges per hour			
b. Isolate the client in a single-client room immediately on arrival in the unit.			
c. Don gloves and gown, even during short visits.			
d. Before and after each visit, use an alcohol-based waterless antiseptic for decontamination of the hands.			
e. Assign this client to a positive-pressure room			
f. Institute contact precautions.			
g. Undergo respirator fit-test and fit-check the LPN's respirator before each use			
h. Use a fresh, sterilized gown for each new task performed on the client during a single visit.			
i. Avoid harsh EPA-registered sporicidal disinfectants for this patient, which will counteract the effective treatment			

Objectives

1. State the principles of body mechanics.
2. Explain the rationale for the use of appropriate body mechanics.
3. Discuss considerations related to mobility for older adults.
4. Discuss the complications of immobility.
5. Demonstrate the use of assistive devices for proper positioning.
6. State the nursing interventions used to prevent complications of immobility.
7. Demonstrate placement of patient in various positions, such as Fowler's, supine (dorsal), Sims, side-lying, prone, dorsal recumbent, and lithotomy positions.
8. State the assessment for the patient's neurovascular status, including the phenomenon of compartment syndrome.
9. Describe and demonstrate range-of-motion exercises and explain their purpose.
10. Identify complications caused by inactivity.
11. Relate appropriate body mechanics to the techniques for turning, moving, and lifting the patient.
12. Discuss use of the continuous passive motion machines.
13. Discuss the nursing process and how it relates to patient mobility.

Key Terms

abduction (ăb-DŬK-shŭn, Table 8.4, p. 173)
adduction (ă-DŬK-shŭn, Table 8.4, p. 173)
alignment (ă-LĪN-mĕnt, p. 163)
base of support (p. 163)
body mechanics (p. 163)
compartment syndrome (p. 171)
contracture (kŏn-TRĂK-chŭr, p. 176)
disuse syndrome (p. 176)
dorsal (supine) (DŎR-săl, sū-PĪN, p. 166)
dorsal recumbent (DŎR-săl rē-KŬM-bĕnt, p. 166)
dorsiflexion (dŏr-sĭ-FLĔK-shŭn, Table 8.4, p. 175)
ergonomics (p. 162)
extension (Table 8.4, p. 173)
flexion (Table 8.4, p. 173)
Fowler's (p. 167)

genupectoral (jĕ-nyū-PĔK-tŏr-ăl, p. 168)
hyperextension (hī-pŭr-ĕk-STĔN-shŭn, Table 8.4, p. 174)
immobility (p. 169)
joint (p. 173)
lithotomy (lĭ-THŎT-ŏ-mē, p. 168)
mobility (p. 169)
orthopneic (ŏr-thŏp-NĒ-ĭk, p. 167)
pronation (prō-NĀ-shŭn, Table 8.4, p. 174)
prone (p. 167)
range-of-motion (ROM) (p. 173)
semi-Fowler's (p. 167)
Sims (p. 167)
supination (sū-pĭ-NĀ-shŭn, Table 8.4, p. 174)
Trendelenburg's (Trĕn-DĔL-ĕn-bŭrgz, p. 168)

The two concepts of body mechanics and patient mobility are directly related to one another. Nursing personnel must learn and practice proper principles of body mechanics to prevent self-injury and injury to their patients. When assisting patients in mobility, nurses must be constantly aware of their own body mechanics. According to the Bureau of Labor Statistics (www.bls.gov), hospital workers were twice other industries with a rate of 68 per 10,000. The injury rate for long-term care facility workers was more than three times as likely as other industries with a rate of 174 per 10,000 (BLS, 2019). The majority of these injuries were a result of manual lifting, moving, and repositioning patients/residents.

Most injuries occur when nursing personnel perform tasks that require repetitive movement, uncomfortable posture, and exertion to assist patients in activities such as feeding, dressing, bathing, toileting, repositioning, and ambulation. Awareness of proper ergonomic principles (ergonomics is the science of matching workplace conditions and job demands to the capabilities of workers, especially in regard to musculoskeletal injuries and their prevention) and good body mechanics help prevent injury.

Mechanical lifting devices (sling and standing lifts) and assistive patient-handling equipment, such as roller boards, sliders, friction-reduction pads, transfer chairs, and gait belts, work by taking on the energy and force that otherwise are imposed on the nurse during the lifting, transferring, or repositioning of a patient. Regular use of lifts and other assistive devices reduces the risk of injury (see the Evidence-Based Practice box). When a mechanical lift with a sling is used, the patient's head must be supported during transfer. To ensure safety, most facilities require that two staff members be present during patient transfer with a mechanical lift. The patient should be informed of what is happening continually during the process because mechanical lifts can be frightening to the patient.

Safe patient transfer requires adequate staffing, the right mix of personnel, and appropriate, readily available, well-maintained patient-lifting equipment. The licensed practical/vocational nurse (LPN/LVN) is responsible for being competent in the appropriate and safe use of equipment and for ensuring that UAP are knowledgeable regarding proper use of assistive devices.

 Evidence-Based Practice

Evaluation of Safe-Lift Programs

EVIDENCE SUMMARY

This study surveyed 200 long-term care facilities that used mechanical lifting devices for a 3-year period. Ninety-five percent of the facilities had mechanical lifts available for use, with an 80% compliance of the staff using the devices. All of the facilities reported a decrease in the number of work-related injuries and worker's compensation claims after implementing a safe-lift program. Safe-lift programs have incorporated the director of nursing (DON) and nursing staff to ensure that mechanical lifts were used consistently, and that all nurses and UAP were trained properly in the use of the devices.

APPLICATION TO NURSING PRACTICE

All nursing personnel must be trained in proper use of
   mechanical lifting devices.
Nursing personnel should strive to use mechanical lifting
   devices 100% of the time that the patient's condition
   warrants a mechanical lift.
DONs must convey the importance of safe-lift programs
   and ensure that all nursing personnel use mechanical
   lifts when necessary.

Sheehan P: Safe-lift programs require commitment, *Long-Term Living* 60(6):46, 2011.

Equally important is the use of appropriate body mechanics or movements that protect large muscle groups from injury and provide safety for patients during ambulation assistance. Special care should be taken in the care of older adults (see the Lifespan Considerations for Older Adults box regarding mobility). Assistive devices such as splints, crutches, braces, canes, gait belts, and walkers are available to aid in promotion of patient activity. Also important is the need to teach the patient appropriate positioning for home care and to help a family member learn how to assist the patient at home.

USE OF APPROPRIATE BODY MECHANICS

Understanding of body mechanics (the area of physiology for the study of muscle action and how muscles function in maintaining the posture of the body and prevention of injury during activity) includes knowledge of how certain muscle groups are used. The nurse uses body mechanics daily in making beds, assisting the patient to walk, carrying supplies and equipment, lifting, providing patient care, and carrying out other procedures.

For prevention of injury to the nurse and the patient, principles of body mechanics for health care workers (Table 8.1) should be followed by all health care professionals and personnel. Patients also should be taught principles of good body mechanics to protect themselves. The appropriate use of body mechanics should be practiced consistently in the workplace and outside the workplace so that MSDs do not occur. Maintenance of appropriate body alignment is the key factor in proper body mechanics. The term alignment refers to the relationship of various body parts to one another. Alignment helps balance and coordinate movements smoothly and effectively.

Maintenance of a wide base of support (a stance with feet shoulder width apart) when standing is one of the basic concepts of good body mechanics and alignment that should be followed because it helps in providing better stability (Fig. 8.1). Better stability prevents the nurse from losing proper balance while carrying out patient care, which could result in strain or injury to muscles.

The skeletal muscles and the nervous system maintain equilibrium, or balance, which facilitates appropriate body alignment when lifting, bending, moving, and performing other activities. Bending the knees and hips before attempting these activities protects the back from the stress and potential injury inherent to the physical work of nursing. When stooping, flex the hips and/or bend the knees and maintain appropriate body alignment (i.e., the back kept straight). Bending from the waist should be avoided because this will, in time, strain the lower back (Fig. 8.2). Work at a height or level that is comfortable to help prevent undue stress and strain on the back muscles. Adjust the height of the bed to a level appropriate for your height.

Use of large muscle groups (such as arm and shoulder muscles, hips, and thigh muscles) helps to perform a bigger workload more safely. The more muscle groups that are used, the more evenly the workload is distributed. If the base of support is widened in the direction of movement, less effort is needed to carry out an activity. To avoid twisting the spine, nurses should stand directly in front of the person or object with which they are working.

Lifespan Considerations

Older Adults

Mobility

The skin of older adults is more fragile and susceptible to injury. When moving or transferring them, avoid pulling them across bed linens because this has the potential to cause shearing or tearing of the skin.

Always support older adults under the joints when moving them in bed. Lifting in any other manner increases the stress on the joint and causes increased pain, particularly if some degenerative joint disease exists. Explain each step in simple language, and avoid jerky, sudden movements.

Aging tends to result in loss of flexibility and joint mobility, which often interferes with normal transfer techniques and necessitates modifications to protect patient and nurse.

Weakness and hypotension are common signs and symptoms noted in an older adult on bed rest. Proceed slowly and cautiously when helping a patient ambulate for the first time after prolonged immobility. While facilitating independence and proper utilization of patient's body mechanics, use assistive devices such as canes, walkers, and trapeze bars. Provide adequate help to ensure patient safety when moving a patient from a lying to a sitting position and from a sitting to a standing position.

Older adults who have many diseases or have undergone prolonged bed rest have greater risk for hypotension with postural change (orthostatic hypotension).

Patients who use medications to reduce blood pressure are at greater risk for orthostatic hypotension.

Older adults, particularly those with altered sensory perception, sometimes become fearful when lifts are used for transfers. Provide eyeglasses and basic instructions.

Limited positioning alternatives are available for the older adult who has arthritis, neuropathies, or other restrictive conditions.

Discourage older adult patients from sitting for prolonged periods of time without stretching and moving. Lack of movement presents a risk for contractures of joints.

Ensuring good body alignment when the patient is sitting is a way to prevent joint and muscle stress.

Provide patient teaching that includes use of strong joints and large muscle groups for activities that require extra strength to prevent strain and pain in joints.

For older adult patients with osteoporosis, encourage appropriate exercise programs that prevent fractures and reduce bone loss.

Encourage exercise programs for those older adults who do not participate in regular exercise. Ensure that patients consult with their health care provider before beginning any exercise program.

Special adjustments to an exercise program are often necessary to prevent any problems for those older adults in advanced age.

Older adults who are not able to participate in a structured exercise program are frequently able to achieve improved circulation and joint mobility by stretching and by exaggerating normal movements.

Data from Potter PA, Perry AG, Stocket PA, et al: *Fundamentals of nursing: Concepts, process, and practice,* ed 9, St. Louis, 2017, Mosby.

Table 8.1 **Body Mechanics for Health Care Workers**

ACTION	RATIONALE
When planning to move a patient, arrange for adequate help. Use mechanical aids if help is unavailable.	Two workers lifting together divide the workload by 50%.
Encourage patient to assist as much as possible.	This promotes patient's abilities and strength while keeping workload to a minimum.
Keep back, neck, pelvis, and feet aligned. Avoid twisting.	Twisting increases risk of injury.
Flex knees; keep feet shoulder length apart.	A broad base of support increases stability.
Position yourself close to patient (or object being lifted).	This minimizes strain and undue stress on the lifter. Holding an object or patient away from the body increases the workload.
Use arms and legs (not back).	The leg muscles are stronger larger muscles capable of greater work without injury.
Slide patient toward yourself using a pull sheet.	Sliding requires less effort than lifting. Pull sheet keeps to a minimum any shearing forces, which can damage patient's skin.
Set (tighten) abdominal and gluteal muscles in preparation for move.	Preparing muscles for the load limits strain to the least possible level.[a]
Person with the heaviest load coordinates efforts of team involved by counting to 3.	Simultaneous lifting keeps the load for any one lifter to a minimum.

[a]Back injuries are still the most common occupational injury among nurses.

Nurses have numerous other ways to protect themselves and the patient from injury. Carrying objects close to the midline of the body (see Fig. 8.2), avoiding reaching too far, avoiding lifting when other means of movement are available (such as sliding, rolling, pushing, or pulling), using devices instead of or in combination with lifting, and using alternating periods of rest and activity are just a few of the ways to prevent injury. Knowing the maximum weight that is safe to carry is also important. Many facilities suggest a 50-lb weight limit on lifting for their staff.

Nurses should assess their own abilities and limitations and those of the person helping, if working in pairs. Correct use of body mechanics is essential to provide efficient care while preventing injury (Box 8.1).

Fig. 8.1 Good position for body mechanics: chin is high and parallel to the floor, abdomen is tightened (internal girdle) in and up with the gluteal muscles tucked in, and feet are spread apart for a broad base of support.

POSITIONING OF PATIENTS

Positioning of patients is a common intervention performed by nursing personnel. Many positions can be used to prevent patients from development of complications (Skill 8.1 and the Patient Teaching box on mobility). Inappropriate positioning poses the risk of causing permanent disability.

Fig. 8.2 Picking up a box with use of good body mechanics. Box is carried close to the nurse's body and base of support.

| Box **8.1** | **Correct Use of Body Mechanics** |

Actions to promote proper body mechanics *(Rationale):*
- Position feet shoulder width apart. *(Provides adequate base of support.)*
- Align and balance weight on both feet. *(Distributes weight evenly.)*
- Flex knees slightly. *(Prevents hyperextension [extreme or abnormal stretching].)*
- Tilt pelvis forward by pulling buttocks inward so that gluteal muscles are contracted in and down. *(Helps straighten the lumbar curve of the spine, increasing power and reducing strain.)*
- Contract abdominal muscles in and up. *(Provides support and reduces muscle strain.)*

- Hold chest up. *(Allows adequate lung expansion.)*
- Keep head erect. *(Helps maintain appropriate alignment of the spine.)*
- Use appropriate body mechanics in all activities: standing, sitting, bending, and lifting. *(Produces most efficient body movement.)*
- Face your work area. *(Prevents unnecessary twisting.)*
- Push, slide, or pull heavy objects. *(Places less strain on body than lifting does.)*
- Lift twice—first mentally, and then physically. *(Helps determine whether assistance is needed.)*
- Do not lift objects higher than chest level. Do not reach above your shoulders. *(Use of a step stool to reach an object higher than chest level is much safer.)*

Skill 8.1 Positioning Patients

NURSING ACTION (RATIONALE)

1. Assess patient's body alignment and comfort level while patient is lying down. (*Provides baseline data concerning body alignment and comfort level. Helps determine ways to improve position and alignment.*)
2. Assemble equipment and supplies. (*Organizes procedure.*)
   - Pillows
   - Footboard
   - Trochanter roll
   - Splinting devices
   - Hand rolls
   - Safety reminder devices
   - Side rails
3. Request assistance as needed. (*Provides for safety.*)
4. Introduce self. (*Decreases patient's anxiety.*)
5. Identify patient. (*Ensures procedure is performed with correct patient.*)
6. Explain procedure. (*Enlists cooperation from patient and decreases patient anxiety.*)
7. Perform hand hygiene. Wear gloves as necessary according to agency policy and guidelines from the Centers for Disease Control and Prevention (CDC) and Occupational Safety and Health Administration (OSHA). (*Reduces spread of microorganisms.*)
8. Prepare patient. (*Prepares for procedure.*)
   a. Close door or pull curtain. (*Provides privacy.*)
   b. Raise level of bed to comfsortable working height. (*Promotes good body mechanics in the nurse and safety for the patient.*)
   c. Remove pillows and devices used in previous position. (*Makes access to patient easier.*)
   d. Put bed in flat position, or as low as patient can tolerate, and lower side rail closest to you. (*Facilitates procedure.*)
9. Position patient.
   a. **Dorsal (supine)** position (lying flat on the back) (see illustration).
      (1) Place patient on back with head of bed flat. (*Necessary for placing patient in supine position.*)
      (2) Place small rolled towel under lumbar area of back. (*Provides support for lumbar spine.*)
      (3) Place pillow under upper shoulder, neck, and head. (*Maintains correct alignment and prevents flexion contractures of cervical lumbar spine.*)
      (4) Place trochanter rolls parallel to lateral surface of thighs. (*Reduces external rotation of hip.*)

   (5) Place small pillow or roll under ankle to elevate heels. (*Reduces pressure on heels, helping to prevent skin impairment.*)
   (6) Support feet in dorsiflexion with firm pillow, footboard, or high-top sneakers. (*Prevents foot drop.*)
   (7) Place pillows under pronated forearms, keeping upper arms parallel to patient's body (see illustration). (*Reduces internal rotation of shoulder and prevents extension of elbows. Maintains correct body alignment.*)
   (8) Place hand rolls in patient's hands. (*Reduces extension of fingers and abduction of thumb.*)

   b. **Dorsal recumbent** position (supine position with patient lying on the back, head, and shoulder with extremities moderately flexed; legs are sometimes extended).
      (1) Move patient and mattress to head of bed. (*Ensures appropriate body alignment.*)
      (2) Turn patient onto back. (*Appropriately positions patient.*)
      (3) Assist patient to raise legs, bend knees, and allow legs to relax. (*Puts patient in dorsal recumbent position.*)
      (4) Replace pillow. Patient sometimes needs a small lumbar pillow. (*Provides comfort.*)
   c. **Fowler's** position (posture assumed by patient when head of bed is raised 45 to 60 degrees) (see illustration).
      (1) Move patient and mattress to head of bed. (*Ensures appropriate body alignment.*)
      (2) Raise head of bed to 45 to 60 degrees. (*Positions patient appropriately.*)
      (3) Replace pillow. (*Provides comfort, maintains proper body alignment, and ensures skin integrity.*)

Skill 8.1   Positioning Patients—cont'd

(4) Use footboard or firm pillow. (*Prevents patient from slipping down in bed.*)

(5) Use pillows to support arms and hands. (*Provides comfort and maintains correct alignment.*)

(6) Place small pillow or roll under ankles. (*Reduces risk of skin impairment over heels.*)

d. Semi-Fowler's position (posture assumed by patient when head of bed is raised approximately 30 degrees).

(1) Move patient and mattress to head of bed. (*Ensures appropriate body alignment.*)

(2) Raise head of bed to about 30 degrees. (*Positions patient appropriately.*)

(3) Replace pillow. (*Provides patient comfort.*) See Step 9c for positioning of pillows.

e. Orthopneic position (posture assumed by the patient sitting up in bed at 90-degree angle, or sometimes resting in forward tilt while supported by pillow on overbed table) (see illustration). Often used for the patient with a cardiac or respiratory condition.

(1) Elevate head of bed to 90 degrees. (*Facilitates positioning.*) Patient sometimes sits on side of bed with legs dangling or propped on a chair.

(2) Place pillow between patient's back and mattress. (*Provides back support.*)

(3) Place pillow on overbed table and assist patient to lean over, placing head on pillow. (*Facilitates ease of breathing. Women are more comfortable with arms on pillow and head on arms.*)

f. Sims position (position in which patient lies on side with knee and thigh drawn upward toward chest) (see illustration). The left Sims position is appropriate for the enema procedure and administration of a rectal suppository.

(1) Place patient in supine position. (*Prepares patient for position.*)

(2) Position patient in lateral position, lying partially on the abdomen. (*Patient is rolled only partially on abdomen.*)

(3) Draw knee and thigh up near abdomen and support with pillows. (*Positions patient appropriately*)

(4) Place patient's lower arm along the back. (*Provides appropriate body alignment.*)

(5) Bring upper arm up, flex elbow, and support with pillow. (*Provides comfort and decreases strain on joints.*)

(6) Allow patient to lean forward to rest on chest. (*Provides maximum comfort.*)

g. Prone position (lying face down in horizontal position) (see illustration).

(1) Assist patient onto abdomen with face to one side. (*Facilitates positioning.*)

(2) Flex arms toward the head. (*Provides appropriate body alignment.*)

(3) Position pillows for comfort. Place a pillow under lower leg to release any "pull" on the lower back, or place a pillow under the head as shown (or both). (*Increases comfort and maintains proper body alignment.*)

Continued

Skill 8.1 Positioning Patients—cont'd

h. Knee-chest **(genupectoral)** position (patient kneels so that weight of body is supported by knees and chest, with abdomen raised, head turned to one side, and arms flexed) (see illustration).

  (1) Turn patient onto abdomen. *(Facilitates positioning.)*

  (2) Assist patient into kneeling position; arms and head rest on pillow while upper chest rests on bed. *(Allows for as much comfort as possible in this position.)*

i. Lithotomy position (patient lies supine with hips and knees flexed and thighs abducted and rotated externally [sometimes feet are positioned in stirrups]) (see illustration).

  (1) Position patient to lie supine (lying on the back). *(Facilitates positioning.)*

  (2) Request patient to slide buttocks to edge of examining table. *(Facilitates positioning)*

  (3) Lift both legs; have patient bend knees and place feet in stirrups. *(Positions patient appropriately.)*

  (4) Drape patient. *(Provides privacy.)*

  (5) Provide small lumbar pillow if desired. *(Provides comfort. Pillow under head also provides comfort.)*

j. Trendelenburg's position (patient's head is low and the body and legs are on inclined plane) (see illustration).

  (1) Place patient's head lower than body, with body and legs elevated and on an incline. Foot of bed is sometimes elevated on blocks (not used if patient has a head or chest injury). Trendelenburg's position was used to treat shock but now is used less often because it causes pressure on the diaphragm by organs in the abdomen and shunts more blood to the brain rather than all of the vital organs. This position is sometimes used to assist in venous distention during central line placement.

k. Lateral position (see Chapter 9).

10. Assess patient for the following: (Provides follow-up with appropriate nursing interventions.)
   • *Proper body alignment:* Small children often need to be propped with pillows to help them maintain a position.
   • *Comfort:* Performing a back massage after turning from one position to another helps prevent impaired skin integrity.
   • *Skin integrity:* Skin of older adults is often thin, lacks elasticity, and needs special care to prevent tearing and further impaired skin integrity.
   • *Breathing:* Additional support is necessary in some positions if patient finds ease of respiratory effort difficult to maintain.
   • *Tolerance of position:* Ongoing observations regarding patient's activity tolerance is provided, and complications of immobility are indicated.
   • *Repositioning:* Reposition debilitated, unconscious, or paralyzed patients at least every 2 h.

11. Perform hand hygiene. (Reduces spread of microorganisms.)

12. Document. (Records procedure, patient's response, and effectiveness of nursing interventions.)
   • Procedure
   • Observations (e.g., skin condition, joint movement, patient's ability to assist with positioning)
   • Patient teaching (see the Patient Teaching and Home Care Considerations boxes).

Patient Teaching

Mobility

Instruct the patient and the family on proper mobility techniques.

Teach the patient ways to assist with positioning.

Provide the opportunity for return demonstration.

Teach the patient and the family signs and symptoms of skin impairment and contractures.

Teach the patient to avoid prolonged sitting. Frequent stretching decreases joint and muscle contractures.

Teach the importance of maintaining skin integrity.

Explain the importance of proper body alignment.

Explain the importance of rising slowly from lying to sitting, from sitting to standing, and after stooping (prevents orthostatic hypotension).

Provide time for questions and answers.

Emphasize the importance of the patient performing active range-of-motion (ROM) exercises when possible.

If the patient's height prevents the feet from touching the floor when sitting, teach the patient to rest feet on a footstool.

For prevention of thrombophlebitis, teach patients not to cross their legs when sitting and to avoid prolonged immobility. Teach those at increased risk the signs and symptoms of thrombophlebitis.

MOBILITY VERSUS IMMOBILITY

Mobility is a person's ability to move around freely in his or her environment. Moving about serves many purposes, including exercising, expressing emotion, attaining basic needs, performing recreational activities, and completing activities of daily living (ADLs; those activities of physical self-care such as bathing, dressing, and eating). In addition, mobility is fundamental to maintaining the body's normal physiologic activities. For normal physical mobility, the body's nervous, muscular, and skeletal systems must be intact, functioning, and used regularly. Although a person may welcome a rare day to lie in bed and rest, the person who is *immobile* (experiencing **immobility**, the inability to move around freely) is predisposed to a wide variety of complications (Box 8.2).

Many types of health problems potentially lead to a decline in a patient's mobility. Patients with certain illnesses, injuries, or surgeries sometimes experience a period of immobilization as a result of changes in medical and physical status. In some cases, immobilization also is used therapeutically to limit the movement of the whole body or a body part, and some patients are under ambulation restrictions.

Box **8.2**   Complications of Immobility and Preventive Measures

COMPLICATIONS

- *Anorexia* (decreased appetite): Lack of mobility slows the digestive process and slows the metabolic rate, causing decreased appetite.
- *Constipation:* Immobility slows peristalsis, resulting in stool remaining in the colon longer and muscle atrophy in the abdominal muscles that aid in expulsion of stool.
- *Contractures:* When muscles, ligaments, and tendons are not shortened and lengthened with movement, a permanent shortening of these structures may occur.
- *Disorientation:* Lack of stimulation, decreased endorphin production, decreased need for thought processes, and decreased socialization may lead to disorientation.
- *Disuse osteoporosis:* Lack of weight bearing on bones causes bone demineralization, allowing fractures to occur more easily.
- *Hypostatic pneumonia:* Decreased aeration and accumulation of secretions lead to inflammation and infection in the lungs.
- *Insomnia:* Decreased stimuli, depression, and frequent napping during the day as a result of immobility may cause difficulty sleeping at night.
- *Muscle atrophy and asthenia* (muscle weakness): Muscles decrease in size and strength when not continually used.
- *Orthostatic hypotension* (drop in systolic blood pressure of 20 mm Hg or a decrease of 10 mm Hg in diastolic blood pressure within 3 min of standing when moving from lying or sitting to standing position): Immobility can lead to a decrease in venous return or decreased cardiac output in response to postural change.

- *Pressure ulcer:* Tissue ischemia (lack of blood flow to an area) from unrelieved pressure results in skin breakdown.
- *Pulmonary embolism* (blood clot that has traveled to the lungs): Deep vein thrombosis (DVT) that has broken loose from vessel and has traveled to the lungs, causing a blockage in a pulmonary vessel.
- *Renal calculi* (kidney stones): Urinary stasis from immobility leads to slowed calcium metabolism, thus leading to stone formation.
- *Thrombophlebitis and DVT* (blood clot with accompanying inflammation of the involved vein, usually of the lower extremity): Decrease in venous circulation allows blood to pool in lower extremities, leading to inflammation of vessels and clot formation.
- *Urinary tract infection:* Urinary stasis causes changes in pH and allows bacterial growth.

INTERVENTIONS

- Reposition at least every 2 h
- Ensure adequate intake; encourage fluids
- Encourage a well-balanced diet
- Prevent deformities (e.g., footboard or other measures to prevent foot drop)
- Handle and transfer patients carefully; maintain proper body alignment
- Position lower extremities properly (a pillow or wedge between the legs, never under knees)
- Early ambulation
- Antiembolism measures (thromboembolic deterrent [TED] hose or decompression boots)
- Progressive ambulation
- Roll up head of bed

| Box 8.2 | **Complications of Immobility and Preventive Measures—cont'd** |

- Dangle over side of bed
- Stand
- Take a few steps
- Sit in the chair
- Up to the bathroom
- Up and about the room
- Up and out in the hallway
- Up as desired

DURING AMBULATION

1. Observe the patient closely.
2. Encourage the patient to do the following:
   - Take slow, deep breaths
   - Keep eyes open and look straight ahead
   - Keep head up

   (These measures aid in preventing vertigo, syncope, weakness, nausea, and vomiting.)
3. If the patient starts to fall, do not attempt to prevent the fall. Ease the patient to the floor. This allows you to break the fall, control its direction, and protect the patient's head. Follow these steps when assisting a patient's fall:
   - Stand with your feet apart. Keep your back straight.
   - Bring the patient close to your body as quickly as possible. Use the gait belt if one is worn. If not, wrap your arms around the patient's waist. Move your leg so that the patient's buttocks rest on it. Move the leg near the patient (see illustration).

- Lower the patient to the floor by letting the patient slide down your leg. Bend at your hips and knees as you lower the patient (see illustration). *(The gravitational pull allows the patient to be lowered to the floor with a minimal amount of strain to your musculoskeletal system.)*
- Call for assistance.
- Assist patient to return to bed.
- Report and document the following:
- How the fall occurred
- How far the patient walked
- How activity was tolerated before the fall
- Any report of symptoms before the fall
- The amount of assistance needed by the patient while walking
- Complete an incident report, if required. *(Know agency policy.)*

4. On a daily basis encourage the following:
   - Deep breathing and coughing exercises (spirometry)
   - Careful use of medications
5. Be certain to provide the following:
   - Suitable diversion
   - Meticulous skin care
   - Range-of-motion exercises
   - Reality therapy

May support the falling patient under the arms as shown.

The patient's buttocks rest on your leg.

Slide the patient down your leg to the floor.

Interventions to prevent complications of immobility are varied, and many do not require a physician's order (see Box 8.2).

Various assistive devices help maintain correct body positioning and prevent complications that commonly arise when a patient needs prolonged bed rest (Table 8.2). Several of the devices are especially useful in the care of patients who have a loss of sensation, mobility, or consciousness (Figs. 8.3 to 8.5).

NEUROVASCULAR FUNCTION

One of the responsibilities of the nurse is frequent monitoring of the patient's neurovascular function, or circulation, movement, and sensation (CMS) assessment.

Table **8.2**	Common Assistive Devices Used for Proper Patient Positioning
ASSISTIVE DEVICE	**COMMON USES**
Pillow	Provides support of body or extremity (e.g., placing behind the patient's back when in lateral position); elevation of body parts (e.g., the arm or leg; splinting of the incision in the postoperative patient during activity or coughing and deep breathing)
Foot drop boots or foot boards	Maintains the foot in dorsiflexion position, which prevents foot drop (plantar flexion)
Trochanter roll (see Fig. 8.3)	Prevents external rotation of legs when patient is in supine position
Hand roll (see Fig. 8.4)	Maintains hand in a normal position; prevents skin-to-skin contact of palm of hand; maintains fingers in slightly flexed position
Hand-wrist splint	Maintains proper alignment of the lower arm and hand; maintains wrist in slight dorsiflexion
Trapeze bar (see Fig. 8.5)	Allows the patient to raise the trunk from bed to assist in movement; allows patient to perform exercises that strengthen upper arms
Side rail	Helps the patient to roll from side to side or to sit up in bed; gives a sense of security in a hospital bed
Bed board	Provides additional firmness to mattress
Abductor splint	Used to maintain the legs in abduction after total hip replacement surgery (see Fig. 8.6)

Fig. 8.3 Trochanter roll.

Fig. 8.4 Hand roll.

Fig. 8.5 Patient using a trapeze bar.

The LPN/LVN checks for skin color, temperature, movement, sensation, pulses, capillary refill, and pain. The affected limb should be compared with the unaffected one (Table 8.3).

This assessment is especially important when compression from external devices, such as casts and bulky dressings, creates the risk of acute **compartment syndrome**, which has the potential to cause extensive tissue damage. Acute compartment syndrome occurs in the extremities, especially the legs, where a sheath of inelastic fascia partitions blood vessel, nerve, and muscle tissue. Normally, the pressure in this compartment is less than capillary pressure. However, compression created by external pressure or the accumulation of excessive tissue fluid from severe burns, fractures, crushing injuries, or severely bruised muscles increases compartmental pressure and in some cases leads to compartment syndrome. Ischemia resulting in necrosis, and/or permanent muscle and nerve damage with irreversible muscle function can occur within 6 hours if the compression of these structures is not reversed (Rasul, 2020).

Symptoms of acute compartment syndrome include pain within the muscle, especially when stretched, which is more intense than expected from the injury or causative factor; tingling and burning or a feeling of pins and needles in the affected area (paresthesias); and a full or tight feeling in the muscle. Numbness and paralysis are late signs of compartment syndrome and may be indicative of permanent damage.

Acute compartment syndrome is an emergency situation. The earlier compartment syndrome is treated, the better the prognosis. If acute compartment syndrome is caused by an external device, such as a cast or tight bandage, the pressure should be removed immediately by cutting away these devices. If the syndrome is caused by other factors, surgical intervention may be required. A fasciotomy may be necessary, in which the surgeon makes an incision into the skin and fascia to release the pressure. This incision is sometimes left open until swelling subsides.

Chronic compartment syndrome is not an emergency situation and usually is caused by exercise that

Fig. 8.6 Abductor splint.

Table 8.3	Assessment of Neurovascular Status	
CHARACTERISTIC	**ASSESSMENT TECHNIQUE**	**NORMAL FINDINGS**
Skin color	Inspect the color of the skin distal to the injury.	The skin color should match that of the unaffected body part.
Skin temperature	Palpate the area distal to the injury to determine whether any change in skin temperature has occurred compared with other body parts.	The skin is warm to touch.
Movement	Ask the patient to move the affected area or the area distal to the injury, unless contraindicated.	The patient is able to move with minimal difficulty and with minimal, if any, discomfort.
	Move the area distal to the injury if the patient is unable to move the body part on his or her own.	No difference in comfort is found compared with the patient actively moving the body part.
Sensation	Ask the patient if numbness or tingling is present (paresthesia), and assess with proper devices as necessary, such as a cotton-tipped applicator or tongue blade.	No numbness or tingling occurs; no difference in sensation is seen in the affected and unaffected body parts.
	Assess sensation with a cotton-tipped applicator, tongue blade, or other device as indicated.	Loss of sensation may indicate nerve or circulatory impairment.
Pulses	Palpate the pulses distal to the site of injury.	Pulses are strong and easily palpated; no difference is found in the affected and unaffected extremities.
Capillary refill	Press the nail beds distal to the injury until blanching occurs (or until the skin near the nail blanches, if nails are thick and brittle); pressure should be applied for approximately 3–5 s.	Blood returns (return to usual color) within 3 s (5 s for older adult patients).
Pain	Ask the patient about the location, the nature, and the frequency of pain and to rate the pain with a pain scale.	The patient should have no or minimal reports of pain.

involves repetitive movement, such as bicycling or running. The symptoms include pain and cramping during exercise, visible muscle bulging, and numbness. These symptoms usually are alleviated by discontinuing the activity and by rest.

PERFORMANCE OF RANGE-OF-MOTION EXERCISES

Regardless of whether the causes of immobility are permanent or temporary, the immobilized patient needs some type of exercise to prevent excessive muscle atrophy and joint contracture. The nurse and other health care personnel, including members of the physical therapy department, help the patient with decreased mobility to perform range-of-motion (ROM) –movement of the body that involves the muscles and joints in natural directional movements) exercises. *Passive* ROM exercise is performed by caregivers, and *active* ROM by patients. The designated joint (any one of the connections between bones) is moved actively or passively to the point of resistance or pain, with avoidance of injury. ROM exercises are increased with subsequent exercises as tolerated (Table 8.4 and Skill 8.2).

| Table **8.4** | Joint Range-of-Motion Exercises |

BODY PART	TYPE OF JOINT	TYPE OF MOVEMENT	BODY PART	TYPE OF JOINT	TYPE OF MOVEMENT
Neck and cervical spine	Pivotal	*Flexion*[a]: Bring chin to rest on chest. *Extension*[b]: Return head to erect position. *Hyperextension*[c]: Bend head back as far as possible. Use caution with older adults. *Lateral flexion:* Tilt head as far as possible toward each shoulder. *Rotation:* Turn head as far as possible to right and left.			*Abduction*[d]: Raise arm to side to position above head with palm away from head. *Adduction*[e]: Lower arm sideways and across body as far as possible.
Shoulder	Ball and socket	*Flexion:* Raise arm from side position forward to position above head. *Extension:* Return arm to position at side of body. *Hyperextension:* Move arm behind body, keeping elbow straight.			*Internal rotation:* With elbow flexed, rotate shoulder by moving arm until thumb is turned inward and toward back. *External rotation:* With elbow flexed, move arm until thumb is upward and lateral to head. *Circumduction*[f]: Move arm in full circle. (Circumduction is combination of all movements of ball-and-socket joint.)

[a]**Flexion**: Movement of certain joints that decreases the angle between two adjoining bones.
[b]**Extension**: Movement of certain joints that increases the angle between two adjoining bones.
[c]**Hyperextension**: Extreme or abnormal extension beyond normal joint ability.
[d]**Abduction**: Movement of the arm or leg away from body.
[e]**Adduction**: Movement of the arm or leg toward axis of body.
[f]**Circumduction**: Movement of a body part in a 360-degree circular motion, usually involves the arm or leg.

Table 8.4   Joint Range-of-Motion Exercises—cont'd

BODY PART	TYPE OF JOINT		TYPE OF MOVEMENT
Elbow	Hinge		*Flexion:* Bend elbow so that lower arm moves toward its shoulder joint and hand is level with shoulder.
			Extension: Straighten elbow by lowering hand.
			Hyperextension: Bend lower arm back as far as possible.
Forearm	Pivotal		*Supination[g]:* Turn lower arm and hand so that palm is up.
			Pronation[h]: Turn lower arm so that palm is down.
Wrist	Condyloid		*Flexion:* Move palm toward inner aspect of forearm.
			Extension: Move fingers so that fingers, hands, and forearm are in same plane, in a straight line.
			Hyperextension: Bring dorsal surface of hand back as far as possible.
			Radial flexion: Bend wrist medially toward thumb.
			Ulnar flexion: Bend wrist laterally toward fifth finger.
Fingers	Condyloid hinge		*Flexion:* Make fist.
			Extension: Straighten fingers.
			Hyperextension: Bend fingers back as far as possible.

BODY PART	TYPE OF JOINT		TYPE OF MOVEMENT
			Abduction: Spread fingers apart.
			Adduction: Bring fingers together.
Thumb	Saddle		*Flexion:* Move thumb across palmar surface of hand.
			Extension: Move thumb straight away from hand.
			Abduction: Extend thumb laterally (usually done when placing fingers in abduction and adduction).
			Adduction: Move thumb back toward hand.
			Opposition: Touch thumb to each finger of same hand.
Hip	Ball and socket		*Flexion:* Move leg forward and up with knee in extension.
			Extension: Move leg back beside other leg while knee joint remains in extension.
			Hyperextension: Move leg behind body.
			Abduction: Move leg laterally away from body.
			Adduction: Move leg back toward medial position and beyond if possible.

[g]**Supination:** Movement of the palm of the hand from facing downward to facing upward.
[h]**Pronation:** Movement of the palm of the hand from facing upward to facing downward.

Continued

Table 8.4   Joint Range-of-Motion Exercises—cont'd

BODY PART	TYPE OF JOINT	TYPE OF MOVEMENT	BODY PART	TYPE OF JOINT	TYPE OF MOVEMENT
		Internal rotation: Turn foot and leg toward other leg.	Ankle	Hinge	*Dorsiflexion¹:* Move foot so that toes are pointed upward.
		External rotation: Turn foot and leg away from other leg.			*Plantar flexion:* Move foot so that toes are pointed downward.
		Circumduction: Move leg in circle.	Foot		*Inversion:* Turn sole of foot medially.
					Eversion: Turn sole of foot laterally.
Knee	Hinge		Toes	Condyloid hinge	*Flexion:* Curl toes downward.
		Flexion: Bring heel back toward back of thigh.			*Extension:* Straighten toes.
		Extension: Return heel to floor.			*Abduction:* Spread toes apart.
					Adduction: Bring toes together.

¹**Dorsiflexion**: Backward flexion of the hand of foot.

Skill 8.2   Performing Range-of-Motion Exercises

CHECK   GATHER   HELLO   ID   PRIVACY   EXPLAIN   WASH   GLOVES

NURSING ACTION (RATIONALE)

1. Refer to medical record or care plan for special interventions. *(Provides basis for care.)*
2. Assemble equipment. *(Organizes procedure.)*
   - Clean gloves, if necessary.
3. Introduce self. (Decreases patient's anxiety.)
4. Identify patient. (Ensures procedure is performed with correct patient.)
5. Explain procedure. (Enlists cooperation and decreases patient's anxiety.)
6. Perform hand hygiene and don clean gloves according to agency policy and guidelines from CDC and OSHA. (Reduces spread of microorganisms.)

7. Prepare patient for intervention:
   a. Close door to room or pull curtain. *(Provides privacy.)*
   b. Drape for procedure if appropriate. (Prevents unnecessary exposure of patient.)
   c. Raise bed to comfortable working level. (Promotes good body mechanics in the nurse and safety for the patient.)
   d. Assist patient to a comfortable position, either sitting or lying down. *(Ensures patient's comfort.)*
   e. Medicate patient as needed for pain. *(Promotes patient comfort.)*

Continued

Skill 8.2   Performing Range-of-Motion Exercises—cont'd

8. Support the body part above (proximal to) and below (distal to) the joint by cradling the extremity or by using cupped hand to support the joint being exercised. *(Protects the weaker joints and muscles.)*

9. Begin by doing exercises in normal sequence (see Table 8.4). Repeat each full sequence five times during the exercise period. *(Exercises are easiest to perform in head-to-toe manner.)* Discontinue exercise if patient reports pain or if resistance or muscle spasm occurs.

10. Assist patient by putting each joint through full range of motion (see Table 8.4). *(Provides baseline for joint movement.)*

11. Position patient for comfort. To prevent **contracture** (an abnormal shortening of a muscle), do not allow patients with joint pain to remain continuously in position of comfort; joints must be exercised routinely. *(Immobility contributes to contractures.)* Periodically provide back massage. *(Provides comfort.)*

12. Adjust bed linen. *(Provides comfort and privacy.)*

13. Remove and dispose of gloves and wash hands. *(Reduces spread of microorganisms.)*

14. Document the following: *(Records procedure and patient's response.)*
    - Joints exercised
    - Presence of edema or pressure areas
    - Any discomfort resulting from the exercises
    - Any limitations of ROM
    - Patient's tolerance of the exercises
    - Patient teaching (see Patient Teaching and Home Care Considerations boxes)

Some patients who are weak or partially paralyzed are able to move a limb partially through ROM, and the nurse then may assist the patient to finish the full ROM. This is referred to as *passive assisted* ROM. *Active assisted* ROM occurs when the patient uses the strong arm to exercise the weaker or paralyzed arm. The LPN/LVN best meets the needs of the patient by encouraging the patient to be as independent as possible.

Assessment by the nurse and the physical therapy department determines the patient's current mobility status. The patient who is able to move about freely independently performs ADLs and active ROM exercises. Patients who are partially immobile or unable to move about freely (from paraplegia, quadriplegia, weakness, or fatigue) need the nurse and other health care personnel to assist with passive ROM exercises.

Encourage and assess active ROM every day (see the Lifespan Considerations for Older Adults box). The total amount of activity required to prevent **disuse syndrome** (a state in which an individual is at risk for deterioration of body systems as a result of prescribed or unavoidable inactivity) is only about 2 hours for every 24-hour period. Schedule this activity throughout the day to prevent the patient from remaining inactive for long periods (Ackley and Ladwig, 2020).

CONTINUOUS PASSIVE MOTION MACHINES

Continuous passive motion (CPM) machines flex and extend joints for passive mobilization without the

 Lifespan Considerations

Older Adults

RANGE-OF-MOTION EXERCISES

Some older adults who have chronic illnesses need to separate range-of-motion (ROM) exercises into two or more sessions to control fatigue.

Inadequate intake of calcium or exposure to sunlight increases older adults' risk of bone loss and increases the need for ROM and weight-bearing exercise.

Older people who fear falling often display reluctance to move about freely. Encouragement, reassurance, and assistance from family members and caregivers decrease anxiety.

Older adult patients who are depressed often prefer to stay in bed, especially when they were accustomed to being very independent and active and now need assistance.

Many older adults with arthritis require additional time in the morning before resuming activities.

Even without arthritis, older adults often need more time in the morning to resume activity.

strain of active exercises (Fig. 8.7). This therapy sometimes is used immediately after total knee replacement surgery (knee arthroplasty), but CPM also can be used in outpatient or home physical therapy programs. The CPM machine's settings must be adjusted according to the health care provider's orders for the degree and the speed of flexion and extension for each individual patient to prevent damage to the joint or surgical site. Some recent studies question the necessity of CPM machines and encourage the use of immediate physical therapy instead. Many orthopedic surgeons have

Fig. 8.7 Continuous passive motion (CPM) machine. (From Cole B: *Surgical techniques of the shoulder, elbow, and knee in sports medicine*, ed 2, Philadelphia, 2013, Saunders.)

adopted the practice of immediate physical therapy over CPM therapy.

CPM machines can be used on joints other than the knee, including the hip, the shoulder, and the ankle. Mobilization of the joint prevents complications, such as joint contracture, atrophy of surrounding muscles, and thromboembolism. Physical therapy typically accompanies CPM therapy. Ongoing CPM therapy can be accomplished in a rehabilitative facility or at home with the oversight of a home care agency.

MOVING THE PATIENT

A common nursing action is assisting patients in movement. Patients may need assistance in various ways, such as moving the patient up in bed, out of bed, or from a chair or wheelchair; turning the patient; and assisting the patient in and out of the bed for ambulation (Skill 8.3). For some situations, the nurse uses mechanical equipment for lifting patients, such as the

Skill 8.3   Moving the Patient

NURSING ACTION (RATIONALE)

1. Refer to the medical record or care plan for special interventions. (*Provides basis for care.*)
2. Assemble equipment. (*Organizes procedure.*)
   - Hospital bed
   - Chair
   - Side rails
   - Patient's slippers
   - Cotton blanket
   - Pillows
   - Extra personnel
   - Lifting devices (see Skill 8.4)
3. Introduce self. (*Decreases patient's anxiety.*)
4. Identify patient. (*Ensures procedure is performed with correct patient.*)
5. Explain procedure. (*Enlists cooperation and assistance from patient and decreases patient's anxiety.*)
6. Perform hand hygiene. (*Reduces spread of microorganisms.*)
7. Prepare patient for interventions.
   a. Close door or pull curtain. (*Provides privacy*)
   b. Adjust bed level for safe working height (*Promotes good body mechanics in the nurse and safety for the patient.*)
   c. Medicate patient as needed. (*Promotes patient comfort.*)

8. Arrange for assistance as necessary. (*Provides for safety.*)
9. Lift and move patient up in bed (sometimes requires one nurse and sometimes more):
   a. Place patient supine with head flat. (Creates less resistance on flat surface.)
   b. Face the patient and establish base of support. (*Protects your back.*)
   c. Use a lift (draw) sheet to assist patient up in bed. (Supports patient, assists staff, and prevents shearing of patient's skin.)
      (1) Roll patient first to one side and then the other, placing lift sheet underneath patient from shoulders to thighs. (*Facilitates the position change.*)
      (2) Flex knees and face body in the direction of the move. The foot farthest away from the bed faces forward for broader base of support.
      (3) With one nurse on each side of patient, grasp lift sheet firmly with hands near patient's upper arms and hips, rolling the sheet material until hands are close to the patient. (*The closer the nurse is to the patient, the less the nurse needs to raise the patient up to clear the bed during the move.*)

Continued

Skill 8.3 Moving the Patient—cont'd

(4) Instruct patient to rest arms over body and to lift head on the count of 3; at the same time, pull the sheet to move the patient up to head of bed.

10. Turning the patient:
    a. Stand with feet slightly apart and flex knees. *(Provides base of support.)*
    b. If the patient is unable to assist in turning, two people should use the lift sheet to turn the patient. *(Provides patient safety and support and protects the back of the persons assisting with the turn.)*
    c. Move patient's body to one side of the bed. *(Allows room for the patient to turn in the bed.)*
    d. If patient is assisting in turning, turn the patient on side facing raised side rail, toward the nurse. *(Prevents patient from falling out of bed.)* If patient is not assisting, then use the lift sheet to turn the patient.
    e. Flex one of patient's legs over the other. Place pad or pillow between legs. *(Reduces pressure on lower leg and prevents skin breakdown by avoiding skin on skin.)*
    f. Align patient's shoulders; place pillow under head. *(Ensures proper body alignment.)*
    g. Support patient's back with pillows as necessary. A "tuck back" pillow is made by folding pillow lengthwise. Tuck smooth area slightly under patient's back. *(Helps keep patient in position.)*
11. Dangling patient:
    a. Assess pulse and respirations. *(Provides baseline for assessing patient's response to dangling.)*
    b. Move patient to side of bed toward the nurse. *(Makes it easier for patient to sit up. Request patient do by self if possible.)*

c. Lower bed to lowest position. *(Provides patient safety when getting up.)*
d. Raise head of bed. *(Patient can swing around more easily to sitting position.)*
e. Support patient's shoulders and help to swing legs around and off bed; do this all in one motion by simply pivoting patient. Ensure patient's feet touch floor. *(Prevents strain on patient, especially if patient has an incision.)*

f. Another way to accomplish this is by rolling the patient onto his or her side before sitting the patient up. *(Decreases the amount the nurse needs to lift because the patient's body weight actually helps the patient to sit upright.)* The nurse then stoops and, when standing, brings the patient along with the nurse. *(This causes less back strain for the nurse and the patient does not feel pulled)*
g. Help patient place slippers on; cover legs. *(Prevents patient from becoming chilled.)* For safety, have patient place slippers on while in bed.
h. Assess patient's pulse and respirations. *(Determines patient's response to procedure.)*
12. Log-rolling the patient (back, neck, or head conditions sometimes necessitate logrolling after injury or surgery):
    a. Enlist the help of at least one additional person. *(Ensures patient safety.)*
    b. Lower the head of the bed as much as the patient can tolerate. *(Maintains alignment of the spinal column.)*
    c. Place a pillow between the patient's legs. Use of a pull sheet placed between shoulders and knees facilitates turning (see Step 9c[4]). *(Maintains position of the lower extremities.)*

Skill 8.3 Moving the Patient—cont'd

d. Extend the patient's arm over the patient's head unless shoulder movement is restricted. *(Prevents rolling over it during the turn.)* If shoulder movement is restricted, keep the arm in extension next to the body.

e. With both nurses on the same side of the bed, one of the nurses places one hand on the patient's shoulder and the other on the hip, while the other nurse places one hand to support the patient's back and the other behind the knee. If a lift sheet is used, space hands in such a way to provide even support for the length of the rolled sheet and to distribute weight evenly.

f. On a count of 3, turn the patient with a continuous, smooth, and coordinated effort. *(Maintains body alignment, preventing stress on any part of the body.)*

g. Support the patient with pillows as previously discussed (see Step 10g). *(Promotes patient comfort.)*

13. Transferring the patient from bed to straight chair or wheelchair:

a. Lower bed to lowest position. *(Provides patient safety when getting up.)*

b. Raise head of bed. *(Patient can more easily swing around to sitting position.)*

c. Support patient's shoulders and help swing legs around and off bed; perform all in one motion (see Step 11e). *(Prevents strain on patient, especially if patient has incision.)*

d. Help patient don robe and slippers (or do this before beginning procedure). *(Prevents chilling.)*

e. Have chair positioned beside bed with seat facing foot of bed. *(Provides easy access to chair.)*

(1) Place wheelchair at right angle to bed and lock wheels after bed is lowered. *(Provides safety.)*

(2) Place straight chair against wall or have another nurse hold the chair. *(Provides safety.)*

f. Stand in front of patient and place hands at patient's waist level or below; allow patient to use his or her arms and shoulder muscles to push down on the mattress to facilitate the move. *(Prepares the patient for movement to chair.)*

Continued

Skill 8.3   Moving the Patient—cont'd

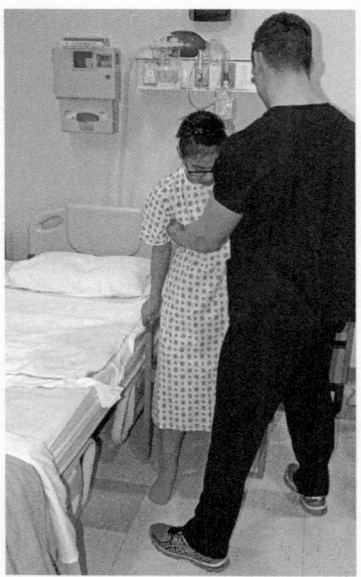

g. Assist patient to stand and swing around with back toward seat of chair. Keep the strong side toward the chair. *(Provides safety.)*

h. Help patient to sit down as the nurse bends his or her knees to assist process. (Prevents patient from slipping and falling. If patient begins to fall, prevent patient injury by holding patient and allowing patient to sit down gently on floor; see Box 8.2, Step 3.)

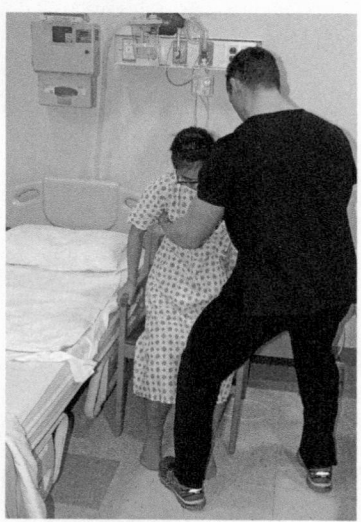

i. Apply blanket to legs. *(Provides extra warmth.)*

j. If transfer belt is used, apply after patient is sitting on side of bed and follow these guidelines:

  (1) Stand in front of the patient. (Permits excellent view of patient.)

  (2) Have the patient hold on to the mattress, or ask the patient to place his or her fists on the bed by the thighs. *(Any assistance from the patient minimizes strain on you.)*

  (3) Be sure the patient's feet are flat on the floor. *(Provides balance and stability for patient.)*

  (4) Have the patient lean forward.

  (5) Instruct the patient to place his or her hands on the nurse's shoulders, not around the nurse's neck or at the side as shown. *(Arms around the neck could result in neck injury to nurse.)*

  (6) Grasp the transfer belt at each side. (Offers stability of patient for the nurse.)

  (7) Brace knees against the patient's knees. (Provides safety and prevents patient's foot from slipping.)

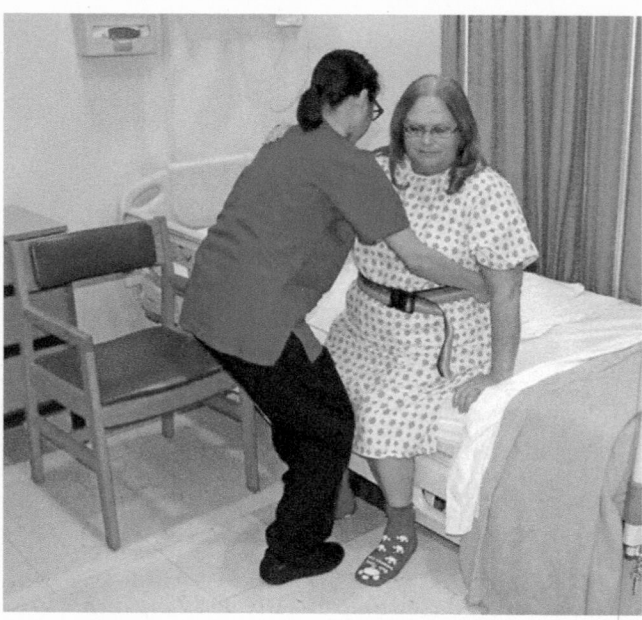

Skill 8.3   Moving the Patient—cont'd

(8) Ask the patient to push down on the mattress and to stand on the count of 3. Pull the patient into a standing position as you straighten your knees. *(Provides for less strain on your back.)*

(9) Pivot the patient so that he or she is able to grasp the far arm of the chair. Back of the legs will be touching the chair. *(Enables patient to assist in the transfer.)*

(10) Continue to turn the patient until the other arm rest is grasped.

(11) Gradually lower the patient into the chair as you bend your hips and knees. The patient assists if able by leaning forward and bending his or her elbows and knees. *(Encourages patient to assist in transfer and increases muscle strength and a sense of control.)*

(12) Ensure buttocks are to the back of the chair. *(Ensures patient safety.)*

(13) Cover patient's lap and legs. (Promotes patient's comfort and privacy.)

14. Transferring from bed to stretcher or gurney back to bed:

   a. Position bed flat and raise to the same height as stretcher or gurney. Lower side rails. *(Facilitates procedure.)*

   b. Cover patient with top sheet or blanket and remove linens without exposing patient. *(Provides privacy.)*

   c. Assess for IV line, Foley catheter, tubes, or surgical drains, and position them to avoid tension during the transfer. *(Prevents accidental tension and possible removal of tubes.)*

   d. Position the gurney as close to the bed as possible, and lock the wheels of the bed and gurney (with side rails lowered). *(Ensures patient's safety.)*

   e. When patient is able to assist, stand near side of gurney and instruct patient to move feet, then buttocks, and finally upper body to the gurney, bringing blanket along. Be certain patient's body is centered on the gurney. *(Promotes safety and security.)*

   f. When patient is unable to assist, place a folded sheet or bath blanket under the patient so that it supports patient's head and extends to mid-thighs. Roll the sheet or bath blanket close to the patient's body. Assist patient to cross arms over chest. Two nurses reach over the bed to the patient, and two more stand as close to the gurney as possible. A fifth nurse stands at the foot to transfer the feet. Using a coordinating count of 3, all five nurses lift the patient to the edge of the bed. With another effort, lift the patient from edge of bed to gurney. Roller devices are available in some facilities to facilitate this transfer.

15. Perform hand hygiene. (Reduces spread of microorganisms.)

16. Assess patient for appropriate body alignment after move. When repositioning, always assess previously dependent skin surfaces (pressure areas). Position pillows for comfort. Do not overtire patient during ambulation. As in all transfers, be certain call device is in easy reach. *(Evaluates, determines, and promotes patient safety and comfort.)*

17. Document procedure. (Notes procedure and patient's response.)
   - Patient's response
   - Expected and unexpected outcomes
   - Patient teaching (see the Patient Teaching and Home Care Considerations boxes)

Continued

hydraulic lift, roller board, and gurney lift. The nurse first should think through the lift to be prepared for lifting the patient and then physically perform the lift. The nurse must ensure that patients do not become too dependent on assistance with mobility. Frequent assessment of the patient's ability to assist with mobility is necessary to prevent overdependence. The LPN/LVN should also assess the patient for pain and administer pain medications before activities that cause further pain (Box 8.3 and the Coordinated Care box).

 Coordinated Care

Delegation

Mobility

The following information is needed when delegating the skill of position changes to UAP:

Have the patient wear shoes with a nonslip surface during transfer or ambulation.

Make slow, gradual position changes.

Help the patient sit in a chair or return to bed if the patient has symptoms of orthostatic hypotension.

When assisting with ambulation:

Do not try to hold patients if they become dizzy or faint. Ease them into a sitting position in a chair or onto the floor.

Use assistive devices such as walkers, crutches, gait belt, or cane when appropriate.

Be sure the area is free of clutter, wet areas, and rugs that may slide.

UAP, Unlicensed assistive personnel.

USE OF THE LIFT FOR MOVING PATIENTS

Mechanical devices, such as the patient lift with a sling (Fig. 8.8), are useful for moving patients safely and protecting the nurse's back and for full-weight lifting of patients who cannot assist. Follow agency policy for use of the lift (Skill 8.4).

❖ NURSING PROCESS FOR PATIENT MOBILITY

The role of the LPN/LVN in the nursing process as stated is that the LPN/LVN:

Participates in planning care for patients based on patient needs.

Reviews the patient's plan of care and recommends revisions as needed.

Reviews and follows defined prioritization for patient care.

Uses clinical pathways, care maps, or care plans to guide and review patient care.

◆ ASSESSMENT

Assessment focuses on ROM, muscle strength, activity tolerance, gait, and posture. Observation during ADLs enables the nurse to estimate the patient's fatigability, muscle strength, and ROM. Further assessment helps determine the type of assistance the patient needs to change position or transfer from bed to chair or

| Box 8.3 | Long-Term Care Considerations for Mobility |

- Patients who have maintained bed rest for a long time sometimes revert to a favorite position. Frequently assess these patients, and turn them more often as needed.
- Use a lift (draw) sheet as often as possible to prevent shearing force on fragile skin.
- Allow the patient to assist with moving and positioning whenever possible to promote independence.
- Perform safety and maintenance checks of ambulation devices on a routine basis.
- Perform periodic assessments to ensure that the patient is using ambulation device properly.
- Consult the physical therapist for additional assistance or exercises and to ascertain the patient's response to the exercise program.
- Group activities (e.g., simple games, walking, tossing a ball in a large circle) are useful in maintaining ROM.

Fig. 8.8 (A) Motorized lift. (B) Use of a mechanical lift to lower patient into chair.

Skill 8.4 Using Lifts for Moving Patients

NURSING ACTION (RATIONALE)

1. Refer to medical records or care plan for special interventions. (*Provides basis for care.*) Read manual for direction.
2. Assemble equipment:
   - Mechanical lift frame (see Fig. 8.8)
   - Seat sling attachment (may be one piece or two) or a standing frame
   - Two cotton bath blankets
3. Introduce self. (*Decreases patient's anxiety.*)
4. Identify patient. (*Ensures procedure is performed with correct patient.*)
5. Explain procedure. (*Enlists cooperation and assistance from patient and decreases patient's anxiety.*)
6. Perform hand hygiene. (*Reduces spread of microorganisms.*)
7. Prepare patient for interventions.
   a. Close door or pull curtains. (*Provides privacy.*)
   b. Adjust bed level to working height (even with level of arm of chair [of lift] if chair is not removable or level with seat if chair is removable). (*Promotes safety.*)
   c. Medicate patient as needed. (*Promotes patient comfort.*)
   d. Place cotton bath blanket over chair for patient's comfort.
   e. Cover patient with remaining bath blanket.
8. Secure adequate number of personnel. (*Provides necessary assistance and patient safety.*)
9. Place chair near bed. (*Prepares seat for patient.*)
10. Appropriately place canvas seat under patient; support head and neck. (*Helps in lifting safely.*)
11. Slide horseshoe-shaped bar under bed on one side. (*Places lift close to bed.*)
12. Lower horizontal bar to level of sling. (*Places lift close to patient.*)
13. Fasten hooks on chain to openings in sling. (*Attaches lift to sling seat.*)
14. Raise head of bed. (*Places patient in sitting position.*)
15. Fold patient's arms over chest. (*Prevents patient injury.*)
16. Pump lift handle until patient is raised off bed. (*Ensures patient safety during lifting.*)
17. With steering handle, pull lift off bed and down to chair. (*Places patient safely in chair provided.*)
18. Release valve slowly to lift and lower patient toward chair. (*Appropriately places patient in chair.*)
19. Close off valve and release straps. (*Prevents patient injury from boom.*)
20. Remove straps and lift. (*Provides safety and comfort.*)
21. Perform hand hygiene. (*Reduces spread of microorganisms.*)
22. Document procedure. (*Note procedure and patient's response.*)
    - Evaluate body alignment to help prevent skin impairment.
    - Evaluate patient's response to movement to help determine patient's mobility potential.
23. Perform patient teaching (see the Patient Teaching and Home Care Considerations boxes).

---

wheelchair. These assessments give the LPN/LVN an understanding of the patient's overall level of mobility and coordination (see the Cultural Considerations box).

◆ PATIENT PROBLEMS

Assessment enables the nurse to cluster relevant data and develop actual or potential (risk) problem statements related to the patient's needs. The patient problems are listed along with the probable causes "related to (r/t)." Identification of the cause of the problem further individualizes the care plan and leads to selection of appropriate care.

Example: Compromised Physical Mobility, r/t left shoulder pain, as evidenced by patient pain 8/10 and patient unable to assist in dressing self.

◆ EXPECTED OUTCOMES AND PLANNING

The nurse should set goals and expected outcomes with the patient to direct interventions. Care planning is individualized to the patient, with the patient's most immediate needs taken into consideration. These goals are based on the patient problem statement formulated.

Goal: Patient will demonstrate ability to assist in dressing self within 3 days.

Expected outcomes: Patient reports pain level decreased to 4/10 for 3 consecutive days and self assists with dressing each of these 3 days.

◆ IMPLEMENTATION

Nursing interventions should be individualized according to the level of risk to the patient. The nurse, the patient, and other members of the health care team work together to determine the most effective interventions (Nursing Care Plan 8.1). While implementing the established goals, the nurse also should assess the patient's readiness to learn and teach appropriate body mechanics (see the Home Care Considerations box on mobility).

Cultural Considerations

Promotion of Patient Mobility

Assess and listen carefully to patient's expressions of health and illness, beliefs, and practices.

Be aware of the patient's personal space; seek permission before intruding in the patient's territory.

The nursing process enables the nurse to provide individualized care; adapt care to be culturally sensitive.

When speaking with a patient (or family member) who does not understand English, many people try to compensate for the lack of understanding by speaking more loudly. Speaking slowly, distinctly, and at a normal volume is more effective (see Chapter 4).

It is acceptable to delegate the skills of safe and effective transfer from bed to chair to UAP who have demonstrated successfully good body mechanics and safe transfer techniques for patients involved.

Teaching patients how to use assistive devices requires critical thinking and knowledge application unique to a nurse. However, UAP are able to assist ambulatory patients with assistive devices.

Have the patient wear shoes with a nonskid surface during ambulation.

Be sure the area is free of clutter, wet areas, and rugs that may slide or buckle.

Ensure UAP knows how to use an intravenous (IV) pole to assist in ambulation for a patient with continuous IV therapy.

Be sure the patient uses the correct gait and weight bearing during ambulation.

Ease the patient to a sitting position in a chair or on the floor if he or she becomes dizzy or faint.

Have UAP alert the LPN/LVN if the patient becomes dizzy or lightheaded or suffers a fall.

The skill of performing ROM exercises can be delegated to UAP. Patients with spinal cord injury or orthopedic trauma or surgery usually require exercise to be performed by nurses or physical therapists. When delegating this skill, instruct UAP to perform exercises slowly and provide adequate support to the joint being exercised. In addition, remind UAP not to exercise joints beyond the point of resistance or to the point of fatigue or pain. In addition, if muscle spasms occur, exercise should stop until the spasms have subsided.

The LPN/LVN may delegate the skill of safe and effective transfer with a mechanical lift to UAP who have demonstrated the ability to use good body mechanics and safe transfer techniques and equipment (mechanical lift).

Nursing Care Plan 8.1   Patient With Activity Intolerance

Mr. D., a 56-year-old patient hospitalized with multiple orthopedic traumas, reports pain in his left shoulder during movement. He also reports difficulty extending his shoulder joint in carrying out activities of daily living. The nurse observes that he limits motion in his left arm. Range of motion (ROM) is reduced 30 degrees during abduction of arm.

PATIENT PROBLEM

Compromised Physical Mobility, related to (r/t) left shoulder pain as evidenced by (AEB) limited mobility of left arm, c/o (complaints of) pain and favoring left arm

Patient Goals and Expected Outcomes	Nursing Interventions	Evaluation
Patient will gain optimal ROM of left shoulder within 4 months. Patient will perform self-care activities using left arm within 2 days. Patient will report decreased pain by at least 2 on a scale of 0–10 within 2 days. Patient will increase ROM in upper extremity joints by 20 degrees. Patient will follow a regular exercise program by discharge.	Offer analgesic 30 min before ROM exercises (peak action of analgesic will occur as patient begins exercises). Schedule active ROM exercises between meals and hygiene activities (promotes frequent exercise to affected joints and reduces risk of contracture development). Teach patient specific ROM exercises for left shoulder and arm. (Teaching provides the patient with opportunity and knowledge to maintain and increase ROM.) (See Patient Teaching and Home Care Considerations boxes on mobility.)	Ask patient to report changes in perception of left shoulder pain, using a scale of 1–10. Observe patient while doing ROM exercises in upper extremities and while doing self-care to determine increase of 20 degrees of upper extremities by time of discharge.

CRITICAL THINKING QUESTIONS

1. The nurse is in the process of transferring Mr. D. from his bed to a chair with use of a mechanical lift. The nurse has prepared the chair and placed it near the bed. The nurse turns Mr. D. to his side, places the sling under Mr. D. to ensure adequate support of his head, returns Mr. D. to his back, and slowly begins to lift him from his bed. What has the nurse forgotten to do, and why is it important?

2. The patient has a trapeze bar across the bed, trochanter rolls, and a footboard. Explain the rationale for use of each of these devices to maintain proper body alignment.

🏠 Home Care Considerations

MOBILITY

Instruct family or caregiver about the rationale for slow, gradual position changes.

Instruct family or caregiver about the use of a gait belt and correct body mechanics for transfer of patient.

Instruct family or caregiver to not attempt ambulation if patient reports dizziness or lightheadedness.

Transfer ability at home is greatly enhanced by prior teaching of family, assessment of home for safety risks and functionality, and provision of applicable aids.

Have family practice transfer in hospital and achieve success before taking patient home.

Alternatively, have the patient who lives alone practice activities he or she will use at home to manage toileting and showering. Teach patients to transfer to armchairs for ease of rising and sitting.

Be sure the home is free of risks (e.g., throw rugs, electric cords, slippery floors). If a wheelchair is used, see that access is possible through all doors and that space for transfer is available in bedroom and bathroom.

Ensure arrangements are made for a home health nurse or support person to continue to assist the family at home.

Instruct patient about how to use the ambulation aids on various terrains (e.g., carpet, stairs, rough ground, inclines).

Instruct patient in how to maneuver around obstacles, such as doors, and how to use the aid when transferring, such as to and from a chair, toilet, tub, and car.

Attach a carrying bag to patient's walker to carry objects; caution patient not to overfill the bag to prevent forward tipping of walker.

Assess family member or primary caregiver's ability, availability, and motivation to assist patient with exercises that patient is unable to perform independently.

Assist family or primary caregiver to arrange home environment to promote exercise program (e.g., space allocation, lighting, temperature, safety precautions).

Teach family members about body mechanics.

In the absence of a hospital bed and equipment, creative adaptation is necessary.

Consider the need for a bed that places the bedridden patient at caregiver's waist level.

Teach caregivers to change patient's position every 1 to 2 h, if possible, to maintain musculoskeletal alignment and to reduce pressure on bony prominences. Develop and post a realistic turning schedule.

The nurse is aware of the patient's motor deficits, ability to aid in transfer, and body weight. As suggested by the National Institute for Occupational Safety and Health's (NIOSH) Division of Safety Research, health care personnel should never attempt to lift more than 35 pounds of a patient's body weight, or should use the Revised NIOSH Lifting Equation (CDC/NIOSH, 2017). For the safety of the staff and the patient, additional assistance always should be secured when the transferability of a patient is in doubt.

Many special problems are to be considered in transfer. Patients who have been immobile for several days or longer may be weak or have vertigo (dizziness) and sometimes have orthostatic hypotension (a drop in blood pressure) when transferred. A patient with neurologic deficits perhaps has paresis (muscle weakness) or paralysis unilaterally or bilaterally, which complicates safe transfer. A flaccid arm easily can sustain injury during transfer if unsupported. The nurse must be creative when necessary in the transfer of trauma patients. As a general rule, a gait (transfer) belt should be used and assistance obtained for mobilization of such patients.

◆ EVALUATION

The success of interventions is evaluated with a comparison of the patient's response with the outcome established for each nursing goal, such as the following:

Ask the patient to rate pain on a scale of 1 to 10 (determines need for additional pain control).

Note the patient's behavioral response to transfer (reveals level of pain, motivation, and self-care potential).

For evaluation of the patient's perception of the interventions, knowledge of the patient's expectations concerning joint mobility, posture, or body alignment is necessary first. What is acceptable or anticipated on the nurse's part is sometimes very different from what the patient and family members anticipate or are able to accept.

Get Ready For The NCLEX® Examination!

Key Points

Protection of the musculoskeletal system is essential to prevent injury to patient and nurse.

Less effort is needed to carry out an activity if the base of support is widened in the direction of movement.

Appropriate body mechanics should be practiced consistently.

Maintenance of correct body alignment is the key to proper body mechanics.

Correct body alignment promotes balance and helps coordinate movements.

Permanent disability can occur from inappropriate positioning.

Proper positioning permits activity, enhances comfort, and prepares patients for procedures.

Immobility sometimes results from illness or trauma, and sometimes it is prescribed for therapeutic reasons. Whatever the reason, immobility poses the risk of serious complications. Interventions to avoid these complications are possible.

The nurse performs range-of-motion exercises to promote circulation, prevent contractures, and provide joint mobility.

When turning, moving, lifting, or carrying a patient, the nurse should secure adequate assistance to reduce strain and prevent injury to the nurse and the patient. The nurse should perform procedures safely and properly, facilitating the patient's independence, and should teach the patient and others safety in moving.

Mechanical devices such as a mechanical lift, roller board, and gurney lift are used for moving patients safely.

Use the nursing process to provide care for patients who are at risk for or are experiencing activity intolerance and impaired mobility.

Additional Learning Resources

SG Go to your Study Guide for additional learning activities to help you master this chapter content.

Be sure to visit the Evolve site at http://evolve.elsevier.com/Cooper/foundations/ for additional online resources.

Review Questions for the NCLEX® Examination

1. The nurse is assigned to care for an 82-year-old patient who weighs 252 pounds (lb) (114.54 kilograms [kg]) and has undergone a bilateral below-the-knee amputation. Which transfer method is the safest for the patient and the nurse?

   1. Logrolling
   2. A gurney lift
   3. A mechanical lift with a sling
   4. Two nurses to lift the patient without assistive equipment

2. The nurse helps ambulate an 84-year-old female patient who has peripheral vascular disease that caused a severe stasis ulcer. The patient becomes very weak, reports feeling faint, and begins to fall. What is the most appropriate action to prevent injury to the patient?

   1. Support her while she is falling and allow her to sit on the floor.
   2. Carefully attempt to return her to her room.
   3. Tell her to hold on to the wall and that you will get more assistance.
   4. Ask her to take deep breaths and look straight ahead.

3. A 56-year-old patient had an open cholecystectomy. The nurse is going to assist the patient with dangling on the side of the bed before ambulation. After sitting the patient on the edge of the bed, which nursing intervention should the nurse perform before proceeding with the ambulation?

   1. Measurement of the patient's temperature
   2. Assessment of the patient's pulse and respirations
   3. Auscultating the patient's lung sounds
   4. Removal of the patient's anti-embolism stockings

4. The patient accidentally knocks the emesis basin to the floor. When picking up the emesis basin, which movement demonstrates proper body mechanics by the nurse?

   1. The nurse lowers the body by flexing the knees and bending the hips.
   2. The nurse bends from the waist and hips.
   3. The nurse flexes the knees and bends at the waist.
   4. The nurse keeps the legs straight and flexes the waist.

5. A patient who was admitted with the diagnosis of a stroke has slid to the foot of the bed. With use of appropriate body mechanics, the nurse maintains a wide base of support and faces the patient in the direction of movement. What do these actions allow the nurse to do?

   1. Use the back muscles
   2. Use the gluteal muscles
   3. Exert less physical effort
   4. Use the large muscles across the scapula

6. An 82-year-old patient has had a cerebrovascular accident that affects her right side. The nurse repositions the patient to her left side, placing a pillow between her legs and another behind her back. What is the primary purpose of this intervention?

   1. Maintaining the patient's comfort
   2. Ensuring the patient's proper body alignment
   3. Keeping the patient in the desired position for at least 2 hours
   4. Preventing the patient from development of contractures

7. It is the patient's first night after an abdominal hysterectomy. She has not voided for 9 hours, and the nurse is to insert a 16-French Foley catheter into her bladder. What patient position best allows insertion of the catheter?

   1. Dorsal recumbent
   2. Lithotomy
   3. Sims
   4. Prone

8. The nurse is assigned to care for a patient who was admitted for exacerbation of chronic obstructive pulmonary disease and pneumonia. The patient is experiencing dyspnea and is unable to rest in a supine position. The nurse elevates the head of the bed to 90 degrees, places a pillow on the overbed table, and

assists the patient to lean forward, placing the patient's head on the pillow. What position should the nurse document the patient as being in?

1. Semi-Fowler's
2. Dorsal
3. Sims
4. Orthopneic

9. The nurse explains to the patient that the log-rolling technique will be used to help the patient change position. The patient asks why this is necessary. Which response is accurate?

1. "Logrolling will help you keep your hips slightly flexed toward your chest."
2. "By having you dangle your legs at the bedside, you will be more comfortable."
3. "Because of your injury, it is extremely important that the head of your bed remain up at all times."
4. "It is important to keep your neck and spine in straight alignment while we help you move onto your side."

10. The nurse and a UAP are to move a dependent patient from the supine to the lateral position. Which action should be performed first?

1. Move the patient to the side of the bed.
2. Turn the patient with use of a lift sheet.
3. Ensure that the upper arm and leg are supported with pillows.
4. Explain to the patient what actions the nurse and UAP are going to perform.

11. An older adult patient has been lying in the supine position for 3 hours and tells the nurse that she is too uncomfortable to move right now. What is the best response by the nurse?

1. The nurse should express concern that she is uncomfortable and promise to come back later.
2. The nurse should assess the patient's need for pain medication before helping her change position.
3. The nurse should explain to the patient that if she does not move now, she will develop pneumonia.
4. The nurse should find another nurse to help move the patient to the lateral position immediately.

12. The nurse is caring for a patient who requires the assistance of one with all activities and ambulation. The patient is going to be transferred home and the patient's spouse will be providing care. The nurse wants to ensure that the spouse practices good body mechanics in order to prevent any injuries to themselves. The nurse asks the spouse to demonstrate assisting the patient with activities and ambulation.

Choose the *most likely* options for the information missing from the statements blow by selecting from the list of options provided.

The spouse keeps their knees in a _____ position when assisting the patient. When the spouse assists the patient from a standing to a sitting position the spouse maintains a _____ base of support. To improve leverage the spouse holds the patient _____ their body when pivoting to the chair.

OPTIONS
Close to
Locked
Narrow

OPTIONS
Away from
Bent
Wide
45 degree angle

1. Keeping the knees in a locked position
2. Maintaining a wide base of support and bending at the knees
3. Bending at the waist to maintain one's balance
4. Holding objects away from the body for improved leverage
5. Asking for help when deemed necessary when assisting a patient with transfers

13. A 73-year-old patient is admitted to a rehabilitation unit in a long-term-care facility following a motor vehicle accident. The accident resulted in a fractured pelvis. The patient is allowed to sit in the chair and ambulate with assistance of one. The patient becomes faint and diaphoretic while sitting on the side of the bed in preparation to ambulate. What action is appropriate for the care of this patient? *(Select all that apply.)*

1. The nurse should call for assistance.
2. The nurse should not allow the patient to get out of bed at this time.
3. The nurse should allow the patient to lower the head to rest on the nurse's abdomen.
4. The nurse should find an emesis basin because the patient will probably vomit.
5. The nurse should continue to assist the patient to a standing position, looking forward and taking deep breaths.
6. The nurse should use a gait belt to assist the patient with any transfers or while walking.
7. The nurse should measure the patient's blood pressure lying, sitting, and standing.
8. The nurse should have the patient remain in bed for the next 24 hours.

14. A patient has been immobilized for 5 days because of extensive abdominal surgery. When this patient is helped out of bed for the first time, which patient problem related to safety applies to this patient? *(Select all that apply.)*

1. Recent Onset of Pain
2. Compromised Skin Integrity
3. Compromised Blood Flow to Tissue
4. Potential for Inability to Tolerate Activity
5. Potential for Falling

15. Which assistive device allows patients to pull with the upper extremities to raise their trunk off the bed, to assist in transfer from bed to wheelchair, and to perform upper arm exercises?

1. Trapeze bar
2. Trochanter roll
3. Hand rolls
4. Footboard

16. In which position is the patient lying face down or chest down?

1. Supine
2. Lateral
3. Prone
4. Fowler's

17. What is a necessary safety precaution when helping a patient who has an unsteady gait to ambulate? *(Select all that apply.)*

    1. Have family members present.
    2. Have patient wear well-fitting nonskid shoes or slippers.
    3. Have at least two people present to assist the patient.
    4. Be sure no pain medication was given for at least 3 hours before ambulation.
    5. Use a gait belt when assisting the patient to stand and to ambulate.

18. What is a major benefit of active ROM exercises? *(Select all that apply.)*

    1. Preventing contractures
    2. Preventing the patient from getting arthritis
    3. Maintaining joint movement and mobility
    4. Preventing atrophy of muscle near the joints
    5. Increasing the patient's self-esteem and motivation

19. The nurse is receiving a report on a patient. The nurse giving the report states that the patient has foot drop. The nurse receiving the report knows that which is the correct terminology for foot drop?

    1. Plantar flexion of the foot
    2. Dorsiflexion of the foot
    3. Ankle extension
    4. Ankle hyperextension

20. When using a lift sheet to assist in moving a patient up in bed, what should the nurse ask the patient to do? *(Select all that apply.)*

    1. Bend the knees to assist in moving
    2. Keep the hands at sides of the body
    3. Raise the arms above the head
    4. Maintain good body alignment
    5. Place the arms across the chest

Hygiene and Care of the Patient's Environment

Objectives

1. Discuss the therapeutic hospital room environment.
2. Describe personal hygienic practices.
3. Discuss variations of the bath procedure determined by a patient's condition and physician's orders.
4. Describe the procedure for a bed bath.
5. Identify nursing interventions for the prevention and treatment of a pressure ulcer/injury.
6. Discuss heat and cold therapy and related procedures.
7. Describe the procedures for oral hygiene, shaving, hair care, nail care, and eye, ear, and nose care.
8. Outline the procedure for a back rub.
9. Summarize the procedure for perineal care for a male patient and a female patient.
10. Discuss the procedures for skin care.
11. Describe the procedure for making an unoccupied bed.
12. Describe the procedure for making an occupied bed.
13. Discuss assisting a patient in the use of the bedpan, the urinal, and the bedside commode.

Key Terms

axilla (ăk-SĬL-ă, p. 197)
bedpan (BĔD-păn, p. 227)
canthus (KĂN-thŭs, p. 197)
cerumen (sĕ-RŪ-mĕn, p. 222)
circumorbital (sŭr-kŭm-ŎR-bĭ-tăl, p. 221)
dentures (DĔN-chŭrs, p. 189)
febrile (p. 209)
hygiene (HĪ-gēn, p. 189)
labia majora (LĀ-bē-ă mă-JŎR-ă, p. 220)
labia minora (LĀ-bē-ă mĭ-NŎR-ă, p. 220)
medical asepsis (ā-SĔP-sĭs, p. 190)
oral hygiene (ŎR-ăl HĪ-gēn, p. 213)
pathogenic (păth-ō-GĔN-ĭk, p. 190)
perineal care (pĕr-ĭ-NĒ-ăl, p. 216)

personal hygiene (PŬR-sŭn-ăl HĪ-gēn, p. 189)
pressure injury (PRĔ-shŭr ĬN-jŭ-rē, p. 203)
pressure ulcer (PRĔ-shŭr ŬL-sĕr, p. 203)
prone (prōn, p. 198)
range of motion (ROM) (rānj ŏv MŌ-shŭn, p. 194)
Sims position (SĬMZ pŏ-zĭ-shŭn, p. 198)
supine (SŪ-pīn [noun], sū-PĪN [adjective], p. 198)
syncope (SĬN-kō-pē, p. 194)
umbilicus (ŭm-BĬL-ĭ-kŭs, p. 197)
urinal (Ū-rĭn-ăl, p. 227)
vasoconstriction (vā-zō-kŏn-STRĬK-shŭn, p. 208)
vasodilation (vā-zō-dī-LĀ-shŭn, p. 208)
vertigo (VŬR-tĭ-gō, p. 194)

Hygiene (the principles of health) includes care of not only the skin but also the hair, the hands, the feet, the eyes, the ears, the nose, the mouth, the back, and the perineum. This chapter discusses the bath, components of the bath, bed making, and assisting the patient in the use of the bedpan, the urinal, and the bedside commode. Many factors influence the practice of an individual's personal hygiene (Box 9.1 and the Cultural Considerations box about personal hygiene).

When assisting with the patient's hygiene needs, the licensed practical/vocational nurse (LPN/LVN) has an opportunity to observe the patient's ability to perform self-care. Assisting a patient with hygiene care gives the nurse an opportune time to perform a complete and thorough physical assessment. During the bath, the nurse is able to assess the patient's physical and emotional state and assess all body systems. Assisting a patient with bathing involves close contact with the patient and offers an opportunity to communicate with the patient to enhance a therapeutic relationship and learn about the emotional needs of the patient.

Patients often are in a dependent role and need assistance from the nurse in carrying out personal hygiene (the self-care measures people use to maintain health and prevent disease). The nurse's responsibility is to preserve the patient's well-being, encourage as much of the patient's independence as possible, and respect the patient's privacy when assisting with hygiene measures.

Sometimes the nurse needs to teach health promotion practices, and the performance of hygienic care provides an excellent opportunity for this. An attitude of acceptance during care for a patient with poor hygiene allows for development of the nurse-patient relationship.

Box 9.1 Factors That Influence a Patient's Personal Hygiene

- *Body image.* Body image is a person's subjective concept of physical appearance. Body image affects the manner in which hygiene is maintained. The nurse must provide education to the unclean patient about the importance of hygiene. Nurses must be careful not to convey feelings of disapproval when caring for the patient whose hygiene practices differ from others.
- *Cultural variables.* Patients from diverse cultural backgrounds follow different self-care practices. In North America, people typically take daily baths (tub or shower), but in many European countries, it is not unusual to bathe completely only once a week. Avoid being judgmental when caring for patients with different hygienic practices (see the Cultural Considerations box).
- *Knowledge.* Knowledge alone is not enough. The patient also must be encouraged to maintain self-care. Often, learning about an illness or condition encourages patients to improve hygienic practices. For example, teaching the patient with diabetes the importance of foot care helps prevent infections. It is important to maintain a nonjudgmental attitude while providing hygiene for the patient.
- *Personal preference.* Individual patients have individual desires and choices as to when to bathe, shave, and shampoo. Patients choose different shampoos, deodorants, and toothpastes according to personal needs or selections. Do not try to change the patient's preferences unless the patient's health is affected.
- *Physical condition.* Patients in the late stages of terminal illness or those who have undergone surgery often lack the physical energy or dexterity to perform personal hygiene. Some disease conditions exhaust or incapacitate patients, thereby requiring the nurse to perform all aspects of hygiene. Other disease conditions, such as serious cardiac or pulmonary problems, cause severe activity intolerance.
- *Social practices.* Social groups, family customs, age, friends, and work groups influence practices of personal hygiene.
- *Socioeconomic status.* The patient's economic resources often influence the type or extent of hygienic practices used.

Cultural Considerations

Personal Hygiene

- Cultural practices vary within a culture. The authors of this text are describing common cultural practices. Please note that these practices are not demonstrated by all members of a particular culture.
- Touch or lack of touch has cultural significance and symbolism and is a learned behavior. Cultural uses of touch vary. Although the rules of touch are typically unspoken and unwritten, they are usually visible to the observer. Stay within the rules of touch that are culturally prescribed.
- Chinese Americans sometimes view tasks associated with closeness and touch as offensive. Vietnamese Americans are likely to feel very uneasy during a back rub. Ask patients what makes them most comfortable during a bath.
- Use touch with discernment and avoid forcing touch on anyone. A momentary and seemingly incidental touch has the capacity to establish a positive, temporary bond between strangers, making them more compliant, helpful, positive, and giving.
- Be mindful of the patient's reaction to touch and avoid being perceived as intrusive.
- Consider the individual patient's beliefs, values, and habits.
- Individual preferences usually do not affect health in any significant manner and usually fit without problem into the plan of care.
- East Indian Hindus consider personal hygiene to be extremely important. A daily bath is part of their religious duty. Some Hindus believe bathing after a meal to be injurious. Likewise, a bath that is too hot has the potential to injure the eyes. Hot water may be added to cold water, but cold water is not to be added to hot water when preparing a bath. Once a bath is completed, the individual carefully dries the body thoroughly with a towel.

Different types of hygienic care usually are performed at certain times throughout the day. These times depend on various factors, including patient schedules and staff responsibilities (Box 9.2). Sometimes scheduling of hygiene measures at the same time as other care measures is most convenient.

The nurse's own conscientious practice of personal hygiene is essential (Box 9.3). Nurses are role models and teach by example. Hygienic practices promote **medical asepsis**, also known as clean technique. This technique inhibits the growth and spread of **pathogenic** (disease-producing) microorganisms (see Chapter 7).

PATIENT'S ROOM ENVIRONMENT

Many patients with limitations such as traction, casts, or monitoring equipment may not leave their rooms as frequently as other patients. Patients who are critically ill may be confined to their rooms for an extended period of time. These rooms must be kept comfortable and safe (Fig. 9.1). By controlling factors such as room temperature, ventilation, noise, and odors, the LPN/LVN creates a more therapeutic environment. Keeping the room clean, neat, and orderly contributes to a sense of well-being.

MAINTAINING COMFORT

Consider the patient's age, severity of illness, and activity tolerance to maintain optimal patient comfort. The recommended room temperature is 68°F to 74°F (20°C to 23°C). Infants, older adults (see the Lifespan Considerations for Older Adults box), and the acutely ill are likely to need warmer temperatures. Physically

Box 9.2	Hygiene Care Schedule

- *Early morning care.* Nursing personnel provide basic hygiene to patients getting ready for breakfast, scheduled tests, or early morning surgery. "a.m. care" includes offering a bedpan or urinal if the patient is not ambulatory, washing the patient's hands and face, and assisting with oral care.
- *Morning care, or after-breakfast care.* This care is performed after breakfast. Offer a bedpan or urinal to patients confined to bed; provide a bath or shower; provide oral, foot, nail, and hair care; give a back rub; change the patient's gown or pajamas; change the bed linens; and straighten the patient's bedside unit and room. This often is referred to as complete a.m. care.
- *Afternoon care.* Because hospitalized patients often undergo many exhausting diagnostic tests or procedures in the morning, they tend to greatly appreciate afternoon care. This is also true for the long-term care resident. Many of these residents have participated in exercise, physical therapy, or activities throughout the day. Afternoon hygienic care includes washing the hands and face, assisting with oral care, offering a bedpan or urinal, and straightening bed linen.
- *Evening care, or hour-before-sleep (HS) care.* Before bedtime, offer personal hygienic care that helps a patient relax to promote sleep. "p.m. care," sometimes referred to as HS care, typically includes changing soiled bed linens, gowns, or pajamas; assisting the patient in washing the face, hands, and back; providing oral hygiene; giving a back massage; and offering the bedpan or urinal to nonambulatory patients.

Box 9.3	Personal Hygiene for Nurses

- Take a daily bath or shower.
- Use a strong, odorless, and effective deodorant every day.
- Wear clean undergarments every day.
- Wear a clean uniform every day.
- Shampoo hair as often as necessary to maintain cleanliness.
- Keep hair off the collar or pulled back away from the face and in a contained hairstyle. Wear ties or fasteners that blend in with the hair.
- Wear clean, comfortable shoes that follow facility policy.
- Keep fingernails short, clean, and well manicured. Artificial nails and nail coverings are prohibited in most facilities. Pathogens get trapped underneath artificial nails and coverings and have the potential to cause serious infections, especially in newborns. Follow agency policy regarding nail polish, and remove if it begins to chip.
- Wear makeup only in moderation.
- Wear only an engagement ring or wedding ring (or both) without stones (stones harbor microorganisms). In departments such as the operating and delivery rooms, rings are not worn at all.
- Wear only small unobtrusive earrings; wear only one pair. Large or dangling earrings are not recommended. These are considered hazardous because they can be pulled out easily and damage the ear.
- Avoid perfumes or colognes (many patients are allergic to these).
- Wear the standard departmental uniform.
- Keep beards and mustaches clean, short, and well trimmed.
- Use breath mints; the smell of coffee, foods, or nicotine is often offensive to patients.

active patients and patients with chronic pulmonary problems tend to be more comfortable in a cooler environment.

Good ventilation is necessary to keep stale air and odors from lingering in the room. Take care to protect the patient from drafts. Ensure that odors are kept to a minimum. Promptly emptying and cleaning bedpans, urinals, and commodes helps to eliminate odors.

Noises are unpleasant intrusions. Ill patients are more sensitive to the noises commonly heard within the hospital environment. Work with other hospital personnel to monitor the noise level that results from the moving of metal equipment on and off the elevator and from televisions and radios, telephones ringing, loud talking, and laughter at the nurses' station. Manage equipment properly, answer phones immediately, and control voice volume. Ask patients to keep televisions and radios turned down.

Proper lighting is necessary for the safety of the nurse and the patient. Reduce lighting levels to encourage sleep, and brighten the room for stimulation. Adjust the lighting by closing or opening the drapes, adjusting overbed and floor lights, and opening or closing room doors.

The nurse must help the patient conserve energy for the recovery process. Controlling stimuli within

Fig. 9.1 A typical hospital room.

Lifespan Considerations

Older Adults

Hygiene Practices

- Older individuals are more likely to become chilled during bathing or when left uncovered. Maintain a warmer room temperature than for younger people and keep drafts to a minimum.
- Drape older adults properly during care to prevent chilling and provide for modesty.
- Older adults with limited mobility may need assistance in perineal care. Use of a side-lying position increases the patient's comfort and provides the nurse with opportunity to provide perineal care and inspect surrounding skin. Perineal care should be performed daily and after each episode of incontinence.
- Impaired circulation or neurologic changes sometimes decrease the older person's ability to sense temperature changes in water, so use caution to prevent burns during tub or shower bathing.
- Too-frequent bathing and use of detergent soaps have harmful effects on the skin of most older adults. Determine the type and frequency of baths and the choice of soap based on individual needs.
- Rehydrate patient's skin with lotions and fluids.
- Immobility, incontinence, and poor nutrition increase the risk of skin impairment in older adults. Adequate diet, frequent change of position, use of pressure-reducing devices, regular toileting, and prompt cleansing of the skin after incontinence reduce the risks.
- Older adults with urinary incontinence need meticulous skin care to reduce skin irritation from urine and feces.
- The aging process contributes to changes in voiding and defecating. Often the aging patient needs immediate response to a request for the bedpan or urinal or assistance to the toilet.
- Incontinence of urine or stool is *not* an expected result of the aging process.
- Decreased production of saliva in aging necessitates more frequent oral hygiene. Good cleaning of the oral cavity and teeth or dentures helps reduce the alteration in taste common with aging.
- Good oral hygiene practices help older adults preserve their ability to eat. Older adults, especially those at risk

- for oral problems, should avoid spicy, coarse, acidic, and sugary foods, which tend to cause dental caries. Patients with diabetes need to visit the dentist a minimum of every 6 months.
- Treat older adults with respect. Keep grooming, including hair care and use of cosmetics, age appropriate.
- Because of normal changes in the nails and an increased incidence of circulatory problems or diabetes mellitus, older individuals are more likely to require special foot care.
- Changes in aging skin include thinning of epidermis and subcutaneous fat, and dryness because of decreased activity of oil and sweat glands. These changes become visible in the feet. In addition, nails become opaque, tough, scaly, brittle, and hypertrophied.
- Individuals who have not participated in regular exercise often experience a laxity of foot ligaments and musculature, which leads to instability and impaired mobility.
- Common foot problems of older adults include heel pain caused by tearing of plantar fascia and foot musculature, metatarsalgia (pain beneath metatarsal head), hammertoes and claw toes, corns and calluses, pathologic nail conditions (e.g., ingrown toenails, fungal infections), arthritis, and neuropathies that cause diminished sensation in the foot.
- Older persons are also more vulnerable to bunions because feet tend to spread with aging.
- Usually the facial hair of the older adult does not grow quickly; thus a shave is not necessarily required every day.
- Older adults have fragile skin and require more protection. Be sure bed linens are clean, dry, and free of wrinkles.
- Encourage older adults to spend as much time out of bed as possible.
- Use draw sheets and waterproof pads with caution. Accumulation of moisture creates a risk for skin maceration and impairment, so these items must be changed as needed.

the patient's personal environment is one way to help conserve energy. This promotes a sense of security and enhances the patient's ability to gain needed rest and sleep (see Chapter 21).

ROOM EQUIPMENT

The usual hospital room contains certain basic furniture: bedside stand, bed, overbed table, chairs, and lights (see Fig. 9.1). In addition, the standard hospital room has either a closet or drawer space. Room equipment and furniture for the long-term care facility differs somewhat, often incorporating more personal furniture and decor (see Chapter 38).

The bedside stand stores the patient's personal articles and hygienic equipment, such as towels, the

emesis and bath basins, toothpaste and toothbrush, and comb and brush. The telephone, the drinking glass, and the water pitcher ordinarily are kept on the patient's bedside stand.

The overbed table is on wheels and is adjustable to various heights over the bed or a chair. Usually a storage area is located under the tabletop. This tabletop is ideal to use as a working space when performing procedures. It also serves as a surface for meal trays, toileting items needed during hygienic care, and other objects frequently used by the patient. The tabletop should be cleaned before and after procedures and before meals.

Chairs are a necessity in the hospital room. Straight chairs and lounge chairs are typical. The patient and visitors make use of the lounge chair. Straight chairs are more maneuverable than lounge chairs. They are also more convenient when temporarily transferring the patient from the bed, such as during bed making. Relatives who sit with the patient are apt to use recliner chairs.

Lights in each patient's room provide comfort, safety, and ease. A call light is available at each bedside. The call signal indicates that a patient needs assistance. Many facilities are designed so that the call light from a patient's bathroom flashes off and on quickly, denoting a call of a more serious nature. In contrast, the bedside call light typically does not flash. Respond as soon as possible when a patient indicates a need for assistance.

Critically ill patients often remain in bed for longer periods of time. Hospital beds are designed for comfort and safety and their capacity to accommodate position changes (Table 9.1). The standard hospital bed has a firm water-repellent mattress on a metal frame that is raised and lowered horizontally as needed. An even surface provides for the greatest comfort. Bariatric beds are available in most facilities to accommodate obese patients. Handles on the sides of the mattress are helpful with removing or turning the mattress.

Different bed positions are used to promote lung expansion, postural drainage, and other interventions.

Most beds are powered by electricity, but some are operated manually. These beds are convenient to raise while working at the bedside and then lower when the patient is being transferred or when leaving the patient's room. Furthermore, the nurse or patient can raise and lower the head or the foot of the bed independently. In most cases, the controls are situated conveniently on the side of the bed or in the side rail. Teach the patient the proper use of the controls, and caution the patient to leave the bed at its lowest level to prevent injuries from falls.

Hospital beds have a number of safety features. Locks on the wheels prevent unwanted movement. Side rails (adjustable metal frames that are raised and lowered by pushing or pulling a knob) are located on both sides of the bed. These side rails protect patients from falling, aid patients in positioning themselves, and provide upper extremity support as the patient gets out of bed. Never leave the bedside of a patient in bed if the side rail is lowered. Full side rails are considered a form of restraint in a long-term care setting (see Chapter 38). Another safety feature is the special removable headboard on some beds, which is important when the medical team needs easy access to the patient's head during cardiopulmonary resuscitation.

Table 9.1   Bed Positions

POSITION	DESCRIPTION	USES
Fowler's to high Fowler's	Head of bed raised to angle of 45 degrees or more (up to 90 degrees); semi-sitting to full upright sitting position	Appropriate position for eating or drinking to prevent aspiration; beneficial during breathing exercises to promote full lung expansion
Semi-Fowler's (also referred to as low Fowler's)	Head of bed raised approximately 30 degrees	Often used for patients who cannot tolerate Fowler's or high Fowler's; position sometimes ordered after lumbar puncture has been performed
Trendelenburg's	Entire bed tilted downward toward head of bed with no break in the middle of the bed	Facilitates removal of secretions with postural drainage; facilitates venous return in patients with poor peripheral circulation; sometimes used to aid in dilation of large vessels for central line placement
Reverse Trendelenburg's	Entire bed frame tilted downward toward foot of bed with no break in the middle of the bed	Not commonly used position; promotes gastric emptying and prevents esophageal reflux; facilitates arterial circulation to lower extremities
Flat	Entire bed frame parallel with floor	For patients with vertebral injuries, immediately after lumbar puncture, and in cervical traction; generally preferred by patients for sleeping

Modified from Potter PA, Perry AG: *Essentials for nursing practice*, ed 8, St. Louis, 2015, Mosby.

BATHING

The extent of the patient's bath and methods used for bathing depend on the patient's capabilities, the degree of hygiene required, and the physician's order, as in the case of therapeutic baths. The types of therapeutic baths are outlined in the following sections. Some hygiene skills are acceptable to delegate to unlicensed assistive personnel (UAP; see the Coordinated Care box on bathing and other hygienic care measures), unless UAP are not available or are not part of the staff of a particular unit or facility.

Maintain a water temperature of 110°F (about 43°C) if the purpose is to apply heat to the affected area. If the purpose is to promote healing or to produce relaxation, use a water temperature of about 98°F to 102°F (34°C to 39°C). Remember to prevent chilling by covering the patient's legs with a bath blanket and the shoulders with a towel. Place a towel behind the patient's back for comfort.

Observe the patient for signs and symptoms of weakness, such as a rapid or weak pulse, tachypnea, **vertigo** (dizziness), or **syncope** (fainting). Never leave the patient alone unless the patient is safe. The call light/signal should be placed within easy reach. Instruct the patient to stay out of drafts and to rest after a sitz bath.

 Coordinated Care

Delegation

Hygiene Care Measures

BATHING

The skilled task of bathing often is delegated to UAP; however, skin and **range of motion (ROM)** (normal movement that any given joint is capable of making) assessment require the critical thinking and knowledge application unique to the nurse.

- Instruct the UAP in what type of bath (e.g., complete, partial assist, tub, shower) is appropriate to the patient's diagnosis and needs.
- Remind the UAP to notify the nurse of any skin integrity problems so that areas of impairment or potential impairment may be inspected.
- Remind the UAP to use an organized approach and reassuring tone of voice so that the patient feels safe and comfortable during bathing.
- Instruct the UAP to encourage the patient to report any concerns or discomfort during the bath.
- Instruct the UAP to encourage as much independence in the patient's self-care skills as appropriate and to provide positive feedback.

ORAL CARE

Skills of oral care, toothbrushing, and denture care are appropriate to delegate to UAP, but the patient's gag reflex should be assessed first.

- Instruct the UAP in the proper way to position the patient if the patient is unconscious or debilitated.
- Remind the UAP to report any changes in oral mucosa.
- Review with the UAP the use of oral suction for cleansing oral secretions (if allowed by facility policy), if the patient is likely to need it.

HAIR CARE AND SHOWERING

The skills of shampooing and shaving are appropriate to delegate to UAP, unless the patient has a trauma or injury of the cervical spine.

- Instruct the UAP how to properly position individual patients and use any special products indicated.
- Be sure the UAP knows how to correctly use medicated shampoos for lice or other conditions and the appropriate steps to prevent transmission to other patients.
- Remind the UAP to report how the patient tolerated the procedure and any changes that indicate possible inflammation or injury.

HAND, FOOT, AND NAIL CARE

The skill of care of the fingernails and foot care for patients without diabetes or any circulatory compromise, anticoagulant therapy, or bleeding disorder is appropriate to delegate to UAP.

- Instruct UAP in the proper way to use nail files and clippers (check agency policy on whether UAP are permitted to use nail clippers on patients).
- Caution UAP to use warm water.
- Remind UAP to report any changes that indicate possible inflammation or injury.

BED MAKING

Bed making usually is delegated to UAP.

- Instruct UAP on whether an unoccupied or occupied bed is to be made.
- Review with UAP the safety precautions or activity restrictions for the patient; stress the use of side rails in the acute care setting and the call system in the event that staff assistance is needed.
- Instruct UAP to notify the nurse immediately if wound drainage, dressing material, drainage tubes, or intravenous (IV) tubing is found in the linen or becomes dislodged.
- Instruct UAP to allow the patient rest periods and notify the nurse if the patient becomes fatigued.

CARE OF THE PATIENT WITH INCONTINENCE

The skill of providing care for patients with incontinence is appropriate to delegate to UAP. The following measures are all particularly important when assisting the patient with incontinence:

- Caution UAP to be aware of the patient's dignity and self-esteem needs and to take measures to prevent violating these needs.
- Ensure that UAP know standard precautions guidelines related to handling of body fluids.
- Be sure UAP report information such as abdominal, flank, or perineal pain, increased episodes of incontinence, changes in appearance, odor, or amount of urine or stool, and evidence of skin irritation or breakdown.
- The nurse is responsible for ensuring that all patients are given adequate privacy for elimination and that cultural modesty standards are observed.

COOL WATER TUB BATH

The cool water tub bath is an option to relieve tension or lower body temperature. Take precautions to prevent the patient from chilling. The water temperature is tepid, 98.6°F (37°C). Cold water should not be used because it causes chilling and shivering.

WARM WATER TUB BATH

A warm water tub bath is given primarily to reduce muscle tension. The recommended water temperature is approximately 110°F (43°C).

HOT WATER TUB BATH

The hot water tub bath helps relieve muscle soreness and muscle spasms. This procedure is not recommended for children. The proper water temperature for adults is 113°F to 115°F (45°C to 46°C). Keep in mind the danger of burns and take precautions to prevent them. This bath is not used for patients with neurologic disorders or circulatory impairment because of the risk of causing burns.

SITZ BATH

A sitz bath cleanses and aids in reducing inflammation of the perineal and anal areas of the patient who has undergone rectal or vaginal surgery or childbirth. Discomfort from hemorrhoids or a fissure also is relieved with a sitz bath. Sitz baths may be cool or warm depending on the need for the treatment. Optimally, the sitz bath lasts from 20 to 30 minutes, and usually is ordered three times daily. The time seems to pass more quickly when the patient has reading material.

The appliance for the sitz bath is shown in Fig. 9.2. Depending on the patient's diagnosis and the health care provider's order, the desired results are possible to obtain from a tub bath. The water in the tub should be kept to a minimum so that the warm water will be concentrated in the perineal area. The tub is the least desirable method because heat also is applied to the legs, thus reducing the effects on the pelvic region.

OTHER BATHS

A complete bed bath is for patients who are totally dependent and require total assistance (Skill 9.1). As the patient's condition improves, only partial assistance

Fig. 9.2 The portable sitz bath.

Skill 9.1   Bathing the Patient and Administering a Back Rub

NURSING ACTION (RATIONALE)

1. Refer to medical record, care plan, or Kardex for special interventions. (*Provides basis for care.*)
2. Assemble the necessary supplies. (*Organizes procedure.*)
   - Bath blanket
   - Bath towels (2)
   - Disposable gloves
   - Drapes
   - Gown or patient's own pajamas or nightgown
   - Hygiene articles, such as lotion, powder, and deodorant
   - Laundry bag or hamper
   - Soap and soap dish
   - Washbasin
   - Washcloths (2)
3. Introduce self. (*Decreases patient's anxiety.*)
4. Identify patient. (*Ensures procedure is performed with correct patient.*)
5. Explain procedure to patient. (*Enlists cooperation and decreases anxiety.*)
6. Perform hand hygiene and, as appropriate, don clean gloves. Know agency policy and guidelines from the Centers for Disease Control and Prevention (CDC) and Occupational Safety and Health Administration (OSHA). (*Reduces spread of microorganisms.*)

Continued

Skill 9.1   Bathing the Patient and Administering a Back Rub—cont'd

7. Prepare patient for intervention.
   a. Close door or pull curtain. (*Provides privacy.*)
   b. Drape for procedure as appropriate. (*Prevents unnecessary exposure.*)
   c. Suggest use of bedpan, urinal, or bathroom. (*Prevents interruptions during procedure and provides for patient's comfort.*)
   d. Arrange supplies. (*Provides convenient access to equipment.*)
   e. Adjust room temperature. (*Prevents patient from chilling.*)
   f. Raise bed to comfortable working position. (*Promotes proper body mechanics.*)
8. Bed bath.
   a. Lower side rail; position patient on side of bed closest to you. (*Ensures proper body mechanics.*)
   b. Loosen top linens from the foot of the bed; place bath blanket over the top linens. Ask patient to hold bath blanket while you remove top linens. If patient is unable, hold bath blanket in place while removing linens. (*Provides warmth and privacy.*)

   c. Place soiled laundry in laundry bag; do not touch uniform with soiled laundry. (*Reduces spread of microorganisms.*)
   d. Assist patient with oral hygiene. (*Prevents mouth diseases, improves self-image, and improves appetite.*) If patient is unable, the nurse performs the procedure (see Skill 9.3).
   e. Remove patient's gown, all undergarments, and jewelry. (*Facilitates a more effective bed bath.*) If an extremity is injured or has reduced mobility, begin removal of the gown from the unaffected side. If the patient has an IV tube, remove gown from the arm without IV first, then lower IV container or remove tubing from pump and slide gown covering down over the affected arm and over tubing and container. Rehang IV container and check flow rate or reset pump. Do not disconnect tubing. (*Undressing the unaffected side first makes manipulating gown over body part easier with reduced range of motion [ROM] [normal movement that any given joint is capable of making].*)

Skill 9.1   Bathing the Patient and Administering a Back Rub—cont'd

f. Raise side rail and fill washbasin two-thirds full with water at 110°F–115°F (43°C–46°C). To prevent spillage, do not overfill basin. *(Maintains patient's safety.)*

g. Remove pillow and raise head of bed to semi-Fowler's position if patient is able to tolerate it. *(The patient's face, ears, and neck are more accessible for cleansing. Patients with breathing difficulties need a pillow or elevation of head of bed during bath.)*

h. Form mitt with bath cloth around your hand (see illustration); dip mitt and hand into bath water. Squeeze out excess water. *(Facilitates handling of bath cloth and prevents corners from brushing against patient. Do not place soap in bath water—too many suds prevent adequate rinsing.)*

i. Wash around patient's eyes, using a different portion of washcloth for each eye. Cleanse from inner to outer canthus (corner of eye; see illustration). Dry gently. *(Prevents irritation, spread of infection, and injury.)*

j. Rinse bath cloth (then continue to use as mitt) and finish washing face. (Ask patient about use of soap on face because some patients, especially female patients, do not use soap on face.) Wash ears and neck. Cleanse pinna (the projecting part of the external ear) with cotton-tipped applicators. *(Rinsing cloth well helps reduce any skin irritation from the soap. Do not place soap in washbasin to keep rinse water from getting soapy.)*

k. Expose arm farthest from you. Place towel lengthwise under patient's arm. To cleanse the hands, the nurse can place washbasin on towel and place patient's hand in basin of water, or the hands can be cleansed with the washcloth

(be sure to clean between the fingers). Bathe arms with long, firm strokes; a firm stroke rather than a light stroke prevents tickling the patient. Supporting arm, raise it above patient's head to bathe the axilla (the underarm area or armpit). Rinse and dry well. In most cases, provide nail care at this time (see next step), although, if desired, it is possible to do separately (see Skill 9.4). Apply deodorant if desired. *(Beginning on far side prevents reaching over clean area; long, firm strokes stimulate circulation. Raising arm promotes ROM and exposes axilla. Deodorant controls body odor. Axilla is bathed last because it is considered less clean than arm.)*

l. When doing nail care, allow patient's hand to soak for 3–5 min; push back cuticles gently with washcloth. Clean under nails and file smoothly as needed. Dry thoroughly. *(Enhances feeling of self-worth and decreases spread of infection. Soaking softens cuticles and loosens debris under nails.)*

m. Bathe arm closest to you. Follow Steps k and l.

n. Cover patient's chest with bath towel; fold bath blanket down to waist and wash chest with circular motion. Be certain to cleanse and dry well in skin folds and under breasts. *(Use of circular motion while bathing chest prevents injury to delicate breast tissue. Covering chest with towel prevents unnecessary exposure. Cleansing well in skin folds and under breasts maintains skin integrity.)* Continue to observe the condition of the patient's skin, degree of mobility, and behavior and encourage the patient to verbalize concerns.

o. Fold bath blanket down to pubic area, keeping chest covered with dry towel. Wash abdomen, including umbilicus (the depressed point in the middle of the abdomen; wash umbilicus with cotton-tipped applicators), and skin folds. Dry thoroughly. *(Maintains privacy. Prevents unnecessary exposure and prevents skin impairment.)*

p. Raise side rail; empty basin into hopper or stool. *(Flushes microorganisms down the stool and does not contaminate sink.)*

q. Rinse basin and washcloth. Refill basin two-thirds full with water at 110°F–115°F (43°C–46°C). *(Promotes patient's safety and comfort.)*

r. Expose leg farthest away from you, keeping *perineum* (the genital area) covered. Place bath towel lengthwise on bed under patient's leg. Place washbasin on towel and place patient's

Continued

Skill 9.1   Bathing the Patient and Administering a Back Rub—cont'd

foot in basin. Patients with diabetes mellitus need special foot care. Be certain to support patient's leg properly; flex knee and grasp heel. If patient is unable to place foot in washbasin, wash leg and foot with mitted washcloth. *(Beginning on the far side prevents reaching over clean area; bath towel prevents wetting bottom linens; supporting patient's leg properly prevents injury.)*

s. With long firm strokes, bathe the leg. *(Promotes circulation.)* However, note that bathing the lower extremities of patients with history of deep vein thrombosis (DVT) or hypercoagulation disorders with long firm strokes is contraindicated; use circular, gentle strokes for these patients so that the clot is not dislodged. After soaking, perform nail care (may be done at a separate time; see Skill 9.4). If skin is dry, apply lotion if desired. Do not massage legs. **Never massage lower extremities.** *(Prevents possible embolus [a moving blood clot].)*

t. Bathe leg and foot closest to you as in Steps r and s.

u. Raise side rail. Be sure patient is covered with bath blanket. Be certain to expose only those body parts being bathed. Change water (see Steps p and q). *(Provides clean water and promotes good hygiene.)* Lower side rail. If patient tolerates, position **prone** (lying face-down) or in **Sims position** (side-lying position). Place towel lengthwise on bed along back. Wash and dry back from neckline down

to buttocks. If patient tolerates a massage action, do so while washing back. *(Promotes circulation, thus preventing skin impairment, and promotes relaxation.)*

v. Reposition patient **supine** (lying face up). Provide basin of water, soap, washcloth, and towel, and instruct patient to cleanse perineal area. (Give patient privacy to do this.) If patient is unable to finish bath, don new gloves and complete this aspect of patient care (see Skill 9.5). *(Completes the bath procedure, decreases infection, and prevents skin impairment.)*

w. Be certain patient is covered with blankets. *(Prevents chilling.)* Raise side rail. *(Promotes safety.)* Empty, wash, and rinse basin. Replace basin in bedside stand. Place washcloth in laundry bag for soiled linen. *(Practice of medical asepsis reduces spread of microorganisms.)*

x. Position patient in Sims or prone position close to you. Place towel lengthwise along patient's back. Give back rub (see Step 14). *(Facilitates back care; provides comfort and promotes skin integrity.)* Never massage reddened areas. *(Potentially causes further skin breakdown.)*

y. Assist patient into clean gown. If ordered, assist patient to ambulate to chair; place towel over shoulders, and comb hair. *(Promotes positive self-image.)* Women sometimes wish to apply makeup at this time. While patient is in chair, make unoccupied bed (see Skill 9.6). If patient is not ambulatory, make the occupied bed (see Skill 9.6). *(Maintains clean environment.)*

z. Place all soiled linen into laundry bag. Be certain all bath equipment is clean and put it away as necessary. *(Reduces spread of microorganisms.)*

Skill 9.1   Bathing the Patient and Administering a Back Rub—cont'd

aa. Place call light, overbed table, nightstand, and telephone within easy reach. (*Promotes safety.*)

bb. Position patient for comfort, and provide warmth. (*Promotes patient's well-being.*)

cc. Remove gloves, if wearing any; discard them in proper receptacle, and perform hand hygiene. (*Reduces spread of microorganisms.*) Maintain a neat, clean work area.

9. The partial bed bath differs from the bed bath only in that the patient does not need assistance bathing many anatomic regions. Help by bathing those areas that the patient cannot reach (e.g., feet, back, perineal area). All steps of the bath are followed, with the same considerations. Place supplies within easy reach. Change water as noted in the bed bath procedure, and give back care, skin care, nail care, and hair care. A partial bath, in which face, neck, hands, axilla, and perineum are washed, is practiced in some agencies. The feet may be included in a partial bed bath if necessary.

10. Towel bath.[a]

   a. Follow Steps 1 and 3–7.

   b. Assemble supplies. (*Organizes procedure.*)

   - Articles for personal hygiene: comb, toothbrush, lotion, toothpaste, and mouthwash
   - Bath blankets (3)
   - Bath towel
   - Clean gown
   - Concentrate or no-rinse solution
   - Disposable gloves
   - Large plastic bag
   - Linens for bed making
   - Measuring device, such as plastic medication cup or liter-calibrated container
   - Towel–bath towel (3 × 7.5 ft)
   - Washcloths (2)

   c. Prepare patient. (*Ensures that bath towel will be warm enough for patient's comfort and for effective towel bath. It is necessary to ready the patient before the bath towel is prepared; the temperature cools down quickly.*)

   (1) Remove patient's clothing and excess bedding (top linens, bedspread). Place patient on bath blanket, and cover patient with bath blanket. (*Provides privacy and prevents unnecessary exposure of patient; provides for patient warmth.*)

   (2) Cover with plastic any surgical dressings, casts, or areas that are not to be gotten wet. (*Maintains integrity of dressing or cast.*)

   (3) Fanfold a clean bath blanket at foot of the bed. (*Provides easy access to clean blankets.*)

   (4) Position patient supine with legs partially separated and arms loosely at sides. (*Facilitates the towel bath.*)

   d. Prepare towel. (*Prevents unnecessary cleanups and promotes effective procedure.*)

   (1) Fold towel in half, top to bottom; fold in half again, top to bottom; fold in half again, side to side. Then roll towel–bath towel with bath towel and washcloths inside, beginning with folded edge.

   (2) Place rolled-up towel–bath towel (with bath towel and washcloths inside) in plastic bag with selvage edges toward open end of bag.

   (3) Draw 2000 mL of water at 115°F–120°F (46°C–49°C) into plastic pitcher. If the towel is not warm, the sauna-like effect is not produced and the patient is chilled. Measure 30 mL of concentrate with a pump (a single stroke measures 30 mL). Mix 2000 mL of water and no-rinse solution.

   (4) Pour mixture over towel in plastic bag.

   (5) Knead the solution quickly into towel; position plastic bag with open end in sink and squeeze out excess water.

   e. Bathe patient with the following procedure. (*Promotes effective towel bath, provides warmth, and keeps bed dry, avoiding chilling the patient.*)

Continued

Skill 9.1   Bathing the Patient and Administering a Back Rub—cont'd

(1) Fold bath blanket down to waist. Remove warm moist towel from plastic bag and place on patient's right or left chest with open edges up and outward. Unroll towel across chest.

(2) Open towel to cover entire body while removing top bath blanket. Tuck towel–bath towel in and around body (leave bath towel and washcloths in plastic bag to keep warm).

(3) Begin bathing at feet, with gentle massaging motion. Use clean section of towel for each part of body as you move toward patient's head.

(4) Fold lower part of towel upward away from feet as bathing continues. Help from an assistant makes the bath process more effective.

(5) Continue to draw clean bath blanket upward and place over patient as you move upward. Leave 3 inches of exposed skin between towel and bath blanket. Skin dries in 2 or 3 seconds. If towel bath is given properly, the patient is refreshed and relaxed.

(6) Wash face, neck, and ears with one of the prepared washcloths.

(7) Turn patient onto side.

(8) Use prepared bath towel for back care. (Give back rub; see Step 14.)

(9) Use second washcloth for perineal care (don disposable gloves). Sometimes you need a basin of warm water, soap, washcloth, towel, and gloves to perform perineal care (see Skill 9.5).

(10) When bath is completed, remove towel and place with soiled linens in plastic laundry bag. (*Promotes medical asepsis.*)

(11) If top bath blanket is not soiled, fold for reuse later.

f. Make occupied bed (see Skill 9.6). (*Provides comfort and promotes practices of medical asepsis.*)

11. Tub bath or shower.

   a. Follow Steps 1 and 3–7.

b. Determine whether activity is allowed by consulting patient's activity order.

c. Be certain tub or shower appliance is clean. See agency policy. Place nonskid mat on tub or shower floor if necessary and disposable mat outside of tub or shower. (*Promotes patient's safety. Conditions that place patients at risk for falls in the bathtub include neurologic impairment, arthritis, and poor balance.*)

d. Assemble all items necessary for bathing. (*Prevents unnecessary interruptions.*)

- Clean gown or patient's own pajamas or nightgown
- Deodorant
- Lotion
- Soap
- Towel
- Washcloth

e. Assist patient to tub or shower. Shower chairs are available in most facilities to transport patients from the bedside to the shower, bathe and dry patients, and return them to bed. Be certain patient wears robe and slippers. (*Promotes patient's safety and prevents patient from chilling.*)

f. Instruct patient on how to use call signal. Place "in use" sign on tub or shower door if not using private bath. (*Provides for patient's safety and privacy.*)

g. If tub is used, fill with warm water, 109.4°F (43°C). Have patient test water, if able, then adjust temperature. Instruct patient on use of faucets—which is hot and which is cold. If shower is used, turn water on and adjust temperature. (*Prevents accidental burns and promotes safety.*)

h. Caution patient to use safety bars. Discourage use of bath oil in water. Safety must be maintained at all times. Check on patient every 5 min (q 5 min). Do not allow to remain in tub more than 20 min. (*Maintains patient's safety and prevents vertigo and syncope.*)

i. Return when patient signals. Make an unoccupied bed while the patient bathes unless patient condition is such that you are required to remain with the patient. Return to the tub or shower room and offer to wash the patient's back. Knock before entering. (*Provides privacy and promotes comfort.*)

j. Assist patient out of tub and with drying. Observe the patient for signs and symptoms of weakness, such as rapid pulse, paleness, diaphoresis, unsteady gait, tachypnea, vertigo, and syncope. If patient reports weakness,

Skill 9.1   Bathing the Patient and Administering a Back Rub—cont'd

vertigo, or syncope, drain tub before patient gets out and place towel over patient's shoulders. (*Prevents falls and promotes comfort.*)

k. Assist patient into clean gown, robe, and slippers. Accompany to room, position for comfort, and give back rub (see Step 14). (*Maintains warmth and safety.*)

l. Make unoccupied bed if patient can tolerate sitting in chair. Perform back, hair, nail, and skin care. (*Maintains clean environment to promote positive self-image and medical asepsis and promotes patient's well-being.*)

m. Return to shower or tub. Clean according to agency policy. Place all soiled linens in laundry bag and return all articles to patient's bedside. (*Promotes orderly environment and reduces spread of microorganisms.*)

n. Perform hand hygiene. (*Reduces spread of microorganisms.*)

12. Give tepid sponge bath for temperature reduction.

a. Follow Steps 1 and 3–7.

b. Assess patient for elevated temperature. (*Provides basis for care.*)

c. Explain to patient; outline steps of the procedure. (*Reduces patient's anxiety.*)

d. Assemble equipment. (*Promotes organization.*)
- Bath basin
- Bath blanket
- Patient thermometer
- Tepid water (98.6°F [37°C])
- Washcloths (4)

e. Cover patient with bath blanket, remove gown, and close windows and doors. (*Prevents chilling and provides privacy.*)

f. Test water temperature. Place washcloths in water, then apply wet cloths to each axilla and groin (the depressed area between the thigh and trunk). If patient is in tub, allow to stay in water for 20–30 min. (*Promotes cooler temperature and allows for more effective heat loss because blood vessels are close to the surface of the body in the axilla and the groin.*)

g. Gently sponge an extremity for about 5 min. If patient is in tub, gently sponge water over upper torso, chest, and back. (*Prevents sudden drop in body temperature.*)

h. Continue sponge bath to other extremities and back, for 3–5 min each. Assess temperature and pulse q 15 min. (*Minimizes risk of patient chilling.*)

i. Change water and reapply freshly moistened washcloths to axilla and groin as necessary. (*Maintains tepid water temperature and continues to promote cooling.*)

j. Continue with sponge bath until body temperature falls to slightly above normal. Keep body parts that are not being sponged covered. (*This prevents shivering, which causes temperature to rise.*) Discontinue procedure according to agency policy. (*Prevents body temperature from falling below normal; body temperature will continue to drop.*)

k. Dry patient thoroughly and cover with light blanket or sheet. (*Prevents chilling.*) Avoid rubbing the skin too vigorously because that may cause an increase in heat production. Leave patient in comfortable position.

l. Clean and return equipment to storage, clean area, and change bed linens as necessary. Perform hand hygiene. (*Reduces spread of microorganisms.*)

13. Give medicated bath.

a. Follow Steps 1 and 3–7.

b. Prepare tub bath (see Steps 11c, f, g). (*Promotes orderly procedure.*)

c. Add agent as ordered by physician. (*Follows physician's orders.*)

d. Don gloves as necessary.

e. Assist patient to tub. (*Maintains patient's safety.*)

f. Allow patient to remain in tub for required time. (*Promotes effective procedure.*)

g. Assist patient out of tub. (*Maintains patient's safety.*)

h. Gently pat dry. (*Allows medication to remain on patient's skin.*) Teach patient not to scratch lesions. (*Avoids further irritation and prevents infection.*)

i. Assist patient into gown, pajamas, or clothes. (*Prevents patient from chilling.*)

j. Assist patient to return to bed, and position for comfort. (*Allows patient to rest and relax. Promotes well-being.*)

k. Remove and dispose of gloves and perform hand hygiene. (*Reduces the spread of microorganisms.*)

14. Give back rub.

a. Prepare supplies. (*Organizes procedure.*)
- Bath blanket (optional)
- Bath towel
- Skin lotion, powder. If powder is used, apply sparingly. (*Lotion lubricates skin, whereas powder absorbs body moisture and clumps, which could result in skin irritation.*)

b. Follow Steps 1 and 3–7 and provide quiet environment.

c. Lower side rail. Position patient with back toward you. Cover patient so that only parts

Continued

Skill 9.1 Bathing the Patient and Administering a Back Rub—cont'd

to massage are exposed. (*Prevents unnecessary exposure.*)

d. Warm hands if necessary. Warm lotion by holding some in hands. Explain that lotion often feels cool. (*Enhances relaxation.*)

e. Begin massage by starting in sacral area using circular motions. Stroke upward to shoulders. Massaging over bony prominences is no longer recommended because this may cause skin breakdown.

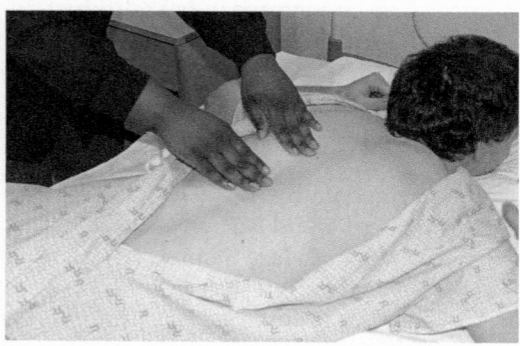

f. Use firm, smooth strokes to massage over scapulae. Continue to upper arms with one smooth stroke and down along side of back to iliac crest. Do not break contact with patient's skin. Complete massage in 3–5 min. (*A firm, gentle pressure promotes relaxation. Use of firm pressure prevents tickling the patient. Continuous contact with skin surface is soothing and stimulates circulation.*)

g. Gently but firmly knead skin by grasping area between thumb and fingers. Work across each shoulder and around nape of neck. Continue downward along each side to sacrum. (*Kneading increases circulation; motion is soothing and relieving.*)

h. With long smooth strokes, end massage, remove excess lubricant from patient's back with towel, and re-tie gown. (*These strokes are relaxing and the most soothing of all massage movements.*) Position for comfort. Lower bed and raise side rail as needed and place call button within easy reach. (*Promotes patient's safety. Excess lotion often irritates skin. Comfortable position enhances the back rub's effect.*)

i. Place soiled laundry in proper receptacle and perform hand hygiene. (*Reduces spread of microorganisms.*)

15. Assess patient. (Determines patient's ability to perform self-care and level of assistance required from staff.)
    - Knowledge of importance of skin hygiene
    - Level of cognitive ability
    - Level of discomfort
    - Musculoskeletal function; extent of joint ROM
    - Risk for compromised skin integrity (e.g., presence of paralysis or large casts or traction, or those patients who are weakened and disabled)
    - Tolerance of activity
    - Vital signs (*Helps detect an unexpected outcome of an elevation in heart rate and systolic blood pressure.*)

16. Document. (*Timely documentation maintains accuracy of patient's record; condition of skin documents response to therapy [e.g., turning and positioning].*)
    - Type of bath (e.g., sitz bath, medicated bath, or tepid sponge bath), water temperature, and solution used, when appropriate
    - Duration of treatment
    - Level of assistance required
    - Condition of skin; any significant findings (e.g., erythematous [pertaining to erythema or redness] skin areas, bruises, nevi [moles], joint or muscle pain, or exudate [drainage])
    - Vital signs if applicable (e.g., sponge bath for temperature reduction)
    - Patient's response
    - Patient teaching (see the Patient Teaching box)

17. Report alterations in skin integrity to nurse in charge or physician. (*Special medical treatment is sometimes necessary.*)

---

[a]An alternative to the towel bath is "bath-in-a-bag." This is similar to the towel bath except the washcloth is presoaked with no-rinse soap. The bag is placed in a warmer, and the patient is bathed. Some facilities use disposable cloths for bath-in-a-bag.

| Box **9.4** | Bathing Patients Who Have Dementia |

- When caregivers maintain a more relaxed demeanor and smile frequently while bathing patients with dementia, the patients demonstrate greater degrees of calmness and cooperation. Use language appropriate to the patient's level of comprehension, and try to determine which words and phrases the patients use in reference to bathing—some say "washing up" rather than "having a bath," for example. Explain what will take place. If the patient reports pain or discomfort, apologize and try to determine and address the cause: for example, "I'm sorry that I hurt you. I won't scrub as hard. Is that better?" Offer reassurance frequently, such as, "You are doing really well; we'll be finished soon," or "As soon as we're finished, I'm going to wrap you in a warm towel and put some of the lotion that you like on your skin."
- Use distraction and negotiation instead of demands.
- Minimize noise in the bathing area.
- Be sure bathing environment is warm.
- Set priorities as to which body parts need bathing and which can be "skipped."
- Use as few staff members as possible.

becomes necessary. Assist with bathing those body parts that are inaccessible to the patient.

If the patient's condition warrants it and ambulation has been ordered, the patient may be allowed to take a tub bath; however, in most facilities, a patient showers.

A tepid sponge bath is administered to reduce the elevated temperature of patients who are **febrile** (condition characterized by an elevated body temperature).

A medicated bath sometimes is ordered. This bath is likely to include agents such as oatmeal, cornstarch, Burow's solution, and sodium bicarbonate (alkaline bath). The medicated bath helps reduce tension, relax the patient, and relieve the pruritus caused by certain skin disorders.

When bathing patients who have dementia, the nurse may find it necessary to adjust the style of interaction (Box 9.4).

BACK CARE AND BACK RUB

The nurse or UAP typically administers the back rub after the patient's bath. Offer this opportunity to the patient because it promotes relaxation, relieves muscular tension, and stimulates circulation. To give an effective back rub, massage for 3 to 5 minutes (see Skill 9.1). During the back rub, observe the skin for abnormalities. Monitor pulse and blood pressure of those patients with a history of hypertension or dysrhythmias. The back rub is contraindicated if the patient has conditions such as fractures of the ribs or vertebral column, burns, pulmonary embolism, or open wounds.

COMPONENTS OF THE PATIENT'S HYGIENE

CARE OF THE SKIN

When a person's physical condition changes, the skin often reflects this by alterations in color, thickness, texture, turgor, temperature, and hydration. As long as the skin remains intact and healthy, its physiologic function remains optimal. Intact skin is the first line of defense against infection by invasion of pathogenic organisms.

Data Collection

Determine the condition of the patient's skin by observing its color, texture, thickness, turgor, temperature, and hydration. Be certain to use ample lighting. Natural or halogen lighting is suggested. Normal skin has the following characteristics:

- Good turgor (elastic and firm); generally smooth and soft
- Intact without abrasions
- Localized changes in texture across surface
- Skin color variations from body part to body part
- Warm and moist

Pressure Ulcers and Pressure Injuries

The National Pressure Injury Advisory Panel (NPIAP) has announced that the term pressure injury will be used to replace the former term, pressure ulcer, in the staging system. The NPIAP has determined that the term pressure injury more accurately describes injuries to intact and ulcerated skin, especially because stage 1 previously was referred to as a pressure injury and the remaining stages were referred to as ulcers. The numbering system also was changed to Arabic numbers (NPIAP, 2016).

The patient problem of *Compromised Skin Integrity,* either *actual* or *risk for,* is a common diagnosis for any patient in a health care facility. Prevention and treatment of skin impairment is one of the nurse's highest priorities of care. Prevention is the ultimate goal, but when this is not possible, good nursing interventions can result in (1) optimal healing of the impaired skin without complications; (2) a decrease in the patient's discomfort; (3) a decrease in length of stay in the facility if a discharge is planned; and (4) a decrease in the cost of ongoing care.

Approximately 2.5 million hospitalized patients develop pressure injuries each year, with 60,000 deaths annually, despite national guidelines regarding their prevention and treatment (Borojeny et al, 2020). The incidence of pressure injuries in acute care facilities is detrimental to the health of patients. The development of pressure injuries leads to longer hospital stays, resulting in increased chance of not only infection to the pressure injury but also other infections related to the extended stay in the facility.

To encourage acute care facilities to become more aggressive in the prevention of pressure injury development, as of October 2008, the Centers for Medicare and Medicaid stopped covering the costs of treatment of pressure injuries that develop during the patient's

Evaluation of Hospital Acquired Pressure Ulcers

(NOTE: This study was conducted before the introduction of the new "pressure injury" terminology.)

Evidence Summary

Lyder et al. conducted a retrospective study of 51,842 randomly selected Medicare patients in hospital settings. The study found that 5.8% of these patients were admitted with pressure ulcers, and 4.5% developed at least one new pressure ulcer during their hospitalization. These patients were hospitalized longer (4.8 vs. 11.2 days) and were 11.2% more likely to die during this stay (increase from 3.3% during normal stay). The study also found that these patients were more likely to die within 30 days of discharge (4.4% vs. 15.3%) and were more likely to be readmitted within 30 days of discharge (17.6% vs. 22.6%), and the facilities incurred significantly more costs resulting from the extended care and stay in the facility.

Reference

Lyder CH, Wang Y, Metersky M, et al. Hospital-acquired pressure ulcers: results from the National Medicare Patient Safety Monitoring System (MPSMS) study, *J Am Geriatr Soc.* 60:1603–1608, 2012.

Fig. 9.3 Diagram of shearing force exerted against sacral area.

hospitalization. The goal is to prevent patients from experiencing the pain, loss of function, complications such as infection, prolonged hospital stays, and the increased costs associated with the development of pressure injuries (Medscape, 2008). The same is true for long-term care facilities.

Pressure injuries occur when sufficient pressure on the skin causes the blood vessels in an area to collapse. The flow of blood and fluid to the cells is impaired, resulting in ischemia, or lack of oxygen and nutrients, to the cells. When the external pressure against the skin is greater than the pressure in the capillary bed (network of capillaries), blood flow decreases to the adjacent tissue. If the pressure continues without relief for more than 2 hours, cells in the involved layers of skin tend to undergo necrosis (death of tissue). Pressure is usually most severe over bony prominences (e.g., sacrum, scapulae, ears, elbows, heels, inner and outer malleoli, inner and outer knees, back of head, ischial tuberosities, trochanteric areas of the hips, and heels).

In addition to unrelieved pressure, two mechanical factors play a common role in the development of pressure injuries. The first is *shearing force*. This occurs when the tissue layers of skin slide on each other, causing subcutaneous blood vessels to kink or stretch and resulting in an interruption of blood flow to the skin (Fig. 9.3).

The second mechanical factor is *friction*. The rubbing of skin against another surface produces friction, which may remove layers of tissue. This may occur when moving patients in bed by sliding them across the bed linen, when improperly lifting patients, and when improperly placing bedpans.

The appearance of pressure injuries is a major manifestation of impaired skin integrity. A patient who stays in one position without relief of pressure, especially over bony prominences, is at risk for development of a pressure injury. Patients especially at risk are chronically ill, debilitated, older, disabled, or incontinent and those with spinal cord injuries, limited mobility, circulatory impairment, or poor overall nutrition.

Those who are incontinent are at risk because continual contact of the skin with urine and feces often causes chemical irritation, which frequently leads to impaired skin integrity. Nutritional factors play a role for those who are overweight and those who are underweight. Obesity increases the risk because fat tissue has less vascularity and resilience, and the added bulk and weight increase the pressure on bony prominences. Obesity also causes increased skin-on-skin contact, especially in skin folds. Being underweight increases the risk because of a lack of cushion over the bones and muscles and lack of nutrition to the skin cells. In addition, any condition that results in a decreased supply of oxygen and nutrients to the cells, such as anemia, atherosclerosis, or edema (swelling), increases the risk of skin impairment because the cells are not adequately nourished.

Medical and non-medical devices such as nasal cannulas, urinary catheter tubing, nasogastric tubing, anti-embolism stockings, splints, and braces, in continuous contact with the skin also contribute to risk for a pressure injury. Nursing interventions to prevent a device-related pressure injury include correct fitting and application of the device, regular repositioning of the device or the patient, maintaining clean and dry skin under the device, ensuring the patient does not lay on the device, and application of a dressing or barrier between the skin and device when appropriate.

Patients who are at increased risk for any reason need careful ongoing assessment and a plan of care aimed at preventing skin impairment (see the Coordinated Care box on skin care).

Definition and staging. The definition of a pressure injury was revised by the NPIAP in 2016. The NPIAP also added definitions to the six-category staging system for pressure injuries. These definitions are for deep tissue injury, medical device pressure-related injury, and mucosal membrane pressure injury. The NPIAP defines a pressure injury as:

Coordinated Care

Collaboration

Skin Care

Although assessment for the presence of skin impairment is a nursing responsibility and is not to be delegated, UAP provide hygienic care in many settings. Therefore UAP should be instructed in the following areas:

- Report any changes in the patient's skin condition, such as redness, irritation, dryness, maceration, or discomfort.
- Provide care to prevent the patient from exposure to body fluids such as urine, feces, wound drainage, and gastric secretions.
- Observe bony prominences (e.g., sacrum, scapulae, ears, elbows, heels, inner and outer malleoli, inner and outer knees, back of head, ischial tuberosities, trochanteric areas of the hips, and heels) for any signs of redness, irritation, or skin breakdown.
- Observe and prevent any areas of pressure from external devices such as oxygen tubing, nasogastric tubing, casts, braces, urinary catheter tubing, or drainage tubing.
- Provide perineal care as needed and observe the area for any signs of skin breakdown. Apply protective barrier creams as allowed by facility policy.

---

localized damage to the skin and/or underlying soft tissue usually over a bony prominence or related to a medical or other device. The injury can present as intact skin or an open ulcer and may be painful. The injury occurs as a result of intense and/or prolonged pressure or pressure in combination with shear. The tolerance of soft tissue for pressure and shear may also be affected by microclimate, nutrition, perfusion, comorbidities and condition of the soft tissue.

Assess any reports from the UAP regarding potential or actual skin integrity issues. If reddened areas are found, assess the area by noting any blanching of the area (by gently pressing on the reddened area with a gloved finger; if the area does not blanch when pressure is applied, injury to the tissue is likely). Document and report such findings to the health care provider. If actual skin impairment has occurred already, measure and document the area according to facility protocol and report the findings to the health care provider.

The following sections summarize the revised stages of pressure injury development according to the NPIAP. Additional information regarding pressure injuries can be found at https://npiap.com/page/PressureInjuryStages

Stage 1. A stage 1 pressure injury is a localized area of skin, typically over a bony prominence, that is intact with nonblanchable redness. Skin with darker tones may not have visible blanching, but its color is likely to differ from the surrounding area. The wound characteristics vary: areas may be painful, firm, soft, warm, or cool compared with adjacent tissue. This stage is typically difficult to detect in patients with dark skin tones.

Stage 2. A stage 2 pressure injury involves partial-thickness loss of dermis. It appears as a shallow open injury, usually shiny or dry, with a red-pink wound bed without slough or bruising. (Bruising raises the suspicion of deep tissue injury.) Some stage 2 injuries manifest as intact or open (ruptured) serum-filled blisters. Do not use the term stage 2 to describe skin tears, tape burns, perineal dermatitis, maceration, or excoriation.

Stage 3. A stage 3 pressure injury involves full-thickness tissue loss, in which subcutaneous fat is sometimes visible, but bone, tendon, and muscle are not exposed. Slough and eschar may be present. Possible features are undermining and tunneling. The depth of a stage 3 pressure injury varies depending on its anatomic location. On the bridge of the nose, the ear, the occiput, and the malleolus, which lack subcutaneous tissue, these injuries are shallow. Extremely deep stage 3 pressure injuries develop in areas with significant layers of deep adipose tissue.

Stage 4. A stage 4 pressure injury involves full-thickness tissue loss with exposed bone, tendon, cartilage, or muscle. Slough or eschar may be present on some parts of the wound bed. The injury often includes undermining or tunneling. As with stage 3 pressure injuries, stage 4 pressure injuries vary in depth depending on their location. Because these injuries extend into muscle and supporting structures, the patient is at risk for osteomyelitis.

Unstageable/unclassified. An unstageable pressure injury involves full-thickness tissue loss, a wound base covered by slough (yellow, tan, gray, green, or brown), or eschar that usually is tan, brown, or black. The true depth and stage of the injury cannot be determined until the base of the wound has been exposed. Stable eschar on the heels provides a natural biological cover; do not remove it.

Suspected deep tissue pressure injury. During this stage, the wound appears as a localized purple or maroon area of discolored intact skin or a blood-filled blister. This is caused by underlying soft tissue damage from pressure or shear. Characteristics of the area range from painful, firm, mushy, boggy, or warm to cool compared with adjacent tissue. In patients with dark skin tones, deep tissue injury is sometimes difficult to detect but often starts with a thin blister over a dark wound bed. The wound sometimes becomes covered with thin eschar. Even with prompt treatment, some wounds evolve rapidly, exposing additional layers of tissue.

Interventions. Nursing interventions for patients with pressure injuries include ongoing assessment and evaluation of improvement. Assessment data include the length, width, and depth of the injury (Fig. 9.4), the presence, direction, and depth of any undermining or tunneling, the amount and the color of any exudate, the presence of pain or odor, and the appearance of the exposed tissue. Healing is a long-term process; therefore be sure the plan of care is consistent over time and evaluate it for effectiveness. Interventions are determined according to the stage of the injury (Boxes 9.5 and 9.6 and Figs. 9.5 through 9.7).

Fig. 9.4 Pressure injuries. (A) Stage 1 pressure injury. (B) Stage 2 pressure injury. (C) Stage 3 pressure injury. (D) Stage 4 pressure injury. (Photos courtesy Laurel Wiersma, RN, MSN, Clinical Nurse Specialist, Barnes-Jewish Hospital, St. Louis. From Potter PA, Perry AG: *Fundamentals of nursing*, ed 7, St. Louis, 2009, Mosby.)

Fig. 9.5 Thirty-degree lateral position to avoid pressure points.

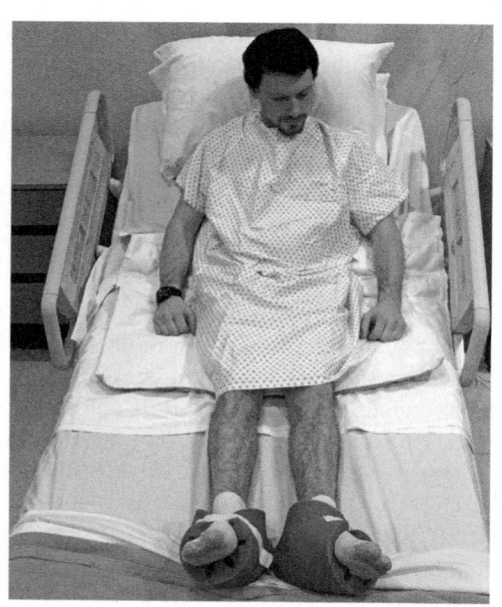

Fig. 9.6 Use of pressure-reducing boots to prevent pressure on heels.

Box 9.5	General Guidelines for Care of Pressure Injuries

- Never massage reddened areas (risk of further skin breakdown). Massage over bony prominences is no longer recommended. *(Massage results in decreased blood flow and tissue damage in some patients.)*
- Nutritional support, which promotes healthy tissue repair, is likely to be as important as local wound care for the patient.
- Observe the patient's hydration. If it is inadequate or if signs of dehydration (decreased skin turgor and recessed eyes) are present, encourage fluid intake, carefully observe and document the patient's intake and output (I&O), and monitor fluid replacement therapy as ordered.
- Turn patients who are on complete bed rest or unable to reposition themselves every 2 hours. It is important to avoid the full lateral position, which results in direct pressure on the trochanteric region. The 30-degree lateral-incline position is preferable (see Box 9.6).
- Reposition chair-bound patients every hour. If chair-bound patients are able to shift their weight, teach them to do so every 15 min.
- Place patients who are at risk for skin impairment on a pressure-relieving mattress or chair cushion. Doughnut types of cushions are not advisable because they sometimes cause a congestion of blood to the area, resulting in edema and decreased blood flow to the area. Placement of a rolled bath blanket under the distal extremity helps prevent pressure injuries on the heel by "floating" the heel (raises the heel off the bed) (see Figs. 9.6 and 9.7).
- Other pressure-relieving devices to try are therapeutic beds and mattresses. Examples of pressure-relieving beds are low-air-loss beds and oscillating support surface beds. In addition, there are the alternating air mattress and the water mattress.
- Many kinds of topical agents to facilitate healing are available to apply to the wound and edges of the wound. Take care to evaluate the effectiveness of any product used on the injury. Use with caution any products that have the capacity to damage fragile skin and prevent epithelialization (formation of new cells), such as hydrogen peroxide or alcohol.

Box 9.6	Moving Dependent Patient to 30-Degree Lateral (Side-Lying) Position

This move removes pressure from bony prominences of the entire back but especially the greater trochanters. (If patient is able to move freely, a side-lying position with upper and lower shoulders aligned is acceptable.)

PROCEDURE (RATIONALE)

1. Lower the head of the bed as much as patient can tolerate, keeping head of bed below 30-degree angle. Lower side rail. *(Reduces shear. Prevents working against gravity.)*
2. Using a pull sheet, move patient to the side of the bed opposite the one toward which the patient will be turned. Raise side rail. Go to opposite side of the bed and lower side rail. *(Ensures that patient is in center of the bed when turned.)*
3. Assist patient to cross arms, or raise arm on the side to be turned above head, adjusting pillow if needed.
4. Grasp patient's shoulder and hip, and assist patient to roll onto side. *(Turning patient toward the nurse promotes patient's sense of security.)*
5. Flex both of the patient's knees after the turn, and support upper leg from knee to foot with a pillow or folded blanket. *(Keeps spine in good alignment.)*
6. Ease lower shoulder forward, and bring upper shoulder back slightly. Assess patient's comfort. *(Prevents excessive pressure directly on shoulder.)*
7. Support upper arm with pillows so that arm is level with shoulder. *(Improves respiratory effort by reducing pressure on chest to a minimum.)*
8. Optional: Place pillow behind and under patient's back so that it is tucked smoothly against back (see Fig. 9.5). *(Provides support and prevents patient from rolling onto back.)*
9. Make certain patient's back is straight without evidence of twisting. Adjust as needed for comfort.
10. Pressure points to assess include the ear, the shoulder, the anterior iliac spine, the trochanter, the lateral side of the knee, the malleolus, and the foot. *(Prevents further skin impairment.)*

HEAT AND COLD THERAPY

Patients who have experienced injury to some part of the body often benefit from the application of heat or cold therapy, or both. The heat or cold can be either dry or moist, depending on the injury, or need, and on the health care provider's order. Because the application of heat or cold affects the blood circulating throughout the body, it is the nurse's responsibility to ensure patient safety during this therapy. Systemic reaction to heat therapy can include a rapid pulse, faintness, or difficulty breathing, and the systemic reaction to cold therapy includes shivering. Therefore, it is important to monitor the patient closely during the administration of heat or cold therapy. The nurse must be able

Fig. 9.7 Pressure injury on heel. (From Cifu DX: *Braddom's physical medicine and rehabilitation*, ed 6, Philadelphia, 2021, Elsevier.)

to evaluate the skin integrity of the body part being treated and determine the patient's ability to perceive temperature variations to the body part affected.

The body's thermoreceptors generally can adapt well to temperatures between 59°F (15°C) and 113°F (45°C). Typically, patients exposed to temperatures below 59°F (15°C) experience numbness followed by pain, and when exposed to temperatures above 113°F (45°C), patients experience pain and burning. Initially, healthy patients are able to sense these temperature changes, but within a short time, the patient's skin adapts to the temperature, and the patient no longer feels sensations of warmth or coolness. This wide range of adaptability, along with decreased sensitivity to temperature extremes, creates the risk of injury. Therefore, it becomes imperative to identify patients at greatest risk for developing injuries related to heat and cold applications (see the Lifespan Considerations box on cold applications).

Lifespan Considerations
Older Adults/Young Children

Cold Applications

- Older adults and young children are more sensitive to cold because skin layers are thin and delicate.
- Remain with the patient for the first 5 minutes of treatment to evaluate subjective response.
- If the patient response to the therapy is poor, shorten the duration of the therapy and notify the health care provider.
- Evaluate skin every 2 to 3 minutes after first 10 minutes of therapy.
- Older adults and young children frequently require more covering for warmth.

Other factors that influence the likelihood of damage to the skin include any diseases or disorders that would impede feeling temperature extremes or changes (e.g., neuropathy, peripheral vascular disease, and spinal cord injury). Damage from heat and cold therapy is also more likely to occur with unconscious or confused patients because they may not be able to report or sense feelings of discomfort. Open wounds should be avoided because heat may cause bleeding and cold may impair circulation because of lack of skin as a barrier.

Local Effects of Heat and Cold

Heat applications generally are used to provide comfort and to speed healing. Patients with musculoskeletal discomfort, such as joint or back pain, may benefit from application of heat to the area. Cold normally is used to decrease swelling and to reduce pain. Cold often is used for sprains, fractures, and nosebleeds or after some surgical procedures, such as tonsillectomies.

Systemic effects of heat application. Heat produces **vasodilation** (dilation of the blood vessels). Vasodilation causes increased blood flow to the area of the body being

Table 9.2	Temperature Ranges for Hot and Cold Applications	
TEMPERATURE	**FAHRENHEIT RANGE**	**CENTIGRADE RANGE**
Very hot	105°F–115°F	41°F–46°C
Hot	98°F–105°F	37°C–41°C
Warm	93°F–98°F	34°C–37°C
Tepid	80°F–93°F	26°C–34°C
Cool	65°F–80°F	18°C–26°C
Cold	50°F–65°F	10°C–18°C

treated; as a consequence, blood flow to the rest of the body decreases, which potentially can result in increased pulse, dizziness, and shortness of breath. In addition, more nutrients are brought to the area, which produces an increase in metabolism and tissue growth. In situations in which infection is involved, the application of heat brings more antibodies and leukocytes to the area to fight infection and speed healing. If heat applications are left in place for more than 1 hour, a heat-conserving mechanism sets in, and vessels begin to constrict, which decreases blood flow to that area. Extended heat application also may cause damage to epithelial cells and produce erythema, tenderness, and blistering. The health care provider's order should include frequency and duration of heat therapy, and it even may specify a temperature (Table 9.2). If it does not, the facility's policy should be followed to prevent systemic complications.

Systemic effects of cold application. Exposure of the skin to cold results in **vasoconstriction** (narrowing of blood vessels). Vasoconstriction decreases blood flow to the area; as a consequence, blood flow to the other organs and tissues increases, which causes the body to shiver in an attempt to produce heat. If the cold application is left in place for too long, or if the temperature is too low, the cold interferes with adequate circulation to the area, and the tissue involved is damaged. Such damage to the skin often is accompanied by a burning type of pain. If exposure to extreme cold continues for an extensive period, the skin could freeze and necrose, as in frostbite. Again, the health care provider's order or facility policy should be followed to prevent complications.

Patient Safety

To prevent injuries related to heat or cold application, it is important for the nurse to determine the patient's ability to distinguish heat and cold temperature variations before application. It is also important for the nurse to check for any contraindications to therapy or intolerance to heat or cold before applying either therapy.

Contraindications to heat therapy include any bleeding because vasodilation increases bleeding; inflammation, which sometimes worsens as a result of the vasodilation; and cardiovascular problems because heat applied to large areas of the body has the potential to interrupt blood flow to vital organs.

| Box **9.7** | Factors Influencing Heat and Cold Tolerance |

The body's response to heat and cold applications depends on the following factors:
- *Age and physical condition:* Tolerance to temperature variations changes with age. Patients who are very young and older adults are most sensitive to the heat and cold. If a patient's physical condition reduces the perception of sensory stimuli, tolerance to temperature extremes is high, but the risk of injury is also high.
- *Body part:* Certain areas of the skin are more sensitive to temperature variations. These areas include the neck, the inner aspect of the wrist and forearm, and the perineal region. The foot and the palm of the hand are less sensitive.
- *Body surface area:* People have less tolerance to temperature changes when a large area of the body is exposed to heat or cold.
- *Damage to body surface:* Exposed skin layers are more sensitive to temperature variations.
- *Duration of treatment:* Short exposure to temperature extremes is better tolerated than is lengthy exposure.
- *Prior skin temperature:* The body responds best to minor temperature adjustments. If a body part is cool and a hot stimulus touches the skin, the response is greater than if the stimulus is warm. (A gradual change in temperature is preferred.)

From Potter PA, Perry AG: *Basic nursing: Essentials for practice*, ed 7, St. Louis, 2011, Mosby.

Cold therapy should not be used if edema has occurred already. The cold decreases circulation to the area, prevents absorption of the interstitial fluid that has accumulated, and prolongs resolution of the edema. Anyone with impaired circulation or an acute injury in which nerve damage is suspected should not receive cold therapy because cold decreases blood supply further and increases complications. Furthermore, cold tends to increase shivering, which results in a significant increase in body temperature; therefore, patients with an already increased temperature may suffer complications from cold therapy.

Patients who have an altered level of consciousness or are disoriented should be observed frequently during heat or cold application because they are at increased risk of injury from either type of application. In addition, the nurse must ensure that the equipment being used for heat and cold applications is in proper working order. Equipment must be checked for leaks, and electrical equipment must be inspected for damaged cords or wires before use. It is also necessary to check for even distribution of temperature of the equipment because uneven temperature distribution may suggest that the equipment is not functioning properly. By making sure the patient and the equipment are prepared appropriately before application of heat or cold therapy, the nurse can determine the effectiveness of therapy and identify any complications after the application of heat or cold (Box 9.7 and see the Coordinated Care box on heat and cold therapy).

 Coordinated Care

Delegation

Heat and Cold Therapy

In some states, the task of applying moist heat, or warm, moist compresses may be delegated to UAP under the supervision of the nurse. When delegating this task, keep in mind that the nurse is responsible for evaluating the condition of the patient's skin and preventing injury to the patient. The nurse should remind the UAP to observe the following guidelines:
- Maintain proper temperature of heat or cold applications.
- Maintain application only for the prescribed length of time.
- Check patient's skin for excessive redness and pain during application and to report any such adverse reactions to the nurse.
- Report to the nurse when the treatment is complete so that the nurse may evaluate the patient's response.

The task of applying cold therapy to intact skin also may be delegated to UAP. Again, the nurse must evaluate the condition of the patient's skin and protect the patient from harm.

Hot, Moist Compresses

When hot, moist compresses are ordered, the solution is heated to the appropriate temperature, gauze or cloth is dipped in the solution, and the damp gauze or cloth then is applied to the designated area. If a wound is open, sterile technique and sterile gauze must be used. Hot, moist compresses increase circulation to the affected area, decrease edema, and consolidate any purulent exudate that may be present.

To maintain the temperature of a compress, it may be necessary to change the compress frequently or wrap the compress in an aquathermia pad (K-pad), a waterproof heating pad, a piece of plastic, or a dry towel. Moist heat is a better conductor of heat than is dry heat; therefore, it may be necessary to lower the temperature settings for moist heat. Because moist heat causes evaporation of heat from the skin, it is important to cover the patient with a blanket and minimize drafts in the room to keep the patient warm, especially for elderly patients (Skill 9.2 and see the Home Care Considerations box on heat and cold applications).

Warm Soaks

Warm soaks are accomplished by immersing a body part in a warm solution or wrapping a body part in dressings that have been saturated with a warm solution. A whirlpool treatment also may be used to apply a warm soak (Fig. 9.8). Warm soaks increase circulation to the affected area, reduce edema, aid in the débridement of wounds, relax muscles, and can be used to apply a medicated solution to large areas.

To administer a warm soak, heat the solution to 105°F to 110°F (40.5°C to 43°C) and then immerse the patient's affected body part in the solution. Place waterproof pads under the container and

Skill 9.2   Applying a Hot, Moist Compress to an Open Wound

NURSING ACTION (RATIONALE)

1. Refer to standard steps 1–9.
2. Assemble equipment:
   - Aquathermia or heating pad (optional)
   - Bath blanket
   - Bath thermometer
   - Commercially prepared compresses (optional)
   - Disposable gloves
   - Dry bath towel
   - Petroleum jelly (optional)
   - Prescribed solution warmed to appropriate temperature, approximately 110°F–115°F (43°C–46°C)
   - Sterile container for solution
   - Sterile cotton swabs
   - Sterile gauze dressings
   - Sterile gloves
   - Tape or ties
   - Waterproof pad
3. Explain purpose of therapy to patient, and describe sensations to be felt (e.g., feeling of warmth and wetness). Explain precautions to prevent burning, and instruct patient to report changes in sensation immediately. (*Promotes patient cooperation, decreases patient's anxiety, and prevents injury to patient.*)
4. Evaluate condition of exposed skin and wound on which compress is to be applied. (*Provides baseline for determination of changes in skin during heat application. Very thin or impaired skin is more susceptible to injury from heat.*)

5. Place waterproof pad under area to be treated. (*Protects bed linens.*)
6. Assemble equipment. Pour warmed solution into sterile container. (If a portable heating source is to be used, keep solution warm. It is acceptable to leave commercially prepared compresses under infrared lamp until just before use.) Open sterile packages, and drop gauze into sterile container to immerse in solution. Set aquathermia pad (if used) to correct temperature and assess fluid level of unit. (*It is necessary for compresses to retain warmth for therapeutic benefit. Refer to health care provider's order or facility policy for appropriate temperature of solution.*)
7. Don disposable gloves. Remove any existing dressings covering wound. Dispose of gloves and dressings in proper receptacle. (*Reduces spread of microorganisms.*)
8. Apply sterile gloves. (*Allows the nurse to manipulate sterile dressing and touch open wound.*)
9. Apply sterile petroleum jelly, if it is ordered, with cotton swab to skin around wound. Do not apply jelly on impaired skin. (*Protects undamaged skin from possible burns and maceration.*)
10. Pick up one layer of immersed gauze and squeeze out excess water. (*Excess moisture macerates skin and increases risk of burns and infections.*)
11. Apply gauze lightly to open wound. Observe patient's response, and instruct patient to report any discomfort. After a few seconds, lift edge of gauze to check site for erythema. (*Enables the nurse to determine appropriate temperature and tolerance of treatment. It also prevents burns.*)
12. If patient tolerates temperature of the compress, pack gauze snugly against wound. Be certain all wound surfaces are covered by hot compress. (*Prevents rapid cooling from underlying air currents and allows all areas to be treated uniformly.*)
13. Wrap or cover moist compress with dry bath towel. If necessary, pin or tie in place. (*Insulates compress to prevent heat loss.*)
14. Change hot compress frequently according to order or facility policy. (*Prevents cooling and maintains therapeutic benefit of compress.*)
15. Apply aquathermia or waterproof heating pad over compress, if applicable, and keep it in place for desired duration of application (20–30 min). (*Promotes consistent temperature of compress. Local application of heat for more than 60 min often results in vasoconstriction. Removing hot compress after 30 min and reapplying in 15 min, if desired, maintains vasodilation and positive therapeutic effects.*)
16. Provide the patient with a timer, clock, or watch. (*Allows patient to assist with timing the treatment; increases independence and compliance.*) Make sure call light is within patient's reach. (*Allows patient to call for assistance if needed and decreases potential for injury.*)

Skill 9.2   Applying a Hot, Moist Compress to an Open Wound—cont'd

17. Instruct patient not to move compress, adjust temperature settings, or touch the wound site. *(Prevents patient injury and infection.)*

18. Check patient periodically for discomfort or burning sensation. Never leave the patient unattended if temperature sensations are impaired. Observe area of skin not covered by compress. *(Helps prevent injury. Continued exposure to heat poses risk of burns to skin.)*

19. Remove pad, towel, and compress in 30 min. Again, evaluate wound and condition of skin. *(Continued exposure to moisture will macerate skin. Action prevents injury.)*

20. Ask patient whether an unusual burning sensation is noticed that was not felt before. *(It is often difficult to determine the presence of a* burn merely by color changes or the presence of inflammation or exudate.)*

21. Apply dry, sterile dressing as ordered. *(Prevents entrance of microorganisms into wound site.)*

22. Refer to standard steps 10–17.

23. Document the following: *(Verifies performance of procedure and ensures continuity of care.)*
- Date and time
- Type of application
- Temperature of application
- Location and duration of application
- Condition of wound and skin before and after application
- Patient's response to therapy.

See Chapter 22b for additional wound care techniques.

Illustration for Step 4 from Ignatavicius DD, Workman ML: Medical-surgical nursing across the health care continuum, ed 6, Philadelphia, 2009, Saunders.

 Home Care Considerations

HEAT APPLICATIONS
- Do not apply heat immediately after an injury; heat will increase bleeding and edema.
- A washcloth or towel soaked in hot or warm water can be used as a moist compress in emergency situations.
- Never put washcloths or linen in the microwave because this may cause a fire.
- Check electrical cords on lamps and heating pads if they are to be used for heat therapy.
- Instruct patient not to lie on heating pads; the heat cannot disperse appropriately and may cause burns.
- Never use the high setting on heating pads.
- Instruct patients not to sleep with a heating pad on; this may increase the risk for burns.
- Use a cloth or towel between the heating device and the skin to prevent burns and skin damage.

COLD APPLICATIONS
- Keeping gel packs in the freezer at home makes at-home cold treatments easy.
- Instruct patients never to use cold packs designed for use in freezer chests for food or beverages on the skin.
- Suggest using a bucket filled with ice and water to immerse foot, hand, or elbow. Use a bath thermometer to test temperature.
- Freeze water in a plastic foam cup, and use it to treat a sprain or strain. Peel off the rim of the cup to or below the level of the ice, and apply ice in a circular motion.
- A bag of frozen vegetables conforms readily to a body part needing cold therapy for a brief time.
- Put ice and water in a zipper-locked bag to quickly make an ice bag for home use.
- Use a cloth or towel between the cooling device and skin to prevent skin damage.

---

cover the container with towels or waterproof pads to minimize heat loss. The solution usually retains the desired temperature for approximately 10 minutes; it is necessary afterward to add more of the heated solution to maintain a constant temperature. To prevent injury to the body part, remove it from the water while the heated solution is added. Upon completion of the soak, dry the body part completely.

Another form of warm soak is a paraffin bath. A paraffin bath consists of a warmed mixture of heated paraffin wax and mineral oil. Patients with painful arthritis or other joint discomforts of the hands and feet may benefit from these baths. In many institutions, physical therapists administer the paraffin bath, but there are now appliances available for home use. It is important to instruct patients not to allow the bath temperature to exceed 128°F to 130°F (53.3°C to 54.5°C), to prevent burns and skin damage.

Aquathermia (Water-Flow) Pads (K-Pads)

In health care institutions, the aquathermia pad, also known as a *water-flow pad* or *K-pad* (Fig. 9.9), is used as a source of moist or dry heat application in lieu of conventional heating pads. Aquathermia pads, which are waterproof, tend to be safer than heating pads because a precise temperature is set by inserting a plastic key into the temperature regulator, or the temperature is preset before use. In aquathermia pads, distilled water is circulated through internal channels in the pad via hoses connected to an electrical unit that houses a heating element and motor.

Fig. 9.8 Whirlpool moist heat therapy. (From Szekeres M, Chinchalkar SJ, King GJW: Optimizing elbow rehabilitation after instability. *Hand Clin.* 24(1):27–38, 2008.)

Fig. 9.9 Aquathermia pad. (From Sorrentino SA & Remmert LN: *Mosby's textbook for nursing assistants*, ed 9, St. Louis, 2017.)

The recommended temperature setting for the aquathermia pad is between 105°F and 110°F (40.5°C and 43°C). To ensure proper functioning and safety of the unit and even distribution of water circulation, make sure the tubing is kept even with the unit and is secured in place. When the water reservoir runs low, the unit should be filled with distilled water rather than tap water to prevent mineral deposits from forming in the unit.

As with all heat or cold applications, a thin towel or pillowcase is placed next to the patient's skin so that the pad is not in direct contact with the patient. The pad may be secured with tape, ties, or gauze rolls. An aquathermia pad must never be secured with safety pins because those may cause the pad to leak. In addition, patients should not be allowed to lie on the pad because this prevents even heat distribution, and burns may occur. Applications typically last for 20 to 30 minutes. Some health care providers may order the application to be applied for longer periods of time, depending on the reason and the patient's condition. No matter how long the application is on, it is always important to check the patient's skin periodically during the application for any signs of burning.

Dry Heat Application

Warm, dry heat can be applied with commercially available disposable hot packs, electric heating pads, or hot water bottles. With the commercially prepared hot packs, the heat is released when the chemicals contained in the pack are mixed by squeezing, kneading, or breaking the internal container according to package directions.

Hot water bottles are not recommended in acute care facilities, but they may be used in the home setting. If they are used in the home, it is essential to instruct the patient to practice extreme caution to prevent burns.

Heating pads also are used frequently in the home setting but are not recommended for use in acute care or long-term care facilities. Heating pads contain an electrical coil surrounded by a waterproof pad covered by cotton or flannel fabric. The temperature regulation for these units is limited to the choice of low, medium, and high settings instead of exact temperatures. Safety precautions include teaching the patient to avoid lying on the pad, to avoid using the high setting, and to avoid securing the pad with a safety pin, which may cause an electrical shock.

Cold, Moist, and Dry Compresses

Cold compresses typically are used to treat inflammation and prevent edema. They can be either clean or sterile and usually are applied for 20 minutes at 59°F (15°C). The procedure for application of cold compresses is similar to that used for warm compresses (see Skill 9.2). A thin towel or cloth should be applied between the skin and the compress, and the health care provider orders frequency and duration of treatment.

Commercially prepared disposable cold packs work like disposable hot packs. They are packaged in various sizes and shapes and permit dry cold application. The nurse is responsible for evaluating the patient for signs of complications from cold therapy, including erythema, burning sensation, numbness, mottling, extreme paleness, and cyanosis. The nurse also must teach the patient the normal progression of sensations experienced during cold therapy; first cold, then pain relief followed by burning skin pain, and finally numbness. Make sure to apply towels (sterile towels over an injured area) between the cold application and the skin (Fig. 9.10). To prevent frostnip or frostbite, remove the cold pack or compress after 20 minutes, and inspect the skin for signs of complications.

Ice Bags or Collars

Ice bags or ice collars can be used to reduce edema formation and bleeding and provide an anesthetic effect to areas of hemorrhage and hematoma formation, as well as for patients who have undergone dental surgery or those with muscle strain. When these devices are used, the nurse must make sure there are no leaks by filling the device with water before use. The device is filled two-thirds full of crushed ice. This allows the

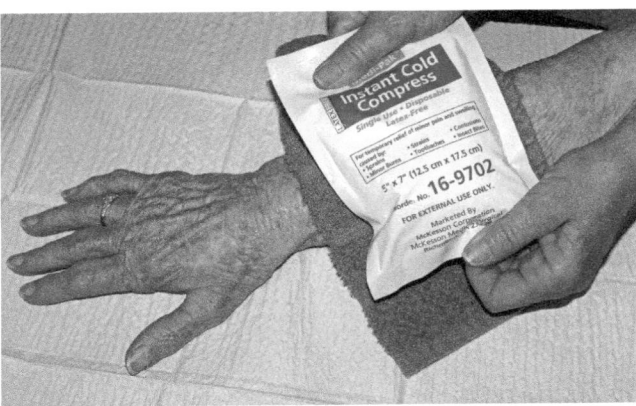

Fig. 9.10 Commercial cold pack used for therapy.

- Alteration in the integrity of teeth and mucosa resulting from disease or treatments
- Inability to perform oral care
- Lack of knowledge about oral hygiene
- Patients in hospitals or long-term care facilities often do not receive appropriate oral care. Patients who are particularly at risk are those experiencing the following:
- Chemotherapy drugs
- Diabetes
- Disorientation
- Nothing-by-mouth (NPO) status
- Paralysis
- Radiation therapy
- Serious illness
- State of unconsciousness
- Upper-extremity activity limitations

device to mold well to the body part, and it does not apply too much pressure on the area being treated. Excess air must be expelled from the device before the cap is secured because conduction of cold is interrupted by excess air in the device. Excess moisture should be dried from the device, and the device is covered with flannel material, a towel, or a pillowcase. The ice pack or collar is applied according to the health care provider's order or facility policy.

ORAL HYGIENE

Oral hygiene (care of the oral cavity) helps maintain a healthy state of the mouth, the teeth, the gums, and the lips. Brushing the teeth removes food particles, plaque, and bacteria; massages the gums; and relieves discomfort that results from unpleasant odors and tastes. Complete oral hygiene gives a sense of well-being and thus can stimulate appetite. Proper care prevents oral disease such as gingivitis or periodontitis and tooth destruction. Certain patients are at risk for oral disorders (Box 9.8).

Patients should brush their own teeth when possible. When the patient is unable to do so, the nurse must perform this procedure (Skill 9.3).

Dentures (a set of artificial teeth not permanently fixed or implanted) are the patient's personal property. Dentures must be handled with care because they easily can be broken and they can be very expensive. Use an enclosed, labeled cup to soak dentures or to store them when they are not being worn (e.g., during surgery or a diagnostic procedure, or at night). Patients who return from surgery or a diagnostic test and patients who have just woken up in the morning usually prefer to have their dentures reinserted as quickly as possible. Many people find the change in appearance that results when dentures are removed to be embarrassing.

Most patients prefer to clean their dentures themselves; encourage them to do so as often as for natural teeth to prevent infection and irritation. However, when the nurse must assist with denture care, always consider the patient's preference of cleanser and soaking (see Skill 9.3).

Provide oral care on a regular basis; frequency of hygiene measures depends on the condition of the patient's mouth. The beneficial outcomes of oral hygiene are probably not seen for several days. Repeated cleansing often is needed to remove tenacious, dried exudate of the tongue and to restore the mucosa's hydration to normal. For patients whose condition warrants turning and repositioning by the staff on a scheduled basis (e.g., every 2 hours), oral care may be provided at these times.

HAIR CARE

Proper hair care is important to the patient's self-image. Combing, brushing, and shampooing are basic hygiene measures needed by all patients. Illness or disability often prevents patients from performing their own daily hair care. A bedfast patient's hair soon becomes tangled. Remember that most patients are always aware of their appearance. Good hair care should be performed routinely, at least daily, to meet the hygiene needs of the patient. If the patient is not able to carry out this part of self-care, the nurse must assist. If the patient is able to take a shower or tub bath, the hair can be shampooed easily at this time. One option is to use a portable chair in the shower, and another is to place a chair in front of a sink.

For the helpless bedfast patient, the shampoo must be performed with the patient in bed. Check whether a health care provider's order is necessary. Most facilities have portable blow dryers and curling irons available and shampoo boards (Skill 9.4). Shampoo caps (Fig. 9.11) are often available (cap with no-rinse shampoo inside). Dry shampoos are also available in most facilities.

SHAVING THE PATIENT

Many patients prefer to shave at the time of bathing. Remember that an electric razor should be used for those

Skill 9.3 Administering Oral Hygiene Care

CHECK GATHER HELLO ID PRIVACY EXPLAIN WASH GLOVES

NURSING ACTION (RATIONALE)

1. Refer to medical record, care plan, or Kardex for special interventions. (*Provides for basis of care.*)
2. Assemble supplies. (*Organizes procedure.*)
   a. For oral care
      - Cleansing solution, such as diluted hydrogen peroxide, toothpaste, normal saline solution, baking soda solution, or mouthwash
      - Dental floss (optional)
      - Disposable gloves
      - Emesis basin
      - Flashlight
      - Toothette, soft-bristled toothbrush, or tongue blade wrapped with gauze
      - Towel
   b. For denture care
      - 4 × 4 gauze
      - Cleansing agent
      - Denture brush
      - Denture cup
      - Disposable gloves
      - Emesis basin or sink
      - Soft-bristled toothbrush
      - Washcloth
      - Water glass
3. Introduce self. (*Decreases patient's anxiety.*)
4. Identify patient. (*Ensures procedure is performed with correct patient.*)
5. Explain procedure to patient. (*Enlists cooperation and decreases patient's anxiety.*)
6. Assess patient for the following: (*Determines special needs and level of assistance required from nurse; wear gloves when in contact with the patient's mucosa or body fluids.*)
   - Ability to perform own oral care (independence is to be encouraged)
   - Aging
   - Chemotherapeutic drugs or radiation therapy to head and neck
   - Diabetes mellitus
   - Integrity of lips, teeth, buccal mucosa, gums, palate, and tongue
   - Oral surgery; trauma to mouth
   - Presence of artificial airway
   - Presence of nasogastric or oxygen (O_2) tubes
   - Risk of dehydration (NPO status)
7. Perform hand hygiene and don clean gloves according to agency policy and guidelines from the CDC and OSHA. (*Reduces spread of microorganisms.*)

8. Prepare patient for intervention.
   a. Close door or pull privacy curtain. (*Provides privacy.*)
   b. Raise bed to comfortable working position. (*Promotes proper body mechanics.*)
   c. Arrange supplies. (*Provides convenient access to equipment.*)
   d. If patient tolerates the activity, provide supplies in the bathroom and allow patient privacy.
   e. If patient is on bed rest but tolerates the activity while remaining in bed, arrange overbed table in front of patient; provide supplies, and allow patient privacy. (*Patient involvement with procedure keeps anxiety to a minimum.*)
   f. If you are performing the procedure with an unconscious patient, position patient's head to the side toward you (dependent side if possible) and close to you (see Step 9a). (*Proper positioning of head prevents aspiration.*)
9. Oral care.
   a. Place towel under patient's face and emesis basin under patient's chin. (*Facilitates procedure and prevents soiling of bed.*)

   b. Carefully separate patient's jaws. (*Protects your fingers.*)
   c. Cleanse mouth using brush, tongue blade, or toothette moistened with cleansing agent. Clean inner and outer tooth surfaces. Swab roof of mouth and inside cheeks. Use flashlight for better visualization of oral cavity. Gently swab tongue. Rinse and repeat. Rinse several times. (*Removes food particles, secretions, and dried exudate. Moistens mucosa; leaves mouth fresh.*)

Skill 9.3   Administering Oral Hygiene Care—cont'd

d. Apply lubricant to lips. (*Provides moisture to prevent drying and cracking [cheilosis].*)

10. Cleaning dentures.

a. Fill emesis basin half full of tepid water or place a washcloth in the bottom of the sink. (*Acts as a cushion for the dentures if accidentally dropped, preventing damage to dentures. Temperature extremes harm dentures.*)

b. Ask patient to remove dentures and place in emesis basin. If patient is unable to remove own dentures, break suction that holds upper denture in place by using thumb and finger. With gauze, apply gentle downward tug and carefully remove from patient's mouth. (*Gauze prevents slipping while handling dentures.*) Next, remove lower denture by carefully lifting up and turning sideways. Remove and place in emesis basin.

c. Cleanse biting surfaces. Cleanse outer and inner tooth surfaces. Be certain to cleanse lower surface of dentures. (*Prevents bacteria, odor, and stain formation from lodged food particles.*)

d. Rinse dentures thoroughly with tepid water. (*Warm water is more effective than cold water.*)

e. Before replacing dentures in patient's mouth or after storing dentures properly, gently brush patient's gums, tongue, and inside of cheeks and rinse thoroughly. (*Cleansing of the oral cavity is also necessary to promote healthy gums and mucosa.*)

f. Replace dentures either in patient's mouth or in container of solution placed in safe place. (*Dentures may become brittle and warped if not kept moist. Dentures are costly and must be handled with care.*)

g. When reinserting the dentures, replace the upper denture first if patient has both dentures. Apply gentle pressure to reestablish the suction. Moisten dentures for easier insertion. Be certain dentures are comfortably situated in patient's mouth before leaving the bedside. (*Promotes comfort.*)

Continued

Skill 9.3   Administering Oral Hygiene Care—cont'd

11. Dispose of gloves in proper receptacle. Clean and store supplies. Perform hand hygiene. *(Reduces spread of microorganisms.)*
12. Position patient for comfort, raise side rail, and lower bed. *(Promotes comfort and safety.)*
13. Assess for patient comfort. *(Helps determine whether dentures are fitting properly.)*
14. Document. *(Timely documentation maintains accuracy of patient's record and communicates interventions given.)*
    • Procedure

• Pertinent observations (bleeding gums, dry mucosa, ulcerations, or crust on tongue)
• Most facilities have flow sheets for documenting activities of daily living (ADLs) but also note condition of oral cavity in nursing notes
• Patient teaching (see the Patient Teaching box)

15. Report bleeding or presence of lesions to nurse in charge or to health care provider. *(Bleeding indicates possibility of serious systemic problems. Certain oral lesions are potentially cancerous.)*

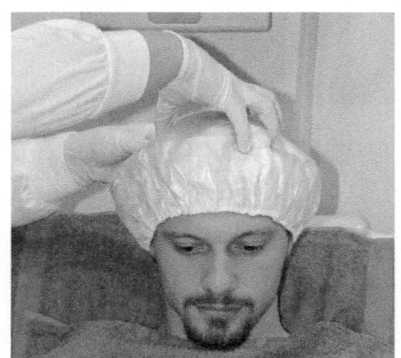

Fig. 9.11 Bed shampoo using a shampoo cap.

patients who have a bleeding disorder or who are undergoing *anticoagulant therapy* (medications that increase the tendency to bleed). Do not allow a disoriented or depressed patient to use a razor with a blade, to prevent accidental or self-inflicted injury. A male patient's beard, mustache, or sideburns are never removed without consent of the patient, except for emergency purposes.

The patient needs to be shaved if unable to perform this himself (e.g., the patient is too ill or has an arm immobilized in traction or a cast) (see Skill 9.4).

HAND, FOOT, AND NAIL CARE

Hands and feet often need special attention to prevent infection, odors, and injury. Problems arise from abuse or poor care of the hands and feet (e.g., biting the nails or wearing ill-fitting shoes).

Assessment of the feet involves a thorough examination of all skin surfaces. Carefully assess the area between the toes. Observe patients with diabetes mellitus or peripheral vascular disease for adequate circulation to the feet. The elderly are also at risk for foot disorders because of poor vision or decreased mobility. Consider whether a podiatry consult is in order; consult the physician.

Administer care of the hands and feet during the morning bath, or at another time if desired (see Skill 9.4).

PERINEAL CARE

Perineal care (pericare, or care of the genitalia) is part of the complete bed bath. Those patients most in need of meticulous pericare are those at risk for acquiring an infection: for example, patients with indwelling catheters, patients recovering from rectal or genital surgery, and postpartum patients. If patients can perform their own pericare, allow them to do so. A professional, dignified attitude helps diminish embarrassment and puts patients at ease when providing this care for patients who are unable to do so themselves. Catheter care is provided at least two times daily, and as needed, for all patients with indwelling catheters, unless otherwise ordered by the health care provider.

Be alert for signs of vaginal or urethral exudate (discharge), skin impairment, unpleasant odors, reports of burning during urination, or localized tenderness or pain of the perineum. Also observe for skin impairment in the perineal area, especially in those patients with urinary or fecal incontinence, rectal and perineal surgical dressings, and indwelling urinary catheters (Skill 9.5).

Perineal Care for the Patient With an Indwelling Catheter

Catheter care is provided twice daily, and as needed, for all patients with indwelling catheters, unless otherwise ordered by the health care provider. Catheter care includes cleansing of the meatal-catheter junction with a mild soap and water, with careful attention to remove any biofilm (colonization of accumulated bacteria). The presence of biofilm is a risk factor in the development of a preventable catheter-associated urinary tract infection. Sometimes application of a water-soluble microbicidal ointment may be applied (only if ordered by the health care provider; this is not routinely performed) (see Skill 9.5).

EYE, EAR, AND NOSE CARE

Special attention is given to cleansing the eyes, the ears, and the nose during the patient's bath. The nurse

Skill 9.4   Care of the Hair, Nails, and Feet

NURSING ACTION *(RATIONALE)*

1. Refer to medical record, care plan, or Kardex for special interventions. *(Provides basis for care.)*
2. Assemble supplies. *(Organizes procedure.)*
   a. Bed shampoo
      - Bath blanket
      - Bath towels (2)
      - Comb and brush
      - Hair dryer and curling iron (optional)
      - Shampoo
      - Shampoo board or shampoo cap
      - Wash basin
      - Washcloth or hand towel
      - Water pitcher
   b. Shaving
      - Aftershave lotion or powder, if desired
      - Basin with hot water, 115°F (46°C), or as patient prefers
      - Bath blanket
      - Bath towel
      - Face towel
      - Mirror
      - Safety razor with sharp blade or electric razor
      - Shaving cream or soap and brush for safety razor
      - Washcloth
   c. Nail and foot care
      - Disposable bathmat
      - Disposable gloves (optional)
      - Emesis basin
      - Hand towel
      - Lotion
      - Nail clippers, emery board, and orangewood stick
      - Wash basin
      - Washcloth
3. Introduce self. *(Decreases patient's anxiety.)*
4. Identify patient. *(Ensures procedure is performed with correct patient.)*
5. Explain procedure. *(Enlists cooperation and reduces patient's anxiety.)*
6. Assess patient for the following: *(Determines special interventions necessary.)*
   - Ability to care for own hair, nails, and feet. *(Encourages independence.)*
   - Condition of scalp, hair, nails, and feet; color and temperature of toes, feet, and fingers.
   - Contraindications to shampooing, shaving, or nail care. *(In some facilities, only RNs are permitted to trim the toenails of a patient with diabetes. Follow agency policy.)*
   - Knowledge of foot and nail care practices.
   - Restrictions to positioning.
7. Perform hand hygiene and don clean gloves according to agency policy and guidelines from the CDC and OSHA. *(Reduces spread of microorganisms.)*
8. Prepare patient for intervention. *(Readies patient for procedure.)*
   a. Close door or pull privacy curtain. *(Provides privacy.)*
   b. Raise bed to a comfortable working height. *(Promotes proper body mechanics.)*
   c. Arrange supplies at bedside or, if patient is able to perform procedure, have supplies available in the bathroom and offer assistance as needed. *(Patient's involvement with procedure reduces anxiety to a minimum.)*
9. Bed shampoo.[a]
   a. Position patient close to one side of bed. Place shampoo board under patient's head and washbasin at end of spout. Ensure spout extends over edge of mattress. *(Prevents wetting of bed linens.)*
   b. Position rolled-up bath towel under patient's neck. *(Reduces discomfort.)* Certain conditions such as cervical neck injuries, open incisions, or tracheostomy place the patient at risk for injury, in which case a modified position is used.
   c. Brush and comb patient's hair. If hair is matted with blood, hydrogen peroxide is effective as a cleansing agent. *(Removes tangles and loosens dried secretions.)*
   d. Obtain water in pitcher at about 110°F (43°C). *(Prevents burns.)*
   e. If patient is able, instruct patient to hold washcloth over eyes. Completely wet hair and apply small amount of shampoo. *(Prevents water and shampoo from getting into eyes.)*
   f. Massage scalp with pads of fingertips, not nails. Shampoo hairline, back of neck (lift head slightly), and sides of hair. *(Ensures thorough cleansing and increases scalp circulation. Use of pads of fingertips prevents injury to scalp.)*
   g. Rinse thoroughly and apply more shampoo, repeating steps e and f. Rinse, and repeat rinsing until hair is free of shampoo. *(Prevents scalp irritation.)*
   h. Wrap dry towel around patient's head. Dry patient's face, neck, and shoulders. Dry hair and scalp with second towel. *(Prevents patient from chilling.)*

Continued

Skill 9.4 Care of the Hair, Nails, and Feet—cont'd

i. Comb hair and dry with hair dryer as quickly as possible. (*Prevents patient from chilling.*)

j. Complete styling hair and position patient for comfort. (*Promotes sense of well-being.*)

10. Shaving the patient.

   a. Assist patient to sitting position if patient is able. (*Simulates the natural position.*)

   b. Observe face and neck for lesions, moles, or birthmarks. (*Cutting poses risk to cause infection, bleeding, or irritation.*)

   c. Use shaving cream or soap. (*Lathering softens beard and facilitates shave.*)

   d. Shave in direction hair grows. Use short strokes. Start with upper face and lips, and then extend to neck. If patient is able, hyperextending (tilting backward) his head is helpful to shave curved areas. (*Provides for closer shave without irritation.*)

   e. Pull skin taut with nondominant hand above or below the area being shaved. (*Promotes uniform shaving.*)

   f. Rinse razor after each stroke. (*Keeps cutting edge clean.*)

   g. Rinse and dry face. (*Removes remnants of lather and shaved hair.*)

   h. If patient desires, apply lotion or cologne. (*Causes cooling sensation that feels refreshing.*)

   i. Dispose of blades in sharps container. (*Protects others from accidental injury.*)

11. Hand and foot care.

   a. Position patient in chair. If possible, place disposable mat under patient's feet. (*Protects bare feet from floor.*)

   b. Fill basin with warm water and test temperature. Place basin on disposable mat and assist patient to place feet into basin. **(Do not soak hands and feet of a patient with diabetes for extended periods of time; soaking increases risk of infection by skin breaking down from maceration.)** Allow to

soak 10–20 min. Rewarm water as necessary. (*Soaking in warm water softens nails and ensures easy manipulation of cuticles. Keeping water warm prevents chilling the patient.*)

   c. Place overbed table in low position in front of patient. Fill emesis basin with warm water and test water temperature. Place basin on table, and place patient's fingers in basin. Allow fingernails to soak 10–20 min. Rewarm water as necessary. (*Soaking loosens foreign particles under nails and ensures easy manipulation of cuticles. Keeping water warm prevents chilling the patient.*)

   d. Using orangewood stick, gently clean under fingernails. (*Orangewood stick removes debris that harbors microorganisms from under nails.*) With clippers, trim nails straight across and even with tip of fingers. With emery board, shape fingernails. Push cuticles back gently with washcloth or orangewood stick. (*Prevents injury to delicate nail beds.*)

   e. Don gloves, and with washcloth scrub areas of feet that are calloused. (*Reduces spread of microorganisms. Scrubbing after soaking helps remove dead skin layers.*)

   f. Trim and clean toenails following Step d instructions.

   g. Apply lotion or cream to hands and feet. Return patient to bed and position for comfort. Dry fingers and toes thoroughly to impede fungal growth and prevent maceration (a softening and breaking down of tissue resulting from prolonged exposure to moisture). (*Creams and lotions lubricate dry skin.*) Do not apply lotion between toes of patients with diabetes. (*Organisms may be harbored and increase the chance of infection.*)

   h. On completion of procedure, observe the nails and the surrounding tissue for condition of skin and any remaining rough edges.

   i. If the patient's nails are extremely hard or if the patient is unable to perform personal nail care, have a podiatrist (a person trained in the treatment of nail and foot problems) provide nail care.

   j. Teach the patient with diabetes about appropriate foot care. The teaching plan includes inspecting the feet daily for breaks, wearing shoes at all times, wearing socks, drying feet completely, and noting any areas of numbness, tingling, or pain.

12. Dispose of gloves in proper receptacle. Clean and store supplies. Place soiled laundry in hamper. Perform hand hygiene. (*Reduces spread of microorganisms.*)

Skill 9.4   Care of the Hair, Nails, and Feet—cont'd

13. Assess for patient's comfort, lower bed level, raise side rails, and place call button within easy reach. (*Promotes safety.*)
14. Document. (*Timely recording maintains accuracy of patient's record and communicates interventions given.*)
    - Procedure
    - Pertinent observations (e.g., breaks in the skin, inflammation, or ulcerations)

- Most facilities have flow sheets for ADLs; shaving, and nail and foot care are usually not recorded in nursing notes; know agency policy
- Patient teaching (see the Patient Teaching and Home Care Considerations boxes)

15. Report abnormal findings (breaks in the skin or ulcerations) to nurse in charge or physician. (*Additional interventions are sometimes required.*)

ᵃ Some facilities use shampoo caps. These caps contain a no-rinse shampoo; they are placed on the patient's head, and the shampoo is massaged into the patient's hair and scalp.

Skill 9.5   Perineal Care: Male and Female and the Catheterized Patient

NURSING ACTION (*RATIONALE*)

1. Refer to medical record, care plan, or Kardex for special interventions. (*Provides basis for care.*)
2. Assemble supplies. (*Organizes procedure.*)
   a. Perineal care
      - Bath blanket
      - Bath towel
      - Bedpan
      - Disposable gloves
      - Mild soap
      - Solution bottle
      - Toilet tissue
      - Washbasin and warm water
      - Washcloths (2)
      - Waterproof pad
   b. Additional supplies that may be needed for the catheterized patient:
      - Antimicrobial ointment (only if ordered by the health care provider)
      - Sterile package of cotton-tipped applicators
3. Introduce self. (*Reduces patient's anxiety.*)
4. Identify patient. (*Ensures procedure is performed with correct patient.*)
5. Explain procedure. (*Enlists cooperation and reduces patient's anxiety.*)
6. Assess patient for the following, wearing gloves when in contact with mucous membranes or secretions: (*Determines whether additional interventions are necessary.*)

- Ability to perform self-care
- Accumulated secretions
- Extent of care required by patient
- Knowledge of importance of perineal care
- Lesions
- Surgical incision

7. Remove and dispose of soiled gloves and perform hand hygiene and don clean gloves according to agency policy and guidelines from the CDC and OSHA. (*Reduces spread of microorganisms.*)
8. Prepare patient for interventions. (*Readies patient for procedure.*) Allow postpartum patients to perform this procedure by themselves while sitting on the stool, using a pericare squeeze bottle. Patients allowed tub or shower baths do this by themselves. Be certain supplies are close by. (*Patient's involvement with procedure reduces anxiety.*)
   a. Close door or pull privacy curtain. (*Provides privacy.*)
   b. Raise bed to comfortable working height and lower side rail. (*Promotes proper body mechanics.*)
   c. Arrange supplies at bedside. (*Facilitates procedure.*)
   d. Assist patient to desired position in bed: dorsal recumbent for female or supine for male. (*Facilitates procedure.*)
   e. Drape for procedure. (*Reduces patient's embarrassment.*)

Continued

Skill 9.5   Perineal Care: Male and Female and the Catheterized Patient—cont'd

9. **Female perineal care**

   a. Raise side rail and fill basin two-thirds full of water at 105°F–109°F (41°C–43°C). (*Promotes patient safety. Filling basin only two-thirds full prevents unnecessary splashing.*)

   b. Position waterproof pad or towel under patient's buttocks with patient lying in the dorsal recumbent position in bed. Drape patient with bath blanket placed in the shape of a diamond. One corner is under the patient's chin; one corner is on each side of the patient, with the bath blanket wrapped around each foot and leg; and the last corner is between the patient's legs. This corner can be lifted to expose the patient's perineum. (*Draping in this manner keeps exposure to a minimum, decreasing the patient's anxiety.*)

   c. With a washcloth or disposable washcloth wrapped around one hand, wash and dry patient's upper thighs. (*Surrounding skin surfaces need cleansing also.*)

   d. Wash labia majora (larger, outer fold or lip) and labia minora (smaller, inner fold or lip). Wash carefully in skin folds. Cleanse in direction anterior to posterior. Use separate corner of washcloth for each skin fold. (*Prevents microorganisms around the anus from entering the meatus or vagina.*)

   e. Separate labia to expose the urinary meatus (opening) and the vaginal orifice. Wash downward toward rectum with smooth strokes. Use separate corner of washcloth for each smooth stroke. (*Reduces spread of microorganisms.*)

   f. Cleanse, rinse, and dry thoroughly. (*Retained moisture harbors microorganisms.*)

   g. Assist patient to side-lying position and cleanse rectal area with toilet tissue, if necessary. Wash area by cleansing from perineal area toward anus. You often may need several washcloths. Many facilities have disposable wipes. If so, use them. Wash, rinse, and dry thoroughly. (*Reduces spread of microorganisms and risk of skin impairment.*)

G

10. **Male perineal care**

   a. Raise side rail and fill basin two-thirds full of water at about 105°F–109°F (41°C–43°C). (*Promotes patient safety and prevents unnecessary spillage.*)

   b. Gently grasp shaft of penis. Retract foreskin of uncircumcised patient. (*Secretions collect under foreskin.*)

   c. Wash tip of penis with circular motion.

   d. Cleanse from meatus outward. (*Prevents microorganisms from entering urethra.*) Two washcloths are often necessary. Wash, rinse, and dry gently.

Skill 9.5   Perineal Care: Male and Female and the Catheterized Patient—cont'd

e. Replace foreskin, and wash shaft of penis with a firm but gentle downward stroke. Replace the foreskin of the uncircumcised male patient after thorough cleansing. (*Prevents edema and discomfort.*)

f. Rinse and dry thoroughly. (*Retained moisture harbors microorganisms.*)

g. Cleanse scrotum gently. Cleanse carefully in underlying skin folds. Rinse and dry gently. (*Pressure on scrotal tissue is often very painful.*)

h. Assist patient to a side-lying position. (*Facilitates procedure.*) Cleanse anal area. Follow Step 9f of female perineal care.

11.   Catheter care

a. Raise side rail and fill basin two-thirds full of water at about 105°F–109°F (41°C–43°C). (*Promotes patient safety and prevents unnecessary spillage.*)

b. Position and drape the patient. (*Supine position with gown to pubic area and bath blanket up over legs, exposing only the perineum.*)

c. Cleanse around urethral meatus and adjacent catheter. Cleanse entire catheter with soap and water. (*Reduces risk of urinary tract infections.*)

d. Repeat cleansing to remove all exudate from meatus and catheter. (*Exudates are often irritating and are medium for infectious organisms.*)

e. If ointment is ordered, open package of sterile cotton-tipped applicators. Do not touch cotton tip. Apply ointment to applicator. Do not touch wrapper to cotton tip. (*Maintains sterility.*)

f. Apply ointment to junction of catheter and urethral meatus. (*Reduces irritation and reduces spread of microorganisms.*)

12. Remove gloves. Clean and store equipment. Dispose of contaminated supplies in proper receptacle. Perform hand hygiene. (*Reduces spread of microorganisms.*)

13. Position patient for comfort. (*Promotes relaxation.*)

14. Document. (*Timely recording maintains accuracy of patient's record and communicates interventions given.*)
   - Procedure
   - Pertinent observations such as the following:
   - Character and amount of discharge and odor if present
   - Condition of genitalia (erythema, edema, or discomfort)
   - Patient's ability to perform own care
   - Patient teaching (see the Patient Teaching and Home Care Considerations boxes)

15. Report abnormal findings to nurse in charge or health care provider. (*Additional interventions are sometimes necessary.*)

---

often has the responsibility of assisting patients in the care of eyeglasses, contact lenses, or artificial eyes. For patients who wear eyeglasses, contact lenses, artificial eyes, or hearing aids, assess the patient's knowledge and methods used to care for the aids, and any problems caused by the aids. Patients who cannot grasp small objects, have limited mobility in the upper extremities, have reduced vision, or are seriously fatigued need the nurse's assistance.

The eyes, ears, and nose are sensitive; therefore, take extra care to prevent injury to these tissues.

Care of the Eyes

The circumorbital (circular area around the eye) area of the eyes usually is cleansed during the bath, typically by washing with a clean washcloth moistened with clear water. Do not use soap because it often causes burning and irritation. Cleanse the eye from the inner to the outer canthus. Use a separate section of the washcloth each time to prevent spread of infection. If the patient has dried exudate that is not removed easily with gentle cleansing, first try placing a damp cotton ball or gauze on the lid margins to loosen secretions. Never apply direct pressure over the eyeball; doing so has the potential to cause injury. Remove any exudate from the eyes carefully and as often as necessary to keep the eye clean.

The eyes are well protected with eyelashes, tearing, and a split-second blink reflex and usually do not need special care. However, the unconscious patient is likely to need frequent special eye care. Secretions often collect along the margins of the lid and the inner canthus when the blink reflex is absent or when the eyes do not completely close.

Many patients wear eyeglasses. They represent a large financial investment; therefore, use care when cleaning glasses and protect them from breakage or other damage when not worn.

Store eyeglasses in the case and place them in the drawer of the bedside stand when not in use to prevent accidental damage. Eyeglasses may require special cleansing solutions and drying tissues. Do not use washcloths, towels, tissue paper, or paper towels when cleaning eyeglasses.

Most patients prefer caring for their own contact lenses. A contact lens is a small, round, sometimes colored disk that fits on the cornea of the eye over the pupil. If the patient's condition does not permit self-removal of the lenses, seek assistance if necessary from someone who is familiar with the procedure (Box 9.9). The lenses need not be reinserted until the patient is more capable of caring for the lenses. Protect those patients who are unable to care for their lenses properly, because prolonged wearing of contact lenses is likely to cause damage to the cornea. A large variety of products are available for lens care.

An artificial eye should be cleaned on a routine schedule based on the type of artificial eye, using the patient's preferred products and method. Before reinserting the artificial eye, assess the patient for pain, inflammation, or any exudate. Gently cleanse the area surrounding the site with a soft cloth and clear water. Artificial tears or specially designed lubricant can provide comfort to some individuals with an artificial eye.

Care of the Ears

The ears are cleaned during the bed bath. A clean corner of a moistened washcloth rotated gently into the ear canal works best. Also, a cotton-tipped applicator is useful for cleansing the pinna. Teach patients never to use bobby pins, toothpicks, cotton-tipped applicators, or any device to clean the internal auditory canal. These objects easily damage the tympanic membrane (eardrum) or cause **cerumen** (wax) to become impacted in the canal.

Hearing aids. Hearing loss is a common health problem. The ability to hear enables patients to communicate and react appropriately to stimuli in their environment. The care of the hearing aid involves routine cleanings, battery care, and proper insertion technique. Assess the patient's knowledge of and routines for cleaning and caring for the hearing aid. Determine whether the patient hears clearly with the use of the aid by talking slowly and clearly in a normal voice tone. Advise restricting initial use of a hearing aid to quiet situations in the home. Patients need to adjust gradually to voices and household sounds. Have the patient suggest any additional tips for care of the hearing aid. When not in use, see that the hearing aid is stored where it will not become damaged. Take care to turn off

---

> ### Box 9.9   Contact Lens Removal and Care
>
> **SOFT LENSES**
> - Wear gloves if exudate is suspected or present.
> - If possible, have patient look straight ahead. Retract lower eyelid and expose lower edge of lens.
> - With pad of index finger, slide lens off cornea to white of eye.
> - Pull upper eyelid down gently with thumb of other hand, and compress lens slightly between thumb and index finger.
> - Gently pinch lens and lift out without allowing edges to stick together.
> - If lens edges stick together, place lens in palm and soak thoroughly with sterile saline or contact solution.
> - Place lens in storage case with contact solution.
> - Follow recommended procedure for cleansing and disinfecting.
>
> **RIGID LENSES**
> - Wear gloves if exudate is suspected or present.
> - Be sure lens is positioned directly over cornea. If it is not, have patient close eyelids. Place index and middle fingers of one hand beside the lens and gently but firmly massage the lens back over cornea.
> - Place index finger on outer corner of patient's eye and draw skin gently back toward ear.
> - Ask patient to blink. Do not release pressure on lids until blink is completed.
> - If lens fails to pop out, gently retract eyelid beyond edges of lens. Press lower eyelid gently against lower edge of lens.
> - If patient is unable to assist, use a specially designed suction cup. Place cup on center of lens, and while applying suction, gently remove lens off patient's cornea.
> - Place lens in storage case.
> - Follow manufacturer's recommended procedure for cleansing and disinfecting.

Fig. 9.12 Hearing aid.

the hearing aid or remove the battery when not in use to prolong the life of the battery, depending on the type of hearing aid and battery. Some hearing aid batteries will begin draining power upon exposure to air; turning off the hearing aid for this type of battery will not prolong the battery life. Clean the outside of the hearing aid with a dry, soft cloth (Fig. 9.12 and see the Coordinated Care box on care of the hearing aid).

Coordinated Care

Delegation

Care of the Hearing Aid

The skill of caring for a hearing aid is appropriate to delegate to assistive personnel.

- Confirm that patient knows proper way to care for prosthetic device.
- Clarify communication tips to use for individual patient while aid is being cleaned.
- Have care provider report presence of any drainage to registered nurse (RN).
- The small size of hearing aids (see Fig. 9.11) frequently makes handling and manipulating the devices difficult for older adults. Have patients with this difficulty contact their hearing aid specialist for assistance. Family members often can assist with care of device.
- High-pitched signals associated with consonants *f, p, t, k, ch, sh,* and *st* are more difficult to hear clearly as people age.
- Inappropriate responses to questions or situations, inattentiveness, difficulty following instructions, and monopolization of conversation often are red flags for hearing loss that may require evaluation. The nurse and family members should remain alert to this possibility, instead of incorrectly assuming that the patient is confused.
- Be alert for patient assessment findings that indicate some possible depression. Hearing loss in association with depression is common, and correction of hearing loss actually resolves depression in some patients.
- Age-related hearing loss, presbycusis, is common. Patients and their families often compensate adequately for this auditory change by speaking slowly and clearly. Not all patients with this type of hearing loss need a hearing aid.
- Avoid exposure of hearing aid to extreme heat or cold. Do not leave it in its case near stove, heater, or sunny window. Do not use with hair dryer on hot settings or with sunlamp.
- Remove hearing aid for bathing and when at hair stylist. Hair spray tends to clog hearing aid.
- Because of the typically high number of hearing aids in long-term care facilities, patients and their families need to clearly mark the hearing aid.
- Always store the hearing aid according to facility policy.
- Instruct family to buy an extra battery to keep in patient's bedside table, whenever possible.
- Instruct patients not to remove their hearing aids in common rooms of the facility (e.g., sunroom, recreation areas).

Care of the Nose

The patient is usually able to remove secretions from the nose by gently blowing into a soft tissue. This is often the only daily hygiene necessary. Teach the patient that harsh blowing causes pressure capable of injuring the tympanic membrane (eardrum), the nasal mucosa, and even sensitive eye structures. If the patient is not able to clean the nose, give assistance, using a saline solution–moistened washcloth or cotton-tipped applicator. Never insert the applicator beyond the cotton tip. If nasal secretions are excessive, suctioning sometimes is necessary. When the patient receives oxygen per nasal cannula or has a nasogastric tube, cleanse the nares every 8 hours with a cotton-tipped applicator moistened with saline solution. Because secretions are more likely to collect and dry around the tube, the tube should be cleansed with water and a mild soap.

BED MAKING

The patient's bed usually is made in the morning after the bath. When possible, make the bed while it is not occupied, when the patient is in the tub, showering, or out of the room for a diagnostic examination or procedure. When the patient is unable to be out of bed, an occupied bed is made (Skill 9.6).

Patient safety is a top priority. Comfort and privacy are also important. Remember to use side rails, to keep the call light within easy reach, and to maintain the bed in the proper position: high position while working at the bedside, and low position when work is completed, to protect the patient from accidental falls.

The nurse's responsibility is to keep the bed as clean and comfortable as possible. This is likely to require frequent inspections to ensure bedding is clean, dry, and wrinkle free. Check the linens for food particles after meals and for urine incontinence or involuntary stool. If linens are soiled with urine, feces, blood, or emesis, change them. Use waterproof pads with caution. Accumulation of moisture creates a risk for skin maceration and impairment.

Follow basic principles of medical asepsis (Box 9.10).

Use proper body mechanics while making the bed: for example, raise the bed to a working level to avoid bending down or stretching. Also, apply the principles of body mechanics while turning and repositioning the patient.

The two ways to make an unoccupied bed are open and closed. In the open bed, the top linens are fanfolded toward the foot of the bed to allow the patient to return to bed more easily. A closed bed is prepared after a patient's dismissal or transfer, or when the patient dies, before another patient is admitted. Closed beds frequently are made in long-term care settings because many patients do not return to bed until nighttime. Housekeeping personnel clean the mattress and bed and apply fresh linens (see Skill 9.6).

The postoperative bed is a form of the open bed. The top sheet and the spread are not mitered or tucked in at the corners. The top linens usually are fanfolded lengthwise or crosswise at the foot of the patient's bed. Arrange the top bed linens in such a way that they allow easy transfer of the surgical patient from the gurney to the bed. A complete linen change is done if the patient is returning from surgery (Fig. 9.13).

Skill 9.6   Bed Making

 CHECK GATHER HELLO ID PRIVACY EXPLAIN WASH GLOVES

NURSING ACTION (RATIONALE)

1. Refer to medical record, care plan, or Kardex to determine potential for orders or specific precautions for mobility and positioning. (*Provides basis for care.*)

2. Assemble supplies. (*Organizes procedure.*)
   - Bedside chair or table
   - Blanket
   - Bottom sheet—many facilities use the contour or fitted sheet
   - Disposable gloves (optional)
   - Laundry bag
   - Linen draw sheet
   - Mattress pad (optional)
   - Pillowcase(s)
   - Protective draw sheet (optional)
   - Spread
   - Top sheet, flat
   - Waterproof cloth or disposable underpad, or bath blanket, or both (2)

3. Introduce self. (*Reduces patient's anxiety.*)

4. Identify patient. (*Ensures procedure is performed with correct patient.*)

5. Explain procedure. (*Enlists cooperation and reduces patient's anxiety.*)

6. Perform hand hygiene and don gloves according to agency policy and guidelines from the CDC and OSHA. (*Reduces spread of microorganisms.*)

7. Prepare patient. (*Readies patient for procedure.*)
   a. Close door or pull privacy curtain. (*Provides privacy.*)
   b. Raise bed to appropriate height and lower side rail on the side closest to you. (*Promotes proper body mechanics.*)
   c. Lower head of bed (HOB) if patient tolerates it. (*Patient with a respiratory disorder frequently is not able to tolerate lying flat. The use of contour sheets makes it easier to make hospital beds with the HOB elevated.*)
   d. Assess patient's tolerance of procedure. Be alert for signs of discomfort and fatigue. (*Use judgment in providing the opportunity for rest and comfort measures.*)

8. Occupied bed.
   a. Remove spread and blanket separately and, if soiled, place in laundry bag. If linens will be reused, fold neatly and place over back of chair. (Keep linens away from uniform.) Do not fan or shake linens. (*Reduces spread of microorganisms.*)
   b. Place bath blanket over patient on top of sheet.

   c. Request patient to hold on to bath blanket while you remove top sheet by drawing sheet out from under bath blanket at foot of bed. If patient is unable to assist, hold bath blanket in place while removing sheet. (*Prevents unnecessary exposure of patient.*)
   d. Place soiled sheet in laundry bag. (*Reduces spread of microorganisms.*)
   e. With assistance from coworker, slide mattress to top of bed. (*If mattress has shifted to foot of bed, it is difficult to tuck in linens.*)
   f. Position patient to far side of bed with the back toward you. Assure patient that he or she will not fall out of bed. Adjust pillow for comfort. Be sure side rail is up. (*Provides for patient's safety.*)
   g. Beginning at head and moving toward foot, loosen bottom linens. Fanfold linen draw sheet, protective draw sheet, and bottom sheet, tucking edges of linens under patient. (*Provides maximal workspace.*)
   h. Apply clean linens to bed by first placing mattress pad (if used). Fold lengthwise, ensuring crease is in center of bed. Likewise, unfold bottom sheet and place over mattress pad. Place hem of bottom sheet (if flat sheet is used) with rough edge down and just even with bottom edge of mattress (see illustration of Step 9g). (*Keeps energy and time you need for bed making to a minimum. Rough edge of hem away from patient prevents skin impairment to patient's heels.*)
   i. Miter corners (if flat sheet) at head of bed. Continue to tuck in sheet along side toward front, keeping linens smooth. (*Prevents linens from becoming easily loosened.*)

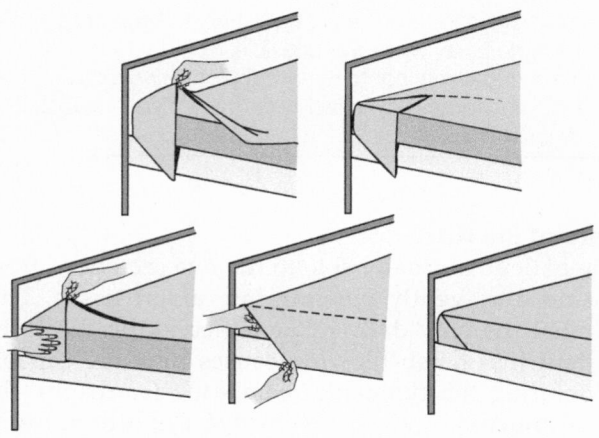

Skill 9.6   Bed Making—cont'd

j. Reach under patient to pull out protective draw sheet (if used), and smooth out over clean bottom sheet. Tuck in. Unfold linen draw sheet and place center fold along middle of bed, smooth out over protective draw sheet, and tuck in. Tuck in folded linens in center of bed so they are under patient's buttocks and torso.

k. Keep palms down as linens are tucked under mattress. *(Provides for patient's comfort.)*

l. Raise side rail and assist patient to roll slowly toward you over folds of linen. Go to opposite side of bed and lower side rail. *(Maintains patient's safety.)*

m. Loosen edges of all soiled linens. Remove by folding into a bundle, and place in laundry bag. *(Reduces spread of microorganisms.)*

n. Spread clean linens, including protective draw sheet, out over mattress and smooth out wrinkles. Assist patient to supine position and position pillow for comfort. *(Maintains patient's comfort.)*

o. Miter top corner of bottom sheet, pulling sheet taut. Tuck bottom sheet under mattress all the way to foot of bed. *(Maintains smooth linens. Avoid lifting mattress too far. Ensures tight fit.)*

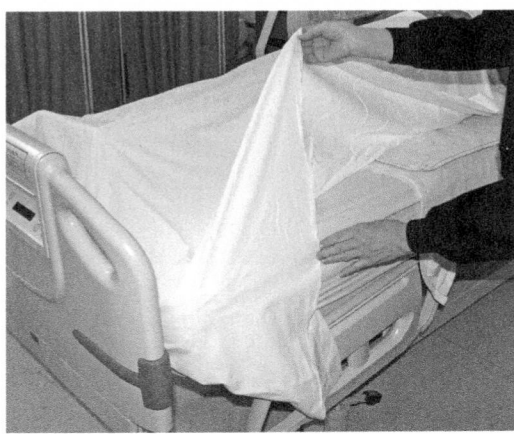

p. Smooth out draw sheets. Pulling sheet taut, tuck in protective draw sheet and then tuck in linen draw sheet, first in center, then top, and bottom last. *(Ensures tight fit.)*

q. Place top sheet over bath blanket that is over patient. Request patient to hold top sheet while you remove bath blanket. Place blanket in laundry bag. (Be sure center fold of sheet is in center of bed.) If blanket is used, place over sheet and place spread over blanket. Form cuff with top linens under patient's chin. *(Provides for patient's comfort and warmth.)*

Continued

Skill 9.6   Bed Making—cont'd

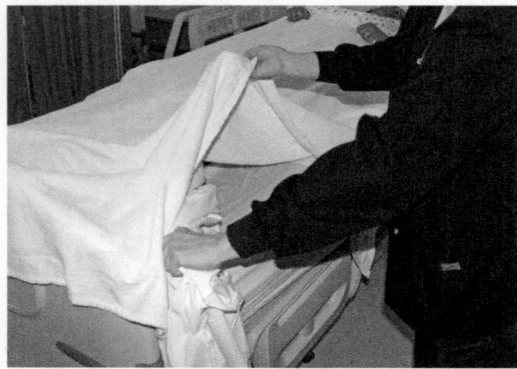

r. Tuck in all linens at foot of bed, making modified miter corner (see illustration). Raise side rail and make opposite side of bed. Remember to allow for toe pleat. Make toe pleat by placing fold either lengthwise down center of bed or across foot of bed. (*Prevents unnecessary pressure on patient's feet, possibly causing foot drop.*)

s. Change pillowcase. Grasp closed end of pillowcase, turning case inside out over hand. Now grasp one end of pillow with your hand in the case and smooth out wrinkles, ensuring pillow corners fit into pillowcase corners. (*Never place pillow on top of patient while changing its cover.*) As pillow is removed from under patient, support neck muscles. (*Prevents injury.*) Never hold pillow under your chin. (*Reduces spread of microorganisms.*)

9. Unoccupied bed

a. Starting at head of bed, loosen linens all the way to foot. Go to opposite side of bed, loosen linens, roll all linens up in ball (see illustration of Step 8m), and place in soiled laundry bag. Do not permit linens to come in contact with uniform. Do not shake or fan linens. Wash hands after handling soiled linens. Perform hand hygiene. (*Reduces spread of microorganisms.*)

b. If blanket and spread are to be reused, fold neatly and place over back of chair. Remove soiled pillowcase.

c. Slide mattress to head of bed. (*It is easier to tuck in linens.*)

d. If necessary, clean mattress with cloth moistened with antiseptic solution, and dry thoroughly. (*Reduces spread of microorganisms.*)

e. Begin to make bed standing on side where linens are placed. Unfold bottom sheet, placing fold lengthwise down center of bed. Be certain rough edge of hem lies down away from patient's heels and even with edge of mattress. Smooth out sheet over top edge of mattress and miter corners (see Step 8i). Tuck remaining sheet under mattress all the way to foot. Keep linens smooth. (*Time is saved if one side of bed is made at a time. Fanfolding all linen lengthwise down bed promotes neatness and prevents wrinkling.*)

f. Place draw sheet on bed so that center fold lies down middle of bed. If protective draw sheet is to be used, place it on first. Smooth out over mattress and tuck in. (*Prevents loosening and wrinkling.*) Keep palms down. (*Prevents stones in wedding rings from catching in bed springs.*)

g. Place top sheet over bed and smooth out. Place blanket over top sheet. Smooth out. Place spread over blanket and smooth out. Make cuff with top linens. (*Provides for patient's comfort.*)

h. Allow for toe pleat. Make modified mitered corner by not tucking tip of sheet under mattress. (*Provides for patient comfort.*)

i. Move to opposite side of bed and complete making bed as described in Steps 9e–9h. (*Saves your time and energy.*) Pull linens tight and keep taut as linens are tucked in.

j. Put on clean pillowcase (see Step 8s). Place pillow at head of bed and position for comfort. Place call light within easy reach and lower bed level. (*Promotes patient's safety.*)

k. If patient is to return to bed, fanfold top linens down to foot of bed. Be sure cuff at top of linens is easily accessible to patient. (*It is easier for patient to return to bed.*)

10. Arrange personal items on bed table or bedside stand and place within patient's easy reach. (*Promotes patient's safety.*)

11. Leave area neat and clean. (*Promotes patient's sense of well-being.*)

Skill 9.6   Bed Making—cont'd

12. Place all soiled linens in proper receptacle. Perform hand hygiene. (*Reduces spread of microorganisms.*)

13. Assist patient to bed, and position for comfort. (*Promotes patient's safety and comfort.*)

14. Documentation.

- Bed making does not have to be recorded in most facilities.
- Record patient's vital signs, signs, and symptoms only if changes occur.

15. Report any abnormal findings to nurse in charge or physician.

Box **9.10**	**Principles of Medical Asepsis for Bed Making**

- Keep soiled linens away from uniform.
- Place soiled linens in hamper or plastic bag.
- Never fan linens in the air. (*This causes air currents, which spread microorganisms.*)
- Never place soiled linens on the floor. If clean linens touch the floor, place in laundry hamper immediately.
- Remove all unnecessary equipment and maintain a neat work area.

Fig. 9.13 The postoperative bed. (From Potter PA, Perry AG, Stockert WR, et al: *Fundamentals of nursing: Concepts, process, and practice,* ed 9, St. Louis, 2016, Elsevier.)

ASSISTING THE PATIENT WITH ELIMINATION

A patient who is unable to get up to the bathroom or bedside commode for the purpose of *urination* (the act of emptying the urinary bladder) or *defecation* (the act of eliminating feces) uses a **bedpan** (device for receiving feces or urine from either male or female patients confined to bed) or **urinal** (a device for collecting urine from male patients; urinals for female patients are also available). Use of a bedpan or urinal is a private and personal procedure. Be sure to afford patients as much privacy as their condition allows.

Offer the bedpan or urinal frequently because patients risk accidentally soiling bedclothes if their elimination needs are not met. Patients often procrastinate using a bedpan because it is uncomfortable and embarrassing. Patients sometimes try to get to the bathroom unassisted even if their condition prohibits ambulation. Remind patients of the possibility of accidents or falls (Box 9.11).

Report and record in the nursing notes any abnormalities in urine or stool (Box 9.12). Flow sheets usually are provided for documentation of normal voiding and stools.

Bedpans are made of plastic. Of the two types of bedpans, one type has a high back, and the second type is flat and smaller and is called a fracture pan (Fig. 9.14A).

A urinal is made of plastic; there are two types of urinals. One type serves the male patient for voiding (see Fig. 9.14B). The other type is called a *female urinal,* which has an adapter that accommodates the female anatomy. If the male patient is unable to place the urinal for himself, assist him.

1. Request that the patient abduct his legs a slight distance.
2. Holding the urinal by the handle and directing the urinal at an angle, place the urinal between the patient's legs, making certain the long flat side, which is opposite the handle of the urinal, is resting on the bed.
3. Gently raising the penis, place it fully within the urinal.

Empty the bedpan and the urinal immediately after use, and cleanse and store it properly. If the patient's intake and output are being monitored, measure urine and record result. Estimate liquid stool on the appropriate form according to the agency's policy. Skill 9.7 for positioning the bedpan.

Another option for elimination, instead of the bedpan or the urinal, is the bedside commode (Fig. 9.15). It is useful at night and for the patient who is not able to safely ambulate as far as the bathroom.

Care of the Incontinent Patient

Incontinence is a very common problem, especially among older adults and adults who are debilitated. Regardless of the cause, incontinence is psychologically distressing and socially disruptive.

Urinary incontinence occurs because pressure in the bladder is too great, because the sphincters are weak, or because neurologic function has been compromised as a result of illness or injury. Collaborate with other members of the health care team to assess

Box 9.11 Assisting the Patient With Elimination

- Allow the patient enough time for elimination. Ignoring the urge to defecate or urinate or not taking time to eliminate completely is a common cause of constipation or urine retention.
- Be prompt when called to assist the patient to the bathroom or onto the bedpan or bedside commode.
- When the patient shares a room with another patient, be certain to curtain off the patient's area. This enables the patient to relax, knowing that interruptions will not occur.
- Close the bathroom door. If it is necessary to remain nearby, stand outside door or curtain.
- For those patients unable to assume the normal squatting position, stool risers can be used, which call for less effort to sit or stand.

Box 9.12 Characteristics of Normal Urine and Normal Stool

NORMAL URINE
- Has a characteristic odor: faintly aromatic
- Is transparent at the time of voiding
- Ranges from a pale to straw color
- Yields negative results when tested for protein, glucose, ketone bodies, red blood cells, white blood cells, and bacteria

NORMAL STOOL
- Brown
- Contains undigested food, dead bacteria, fat, bile pigment, living cells, intestinal mucosa, and water
- Frequency ranges from once a day to two or three times a week
- Has soft, formed consistency
- Odor is affected by food types
- Resembles the shape of the rectum

the cause and the extent of incontinence and to assist in managing the problem. The physical therapist, for example, is prepared to assess the extent of musculoskeletal involvement and determine methods of treatment.

Incontinence sometimes involves a small leakage of urine that occurs when a person laughs, coughs, or lifts something heavy. This type of incontinence is referred to as stress incontinence. Teach the patient exercises to strengthen muscles around the external sphincters to help manage this type of incontinence. Pelvic floor exercises (Kegel exercises) involve tightening the ring of muscle around the vagina and anus and holding the muscle contraction for several seconds. Have the patient do this a minimum of 10 times, 3 times a day.

Alert patients need an incontinence product that is discreet and promotes self-care. Some incontinence

Fig. 9.14 Selected equipment and supplies for elimination. (A) Regular bedpan *(left)* and fracture pan *(right)*. (B) Male urinal.

Skill 9.7 Positioning the Bedpan

CHECK   GATHER   HELLO   ID   PRIVACY   EXPLAIN   WASH   GLOVES

NURSING ACTION *(RATIONALE)*

1. Refer to medical record, care plan, or Kardex. *(Provides basis for care.)*
2. Assess patient's needs. *(Allows nurse to note any potential problems with patient's environment.)*
3. Assemble supplies according to patient's needs (see Fig. 9.10). *(Organizes procedure.)*
4. Introduce self. *(Reduces patient's anxiety.)*
5. Identify patient. *(Ensures procedure is performed with correct patient.)*
6. Explain procedure. *(Enlists cooperation and reduces patient's anxiety.)*

7. Prepare patient. *(Facilitates procedure.)*
   a. Close door or pull privacy curtain. *(Elimination is a personal function and is greatly facilitated by providing privacy.)*
   b. Arrange supplies close to the bedside. *(Provides easy access to supplies.)*
   c. Place protective pad under patient's buttocks, if necessary. *(Protects linens from soiling.)*
8. Perform hand hygiene and don clean gloves according to agency policy and guidelines from the CDC and OSHA. *(Reduces spread of microorganisms.)*

Skill 9.7   Positioning the Bedpan—cont'd

9. When patient is able to assist self onto bedpan, nurse positions patient in supine position with knees flexed and bottom of feet flat on bed surface. As patient raises hips, nurse supports patient's lower back with arm and positions bedpan under patient. When patient has finished with elimination, nurse removes bedpan in same manner. (*Allows for some measure of independence.*)
10. For patient unable to assist self on bedpan.
    a. Turn patient away from nurse toward opposite side rail, moving linens out of way. (*Provides for patient safety and maintains clean linens.*)
    b. Fit bedpan to patient's buttocks. (*Prevents injury to patient's skin.*)

c. Assist patient to turn over onto bedpan while nurse secures bedpan. (*Allows nurse to use appropriate body mechanics.*)

d. Raise head of bed 30 degrees. (*Promotes patient's comfort.*)
    e. Place toilet tissue and call light within easy reach. (*Provides for patient's convenience and promotes certain measure of independence.*)
11. For those patients who can be out of bed but are unable to ambulate far, the bedside commode can be used (see Fig. 9.14). Some are equipped with wheels, which allow the patient to be moved to the bathroom. (*Provides privacy.*)
12. When transferring a patient to the commode, assist the patient in the same manner as if assisting to a chair. (*Maintains proper body mechanics.*)
13. Provide a means for the patient to wash hands, either assisting to the sink or providing hand washing while patient is in the bed.
14. Document according to agency policy: (*Verifies patient's care.*)
    • Amount
    • Color
    • Consistency
    • Abnormal findings such as blood, unusual odor, or color
15. Report unusual findings. (Further interventions may be necessary.)

products are designed for small amounts of leakage. Persistent urge, stress, or overflow incontinence most likely necessitates referral for urologic evaluation (refer to Chapter 15 for types of incontinence).

Incontinence characterized by urine or fecal flow at unpredictable times necessitates the use of disposable adult undergarments or underpads as the primary means of management. Urine and feces are very irritating to the skin. Skin that is continually exposed quickly becomes inflamed and irritated. Cleanse the skin thoroughly after each episode of incontinence with warm, soapy water and dry it thoroughly to help prevent skin impairment.

Fig. 9.15 The bedside commode has a toilet seat with a container underneath. The container slides out from under the toilet seat for emptying and cleaning.

Many facilities use a protective barrier cream for patients with incontinence to prevent skin breakdown.

When urinary incontinence results from decreased perception of bladder fullness or impaired voluntary motor control, bladder training may be helpful. Bladder training consists of assisting the patient to the bathroom or commode at certain time intervals in an attempt to strengthen the urinary sphincter muscles, typically every 2 hours initially for the first several times, then at increased time intervals as the patient tolerates until the point of bladder control is reached.

❖ NURSING PROCESS FOR HYGIENE

The role of the LPN/LVN in the nursing process as stated is that the LPN/LVN:
- Participates in planning care for patients based on patient needs
- Reviews patient's plan of care and recommends revisions as needed
- Reviews and follows defined prioritization for patient care
- Uses clinical pathways, care maps, or care plans to guide and review patient care

◆ ASSESSMENT

Nursing assessment is an ongoing process. It is important to determine whether the patient can perform hygienic care independently or whether assistance is required. Also, observe the patient's physical condition and the integrity of the patient's skin, oral cavity, and sensory organs. Explore any developmental factors that influence the patient's hygiene needs. Note the patient's self-care ability and hygiene practices. Determine the patient's cultural preferences as well.

◆ PATIENT PROBLEMS

Nursing assessment helps identify the patient's need for and ability to maintain personal hygiene. Interventions are based on the identified patient problem. Patient problem statements possibly include the following:
- Compromised Oral Mucous Membranes
- Compromised Physical Mobility
- Compromised Skin Integrity (Nursing Care Plan 9.1)
- Inability to Bathe Self
- Inability to Dress Self

◆ EXPECTED OUTCOMES AND PLANNING

Considering the patient's preferences before planning is important. The hygiene measures that the patient desires or requires determine the supplies and equipment that are necessary. In some cases, hygiene measures must be scheduled around laboratory tests and diagnostic procedures and involve the family in planning and adapting approaches for home care, and in hygiene instruction. Be aware of community resources that will be of assistance to meet the patient's needs.

Nursing interventions are focused on specific goals and outcomes that pertain to the identified patient problems, such as the following:

Goal: Patient's skin integrity will remain intact during stay in facility.

Outcome: Patient's skin remains pink and warm and with good turgor and no open areas noted.

Goal: Patient will assist with hygienic measures by washing face, neck, and hands.

Outcome: Patient was able to wash face, neck, and hands without difficulty.

◆ IMPLEMENTATION

Nursing interventions that promote the patient's personal hygiene include bed making, bathing, and care of hair, eyes, ears, nose, nails, and skin.

Hygiene is a basic part of a patient's care. Learn and use care practices that help alleviate the patient's anxiety and promote comfort and relaxation while performing each hygiene measure. For example, while giving a patient a bath and changing a gown, use a gentle approach in turning and repositioning. Use of a soft, gentle voice while conversing with the patient helps relieve any fears or concerns. Inform the patient of all care being performed. For patients experiencing symptoms such as pain or nausea, administering

Nursing Care Plan 9.1 | **Skin Care**

Mr. P. is a 48-year-old patient immobilized because of trauma to the spinal cord. He has periods of diaphoresis. He has had liquid diarrhea for the past 48 h. The skin on Mr. P.'s back, sacral regions, and buttocks is dry and intact, with a 2-cm area of erythema around the sacrum.

PATIENT PROBLEM

Compromised Skin Integrity, related to immobilization and secretions

Patient Goals and Expected Outcomes	Nursing Interventions	Evaluation
Skin will remain intact during hospitalization Skin will remain free of pressure Skin will have reduced or absent secretions Skin will be dry, warm, and smooth	Provide perineal care after each diarrheal episode. Change linen after diaphoresis or diarrheal episode. Apply lotion to areas that easily become dried and chapped. Monitor length of time any areas of erythema persist. Determine turning interval (e.g., 2 h). Place oscillating air mattress on patient's bed. Do not massage erythemic (reddened) area or bony prominences. Reassess skin area daily. Assess for history of preexisting chronic diseases (diabetes, malignancy, acquired immunodeficiency syndrome [AIDS], peripheral or cardiovascular conditions). Assess surface that patient spends majority of time on (mattress for bedridden patient, cushion for wheelchairs). Specifically assess skin over bony prominences (sacrum, scapulae, ears, elbows, heels, inner and outer malleoli, inner and outer knees, back of head, ischial tuberosities, trochanteric areas of the hips, and heels).	Observe and time the duration of erythemic area after each position change; palpate underlying and adjacent tissues after each position change.

CRITICAL THINKING QUESTIONS

1. Mr. P. has a poor appetite, and his chemistry profile reveals low protein, low albumin, and low anion gap (A/G) ratio. Explain why poor nutrition predisposes to impairment of skin integrity and poor tissue healing.
2. With Mr. P.'s history of diarrhea, explain the possible complication that could evolve if the dry intact skin develops an open lesion.

symptom relief before hygiene procedures better prepares the patient.

The nurse is in a unique position to assess the patient's readiness to learn, and to teach health promotion practices whenever possible (see the Patient Teaching and Home Care Considerations boxes). This includes educating patients on proper hygiene techniques and connecting patients with the community resources necessary to enable them to perform hygienic care in the home setting when assistance is required. The nurse should always encourage the patient's independence and privacy and foster the patient's physical well-being.

◆ **EVALUATION**

Assess the success of the nursing interventions on completion of the hygienic measures. Reassess the condition of the patient's skin, nails, oral cavity, and sensory organs. Determine whether the patient's comfort level has improved. Ask the patient to demonstrate hygiene self-care skills, and ask the patient whether expectations are being met.

Always be prepared to revise the care plan based on the evaluation. Systematic evaluation requires the nurse to determine whether expected outcomes have been met. Refer to the identified goals and outcomes when planning interventions.

Goal: Patient's skin integrity will remain intact during stay in facility.

Evaluative measure: Assess for pink skin that is warm, moist, without abrasions, and with immediate color return on blanching.

Goal: Patient will assist with hygienic measures by washing face, neck, and hands.

Evaluative measure: Evaluate patient's ability to assist with hygienic measures.

Patient Teaching

Hygiene

GENERAL PRINCIPLES
- Initiate patient teaching at the beginning of the hygienic procedure and continue throughout the intervention.
- Teach and encourage independence no matter how minimal it seems to be (e.g., washing the face and perineal area, brushing teeth, combing hair).
- Explain steps of procedure in which patient will be participating.

Teaching Points
Teaching points include the following:
- How to assess temperature of the bath water, especially for elderly and other patients with reduced sensation (e.g., bath thermometer).
- How to inspect surfaces between skin folds for signs of irritation or impairment (breakdown; e.g., erythema, scalding).
- Proper cleansing of the perineum (e.g., female patients: cleansing from front to back; uncircumcised males: retracting foreskin to adequately cleanse underneath, then replacing foreskin).
- How to use a trapeze bar on beds to assist in bed mobility.
- Importance of washing hands before and after performing catheter care or after urinating and defecating.
- If patient achieves relaxation from back rub, teaching family members how to perform procedure.
- Stressing importance of consistent use of sunscreen with a protective factor of at least 15 and avoidance of unnecessary sun exposure.
- Methods to prevent tooth decay (e.g., reduce intake of carbohydrates between meals [sweet snacks], brush within 30 minutes of eating sweets, rinse mouth thoroughly with water or eat acid-containing fruit such as an apple, use fluoridated water).
- How to prevent or heal dry lips by applying lip ointment or lubricant and avoiding licking the lips.
- Proper storage methods for dentures, stressing techniques of cleaning that avoid damage to dentures (e.g., use brush with soft bristles; carry dentures in a container; hold dentures with cloth to avoid dropping).
- How to remove dentures at bedtime to give gums a rest and to store dentures in water or cleansing solution to prevent drying and warping.
- Signs and symptoms of oral infection or irritation (e.g., erythematous or whitened areas, bleeding, lesions).

- Advise patient to brush teeth at least two times daily and to rinse well after brushing.
- Advise patients with diabetes to visit their dentist every 3–4 months and to handle tissues gently. *(Diabetes depresses the immune system and decreases circulation to the mucosa.)*
- Proper hair care: regular shampooing, avoidance of chemicals and hot combs for straightening hair. *(May result in scalp burns, hair loss, or allergic reaction.)*
- Primary caregiver safety precautions for shaving, especially if patient is receiving anticoagulant therapy, and the technique to follow in the event a patient is nicked accidentally.
- Proper foot care:
- Wash and soak feet daily with lukewarm water; thoroughly pat feet dry and dry well between toes. Soaking the feet of a patient with diabetes or a patient with peripheral vascular disease is not recommended. This potentially leads to maceration (excessive softening of the skin), skin breakdown, and infection.
- File nails; never clip them if patient is diabetic or has circulatory issues.
- Caution against self-treating corns or calluses. Consult a physician or podiatrist.
- If needed, apply a mild foot powder.
- Inspect feet daily.
- Wear clean socks or stockings daily (change twice a day if feet perspire).
- Do not walk barefoot.
- Wear properly fitting shoes.
- Wash and dry minor cuts immediately. Use only mild antiseptic (e.g., triple antibiotic ointment).
- Cleansing the eye by going from the inner corner or canthus to the outer corner or canthus.
- Never inserting hairpins, toothpicks, cotton-tipped applicators, or any device into the ear canal. If necessary, consult a physician.
- Skin care:
- Process of wound healing and expected wound appearance.
- Signs and symptoms of pressure ulcers to report to health care team.
- Prevention guidelines to halt further breakdown.
- Importance of good nutrition and adequate fluid intake.

 Home Care Considerations

Hygienic Care

BATHING
- Include family members in discussion about patient's hygienic care, before discharge if possible.
- Set up equipment according to established routine.
- Advise installing grab bars around tub, carpeting bathroom floor, and using a portable shower seat for safety.

- The three types of baths for the home-bound patient are the complete bed bath; the abbreviated bed bath, during which only the parts of the patient's body are washed whose neglect will potentially cause illness, odor, or discomfort; and the partial bath, which takes place at the sink, in the tub, or in the shower with a shower chair.

⌂ Home Care Considerations—cont'd

- The kind of bath chosen depends on assessment of the home, availability of running water, and condition of the bathing facilities, as well as the patient's health status, mobility status, and ability to participate.
- If beds do not have side rails, positioning is possible with pillows or by placing bed against the wall.
- Never leave bathing patient unattended. Adhesive strips on bottom of tub or shower, handrails, chairs, or stools in tub or shower further protect patient.
- Follow patient's usual bathing and skin care routines.
- Assess patient to see whether a home health aide or other assistance is needed after discharge.

SKIN CARE
- Assess perineum at every visit because of risk for infection and skin breakdown.
- Protect patient from falling off bed during back rub.
- The 30-degree lateral position or the prone position is sometimes useful at night to prolong the time needed between position changes, resulting in less sleep disruption for the patient and the caregiver.
- Identify community resources such as neighbors and relatives for assistance should patient need help with position changes.
- Customize pressure-relief maneuvers for the independent patient. Some individuals find it useful to use a watch with timer, mark even or odd hours, and use television commercials as guidelines to remember when to complete pressure-relief techniques.
- Identify clean storage area for dressing supplies.
- Determine availability of required supplies.
- Discuss need for home pressure-relief surface or bed.
- Identify adaptive equipment needed to care for patient at home, such as a stool riser.

ORAL CARE
- Assess state of dental health of patient and family members and attitudes toward oral hygiene.
- Family members need instruction in oral care so that family understands how to protect the patient from aspirating while ensuring thorough cleansing of the oral cavity.
- Irrigate oral cavity with a bulb syringe; if unavailable, a clean gravy baster is acceptable to use as a substitute. A large syringe is another possibility.
- Cleanse mouth at least twice a day. If patient breathes through mouth, use a sponge-tipped applicator or wrap gauze or soft linen around a tongue blade, moisten, and use every 1–2 h to keep mouth moist and fresh.
- On regular visits, assess for signs and symptoms of infection or irritation, including erythematous, bleeding lesions of the gums.
- Provide special care to patients undergoing head and neck radiation because the gums are usually dry and edematous and are likely to interfere with proper denture fit.

HAIR CARE
- Assess temperature of the room, availability of water, and the most satisfactory position of the patient for the procedure.
- Provide extra protection from wetness for patients with casts.
- Obtain dry shampoo preparations or a shampoo cap when a wet shampoo is contraindicated.
- Construct a trough by arranging a plastic shower curtain or tablecloth under the patient's head and then tapering the cloth to form a narrow end that can drain into a container or basin next to the patient's bed.
- In the home setting, find ways the patient can shampoo the hair without causing injury. Some patients with a long leg cast need to wash the hair at a sink until it is safe to shower or until the cast is removed and resumption of tub baths is permitted.
- Caution patients about use of chemicals and hot combs for straightening hair. Such practices often cause considerable damage to the hair. Misuse results in possible scalp burns, hair loss, and allergic reactions that cause severe skin rashes, urticaria, and conjunctivitis.

SHAVING AND FACIAL HAIR REMOVAL
- Provide enough towels around the patient's neck to help prevent spilling shaving cream or water on chest or bed.
- Provide adequate lighting for the procedure.
- Perform the procedure in a comfortable setting, such as the bathroom or bedroom.
- Usually the facial hair of the older patient does not grow quickly, so a shave may not be necessary every day.
- If patient is on anticoagulant therapy, use an electric razor.
- Facial hair for females should be addressed according to the patient's preference. Methods of facial hair removal include clipping, tweezing, shaving, hair removal lotions, and use of a depilatory.

NAILS AND FEET
- Alternative therapies: moleskin applied to areas on feet that are under friction is less likely to cause local pressure than corn pads; spot adhesive bandages guard corns against friction but do not have padding to protect against pressure; wrapping small pieces of lamb's wool around toes reduces irritation of soft corns between toes.
- Assess use of patient's bathroom sink for soaking patient's hands, and tub for soaking patient's feet.
- Financial constraints are often why patients wear poorly fitted shoes, which can cause foot problems.

BED MAKING
- Assess primary caregiver's ability and willingness to maintain a clean environment for the patient.
- Assess home laundry facilities to plan with the primary caregiver the most reasonable frequency with which linens will be laundered.
- Assess amount of linens in the home to establish with the primary caregiver the number of changes of sheets that it is possible to reserve for the patient's use.

Get Ready for the NCLEX® Examination!

Key Points

- Hygiene is a personal matter; all factors that influence the personal hygiene routine must be considered.
- Be sure the patient's room is comfortable, safe, and large enough to allow the patient and visitors to move around freely.
- Assume the responsibility for providing the daily hygienic needs of patients if they are unable to care for themselves adequately.
- Providing hygienic care gives the nurse the opportunity to assess all external body surfaces and the patient's emotional state.
- Assisting or providing the patient with daily hygienic needs allows the nurse to use teaching and communication skills to develop a meaningful relationship with the patient.
- Consider the patient's personal preferences when planning the daily hygienic care.
- Be sure to maintain the patient's privacy and comfort when providing daily care.
- Various sociocultural, economic, and developmental factors influence patients' hygiene practices.
- During assessment of the skin, observe the characteristics most influenced by hygienic measures.
- Patients who are immobilized, who are poorly nourished, and who have reduced sensation are at risk for impaired skin integrity.
- External pressure, shearing force, moisture, impaired peripheral circulation, edema, poor nutrition, immobility, and obesity contribute to the development of pressure injuries.
- When the external pressure against the skin is greater than the pressure in the capillary bed, blood flow decreases to the adjacent tissues.
- Pressure injuries tend to occur initially in the superficial layers of the skin.
- Meticulous assessment of the skin and underlying tissue and identification of risk factors are important in preventing the circumstances favorable to development of pressure injuries.
- Preventative skin care is aimed at controlling external pressure on bony prominences and keeping the skin clean, well lubricated, hydrated, and free of excess moisture.
- Proper positioning reduces the effects of pressure and guards against shearing force.
- Cleansing and topical agents used to treat pressure injuries vary according to the stage of the injury.
- When applying heat or cold therapy, properly assess the patient's ability to sense variation in temperatures, know factors that place the patient at risk for complications, and understand the physiologic effects of the applications to use the therapies safely.
- Patient teaching is important in assisting the patient to take responsibility for his or her own care.
- Wear gloves during hygienic care when there is risk of contacting body fluids.
- Techniques used during tepid sponging are designed to minimize the risk of a patient becoming chilled.
- Patients with diabetes mellitus need special consideration when providing nail and foot care.
- When administering oral care to unconscious patients, take measures to prevent aspiration.
- The evaluation of hygienic care is based on the patient's expression of a sense of relaxation and well-being and an understanding of personal hygienic techniques.

Additional Learning Resources

SG Go to the Study Guide for additional learning activities to help master this chapter content.

Be sure to visit the Evolve site at http://evolve.elsevier.com/Cooper/foundations/ for additional online resources.

Review Questions for the NCLEX® Examination

1. The nurse is supervising a new UAP providing hygiene care to a patient. Which action by the UAP requires the nurse to provide additional instruction regarding hygiene care? *(Select all that apply.)*

   1. The UAP performs hand hygiene before providing care.
   2. The UAP holds the clean linens against the uniform.
   3. The UAP places soiled linens on the floor.
   4. The UAP places clean linens on the patient's clean overbed table.
   5. The UAP places soiled linens in a linen bag for transport.

2. During the bed bath, the nurse covers the patient with a bath blanket. The patient asks what the bath blanket is for. What is the nurse's best response?

   1. "The bath blanket helps to prevent skin irritation."
   2. "The bath blanket is part of our bathing procedure."
   3. "The bath blanket helps to prevent chilling during the bath."
   4. "The bath blanket is used to prevent the spread of microorganisms."

3. A patient with severe crippling rheumatoid arthritis is confined to bed for extended periods. An erythematous area over the coccyx that has the potential to become an open lesion is noted. The nurse is correct in reporting this area to the health care provider as having the potential to become what?

   1. An inflammatory injury
   2. A pressure injury
   3. A stasis injury
   4. An arterial injury

4. A patient is too weak to perform her own perineal care. The student nurse includes bathing which areas as part of perineal care?

   1. Back and buttocks
   2. Lower back, upper thighs
   3. Upper torso and thighs
   4. Upper thighs, genitalia, and anal area

5. Which patient is at greatest risk for skin impairment?

   1. A 12-year-old on bed rest
   2. A 7-month-old with cool skin temperature
   3. A 26-year-old with diarrhea
   4. A 60-year-old in a body cast

6. A patient is in her second postoperative day after an abdominal hysterectomy. The nurse plans to give the patient a bed bath. Which action is appropriate when caring for the patient's face? *(Select all that apply.)*

   1. Use only water on the patient's face.
   2. Ask the patient if she prefers soap or plain water.
   3. Use soap in all areas of the face except the eyes.
   4. Use a cleansing cream to cleanse her face and neck.
   5. Use a different area of the washcloth for each eye.

7. The nurse is teaching the patient proper hygiene measures. What should the nurse include when teaching the patient about eye care?

   1. Wash from the inner canthus to the outer canthus.
   2. Cleanse dried exudate with hot water.
   3. Avoid drying the circumorbital area after washing.
   4. Use a cotton-tipped applicator for each eyelid.

8. An 11-month-old infant is admitted with a tympanic temperature of 105°F (40.6°C). The physician orders a tepid sponge bath. The infant's mother asks, "What is the purpose of this bath?" Which is the best response by the nurse?

   1. "The bath helps reduce your baby's body temperature."
   2. "The bath is used to help prevent febrile seizures."
   3. "The bath stimulates circulation to the skin."
   4. "The bath helps calm and relax your baby."

9. An uncircumcised man is in the first postoperative day after a transurethral prostatectomy. When administering perineal care, which action by the nurse is correct?

   1. Retract the foreskin, cleanse the penis, and allow the foreskin to return to its former position.
   2. Retract the foreskin, cleanse the penis, and sprinkle powder under the foreskin to facilitate retraction.
   3. Retract the foreskin, cleanse the penis, and leave the foreskin slightly damp to allow retraction to its former state.
   4. Retract the foreskin, cleanse the penis, and return the foreskin with a gentle forward motion.

10. A patient was discharged home with a Foley catheter. The student nurse instructs the patient in the proper procedure for cleansing the female perineal area. What teaching point should the nurse include in discharge instructions?

    1. Cleanse the area in circular motions around the rectum.
    2. Cleanse from the rectum toward the pubis.
    3. Cleanse from the pubis toward the anal area.
    4. Cleanse in circular motions around the vaginal area.

11. The nurse is reviewing the teaching plans of several patients on a medical unit. Which patient does the nurse correctly identify as most at risk for development of complications of the feet?

    1. A 55-year-old disoriented patient
    2. A 30-year-old patient whose career requires extensive standing
    3. A 60-year-old patient with a 30-year history of diabetes mellitus
    4. A 62-year-old patient who had a total hip replacement 2 years ago

12. The nurse is providing oral care to a patient who is unconscious. The optimal position for providing oral hygiene to this patient is _____ to prevent choking.

    1. High Fowler's position
    2. High Fowler's position with head hyperextended
    3. Supine with the head lowered
    4. Side-lying with head facing to the side

13. A patient has diffuse pancreatitis causing severe weakness. The CNA is bathing the patient. While the CNA cleanses the patient's ears, which action by the CNA will prompt the nurse to intervene? *(Select all that apply.)*

    1. Cleansing the outer ear with the washcloth during the bath
    2. Retracting the outer ear downward to loosen visible cerumen
    3. Irrigating the ear with cool water to remove tenacious cerumen
    4. Using cotton-tipped applicators to cleanse the pinna of each ear
    5. Placing an otoscope in the ear canal to visualize any areas that need cleaning

14. The student nurse has completed her educational instructions on the correct procedures for bed making. Which intervention is correct for bed making? *(Select all that apply.)*

    1. Preparing a closed bed for receiving postoperative patients
    2. Shaking soiled linen before placement in the hamper
    3. Mitering the corners of the bottom fitted sheet
    4. Washing hands thoroughly after making a patient's bed
    5. Folding and reusing the patient's bedspread if it is not soiled

15. A patient is in his first postoperative day. As part of his morning care, the nurse removes and cleanses his dentures. Which action demonstrates proper denture care?

    1. Brushing the dentures over an open sink with the water running
    2. Rinsing dentures thoroughly with hot water before brushing
    3. Brushing dentures with a soft toothbrush or denture brush
    4. After cleaning, storing dentures in a dry denture cup

16. The nurse is providing instruction to the UAP who is assisting with caring for an immobile patient who requires turning every 2 hours. The UAP asks the nurse why it is best to place the patient in the 30-degree lateral position. Which response by the nurse is correct?

    1. "This position helps prevent pressure injuries on spinous processes."
    2. "This position helps prevent pressure injuries on the ischial tuberosities."
    3. "This position helps prevent pressure injuries on the greater trochanters."
    4. "This position helps prevent pressure injuries on the occipital prominence."

17. The nurse is reviewing documentation from the previous shift. The nurse is correct when determining the patient has a stage 3 pressure injury based on which note?

1. Nonblanchable reddened areas where the skin is intact
2. Full-thickness tissue loss extending through subcutaneous tissue and muscle
3. Extensive destruction of skin and adipose tissue with possible tunneling
4. Areas of full-thickness skin loss with extension to the bone

18. The patient has been changing a dressing on a pressure injury for several days and is now being seen in the physician's office. The patient states, "There is a lot of pink tissue at the base of the wound." The nurse explains to the patient that this is the result of what process?

1. Improper dressing technique and probable infection
2. Presence of a layer of eschar that has to be removed
3. Development of a fungal overgrowth interfering with healing
4. The normal process of healing with healthy granulation tissue

19. The nurse is most concerned when applying heat therapy to which patient?

1. A patient who has been diagnosed with high blood pressure
2. A patient who is unconscious as the result of an automobile accident
3. A patient who has just returned from physical therapy for back pain
4. A patient who was recently diagnosed with type 2 diabetes mellitus

20. The nurse is providing discharge instructions for a patient who will be using cold therapy after knee replacement surgery. What statement by the patient indicates the need for further instruction? *(Select all that apply.)*

1. "I don't have a cold pack at home like the one I had in the hospital. I will use the cold pack I use in my cooler to ice my knee."
2. "I will use a cloth or towel to wrap my cold pack in when I get home so that I don't damage my skin when I'm applying it to my knee."
3. "My friend says that using a bag of frozen vegetables works well as an ice pack as long as you wrap it in a cloth."
4. "I will leave the cold pack on my knee for 1 hour, leave it off for 30 minutes, and then apply it again for 1 hour all day long so that my knee won't swell."
5. "The cold pack really helps the pain in my knee. I will use it at home so that I hopefully won't have to take a lot of pain medication."

21. A woman, 74, has been hospitalized for three and a half weeks after suffering a partial stroke at home in her bed, where she had been mostly confined for the past year due to her excess weight. She has pressure injuries on her heels and back. Her sister, who is healthy but frail, says, "I haven't been able to get her out of bed or the wheelchair by myself these past weeks, and Lily can't help me move herself much because of the painful swelling in her left leg. For the past couple of weeks, she's eaten most of her meals in bed, and we watch TV together in her room." The client has a history of type 2 diabetes, deep vein thrombosis (DVT), and congestive heart failure. Pitting edema is observed in the lower left calf, localized tenderness along the distribution of the deep venous system, collateral superficial veins (non-varicose), and the calf swelling is 3 to 4 cm greater than the asymptomatic side. The LPN assigned to this client is asked to give her a bed bath. Given this client's condition, identify which procedures should be followed before, during, and after her bed bath?

ACTIONS	PLAN OF CARE
a. When preparing this client for a bed bath, remove the gown from the arm without the IV first.	
b. Cleanse the eye by wiping from the outer to inner canthus, then away from the eye.	
c. Bathe each leg with circular strokes, but don't massage the lower extremities.	
d. Clip the client's nails after soaking.	
e. After bathing, favor the 30-degree lateral-incline position for this client.	
f. Use a doughnut type cushion to relieve pressure on fragile skin.	
g. Massage all reddened areas, applying lotion.	
h. Secure aquathermia pad securely with safety pins, tape, ties, or gauze rolls.	

Safety

Objectives

1. Summarize safety precautions to help prevent falls.
2. Relate specific safety considerations to the developmental age and needs of individuals across the lifespan.
3. Identify nursing interventions that are appropriate for individuals across the lifespan to ensure a safe environment.
4. Describe safe and appropriate methods for the application of safety reminder devices and nursing interventions when caring for patients.
5. Discuss nursing interventions that promote a restraint-free environment.
6. Discuss safety concerns in the health care environment.
7. Cite the steps to be taken during a fire.
8. Describe nursing interventions to treat accidental poisoning.
9. Discuss the role of the nurse in disaster planning and active shooter situations.
10. Discuss terrorism.
11. Discuss high-risk syndromes of bioterrorism and the role of the nurse.

Key Terms

bioterrorism (p. 255)

Centers for Disease Control and Prevention (CDC) (SĔN-tĕrz fŏr dĭ-ZĒZ kŏn-TRŌL ănd prē-VĔN-shŭn, p. 250)

codes (p. 254)

disaster manual (p. 254)

disaster situation (p. 253)

elopement (ē-LŌP-mĕnt, p. 245)

endemic (ĕn-DĔM-ĭk, p. 256)

epidemic (ĕp-ĭ-DĔM-ĭk, p. 257)

Hazard Communication Act (p. 250)

Occupational Safety and Health Administration (OSHA) (p. 250)

PASS (p. 252)

poison (p. 253)

RACE (p. 252)

safety reminder device (SRD) (p. 244)

sentinel event (SĔN-tĭ-nĕl, p. 237)

terrorism (p. 254)

Safety of the patient is the primary concern of the nurse. Ensuring a safe physical environment, administering medications safely, and helping patients feel safe in their environment are goals for nurses within a health care facility. The nurse also is concerned with the safety of patients within the community setting. Numerous factors can endanger the patient's safety both physically and psychologically. This chapter explores potential threats to a patient's safety in various environments as well as how the nurse can meet the safety needs of the patient.

SAFETY IN THE HOSPITAL OR HEALTH CARE ENVIRONMENT

Traditionally, the patient's overall safety in the hospital or any other health care environment has been the primary concern of nursing. Today, the focus on a safe environment has expanded as we have come to recognize and identify potential hazards and threats faced by hospital and long-term care facility personnel, patients, and visitors (Box 10.1).

A safe environment implies freedom from injury as well as the prevention of falls, electrical injuries, fires, burns, and poisoning. The nurse must be alert to potential safety problems, such as workplace violence, and must know how to report and respond when someone's safety is threatened.

Providing and maintaining a safe environment involves the patient, visitors, and members of the health care team. Protection and education are primary nursing responsibilities, as the nurse is involved directly and actively in ensuring and maintaining a safe health care environment; for example, checking to see that the call light or signal system is working and accessible.

Each year, The Joint Commission releases national patient safety goals for health care facilities. These goals are based on evidenced-based practices and developed from a review of national databases and assist facilities in maintaining patient safety. A component of these goals includes the identification of sentinel events. The Joint Commission defines a sentinel event as "a patient safety event that results in death, permanent harm, or

Box 10.1   Precautions to Promote Safety

- Assist patients when they get out of bed if they have had surgery, have received narcotics for analgesia, have an unsteady gait, or have been in bed for an extended period.
- Demonstrate the proper use of emergency call buttons or cords.
- Encourage patients to wear nonslip slippers or shoes when ambulating.
- Encourage the use of handrails in the bathrooms and halls.
- Follow facility policies regarding the use of side rails.
- If bed is equipped with an alarm, turn on for the restless, disoriented patient.
- Instruct patient to use the call bell for assistance.
- Keep adjustable beds in the low position except when giving care.
- Keep environment free of clutter, as items such as books, magazines, and shoes sometimes cause the patient to trip and fall.
- Lock wheels on beds, wheelchairs, and gurneys.
- Orient patient to the environment to provide familiarity.
- Place bedside table and overbed table within reach. Ensure that frequently used items, such as the telephone, eyeglasses, or other personal belongings, are easily accessible.
- Provide adequate lighting.
- Some institutions have adopted "fall precaution" policies in which every patient is evaluated on admission to determine the degree of likelihood for a potential fall (see Box 10.2).
- Wipe or mop up spilled liquids promptly. Personnel and patients must be alert to signs warning of wet or slippery floors.

Box 10.2   Sample Questions Found on a Fall Assessment Tool

	YES	NO
1. Is there a history of a fall(s) in the past year?		
2. Does the patient have an unsteady gait or difficulty ambulating?		
3. Is the patient on any high-risk medications?		
4. Does the patient require equipment to assist in ambulating?		
5. Does the patient have an altered mental status?		
6. Is the patient experiencing blood pressure problems, dizziness, or vertigo?		
7. Is the patient age 70 years or older?		
8. Does the patient experience bowel or bladder incontinence?		
9. Does the patient have an intravenous (IV), chest tube, oxygen line, or attachment to any other tubing?		
10. Does the patient have any vision or other sensory problems?		

severe temporary harm. Sentinel events are debilitating to both patients and health care providers involved in the event" (TJC, n.d.). The reporting of certain sentinel events to The Joint Commission is required; it should include a thorough review of the event as well as the plan for improvements that will prevent the event from occurring again. Examples of sentinel events include medication errors, errors in procedures and treatments that lead to the death of an individual, and inappropriate application of safety reminder devices (SRDs; formerly referred to as *restraints*).

FALLS

Falls are a common problem in health care facilities, requiring the nurse to be alert to patients who are at an increased risk for falls. A fall risk assessment is important to perform upon the patient's admission to the unit and whenever a significant change in their condition has occurred. Patient falls are a major safety consideration for *all* institutions (see the Coordinated Care box). The very young and older adults are not the only individuals at risk in the health care environment; individuals who become ill or who are injured are also at risk. An unfamiliar environment and the various symptoms and

signs associated with the patient's diagnosis often place an individual at risk. The use of anesthesia, sedatives, or narcotics increases the risk of falling, as does an unstable gait or a problem with balance. A fall risk assessment is necessary on admission to a facility or if a significant change in the patient's condition has occurred. Box 10.2 is a sample list of questions found on a fall risk assessment tool. Facilities require fall precautions if the answer is "yes" to a specified number of questions on a fall risk assessment tool.

 Coordinated Care

Delegation

Patient Safety and Fall Prevention

Although preventing falls is the responsibility of all caregivers, including unlicensed assistive personnel (UAP), assessment for risk of fall or injury requires the critical thinking and knowledge application unique to the nurse and is not delegated. When delegating safety measures, stress the importance of the following:
- The patient's mobility limitations and any specific measures to minimize risks
- Environmental safety precautions (e.g., bed is locked and in low position, call bell and personal items are within reach, pathway is clear, patient has nonskid footwear)
- What to do when a patient starts to fall while being assisted with ambulation (i.e., ease patient into a sitting position in a chair or on the floor and alert the nurse)

Monitoring patient behavior for risk of injury and promoting a safe environment are acceptable to delegate as a responsibility of UAP and of nursing staff. Assessment of a patient's behaviors and decisions about less restrictive interventions require the critical thinking and knowledge application unique to the nurse.

Although the application of SRDs is acceptable to delegate to UAP, assessment of when SRDs are needed and the appropriate type to use requires the critical thinking and knowledge application unique to the nurse and is not delegated. The importance of the following factors should be emphasized:

- Correct placement of the SRD
- Observation for constriction of circulation, skin integrity, and adequate breathing
- When and how to change position and provide range-of-motion exercises, skin care, toileting, and opportunities for socialization

Care of the patient receiving internal radiation therapy is acceptable to delegate to UAP. Care measures that should be highlighted include the following:

- Patient's activity limitations
- Safety regulations (e.g., use of dosimeter, time and distance limits)
- Use of protective equipment (e.g., shields, gloves)
- Visitor restrictions (no one younger than 18 years of age, no one who is or may be pregnant)
- Handling of patient care–related items and substances (e.g., linen, trash, dietary tray, specimens, urine, feces)

The setting up of seizure precautions and protection for patients at risk for seizures is acceptable to delegate to UAP if they have been trained appropriately. Stress the importance of protection from falls, avoiding attempts to restrain, and not placing anything in the patient's mouth.

Interventions for a patient experiencing a seizure are not to be delegated. Assessment of the patient's airway patency, breathing, and circulatory status requires the critical thinking and knowledge application unique to the nurse and cannot be delegated. Refer to *Adult Health Nursing*, Chapter 14, for further care of the patient with seizures.

Gait belts are an effective way to help patients ambulate safely. A gait belt is a canvas (or other very strong material) belt that encircles the patient's waist (some belts have handles attached for the staff to grasp) while the patient ambulates. Correct technique in the use of the gait belt is as follows:

1. Apply gait belt securely around the patient's waist. The health care worker should be able to fit two fingers between the gait belt and the patient's waist.
2. Walk to the side of patient, grasping the gait belt at the patient's back. The other hand may either support the patient's arm or grasp the gait belt at the patient's side. Unless the patient has a tendency to lean toward one particular side, walk on the patient's weaker side so that you are able to give assistance if the patient starts to fall. See the illustration for Skill 10.1, Step 6d(1).
3. Have patient support self by leaning on or holding your arm.
4. Walk slightly behind the patient for better support.
5. Walk with your knees and hips flexed.
6. After ambulation, loosen or remove the gait belt.
7. Document procedure.

INFANTS AND CHILDREN

Ensuring the safety of an environment for infants and children requires protecting the child and educating the parents to do so. The nurse is responsible for anticipating potential injuries and individualizing patient care and teaching. Accidents involving children are largely preventable, but parents and caregivers need to be aware of specific dangers at each stage of growth and development. Growth and the acquisition of new motor skills place the child at great risk for injury. See Chapters 24, 30, and 31 for a more detailed discussion.

Many dangers exist in a child's environment. All household cleaning items are potentially poisonous when ingested and must be kept out of children's reach. Remind parents that most younger children are not able to read or understand labels on cleaning materials or medication containers. Educate parents that infants in the oral stage of development put almost anything into their mouths, and as infants learn to crawl, electrical sockets and cords will become a danger. Toddlers and young children can be protected from burns by turning pot handles on a stove away from the child's reach. Bath water can be another potential hazard for children, either because of the temperature of the water or from leaving children unattended for any length of time. Pool safety should also be emphasized to parents and caregivers. Protecting infants and toddlers from falling out of bed while in the health care facility is a concern. Keeping side rails up or using a pediatric crib are important safety measures to prevent falls. When giving care, place your hand on the infant or toddler when you turn to obtain supplies; this prevents the infant or child from falling off a bed or examination table. See Chapters 24, 30, and 31 for a more detailed discussion.

OLDER ADULTS

Changes associated with aging affect the ability of older adults to protect themselves from injury (see the Lifespan Considerations for Older Adults box). Unsteady gait, age-related vision changes, and medication side effects (such as vertigo) pose a threat to the older adult's safety. Ensuring that older adults wear their eyeglasses and hearing aids and use assistive devices for ambulating when necessary are important nursing interventions to promote patient safety.

Skill 10.1   Applying Safety Reminder Devices

 CHECK   GATHER   HELLO   ID   PRIVACY   EXPLAIN   WASH   GLOVES

NURSING ACTION (RATIONALE)

1. Refer to medical record or care plan. Review the agency policy. (*Provides basis of care; a physician's order is required before SRDs are applied.*)
2. Perform hand hygiene. (*Reduces spread of microorganisms.*)
3. Introduce self. (*Decreases patient's anxiety.*)
4. Identify patient. (*Identifies correct patient for procedure.*)
5. Procedure:
   a. Explain procedure. (*Enlists cooperation or assistance from patient and family and decreases anxiety.*)
   b. Prepare for procedure by providing privacy and assembling necessary supplies. (*Organizes procedure and decreases patient's anxiety.*)
   c. Assess patient for need of SRD (a comprehensive nursing assessment of the patient's potential for injury and treatment in relation to the need for an SRD is crucial before applying SRD). (*Restraining a patient without a physician's order or without reasonable cause incurs risk of charges of false imprisonment. Some facilities have specific requirements for SRD use in certain situations [e.g., the presence of an endotracheal tube].*)
6. Apply appropriate type of SRD:
   a. Wrist or ankle (extremity) SRD designed to immobilize one or more extremities
      (1) If using Kerlix gauze, make a clove hitch by forming a figure-8 and picking up the loops. (*The clove hitch does not tighten when pulled.*)
      (2) Place gauze or padding around the extremity. (*Decreases risk of injury to underlying skin.*)
      (3) Slip the wrist(s) or ankle(s) through loops directly over the padding; if using a commercially made SRD, wrap the padded portion of the device around affected extremity, thread tie through slit in device, and fasten to second tie with a secure knot. (*Decreases risk of injury to underlying skin.*)

(4) Secure ends of ties to the portion of the bed frame that moves with the patient when the bed is adjusted, **not to side rails.** (*If side rails are lowered with the SRD attached, injury is a possible result.*)

(5) Leave as much slack as possible (1–2 inches). (*Provides for movement.*)
(6) Palpate pulses below the SRD. (*Ensures that the device is not so tight as to occlude circulation.*)

   b. Elbow SRD
      (1) Place SRD (a piece of fabric with slots for the insertion of tongue blades to keep the elbow straight) over the elbow or elbows. (*Elbow SRDs often are used with children to prevent elbow flexion so that they cannot disturb tubes, catheters, and dressings.*)

Skill 10.1   Applying Safety Reminder Devices—cont'd

(2) Wrap SRD(s) snugly, tying them at the top. For small infants, tie or pin SRDs to their shirts. (*Tying or pinning the restraint to the infant's shirt ensures a secure fit.*)

c. Vest (sometimes referred to as a wrap jacket or chest SRD)

   (1) Apply device over the patient's gown. (*Protects the skin.*)

   (2) Put vest on patient with V-shaped opening in the front. (If vest is on backward and patient becomes restless, choking is possible result.)

(5) With a proper fit, there is room for a fist in the space between the vest and the patient. (*This determines that the vest is not too tight.*)

d. Gait or safety reminder belts

   (1) Apply belt over the patient's gown. (*Protects the skin.*)

(3) Pull tie at end of vest flap across the chest and slip tie through slit on opposite side of vest.

(4) Wrap the other end of the flap across patient and tie the straps to frame of bed or behind wheelchair. (*Helps secure vest SRD to the patient.*) Use the quick-release knot. (*A tight restraint potentially causes constriction and impedes circulation. Assessment for constriction prevents neurovascular injury.*)

(2) If patient is ambulating, place belt around the patient's waist. The belt usually has a buckle to secure it in place. (*Provides a snug fit and prevents slipping.*)

(3) If the belt does not have a buckle, use a slip knot. (*Allows for quick removal in case of emergency.*)

7. Use a quick-release knot rather than a regular knot to secure the safety reminder device to bed frame. (*A quick-release knot is quick to undo in an emergency.*)

Continued

Skill 10.1 Applying Safety Reminder Devices—cont'd

8. Secure SRDs so that the patient cannot untie them. (*Prevents patient injury.*)
9. Apply SRD gently and with compassion.
10. Perform hand hygiene. (Reduces spread of microorganisms.)
11. Document procedure. (Notes procedure and patient's response.)
    - Reason(s) SRD is needed
    - If appropriate, the notification of the physician and time order obtained
    - The time and type of SRD applied
    - The ongoing assessment and monitoring of the patient's skin, extremity circulation, and mental status
    - The response(s) of the patient
    - The periodic removal of the SRD and any skin care performed
    - If SRD removed, note time and follow-up assessments
    - If reapplication is needed, note reasons, time, and patient assessment
    - A flow sheet is an excellent tool for this documentation (see Fig. 3.8 for an example of a flow sheet)
12. Follow-up
    a. Monitor for skin impairment. (Excessive pressure potentially leads to loss of skin integrity.)
    b. With the use of extremity SRD, assess extremity distal to SRD every 30 min or more often according to agency policy. (Identifies any problems or need to remove or adjust SRD.)

    (1) Remove SRD on one extremity at a time at least every 2 h (know agency policy) for 5 min. (Allows supervised movement of extremity, enhances circulation, and reduces apprehension.)
    c. Monitor position of SRD, circulation, skin condition, and mental status frequently. (Ensures patient safety.) Remove SRD when no longer needed.
    d. With the use of vest SRD, monitor respiratory status. (Respiratory distress is possible if there is restriction from the vest.)
    e. Do NOT leave the patient unattended during temporary removal of SRD. (An unattended patient is at risk for injury.) Do take advantage of removal to change patient's position and inspect skin.
    f. Gently massage the skin beneath SRD; apply lotion or powder if desired. (A gentle massage of the skin increases circulation to area.)
    g. Change SRD when soiled or wet. (Reduces risk of skin impairment and infection.)
    h. Assess frequently for tangled ties or pressure points from knots; adjust SRD device(s) as needed. (Excess pressure leads to loss of skin integrity and impaired circulation.)
13. Evaluation
    a. The SRD is adequate and appropriate for the individual patient's condition. (Prevents interruption of treatment or therapy; prevents patient from falling from bed, chair, or wheelchair, and possibly from harming others.)
    b. SRDs are applied correctly. (Correct application prevents injury to the patient or to others.)
    c. Quick-release knots are released easily. (Ensures quick access to the patient in case of an emergency.)
    d. Related problems (e.g., of the skin or of the musculoskeletal system) are identified. (*Complications are prevented by performing timely interventions.*)
14. Provide patient teaching (see the Patient Teaching box on safety promotion).
15. Pediatric considerations
    a. When a child must be restrained for a procedure, it is best that the person applying the restraint is not the child's parent or guardian.
    b. A mummy restraint is a safe, efficient, short-term method to restrain a small child or infant for examination or treatment.
    (1) Open a blanket, and fold one corner toward the center. Place the infant on the blanket with shoulders at the fold and feet toward the opposite corner.

Skill 10.1   Applying Safety Reminder Devices—cont'd

(2) With infant's right arm straight down against body, pull the right side of the blanket firmly across the right shoulder and chest, and secure beneath the left side of body.

(3) Place the left arm straight against the body, bring the left side of the blanket across the shoulder and chest, and lock beneath the infant's body on the right side.

(4) Align the infant's legs, pull the corner of the blanket near the feet up toward the body, and tuck snugly in place or fasten securely with safety pins.

(5) Remain with the infant during restraint and remove the restraint immediately after treatment is complete. If restraint is required for an extended period, remove it at least every 2 h and perform range-of-motion exercises on all extremities.

Lifespan Considerations
Older Adults

Safety

Physiologic changes in aging that increase the need for safety precautions:

- Changes in vision, including altered depth perception, increased sensitivity to glare, and decreased visual acuity in dim light, increase the risk of falls because of misperception of visual cues.
- Changes in hearing, including varying degrees of deafness and tinnitus (ringing in the ears), increase the risk of injury from hazards in the environment because certain warnings that commonly are detected with auditory cues, such as motor vehicle horns, alarms, or even spoken warnings, are not heard.
- Prevent sensory overload in older adults because reflexes and the ability to respond to multiple stimuli slow with aging.
- Changes in muscle strength and joint function that result in slowed reaction time, altered gait, and altered sense of balance make it more likely that stumbling will result in a fall.
- Changes in the cardiovascular system such as anemia, orthostatic hypotension, and heart block increase the risk of syncope, which increases the risk of falls.
- Changes in the peripheral vascular system sometimes result in loss of sensitivity to heat, cold, or foreign objects, which increases the risk of tissue damage from burns, frostbite, and pressure.
- Older adults take many medications that increase the need for safety precautions. Sedatives, hypnotics, and tranquilizers affect reaction time and increase the risk of injury. Similarly, antihypertensives, diuretics, and antihistamines increase the risk of orthostatic hypotension (a drop of 25 mm Hg in systolic pressure and 10 mm Hg in diastolic pressure), which increases the risk of falls.
- Keep the use of SRDs and the amount of any restraint used to a minimum. SRDs reduce mobility and result in a loss of strength that can increase the risk of falls or injury.
- Accidental poisoning is a significant problem in older adults. Visual changes raise the potential for misreading of labels on medication or other packages and can lead to overdose or other errors in administration. Medication organizers or dispensers help reduce the risk of medication errors in the home. In addition, many older adults do not consider over-the-counter medications to be "real" medicine, so they take them freely and fail to mention them when questioned regarding drug use. Many over-the-counter medications increase the risk of injury to the older adult by potentiating or interfering with the effects of prescription drugs.

Assisting weak or disoriented older patients when drinking hot liquids such as soups, coffee, or tea can prevent burns. People in this age group are more vulnerable to burns from spilled hot liquids or heating pads and electric blankets.

SAFETY REMINDER DEVICES

A **safety reminder device (SRD)** is defined as any of the numerous devices used to immobilize a patient or part of the patient's body, such as arms or hands. Many facilities have adopted a restraint-free environment, thus eliminating the use of any type of SRD. This is especially true in long-term care facilities; they are a permanent home for many residents, so maintaining a safe environment while protecting the individual's dignity is a priority.

The use of SRDs also tends to result in increased restlessness, disorientation, agitation, anxiety, and a feeling of powerlessness. It contributes to patient immobility and associated problems with immobility such as dehydration, health care–associated infection, and incontinence. The resulting disuse of body parts has the potential to increase disability and lead to further patient weakness and unsteadiness. Patients often pull against the SRDs, causing skin and circulation problems.

SRDs may be used for various reasons but are primarily for considerations of patient safety. SRDs that restrain the use of a limb (e.g., a wrist restraint) are used primarily in the mental health setting to protect the patient and the staff from harm, the pediatric setting to prevent incidents such as displacement of intravenous lines by the patient, and the intensive care setting to prevent the patient from pulling out medical devices such as an endotracheal tube. Certain patient populations, such as the disoriented patient, are more likely to need SRDs in the forms of bed or chair alarms. A bed or chair alarm alerts the staff if a patient attempts to get out of a bed or chair without assistance. This helps reduce the risk of the patient falling from a bed, chair, or wheelchair (Fig. 10.1). However, bed

Fig. 10.1 (A) Weight-sensitive alarm. (B) Chair alarm.

and chair alarms are now viewed by some long-term-care facilities as a form of restraint. For patients or residents in a long-term care setting who are at risk for elopement (leaving the health care facility without permission or necessary supervision), a device referred to as a wander guard may be needed. This device is worn on the wrist or ankle and sets off an alarm when the person leaves the facility. These devices are especially beneficial for the confused or disoriented patient or resident who would be at risk for attempting to leave the facility.

The focus of patient care is on attempting alternative strategies before turning to the use of SRDs (Box 10.3). By assessing individual patient needs, characteristics of the environment, and organizational change, the licensed practical/vocational nurse (LPN/LVN) is able to plan interventions that reduce or eliminate the need for SRDs. Patient safety and the safety of others are the only reasons an SRD is used. Most health care facilities have specific policies and procedures related to their use (Box 10.4 and see Skill 10.1), and most require a specific order from a health care provider. Some facilities require that a health care provider order for SRDs be renewed every 24 h. Explain to the patient the need for the devices, even if the patient does not seem to understand the explanation. Inform family members about the need for SRDs (see the Cultural Considerations box and the Patient Teaching box). Include information about the specific device used and the approximate period for use.

Box 10.3 Designing a Restraint-Free Environment

Care of the patient who may be prone to threats to safety and security requires a creative, systematic, and attentive approach. A wide variety of electronic devices have been developed to alert staff to a patient's need for assistance. A weight-sensitive alarm can be placed under a patient in bed or in a chair. When the patient tries to get up, an alarm sounds (see Fig. 10.1A). A chair alarm may be used to remind the patient or to alert the staff when a patient who requires assistance when standing or ambulating tries to get up without assistance (see Fig. 10.1B).

To design a restraint-free environment:
- Orient patient and family to surroundings; explain all procedures and treatments.
- Encourage family and friends to stay or use sitters for patients who need supervision.
- Assign confused or disoriented patients to rooms near the nurses' station. Observe these patients frequently.
- Provide appropriate visual and auditory stimuli (e.g., family pictures, clocks, radio).

- Eliminate bothersome treatments as soon as possible. For example, discontinue tube feedings and begin oral feedings as quickly as the patient's condition allows.
- Use relaxation techniques (e.g., massage).
- Institute exercise and ambulation schedules as the patient's condition allows.
- Encourage participation in diversional activities (e.g., long-term care facilities typically have daily activities planned for the residents, such as games, movies, entertainment).
- Maintain toileting routines.
- Consult with physical and occupational therapists to enhance patient's abilities to carry out activities of daily living.
- Evaluate all medications patient is receiving to determine whether the medication is having the desired therapeutic effect.
- Conduct ongoing assessment and evaluation of patient's care and patient's ongoing response to care.

Box 10.4 Long-Term Care Variations for Safety Reminder Devices

Legislation has affected greatly the use of safety reminder devices (SRDs) in the long-term care facility. Under the Omnibus Budget Reconciliation Act (OBRA) of 1987, residents' rights are addressed specifically in terms of SRDs. This act, effective October 1, 1990, mandates specific guidelines and prohibits routine use of SRDs in long-term care facilities. The act regulates the use of extremity SRDs, hand mitts, safety vests, and wheelchair safety bars. SRDs may be used only to ensure the physical safety of the patient or other residents. A written order by the physician must detail the duration and circumstances under which the SRDs are to be used.

OBRA states the following as acceptable reasons for the use of physical restraints:
- All other interventions have been attempted before the use of restraints.
- Other disciplines have been consulted for their assistance.
- Supporting documentation has been completed.

ESSENTIALS OF SRD DOCUMENTATION
- Reason for the physical restraint
- Explanation given to patient and family
- Date and time of the patient's response to treatment
- Duration
- Frequency of observation and patient's response
- Safety
- Release the physical restraint at least every 2 h
- Routine exercise of extremities, including range-of-motion exercises
- Assessment for circulation and skin integrity
- Assessment for continued need for the physical restraint
- Patient outcome

🌐 Cultural Considerations

Safety in Health Care Settings

- Cultural heritage affects all dimensions of health; the nurse must consider cultural background when planning for patient safety.
- The way that culture influences behaviors, attitudes, and values depends on many factors and thus may not be the same for individual members of a cultural group.
- Before assessing the cultural background of a patient, assess the influence of the nurse's own culture.
- Adapt the planning and implementation of nursing interventions for safety as much as possible to a patient's cultural background.
- Evaluate attitudes and emotions toward providing nursing interventions for safety to patients from diverse sociocultural backgrounds.
- Patients from some cultures may seem unfriendly and distant in terms of space. It is often very difficult for them to have an outsider in their home who is suggesting changes with regard to their personal belongings, even though the purpose is to reduce physical hazards.
- Determination of a patient's attitude toward the home is particularly difficult when another language is spoken. Use an interpreter or engage the patient's family to interpret if available. Attentiveness to the patient's nonverbal communication becomes extremely important as you assess the home.
- Another culturally sensitive issue is the patient's sense of environmental control. Be aware of health beliefs and practices that affect the outcome of interventions. For example, reliance on family and religious organizations, as opposed to community resources, is likely to affect compliance with nursing interventions and referrals.

👥 Patient Teaching

Safety Promotion

- Teach the primary caregiver the dangers associated with restraining a patient who has a history of seizures; show them how to modify the environment for the patient's protection.
- Teach the primary caregiver how to correctly position a patient who is nauseated and vomiting if a restraint is in use.
- Teach the primary caregiver how to routinely change the patient's position and use passive range of motion.
- Explain to the patient and members of the family why SRDs are necessary.
- Provide information about the type of SRD being prescribed and the approximate time frame for use.
- Inform the patient and family that the patient will still receive comfort measures such as repositioning and limb exercises.
- Inform patients and parents about potential sources of poisoning found in the home as well as appropriate safety precautions (see Box 10.11).
- Inform patients and parents about poison control centers. Provide a number for the closest center or instruct them to call 911.
- Teach basic interventions to follow in the case of a poisoning.
- See that safety items, such as stickers with poison center information, are available.
- Teach parents and caregivers not to try home remedies. When ingestion of a dangerous substance is suspected, appropriate medical intervention must be sought immediately (see the Cultural Considerations box).
- Removal of poisonous and toxic substances does not take the place of education as a means to prevent accidental poisoning.
- Instruct family to place bedside tables and overbed tables close to the patient.
- Encourage the patient to rise from the bed or chair slowly to prevent vertigo (dizziness) that results from postural hypotension.
- Advise the family to remove clutter from bedside tables, hallways, bathrooms, and grooming areas.
- Encourage family to mount grab bars around toilets and showers; teach the patient how to use them.
- Recommend that rugs and carpets be attached securely to floors and stairs.
- Recommend that bathmats and nonskid strips be attached to bathtubs and the floors of shower stalls.
- Recommend that electrical cords be secured against baseboards so that the patient will not trip over them.
- Ensure that the call bell is within easy reach of the hospitalized patient; show the patient the location of emergency call bells in bathrooms. (The nurse must respond to call lights quickly, especially for patients who need assistance to the bathroom.)
- See that wheelchairs remain locked when transporting a patient from bed to wheelchair or back to bed.
- Instruct caregivers to check that side rails are up and safety straps secured around a patient who is on a gurney (stretcher; see the Coordinated Care box).
- Use the fire drill procedure as an opportunity to talk about fire safety.

Documentation about the need for the SRDs, the type of device used, and the patient's response is crucial (see Box 10.4). Perform a comprehensive assessment that focuses on the patient's behavior, activity, and skin condition. Note all nursing interventions, including patient and family teaching about the SRDs.

LATEX SENSITIVITY

Question all patients regarding allergies and ask specifically about latex allergies. A latex allergy can precipitate a respiratory arrest, which is a life-threatening event (Box 10.5). This potential reaction must be kept in mind at all times. Do not wear, or permit others to

Box 10.5	Levels of Latex Sensitivity

- *Contact dermatitis:* A nonallergic response characterized by skin redness and itching.
- *Type IV hypersensitivity:* Cell-mediated allergic reaction to chemicals used in latex processing. Delayed reaction including redness, itching, and hives for up to 48 h is possible. Localized swelling, red and itchy or runny eyes and nose, and coughing often develop.
- *Type I hypersensitivity:* A true latex allergy that is possibly life threatening. Reactions are likely based on type of latex protein and degree of individual sensitivity, including local and systemic. Symptoms include hives, generalized edema, itching, rash, wheezing, bronchospasm, difficulty breathing, laryngeal edema, diarrhea, nausea, hypotension, tachycardia, and respiratory or cardiac arrest.

From Asthma and Allergy Foundation of America: Latex allergy. Retrieved from www.aafa.org/latex-allergy.

Box 10.6	Mercury Spill Cleanup Procedure

In the event of a mercury spill, follow these steps while waiting for trained personnel to arrive:
1. Evacuate the room except for a housekeeping crew (if available).
2. Ventilate the area. Close interior doors and open any outside windows.
3. Do not vacuum the spill.

After the mercury has been recovered:
4. Mop the floor with a mercury-specific cleanser (see agency policy).
5. Dispose of collected mercury according to local environmental safety regulations.

wear, latex gloves when caring for patients with latex allergies. For individuals at high risk of or with suspected sensitivity to latex, use exclusively latex-free products, including gloves, and inspect the contents of all patient care supply kits for items that contain latex (e.g., catheters, tubing). Institutions have latex-free procedure kits available for use.

ELECTRICAL HAZARDS

Much of the equipment used in health care settings is electrical and requires maintenance. Use of properly grounded and functional electrical equipment decreases the risk of electrical injury and fire. Teaching patients and family how to reduce their risk of electrical injury in the home (e.g., prevention of electrical shock, avoidance of use of electrical appliances near water source, methods of grounding appliances, avoidance of operating unfamiliar equipment) is a responsibility of the home health nurse.

RADIATION

Radiation presents a health hazard, if used incorrectly, in health care settings and the community. Radiation and radioactive materials are used in the diagnosis and treatment of patients. Hospitals have strict guidelines on the care of patients who are receiving radiation and on the handling of radioactive materials. To reduce the amount of exposure to radiation, the nurse must limit time spent near the source, keep as great a distance from the source as possible, and use shielding devices such as lead aprons. Staff members who work near radiation on a routine basis are required to wear devices that track their cumulative exposure to radiation. After collection and processing of these devices, those staff members whose radiation exposure readings fall above a set limit frequently are assigned to an alternative work area away from radiation exposure. Follow-up medical attention is often mandated for them as well.

The community is put at risk for radiation exposure if radioactive waste products are disposed of or transported incorrectly. Community health agencies, the Environmental Protection Agency (EPA), the Nuclear Regulatory Commission (NRC), the Department of Energy (DOE), and the Department of Transportation (DOT) have established specific, strict guidelines for the disposal of radioactive waste (NRC, 2020). If a radioactive leak occurs, these agencies institute measures to prevent exposure of surrounding neighborhoods, clean up radioactive leaks as quickly as possible, and ensure that anyone injured receives prompt medical care.

MERCURY SPILL

The nurse must know whom to contact when exposure to a hazardous chemical (such as mercury) occurs in the health care setting. Exposures in a health care facility include broken thermometers or sphygmomanometers, although these devices are seldom used or allowed in most health care facilities. Mercury enters the body through inhalation and absorption through the skin. Exposures that occur in a health care facility setting are usually brief but still have the potential to affect the brain or kidney. Full recovery is likely once the body cleans itself of the contamination. Box 10.6 summarizes steps to take in the event of a mercury spill. Although a mercury spill is not likely to occur in the health care setting, it is important to be aware of the facility's policy for proper cleanup of a mercury spill. Mercury-containing equipment may be used in factory settings, so the occupational health nurse should be aware of mercury spill safety in case an employee comes into contact with mercury while on the job.

WORKPLACE SAFETY

The health care environment is a source of potential safety hazards to health care workers. Of significant impact is the threat of workplace violence (Box 10.7). Active shooters are also a concern in the health care setting. An active shooter is defined by the US Department of Homeland Security (2008) as "an individual actively engaged in killing or attempting to

Box 10.7   Workplace Violence

Violence does not always involve physical injury, especially in relation to workplace violence. The term workplace violence refers to any extreme behavior used to frighten, intimidate, threaten, or injure a person or damage or destroy property. The behavior is sometimes physical, sometimes verbal, and sometimes even nonverbal, such as a gesture. Legally, if by either threat or gesture, someone causes a person to fear being struck, an assault has occurred. Any unwelcomed physical contact from another person is battery. In other words, one does not have to be physically "hurt" to be protected under the law.

According to the most recent statistics from the US Bureau of Labor Statistics in 2018, the days away from work due to workplace violence was 10.4 per 10,000 full-time workers, compared to the all-worker incidence rate of 2.1 days per 10,000 full-time workers (BLS, 2020). Most workplace violence, including in the health care setting, results in nonfatal injuries.

Unfortunately, these statistics do not provide the full picture. because many workplace violence incidents are not reported. Sometimes nurses do not report a violent incident because they are unsure what constitutes violence, do not know of the requirement to report the incident, or do not know whom to inform; sometimes they do not file a report because the injuries do not require emergency treatment or time off from work.

Risk factors for work-related assaults in health care agencies include the following:

- On-site presence of patients, families, friends, and coworkers in the possession of handguns
- Patients who are hospitalized and under police custody at the same time (people arrested or convicted of crimes)
- On-site presence of acutely disturbed and violent people seeking health care
- On-site presence of mentally ill people who do not take medicine, do not receive follow-up care, and are not hospitalized unless they are an immediate threat to themselves or others
- On-site presence of upset, agitated, or disturbed family members and visitors
- Long emergency department waits that increase a person's agitation and frustration
- On-site agency pharmacies that are a source of drugs and therefore a target for robberies
- Gang members and substance abusers having access to agencies as patients or visitors
- Staff being alone with patients during care or transport to other agency areas during examination or treatment

- Low staffing levels during meals, during emergencies, and at night
- Poorly lit or distant parking areas
- Lack of staff training in recognizing and managing potentially violent situations

OSHA provides guidelines for violence identification and prevention programs with a goal of eliminating or reducing employee exposure to situations that have potential to cause death or injury. These guidelines can be found at the OSHA Workplace Violence Safety and Health Topics page. The worksite is analyzed for hazards. Prevention strategies are developed and implemented. Furthermore, employees are required to receive safety and health training per facility protocol. The nurse's responsibility in violence prevention programs include the following:

- Understand and follow the workplace violence prevention program.
- Understand and follow safety and security measures.
- Voice safety and security concerns.
- Report violent incidents promptly and accurately.
- Serve on health and safety committees that review incidents of workplace violence.
- Take part in training programs that focus on recognizing and managing agitation, assaultive behavior, and criminal intent.
- Practice the following safety measures when dealing with agitated or aggressive people:
- Stand away from the person. Judge the length of the person's arms and legs. Stand far enough away that the person will not be able to hit or kick you.
- Position yourself close to the door. Do not allow yourself to become trapped in the room.
- Note the location of panic buttons, call bells, alarms, closed-circuit monitors, and other security devices.
- If you wear your identification badge around your neck, be sure it will break away if pulled.
- Keep your hands free.
- Stay calm. Talk to the person in a calm manner. Do not raise your voice at, argue, scold, or interrupt the person.
- Do not touch the person.
- Tell the person that you will get the supervisor to speak to them.
- Leave the room as soon as you are able. Be sure the person is safe.
- Notify the supervisor or security officer of the situation.
- Complete an incident report according to agency policy.

From the US Department of Labor Occupational Safety and Health Administration (OSHA): Workplace violence. Retrieved from https://www.osha.gov/SLTC/healthcaref acilities/violence.html.

---

kill people in a confined and populated area; in most cases, active shooters use firearms(s) and there is no pattern or method to their selection of victims." In July 2016, The Joint Commission issued Planning and Response Guidelines in Health Care Settings from the FBI. It was recognized that active shooter guidelines were geared toward schools, government, and business settings but not toward the health care setting. In 2017, the guidelines were updated by the International Association of Emergency Medical Services Chiefs (IAEMSC) (TJC, 2017). The environment within the health care setting has several potentially dangerous

areas in the presence of an active shooter. The patient population is a vulnerable and potentially large target for an active shooter. Another area of concern is departments that house hazardous materials. Suggested response guidelines to an active shooter can be found at https://www.jointcommission.org/-/media/tjc/docu ments/resources/workplace-violence/2017_active_sho oter_planning_response_healthcare_settingpdf.pdf

Workplace safety also addresses other various biological, chemical, radiologic, and physical hazards. The increased use of lasers in the health care setting requires specific safety precautions because a laser has

Box 10.8 **Centers for Disease Control and Prevention Health Care Personnel Vaccination Recommendations**

VACCINES	RECOMMENDATIONS IN BRIEF
Hepatitis B	If you do not have documented evidence of a complete hepatitis B (HB) vaccine series, or if you do not have an up-to-date blood test that shows you are immune to hepatitis B (i.e., no serologic evidence of immunity or prior vaccination) then you should • Get the 3-dose series (dose #1 now, #2 in 1 month, #3 approximately 5 months after #2). • Get anti-HBs serologic tested 1–2 months after dose #3.
Flu (influenza)	Get 1 dose of influenza vaccine annually.
MMR (measles, mumps, and rubella)	If you were born in 1957 or later and have not had the MMR vaccine, or if you do not have an up-to-date blood test that shows you are immune to measles or mumps (i.e., no serologic evidence of immunity or prior vaccination), get 2 doses of MMR (1 dose now and the 2nd dose at least 28 days later). If you were born in 1957 or later and have not had the MMR vaccine, or if you do not have an up-to-date blood test that shows you are immune to rubella, only 1 dose of MMR is recommended. However, you may end up receiving 2 doses, because the rubella component is in the combination vaccine with measles and mumps. For health care workers (HCWs) born before 1957, see the MMR Advisory Committee on Immunization Practices (ACIP) vaccine recommendations.
Varicella (chickenpox)	If you have not had chickenpox (varicella), if you have not had varicella vaccine, or if you do not have an up-to-date blood test that shows you are immune to varicella (i.e., no serologic evidence of immunity or prior vaccination), get 2 doses of varicella vaccine, 4 weeks apart.
Tdap (tetanus, diphtheria, pertussis)	Get a one-time dose of Tdap as soon as possible if you have not received Tdap previously (regardless of when previous dose of Td was received). Get Td boosters every 10 years thereafter. Pregnant HCWs need to get a dose of Tdap during each pregnancy.
Meningococcal	All preteens and teens at 11 to 12 years of age, with a booster dose at 16 years of age. Also, children and adults at increased risk for meningococcal disease.
Covid-19	Depending on the kind of COVID-19 vaccine you get, you might need a second shot 3 weeks (or 21 days) or 4 weeks (or 28 days) after your first shot.

Modified from Centers for Disease Control and Prevention (CDC): Vaccine information for adults: Recommended vaccines for healthcare workers. Retrieved from https://www.cdc.gov/vaccines/adults/rec-vac/hcw.html.
Covid-19 vaccine. Retrieved from: https://www.cdc.gov/coronavirus/2019-ncov/vaccines/recommendations/hcp.html.

the potential to cause skin and eye injury and start a fire, if used improperly. Eye protection is necessary for the patient and the staff working with the laser. Personnel involved with laser-based procedures wear specially designed eyewear. Because a laser beam generates an enormous amount of energy, dry combustibles in the surgical field can accidentally ignite, posing a threat to the patient and staff. Ensure that water and a halon fire extinguisher are readily available. For prevention of injury to patients, staff, and equipment, sufficient and appropriate fire extinguishers must be located in magnetic resonance imaging (MRI) areas.

Hospital workers frequently are exposed to blood and body fluids, contaminated needles, radiation, and vaccine-preventable diseases. Immunization programs help protect hospital personnel and, in turn, patients at risk of being infected by hospital personnel. The Centers for Disease Control and Prevention (CDC, n.d.) have published health care personnel vaccination recommendations (Box 10.8). These recommendations also apply to student nurses because they are fulfilling clinical requirements in health care facilities.

Needlesticks are another source of potential injury to health care personnel. Intravenous tubing and accessories that do not require needles are available, thus reducing the risk of needlesticks. Needlesticks can be reduced further by never recapping needles and following proper disposal of needles into sharps containers after use. A stray needle lying in bed linens or carelessly thrown into a wastebasket is a prime source of exposure to bloodborne pathogens, not only for the direct care giver, but for housekeeping and laundry personnel. Overfilling a sharps container is another source of needlestick injuries. A staff member may try to deposit a needle into the overfilled container, thus causing a stick to occur. Many facilities use safety devices that prevent the need to recap needles (see Fig. 9c). Bloodborne diseases that can be transmitted through accidental needlesticks include hepatitis B and C as well as HIV. While needleless safety devices drastically reduced the number of needlesticks when the devices were introduced from the early 1980s to early 2000s (Stobart-Gallagher, 2019), recent studies have shown an increase in needlestick injuries. Some of the reasons cited for this increase include injuries occurring prior to activating the safety device and improper disposal of the needle (CDC/NORA, 2019), as well as problems in operating the safety device (King and Strony, 2021). It is important for students and nurses to make themselves familiar with how specific needle safety devices work in a facility in order to avoid such injuries.

The National Institute for Occupational Safety and Health (NIOSH) focuses on safety and issues related to health. Identifying risks associated with the preparation of certain drugs and looking at ways to control exposure during preparation and administration is just one example of how this group works to ensure a safe health care environment for health care workers. The **Hazard Communication Act** of the **Occupational Safety and Health Administration (OSHA)** (a federal organization that provides guidelines to help reduce safety hazards in the workplace) requires health care facilities to inform employees about the presence of or potential for harmful exposures and how to reduce the risk of exposure. The **Centers for Disease Control and Prevention (CDC)** (a federal agency that provides facilities and services for the investigation, identification, prevention, and control of disease) also provides guidelines for working with infectious patients (e.g., standard precautions; see Chapter 7). Referring to this information and following recommended guidelines for reducing exposure to the variety of hazards present in the health care environment is the responsibility of the nurse.

FIRE SAFETY

In 2016, the National Fire Protection Association reported that from 2009 to 2013, fire departments in the United States responded to 5650 health care facility structural fires; 65% of those were caused by cooking. Only 4% of health care facility fires spread beyond the room in which the fire originated. The reports indicate that 4 deaths and 160 injuries resulted from these fires (Campbell, 2017).

An established fire safety program is mandatory for all health care facilities (Box 10.9). Most facilities have a safety committee that is actively involved in establishing and monitoring prevention as well as fire education programs. Fire prevention includes good housekeeping, maintenance, and employee discipline (Box 10.10).

Box 10.9   Fire Safety Interventions and Safe Evacuation of Patients

ACTION (RATIONALE)

1. Follow facility fire plan in the event of a fire. *(Fire plan outlines procedures to follow.)*
   a. Ascertain patient's age, sensory impairments, level of mobility, ability to comprehend instructions, and overall need for protection. *(Protects and assists patient in interpreting environmental stimuli relevant to safety.)*
   b. If indicated, assess patients for type of evacuation assistance needed. *(Move individuals at risk for injury to a safer area.)*
   c. Provide clear explanations to patients and visitors in a calm manner. (Anxiety hinders understanding of situation and ability to follow instructions.)
   d. Assist with evacuations if needed:
      (1) Usually patients are moved horizontally (e.g., out of rooms, across halls, and through the next set of fire doors). (The fire and its potential for spreading often necessitate movement to a safer area. Some agencies have fire doors that are normally held open by magnets and close automatically when a fire alarm sounds. It is important to keep equipment away from these doors.)
      (2) If smoke or fire prevents you from moving patients across the hall, proceed vertically down to a lower level. **Never use elevators as an exit route. A fire spreads very quickly up through the elevator shaft.**
      (3) If a patient cannot walk or be moved by bed, stretcher, or wheelchair from the fire area, the patient often must be carried. (Use the carrying method that is safe for you and the patient; fire department personnel will help with the evacuation.)
      (4) Infant and child removal.
         (a) Place a blanket or sheet on floor.
         (b) Place two infants in each bassinet, using diapers or small blankets for padding.
         (c) Place the bassinet in the middle of the blanket.
         (d) Use the baby vest if available or fold the blanket over one end, fold the corners in, then roll the sides in to form a pocket.
         (e) Grasp the folded corners of the blanket and pull the infants to safety. Two people (or, if necessary, one person) are able to drag eight babies to the prescribed area.
         (f) Alternatively, place as many children as possible in one crib and pull the crib to the prescribed area.
      (5) Universal carry: The universal carry is a method of removing a patient from a bed to the floor. It is a quick and effective method for removing a patient who is in immediate danger. This carry can be used by anyone, regardless of patient size.
         (a) Spread a blanket, sheet, or bedspread on the floor alongside the bed, placing one-third of it under the bed and leaving about 8 inches to extend beyond the patient's head.
         (b) Grasp the patient's ankles and move the patient's legs until they fall at the knee over the edge of the bed.
         (c) Grasp each shoulder, slowing pulling the patient to a sitting position.
         (d) From the back, encircle the patient with your arms, place your arms under the patient's armpits, and lock your hands over the patient's chest.
         (e) Slide the patient slowly to the edge of the bed and lower the patient to the blanket. If the bed is high, instruct the patient to slide down one of your legs.
         (f) Taking care to protect the patient's head, gently lower the head and upper torso to the blanket and wrap the blanket around the patient.
         (g) At the patient's head, grip the blanket with both hands, one above each shoulder, holding the patient's head firmly in the 8 inches of blanket. Do not let the patient's head snap back.
         (h) Lift the patient to a half-sitting position and pull the blanketed patient to safety.

Box 10.9 **Fire Safety Interventions and Safe Evacuation of Patients—cont'd**

(6) Blanket drag: If vertical or downward evacuation by an interior stairway is necessary, in many cases one person can handle a helpless patient by using the blanket drag.

   (a) Double a blanket lengthwise and place it on the floor parallel and next to the bed, leaving 8 inches to extend above the patient's head.

   (b) Using cradle drop, kneel drop, universal carry, or other suitable means, remove the patient from the bed to the folded blanket on the floor alongside the bed.

   (c) Grasp the blanket above the patient's head and pull to the stairway; start down the stairs with patient coming headfirst onto the stairway.

   (d) Position yourself one, two, or three steps lower than the patient, depending on your height and the patient's height. The patient's lower body inclines upward.

   (e) Place your arms under the patient's arms and clasp your hands over the patient's chest.

   (f) Back slowly down the stairs, constantly maintaining close contact with the patient, keeping one leg against the patient's back.

(7) When considering the two-person swing, and all evacuation methods, take into consideration the patient's size and weight.

   (a) Two staff members grasp each other's forearms to form a seat for the patient to sit in (Fig. 10.2A).

   (b) Other personnel lift the patient into the seat formed and patient is removed from area (see Fig. 10.2B).

2. Follow-up

   a. Listen to the "All clear" announcement after a drill or follow specific instructions from the fire department or supervisor regarding the return of patients. ("This area is safe for patients and staff.")

   b. Reduce the potential for fire-related injuries by doing the following:

      (1) Follow and enforce the smoking policy. Most facilities have adopted a *No Smoking* policy to promote a smoke-free environment for patients and employees.

      (2) Know the location of fire alarm boxes and type of fire extinguishers available.

      (3) Know the location of the fire exits.

      (4) Be familiar with the hospital fire safety program and protocols for evacuation.

      (5) Keep hallways free of unnecessary supplies, furniture, and other obstacles.

      (6) Check to see that electrical equipment is operating safely. *(Planning saves valuable time and improves overall performance.)*

   c. Participate, when possible, in fire drills. Fire safety education programs are necessary to meet the requirements of accrediting agencies, such as The Joint Commission. *(Learning experiences are provided through participation in fire drills and formal critiques of the activity.)*

3. Evaluation

   a. The immediate environment of the patient is safe from potential fire hazards. *(Fire safety practices help prevent fires.)*

   b. In the event of a fire, established protocols are followed. *(The emergency will be handled rapidly and appropriately.)*

Box 10.10 **Fire Prevention Guidelines for Nurses**

- Keep the phone number for reporting fires visible on the telephone at all times.
- Know the agency's fire drill and evacuation plan.
- Know the location of all fire alarms, exits, and fire extinguishers.
- Use the mnemonic *RACE* to set priorities in case of fire:
  R: Rescue and remove all patients in immediate danger.
  A: Activate the alarm. Always do this before attempting to extinguish even a minor fire.
  C: Confine the fire by closing doors and windows and turning off all oxygen and electrical equipment.
  E: Extinguish the fire using an extinguisher.
- Memorize the mnemonic *PASS* to operate the fire extinguisher:
  P: Pull the pin to unlock the handle.
  A: Aim low at the base of the fire.
  S: Squeeze the handle.
  S: Sweep the unit from side to side.

Housekeeping responsibilities include eliminating all unnecessary combustible material; maintenance responsibilities include ensuring the proper functioning of fire protection devices, such as alarms, extinguishers, and sprinklers. It is mandatory to identify, light, and unlock exits. Cooking and laundry equipment, filters, and air ducts are to be kept free of lint and grease. It is obligatory to inspect and maintain all mechanical and electrical equipment regularly to keep fire hazards to a minimum.

All employees need to know the telephone number or procedure for reporting a fire and the location of the nearest alarms and firefighting equipment. In addition, health care workers must know their roles in the overall hospital evacuation plan. Checking for fire hazards on an ongoing basis is a must.

An important element in any fire safety program is an understanding of what type of fire extinguisher to use on different types of fires. Use the appropriate fire extinguisher for each type of fire:

- Paper, wood, and cloth fires require a type A fire extinguisher.
- Flammable liquid fires, such as those caused by grease and anesthetics, require a type B fire extinguisher.
- Electrical fires require a type C fire extinguisher.

Fig. 10.2 The two-person evacuation carry. (A) Hands positioned to form two-person evacuation swing. (B) Patient is seated firmly on swing and holds nurses by shoulders for emergency evacuation.

- Fire extinguishers marked ABC are acceptable for use on any type of fire.

Knowledge of which type of extinguisher is on the unit before a fire occurs is vital. Most fire safety programs afford health care workers the opportunity to handle the different types of fire extinguishers.

Certain areas of the health care facility require additional fire safety programs and precautions. Fire and smoke inhalation are potential problems associated with the use of lasers in surgery and with oxygen therapy. Other common ignition sources in the operating area are electric cautery equipment and high-intensity light cords. In the event of a fire, patients on life-support systems may need manual respiratory support with an Ambu bag.

By remembering the mnemonic **RACE** (**R**escue patients, sound the **A**larm, **C**onfine the fire, and **E**xtinguish or **E**vacuate), the LPN/LVN is prepared when safety is threatened by fire. In the event of fire, rescue patients who are in *immediate* danger, and then follow the facility's procedure for activating the fire alarm and reporting the location and extent of the fire. Take measures to contain or extinguish the fire if no immediate threat to safety exists; these measures include closing doors and windows, turning off oxygen and electrical equipment, and using the appropriate fire extinguisher (Fig. 10.3).

Fig. 10.3 Fire extinguisher.

The mnemonic **PASS** (**P**ull the pin, **A**im low, **S**queeze handle, **S**weep the unit) will help the nurse remember how to operate the fire extinguisher (see Box 10.10).

 Home Care Considerations

Fire Safety

- Today, as more patients are discharged with follow-up care to be provided in the home, the nurse has an excellent opportunity to evaluate fire safety practices in the home environment. Patients who are elderly or who have mobility limitations often need your assistance to achieve an environment free of potential fire hazards.
- Give instructions about the proper use of monitoring or therapy equipment used.
- See that several electrical circuits are used to prevent overloading of any single one.
- Do not use electrical appliances and equipment near sinks, bathtubs, or showers.
- Review smoking practices and give instructions to not smoke in bed or when sleepy.
- Do not permit smoking by the patient, family, or visitors in areas where oxygen is used.
- Advise against the use of electrical appliances (e.g., electric razors) around oxygen.
- Encourage the installation of fire alarms, smoke detectors, and carbon monoxide detectors, and the purchase of a portable fire extinguisher.
- Have the family plan fire escape routes from each room and practice exit drills. Establish a place to meet outside to verify that everyone is safe.
- Teach *stop*, *drop*, and *roll* to extinguish fire on clothing.
- Do not place electrical cords under carpeting.
- Allow only certified electricians to work on wiring.
- Avoid using candles for light or heat, and never leave a burning candle unattended.

Enforcement of the facility's smoking policy and monitoring for potential electrical hazards help prevent fires. Frayed or broken electrical cords or a faulty piece of equipment should never be used. Notify the maintenance department of any defects in the equipment, and report any shocks felt while using equipment. The nurse must enforce no-smoking policies. The safety of patients and caregivers depends on the staff's knowledge of fire prevention guidelines and procedures (see the Home Care Considerations box).

ACCIDENTAL POISONING

The CDC defines a poison as "any substance, including medications, that is harmful to your body if too much is eaten, inhaled, injected, or absorbed through the skin. An unintentional poisoning occurs when a person taking or giving too much of a substance did not mean to cause harm" (CDC, 2015). According to the National Capital Poison Center, the 2018 poison statistics show that approximately 2.1 million Americans contacted poison control centers by phone. Of those calls, 6.4 poison exposures/1000 population occurred with 37.4 poison exposures in children younger than 6 years/1000 children (National Capital Poison Center, 2019). Although legislation passed in the early 1970s required the use of child safety packaging for certain substances, a significant number of accidental poisonings continue to occur. Emergency department visits for medication poisoning are twice as common as household substance poisonings among children. Statistics for children under the age of 6 years indicate that the most frequent age group affected by poisoning are 1- and 2-year-olds. Specific antidotes and treatments are now available for all types of poisons; note that syrup of ipecac is no longer recommended for use (see the Patient Teaching box on nonuse of ipecac). The 2019 statistics from the National Capital Poison Center also indicate that teens and adults saw the highest death rate caused by unintentional poisonings. Ninety-one percent of all unintentional poisonings are related to drugs (over-the-counter and prescription).

 Patient Teaching

Nonuse of Ipecac at Home

According to the National Capital Poison Center:

- The American Academy of Pediatrics and the American Association of Poison Control Centers recommend that ipecac syrup not be kept in homes for available use.
- The US Food and Drug Administration (FDA) is considering making ipecac syrup available to the public by prescription only.
- Most pharmacies no longer carry ipecac syrup.
- The first action recommended in the event of ingestion of a poison is to call the poison control center at 1-800-222-1222.

From National Capital Poison Center: Ipecac syrup. Retrieved from www.poison.org/prepared/ipecac.asp.

The older adult is also at risk. Changes associated with aging interfere with the individual's ability to absorb and excrete drugs. Some older adults share medications with friends or limit their medications because of the expense. Changes in eyesight sometimes lead to an accidental ingestion. If elderly patients have any memory impairment, they are likely to forget when they last took either prescribed or over-the-counter medication.

Hospitalized patients and those in other types of health care facilities are at risk for accidental poisoning because of poisonous substances in the environment. Cleaning solutions and disinfectants must be labeled and stored properly. To prevent poisoning, toxic agents are removed from areas where accidental poisoning is possible. Do not remove toxic or poisonous substances from their original containers because incorrect labeling is one of the likely results, and never use substances from unmarked containers.

Drugs are potentially hazardous if prepared or administered inappropriately. Human carelessness causes errors of both types. Always follow medication administration procedures (see Chapter 17). Be sure to attend staff in-service programs that present new drugs or provide updated information on frequently used drugs.

Poison control centers are valuable sources of information when poisoning occurs or is suspected. Nurses must ensure that the closest poison control center phone number is posted clearly in the patient's home and in the health care facility. Information received from the center helps in treatment and in referral. Most health care facilities also have posted instructions about how to handle poisoning cases (Box 10.11). Additional information on poisoning can be found in Chapter 16.

DISASTER PLANNING

Disaster planning, or emergency preparedness, enables rescuers to respond effectively and efficiently when confronted with a disaster situation. A disaster situation is an uncontrollable, unexpected, psychologically shocking event that is unique and likely to have a significant impact on a variety of health care facilities. Examples of natural threats to safety are earthquakes, hurricanes, floods, and tornados. Bombings, arson, riots, shootings, and hostage taking are acts of violence carried out by people and do not always affect a facility's day-to-day operations.

Factors that affect disaster response include the time of the day; the scope and duration of the triggering event; readiness of the health care facility, personnel, and equipment; preparations for appropriate procedures; and the extent to which the various community agencies and institutions collaborate with one another. Health care facilities are expected to receive victims and survivors and to assist rescuers.

Box 10.11   Accidental Poisoning Interventions

ACTION (RATIONALE)

1. When a poisoning occurs:
   a. Obtain an accurate history. (Identifies possible antidote[s] and method of treatment needed.)
      (1) Identify the route (e.g., injected, ingested, inhaled), type, and amount of poisonous substance(s) received.
      (2) Determine how long ago the poisoning happened.
      (3) Obtain a history of allergies, prescribed medications, medical problems, and general state of physical and mental health.
   b. Assess for changes in mental status and the presence of motor and sensory deficits. (Incomplete data possibly result in incorrect identification of patient's health needs.)
   c. Notify the poison control center and follow facility protocols (see the Patient Teaching box on nonuse of ipecac). *(Treatment guidelines will be furnished.)*
   d. Do not induce vomiting if poisoning is related to the following substances: household cleaners, lye, furniture polish, grease, or petroleum products. *(Vomiting increases risk of internal burns.)*
   e. Do not induce vomiting in an unconscious individual. *(Vomiting increases danger of aspiration.)*
2. Perform hand hygiene. (Reduces spread of microorganisms.)
3. Document procedure. (Note procedure and patient's response.)
4. Follow-up
   a. Continue to monitor vital signs and response to treatment. *(Ongoing assessment is a part of the treatment.)*
   b. Reduce the potential for accidental poisoning by doing the following:

   (1) Be aware of potentially poisonous substances (e.g., drugs, plants, and cleaning solutions).
   (2) Inform patients and families about how to handle a poisoning emergency.
   (3) Ensure that poisonous substances are labeled, locked, and out of the reach of children. (It is possible to greatly reduce the risk of accidental poisoning. Quick and appropriate action often decreases the effects of the poisoning.)
   c. Know where emergency instructions are located. (Procedures and guidelines for handling the emergency are outlined.)
   d. Know the number of the poison control center (National Poison Control Center: 1-800-222-1222; www.poison.org) or call 911 and be prepared to provide information about the poison. *(The poison control center provides information needed to treat the patient, and all dispatchers offer referral assistance.)*
   e. The immediate environment is safe from potential poisoning hazards when poisonous substances are labeled, locked, and properly stored. *(Safety practices reduce the risk of accidental poisoning.)*

SPECIAL CONCERNS

- Always follow drug administration policies and procedures. Have your dosage calculations checked, especially if a mixed or prepared drug is to be infused.
- Keep informed of new medications and recommended dosages.
- Properly label and store cleaning solutions and disinfectants.
- Never use substances from unmarked containers.

Disasters are referred to as external or internal. The external disaster originates outside the health care facility and results in an influx of casualties brought to the facility (e.g., an explosion in a chemical plant, a tornado, a train accident). The emergency department is the main focus of activity. Typically, there is no immediate safety threat to staff, patients, or hospital property.

The internal disaster represents an extraordinary situation that is brought about by events within the health care facility, such as a fire. In many cases, the organization's ability to function normally is threatened. An internal disaster has the ability to threaten the safety of patients, visitors, staff, and facility property.

Disaster planning consists of putting appropriate measures into place to ensure that health care facilities and personnel have the capacity to manage a disaster effectively (Boxes 10.12 and 10.13). Most state and federal regulators require health care personnel to conduct disaster drills on a routine basis to prepare to meet their responsibilities effectively. Personnel must be familiar with the location and the contents of the facility's **disaster manual** (sometimes called the Emergency Response Plan or Emergency Management

Plan). This manual specifies chain of command, callback procedures, assignment procedure, departmental responsibilities, patient evacuation procedure and routes, procedures for the receipt and management of casualties, and policies related to the overall management of supplies and equipment.

Various **codes** (a system of notification to be transmitted rapidly) are used by health care facilities to alert personnel to the various emergencies affecting the facility. All personnel in a health care facility must be knowledgeable of the code system and how to act in response to codes.

TERRORISM

Terrorism, or the possibility of a terrorist attack, is viewed as an environmental health threat. **Terrorism** is a violent or dangerous act used to intimidate or coerce a person or government to further a political or social agenda. Before 1990 and the Gulf War, the possibility of the United States coming under attack from terrorist groups using biological, chemical, or nuclear weapons seemed remote. After the terrorist attacks on the World Trade Center in New York City and the Pentagon on

Box 10.12 Disaster Planning Interventions

ACTION (RATIONALE)

1. Planning
   a. Review facility disaster plan frequently to update knowledge. The development of the disaster preparedness plan is an evolving and ongoing process. The purpose of disaster preparedness planning is to prepare the facility and health care workers for external and internal disasters. *(Information helps health care workers anticipate their roles in the event of a disaster.)*
   b. Know your own particular responsibilities in a disaster emergency. *(Valuable time is saved and overall performance improved.)*
   c. Participate, when possible, in disaster drills. Learning experiences are provided through disaster drills and formal critiques of the responses. *(Drills are helpful in evaluating the overall safety program and are required by accrediting agencies.)* Disaster drills may be initiated on a particular nursing unit, facility wide, community wide, or even statewide.
   d. Participation in a crisis support group is desirable if directly involved in a disaster or a disaster response. Individuals often experience some level of emotional or critical incident stress. *(Crisis support teams or groups encourage staff to share thoughts and feelings related to the experience [debriefing].)*
2. **Follow facility disaster plan in the event of a disaster.** (Disaster plan outlines procedures to follow and is most effective when personnel respond appropriately.)
   a. Identify the type of disaster emergency by recognizing the code that is used to announce it. (Unfamiliarity with the codes tends to result in loss of valuable time and injury to patients or personnel.)

   b. Identify each patient's age, sensory impairments, level of mobility, ability to comprehend instructions, and overall need for protection. *(Helps you to protect and assist patients in interpreting environmental stimuli relevant to safety.)*
   c. If indicated, assess patients for possible discharge or transfer. Protection of inpatients, and casualties from a disaster, is a top priority. *(Space may be needed for disaster victims.)*
   d. Provide clear explanations to patients and visitors in a calm manner. (The amount of information patients and families have about the situation [drill, disaster event] affects their ability to cooperate and participate in any planned or unplanned activity.)
   e. If a disaster occurs when you are off duty, follow your facility protocols for reporting in (i.e., some facilities require you to report for duty at your regularly scheduled times, whereas others require you to contact your manager for instruction). Community agencies and resources are incorporated into the overall plan. *(Additional personnel [e.g., student nurses and clinical faculty] in some cases assist with inpatient care to free staff for more critical disaster victims.)*
   f. If an internal disaster occurs, assist with planned evacuations as needed. *(Some disasters necessitate moving patients to a safer area.)*
   g. Listen for the "All clear" announcement after a disaster drill. *(This indicates that the drill is over.)*
3. **Evaluation.** Compare actual outcomes and performances with disaster preparedness plan (usually a critique session is held). *(Evaluation allows facility to examine whether plan accomplished goals and objectives; permits necessary changes to be made.)*

Box 10.13 Variations for Disaster Planning: Nursing Home

Nursing home residents also sometimes need evacuation and relocation in the case of an internal disaster. The successful nursing home disaster preparedness plan, like those for hospitals, outlines the sequence of events to be followed:

- Residents need some type of identification (picture identification or identification bracelet, such as those used in the memory support unit for patients diagnosed with Alzheimer disease).
- At the designated triage site, nurses decide where residents will go.

- Residents sometimes need admission to a hospital or other building, such as a school or church, for temporary shelter and care.
- The disaster plan must include instructions and guidelines for what is to be done after the relocation is completed.
- Notification of families and physicians is critical.
- A log is kept to document events. List the name of the patient, who and how they were transported, and where patient was sent so family and physicians are aware of their location and transfers as they occur.

September 11, 2001, the government implemented the Homeland Security Act of 2002. Its purpose was to have a single agency to oversee the development of a comprehensive approach to a large domestic incident. The Department of Homeland Security is concerned primarily with preventing and managing potential attacks by an individual or small group on one of our cities, large sporting events, schools, or units of our military forces.

BIOTERRORISM

Bioterrorism is the use of biological agents to create fear and to threaten. Health care facilities must be prepared to treat mass casualties from such an attack. A facility's emergency management plan provides details on how to respond to a terrorist attack: for example, determining the agent used, determining the time and location of the attack and the affected population, obtaining and delivering supplies, and providing treatment. Education and training are required to prepare nurses to respond to an attack by taking the necessary steps to initiate an agency's emergency management plan.

Bioterrorist Attacks

The nurse must be prepared to make accurate and timely assessments in any type of setting in the event of a bioterrorist attack. OSHA has health safety and topics information concerning the biological agents plague, ricin, anthrax, tularemia, smallpox, and viral hemorrhagic fever (VHF). A bioterrorist attack may resemble a natural outbreak initially, but sometimes the microorganism used is modified to obtain increased virulence or have resistance to antibiotics or vaccines. Biological attacks can be *overt* (announced) or *covert* (unannounced). In the case of an overt attack, rapid assessment of its real scope is necessary, followed by an appropriate response. Covert attacks become obvious only after victims seek medical care, that is, after the incubation period has passed and clinical signs begin to appear. In both cases, the nurse must recognize and understand how to manage high-risk syndromes (groups of signs and symptoms that result from a common cause or appear together to present a clinical picture of a disease) (Box 10.14). Acutely ill patients representing the earliest cases after a covert attack usually seek care in emergency departments. Less ill patients or those at the onset stage of an illness sometimes seek care in primary care settings or try to manage the signs and symptoms on their own.

Basic epidemiologic (the distribution and determinants of health-related states and events in populations) principles are used to assess whether a patient's presentation of symptoms is typical of an endemic (the expected or normal incidence native to or occurring naturally

---

Box 10.14   High-Risk Syndromes for Bioterrorism

1. **Anthrax** (acute infectious disease caused by *Bacillus anthracis*, a spore-forming, gram-positive bacillus). Humans become infected through skin contact, ingestion, or inhalation. Person-to-person transmission of inhalational disease does not occur. Direct exposure to vesicle secretions of skin anthrax potentially results in secondary cutaneous infection.
   Clinical Features. Inhalation: Incubation period is usually less than a week but can be up to 2 months. Symptoms include flulike symptoms (e.g., low-grade fever, nonproductive cough, fatigue, diaphoresis) with possible brief interim improvement; within 2–4 days, abrupt onset of respiratory failure and hemodynamic collapse occur. Gram-positive bacilli are found on blood culture tests. *Cutaneous:* Local skin involvement is common on head, forearms, and hands; localized itching is followed by a papular lesion that becomes vesicular and within 2–6 days becomes a depressed black eschar. *Gastrointestinal:* Incubation period is usually 1–7 days; it causes abdominal pain, nausea, vomiting, anorexia, and fever after eating contaminated food (usually meat), bloody diarrhea or hematemesis, and gram-positive bacilli are found on blood culture. Abdominal pain becomes severe as symptoms progress.

2. **Botulism** (caused by *Clostridium botulinum,* an encapsulated anaerobic gram-positive, spore-forming bacterium that produces a potent neuroparalytic). Food-borne botulism is the most common form. Airborne and wound are other forms of botulism that may occur.
   Clinical Features. Food-borne botulism symptoms can occur within 6 h to 10 days after exposure and cause abdominal cramping, diarrhea, and other gastrointestinal symptoms. Food-borne and inhalation botulism cause the following: drooping eyelids, weakened jaw clench, difficulty swallowing or speaking; blurred vision and double vision; symmetric paralysis of arms first, followed by respiratory muscles, then legs; respiratory dysfunction from

respiratory muscle paralysis; *no sensory deficits or change in alertness or body temperature.* Neurologic symptoms often begin 12–36 h after ingestion of food-borne botulism and 24–72 h after inhalation of the airborne form. The disease is not transmitted from person to person.

3. **Plague** (an acute bacterial disease caused by the gram-negative bacillus *Yersinia pestis).* Bubonic plague occurs from a flea bite or through a break in the skin. A bioterrorism-related outbreak is likely to be airborne (pneumonic plague) and can spread among people via large aerosol droplets.
   Clinical Features. Features include fever, cough, headache, chest pain, weakness, hemoptysis, and mucopurulent or watery sputum with gram-negative rods in a Gram stain test. Pneumonia develops rapidly after exposure to the bacteria and may cause respiratory failure and death if early treatment is not initiated.

4. **Smallpox** (an acute viral illness caused by the variola virus). Disease has the potential to cause severe morbidity in a nonimmune population. Transmission via the airborne route is most common, but transmission can occur through direct contact. A single case of smallpox is a public health emergency.
   Clinical Features. Incubation period is 7–17 days, in which time the infected person is not contagious. Initial symptoms last 2–4 days and include fever, malaise, and myalgia (muscle aches). The symptoms then progress to a rash that starts on the tongue and in the mouth and throat. The rash progresses into pustules and spreads to the face and extremities (including palms and soles). During this time, the infected person is most contagious. The rash typically scabs over in 1–2 weeks. Smallpox is transmitted by large and small respiratory droplets. Patient-to-patient transmission is likely from airborne and droplet exposure and by contact with skin lesions or secretions.

Data from Centers for Disease Control and Prevention (CDC): *Bioterrorism agents/diseases.* Retrieved from http://emergency.cdc.gov/agent/agentlist.asp#.

to a specific area or environment) disease or is an unusual event that calls for investigation. The possibility of a bioterrorism-related outbreak should be considered if trends or events such as the following are observed:

- A rapidly increasing incidence of a disease (e.g., within hours or days) in a normally healthy population
- An unusual increase in the number of people seeking care, especially with fever, respiratory, or gastrointestinal symptoms
- An epidemic disease, or a disease that emerges rapidly at an uncharacteristic time or in an unusual pattern
- Lower incidence among patients who were indoors, in areas with filtered or closed ventilation, compared with people who were outdoors
- Clusters of patients arriving from a single locale
- Large numbers of rapidly fatal cases
- Any patient with development of a disease that is relatively uncommon and has bioterrorism potential

The nurse must have the ability to recognize a casualty of a biological attack and carry out roles and responsibilities quickly and efficiently. Timely communication is critical for alerting the medical and general community to a bioterrorist attack. Health care agencies' emergency plans outline the departments to contact in the event of an attack and who is responsible for reporting the suspected occurrence to the local public health authorities.

Infection prevention and control practices are critical in the event of a biological attack. Manage all patients with suspected or confirmed bioterrorism-related illnesses with standard precautions (see Chapter 7). For certain diseases, such as smallpox or pneumonic plague, airborne and contact isolation precautions are needed. Although a number of infections associated with biological agents are not transmissible from patient to patient, in general, be sure to limit the transport and movement of patients to what is essential for treatment and care. Also ensure that staff uses all safety precautions necessary to protect themselves and those in the immediate surroundings.

TERRORISM BY NUCLEAR EXPOSURE

One example of how the threat of nuclear terrorism possibly would manifest is an attack on a domestic nuclear weapon facility. Another is the use of a so-called "dirty bomb," which is a radiation-dispersal device that couples nuclear waste with a conventional bomb.

A patient is contaminated by radiation from a source on the body or the clothing, from ingesting it, or by absorbing it through a skin opening. The effects on the patient are determined by the amount of radiation absorbed (absorbed radiation is measured by the gray [Gy], equal to 100 rads). When less than 0.75 Gy is absorbed, patients usually do not have any symptoms. Patients who absorb 8 Gy usually die, and an absorption of 30 Gy is always fatal.

The patient who absorbs more than 0.75 Gy is at risk for development of acute radiation syndrome; the severity and nature of symptoms vary, depending on the amount of radiation absorbed:

- *Cerebrovascular and central nervous systems:* Cerebral edema, hyperpyrexia, hypotension, confusion, and disorientation.
- *Gastrointestinal:* Loss of mucosal barrier and cells that line the intestine, which results in fluid and electrolyte loss, vomiting, hematemesis, diarrhea, melena, loss of normal flora, and sepsis.
- *Hematopoietic:* Deficiency of white blood cells and platelets, which leads to bleeding, anemia, infections, impaired wound healing, and immunodeficiency.
- *Skin:* Loss of epidermis and possibly the dermis.

During the prodromal phase immediately after exposure, signs and symptoms in more than one of these areas typically appear. The latent phase, when all symptoms generally disappear for a few days to a few weeks, follows in 1 or 2 days. Then, in the illness phase, the signs and symptoms reappear and intensify. After this peak, the patient either begins to recover or dies. Death typically occurs from infection or other complications related to the exposure. OSHA requires that hospitals have an emergency plan for treating patients contaminated with radioactive substances. A decontamination unit is set up near the emergency department.

CHEMICAL TERRORISM

Chemical terrorism or exposure occurs by several different methods. Health care facilities have specific guidelines that must be followed in the event of patient exposure to chemical agents. Gross decontamination and formal and fine decontamination are methods that the nurse may be involved in implementing in the event of chemical exposure. *Gross decontamination* refers to a continuous shower of low-volume and high-volume water and removal of the patient's clothing. *Formal decontamination* and *fine decontamination* follow gross decontamination. Formal decontamination may incorporate several steps in the cleaning process, including water spray, cleaning solution, and scrubbing the patient with brushes. Fine decontamination is performed in specific isolated areas of the facility and includes cleaning of the eyes, ears, and fingernails and inspecting body orifices, and swabbing mucous membranes of the nose and mouth (OSHA, n.d.).

The following are several types of agents that may possibly be used in chemical terrorism:

- *Pulmonary agents:* Include the gases chlorine (Cl), phosgene, ammonia, and hydrochloric acid. These agents cause shortness of breath, chest tightness, wheezing, and, in some cases, pulmonary edema. Symptoms sometimes take 2 to 24 hours to appear. Fluid in the lungs leads to hypovolemia and hypotension. Patients often need mechanical ventilation and supportive care.
- *Incapacitating agents:* Include 3-quinuclidinyl benzilate, a glycolate anticholinergic compound typically known by its NATO code *BZ* and *agent 15* (an Iraqi version of BZ). These agents impair rather than kill or seriously injure victims. The effects include decreased organ function, hyperthermia, hallucinations, altered perceptions, and erratic behavior.

- *Cyanide agents:* Hydrogen cyanide is one example; these agents form cyanide when metabolized and are either ingested or inhaled. A patient in severe respiratory distress without cyanosis has probably been exposed to cyanide. Cyanide has a pungent odor similar to bitter almonds or peaches. When an individual is exposed to a high concentration, death occurs within 5 to 10 minutes.
- *Nerve agents:* Taubin, sarin, soman, and V-agents are some of the most toxic nerve agents, and they cause death in a matter of minutes. Symptoms include increased saliva production, chest pressure, rhinorrhea, vomiting, muscle weakness, incontinence, and convulsions. Symptoms usually appear up to 10 hours after exposure to a low concentration.
- *Vesicant agents:* Sulfur mustard (H), distilled mustard (HD), nitrogen mustard (HN 1, 3), mustargen (HN 2), lewisite (L), and phosgene oxime (OX) are in this group. Vesicants are more lethal than pulmonary agents and cyanide agents because they sometimes remain in the environment for weeks, which results in a continuing source of exposure. Sulfur mustard smells like mustard or garlic, whereas another agent smells like geraniums, and yet another has a peppery smell. Vesicants affect the skin, the eyes, and the airway, and large doses damage the bone marrow. These agents have the capacity to cause the formation of vesicles that progress to severe tissue necrosis and sloughing. Symptoms of sulfur mustard exposure appear in 4 to 8 hours, but cellular damage occurs in 2 minutes with agents such as lewisite and phosgene.

The CDC classifies chemical agents according to their ease of dissemination, likelihood of morbidity and mortality, panic potential, and level of public health requirement. These classes include category A (high risk), category B (low risk), and category C (agents identified as being able to be engineered for widespread dissemination). Examples include:

Category A: Anthrax, botulism, bubonic plague, smallpox, tularemia or rabbit fever, and viral hemorrhagic fever

Category B: Abrin toxin from Abrus Precatorius, food bacterium, Ricin, water supply threats, viral encephalitis, and Glanders

Category C: H1N1 influenza, SARS, Coronavirus, chemical weapons (i.e., VX, mustard gas, hydrogen cyanide)

❖ NURSING PROCESS FOR PATIENT SAFETY

The role of the LPN/LVN in the nursing process as stated is that the LPN/LVN will:

- Participate in planning care for patients based on patient needs.
- Review patient's plan of care and recommend revisions as needed.
- Review and follow defined prioritization for patient care.

- Use clinical pathways, care maps, or care plans to guide and review patient care.

◆ ASSESSMENT

Using the nursing process, the LPN/LVN can reduce the risk of injury to patients and staff. Seek to determine which patients are at risk for injury as soon as possible. Identify actual and potential threats to the patient's safety, the effect of the underlying illness on the patient's safety, and the risks for the patient's developmental stage. Specific interventions help ensure a safe environment. If safety is threatened, follow established guidelines to resolve the situation (Nursing Care Plan 10.1).

◆ PATIENT PROBLEMS

Identification of defining characteristics from the data directs the LPN/LVN's efforts to identify appropriate patient problems. Include specific causes of a patient's safety risk among the patient problems to individualize nursing care. For example, a patient with an unsteady gait is at risk for falling or injury. Patient problems related to patient safety could include the following:

- Compromised Physical Mobility
- Potential for Falling
- Potential for Harm or Damage to the Body

◆ EXPECTED OUTCOMES AND PLANNING

In the plan of care, identify nursing interventions that prevent threats to safety and meet safety needs. Perform planning and goal setting with the patient, the family, and other members of the health care team. Goals and priorities are based on the risk to patient safety and health promotion. The overall goal for a patient with a threat to safety is remaining free from injury (see Nursing Care Plan 10.1).

◆ IMPLEMENTATION

Nursing interventions are designed to promote the safety of the patient in the home and the health care setting. These interventions include health promotions, developmental considerations, environmental protection, and education of family members or patient caregivers (see Nursing Care Plan 10.1).

◆ EVALUATION

Evaluate nursing interventions for reducing threats to safety by comparing the patient's response to the expected outcomes for each goal of care. Assess patient for signs and symptoms of injury and assess the environment for physical hazards continually throughout hospitalization. Remove the hazards and modify the environment as necessary.

Observe for correct application of SRDs. Observe skin, monitor pulses, assess the restrained body part every 30 minutes, and release the restrained body part every 2 hours. Continuously monitor for complications of immobility.

Nursing Care Plan 10.1 | **Patient Safety**

This care plan has been adapted for the patient who is at risk for injury.

PATIENT PROBLEM

Potential for Harm or Damage to the Body, related to disease process, weakness, lack of mental acuity, medications, or age.

Patient Goals and Expected Outcomes	Nursing Interventions	Evaluation
Patient or caregiver will demonstrate knowledge and understanding of potential hazards and will practice preventive measures, or will be protected from injury as necessary during hospitalization	Assess the following: 1. Patient's mental, visual, and auditory acuity (fall assessment, see Box 10.2). 2. Patient's level of consciousness. 3. Patient's ability to perform activities of daily living (ADLs), exercise, and ambulation. Prevent clutter; wipe up spills; provide adequate lighting. Orient patient to surroundings and assess effectiveness of reality orientation. Maintain side rails (depending on facility policy) and bed alarm. Maintain bed in low position when care is not being given. Place patient in room close to nurses' station. Assist patient with ADLs as needed. Determine the need for assistive devices such as a walker, cane, or wheelchair. Obtain medication history and administer medications according to agency policy. Document nursing interventions for medications and monitor side effects. Offer fluids q 2 hr while awake unless contraindicated. Offer use of commode, bedpan, or urinal q 2 hr while awake.	Patient demonstrates understanding of potential health hazards. Patient practices injury prevention for self. Patient remains injury free.

CRITICAL THINKING QUESTIONS

1. The nurse walking down the hall hears a patient calling out for help. The nurse assesses the situation and realizes that the patient does not remember how to use the call light. What factors possibly contribute to the patient's inability to remember, and how should the nurse teach the patient to use the call light?
2. The nurse enters the patient's room to answer the call bell and sees the patient frantically pointing to the trash can next to the bed. The nurse smells smoke and sees small flames. What should be done to help prevent fires, and what should the nurse do in this situation?

Get Ready For The Nclex® Examination!

Key Points

- Discuss safety measures for coping with violence in the workplace.
- Prevention of falls, electrical injuries, fires, burns, and accidental poisoning is key to maintaining a safe environment.
- Infants, young children, older adults, and the ill or injured are at risk for falling.
- Proper patient orientation includes information about the use of the call light and bed controls. Place frequently used items within reach of patients.
- Question all patients regarding allergies. Ask specifically about food and latex allergies.
- Keep adjustable beds in the low position except when care is given.
- Gait belts are an added safety feature to use when assisting patients to ambulate.
- Consider designing a restraint-free environment before applying an SRD.

- Ensure your priority is patient safety or the safety of others when applying an SRD.
- SRD use has the potential to result in increased restlessness, disorientation, agitation, anxiety, and feelings of powerlessness.
- Once SRDs are applied to a patient, document the position of the device, circulation, physical and mental status, and ongoing need for the device.
- When extremity SRDs are applied, place gauze or padding around the extremity and secure the ends of the ties to the bed frame, not to the side rails.
- Remove SRDs at least every 2 hours and assess the skin. Do not leave the patient unattended during this time.
- Know agency policy and procedures regarding SRD use and documentation.
- Electrical accidents often are prevented by reporting frayed or broken electrical cords or any shocks felt while using equipment.
- Fire-related injuries can be reduced by knowing the location of exits, fire alarm boxes, and fire extinguishers.

- By remembering the mnemonic RACE (**R**escue patients, sound the **A**larm, **C**onfine the fire, and **E**xtinguish or **E**vacuate), you will be prepared when safety is threatened by a fire.
- Participation in fire and disaster drills helps staff become familiar with established protocols.
- Poison control centers are valuable sources of information when poisoning is suspected or has occurred.
- A terrorist attack is a potential environmental health threat.
- Bioterrorism, or the use of biological agents to create fear and threat, is the most likely form a terrorist attack will take.
- Several national organizations, including OSHA, NIOSH, and the CDC, provide guidelines that help reduce safety hazards in the workplace.

Additional Learning Resources

SG Go to your Study Guide for additional learning activities to help you master this chapter content.

Be sure to visit the Evolve site at http://evolve.elsevier.com/Cooper/foundations/ for additional online resources.

Review Questions FOR THE NCLEX® Examination

1. **The nurse is caring for a patient on a ventilator and reads the order "restrain prn." The nurse considers which factor when caring for this patient?** *(Select all that apply.)*
   1. SRDs often decrease anxiety because the patient feels safer.
   2. All older adult patients need some type of SRD at night.
   3. Allow as much freedom of movement as possible when applying SRDs.
   4. When using soft SRDs to prevent pulling of the ventilator tubing, tie them to the side rail.
   5. Ensure that the nurse's two fingers can be inserted between the SRD and the patient's skin.
   6. Assign confused or disoriented patients to rooms near the nurses' station.
   7. Release the physical restraint at least every 4 hours.
   8. Ensure an order is renewed a minimum of every 48 hours while the restraints are necessary.

2. **The LPN/LVN is reviewing the care plan of the patient who has an SRD applied for personal safety. Which is the highest priority goal for this patient?**
   1. Patient will remain free of injury.
   2. Patient will allow SRDs to be used.
   3. Nurse will check SRD every 30 minutes.
   4. Use least restrictive form of SRD possible.

3. **The nurse is documenting on a patient with an SRD. What information must the nurse include in this documentation?**
   1. The nurse's feelings about having used the SRD.
   2. The specific type of SRD used and an assessment of the patient.
   3. Confirmation of a prn order for use of the SRD.
   4. Evidence that the patient was assessed every 8 hours.

4. **When caring for the patient who requires the use of an SRD, what should be included in the patient's plan of care?** *(Select all that apply.)*
   1. Monitor the skin for signs of impairment.
   2. Remove the SRD once every 2 hours.
   3. Secure the ends of the ties to the side rails.
   4. Ensure that the SRD is in place at all times.
   5. Reevaluate the need for the SRD frequently.

5. **The nurse discovers smoke in a soiled utility room across the hall from a patient's room. What should the nurse's initial action be?**
   1. Sound the fire alarm.
   2. Disconnect the oxygen supply.
   3. Use any extinguisher on the fire.
   4. Remove the patient from the area.

6. **The nurse is observing the UAP who is assisting a resident in a long-term care facility to ambulate with a gait belt. Which action by the UAP indicates to the nurse that further instruction is necessary?** *(Select all that apply.)*
   1. The UAP loosely fastens the gait belt around the patient's waist.
   2. The UAP places the gait belt on the resident before assisting the resident to a standing position.
   3. The UAP grasps the gait belt while assisting the resident out of bed.
   4. The UAP fastens the belt around the arm of the chair to prevent the resident from slipping out of the chair.
   5. The UAP explains to the resident that the gait belt is used to prevent injury to the resident and the UAP when assisting with ambulation.

7. **A type C fire extinguisher is required for which type of fire?**
   1. Paper
   2. Cloth
   3. Grease
   4. Electrical

8. **When the staff's knowledge of the fire safety precautions is assessed, which action indicates the need for further fire safety instruction?** *(Select all that apply.)*
   1. Fire exits and corridors are kept clear.
   2. A *No Smoking* sign is posted when oxygen is in use.
   3. A heating pad cord is taped when a frayed area is noted.
   4. Facility smoking policies are a part of the admission procedure for patients.
   5. A UAP evacuated critically ill patients on the elevator during a fire drill.

9. **The home health nurse is assessing a child for the risk of injury. Which factor places a child at greatest risk for specific types of injuries?**
   1. Gender of the child
   2. Overall health
   3. Educational level
   4. Developmental level

10. During the 7 a.m. to 3 p.m. shift on the adult surgical unit, the code is announced for an external disaster emergency. Which event best represents this type of situation?

   1. A school bus accident
   2. A bomb threat in the mail room
   3. A hostage-taking event in the emergency department
   4. An electrical fire in the maintenance department

11. The nurse is providing home poison control instruction to the parent of a 2-year-old boy. Which statement by the parent indicates the need for further teaching?

   1. "I will call the national poison control center if my child ingests a poisonous substance."
   2. "I will call 911 immediately if my child ingests medication that is not intended for him."
   3. "Child safety caps on household cleaner can still be opened by some children."
   4. "I will give my child syrup of ipecac if he ingests a poisonous substance that is not caustic."

12. A 6 year-old patient is brought to the emergency department, by their parents, for treatment of an unintentional poisoning from a cleaning product. When providing care to this patient which actions are appropriate?

   Choose the most likely options for the information missing from the statements below by selecting from the list of options provided.
   The nurse's first action should be to _____ the patient's parents. The _____ should be contacted for recommendations. _____ is no longer a suggested treatment for ingested poisonings of this type.

OPTIONS
Syrup of Ipecac
Obtain a health history from
Patient's family
Poison control center
Contact child protective services
Counteracting medication
Restrain

13. The home health nurse is visiting an older adult patient and her husband. What safety concern is of the highest priority when the nurse is assessing this patient's home environment?

   1. Accidental poisoning
   2. Electrical shock
   3. Accidental falls
   4. Thermal burns

14. The LPN/LVN is reviewing the admission information of a patient. Which information is of most concern to the nurse that this patient is at high risk for falling?

   1. The patient has diabetes.
   2. The patient had a stroke 3 years ago with no complications.
   3. The patient becomes disoriented in the evening hours.
   4. The patient wears eyeglasses and a hearing aid.

15. The occupational health nurse learns of a mercury spill that occurred in the factory in which she is employed. Which action by the nurse is correct?

   1. The nurse cleans the mercury spill with alcohol and ordinary cleaning cloths.
   2. The nurse closes all windows and doors to prevent the mercury spill from spreading out of the area.
   3. The nurse instructs the housekeeping staff to vacuum up the spill.
   4. The nurse evacuates the area and contacts trained personnel to clean up the spill.

Objectives

1. Identify guidelines for admission, transfer, and discharge of a patient.
2. Discuss the concepts of the Health Insurance Portability and Accountability Act (HIPAA).
3. Describe common patient reactions to hospitalization.
4. Identify nursing interventions for common patient reactions to hospitalization.
5. Discuss the nursing process and how it pertains to admitting, discharging, and transferring the patient.
6. Discuss the nurse's responsibilities in performing an admission.
7. Describe how the nurse prepares a patient for transfer to another unit or facility.
8. Discuss discharge planning.
9. Explain how the nurse prepares a patient for discharge.
10. Identify the nurse's role when a patient chooses to leave the hospital against medical advice.

Key Terms

admission (p. 262)
against medical advice (AMA) (p. 277)
continuity of care (p. 271)
discharge (p. 272)
discharge planning (p. 272)
disorientation (dĭs-ŏr-rē-ĕn-TĀ-shŭn, p. 262)

empathy (ĔM-pă-thē, p. 263)
health care facility (p. 262)
home health agency (p. 275)
separation anxiety (p. 262)
third-party payers (p. 271)
transfer (p. 271)

COMMON PATIENT REACTIONS TO ADMISSION TO A HEALTH CARE FACILITY

Admission (entry of a patient into the health care facility) to a hospital or other health care facility (any agency that provides health care) is an anxious time for patients and their families. The patient usually is concerned about health problems or possible health problems and the potential outcome of treatment. Often the patient is having pain or other discomfort. The first contact with nurses and health care workers is important. It provides an opportunity to lessen anxiety and fears and initiate a positive attitude regarding the care to be received.

A way to significantly ease the patient's anxiety and promote cooperation and positive response to treatment is to convey concern for the patient while implementing efficient admission routines. Admission routines that the patient perceives as careless or excessively impersonal tend to heighten anxiety, reduce cooperation, impair response to treatment, and possibly aggravate symptoms.

The nurse's responsibility is to assist the patient in maintaining dignity and a sense of control and in becoming comfortable in the new environment of the health care facility. This environment differs from a patient's home and has new sights, sounds, and smells that may interfere with the patient's comfort.

Each person's reaction to admission to a health care facility is unique. Some common reactions include fear of the unknown, loss of identity, disorientation (mental confusion characterized by inadequate or incorrect perception of place, time, and identity), separation anxiety (fears and apprehension caused by separation from familiar surroundings and significant people), and loneliness. These reactions are related to some of the needs described by Maslow (1970) (see Fig. 1.8).

Fear of the unknown, which causes insecurity, is often the most common reaction. This relates to the need Maslow calls safety. Explanations about facility policies, information about medical orders and procedures, and simple direct answers to common questions from the patient or family help the person to feel more comfortable and in control of the situation. Questions the patient may have include: "How do I work the bed?"; "How do I call the nurse?"; "How or when do I get some food?"; "When can my family visit?"; and "What are they going to do to me next?" Orienting the patient to the new environment and answering these simple questions can alleviate much of the fear and anxiety felt by the patient on admission to the facility.

During the admission process to a health care facility, many patients feel a loss of identity that reflects a need for esteem, love, and belonging. Recognition, as described by Maslow, is part of this need. Sometimes putting the identification (ID) band on the patient's wrist reduces the patient to feeling like the number and name on the ID rather than a person. Explain that the ID is a necessary procedure to provide a positive means of identification and maintain the safety of the patient.

Learn new patient names quickly. Address patients with Mr., Mrs., Ms., or Miss with the last name, and use a first name only at the patient's request. Use of terms such as "honey," "dear," "Gramps," and "Grandma" is never appropriate.

 Lifespan Considerations

Older Adults

Admission, Transfer, and Discharge

- The older adult admitted to the health care facility today is likely to be seriously ill.
- In a normally alert and oriented older adult, medical conditions that necessitate admission to a health care facility often result in some level of disorientation.
- Older adults, who often have some limitation of vision or hearing, are more likely to become agitated or fearful on admission to a health care facility. Many experience relocation stress.
- Transfers, even within the facility, tend to be confusing and upsetting to older adults.
- Hospitalized older adults frequently are concerned that they will be unable to return to their homes and will need institutional placement.
- Appropriate referrals for home nursing, therapy, homemaking, home nutrition programs, or other services are essential for older adults.
- Older adult patients need health care professionals to converse with them slowly and clearly because hearing may be less acute and information may take longer to process. Do not rush older patients; wait for patients to answer questions rather than letting family members answer.
- The change in environment and daily routine sometimes causes disorientation, loss of appetite, or reversal of sleeping-waking patterns.
- The stress of being in a health care facility sometimes is serious for the older patient because of a reduction in adaptive capacity. Helplessness, lack of control, and dependency often emerge, although a large degree of personal control possibly can be restored.
- When an older adult patient is transferred to a new facility, the relocation is also stressful. Ensure that significant support people are still accessible, the patient is oriented thoroughly to new surroundings, the patient is allowed to take along important memorabilia, and the patient has an opportunity to make decisions about care.

Separation anxiety and loneliness are reactions that reflect the needs Maslow identified as belongingness and love. Separation anxiety is very common in young children, but adults and older adults often have this reaction as well. In children, it generally is expressed by crying; with adults, behaviors may include the patient being withdrawn or being very talkative; the older adult sometimes exhibits disorientation or depression.

The company of friends and loved ones is the best antidote to separation anxiety. Liberal visiting hours in health care facilities encourage family and friends to visit. Many facilities allow small children to visit relatives (facility policy and the patient's condition must be considered). Parents should be encouraged to stay with their hospitalized child to prevent the anxiety separation causes and to give the child a feeling of security. In some facilities, pets are allowed to visit. Many long-term facilities have pet therapy visits from organizations or actually have pets that live in the facility.

The licensed practical/vocational nurse (LPN/LVN) has the ability to help reduce the severity of these common reactions to hospitalization with a warm, caring attitude and with courtesy and empathy (ability to recognize and to some extent share the emotions and state of mind of another and to understand the meaning and significance of that person's behavior). To help patients adapt, treat them with respect; maintain their dignity; involve them in the plan of care; and, whenever possible, adjust facility routines to meet their desires. Special considerations for the older adult are listed in the Lifespan Considerations for older adults box.

CULTURAL CONSIDERATIONS FOR THE HOSPITALIZED PATIENT OR LONG-TERM CARE RESIDENT

If the patient does not speak English and is not accompanied by a bilingual family member on admission, contact the appropriate resource (usually the social services department) to secure an interpreter. Culture plays a vital role in the patient's ability to cope with stress and illness. Assist the patient with maintaining cultural practices as much as possible (see Chapter 6 for an in-depth discussion of cultural issues in health care).

ADMITTING A PATIENT

The admission procedure generally begins in the admitting department. The admission department representative is responsible for obtaining vital information from the patient, such as demographic information, insurance information, identifying information (social security number), and emergency contacts. Privacy and confidentiality must be maintained while this information is obtained. An interpreter should be used if the patient does not speak English. Depending on the facility and the time of admission, the collection of this information may become the responsibility of the nurse.

Once the necessary identifying information has been collected, an ID band is placed on the patient's

Cultural Considerations

Admission, Transfer, and Discharge

- It should be noted that any reference to cultural practices among a specific culture are commonalities. Individuals within a culture may or may not possess the same practices, beliefs, or values.
- Consider the decision-making process of the family. Some patients may need extra time for decisions regarding care and procedures if the family unit is important in this process. Other patients may refer to whomever is the authority figure for decision making.
- Some cultures often intertwine religion and culture; therefore, in the interests of cultural sensitivity, include the assessment of the patient's religious beliefs on admission to the health care system.
- Some cultures often value personal relationships over rules and procedures. Be sure to consider the importance of the patient's loved ones when planning care.
- Some cultures believe that leaves have a special significance in healing. The nurse may sometimes find leaves in the clothes and on various parts of the body. Leaves are thought to have mystical power related to regaining or keeping health.
- Some cultures are more likely to feel they are receiving effective treatment when a nurse is seen. In these cultures, a nurse is given more authority and status than a physician, and the patient may be more cooperative with directions given by a nurse. When nursing measures are implemented (e.g., taking the patient's blood pressure), tell the patient what you are doing and that it is for the patient's benefit. Nursing actions are seen as caring and helpful.
- Some cultures associate wheelchairs with sickness. Therefore the patient who is allowed to walk out of the hospital at discharge is more likely to feel that care has been effective.
- A belief with some cultures is that contact with blood, skin disease, and corpses causes illness. These cultures may also believe improper care of the body, including poor diet and lack of sleep, causes illness.
- Some religions observe sundown Friday to sundown Saturday as the Sabbath, which is a time of rest. These patients may avoid the use of any electronic equipment during that time, so the nurse should find alternatives to the use of this equipment if possible.

wrist. The ID band usually contains the patient's full name and date of birth. Some facilities may assign a facility number that also is included on the ID band. Patient allergies typically are identified on a separate red wrist band. This information should be checked and verified by looking at the ID band and asking the patient to state this information (if capable) before procedures and medication administration. Identification of the patient who is unconscious on admission to the facility is delayed until a family member or legal guardian is present.

On admission to a health care facility, the patient signs a consent form that gives permission for general treatment. The Joint Commission (TJC) and Medicare and Medicaid Services require that all hospitals and other health care facilities present a Patient's Bill of Rights to the patient or the patient's legal guardian at the time of admission. Facilities also may have other written forms that are presented, which contain policies and procedures that further inform patients of their rights and of the nurse's responsibilities in ensuring these rights are honored.

The Patient Self-Determination Act of 1991 and the Health Insurance Portability and Accountability Act (HIPAA) also are presented on admission to a health care facility. Facilities that accept Medicare and Medicaid reimbursement are required to present information on The Patient Self-Determination Act. It addresses the patient's right to refuse or accept medical treatment and information regarding advance directives. The facility must refer the patient who requests information about advance directives to the appropriate resources. All patients, regardless of the type of health care facility, must be given and sign a document that verifies receipt of information regarding HIPAA (see Chapter 2 for an explanation of HIPAA).

Some hospitals or surgery centers have telephone admitting. The day before a planned admission, a representative from the admitting office calls the patient at home and gathers all the information needed to begin the records. Instructions are given regarding time to arrive at the facility, items to bring to the facility, and items that are better to leave at home (e.g., jewelry and large sums of money). When the patient arrives the next day, the records and ID band must be verified with the patient for accuracy.

People brought to the emergency department of a hospital sometimes are admitted directly to a patient care room or a special care unit (SCU), intensive care unit (ICU), coronary care unit (CCU), or burn unit. In these situations, a family member, usually the next of kin or the patient's health care representative, provides the admitting office with the necessary information.

When the unit staff are notified that a new patient is en route, they prepare the room for admission of the patient. A room that is neat and clean, of appropriate temperature, with lighting and personal care items in place, makes the patient feel expected and welcome. This makes a good first impression and facilitates the development of a therapeutic nurse-patient relationship.

If special equipment is needed by the new patient, such as oxygen, have it in place and ready when the patient arrives. A patient who arrives on a stretcher needs the bed in the high position; the low bed position is best for a patient who arrives by wheelchair or walking.

Greeting the patient by name and making the patient feel welcome is one of the most important aspects

Box 11.1	Patient Room Orientation

Orientation should include the following:
- Explanation of policies applicable to the patient
- How to adjust the bed and the lights
- How to call the nurse from the bed and the bathroom
- How to operate the telephone and the radio
- How to operate the television
- How to use the intercom system if one is present
- The location of lounge areas
- The location of shower and bathroom facilities
- The relationship of the room to the nurses' station

of the admission procedure. Call patients by their surname unless otherwise directed by the patient. To introduce yourself, give your first name and title. A person who is warmly welcomed is more at ease in this new environment.

Remember that patients do not get ill and need hospitalization at the nurse's convenience. The patient's admission to the unit may occur at any time. Regardless of the time or the activity occurring on the nursing unit, the staff must be courteous to, interested in, and receptive of the new patient. The new patient needs an orientation to the unit and the room (Box 11.1).

The routine of the facility must be explained to the patient and family. Knowledge of when meals are served (or in some facilities the time frame for the patient to call the dietary department to order food to be delivered), when family and friends are allowed to visit, when laboratory tests or diagnostic imaging evaluations are scheduled, when the health care provider usually makes rounds, and the policy on side rails gives the patient a sense of security and lessens anxiety. Many facilities have booklets for patients that explain these routine activities so that patients have a reference for this information. Some booklets include information about the availability of various social services, religious services, and facilities such as cafeteria, library, and gift shop. Some degree of patient teaching also may occur during the admission process (see the Patient Teaching box).

The electronic health record (EHR) may expedite the admission process in the admitting department and on the nursing unit. Information in the EHR is transferred into the admission form used by the admitting department and the nursing admission form. The admission department and the admitting nurse must verify information found in the EHR with the patient to verify that the data are current and accurate. This time-efficient practice benefits staff and the patient.

The admitting procedure on the patient care unit is much more extensive than that in the admitting department (Skill 11.1). Check the ID band and verify the information with the patient. Assess immediate needs such as pain, shortness of breath, or severe anxiety, and report the results. If another patient is in the room, introduce the two patients.

Patient Teaching

Patient Admission to the Health Care Facility

- Some teaching occurs during the admission process. The nurse provides information regarding physical assessment findings, planned diagnostic procedures, and facility routines. A formal teaching plan does not begin until assessment is completed and a care plan is developed.
- In an emergency situation, instruct family members on the rationale for any procedures and routines to expect in the patient's care.
- Teaching begins early in a patient's admission to a facility. Introduce instruction when the patient is able to be attentive and learn from the information. This is sometimes difficult in an acute care setting. Keep information specific, and focus on topics such as nature of the patient's illness, medications needed for treatment, and use of equipment in self-care (e.g., dressing, ambulatory devices).
- Explain shift times and shift changes to the patient.
- Consider how hospitalization influences an adult patient's occupational status. Will the illness seriously delay work that the patient is assigned to complete? Will there be a considerable delay before the patient can return to work?
- Confirm the patient's understanding of transfer and procedures through discussion and questions. Explain the reason for the transfer, the time it is to occur, and what procedures are planned.
- Be prepared to repeat information and instructions to the patient and significant others during the transfer of a patient because transfers often elicit feelings of anxiety.
- Before the patient leaves the facility, provide for return demonstration of any skills taught.
- Patients who have short stays in health care facilities often do not receive teaching until the day of discharge.
- Anticipation of some prescriptions is not always possible. The day of discharge is sometimes the only opportunity to teach patient about medications. Some facilities have standardized information material that provides specific information about individual medications (see Fig. 11.4).
- Obtain the help of social services or discharge planners to ensure the transfer of a patient to a long-term care facility or home care agency is appropriate in meeting the patient's physical and mental needs.

Encourage the patient to give jewelry, money, and medications to the family to take home as long as the patient feels comfortable with doing so. If no family member is present, valuables are placed in the facility safe. Carefully follow the facility policy for patient valuables. Loss of a patient's valuables incurs serious legal implications for the nurse and the facility. Documentation of disposition of valuables must be in the medical record. In an Alzheimer unit of a long-term care (LTC) facility or in a mental health unit, the facility does assume some responsibility for patient belongings because the patient is not competent to do so. In this case, the careful listing and description of the patient's property become even more important.

Skill 11.1 Admitting a Patient

NURSING ACTION (RATIONALE)

1. Perform hand hygiene. (*Reduces spread of microorganisms.*)
2. Prepare the room before the patient arrives: care items in place; bed at proper height and open; light on. (*This makes patient feel expected and welcome.*)
3. Courteously greet the patient and family. Introduce yourself. Project interest and concern. Introduce roommate. (*The patient and family are more at ease when they know the people around them.*)
4. Check the identification (ID) band, and verify its accuracy. (*Ensures identification before tests or surgery are performed or medication is given. In long-term care facilities, the residents may not wear ID bands. A picture of the resident is used for identification purposes.*)
5. Assess immediate needs. (*Establishes trust when needs are recognized and met.*)
6. Orient the patient to the unit, the lounge, and the nurses' station. (*Promotes safety.*)
7. Orient the patient to the room. Explain the use of equipment, call system, bed, telephone, and television. (*Allows the patient some control over the environment and promotes safety.*)
8. Explain facility routines, such as visiting hours and meal times. (*Decreases fear of unknown and gives a feeling of security.*)
9. Provide privacy if the patient desires or if abuse is suspected. Family members are sometimes asked to leave the room. (*This allows the patient to answer questions openly and honestly without fear of the family member hearing the answers.*) Admission of an infant or small child requires emotional support for child and parents. Parents generally are encouraged to stay with their child to prevent separation anxiety. The most reliable source of admission information is the parent. Assist the patient to undress if necessary. (*Helps maintain dignity and shows respect for the patient. Helping the patient undress prevents fatigue and falls. Provides opportunity to assess range of motion and the skin.*)
10. Follow facility policy for care of valuables, clothing, and medications. (*Helps prevent loss of valuables, clothing, or medications, which is disturbing to the patient and family and potentially results in legal problems.*)
11. Obtain the patient's health history and perform the initial nursing assessment. (*Provides a basis for individualized care.*) When a patient is admitted in critical condition, only the most pertinent information must be collected immediately. The remaining information can be obtained later. Young children are very curious about what is happening to them and the environment around them. Encourage the child to use equipment on dolls to help reduce anxieties. Encourage children to express how they feel. Invasive procedures (e.g., obtaining blood specimens, starting intravenous lines) generally are performed best in a treatment room. (*Enables children to perceive their room as a safe area.*)
12. Provide for safety: bed in low position, side rails up (unless admission is to a long-term care facility), and call light within easy reach. (*Promotes patient safety.*)
13. Begin care as ordered by the health care provider. (*The patient and family develop a positive attitude about the institution when care is started immediately.*)
14. Invite family back into the room if they left earlier. (*Decreases family anxiety when they observe the patient is settled.*)
15. Perform hand hygiene. (*Reduces spread of microorganisms.*)
16. Record the information on the patient's health care record according to agency policy. (*Provides information that also can be used by other health professionals. It is the beginning of the permanent record.*)
17. Allow patient and family time alone together, if desired. (*Admission procedure is often stressful and fatiguing. Allows time for decision making.*)
18. Perform patient teaching (see the Patient Teaching box).

In some cases, hospitals are required to reimburse the patient for lost items. In these units, patients generally are not allowed to keep any jewelry (other than a wedding ring) or any money at the bedside. Medications brought in by the patient should be sent home if possible. If this is not possible, these medications typically are locked in a designated area following the same process as valuables.

 Coordinated Care

Delegation

ASSESSMENT AND DATA COLLECTION

TJC requires each hospitalized patient to have an admission assessment prepared by a registered nurse (RN) within 24 hours of admission (TJC, n.d.). The RN then is allowed to delegate aspects of data collection, for example, to the LPN/LVN. Preadmission assessment and screening for a patient who is hospitalized with a planned admission to an LTC setting usually is performed by the LTC's admissions coordinator, who is typically an RN. Admission requirements for LTC facilities are directed by each state's governing agency.

The patient usually is asked to put on a hospital gown for the admission process so that a physical assessment can be completed. If the patient does not need help with dressing, the nurse provides privacy for the patient to change. An inventory is made of clothing along with other personal items the patient uses, such as glasses, contacts, dentures, prostheses, canes, or hearing aids. If the patient is keeping any jewelry or money in the room, these items also must be recorded. Fig. 11.1 shows sample clothing and valuables on an inventory checklist.

Once the patient is established in the room, the nurse obtains the health history and the initial nursing assessment (see the Coordinated Care box). The health history generally includes the reason for admission; signs and symptoms the patient is experiencing; past illnesses, surgical procedures, and hospitalizations; medications (prescription and nonprescription); allergies (food, medications, other); eating habits; urinary and bowel patterns; sleep routine; and activity and exercise habits and routine. Other information to be included in a history is the language spoken (and languages understood), family members or significant others, home situation, interests, abilities, activities of daily living, and occupation.

It should be noted that the admission and discharge process, as well as visitor rules, were greatly impacted during the 2020 Covid-19 pandemic and may well effect how these processes are carried out in the future. At the time this text edition was published, visitor rules have ranged from no visitors being allowed in acute, LTC, and provider office/clinic settings to one consistent visitor being allowed during specific hours. These visitor rules were initiated to decrease the chance of spread of the virus. For a time period, elective surgeries were postponed. Once this ban was lifted, patients being admitted for elective surgeries were required to have Covid-19 testing prior to their surgery. The inability for family members/significant others to visit patients/residents greatly impacted the love and belonging and safety and security needs of both the patients/residents and family members/significant others. Communication in some units or facilities occurred only with nursing personnel using smart phones to voice call or video call for patient/resident and their significant others. Patients/residents, in some instances, even died without family or significant others by their side. This has taken an emotional toll not only on family and significant others but also on nurses for being required to uphold these rules and be the support system for the patient/resident.

The initial assessment includes level of consciousness, vital signs, height, weight, and a review of body systems (see Chapter 13). Fig. 11.2 is an example of a record used to collect this information. Fig. 11.3 shows a typical medication record to keep track of the medications a patient is taking on admission.

The health care provider is notified when the patient has been admitted. If no orders have been received yet, the health care provider gives orders at this time. In some acute care settings, a hospitalist is assigned to the patient's care if the primary health care provider chooses not to follow patient care in the hospital setting.

Skill 11.1 identifies the general steps to follow in admitting a patient. Specific facility policies and the patient's condition may necessitate some alterations to these steps. See Box 11.2 for managing emergency admissions.

❖ NURSING PROCESS FOR PATIENT ADMISSION

The role of the LPN/LVN in the nursing process as stated is that the LPN/LVN will:

- Participate in planning care for patients based on patient needs
- Review patient's plan of care and recommend revisions as necessary
- Review and follow defined prioritization for patient care
- Use clinical pathways, care maps, or care plans to guide and review patient care

◆ ASSESSMENT

Assessment of the patient begins at admission. Subjective and objective data are collected during the assessment. Most facilities have a patient database form to assist in organizing these data (see Figs. 11.2 and 11.3). Facility policy mandates the time frame in which the admission assessment must be completed and what the RN and LPN/LVN responsibilities are concerning the admission process.

CLOTHING LIST		
[ ] Clothing	[ ] Hose/socks	[ ] Slippers
[ ] Belt	[ ] Jeans/slacks	[ ] Sweatpants
[ ] Blouse	[ ] Luggage	[ ] Sweatshirt
[ ] Boots	[ ] Nightgown/pajamas	[ ] Sweater
[ ] Bra	[ ] Robe	[ ] Tie
[ ] Coat/jacket	[ ] Shirt	[ ] Underwear
[ ] Dress/skirt	[ ] Shoes	[ ] Other clothing
[ ] Hat/cap gloves	[ ] Shorts	
	[ ] Slip	[ ] Clothing sent with family
		[ ] No clothing items
[ ] Personal items	[ ] Prosthesis	[ ] Personal items sent with family
[ ] Bible/book	[ ] Radio/tape player	
[ ] Crutches	[ ] Razor	
[ ] Curling iron	[ ] Toothbrush	
[ ] Dentures, upper	[ ] Walker	[ ] All personal items sent with family
[ ] Dentures, lower	[ ] Other personal items	
[ ] Dentures, partial		[ ] No personal items
[ ] Hair dryer		
[ ] Right hearing aid		
[ ] Left hearing aid		
[ ] Valuables	[ ] Necklace	[ ] Valuables sent with family
[ ] Bracelet		
[ ] Contacts	[ ] Purse	[ ] All valuables sent with family
	[ ] Rings	
[ ] Earrings		[ ] Valuables sent to safe (receipt on
	[ ] Wallet	chart)
[ ] Glasses/case	[ ] Wrist watch	
		[ ] Valuables in Same Day Surgery
[ ] Medals/rosary	[ ] Other valuables	locker number
[ ] Money		

I take full responsibility for retaining in my possession the items/clothing listed above and any others brought to me while I am a patient at Regional Medical Center.

Admission signatures completed at time admission		Discharge signatures completed at time of discharge	
Patient/Family:	Date/Time:	Patient/Family:	Date/Time:
Staff 1:	Date/Time:	Nurse:	Date/Time:
Staff 2:			

Fig. 11.1 Example of a clothing and personal belongings list.

◆ PATIENT PROBLEM

The patient being admitted to most health care facilities is required to have a nursing care plan initiated by the RN within the first 24 hours of admission. Although care plans must be individualized, common patient problems for a newly admitted patient include *Anxiousness and Potential for Injury, Insufficient Knowledge Regarding Admission Process/ Illness,* and *Fearfulness, related to admission to health care facility.*

◆ EXPECTED OUTCOMES AND PLANNING

Planning involves the development of patient-centered goals based on the patient problem statements formed.

Expected outcomes and planning are discussed further in Chapter 5.

Goal 1: Patient will voice understanding of care planned while in facility.

Goal 2: Patient will not suffer accidental injury while in facility.

◆ IMPLEMENTATION

Nursing interventions related to admission include the following:

- Orient or acquaint the patient to the facility to ease the patient's anxiety.
- Establish nurse-patient rapport directed at fostering a therapeutic nurse-patient relationship.

NURSING ADMISSION STATEMENT

Admitted: Ambulatory, Cart, Wheelchair, Arms, Ambulance

From: Office, ER, Surgery, Radiology, Recovery Room Transferred From: _____

Oriented to Room: Call Light, Side Rails, TV, Phone, Safety/Smoking Policy: Yes _____ No _____

Vital Signs: T _____ P _____ R _____ BP _____ HT _____ WT _____ Dentures _____

Diet at Home _____

Allergies: Drug _____ Reaction _____

Other _____ Organ Donor: Yes _____ No _____

Reason for Admission _____ Signature _____

Date: _____ Time: _____

EYES: Impaired vision, blind, cataract, glaucoma, contacts, glasses, prosthesis R.L.
Comments: _____

EARS, NOSE, THROAT: Hard of hearing, deaf, lesions, hearing aid R.L., tracheotomy
Comments: _____

RESPIRATORY: Pain, dyspnea, wheeze, asthma, sinusitis, COPD, cough,
Productive _____ Nonproductive _____
Oxygen needed, smoker
Comments: _____

CIRCULATION: Apical, radial, strong, weak, thready, bounding, regular, palpitations, chest pain, numbness, bruising, edema, hypertension, Hx MI, CHF, pacer, bypass surgery
Comments: _____

ENDOCRINE: Thyroid, diabetes
Comments: _____

GI TRACT: Heartburn, ulcers, pain, hernia, dysphagia, nausea, vomiting, loss of appetite, distention, diverticulitis
Comments: _____

ELIMINATION: Last BM _____ Normal, constipated, diarrhea, tarry, bright red, clay colored, hemorrhoids, involuntary, use of laxatives: Yes/No, enema: Yes/No, ileostomy, colostomy
Comments: _____

URINARY: Incontinence, nocturia, hematuria, dysuria, burning, frequency, urgency, dribbling, infections, cath: Yes/No
Comments: _____

NEUROLOGIC: Convulsions, paralysis, syncope, paresthesia, dizziness, coordination, weakness, headaches
Comments: _____

SKIN: Color _____ Turgor _____ Temp _____
Describe any rashes, lesions, ecchymosis, petechiae, scars, diabetic sores
Comments: _____

MUSCULOSKELETAL: Pain, stiffness, contractures, deformities, tremors, backaches, weight bearing, amputation
Comments: _____

FEMALE REPRODUCTION: L MP _____ EDC _____
Menopause, breast pain, breast tenderness, vaginal discharge
Comments: _____

PREVIOUS SURGERIES:
_____
_____
_____

MEDS TAKEN AT HOME:
Med: _____ Dose: _____ Last taken: _____
_____
_____
_____

DISPOSAL OF MEDS:
Did not bring _____
Pt. has _____ Family took home _____
Retained/taken to pharmacy _____
Other: _____
Signature: _____
Time: _____

Fig. 11.2 Nursing admission assessment form.

MEDICAL INFORMATION

Medical Conditions: *HF and Hypertension*

My Doctor(s): *Dr. J. Bernard*

Allergies: *Darvocet-N 100*

Pharmacy or Pharmacist:
James Manning

MEDICATION RECORD

Mable Lauritsen
Name

28 West Park
Address (street)

Spencer,	*Iowa*	*59101*
City	State	Zip

8-28-1933

My Birth Date

262 lb	*5'-4"*
My Weight	My Height

MEDICATION (Prescription and Over-the-Counter)	FOR WHAT CONDITION	DOSAGE	WHEN and HOW TO TAKE
1. *Furosemide*	*HF*	*40 mg*	*by mouth every AM*
2. *Digoxin*	*HF*	*0.125 mg*	*by mouth every AM*
3. *Potassium supplement*	*HF*	*8 mEq*	*by mouth twice a day*
4. *Psyllium*	*constipation*	*$\bar{\Pi}$ Tbs.*	*at bed time*
5. *Nystatin*	*leg ulcers*	*topical*	*apply to lesions daily*
6.			
7.			
8.			
9.			
10.			
11.			
12.			

Fig. 11.3 Example of a patient's medication record.

Box 11.2 Managing Emergency Admissions

- For the patient admitted through the emergency department (ED), immediate treatment takes priority over routine admission procedures. After ED treatment, the patient arrives on the nursing unit with a temporary identification (ID) bracelet, a physician's order sheet, and a record of treatment. Read this record and confer with the nurse who cared for the patient in the ED to gain insight and to ensure continuity of care.
- Document any ongoing treatment, such as an intravenous infusion, in the nursing notes. Obtain and record the patient's vital signs, and follow the health care provider's orders for treatment. If the patient is conscious and not in great distress, explain any treatment orders. If family members accompany the patient, ask them to wait in the lounge while assessing the patient and beginning treatment. Permit them to visit the patient after the patient is settled in the room. When the patient's condition allows, proceed with routine admission procedures.

- Identify risk behaviors or limitations to assist the staff in making the environment safe (see Skill 11.1).
- Confirm through discussion and questions that the patient understands the diagnostic tests and procedures.
- Monitor the patient's ability to ambulate alone.
- Monitor the patient's ability to operate the hospital bed, the call light, and the emergency button.

◆ EVALUATION

Determine whether the patient has met the previously established goals.

Goal 1: Patient demonstrates understanding of procedure (specify).

Goal 2: Patient has remained injury free.

TRANSFERRING A PATIENT

The changing condition of a patient, whether improving or becoming more critical, frequently necessitates

Long-Term Care Considerations

Admission to a long-term care facility sometimes occurs as a transfer from the hospital (see Skill 11.2) and sometimes as a direct admission. Perform a health history and initial nursing assessment to determine the patient's condition. Encourage the patient to bring clothing and other personal items, such as pictures; even personal furniture may be brought to place in the room to give a feeling of familiarity (see Chapters 33, 38, and 39). Agency policies and requirements of **third-party payers** (entities [people or elements] other than the giver or receiver of service responsible for payment; e.g., Medicare or insurance company) must be followed so that benefits are not lost. Discharge from a nursing home is essentially the same as discharge from a hospital. There are more personal belongings to gather and pack.

Special Considerations for Transferring Patients

- Arrange transportation via ambulance with social services department, if the patient requires it, for transfer to another facility. Ensure that the necessary equipment is assembled to provide care during transport.
- Be especially careful that all documentation is complete when the patient is being transferred to another facility. (A communication breakdown carries high potential to interfere with continuity of the patient's care.)
- If the patient is being transferred to a different facility, be sure that all of the appropriate patient care measures have been performed (e.g., suctioning of airway, administration of prescribed medication, changing of soiled dressings, bathing of an incontinent patient, and emptying of collection devices).

transfer (moving a patient from one unit to another [intra-agency transfer] or moving a patient from one health care facility to another [interagency transfer]). Transfers are sometimes to another unit in the hospital and sometimes to another health care institution, such as an LTC facility or rehabilitation hospital (Box 11.3 and Fig. 11.4).

Often a patient whose condition becomes critical while in the hospital is moved to special care areas, such as the ICU or CCU. A patient whose condition improves is likely to be moved from a special care area to a general care area or a step-down unit. Other patients are transferred to an LTC facility if they need continued care. Transfers also may be done at the patient's request; for example, some patients wish to have a private room or a quieter room.

The patient transfer requires thorough preparation and careful documentation. Preparation includes an explanation of the transfer to the patient and family, discussion of the patient's condition and plan of care with the staff of the receiving unit or facility, and arrangements for transportation, if necessary. Documentation of the patient's condition before and during transfer and adequate communication among nursing staff ensures **continuity of care** (continuing of established patient care from one setting to another) and provides legal protection for the transferring facility and its staff.

Transfer combines admission and discharge. The patient is discharged from one unit and received on the new unit, much like an admission. An order from the health care provider is necessary to begin the transfer process. An interagency transfer requires documentation from the accepting facility and health care provider and a signed consent from the patient indicating an understanding of the risks and benefits associated with the transfer. Failure to follow these procedures instituted by COBRA and EMTALA (discussed in Chapter 2) may result in monetary fines to both facilities. Skill 11.2 gives general steps to follow when transferring a patient. Box 11.4 lists special considerations for transferring patients.

❖ NURSING PROCESS FOR PATIENT TRANSFER

◆ ASSESSMENT

The nurse determines the patient's understanding of the reason for the transfer and gives explanations as necessary. The patient's condition must be assessed before transfer to determine the necessary method of transfer. The nurse receiving the patient after a transfer also assesses the patient because the patient is now his or her responsibility.

◆ PATIENT PROBLEM

Patient problems that the patient had before the transfer may still be current after the transfer. The nurse's assessment helps in determining whether revisions to the care plan are necessary. If the patient has been transferred from one facility to another, new patient problem statements are likely to be necessary. As with admission, the patient commonly has the nursing problem of *Anxiousness* and *Potential for Injury* because of the new environment.

◆ EXPECTED OUTCOMES AND PLANNING

Transfer planning involves the development of patient-centered goals based on the nursing diagnosis formed.

Goal 1: Patient will voice an understanding of the reason for and the process involved with the transfer.

Goal 2: Patient will incur no injury during or after transfer.

◆ IMPLEMENTATION

Nursing interventions include the following:
- Explain to patient and family the reason for the transfer, when it is to occur, and what procedures are planned.
- Encourage questions (see Skill 11.2).
- Confirm the patient understands the transfer and procedures through discussion and questions.
- Inspect the patient's positioning in or on transport vehicle.
- During final assessment, compare present data with previous findings.

Patient Transfer Form		Date *1-31-22*	Medical record no. *432-612-1111*
Patient's name *Sandra Knox* Phone # *555-1263*		Diet on transfer *Low sodium*	Date of transfer *1-31-22*
Address *28 West Park, Spenser, Iowa*		Attending physician at time of transfer *Dr. J.W. Short*	

Diagnosis:
Primary ___*myocardial infarction*___
Secondary ___*heart failure*___
All other conditions _____   Allergies: *penicillin*

Current medications: (date and time last dose)

Bumetanide 1 mg po daily

Digoxin 0.25 mg po daily

Docusate tabs po H.S.

Potassium supplement 10 mEq po B.I.D.

Nifedipine XL 30 mg po B.I.D.

Nitroglycerine 6.5 mg po daily

Nursing evaluation

a. Speech	☒ Normal	☐ Impaired	☐ Unable to speak
b. Hearing	☐ Normal	☒ Impaired	☐ Deaf
c. Sight	☐ Normal	☒ Impaired	☐ Blind
d. Mental status	☒ Always alert	☐ Occasionally confused	☐ Always confused
e. Feeding	☒ Independent	☐ Help with feeding	☐ Cannot feed self
f. Dressing	☒ Independent	☐ Help with dressing	☐ Cannot dress self
g. Elimination	☐ Independent	☒ Help to bathroom	☐ Bedpan or urinal required ☐ Incontinent
h. Bathing	☒ Independent	☒ Help with bathing	☐ Bed bath with help ☐ Bed bath
i. Ambulatory status	☐ Independent	☒ Walks with assistance	☐ Help from bed to chair ☐ Bed bound

Appliances or support: _*walker, up c̄ assistance*_____

Physical activity: _____

Nursing assessment and other pertinent information: *grieving the loss of husband 2 months ago, alert and oriented × 3,*
crackles in right apex, last BM this AM - brown semiformed stool, last set of vitals = 97°-80-22 100/60. Abdomen soft and
nondistended, pedal pulse + 2 bilaterally

Nurse's signature: *Kelly J. Russell*   Title: *RN, MSN*   Date: *1-31-22*

Fig. 11.4 Example of a patient transfer form.

◆ EVALUATION

Goal 1: Patient states the reasons for the transfer.
Goal 2: Patient is secured into wheelchair or gurney and remains injury free.

DISCHARGING A PATIENT

DISCHARGE PLANNING

Planning for a patient's discharge is just one aspect that aids in providing continuity of care for a patient in a health care facility. Discharge planning is defined as the systematic process of planning for patient care after discharge from a hospital or health care facility.

Although discharge from a facility usually is considered routine, effective discharge requires careful planning and continued assessment of the patient's needs during the stay in the facility. Ideally, discharge planning begins shortly after admission. Discharge planning has several purposes, including teaching the patient and the family about the patient's illness and its effect on lifestyle; providing instructions for home care; communicating dietary or activity instructions; and explaining the purpose, adverse effects, and scheduling of medication treatment. It also can include arranging for transportation, follow-up care when necessary, and coordination of outpatient or home health care services.

Skill 11.2   Transferring a Patient

NURSING ACTION (RATIONALE)

1. Perform hand hygiene. (Reduces spread of microorganisms.)
2. Check health care provider's order for transfer. (Verifies if and when a patient is to be transferred.)
3. Inform patient and family of the transfer. (Reduces the fear of the unknown and strengthens the nurse-patient relationship.)
4. Notify the receiving unit of the transfer and when to expect the patient. (Allows preparation time to best welcome the new patient and begin care in a courteous, thoughtful, and unhurried manner.)
5. Gather all the patient's belongings and necessary care items to accompany the patient. (Builds trust and prevents loss of items.)
6. Assist in transferring the patient, usually via stretcher or wheelchair. (Ensures patient safety. The patient's condition determines mode of transportation.)
7. Introduce patient and family to nurses on new unit and to roommate. (Establishes the beginning of new therapeutic nurse-patient relationship and gives a sense of belonging.)
8. Provide a brief summary of medical diagnosis, treatment care plan, and medications. Review medical orders with nurse assuming care. Situation, background, assessment, and recommendation (SBAR) is the common format used for reporting this information (see Chapter 3 for information regarding SBAR). If transfer is to another facility, complete an interagency transfer form. (Gives personnel on the receiving unit pertinent information for continuing care. Reviewing records together prevents errors.)
9. Explain equipment, policies, and procedures that are different on the new unit. (Gives the patient some control and reduces anxiety.)
10. Perform hand hygiene. (Reduces spread of microorganisms.)
11. Record condition of patient and means of transfer. The nurse on the new unit also records an assessment of the patient's condition on arrival. (Properly executed, the patient's medical record reflects all care given and the patient's response to that care while in the facility.)
12. For an intra-agency transfer, other departments, such as diagnostic imaging, laboratory, admission department, physical therapy, dietary, and business offices, must be notified of the transfer. (Keeps records current and prevents errors.)
13. An interagency transfer usually is made via air or ground ambulance or via private car. Be sure the patient is dressed or covered appropriately for environmental comfort. If oxygen is necessary, a small transport tank usually is used. A nurse generally accompanies a critically ill patient who is being transferred. (Promotes continuity of care.)
14. Infants generally are transported in an isolette that is later returned to the sending health care facility. Parents usually accompany their child during transfer unless the transfer is via air ambulance. In this case, the parents generally follow in family transportation. (Promotes continuity of care.)
15. Perform patient teaching (see the Patient Teaching box). See Box 11.4 for special considerations for patient transfer.

Good discharge planning involves the patient from the beginning, uses the strengths of the patient and caregivers in planning, provides resources to meet the patient's limitations, and is focused on improving the patient's long-term outcomes.

TJC (Kind and Smith, n.d.) suggests the following instructions be given to patients upon discharge from a health care facility:

- Reason for the admission
- Safe and effective use of medications and medical equipment
- Instruction on nutrition and modified diets
- Rehabilitation techniques to support adaptation to or functional independence in the environment
- Access to available community resources as needed
- When and how to obtain further treatment

- The patient's and family's responsibilities in the patient's ongoing health care needs and the knowledge and skills needed to carry out those responsibilities
- Maintenance of good standards for personal hygiene and grooming
- It is also necessary to identify risk factors for discharge planning, such as the following:
  - Older adult age group
  - Multisystem disease process
  - Major surgical procedure
  - Chronic or terminal illness

Discharge planning is a multidisciplinary process that involves participation by all members of the health care team, the patient, and the patient's family or significant others. Most hospitals have discharge planners/coordinators or case managers. The social worker is often in charge of discharge planning for the LTC resident. Considered part of the health care team, these people orchestrate the discharge planning. This is especially important when the patient is considered at risk. Depending on the facility or acuity level of the patient, the staff or the charge nurse may be responsible for discharge planning. With the assistance of social workers or community-based nurses, the staff identifies and anticipates patient needs after discharge from the hospital and formulates a plan for meeting those needs (Box 11.5, Fig. 11.5, and the Home Care Considerations box).

Another approach to discharge planning is to perform transitional care with transition specialists. This role was developed to facilitate the transition from hospital (where discharge planning is initiated) to recovery (in the home). The transition specialist begins

---

Box 11.5 Discharge Teaching Goals

THE GOALS OF DISCHARGE TEACHING HELP TO ENSURE THAT PATIENTS DO THE FOLLOWING:
- Carefully follow their diet
- Comply with their medication therapy
- Know about possible complications
- Know when to seek follow-up care
- Manage their activity level
- Recognize their need for rest
- Understand their illness
- Understand their treatments

Be certain that the discharge teaching includes the patient's family or other caregivers to ensure that the patient receives proper care at home.

DISMISSAL INSTRUCTION SHEET

Name _Marjorie Oden_   Allergies _NKA_

1. Diet: Regular _____   Soft __X__   Liquid _____   Special instructions: _____

2. Activity: Walking __X__   Rest __X__   Lifting _10 lb._   Driving _no_ _____
   Work _____   Other _____

3. Bowels: _Laxative of choice_ _____

4. Bathing: Shower __X__   Tub _no_   Sponge __—__

5. Wound care: Incision care _____
   Dressing change _____
   Special instructions _____

6. Tubes, drains, saline lock, appliances: Special instructions _Leave Steri-Strips in place on abdomen until physician's visit_

   Saline lock patient instruction sheet given: yes _____ NA __X__   Prescriptions sent: yes __X__ NA _____
   Physician's instruction sheet given: yes __X__ NA _____   Home med sent: yes __X__ NA _____

7. Medications:

Drug	Dose	Frequency	Route	Special Instructions
Cephalexine	250 mg	three times daily	by mouth	Take with food or milk
Acetaminophen	tabs 2	every 4 hr	by mouth	As needed for pain control
Docusate	caps 2	daily	by mouth	At hours of sleep
Zolpidem	5 mg	daily	by mouth	As needed for sleep

8. Other instructions: _Call physician if any redness, pain, or swelling of incision or temperature greater than 100° F_
   _____
   _____
   _____

9. Office visit: Call for an appointment on _5-9-14 at 2 PM_ _____ (date)
   Doctor _Edward Roberts_   Address _1402 Indiana Street_   Phone number _308-2890_

Please bring this instruction sheet to your first appointment with your doctor.

Instructions received and understood,
Patient or responsible party _Kinsey Nicoley_
Nurse signature _Kimberly Horrall, RN, MSN_ Signature   _Daughter_   Date _5-2-22_

Label

Fig. 11.5 Example of a dismissal instruction sheet.

Home Care Considerations

The Discharged Patient

- A patient who needs care at home after discharge from a health care facility often is referred to a **home health agency** (an organization that provides health care in the home; see Chapter 37). Typical services include skilled nursing care or simply assistance with activities of daily living. A health care provider's order is necessary for these services to be reimbursable from insurance or Medicare and Medicaid. A health history and initial assessment are performed, just as in the hospital.

- Discharge from a home health agency involves the same kind of teaching as discharge from the hospital. The nurse is responsible to ascertain whether the patient or family is able to provide any care still needed.

- Assess availability and skill of the primary caregiver; assess time availability, ability, willingness, emotional and physical stamina, and knowledge.

- Perform the following assessments of immediate family members: attitude; ability to adjust to demands of patient care; impact of care demands on their lives; and impact of potential ongoing nature of the patient's needs. Family members who are not properly prepared for their role as caregivers are more likely to be overwhelmed by the patient's needs, resulting in caregiver role strain or readmission to a health care facility.

- Assess additional resources that may be available to help, such as close friends.

- Evaluate emergency preparations: for example, signaling device or phone is set up within patient's reach, and appropriate protocol is written out.

discharge planning and usually makes a home visit before the patient is discharged. After discharge to the home, this specialist is available to the patient and family. This type of transitional care and coordination is cost effective and has improved the quality of care.

Communication among the patient, the family or caregivers, and health care agencies is essential for effective discharge planning. The nurse establishes a dialogue between these various people and coordinates the discharge plan before the patient leaves the facility. Any necessary referrals to other agencies are initiated before the patient is discharged. The nurse, if no discharge planner is available, is responsible for coordinating such referrals, including signed health care provider's orders for specific care, treatments, or medications, to enable the patient to obtain reimbursement from third-party payers.

A discharge summary is part of the discharge plan. This summary includes the patient's learning needs, how well they have been met, the patient teaching completed, short-term and long-term goals of care, referrals made, and coordinated care plan to be implemented after discharge.

REFERRALS FOR HEALTH CARE SERVICES

Often a patient who is discharged needs the further services of various disciplines (departments) within a facility, such as dietary, social work, or physical therapy. The nurse is often the first to recognize the patient's needs, so it is important to recognize the specialized skills and knowledge of other health professionals. They are often in a position to give a patient services that the nurse is unable to offer. Referrals should be made as soon as possible after the patient's need is identified. In many facilities, a health care provider's order is needed for a referral, especially when specific therapies are planned (e.g., physical therapy) (see the Health Promotion box).

 Health Promotion

Referrals and Discharge Planning

Continuity of care for the patient can be enhanced by approaching discharge planning with an interdisciplinary approach. The following list summarizes the role that various health disciplines play in referrals during discharge planning.

Dietitian
- Provides proper nutrient and food source requirements in patients' diets
- Instructs patients on meal planning and diet restrictions

Social Worker
- Provides counseling for major life crises, such as terminal illness and family problems
- Assists in finding community resources, such as equipment for home health care or an agency that accepts patients after discharge from a facility
- Assists in finding financial resources to cover medical costs

Physical Therapist
- Assists in the examination and treatment of physically disabled people
- Assists in rehabilitating patients and restoring musculoskeletal function to a patient's greatest potential

Occupational Therapist
- Teaches patients to adapt to physical or cognitive challenges by learning new vocational skills or performing activities of daily living

Speech Therapist
- Assists patients with disorders that affect normal oral communication
- Assists patients with techniques that address swallowing disorders

Clinical Nurse Specialist
- Consults with nursing staff on appropriate nursing interventions for complex nursing diagnoses
- Provides instruction to patients and family members who will assume patient care

Home Health Care Nurse
- Provides follow-up discharge visits to a patient's home for the delivery of nursing services

DISCHARGE PROCESS

Many facilities have a form with written instructions and teaching documentation for the patient to sign acknowledging understanding of the instructions. These instructions serve as a guide for the patient to use at home (see Fig. 11.5). Skill 11.3 outlines the steps for discharging a patient. Box 11.6 discusses what to do if a patient decides to leave hospital facility against medical advice (Fig. 11.6).

Skill 11.3 Discharging a Patient

NURSING ACTION (RATIONALE)

1. Perform hand hygiene. (Reduces spread of microorganisms.)
2. Be certain there is a discharge order. (Verifies health care provider's decision regarding time for the patient to be discharged.)
3. If no discharge order has been written and the patient insists on leaving the facility, have the patient sign against medical advice (AMA) form (see Fig. 11.6). (In general, patients cannot be held against their wishes.) The patient's signature acknowledges full responsibility for what happens after the patient leaves. Be sure the health care provider is notified. Every effort should be made to encourage the patient to stay until speaking with the health care provider.
4. Notify the family or the person who will be transporting the patient home. (Prevents delay in discharge.)
5. Verify that the patient and the family or caregiver understand the instructions for care (e.g., medications, special diet, exercise, follow-up care). (Ensures appropriate home care.)
6. Gather equipment, supplies, and prescriptions that the patient is to take home. (Provides service patient and family are unable to perform for themselves.)
7. Assist the patient in dressing and packing items to go home. (Conserves patient's strength.)
8. Check clothing and valuables list made on admission according to policy. (Prevents patient from leaving personal items at facility.)
9. Transfer the patient and belongings to the vehicle outside.
   a. Many facilities escort the patient via wheelchair.

b. Many patients are discharged via gurney.

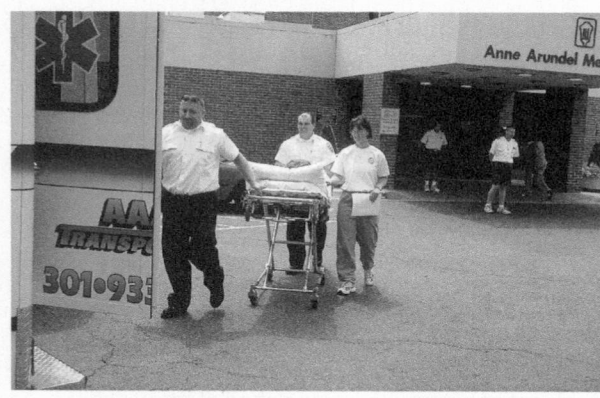

c. Assist the patient into the vehicle. Help the family place personal belongings into car. As with all procedures, use good communication skills and wish patients well as they leave the facility. (Provides patient safety and complies with policy of most health care facilities. Agency's liability ends once patient is safely in vehicle.)
10. Perform hand hygiene. (Reduces spread of microorganisms.)
11. Document entire discharge procedure. (Completes the record. Legally this is necessary to verify what occurred during the discharge process.) Document the following:
    - Teaching
    - Patient's condition
    - Method of discharge
12. When the patient is a child, the parents must be included in all aspects of teaching and in the entire discharge procedure. Some facilities have a special form to be signed by the person legally responsible for taking the child away from the facility.

STATEMENT OF PATIENT LEAVING HOSPITAL AGAINST ADVICE

This is to certify that I am leaving ————————————————————————————————— Hospital at my own insistence and against the advice of the hospital authorities and my attending physician. I have been informed by them of the dangers of my leaving the hospital at this time. I release the hospital, its employees and officers, and my attending physician from all liability for any adverse results caused by my leaving the hospital prematurely.

Signed ————————————————————————

I agree to hold harmless the ————————————————————————————————— Hospital, its employees and officers, and the attending physician from all liability, with reference to the discharge of the patient named above.

————————————————————————
(Husband, wife, parent, etc.)

Date ————————————————————

Witness ————————————————————

Fig. 11.6 Example of form used when a patient leaves the hospital against medical advice.

Box 11.6   Discharge Against Medical Advice

Occasionally, the patient or the patient's family may demand discharge **against medical advice (AMA**; when a patient leaves a health care facility without a health care provider's order for discharge). If this occurs, notify the health care provider immediately. If the health care provider fails to convince the patient to remain in the facility, the provider asks the patient to sign an AMA form (see Fig. 11.6) releasing the facility from legal responsibility for any medical problems the patient experiences after discharge.

If the health care provider is not available, discuss the discharge form with the patient and obtain the patient's signature. If the patient refuses to sign the AMA form, do not detain the patient. Doing so is a violation of the patient's legal rights.[a] After the patient leaves, document the incident thoroughly in your notes and notify the health care provider.

[a]Forcible detainment of a rational adult patient who will not sign the form is not permitted. Only if a court order was issued for the admission, as in some cases of mental illness, is it possible to forcibly detain a patient. A lawsuit for false imprisonment can be filed against the hospital or personnel for keeping patients against their wishes. The refusal to sign the form and the information given about the risks of leaving must be documented in the patient's health care record.

❖ NURSING PROCESS FOR PATIENT DISCHARGE

◆ ASSESSMENT

Every patient requires discharge planning, which is initiated on admission. Some conditions place a patient at greater risk for being unable to meet continuing health care needs after discharge. These conditions include multiple disease processes, major surgical procedures, chronic or terminal illness, emotional or psychologic instability, and advanced age.

Assess the patient's and family's needs for health teaching and collaborate with health care providers and staff in other disciplines to assess any needs for referral. This assessment is important in providing continuity of care to the patient.

◆ PATIENT PROBLEM

When patients are discharged, they may still have nursing diagnoses that must be addressed. Common nursing diagnoses for the patient being discharged include *Compromised Maintenance of Health* and *Inability to Bathe Self.*

◆ EXPECTED OUTCOMES AND PLANNING

Planning involves the development of patient-centered goals based on nursing diagnoses.

Goal 1: Patient or family member will be able to care for individual needs.

Goal 2: Health care resources regarding bathing and hygiene will be available at home.

◆ IMPLEMENTATION

On the day of discharge, nursing interventions include the following:

- All equipment, supplies, and prescriptions that the patient is to take home are gathered.
- The nurse verifies that the patient and the caregiver understand the instructions for care.
- Have patient or family member perform any treatments to be continued in the home (return demonstration).
- Home health nurse inspects home environment to assess for obstacles or risks.

◆ EVALUATION

Goal 1: Home health agency has been notified of patient's needs on arrival at home.

Goal 2: Home health agency's initial visit is completed before discharge or soon thereafter.

Get Ready for the NCLEX® Examination!

Key Points

- Admission into a health care facility begins with ensuring that patients are knowledgeable about routine procedures and activities that will occur during their stay.
- The Patient Self-Determination Act requires all Medicare-recipient and Medicaid-recipient hospitals to provide patients with information about their right to accept or reject medical treatment.
- The patient has the right to be treated with dignity, courtesy, and respect.
- The nurse's attitude often influences the patient's feelings about the care received.
- Common reactions to admission to a health care facility are fear of the unknown, loss of identity, disorientation, separation anxiety, and loneliness.
- An adult patient always should be addressed as Miss, Ms., Mrs., or Mr. (last name), unless the patient grants permission to do otherwise.
- Transfers may be intra-agency (patient is discharged from one unit and received on the new unit, much like an admission).
- Transfers also may be interagency (patient leaving one health care facility to enter another health care facility).
- Coordination is the key to the efficient and safe transfer of a patient.
- Discharge planning begins when a patient is admitted to a health care facility.
- Multiple medical conditions sometimes place a patient at risk for needing more thorough discharge planning.
- Nurses may find involvement of other health care professionals in discharge planning necessary when the expertise of those professionals is needed to help plan or provide ongoing care.
- Although discharge from a health care facility usually is considered routine, effective discharge requires careful planning and continuing assessment of patients' needs during their stay in the facility.
- Every patient in a health care facility requires discharge planning.
- Successful discharge planning is a centralized, coordinated, multidisciplinary process that ensures the patient has a plan for continuing care after leaving the health care facility.
- The ultimate goal of discharge planning is to give patients and families the knowledge, skills, and resources needed to assume self-care or patient care after discharge.
- When the patient is leaving without a health care provider's discharge order, the appropriate forms (AMA) must be signed and the health care provider notified.
- In general, a person cannot be kept in a health care facility against his or her will.

Additional Learning Resources

SG Go to your Study Guide for additional learning activities to help you master this chapter content.

Be sure to visit the Evolve site at http://evolve.elsevier.com/Cooper/foundations/ for additional online resources.

Review Questions for the NCLEX® Examination

1. A patient is being admitted to the hospital for stabilization of a heart condition. Before the patient arrives on the nursing unit, what tasks will the admissions department complete? *(Select all that apply.)*
   1. The patient has been informed of the Patient's Bill of Rights.
   2. A list of patient allergies has been recorded in the patient's record.
   3. The patient has been informed of current health care provider's orders.
   4. The patient has an allergy band in place.
   5. The patient has an ID band in place with proper identification information.

2. A patient is admitted for observation and various diagnostic tests. What is the initial nursing action in the admission process?
   1. The nurse introduces self and roommates.
   2. The nurse measures vital signs.
   3. The nurse helps the patient get undressed and into bed.
   4. The nurse notifies the physician.

3. A 90-year-old patient has been hospitalized with pneumonia and needs reorientation to his surroundings periodically. The nurse assisting him with his morning care hears the unlicensed assistive personnel (UAP) refer to the patient as "Gramps." What action should the nurse take?
   1. Tell the UAP it is okay to call him "Gramps" if he has grandchildren.
   2. Inform the UAP that it is acceptable if the UAP cannot remember his name.
   3. Explain that it is acceptable if the UAP feels comfortable calling him "Gramps."
   4. Educate the UAP that it is not acceptable to call the patient "Gramps" unless the patient has requested to be called this.

4. A patient has been transferred out of the ICU to a medical unit. A nurse has been assigned to complete the transfer. Which type of transfer is this?
   1. Patient-initiated transfer
   2. Interagency transfer
   3. Business office transfer
   4. Intra-agency transfer

5. A patient is being transferred to the surgical unit from the recovery room after extensive surgery as the result of trauma from an automobile accident. What concept should the nurse remember when transferring this patient?
   1. The patient is a human who deserves dignity, courtesy, and respect.
   2. The patient is ill and unable to make decisions or give accurate information.
   3. The nurse knows best and should tell the patient what to do.
   4. Families get in the way and should be encouraged not to get involved in the patient's care.

6. A patient has been recently diagnosed and hospitalized for type 1 diabetes. The multidisciplinary health care team has been preparing her for discharge. What is the primary purpose of discharge planning?

   1. Verifying prescribed medications
   2. Providing accurate medical treatment
   3. Supplying ongoing patient education
   4. Ensuring continuity of care

7. A patient has been hospitalized for 6 days with a diagnosis of a stroke. When should the nurse begin the patient's discharge planning?

   1. When his condition has stabilized
   2. On his admission to the hospital
   3. When he begins to ask questions
   4. When his family asks for information

8. A patient (who is alert and oriented to person, place, and time) is being treated with intravenous (IV) antibiotic therapy for acute pancreatitis insists on leaving the hospital. His health care provider is not aware of his intent, nor is it in his best interest to be discharged at this time. What nursing actions would be appropriate in this situation? *(Select all that apply.)*

   1. Call the family so that they can expect the patient at home.
   2. Allow the patient to leave because no one can be held against his or her will.
   3. Call security because a physician's order is necessary before a patient may leave.
   4. Notify the physician as soon as possible regarding the patient's intent.
   5. Explain the risks of leaving because the patient's diagnosis requires acute care.
   6. Ask the patient to sign an AMA (against medical advice) form, to protect the provider and hospital.
   7. Arrange for the patient to speak with their health care provider on the phone until the provider can visit the patient.
   8. Use a soft wrist restraint to prevent the patient from leaving the facility.
   9. Talk to the patient about why they are insisting to leave the facility.

9. The nurse is admitting a patient to the long-term care facility. What nursing problem statement is most appropriate at this time?

   1. Impaired self-care, activities of daily living related to necessary admission to a long-term care facility
   2. Anxiousness related to new living environment
   3. Impaired coping related to admission to a long-term care facility
   4. Lonesomeness related to separation from family and friends.

10. The patient is being discharged from the hospital to home and will be assisted with abdominal bandage changes by his wife. Which nursing action is most important?

   1. Ask the patient if he has any questions.
   2. Have the patient and wife read all discharge instructions.
   3. Demonstrate how to change the bandage every time the wife visits.
   4. After teaching, ask the patient and his wife to perform the bandage change and observe their technique.

11. During the admission of a patient to a long-term care facility, for what is the LPN/LVN most likely responsible?

   1. Admission charting
   2. Admission interview
   3. Initiating the care plan
   4. Obtaining vital signs and assisting with assessment

12. The nurse is discharging a patient for the first time. What documentation demonstrates that the nurse understands the discharge process? *(Select all that apply.)*

   1. A summary of the patient's stay
   2. An account of all financial obligations
   3. The method of discharge
   4. A summary of personnel who cared for the patient
   5. Where the patient is being discharged to

13. The services of a transition specialist for patient discharge are most important for which reason?

   1. Increasing insurance reimbursement rates for facilities
   2. Improving continuity of care from facility to home
   3. Ensuring completion of facility documentation requirements
   4. Preventing readmitting of patients to hospitals

14. What is the correct order of the steps for discharging a patient from a long-term care facility?

   1. Asking the patient what the home situation is in regard to people who can assist in care, levels of floors, and number of steps
   2. Giving the patient written discharge instructions
   3. Obtaining the order for the resident to be discharged
   4. Meeting with members of the health care team, such as the physical therapist or dietitian, to discuss the patient's discharge

12

Vital Signs

http://evolve.elsevier.com/Cooper/foundations/

Objectives

1. Discuss the importance of accurate assessment of vital signs.
2. Identify the guidelines for measurement of vital signs.
3. Accurately assess oral, rectal, axillary, and tympanic temperatures.
4. List the various sites for pulse measurement.
5. Accurately assess an apical pulse, a radial pulse, and a pulse deficit.
6. Describe the procedure for determining the respiratory rate.
7. Accurately perform a pulse oximetry measurement.
8. Accurately assess the blood pressure.
9. State the normal limits of each vital sign, including the oxygen saturation.
10. List the factors that affect vital sign readings.
11. Accurately assess height and weight measurements.
12. Discuss optimal frequency of vital sign measurements.
13. Discuss methods by which the nurse can ensure accurate measurement of vital signs.
14. Identify the rationale for each step of the vital sign procedures.
15. Describe the benefits of and the precautions for self-measurement of blood pressure.
16. Accurately record and report vital sign measurements.

Key Terms

apical pulse (ĂP-ĭ-căl PŬLS, p. 295)
auscultate (ĂW-skŭl-tāt, p. 291)
blood pressure (p. 297)
bradycardia (brăd-ĭ-KĂR-dē-ă, p. 292)
bradypnea (brăd-ĭp-NĔ-ă, p. 296)
Cheyne-Stokes respirations (CHĀN STŌKS, p. 297)
diastolic (dī-ă-STŎL-ĭk, p. 297)
dyspnea (DĬSP-nē-ă, p. 297)
dysrhythmia (dĭs-RĬTH-mē-ă, p. 292)
febrile (FĔB-rīl, p. 284)
hypertension (hī-pŭr-TĔN-shŭn, p. 298)
hyperthermia (hī-pŭr-THŪR-mē-ă, p. 284)
hypotension (hī-pō-TĔN-shŭn, p. 299)
hypothermia (hī-pō-THŪR-mē-ă, p. 285)
Korotkoff sounds (kŏ-RŎT-kŏf, p. 300)

orthostatic hypotension (ŏr-thō-STĂT-ĭk hī-pō-TĔN-shŭn, p. 299)
oxygen saturation (p. 303)
pulse (p. 292)
pulse deficit (p. 295)
pulse oximeter (p. 303)
pulse pressure (p. 298)
respiration (p. 295)
sphygmomanometer (sfĭg-mō-mă-NŎM-ĕ-tŭr, p. 300)
stethoscope (STĔTH-ō-skōp, p. 290)
systolic (sĭs-TŎL-ĭk, p. 297)
tachycardia (tăk-ĭ-KĂR-dē-ă, p. 292)
tachypnea (tăk-ĭp-NĔ-ă, p. 296)
temperature (p. 283)
tympanic (tĭm-PĂN-ĭk, p. 286)
vital signs (p. 280)

Vital signs include temperature, pulse, respirations, blood pressure, and, per some facilities, oxygen saturation. The ability to obtain accurate measurements of vital signs is critical. Because vital signs are an indication of basic body functioning, it is appropriate to begin the physical assessment by obtaining these data. These data are called vital signs because of their importance.

The skills required to measure vital signs are simple, but simplicity should never reduce the critical value of the task. Vital signs and other physiologic measurements often provide the basis for problem solving. Careful technique ensures accurate findings.

Many facilities now include pain level or comfort level as a vital sign assessment (see Chapter 21; Fig. 21.3 provides an example of a pain assessment guide). Nurses use a more descriptive format for documentation in their notes.

Assessment of vital signs enables the identification of nursing diagnoses, implementation of planned interventions, and evaluation of success when vital signs have returned to acceptable values (see the Health Promotion box).

A cultural assessment should be included in the overall assessment for all patients. This provides a

Health Promotion

Vital Signs

- Demonstrate measurement of vital signs on self or a family member. (Demonstrating on the patient prevents the patient from being able to observe entire procedure.)
- Explain rationale for each step during demonstration.
- Instruct patient and family in proper cleaning and storage of the thermometer in the home.
- Patient should be instructed to wait at least 20 min after smoking or eating before measuring their vital signs.
- Instruct patient or primary caregiver to use fingertips, never thumbs, for counting the pulse (as the thumb has its own pulse).
- Instruct in use of gentle pressure; reinforce not to press hard over the pulses because this obliterates (blocks) the pulse.
- Instruct in use of a watch with a second hand to assess pulses.
- Patients who demonstrate decreased ventilation often benefit from being taught deep-breathing and coughing exercises.
- Advise a family member to count patient's respiratory rate when the patient is unaware of being observed. (If the patient is aware of the assessment, respiratory rate can be altered.)
- Instruct family member to notify health care provider if unusual fluctuations in respiratory rate occur.
- Educate patient about risks for hypertension. People with family history of hypertension are at significant risk. Obesity, cigarette smoking, heavy alcohol consumption, high blood cholesterol levels, high sodium diets, and continued exposure to stress are factors linked to hypertension.
- Patients with hypertension should learn about blood pressure values, long-term follow-up care and therapy, the usual lack of symptoms that is responsible for hypertension's nickname (*the silent killer*), therapy's ability to control but not cure it, and the benefits of a consistent treatment plan.
- Patients often learn to take their own blood pressure.
- Instruct patient or primary caregiver to take blood pressure at the same time each day after the patient has had a brief rest. The blood pressure should be taken with the patient sitting or lying down; use the same position and arm each time pressure is taken. Advise the patient not to cross their legs.
- Body position and the selection of the site on the arm are potential causes of inaccurate readings.
- Place arm on a table or desk that is raised to the level of the heart.
- Instruct caregiver that if the pressure is difficult to hear, the cuff may be too loose, not big enough, or too narrow, the stethoscope may be misplaced or 'open' to the wrong side (if a dual headed stethoscope), the cuff may have been deflated too quickly or too slowly, or the cuff may not have been pumped high enough for systolic readings. Wait 1 minute and try again.
- Teach patient risk factors for hypothermia and frostbite: fatigue; malnutrition; hypoxemia; cold, wet clothing; and alcohol intoxication.
- Teach patient risk factors for heat stroke: strenuous exercise in hot, humid weather; tight-fitting clothing in hot environments; exercising in poorly ventilated areas; sudden exposure to hot climates; and poor fluid intake before, during, and after exercise.
- Patients undergoing cardiac rehabilitation should learn to assess their own pulse rates to determine their response to exercise. Pulses should be taken before, during, and after exercise.
- Instruct patients on the importance of appropriate size and placement of blood pressure cuff for home use.
- Teach the patient signs and symptoms of hypoxemia: headache, somnolence, confusion, dusky color, shortness of breath, and dyspnea.
- Inform the patient of the effects of high-risk behaviors, such as cigarette smoking on oxygen saturation.

better understanding of each patient as an individual and assists with administering appropriate nursing care to the patient. See Chapters 6 and 13 for a more thorough discussion (see the Cultural Considerations box).

GUIDELINES FOR OBTAINING VITAL SIGNS

Vital signs are a part of the database obtained during assessment. The procedure for assessing vital signs is not routine; part of the nurse's task is to individualize the procedure to each patient's needs and condition. Nurses must ensure their skills include all of the following:
- Measuring vital signs correctly
- Understanding and interpreting the values
- Communicating findings appropriately
- Documenting vital signs correctly
- Beginning interventions as needed

Cultural Considerations

Vital Signs

- Many cultures believe that certain natural or herbal products can protect one's health or treat certain health conditions.
- Provide privacy when measuring vital signs.
- Procedures that may be considered routine in some cultures can produce anxiety due to cultural variables regarding touch, privacy, and gender of the health care worker.
- If the patient speaks a different language than the nurse, take extra steps to ensure that the patient understands the vital sign measurement procedure and findings.
- Use an interpreter if needed; demonstrate the procedure to promote patient understanding.

Whether and how frequently vital signs are measured (Box 12.1) depends on the nurse's judgment of

Box 12.1 Guidelines for Measurement of Vital Signs

- The nurse who cares for the patient is ideally the one to assess vital signs, interpret their significance, and participate in decisions about care.
- Be sure equipment used to measure vital signs (e.g., thermometer, stethoscope, sphygmomanometer) is in proper working condition to ensure accuracy of findings.
- Use standard precautions and ensure equipment is clean. Be aware of the normal range for all vital signs; this knowledge helps detect abnormalities.
- Be aware of the patient's normal range of vital signs. The normal range of some patients differs from the standard range. These values serve as a baseline for comparison with findings obtained later.
- It is wise to know the patient's medical history, therapies, and medications prescribed. Some illnesses or treatments cause predictable changes in vital signs.
- Keep environmental factors that have potential to affect vital signs to a minimum. If you are not able to control these factors, values that are not true indicators of the patient's condition are likely to result (e.g., if assessing the patient's pulse after ambulation or an emotional trauma, or obtaining a temperature reading in a warm, humid room).
- Approach the patient in a calm and caring manner while demonstrating proficiency in handling supplies needed for vital sign measurements.
- Use an organized, systematic approach when obtaining vital signs.

- The nurse and the healthcare provider decide the frequency of vital signs measurement on the basis of the patient's condition. Most acute care facilities have a policy of assessing a patient's vital signs at least once every shift. However, certain conditions dictate more frequent measurement of vital signs; for instance, after a patient has had surgery or a major diagnostic procedure, take frequent measurements until vital signs stabilize to the patient's baseline before the procedure. If a patient's physical condition begins to worsen, take vital signs more frequently, perhaps every 5–10 min.
- Evaluate the results of vital sign measurement. Vital signs are only one measurement of the patient's condition. It is also necessary to assess other signs and symptoms and be aware of the patient's ongoing health status. Vital signs are only a part of the assessment of the patient's physical and psychologic condition.
- Verify and communicate significant changes in vital signs. The baseline measurement allows the nurse to identify changes in vital signs. Report significant changes in vital signs to the healthcare provider. Also record and report any changes to the nurses working the oncoming shift.
- Before examination of a patient by the primary provider in an outpatient setting, the nurse or appropriate healthcare personnel measure the vital signs.
- Report abnormalities in vital signs to the healthcare provider.

---

the need, the patient's condition, and the orders of the health care provider.

If a possibility of contact with body secretions exists, gloves should be worn while obtaining vital signs.

WHEN TO ASSESS VITAL SIGNS

Although this chapter presents assessing temperature, pulse, respiration, and blood pressure as separate procedures, they usually are assessed at the same time and at set intervals. A set of vital signs is taken when a patient is admitted to a facility, when the patient is discharged, and when a condition change is observed. The nurse is able to assess vital signs without a provider order, but also must assess vital signs as prescribed by the healthcare provider or as policy dictates (e.g., every 4 hours, once a shift, every 8 hours) (Box 12.2). In some critical care units and post anesthesia units, vital signs such as blood pressure may be assessed as often as every 5 minutes, and the pulse and oxygen saturation may be continuously monitored. In long-term care facilities and in the home setting, vital signs may be assessed weekly.

The more ill the patient, the more frequently the nurse takes vital signs. The nurse must use judgment in cases when the patient's condition worsens, at which time it is necessary to obtain vital signs more frequently. Vital sign readings are interrelated; a rise in temperature of

Box 12.2 When to Assess Vital Signs

- During admission and discharge to a health care facility
- On a routine schedule as determined by health care provider's order or agency policy
- Before and after surgical procedures
- Before and after invasive diagnostic procedures
- Before and after administering certain medications, especially those that affect cardiovascular, respiratory, and temperature control function
- When the patient's general condition changes (loss of consciousness, hemorrhage, cardiac dysrhythmias, or the onset of intense pain)
- Before and after certain nursing interventions (when a patient ambulates for the first time or after tracheal suctioning)
- When the patient reports nonspecific symptoms of physical distress (reports of "feeling funny" or "different")
- Routinely as part of a procedure (e.g., blood transfusion, liver biopsy, paracentesis, thoracentesis)
- When assessing a patient during a home health visit
- Pain is considered the fifth vital sign. Pain must be evaluated and documented each time other vital signs are taken. Refer to Chapter 21 for a more in-depth discussion of pain and the interventions available for pain control.

Table **12.1**	Age-Related Variations in Vital Signs		
AGE GROUP	**HEART RATE (PER MINUTE)**	**RESPIRATORY RATE (PER MINUTE)**	**BLOOD PRESSURE (MM HG)**ᴬ
Neonate	120–160	36–60	Systolic 20–60
Infant	125–135	40–46	Systolic 70–80
Toddler	90–120	20–30	Systolic 80–100
School-age (6–10 yr)	65–105	22–24	Systolic 90–100 Diastolic 60–64
Adolescent (10–18 yr)	65–100	16–22	Systolic 100–120 Diastolic 70–80
Adult	60–100	12–20	Systolic 100–120 Diastolic 70–80
Older adult	60–100	12–18	Systolic 130–140 Diastolic 90–95

ᵃA blood pressure reading of 120/80 mm Hg is now considered prehypertension.

1°F has potential to cause an increase in pulse rate by 4 beats per minute. Respiratory rate and blood pressure readings likewise increase with a rise in temperature; however, when blood pressure falls because of hemorrhage, the pulse and respirations rates increase, and the temperature usually decreases. Age-related differences in vital signs are also important to recognize (Table 12.1 and the Home Care Considerations and Lifespan Considerations for Older Adults boxes).

🏠 Home Care Considerations

Vital Signs

- Assess temperature and ventilation of environment to determine existence of any conditions that have the potential to influence the patient's temperature.
- Assess home noise level to determine the room that provides the quietest environment for assessing pulse and blood pressure (BP).
- Assess family's financial ability to afford a sphygmomanometer for performing BP evaluations on a regular basis.
- Consider an electronic BP cuff with a large digital display if the patient or caregiver has hearing or vision difficulties.
- It is wise for patients taking certain prescribed cardiotonic or antidysrhythmic medications to learn to assess their own pulse rates in order to detect side effects of medications.
- Assess for environmental factors in the home that have the potential to influence patient's respiratory rate, such as secondhand smoke, inadequate ventilation, or gas fumes.
- Instruct patients who are using mercury-in-glass thermometers at home on their proper use, safety factors, and hazards (see Box 12.8).
- Monitor the effectiveness of home oxygen therapy with the noninvasive method of pulse oximetry.

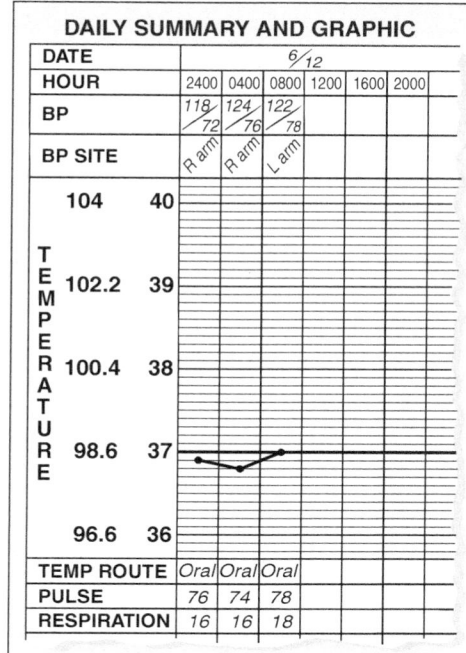

Fig. 12.1 Vital signs documented on flow sheet.

RECORDING VITAL SIGNS

Accuracy in documentation is important; most facilities have graphic flow sheets for charting vital signs, such as Fig. 12.1. In some facilities, a rectal temperature is indicated with a small, circled *R*, and axillary temperature with a small, circled *Ax* (see Fig. 12.1) next to the reading. The blood pressure is always written with the systolic first and the diastolic beneath: 120/80 mm Hg. A final /0 may be added (120/80/0) if the beat is clearly heard until the end. All abnormal findings must be reported immediately to the nurse manager or health care provider. In addition to actual vital signs values, any accompanying or precipitating signs and symptoms such as chest pain, vertigo, shortness of breath, flushing, and diaphoresis should be noted in the nurse's notes. Any interventions initiated as a result of vital sign measurements, such as tepid sponging (for temperature elevation), also should be documented.

TEMPERATURE

BODY'S REGULATION OF TEMPERATURE

The body strives to maintain a **temperature** (a relative measure of sensible heat or cold) of 98.6°F (37°C) (Box 12.3), which has historically been considered normal. Variations from 97°F to 99.6°F (36.1°C to 37.5°C) are considered to be within normal range. Many factors have the potential to cause body temperature variances, including the environment, the time of day, the patient's state of health and activity levels, and the stage of the patient's monthly menstrual cycle (Box 12.4).

Lifespan Considerations

Older Adults

Taking Vital Signs

- An active older adult generally maintains a core body temperature within the accepted norms for younger adults. After 75 years of age, core temperature averages 97.2°F (36°C).
- Older adults often have a baseline temperature that is not typical of the adult patient, so knowledge of each patient's baseline is important.
- Environmental temperature has more of an effect on body temperature in older than in younger adults and is more likely to contribute to hypothermia and hyperthermia.
- Older adults often have occlusive amounts of earwax in one or both ear canals. Consider this when assessing an older adult's tympanic temperature reading.
- The older adult with an infection is often afebrile; be aware of other signs and symptoms of infection in the older adult.
- Manifestations of delayed or diminished febrile response to infection are subtle and variable and very difficult to assess. Be especially attentive to subtle temperature changes and other manifestations of fever, such as tachypnea, anorexia, falls, delirium, and overall functional decline.
- The older adult has a decreased resting heart rate.
- Once elevated, the pulse rate of an older adult takes longer to return to normal resting rate.
- Pulses can be occluded easily in older adults; apply only gentle pressure.
- Pulse irregularities are seen more commonly in older adults; apical pulses should be auscultated as part of a thorough assessment.
- When assessing older women with sagging breasts, gently lift the breast tissue and place the stethoscope at the fifth intercostal space (ICS) or the lower edge of the breast.
- Heart sounds are often muffled or difficult to hear in older adults due to an increase in air space in the lungs.
- With aging, depth of respirations typically decreases; respiratory rate often increases to compensate.

- Decreased efficiency of respiratory muscles results in breathlessness at low exercise levels.
- Responses to hypoxia are reduced in older adults, which limits their ability to respond to hypoxia with respiratory changes.
- Often a standard adult cuff is too large for an older individual who has lost upper arm mass; incorrect cuff sizing potentially results in significant errors.
- The skin of many older adults is more fragile and susceptible to cuff pressure when blood pressure measurements are frequent, as during the use of repeated electronic measurement. Perform more frequent assessment of the skin area under the cuff or increase rotation of blood pressure sites.
- Accurate measurement of blood pressure is essential for older adults receiving antihypertensive medication.
- Orthostatic hypotension (a sudden drop in blood pressure with positional change) commonly is observed in inactive older adults, particularly when rising after a period of bed rest.
- Closely monitor older adults receiving antihypertensives and vasodilators for orthostatic hypotension.
- An older adult's blood pressure often elevates with age. Do not consider such elevations a normal aspect of aging; monitor minor elevations.
- Older adults have an increase in systolic pressure related to decreased vessel elasticity. The diastolic pressure remains the same, resulting in a wider pulse pressure.
- Older adults are instructed to change position slowly and wait after each change to avoid postural hypotension and prevent injuries.
- Identification of an acceptable pulse oximeter probe site on older adults is often difficult because of the possible presence of peripheral vascular disease, decreased cardiac output, cold-induced vasoconstriction, and anemia. Alternate pulse oximetry sites include the earlobe and toes.

Box 12.3	Normal Body Temperatures According to Measurement Sites			
	ORAL	**RECTAL**	**AXILLARY**	**TYMPANIC/ TEMPORAL**
Fahrenheit (F)	98.6°F	99.6°F	97.6°F	98.6°F
Celsius (I)	370°C	37.5°C	36.4°C	37.0°C

When it is necessary to convert temperature readings, formulas are available to use. To convert Fahrenheit to centigrade, subtract 32° from the Fahrenheit reading and multiply the results by 5/9: (98.6–32) × 5/9 = 37. To convert centigrade to Fahrenheit, multiply the Celsius reading by 9/5 and add 32° to the reading: 37 × 9/5 + 32 = 98.6. While the nurse should be able to convert patient temperatures from Fahrenheit to Celsius, most units have a conversion chart available for easy conversion. By remembering the 37°C is equivalent to 98.6°F, the student nurse can easily determine if the patient is above normal or below normal temperature. For example, if the body temperature is reported as "37.6°C," the nurse would know the patient is above normal. This technique of remembering provides a quick reference point only; knowing the conversion formula is important.

Regulation of body temperature is the job of the hypothalamus, which is located in the brain and forms the floor and part of the lateral wall of the third ventricle. The hypothalamus helps maintain a balance between heat lost and heat produced by the body. A rise in metabolism, as occurs with exercise and digestion, is the primary mechanism the body uses to generate heat. Constriction of peripheral vessels prevents loss of heat through the skin surface and thus helps conserve heat.

Body temperature falls into two categories: *core temperature,* which is the temperature of the deep tissues of the body; and *surface temperature,* which is the temperature of the skin. Apart from pathologic disturbances, core temperature remains relatively constant unless a person is exposed to severe extremes in environmental temperature. Surface temperature, on the other hand, often varies a great deal in response to the environment.

Temperature elevations are frequently the first sign of illness (Box 12.5). The terms *pyrexia,* **febrile,** and **hyperthermia** are used to describe the condition of having above-normal body temperature. Fever is actually

Box 12.4 Factors That Affect Body Temperature

AGE
The neonate's temperature normally ranges from 96°F to 99.5°F (35.5°C to 37.5°C). Temperature regulation is labile (unstable) during infancy because of immature physiologic mechanisms. This often continues to be the case until puberty. In older adults, the normal range commonly lowers; a body temperature of 95°F (35°C) is not unusual for some older patients in cold weather. With aging, sensitivity to temperature extremes develops because of deteriorating control mechanisms.

EXERCISE
Any form of exercise can increase body temperature. Prolonged strenuous exercise has the potential to temporarily raise body temperatures to as high as the 103.2°F–105.8°F (40°C–41°C).

HORMONAL INFLUENCES
Women generally have greater variations in body temperature than men. Hormonal changes during ovulation and menopause cause body temperature fluctuations.

DIURNAL (DAILY) VARIATIONS
Body temperatures normally change throughout the day, with the lowest occurring between 1 a.m. and 4 a.m. (97.7°F [36.5°C] on average). The temperature usually peaks around 4–6 p.m. The temperature patterns in people who work at night and sleep during the day do not reverse automatically; it generally takes 1–3 weeks for the cycle to reverse.

STRESS
Physical or emotional stress, such as anxiety, often raises body temperature.

ENVIRONMENT
Environmental temperature extremes have the potential to raise or lower the body temperature. The changes depend on the extent of exposure, air humidity, and the presence of convection currents.

INGESTION OF FOOD AND HOT AND COLD LIQUIDS
Drinking hot or cold liquids or ingestion of food can cause variations in oral temperature readings (e.g., by 2.2°F–2.6°F after drinking iced water).

SMOKING
Smoking cigarettes or cigars sometimes alters body temperature measurement (±0.2°F).

Box 12.5 Signs and Symptoms of Elevated Body Temperature

- Anorexia
- Disorientation, confusion, or convulsions in infants and children
- Elevated pulse and respiratory rates
- Flushed, warm skin
- Glassy eyes, photophobia (sensitivity to light), or both
- Headache
- Increased perspiration
- Irritability
- Restlessness or excessive sleepiness
- Thirst

Box 12.6 Nursing Interventions for the Patient With an Abnormal Body Temperature

- If temperature reading is abnormal, repeat measurement. If indicated, select another site.
- Remove or reduce the patient's external coverings.
- Keep patient's clothing and bed linens dry.
- Monitor patient's temperature at least every 4 h or prn.
- Administer medication (usually acetaminophen) as ordered by the healthcare provider.
- Limit patient's physical activity. Increase frequency of rest periods.
- Increase or encourage oral fluid intake if not contraindicated (i.e., heart failure [HF]). If temperature is elevated, assess for additional related data that suggest systemic infection such as anorexia, headache, thirst, or chills.
- If temperature is above normal, further assess for the possible site of localized infection such as pain or tenderness, purulent exudates, erythema, edema, or an area of unusual warmth. Monitor urine for cloudiness or odor, assess lungs for adventitious lungs sounds, monitor for gastrointestinal symptoms indicating bowel infection (C-diff etc.). In children, monitor for any signs of an ear infection (pulling at ears, etc.) and assess them for signs of a sore throat (drooling, resistance to swallow, etc.)
- If temperature continues to be elevated, encourage oral hygiene because oral mucous membranes dry easily from dehydration.
- If patient's temperature is subnormal, cover patient with more blankets, close room doors or windows to eliminate drafts, encourage warm liquids, and remove wet clothes to be replaced with dry ones.

a body defense; elevated body temperature helps destroy invading bacteria. Typically, a temperature greater than 100.4°F (38°C) is considered a fever, indicating an infection or an illness (NLM, n.d.). Temperatures exceeding 105°F (40.5°C) also have the potential to damage normal body cells, and intervention is often necessary (Box 12.6).

Fevers are classified as constant, intermittent, or remittent. Constant fevers remain elevated consistently and fluctuate very little. Intermittent fevers rise and fall; for example, temperature is normal or subnormal in the morning and "spikes" (is elevated) in the afternoon. Remittent fevers are similar to intermittent

fevers, except the temperature does not return to normal at all until the patient becomes well (Fig. 12.2).

When the body temperature is abnormally low, the condition is called **hypothermia.** Death is a risk when the body temperature falls below 93.2°F (34°C); however, cases of people surviving with much lower temperatures have been documented. Patients may be placed intentionally in hypothermia for a surgical procedure. Certain conditions, such as hypothyroidism, produce a subnormal temperature.

GRAPHIC RECORD

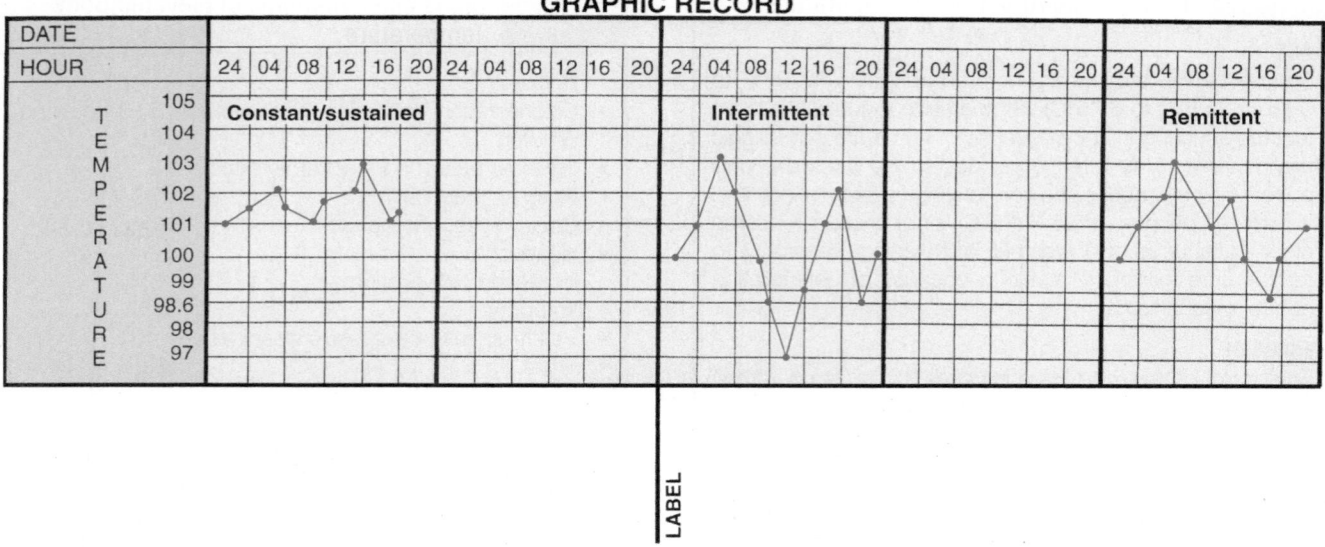

DATE																														
HOUR			24	04	08	12	16	20	24	04	08	12	16	20	24	04	08	12	16	20	24	04	08	12	16	20	24	04	08	12	16	20

Fig. 12.2 Temperature measurements recorded on a flow sheet showing types of fevers.

OBTAINING TEMPERATURE MEASUREMENTS

Temperature measurements are obtained by several methods (Skill 12.1). When a patient has a normal body temperature, a peripheral temperature gives a good estimate of core temperature. Touch the patient's skin and observe its moisture and warmth. For an actual reading of surface temperature, one may use heat-sensitive patches (Fig. 12.3A). Place the patch on an area of skin, such as the forehead, and the color change on the patch will indicate the temperature.

If the patient's temperature is rising or falling rapidly, the body's thermoregulatory system affects peripheral sites, and temperatures can lag significantly behind true core temperature. Remember this when using one of the various types of thermometers to assess a patient's core temperature (Box 12.7). Experts no longer recommend the use of mercury-containing thermometers (Box 12.8). Electronic thermometers (see Fig. 12.3B) consist of a rechargeable battery-powered display unit, a thin wire cord, and a temperature-processing probe that should be used only with a disposable cover. Separate probes are available for oral temperature measurement (blue tip) and rectal temperature measurement (red tip). Specially designated electronic thermometers are used to obtain the **tympanic** temperature by scanning the tympanic (eardrum) membrane (see Fig. 12.3C).

Tympanic thermometers have been available for many years and are now widely accepted. They are very likely more accurate than traditional thermometers when placed correctly, because measurement is from an enclosed cavity unaffected by environmental temperatures. The tympanic membrane shares its blood supply with the hypothalamus, the body's temperature control center, and thus is a good source for obtaining core-temperature readings. To obtain

Fig. 12.3 (A) Disposable, single-use thermometer. (B) Electronic thermometer. (C) Tympanic thermometer.

the reading, place the sensor probe on the tympanic thermometer in the external ear; the sensor measures infrared heat. These thermometers boast many advantages: they are easy to use and produce readings in a few seconds, they are suitable for patients of all ages (except infants less than 6 months old), they virtually eliminate the risk of cross-contamination, and they are cost effective (see Skill 12.1). In contrast to rectal and oral measurement, they necessitate neither the exposure of the patient nor the patient's active participation. An additional means of measuring core temperature is the temporal artery method, which provides a reliable noninvasive measurement. It uses an infrared sensor that is brushed over the temporal artery to measure the core temperature that is present in the blood passing through the temporal artery (see Skill 12.1).

Skill 12.1 Measuring Body Temperature

NURSING ACTION *(RATIONALE)*

1. Perform hand hygiene. *(Reduces spread of microorganisms.)*
2. Assess for signs and symptoms of temperature alterations and for factors that influence body temperature. *(Enables the nurse to more accurately assess nature of variations.)*
3. Introduce self to patient. *(Decreases patient's anxiety.)*
4. Identify patient by identification band. *(Ensures correct patient for procedure.)*
5. Explain the procedure to patient: site of temperature reading and importance of maintaining proper position until reading is complete. *(Gains patient's cooperation.)*
6. Prepare for procedure.
   a. Assemble the thermometer, soft disposable tissues, lubricant (for rectal temperature only), pen and note pad, disposable gloves, plastic sleeve, or disposable probe cover. *(This promotes an efficiently completed procedure.)*
   b. Provide for patient privacy. *(This will decrease patient's anxiety level.)*
   c. Determine whether patient has consumed hot or cold beverages or food or has been smoking; if so, wait 20–30 min before measuring oral temperature. *(Ensures accuracy.)*
7. Obtaining an oral temperature reading with an electronic thermometer:
   a. Follow Steps 1 through 6.
   b. Perform hand hygiene and don disposable gloves (optional). *(Reduces spread of microorganisms.)*
   c. Remove thermometer pack from charging unit. *(Adds maneuverability; battery power is available.)* Remove probe from storage well of recording unit. Grasp top of stem, being careful not to apply pressure to eject button. *(Ensures proper working order.)*
   d. Insert probe snugly into probe cover: red probe for rectal readings, blue probe for oral and axillary readings (see Fig. 12.3). *(Using the probe cover helps reduce spread of microorganisms.)*
   e. Inspect digital display. *(Ensures that unit is ready for use.)*
   f. Request patient to open their mouth; gently insert probe into the posterior sublingual pocket. Request patient to hold thermometer in place with lips closed. *(Ensures an accurate reading.)*

g. Wait for audible signal. *(Indicates temperature reading is complete.)*
h. Remove probe from patient's mouth and remove probe cover by pressing the eject button, directing probe cover into trash receptacle. *(Reduces spread of microorganisms.)*
i. Provide for patient comfort.
j. Read and write down reading from digital display before reinserting probe into holder. *(Ensure accurate recording.)*
k. Perform hand hygiene. *(Reduces spread of microorganisms.)* Return electronic unit to charger. *(Maintains battery charge.)*
l. Complete procedure by following Step 12, a through d.

8. Measuring rectal temperature with an electronic thermometer. CAUTION: If unable to insert thermometer adequately into the rectum, remove thermometer and consider alternative method for obtaining temperature. Never force thermometer.
   a. Follow Steps 1 through 6b.
   b. Don gloves. *(Maintains standard precautions.)*
   c. Assist patient to the Sims position with upper leg flexed. Move aside the bed linens to expose only the rectal area. *(Ensures correct thermometer placement and prevent unnecessary exposure of patient.)*
   d. Remove thermometer pack from charging unit. Be certain rectal (red) probe is attached to the unit and slide disposable plastic cover over thermometer probe until it locks into place. *(Reduces spread of microorganisms.)*
   e. With thermometer in probe cover, lubricate 1 inch of tip. *(Eases insertion.)*
   f. For an adult, with patient in the Sims position, gently spread buttocks and insert thermometer probe 1.5 inches into rectum. Hold on to thermometer throughout procedure. *(Ensures safety.)*

Continued

Skill 12.1   Measuring Body Temperature—cont'd

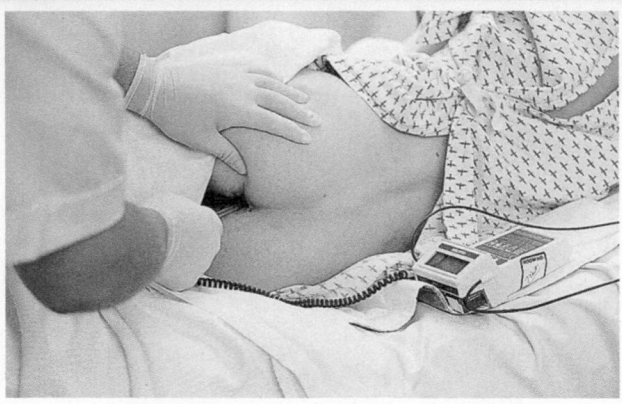

g. Hold electronic probe until audible signal occurs; only then read temperature on digital display (keep probe in place until signal occurs). (*Ensures accurate reading.*)

h. Carefully remove probe from rectum; push eject button to remove probe cover and dispose into appropriate receptacle. (*Reduces spread of microorganisms.*)

i. Return probe to storage unit, and later return the unit to its charging device. (*Prevents damage to the unit and ensures accurate working for the next assessment.*)

j. Clean anal area of lubricant and possible feces. Remove and dispose of gloves and perform hand hygiene. (*Provides comfort and hygiene and reduces the spread of microorganisms.*)

k. Assist patient to position of comfort. (*Restores self-esteem.*)

l. Write down reading for later documentation. (*Ensures accurate recording.*)

m. Complete procedure by following Step 12, a through d.

9. Measuring axillary temperature with an electronic thermometer.
   a. Follow Steps 1 through 6b.
   b. Don gloves. (*Maintains standard precautions.*)
   c. Assist patient to supine or sitting position. (*Provides easy access to axilla.*)
   d. Expose axilla; be certain the area is clean and dry. (*Ensures accurate reading.*)
   e. Prepare electronic thermometer following Step 7, c through e.
   f. Insert probe into center of axilla; lower arm over thermometer, placing arm across patient's chest. In an infant or young child, it is sometimes necessary to hold the arm against the child's side when using the

axillary method. If the infant is in a side-lying position, the lower axilla records the higher temperature. (*Maintains proper positioning of temperature probe.*)

g. Hold electronic probe until audible signal occurs. Reading appears on digital display. Probe must stay in place for accurate reading to occur.

h. Remove probe from patient's axilla. Push eject button to remove probe cover and dispose into trash container. (*Reduces spread of microorganisms.*)

i. Return electric probe to storage well of recording unit. (*Prevents damage to unit.*)

j. Assist patient to re-gown and position for comfort. (*Restores a sense of well-being.*)

k. Remove and dispose of gloves in proper receptacle and perform hand hygiene. (*Reduces spread of microorganisms.*)

l. Return thermometer to charger base. (*Maintains battery charge.*)

m. Write down reading for later documentation. (*Ensures accurate recording.*)

n. Complete procedure by following Step 12, a through d.

Skill 12.1   Measuring Body Temperature—cont'd

10. Measuring tympanic temperature with an electronic thermometer.
    a. Follow Steps 1 through 6a.
    b. Assist patient to a comfortable position with head turned toward the side, away from you. (*Ensures comfort and exposes auditory canal for accurate temperature reading.*)
    c. Remove thermometer handheld unit from charging base. (*Provides easy access to thermometer.*)
    d. Slide disposable plastic speculum cover over otoscope-like tip until it locks into place. (*Prepares the unit to measure temperature; the plastic speculum reduces spread of microorganisms.*)
    e. Follow manufacturer's instructions for tympanic probe positioning.
        (1) Gently tug ear pinna upward and back for an adult, down and back for a child . (*Difference is because of age-related anatomic differences*).
        (2) Gently insert thermometer into ear. (*Ensures correct placement.*)
        (3) Fit ear probe snugly into canal. Do not allow further movement. (*Ensures correct reading.*)
        (4) Point digital readout toward you, following manufacturer's positioning recommendations. (*Steps [1] through [4] ensure correct positioning of the probe with respect to ear canal; the ear tug straightens the external auditory canal, allowing maximum exposure of the tympanic membrane.*)
    f. Depress scan button on handheld unit and read assessment. Temperature reading appears on digital display.
    g. Carefully remove sensor from ear and push release button to eject plastic speculum cover; discard into proper receptacle. (*Reduces spread of microorganisms.*)
    h. Return handheld unit to charging base. (*Maintains battery charge.*)
    i. Assist patient to a comfortable position. (*Restores sense of well-being.*)
    j. Perform hand hygiene. Dispose of gloves, if worn, into proper receptacle. (*Reduces spread of microorganisms.*)
    k. Write down reading (for documentation later).
    l. Complete procedure by following Step 12, a through d.

11. Measuring temporal artery temperature. (This skill can be delegated to unlicensed assistive personnel who are knowledgeable in the procedure, but it is the nurse's responsibility to assess the significance of the findings.)
    a. Follow Steps 1 through 6a.
    b. Ensure that forehead is dry. (*Decreases chance of moisture interfering with temperature measurement.*)
    c. Place probe flush on patient's forehead. (*Prevents measuring ambient temperature by mistake.*)
    d. Press the scan button. (*Continuous scanning for the highest temperature occurs until you release the scan button.*)
    e. Keeping the probe flush on the skin, slowly brush the thermometer straight across forehead. (*Promotes accuracy in measurement.*)
    f. Keeping the scan button pressed, sweep the probe across the forehead and continue to just behind the earlobe.
    g. The thermometer makes a clicking sound when highest temperature is reached. Read and document temperature.
    h. Wipe probe with alcohol, or remove and dispose of probe cover.
    i. Complete procedure by following Step 12, a through d.

12. Complete the procedure for body temperature measurement.
    a. Compare temperature findings with baseline and normal temperature range for patient's age group. (*Comparison reveals presence of abnormalities.*)
    b. If temperature is abnormal, repeat procedure. If indicated, choose an alternate site or instrument. (*Second reading confirms initial findings of abnormal body temperature.*)
    c. Record temperature on vital sign flow sheet, graphic flow sheet, or nurse's notes and report abnormal findings to nurse in charge or health care provider (see Fig. 12.1 and Box 12.5). (*Recording promptly prevents omissions from the record. Abnormalities often necessitate immediate therapy.*) When recording an axillary temperature, write *Ax* above your documentation. When recording a rectal temperature, write *R* above the reading.
    d. Do patient teaching (see patient teaching in the Health Promotion box on vital signs).

An assessment of the patient guides the choice of method to measure the temperature (Table 12.2). The method chosen to check the temperature must be documented along with the reading. Obtaining an oral temperature should not be attempted on the comatose or disoriented patient, or in small infants, because this method requires the patient's cooperation. Rectal measurements are contraindicated for patients with recent rectal surgery or certain conditions of the perineum. Axillary measurement is considered the least accurate method and is used less frequently since the advent of the tympanic thermometer (see Skill 12.1). Rectal

readings are normally 1°F higher, and axillary readings 1°F lower, than oral readings. When obtaining an oral or a tympanic reading, the nurse typically does not need to provide privacy for the. Use of the temporal artery scanner is appropriate in almost all situations. If the patient has diaphoresis, to increase the accuracy of the measurement, brush the scanner all the way across the forehead through to behind the ear.

AUSCULTATING WITH THE STETHOSCOPE

A **stethoscope**, an instrument that is placed against the patient's chest or back to hear heart and lung sounds (Fig. 12.4), is used to measure the apical rate of the heart (see definitions of *apical* and *radial* in the following section on the pulse). The major parts of the stethoscope are the earpieces, binaurals, tubing, and chest piece.

The plastic or rubber earpieces should fit snugly and comfortably in the ears. If the fit is proper, the binaurals are angled and strong enough that the earpieces stay firmly in the ears without causing discomfort. For the best reception of sound, the earpieces follow the contour of the ear canal, pointing toward the user's face when the stethoscope is in place.

The proper polyvinyl tubing is flexible and measures 12 to 18 inches (30 to 40 cm) long (longer tubing decreases the transmission of sound waves). The tubing is thick-walled and moderately rigid to eliminate transmission of environmental noise and prevent the tubing from kinking, which distorts sound wave transmission. Some stethoscopes have single tubes, and some have dual tubes.

The chest piece consists of a bell and a diaphragm. According to which is chosen for use, the bell or the diaphragm is rotated into proper position on the chest piece so that the sounds are heard through the stethoscope. To test, lightly tap to determine which side is functioning.

The diaphragm is the circular, flat-surfaced portion of the chest piece covered with a thin plastic disk

---

Box 12.7	**Assessing Tympanic Temperature Accurately**

- Be certain the patient has been indoors for at least 10 min. Also be certain the patient has not been lying on the ear, which could warm it artificially. Remove hearing aids and assess temperature after they are out for a few minutes.
- The base of the thermometer provides battery power.
- If the reading seems too low, replace the probe cover and repeat the procedure. Be certain that the lens and the probe cover are clean and intact. Reassess the temperature, paying close attention to technique. Follow manufacturer's recommendations.
- The eject button releases the plastic probe cover from the tip of the thermometer.
- Be alert to temperature variations from ear to ear, especially if the temperature does not fit the patient's clinical picture. Sometimes different readings are obtained in the patient's left and right ears; document which ear was used for the temperature assessment.
- Fluctuations in normal body temperature are minimal, so if a significant variation from normal is seen, a second measurement is necessary for comparison. Ensure that the probe is not placed improperly or moved during temperature measurement.
- Clean the unit between patients with facility or manufacture recommended product.

Box 12.8	Elimination of Mercury-Containing Devices

- In 1714, Fahrenheit invented the constant reference point thermometer using mercury in glass.
- In 1868, Wunderlich established the normal range of body temperatures in humans as 97.25°F–99.5°F, using Fahrenheit's constant reference point thermometer. This remains the standard today.
- The mercury-in-glass thermometer was the only instrument available for use for more than 200 years. It was portable, accurate, and easy to use. However, we now know these thermometers are potentially dangerous if they break, posing a serious threat to not only the patient but also the environment. One gram of mercury, the amount contained in a mercury-in-glass thermometer, is enough to contaminate a lake with the surface area of 20 acres.

- A technical report from the American Academy of Pediatrics (Goldman, 2001) addresses the hazards of mercury and discusses possible measures for pediatricians to reduce children's exposure. One of the chief findings was the recommendation for pediatricians to stop using all mercury-containing devices, including thermometers, and encourage parents to do the same. If the thermometer breaks, the mercury vaporizes and can be inhaled, causing toxicity. The statement calls for an end to the use of all mercury-containing thermometers. **In the United States, healthcare facilities, clinics, and healthcare provides' offices have discontinued the use of glass mercury thermometers and mercury-calibrated sphygmomanometers.**

Table **12.2**	Selection of Sites for Temperature Measurement
ADVANTAGES	**DISADVANTAGES AND LIMITATIONS**
Oral	
Most accessible site; comfortable for patient; necessitates no position change	Do not use for patients who could be injured by thermometer, who are unable to hold thermometer properly, or who may bite down on thermometer (glass thermometer); infants or small children; disoriented or unconscious patients; patients who have had oral surgery; patients with trauma to face or mouth; patients experiencing oral pain; patients who breathe only with mouth open; patients with history of convulsions; or patients experiencing a shaking chill.
Rectal	
Argued to be more reliable when oral temperature cannot be obtained	Use sensitivity because use is embarrassing for the patient. Do not use for patients after rectal surgery; patients who have a rectal disorder, such as tumor or hemorrhoids; or patients who cannot be positioned for proper thermometer placement, such as those in traction. There is a risk of body fluid exposure, and lubrication is required.
Axilla	
Safe method because noninvasive	This is the least accurate method.
Tympanic	
Noninvasive, accurate, safe; provides core reading	Excessive cerumen (earwax) has the possibility to interfere with accurate reading; continuous measurement of temperature is not possible; new disposable probe cover is necessary for each patient, which raises the cost; patients must remove hearing aid in the ear that temperature is being measured.
Temporal Artery	
Provides core temperature; rapid, noninvasive method; tolerated well by children; lessens need to handle newborns, which aids in preventing heat loss	Diaphoresis and airflow across the face may affect the accuracy; possible for any bandages or dressings on the face or head to prevent measurement with the device.

Fig. 12.4 Parts of a stethoscope. Chest piece must be placed firmly against the chest wall.

(see Fig. 12.4). It transmits the high-pitched sounds created by the high-velocity movement of air and blood. **Auscultate** (listen for sounds within the body to evaluate the condition of heart, lungs, pleura, intestines, or other organs or to detect fetal heart tones) bowel, lung, and heart sounds with the diaphragm. Position the diaphragm to make a tight seal against the patient's skin and exert enough pressure to leave a temporary red ring on the patient's skin when removed.

The bell is the bowl-shaped chest piece, usually surrounded by a rubber ring (see Fig. 21.4). The ring prevents the cold metal from chilling the patient's skin. The bell transmits low-pitched sounds created by the low-velocity movement of blood. Auscultate heart and vascular sounds using the bell. Apply the bell lightly, resting the chest piece on the skin; compressing the bell against the skin reduces low-pitched sound amplification and creates a "diaphragm of skin."

When listening through the stethoscope, maintain a position that allows the tubing to extend straight and hang free. Movement creates the potential for tubing to rub or bump objects, creating extraneous sounds, and kinked tubing muffles sounds. When the nurse is using the stethoscope, the nurse and the patient should remain quiet.

The stethoscope is a delicate instrument and requires proper care for optimal function. Remove the earpieces regularly and clean them of cerumen (earwax). Clean the bell and diaphragm of dust, lint, and body oils after each patient contact for infection control purposes. Keep the tubing away from your body oils. Do not drape the stethoscope around your neck next to the skin. Cleaning the tubing or head with alcohol can dry and crack the material and is not recommended; mild soap and water are preferred.

PULSE

BODY'S REGULATION OF PULSE

A **pulse** is a rhythmic beating or vibrating movement. In the body, it signifies the regular, recurrent expansion and contraction of an artery produced by the waves of pressure. The waves of pressure are caused by the ejection of blood from the left ventricle of the heart as it contracts. Each pulse beat corresponds to a contraction of the heart; the adult pulse rate is normally between 60 and 100 beats per minute, with the approximate average being 80.

The patient's age, gender, emotional state, size, temperature, amount of physical activity, and condition of the heart can influence the pulse rate. If the pulse is faster than 100 beats per minute, the adult patient has **tachycardia**; if it is slower than 60 beats per minute, the patient has **bradycardia**. Tachycardia has many potential causes: shock, hemorrhage leading to hypovolemia (an abnormally low circulating blood volume), exercise, fever, medication or substance abuse, and acute pain. Some drugs, such as epinephrine, increase the pulse rate. One cause of bradycardia is unrelieved severe pain. Pain stimulates the parasympathetic nervous system, which slows the heart rate. Cardiac issues such as heart blocks also may cause bradycardia (see *Adult Health Nursing,* Chapter 8). Some drugs, such as beta blockers, lower the heart rate. Resting in a supine position also has the potential to decrease the heart rate, as does the cardiac condition called *heart block* (Box 12.9).

If the amount of time between beats varies, there is an irregular pulse or **dysrhythmia** (any disturbance or abnormality in a normal rhythmic pattern; specifically irregularity in the normal rhythm of the heart). In a normal pulse, the amount of time between beats is even.

The volume of the pulse refers to the amount of blood pushing against the artery wall with each beat. A weak pulse is difficult to palpate; a bounding pulse is easily felt with light palpation. A pulse that you are unable to feel at all is imperceptible. Another means to communicate the volume of the pulse is by the use of numbers (Table 12.3). Follow agency policy when describing the pulse, because some agencies may use a slightly different scale.

OBTAINING PULSE MEASUREMENTS

When taking the pulse, note the rate, the rhythm, and the volume, or strength. Palpate pulses using the pads of the index and middle fingers (Skill 12.2); apply only slight pressure over the artery to avoid obliterating the pulse (by occluding blood flow). Assess pulses on both sides of the peripheral vascular system. Assess both radial pulses, for example, to compare the characteristics of each and compare the left with the right pulse. In many disease states (e.g., thrombus [clot] formation, aberrant [abnormal] blood vessels, cervical rib syndrome, or aortic dissection), a pulse in one extremity is

---

Box 12.9   **Factors That Influence Pulse Rates**

ACUTE PAIN, ANXIETY
These increase the pulse rate because of sympathetic stimulation.

AGE
The pulse rate decreases as the aging process progresses from infancy through adulthood. Pulse rate in the older adult is sometimes greater than 80 beats/min because of weakened heart muscle or medication.

EXERCISE
Short-term exercise increases pulse rate, while long-term exercise strengthens heart muscle, resulting in a lower-than-normal rate at rest and a quicker return to resting rate after exercise.

FEVER, HEAT
Both increase the pulse rate because of increased metabolic rate. Hypothermia decreases pulse rate.

HEMORRHAGE
Loss of blood increases the pulse rate because of the sympathetic stimulation. The heart is trying to maintain perfusion to all the organs in the body and has too little blood to do that, so the heart beats faster to make up for the demand.

MEDICATIONS
Various medications alter pulse rate. For example, digitalis and beta-blockers decrease the pulse rate, while atropine and epinephrine increase the pulse rate.

METABOLISM
Certain diseases such as hyperthyroidism can cause an elevated pulse rate, while hypothyroidism may cause a slowing of the pulse.

POSTURAL CHANGES
Lying down initially decreases the pulse rate, while standing or sitting increases the pulse rate.

PULMONARY CONDITIONS
Pulmonary conditions increase pulse rate because these diseases cause poor oxygenation.

UNRELIEVED SEVERE PAIN, CHRONIC PAIN
These decrease the pulse rate because of parasympathetic stimulation.

Dehydration
Dehydration causes less blood volume to be available for circulation, so the heart works faster to compensate.

Fluid Volume Excess
When the heart is taxed with pumping extra fluid, it must work harder to pump. An elevated heart rate may indicate too much fluid causing the heart to beat faster to try to manage the fluid.

---

unequal in strength or absent. Assessment of all symmetric pulses simultaneously is acceptable, except for the carotid pulse. Never measure both carotid pulses simultaneously, because excessive pressure has the potential to occlude blood supply to the brain. Do not reach across the patient's neck to count the carotid pulse (the patient's airway can be occluded with the pressure of your arm); measure the carotid pulse in the patient's neck on the side facing you.

Table **12.3**		Pulse Volume Variations
NUMBER	TYPE	DESCRIPTION
0	Absent pulse	None felt
1+	Thready pulse	Difficult to feel; not palpable when only slight pressure applied
2+	Weak pulse	Somewhat stronger than a thready pulse but not palpable when light pressure applied
3+	Normal pulse	Easily felt but not palpable when moderate pressure applied
4+	Bounding pulse	Feels full and springlike even under moderate pressure

Any artery can be assessed for pulse rate, but the radial and carotid arteries are the most easily palpated peripheral pulse sites (Fig. 12.5). People learning to monitor their own heart rates, such as athletes, often use these sites. When a patient's condition suddenly deteriorates (Box 12.10), the carotid site is the best for finding a pulse quickly. The heart continues delivering blood through the carotid artery to the brain as long as possible. When cardiac output declines significantly, peripheral pulses weaken and are difficult to palpate. (See Chapter 13 for further identification of the pulse sites.)

The radial pulse is obtained at the radial artery, which is located on the thumb side of the inner wrist.

Skill 12.2 Obtaining a Pulse Rate

CHECK GATHER HELLO ID PRIVACY EXPLAIN WASH GLOVES

NURSING ACTION (RATIONALE)

1. Perform hand hygiene. (*Decreases spread of microorganisms.*)
2. Introduce self to patient. (*Decreases patient's anxiety.*)
3. Identify patient by identification band. (*Verifies correct patient for procedure.*)
4. Explain procedure. (*Seeks cooperation and assistance from the patient and decreases patient's anxiety.*)
5. Prepare for procedure by doing the following:
   a. Assemble all necessary supplies, including a wristwatch with second hand. (*Organizes procedure.*)
   b. Provide privacy for the patient if necessary. (*Decreases patient's anxiety.*)
6. Implement procedure: count pulse for 60 s.
   a. Palpate pulse:
      (1) For *radial pulse*, lightly place tips of first and second fingers in groove formed along radial side of forearm, lateral to flexor tendon of wrist. (*Pulse is relatively superficial and should not require deep palpation.*)

   (2) For ulnar pulse, place fingertips along ulnar side of forearm. (*Palpated when arterial insufficiency to hand is expected or when nurse assesses effects radial occlusion might have on circulation to hand.*)

   (3) For *brachial pulse*, locate groove between biceps and triceps muscles above elbow at antecubital fossa. Place tips of first three fingers in muscle groove. (*Artery runs along medial side of extended arm, requiring moderate palpation.*)

Skill 12.2   Obtaining a Pulse Rate—cont'd

(4) For *femoral pulse,* with patient supine, place first three fingers over inguinal area below inguinal ligament, midway between pubic symphysis and anterosuperior iliac spine. *(Supine position prevents flexion in groin area, which interferes with artery access.)*

(5) For *popliteal pulse,* instruct patient to slightly flex knee with foot resting on table or bed. Instruct patient to keep leg muscles relaxed. Palpate deeply into popliteal fossa with fingers of both hands placed just lateral to midline. It is also possible for patient to lie prone to achieve exposure of artery. *(Flexion of knee and muscle relaxation improve accessibility of artery. Popliteal pulse is one of the more difficult pulses to palpate.)*

(6) For *dorsalis pedis pulse,* instruct patient to lie supine with feet relaxed. Gently place fingertips between great and first toes and slowly move them along the groove between extensor tendons of great and first toes until pulse is palpable. *(Artery lies superficially and does not require deep palpation. Pulse is sometimes congenitally absent in healthy adults.)*

(7) For *posterior tibial pulse,* instruct patient to relax and slightly extend feet. Place fingertips behind and below medial malleolus (ankle bone). *(Artery is easily palpable with foot relaxed.)*

b. Determine strength of the pulse. Note thrust of vessel against fingertips. Strength equals volume of blood ejected against arterial wall with each heart contraction.

7. Write down radial pulse rate for documentation later.
8. Perform hand hygiene. *(Reduces spread of microorganisms.)*
9. Document rate on graphic flow sheet (see Fig. 12.1). *(Records procedure.)*
10. Follow up by reporting any abnormal pulse rates. *(Rate sometimes has to be reassessed.)*
11. Do patient teaching (see patient teaching in Health Promotion box on vital signs and Skill 12.1).

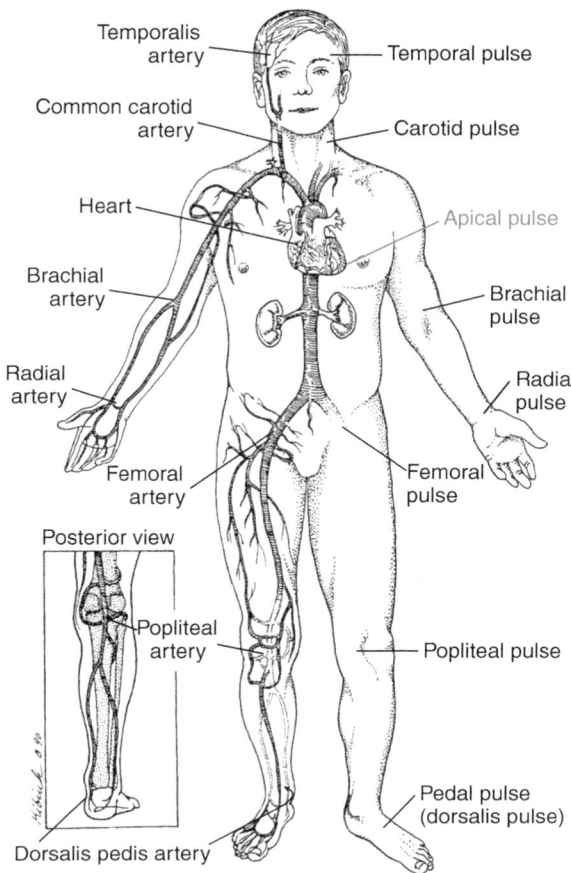

Fig. 12.5 Pulse sites.

Box **12.10** **Nursing Interventions for the Patient With an Abnormal Pulse**

- If the patient's pulse is weak or difficult to palpate, perform complete assessment of all peripheral pulses.
- If the nurse cannot palpate the pulse, a Doppler should be used to verify blood flow and pulse is present. Some things make the pulse difficult to palpate, such as excess edema at the pulse point.
- If a Doppler is not available (such as in the home care setting), the nurse would document additional assessment factors indicating circulation is intact (pink extremities, sensation and movement intact, capillary refill is <3 s, etc.) or not intact (toes are cool to touch, cyanotic, patient has decreased sensation/movement). If circulation is thought to be less than adequate, the provider should be notified for further evaluation.
- Observe for symptoms associated with altered tissue perfusion, such as pallor or cyanosis of tissue distal to weak pulse, and for coldness of extremity and any change in level of consciousness (LOC).
- Observe for factors associated with a decrease in cardiac output, such as hemorrhage, hypothermia, or heart muscle damage, that result in diminished peripheral pulses.
- If pulse is above normal, assess for related data such as pain, fear, anxiety, recent exercise, low blood pressure, elevated temperature, inadequate oxygenation, or dehydration.
- Observe for symptoms such as dyspnea, fatigue, chest pain, orthopnea, syncope, cyanosis, or pallor of skin.
- If pulse is below normal, assess apical pulse and ascertain the presence of such factors as digoxin, beta-blockers, and antidysrhythmic medications. It is sometimes necessary to withhold medication pending the healthcare provider's evaluation of the situation.
- If the pulse is weak or irregular, assess apical pulse for a pulse deficit. Sometimes the healthcare provider will order an electrocardiogram or 24-h heart monitor.
- When assessing for a pulse deficit, which sometimes indicates alteration in cardiac output, count the apical pulse while your colleague counts the radial pulse. Begin the assessment, counting out loud so that you assess pulses simultaneously. The nurse with the watch should indicate when to begin counting, either by counting out loud or by another predetermined signal. This same nurse indicates when to stop counting. If pulse count differs by more than two, a pulse deficit exists.

On initial assessment, palpate all major pulses and auscultate the apical rate. Major pulses include temporal, facial, carotid, brachial, radial, femoral, popliteal, posterior tibial, and dorsalis pedis (see Fig. 12.5); the pulses provide general and specific information. A pulse palpated at the dorsalis pedis, for example, indicates blood flow to the foot.

Auscultation of the apical rate is essential on all cardiac patients as well as when the radial pulse is irregular, is difficult to palpate, or when the patient is taking certain medications such as digoxin (Skill 12.3). *Apical* refers to apex (the tip, the end, or the top of a structure) of the heart. The apical pulse represents the actual beating of the heart, and the apical site is the best site to use when taking the pulse of an infant. In auscultation of the apical rate, the "lub-dub" that is heard represents one cardiac cycle (heartbeat) (Figs. 12.6 and 12.7).

At times, a difference is found between the radial and the apical rates. This is called a pulse deficit. A *pulse deficit* is confirmed by one nurse listening to the apical rate and a second nurse palpating the radial pulse at the same time, using the same watch, for 1 full minute. A deficit exists when the radial rate is less than the apical rate. For example, an apical rate of 92 beats per minute and a radial rate of 88 beats per minute means there is a pulse deficit of 4. A pulse deficit signifies that the pumping action of the heart is faulty or there is a peripheral vascular issue. This is often seen in atrial fibrillation because the heart is not pumping effectively to distribute blood throughout the body (see *Adult Health Nursing*, Chapter 8).

RESPIRATION

RESPIRATORY FUNCTION

Respiration (the taking in of oxygen, its utilization in the tissues, and the giving off of carbon dioxide; the

Skill 12.3   Obtaining an Apical Pulse Rate

NURSING ACTION (RATIONALE)

1. Perform hand hygiene. (*Reduces spread of microorganisms.*)
2. Introduce self to patient. (*Decreases patient's anxiety.*)
3. Identify patient by identification band. (*Ensures correct patient for procedure.*)
4. Explain procedure. (*Seeks cooperation and assistance from patient and decreases patient's anxiety.*)
5. Prepare for procedure by doing the following:
   a. Assembling all necessary supplies: stethoscope and watch with second hand. (*Organizes procedure.*)
   b. Providing privacy for patient if necessary. (*Decreases patient's anxiety.*)
6. Implement procedure:
   a. Clean earpiece and diaphragm of stethoscope with alcohol swab as necessary. (*Ensures instrument is clean and promotes auscultation.*)
   b. With patient in supine or sitting position, expose sternum and left side of chest. (*Exposes portion of chest wall for selection of auscultation site.*)
   c. Palpate angle of Louis located just below suprasternal notch at the point where horizontal ridge is felt along body of sternum. Place index finger just to right (patient's left) of sternum and palpate second intercostal space. Place next finger in intercostal space below and proceed downward until fifth intercostal space is located. Move index finger horizontally along fifth intercostal space to left midclavicular line. Palpate point of maximal impulse (PMI), also

called the apical area. (*Use of anatomic landmarks allows correct placement of stethoscope over apex of heart. Position enhances ability to hear heart sounds clearly. PMI is over apex of heart.*)
   d. Place bell or diaphragm of stethoscope over PMI (apical area).
      (1) Count pulse rate for 60 s . (*Ensures accuracy.*)
      (2) Assist patient to dress. (*Provides for patient's comfort.*)

7. Write down pulse rate (for later documentation).
8. Perform hand hygiene. (*Reduces spread of microorganisms.*)
9. Document pulse rate on graphic flow sheet (see Fig. 12.1).
10. Follow up by reporting an abnormal pulse rate (see Box 12.9).
11. Do patient teaching (see patient teaching in the Health Promotion box on vital signs).

---

act of breathing [i.e., inhaling and exhaling]) is internal and external. Internal respiration refers to the exchange of gas at the tissue level caused by the process of cellular oxidation (any process in which the oxygen content of a compound is increased) and the gas exchange that occurs in the alveoli (plural for alveolus, an air sac in the lungs where gases are exchanged during respirations) of the lungs. The breathing movements of the patient that are observed are called *external respirations*. The cycle of external respirations has two parts: inspiration and expiration. *Inspiration* is inhaling air with oxygen into the lungs, and *expiration* is exhaling air with carbon dioxide out of the lungs. The rate of respiration is controlled by the medulla oblongata in the brain.

Any activity that increases metabolism (the aggregate of all chemical processes that take place in living organisms resulting in growth, generation of energy, elimination of wastes, and other bodily functions as they relate to the distribution of nutrients in the body after digestion) also increases the need for oxygen by the body as well as the respiratory rate.

The normal respiratory rate for an adult is between 12 and 20 respirations per minute (Boxes 12.11 and 12.12). A rapid respiratory rate is called tachypnea. Exercise and fever increase respiratory rate. A slow respiratory rate, below 10 per minute, is called bradypnea. The depth of respiration is determined by the amount of air taken in with inhalation. Normally, 500 mL of air is inspired with each breath. The diaphragm (a dome-shaped fibrous muscle partition that separates the thoracic and abdominal cavities) aids respirations by moving down during inspiration and up during expiration. The proper rhythm of respiration is regular and uninterrupted. Occasional sighing is normal and allows all alveoli to be aerated. Normal respirations are not audible except with the aid of a stethoscope.

ASSESSMENT OF RESPIRATION

When assessing respirations, note the rate, the depth, the quality, and the rhythm (Skill 12.4). Assessment of the depth of respirations requires observing the movement by the diaphragm and the intercostal muscles. Shallow respirations make ventilation difficult to observe, and only a small amount of air is exchanged in the lungs. Dyspnea is breathing with difficulty; the patient may be laboring to get enough oxygen, with pursed lips, flared nostrils, and clavicular and costal retractions (the visible sinking in of the soft tissues of the chest between and around the firmer tissues of the cartilaginous and body ribs, as occurs with increased inspiratory effort).

Fig. 12.6 Taking an apical or radial pulse. One worker takes the apical pulse, and the other takes the radial pulse. NOTE: Two nurses are using the same watch.

Assessing patterns of breathing is another part of checking the respiratory status (Fig. 12.8). Apnea is a lack of spontaneous respirations. Cheyne-Stokes respirations are an abnormal pattern of respiration characterized by alternating periods of apnea and deep rapid breathing. The periods of apnea increase as time goes on. Cheyne-Stokes respirations are noted in the critically or terminally ill patient. Hyperventilation is when the rate of ventilation exceeds normal metabolic requirements for exchange of respiratory gases, such as during emotional trauma; volume and depth of respirations increase. Hypoventilation occurs when the rate of ventilation entering the lungs is insufficient for metabolic needs. Respiratory rate is below normal, and depth of ventilation is depressed. A patient may experience hypoventilation after certain surgical procedures, such as a cholecystectomy; in these cases, deep breathing results in discomfort.

The best time to assess respirations is immediately after counting a radial or an apical pulse. The patient is unaware you are doing so and is less likely to consciously alter respirations.

BLOOD PRESSURE

FACTORS THAT DETERMINE BLOOD PRESSURE

The blood pressure is the pressure exerted by the circulating volume of blood on the arterial walls, veins, and chambers of the heart. Blood pressure is measured in millimeters of mercury (mm Hg). Two pressures are actually elements of what we call *blood pressure*; the systolic pressure is the higher number and represents the ventricles contracting, forcing blood into the aorta and the pulmonary arteries. The occurrence of systole is indicated by the first sound heard on auscultation. The lower number of the blood pressure reading is the diastolic pressure. It represents the pressure within the artery between beats (that is, between contractions of the

Fig. 12.7 (A) Point of maximal impulse is at fifth intercostal space. (B) Assessing apical pulse. *MCL*, Midclavicular line; *PMI*, point of maximal impulse.

Box 12.11	Factors That Influence Respiration

ACUTE PAIN

Pain increases the rate and the depth of respirations as a result of sympathetic stimulation; breathing becomes shallow.

AGE

With growth from infancy to adulthood, the lung's capacity increases and respiratory rate gradually declines. In older adults, lung capacity and depth of respirations decrease, and respiratory rate increases.

BODY POSITION

In slumped or stooped positions, ventilation often is impaired, with a reduced depth of respirations. A straight, erect posture promotes full chest expansion. Lying flat should be avoided as full chest expansion is limited in this position.

BRAINSTEM INJURY

Injury to the brainstem impairs the respiratory center and inhibits respiratory rate and rhythm.

DISEASE OR ILLNESS

Chronic lung disease (e.g., emphysema or bronchitis) alters the normal stimulus for ventilation. Lung tissue disease, reduced red blood cell levels, chest pain, kidney disease, febrile disease, and diseases of the heart are a few of the conditions that alter the rate and the depth of respirations.

EXERCISE

Exercise increases the rate and the depth of respirations.

FEVER

Hyperpyrexia (greatly elevated temperature) results in an abnormally rapid rate of breathing.

GENDER

Men have a greater lung capacity than women.

HEMOGLOBIN FUNCTION

Respiratory rate and depth are increased by conditions caused by decreased hemoglobin function. Examples include anemia, in which the blood's oxygen-carrying capacity is limited, and increased altitude, in which the amount of saturated hemoglobin is reduced.

MEDICATIONS

Narcotic analgesics depress the patient's ability to increase the volume of air inspired, and the rate of respirations is decreased. Other medications have the potential to increase or decrease the rate and depth of respirations and affect the rhythm. The rate and depth of respirations is increased with the use of amphetamines and cocaine. Conversely, bronchodilators cause dilation of the airways, causing the respiratory rate to decrease.

SMOKING

Long-term smoking changes the lung's airways, resulting in an increased respiratory rate.

STRESS

An anxious or fearful patient likely has increases in the rate and depth of respirations, and as a result, hyperventilation can occur.

Box 12.12	Nursing Interventions for the Patient With Abnormal Respirations

- Occasional periods of apnea are a symptom of underlying disease in the adult and must be reported to the healthcare provider or nurse in charge. Irregular respirations and short apneic spells of less than 20 s are normal in a newborn.
- Positions of discomfort may cause patient to breathe more rapidly. Assess patients with difficulty breathing (dyspnea), such as those with heart failure or abdominal ascites or who are in late stages of pregnancy, in the position of greatest comfort.
- Repositioning may increase the work of breathing, which increases respiratory rate; allow for a period of rest. Typically, an orthopneic position is tolerated well, such as sitting the patient upright, or in an upright position while slightly leaning over a bedside table.
- Respiratory rates of <10 or >20 breaths/min or shallow and slow respirations (hypoventilation) are likely to necessitate immediate intervention.
- See *Adult Health Nursing*, Chapter 2, for discussion of inspirometry.
- See *Adult Health Nursing*, Chapter 9, for discussion of pulse oximetry and assessment of adequate oxygenation.
- Observe for related factors such as obstructed airway or stertorous (snoring) respirations.
- Observe for related signs and symptoms such as cyanotic nail beds, lips, or mucous membranes, restlessness, irritability, confusion, dyspnea, shortness of breath, productive cough, or abnormal breath sounds.
- Consider possible effects of anesthesia or medications such as opioids.
- Provide oxygen as ordered by healthcare provider (see Chapter 14) if the patient shows signs of respiratory distress.

atria or the ventricles, when blood enters the relaxed chambers from the systemic circulation and the lungs). The difference between the two readings is called the **pulse pressure**. A reading of 120/80 mm Hg reveals a pulse pressure of 40, which is a normal pulse pressure. Pulse pressure is an indication of cardiac function.

Blood pressure reflects *cardiac output* (the amount of blood discharged from the heart per minute), quality of the arteries, blood volume, and blood viscosity. When blood is pumped by the heart into the arteries, the pressure within the arteries rises. The greater the amount of blood pumped by the heart, the greater the pressure.

Likewise, if the blood volume is increased, the pressure within the artery increases. When the arteries' lumens (channels within the arteries) narrow and become less flexible, blood pressure rises because there is less space for the blood to enter. Increased viscosity (thickness) of the blood causes a slower flow of blood in the capillaries, which causes backup pressure in the larger vessels. See Box 12.13 for factors that influence blood pressure.

The optimal blood pressure reading for a healthy middle-aged adult is less than 120/80 mm Hg. Values of 120–139/80–89 mm Hg are considered *prehypertensive*. **Hypertension** occurs when the elevated pressure is

Skill 12.4 Obtaining a Respiratory Rate

NURSING ACTION *(RATIONALE)*

1. Perform hand hygiene. *(Reduces spread of microorganisms.)*
2. Introduce self to patient. *(Decreases patient's anxiety.)*
3. Identify patient by identification band. *(Verifies correct patient for procedure.)*
4. Explain procedure. *(Seeks cooperation and assistance from patient and decreases patient's anxiety.)*
5. Prepare for procedure:
   a. Assemble all necessary supplies, including a wristwatch with a second hand. *(Organizes procedure efficiently.)*
   b. Provide privacy for patient if necessary. *(Decreases patient's anxiety.)*
   c. If patient has been active, wait 5–10 min. *(Exercise increases respiratory rate and depth.)*
   d. Be certain patient is in a position of comfort, preferably sitting or lying supine with the head of the bed elevated 45–60 degrees if patient can tolerate it. *(Discomfort causes the patient to breathe more rapidly. The erect, sitting position promotes full ventilation.)*
6. Implement procedure:
   a. Place fingertip as if to obtain a radial pulse (see illustration). Because patients sometimes unconsciously alter the respiratory rate when being observed, it is best to obtain the respiratory rate at the same time as the radial pulse reading.

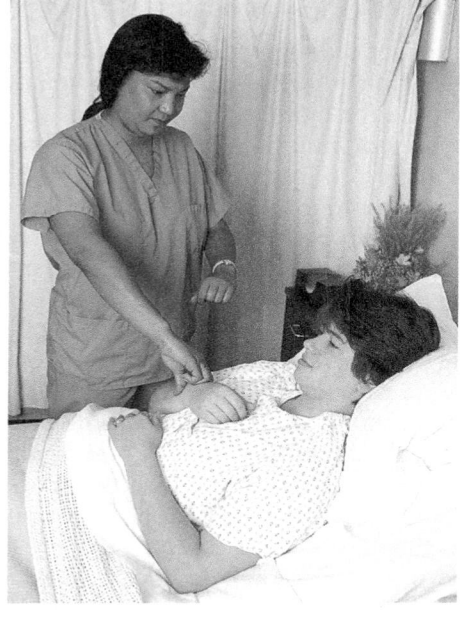

   b. Observe respiratory rate for 60 s. *(Ensures accuracy.)* Count each rise of the chest wall. One inhalation and exhalation = one respiration.
   c. Provide for patient comfort. *(Promotes patient's self-esteem.)*
7. Write down rate (for documentation later).
8. Perform hand hygiene. *(Reduces spread of microorganisms.)*
9. Document the rate on the graphic flow sheet (see Fig. 12.1).
10. Follow up by reporting any abnormal respiratory rates (see Box 12.11). *(Rate sometimes has to be reassessed.)*
11. Do patient teaching (see patient teaching in Health Promotion box on vital signs).

---

sustained above 140/90 mm Hg. The diagnosis of hypertension in adults is not made with only one random elevated reading; for this diagnosis, an average of 90 mm Hg or higher of two or more diastolic readings on at least two subsequent visits is necessary, or an average higher than 140 mm Hg of two or more systolic readings on at least two visits. Primary (essential) hypertension is the most common form. The cause for this type of hypertension is unknown, but risk factors also contribute; consider their significance when doing patient teaching. These risk factors include family history of hypertension, obesity, smoking, heavy alcohol consumption, elevated blood cholesterol level, and continued exposure to stress. Table 12.4 lists normal and hypertensive values. If an individual's blood pressure is normal, the blood pressure

should be monitored once every 2 years starting at the age of 20. For prehypertension and hypertension, individuals should follow the recommendations of their healthcare provider for how often they should be monitored (American Heart Association, 2017).

A blood pressure below normal is **hypotension**. A low blood pressure is considered healthy, provided there are no ill effects, such as vertigo (dizziness) or syncope (fainting). **Orthostatic hypotension** (a drop of 25 mm Hg in systolic pressure and a drop of 10 mm Hg in diastolic pressure when a person moves from a lying to a sitting or from a sitting to a standing position) occurs when a person rises too quickly, usually from a supine position. The patient frequently feels lightheaded and unstable. Advise the patient to rise slowly from lying to sitting to standing in order to prevent blood volume from shifting suddenly (Box 12.14). Hypotension resulting from shock or massive hemorrhage is very serious and necessitates immediate medical intervention. See Table 12.5 for conditions that cause alterations in blood pressure.

OBTAINING BLOOD PRESSURE MEASUREMENTS

Blood pressure readings are taken with a sphygmomanometer and a stethoscope. A sphygmomanometer (a device for measuring the arterial blood pressure) consists of an inflatable cuff and a gauge. The gauge is aneroid (Figs. 12.9 and 12.10; see Box 12.8). Inflate the cuff around the patient's arm to compress the artery, which occludes blood flow; then, slowly deflate it, allowing blood flow to resume (see the Evidence-Based Practice box). While doing this, listen at the brachial artery with the stethoscope to hear pulsating sounds. These are called Korotkoff sounds, and they go through five phases (Fig. 12.11). At the first audible sound, make a mental note of the point on the sphygmomanometer gauge at which it occurs, and note again the point at which the sound disappears. That first point is the systolic pressure, and the second is the diastolic pressure.

As the pressure is lowered, the Korotkoff sounds sometimes seem to disappear temporarily. In this case, listen for a subtle difference in the quality of what you hear as the manometer approaches the diastolic reading. In patients with hypertension, the sounds usually heard over the brachial artery disappear as pressure is reduced and then reappear at a lower level. This temporary disappearance of sound is the auscultatory gap; it typically occurs between the first and the second Korotkoff sounds. The gap in sound sometimes covers a range of 40 mm Hg and thus has the potential to cause an underestimation of systolic pressure or overestimation of diastolic pressure. Be certain to inflate the cuff enough to hear the true systolic pressure before the auscultatory gap. Palpation of the radial artery helps determine how high to inflate the cuff. Inflate the cuff 30 mm Hg above the pressure at which the radial pulse was palpated and disappeared. The range of pressures in which the auscultatory gap occurs is recorded (e.g., "blood pressure 190/94, with an auscultatory gap from 190 to 160").

If sounds are heard immediately after inflation of the cuff and the beginning of listening, the pressure should be released immediately and completely. After 60 seconds, the cuff then may be reinflated to a point 30 mm Hg above where the sounds were heard the first time. Reinflation of a partially deflated cuff is uncomfortable for the patient and often yields an inaccurate reading.

If sounds cannot be auscultated because of a weakened arterial pulse, use of a Doppler ultrasonic stethoscope may be possible. This stethoscope allows low-frequency sounds to be heard and is used commonly with adults who have very weak blood pressure as well as with infants and children (Fig. 12.12).

For the blood pressure reading to be accurate, the environment must be quiet, the equipment should be in good working order, and the cuff must fit correctly on the arm and be at the level of the heart. The gauge must be in plain view, not off to the side of the arm. The patient should be lying down or sitting up with both feet flat on the floor (legs not crossed) (Skill 12.5). See Box 12.15 for nursing interventions for the patient with an abnormal blood pressure reading. See Box 12.16 for assessment of blood pressure in both arms.

Assessment of Blood Pressure in the Lower Extremities

Occasionally, dressings, casts, intravenous catheters, or other devices make the upper extremities

---

🔍 **Evidence-Based Practice**

Forearm Versus Upper Arm Blood Pressure Measurements

EVIDENCE SUMMARY

Blood pressure measurement is an important factor in determination of the diagnosis of hypertension and evaluation of therapies. Because hypertension leads to serious complications, eliminating errors in measuring blood pressure is important. When the upper arm is not accessible or when the blood pressure (BP) cuff does not fit the patient's upper arm, the forearm has been used for BP measurement. In this research study, BP measurements taken on the forearm and the upper arm were compared when patients were supine and when the head of the bed was elevated at 45 degrees. The researchers wanted to know whether placement of the BP cuff affected systolic and diastolic BP. The BP of 221 medical surgical inpatients was measured at both arm locations in the supine and head-elevated positions. Researchers selected cuff size based on forearm and upper arm circumference. Results indicated a significant difference between upper arm and forearm blood pressures in both positions.; systolic and diastolic blood pressure differed as much as 33 mm Hg.

APPLICATION TO NURSING PRACTICE
- A consistent approach to the placement of upper extremity blood pressure cuff allows accurate assessment of a change in condition.
- Appropriate cuff size is essential for accurate measurement.
- Forearm BP measurements cannot be substituted for upper arm blood pressure measurements and are considered inaccurate.

From Schrauf CM: Monitoring blood pressure: Do method and body location matter? *Nephrol Nurs J* 39(6):502–512, 2012.

Normal

Regular and comfortable at a rate of 12-20 per minute

Hyperventilation (hyperpnea)

Faster than 20 breaths per minute, deep breathing

Bradypnea

Slower than 12 breaths per minute

Sighing

Frequently interspersed deeper breath

Tachypnea

Faster than 20 breaths per minute

Cheyne-Stokes

Varying periods of increasing depth interspersed with apnea

Kussmaul

Rapid, deep, labored

Fig. 12.8 Patterns of respirations.

Box 12.13	Factors That Influence Blood Pressure

Normal blood pressure levels vary throughout life.

AGE	BLOOD PRESSURE (MM HG)
Newborn (3000 g [6.6 lb])	Mean 36–40
1 months	85/54
1 year	95/65
6 years	105/65
10–13 years	110/65
14–17 years	<120/75
18 years and up	<120/80

In children and adolescents, hypertension is defined as blood pressure that is, on repeated measurement, at the 95th percentile or greater, adjusted for age, height, and gender.

Alcohol and tobacco use. Excessive use of alcohol and any use of tobacco raises the blood pressure.

Anxiety, fear, pain, and emotional stress. May increase blood pressure because of increased heart rate and increased peripheral vascular resistance. Stress can also lead to other activities that increase blood pressure, such as using tobacco or alcohol.

Diet. Eating a healthy diet can help maintain the blood pressure at normal levels; switching from an unhealthy to a healthy diet can sometimes lower the blood pressure. Diets high in sodium, fats, and sugars tend to raise the blood pressure.

Diurnal (happening daily). The blood pressure tends to vary through the day, starting low in the morning, rising during the day, then lowering at night.

Gender. Men are more likely to be hypertensive until the age of 45. From the age of 45 to 64 there is no difference in the rate of hypertension. After the age of 65 women have a higher rate of hypertension.

Hormones. Variations in blood pressure may be manifested as a person ages because of hormonal alterations. Pregnancy may cause mild to severe elevations in blood pressure.

Medications. Can either lower or increase blood pressure depending on their pharmacologic action. Common medications that raise blood pressure are over-the-counter cold medications, while diuretics lower blood pressure.

Obesity and being overweight. Excess weight places extra workload on the heart, resulting in hypertension.

Race. The occurrence of hypertension is higher in African Americans than any other populations, and hypertension starts at an earlier age. The incidence of hypertension-related deaths is high in African Americans.

Data from the American Heart Association: Know your risk factors for high blood pressure, 2017. Retrieved from http://www.heart.org/HEARTORG/Conditions/HighBloodPressure/UnderstandYourRiskforHighBloodPressure/Understand-Your-Risk-for-High-Blood-Pressure_UCM_002052_Article.jsp#.Wl0aWflsOSo.

inaccessible, so you have to measure blood pressure in the lower extremities. In patients with certain circulatory abnormalities, a comparison of blood pressure in the upper extremities with that in the legs is helpful. The popliteal artery, located behind the knee in the popliteal space, is the site for auscultation. With a cuff that is wide and long enough to allow for the larger girth of the thigh, position the cuff with the bladder over the posterior aspect of the mid-thigh. Placing the patient in a prone position is best, but if such a position is impossible, ask the patient to flex the knee slightly for easier access to the artery. The procedure is the same as that for brachial artery auscultation. Systolic pressure in the lower extremities is usually higher by 10 to 40 mm Hg than in the brachial artery, but the diastolic pressure is essentially the same (Fig. 12.13A and B).

Electronic Measurement Devices

Many electronic devices determine blood pressure automatically (Figs. 12.14 and 12.15). The devices may be programmed to check blood pressure continuously or at set intervals. On medical-surgical floors and in operating rooms, post-anesthesia care units, intensive care units, and postpartum units (see the Coordinated Care box), their use is now frequent.

Once the cuff is applied, the device can be programmed to obtain and record blood pressure readings at preset intervals. Alarm limits can be programmed to alert the nurse if the blood pressure measurement is outside desired parameters; the system includes either a microphone or a pressure sensor built into the inflatable cuff. The microphone or acoustic system picks up Korotkoff sounds and registers systolic and diastolic readings. The pressure

Table 12.4 Values for Normal Blood Pressure and Hypertension Categories

BLOOD PRESSURE CATEGORY	SYSTOLIC MM HG (UPPER NUMBER)		DIASTOLIC MM HG (LOWER NUMBER)
Normal	<120	and	<80
Elevated	120–129	and	<80
High blood pressure (Hypertension) stage 1	130–139	or	80–89
High blood pressure (Hypertension) stage 2	140 or higher	or	90 or higher
Hypertensive crisis (Emergency care needed)	>180	or	>120

Source: American Heart Association, Inc.

Box 12.14 Measurement of Orthostatic Blood Pressure

Some patients, especially those who are older or taking certain medications, experience a drop in blood pressure or an increase in pulse when changing from a lying to a sitting or from a sitting to a standing position.[a]

Certain medications, including many antiseizure medications, antipsychotics, and antihypertensives, commonly cause orthostatic hypotension. Patients taking these medications often have a routine order to have orthostatic blood pressure readings taken.

1. Obtaining orthostatic blood pressure measurements requires critical thinking and ongoing nursing judgment; do not delegate this task.
2. Obtain supine patient's blood pressure in each arm. Select arm with highest systolic reading for subsequent measurements.
3. Leaving blood pressure cuff in place, assist patient to sitting position. After 1–3 min with patient in sitting position, obtain blood pressure. If orthostatic symptoms occur, such as dizziness, weakness, lightheadedness, faintness, or sudden pallor, terminate blood pressure measurement and assist patient to a supine position.
4. Leaving blood pressure cuff in place, assist patient to standing position and obtain blood pressure. If orthostatic symptoms occur (see previous), terminate blood pressure measurement and assist patient to a supine position. In most cases, orthostatic hypotension is detectable within 1 min of standing.
5. Record patient's blood pressure in each position; for example, 140/80 supine, 132/72 sitting, 108/60 standing. Note any additional symptoms or reports.
6. Report findings of orthostatic hypotension or orthostatic symptoms to healthcare provider or nurse in charge. Instruct patient to obtain assistance when getting out of bed if orthostatic hypotension is present or orthostatic symptoms occur.

[a]Although the pulse is not technically part of the Orthostatic Blood Pressure reading, it would be wise to obtain the pulse with each blood pressure reading. The provider will use the pulse and blood pressure readings to further evaluate the patient.

The advantages of automatic devices are the ease of use and efficiency when repeated or frequent measurements are needed. The automatic blood pressure cuff is also useful for home use if the patient or caregiver has hearing difficulties, as the ability to use a stethoscope is not required. Automatic devices are sensitive to outside interference and are susceptible to error. For proper function, the microphone or the pressure sensor must be positioned directly over the artery. Patient movements, vibration, or outside noise may interfere with the microphone or the sensor signal. Most automatic blood pressure devices are unable to process sounds or vibrations of low blood pressure (Box 12.17). In addition, the range of device quality sometimes makes comparing blood pressure measurements difficult.

The use of automatic blood pressure devices permits assessment of blood pressure during interpersonal interactions; nonetheless, avoid speaking to the patient for at least a minute before initiating a blood pressure recording. Talking to a patient when the blood pressure is being assessed has the potential to increase readings.

Self-Measurement

More people today measure their own blood pressure, thanks to improved technology in home monitoring devices and a greater interest in their health. Two of the more common types of devices the general public uses are portable home devices and stationary automated machines.

The portable home devices include the aneroid sphygmomanometer (see Fig. 12.9) and electronic digital readout devices that do not require use of a stethoscope. The electronic devices inflate and deflate cuffs with the push of a button (see Fig. 12.15). Although the electronic devices are easier to manipulate, there are some disadvantages. They easily become inaccurate and require recalibration more than once a year. Because of their sensitivity, improper cuff placement or movement of the arm frequently causes electronic devices to give incorrect readings. A useful blood pressure device that overcomes these

sensor or the ultrasonic system responds to the pressure waves generated by the movement of blood through the artery.

Table 12.5   **Conditions That Cause Alterations in Blood Pressure**

CONDITION	EFFECT	CAUSE
Hemorrhage	Lowers pressure	Decreased blood volume
Increased intracranial pressure	Raises pressure	Disturbance of cardiovascular control mechanisms in brainstem resulting from pressure exerted on the medulla oblongata
Acute pain	Raises pressure	Increased vasomotor tone and peripheral vascular resistance as a result of sympathetic stimulation
End-stage renal disease	Raises pressure	Increased blood volume resulting from increased retention of sodium and water; release of renin, a vasopressor that increases peripheral vascular resistance
Primary essential hypertension	Raises pressure	Increased peripheral vascular resistance resulting from progressive thickening of arterial walls
General anesthesia	Lowers pressure	Decreased vasomotor tone resulting from depression of vasomotor center in brainstem
Exercise	Raises pressure	Increased cardiac output
Postural change	Lowers pressure	Decreased blood volume as person moves from lying to sitting or standing; normally variations are minimal
Smoking	Raises pressure	Increased vasoconstriction

Fig. 12.9 Aneroid manometer and cuff.

difficulties fits around the wrist, does not require a stethoscope, is easy to use, and is well adapted for home use. This device also inflates and deflates at the push of a button.

Stationary automated machines often are located in public places such as grocery stores, pharmacies, fitness clubs, banks, airports, and work sites. Users simply rest the arm within the machine's inflatable cuff, which contains a pressure sensor. The cuff fits over the clothing. A visual display tells users their blood pressure within 60 to 90 seconds. The reliability of the stationary machines is limited; blood pressure values sometimes vary by 5 to 10 mm Hg or more (for the systolic and diastolic values) compared to the pressures taken with a manual sphygmomanometer.

If they have the information that they need to perform the procedure correctly, and if they know when to seek medical attention, consumers can learn to use self-measurement devices to their benefit. Patients should be advised of possible inaccuracies in the machines, how to understand the meaning and

Fig. 12.10 Wall-mounted aneroid sphygmomanometer. (From Potter PA, Perry AG: *Fundamentals of nursing: Concepts, process, and practice*, ed 8, St. Louis, 2013, Mosby.)

implications of readings, and the proper measurement techniques.

PULSE OXIMETRY

A facility may include the measurement of **oxygen saturation** (measurement of how much oxygen has combined with hemoglobin in the red blood cell) with the use of the **pulse oximeter** (device used to measure the oxygen saturation) when obtaining

Fig. 12.11 The sounds auscultated during blood pressure measurement can be differentiated into five Korotkoff phases. In this example, blood pressure is 140/90 mm Hg.

Korotkoff phases

A sharp thump	Phase 1
A blowing or whoosing sound	Phase 2
A softer thump than phase 1	Phase 3
A softer blowing sound that fades	Phase 4
Silence	Phase 5

Fig. 12.12 Doppler stethoscope over brachial artery to measure blood pressure.

vital sign measurements (Skill 12.6). The pulse oximeter is a noninvasive device; the probe is usually placed on the patient's finger (see Skill 12.6, step C). LED and infrared light is emitted and determines the oxygen saturation. Hemoglobin that is oxygenated absorbs more infrared light and allows more red light to pass through, while hemoglobin that is deoxygenated (lacks oxygen) allows more infrared light to pass through the hemoglobin molecules and absorbs more red light. Oxygen saturation is measured in percentage, based on how much hemoglobin is saturated with oxygen. For the person without chronic lung disease, normal oxygen saturation is 95% to 100%. Individuals with chronic lung disease, such as chronic obstructive pulmonary disease (COPD), may have adjusted to different amounts of oxygenated blood, so their normal may vary (see

Adult Health Nursing, Chapter 9). Nail polish and artificial nails interfere with oxygen saturation measurements and should be removed. Cold hands and thick nails can also interfere with measurements. If the fingers cannot be used, there are probes for ears and toes. The pulse is also measured with the pulse oximeter; however, it is advisable to obtain a manual pulse in order to assess the strength and rhythm. Comparing the manual pulse to the oximeter also ensures the accuracy of the oximeter measurement.

HEIGHT AND WEIGHT

With the initial measurement of vital signs, the patient's height (the vertical measurement of a structure, organ, or other object from bottom to top, when it is placed or projected in an upright position) and weight (the force exerted on a body by the gravity of the earth; normal weight depends on the frame of the individual) should be measured. Height and weight determination is important because it helps assess normal growth and development, aids in proper drug dosage calculation, and is used to assess the effectiveness of drug therapy (such as diuretics). Only in cases of extreme illness is it acceptable to delay obtaining these valuable assessments. Because of the importance placed on these measurements, a stated height and weight should not be relied on. Malnourished patients, patients who are undergoing diuretic therapy, and patients who have diseases that increase fluid retention, such as heart, liver, and kidney disease, may need to be weighed frequently (weekly or daily).

OBTAINING WEIGHT MEASUREMENTS

Patients are weighed to give the health care provider information for prescribing medication dosages and to determine nutritional status and water balance.

Skill 12.5   Obtaining a Blood Pressure Reading

CHECK GATHER HELLO ID PRIVACY EXPLAIN WASH GLOVES

NURSING ACTION (RATIONALE)

1. Perform hand hygiene. (*Reduces spread of microorganisms.*)
2. Introduce self. (*Decreases patient's anxiety.*)
3. Identify patient by identification band. (*Verifies correct patient for procedure.*)
4. Explain procedure. (*Seeks cooperation and assistance from patient and decreases patient's anxiety.*)
5. Determine whether patient has ingested caffeine or has been smoking. (*If so, wait 30 minutes before assessment, because caffeine and smoking can cause false elevations.*)
6. Prepare for procedure:
   a. Assemble all necessary supplies, sphygmomanometer, and stethoscope. (*Organizes procedure efficiently.*) Determine the correct cuff size. (*An improper size gives an inaccurate reading.*) The cuff should be approximately 40% of the circumference of the extremity on which the cuff is to be used. (*A higher, inaccurate reading is obtained if too small a cuff is used; a lower, inaccurate reading is obtained if too large a cuff is used.*)
   b. Provide privacy. (*Decreases patient's anxiety.*)

   c. Request that patient assumes sitting or lying position. Be certain room is quiet and warm. (*Maintains comfort.*)
   d. Determine site for blood pressure measurement. Do not apply cuff to arm when in the following situations: (*Applying the cuff complicates these preexisting conditions.*)

(1) Catheter is in antecubital fossa and fluids are infusing.
(2) Arteriovenous shunt is in place.
(3) Breast or axillary surgery has been performed on that side.
(4) An arm or hand has been traumatized or is diseased.
(5) A lower arm cast or bulky bandage is in place.

7. Implement procedure:
   a. Apply cuff to bare arm with patient's palm facing upward. Do not hyperextend. The cuff is applied 1–2 inches above the antecubital space. The cuff is centered over the brachial artery. The patient's upper arm is held at the level of the heart, and the lower arm is rested on a firm surface. (*Ensures accuracy of procedure.*)
   b. Palpate radial artery (see illustration in Skill 12.2).
   c. Inflate cuff. Note the point on the manometer gauge when the radial pulse is obliterated. (*This is the approximate systolic pressure.*)
   d. Deflate the cuff. (*Deflating the cuff allows congestion to leave the arm, preventing a false-high reading.*) Rest arm for 1 min.

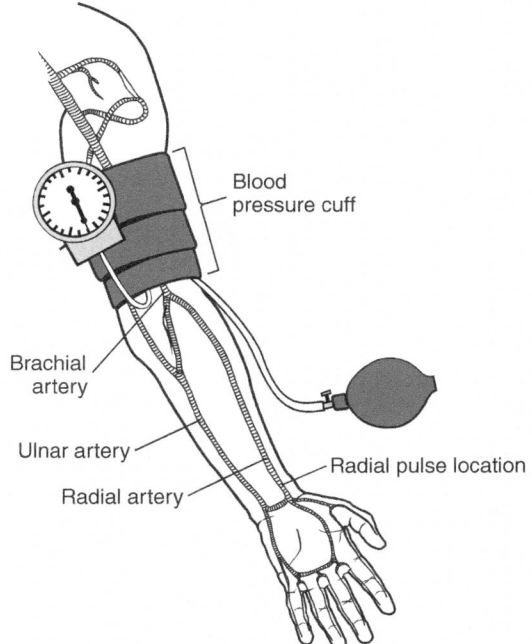

Blood pressure cuff

Brachial artery

Ulnar artery

Radial artery

Radial pulse location

   e. Palpate the brachial artery and place the bell or the diaphragm of the stethoscope over it.

Continued

Skill 12.5   Obtaining a Blood Pressure Reading—cont'd

f. Reinflate cuff to 30 mm Hg above point at which radial artery was obliterated. (*Avoids the auscultatory gap.*) Estimating prevents false low readings that possibly result from the presence of this auscultatory gap (inaudible sounds below the systolic pressure). This phenomenon occurs in about 5% of adults and is prevalent in individuals with hypertension.

g. Slowly deflate cuff. Cuff is deflated at a rate of 2 mm Hg/s. Note the point at which the pulse is heard. (*This is the systolic pressure.*) Note the point at which no pulse is heard. (*This is the diastolic pressure.*)

h. When the Korotkoff sounds are no longer audible, continue to listen for another 10–20 mm Hg. (*Confirms blood pressure reading. Too-rapid deflation often causes a measurement error.*)

i. Completely deflate and remove the cuff.

j. Assist the patient to dress. (*Provides patient comfort.*)

8. Write down reading (for documentation later).

9. Perform hand hygiene. (*Reduces spread of microorganisms.*)

10. Document reading on graphic flow sheet (e.g., blood pressure 120/80 mm Hg; see Fig. 12.1).

11. Follow up by reporting abnormal readings immediately (see Box 12.16 for assessment of blood pressure in both arms and Box 12.14 for assessment of orthostatic blood pressure). (*Reading sometimes has to be reassessed.*)

12. Do patient teaching (see patient teaching in the Health Promotion box on vital signs).

| Box 12.15 | **Nursing Interventions for the Patient With Abnormal Blood Pressure Reading** |

- Repeat assessment, but first eliminate extraneous noise, such as television and conversation, as noise interferes with accuracy. Falsely elevated readings are obtained if patient moves, talks, or coughs during blood pressure measurement.
- If you hear Korotoff sounds (the pulse) immediately when releasing the valve, the patient's systolic blood pressure is higher than the cuff has been inflated. To obtain an accurate reading, release the pressure, wait 60 s, and estimate systolic pressure at higher reading. Reinflate cuff 30 mm Hg above the sound first heard. Reinflation of a partially deflated cuff is uncomfortable for the patient and often yields an inaccurate reading.
- Patient should be seated or lying in a quiet environment, free from temperature extremes, for at least 5 min before blood pressure is obtained. This is a good time to discuss the benefits of exercise and weight control in reducing the risks for hypertension and coronary artery disease or lowering an existing blood pressure elevation.
- Electronic blood pressure cuff and machine must be matched by the manufacturer. Do not interchange blood pressure cuffs from machines of different manufacturers.
- Because blood pressure measurement can frighten children, this is a good time to prepare the child for the squeezing feeling of the inflated blood pressure cuff by saying, "This will feel like a tight hug for a minute."
- If using an electronic blood pressure machine, tell the patient and family that these machines have audible alarm systems. Explain and allow the patient to hear the sound. Inform patient that the alarms do not always mean you have a problem, but also show that the machine needs attention.
- If an abnormal blood pressure reading is obtained, measure blood pressure on the other arm or on a lower extremity or use an ultrasonic Doppler instrument (see Fig. 12.12). Ask another nurse to reassess abnormal readings.
- If blood pressure is above normal, observe for related symptoms such as headache (usually occipital), flushed face, and epistaxis (nosebleed). Older patients may notice fatigue.
- Be certain size of cuff is appropriate. A cuff that is too big will result in an inaccurate low reading, and a cuff that is too tight will result in an inaccurate high reading.
- Positioning and comfort of the extremity should be maintained. For forearm measurements, the arm should be supported or permitted to be on a table or pillow at approximately heart level. For wrist measurements taken with a digital device, the wrist should be placed across the chest or on a table at heart level, depending on manufacturer guidelines.
- Administer medications as ordered.
- Compare your current reading with the patient's baseline.
- If blood pressure is below normal, observe for symptoms such as weak, thready pulse, weakness, vertigo, confusion, pale, dusky, or cyanotic skin, or cool, mottled skin.
  - Position patient in supine position and limit activity.
  - Increase rate of intravenous fluid if infusing, per order

Box **12.16**   **Assessing Blood Pressure in Both Arms**

- For the initial assessment, measure blood pressure in both arms, especially if the patient has heart disease or if the reading in the first arm is abnormal.
- Normally, a difference of 5–10 mm Hg exists between the arms. In subsequent assessments, the blood pressure should be measured in the arm with the higher pressure.
- Pressure differences higher than 10 mm Hg indicate conditions such as aortic stenosis or an arterial occlusion in the arm with the lower pressure.

Fig. 12.14 Monitor displays blood pressure reading.

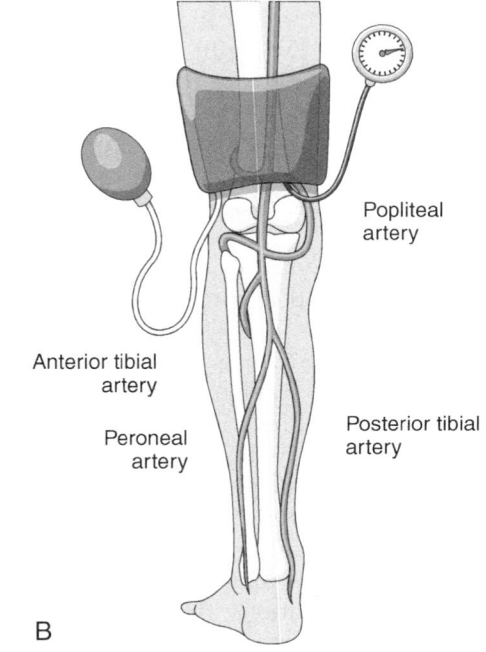

Fig. 12.13 (A) Lower-extremity blood pressure cuff positioned above popliteal artery at mid-thigh. (B) Location of the popliteal artery and placement of the cuff.

Fig. 12.15 Electronic sphygmomanometer.

Because 1 L of fluid equals 1 kg (2.2 lb), a weight change of 1 kg (2.2 lb) often reflects a loss or gain of 1 L of body fluids. A significant loss of weight frequently points to an underlying disease.

Patients should be weighed at the same time of day, on the same scale, and in the same type or amount of clothing to allow an objective comparison of subsequent weighings. An ideal time to weigh

patients is in the morning after voiding and before breakfast.

Various types of weighing scales are available to meet the patient's needs. Patients capable of bearing their own weight use a standing scale (see Skill 12.7); the patient must stand on the scale platform and remain still. Manual scales are calibrated by setting the weight at zero and noting whether the balance beam registers in the middle of the mark. To obtain the patient's weight, slowly adjust the scale weight on the balance beam until the tip of the beam registers in the middle of the mark. Scales with a digital display must read zero before each use, and readouts will display in a matter of seconds.

Chair and sling scales are available for patients unable to bear weight (Fig. 12.16). The sling is placed under the patient and connected to the arms of the scale. The patient is lifted above the bed by a hydraulic device, and the weight is measured on a balance beam or digital display. Caution must be used to promote patient safety when transferring them to and from the scales.

Bed scales may be available in some facilities for those patients who are unable to get out of bed. The nurse should ensure that the patient is not placed in the bed before the scale is zeroed. The patient should always be weighed in the same clothing and, if possible, at the same time of the day.

OBTAINING HEIGHT MEASUREMENTS

Height measurement is recorded in inches or centimeters, depending on agency policy. The calculation to use if transferring height from inches into centimeters

Box 12.17	**Patient Conditions That Make Use of Electronic Blood Pressure Measurements Inappropriate**

- Arrhythmias
- Excessive tremors
- Inability to cooperate to minimize arm motions
- Irregular heart rate
- Obese extremity
- Older adults
- Peripheral vascular obstruction (e.g., clots, narrowed vessels)
- Seizures
- Shivering

is 1 inch equal to 2.54 cm. For example, a person who is 68 inches is 172.72 cm.

When measuring the height of a patient (see Skill 12.7) on a standing scale, ensure that the patient is standing upright with shoes removed. Most standing scales have a metal bar that is placed over the top of the patient's head. For the patient who is unsteady, there is often a handrail attached to the wall for safety. Assist patients on and off the scale. Disinfect the scale after patient use.

Coordinated Care

Supervision

VITAL SIGNS

The skill of vital signs measurement can be delegated to unlicensed assistive personnel (UAP). It is important to remember that even though this task can be delegated, it is ultimately the nurse's responsibility to ensure the accuracy of vital sign measurements. The nurse is also responsible for assessing the effect of changes in the body's vital signs.

- Inform UAP of the following:
  - Appropriate route and device to measure temperature
  - Specific factors related to the patient that can falsely raise or lower temperature
  - The frequency of temperature measurement for a specific patient
  - Any factors that will affect the positioning of a patient when measuring a rectal temperature
  - The patient's history or risk of irregular pulse
  - Frequency of pulse measurement for a specific patient
  - The proper positioning of the patient when measuring the apical pulse
  - The patient's history or risk for increased or decreased respiratory rate or irregular respirations
  - Frequency of respiration measurement for a specific patient
  - If the patient has alterations that affect the appropriate limb for blood pressure measurement
  - Appropriately sized blood pressure cuff for designated extremity
  - Frequency of blood pressure measurement for a specific patient
  - If the patient is at risk for experiencing orthostatic hypotension (before blood pressure measurement)
- Determine that UAP is aware of the usual values of each vital sign for patient.
- Inform UAP of abnormalities of each vital sign that should be reported and reconfirmed by the nurse.
- The UAP is not responsible for using the Doppler. This is a skill for the registered nurse (RN) or licensed practical/vocational nurse (LPN/LVN) to perform.
- Explain which weight device to use for a specific patient.

❖ NURSING PROCESS

The role of the LPN/LVN in the nursing process as stated is that the LPN/LVN will:

- Participate in planning care for patients based on patient needs
- Review patient's plan of care and recommend revisions as needed
- Review and follow defined prioritization for patient care
- Use clinical pathways, care maps, or care plans to guide and review patient care

◆ ASSESSMENT

At initial contact with a patient, a baseline measurement of vital signs routinely is obtained to provide a means for comparison with subsequent vital signs values. These findings aid in determining whether a more thorough assessment of specific body systems is necessary. For example, after assessment of an abnormal respiratory rate, the lung sounds should be auscultated. In certain situations, the assessment of vital signs may be limited to measurement of a single vital sign for the purpose of reviewing a specific aspect of a patient's condition; for example, after the administration of an antihypertensive medication, measurement of the patient's blood pressure to evaluate the medication's effects is essential. Part of a nurse's clinical judgment involves deciding which vital signs to assess and measure and when and how frequently.

This assessment includes the following:

- Normal daily fluctuations
- Factors likely to interfere with accuracy of vital signs reading
- Medications that may influence vital signs

Skill 12.6   Measuring Oxygen Saturation With a Pulse Oximeter

CHECK   GATHER   HELLO   ID   PRIVACY   EXPLAIN   WASH   GLOVES

NURSING ACTION *(RATIONALE)*

1. Perform hand hygiene. *(Reduces spread of microorganisms.)*
2. Introduce self. *(Decreases patient's anxiety.)*
3. Identify patient by identification band and date of birth. *(Verifies correct patient for procedure.)*
4. Explain procedure to patient. *(Gains cooperation and assistance and decreases patient's anxiety.)*
5. Prepare for procedure:
   a. Assemble supplies: Pulse oximeter and alcohol swab. *(Organizes procedure efficiently.)*
   b. Provide privacy. *(Decreases patient's anxiety.)*
6. Implement procedure:
   a. Clean the pulse oximeter probe with alcohol. *(Eliminates microorganisms.)*
   b. If using the patient's finger, ensure that there is not wearing nail polish or artificial nails. *(Nail polish or artificial nails will prevent an accurate measurement of oxygen saturation.)*
   c. Place the probe on the patient's finger. *(Area of measurement for oxygen saturation to be obtained.)*

d. Keep the probe on the finger until a consistent reading is obtained. This may take approximately 15–30 s. *(Taking the measurement too quickly may lead to an inaccurate measurement.)*
e. If unable to obtain a consistent measurement, change to another finger. If still unable to obtain a consistent measurement a toe or earlobe probe may be necessary. *(Changing to a different finger may allow for an accurate measurement. Oxygen saturation can be obtained with a different probe if the toe or earlobe is needed to obtain the measurement.)*
f. If continuous pulse oximetry is ordered, the probe may need to be secured to the patient's finger, toe, or earlobe using tape or Velcro band. *(If a continuous pulse oximeter is not secured to the finger, toe, or earlobe, it may become dislodge easily.)*
g. The pulse can also be obtained using the pulse oximeter; obtaining the pulse manually can assist in ensuring that the pulse oximetry measurement is accurate. *(The pulse oximeter measures the pulse and oxygen saturation level. Obtaining a manual pulse and comparing it to the pulse oximeter ensures that the pulse oximeter is working properly.)*
7. Write down measurement or document the measurement in the electronic record immediately. *(If not immediately documenting the measurement in the electronic record, the measurement should be written down to ensure correct documentation later.)*
8. Clean the probe with alcohol. *(Removes microorganisms from the probe for later use).*
9. Perform hand hygiene. *(Reduces spread of microorganisms.)*
10. Document measurement (e.g., O_2 saturation [O_2 sat] 97%).

Follow up by reporting measurement and remeasuring as ordered or warranted by the patient's condition. *(Reading often varies and must be reassessed.)*

- Other factors that influence vital signs
- Conditions that precipitate fever, such as infections
- Previous baseline vital signs from patient's record; baseline information provides basis for comparison and assists in assessment of current status

◆ PATIENT PROBLEM

A review of all data gathered during assessment is required to determine the patient problem; defining characteristics, when clustered, will reveal this problem. The following are possible patient problems related to vital signs:

- Inadequate fluid volume
- Elevated body temperature
- Below normal body temperature
- Potential for inability to regulate body temperature
- Inefficient oxygenation

◆ EXPECTED OUTCOMES AND PLANNING

The appropriate focus for the plan of care is on those nursing interventions that identify abnormalities and restore homeostasis (a relative constancy in the internal environment of the body, naturally maintained by adaptive responses that promote healthy survival).

A possible patient-centered goal is often "patient's vital signs will be within normal range" or, for patients with chronic diseases that alter vital signs, such as chronic obstructive pulmonary disease (COPD), "baseline will be established."

Expected outcomes often include the following:
- Patient's vital signs are within normal range for age group.
- Baseline is established for patients with chronic diseases such as COPD.

◆ IMPLEMENTATION

The severity of an alteration in a vital sign influences the priorities in the care of the patient.

What procedures the health care team uses to intervene and treat an abnormal vital sign depends on the cause, any adverse effects, the strength and intensity of the abnormal vital signs, and how long the abnormality persists. Direct interventions toward providing comfort to the patient and to keeping complications to a minimum (see Boxes 12.6, 12.10, 12.12, and 12.15).

◆ EVALUATION

Evaluate all nursing interventions by comparing the patient's actual responses with the outcome of the care plan; for example:

Outcome: Patient's blood pressure, pulse, respirations, and temperature are within normal range for age group.

Evaluative measures: Assess vital signs on a regular basis, such as every 4 hours and after activity.

Fig. 12.16 Types of scales. (A) Standing scale. (B) Chair scale. (C) Lift scale. (D) Bed scale. (B and C, From Sorrentino SA, Remmert LN: *Mosby's textbook for nursing assistants*, ed 9, St. Louis, 2017, Elsevier.)

Skill 12.7   Measuring Height and Weight

NURSING ACTION *(RATIONALE)*

1. Perform hand hygiene. *(Reduces spread of microorganisms.)*
2. Introduce self. *(Decreases patient's anxiety.)*
3. Identify patient by identification band. *(Verifies correct patient for procedure.)*
4. Explain procedure to patient. *(Gains cooperation and assistance and decreases patient's anxiety.)*
5. Prepare for procedure:
   - c. Assemble supplies, including scale: standing, chair, or bed type. *(Organizes procedure efficiently.)*
   - d. Provide privacy. *(Decreases patient's anxiety.)*
6. Implement procedure:
   - h. Balance scale at zero. *(Ensures accurate reading.)*
   - i. Place paper towel over base of scale where patient will stand, if patient is barefoot. *(Promotes medical asepsis.)*
   - j. Have patient step onto scale. Patient should be weighed in same amount of clothing each time—preferably gown; slippers are optional. *(Promotes an accurate comparison.)*
   - k. Measure height with patient standing upright, if patient can tolerate this. *(Promotes accurate measurement.)*
   - l. Measure weight. *(Provides accurate measurement.)*
   - m. Assist patient off scale by having patient step to side. *(Safer than stepping backward.)*
   - n. Assist to bed or chair to provide for patient's comfort. *(Promotes patient's self-esteem.)*
7. Write down measurement (for documentation later).
8. Perform hand hygiene. *(Reduces spread of microorganisms.)*
9. Document measurements (e.g., height: 64 inches [162.56 cm], weight: 136 lb) (see Fig. 12.1).
10. Follow up by reporting measurement. *(Reading often varies and must be reassessed.)*

Get Ready for the NCLEX® Examination!

Key Points

- Vital signs include the physiologic parameters of temperature, pulse, respiration, and blood pressure.
- Vital signs often are measured as part of a complete physical examination or, more commonly, in a review of the patient's condition.
- Obtain vital signs whenever the patient's condition changes adversely.
- Knowledge of the factors that influence vital signs can assist in interpreting abnormal values.
- Vital signs' measurements provide a basis for evaluating the patient's response to medical and nursing interventions.
- Approach the patient in a calm and caring manner while demonstrating proficiency in handling supplies needed for vital sign measurement.
- Vital signs are best measured when the patient is inactive (at rest) and the environment is controlled for comfort.
- A fever is one of the body's normal defense mechanisms.
- Temperatures are obtained via oral, rectal, axillary, and tympanic routes.
- The use of in-glass mercury thermometers and all mercury-containing devices for patient care is no longer advisable due to the danger of mercury toxicity.

- Do not perform rectal temperature measurements on newborns, infants, or adults with rectal alterations.
- The tympanic route is the most accessible and acceptable site for measuring core body temperature.
- Assess the presence and character of peripheral pulses to determine the adequacy of peripheral blood flow.
- For blood pressure assessment, having the proper equipment is as important as using the correct technique.
- Self-measurement of blood pressure is useful when it leads to the detection of an elevated blood pressure in people previously unaware of a problem. It is also useful in monitoring blood pressure in people already diagnosed with hypertension.
- No clinically significant difference in blood pressure levels is found between boys and girls. After puberty, males tend to have higher blood pressure readings. After menopause, women tend to have higher levels of blood pressure than men of similar age.
- The automatic blood pressure cuff is useful for home use if the patient or caregiver has hearing difficulties.
- Most facilities have developed a fifth vital sign: pain control or comfort level. Pain has an observable effect on vital signs.
- Temperature, pulse, respiration, and blood pressure are interrelated; a change in one has the potential to alter the others.

- Oxygen saturation (O_2 sat) is a measurement of the amount of oxygen that has combined with hemoglobin in the red blood cell.
- Normal oxygen saturation is 95% to 100%.

Additional Learning Resources

SG Go to your Study Guide for additional learning activities to help you master this chapter content.

Be sure to visit the Evolve site at http://evolve.elsevier.com/Cooper/foundations/ for additional online resources.

Review Questions for the NCLEX® Examination

1. A patient is undergoing antibiotic therapy for pneumonia, and his rectal temperature reading is 101.6°F. What is the expected oral temperature reading?

   1. 101.6°F (38.7°C)
   2. 100.6°F (38.1°C)
   3. 99.6°F (37.5°C)
   4. 97.6°F (36.4°C)

2. A patient has a postpartum temperature that is elevated in the evening but returns to a normal reading in the morning. This has occurred for several days. What is this type of fever classification?

   1. Constant
   2. Intermittent
   3. Remittent
   4. Crisis

3. A patient has a 10-year history of coronary artery disease. The patient is recovering from a myocardial infarction. What is the most accurate way for the nurse to assess the pulse rate?

   1. Carotid pulse
   2. Radial pulse
   3. Apical pulse
   4. Brachial pulse

4. An adult patient is admitted to the emergency department with an exacerbation of asthma. Respirations are 40 breaths per minute. After treatment, the rate returns to normal limits. What respiratory range is considered to be normal?

   1. 30 to 60
   2. 12 to 20
   3. 16 to 22
   4. 24 to 30

5. During a routine physical examination, a patient's blood pressure is noted at 180/90 mm Hg. The patient states, "Oh no, I didn't know I had high blood pressure." The nurse is aware that the patient's blood pressure must measure above what level at two separate office visits for the patient to be diagnosed with hypertension?

   1. 160/100 mm Hg
   2. 140/90 mm Hg
   3. 130/70 mm Hg
   4. 120/80 mm Hg

6. A 65-year-old man has a history of emphysema resulting from 30 years of cigarette smoking. He frequently reports dyspnea. What is dyspnea?

   1. Pallor
   2. Absence of retractions
   3. Cyanosis
   4. Difficulty breathing

7. A patient reports palpitations that result from anxiety over an impending surgery. The pulse rate is found to be 110 beats per minute. How will the nurse describe this heart rate?

   1. Bradycardia
   2. Tachycardia
   3. Tachypnea
   4. Hypertension

8. The nurse obtains a supine blood pressure reading of 130/64 mm Hg. One hour later, the nurse obtains a supine blood pressure reading of 134/62 mm Hg and a sitting blood pressure reading of 95/62 mm Hg. What should be the immediate action of the nurse?

   1. Assist the patient to return to a supine position.
   2. Obtain a blood pressure reading in the other arm.
   3. Report the findings to the nurse in charge.
   4. Question the patient about any symptoms.

9. The nurse is assessing a patient's blood pressure for the first time as part of the patient's postoperative assessment. After reaching the point at which the radial pulse is obliterated, what is the next action of the nurse?

   1. Deflate the cuff slowly and wait 15 to 20 seconds before reinflating.
   2. Deflate the cuff rapidly and wait 15 to 30 seconds before reinflating.
   3. Deflate the cuff slowly and wait 1 minute before reinflating.
   4. Deflate the cuff rapidly and wait 1 minute before reinflating.

10. The nurse has been assigned several patients. Which patient is most likely to have a higher-than-normal temperature? *(Select all that apply.)*

    1. A depressed, apathetic patient
    2. A patient assessed with hemorrhage
    3. A patient who is recovering from surgery
    4. A patient who just finished eating
    5. A patient who has a temperature of 101.4°F

11. A patient is admitted after a motorcycle accident. The nurse is assessing the pulse pressure. The blood pressure reading is 140/102 mm Hg. What is the correct pulse pressure?

    _____

12. The nurse is preparing to assess a 2-day-old infant's pulse rate. Which site should be used?

    1. Scalp artery
    2. Femoral artery
    3. Apical site
    4. Radial site

13. The nurse is assessing a postoperative patient's apical and radial pulses. Which statement is correct concerning this assessment of the patient's apical and radial pulse measurements?

    1. The apical pulse and radial pulse should be taken for 1 full minute each.
    2. The apical and radial pulse rates are lower when the temperature is elevated.
    3. The apical and radial pulses are taken at the same time for 30 seconds.
    4. The apical and radial pulses are taken at the same time for 60 seconds.

14. The healthcare provider has ordered an orthostatic blood pressure measurement. Place the following statements in the correct order concerning the orthostatic method of assessing blood pressure.

    1. The measurement is taken when the patient is standing.
    2. The measurement is taken with the patient lying down.
    3. The nurse assesses the blood pressure in the sitting position.
    4. The nurse documents the blood pressure readings.

15. The patient's oral temperature is 37°C. What is the appropriate reporting of this temperature?

    1. Febrile
    2. Afebrile
    3. Hypotensive
    4. Hypertensive

16. Which is an important factor in the measurement of vital signs? *(Select all that apply.)*

    1. Ranges of normal for vital signs are very narrow and apply to all patients.
    2. The most significant aspect of measuring vital signs is their documentation.
    3. Environmental factors have an insignificant effect on the patient's vital signs.
    4. All measuring equipment is chosen on the basis of the patient's conditions and characteristics.
    5. Smoking can alter the temperature, pulse, respirations, and blood pressure by increasing each vital sign.

17. The patient has been hospitalized after a severe head injury. What is the most likely reason for the patient having difficulty in maintaining a normal body temperature when there is no infection present?

    1. Choosing the wrong time of day to obtain vital signs
    2. Errors by the nurse in measuring temperature
    3. Increased vasodilation of the superficial vessels contributing to excess heat loss
    4. The patient's head injury causing interference with the function of the hypothalamus

18. A pulse deficit provides information about the heart's ability to adequately perfuse the body. What is the definition of a pulse deficit?

    1. The difference between the radial and the apical pulse rates
    2. The digital pressure felt when taking radial and ulnar pulses

    3. The amount of pressure felt when taking radial and ulnar pulses
    4. The difference between the systolic and the diastolic blood pressure readings

19. The nurse finds that the patient's oral temperature is 98.8°F (37.1°C). What is the nurse's next action?

    1. Administer an antiemetic drug.
    2. Offer the patient an additional blanket.
    3. Report that the patient's temperature is normal.
    4. Compare this with the patient's baseline.

20. The unlicensed assistive personnel reports that the patient is feeling "funny." What is the nurse's first action?

    1. Notify the health care provider.
    2. Obtain the patient's vital signs yourself.
    3. Delegate the assistant to retake the vital signs.
    4. Tell the assistant to keep assessing the patient and report any further symptoms.

21. The nurse is taking vital sign measurements and notes that the patient has a strong radial pulse that diminishes in intensity, and that there are interruptions in rhythm about every four to six beats. What is the nurse's next action?

    1. Report the findings to a health care provider.
    2. Measure a 60-second apical pulse.
    3. Connect the patient to a cardiac monitor.
    4. Obtain a 60-second apical-radial pulse.

22. When documenting a patient's blood pressure, at what point is the systolic pressure recorded?

    1. At the first Korotkoff sound
    2. At the second Korotkoff sound
    3. At the fourth Korotkoff sound
    4. At the fifth Korotkoff sound

23. Which method of measuring temperature reveals core temperature? *(Select all that apply.)*

    1. Skin
    2. Temporal
    3. Oral
    4. Axillary
    5. Tympanic

24. The nurse is providing discharge teaching to a patient who has recently been diagnosed with a cardiac condition. In teaching this patient how to assess the pulse, which is the best location for the nurse to advise?

    1. Radial artery
    2. Pedal artery
    3. Brachial artery
    4. Femoral artery

25. When teaching the patient about monitoring his own pulse, the nurse informs the patient that the pulse may be elevated by which of the following? *(Select all that apply.)*

    1. Taking beta blockers
    2. Fever
    3. Sleeping
    4. Standing up too quickly
    5. Acute pain

26. The nurse begins to measure the blood pressure of an adult. The patient says that his doctor has instructed him to always use a large cuff. What is a reason for using a large cuff?

    1. A blood pressure cuff that is too small gives inaccurately high readings.
    2. A blood pressure cuff that is too small likely injures the brachial artery.
    3. Large cuffs are typically more accurate on adults than normal-size cuffs.
    4. Normal-size cuffs should be used for pediatric patients.

27. The nurse is developing a care plan for a patient taking a diuretic to treat fluid retention. The nurse knows that weighing the patient on a daily basis will assist in monitoring the effectiveness of the medication, because a weight loss of 1 kg indicates a fluid loss of how much? _____

28. A man, 76, came to the ER after passing out while getting up from his chair. His wife mentions noticing his speech sounding slurred and somewhat garbled that afternoon as they were chatting while putting a puzzle together, just minutes before he collapsed. While the patient is unable to recall the moment of passing out, the patient remembers that his vision felt "off" leading up to the incident, as if he were seeing double while trying to sort through the puzzle's edge pieces. The patient reports that his vision now feels normal, and his wife affirms that his speech sounds clear again, but he describes still feeling "dizzy" and "off balance." The staff take his vitals and find slightly elevated BP and mild fatigue. He is concerned that he is having some difficulty opening and closing his hand. The medical team suspects the patient had a transient ischemic attack (TIA), often called a ministroke. Because he is stable, a decision is made to release him to home. In addition to guiding the couple in how to monitor for after-effects of TIA, the nurse gives them instructions on how to take vital signs at home.

Place a check mark to indicate each teaching point in the left column that applies to the guidelines for vital signs measurement. Check all that apply.

TEACHING POINT	APPROPRIATE GUIDELINES FOR VITAL SIGNS MEASUREMENT
Use fingertips, never thumbs, for counting the pulse.	
Vary time of blood pressure measurements to get an an accurate assessment.	
Measure vital signs before eating or smoking.	
Use gentle pressure when taking the pulse.	
Alert patient before taking respiratory rate.	
Raise patient's arm to heart level for BP measurement.	

Physical Assessment

Objectives

1. Discuss the difference between a sign and a symptom.
2. Compare and contrast the origins of disease.
3. List the four major risk categories for development of disease.
4. Discuss frequently noted signs and symptoms of disease conditions.
5. List the cardinal signs of inflammation and infection.
6. Describe the nursing responsibilities when assisting a physician with the physical examination.
7. List equipment and supplies necessary for the physical examination/assessment.
8. Explain the necessary skills for the physical examination/nursing assessment.
9. Discuss the nurse-patient interview.
10. List the basic essentials for gathering a patient's health history.
11. Discuss the sequence of steps when performing a nursing assessment.
12. Discuss normal and abnormal assessment findings in the head-to-toe assessment.
13. Describe documentation of the physical examination/nursing assessment.
14. Explain ways to develop cultural sensitivity.

Key Terms

acute (p. 317)
anorexia (p. 318, table 13.1)
assessment (p. 319)
auscultation (ăw-skŭl-TĂ-shŭn, p. 322, box 13.4)
borborygmi (bŏr-bō-RĬG-mē, p. 336)
bruits (BRŪ-ē, p. 315)
chronic (p. 317)
crackles (p. 332)
disease (p. 316)
drainage (p. 315)
dullness (p. 322, box 13.4)
edema (p. 317)
erythema (ĕr-ĕ-THĒ-mă, p. 317)
etiology (ē-tē-ŎL-ĕ-jē, p. 316)
exudate (ĔKS-ū-dāt, p. 316)
flatness (p. 322, box 13.4)
focused assessment (p. 328)
functional disease (p. 317)
infection (p. 317)
inflammation (p. 317)

inspection (p. 322, box 13.4)
level of consciousness (LOC) (p. 326)
neoplastic (nē-ō-PLĂS-tĭk, p. 316)
nursing health history (p. 320)
nursing physical assessment (p. 326)
objective data (p. 315)
organic disease (p. 317)
palpation (p. 315, box 13.4)
percussion (pŭr-KŬ-shŭn, p. 322, box 13.4)
pruritus (prū-RĪ-tŭs, p. 316)
purulent (PYŪ-rū-lĕnt, p. 317)
remission (p. 317)
signs (p. 315)
subjective data (p. 316)
symptoms (p. 316)
thrill (p. 331)
turgor (TŬR-gŏr, p. 330)
tympany (TĬM-pă-nē, p. 322, box 13.4)
wheezes (p. 332)

Assessment of the patient is a key element of nursing care. The patient's baseline condition and changes in condition are monitored by the nurse. The patient's well-being relies on accurate nursing assessments.

SIGNS AND SYMPTOMS

In a nursing assessment, signs are objective data as perceived by the nurse. What the nurse sees, hears, measures, and feels are considered objective data. More than one person can verify objective data with observation and measurement. Examples of signs are rashes, altered vital signs, abnormal lung or heart sounds, and visible drainage or exudate. Drainage refers to the passive or active removal of fluids from a body cavity, wound, or other source of discharge by one or more methods. Examples are the closed urinary drainage system or an open drainage system, such as a Jackson-Pratt drain. Exudate is fluid that leaks out of blood vessels into nearby tissues. The fluid is made of cells, proteins, and solid materials. Exudate may ooze from cuts or from areas of infection or inflammation. It is also called pus.

The senses of sight, hearing, touch, and smell are used to gather the objective data or signs. Objective data also include laboratory findings and diagnostic imaging and other diagnostic studies.

Symptoms are subjective indications of illness that the patient perceives. Examples of symptoms are pain, nausea, vertigo, pruritus, diplopia, numbness, and anxiety. Subjective data are what the patient tells the nurse about a symptom. An example is, "I feel like a knife is stabbing me in my stomach" as the patient points to the upper abdominal area.

In subjective data collection, the nurse encourages a full description by the patient of the onset, the course, and the character of the problem and any factors that aggravate or alleviate it. Many signs accompany symptoms; for example, the nurse often sees erythema and a rash when a patient reports pruritus (itching). Objective confirmation of some symptoms is possible; for example, absence of response to a pinprick confirms patient reports of numbness of a body part.

DISEASE AND DIAGNOSIS

Disease, a pathologic condition of the body, is any disturbance of a structure or function of the body. A recognized set of signs and symptoms characterizes a given disease. How the signs and symptoms are clustered or grouped allows the health care provider to make a medical diagnosis. The nurse relies on assessment of signs and symptoms in this case to formulate a patient problem statement. Unlike the medical diagnosis, which deals with pathophysiologic factors and the cure of disease, the patient problem statement recognizes holistic needs of the patient that will be treated with nursing interventions. Some nursing interventions are made independently. To accomplish others, the nurse depends on or collaborates with other members of the health care team.

ORIGINS OF DISEASE

Disease or illness originates from many causes; these are sometimes hereditary and sometimes congenital, inflammatory, degenerative, infectious, deficiency, metabolic, neoplastic, traumatic, environmental, or some combination of these. For other diseases, no apparent cause is known. These illnesses, such as autoimmune diseases, are said to have an unknown etiology, or cause.

Hereditary diseases are transmitted genetically from parents to children. Some examples are cystic fibrosis, sickle cell anemia, color blindness, and hemophilia.

Congenital diseases appear at birth or shortly thereafter but are not caused by genetic abnormalities.

Congenital diseases result from some failure in development during the embryonic stage, or the first 2 months, of pregnancy. Contributing factors include inadequate oxygen, maternal infection, drugs, alcohol, malnutrition, and radiation. Structural and functional defects occur. Examples include absence of limbs (structural) and blindness (functional).

Inflammatory diseases are those in which the body reacts with an inflammatory response to some causative agent. Microorganisms are the cause in many instances, such as with pharyngitis or bronchitis. Other inflammatory diseases, such as hay fever, are manifestations of an allergic reaction. Still others have an unknown cause.

Degenerative disease implies degeneration, often progressive, of some part of the body. The aging process may play a role in degenerative diseases. Osteoarthritis is a common example.

Infectious diseases result from the invasion of microorganisms into the body. Examples of infectious diseases include acquired immunodeficiency syndrome (AIDS), tuberculosis, measles, and pneumonia.

Deficiency diseases result from the lack of a specific nutrient. Nutrients are minerals, vitamins, proteins, fats, and carbohydrates. Iron deficiency anemia sometimes results from a severe deficiency of iron in the diet.

Metabolic disease is caused by a dysfunction that results in a loss of metabolic control of homeostasis in the body. The dysfunction usually involves endocrine glands, which secrete hormones to regulate body processes. Diabetes mellitus results from the dysfunction of the pancreatic islets. Other examples of metabolic disease are hypothyroidism and acromegaly, which involve the thyroid and pituitary glands.

Neoplastic disease is described as an abnormal growth of new tissues. The new growth is sometimes benign and sometimes malignant (cancerous). Malignant neoplasms are a serious threat to health because of the rapid growth of the cells and their ability to invade and metastasize.

Traumatic conditions result from physical and emotional trauma. Physical trauma, such as a motor vehicle accident, has the potential to result in traumatic brain injury (TBI). TBI frequently leaves the individual mentally and physically impaired. Individuals who suffer emotional trauma, such as the loss of a loved one, sometimes become unable to manage the activities of daily living (ADLs) they participated in before the trauma. Other examples of traumatic conditions include physical, psychosocial, and sexual abuse.

Environmental diseases are a group of conditions that develop from exposure to a harmful substance in the environment. Carbon monoxide (CO), an odorless, colorless gas that can cause sudden illness and death, is produced any time a fossil fuel is burned and is produced by cars and trucks, generators, stoves, lanterns, burning charcoal and wood, gas ranges, and heating systems (CDC, 2020). Asbestos is another substance in the environment that potentially leads to lung problems and various cancers.

Many diseases with an unknown cause are now considered to result from *autoimmune responses*. In an autoimmune response, the body develops immunoglobulins (antibodies) against its own tissues or body substances. Autoimmune diseases include rheumatoid arthritis and ulcerative colitis.

RISK FACTORS FOR DEVELOPMENT OF DISEASE

A risk factor is any situation, habit, environmental condition, genetic predisposition, physiologic condition, or other variable that increases the vulnerability of an individual or group to illness or accident. Risk factors for the development of coronary artery disease include heredity, cigarette smoking, high blood levels of cholesterol, diabetes, obesity, and stress. The presence of risk factors does not necessarily mean a person will develop a disease, only that the chance is higher. The nurse assesses the patient's risk factors and uses the risk factors to help formulate nursing diagnoses. Nursing diagnoses are utilized for the patient's potential, and actual, health problems.

Risk factors fall into four major categories: genetic and physiologic, age, environment, and lifestyle (Box 13.1). Many environmental and lifestyle risk factors are modifiable; others, such as age and family history, are not.

TERMS USED TO DESCRIBE DISEASE

Diseases are described in terms of duration. Chronic disease develops slowly and persists over a long period, often for a person's lifetime. Diabetes mellitus (inability of the body to use glucose) is an example of a chronic disease. Chronic disease frequently is described further as early, late, or terminal; another possibility is that it is in remission. Remission means a partial or complete disappearance of clinical and subjective characteristics of the disease has occurred. Remission is sometimes spontaneous and sometimes a result of therapy.

In comparison, a disease described as acute begins abruptly with marked intensity of severe signs and symptoms and then often subsides after a period of treatment. An episode of appendicitis is considered acute.

Disease is often described as organic or functional. An organic disease results in a structural change in an organ that interferes with its functioning. Stroke is an organic disease of the brain. Manifestations of functional disease often appear to be those of organic disease, but careful examination fails to reveal evidence of structural or physiologic abnormalities. Many nervous and mental diseases are classified as functional.

FREQUENTLY NOTED SIGNS AND SYMPTOMS OF DISEASE

Although signs and symptoms of inflammation and infection are similar, it is important not to confuse the

---

Box **13.1** Risk Factors for Disease

GENETIC AND PHYSIOLOGIC
- A family history of cancer increases the risk that an individual will have cancer develop (genetic).
- Malnourishment predisposes an individual to illness (physiologic).

AGE
- Osteoporosis makes the older adult more prone to fractures, especially of the hip.
- Thinning skin in older adults makes this group more susceptible to skin trauma.

ENVIRONMENT
- Air, water, and noise pollution increase the risk of illness.
- Asbestos in building structures increases the risk of cancer of the pleura (in lung).
- Carbon monoxide (CO) with the burning of fossil fuels in generators, gas stoves, and heaters may lead to sudden illness and death.
- Extremes of heat and cold have potential to damage or destroy body cells.
- High crime rates and overcrowding also lead to stress, which makes individuals more susceptible to disease.
- Within the family, conflicts or other problems have the potential to create stressors that put individual members or the family as a whole at increased risk of illness.

LIFESTYLE
- Other habits that place a person at risk for illness include alcohol and substance abuse.
- Overeating or poor nutrition, insufficient rest and sleep, and poor personal hygiene also add to increased risk for illness for the individual.
- Prolonged emotional stress, especially with ineffective coping mechanisms, increases the risk of the development of illness and disease.
- Smoking increases the risk of many diseases, including oral (mouth) cancer, pharyngeal cancer, laryngeal cancer, lung cancer, renal cancer, esophageal cancer, pancreatic cancer, bladder cancer, uterine and cervical cancer, cardiovascular disease, and osteoporosis. Smoking is the most preventable cause of death in our society.
- Sunbathing increases the risk of skin cancer.

---

two. Infection is caused by an invasion of microorganisms, such as bacteria, viruses, fungi, or parasites, that produce tissue damage. Inflammation is a protective response of body tissues to irritation, injury, or invasion by disease-producing organisms. The cardinal signs of infection and inflammation include erythema (redness), edema (swelling), heat, pain, purulent drainage (pus), and loss of function (Table 13.1).

The inflammatory response is the body's defense against some causative agent. Erythema and heat are the result of increased blood flow to the area. The damaged tissue releases chemical substances that cause the capillary walls to become more permeable. This enables white blood cells and plasma to move from

Table 13.1 Frequently Noted Signs and Symptoms of Disease Conditions

TERM	DEFINITION
Anorexia	Lack of appetite that results in the inability to eat. This symptom can occur in many disease conditions.
Asthenia	A condition of debility, loss of strength and energy, and depleted vitality.
Bradycardia	A circulatory condition in which the myocardium contracts steadily but at a rate of less than 60 contractions per minute.
Constipation	Difficulty in passing stools or an incomplete or infrequent passage of hard stools. There are many organic and functional causes.
Coughing	A sudden audible expulsion of air from the lungs. Coughing is an essential protective response that clears the lungs, the bronchi, and the trachea of irritants and secretions and prevents aspiration of foreign material into the lungs. It is a common sign of diseases of the larynx, bronchi, and lungs.
Cyanosis	Bluish discoloration of the skin and mucous membranes caused by an increase of deoxygenated hemoglobin in the blood.
Diaphoresis	The secretion of sweat, especially the profuse secretion associated with an elevated body temperature, physical exertion, exposure to heat, and mental or emotional stress.
Diarrhea	Frequent passage of loose, liquid stools; generally results from increased motility in the colon. This is usually a sign of an underlying disorder. The characteristics of the diarrhea give evidence as to the source. Dark black, tarry stools sometimes mean there is bleeding in the intestines. Bright red blood in the feces indicates active bleeding from the lower portion of the intestinal tract.
Dyspnea	A shortness of breath or difficulty in breathing that is sometimes caused by certain heart and lung conditions, strenuous exercise, or anxiety.
Ecchymosis	Discoloration of an area of the skin or mucous membrane caused by the extravasation of blood into the subcutaneous tissues as a result of trauma to the underlying blood vessels or by fragility of the vessel walls (also called a *bruise*).
Edema	An abnormal accumulation of fluid in interstitial spaces. Some causes include overhydration, excess sodium intake, capillary hyperpermeability, and loss of serum albumin (a protein), which causes fluid to leave the vessels and collect in the interstitial space. Skin that is edematous is taut and shiny. Pitting sometimes occurs when the skin is pressed; a small indentation remains after the finger is removed.
Erythema	Redness or inflammation of the skin or mucous membranes that is the result of dilation and congestion of superficial capillaries; erythema is seen in a mild sunburn.
Fetid	Pertaining to something that has a foul, putrid, or offensive odor. Also called *malodorous*.
Fever	An abnormal elevation of the temperature of the body above 98.6°F (37°C) because of disease; also called *pyrexia.* It results from an imbalance between the elimination and production of heat. Infection and many different diseases often lead to febrile condition, or elevated temperature.
Inflammation	The protective response of the tissues of the body to irritation or injury.
Jaundice	Yellow tinge to the skin; often indicates obstruction in the flow of bile from the liver.
Lethargy	The state or quality of being indifferent, apathetic, or sluggish.
Nausea	A sensation that often leads to the urge to vomit. Common causes include intense pain, gallbladder disease, inflammation of the stomach, paralytic ileus, and food poisoning.
Orthopnea	An abnormal condition in which a person has to sit or stand to breathe deeply or comfortably. Occurs in many disorders of the respiratory and cardiac systems.
Pain	An unpleasant sensation caused by noxious (extremely destructive or harmful) stimulation of the sensory nerve endings. It is a cardinal symptom of inflammation and is valuable in the diagnosis of many disorders and conditions. Pain has varied manifestations: mild or severe, chronic, acute, burning, dull or sharp, precisely or poorly localized, or referred.
Pallor	An unnatural paleness or absence of color in the skin; often results from a decrease in hemoglobin and erythrocytes (red blood cells).
Pruritus	A symptom of itching and an uncomfortable sensation that leads to an urge to scratch. Some causes are allergy, infection, jaundice, elevated serum urea, and skin irritation.
Purulent drainage (pus)	A creamy, viscous, pale yellow, or yellow-green fluid exudate that is the result of fluid remains of liquefied necrosis of tissues. Bacterial infection is the most common cause. The character of the pus, including its color, consistency, quantity, or odor, often has diagnostic significance.
Sallow	Pertaining to an unhealthy, yellow color; usually said of a complexion or skin.
Scleral icterus	The color of the sclera is yellow. This jaundice is the result of coloring of the sclera with bilirubin that infiltrates all tissues of the body.

Table **13.1**	Frequently Noted Signs and Symptoms of Disease Conditions—cont'd
TERM	**DEFINITION**
Tachycardia	An abnormal condition in which the heart contracts regularly but at a rate greater than 100 beats/min. The heart rate accelerates in response to fever, exercise, or nervous excitement.
Tachypnea	An abnormally rapid rate of breathing seen in many disease conditions.
Vomit	To expel the contents of the stomach through the esophagus and out of the mouth. The quality of the vomitus often gives a clue to the underlying cause. "Coffee-ground" vomitus indicates bleeding in the stomach. The blood takes on a coffee-ground appearance because of the effect of the digestive juices. Vomiting of bright red blood is potentially a sign of gastric hemorrhage.

Fig. 13.1 Equipment used during a physical examination *(clockwise from upper left):* disposable gloves, ophthalmoscope, otoscope attachment, sterile safety pin, tuning fork, cervical spatulas, tongue depressor, cotton-tipped swab, lubricant, vaginal speculum, reflex hammer, tape measure, penlight, specimen cup, sphygmomanometer, and stethoscope *(bottom).* (From Bonewit-West K, Hunt S: *Today's medical assistant*, ed 4, St. Louis, 2021, Elsevier.)

the blood to the affected area. The white blood cells (neutrophils) digest microorganisms and cellular debris, and the excess of fluid in the tissues, or edema, increases pressure on sensitive nerve endings, causing pain. Loss of function imposes a period of rest for the injured area. Purulent exudate is the accumulation of neutrophils, dead cells, bacteria, and other debris from the infectious process.

ASSESSMENT

A complete health **assessment** is an evaluation or appraisal of the patient's condition. The process involves the orderly collection of information concerning the patient's health status. It is performed by the health care provider and nursing personnel and usually involves taking a medical history and performing a physical examination. The data collected establish a baseline. This baseline allows the health care provider or the nurse to identify problems and plan care; in addition, ongoing assessments produce contrasting data that permit the evaluation of the effectiveness of care.

MEDICAL ASSESSMENT

When the health care provider conducts a physical examination, the licensed practical nurse (LPN) often is expected to carry out certain assistive functions. Preparing the examining room, assisting with equipment, preparing the patient, and collecting specimens are a few examples of the nurse's responsibilities to facilitate the physical examination. The nurse has both pre-examination and post-examination responsibilities.

When preparing the patient for the physical examination, verify that certain data have been obtained and specific requirements have been addressed. The following list addresses the requirements and data:

- Ensure that an informed consent has been obtained by the health care provider for necessary procedures and that the consent form contains appropriate signatures.
- Verify that all prerequisite tests have been completed and that results are available.
- Confirm that all necessary supplies and equipment have been obtained for the health care provider to perform the examination (Fig. 13.1 and Box 13.2).

Box 13.2	**Equipment and Supplies for Physical Examination and Assessment**

- Cotton applicators
- Cytobrush
- Disposable pad
- Drapes
- Eye chart (e.g., Snellen chart)
- Flashlight and spotlight
- Forms (e.g., physical examination results, laboratory requisitions)
- Gloves (sterile and clean)
- Gown for patient
- Lubricant
- Ophthalmoscope
- Otoscope
- Papanicolaou (Pap) smear slides
- Paper towels
- Percussion hammer
- Safety pins
- Scale with height measurement rod
- Spatula
- Specimen containers and microscope slides
- Sphygmomanometer and cuff
- Stethoscope
- Swabs or sponge forceps
- Tape measure
- Thermometer
- Tissues
- Tongue depressor
- Tuning fork
- Vaginal speculum
- Wristwatch with second hand

Box 13.3	**Psychological Preparation for a Physical Examination**

Psychological preparation often is the nurse's highest priority before the examination. Patients become embarrassed when required to answer sensitive questions about body functions or when certain body parts are exposed and examined. The possibility of the examiner finding something abnormal also creates anxiety. Give the patient information about the examination in general terms. As each body system is examined, provide a more detailed explanation. Simple terms are used when describing the steps of the examination because complicated terminology confuses some patients and easily adds to their fears.

- A full set of vital signs should be measured and the results made available to the health care provider before the examination is performed.
- Explain what will occur during the examination to the patient. Determine whether the patient has any unanswered questions (Box 13.3).
- Determine whether the physical examination will be performed in the patient's room (when in the hospital or long-term care setting) or if an examination room must be reserved. If the examination is occurring in a health care provider's office, ensure

that the room is appropriate for the examination (e.g., if a gynecologic examination is planned, an examination table with stirrups is necessary).
- Consider the patient's ability to assume the necessary positions (Table 13.2) for the examination and determine what assistance will be needed.
- Determine whether the nurse's assistance will be required during the examination. The nurse should not leave the patient alone. Most examiners appreciate a nurse in attendance. Many facilities require a female nurse to be present when a male health care provider is performing a gynecologic examination.
- If specimens are being obtained, determine what supplies will be necessary and where the specimens are being sent for testing (see Chapter 23).
- Document information regarding the procedure, including vital signs, pertinent signs and symptoms, reports of pain, anxiety level, and specimens; obtain the necessary specimens and send them to the laboratory.

Perform an assessment to determine the actual or potential (risk for) patient problems that will require nursing interventions for the safety and well-being of the patient. For example, if during the examination you observe that the patient has a need for oxygen (a basic human need), take steps to ensure placement of oxygen, positioning, deep breathing, and coughing to meet this need.

The nurse is in constant contact with the patient and must perform accurate assessments to discover developing complications and to evaluate medical treatments.

NURSING ASSESSMENT

Nursing assessment comprises the gathering, verifying, and communicating of data about the patient. The purpose of the assessment is to establish a baseline database about the patient's level of wellness, health practices, past illnesses, related experiences, and health care goals. The information contained in the database is the basis for an individualized plan of nursing care developed throughout the nursing process.

Data collected during this process include the **nursing health history**, physical examination findings, results of laboratory and diagnostic tests, and information from health care team members and the patient's family or significant others. Obtain the health history while initiating the nurse-patient relationship by interviewing the patient. Various techniques are used to progress through the interview (see Chapter 4). When assessing the patient, always pay special attention to areas about which the patient has expressed concern.

Once the interview is completed, proceed to the physical assessment. Use inspection, palpation, auscultation, and percussion to collect physical examination data (Box 13.4). Laboratory and diagnostic tests

Table **13.2**	Positions for Examination			
POSITION	**AREAS ASSESSED**	**RATIONALE**	**LIMITATIONS**	
Sitting	Head and neck, back, posterior thorax and lungs, anterior thorax and lungs, breasts, axillae, heart, vital signs, and upper extremities	Sitting upright provides full expansion of lungs and provides better visualization of symmetry of upper body parts.	Some physically weakened patients are unable to sit. Use supine position with the head of the bed elevated instead.	
Supine	Head and neck, anterior thorax and lungs, breasts, axillae, heart, abdomen, extremities, pulses	This is the most normally relaxed position. It provides easy access to pulse sites.	If a patient becomes short of breath easily, consider raising the head of the bed.	
Dorsal recumbent	Head and neck, anterior thorax and lungs, breasts, axillae, heart, abdomen	Position is used for abdominal assessment because it promotes relaxation of abdominal muscles.	Patients with painful disorders are more comfortable with knees flexed.	
Lithotomy[a]	Female genitalia and genital tract	This position provides maximal exposure of genitalia and facilitates insertion of vaginal speculum.	Lithotomy position is embarrassing and uncomfortable, so minimize the time that a patient spends in it. Keep the patient well draped.	
Sims	Rectum and vagina	Flexion of hip and knee improves exposure of the rectal area.	Joint deformities may hinder a patient's ability to bend hip and knee.	
Prone	Musculoskeletal system	This position is used only to assess extension of hip joint.	Patients with respiratory difficulties tolerate this position poorly.	
Lateral recumbent	Heart	This position aids in detecting murmurs.	Patients with respiratory difficulties tolerate this position poorly.	
Knee-chest[a]	Rectum	This position provides maximum exposure of rectal area.	This position is embarrassing and uncomfortable.	

[a]A patient with severe arthritis or other joint deformity may be unable to assume this position.

validate findings from the history and physical examination and often lead to identification of problems not previously noted (Box 13.5).

Initiating the Nurse-Patient Relationship

Perhaps the most challenging patient interview the nurse ever has to conduct is the first one with every patient. For some patients, being interviewed by a nurse is a new experience. The nurse's first task is to establish an effective nurse-patient relationship before proceeding to the nursing health history.

 Communication

Before Assessment

Nurse: Good morning, Mr. C. I'm Ms. A., a student nurse. I'll be caring for you today. A portion of my nursing care is to conduct an assessment. My assessment will help me plan your nursing care. I will be including temperature, pulse, respirations, blood pressure, heart rate, orientation, pain scale, lung sounds, O_2 saturations, abdominal sounds, arterial pulses, and skin color in my assessment. It will take me about 30 minutes. Do you have any questions? (pause) May I begin now? (pause) I will start with your vital signs.

Box 13.4   Physical Assessment Techniques

INSPECTION

Visually inspect the patient's body and observe moods, including all responses and nonverbal behaviors. This **inspection**, or purposeful observation, is the technique the nurse uses most frequently. It begins with the nurse's first contact with the patient and continues throughout the gathering of the nursing history. Use inspection to collect data systematically about significant behaviors or physical features. It is important to be accurate and thorough using a systematic approach such as a head-to-toe assessment.

PALPATION

With **palpation**, the nurse uses the hands and sense of touch to gather data. Hands are highly sensitive to texture, temperature, and moisture and thus help determine the quality of an area. Use palpation to detect tenderness, temperature, texture, vibration, pulsations, masses, and other changes in structural integrity. Palpate each body part, usually according to a systematic assessment pattern. Palpation rules out or confirms suspicions raised during interview and inspection. Because touching has the potential to elicit fear, embarrassment, pain, or other strong emotions, explain the nurse's actions and the reasons for them. In addition, instruct the patient to let the nurse know whether palpation produces sensations of tenderness, pressure, or pain. The three palpation techniques are light, moderate, and deep. Light and moderate palpations are illustrated in Figs. 13.10A and B.

When using palpation, be sure the fingernails are short, and warm the hands before touching the patient. Social conversation during palpation is appropriate at times to distract patients and help them relax. Use the pads of the fingers; place them flat against the patient's skin with slight pressure and gentle rotation of the area under examination. The thumb and forefinger can be used to palpate muscle mass on arms and legs. Palpate pulses with the pads of the fingers. Someone who is not appropriately trained to perform palpation can cause internal injuries. During palpation, also observe the patient's facial expressions; if you see a grimace indicating pain, for instance, ask the patient to describe it.

AUSCULTATION

Auscultation is the process of listening to sounds produced by the body. Three systems produce sounds the nurse will auscultate: the cardiovascular system, the respiratory system, and the gastrointestinal system. For auscultation of these systems, the nurse uses a stethoscope, an instrument that amplifies sounds produced by internal organs. The nurse also uses the technique of auscultation to detect the fetal heart sound.

To master the auscultation technique and gain experience at interpreting the sounds the nurse hears, the nurse needs repeated practice on healthy and ill patients. Accurate assessment requires a quiet environment. Television, sounds from nasogastric suction, movement of bed linen, and conversation can interfere with accurate auscultation. Try closing the eyes while listening to reduce visual distractions. Never rush auscultation. Take time to assess each area properly.

Place the diaphragm of the stethoscope gently over the patient's skin. If the area is hairy, dampening it sometimes decreases the sound of the hair rubbing against the diaphragm.

PERCUSSION

Percussion is the use of the fingertips to tap the body's surface to produce vibration and sound. The sounds indicate the density of the underlying tissue and thus help the nurse detect the location of body organs and structures. For example, percussion over a hollow organ such as the stomach produces a high-pitched, drumlike sound called **tympany**. Percussion over a dense organ such as the liver produces a low-pitched, thudlike sound called **dullness**. Percussion over a muscle produces a soft, high-pitched, flat sound called **flatness**. To perform percussion, place the palmar surface of one hand against the patient's body while tapping with the fingers of the other hand. Tap each area two or three times. Properly performed, percussion is not painful for the patient, but if it does cause discomfort, discontinue it and document the results. This assessment technique is the one the nurse uses least frequently.

The first step in initiating the nurse-patient relationship is to introduce oneself, including name, position, and the purposes of the interview. In the Communication box, the nurse introduces herself, gives an estimate of the time needed for the assessment, and tells the patient the reason for the assessment. Indicating the length of time is important because it helps ensure cooperation. Do not consider the patient, even one in a hospital, a captive audience. Take steps to ensure that the patient's time is used appropriately. In the example, the nurse gives the patient an opportunity to ask questions. Whether the patient has any pressing questions is important to determine before beginning the more targeted part of the interview. By answering questions, the nurse meets some of the patient's immediate needs, and the patient may feel more comfortable answering the nurse's questions. For example, sometimes a patient who is unsure of how the hospital bed

operates is distracted and thinks more about the bed than about the questions being presented; this patient is less likely to provide complete information for the database. Finally, the nurse asks whether it is acceptable to conduct the interview at that time, thereby giving the patient a choice.

The next step in initiating the nurse-patient relationship is to communicate the nurse's trustworthiness and discretion to patients. Illnesses causing people to seek help often are accompanied by anxiety, powerlessness, altered family processes, economic concerns, and changes in self-image. Patients frequently are asked to provide highly personal information about themselves and their families. Generally, people share such information only with family members or close friends. To be able to do so with the nurse, the patient must be comfortable that the information will be shared only with caregivers who need it to provide proper care.

Box 13.5   Common Laboratory and Diagnostic Tests

BLOOD ANALYSIS
- Arterial blood gas (ABG) analysis
- Blood chemistry profile
- Complete blood count (CBC), includes red blood cell (RBC), hemoglobin (Hgb), hematocrit (Hct), erythrocyte indices, platelets, white blood cell (WBC) with differential, and examination of peripheral blood cells
- Electrolyte tests: sequential multiple analysis–6 (SMA-6), SMA-12
- Fasting blood sugar (FBS) test
- International normalized ratio (INR)
- Megaloblastic anemia profile
- Partial thromboplastin time (PTT)
- Prothrombin time (PT)

URINE ANALYSIS
- 24-hour urine collection for creatinine clearance, protein content
- Urinalysis (UA)
- Urine culture and sensitivity test

DIAGNOSTIC IMAGING EXAMINATIONS
- Barium enema (BE) examination
- Chest roentgenogram (chest x-ray [CXR])
- Computed tomography (CT): scans of the body, the head, the chest, the abdomen, the pelvis, and the bones
- Intravenous pyelogram (IVP)
- Magnetic resonance imaging (MRI)
- Upper gastrointestinal (UGI) examination

STOOL ANALYSIS
- Clostridium difficile
- Culture and sensitivity
- Escherichia coli strain O157:H7
- Guaiac tests (Hematest stools)
- Ova and parasite tests

SPUTUM ANALYSIS
- Acid-fast bacilli (AFB) test
- Culture and sensitivity test
- Cytology tests

OTHER
- Colonoscopy examinations
- Endoscopy examinations
- Electrocardiogram (ECG), echocardiogram, transesophageal echocardiogram
- Stress test
- Tuberculosis (TB) skin test

Assure patients that information concerning past or present levels of wellness or family relationships is strictly confidential. A sense of trust is essential for open communication and identification of the patient's health care needs and goals. The nurse's professionalism promotes development of a therapeutic relationships with patients and families.

Interview

Conduct the interview in a private setting that is well lit. Convey feelings of compassion and concern while remaining objective. The patient must feel the information being sought is important and that the nurse demonstrates an interest in the patient's state of wellness.

Ask the patient how he or she wishes to be addressed, and use that name during the interview. The nurse should have a calm demeanor and sit at eye level with the patient to enhance the patient's comfort during the interview. A pleasant facial expression promotes communication, and eye contact conveys the nurse's full attention.

One way to enhance communication is by using nonjudgmental language. Statements such as "Yes, I see," or "What happened next?" encourage the patient to communicate without feeling threatened. Reflecting what the patient has stated clarifies statements, as does summarizing and restating. Approving nods and gestures facilitate the exchange of information. The nurse must be responsive to the patient's condition. Pause the interview if necessary, stabilize the patient's condition, and ensure comfort and safety before proceeding. (Read more about interviewing in Chapter 4.)

HEALTH HISTORY

Collecting the patient's health history is the initial step of the nursing assessment. Data collected provide the nurse with information about the patient's level of wellness, changes in life patterns, sociocultural role, and mental and emotional reactions to illness. The objective is to identify patterns of health and illness, risk factors for physical and behavioral health problems, deviations from normal, and available resources for adapting to changes in health status.

Biographic Data

In most facilities, the admitting department obtains the biographic data; begin the interview by referring to this information. It generally includes data such as date of birth, gender, address, family members' names and addresses, marital status, religious preference and practices, occupation, current primary care provider, and insurance, Medicare, and Medicaid benefits. Verify this information with the patient to ensure that it is correct.

Reasons for Seeking Health Care

Determine why the patient is seeking health care. This often is referred to as the *chief complaint*. The nurse can ask, "What brings you to the hospital today?" This allows the patient to describe the reason for admission and gives the patient an opportunity to discuss expectations of care. To get the most information from the patient about health concerns, use the OPQRSTUV method (Box 13.6). Document information in the patient's own words, using quotation marks. This helps remove the possibility of bias from later interpretation of the data.

Determine whether patients expect to be "cured" or become "free of pain" or "able to care for self." This information assists in establishing goals for care and

---

Box 13.6 **History of Present Illness**

When discussing the history of the present illness with the patient, be sure the patient describes the problems fully. To do this, ask the patient the following questions about each symptom:

Time of onset. When was the first date (the problem) happened? What time did it begin?

Type of onset. How did (the problem) start: Suddenly? Gradually?

Original source. What were you doing when you first experienced or noticed (the problem)? What seems to trigger it: Stress? Position? Certain activities? Arguments?

Characteristics. What is (the problem) like? If describing a discharge: Thick? Runny? Clear? Colored? If describing a psychological problem: Do the voices drown out other sounds? Whose voice does it sound like?

Severity. How bad is (the problem) when it is at its worst? Does it interfere with your normal activities? Does it force you to lie down, sit down, slow down?

Radiation. In the case of pain, does it travel down your back or arms, up your neck, or down your legs? What is the pain intensity on a scale of 0–10?

Time relationship. How often do you experience (the problem): Hourly? Daily? Weekly? Monthly? When do you usually experience it: Daytime? At night? In the early morning? Are you ever awakened by it? Does it ever occur before, during, or after meals? Does it occur seasonally?

Duration. How long does an episode last?

Course. Does (the problem) seem to be getting better or getting worse, or does it remain the same?

Associations. Does (the problem) lead to anything else? Is it accompanied by other signs and symptoms?

Source of relief. What relieves it: Changing diet? Changing position? Taking medications? Being active?

Source of aggravation. What makes it worse?

The nurse can remember all these questions using the letters OPQRSTUV:

O Onset-Timing
  Onset, duration
P Precipitating-Provocative-Palliative
  What causes it? What makes it worse? What makes it better?
Q Quality-Quantity: describe it: sharp, dull …
  How does it feel, look, or sound, and how much of it is there? How often, when, how long?
R Region-Radiation
  Where is it? Does it spread?
S Severity scale
  Does it interfere with activities? How does it rate on a severity scale of 0–10?
T Treatments
  What helps? For how long?
U Understanding
  What do you think is causing it? How does it affect you?
V Values
  Goals of care; expectations

---

nursing interventions. In addition, such expectations provide the nurse with information on patient perceptions about health and illness.

Present Illness or Health Concerns

The data collected relate to the progression of the present illness from the onset to the current signs and symptoms. The data must be detailed and comprehensive to allow the nurse to plan appropriate interventions. To ensure data collection is complete, examine the guidelines in Box 13.7.

Health History

Information from the health history provides data on the patient's health care experiences. Determine if the patient has ever been hospitalized or undergone surgery. Ask the patient if allergies to medications, food, or environmental pollutants exist. If an allergy to any substance is identified, document the allergy, specific reaction, and treatment on the assessment form.

Use the health history to identify habits and lifestyle patterns. The use of alcohol, tobacco, illegal drugs, caffeine, herbal products, over-the-counter drugs, or prescription medication has the potential to place the patient at risk for diseases involving the liver, the kidneys, the lungs, the heart, the nervous system, and thought processes. Document the type of habit, frequency, and duration of use in the medical record. This is sometimes an uncomfortable area for the patient and the nurse. To have a better chance of obtaining an accurate response, ask the patient, "How much alcohol do you drink?" rather than asking whether the patient drinks alcohol.

Assess the patient's ability to perform ADLs, patterns of sleep, exercise, and nutrition. This data will assist the nurse in planning interventions. If possible, accommodate variations in sleep, activity, and nutrition.

Family History

The purpose of the family history is to obtain health data about the patient's immediate family members and blood relatives. Data include history of illnesses (e.g., diabetes mellitus, hypertension, heart disease, cancer) and cause of death. The objectives are to determine if the patient is at risk for illnesses of a genetic or familial nature and to identify areas of health promotion and illness prevention. The family history provides information about family structure, interaction, and function that are often useful in planning care. For example, a cohesive, supportive family is a possible resource in assisting a patient to adjust to an illness or disability; it is important in this case to incorporate the family into the plan of care. Conversely, if the patient's family is not supportive, it is often more therapeutic to refrain from involving them in care, particularly if the family history reveals the patient is experiencing stress related to familial relationships.

Box 13.7   Review of Systems

The nurse probably will not include questions pertaining to all the aspects of each system every time a nursing health history is taken. Nevertheless, include some questions regarding each system in every history. These essential areas are listed in italic type in the outline that follows. Whenever the patient gives positive responses to the first questions for that system, include questions about the more comprehensive and detailed areas relating to each system listed afterward. Keep in mind that these lists do not represent an exhaustive enumeration of questions; even more details are required frequently within an organ system, depending on the patient's problem.

A. *General constitutional symptoms:* Fever, chills, malaise, fatigability, night sweats; weight (average, preferred, present, change, appetite)

B. *Skin:* Rash or eruption, pruritus, pigmentation or texture change; diaphoresis (excessive sweating); abnormal nail or hair growth or loss; new growths or changes in moles

C. *Skeletal:* Joint stiffness, pain, restriction of motion, edema, erythema, heat, bone deformity

D. *Head*
  1. *General:* Frequent or unusual headaches, vertigo (sensation of the room spinning), dizziness (sensation of themselves spinning), syncope (fainting), severe head injuries
  2. *Eyes:* Visual acuity, blurring, diplopia (double vision), photophobia (abnormal sensitivity to light), scotomas (spots before the eyes), nystagmus (involuntary rhythmic movements of the eye), pain, recent changes in appearance or vision, glaucoma, use of eye drops or other eye medications, history of trauma or familial eye disease
  3. *Ears:* Hearing loss, pain, discharge, tinnitus (ringing in ears), vertigo
  4. *Nose:* Sense of smell, frequency of colds, obstruction, epistaxis (nosebleed), postnasal discharge, sinus pain
  5. *Mouth:* Bleeding or edema of gums; recent tooth abscesses or extractions; soreness of tongue or buccal mucosa, ulcers; disturbance of taste; throat: hoarseness or change in voice; dysphagia (difficulty swallowing); frequent sore throats

E. *Endocrine:* Thyroid enlargement or tenderness, heat or cold intolerance, unexplained weight change, diabetes mellitus (changes in thirst, urination, and hunger), nervousness or depression, and fatigue

F. *Reproduction*
  1. *Males:* Onset of puberty, erections, emissions, testicular pain, libido, infertility
  2. *Females*
    a. *Menses:* Onset, regularity, duration of flow, dysmenorrhea (pain associated with menstruation), last period, intermenstrual discharge or bleeding, pruritus, date of last Papanicolaou (Pap)

smear, age at menopause, libido, frequency of intercourse, sexual difficulties
    b. *Pregnancies:* Number, miscarriages, abortions, duration of pregnancy in each and any complication during any pregnancy or postpartum period; use of oral or other contraceptives
    c. *Breasts:* Pain, tenderness, discharge, lumps, mammograms; family history of breast cancer

G. *Respiratory:* Pain relating to respiration, dyspnea, cyanosis, crackles, wheezing, cough, sputum (character and quantity), hemoptysis (expectorating blood from respiratory tract), night sweats; date and result of last chest x-ray examination; dependence on supplemental oxygen, smoker (include how much and how long)

H. *Cardiac:* Chest pain or distress, precipitating causes, timing and duration, relieving factors, palpitations, dyspnea, orthopnea (number of pillows needed), edema, claudication (weakness of legs accompanied by cramplike pain), hypertension, previous myocardial infarction, heart failure, estimate of exercise tolerance, past electrocardiogram (ECG) or other cardiac tests; history of coronary artery bypass surgery, percutaneous transluminal coronary angioplasty, or percutaneous balloon valvuloplasty

I. *Hematologic:* Anemia, tendency to bruise or bleed easily, thromboses, thrombophlebitis, any known abnormality of blood cells, transfusions

J. *Lymph nodes:* Enlargement, tenderness, suppuration (to produce purulent material [pus])

K. *Gastrointestinal:* Appetite, digestion, intolerance for any type of foods, dysphagia (difficulty swallowing), heartburn, nausea, vomiting, hematemesis, regularity of bowels, constipation, diarrhea, change in stool color or contents (clay colored, tarry, fresh blood, mucus, undigested food), flatulence, hemorrhoids, hepatitis, jaundice, dark urine; history of ulcer, gallstones, polyps, tumor; previous x-ray examinations (where, when, findings)

L. *Genitourinary:* Dysuria, flank or suprapubic pain, urgency, frequency, nocturia, hematuria, polyuria, hesitancy, dribbling, loss in force of stream, passage of stone, edema of face, stress incontinence, hernias, sexually transmitted infection (inquire what kind and signs and symptoms, and list results of serologic test for syphilis [STS], if known)

M. *Neurologic:* Syncope (brief lapse in consciousness caused by transient cerebral hypoxia); history of stroke, seizures, weakness or paralysis, abnormalities of sensation or coordination, tremors, loss of memory; unusual frequency, distribution, or severity of headaches; serious head injury in past

N. *Psychiatric:* Depression, mood changes, difficulty concentrating, nervousness, tension, suicidal thoughts, irritability, sleep disturbances

Environmental History

The environmental history provides data about the patient's home and work environments. The environmental history identifies areas of concern such as exposure to pollutants that can affect health, high crime rates that prevent patients from walking around neighborhoods, and resources available to assist patients in returning to the community.

Psychosocial and Cultural History

The psychosocial and cultural history includes data about the patient's primary language, cultural group, educational background, attention span, and developmental stage. It provides information about the patient's and family's coping skills and support systems. It can help in identifying potential or actual problems in dealing with the present illness and in the planning of appropriate interventions. Be certain to identify major values, beliefs, and behaviors related to particular health concerns. Individualize assessments and interventions to the patient and family. Avoid making assumptions about cultural beliefs and behaviors without receiving validation from the patient (see the Cultural Considerations box).

 Cultural Considerations

Developing Cultural Sensitivity

Cultures are complex, integrated systems that include knowledge, skills, art, morals, law, customs, and any other acquired habits of a group of people. Cultural beliefs and personal characteristics determine health behavior in individuals and families. More than half of all health problems are the result of lifestyle behaviors. If nursing's goal is to promote health while respecting individual value systems and lifestyles, culture-based behavior must be understood (see Chapter 6).

The following are ways to develop cultural and ethnic sensitivity:

- Recognize cultural and ethnic diversity exists.
- Nurses identify and examine personal cultural and ethnic beliefs.
- Demonstrate respect for people as unique individuals.
- Respect the unfamiliar.
- Recognize some cultural and ethnic groups have definitions of health and illness and practices aimed at promoting health and curing illness that differ from the nurse's own.
- Interpret patients' signs and symptoms and respond in accordance with cultural norms.
- Be willing to modify health care delivery in keeping with the patient's cultural background.
- Do not expect all members of one cultural group to behave in the same manner.

Review of Systems

The review of systems (ROS) is a systematic method for collecting data on all body systems (see Box 13.7). During the ROS, the nurse asks the patient about the normal functioning of each system and any changes the patient has noted. The patient's statements and descriptions of changes in body systems are subjective data.

As you proceed through the health history, document the data obtained in a clear, concise manner with appropriate terminology. A clear, concise record is necessary because other health care professionals are likely to use the nursing health history when delivering health care. Fig. 13.2 illustrates the correct way to record such information.

When determining the status of each body system, ask the patient specific questions relating to the functioning of the system. For example, you may begin assessment of the respiratory system with the question, "Are you having any difficulty with breathing?" Remember to be alert to the patient's comfort and well-being in the moment; if the answer is "yes," the focus of the assessment may shift to the current situation before continuing with questions. Once the patient's respiratory status is stable, continue the questioning with, "Please tell me more about….," or more specific questions, such as, "Do you have shortness of breath?" An ROS guide can be used to guarantee a complete interview.

The Communication box on admission assessment shows an example of an interview using the OPQRSTUV technique. However, the ROS carried out during the patient interview at the beginning of the physical assessment may give much more information about the patient than the content of the words spoken. The nurse observes patient mobility and gains insight about the patient's intellect, level of orientation, and emotional and psychological states.

 Communication

Admission Assessment

Mr. J. is admitted to the hospital with a diagnosis of a possible peptic ulcer.

Nurse: Mr. J., can you tell me about your pain? What brings on your pain?

Patient: I get the pain several times a day after I eat. *(Provocative) (Timing)*

Nurse: What does it feel like?

Patient: It feels like burning. *(Quality)*

Nurse: Where does the pain occur?

Patient: In my stomach. *(Region)*

Nurse: How does the pain rate, on a scale of 0 to 10?

Patient: About an 8. *(Severity)*

Nurse: How long have you had this pain?

Patient: It began about 6 months ago. *(Timing)*

See the description in Box 13.6 of the OPQRSTUV method of interviewing.

Assess the appropriateness of the patient's answers. By asking questions such as "Can you tell me your name?" "Why are you here?" "What is the date?" and "Can you tell me where we are right now?" determine the patient's **level of consciousness (LOC)** and orientation. Assess and document the patient's orientation to person, place, time, and purpose.

NURSING ASSESSMENT

The **nursing assessment** consists of subjective and objective data collection. Nurses are usually the first to detect changes in the patient's condition. The skills of physical assessment provide the nurse with powerful tools to detect subtle and obvious changes in a patient's

NURSING ADMISSION ASSESSMENT

Admitted: Ambulatory, Cart, (Wheelchair) Arms, Ambulance

From: (Office) ER, Surgery, Radiology, Recovery Room   Transferred From: __physician's office__

Oriented to Room: Call Light, Side rails, TV, Phone, Safety/Smoking Policy: Yes __✓__   No _____

Vital Signs: T __101^2__ P __92__   P __24__ BP __160/92__ HT __5'4"__ WT __190__ Dentures __upper/lower__

Diet at home: __2 g sodium__

Allergies: Drug __penicillin__   Reaction __hives__

Other: __none__   Organ Donor: Yes _____   No __X__

Reason for Admission __Elevated temperature & fluid retention__   Signature __J.Doe, LPN__   Date: 12/20/2022   Time: _____2010_____

EYES: Impaired vision, Blind, (Cataract) (Glaucoma)
Contacts, (Glasses) Prosthesis R. L.
Comments: _____
   __cataract surgery (rt eye)__
   __2012   OD__

EARS, NOSE, THROAT: (Hard of hearing) Deaf,
Lesions (Hearing Aid,) (R) L., Tracheotomy
Comments: _____

RESPIRATORY: Pain, (Dyspnea) (Wheeze) Asthma,
Sinusitis, COPD, Cough,
Productive ____ Nonproductive __X__
Oxygen needed, Smoker
Comments: __c/o shortness__
   __of breath upon exertion__
   __crackles right base__

CIRCULATION: Apical, Radial, Strong, Weak, Thready,
(Bounding,) Regular, Palpitations, (Chest pain,)
Numbness, Bruising, (Edema) (Hypertension,)
Hx MI, (CHF) Pacer, Bypass Surgery
Comments: __st" 4 pound weight__
   __gain in the last 3 days__
   __3+ pitting edema bilaterally__

ENDOCRINE: Thyroid, Diabetes
Comments: __no problems__

GI TRACT: Heartburn, Ulcers, Pain, Hernia, Dysphagia,
(Nausea) Vomiting, (Loss of Appetite) Distention,
Diverticulitis
Comments: _____

ELIMINATION: Last BM 2 days ago, Normal, (Constipated)
Diarrhea, Tarry, Bright red, Clay colored,
(Hemorrhoids) Involuntary, Use of laxatives, (Yes)/No
enema, Yes/(No) Ileostomy, Colostomy
Comments: _____

URINARY: Incontinence, (Nocturia) Hematuria, (Dysuria)
Burning, (Frequency) Urgency, Dribbling, infections,
Cath: Yes/No
Comments: _____

NEUROLOGICAL: Convulsions, Paralysis, Syncope,
Paresthesia, (Dizziness) Coordination, Weakness,
(Headaches)
Comments: _____

SKIN: Color __pale__ Turgor __poor__ Temp __warm__
Describe any Rashes, Lesions, Ecchymosis,
Petechiae, (Scars) Diabetic sores,
Comments: __central abdominal scar__

MUSCULOSKELETAL: (Pain) (Stiffness) Contractures
Deformities, Tremors, Backaches,
Weight bearing, Amputation
Comments: _____

FEMALE REPRODUCTION: LMP   EDC
(Menopause) Breast pain, Breast tenderness,
Vaginal discharge
Comments: __post__

PREVIOUS SURGERIES: __herniorrhaphy__
__ventral__   __2009__
__Rt eye Cataract surgery__
__2008__

MEDS TAKEN AT HOME:

Med:	Dose:		Last Taken:
Cozaar	- 50 mg hour of sleep	-	Last PM
Coreg	- 12.5 mg BID	-	AM
Lasix	- 40 mgm qAM	-	AM
K-Lor	- 10 mEq BID	-	AM
Restoril	- 15 mg hour of sleep	-	Last PM

DISPOSAL OF MEDS:
Did not bring __✓__
Pt. has _____ Family took home _____
Retained/taken to Pharmacy _____
Other: _____

Signature: __S.Smith RN__
Time: _____

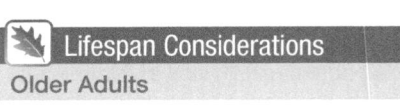

Fig. 13.2 Nursing admission assessment.

health. The data collected comprise the first step of the nursing process. Remember the purpose of the nursing assessment is to determine the patient's state of health or illness. It is the initial step used to form the nursing care plan, just as the physician performs a physical examination to determine the medical diagnosis and proposed course of treatment. Special considerations for assessing older adults are listed in the Lifespan Considerations box.

Lifespan Considerations
Older Adults

Assessment

- All body systems change with aging. An awareness of how aging affects an older adult helps sort out expected changes from pathologic processes. Adapt assessments to uncover problems and intervene effectively. All older adults do not show the physical signs of aging at the same rate.
- Adequate time must be allowed for a thorough assessment. Several shorter sessions are likely to be better tolerated than one long session.
- During the assessment, monitor for signs of fatigue, such as slumping, sighing, or irritability.

- For comfort during the assessment, do the following:
  - Ensure privacy. If the older person has cognitive difficulty or wishes a family member's assistance, allow it. Be careful that the family member does not dominate the conversation.
  - Encourage the older person to void before the assessment.
  - Conduct the assessment in a room where bathroom facilities are readily available.
  - Verify that the temperature of the room is warm enough for the older person and free from drafts.
- Explain what is going to occur in terms the older person can understand and avoid the use of medical jargon. Speak slowly and clearly so that the older person is able to hear what is being said and has the opportunity to process the information.
- Be patient and listen. Older people often take longer to reply, but they should be allowed to complete ideas in their own words without interruption.
- Obtain objective and subjective data during the assessment.

When to Perform a Nursing Physical Assessment

The best time to assess the patient is as soon after admission as possible. In some facilities, policy dictates that the assessment be completed within 24 hours of admission. A registered nurse (RN) performs the initial baseline nursing assessment. The ongoing assessment is the responsibility of the RN and the licensed practical/vocational nurse (LPN/LVN).

The formal head-to-toe assessment is completed when the patient is admitted and at the beginning of each shift. A focused assessment is performed when the nurse assesses a change in the patient's condition. During a *focused assessment*, attention is directed to a particular part of the body where signs and symptoms are localized or most active. Performing the assessment at the beginning of each shift allows the nurse to identify changes in the patient's condition, anticipate potential problems, communicate changes to health care providers, and alter the nursing plan of care accordingly.

Where to Perform a Nursing Physical Assessment

Regardless of the setting—hospital, clinic, extended care facility, or the patient's home—the location for performing the nursing assessment must be comfortable and safe for the patient. Ensure an adjustable table or bed is available and consider the patient's privacy. Ascertain the location is free of distracting sights, sounds, and odors. Keep the ambient temperature comfortable, since the patient's body is exposed during the assessment. In most cases, the patient's own room works very well and is convenient for the nurse and the patient.

Methods of Performing a Nursing Physical Assessment

The assessment can be organized in head-to-toe order or system by system. In either case, proceed systematically. By performing the assessment in the same manner each time, the nurse can avoid inadvertently omitting a portion of the assessment. Box 13.8 is an example of a pocket guide to follow during the physical assessment, which can be useful when charting the assessment in the nursing notes.

If the patient expresses special concerns, or observation of changes in a patient's status is assessed, it might be necessary to perform a focused assessment first. During the head-to-toe assessment, any painful areas are best assessed last. This ensures better cooperation from the patient.

Performing the Nursing Physical Assessment

Items essential to the nurse's assessment are a penlight or flashlight, stethoscope, blood pressure cuff, thermometer, gloves, watch with second hand, scissors, black pen, and a tongue blade (see Fig. 13.1 and Box 13.2). The nurse uses the sense of touch, smell, sight, and hearing. Thorough washing of the hands should be completed before beginning the physical assessment. Follow the Centers for Disease Control and Prevention (CDC) guidelines on standard precautions

and hand hygiene guidelines (Centers for Disease Control, 2016). Provide the patient the opportunity to empty the bladder before the examination. This makes the patient more comfortable and allows easier assessment of the bladder.

Obtain the patient's vital signs, including temperature, pulse, respirations, and blood pressure. Perform pain assessment to obtain the fifth vital sign (Box 13.9). The vital signs often provide clues to areas that warrant more critical evaluation. The beginning of the examination is a good time to measure the patient's height and weight. For accuracy, measure height and weight on admission and then compare the results with the patient's stated height and weight. If a significant difference is found between the measurements, possible causes must be explored.

Head-to-toe assessment. When performing a head-to-toe assessment, begin with a neurologic assessment, followed by an assessment of the skin, the hair, the head, and the neck. The assessment of the head includes the eyes, ears, nose, and mouth. Examine the chest, the back,

---

Box 13.8 **Physical Assessment Guide**

1. *Neurologic:* Level of consciousness: alert, drowsy, lethargic, oriented to: 1 (person); 2 (person, place); 3 (person, place, and time); 4 (person, place, time, and purpose)
2. *Integumentary:* Skin condition, color, temperature, turgor, skin impairments, moist, dry
3. *Cardiovascular:* Apical pulse (strength and regularity), capillary refill (less than 3 seconds) in upper and lower extremities, pedal pulses (1+ to 4+), pitting edema (1+ to 4+; see Box 13.10), nonpitting edema, type of intravenous fluid with rate, site condition (without edema or erythema)
4. *Respiratory:* Posteriorly (lower lobes), anteriorly (upper lobes), right axilla (right middle lobe); auscultate for crackles, wheezes (sibilant and sonorous), pleural friction rub, respiration characteristics (tachypnea, orthopnea, dyspnea [resting or exertional]); assess arterial oxygen saturation (SaO_2) via pulse oximeter; oxygen therapy with route (cannula, mask), and liters per minute of oxygen flow (e.g., O_2 2 L/min per nasal cannula)
5. *Gastrointestinal:* Diet, appetite, fluid intake; observe for distention; auscultate for presence of bowel sounds × 4 quadrants (active, hypoactive, hyperactive, absent by quadrants); palpate masses, tenderness, bowel movement with description, including colostomy or ileostomy stoma assessment, amount and consistency; nasogastric suction (color and amount)
6. *Urinary:* Urine amount, color, odor; presence of catheters (Foley, nephrostomy, suprapubic, ureteral); voiding; include ureterostomy stoma assessment
7. *Mobility:* Activity level: bed rest, chair, up ad lib; gait and level of tolerance; ambulation aids needed, such as walker, cane, or crutches

the arms, the abdomen, the perineal area, the legs, and the feet (in that order).

Note the assessment does not stop after completion of the head-to-toe assessment. It is a continuous process.

Neurologic. The neurologic assessment can be integrated into the rest of the assessment. For instance, after taking the radial pulse, have the patient grasp your hands to test for equal grip. Always begin the neurologic assessment with the patient's level of consciousness and level of orientation.

Consciousness is awareness of one's thoughts and feelings and of the environment. The levels of consciousness generally are described according to the behavior exhibited by the individual (Table 13.3).

Box **13.9** Pain Assessment Scale

Use a pain rating scale to assess pain intensity systematically and manage pain. The most used numeric scale is 0–10. Ask the patient to rate pain from 0 (no pain) to 10 (worst pain). Ratings of 3–5 are considered mild pain, ratings of 5–7 are considered moderate pain, and ratings greater than 7 are considered severe pain. Some agencies use a scale of 0–5. For children, use happy and sad faces to rate the pain. For clinical assessment, any of these scales is adequate and appropriate. However, always use the same scale with the same patient. See Fig. 21.8 for sample pain intensity scales.

Careful assessment is critical of the neurologic status of patients who have a head injury or signs or symptoms of a neurologic deficit from a neurologic disease (Jarvis, 2020). Neurologic assessment includes the following:

1. *Level of consciousness.* A change in the level of consciousness is one of the first signs of an alteration in a person's neurological status. Patients are alert if they can open their eyes spontaneously. See Table 13.3 for a complete assessment of the level of consciousness

2. *Orientation.* Determine whether the patient is oriented to person, place, and time. This is considered "oriented x 3." Some facilities also require the nurse to determine and document if the patient is oriented to purpose. When purpose is also assessed the patient is considered "oriented x 4."

3. *Motor function.* Ask the patient to move each extremity. Have the patient smile, frown, and lift the eyebrows.

4. *Pupillary response.* Check the pupils for size, equality, and shape. Use a penlight to shine into each pupil. Each pupil should constrict quickly. Pupils should be equal in size (3 to 7 mm in diameter). When the pupils are assessed and the reaction is normal in all examinations, record the letters PERRLA (pupils equal, round, reactive to light, and accommodation).

5. The third cranial nerve, the oculomotor nerve, runs parallel to the brainstem. The function of the

Table **13.3** **Level of Consciousness**

LEVEL	BEHAVIORS
Consciousness	Level of awareness of oneself and the environment. Appropriate response to external stimuli; oriented to time, place, person, and purpose.
Confusion	Inappropriate response to stimuli and decreased attention span and memory; inappropriate reactions to simple commands.
Lethargy (hypersomnia)	Drowsiness or increased sleep time; is able to be aroused; responds appropriately; possibly falls asleep again immediately.
Delirium	Confusion, disordered perception, and decreased attention span; motor and sensory excitement; inappropriate reactions to stimuli; marked anxiety.
Coma	Loss or lowering of consciousness.
Stage I (stupor)	Arousable with vigorous repeated stimuli. See slowed verbal responses but deep tendon and superficial reflexes are intact.
Stage II (light coma)	Simple motor and verbal (moaning) response to painful stimuli; mass motor movement or flexion (avoidance) response.
Stage III (deep coma)	Decerebrate posturing to painful stimuli (extension of body and limbs and pronation of arms).
Stage IV	Flaccid muscles; papillary reflex absent, apneic; on ventilator; superficial and some deep tendon reflexes present.
Brain death	No responses noted, and reflexes are abnormal or absent.
Syncope	Temporary loss of consciousness (partial or complete) associated with increased rate of respiration, tachycardia, pallor, perspiration, and coolness of skin.
Fugue state	Dysfunction of consciousness (hours or days) in which the individual carries on purposeful activity that he or she does not remember afterward.
Amnesia	Memory loss over time or for specific subjects; individual affected responds appropriately to external stimuli.

From Estes MEZ: *Health assessment and physical examination,* ed 4, Clifton Park, NY, 2010, Delmar.

oculomotor nerve is essential for eye movements. It supplies the extrinsic and intrinsic eye muscles. The intrinsic muscle affects the size and the equality of the pupils. A TBI often results in increased intracranial pressure and edema of the brainstem with pressure on the oculomotor nerve causing the ominous sign of a unilateral, dilated, and nonreactive pupil (Jarvis, 2020).

Other major areas of neurologic examination include the following:

1. Proprioception (pertaining to the sensations of body movements and awareness of posture) and cerebellar function
2. Deep tendon reflexes
3. Cranial nerve assessment (performed by the RN)
   Vital signs.
4. (Jarvis, 2020). Vital signs help determine the overall condition of the patient. A change in vital signs can be an early indication of conditions such as shock or infection. Pain can also alter the vital signs.
   Glasgow Coma Scale.
5. The Glasgow Coma Scale (GCS) is a standardized, objective measurement of the level of consciousness (Table 13.4). The scale has a numeric value. The scale is divided into three areas: eye opening, verbal response, and motor response. Assess each of the three areas separately, and give a number for the patient's correct response. Sum the three numbers. A normal GCS demonstrating no brain trauma is 15. A score of 8 or less indicates severe brain injury (Jarvis, 2020).

Clues to areas of neurologic abnormality are sometimes evident during the patient's history, such as orientation, speech, and ability to interact with the examiner. Continue to evaluate the patient throughout the assessment. (Refer to *Adult Health Nursing,* Chapter 14 for a more detailed description of the neurologic system.)

Skin and hair. Observe the skin for color, temperature, moisture, texture, turgor, and evidence of injury or skin lesions. Normal skin tones vary with race, heredity, and sun exposure. Note the overall appearance and the color in the sclera, the mucous membranes, the tongue, the lips, the nail beds, and the palms and soles. A general uniformity of color from dark brown to light tan with pink or yellow overtones, depending on the patient's race, is normal. Changes in skin color that may provide evidence of systemic disease include pallor, cyanosis, jaundice, erythema, and ecchymosis. The appearance of cyanotic or dusky blue fingers, lips, or mucous membranes is abnormal in light-skinned and dark-skinned individuals. Jaundice in dark-skinned individuals sometimes appears as yellow staining in the sclera, hard palate, and palmar or plantar surfaces.

Normally, the skin is warm, dry, and smooth, with good turgor. **Turgor** refers to the elasticity of the skin caused by the outward pressure of the cells and interstitial fluid (Fig. 13.3). Dehydration results in *decreased* skin turgor and is manifested by lax skin that, when grasped and raised between two fingers, slowly returns to its previous position, called skin tenting. Marked edema results in *increased* turgor, manifested by smooth, taut, shiny skin that cannot be grasped and raised.

Table 13.4   Glasgow Coma Scale: Demonstrating Measurement of Level of Consciousness[a]

STIMULUS	RESPONSE	SCORE
Eye opening	Spontaneous—open with blinking at baseline	4
	To verbal stimuli, command, speech	3
	To fingertip stimulus	2
	None	1
	Closed by local factor	NT
Verbal response	Oriented	5
	Confused conversation, but able to answer questions	4
	Intelligible single words	3
	Only moans or groans	2
	No response	1
	Factor interfering with communication	NT
Motor response	Obeys commands for movement	6
	Brings hand above clavicle to stimulus on head neck	5
	Bends arm at elbow rapidly but features not predominantly abnormal (normal flexion)	4
	Bends arm at elbow, features clearly predominantly abnormal (abnormal flexion)	3
	Extends arm at elbow	2
	No response	1
	Paralyzed or other limiting factor	NT

[a]The Glasgow Coma Scale provides a score in the range 3 to 15; patients with scores of 3 to 8 are usually said to be in a coma. The total score is the sum of the scores in three categories. *NT,* Non testable.
Please refer to glasgowcomascale.org for more information (https://www.glasgowcomascale.org/downloads/GCS-Assessment-Aid-English.pdf?v=3)

Note any skin lesions or evidence of other skin impairments. Document their size, shape, color, pattern, and location and any presence of exudate.

Examine the hair over the entire body to determine the distribution, quantity, and quality. Hairless lower extremities sometimes signify an arterial disorder with reduced arterial blood flow. The hair is normally of a smooth texture and not oily or dry. A healthy scalp is free of dandruff, lesions, and parasites. Wear gloves if you wish to inspect the hair and scalp. Abnormalities are sometimes related to external factors, such as the use of beauty products, and sometimes to internal factors, such as systemic or localized illnesses.

Head and neck. Assessment of the head includes the eyes, the ears, the nose, and the mouth. The neck assessment involves the arteries, the veins, and the lymph nodes. Facial expression and appearance are likely to be the first observations the nurse makes and often give clues to the emotional state of the patient. Note the symmetry of the face; normal facial movements are asymmetric and appropriate. The head is normally upright and still.

A gross assessment of the range of motion (ROM) can be made by having the patient move the head from side to side and in a nodding motion. The patient should be able to move the head comfortably through the motions. With the pads of the fingers, palpate beneath the jaw and down each side of the neck to feel for enlarged lymph nodes. Although having an enlarged node may not be abnormal, tenderness is not normal. Palpate the carotid arteries gently and one at a time (Fig. 13.4). The normal carotid pulse is regular and palpable without a **thrill**, a vibrating sensation the nurse perceives during palpation along the artery.

Inspect for jugular venous distention. The jugular veins give information about activity on the right side of the heart. Specifically, reflecting filling pressure and volume changes. Distention results when ineffective pumping action of the right ventricle causes increased volume and pressure within the veins (Jarvis, 2020). Normally, the veins are not observable with the patient in a sitting position. Jugular venous distention is seen in venous hypertension or right-sided heart failure. Auscultation of the carotid artery can be performed by listening with the bell of the stethoscope. Normally, no bruits are audible. **Bruits** are abnormal "swishing" sounds heard over organs, glands, and arteries. A bruit results from an abnormality in an artery that results from a narrow or partially occluded artery, such occurs in atherosclerosis (Jarvis, 2020).

Mouth and throat. Inspect the lips and the mucous membranes of the mouth with a tongue blade and penlight, assessing all surfaces of the oral cavity. Normal mucous membranes are moist, pink, and free of lesions. With dehydration, mucous membranes look dry. The lips should be smooth, moist, and free of cracking. The condition of the teeth and gums gives the nurse insight into the health habits of the patient. Breath odors often indicate disease; foul, fruity, or musty breath is not normal.

Eyes. Note whether the eyes are symmetric. No exudate from the eyes is normally seen, and the lids should be open. The normal sclera of the eye is white, and the conjunctiva is pink. The conjunctiva is observed by gently depressing the lower lid. Periorbital edema, edema around the eyes, is abnormal.

Assess both eyes individually. Observe the eyes for pupillary reflex. Do this by darkening the room and using the penlight to shine light into the pupil. Have the light come from the side of the eye; shine the light across the eye, with the patient looking straight ahead at a focal point. The normal eye shows the pupil constricting when the light is applied. The pupil toward which the light is directed normally constricts; this reaction is the direct papillary response to light. If normal, the other pupil also constricts; this reaction is the consensual response to light. When assessing accommodation, ask the patient to follow his or her finger when it is brought in toward the patient's eyes, directly between the eyes. A normal accommodation response is that both pupils constrict equally. The rate and degree of constriction should be equal. Use the acronym PERRLA, which stands for *pupils equal, round, reactive to light, and accommodation*, to document the findings.

Fig. 13.3 Assess skin turgor by first grasping fold of skin on back of the patient's hand, sternum, forearm, or abdomen. Note ease and speed with which skin returns to place.

Fig. 13.4 Palpation of carotid artery.

Ears. First, note whether the ears are symmetric. Pull back and up gently on the external ear to straighten and examine the ear canal with help from the penlight. With a child younger than 3 years of age, pull the pinna back and down. Normally no pain is associated with this movement. The ear canal is normally free of excess cerumen or earwax, blood, and any other discharge. During this assessment, note whether the patient is following commands appropriately, indicating an ability to hear.

Nose. The nose is usually symmetric, although variation in size is considered normal. To test for patency, press against one nostril and ask the patient to breathe. Air should flow through the nose. Assess both nostrils, observing for bleeding or drainage. Also note the appearance of a deviated septum.

Chest, lungs, heart, and vascular system. Perform assessment of the chest and lungs with the patient in a sitting position. Inspect the chest for bilateral chest expansion, which is normally symmetric. Assess the rate and depth of respirations. The normal rate for an adult is 12 to 20 breaths/min. Normal breathing is quiet.

6. Tachypnea is a rapid rate of breathing at a rate greater than 20 breaths/min. Tachypnea occurs in fever, fear, exercise, pneumonia, alkalosis, and respiratory insufficiency. Bradypnea, less than 10 breaths/min, refers to slow breathing. Bradypnea occurs in increased intracranial pressure or depression of the respiratory center in the medulla oblongata from the action of opioids. Cheyne-Stokes is an irregular cycle of respirations that begins with slow, shallow respiration, becomes rapid, then slows, and are followed by periods of apnea before the cycle repeats. The most common causes of Cheyne-Stokes respiration are heart failure, opioid overdose, renal failure, meningitis, severe head injury, and when a client is near the end of life (Jarvis, 2020).

Note any sounds that are audible without the stethoscope; later, auscultate and determine the origin. Posture is often indicative of acute or chronic respiratory disease. The patient who is unable to lie supine or who must lean forward to breathe is showing signs of respiratory distress. A large, rounded "barrel chest" is diagnostic for adults with pulmonary disease such as emphysema. Assess arterial oxygen saturation via pulse oximetry, a noninvasive method of monitoring in which a sensor is attached to the person's finger or earlobe. An SPO_2 of 90% to 100% is needed to replenish O_2 in plasma.

Breasts. The breasts can be examined during a lung assessment. Many patients complete a self-breast examination on a monthly basis. Teach breast self-examination to male and female patients. Recommendations regarding breast self-examination are available at the National Breast Cancer Foundation *(www.nationalb reastcancer.org/breast-self-exam)*. Note any changes in how the breast feels, appearance of the nipples, or discharge from the nipples and teach the patient to report any abnormal finding.

Lung sounds. Auscultation provides information about the functioning of the respiratory system and about the presence of any obstruction in the air passages. The nurse should use the diaphragm of the stethoscope, which is designed to transmit the usually higher pitch of abnormal breath sounds.

Place the patient in a sitting position, leaning forward with arms across the lap. Instruct the patient to breathe through the mouth quietly and more deeply and slowly. Place the stethoscope firmly but not tightly on the skin and listen for one full inspiratory–expiratory cycle at each point. Never listen with a stethoscope over clothing. Systematically auscultate the posterior, lateral, and anterior chest using a zigzag approach from lung apices to bases. Compare the findings at each point with the corresponding point on the opposite side (Figs. 13.5 and 13.6).

Adventitious breath sounds are classified as either crackles or wheezes (Fig. 13.7). **Crackles,** produced by fluid in the bronchioles and the alveoli, are short, discrete, interrupted, crackling, or bubbling sounds that are usually heard during inspiration. The sound of crackles is similar to the sound produced by hairs being rolled between the fingers while close to the ear. Crackles are described further as fine or coarse. **Wheezes** are sounds produced by the movement of air through narrowed passages in the tracheobronchial tree. Wheezes predominate in expiration because bronchi are shortened and narrowed during this respiratory phase. Sometimes wheezes occur in the inspiratory and expiratory phases of respiration. Wheezes are classified as sibilant or sonorous (see the Coordinated Care box).

📷 Coordinated Care

Leadership

Assessing Lung Sounds

Assessment of the lung and thorax requires the application of skills and knowledge unique to a nurse. For these skills, delegation is inappropriate. If a patient has abnormal lung sounds, instruct certified assistive personnel (CAP) to observe a patient's respirations and report any changes in rate and depth to the nurse immediately and to keep the head of the bed elevated to assist the patient to breathe easier.

Sibilant wheezes have a high-pitched squeaking and musical quality and are produced by airflow through narrowed airways. *Sonorous* wheezes have a lower-pitched, coarser, gurgling, snoring quality and usually indicate the presence of mucus in the trachea and the large airways. *Stridor* is a high-pitched, inspiratory, crowing sound, louder in the neck than over the chest wall. Stridor originates in the larynx or the trachea and indicates upper airway obstruction from edematous, inflamed tissues or a foreign body. *Pleural friction rubs* are produced by inflammation of the pleural sac; the

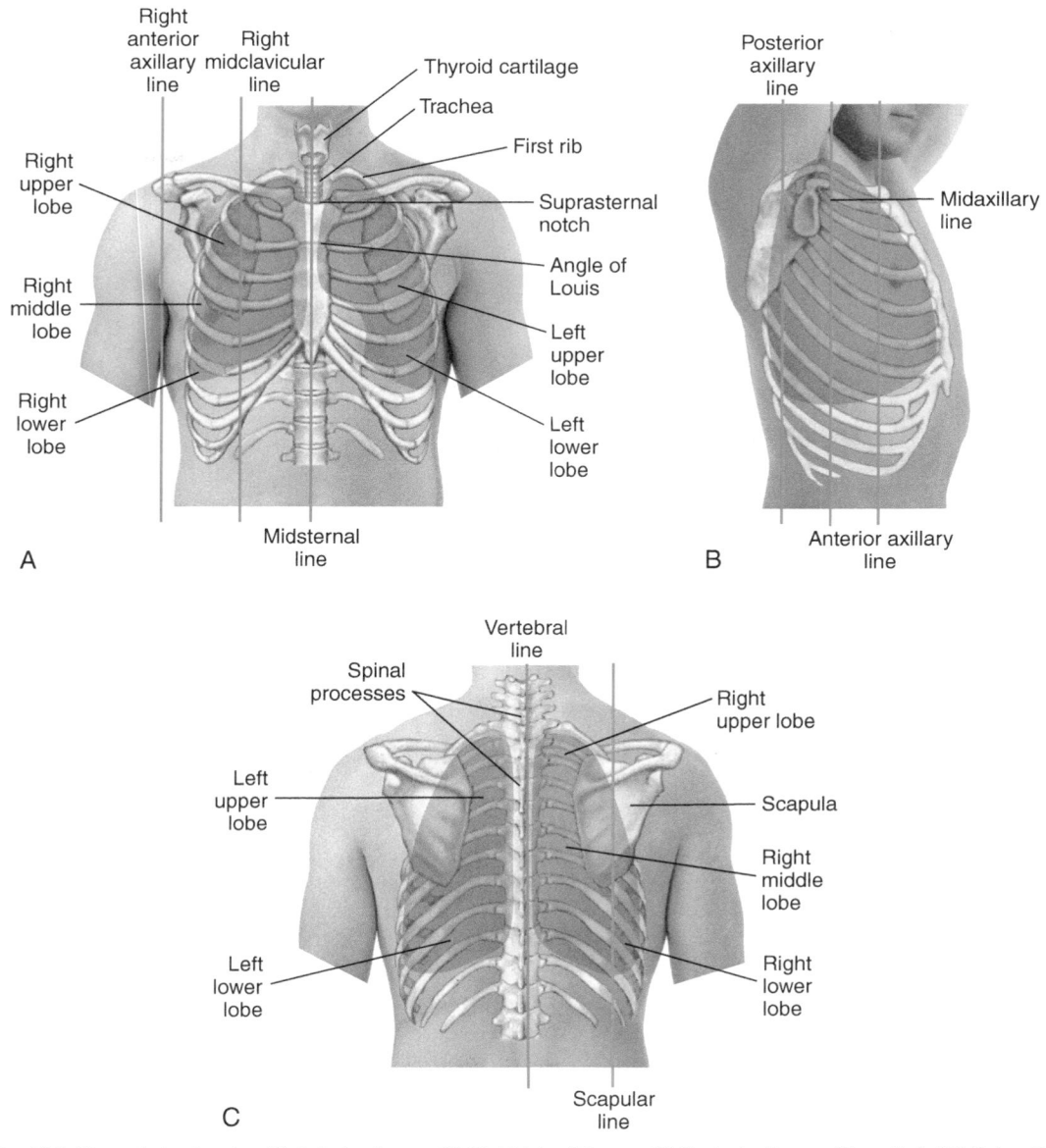

Fig. 13.5 Thoracic landmarks. (A) Anterior thorax. (B) Right lateral thorax. (C) Posterior thorax. (From Ball JW, Dains JE, Flynn JA, et al: *Seidel's guide to physical examination*, ed 9, St. Louis, 2019, Elsevier.))

nurse hears a rubbing, grating, or squeaky sound on auscultation. The grating sounds as if two pieces of leather are being rubbed together.

Whenever you hear adventitious breath sounds during auscultation, instruct the patient to cough, and then listen again. Sonorous wheezes are the most likely to clear, at least somewhat, with cough. However, crackles, especially when patients are on bed rest, sometimes also clear somewhat with cough. Document this finding with the breath sounds.

Spine. With the patient in a sitting position, note the curvature of the spine. Assess the patient's posture when standing. Run the fingers down the patient's spine, which should be straight, assessing for the normal lumbosacral curve. The shoulders and hips should be evenly aligned. Common postural abnormalities include lordosis, kyphosis, and scoliosis. Kyphosis, or humpback, is an exaggeration of the posterior curvature of the thoracic spine. Lordosis, or swayback, is an increased lumbar curvature. Scoliosis is a lateral spinal curvature. Check that the skin of the back has normal color, temperature, and moisture.

Heart sounds.

7. Heart sounds are auscultated with the stethoscope using both the bell and the diaphragm. The normal "lub-dub" sound of the heart is caused by the closure of the atrioventricular and the semilunar valves, respectively. The first normal heart sound, S_1, occurs with closure of the atrioventricular valves (AV) and thus signals the beginning of systole. S_1 usually is auscultated most clearly at the apex. The second normal heart sound, S_2, occurs with closure

Fig. 13.6 Suggested sequence for systematic percussion and auscultation of the thorax. (A) Posterior thorax. (B) Right lateral thorax. (C) Left lateral thorax. (D) Anterior thorax. The pleximeter finger or the stethoscope is moved in the numeric sequence suggested; however, other sequences are possible. It is beneficial to be systematic. (From Ball JW, Dains JE, Flynn JA, et al: *Seidel's guide to physical examination,* ed 9, St. Louis, 2019, Elsevier.))

Fine crackles:
High-pitched, discrete, discontinuous crackling sounds heard during the end of inspiration; not cleared by a cough

Rhonchi (sonorous wheeze):
Loud, low coarse sounds like a snore most often heard continuously during inspiration or expiration; coughing may clear sound (usually means mucus accumulation in trachea or large bronchi)

Medium crackles:
Lower, more moist sound heard during the midstage of inspiration; not cleared by a cough

Wheeze (sibilant wheeze):
Musical noise sounding like a squeak; most often heard continuously during inspiration or expiration; usually louder during expiration

Coarse crackles:
Loud, bubbly noise heard during inspiration; not cleared by a cough

Pleural friction rub:
Dry, rubbing, or grating sound, usually caused by inflammation of pleural surfaces; heard during inspiration or expiration; loudest over lower lateral anterior surface

Fig. 13.7 Adventitious breath sounds.

of the semilunar valves and signals the end of systole. S_2 is auscultated most clearly at the base (Jarvis, 2020).

8. Extra heart sounds are S_3 and S_4. S_3, which sounds after S_2, is heard best at the apex. S_3 is sometimes normal in children but is usually abnormal in adults. S_3 has a dull, soft sound and is sometimes an early sign of heart failure. S_4 is heard late in diastole when the atria contract. It is auscultated most clearly at the apex and is heard immediately before S_1. The sound is soft with a low pitch. S_4 is sometimes normal and sometimes pathologic; it is heard in patients with coronary artery disease after myocardial infarction (MI) or cardiomyopathy (Jarvis, 2020).

With the patient in various positions (Fig. 13.8), listen to the heart sounds for several cardiac cycles. Listen for the intensity of the sound, ranging from faint to strong. Determine the regularity of the rhythm: regular, regularly irregular, or irregularly irregular. For patients with faint heart sounds, very irregular rhythms, very rapid heart rates, or noisy respirations, palpation of the carotid or the radial pulses simultaneously with auscultation of the heart sounds is helpful.

Peripheral vascular system. Arteries provide oxygen and nutrients to the tissues. The nurse assesses the peripheral arteries by palpating peripheral arterial pulses. An arterial pulse is a pressure wave transmitted through the arterial system with each contraction of the heart. Nurses should assess radial, brachial, ulnar,

femoral, popliteal, dorsalis pedis, and posterior tibial pulses *(see Chapter 12, Skill 12.2 and Figure 12.5).*

Using the pads of the fingertips, apply enough pressure at the pulse site to gather information on the pulse rate, rhythm, and strength. Do not press so hard that the artery is occluded. If difficulty in locating the pulse is encountered, carefully move the fingers to slightly different positions in the area and vary the pressure exerted. Assess the pulse rate by counting the pulsation for 60 seconds. Check the rhythm for regularity. Measure the strength of the pulse by using the following scale: 0, absent; 1+, thready; 2+, weak; 3+, normal; and 4+, bounding. Follow agency policy when describing the pulse.

9. Begin with the most distal pulses to assess the arterial circulation at the farthest palpable point. Palpate the brachial pulse over the antecubital fossa (anterior surface of the elbow joint). Palpate the radial pulse by placing the pads of the first and second fingers on the palmar surface of the patient's relaxed and slightly flexed wrist medial to the radius bone. Palpate the femoral pulse midway between the anterosuperior iliac crest and the symphysis pubis, below and medial to the inguinal ligament. Palpate the popliteal pulse by pressing deeply into the dorsal aspect of the knee while the knee is slightly bent. Palpate the dorsalis pedis pulse by applying light touch between the first and second toes and slowly moving up the dorsum of the foot.

Fig. 13.8 Sequence of patient positions for auscultation of heart sounds. (A) Sitting up, leaning slightly forward. (B) Supine. (C) Left lateral recumbent.

The dorsalis pedis artery runs along the top of the foot in line with the groove between the extensor tendons of the great toe and the first toe. Palpate the posterior tibial pulse slightly below and posterior to the medial malleolus of the ankle. Ischemia results if there is a decreased supply of oxygenated blood to the tissues; often, this is caused by a narrowing of an artery. An embolism sometimes results in complete occlusion of an artery and death of tissue distal to the occlusion. Atherosclerosis has the potential to cause partial occlusion of an artery and thus insufficient delivery of oxygenated blood to the tissues. Atherosclerosis in the peripheral arteries of the lower extremities can cause a condition called claudication, which induces cramplike pain in the lower extremities, usually after walking. The pain is caused by insufficient delivery of oxygenated blood to the muscles of the lower extremities (Jarvis, 2020).

Inspect the extremities for symmetry, color, and varicosities. The extremities are normally symmetric and without edema or discoloration. Palpate the hands and feet for temperature; normally, they are warm. Peripheral veins should be fairly flat and barely visible.

Assess capillary refill by pressing firmly for 5 seconds on the fingernail or toenail and estimating the speed at which the blood returns. The tips of the fingers and toes can be used if the person has thick, unblanchable nail beds. In a person with good cardiac function and distal perfusion, capillary refill usually takes less than 3 seconds. A capillary refill of more than 3 seconds is considered a sign of sluggish circulation, and a time of 5 seconds is considered abnormal. Poor cardiac function, dehydration, and peripheral vascular diseases are examples of conditions that often cause delays in capillary refill.

Gastrointestinal system. During the remaining portion of the examination, the patient may remain in the supine position with knees elevated. During this portion of the assessment, be sure the patient is properly draped to decrease exposure of the pubic area and the breasts. When interviewing the patient, ask about the last bowel movement, frequency of bowel movements, and determine if the patient is experiencing nausea, vomiting, an altered or decreased appetite (anorexia). After the interview, examine the abdomen. First inspect the abdomen for shape, contour, lesions, scars, lumps, or rashes. Normally, the abdomen's contour is even, and skin color is the same as that of the thorax. Before palpating the abdomen auscultate for bowel sounds. Palpating first can alter the bowel sounds. Place the diaphragm of the stethoscope over the divisions of the abdomen (Fig. 13.9) and listening for the sounds of peristalsis, wavelike movements of the intestine. It is helpful, before beginning, to make sure the room is quiet. Light pressure on the stethoscope is enough to detect bowel sounds. Since peristalsis is continuous, bowel sounds are normally heard in all

Fig. 13.9 Anatomic divisions of the abdomen (quadrants). (From Wilson SF, Giddens J: *Health assessment for nursing practice*, ed 6, St. Louis, 2016, Elsevier.)

quadrants. Bowel sounds occur every 15 to 60 seconds and are classified as active, hyperactive, hypoactive, or absent. The normal rate of bowel sounds is 4 to 32 per minute.

Listen to bowel sounds for 1 minute in all quadrants to ensure you do not miss any sounds and to localize specific sounds. It is especially important to be thorough and take time when evaluating for a silent abdomen, the absence of bowel sounds, which indicates the arrest of intestinal motility, a medical problem. Bowel sounds can be highly irregular, listen for at least 4 minutes before concluding the absence of bowel sounds.

The two significant alterations in bowel sounds are the absence of any sound or extremely soft and widely separated sounds and increased sounds with a characteristically high-pitched, loud, rushing sound (borborygmi):

- *Decreased bowel sounds.* Diminished or absent bowel sounds accompany inhibition of bowel motility. Decreased motility occurs with inflammation, gangrene, or paralytic ileus. Decreased peristalsis frequently accompanies peritonitis, electrolyte disturbances, the aftermath of surgical manipulation of the bowel, and late bowel obstruction. In addition, diminished bowel sounds often are correlated with lower lobe pneumonia.
- *Increased bowel sounds.* Loud, gurgling borborygmi often accompanies increased motility of the bowel, such as with diarrhea. Sounds of loud volume are heard over areas of stenotic bowel. Sounds from an early bowel obstruction are high pitched, usually like splashing sounds or the emptying of a bottle into a hollow vessel. Fine, metallic, tinkling sounds are emitted as tiny gas bubbles break through the surface of intestinal juices. Common

Fig. 13.10 (A), Light palpation of the abdomen to assess for distention, masses, or tenderness. (B) Palpation of the liver using moderate palpation.

pathologic conditions associated with increased bowel sounds are gastroenteritis and subsiding ileus. Increased motility can be caused by laxative use or gastroenteritis.

Assessment of the abdomen for distention, firmness, and tenderness is important. After auscultating bowel sounds, palpate the underlying structures. Palpation comes after auscultation since the manipulation has potential to stimulate intestinal activity and thus alter bowel sounds. Use light palpation and note texture, temperature, and moisture of the skin in all abdominal quadrants (Fig. 13.10A). Normal skin of the abdomen is smooth, dry, and warm. Light palpation enables the nurse to detect superficial lesions just below the skin. Advanced practice nurses use deep palpation to detect tenderness or masses of the abdomen. In the upper right quadrant just below the rib cage, palpation of the liver is sometimes possible (Fig. 13.10B). If the liver is felt, it may be enlarged. The normal liver is smooth and nontender. The abdomen is normally free of masses, and nontender.

To ensure the patient is relaxed during palpation, warm your hands and use conversation to distract the patient. Assess the patient's face when palpating and check for grimacing. Patients may guard a tender area, which means the patient will tighten up abdominal muscles when the area is touched. If a pulsating mass is detected in the abdomen, stop palpation immediately and notify the health care provider. A pulsating mass in the abdomen can indicate the presence of an aneurysm.

Percussion of the abdomen is used to note the density of underlying tissue and to locate the margins of internal organs. The normal abdomen has a tympanic or drumlike sound, with dullness noted over the liver. A hollow sound heard over the stomach or intestines indicates flatus. Percussion generally is performed by the physician or an advanced practice nurse.

Genitourinary system. Nurses do not perform the vaginal examination with a speculum. Assessment of the urinary system is performed using inspection and palpation. It is most convenient for the nurse to perform this inspection during the perineal care of the patient. Wear gloves when inspecting the labia for lesions. Inspect the pubic hair for lice and note any vaginal discharge. Normal labia are pink, moist, and free of lesions. A normal white vaginal discharge known as leukorrhea is sometimes present.

Inspect the male genitalia for lesions and lice; look for discharge from the penis. Palpate the scrotum for lumps or hernias. If the male is uncircumcised, gently retract the foreskin to inspect for lesions on the glans penis.

While inspecting the genitalia on male and female patients, palpate the femoral artery in that area (see Skill 12.2). Use palpation of the suprapubic area to determine if the bladder is distended.

Rectum. The rectal area is best examined with the patient in a Sims position. Spread the buttocks to look for hemorrhoids or lesions. Normal skin around the anus is darker than the surrounding skin. To further assess the intestinal system, the health care provider may order a hemoccult test of occult blood (see Chapter 15). The results of the test can indicate if gastrointestinal bleeding is present.

Legs and feet. The legs and feet are the final area of assessment. Palpate femoral, popliteal, dorsalis pedis, and posterior tibial as described earlier (see Skill 12.2). Assess the extremities for temperature. Cold extremities signal possible peripheral vascular disease with inadequate arterial perfusion. Inspect the legs and feet and palpate for edema. *Edema* is an excessive accumulation of fluid in the interstitial spaces caused by leakage of fluid from veins and capillary beds. Edema occurs as a result of many disease processes, such as heart failure, pathologic conditions of the kidneys, burns, lymphatic stasis, and trauma. Assess for edema in dependent parts of the body including the feet, legs, scrotum, and sacral area.

Box 13.10   Pitting Edema Scale

1+   *Trace:* A barely perceptible pit (2 mm)

2+   *Mild:* A deeper pit (4 mm), with fairly normal contours, that rebounds in 10–15 s

3+   *Moderate:* A deep pit (6 mm); lasts for 30 s to more than 1 min

4+   *Severe:* An even deeper pit (8 mm), with severe edema that possibly lasts as long as 2–5 min before rebounding

To assess for pitting edema, press against a bony prominence for 5 seconds and then lift the finger. Observe the skin for rebounding and for the presence of an indentation. If the tissue rebounds immediately, the patient does not have pitting edema. An indentation indicates pitting edema, which is usually graded on a scale of 1 to 4, as shown in Box 13.10.

If edema is not pitting, it cannot be given a grade on this scale. Edema without pitting often arises from arterial disease and arterial occlusion. Unilateral edema is likely the result of occlusion of a major vein.

Assess the color, motion, sensation, and temperature (CMST) of both feet. A normal skin color on the legs is similar to that of the rest of the body. Test for sensation by asking the patient to close the eyes; then, touch the patient's toes and ask whether the patient feels it. Ask patients if they have pain or decreased sensation in the lower extremities, which sometimes indicates peripheral neuropathy. Normally, both feet are equally warm and pedal pulses are present. Direct the patient to flex the knees and ankles to test for ROM, although a better assessment of ROM is by observing the patient's gait. Varicosities, enlarged veins, are not normally present.

Documenting the Interview and the Assessment

Most institutions have a designated flowsheet in the electronic medical record or a standardized form to

Box 13.11   Telephone Communication: SBAR

SBAR stands for **S**ituation, **B**ackground, **A**ssessment, and **R**ecommendation. SBAR was initiated by Michael Leonard, MD, Physician Leader for Patient Safety, along with colleagues Doug Bonacum and Suzanne Graham at Kaiser Permanente of Colorado (Evergreen, Colorado, USA). SBAR is a communication tool and has seen improved patient safety during routine care and transfer and in complex cases. A copy of this tool may be found at the website for the Institute for Healthcare Improvement *(www.ihi.org/resources/Pages/Tools/SBARToolkit.aspx).*

This tool meets The Joint Commission safety goals and allows for the standardized communication during the hand-off of patient care between the sender and receiver. This can be a combination of verbal and written communication. (see Box 3.1 for an example of SBAR communication).

follow when completing the patient history and physical assessment. This serves as the baseline for evaluation of subsequent changes in the patient's condition and for decisions related to medical therapy (see Fig. 13.2). The documentation must be objective, clear, complete, and concise.

Telephone Consultation

With the rapid changes taking place in health care, nurses work in a variety of new settings. One example is telephone consultation, especially in the health care provider's office or clinic. When patients call a health care providers office to report a health problem, the nurse is usually the person the patient speaks with. The nurse can advise, direct the patient to come in for a visit, instruct the client to call a specialist that is already part of the patient's health care team, or instruct the patient to seek care in the emergency department. Interventions are based on the nurse's assessment of the patient, even though the assessment data the nurse uses comes directly from the patient. In some instances, the nurse will need to collaborate with another health care provider in order to advise the patient, which typically requires calling the patient back with recommendations from a physician or nurse practitioner. Several publications are currently available to use as a guideline to assist the nurse. Box 13.11 is an example of a tool to use when communicating between patient and health care providers and health care facility to health care facility. Health Insurance Portability and Accountability Act (HIPAA) guidelines must be followed to protect the privacy of patient information.

Get Ready for the NCLEX® Examination!

Key Points

- The health care provider assesses patients by using the senses of sight, touch, smell, and hearing.
- The patient feels symptoms, which are sensations such as pruritus (itching), pain, and dizziness.
- Diseases originate from various causes including hereditary, congenital, traumatic, neoplastic, infectious, inflammatory, degenerative, deficiencies, or environmental factors.
- Risk factors for acquiring a disease include age, genetics, environment, and lifestyle variables.
- The universal signs of infection are erythema, edema, pain, heat, loss of function, and purulent, malodorous drainage.
- Some frequently noted signs and symptoms of disease are cyanosis, pallor, erythema, edema, pain, nausea, vomiting, diarrhea, dyspnea, tachycardia, and fever.
- When a physician conducts a physical examination, the nurse often is requested to assist the examiner. The nurse has certain responsibilities, such as preparing the examining room, assisting with equipment, and preparing the patient.
- Laboratory results of blood, urine, and stool specimens often add to the information about the patient.
- Optimally a complete nursing physical assessment is performed as soon after admission as possible.
- Interviewing the patient initially helps to identify signs, symptoms, and areas of patient concern.
- Properly performed, the physical assessment proceeds in an orderly fashion: head to toe or system by system.
- Perform assessment using specific skills; inspection, palpation, percussion, and auscultation.
- The nurse's role requires the nurse to be familiar with normal assessments findings in order to identify abnormalities.
- Perform a physical assessment of each patient at the beginning of each nursing shift to determine actual or potential patient problems requiring medical or nursing interventions to promote the safety and well-being of the patient.

Additional Learning Resources

SG Go to the Study Guide for additional learning activities to help you master this chapter content.

Be sure to visit the Evolve site at http://evolve.elsevier.com/Cooper/foundations/ for additional online resources.

Review Questions for the NCLEX® Examination

1. When preparing to perform an assessment, which elements need to be included to ensure the integrity of the nurse-patient relationship?

   1. Introduction of the nurse to the patient, which includes title (LPN/LVN) and purpose of visit
   2. Explanation of what the nurse will need to accomplish (i.e., vital signs, body system review) during the time with the patient
   3. An estimated time frame to complete the assessment
   4. Standing at the foot of the bed to get the best look at the patient and his and her responses
   5. Preparation of the room for the least amount of distractions so that the patient can remain focused to questions offered by the nurse

2. A patient has been admitted with acute bronchitis. When performing a lung assessment, the nurse is best able to auscultate the lower lobes by listening to what location on the body?

   1. Posterior
   2. Anterior
   3. Lateral
   4. Superior

3. A 90-year-old patient is having difficulty answering the nurse's questions while completing the patient history. What should the nurse keep in mind about caring for older adults?

   1. All older adults age at the same rate.
   2. The nurse should write down all the questions and have the patient's family complete the information.
   3. The nurse should sit down at eye level with the patient and allow a longer period to answer each question.
   4. The nurse should talk more loudly and raise the pitch of the voice.

4. The nurse documents which finding while assessing a patient with heart failure where it is noted that the lower extremities have deep indentations that remain for 30 seconds when pressed?

   1. Nonpitting edema
   2. 2+ pitting edema
   3. 3+ pitting edema
   4. 4+ pitting edema

5. The patient reports severe abdominal pain. What type of assessment should the nurse perform?

   1. Head-to-toe assessment
   2. Focused assessment
   3. System-by-system assessment
   4. Complete assessment

6. An elderly male patient is admitted for chest pain. How does the nurse best document the information the patient gives about his symptoms?

   1. Use the patient's own words in quotation marks.
   2. Briefly summarize what the patient says.
   3. Interpret the patient's comments using medical terminology.
   4. Use the information for the chief complaint from the admission sheet.

7. The nurse asks the patient about which signs and symptoms experienced when reviewing the elderly patient's gastrointestinal system? *(Select all that apply.)*

   1. Changes in bowel habits
   2. Pyrosis (heartburn)
   3. Firmness of the abdomen
   4. Dyspnea
   5. Anorexia

8. What is the first area to be assessed after taking vital signs when performing a nursing assessment?

   1. Assess for level of consciousness and orientation.
   2. Assess the skin.
   3. Listen to lung sounds.
   4. Check for pitting edema.

9. A patient has been admitted for dehydration after a prolonged period of diarrhea. Which finding does the nurse expect to observe in this patient?

   1. Skin warm, moist, pink with good skin turgor
   2. Skin warm, dry, pale with decreased skin turgor
   3. Skin cool, dry, pink with increased skin turgor
   4. Skin cool, moist, pale with decreased skin turgor

10. The nurse assesses a vibration felt along the patient's carotid artery with palpation. How should the nurse describe this assessment finding?

    1. Palpation
    2. Thrill
    3. Bruit
    4. Aneurysm

11. The nurse is preparing a female patient for a gynecologic examination. Which patient position best assists the health care provider in this examination?

    1. High Fowler's
    2. Dorsal recumbent
    3. Lithotomy
    4. Sims

12. Which risk factor for cardiovascular disease can be modified? *(Select all that apply.)*

    1. Age
    2. Race
    3. Diet
    4. Family history
    5. Smoking

13. What is the term used to describe a patient's respiratory rate that exceeds 36 breaths/min?

    1. Sonorous
    2. Bradypnea
    3. Tachypnea
    4. Apnea

14. The nurse is auscultating breath sounds on a patient and detects adventitious breath sounds. The nurse describes them as a loud, bubbly noise heard during inspiration. The nurse is correct when using which term for documenting this finding?

    1. Coarse crackles
    2. Sonorous wheezes
    3. Pleural friction rub
    4. Sibilant wheezes

15. The nurse is documenting a patient assessment. The nurse correctly identifies which information as being objective data? *(Select all that apply.)*

    1. "I have a headache and feel like the room is spinning."
    2. "When I eat I have horrible pain in my stomach."
    3. "It burns when I use the bathroom; what do you think is wrong with me?"
    4. "It is noted that the blood pressure (B/P) is high at 156/96."
    5. "Abdomen is distended, and hypoactive bowel sounds are noted."

16. The nurse is performing a cardiovascular system assessment on a patient. Which is included in an assessment of the peripheral vascular system? *(Select all that apply.)*

    1. Assessment of the apical pulse rate by counting the pulsations for 60 seconds
    2. Assessment of the brachial, radial, ulnar, femoral, popliteal, dorsalis pedis, and posterior tibial pulses
    3. Assessment of capillary refill in the nail beds of the fingers and toes
    4. Determination of the rate, rhythm, and strength of the dorsalis pedis pulse
    5. Assessment of the patient's skin turgor by counting the amount of time the skin remains tented

17. The patient has been admitted to the medical unit with a wound to the left lower extremity from a mowing accident 2 days ago. The inflammatory response present at this stage includes which signs and symptoms? *(Select all that apply.)*

    1. Swelling
    2. Pain
    3. Coolness
    4. Purulent drainage
    5. Pale skin at injury site

18. The patient asks the nurse why all the nurses always listen to his abdomen with the stethoscope before pressing on it. Which response is correct?

    1. This prevents distortion of vascular sounds.
    2. This prevents distortion of bowel sounds.
    3. This determines any areas of tenderness or pain.
    4. This allows the patient to relax and be comfortable.

19. A woman, 27, has come to the urgent care clinic with red circles erupting on her lower extremities that itch and burn and "look like spider bites. They are driving me crazy," she says, wincing as she tries to avoid scratching them. The woman explains that she was camping and hiking in a nearby state park with friends all weekend. "I don't know if I walked into a patch of poison oak, or kicked my way through too many spider webs, or maybe stepped on a red ant hill. I have no idea. All I know is, I came home, threw my clothes straight into the wash, and immediately took a long, hot shower, but I'm *still* breaking out

in this hideous rash, and no ointment or cream seems to make any difference." In addition to the itching, burning red circles on her lower extremities, the skin on her calves is red, shiny and swollen, almost tight. Her vital signs are as follows: Oral temp: 101.2; Pulse: 90; Resp: 18; White blood cellcell count: 12,000/mm^3. A wound culture test is swabbed for bacterial analysis and to identify the type of infection. From this same sampling, the physician orders a susceptibility test to help determine which antibiotic will be most effective in treatment—provided the infection is bacterial.

Place an X (or drag and drop) to indicate *objective* assessment findings that may indicate inflammation or infection.

ASSESSMENT FINDINGS	OBJECTIVE SIGN
a. Edema	
b. Nausea	
c. Pruritis	
d. Erythema	
e. Purulent exudate	
f. Tachypnea	
g. PERRLA	
h. Dysphagia	

14

Oxygenation

Objectives

1. Discuss nursing interventions and related procedures for the patient receiving oxygen therapy.
2. Identify safety precautions necessary when oxygen therapy is in use.
3. Differentiate the various types of oxygen therapy delivery devices.
4. Discuss transtracheal oxygen delivery.
5. Develop patient problem statements for the patient receiving oxygen therapy to direct nursing care.
6. Describe the process of suctioning a patient with a tracheostomy.
7. Describe the process of providing tracheostomy care.
8. Differentiate and describe oropharyngeal, nasopharyngeal, and nasotracheal suctioning.

Key Terms

apnea (ĂP-nē-ă, p. 350)
arterial partial pressure oxygen (PaO$_2$) level (p. 342)
endotracheal tube (ĕn-dō-TRĂ-kē-ăl tūb, p. 342)
flowmeter (p. 343)
fraction of inspired oxygen (FiO$_2$) (p. 343)
hypoxia (hī-pŎK-Sē-ăh, p. 342)
nasal cannula (NĂ-zŭl KĂN-yū-lă, p. 344)

nonrebreather mask (Table 14.1, p. 342)
oxymizer (Table 14.1, p. 343)
partial rebreather mask (Table 14.1, p. 343)
patency (PĂ-tĕn-cē, p. 356)
simple face mask (Skill 14.1, p. 348)
tracheostomy (trā-kē-ŎS-tō-mē, p. 350)
Venturi mask (vĕn-TŪ-rē măsk, Skill 14.1, p. 348)

Oxygen is needed by all cells of the body to metabolize nutrients and produce the energy needed to function. When hypoxia (reduced oxygen content in tissue and cells) occurs, cell metabolism slows down, and cells begin to die. Oxygen therapy is one method of preventing or relieving tissue hypoxia. Oxygen therapy must be ordered by a health care provider and closely monitored by the nurse to ensure proper administration (see the Coordinated Care box on oxygen administration). Oxygen is treated as a drug; therefore, it is important to follow the six rights of drug administration when administering oxygen (see Chapter 17).

An accurate and thorough assessment of the respiratory system (see Chapter 13) is necessary when administering oxygen therapy to determine the need and the effectiveness of the treatment ordered. Knowledge of the respiratory system and related disorders (see *Adult Health Nursing,* Chapter 9) also helps the nurse care for the patient requiring oxygen therapy. Some oxygen delivery devices, such as the continuous positive airway pressure (CPAP) device, are discussed in *Adult Health Nursing,* Chapter 9.

STANDARD STEPS IN SELECTED SKILLS

To ensure patient safety, as well as nurse safety, during nursing procedures, it is important to understand the steps involved in specific skills. The skill boxes in this chapter list those steps for a variety of nursing procedures

related to oxygen therapy. Certain steps performed before and after every procedure are listed as follows. The skill boxes that follow refer to them as *Standard Steps.* These steps must be followed before and after every procedure to provide the patient with safe, effective nursing care.

BEFORE THE PROCEDURE

The rationales for these steps are listed in italics in parentheses.

1. Check the health care provider's order. (*Provides a basis for care. Many nursing interventions require a health care provider's order. Verification is essential before any procedure is started.*)
2. Introduce yourself to the patient; include your name and title or role. (*Decreases patient anxiety and aids in establishing rapport with the patient.*)
3. Identify the patient by checking his or her identification bracelet and requesting that the patient state his or her full name or birth date, or both (facility policy will determine the methods for patient identification). (*Ensures that the procedure is performed on the correct patient.*)
4. Explain the procedure and the reason it is to be done in terms that the patient is able to understand. Advise the patient of any unpleasantness that may be involved with the procedure. Give the patient time to ask questions. (*Promotes cooperation, decreases patient's anxiety, and prepares patient.*)

5. Determine the need for and provide patient education before, during, and after the procedure. (*Promotes patient's independence and compliance.*)
6. Evaluate the patient. Each skill box contains an assessment section that includes specific data to evaluate. (*Provides baseline information for later comparisons.*)
7. Perform hand hygiene. Don clean or sterile gloves and personal protective equipment as needed according to the procedure, agency policy, and guidelines from the Centers for Disease Control and Prevention (CDC) and the Occupational Safety and Health Administration (OSHA) (see Chapter 7). (*Reduces the spread of microorganisms and protects the patient and the nurse.*)
8. Assemble equipment, and complete necessary charges. Each skill box lists the specific equipment required. (*Organizes procedure so that it will go more smoothly. Some equipment is reusable and is kept at the patient's bedside. Some of the equipment is disposable and charged to the patient when used. Know agency policy.*)
9. Prepare the patient for the procedure:
    a. Close the door or pull the privacy curtain around the patient's bed. (*Provides privacy and promotes patient comfort.*)
    b. Raise the bed to a comfortable working height, and lower the side rail on the side nearest the nurse. (*Promotes proper body mechanics by minimizing nurse's muscle strain and preventing injury and fatigue.*)
    c. Position and drape the patient as necessary. Descriptions of specific positions are included in each skill. (*Shows respect for patient's privacy and dignity.*)

DURING THE PROCEDURE

10. Promote patient involvement as much as possible. (*Participation encourages the patient's cooperation and increases the patient's knowledge of condition and care. It also may increase the patient's sense of independence and importance and increase the patient's compliance with treatment.*)
11. Determine the patient's tolerance of the procedure, being alert for signs and symptoms of discomfort and fatigue. If the patient cannot tolerate a procedure, describe this inability in the nursing notes. (*Patients' ability to tolerate interventions varies, depending on the severity of illness and disability. It is necessary to determine when to provide the patient with an opportunity to rest and when to provide comfort measures.*)

AFTER THE PROCEDURE

12. Assist the patient to a position of comfort, and place needed items within easy reach. Ensure that the patient has a means to call for help and knows how to use it. (*Promotes comfort and safety. Patients often try to reach items and risk falling or injury.*)
13. Raise the side rails in the acute care setting, and lower the bed to the lowest position. (*This minimizes the patient's risk of getting out of bed unattended. Use nursing judgment and facility policy to safely allow alert, cooperative patients to have their side rails down.*)
14. Remove gloves and all protective barriers such as gown, face shield, and masks. Store appropriately or discard. Remove and dispose of soiled supplies and equipment according to agency policy and guidelines from the CDC and OSHA. (*Reduces spread of microorganisms, maintains cleanliness of the environment, and enhances patient comfort and safety.*)
15. Perform hand hygiene after removing gloves. (*Wearing gloves does not eliminate the need to perform hand hygiene. Hand hygiene is the most important technique for preventing and controlling the spread of microorganisms.*)
16. Document the patient's response to the procedure, expected or unexpected outcomes, and all patient teaching. Specific areas of documentation are indicated in each skill box. (*Timely and accurate documentation is legally required, records patient's progress, and promotes continuity of care.*)
17. Report any unexpected outcomes. Specific notes for reporting unexpected outcomes are included in each skill. (*Additional procedures or treatments may be necessary.*)

SKILLS FOR RESPIRATORY DISORDERS

OXYGEN THERAPY

Oxygen therapy consists of various devices, depending on the respiratory needs of the patient. The skill of the nurse with these therapies directly affects the patient's outcome of the prescribed therapy, as well as the confidence the patient has in the nurse's ability to perform a procedure. Being familiar with the various devices used in oxygen therapy is critical for the nursing student before providing care to the patient. The flow rate of oxygen is ordered in liters per minute (L/min). This determines how much oxygen the patient will receive; however, these numbers do not correlate directly with the percentage of oxygen delivered. The percentage or concentration of oxygen delivered is called the fraction of inspired oxygen (FiO_2). The amount of oxygen delivered will depend on the type of device used (Table 14.1). An oxygen flowmeter (Fig. 14.1) is the device used to set the prescribed rate of oxygen.

Table 14.1	Oxygen Delivery Devices With Percentage of Oxygen Delivered
DELIVERY DEVICE	**AMOUNT OF DELIVERED FiO_2**
Nasal cannula	1–6 L/min = 24%–44% O_2
Oxymizer	1–15 L/min = 29%–50% O_2
Simple face mask	5–8 L/min = 35%–55% O_2
Venturi mask	4–10 L/min = 24%–55% O_2
Partial rebreather mask	6–12 L/min = 60%–90% O_2
Nonrebreather mask	6–15 L/min = 70%–100% O_2

Coordinated Care

Collaboration

Oxygen Administration

- Oxygen administration requires the critical thinking skills of a nurse. The nurse is responsible for ensuring that the oxygen is administered in the correct manner, adjusting the oxygen flow rate, and evaluating the patient's response to oxygen therapy.
- Correct placement and adjustment of oxygen devices may be delegated to unlicensed assistive personnel (UAP) after the care provider is instructed about the possible complications and outcomes associated with oxygen delivery and the need to report these to the nurse immediately if they occur. Adjustment of the oxygen flow rate is not delegated to UAP.

There are many safety issues involved in the administration of oxygen. It is a colorless, odorless, and tasteless gas that does not burn or explode, but it does support combustion; that is, if it is combined with other factors, such as an electrical spark or fire, oxygen enables combustion, and nearby objects ignite. Therefore smoking, wool blankets, electric razors, and friction toys should be avoided when oxygen is administered. The nurse must observe all safety precautions (Box 14.1). It also can be very drying to mucous membranes, which increases the risk of tissue cracking and opening, leaving the patient at risk for infection; humidification may be necessary. In addition, oxygen toxicity can cause scarring of the respiratory tract tissue and blindness.

Oxygen therapy may be initiated by a respiratory therapist, a nurse, an emergency medical technician (EMT), or any other licensed health care provider with an appropriate order for the oxygen. In some facilities, there is a respiratory care department staffed by respiratory therapists who assume the responsibility of administering oxygen and delivering treatments that will improve a patient's ventilation and oxygenation.

Patients in need of oxygen may exhibit various symptoms in accordance with the degree of oxygen deprivation they are experiencing (Boxes 14.2 and 14.3). In caring for a patient having difficulty breathing or exhibiting any symptoms of hypoxia, the nurse must recognize the symptoms quickly and administer the oxygen via the appropriate mechanism as soon as possible. There are several ways to deliver oxygen. Delivering through a **nasal cannula** (device consisting of small tubes inserted into the nares) is the most common way to administer oxygen, but it also can be delivered by an oxymizer, Venturi mask (Fig. 14.2), oxygen hood or halo, or oxygen tent (Skill 14.1). Many elderly patients and patients with chronic lung disease require oxygen in the home setting. See the Lifespan Considerations for Older Adults, Patient Teaching, and Home Care Considerations boxes for special considerations and instructions for these patients.

Fig. 14.1 Oxygen flowmeter.

Box 14.1	Safety Precautions During Oxygen Use

- Place "No Smoking" or "Oxygen in Use" signs, or both, in the patient's room and where easily seen.
- Instruct the patient, the family, and visitors that smoking is not permitted because oxygen supports combustion (burning).
- Avoid the use of electrical appliances such as razors, blankets, and heating pads while oxygen is administered.
- Avoid the use of petrolatum products such as petroleum jelly when oxygen is administered because of the combustibility of oxygen.
- Secure portable oxygen delivery systems, such as cylinders or portable tanks, into proper portable oxygen-carrying equipment to prevent falling or tipping because these delivery devices can become projectiles.
- Avoid placing oxygen cylinders near sources of heat, such as lamps or radiators.
- Avoid clothing that is not fire resistant.
- Ensure that all electrical equipment is functioning appropriately and is well grounded (three-prong plug). Avoid frayed, tangled, or cluttered cords, and do not overload circuits.
- Know the facility's fire procedure and the locations of fire extinguishers.
- Administer oxygen by the method and rate ordered by the health care provider.
- Ensure that the patient is aware if extension tubing is in use to prevent falls from tripping over the tubing.

Lifespan Considerations

Older Adults

Oxygen Therapy

- Normal arterial oxygen levels sometimes decrease with age but are not usually low enough to fall outside the normal range. It may be possible for a 70-year-old person to have an **arterial partial pressure oxygen (PaO_2) level** (the amount of oxygen found in the arterial circulation) between 80 and 85 mm Hg (normal range is 80 to 100 mm Hg) without experiencing significant alterations in health. Lower than normal levels of PaO_2, even below 80 mm Hg, are common in the patient with chronic obstructive pulmonary disease (COPD; see Chapter 9, *Adult Health Nursing*).
- The respiratory drive normally is initiated by arterial carbon dioxide ($PaCO_2$) levels rising, but in patients with COPD, hypoxia tends to be the driving force behind respiratory effort (hypoxic drive). If the hypoxia is corrected in a patient with COPD, then the respiratory drive is reduced, and respiratory difficulty will occur. For this reason, oxygen flow rates greater than 2 L/min are to be given with great caution in these individuals. Flow rates higher than 2 L/min could eliminate the respiratory drive, and breathing may stop.
- The older adult is often at increased risk for skin impairment. Therefore, frequent monitoring for erythema and skin breakdown over the ears is necessary when a nasal cannula is being used for oxygen delivery. Early interventions such as loosening the straps, repositioning the tubing, or adding padding over the ears often prevent impairment.

 Patient Teaching

Oxygen Therapy

- Teach the patient how to apply the oxygen equipment, such as the nasal cannula or oxygen mask, appropriately.
- Discuss safety precautions for oxygen use (see Box 14.1).
- Stress the dangers of adjusting the oxygen flow rate without notifying the health care provider. Emphasize that it is possible for the patient to be short of breath because of reasons other than hypoxia and to contact the health care provider if shortness of breath increases.
- Instruct patient to ambulate or change positions frequently to mobilize secretions.
- Teach the patient to cough and practice deep breathing, and encourage practicing these techniques frequently, as directed by the patient condition or provider's orders, to facilitate air exchange.
- Teach the patient to maintain adequate fluid intake to help liquefy secretions. Recommend fluids that are free of caffeine and sugar because drinks high in caffeine and sugar sometimes cause dehydration. Teach the patient to avoid dairy products, which tend to thicken secretions.
- Teach the rationale for prescribed medications, as well as side effects. This helps increase compliance.
- Teach that performing oral hygiene at regular intervals helps rid the mouth of any bad taste from secretions coughed up or expectorated.

 Home Care Considerations

Oxygen Therapy

- If oxygen is used at home, instruct the patient's family to post a "No Smoking" sign on all entry doors of the house.
- When oxygen cylinders are used, it is necessary to secure them so that they will not fall over. Oxygen cylinders are stored upright, chained on appropriate holders.
- In home settings, oxygen tubing is sometimes as long as 50 feet (15.2 m), which presents a tripping hazard. Instruct patient on risks for falling that are associated with this length of tubing.
- Instruct patient's family on safety measures of oxygen therapy (see Box 14.1).
- Teach the patient and family members how to use home equipment.
- Instruct patient and family members to observe the level of oxygen in canister tanks and to use portable tanks when the patient is not at home.
- Instruct patient and family members to fill plastic humidifier bottles with distilled water every 24 h. Instruct patient and family members to use only distilled water, not tap water.
- Provide two complete sets of tubing so that one set of equipment is available for use while the other is being cleaned or repaired.
- Evaluate home for availability of a three-pronged outlet for the compressor to prevent electric shock.
- Teach the patient to maintain a constant flow rate and to change the flow rate only with the health care provider's knowledge and advice.
- Evaluate home for appropriate storage of equipment.
- Evaluate family's willingness to assist the patient with a home delivery system.
- Teach the patient and family deep breathing and coughing exercises.
- Teach the patient and family adequate nutritional and hydration needs based on the patient's diagnosis and current condition.

Box **14.2**	Signs and Symptoms of Hypoxia

- Apprehension, anxiety, restlessness
- Behavioral changes
- Cardiac dysrhythmias
- Cyanosis
- Decreased ability to concentrate
- Decreased level of consciousness
- Digital clubbing (with chronic hypoxia)
- Dyspnea
- Elevated blood pressure
- Increased fatigue
- Increased pulse rate: As hypoxia advances, bradycardia results, which in turn results in decreased oxygen saturation
- Increased rate and depth of respiration: As hypoxia progresses, respirations become shallow and slower, and apnea develops
- Pallor
- Vertigo

TRANSTRACHEAL OXYGEN DELIVERY

A method of oxygen delivery for the patient with a tracheostomy is the transtracheal catheter, which is inserted directly into the trachea between the second and third tracheal cartilages.

Box **14.3**	Identifying Patient Problem Statements to Promote Oxygenation

Inability to Clear Airway
- Related to ineffective cough
- Related to excessive secretions

Inability to Maintain Adequate Breathing Pattern
- Related to respiratory muscle weakness
- Related to fatigue
- Related to abnormal breathing patterns

Inability to Tolerate Activity
- Related to an imbalance between oxygen supply and demand

Anxiousness, Fearfulness, or Despair
- Related to dyspnea and feelings of suffocation
- Related to fear of dying

Compromised Verbal Communication
- Related to the presence of tracheostomy
- Related to intubation

Unlike a tracheostomy tube, a transtracheal catheter (Fig. 14.3) does not interfere with drinking, eating, or talking. With a nasal cannula, oxygen is delivered only during inhalation. With the transtracheal oxygen delivery system, oxygen is delivered throughout the entire respiratory cycle. No oxygen is lost to the atmosphere; therefore, oxygen delivery is less expensive. Additional humidification is unnecessary because the nasopharynx, the area most in need of supplemental humidity, is bypassed. This delivery system also allows the flow rate to be decreased for some patients. Patients who require 2 L/min with a cannula may need only 1 L/min with a transtracheal catheter. The low flow rates also enable patients to use portable oxygen delivery systems longer between refills.

For transtracheal oxygen delivery, a small oxygen tube (8-French [Fr] or 9-Fr) is inserted through the transtracheal tract opening through which oxygen is administered. After the insertion tract has matured (healed), it is possible for the patient or a family member to remove the tube for cleaning. A single transtracheal catheter may last up to 3 months. After that period, the catheter is likely to become brittle and must be replaced. This method of oxygen delivery is suited especially for home use. It allows the individual to be more active and can be concealed under a shirt. Some transtracheal oxygen

Adjustable nose clip

Opening for exhaled air

Venturi barrel

Room air

100% oxygen

Fig. 14.2 Venturi mask.

Skill 14.1   Oxygen Administration

NURSING ACTION (RATIONALE)

1. Refer to Standard Steps 1–9.
2. Assemble equipment:
   - Specific oxygen delivery system (e.g., mask, cannula, or tent, the last of which is used primarily for pediatric patients)
   - Oxygen tubing (consider extension tubing)
   - Source of oxygen
   - Flowmeter
   - Humidifier bottle and distilled water
   - "Oxygen in Use" sign
   - Clean gloves
   - Stethoscope
3. Explain necessary precautions during oxygen therapy (see Box 14.1). *(Increases patient knowledge and compliance and promotes safety.)*
4. Position the patient in Fowler's or semi-Fowler's position. *(Allows for maximum lung expansion.)*
5. Auscultate lung sounds and observe for signs and symptoms of hypoxia or respiratory distress (see Box 14.2). Review arterial blood gas results. *(Enables the nurse to confirm patency of the airway and to determine the need for oxygen.)* Suction any secretions obstructing the airway and listen to lung sounds after suctioning (see Skill 14.2 and 14.5). *(Assists in clearing the airway and increasing oxygenation.)*
6. Use a prefilled humidification container or fill the humidifier container with distilled water to a designated level, if necessary. Humidify oxygen if the flow rate is greater than 4 L/min. Use only distilled water in the humidifier. *(Provides moisture to prevent drying of the nasal and oropharyngeal mucosa. Distilled water provides bacteria- and mineral-free water.)*
7. Attach flowmeter to the humidifier and insert in a proper oxygen source: central oxygen outlet, portable oxygen cylinder, or oxygen concentrator. The oxygen then is turned on to the prescribed liter flow. If the flowmeter has a metal ball, the oxygen is turned on until the middle of the metal ball is positioned on the line on the flowmeter for the prescribed oxygen flow. *(It is necessary to secure flowmeter properly to oxygen source for adequate delivery of oxygen.)* Verify that water is bubbling. *(Presence of bubbling indicates that oxygen is humidified before delivery to the patient.)*
8. Administer oxygen therapy:
   a. A *nasal cannula* allows the patient to eat and talk normally, and its use is appropriate for all age groups.

(1) Attach nasal cannula tubing to the flowmeter. *(Oxygen delivery system must be continuous to ensure adequate supply of oxygen.)*

(2) Adjust flowmeter to 6–10 L/min to flush tubing and prongs with oxygen. Feel the oxygen on your skin to ensure flow. *(Enables the nurse to determine patency and removes any microscopic particles possibly in the tubing.)*

(3) Adjust the flow rate to a prescribed amount; 1–6 L/min may be ordered. *(Ensures delivery of oxygen flow rate as directed by the health care provider.)*

(4) Place a nasal prong into each nostril of the patient in the direction that the prongs are curved (see illustration). *(Directs flow of oxygen into the patient's upper respiratory tract.)*

Continued

Skill 14.1   Oxygen Administration—cont'd

(5) Place cannula tubing over the patient's ears and tighten under the chin (see illustration). *(Proper fit is snug and comfortable to prevent displacement of prongs.)*

(6) Place padding between strap and ears if needed. Use lamb's wool, gauze, or cotton balls. Some nasal cannula tubing already has protective devices in place. *(Prevents skin irritation and breakdown.)*

(7) Ensure that the cannula tubing is long enough to allow for patient movement. *(Reduces the risk that one or both prongs will cause pressure on the nares, as well as the risk of displacement, as the patient moves or is repositioned.)*

(8) Regularly evaluate equipment and patient's respiratory status. *(Ensures delivery of prescribed oxygen flow rate. Determines whether the patient needs further respiratory interventions.)*

    (a) Evaluate cannula frequently for possible obstruction.

    (b) Observe external nasal area, nares, and superior surface of both ears for skin impairment every 6–8 h.

    (c) Observe nares and cannula prongs at least once a shift for irritation or breakage. Cleanse skin with a cotton-tipped applicator as needed. *(Prevents skin irritation or trauma to the nares from damaged cannula prongs.)*

    (d) Apply water-soluble lubricant to nares if needed. *(Prevents drying and irritation of nares. Water-soluble lubricant will not occlude the nasal cannula.)*

    (e) Refer to health care provider's orders for any prescribed changes in flow rate.

    (f) Maintain solution in humidifier container, if used, at an appropriate level at all times. *(Prevents inhalation of dehumidified oxygen.)*

    (g) Auscultate lung sounds. *(Verifies adequate oxygenation and patency of the airway.)*

    (h) Consult with health care provider regarding need for pulse oximetry if the patient's oxygen level is unstable. *(Assists in determining oxygenation needs and helps prevent oxygen toxicity.)*

    (i) Oxymizer: the oxymizer is similar to the nasal cannula in delivery. The steps for initiating oxygen via this device are the same as a nasal cannula. The difference lies in the amount of oxygen delivered (FiO$_2$). The reservoirs of the oxymizer collect and conserve oxygen, allowing a higher percentage of oxygen to be delivered. It is important to check the reservoirs to ensure that they do not deflate, as this would lower the percentage of oxygen delivered. When comparing the nasal cannula to the oxymizer, at 6 L/min, the oxymizer delivers 7% more FiO$_2$ than the nasal cannula, and the oxymizer can be set as high as 15L/min.

b. *Face mask:* Depending on the patient's respiratory condition, the health care provider may prescribe delivery of oxygen by a mask. The mask is designed to fit snugly over the patient's nose and mouth. Different types of masks are used according to the patient's needs, such as the Venturi mask (see Fig. 14.2), partial rebreather mask (Step 8b[5a]), nonrebreathing mask (Step 8b[5b]), and simple face mask.

(1) Explain to the patient the need for an oxygen mask. *(Decreases patient's fear and increases compliance.)*

(2) Adjust flow rate of oxygen per health care provider's order. Usually, 6–10 L/min, which is measured in percentages (35%–95%), is prescribed. In some facilities, the respiratory therapist assumes responsibility for maintaining proper flow. Observe for a fine mist or bubbling in the humidifier.

Skill 14.1 Oxygen Administration—cont'd

(3) Allow the patient to hold the oxygen mask over the bridge of the nose and mouth, if he or she is able. Assist as necessary. *(Placing a mask over a patient's face sometimes causes a feeling of suffocation and apprehension. Allowing the patient to place the mask helps the patient become accustomed to it and to have some control over placing it on their face.)*

(4) Adjust straps around patient's head and over ears. Place a cotton ball or gauze over the ears under elastic straps. *(Provides comfort and prevents skin impairment.)*

(5) Cover the reservoir hole in the mask and allow the reservoir bag to completely fill BEFORE placing it on the patient. Observe the reservoir bag for appropriate movement if one is attached to the mask. *(Mask's expanding and collapsing with patient's breathing confirm the appropriate fit and that oxygen delivery is maintained.)*

(a) Partial-rebreathing mask: When functioning properly, the reservoir fills on exhalation and almost collapses on inhalation.

(b) Nonrebreathing mask: When functioning properly, the reservoir fills on exhalation but never totally collapses on inhalation.

(6) Evaluate equipment function regularly. *(Ensures that mask is working properly and that the patient is receiving an appropriate amount of oxygen.)*

(a) Remove mask and evaluate skin every 2–4 h. Clean and dry skin as needed. *(Removes condensation and other debris that may form and prevents skin breakdown.)*

(b) Refer to health care provider's orders for prescribed flow rate and any changes.

(c) Maintain solution in humidifier container, if used, at an appropriate level at all times. Always use distilled, never tap, water. *(Prevents the inhalation of dehumidified oxygen. Distilled water decreases the growth of microorganisms.)*

9. Refer to Standard Steps 10–17.

10. Document the following. *(Verifies performance of procedure and ensures continuity of care.)*
- Date
- Time
- Flow rate
- Method of oxygen delivery
- Evaluation of respiratory status
- Patient's response to oxygen therapy
- Changes in health care provider's orders
- Adverse reactions or side effects of oxygen therapy
- Assess the condition of the skin around the oxygen device
- Patient teaching (see the Patient Teaching and HomeCareConsiderationsboxesonoxygentherapy)

8b(5)(a) from Perry AG, Potter PA, Ostendorf WR, et al: *Clinical nursing skills and techniques,* ed 9, St. Louis, 2018, Elsevier.

Fig. 14.3 A transtracheal catheter is inserted into the trachea between the second and third tracheal cartilages.

delivery systems even have a beaded chain necklace attached to help disguise the catheter. The patient should be instructed to inspect the transtracheal tract opening regularly for erythema, edema, or excessive exudate. (Small amounts of clear exudate are expected.) The area is cleaned twice daily with a cotton-tipped applicator. Hydrogen peroxide may be used to wash the neck and remove dried exudate. The transtracheal tract (like a tracheostomy) never truly heals as long as it is kept open with an oxygen delivery catheter. If the catheter is removed and not replaced within a timely manner, the opening may close over. If this occurs, the surgical procedure must be repeated.

ENDOTRACHEAL TUBES

An **endotracheal** (ET) **tube** (Fig. 14.4) is a tube inserted through the patient's mouth and into the upper airway to provide a patent airway. Oxygen is administered through an ET tube via an oxygen setup or through a ventilator. Suctioning of secretions also can be performed through an ET tube. An ET tube typically is used in an emergency situation to establish a patent airway or to provide an airway and oxygenation of a patient undergoing general anesthesia. ET tubes are used for short-term management of the airway. Typically an ET tube is replaced by a tracheostomy if an artificial airway is needed for longer than 2 weeks.

Care of the Tracheostomy

A **tracheostomy** is an artificial opening made by a surgical incision into the trachea. A tracheostomy may be created for patients who are experiencing **apnea** (cessation of breathing) or some form of respiratory obstruction. It also may be used to prevent aspiration of secretions and blood or to provide easier access to the lower airways. Many types of tracheostomy tubes are available; the one chosen depends on why it is being used and the condition of the patient. During a sterile surgical procedure, the health care provider makes an incision into the patient's trachea and inserts a tracheostomy tube into the opening. The tube then is secured in place by cotton tape or a specifically designed tie/strap wrapped around the patient's neck. This provides the patient with a patent airway. Sterile 4 × 4 precut drain gauze is placed around the opening in the

neck under the flange of the outer tube. This protects the skin during the healing process and decreases the risk of infection. An endotracheal or a tracheostomy tube provides a direct route for the introduction of pathogens into the lower airway, increasing the risk of infection.

The primary nursing responsibilities for maintaining a tracheostomy tube are to keep the airway clear, keep the inner cannula clean, prevent impairment of surrounding tissue, and provide the patient with a means of communication (Skill 14.2 and see Fig. 14.4). The nursing interventions that follow enable the nurse to meet those responsibilities and adequately care for a patient with a tracheostomy tube.

- Minimize infection risk:
  - Evaluate the patient for excess secretions and suction as often as necessary.
  - Provide constant airway humidification.
  - Change or clean all respiratory therapy equipment every 8 hours.
  - Remove water that condenses in equipment tubing.
  - Provide frequent mouth care (apply moisturizing agents to dry, cracked lips).
- Maintain nutritional levels:
  - Patients with ET tubes are allowed nothing by mouth (NPO). It is necessary to provide parenteral or enteral nourishment.
  - Patients with a tracheostomy may not be limited in regard to drinking fluids and eating once the initial healing phase of the new tracheostomy

A — Endotracheal tube / Inflated cuff

B

Fig. 14.4 (A) Endotracheal tube with inflated cuff. (B) Endotracheal tubes with inflated cuffs and syringe for inflation. The patient is unable to speak while the tube is in place because air cannot flow through the vocal cords.

Skill 14.2   Tracheostomy Suctioning and Care

 CHECK GATHER HELLO ID PRIVACY EXPLAIN WASH GLOVES

NURSING ACTION (RATIONALE)

Tracheostomy Suctioning

1. Refer to Standard Steps 1–9.
2. Assemble equipment:
   - Sterile suction catheter kit
   - Sterile water or normal saline if not contained in the kit
   - Sterile gloves
   - Clean gloves
   - Clean, water-repellent gown, and mask with face shield (if indicated)
   - Stethoscope
3. Check the patient's tracheostomy for exudate, edema, and respiratory obstruction; check that the tracheostomy phalange is secure with the ties/strap. *(Allows the nurse to identify the potential need for further nursing interventions.)*
4. Position the patient in the semi-Fowler's position. *(Allows for optimal lung expansion; during suctioning, the patient may cough forcefully and dislodge the tracheostomy if it is not secure.)*
5. Provide paper and pencil or a communication board for the patient. *(Because the patient cannot speak, this offers a means of communication.)*
6. Position self at the head of the bed facing the patient. Always face the patient while cleaning or suctioning a tracheostomy. *(Enables close observation for respiratory difficulty and coughing, which could expel the tracheostomy cannula.)*
7. Auscultate lung sounds. *(Provides baseline information regarding airway for comparison after suctioning.)*
8. Place towel or prepackaged drape under tracheostomy and across the chest. *(Protects patient's gown and the bed linens and provides a sterile field on the chest.)*
9. Perform hand hygiene. Prepare equipment and supplies on the overbed table. *(Organizes procedure.)*

a. Open suction catheter kit but maintain sterility of contents, leaving the catheter in its wrapper. *(Maintains sterility.)* The order of steps depends on how the equipment is placed in the kit and if there is a prefilled container of sterile saline or water. Don sterile gloves if there is a prefilled container of saline or water. Open the container. If there is only an empty basin for saline to be added, open the basin and remove the lid from the bottle of sterile saline or water outside of the kit, then don sterile gloves. Fanfold or wrap suction catheter around dominant hand. *(Helps protect the sterility of the catheter tip.)* Pick up tubing from the machine with the nondominant hand and attach the end of the suction catheter to the suction machine tubing. *(This hand will no longer be sterile for the remainder of the procedure.)*

Skill 14.2   Tracheostomy Suctioning and Care—cont'd

b. If sterile saline or water is to be added to an empty basin inside the suction kit, use the nondominant hand to pour the sterile saline or water into the basin. *(Sterile saline or water is used to rinse the suction catheter. The nondominant hand is no longer sterile and can be used to pour solution.)*

c. Turn on the suction machine with the nondominant hand and check that suction is working by suctioning a small amount of the sterile saline or water. This is accomplished by covering the port on the suction tubing with the thumb of the nondominant hand.

10. Preoxygenate the patient by having the patient take several deep breaths by setting the ventilator to deliver 100% oxygen with sigh breaths, or by having an assistant use a resuscitator bag. If the patient is receiving oxygen, wait to remove the oxygen delivery system until just before suctioning. *(Prevents oxygen depletion during the procedure.)*

11. Suction tracheal cannula. *(Aids in maintaining a patent airway.)*

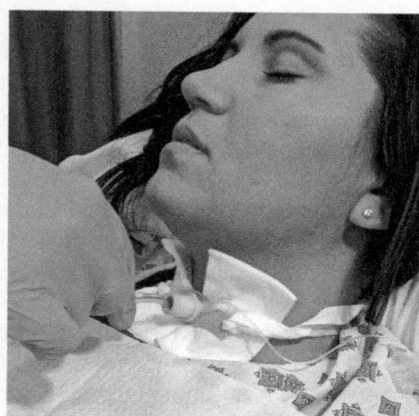

a. Place thumb over suction control vent; place tip of the suction catheter in the container of sterile rinse solution. Withdraw sterile rinsing solution through the catheter by placing a thumb over the suction control. *(Moistens catheter and clears any mucus from the catheter tip.)*

b. Remove the thumb from suction control; advance catheter gently through the tracheostomy while maintaining sterility until resistance is met, and then withdraw catheter approximately 1 cm. (Depth of the catheter approximately equals the length of the outer cannula, and the distal end of which protrudes from the opening approximately 1 to 2 inches.) *(Keeping thumb off of suction vent prevents suctioning while inserting the catheter, which has the potential to damage the mucosa. Resistance is met when the catheter reaches the junction of the main bronchi.)*

c. Apply intermittent suction by placing a thumb on and off suction control and gently rotate the catheter as it is withdrawn. *(Secretions are suctioned around the circumference of the trachea.)*

d. Suction for a maximum of 10 s at a time, never longer. *(Prolonged suctioning depletes oxygen supply.)*

e. Rinse the catheter with a sterile solution by suctioning the sterile solution through it. Repeat Steps 11b through 11e if needed. Most facilities' policies indicate no more than three suction attempts during the suctioning procedure.

f. Allow the patient to rest between each suctioning effort. If the patient was receiving oxygen previously, reapply it at the prescribed rate between each suctioning episode. *(Suctioning is often exhausting and frightening for the patient. Resting helps the patient regain depleted oxygen and decreases fear.)*

g. Turn off suction, and dispose of catheter appropriately by rolling the catheter up into one gloved hand and pulling the glove off over the catheter; then, place the glove with the catheter into the other hand and pull the glove off over the glove with the catheter.

h. Perform hand hygiene.

i. Auscultate lung sounds. *(Evaluate the effectiveness of suctioning.)*

12. Refer to Standard Steps 10–17.

13. Document the following. *(Verifies performance of procedure and ensures continuity of care.)*
- Date
- Time
- Respiratory evaluation before suctioning
- Tracheostomy suctioned
- Characteristics of material that was suctioned
- Amount (it will not be possible to determine the exact amount suctioned because the sterile saline for rinsing the catheter is in the suction canister along with the respiratory secretions. This is a subjective measure noting the amount as small/moderate/large or copious.)
- Color
- Consistency
- Respiratory evaluation after suctioning
- Adverse reactions
- Patient's response
- If oxygen is administered, note flow rate and method used
- Patient teaching

Skill 14.2   Tracheostomy Suctioning and Care—cont'd

Tracheostomy Care

1. Refer to Standard Steps 1–9.
2. Check the patient's tracheostomy for exudate, edema, and respiratory obstruction. (*Allows the nurse to identify the potential need for further nursing interventions.*)
3. Perform suctioning if it is needed before performing tracheostomy care. (*Removes excess secretions and prevents soiling new dressing.*)
4. Position the patient in the semi-Fowler's position. (*Provides for optimal lung expansion.*)
5. Perform hand hygiene; then position self at the head of the bed, facing the patient. Always face the patient while cleaning or suctioning a tracheostomy. (*Hand hygiene prevents the spread of microorganisms. Facing patient enables a close observation for respiratory difficulty and coughing.*)
6. Don clean gloves. Remove old dressing from around tracheostomy stoma, and discard it in an appropriate receptacle. (*Removes any exudate or drainage from the stoma site.*)
7. Prepare equipment and supplies on the overbed table (see Step 9 illustration under "Tracheostomy Suctioning"). (*Organizes procedure.*)
   a. Open tracheostomy cleaning kit with an aseptic technique. (*Prevents contamination of supplies.*)

   b. If basins are packed with sterile gloves, apply one sterile glove to the dominant hand. Separate basins with the dominant hand. Use

the nondominant hand to pour cleansing solution (hydrogen peroxide) in one basin and rinsing solution (sterile saline) in another basin. (*Cleanses mucus and secretions from the inner cannula and to rinse the cannula.*) In some facilities, a third solution of half hydrogen peroxide and half normal saline is used to clean around the tracheostomy stoma. Check facility policy.

8. With the nondominant hand, unlock and remove the inner cannula; place in a hydrogen peroxide cleansing solution. (*The nondominant hand has a clean glove on it and can remove contaminated inner cannula without breaking sterile technique.*) Never remove the outer cannula. If it is expelled by the patient, use a hemostat to hold the tracheostomy open and call for assistance. Always have a sterile packaged hemostat, as well as an extra sterile tracheostomy set, available at the bedside. (*Prevents closure of stoma until new outer cannula can be inserted.*)
9. Apply a second sterile glove or apply new pair of sterile gloves if contamination has occurred. (*Reduces spread of microorganisms.*)
10. Clean the inner cannula. (*Removes secretions and hydrogen peroxide from the inner cannula.*)
    a. Use a brush to clean the inside and outside of the inner cannula.
    b. Place the inner cannula in sterile normal saline solution. (*Rinses away the hydrogen peroxide.*)
    c. At some facilities, pipe cleaners are used to dry inside of the inner cannula. Check facility policy.
    d. Inspect inner and outer areas of the inner cannula. Remove excess liquid (see Step 13a).
    e. Insert inner cannula in the direction of the tracheostomy and lock it in place. (*Secures inner cannula and reestablishes oxygen supply.*)

11. Clean skin around tracheostomy and tabs of an outer cannula with hydrogen peroxide (or half-and-half mixture) and cotton-tipped swabs; clean

Continued

Skill 14.2   Tracheostomy Suctioning and Care—cont'd

away from the opening. Use wipes that are free of lint around the tracheostomy opening. (*Removes any remaining exudate or drainage. Inhaled lint [e.g., from cotton balls] irritates the respiratory passages and tends to cause undue coughing. Special tracheostomy dressings are available.*)

12. It may be necessary to rinse cleansing solution from the skin. If so, use sterile 4 × 4 gauze. (*Aseptically removes secretions from stoma site.*) Place dry, sterile 4 × 4 drainage sponge around the tracheostomy opening. (*Prevents skin impairment caused by rubbing of the flange of tracheostomy tube against the skin.*)

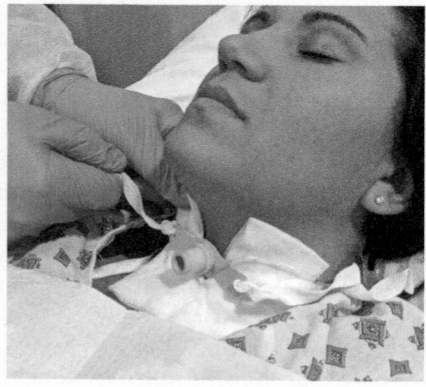

13. Change ties/straps holding tracheostomy in place if necessary. (*Always do this after cleaning the inner and outer cannula to prevent the cannula from being expelled.*)
    a. If assistance is not available, thread clean tie through an opening in a flange of the outer cannula along an old tie. If assistance is available, untie one side of cotton tape from the outer cannula and replace it with a clean one while the assistant stabilizes the tracheostomy tube. (*Prevents accidental expulsion of the outer cannula.*)

b. Bring the clean tape under the back of the neck. (*Securely holds the tracheostomy tube in place to prevent movement of the cannula.*)
c. If assistance is not available, thread tie through the opening in the opposite flange of the outer cannula along the old tie. If assistance is available, remove the other side from the outer cannula and replace it with clean tape.
d. Tie ends of clean cotton tapes together in a knot at the side of the neck. (*Secures ties and cannula in place. Putting a knot at the side of the neck avoids pressure and skin irritation at the back of the neck.*)

14. Auscultate lung sounds. (*Enables the nurse to determine any change from baseline.*)
15. Provide mouth care. (*Promotes good oral hygiene. Patients with tracheostomies often have halitosis.*)
16. Refer to Standard Steps 10–17.
17. Place call light, paper, and pencil within easy reach of the patient. (*Enables patient to communicate needs.*)
18. Reassess the patient's tracheostomy for signs of bleeding, edema, and respiratory obstruction. (*Patients with tracheostomy frequently have bloody secretions for 2–3 days after the procedure or for 24 h after each tracheostomy tube change.*)
19. Document the following: (*Verifies performance of procedure and ensures continuity of care.*)
    • Date/time of tracheostomy care
    • Type of tracheostomy care performed and solution used to clean around the stoma
    • Patient's response
    • Evaluation of respiratory status
    • Adverse reactions
    • Condition of tracheal stoma and peristomal skin
    • If oxygen is administered, note flow rate and method used
    • Patient teaching (see the Home Care Considerations box on tracheostomy care)

has passed. If a patient is able to eat, a cuffless tracheostomy tube is best. Not all patients have cuffless tracheostomy tubes. The patient may have a tracheostomy tube with a cuff to provide maximum sealing of the airway. Cuffed tracheostomy tubes generally are used for patients who are at risk for aspiration because of swallowing difficulties or who are receiving mechanical ventilation. The cuff must be deflated at prescribed intervals to prevent tissue necrosis of the trachea. Noncuffed tracheostomy tubes often are used to maintain the patient's airway when a ventilator is not needed or when the patient is being prepared to have the tracheostomy discontinued. The physician, often with

consultation with the respiratory therapist, chooses the tube based on the patient's condition, neck shape, and size and purpose of the tracheostomy.
• Ensure adequate ventilation and oxygenation:
    • Listen to lung sounds regularly.
    • Elevate the head of the bed to assist with ventilation.
    • Turn and reposition the patient every 2 hours for maximal ventilation and lung expansion.
    • Evaluate the effects of respiratory therapy regularly.
• Provide safety and comfort:
    • Check tube placement at regular intervals; tracheostomy tubes are secured around the neck

Fig. 14.5 (A) Tracheostomy tube (fenestrated) with inner cannula removed and cap in place to allow speech. (B) Tracheostomy tube with obturator for insertion and syringe for inflation of the cuff.

with tapes or specially designed ties/strap. Make sure they are snug and the tube is securely in the neck stoma.

- Change the tapes or ties/strap whenever they are soiled to lessen the chances of skin impairment.
- Always keep a spare sterile tracheostomy tube at the bedside.
- Enhance communication:
  - Organize questions so that the patient can give simple "yes" or "no" responses by nodding the head or using hand signals.
  - Assess whether the patient can use an erasable board or notepad to communicate.
  - Talk to the patient and explain all procedures.
  - Reorient the patient frequently if necessary.
  - Encourage family and friends to talk to the patient.
  - Keep a call light (or tap bell) within the patient's reach.

Currently, many types of tracheostomy tubes are available; tube types can be specific to the patient who needs them. Tubes are available in cuffed and cuffless styles; some have only a single cannula, and others have an outer cannula and an inner cannula that can be removed easily for cleaning. Being able to remove and clean the inner cannula reduces the risk of occlusion from a buildup of secretions (see Fig. 14.4).

Cuffed tracheostomy tubes are used routinely in patients who require mechanical ventilation (Fig. 14.5 a and b). Step 14.3 describes how to care for a cuffed tracheostomy tube. A cuffless tube may be used for patients who require a long-term tracheostomy and for those in the process of being weaned from a

tracheostomy tube. A single-cannula tracheostomy tube has one tube or cannula for airflow and suctioning of secretions. Uncuffed, single-cannula tubes are usually for neonates, infants, and young children. A double-cannula tube has a hollow outer cannula and a removable inner cannula. A fenestrated tube has holes (fenestrations) for air to flow upward through the vocal cords and mouth. This type of tracheostomy tube lets the patient talk and breathe naturally.

Although nursing interventions for patients with endotracheal and tracheostomy tubes are similar, patients with tracheostomies have additional nursing care needs and considerations related to respiratory status and suctioning (see Skill 14.2 and Skill 14.3 the Home Care Considerations and Coordinated Care boxes on suctioning for tracheostomy care). Some of these considerations are as follows:

- To prevent depression of the respiratory center, it is advisable to give analgesics and sedatives with caution.
- Suction is performed as often as necessary, possibly every 5 minutes during the first few postoperative hours. (Whenever respirations are noisy and the pulse and respiratory rates are increased, the patient needs suctioning.)
- Patients who are conscious are usually able to indicate when they need suctioning.
- A patient who is able to expectorate secretions requires less suctioning.
- The amount of mucus decreases gradually, and the nurse performs suctioning less frequently. A patient who remains apprehensive may require constant attendance and reassurance.

Skill 14.3   Care of a Cuffed Tracheostomy Tube

NURSING ACTION (RATIONALE)

1. Refer to Standard Steps 1–9.
2. Perform suction for the patient as in Skill 14.2, Steps 1–11.
3. Connect the syringe to the pilot balloon valve. (*Provides inflation and deflation of tube balloon.*)
4. Clean the diaphragm of the stethoscope and position the stethoscope in the sternal notch or above the tracheostomy tube and listen for a minimal amount of air leak at the end of inspiration. (*Allows the nurse to confirm proper cuff inflation.*)

5. Remove all air from the cuff if no air leak is auscultated. (*Releases excessive air pressure.*)
6. While you listen with a stethoscope, slowly inflate the cuff with 0.5–1 mL of air at a time. When no air leak is heard, stop injecting air and slowly withdraw up to 0.5 mL of air until air leak is auscultated with a stethoscope.
7. If excessive air leak is heard, slowly add air as in Step 6. (*Air leak will sometimes prevent lung expansion and increases the risk of aspiration.*)
8. Remove the stethoscope and cleanse the diaphragm with an alcohol swab. (*Reduces spread of microorganisms.*)
9. Remove the syringe from the pilot balloon valve and discard in an appropriate receptacle. Do not leave the syringe attached to the pilot balloon valve. (*Leaving the syringe attached may cause the valve to break or stick open.*)
10. Follow Steps 17–19 in Skill 14.2.

 ### Home Care Considerations

Tracheostomy Care

- Some patients with an artificial airway who are at home have a permanent tracheostomy, as well as a T piece or T tube or tracheostomy collar (Figs. 14.6 and 14.7).
- Determine the patient's ability to perform tracheostomy care and suctioning techniques.
- Evaluate the patient's home environment for the presence of respiratory irritants, cleanliness, and location in which to clean suctioning equipment and hang it up to drain.
- Ensure that a humidifier is present: added moisture is important.

Flexible tubing from oxygen source   T piece adapter   Reservoir tube

15-mm adapter

Endotracheal tube

Fig. 14.6 T piece or T tube.

 ### Coordinated Care

Collaboration

Suctioning a Tracheostomy

- The skill of suctioning, other than oropharyngeal suctioning, requires the critical thinking and knowledge of a nurse or other licensed health care professionals.
- The task of oropharyngeal suctioning can be delegated to unlicensed assistive personnel (UAP), including the patient and family, when in the home setting, after receiving instruction.
- In special situations, the task of performing a permanent tracheostomy tube suctioning can be delegated to UAP, including the patient and family, when in the home setting. These situations include those in which stable patients have a well-established permanent tracheostomy tube and patients are receiving mechanical ventilation at home.
- The nurse is responsible for evaluating the patient's airway **patency** (openness) and response to airway suctioning.

Care of the Patient With a Tracheostomy Collar and T Piece or T Tube

In a healthy person, the upper airway normally filters and humidifies air upon inspiration. The air taken in by a patient with a tracheostomy bypasses the upper airway and is not humidified. For this reason, patients

Fig. 14.7 Tracheostomy collar.

with artificial airways must have constant humidification. To humidify the air, or oxygen being given, a T piece (T tube) or a tracheostomy collar (Fig. 14.7) is attached to the tracheostomy tube to deliver moisture, oxygen, or both.

The T piece or T tube is a T-shaped device that is connected to large-bore tubing and then can deliver humidification, oxygen, or both (see Fig. 14.6). A tracheostomy collar also is designed to supply humidification and humidified oxygen to the lower respiratory tract. The collar covers the open end of the tracheostomy tube and has an adjustable strap that extends around the patient's neck (see Fig. 14.7). Refer to Skill 14.4 for procedures used to ensure adequate oxygenation and humidification via a T tube or tracheostomy collar. Refer to Skill 14.5 for the steps involved in clearing a patient's airway.

Skill 14.4 Care of the Patient With a T Tube or Tracheostomy Collar

NURSING ACTION (RATIONALE)

1. Refer to Standard Steps 1–9.
2. Perform hand hygiene. (*Reduces transmission of microorganisms.*)
3. Position the patient for comfort, usually in a semi-Fowler's position. (*Helps the patient relax and allows adequate access to tracheostomy and to the T tube or tracheostomy collar.*)
4. Inspect the rate of flow and the solution level for humidification at regular intervals during the course of the patient's oxygen therapy. (*Ensures adequate oxygenation and humidification.*)
5. Provide nose and mouth care regularly during the course of the patient's therapy. (*Keeps the mucosa lubricated, moist, clean, and fresh.*)
6. Secure the collar or T piece at the neck over the tracheostomy. Make certain all tubing connections are secure. (*Prevents the T piece or collar from dislodging and depriving the patient of oxygen, humidification, or both.*)
7. Adjust the oxygen flow rate according to the health care provider's order. (*Provides adequate oxygenation for the patient.*)
8. Adjust the temperature of the humidified oxygen. (*Higher temperatures create more moisture and condensation.*)
9. Use large-lumen tubing from the oxygen source to the patient. (*Allows for adequate oxygenation and fewer complications from condensation.*)
10. Condensation occurs within the tracheostomy collar or T piece, so observe frequently. (*Too much condensation can create problems with oxygen delivery and cause respiratory distress in the patient.*)
11. The collar or T piece and tubing should be removed frequently to be drained and cleaned. (*Decreases risk of aspiration of the moisture and infection.*)
12. As moisture collects, suction the tracheostomy, and provide tracheostomy care as often as necessary. (*Helps to prevent excess moisture buildup and aspiration.*)
13. Make sure the nurse is always able to see the mist of the humidified oxygen. (*A visual way to determine whether the oxygen is being humidified.*)

Continued

Skill 14.5 Clearing the Airway

CHECK · GATHER · HELLO · ID · PRIVACY · EXPLAIN · WASH · GLOVES

NURSING ACTION (RATIONALE)

1. Refer to Standard Steps 1–9.
2. Assemble equipment:
   - Appropriate suction catheter
   - Sterile gloves if not in the kit
   - Clean gloves as indicated
   - Sterile equipment (suction kit)
   - Unsterile equipment (unsterile basin or cup)
   - Sterile water, or normal saline
   - Towel
   - Portable or wall suction apparatus
   - Connecting tubing
   - Face shield, if splashing is anticipated
3. Evaluate the need for suctioning. (*Physical signs will indicate the need for this procedure.*)
   - Gurgling respirations
   - Restlessness
   - Vomitus in mouth
   - Drooling
4. Explain the procedure to the patient and that coughing, sneezing, or gagging is expected. (*Encourages patient's cooperation and reduces patient's anxiety.*)
5. Position patient.
   a. If the patient is alert and conscious, place them in the semi-Fowler's position with the head to one side. (*Promotes drainage of secretions.*)
   b. If the patient is unconscious, place them in a side-lying position facing the nurse. (*Promotes drainage of secretions.*)
      (1) Place towel lengthwise under patient's chin and over the pillow. (*Protects bed linens from contamination.*)
6. Pour sterile normal saline solution into a sterile container. (*For moistening and cleansing catheter.*)
7. Perform hand hygiene and don clean gloves. Turn on the suction machine, and select appropriate suction pressure. (Check facility policy.) Never suction with any more vacuum pressure than needed to remove the secretions, and use the smallest catheter that will remove the secretions well. (*Elevated pressure setting or using a too-large catheter increases the risk of trauma to the oral and nasal mucosa.*) Connect suction catheter to tubing.
   a. Common vacuum settings for wall suction units:
      (1) Infants: 60–80 mm Hg
      (2) Children: 100–120 mm Hg
      (3) Adults: 120–150 mm Hg
   b. Common catheter sizes:
      (1) Infant: 6-Fr to 8-Fr
      (2) Children: 10-Fr to 12-Fr
      (3) Adults: 12-Fr to 14-Fr
8. Suction solution through the catheter by placing thumb over the open end of the connector or over the vent. (*Enables the nurse to check patency of suction catheter and suction pressure and moistens catheter for ease of insertion.*)

9. Remove the thumb from the open end of the connector or vent, or pinch the catheter with a thumb and index finger if a continuous suction catheter is used. (*Stops suctioning and prevents injury to the mucous membrane while the catheter is being inserted.*)
10. Proceed with suctioning. (See specific suction guidelines.)
    a. Oropharyngeal suctioning:
       (1) Don clean gloves if those are not already on. (*Prevents spread of microorganisms.*)
       (2) Gently insert Yankauer or tonsillar tip suction catheter into one side of the mouth and glide it toward the oropharynx without suction. (*Prevents tissue trauma.*)

Skill 14.5   Clearing the Airway—cont'd

Trachea   Carina

(3) Move Yankauer or tonsillar tip catheter around the mouth until secretions are cleared. (*Removes secretions without damaging tissue.*)

(4) Encourage the patient to cough. (*Moves secretions from the lower airway into the mouth and upper airway so that they can be suctioned.*)

(5) Rinse Yankauer or tonsillar tip catheter with water in cup or basin until connecting tubing is cleared of secretions. Turn off suction. (*Rinses catheter and reduces the probability of transmission of microorganisms.*)

(6) Repeat procedure as necessary.

b. Nasopharyngeal suctioning:

(1) Ask the patient if either side of the nose is obstructed; use an unobstructed side. If the patient is unable to answer this question cover one nostril and feel for air from the other nostril.

(2) Open suction catheter kit and don sterile gloves. (*Prevents spread of microorganisms.*) Holding suction catheter with thumb and index finger, place nasal catheter near region between patient's earlobe and the tip of the nose. Do not touch the side of the face, nose, or earlobe. (*Marks correct length of the catheter for insertion. Distance from earlobe to the tip of nose approximates the depth of insertion.*) Approximate length of insertion:

   (a) Adults: 16 cm

   (b) Older children: 8–12 cm

   (c) Infants and young children: 4–8 cm

(3) Lubricate the catheter with water-soluble jelly or dip the tip of the catheter into the sterile saline or water, depending on facility policy. (*Water-soluble lubricant dissolves, thus preventing possible buildup that could hinder airway. Lubricating catheter allows for easier insertion.*)

(4) Hold catheter angled up then downward with the anatomy of the nasopharyngeal area. Gently insert the catheter into one side of the nasal passage. (*Using the natural curvature of the catheter and gentleness facilitates easier and less traumatic insertion.*)

c. Nasotracheal suctioning:

(1) Ask the patient if either side of the nose is obstructed; use an unobstructed side. If the patient is unable to answer this question, cover one nostril and feel for air from the other nostril.

(2) Open suction catheter kit and don sterile gloves. Holding suction catheter with a thumb and index finger, place nasotracheal catheter near region between earlobe to the tip of the nose and extend to the trachea. Do not touch the patient's side of the face, nose, or earlobe. (*Maintains sterility. Marks correct length of the catheter for insertion.*) Length of insertion:

   (a) Adults: 20–24 cm

   (b) Older children: 14–20 cm

   (c) Young children and infants: 8–14 cm

(3) Lubricate the catheter with a water-soluble jelly or dip the tip of the catheter into the sterile saline or water, depending on facility policy. (*Water-soluble lubricant dissolves, thus preventing possible buildup that could hinder airway. Lubricating catheter allows for easier insertion.*)

(4) Hold catheter angled up then downward with the anatomy of the nasopharyngeal area. Gently insert the catheter into one side of the nasal passage. (*Using the natural curvature of catheter and gentleness facilitates easier and less traumatic insertion.*)

(5) Stimulate coughing reflex, or ask patient to cough, to guide the catheter into the trachea. If no cough reflex is present or if the patient is not able to assist, insert the catheter when the patient inhales (see illustration of Step 10b[4]). (*Helps prevent displacement of the catheter into the esophagus.*)

11. Apply intermittent suction by placing a thumb over the suction opening; withdraw the catheter while rotating it gently. (*Intermittent suction and*

Continued

Skill 14.5 Clearing the Airway—cont'd

gentle rotation of the catheter prevents injury to mucosa.)

12. Observe the patient closely, and limit suction to 10–15 s. *(Suctioning longer than 10–15 s risks causing cardiopulmonary compromise.)*
13. Repeat suctioning if it is needed.
14. Allow 1–2 min of rest between suctioning if it is necessary to repeat the procedure. If oxygen is administered by nasal cannula, mask, or other means, reapply oxygen during the rest period. *(Provides rest and comfort and allows patient to regain oxygen supply. The time needed for the patient to rest between suctioning varies depending on the patient's ability to tolerate the procedure.)*
15. If the patient is alert and is able to cooperate, instruct the patient to breathe deeply and cough between suctioning attempts. *(Coughing moves secretions from the lower airway into the mouth and upper airway and allows them to be removed more easily.)*
16. When suctioning of the catheter is complete, suction between cheeks and gum line and under the tongue; suction mouth last to prevent contaminating the catheter. *(Ensures that all secretions have been removed.)*
17. Place the catheter in solution and apply suction. *(Flushes secretions from catheter and tubing to maintain patency in the event it is necessary to repeat the procedure.)*
18. Discard the catheter and used suction catheters: wrap the catheter around the gloved hand; pull the glove off the hand and over the catheter. Remove face shield, if worn. Perform hand hygiene. *(Reduces the transmission of microorganisms and prevents direct contact with equipment and secretions.)*
19. Place the sterile, unopened catheter at the patient's bedside. *(Provides quick access to suction equipment if the patient needs suctioning immediately.)*
20. Provide mouth care. *(Promotes patient comfort.)*
21. Evaluate the patient's breathing patterns, fatigue, vital signs, level of consciousness, and color. Determine whether the patient has a decrease in anxiety. *(Identifies successful suctioning attempt and patient's response to the suction procedure.)*
22. Refer to Standard Steps 10–17.
23. Document the following. *(Verifies performance of procedure and ensures continuity of care.)*
    • Date
    • Time
    • Method of suctioning
    • Amount, consistency, color, and odor of secretions
    • Respiratory assessment before and after the procedure
    • Patient's response
    • Patient teaching

Get Ready for the NCLEX® Examination!

Key Points

• Oxygen therapy improves tissue oxygenation. Delivery devices include, but are not limited to, nasal cannulas, nasal catheter, and various types of oxygen masks.
• Teaching the patient effective coughing techniques and the implementation of suctioning will help keep the patient's airway patent.
• The Venturi mask offers a precise concentration of oxygen and is used for patients requiring a more controlled concentration of oxygen.
• Safety precautions must be followed in the clinical setting and in the home setting.
• Hypoxia signs and symptoms include neurologic changes, changes in vital signs, cardiac dysrhythmias, and changes in the color of the mucous membranes. Early and later signs of hypoxia differ.
• COPD patients require a lower concentration of oxygen therapy to not suppress their respiratory center.

• Endotracheal tubes are used for short-term airway maintenance.
• Tracheostomy is used for long-term airway maintenance.
• Tracheostomy tubes may be cuffed or non-cuffed, depending on the patient's need.
• Tracheostomy care and suctioning can be performed by the nurse, or by the patient or caregivers.
• Tracheostomy care and suctioning requires a sterile technique.
• The tracheostomy collar is used to supply oxygen to a patient with a tracheostomy.
• The Yankaur suction catheter is used to perform oropharyngeal suctioning.

Additional Learning Resources

SG Go to your Study Guide for additional learning activities to help you master this chapter content.

Be sure to visit the Evolve site at **http://evolve.elsevier.com/Cooper/foundations/** for additional online resources.

Review Questions for the NCLEX® Examination

1. The LPN/LVN is suctioning a patient through an endotracheal tube. What indicates proper technique? *(Select all that apply.)*

   1. Preoxygenating the patient before suctioning
   2. Dipping the suction catheter into sterile saline before suctioning
   3. Using a clean catheter with each suctioning attempt
   4. Withdrawing the catheter with the thumb continually covering the suction control vent
   5. Suctioning the tube for at least 30 seconds with each suctioning attempt

2. A patient's physician told the patient that she was suffering from hypoxia. The patient asks the nurse what that means. Which statement by the nurse is most accurate?

   1. "Hypoxia means that there is a deficient amount of oxygen in your blood."
   2. "It would be best if you asked your physician to explain hypoxia."
   3. "There is too much carbon dioxide in your blood."
   4. "Hypoxia means that the cells in your body's tissues are not receiving enough oxygen."

3. What is the maximum time suction should be applied during nasotracheal suctioning?

   1. 15 seconds
   2. 20 seconds
   3. 30 seconds
   4. 45 seconds

4. If a patient's condition requires a very precise delivery of oxygen concentration, the nurse anticipates that the health care provider will order oxygen to be delivered via which device?

   1. Venturi mask
   2. Simple face mask
   3. Nasal cannula
   4. Transtracheal cannula

5. A patient is being discharged to home with an order for oxygen. The order reads, "Continuous O_2 at 2 L per N/C." What is the best explanation of this order for the nurse to give the patient?

   1. "You will have oxygen on 24 hours a day at home by use of a nasal cannula, with the flow meter set at 2 liters."
   2. "You will need to wear your oxygen during the hours you are awake, since your body uses more oxygen during the day. Your order is for 2 liters by nasal cannula."
   3. "Your doctor has ordered oxygen for you to use at home to keep your blood oxygen levels at a good level."
   4. "You will need to wear oxygen at home whenever you are feeling short of breath. Be sure to set your flowmeter at 2 liters and use your nasal cannula."

6. The home health nurse is visiting a patient who is on home oxygen therapy. The patient's oxygen is being delivered via a nasal cannula. The patient has a diagnosis of COPD, and the nurse notes that the patient becomes short of breath if the oxygen is not being worn at all times. What action by the patient and family members alerts the nurse that further teaching about home oxygen therapy is necessary? *(Select all that apply.)*

   1. The nurse notes a fire extinguisher in the kitchen.
   2. The patient's brother-in-law is in a separate room smoking a cigarette.
   3. The patient states that when shaving, an electrical razor is used.
   4. The patient is using a water-soluble gel to help with lubricating dry mucous membranes.
   5. The oxygen tubing is coiled and secured with a rubber band to prevent the patient from tripping over the tubing.
   6. The oxygen liter flow is set at 12 L when the nurse arrives to care for the patient.
   7. The patient removes their oxygen when eating and bathing.
   8. The patient's wife states that she turns up her husband's oxygen when he becomes short of breath.
   9. The patient's front and back door have signs displayed stating "No Smoking, oxygen in use."
   10. The patient cleans the nasal cannula tubing with a washcloth with warm water.

7. The nurse encourages the patient to drink an adequate amount of fluids to help with dry mucous membranes and to liquefy secretions. What fluids should the nurse include in this teaching? *(Select all that apply.)*

   1. Coffee
   2. Milk
   3. Water
   4. Juice
   5. Tea

8. The nurse is reviewing the arterial partial pressure of oxygen (PaO_2) level on the patient's arterial blood gas report. Which level is most concerning to the nurse?

   1. PaO_2 75 mm Hg
   2. PaO_2 80 mm Hg
   3. PaO_2 85 mm Hg
   4. PaO_2 90 mm Hg

9. The home health care nurse is observing the patient while he is filling the humidifier bottle attached to the oxygen tank. Which action by the patient demonstrates knowledge of this procedure?

   1. The patient fills the bottle with distilled water.
   2. The patient fills the bottle with tap water.
   3. The patient fills the bottle sterile normal saline.
   4. The patient fills the bottle with spring water.

10. The nurse observes the student nurse suction the patient with a tracheostomy. Which action by the student nurse requires the nurse to intervene? *(Select all that apply.)*

    1. The student preoxygenates the patient before beginning suctioning.
    2. The student suctions the patient for 30 seconds during each suctioning attempt.
    3. The student uses tap water to clear the catheter tubing between suction attempts.
    4. The student applies intermittent suction when withdrawing the suction catheter from the airway.
    5. The student places the thumb over the suction control vent when advancing the catheter into the patient's airway.

11. The health care provider has ordered oxygen at 100% via a nonrebreathing mask. The nurse evaluates that the mask is working properly when making which observation?

1. The reservoir bag collapses 50% when the patient inhales.
2. The reservoir bag collapses completely when the patient inhales.
3. The reservoir bag remains nearly full when the patient inhales.
4. The reservoir bag inflates when the patient inhales.

12. The nurse is preparing to perform tracheostomy care and suctioning. What is the best order of actions when performing these two procedures? Place the steps in the correct order.

1. The nurse performs tracheostomy suctioning.
2. The nurse changes the tracheostomy ties/strap.
3. The nurse changes the dressing around the tracheostomy.
4. The nurse cleans around the tracheostomy with the prescribed solution.

13. The nurse has just performed oropharyngeal suctioning. Which documentation is the most complete after this procedure?

1. "Suctioned patient using a Yankaur suction catheter. Large amount of mucus suctioned. Patient tolerated procedure well and is breathing better."
2. "Performed oropharyngeal suctioning using Yankaur suction catheter. Moderate amount of thick green, odorless, mucus suctioned. Tolerated procedure well and respirations are nonlabored."
3. "Oropharyngeal suctioning performed due to patient being unable to expectorate secretions. Used Yankaur suction catheter to perform procedure. Patient breathing better following suctioning."
4. "Patient requiring suctioning. Oropharyngeal suctioning performed. Patient unable to cough up thick mucus. Breathing improved after suctioning. Used a Yankaur suction catheter for procedure."

14. The health care provider has ordered a patient diagnosed with pneumonia to have oxygen via a simple face mask. The nurse is aware that the patient will be receiving a FiO_2 of what percentage depending on the flowmeter setting?

1. 24% to 44%
2. 35% to 55%
3. 24% to 55%
4. 60% to 90%

15. The nurse is assessing a patient who is displaying early signs of hypoxia. What signs and symptoms will the nurse observe? *(Select all that apply.)*

1. Restlessness
2. Increased pulse rate
3. Decreased blood pressure
4. Irregular apical pulse
5. Dyspnea

15

Elimination and Gastric Intubation

Objectives

1. Discuss management of the patient with an indwelling catheter or urinary diversion:
   - Male catheterization
   - Female catheterization
   - Discontinuing an indwelling catheter
   - Catheter irrigation
2. Explain the procedure for external and internal vaginal irrigation (douche).
3. Explain nursing interventions for the patient with nasogastric intubation.
4. Discuss gastric and intestinal suctioning care.
5. Describe the procedure for nasogastric tube removal.
6. Identify the procedures for promoting bowel elimination:
   - Administering an enema
   - Inserting a rectal tube
   - Removing a fecal impaction
7. Describe nursing care necessary to maintain structure and function of a bowel diversion.
8. Discuss the need for and nursing care necessary to maintain an ostomy.

Key Terms

bladder training (BLĂD-ŭr TRĀ-nĭng, p. 375)
catheterization (kă-thĕ-tŭr-ĭ-ZĀ-shŭn, p. 365)
colostomy (kŏl-ŎS-tō-mē, p. 388)
defecation (dĕf-ĕ-KĀ-shŭn, p. 383)
dumping syndrome (DŬMP-ĭng SĬN-drōm, p. 378)
enema (ĔN-ŭ-mŭ, p. 387)
fecal impaction (FĒ-căl ĭm-PĂK-shŭn, p. 387)
flatulence (FLĂCH-yŭ-lĕns, p. 387)

ileostomy (ĭl-ē-ē-ŎS-tō-mē, p. 387)
incontinence (ĭn-KŎN-tĭ-nĕns, p. 373)
irrigation (ĭr-ĭ-GĀ-shŭn, p. 365)
nasogastric (NG) tube (nā-zō-GĂS-trĭk TŪB, p. 378)
ostomy (ŎS-tō-mē, p. 388)
urinary catheter (YŪ-rĭn-ăr-ē KĂ-thĕ-tŭr, p. 365)
urostomy (yŭr-ŎS-tō-mē, p. 388)

Elimination includes the urinary system and the gastrointestinal system. Elimination is essential for the body to function properly. Both systems help the body to detoxify and eliminate waste products. Disease, tumors, surgery, medications, or trauma may interfere with normal elimination. When elimination is interrupted, certain procedures may be ordered by the health care provider.

An accurate and thorough assessment of the urinary and gastrointestinal systems (see Chapter 13) is necessary when implementing ordered procedures to determine the effectiveness of the treatment ordered. Knowledge of these systems and related disorders (see *Adult Health Nursing,* Chapters 5 and 10) also helps the nurse to care for the patient.

Nasogastric (NG) intubation procedures also are discussed in this chapter because they involve the gastrointestinal system. Insertion of an NG tube, procedures involving an NG tube, and care of an NG tube are discussed. Mastering these skills is necessary for the nurse to provide competent care for the patient.

STANDARD STEPS IN SELECTED SKILLS

To ensure patient safety, as well as nurse safety, during nursing procedures involving elimination and gastric intubation, it is important to understand the steps involved in specific skills. The skill boxes in this chapter list those steps for a variety of nursing procedures. Certain steps performed before and after every procedure are listed in the next section. The skill boxes that follow refer to them as *Standard Steps.* These steps must be followed before and after every procedure to provide the patient with safe, effective nursing care.

STANDARD STEPS BEFORE THE PROCEDURE

The rationales for these steps are listed in italics in parentheses.

1. Check the health care provider's order, and review facility policy. (*Provides basis for care. Many nursing interventions require a health care provider's order. Verification is essential before any procedure is begun.*)
2. Introduce yourself to the patient; include your name and title or role. (*Decreases patient anxiety and aids in establishing rapport with the patient.*)
3. Identify the patient by checking his or her identification bracelet and requesting that the patient state his or her name or birth date, or both. (*Ensures that procedure is performed on correct patient.*)
4. Explain the procedure and the reason it is to be done in terms that the patient is able to understand. Advise the patient of any unpleasantness that may be involved with the procedure. Give the patient time to ask questions. (*Promotes cooperation, decreases patient's anxiety, and prepares patient. Also helps determine whether procedure is still appropriate.*)
5. Determine need for and provide patient education before and during procedure. (*Promotes patient's independence and compliance.*)
6. Evaluate the patient. Each skill box contains an assessment section that includes specific data to evaluate. (*Provides baseline information for later comparisons.*)
7. Perform hand hygiene and don clean gloves according to agency policy and guidelines from the Centers for Disease Control and Prevention (CDC) and the Occupational Safety and Health Administration (OSHA) (see Chapter 7). (*Reduces the spread of microorganisms and protects the patient and the nurse.*)
8. Assemble equipment, and complete necessary charges. Each skill box lists the specific equipment required. (*Organizes procedure so that it will go more smoothly. Some equipment is reusable and is kept at the patient's bedside. Some of the equipment is disposable and charged to the patient when used. Know agency policy.*)
9. Prepare the patient for the procedure:
   a. Close the door or pull the privacy curtain around the patient's bed. (*Provides privacy and promotes patient comfort.*)
   b. Raise the bed to a comfortable working height, and lower the side rail on the side nearest the nurse. (*Promotes proper body mechanics by minimizing nurse's muscle strain and preventing injury and fatigue.*)
   c. Position and drape the patient as necessary. Descriptions of specific positions are included in each skill. (*Shows respect for patient's privacy and dignity.*)

DURING THE PROCEDURE

10. Promote patient involvement as much as possible. (*Participation encourages the patient's cooperation and increases patient's knowledge of condition and care. It also may increase patient's sense of independence and importance and increase patient's compliance with treatment.*)
11. Determine the patient's tolerance of the procedure, being alert for signs and symptoms of discomfort and fatigue. If the patient cannot tolerate a procedure, describe this inability in the nursing notes. (*Patient's ability to tolerate interventions varies, depending on severity of illness and disability. It is necessary to determine when to provide the patient with an opportunity to rest and when to provide comfort measures.*)

STANDARD STEPS AFTER THE PROCEDURE

12. Assist the patient to a position of comfort, and place needed items within easy reach. Ensure that the patient has a means to call for help and knows how to use it. (*Promotes comfort and safety. Patients often try to reach items and risk falling or injury.*)
13. Raise the side rails, and lower the bed to the lowest position. (*This minimizes the patient's risk in getting out of bed unattended. Use nursing judgment and facility policy to safely allow alert, cooperative patients have their side rails down.*)
14. Remove gloves and all protective barriers such as gown, goggles, and masks. Store appropriately or discard. Remove and dispose of soiled supplies and equipment according to agency policy and guidelines from the CDC and OSHA. (*Reduces spread of microorganisms, maintains cleanliness of environment, and enhances patient comfort and safety.*)
15. Perform hand hygiene after removing gloves. (*Wearing gloves does not eliminate the need to perform hand hygiene. Hand hygiene is the most important technique for preventing and controlling the spread of microorganisms.*)
16. Document the patient's response to the procedure, expected or unexpected outcomes, and all patient teaching. Specific areas of documentation are indicated in each skill box. (*Timely and accurate documentation is legally required, records patient's progress, and promotes continuity of care.*)
17. Report any unexpected outcomes. Specific notes for reporting unexpected outcomes are included in each skill. (*Additional procedures or treatments may be necessary.*)

SKILLS FOR URINARY TRACT PROCEDURES

URINARY ELIMINATION

Urinary elimination is a natural process that clears the body of waste material and helps to maintain electrolyte balance. Therefore conditions that interfere with urinary function have the potential to create a health crisis. The urinary tract can be affected by a problem with the kidneys, the ureters, the bladder, the urethra, or surrounding organs. It is also very susceptible to infection. Neurologic deficits also may lead to problems with the urinary system.

Patients at risk for problems with urine elimination include those who have undergone surgical procedures of the bladder, the prostate, or the vagina; patients with primary urologic problems, such as urethral stricture or tumor; those with neurologic trauma; and those who are critically ill with multisystem problems. When there is a problem with the urinary system, the health care provider often orders a urinary catheter to be inserted to monitor urinary output and the urinary system. Most often the nurse caring for the patient is responsible for inserting and monitoring the catheter and output (see the Coordinated Care box).

Coordinated Care
Delegation

Urinary Catheterization

- Urinary catheterization is a task that can be delegated to unlicensed assistive personnel (UAP) in few settings (check facility policy). In most facilities, first-time catheterization, catheterization of patients in an acute care and long-term care settings, or catheterization of patients with urethral trauma requires the critical thinking and knowledge of a nurse, and delegation of this task to UAP is inappropriate.
- The task of removing a urinary catheter can be delegated to UAP in few facilities (check facility policy); however, patient evaluation and teaching must be performed by the nurse. After removal of the catheter, instruct UAP to measure amount of urine in patient's first voiding and to report time and amount to the nurse.
- It is acceptable to delegate the task of obtaining urine specimens from a catheter to UAP in some settings (check facility policy). Initial patient evaluation and coordination of repeated specimens require the knowledge of a nurse, and delegation of this task to UAP is inappropriate.
- The skill of catheter irrigation requires knowledge of a nurse. Delegation of this task to UAP is inappropriate.
- The skill of caring for a newly established suprapubic catheter requires the knowledge of a nurse. Delegation of this task to UAP is inappropriate.
- Performing catheter care (providing perineal care and cleansing the catheter tubing) can be delegated to UAP. Catheter care does not involve sterile technique and can usually be performed during the bath, when the patient is incontinent of stool, and during care before bed.

Urinary Catheters

Most urinary catheters are made of soft plastic or rubber and can be used for treatment and diagnosis. Urinary catheters are used to maintain urine flow, to divert urine flow to facilitate healing postoperatively, to introduce medications by irrigation, and to dilate or prevent narrowing of some portions of the urinary tract. Catheters are used for intermittent and continuous urinary drainage. Urinary catheters can be placed

in the bladder, the ureter, or the kidney. **Catheterization** of the bladder, which is usually the responsibility of the nurse, involves introducing a rubber or plastic tube (a **urinary catheter**) through the urinary meatus and the urethra into the urinary bladder. Catheterizing the ureters or kidneys is the responsibility of the primary care provider. Catheters are measured by the French (Fr) system and range in size from 3 to 34 Fr. Children's catheter range from 3 to 8 Fr, and adult catheter sizes range from 14 to 18 Fr. Teenagers (depending on body size) range from 8 Fr up to 14 Fr. Catheters larger than 18 Fr are typically used for patients such as postoperative surgeries that involve the urinary system, prostate surgery or for patient's whose urethra has stretched due to repeated catheterizations. Most facilities require a provider's order if using catheter sizes larger than an 18 Fr.

Types of Catheters
Several types of catheters are used for different purposes (Fig. 15.1). The type and size of urinary catheter used are determined by the location being catheterized and the cause of the urinary tract problem. The coudé catheter has a tapered tip and is used when enlargement of the prostate gland is suspected. The curved stylet of the coudé catheter is used to assist the health care provider in the insertion of a urethral catheter in a male patient with prostate enlargement. The Foley catheter has a balloon near its tip that is inflated after insertion to hold the catheter in the urinary bladder for continuous drainage. Malecot and de Pezzer (mushroom) catheters are used to drain urine from the renal pelvis of the kidney, and the Robinson catheter has multiple openings in its tip to facilitate intermittent drainage. Catheters designed to be inserted into the ureters are long and slender to pass into the ureters more easily. In patients with blood in their urine, a

Fig. 15.1 Different types of commonly used urinary catheters. (A) Simple urethral catheter. (B) Mushroom, or de Pezzer, catheter (can be used for suprapubic catheterization). (C) Winged-tip, or Malecot, catheter. (D) Indwelling catheter with inflated balloon. (E) Indwelling catheter with coudé tip, or Tiemann catheter. (F) Three-way indwelling catheter (the third lumen is used for irrigation of the bladder).

Fig. 15.2 (A) Condom catheter. (B) Condom catheter attached to leg bag. (C) Purewick female external catheter

whistle-tip catheter may be used because it has a slanted, larger orifice at its tip. The cystostomy, the vesicostomy, or the suprapubic catheter is inserted through the abdominal wall above the symphysis pubis to create a urinary diversion in cases of obstruction, strictures, or injury to the bony pelvis, the urinary tract, or surrounding organs. The catheter is inserted surgically, is connected to a sterile closed drainage system, and is secured to avoid accidental removal; the wound is covered with a sterile dressing. When the lower urinary tract has healed, the patient's ability to void is tested, and when the patient's residual urine is low enough, according to the health care provider, the catheter can be removed. Sometimes, the problem causing the need for a suprapubic catheter is permanent, and the catheter is left in place.

Another form of urinary drainage system that many refer to as a catheter is the condom catheter. This device is not a catheter but rather a drainage system connected to the external male genitalia (Fig. 15.2A and B). This noninvasive appliance is used for incontinent men to minimize skin irritation from urine. Use of the external condom catheter allows for a more normal lifestyle for the patient and limits the risk for infection that an indwelling catheter may cause. Disadvantages

to using this device is that it can become too constrictive or it slips off too easily. It is therefore important to remove the appliance daily for cleansing and inspection of the skin.

Like the condom catheter for males, there is also an external catheter that can be used for female urinary incontinence. The Purewick female external catheter (see Fig. 15.2 C) is a system that is used for this purpose. This system is a noninvasive method of collecting urine using low continuous suction. The device is used in instances when a patient is either less mobile or nonmobile, such as after surgery or when ordered to be on bedrest. The device should not be used for patients who have urinary retention or whose urinary output needs to be closely monitored. The soft gauze portion is placed against the patient at the urinary meatus. Clear directions for proper placement are on the Purewick package and should be followed for best results. The device should be changed every 8 to 12 hours or when soiled. It is important to monitor the patient's skin condition when this system is used.

Nursing Interventions

Nursing interventions for the patient with a urinary drainage system are aimed at early detection and

Fig. 15.3 (A) Catheter kit with urinary drainage device, sterile specimen cup, sterile drape, sterile gloves, indwelling catheter, sterile cleansing swabs, sterile saline or water in syringe, and sterile lubricant. (B) Catheter kit with straight catheter, sterile specimen cup, sterile drape, sterile gloves, sterile lubricant, sterile collection device.

Fig. 15.4 Urinary drainage system. (A) Balloon inflation in male and female patients. (B) It is essential to keep drainage system below the level of the bladder. Do not place bag on side rails or allow it to rest on the floor. Attach drainage bag to bed or, while patient is ambulating, to intravenous pole.

prevention of infection and trauma (Fig. 15.3 and see Skills 15.1, 15.2, and 15.3). When caring for urinary drainage systems, take the following actions:

1. Follow aseptic technique when inserting the catheter and keep the collection bag off the floor. This prevents the introduction of microorganisms into the body from the environment (Fig. 15.4).
2. Record fluid intake and urinary output (I&O), and check the drainage system for proper placement and function regularly (Fig. 15.5). For precision monitoring, such as hourly urine output, add a urometer to the drainage system.
3. Encourage the patient to drink plenty of fluids to flush the urinary tract.
4. Do not open the drainage system after it is in place unless an open irrigation of the catheter is necessary, and then only with a specific order from the

health care provider. It is important to maintain a closed system to prevent urinary tract infections (Fig. 15.6).

5. Perform catheter care twice daily and as needed, according to standard precautions (see Skill 15.2). Inspect insertion site for blood or exudate that could indicate infection or trauma.
6. Check the drainage system daily for leaks. Know facility policy on replacing the system. Observe characteristics of the urine, noting blood or sediment. Note odor when draining collection bag.
7. Avoid placing the urinary drainage bag above the level of the catheter insertion. This will cause backflow of urine and potentially contaminate the urinary tract (see Fig. 15.4).
8. Secure the catheter to the patient to prevent tension on the system or backflow of urine.

Fig. 15.5 Empty and record urine output from Foley catheter into clean graduated container. Clean the drainage port before draining and before recapping.

9. Have the patient ambulate, if possible, to facilitate urine flow. If it is necessary to restrict the patient's activity, turn and reposition patient every 2 hours.

10. Avoid kinks or compression of the drainage tube to prevent pooling of urine within the system. Gently coil excess tubing and secure to the bottom bed linens with a clamp to avoid dislodging the catheter. Remember to release the tubing before transferring or repositioning the patient.

11. When urine specimens are ordered, collect specimens from the catheter by cleansing the drainage port with alcohol, then withdrawing the urine by using a sterile needle and 10-mL syringe according to standard precautions.

12. Be sensitive to the patient's feelings regarding the catheter and the constant drainage from the system, and answer patient's questions and concerns when presented (see the Lifespan Considerations for older adults box on catheterization and the Home Care Considerations box on urinary catheter care).

After the urinary catheter is removed, some patients may have difficulty voiding as a result of poor bladder tone and decreased sensation. If the patient complains of urinary retention, try stimulating urination by running water, placing the patient's hands in warm water, or pouring warm water over the perineum. Female patients should be encouraged to sit on a bathroom stool or commode and male patients to stand to void. Some patients may experience some dribbling of urine after voiding as a result of dilation of the sphincter from

 Lifespan Considerations
Older Adults

Catheterization

- A patient with a catheter is especially vulnerable to urinary tract infections. Older adult patients who are physically compromised run the additional risk of developing septicemia, a potentially life-threatening infection that has spread to the blood. Therefore routine catheterization of an older patient who is incontinent is not recommended.

- Encourage adequate oral fluid intake of at least 2000 mL/day, and assist the older adult to the bathroom on a regular, timed basis. This will help with bladder retraining and may prevent the need for excessive catheterization.

- When catheters are required, an older adult may be more cautious when ambulating. Encourage as much ambulation as tolerated and remove the urinary drainage device as soon as possible, per provider's orders.

- Suggest to patients who are at home or in long-term care that they use a leg bag during the day and switch to a large-volume bag at night so that sleep is not interrupted.

- Intermittent self-catheterization may be an option for some patients at home or in long-term care facilities. Discuss this option with the health care provider. Self-catheterization can be successful in maintaining continence and may enable more independence. Self-catheterization in the home setting often only requires clean technique since the patient is in their own environment.

- External catheters may work well for male patients with urinary incontinence. An internal catheter increases the risk of infection.

- Carefully evaluate patients with neuropathy before application of an external catheter; such patients may require more frequent monitoring related to the tissue damage that could occur.

- If a condom catheter is used on an older person, close monitoring is necessary. The skin of an older patient may be frail and delicate, leading to skin breakdown.

the catheter. Such patients should be reassured that this is normal and should improve as sphincter tone improves. Record the time of urination, the amount of urine output, and the color of the urine.

Self-Catheterization

Self-catheterization is a potential option for the patient who has had a spinal cord injury or other neurologic disorders that interfere with urinary elimination. Intermittent self-catheterization promotes independence for the patient and eliminates the need for an indwelling urinary drainage system. In the home, there are fewer foreign microorganisms and therefore less risk of cross-contamination. For this reason, it is possible to perform the catheterization procedure with clean technique rather than sterile technique. It is necessary to instruct the patient to be alert for signs of infection, and the patient should be encouraged to have periodic evaluations by the health care provider.

![home icon] **Home Care Considerations**

Urinary Catheter Care

- Determine patient and primary caregiver's ability and motivation to perform the following actions:
  - Maintain accurate records of intake and output (I&O)
  - Participate in routine catheter care
  - Perform catheter irrigation when necessary
- Demonstrate proper method for measuring I&O, and provide appropriate receptacles for measuring urinary output if needed. Allow for questions and return demonstrations.
- Instruct on appropriate catheter care (see Skill 15.2).
- Teach signs and symptoms of urinary tract infection:
  - Urgency
  - Frequency
  - Hesitancy
  - Burning sensation
  - Bladder spasms
- Disposable supplies are best, and most insurance companies will cover disposable catheters. If it is necessary to reuse catheters, teach patient and primary caregiver to cleanse the catheter according to manufacturer guidelines.
- Teach catheterization techniques if necessary (see Skill 15.1).
- Evaluate patient's environment for appropriate space to store required materials and to perform procedure.
- Consult with health care provider for a home care agency referral for follow-up and to reinforce teaching concepts.

Routine Catheter Care

Routine catheter care is an important aspect of an indwelling urinary drainage system. Patients should receive routine catheter care and perineal hygiene at least two times per day to prevent urinary tract infections (see Skill 15.2). During catheter care, cleanse the first 2 inches of the catheter to remove any secretions or encrustations from the catheter. Look for inflammation at and around the urethral meatus, and check for swelling or discharge from the urethra. Some facilities discourage the use of powders and lotions in the perineal area of patients with catheters because these can lead to the growth of microorganisms that could enter the urinary tract and cause urinary tract infections. Perform perineal and catheter care after bowel movements, especially if the patient is incontinent of stool.

If a catheter strap or adhesive tape is used to secure the tubing to the abdomen or leg, it should be replaced after catheter care is given. If the tubing and collection device must be changed because of leakage, odor, or collection of sediment in the tubing or collection device, follow sterile technique (see the Patient Teaching and Home Care Considerations boxes). If patency of the catheter itself becomes interrupted by mucus, blood clots, or sediment, catheter irrigation may be necessary. This procedure requires a physician's order in most facilities (see Skill 15.3).

![patient teaching icon] **Patient Teaching**

Indwelling Urinary Drainage System Care

- Explain the procedure and expected sensations associated with the procedure to the patient before you insert the catheter.
- Answer the patient's questions about the procedures.
- Explain the need for the patient to drink fluids to flush the urinary system.
- Instruct the patient about proper transfer from a bed, chair, or stretcher.
- Teach the principles of, and need for, catheter and perineal care.
- Instruct the patient how to perform Kegel exercises to strengthen the urethral sphincters to prepare for potential removal of the catheter.
- Teach the patient the side effects that are possible with an indwelling catheter and symptoms of an infection. Encourage the patient to report symptoms immediately.
- Caution the patient not to lie on tubing and to keep the drainage bag below the level of the bladder.
- Discourage the use of lotions or powder during perineal care.
- Encourage using a leg bag during the day to promote mobility and a bedside drainage bag at night.
- Instruct patient to wear loose-fitting clothing to promote adequate drainage.

Fig. 15.6 Bladder irrigation. (A) Triple-lumen catheter with sterile syringe to inflate catheter balloon. Note the port for inflating the balloon. (B) Continuous sterile bladder irrigation setup.

Skill 15.1 Catheterization: Male and Female Patients

CHECK GATHER HELLO ID PRIVACY EXPLAIN WASH GLOVES

NURSING ACTION (RATIONALE)

1. Refer to Standard Steps 1–9.
2. Assemble equipment:
   - Sterile indwelling catheterization or straight catheterization tray:
     - Antiseptic cleansing unit
     - Bed protector
     - Catheter of correct size and type for procedure
     - Cotton balls and pickup forceps
     - Drape
     - Lubricant
     - Prefilled syringe of sterile water
     - Receptacle or basin (usually bottom of catheterization tray)
     - Catheter securing strap
     - Specimen container (optional)
     - Sterile drainage tubing and collection bag
     - Sterile gloves (may not be included in tray)
   - Light (flashlight or penlight)
   - Bath blanket
   - Disposable gloves, basin of warm water, soap, towel, and disposable washcloth
3. Determine the following. (*Enables the nurse to determine need for procedure and special interventions.*)
   a. When patient last voided
   b. Patient's level of awareness
   c. Mobility and physical limitation of patient
   d. Patient's sex and age
   e. Whether patient's bladder is distended
   f. Presence of any pathologic conditions that are likely to impair passage of catheter (especially enlarged prostate gland in men)
   g. Allergies (to antiseptic [iodine], catheter material, and lubricant)
   h. Patient's knowledge of the purpose of catheterization
4. Arrange for extra nursing personnel to assist if needed. (*Patients are not always able to assume positioning for procedure.*)
5. Position patient.
   a. Male patient: Supine position with thighs slightly abducted. (*Allows relaxation of muscles and easy access to urinary meatus.*)
   b. Female patient: Supine position with knees flexed and approximately 2 feet apart (see illustration). (*Allows relaxation of muscles and easy access to urinary meatus.*)

6. Drape patient with bath blanket, covering upper body and shaping over both knees and legs but leaving genital area exposed. (*Prepares patient for procedure and provides for patient's privacy.*)
7. Place waterproof absorbent pad under patient's buttocks. (*Protects bed linens.*)
8. Arrange supplies and equipment on bedside table. Provide a good light. (*Easy access prevents possible contamination.*)
9. Don clean gloves, and wash perineal area with mild soap and warm water. (*Decreases microorganisms at the site.*)
10. Remove disposable gloves, and place them in proper receptacle. (*Reduces the spread of microorganisms.*)
11. Facing patient, stand on left side of bed if right-handed (on right side if left-handed). (*Successful catheter insertion requires the nurse to assume comfortable position with all equipment close by.*)
12. Open packaging with the use of sterile technique. Don sterile gloves. (*Allows the nurse to handle sterile supplies without contamination and decreases spread of microorganisms.*)
13. If indwelling catheter is used, test balloon, only if directed by the manufacturer's guidelines, by injecting normal saline or sterile water into balloon lumen until balloon is inflated if directed by manufacturer's guidelines; then aspirate saline or sterile water out of balloon.

Skill 15.1   Catheterization: Male and Female Patients—cont'd

(Determines integrity of balloon. If balloon fails to inflate, obtain another sterile catheter. This step is omitted if the manufacturer indicates that balloon testing has already occurred before shipment of the equipment.)

14. Add antiseptic to cotton balls or open antiseptic swab package; open lubricant container. Lubricate catheter approximately 1.5–2 inches (3.5–5 cm) for female patient and approximately 6–7 inches (15–18 cm) for male patient. *(Maintains sterility of supplies. Lubricating catheter reduces the chance that friction will cause trauma to the delicate mucous membranes of the urethra.)*

15. Wrap edges of sterile drape around gloved hands, and request patient to raise hips; then slide drape under patient's buttocks. *(Protects hands from contamination while towel is placed under edge of patient's buttocks.)*

16. Cleanse perineal area with forceps to hold cotton balls soaked in antiseptic solution or with antiseptic swabs. *(Cleansing reduces number of microorganisms at urethral meatus and decreases risk of urinary tract infection.)*

    a. Male: If male patient is not circumcised, retract foreskin with nondominant hand. Be certain to replace foreskin when procedure has been completed. If erection occurs, discontinue procedure momentarily. This is normal but often embarrassing to patient. React in a professional manner. *(Release of foreskin or letting go of the penis during cleansing requires process to be repeated because area has been contaminated.)*

    (1) Grasp penis at shaft below glans with nondominant hand; continue to hold throughout insertion of catheter. The nondominant hand is no longer sterile and must not come in contact with sterile supplies.

    (2) With other hand, use forceps to pick up cotton balls soaked in antiseptic solution.

    (3) Cleanse meatus by beginning at top of penis and moving in a circular motion down and around meatus one time. Discard cotton ball in appropriate receptacle. *(Decreases introduction of organisms into bladder.)*

    (4) Repeat cleansing two more times with sterile cotton balls or antiseptic swabs each time. *(Cleansing in this manner ensures optimal reduction of microorganisms from the area.)*

    b. Female:

    (1) Spread labia minora with thumb and index finger of nondominant hand to expose meatus; continue to hold throughout insertion of catheter. The nondominant hand is no longer sterile and must not come in contact with sterile supplies.

    (2) With other hand, use forceps to pick up cotton balls soaked in antiseptic solution or open antiseptic swab package.

    (3) Cleanse area from clitoris toward anus. Use a different sterile cotton ball each time: first to the right of the meatus, then to the left of the meatus, then down the center over meatus. *(Full separation of labia prevents contamination of meatus during cleansing. If the labia close, it is necessary to repeat the procedure.)*

Continued

Skill 15.1   Catheterization: Male and Female Patients—cont'd

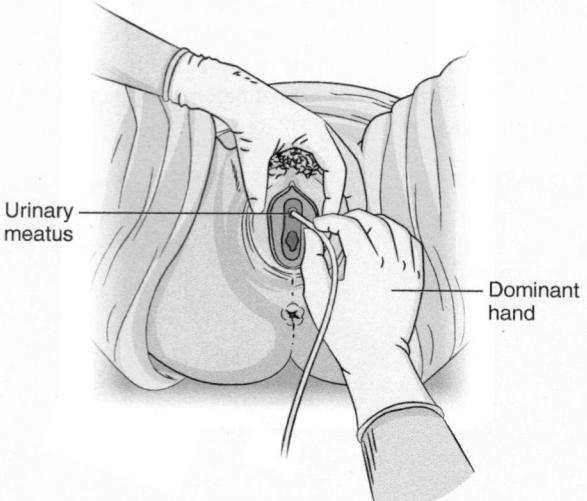

Urinary meatus

Dominant hand

17. Pick up catheter with dominant sterile-gloved hand near the tip; hold remaining part of catheter coiled in hands; place distal end in basin. (*Placing distal end of catheter in basin allows for urine collection. Coiling catheter in hand and holding near the tip allows easier manipulation during insertion.*)

18. Insert catheter gently, approximately 6–7 inches (15–18 cm) for male patient or 2–4 inches (5–10 cm) for female patient. (*Asking patient to bear down gently as if to void causes relaxation of external sphincter, which aids in insertion of catheter.*) Once urine flow is established, insert catheter least 1½ inches (3.5 cm) farther. (*Advancement of catheter ensures correct bladder placement.*) Inflate balloon with 10 mL of sterile water. Gently pull back on catheter until resistance is felt as balloon rests at orifice of urethra (see illustration and Fig. 15.5A). In a female patient, if no urine returns in a few minutes, observe whether catheter has been inserted by mistake into vagina. If so, leave catheter in place as landmark indicating where not to insert, and insert another sterile catheter. (*Use of the same catheter will introduce microorganisms into the bladder.*)

a. Indwelling catheter:
  (1) Inflate balloon with required amount of normal saline or sterile water (see Fig. 15.4A).
  (2) Pull gently to feel resistance.
  (3) Collect urine specimen, if needed, by placing open lumen end of catheter into specimen container. (*Allows for sterile specimen to be obtained for testing.*)
  (4) Attach open lumen of catheter to collecting tube of drainage system, holding drainage bag below bladder level. (Some catheters are presealed to the collecting tube of the drainage system. If catheter is not presealed, clean both the catheter and tubing end with antiseptic before reconnecting them, to maintain sterility of catheter and tube.)
  (5) Attach collection bag to a nonmovable part on the side of bed (see Fig. 15.4B).
  (6) Secure catheter to patient. (Minimizes tension and trauma to urethral opening.)
    (a) Male patient: Tape catheter to inner aspect of thigh or up over pubis, or apply leg strap (depends on health care provider's order); allow slack for body movement.
    (b) Female patient: Tape catheter to inner thigh or apply leg strap; allow slack for body movement.

Skill 15.1   Catheterization: Male and Female Patients—cont'd

(7) Clip drainage tubing to bed linen; allow slack for body movement.
b. Straight catheter:
(1) Once urine flow is established, hold open lumen of catheter over basin.
(2) Empty bladder (approximately 700–1000 mL). Refer to facility policy to determine whether urine should be allowed to

continue draining. *(If a distended bladder is drained too rapidly, the bladder may collapse into spasms, which are painful.)*
(3) Collect urine specimen, if needed, by placing open lumen end of catheter into specimen container. *(Allows for sterile specimen to be obtained for testing.)*
(4) Withdraw catheter slowly. (Minimizes patient discomfort.)
19. Wash and dry perineal area. *(Maintains patient comfort.)*
20. Refer to Standard Steps 10–17.
21. Label urine specimen with patient's name, date, health care provider's name, and other information as required by facility. *(Verifies correct specimen for laboratory.)* Ensure urine is transported to laboratory.
22. Check flow of urine and drainage tubing. *(Checks for proper drainage of urine.)*
23. Document the following. (Verifies performance of procedure and ensures continuity of care.)
- Date and time of procedure
- Type and size of catheter
- Amount of solution used to inflate balloon
- Characteristics of urine
- Amount of urine
- Color of urine and consistency of urine (note particles in urine)
- Reason for catheterization
- Specimen collected
- Patient's response to procedure (any resistance met)
- Patient teaching (see Lifespan Considerations for older adults box on catheterization)
24. Report any unusual findings immediately:
- No urine output
- Bladder discomfort despite catheter patency
- Leakage of urine from catheter
- Inability to insert catheter (If it is not possible to advance catheter, report immediately. Discomfort indicates possible infection or trauma. Leakage around catheter indicates possibility of improper catheter placement or inflation of balloon.)

Incontinence and Its Management

Incontinence—the inability to control urine or bowel elimination—can be a psychologically distressing and socially disruptive problem, especially among older adults.

Urinary incontinence can occur because pressure in the bladder is too great or because the sphincters are too weak. It can involve a small leakage of urine when the person laughs, coughs, or lifts something heavy (stress incontinence), or it can be a constant leakage whenever the bladder contains urine (urge incontinence). Collaborating with other members of the health care team is important to identify the cause and the extent of incontinence and to assist in managing the problem.

Skill 15.2 Performing Routine Catheter Care

NURSING ACTION *(RATIONALE)*

1. Refer to Standard Steps 1–9.
2. Assemble equipment:
   - Bath blanket
   - Bed protector
   - Catheter care kit (if not using a kit, the following supplies are necessary):
     - Basin of warm water and mild soap
     - Towel and washcloth (disposable washcloths are acceptable)
     - Small plastic bag for trash
   - Disposable gloves
3. Evaluate patient for the following. *(Enables the nurse to determine patient's condition.)*
   a. Length of time catheter has been in place (follow facility policy)
   b. Encrustations or discharge around urethral meatus
   c. Complaints of pain and for allergies to antiseptic ointment
   d. Patient's temperature (check temperature every 4 h for 24 h if odor or exudate is present)
   e. Patient's intake (maintain adequate fluid intake to ensure free-flowing urine)
4. Position patient.
   a. Male: supine position in bed with thighs slightly abducted
   b. Female: supine position in bed with knees flexed and about 2 feet apart
5. Place waterproof disposable pad under patient's buttocks. *(Keeps bed linens dry.)*
6. Drape patient with bath blanket, exposing only perineal area. *(Keeps patient warm and protects privacy.)*
7. If sterile catheter care kit is to be used:
   a. Open supplies with sterile technique, and arrange them on bedside table. *(Organizes procedure.)*
   b. Don sterile gloves. *(Prevents transmission of microorganisms.)*
   c. Place cotton balls in sterile basin near the nurse, and saturate with antiseptic solution. *(Having supplies nearby prevents accidental contamination. Maintaining sterility of supplies reduces the possibility of introducing pathogens into the urinary tract.)*
   d. With one hand, expose urethral meatus:
      (1) Male: Retract foreskin if it is present, then hold penis erect; hold position.

   (2) Female: Gently retract labia minora away from urinary meatus and hold in position.
   e. Wash the area at the meatus and around catheter with cotton balls soaked in antiseptic solution.
      (1) Male:
         (a) With one cotton ball, cleanse around meatus and catheter in a circular motion, starting at top of penis.
         (b) Repeat twice more, using different cotton balls each time.
      (2) Female:
         (a) With one cotton ball, swab to one side of labia minora from anterior to posterior. *(Prevents microorganisms from rectum entering the urinary system.)*
         (b) Repeat with second cotton ball on opposite side.
         (c) Repeat with third cotton ball down middle over meatus and around catheter; do not bring cotton ball back up once descent has begun.
      (d) Discard soiled cotton balls in other basin in kit.
      (e) With forceps, pick up cotton ball soaked in antiseptic solution, or use mild soap and water, and cleanse around catheter from urethral opening to approximately 4 inches (10 cm) of the catheter from the urethral opening. *(Cleans catheter of exudate. The urethral opening is considered less contaminated than the catheter tube.)*
8. If a collection of sterile supplies is to be used:
   a. Open separate sterile packages, observing sterile technique.
   b. Don clean gloves. *(Prevents accidental contamination. Maintaining sterility of supplies reduces the possibility of introducing pathogens into the urinary tract.)*
   c. Arrange small plastic bag for used, contaminated supplies.
   d. Cleanse the perineal area with mild soap and warm water. Pat dry.
      (1) Male: Retract foreskin if it is present; then hold the penis erect.
      (2) Female: Gently retract labia away from urinary meatus.
   e. Release labia of female patient; replace foreskin of male patient after cleaning.

Skill 15.2   Performing Routine Catheter Care—cont'd

9. Observe meatus, catheter, and surrounding tissue to determine normal or abnormal condition. Note presence or absence of inflammation, edema, malodorous exudate, color of tissue, or burning sensation. (*Determines need for more aggressive therapy.*)
10. Dispose of equipment and linens, according to standard precautions and facility policy; remove gloves and dispose of them in proper receptacle. Perform hand hygiene. (*Reduces spread of microorganisms.*)
11. Retape catheter to thigh or use a catheter strap. (*Prevents trauma and pain from tension and pulling.*)
12. Refer to Standard Steps 10–17.
13. Observe flow of urine through drainage tubing; note the accumulation of urine in the collecting receptacle. (*Promotes accurate evaluation of urine.*) If the drainage tubing becomes cloudy or stained, change the tubing to aid accurate observations of urine. Empty drainage receptacle at least every 8 h or as necessary to prevent backup of urine into the tubing or bladder (see Fig. 15.6).
14. If sterile catheter care kit is not used, follow same steps as for sterile catheter care kit but use a washcloth with soap and water. Follow agency policy for which method is used.
15. Document the following. (*Verifies performance of procedure and ensures continuity of care.*)
    - Date and time
    - Procedure
    - Assessment of urinary meatus
    - Character of urine
    - Patient's response
    - Patient teaching
16. Report any unusual findings immediately. (*Further therapy may be required.*)

Patients with urinary incontinence may be referred to a urologist for evaluation, and treatment may involve teaching the patient exercises to strengthen muscles around the external sphincters or using bladder training. If a paralyzed patient has overflow incontinence or incontinence related to an overfull bladder, the Credé maneuver may be helpful. This involves applying manual pressure over the lower abdomen from the umbilicus towards the bladder to aid in expressing urine from the bladder at regular intervals. When this technique is used, care must be taken to prevent injury to the bladder from excess pressure. This technique should be performed only if the provider approves its use.

Fecal incontinence may result from diarrhea or constipation, muscle damage or weakness, nerve damage, a rectocele, or even inactivity. Patients with urinary or fecal incontinence may require disposable adult undergarments or underpads to help prevent soiling of clothing and embarrassment. Use of discreet incontinence products helps to promote self-care and self-esteem.

Urine and feces are also very irritating to the skin. Skin that is exposed continuously becomes inflamed and irritated quickly. To help prevent skin impairment, make sure to change the undergarments or underpads frequently; cleanse the skin thoroughly after each episode of incontinence with warm, soapy water; and dry it completely (Box 15.1). Cleanse the perineum in a professional, caring, and matter-of-fact manner. It is important that the patient is not meant to feel as though they are a burden for requiring extra care by the nursing staff.

Box 15.1   Patient Problem Statements for the Patient With a Urinary Tract Disorder

Functional Inability to Control Urination:
- Related to cognitive deficits
- Related to mobility deficits
- Related to sensory deficits

Potential for Compromised Skin Integrity:
- Related to presence of urine on skin

Impaired Self-Esteem due to Current Situation:
- Related to inability to control passage of urine

Inability to Control Urination due to Physical Stress:
- Related to changes in muscles and structure of urinary system associated with increased age

Inability to Control Urination due to Urgency:
- Related to decreased bladder capacity

Potential for Infection:
- Related to inadequate personal hygiene
- Related to lack of knowledge of care of a urinary stoma

Bladder training. Bladder training is the achievement of voluntary control over voiding; it often involves developing the use of muscles in the perineum. When urinary incontinence results from decreased perception of bladder fullness or impaired voluntary motor control, bladder training is often helpful.

Before the removal of a urethral catheter, bladder training may be ordered by the health care provider and involves a clamp-unclamp routine to improve bladder tone. Kegel exercises also may be used to improve perineal muscle tone and sphincter control as part of a bladder training regimen. The patient is

Skill 15.3 Catheter Irrigation

NURSING ACTION *(RATIONALE)*

1. Refer to Standard Steps 1–9.
2. Assemble equipment (exact equipment depends on method used):
   - Antiseptic cleanser
   - Clean gloves
   - Irrigation setup
   - Medication for instillation
   - Sterile basin
   - Sterile calibrated container
   - Sterile gloves
   - Sterile plug
   - Sterile solution
   - Sterile syringe
   - Waterproof pad
3. Observe the following. *(Enables the nurse to determine patient's condition.)*
   a. Color of urine and presence of mucus or sediment
   b. Patency of drainage tubing
   c. Patient's intake and output record
   d. Patient for presence of bladder spasms and discomfort
   e. Patient's knowledge regarding purpose of the catheter irrigation
4. Position patient:
   a. Male: supine position in bed
   b. Female: supine position in bed
5. Drape patient with bath blanket, exposing only perineal area; remove and dispose of gloves. *(Exposes catheter.)*
6. Place waterproof absorbent pad under patient's buttocks and perform catheter care (see Skill 15.2). *(Protects bed linens from soiling and cleans area before procedure.)*
7. Arrange supplies and equipment at bedside on overbed table. *(Easy access prevents possible contamination.)*
8. Perform irrigation:
   a. Open method:
      (1) Pour sterile irrigating solution (sterile normal saline unless otherwise specified) into sterile graduated container, and recap solution bottle. Have irrigating solution at room temperature.
      (2) Don sterile gloves. *(Maintains the sterile field.)*
      (3) Place sterile basin between patient's legs, close to perineal area.
      (4) Kink catheter and disconnect catheter from drainage system. Plug drainage

tubing with sterile plug. *(Prevents urine from draining from catheter before procedure. Sterile plug maintains sterility of drainage tube during procedure.)*

   (5) Draw 30 mL of sterile solution into syringe.
   (6) Cleanse catheter end with antiseptic swab. *(Maintains sterility of equipment.)*
   (7) Place tip of syringe into end of catheter, and gently insert solution. *(A gentle approach reduces incidence of bladder spasms and clears catheter of obstruction.)*
   (8) Withdraw syringe, and allow solution to drain into basin by gravity.
   (9) If solution does not return, turn patient on side, facing the nurse. If solution still does not return, refer to facility policy for further action. *(Change in position sometimes moves tip of catheter in bladder, increasing the likelihood that instilled fluid will flow out.)*
   (10) Repeat injection of solution until amount ordered is instilled and returned; maintain sterility of equipment.
   (11) Clean end of catheter with antiseptic solution. Remove plug from drainage tubing, and connect tubing to catheter. Do not touch ends of catheter and tubing. *(Prevents contamination of the system.)*
   (12) Measure solution. *(Determines amount returned and amount of urine expelled.)*

   b. Closed intermittent method (repeat Steps 1 through 7 as described). *(Maintaining a closed system ensures against contamination that could result in a urinary tract infection.)*
   (1) Pour sterile irrigating solution into graduated container. (Sterile normal saline is used unless otherwise specified.)
   (2) Draw up sterile solution into syringe.
   (3) Clamp catheter below injection port.
   (4) Cleanse port with antiseptic. *(Decreases spread of microorganisms.)*
   (5) Insert needle of syringe into port. (Needleless ports may also be present.)
   (6) Inject solution into catheter slowly. *(Helps to prevent bladder spasm while dislodging clots, sediment, or other material.)*

   c. Closed continuous method (continuous bladder irrigation). The health care provider must order the solution, the strength, and the flow rate of a continuous bladder irrigation. If the health care provider specifies only

Skill 15.3   Catheter Irrigation—cont'd

solution, check with facility policy for protocol for strength and rate. The irrigation solution infuses continuously through one port of a triple-lumen catheter, and the second port drains urine and irrigation solution.

(1) Set up irrigating solution by attaching tubing to bag.

(2) Clamp off tubing so that no solution flows through.

(3) Suspend bag on intravenous pole.

(4) Open clamp and allow solution to flow through tubing. (*Primes tubing to prevent air from entering the bladder and causing patient pain or discomfort.*)

(5) Cleanse irrigating lumen on end of triple-lumen catheter (see Fig. 15.6A). (*Necessary for system to remain sterile.*)

(6) Connect irrigating solution tubing to catheter lumen; maintain sterility of equipment.

(7) Open clamp on irrigation tubing and calculate drip rate. (*Ensures continuous, even irrigation of catheter system. Prevents accumulation of solution in bladder, which can cause bladder distention and injury.*)

(8) When drainage bag is emptied, the amount of irrigation solution infused should be subtracted from total amount returned. (*Allows the nurse to compute accurate urine output.*)

d. Bladder instillation:

(1) Disconnect catheter from tubing; stabilize tubing to prevent touching the floor. NOTE: Using triple-lumen catheter makes it unnecessary to disconnect catheter from drainage tubing (see Fig. 15.6B).

(2) Cleanse end of catheter with antiseptic swab. (*Maintains sterility of equipment and decreases spread of microorganisms.*)

(3) Draw medication or solution into syringe. (*Prepares for instillation.*)

(4) Place tip of syringe into end of catheter, and slowly inject medication or solution. (*Proceeding slowly prevents trauma to bladder mucosa.*)

(5) Clamp off end of catheter for necessary period. (*Allows medication or solution to be absorbed by bladder.*) Clean catheter and tubing ends with antiseptic solution; then reconnect catheter and tubing, making certain the system is tightly connected. (*Decreases risk of infection.*)

(6) Measure solution returned. (*Enables the nurse to determine amount returned and amount of urine for accurate recording of input and output [I&O].*)

9. Observe flow of urine through drainage tubing (see Fig. 15.6B). (*Determines urine flow and effectiveness of therapy.*)

10. Refer to Standard Steps 10–17.

11. Record urine output on I&O sheet, and document the following:

- Date and time
- Solution used as irrigant
- Amount of solution used
- Amount returned as drainage
- Character of drainage
- Patient teaching (see the Patient Teaching boxes on catheter care and removing a urinary catheter)

12. Report any unusual findings immediately. (*More aggressive therapy may be necessary.*)

- If irrigant does not return
- Increased pain
- Occlusion
- Signs or symptoms of infection
- Sudden bleeding
- Unrelieved bladder spasms

---

instructed to perform Kegel exercises by trying to stop the flow of urine during voiding. Once the patient has identified the correct muscles and the feeling of their contraction, the patient can perform these exercises when not voiding by tightening the muscles of the perineum, holding the tension for 10 seconds, and then relaxing for 10 seconds. This should be done multiple times, several times a day. Because muscle control develops gradually, it sometimes takes 4 to 6 weeks to slow or stop urinary leakage.

Habit training is also a part of bladder training and involves establishing a voiding schedule. This provides cooperative patients with the opportunity to achieve continence by voiding at regular intervals beginning with every 1.5 to 2 hours, then increasing the time interval as tolerated. Monitor the patient's voiding for a few days to identify patterns, or schedule voiding times to correlate with the patient's activities. Typical voiding times are upon rising, before each meal, and at bedtime. Assist the patient to void as scheduled, check the patient for wetness periodically, and remind or assist the patient to the toilet as scheduled. After a few days, evaluate the scheduled voiding pattern by identifying its effectiveness in keeping the patient continent. Then the schedule is modified until continence is established. Fluid intake and medications typically influence voiding patterns. Limiting fluids after the evening meal reduces the need for nighttime voiding and helps keep the patient dry.

REMOVAL OF AN INDWELLING CATHETER

It is always best to remove an indwelling catheter as soon as possible because its presence increases the risk for urinary tract infection (Skill 15.4). After surgery, the health care provider usually orders the catheter removed after 8 to 24 hours, depending on the type of surgery. In some situations, the catheter remains in place for days or even weeks. The longer a catheter has been in place, the greater is the risk that an infection will develop. Urinary tract infections are one of the most common types of *iatrogenic* (caused by treatments or diagnostic procedures) infections in health care. Symptoms of a urinary tract infection may not appear for 2 or more days after the catheter is removed. That means the patient may already be home before he or she begins displaying symptoms. For that reason, it is necessary to inform the patient of the risk for infection, how to prevent it, signs and symptoms to watch for, and when to call the health care provider.

Sometimes patients have difficulty voiding after the removal of a urinary catheter because the sphincter muscles are weakened. Patients with an overdistended bladder or who have altered sensory perception because of regional anesthesia, such as a spinal or epidural block, are likely to have difficulty voiding after catheter removal. Most patients should void adequately within 8 hours after catheter removal. If they do not, the health care provider must be notified and further orders received (see the Patient Teaching box on removing a urinary catheter).

👥 Patient Teaching

Removing Urinary Catheter

- Instruct the patient that it will take time for the urinary bladder to reestablish voluntary control of urine.
- Explain the need for collecting and measuring urine output, and teach the patient how to do so.
- Explain the need to drink at least 2 L (eight 8-oz glasses/cups) of fluid per day (to reduce risk of infection) unless this is contraindicated by the patient's condition.
- Explain that it is common to feel some burning sensation or discomfort when first voiding.
- Identify the side effects that are possible and explain the need to report them immediately.
- Instruct patients that the use of over-the-counter medications, such as nasal decongestants and anticholinergic medications (e.g., diphenhydramine, acetaminophen PM), has the potential to cause urinary retention and should be limited.

SKILLS FOR GASTROINTESTINAL PROCEDURES

INSERTING AND MAINTAINING NASOGASTRIC TUBES

A nasogastric (NG) tube is a flexible, hollow tube that is passed into the stomach via the nasopharynx. It can be used to remove gas, fluids, or toxic substances from the stomach; to diagnose gastrointestinal problems; to obtain secretions; or to administer fluids and nutrients into the stomach. It also can help to prevent vomiting and abdominal distention and allow the digestive tract to rest and heal. There are various types of NG tubes, including percutaneous endoscopic gastrostomy (PEG), button, and jejunal tubes. The physician determines which tube is best suited for the patient.

Gastric Gavage

When used to deliver fluids or nutrients (gastric gavage), the NG tube can be attached to a feeding pump, or the feeding can be allowed to flow in by gravity via a bag or a syringe. If a patient is receiving feedings by way of an NG tube, it is essential to keep the head of the bed elevated at least 30 degrees to help prevent aspiration or gastric reflux.

Tube feedings usually are started slowly and gradually increased, or they may be diluted and gradually strengthened, to prevent dumping syndrome. Dumping syndrome is caused by too rapid an infusion of highly concentrated feedings. The symptoms are similar to those of shock and can be very disturbing to the patient. During tube feedings, the health care provider also may order additional water to be given through the tube. This helps to meet the fluid needs of the patient, keeps the tube patent, and helps to dilute the tube feeding.

Before introducing anything into an NG tube, verify placement of the tube to prevent contents from entering the lungs. The most definitive way to verify NG tube placement is by x-ray. Aspirating gastric contents is another method used to verify NG tube placement. There are two ways that aspirating stomach contents can verify placement. One method is by observing the aspirated contents for color and consistency of the fluid. Gastric juices may be a clear liquid or watery yellow in color. A second method is by testing the aspirated gastric juices for pH. Gastric juice pH is less than 4. While the nurse monitors patients receiving nutrients through an NG tube, it is also necessary to check occasionally for residual feeding left in the stomach. Excess residual formula could indicate a problem with peristalsis, and the health care provider must be notified. It also could cause gastric reflux, aspiration, or both. Each facility and health care provider has a policy for how often to check residual formula and how much is considered excessive.

Gastric Lavage

Gastric lavage often is used in cases of poisoning or to stop gastrointestinal bleeding. It involves instilling

Skill 15.4   Removing an Indwelling Catheter

CHECK   GATHER   HELLO   ID   PRIVACY   EXPLAIN   WASH   GLOVES

NURSING ACTION (RATIONALE)

1. Refer to Standard Steps 1–9.
2. Assemble equipment:
   - 10-mL syringe or larger (depending on volume of fluid used to inflate balloon) without a needle.

3. Determine the following:
   a. Length of time catheter has been in place. (*The longer the catheter has been in place, the greater the risk for decreased bladder muscle tone and inflammation of the urethra.*)
   b. Patient's knowledge of procedure and what to expect. (*Many patients anticipate discomfort or have fears about ability to void successfully after removal of the catheter.*) Educate patient if necessary.
4. Provide privacy. Position the patient supine, and place a waterproof pad under the patient's buttocks. (*Protects the bed linens.*) Female patients need to abduct their legs with the drape between their thighs (see Step 5b of Skill 15.1). For male patients, it is acceptable for drape to lie on the thighs.
5. Insert hub of syringe into inflation valve (balloon port), and aspirate until tubing collapses or resistance is felt. (*Indicates that entire contents of balloon have been removed.*)
6. Remove catheter steadily and smoothly (in female patients, the catheter is in approximately 2–3 inches [5–7.5 cm] and in male patients, approximately 6–7 inches [15–18 cm]). (*Decreases discomfort.*) Catheter usually slides out very easily.

Do not use force. If any resistance is noted, repeat Step 5 to remove remaining water. (*Prevents trauma to the urethra.*)

7. Wrap catheter in waterproof pad. Unhook collection bag and drainage tubing from the bed. (*Prevents any leakage from the catheter onto the patient, the nurse, or bed linens.*)
8. Measure urine, and empty drainage bag. (*Promotes accurate reporting and recording.*)
9. Record output. (*Communicates patient care.*)
10. Cleanse the perineum with soap and warm water, and dry area thoroughly. (*Promotes comfort and a feeling of cleanliness.*)
11. Explain the following to patient:
    a. It is important to have a fluid intake of 1.5–2 L/day unless contraindicated.
    b. The patient must void within 8 h, and each voiding should be measured. Some facilities and health care providers determine how much the patient should void to verify adequate emptying of the urinary bladder. (*Confirms the ability of the patient to empty the bladder adequately.*)
    c. Mild burning sensation or discomfort with first voiding is anticipated. Instruct patient to notify the nurse if it does not subside with subsequent voidings. (*Infection may be present, and treatment may have to be initiated.*)
    d. Signs of urinary tract infection are urinary urgency, burning sensation, urinary frequency, excretion of only small amount, and continued pain or discomfort. These symptoms may develop 2–3 days after removal of catheter.
12. Place the urine measuring device on the toilet seat. (*Facilitates accurate assessment of patient's output.*)
13. Refer to Standard Steps 12–17.
14. Document and report the following. (*Promotes continuity of patient care.*)
    - Date and time of catheter removal
    - Patient teaching related to increasing fluid intake and signs and symptoms of urinary tract infection
    - Time, amount, and characteristics of first voiding after catheter removal
    - Complete input and output record

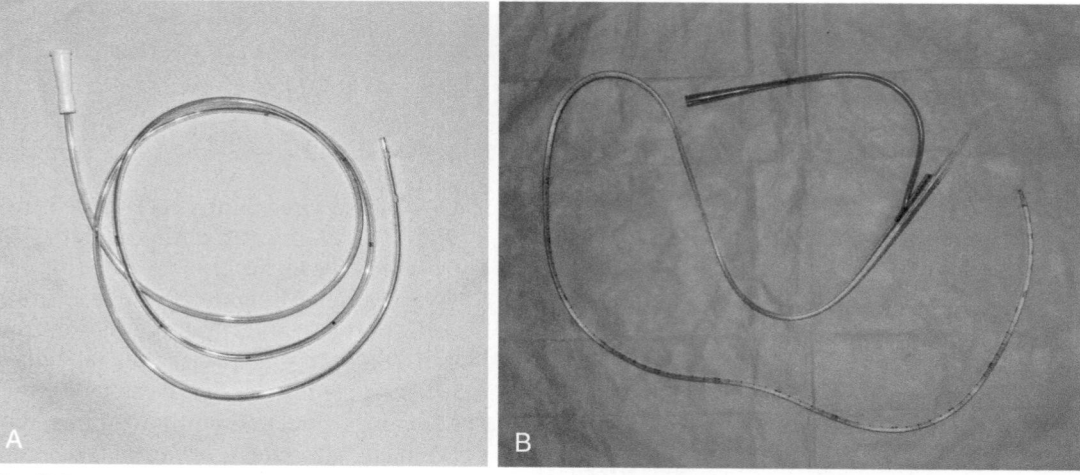

Fig. 15.7 Types of nasogastric tubes. (A) Small-bore feeding tube. (B) Salem sump tube. Note the blue "pigtail." This pigtail is an air vent that helps to prevent the tube from adhering to the gastric mucosa.

room temperature medications or solutions into the stomach and then suctioning it back out. Iced or cooled solutions should not be used, especially when copious amounts are needed, as with gastrointestinal bleeding, because they may cause hypothermia, impair platelet production, and cause increase in bleeding.

When performing gastric lavage, the health care provider orders the type of solution, as well as the amount, to be instilled. Usually 500 mL of the solution is administered at a time and then siphoned back out of the stomach. This process is repeated until the ordered amount of solution has been used or the anticipated results have been achieved. Every time the solution is removed from the stomach, it must be measured and evaluated, and the results documented. Sometimes the health care provider orders a specimen of the removed solution to be sent to the laboratory for analysis.

Gastric Decompression

The purpose of gastric decompression is to remove the air and fluids that build up when gastrointestinal motility is slowed. It is used frequently after surgery to help with the distention that may occur and to prevent nausea and vomiting. When used for decompression, the NG tube usually is connected to an intermittent gastric suction device, and the nurse must routinely measure and evaluate the contents of the suction canister. The tubes most commonly used for decompression are the Levin and Salem sump tubes. The Levin tube has one lumen and several openings near the tip. The Salem sump tube is a double-lumen tube: one lumen provides an air vent, and the other is for removal of gastric contents (Fig. 15.7).

The patient with an NG tube presents several nursing challenges. Maintaining patient comfort is sometimes the biggest challenge. NG tubes continually irritate the nasal mucosa and can cause trauma to the tissue. To lessen this discomfort and potential trauma,

the tube should be secured to the patient's nose with tape or a nose guard and then secured to the patient's gown with a pin to prevent unnecessary movement (Skill 15.5 and the Patient Teaching box on nasogastric tubes). Other comfort measures include removing excess secretions from around the nares and then lubricating the nostrils and the tube with a water-soluble lubricant to prevent crusting of secretions. Box 15.2 lists selected patient problem statements for the patient with a gastric tube.

Patient Teaching

Nasogastric Tube

- Explain the need for a nasogastric tube.
- Explain how the tube will prevent nausea, vomiting, and abdominal distention.
- Teach patient and family how to care for the nasogastric tube at home, if this is appropriate.
- Explain the need to maintain moistness of mucous membranes with special mouth care.
- Explain to patient how to relax and communicate during tube insertion.
- Before insertion, explain the technique and sensations that the patient may feel.
- Allow time for, and address, patient's questions and concerns.
- Ensure adequate lubrication of the tube to decrease discomfort, especially with older adults.

After an NG tube is inserted, patients tend to breathe through their mouths because of the nasal occlusion by the tube, and the lips and tongue often become dry and cracked. Provide mouth care at least every 2 hours to increase comfort. Rinsing the mouth with cool water or oral swabs provides some comfort. Ensure that the patient does not swallow any water. Check the health care provider's orders to see whether the patient is permitted to chew gum to increase

Skill 15.5   Inserting a Nasogastric Tube

NURSING ACTION (RATIONALE)

1. Refer to Standard Steps 1–9.
2. Assemble equipment:
   - 14- or 16-Fr nasogastric (NG) tube (smaller bore for child) or feeding type of tube (see Fig. 15.7)
   - Bath towel
   - Clamp
   - Clean gloves
   - Facial tissues
   - Felt tip marker
   - Flashlight
   - Glass of water with straw
   - Normal saline or tap water
   - Safety pin and rubber band
   - Stethoscope
   - Suction container
   - Suction machine
   - Syringe
   - Tape, nose guard, or both
   - Tincture of benzoin (optional)
   - Tongue blade
   - Water-soluble lubricating jelly
3. Evaluate condition of patient's oral cavity. (*Enables the nurse to determine need for special nursing measures and for oral hygiene after tube placement.*) Palpate patient's abdomen. (*Provides baseline data for later comparison after tube is inserted.*)
4. Position patient in high Fowler position with pillow behind head and shoulders. (*Promotes patient's ability to swallow during procedure.*)
5. Stand at right side of bed if you are right-handed and left side if you are left-handed. (*Allows for easy manipulation of tubing.*)
6. Place bath towel over patient's chest; give tissues to patient. (*This prevents soiling of gown. Tube insertion through nasal passages sometimes causes eyes to tear up.*)
7. Instruct patient to relax and breathe normally while one nostril is occluded. Repeat this action for other nostril. Select nostril with greater airflow. (*The tube passes more easily through nostril that is more patent.*) Some institutions suggest nasogastric tubes be cooled in ice or saline, which stiffens them to facilitate passage. Know facility policy.
8. Measure distance to insert tube. Measure total distance from tip of nose to earlobe and from there to xiphoid process of sternum. Tube should extend from nostril to stomach; distance varies with each patient. (*Allows tube to be inserted completely into stomach and not end in esophagus.*)

9. Mark off length of tube to be inserted with piece of tape or felt tip marker or note distance from next tube marking. (*Helps to ensure correct length of tubing will be inserted.*)
10. Curve 14–16 inches (10–15 cm) of tube tightly around fingers; release. (*Curving tube tip aids insertion.*)
11. Lubricate 3–4 inches (7.5–10 cm) of end of tube with water-soluble lubricating jelly. (*Minimizes friction against nasal mucosa.*)
12. Instruct patient to extend head against pillow; insert tube slowly through nostril with curved end pointing downward (see illustration). (*Facilitates initial passage of tube through nostril and maintains clear airway for open nostril.*)

13. Continue to pass tube along floor of nasal passage, aiming down toward ear. When resistance is felt, apply gentle downward pressure to advance tube (do not force past resistance). (*Reduces discomfort of tube rubbing against upper nasal turbinates. Resistance is caused by posterior*

Continued

Skill 15.5   Inserting a Nasogastric Tube—cont'd

nasopharynx. *Downward pressure helps tube to curl around corner of nasopharynx.*)

14. If resistance continues, withdraw tube, allow patient to rest, relubricate tube, and insert into other nostril. (*Forcing against resistance has potential to cause trauma to mucosa. Pause also helps to relieve anxiety.*)

15. Continue insertion of tube until just past nasopharynx by gently rotating tube toward opposite nostril.
    a. Stop tube advancement, allow patient to relax, and provide tissues. (*Relieves anxiety; tearing is natural response to mucosal irritation.*)
    b. Explain that the next step requires swallowing. (*Tube is about to enter esophagus.*)

16. With tube just above oropharynx, instruct patient to flex head forward and dry swallow or suck in air through straw. Advance tube 1–2 inches (2.5–5 cm) with each swallow. While advancing the tube in an unconscious patient (or in a patient who cannot swallow), stroke the patient's neck. (*Encourages the swallowing reflex and facilitates passage down the esophagus.*) If patient has trouble swallowing and is allowed fluids, offer glass of water. Advance tube with each swallow of water. (*The flexed position closes off upper airway to trachea and opens esophagus. Swallowing closes epiglottis over trachea and helps to move tube into esophagus. Swallowing water reduces gagging or choking.*)

17. If patient begins to cough, gag, or choke, stop tube advancement. Instruct patient to breathe easily and take sips of water. (*Tubing sometimes accidentally enters larynx and initiates cough reflex. Gagging is eased by swallowing water.*)

18. If patient continues to cough, pull tube back slightly. (*It is possible for tube to enter the larynx and obstruct airway.*)

19. If patient continues to gag after tube is pulled back, check back of pharynx with flashlight and tongue blade. (*It is possible for tubing to accidentally enter larynx and initiate cough reflex.*)

20. After patient relaxes, continue advancing tube to desired distance. (*Tip of tube must be in the stomach to provide proper decompression.*)

21. Ask patient to talk. (*Patient is unable to talk if tube is passed through vocal cords.*)

22. Observe posterior pharynx for coiling of tube. (*The tube is pliable, and there is potential for it to coil up in back of pharynx instead of advancing into esophagus.*)

23. Attach syringe to end of tube. Aspirate gently back on syringe to obtain gastric contents. (*Begins determination of whether tube is correctly in place in the stomach.*)

24. Measure pH of aspirate with color-coded pH paper. Gastric aspirates have acidic pH values of 4 or less. (*Determines whether tube is correctly placed in the stomach.*) While returning gastric aspirates to stomach, place stethoscope over stomach area on abdomen and listen for swishing or gurgling sounds. (*Another check to determine correct placement of tube.*)

25. If tube is not in the stomach, advance another 1–2 inches (2.5–5 cm) and repeat Steps 23 and 24. (*Assesses for tube placement.*)

26. After tube is properly inserted, clamp end or connect it to suction. (*Refer to health care provider's order determining suction or clamp.*)

27. Secure tube to nose with tape or nose guard. Avoid putting pressure on nares. (*Anchors the tube securely.*) Clean the skin over the nose with alcohol to remove any skin oils or soil and coat with skin protectant solution before applying the tape or nose guard.

28. Fasten end of tube to gown by looping rubber band around tube in slip knot. Pin rubber band to gown. Provide slack in tubing to allow for movement. (*Reduces chance of putting pressure on nares by tube moving. Pinning provides slack for movement.*)

Skill 15.5   Inserting a Nasogastric Tube—cont'd

29. Unless health care provider orders otherwise, elevate head of bed 30 degrees. (*Helps to prevent esophageal reflux and minimizes irritation caused by tube against posterior pharynx.*)
30. Refer to Standard Steps 10–17.
31. Document the following. (*Verifies performance of procedure and ensures continuity of care.*)
    - Date, time, and type of tube inserted
    - Patient's tolerance of procedure
    - Confirmation of placement
    - Character and amount of gastric contents
    - Whether tube is clamped or connected to suction
    - Patient teaching (see the Patient Teaching box on nasogastric tubes)
32. Report abnormalities:
    - Inability to advance tube (Additional interventions or therapies may be necessary.)

Box 15.2	Patient Problem Statements for the Patient With a Gastric Tube

Deficient Nutrition:
- Related to insufficient intake

Compromised Swallowing Ability:
- Related to neuromuscular impairment

Potential for Aspiration Into Airway:
- Related to inability to swallow effectively

Frequent, Loose Stools:
- Related to altered intake associated with tube feedings

Infrequent or Difficult Bowel Elimination:
- Related to altered intake associated with tube feedings

---

salivation or to suck on small ice chips to help relieve throat dryness.

Another nursing concern is maintaining patency of the tube. Sometimes the tube becomes occluded with secretions, or the internal tip of the tube becomes occluded if the end of the tube is pressing against the gastric mucosa. Irrigate the NG tube regularly with normal saline or tap water and a syringe if necessary (Skill 15.6). Turning the patient helps to drain the stomach and may help to reposition the tube so that it is not against the wall of the stomach. If necessary, try advancing the tube further or withdrawing it a little to reposition it. However, keep in mind that only a health care provider is permitted to reposition the tube when the patient has had gastric or esophageal surgery.

States and facilities vary on policy for who is authorized to insert NG tubes (see the Coordinated Care box on nasogastric tubes). Some states and facilities allow a licensed practical nurse or licensed vocational nurse (LPN/LVN) to insert NG tubes (see Skill 15.5). Most facilities allow the LPN/LVN to irrigate the NG tube (see Skill 15.5), administer feedings (see Chapter 19, Skill 19.1), care for the NG tube (Skill 15.7), and remove the NG tube (Skill 15.8). Check your state's scope of practice for the LPN/LVN and facility policy.

 Coordinated Care

Collaboration

Nasogastric Tube

- The skill of inserting a nasogastric (NG) tube requires the critical thinking and knowledge of a nurse. Unlicensed assistive personnel (UAP) may be permitted to measure and record the drainage from the NG tube and provide oral and nasal hygiene. Teach UAP how to properly secure the NG tube.
- The skill of irrigating an NG tube requires the critical thinking and knowledge of a nurse; this task should not be delegated to UAP.
- The skill of removing an NG tube requires the critical thinking and knowledge of a nurse; this task should not be delegated to UAP.

BOWEL ELIMINATION

Elimination of bowel wastes (defecation) is a basic human need and is essential for normal body function.

Skill 15.6 Nasogastric Tube Irrigation

NURSING ACTION *(RATIONALE)*

1. Refer to Standard Steps 1–9.
2. Assemble equipment:
   - Clamp
   - Clean gloves
   - Container for irrigant
   - Irrigation set with syringe
   - Irrigation solution (usually normal saline)
   - Stethoscope
   - Syringe
   - Towel or waterproof pad
3. Place patient in semi-Fowler position. *(Facilitates procedure.)*
4. Verify that tube is in right place:
   a. Attach syringe to end of tube and aspirate for stomach contents. Listen with stethoscope over stomach area on abdomen while returning aspirate for gurgling or swishing sounds. *(Confirms that tip of tube is in the stomach.)*
5. Evaluate abdomen. *(Provides baseline data for later comparison.)*
6. Pour normal saline or tap water into container; draw 30 mL (or amount ordered) into syringe. *(Use of saline minimizes loss of electrolytes from stomach fluid.)*
7. Clamp connection tubing distal to connection site. Disconnect tubing, and lay end on a towel. *(Reduces backflow of secretions and minimizes soiling of patient's gown and bed linens.)*
8. Insert tip of irrigating syringe into end of nasogastric (NG) tube. Hold syringe with tip pointed toward the floor, and instill 30 mL or ordered amount of saline or tap water slowly and evenly. Do not force solution; allow it to flow in by gravity. Never use air vent or pigtail on tubing of Salem sump for irrigation. *(Position of syringe prevents introduction of air into vent tubing, which has potential to cause gastric distention. Introducing solution under pressure may cause gastric trauma.)*

9. If resistance is met, check tubing for kinks, change patient's position, and repeat attempt; if resistance continues, confer with registered nurse (RN) or health care provider. *(Ensures that tip of tubing is not lying against wall of stomach. Buildup of secretions will cause distention.)*
10. Withdraw fluid into syringe and measure; continue irrigating with ordered amount of saline until purpose of irrigation has been accomplished. *(Clears the tubing.)*
11. Reconnect NG tube to suction or drainage tubing. To prevent leakage of fluid from airway vent of Salem sump tubes, introduce 30 mL of air into airway lumen to clear air vent tubing. Secure airway lumen above level of stomach to prevent siphoning effect. *(Reestablishes drainage collection.)*
12. Note amount of saline instilled and withdrawn. Subtract amount instilled from amount withdrawn and record difference as output. *(Fluid remaining in stomach is measured as intake.)*
13. Refer to Standard Steps 10–17.
14. Document the following. *(Description of gastric contents provides baseline to determine any change.)*
    - Date and time
    - Type and amount of solution
    - Character and volume of aspirate
    - Patient teaching (see the Patient Teaching box on nasogastric tubes)
    - Record balance of fluid instilled and aspirated on intake and output (I&O) sheet *(Balance reflects fluid gain or loss.)*
15. Report abnormalities. *(Abnormal findings indicate need to reposition tube or administer additional therapies.)*
    - Failure of tube to drain
    - Abdominal distention
    - Unusual characteristic of drainage (blood)

Normal bowel elimination depends on several factors: a balanced diet, including high-fiber foods; a daily fluid intake of 2000 to 3000 mL; and activity to promote muscle tone and peristalsis. Each patient has an individual pattern of defecation, but every patient should have a bowel movement at least every 1 to 3 days. This pattern should be determined on hospital admission, and an abdominal evaluation should be completed. Ask about any alterations in bowel elimination to determine patient problems related to elimination (Box 15.3).

To promote a normal pattern of elimination, establish a routine time for defecation, encourage the patient to heed the urge to defecate, and allow the patient to sit on a commode or, if he or she is in bed, in a Fowler position because this is the customary position for defecation. Bowel elimination is a private activity. Afford the patient as much privacy as

Skill 15.7   Care of Gastric and Intestinal Suctioning

 CHECK GATHER HELLO ID PRIVACY EXPLAIN WASH GLOVES

NURSING ACTION (RATIONALE)

1. Refer to Standard Steps 1–9.
2. Assemble equipment:
   - Clean gloves
   - Emesis basin
   - Stethoscope
   - Suction apparatus (if used)
   - Syringe
   - Towel
3. Determine that suction apparatus is working correctly.
   a. For suction machine (Gomco), check the following:
      (1) Machine is plugged in securely.
      (2) Light is blinking on and off.
      (3) Tubing connections are secured.
      (4) Setting is correct.
   b. For wall suction, check the following:
      (1) Pressure gauge connections are tight.
      (2) Pressure indicated on gauge is as ordered or according to facility policy. (*High pressure could lead to gastric bleeding.*)
      (3) Suction is set on intermittent or continuous as ordered.
4. Evaluate the following. (*Enables the nurse to determine need for any special care before or after procedure.*)
   a. Patient's oral and nasal cavities
   b. Patient's abdomen for bowel sounds and extent of distention. (*Provides baseline data for further assessments and may indicate tube malfunction.*)
   c. Patient's oral intake; nothing-by-mouth (NPO) status should be ordered
   d. Patient's lips and oral mucosa for dryness and cracking
5. Ensure that tubing is not kinked and that patient is not lying on tubing. (*Verifies that the patient or tube is not causing obstruction.*)
6. Pin nasogastric (NG) tube to patient's gown with enough slack to allow movement (see illustration for Step 28 of Skill 15.5). (*Prevents dislodging tube and patient discomfort.*)
7. Verify that drainage is moving through tubing to drainage collection bottle. (*Indicates that stomach or intestinal contents are being removed.*)
8. For Salem sump tube, ensure that vent is pointing upward. (There is potential that vent pointing downward will promote drainage through vent via gravity.) Listen at opening of blue air vent. (Hissing sound indicates air vent is patent.) If no hissing sounds are heard, instruct patient to cough, or reposition patient in the right or left Sims position or the supine position. (*Helps to move distal opening of tube in the stomach away from the mucosa wall and enables the suction to resume.*) It may be necessary to momentarily disconnect the NG tube from the suction tubing; be certain to reconnect immediately.
9. Measure amount of drainage in bottle, noting color; empty when it becomes full and at end of each shift. (*Provides baseline data for further assessments, prevents overflow, and ensures accurate measurement.*)
10. Refer to Standard Steps 10–17.
11. Document the following. (*Description of gastric contents provides baseline data to determine any change.*)
    - Date and time
    - Procedure
    - Observations
    - Amount, color, and consistency of drainage
    - Abnormalities
    - Patient teaching (see the Patient Teaching box on nasogastric tubes)
12. Report any abnormalities to health care provider. (*Abnormal findings indicate need to reposition tube or administer additional therapies.*)
    - Failure of tube to drain
    - Abdominal distention
    - Unusual characteristics of drainage (blood)

possible, and avoid continually "checking on" the patient, because this may make the patient uncomfortable and not provide an environment conducive for defecation. Some patients may resist using a bedpan because of discomfort and lack of privacy. Reassure the patient as much as possible, and make sure the bed is in Fowler position.

Many people have their own established ritual to promote elimination, such as drinking warm water with lemon juice or drinking black coffee with breakfast. Be alert to patient habits that are detrimental to normal bowel function, such as long-term, routine use of laxatives and cathartics. Eventually these may cause the intestines to lose the ability to respond to

Skill 15.8   Nasogastric Tube Removal

NURSING ACTION (RATIONALE)

1. Refer to Standard Steps 1–9.
2. Assemble equipment:
   - Clamp (optional)
   - Clean gloves
   - Facial tissues
   - Mask and goggles if splashing is expected (optional)
   - Plastic bag
   - Towel or waterproof pad
3. Reassure patient that nasogastric (NG) tube removal is less distressing than tube insertion. (*Reduces patient's anxiety and promotes cooperation.*)
4. Evaluate the following:
   a. Patient's abdomen for bowel sounds. (*Provides baseline abdominal data for future comparison.*)
   b. Patient's nasal and oral cavities. (*Enables the nurse to determine need for special interventions before or after procedure.*)
5. If tube is attached to suction, turn off suction and disconnect tubing, remove tape or nose guard from nose, and unfasten pin from patient's gown. (*Prevents pulling on tape or nose guard and damaging tissue on nose.*)
6. Place towel or waterproof pad across patient's chest and give patient tissues. (*Protects bed linens and patient's gown. Patients often wish to wipe eyes and blow nose after tube removal.*)
7. Instruct patient to take deep breath and hold it; pinch tube with fingers or clamp. (*Prevents aspiration from any leakage and prevents tube from leaking during procedure.*) Quickly and smoothly remove tube while patient is holding breath. (*If patient begins to gag, continue to remove tubing. It is the tubing that is causing the patient to gag.*)
8. Place tubing in plastic bag or towel. (Plastic bag or towel covers and conceals tube, which is not usually a pleasant sight.)
9. Provide oral and nasal care; position patient for comfort. (*Promotes comfort.*)
10. Dispose of tube and equipment; measure drainage and note characteristics of drainage. (*Reduces transfer of microorganisms. Ensures accurate measure of fluid output.*)
11. Inspect condition of nares and oral cavity. Report abnormalities. (*Abnormal findings indicate need for additional therapies.*)
    - Absence of bowel sounds
    - Complaints of severe sore throat
    - Erythema
    - Excoriation
    - Irritation during swallowing
    - Nasal fullness
    - Tenderness
12. Palpate abdomen periodically, noting any distention, pain, or rigidity; auscultate abdomen for bowel sounds. (*Determines success of abdominal decompression and the return of peristalsis.*)
13. Refer to Standard Steps 10–17.
14. Document the following. (*Verifies performance of procedure and ensures continuity of care.*)
    - Date and time
    - Removal of NG tube and condition of tube
    - Characteristics of drainage
    - Condition of nasal cavity
    - Presence of bowel sounds
    - Abdominal distention
    - Patient's tolerance of procedure

Box 15.3   Patient Problem Statements for the Patient With Altered Bowel Elimination

Anxiousness:
- Related to bowel function
- Related to rejection by friends

Distorted Body Image:
- Related to presence of ostomy

Impaired Coping:
- Related to daily ostomy care requirements

Infrequent or Difficult Bowel Elimination:
- Related to decreased activity
- Related to decreased peristalsis
- Related to dehydration
- Related to inadequate dietary fiber

Insufficient Knowledge Regarding Condition, Treatment Program, and Self-Care:
- Related to lack of exposure and information
- Related to misinterpretation of information
- Related to unfamiliarity with information

Potential for Compromised Skin Integrity:
- Related to irritation of skin around stoma

Recent Onset of Pain:
- Related to bowel distention

the presence of stool in the rectum, which often results in chronic constipation. Overcoming dependency on these medications is often difficult to accomplish and requires cooperation and compliance from the patient (see the Lifespan Considerations box on altered bowel elimination in older adults).

 Lifespan Considerations

Older Adults

Altered Bowel Elimination

- Many older adult patients are especially prone to dysrhythmias and other problems related to vagal stimulation associated with defecation. Therefore it is important to monitor heart rate and rhythm closely.
- In many older adults, constipation results from insufficient dietary bulk, inadequate fluid intake, laxative abuse, diminished muscle tone and motor function, decreased defecation reflex, mental or physical illness, and the presence of tumors or strictures.
- For an older adult, a diet containing at least 6–10 g of dietary fiber per day adds bulk, weight, and form to stool and improves defecation.
- Older adults should develop a regular toileting routine in response to the urge to defecate.
- The older adult patient or a family member should keep a week's diary of meals and fluid intake. The nurse should determine whether dietary pattern contributes to constipation. The nurse should recommend an increase in fiber if it is needed.
- The nurse should encourage as much activity as tolerated to maintain peristalsis and decrease the risk for constipation.

CARE OF THE PATIENT WITH HEMORRHOIDS

Hemorrhoids are swollen and inflamed veins in the anus and lower rectum. They may result from straining during bowel movements or from increased pressure during pregnancy or with heavy lifting. Hemorrhoids can be internal (inside the rectum) or external (around the anus). They are frequently a source of discomfort and have the capacity to cause an alteration in elimination. The goal for patients with hemorrhoids is to decrease pain, prevent elimination problems, and prevent damage to the already swollen tissue. To facilitate these goals, it is necessary for the patient to maintain a proper diet high in fiber, ensure adequate fluid intake, and participate in regular exercise. If the hemorrhoids are particularly troublesome, localized heat in the form of a sitz bath, or witch hazel pads often provide some relief. Use extreme caution when inserting rectal suppositories for patients with hemorrhoids. Use a liberal amount of lubricant during insertion to prevent pain or trauma to the rectal tissue. In such patients, rectal thermometers and rectal tubes should not be used.

FLATULENCE

Flatulence, or the presence of air or gas (flatus) in the intestinal tract, typically occurs when a person consumes gas-producing liquids and foods such as carbonated beverages, and foods such as cabbage or beans; swallows excessive amounts of air; or is constipated. It also can be caused by decreased peristalsis, abdominal surgery, some narcotic medications, and decreased physical activity. Flatulence may cause distention of the stomach and abdomen and, in some cases, mild to moderate abdominal cramping, which can be painful. To promote peristalsis and passage of flatus, encourage the patient to ambulate. If ambulating does not help to relieve the flatulence and the possible cause is not found, use of a rectal tube may be necessary. The presence of the tube in the rectum stimulates peristalsis and the movement of flatus, thus eliminating the discomfort (Skill 15.9).

ADMINISTERING AN ENEMA

An **enema** is the instillation of a solution into the colon via the anus. The primary reason for an enema is promotion of defecation in a patient with constipation. Enemas can be given for a number of reasons, such as cleansing the colon before a diagnostic procedure or abdominal surgery, management of constipation or fecal impaction, and administration of medication. The volume and type of enema administered depends on the reason for it and the health care provider's order.

A cleansing enema stimulates peristalsis by introducing large volumes of fluid to distend the bowel. This type of enema helps to empty the colon completely and is used frequently before surgery or a GI diagnostic procedure.

An oil retention enema is used to soften the stool and lubricate the bowel to make defecation easier. It is used when a fecal impaction is suspected. A **fecal impaction** is a collection of feces in the rectum in the form of a mass that becomes so large or hard that the patient is unable to pass it voluntarily. Medicated enemas can be used for a variety of reasons but are used most frequently to bring down an extremely high potassium level (polystyrene sulfonate enema).

No matter what type of enema is used, caution patients to limit the number of enemas they use. The defecation reflex may become dependent on enemas with repeated use, which can cause constipation. It is better to determine the cause of bowel irregularity or constipation and treat the cause rather than relying on enemas (Skill 15.10).

OSTOMIES

An **ostomy**, by definition, is an artificial opening. The site of the opening is called a *stoma*. Ostomies can be created because of trauma to the intestine, severe inflammation, or diseases such as cancer that involve part of the intestine. They can be temporary or permanent, depending on the reason they are present, and the characteristics of the fecal material vary according to where the ostomy is located along

Skill 15.9 Inserting a Rectal Tube

NURSING ACTION *(RATIONALE)*

1. Refer to Standard Steps 1–11.
2. Assemble equipment:
   - Clean gloves
   - Commercial kit with water-soluble lubricant, gloves, rectal tube, sponges, basin, and waterproof pad (if available)
   - Protector pad (Chux)
   - Stethoscope
   - Water-soluble lubricant
3. Auscultate bowel sounds. (*Provides basis for determining effectiveness of therapy.*)
4. Assist the patient to the left Sims position. Arrange gown and top linens to prevent soiling while still covering patient. (*Facilitates procedure and provides for patient privacy.*)
5. Place waterproof pad under buttocks. (*Protects bottom linen.*)
6. Don clean gloves. Lubricate tube well with water-soluble lubricant. (*Reduces spread of microorganisms and facilitates the insertion of tube.*)
7. Expose patient's anus. Insert tube 4–6 inches (10–15 cm) in the same manner as for an enema (see Skill 15.10).

8. Insert drainage end into receptacle or use commercially prepared set. (*The receptacle will contain any expelled stool.*)
9. Instruct the patient to lie quietly to prevent dislodging tube; leave tube in place no more than 30 min. If flatulence persists, notify the health care provider.
10. Remove tube, and assist patient to bedpan, bedside commode, or toilet as necessary; stimulation of peristalsis often results in bowel movement.
11. Provide for patient hygiene; auscultate bowel sounds, and assist patient to bed or chair.
12. Refer to Standard Steps 12–17.
13. Document the following. (*Verifies performance of procedure and ensures continuity of care.*)
    - Date and time of tube insertion
    - Results
    - Patient's response to procedure
14. If flatulence, abdominal discomfort, or distention continues, reinsert tube as required or as ordered by health care provider. (*Continued use of rectal tubes has potential to cause irritation and eventual skin impairment of the anus and the rectal mucosa.*)

the intestine. Fecal material in the ileum is liquid, and fecal matter in the rectum is solid. The closer the ostomy is to either end determines what type of stool will be in the ostomy. Material coming out of the stomach contains many enzymes that increase the acidity of the material. Stool in the ileum, cecum, and ascending colon tends to be more acidic and irritating to the skin surrounding the ostomy. As the material moves through the large intestine, water is removed, and the material becomes more solid and less acidic, causing less irritation to the skin surrounding the stoma.

An ileostomy is an opening in the ileum (the distal part of the small intestine). An ileostomy is needed when the entire colon must be removed or bypassed, as in cases of congenital defects, cancer, inflammatory bowel disease, or bowel trauma.

A colostomy is the surgical creation of a stoma on the abdominal wall to where the colon is normally attached. The colostomy then diverts stool through the stoma. Again, the stool may be liquid, semiformed, or formed, depending on the area of the colon incised. The procedure is performed for patients with cancer of

the colon, intestinal obstructions, intestinal trauma, or inflammatory diseases of the colon. Some colostomies are permanent, and some are temporary measures used until intestinal healing occurs.

A urostomy is the diversion of urine away from a diseased or defective bladder through a surgically created opening or stoma in the skin. This may be necessary in the presence of a congenital anomaly or when the bladder must be removed because of disease, trauma, or obstruction.

Colostomy Care

To be able to provide the patient with optimal colostomy care, it is important for the nurse to know the correct use of various products used for colostomy care and to educate the patient about appropriate care and use of these products. There are various types of pouching systems and skin barriers available to patients. One-pouch systems have a skin barrier (wafer) that is preattached to the pouch; two-piece systems have a pouch that is separate from the wafer. Some skin barriers are precut, whereas others must be cut to fit the stoma. When skin barriers are cut to fit the

Skill 15.10   Administering an Enema

CHECK   GATHER   HELLO   ID   PRIVACY   EXPLAIN   WASH   GLOVES

NURSING ACTION (RATIONALE)

1. Refer to Standard Steps 1–9.
2. Assemble equipment:
   - Bath blanket
   - Bedpan, bedside commode, or access to toilet
   - Clean gloves
   - Intravenous (IV) pole
   - Pre-prepared small volume enema or enema set
   - Solution
   - Toilet tissue
   - Wash basin, washcloth, towel, soap
   - Water-soluble lubricant

Pre-prepared small volume enema

3. Determine the following. (*Determines need for enema.*)
   a. Most recent bowel movement
   b. Presence or absence of bowel sounds
   c. Ability to control rectal sphincter (It is necessary to place patients with no sphincter control on a bedpan before the procedure because such patients cannot retain enema solution.)
   d. Presence or absence of hemorrhoids (*Hemorrhoids may obscure the rectal opening and cause discomfort or bleeding.*)
   e. Presence of abdominal pain (May preclude the use of enema. Never give an enema to patients with possible appendicitis because the appendix can rupture.)
   f. Patient's level of understanding and previous experience with enemas (*Enables the nurse to provide for appropriate teaching and reassurance.*)
4. Prepare solution. There are several types of enema solutions. Cleansing enemas include tap water, normal saline, low-volume hypertonic solutions, and soapsuds solution. (*Prepares equipment for procedure.*)
5. Arrange equipment at patient's bedside. (*Organizes procedure.*)
6. Assist patient to the Sims position. (*Allows enema solution to flow downward by gravity along natural curve of sigmoid colon and rectum, thus improving retention of enema.*) When an enema is given to a patient who is unable to contract the external sphincter, position the patient on the bedpan. Avoid giving the enema with the patient sitting on the toilet; it is possible for the inserted rectal tubing to abrade the rectal wall, and the enema solution is forced uphill, which makes the enema less effective.
7. Place waterproof pad under patient. (*Protects bed linens.*)
8. Place bath blanket over patient, and fanfold linen to foot of bed; adjust patient's gown to keep it from being soiled while it still provides privacy. (*Protects bed linens and patient's gown from soiling and provides warmth and privacy.*)
9. Clamp tubing; fill container with correctly warmed solution (usually 750–1000 mL at 105°F [41°C]) and any additives ordered. Administer a child's enema using appropriate equipment at 100°F to avoid burning rectal tissue (see illustration for Step 2, *top*); read disposable package for instructions. (*Hot water has capacity to burn intestinal mucosa. Cold water has capacity to cause abdominal cramping and is difficult to retain.*) Release clamp, allowing solution to flow through tubing to remove any air from the tubing; reclamp. Suggested maximal volumes are as follows:
   - Infant: 150–250 mL
   - Toddler: 250–500 mL
   - School-age child: 500 mL
   - Adolescent: 500–700 mL
   - Adult: 750–1000 mL
   a. For commercially prepared enema (see illustration for Step 2, *bottom*)
      (1) Remove cover from tip of enema (tip is prelubricated, but add additional lubricant if needed); insert entire tip into anus.

Continued

Skill 15.10 Administering an Enema—cont'd

(2) Squeeze container until it is empty. Usually a small amount of solution will remain in container. Most containers hold approximately 250 mL. Continue to squeeze the container to prevent siphoning solution back into the container.

(3) Encourage patient to retain solution at least 5 min. (*Retention of solution promotes peristalsis and enhances defecation.*)

b. For standard enema:

(1) Lubricate 4 inches (10 cm) at end of tubing; spread patient's buttocks to expose anus; while rotating tube, gently insert it 3–4 inches (7–10 cm). Instruct patient to breathe out slowly through mouth. (*Breathing out promotes relaxation of external rectal sphincter.*)

(2) Elevate container 12–18 inches (30–45 cm) above level of anus (see illustration). (*Allows solution to flow at appropriate rate. Raising container too high causes rapid infusion and possible painful distention of colon. Holding container too low leads to inadequate instillation of enema solution.*)

(3) Release clamp and allow solution to flow slowly. Usually solution will flow for 5–10 min. (*Allowing solution to instill slowly enables patient to retain all of solution and minimizes discomfort.*)

(4) Lower container or clamp tubing to slow the flow of solution if patient complains of cramping; encourage slow, deep breathing. Do not remove tubing tip. (*Temporary cessation of infusion reduces cramping and promotes ability to retain all of the solution.*) If severe cramping, bleeding, or sudden severe abdominal pain occurs and is unrelieved by temporarily stopping or slowing flow of solution, stop enema and notify health care provider.

(5) Clamp and remove tube when all the solution has been administered. Encourage patient to retain solution at least 5 min. (*Retention of solution promotes peristalsis and enhances defecation.*)

15. When patient is no longer able to retain solution, assist patient to bedpan, bedside commode, or bathroom. (*Normal squatting position promotes defecation; longer retention promotes more effective stimulation of peristalsis and defecation.*)

16. Instruct patient to call the nurse to inspect results before stool is flushed. Observe characteristics of feces or solution. (*Allows nurse to evaluate effectiveness of procedure.*) When enemas are ordered "until clear" in preparation for surgery, enemas are repeated until patient passes fluid that is clear and contains no fecal matter. Usually three consecutive enemas are adequate. If after three enemas the water is highly colored or contains solid fecal material, notify health care provider before continuing. (*Excessive loss of electrolytes is a dangerous possibility.*)

17. Refer to Standard Steps 10–17.

18. Provide for patient hygiene; assist patient to bed or chair. (*Patients sometimes need assistance to clean anal area. Fecal contents tend to irritate skin. Hygiene promotes patient comfort and decreases the risk of skin impairment.*)

19. Document the following. (*Verifies performance of procedure and ensures continuity of care.*)
- Date and time
- Type and volume of enema
- Temperature of solution
- Characteristics of results
- How patient tolerates procedure

stoma, ensure the ostomy appliance opening is small enough to form a proper seal, 1/16 inch larger than the stoma. In addition, the appliance must not cause pressure on the stoma, because there is a blood and nerve supply in the stoma but no sensation. An ill-fitting appliance can cause a pressure sore and lead to gangrene (Fig. 15.8 and Skills 15.11 and 15.12; see also the Patient Teaching boxes on ostomy care and on urostomy care, and the Home Care Considerations, Lifespan Considerations, and Coordinated Care boxes on ostomy care).

Colostomy Irrigation

Colostomy irrigation sometimes is used to maintain a regular elimination pattern. It is used less frequently now than in the past: many patients have regular

Fig. 15.8 Ostomy pouches and skin barriers.

Skill 15.11   Performing Colostomy, Ileostomy, and Urostomy Care

NURSING ACTION (RATIONALE)

Ostomy Care

1. Refer to Standard Steps 1–9.
2. Assemble equipment (see Fig. 15.8):
   - 1-inch–wide paper tape (optional)
   - Barrier paste
   - Basin with warm water
   - Bedpan or trash bag
   - Clean gloves
   - Measuring guide (if used)
   - Pouch clamp
   - Pouch with attached wafer seal
   - Scissors
   - Skin sealant wipes
   - Washcloth (disposable washcloth is acceptable)
3. Observe for the following. (*Enables the nurse to determine need for pouch change.*)
   a. Pouch leakage and length of time in place (*Pouches must be changed every 3–7 days to prevent skin impairment.*)
   b. Stoma for healing and color (*Proper stoma appearance is moist and reddish pink.*)
   c. Abdominal incision
4. Arrange supplies and equipment at patient's bedside or in bathroom (see Fig. 15.8). (*Promotes smooth flow of procedure.*)
5. Position patient supine and comfortable. (*When patient is in the supine position, there are fewer skinfolds and wrinkles, and it is easier to position and affix wafer.*)
6. Carefully remove wafer seal from skin (adhesive solvent is sometimes needed). (*Reduces trauma;*

jerking irritates the skin and sometimes causes skin impairment.)
7. Place reusable pouch in bedpan or disposable pouch in plastic bag. (*Reduces the transmission of microorganisms.*)
8. Cleanse skin around stoma with warm water; pat dry. (To prevent skin impairment, do not rub. Avoid use of soap because it leaves a residue on the skin that interferes with pouch adhesion to skin.)
9. Measure stoma opening. (*Ensures proper fit.*)
10. Place toilet tissue over stoma; use gauze for ileostomy. (*Prevents expelled stool from leaking during procedure.*) Note color and viability of stoma. If skin sealant is to be used, apply to skin and allow to dry.
11. Apply protective skin barrier approximately 1/16 inch from stoma. (*Creates wrinkle-free, secure seal; decreases chance of skin irritation from adhesive on skin.*)
12. Cut an opening in the center of wafer to {1/16} inch larger than stoma and apply protective wafer with flange. (*Ensures proper fit.*)
13. Gently attach pouch to flange by compressing the two together. (Ensures appropriate collection of feces and application of pouch reservoir.)
14. Remove tissue or gauze from stoma and backing from protectant wafer; center opening over stoma, and press against skin for 1–2 min. (*Establishes contact between barrier adhesive and skin and ensures pouch adherence.*)

Continued

Skill 15.11   Performing Colostomy, Ileostomy, and Urostomy Care—cont'd

15. Fold over bottom edges of pouch once to fit clamp. Secure clamp. If bottom edge of pouch is folded over more than once, the plastic will be too thick for the clamp, thus springing the clamp and causing spillage of fecal matter. (*Creates secure seal to prevent leaking.*)

16. If patient uses belt, attach at this time. (*Supports pouch and enhances feelings of security.*)

17. Assist patient to comfortable position in bed or chair; remove equipment from bedside. (*Promotes comfort.*)

18. Empty, wash, and dry reusable pouch. (*Reduces odor and extends usefulness.*)

19. Refer to Standard Steps 10–17.

20. Document the following. (*Verifies performance of procedure and ensures continuity of care.*)
    - Date and time
    - Procedure
    - Type of pouch
    - Type of skin barrier
    - Amount and appearance of feces
    - Condition of stoma and peristomal skin
    - Patient's level of participation
    - Patient teaching (see the Patient Teaching boxes on urostomy and ostomy care and Home Care Considerations box on ostomy care)

UROSTOMY CARE

Follow Steps 1–5 of ostomy care procedure. Then perform the following actions:

1. Empty urine into graduated pitcher; note amount and characteristics of urine. (*Provides nurse with data to determine further needs.*)

2. Carefully remove wafer seal from skin (use adhesive solvent if necessary), and place pouch in plastic bag. (*Reduces trauma; jerking movements irritate the skin and tend to cause skin impairment.*)

3. Cleanse skin with warm water and pat dry. (To prevent skin impairment, do not rub. Avoid using soap because it may irritate the skin.)

4. Measure stoma. Note color and viability of stoma. (*Ensures accurate fit. Careful observation provides data for later comparison.*)

5. Place gauze over stoma. (*Prevents urine from contacting skin.*)

6. If skin sealant is to be used, apply to skin and allow to dry; apply protective stoma paste approximately {1/16} inch from the stoma. (*Ensures a snug fit.*)

7. Cut an opening in the center of wafer {1/16} inch larger than stoma. Apply protective wafer with flange. (*Creates wrinkle-free seal; decreases chance that skin impairment will occur.*)

8. Refer to Steps 13 through 20 of ostomy care procedure to complete urostomy care.

Skill 15.12   Performing Colostomy Irrigation

NURSING ACTION (RATIONALE)

Note that colostomy irrigation is no longer performed on a routine basis, but it may help patients to achieve some regularity of elimination.

1. Refer to Standard Steps 1–9.

2. Assemble equipment and supplies:
    - Bed protector
    - Bedpan or toilet
    - Catheter with cone
    - Clamp
    - Clean gloves
    - Container
    - Irrigation set
    - Irrigation sleeve with or without belt
    - New pouch and wafer seal with flange
    - Tubing with clamp
    - Warm water and basin
    - Washcloth and towel (disposable washcloth is acceptable)
    - Water-soluble lubricant

3. Determine the following. (*Enables the nurse to determine need for procedure.*)
    a. Level of comfort (on a scale of 0–10) and need for pain management

Skill 15.12   Performing Colostomy Irrigation—cont'd

   b. Appropriateness of patient's condition for irrigation (Only patients with a descending or sigmoid colostomy are appropriate candidates because stool is more formed and less liquid.)

   c. Patient's ability to manipulate irrigation equipment and to understand concepts of bowel management

   d. Patient's readiness to learn self-irrigation of colostomy

4. Position patient.

- Bathroom: Instruct patient to sit on toilet or on a chair in front of the toilet.
- Bed: Have patient lie comfortably with head of bed slightly elevated. (*Do not overexpose patient.*)
- NOTE: Allow the patient to perform as many of these steps as possible independently; provide teaching and assistance as needed. Be alert to patient's readiness to learn and perform self-care.

5. Remove pouch, cleanse skin, and place irrigation sleeve over stoma; attach belt if patient uses one; place end of sleeve in toilet. (*Provides for patient cleanliness and decreases risk for skin breakdown. Make sure irrigation sleeve is correctly attached. End of sleeve must be in toilet or bedpan to prevent spillage of feces.*)

6. Close clamp on irrigation tubing; fill irrigation container with 1000 mL of tepid water (or as otherwise ordered). It is acceptable to hang container on a hook at patient's shoulder level. (*This position prevents too high a pressure and reduces possibility of bowel damage.*) Allow a small amount of water to flow through tubing. (*Allow some solution to fill tubing to express air, which is otherwise forced into the bowel and causes cramps.*)

7. Attach cone to tubing; lubricate cone; insert cone into stoma through top of sleeve. Do not force cone into stoma. Use gentle pressure to hold tip in place in stoma. (*To prevent trauma to bowel, do not insert entire length of cone into stoma. Too little pressure causes the irrigation solution to flow out alongside of cone and not into patient. Too much pressure has capacity to block flow of irrigation solution into patient.*)

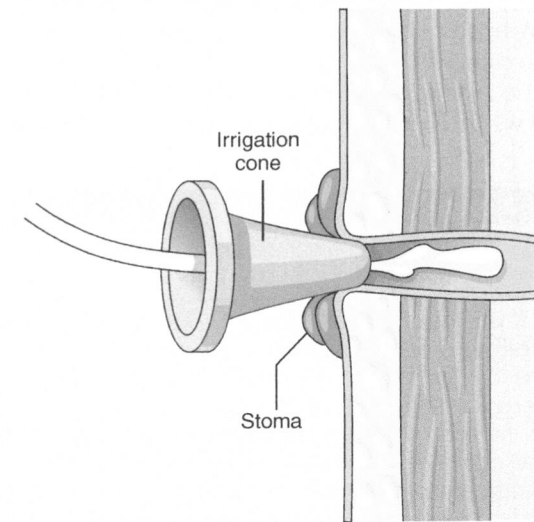

Irrigation cone

Stoma

8. While you hold cone in place, allow solution to flow slowly into colon (500–1000 mL over 15 min). If patient complains of cramping, stop flow without removing cone until cramps subside. (*Stopping or slowing infusion allows patient to adjust to irrigation and tolerate the procedure better.*)

9. After all solution is instilled, remove cone and close top of sleeve. (*Prevents spillage of feces.*)

10. Instruct patient to sit about 15–20 min while the returning solution flows into toilet. (If patient cannot sit this long, it is acceptable to close the end of the irrigation sleeve with a clamp and allow the patient to be up and walk around the room. Exercise stimulates the bowel.)

11. Drain sleeve; rinse and remove it. (Some irrigation sleeves are reusable and should be cleaned as directed by manufacturer.)

12. Observe patient and results of irrigation; flush toilet. (*Provides data for comparison.*)

13. Perform colostomy care (see Skill 15.11). (*Provides for patient comfort.*)

14. Refer to Standard Steps 10–17.

15. Document the following. (*Verifies performance of procedure and ensures continuity of care.*)

- Date and time
- Solution used
- Amount of solution
- Results
- Observations
- Patient's tolerance of procedure

bowel movements without irrigation. If the patient desires irrigation, the patient must be prepared to devote 60 to 90 minutes per day in the bathroom for the procedure.

Colostomy irrigation requires special equipment and is not without complications. The patient needs a cone-tipped irrigation device (see Step 7 of Skill 15.12), an irrigation sleeve, and irrigation solution or access to tap water. The patient places the cone-tipped irrigation device in the stoma through the sleeve. The sleeve is used to contain the drainage from the stoma as it passes into the commode. Approximately 500 to 1000 mL is instilled slowly into the stoma, and the patient must sit on the commode while it drains out (approximately 30 minutes).

Complications associated with colostomy irrigation include damage or perforation of the bowel, which can lead to peritonitis. Other complications range from tissue damage as a result of the temperature of the irrigating solution to fluid and electrolyte imbalances if too much tap water is used.

Lifespan Considerations

Older Adults

Ostomy Considerations

- Evaluate the older adult's cognitive status and capacity to understand ostomy self-care instructions.
- Evaluate the older adult's motor and visual ability to prepare ostomy equipment.
- For patients who are unable to custom-cut the size of their skin barriers, consider having barriers precut by the ostomy equipment supplier or a family member/friend.
- Avoid hot water and harsh soaps when washing the skin around the ostomy.

- Teach patients about the change in the number of bowel movements that may occur on a daily basis. With some irrigation routines, irrigation is not performed daily; in this case the patient may not have a daily bowel movement.
- The cost of ostomy supplies and reimbursement are often an important concern for older patients on limited incomes; referral to community resources may be necessary.

Patient Teaching

Ostomy Care

- Include family members or significant others in teaching; this tends to facilitate the patient's readiness to learn.
- Use every pouch change as an opportunity to teach even if the patient does not appear interested. Do not force the patient to look at the stoma; allow for a period of adjustment.
- Reinforce positive performance. Some patients are not willing to learn ostomy care for a period of time after receiving one. The patient may refuse to look at or touch the stoma and may not participate in ostomy care until he or she has accepted the ostomy.
- Many nurses are able to judge a patient's readiness to learn by the patient's willingness to look at the stoma and by the patient's asking questions. If the patient is apprehensive about touching or looking at stoma, have the patient hold a gauze pad over the stoma and clean around the stoma.
- Some patients acknowledge a stoma with minimal emotional difficulty; some never completely adjust to it.

Individualize care according to the patient's situation and circumstances.
- Teach the patient to avoid constipation by eating a balanced diet or using a daily stool softener.
- If the patient has limitations affecting dexterity, select a pouching system that can be most easily managed.
- A teaching manual with clearly stated steps or audiotaped instructions may be helpful for the patient. Patients with a learning disability may benefit from a picture book of the steps involved in ostomy care.
- Give the patient a list of equipment and the name, address, and phone number of a supplier in the patient's community.
- In most cases, patients are able to wear their normal clothes; snug clothing does not interfere with ostomy function.
- Instruct patients not to leave pouches in extremely hot or cold locations, because temperature has the potential to affect the barrier and adhesive materials.

Patient Teaching

Urostomy Care

- Teach the patient and caregivers to avoid touching the stoma with adhesive solvents to prevent irritating the stoma.
- Teach the patient and caregivers to wick the urine with an absorbent, lint-free material to prevent a constant flow of urine while they change the appliance.
- Teach the patient and caregivers to remove hair from the stoma area with scissors or an electric razor to prevent hair follicles from becoming irritated when the pouch is removed.
- Teach the patient and caregivers that the appliance should be able to remain in place 5–7 days.

- Teach the patient and caregivers to empty appliance through the drain valve when it is one-third to one-half full to prevent the weight of the urine from loosening the seal around the stoma.
- Teach the patient and caregivers to connect the appliance to a urine-collection container at night to prevent urine from stagnating in the appliance.
- Teach sanitary and dietary measures that will protect the skin around the ostomy and control odor.
- Offer positive reinforcement and written instructions or videos.

See the Patient Teaching box on ostomy care for further instructions.

Coordinated Care

Collaboration

Ostomy Care

- The skill of applying a pouch to a fresh stoma requires the critical thinking and knowledge of a nurse. Some facilities permit delegation of the task of pouching of an established ostomy. Instruct the care provider about the expected amount, color, and consistency of drainage from the ostomy. In addition, teach the care provider to report changes in the stoma and surrounding skin integrity.
- The skill of applying a pouch to an incontinent urinary diversion requires the critical thinking and knowledge of a nurse. In some facilities, a stoma nurse specialist is available to provide this care. Unlicensed assistive personnel (UAP) who provide personal care are instructed to report any leakage of urine and breakdown of skin to the nurse.
- The skill of irrigating a newly established colostomy requires the critical thinking and knowledge of a nurse. In some settings, UAP are trained to perform irrigations on established ostomies. Review facility policy.

 Home Care Considerations

Ostomy Care

- Consult with the health care provider to obtain a referral to a home health agency or a visiting nurse before patient's hospital discharge.
- Pouches that wear well in the hospital will not necessarily wear well when the patient resumes a normal routine.
- If an irrigation routine is required, assist the patient to adapt the procedure to the home setting. Suggest hanging the irrigation solution container from a hook on the wall or from a shower curtain rod instead of an intravenous (IV) pole.
- Urostomy, colostomy, and ileostomy products are usually available for purchase online or at local pharmacies or medical supply companies.
- Encourage the patient to become involved with local ostomy organizations or support groups found on social media.
- Teach the patient and caregivers to routinely inspect the stoma and the surrounding skin. The proper appearance of the stoma is moist, shiny, and dark pink to red, with minimal if any bleeding around it. Teach the patient and caregivers to report excessive bleeding, abnormal color, or swelling to the nurse or the health care provider.
- Teach the patient and caregivers to avoid using alcohol around the stoma because alcohol dilates capillaries, causing bleeding, and may dry the skin excessively.
- Teach the patient and caregivers not to use lotions or creams around the stoma because they may prevent pouches from adhering.
- Teach the patient and caregivers not to use peroxide on or around the stoma because it may irritate the tissue.

- Instruct the patient and caregivers to wash the skin around the stoma with mild soap and water and rinse thoroughly. If the patient finds that soap is irritating to the skin, they can use water only. Pat or blot the skin dry.
- Evaluate the patient's home toileting facilities for the following:
  - The presence of adequate functioning and accessible toileting facilities
  - Number and location of toileting facilities
  - Number of other people living in the home who have to share the toileting facilities
  - The pattern of use of the toileting facilities by the other people living in the home (time of day and amount of time spent in bathroom)
- Evaluate the patient's ostomy routine in relation to his or her usual lifestyle after discharge.
- Caution the patient not to flush ostomy pouches and barriers down the toilet; they clog the pipes. Dispose of used ostomy pouches according to local sanitation regulations.
- Make sure the patient understands that it is not necessary to use sterile gauze to cleanse the stoma. Using a washcloth made of any soft material is fine.
- Review the patient's dietary pattern. Help patient and family members to learn the types of foods to avoid to prevent problems with stoma drainage or odor.
- Teach patients that if water is not drinkable, they should not use it for irrigations (e.g., as in another country).

Get ready for the NCLEX® Examination!

Key Points

- Closed bladder drainage systems necessitate the use of aseptic technique during care.
- Intermittent urinary catheterization has a lower risk of infection than indwelling urinary catheterization because of the relatively shorter time the intermittent catheter remains in the bladder.

- Strict asepsis is necessary in caring for a closed urinary drainage system.
- It is possible to use closed urinary drainage systems for instillation of sterile solutions or medications into the bladder.
- When a nasogastric tube is to be inserted, it is necessary to lubricate the tube well with a water-soluble lubricant to prevent trauma to the mucous membranes.

- It is imperative for the nurse to check for proper nasogastric tube placement before an irrigation or a tube feeding.
- Proper administration of an enema consists of the slow instillation of the correct volume of a warm solution.
- Emotional support of the patient with an ostomy is important to foster eventual acceptance of the change in body image.
- Consistency of the feces is affected directly by which portion of the colon is brought out to the stoma.
- Even when an ostomy pouch is adhering well, it is best to change it at least every 5–7 days or according to pouch recommendations to allow for observation of the stoma and the skin around the stoma.
- Patients with urostomies are at high risk for skin impairment at the site because of the nearly continuous urine drainage.
- Irrigation of an ostomy follows the same principles as an enema administration, except that a special irrigating tube is needed and the patient is not able to control the passage of feces.
- Skin impairment is possible after repeated exposure to liquid stool. This is especially true in patients who have a stoma.

Additional Learning Resources

SG Go to your Study Guide for additional learning activities to help you master this chapter content.

Be sure to visit the Evolve site at http://evolve.elsevier.com/Cooper/foundations/ for additional online resources.

Review Questions for the NCLEX® Examination

1. **What would the nurse do to determine the correct distance to insert a nasogastric tube?**
   1. Measure from center of forehead to top of nose to end of sternum.
   2. Measure from tip of nose to tip of earlobe to the xiphoid process.
   3. Measure from lips to tip of ear to just below the umbilicus.
   4. Measure from tip of ear to midway between end of sternum and umbilicus.

2. **A patient is transferred from the postanesthesia care unit (PACU) to the postoperative unit following abdominal surgery for placement of a transverse colostomy. The patient has a nasogastric tube to medium intermittent suction. What actions can the nurse perform to verify correct placement of the nasogastric tube?** *(Select all that apply.)*
   1. Assess the patient for complaints of abdominal pain or nausea.
   2. The nurse injects 30 mL of normal saline through the nasogastric tube with ease.
   3. The nurse auscultates a gurgling or a swishing sound heard with a stethoscope over the stomach when air is injected into the tube.
   4. The nurse aspirates gastric contents with the appearance of being a watery yellow or green tint with a syringe.
   5. The nurse places the end of the tube in a glass of water and watches for bubbling.
   6. The nurse contacts the x-ray department to perform an x-ray for placement verification according to provider's orders.
   7. The nurse aspirates contents from the nasogastric tube and checks the pH to determine if the pH is below 4.
   8. The nurse asks the patient if they can feel suction in their stomach when initiating the suction.
   9. The nurse assesses the amount of drainage in the nasogastric tube to determine if it is in the stomach.

3. **If the patient is suspected of having a fecal impaction, which type of enema would the nurse anticipate the health care provider to order?**
   1. Soapsuds enema
   2. Polystyrene sulfonate enema
   3. Oil retention enema
   4. Tap water enema

4. **Bladder training instructions are being given to a patient who has a history of urinary incontinence. The nurse should give the patient which instruction?**
   1. "Wait until you feel the urge to void."
   2. "Don't void any more often than every 4 to 6 hours."
   3. "Void every 1.5 to 2 hours while you are awake."
   4. "Void any time you feel the urge."

5. **A nurse is preparing to insert a nasogastric tube. The nurse should place the patient in which position?**
   1. On the right side.
   2. Low Fowler position.
   3. High Fowler position.
   4. Supine with head of bed flat.

6. A male patient with urinary incontinence has been using an external (condom) catheter. The nurse is evaluating the patient's technique of applying the device. Which finding would indicate that the nurse should give the patient further instructions? *(Select all that apply.)*

   1. Washing the penis with warm, soapy water and drying the area well before applying the device
   2. Using tape around the penis to secure the device
   3. Using a narrow width elastic bandage to wrap in a spiral pattern to secure the device
   4. Checking the penis carefully for any signs of irritation before applying the device
   5. Changing the catheter after each episode of urinary incontinence
   6. Applying a leg bag to the condom catheter during the day and changing to a larger drainage bag at night
   7. Removing the condom catheter at night and using an incontinent pad for urine incontinence
   8. Using a foam skin applicator that has adhesive on the outside to hold the condom catheter in place

7. What is considered a noninvasive method of collecting urine for the incontinent patient?

   1. Suprapubic catheterization
   2. Reinsertion of a Foley catheter
   3. Catheter irrigation
   4. Condom catheterization

8. A patient with a colostomy continues to worry about odor. Which statement would be appropriate for the nurse to tell the patient about colostomy odor?

   1. "It occurs only when the colostomy appliance is changed."
   2. "It is caused by certain foods that can be omitted from the diet."
   3. "It is mainly caused by poor hygiene and can be remedied."
   4. "It is far more noticeable to the patient than to others."

9. The nurse is instructing the patient in performing Kegel exercises. The patient should be instructed to contract the muscles he or she would use to stop the flow of urine. What is the proper technique for performing Kegel exercises?

   1. Contract for 3 to 4 seconds and relax for 3 to 4 seconds.
   2. Contract for 3 to 4 seconds and relax for 10 seconds.
   3. Contract for 10 seconds and relax for 3 to 4 seconds.
   4. Contract for 10 seconds and relax for 10 seconds.

10. A bladder retraining program for a patient in an extended-care facility should include which intervention? *(Select all that apply.)*

    1. Providing negative reinforcement when the patient is incontinent.
    2. Having the patient wear clothing protectors to help decrease embarrassment.
    3. Initiating a toilet schedule of every 2 hours during the day.
    4. Promoting the intake of caffeine to stimulate voiding.
    5. Encouraging the use of the bedpan.

11. The nurse is caring for a patient with a new ostomy. What is the **best** nursing strategy for encouraging patient self-care of an ostomy?

    1. Plan to change the pouch when family members will be present, have the patient watch, and have the patient and family listen to the procedure.
    2. Frequently tell the patient that if he or she does not learn stoma self-care, no one is going to do it for him or her.
    3. Encourage the patient to watch the stoma care procedure, gradually encouraging participation.
    4. Shield the patient from sight of the stoma until the patient actually asks to see it.

12. A patient has a nasogastric tube inserted. What type of patient teaching should the nurse give the patient about the nasogastric tube? *(Select all that apply.)*

    1. "Be careful to not pull on the tube."
    2. "Call the nurse if you feel as if you are going to vomit."
    3. "Turn the suction off if you feel as if you are going to vomit."
    4. "Refrain from coughing while the tube is in place."
    5. "Let the staff know if the tape holding the tube is irritating your skin."

13. To maintain proper drainage of an indwelling catheter, it is important to perform which action?

    1. Irrigate the catheter every 2 to 4 hours.
    2. Ensure that the collection device is below bladder level.
    3. Place the tubing under the patient's leg to prevent pulling on the bladder neck.
    4. Demonstrate to the patient how to disconnect the device while ambulating.

14. The nurse instructs the patient to be diligent in cleaning fecal matter from around the stoma because the fecal matter can cause which complication? *(Select all that apply.)*

    1. Fungal infection
    2. Bacterial infection
    3. Yeast infection
    4. Irritation of the stoma
    5. Skin breakdown around the stoma

15. The nurse is administering a cleansing enema. Before administering the enema, the nurse assists the patient into which position?

    1. Supine
    2. On right side
    3. Left Sims position
    4. Left side with head of bed elevated 45 degrees

16. The nurse caring for a patient with an indwelling catheter should perform which actions to lower the risk for infection? *(Select all that apply.)*

    1. Keep drainage bag below the level of the bed.
    2. Provide perineal care twice a day.
    3. Coil tubing on the bed.
    4. Keep the drainage system closed.
    5. Limit fluid intake to 300 mL per shift.

17. The nurse is administering a cleansing enema to an adult patient. The patient complains of cramping and the urge to defecate. Which nursing intervention is the best to carry out?

   1. Quickly finish instilling the rest of the solution.
   2. Slow the flow and encourage the patient to take deep breaths.
   3. Instruct the patient to hold his or her breath and bear down.
   4. Immediately discontinue the instillation and withdraw the enema tubing from the rectum.

18. When providing routine indwelling catheter care, the nurse should be most diligent in cleaning which areas?

   1. The perineal area
   2. The area surrounding the urinary meatus
   3. The labia majora and the labia minora
   4. The perineal area and 2 inches of the catheter

Care of Patients Experiencing Urgent Alterations in Health

Objectives

1. List the priorities of assessment to be performed in a situation in which first aid is necessary.
2. Discuss moral, legal, and physical interventions/implications involved in performing first aid.
3. List the reasons for performing cardiopulmonary resuscitation (CPR).
4. List the steps in performing one-rescuer and two-rescuer CPR on an adult, child, and infant victim.
5. Identify the steps in performing the abdominal thrusts on conscious and unconscious victims and pregnant victims.
6. Compare management of airway obstruction in a child and an infant.
7. Determine the signs and symptoms of shock and interventions to treat shock.
8. Examine methods of controlling bleeding.
9. Explain the five general types of open wounds: abrasions, incisions, lacerations, punctures, and avulsions.
10. Discuss treatment of the various types of wounds, general principles of bandaging, and bandage application.
11. Explore methods of assessing and treating four common types of poisonings.
12. Summarize appropriate methods for assessing and treating drug and alcohol emergencies.
13. Describe the nursing interventions used when treating heat and cold emergencies.
14. List characteristics and first aid treatment of bone, joint, and muscle injuries.
15. Define the classifications of burns and list nursing interventions used in the first aid treatment of burns.

Key Terms

air embolism (ār ĔM-bŏ-lĭzm, p. 409)
biological death (p. 401)
brain death (p. 401)
CAB (circulation, airway, breathing) (p. 402)
cardiac arrest (p. 402)
cardiopulmonary resuscitation (CPR) (kăr-dē-ō-PŬL-mō-nā-rē rē-sŭs-ĭ-TĀ-shŭn, p. 400)
clinical death (p. 401)
contusions (kŏn-TŪ-zhŭnz, p. 412)
crepitus (KRĔP-ĭ-tŭs, p. 421)
cyanosis (sī-ă-NŌ-sĭs, p. 408)
ecchymoses (ĕk-ĭ-MŌ-sēz, p. 412)
emergency medical services (EMS) (p. 399)
epistaxis (ĕp-ĭ-STĂK-sĭs, p. 410)
epistaxis digitorum (ĕp-ĭ-STĂK-sĭs dĭj-ĭ-TŌR-ŭm, p. 410)

flail chest (p. 413)
Good Samaritan laws (p. 400)
hematemesis (hē-mă-TĔM-ē-sĭs, p. 411)
hematuria (hē-mă-TŪ-rē-ă, p. 411)
hemoptysis (hē-MŎP-tĭ-sĭs, p. 411)
hemothorax (hē-mō-THŎ-răks, p. 413)
melena (MĔL-ē-nă, p. 411)
oliguria (ŏl-ĭ-GŪ-rē-ă, p. 408)
pleural space (PLŪR-ăl spās, p. 413)
pneumothorax (nū-mō-THŎ-răks, p. 413)
shock (shŏk, p. 408)
stridor (STRĪ-dŏr, p. 407)
tachycardia (tăk-ē-KĂR-dē-ă, p. 408)
tetanus toxoid (TĔT-ă-nŭs TŎKS-ŏyd, p. 412)
triage (TRĒ-ăhzh, p. 399)

First aid is the immediate, initial assistance given to a person who is injured or has become ill. First aid education should be universally available and is useful in improving morbidity and mortality rates. First aid includes assessing the victim for life-threatening conditions, performing appropriate interventions to sustain life, and keeping the person in the best possible physical and mental condition until the assistance of emergency medical services (EMS) is obtained. EMS is a national network of services that provides coordinated aid and medical assistance from primary response to definitive care. First aid does not replace medical care but is used to preserve life until medical help is obtained. Because permanent disability and injury can occur within minutes, the nurse should be prepared to handle emergency conditions and administer first aid. In the case of multiple injuries, patients are surveyed quickly for severity of injuries so that health care providers can treat life-threatening problems first. This process of classifying a group of patients according to the severity of injury and need of care is called triage. The triage process is based on the premise that patients who have a threat to life, vision, or limb should be treated before other patients. In a disaster, triage is a process in which numerous patients are "sorted" so that it is possible to concentrate care and resources on those who are more likely to survive. In this chapter, the rescuer often is referred to as the nurse or you, the reader. However, any person certified to perform cardiopulmonary resuscitation (CPR) and first aid may assist with these activities.

OBTAINING MEDICAL EMERGENCY AID

The nurse's ability to recognize the need for medical assistance and understanding of how to obtain medical emergency aid can sometimes mean the difference between life and death to an injured or ill person. It is important for the nurse to know the right phone number to call in the community and in the institutional setting. In most communities, the emergency medical number is 911. However, in some areas and in some situations, it may be best to call the number for the fire department, police department, or local hospital. Box 16.1 provides information to convey when calling in a medical emergency from the community.

Health care providers must be prepared to provide cardiopulmonary resuscitation (CPR) (basic emergency procedure for life support) if needed until emergency medical assistance arrives. All health care providers should maintain CPR certification. Most health care institutions provide training. CPR certification is also available from local fire departments and local chapters of the American Red Cross and the American Heart Association.

The guidelines for administering CPR undergo periodic review and are subject to change. This chapter discusses CPR in accordance with the most current

guidelines provided by the American Heart Association at the time of this text's publication. Further information on CPR can be found at www.heart.org.

MORAL AND LEGAL RESPONSIBILITIES OF THE NURSE

Good Samaritan laws (legal protection for those who give first aid in an emergency situation) have been enacted in most states to protect health professionals from legal liability when they provide emergency first aid. If a nurse follows a reasonable and prudent course of action, the chances of resulting legal problems are very small. Nurses are obliged to obtain permission to treat any conscious patient, even in an emergency situation. Before first aid is administered, verbal permission should be obtained from the victim because the victim has the right to refuse first aid. The law assumes consent from an unconscious person. After the nurse has initiated first aid, they have a moral and legal obligation to continue the aid until someone with comparable or better training is able to care for the victim; for example, an emergency medical technician (EMT), or paramedic, or a health care provider may arrive at the scene and assume first aid care of the victim.

ASSESSMENT OF THE EMERGENCY SITUATION

Assessment of life-threatening problems is the priority in an emergency situation. Assess the scene for potential safety hazards. Sometimes the nurse will need the aid of another person, whether to help care for victims with some injuries or illnesses or to call EMS. If necessary, shout to get someone's attention or request that someone call 911 or another emergency number. While seeking help, continue the primary survey by assessing the patient's circulation, airway, and breathing (CAB). An immediate life-threatening situation of highest priority is abnormal circulation; an absent or abnormal pulse is a life-threatening situation. Assess the rate, rhythm, and strength of the carotid pulse for no longer than 10 seconds. Monitor the victim for signs of external bleeding and internal bleeding, which may lead to shock. Additional assessment includes the person's skin color, temperature, pupil reaction, pulse, and respiration. Poisonings also may be life threatening. Observe for burns or stains in and around the person's mouth or hands. Depressed respirations and circulatory collapse are other possible results of poisoning.

Ensure that the victim's airway is open. The airway is opened with a head-tilt/chin-lift maneuver unless a neck injury is suspected. If a cervical spine injury is suspected, use a jaw-thrust maneuver without tilting the head to open the airway. Use caution not to move the neck out of proper alignment. Because of the potential for causing or exacerbating a cervical spine injury, do not hyperextend the patient's neck to establish an airway.

Box 16.1	Information to Convey in a Medical Emergency

1. Name of the person making the call
2. Location of the emergency
3. What has happened (either by direct observation or by gathering data from other people)
4. Whether an immediate threat, such as fire or flood, or physical threat by someone, such as use of a gun or knife, still exists
5. Number of people who need assistance
6. Each victim's name and age
7. Obvious injuries and each victim's apparent condition
8. First aid measures that have already been administered
9. Presence of medical-alert bracelet or any known history
10. The physical characteristics of the scene of the rescue (stairs, elevators)

Note: Only hang up when instructed to do so by the emergency services operator.

Assess the victim's ability to breathe by determining whether the chest is rising, listen for breath sounds, and place your cheek near the victim's mouth to feel the passage of air from the victim's breathing. Assess rhythm, depth, and rate of respirations. The following clinical manifestations indicate that the victim is having trouble breathing: cyanosis, gasping, wheezing, stridor, and snoring.

After the initial assessment for life-threatening problems, assess the victim for indications of skull injury and brain or spinal cord damage, all of which necessitate immediate interventions. A decreasing level of consciousness, abnormal pupil reaction, and lack of movement in the arms or the legs are indicative of a possible injury to the head or spinal cord. Focus on the victim's fractures, dislocations, and superficial ecchymoses or wounds only after treating the more serious conditions.

CARDIOPULMONARY RESUSCITATION

ETHICAL IMPLICATIONS

Reasons that individuals choose not to become involved in performing CPR include feeling panicked, fear of incorrectly administering CPR, and fear of hurting the patient. However, once the nurse or anyone starts CPR, it should not be discontinued *except* for the following reasons:

- The victim recovers.
- An automated external defibrillator (AED) is available, and CPR is discontinued before the equipment is applied.
- The scene becomes unsafe, and evacuation of the victim is necessary.
- The rescuer is exhausted and is not able to continue CPR.
- Trained medical personnel arrive on the scene and take over CPR.
- A licensed health care provider arrives on the scene, has the authority to pronounce the victim dead, and orders CPR to be discontinued.

When a licensed practical nurse/licensed vocational nurse (LPN/LVN) is providing emergency care to a patient, this nurse should stay with the patient until care is taken over by a registered nurse (RN), a health care provider, or emergency medical personnel.

EVENTS NECESSITATING CARDIOPULMONARY RESUSCITATION

Many situations necessitate resuscitation efforts (Box 16.2). CPR is indicated when the patient is not responsive and not breathing. There are two purposes of CPR:

1. To keep the blood circulating and carrying oxygen to the brain, the heart, and other parts of the body
2. To keep the airway open, and the lungs supplied with oxygen when breathing has stopped

   Clinical death means that heartbeat and respiration have stopped. **Biological death** results from permanent

---

Box 16.2	Events Necessitating Cardiopulmonary Resuscitation

- *Anaphylactic reaction:* Exposure to a known allergen (e.g., food, poisons, and drugs) or an insect bite has the capacity to produce the severe allergic reaction known as *anaphylaxis.* This reaction often causes spasms or edema of the upper airway and, in some cases, progresses to cardiovascular collapse. It is necessary to initiate cardiopulmonary resuscitation (CPR) immediately, as with any other emergency situation.
- *Asphyxiation:* Asphyxiation or suffocation caused by inhaling a gas other than oxygen is possible as a result of fires, chemical spills, or gas leaks. In addition, children and adults sometimes suffer respiratory arrest and ultimately cardiac arrest from choking on food or small objects that are placed in the mouth. Abdominal thrusts and CPR are performed in this instance.
- *Cardiac arrest:* The most common cause of cardiac arrest is myocardial infarction (MI). In addition, shock from hemorrhage, trauma to the heart, respiratory arrest, and drugs have the potential to precipitate a cardiac arrest.
- *Drowning:* Children are common victims of drowning and boating accidents. People using alcohol or other drugs near bodies of water are often victims of drowning. It is important to note that near-drowning victims sometimes recover completely after long periods of submersion. The low water temperature that produces hypothermia reduces the metabolic rate and decreases oxygen demands. Because of this, it is necessary to initiate CPR even when 4 to 6 min of cardiac or respiratory arrest is known to have elapsed.
- *Drug overdose:* Intentional or accidental abuse of alcohol and drugs poses a risk for respiratory and cardiac arrest. Besides treating this as a poisoning emergency, perform CPR as necessary.
- *Electrical shock:* People who come near sources of high-voltage electricity run the risk of accidental electrocution. Electrical shock sometimes paralyzes the breathing muscles and causes cardiac arrest by interfering with the normal rhythm of the heart. It is essential for the rescuer who is initiating CPR to be careful not to inadvertently come into contact with the electric current. The rescuer must ensure that the current is de-energized before beginning CPR.
- *Sudden infant death syndrome (SIDS):* SIDS is the unexpected and sudden death of an apparently normal and healthy infant that occurs during sleep and with no evidence of disease on physical examination or autopsy. Aspects of prevention include readiness to perform early CPR and home monitoring systems.

---

cellular damage caused by lack of oxygen. The brain is the first organ damaged by this lack of oxygen. If CPR is started within 4 minutes of cardiopulmonary arrest, it may help reverse clinical death. After 10 minutes without CPR, brain death most likely occurs. Therefore, it is extremely important to begin CPR as quickly as possible. **Brain death** is an irreversible form of unconsciousness characterized by a complete loss of brain stem function while the heart may continue to beat. The legal definition of this condition varies from state to state. Brain death statutes, tests to determine brain death, and who is qualified to determine brain death in the United States differ by state and institution. Criteria regarding these variables can be found in the article *Brain Death Criteria* on the NCBI website (Aboubakr, 2021). Because hypothermia, anesthesia, poisoning, and drug intoxication have the capacity to cause a deep physiologic depression that resembles brain death, a diagnosis of brain death requires testing and evaluation according to the required criteria within the state and institution. Apnea testing, physical examination, and ancillary tests such as cerebral blood flow studies are permitted in some states to evaluate whether brain death has occurred. Brain death is sometimes referred to as *irreversible coma*. The LPN/LVN should refer to the state law and to facility policy and procedure manuals.

INITIAL ASSESSMENT AND RESPONSE

The initial assessment task in determining the need for CPR is to determine responsiveness. The trained rescuer—the nurse—should do this by gently shaking the victim and loudly asking, "Are you OK?" This precaution will prevent the nurse from injuring a person who is sleeping.

The nurse, or layperson, should call for help immediately when beginning a rescue. It is imperative to access the EMS as quickly as possible. Shout for help, make a phone call for help, or direct another person to make a phone call if another person is available. The American Heart Association (AHA) (Rumsfeld, 2016) guidelines indicate that it may be reasonable for communities to incorporate social media technologies that summon rescuers who are in proximity to a victim of suspected out of hospital cardiac arrest (OHCA) and are willing and able to perform CPR. It is vital to obtain an AED if one is available. Use the AED to treat defibrillation if necessary.

For the most successful treatment of cardiac arrest, CPR and the use of an AED should be initiated within the first 3 to 5 minutes. AEDs are available in numerous nonhospital settings such as airports, schools, and business locations for use by laypersons who determine that someone has suffered cardiac arrest (Fig. 16.1). Basic life support education for health care providers, as well as for non–health care providers, includes instruction in CPR and in how to use an AED.

CABS OF CARDIOPULMONARY RESUSCITATION

To remember the steps of one-rescuer or two-rescuer CPR, remember to spell **CAB**, a mnemonic for assessing the status of patients in an emergency:

Circulation
Airway
Breathing

Fig. 16.1 A portable automatic external defibrillator (AED). (Copyright Thinkstock Photos.)

CPR performed by the health care provider differs slightly from that performed by the layperson. The health care provider and layperson verify unresponsiveness, activate the EMS, and retrieve an AED. Both determine whether there is no breathing or abnormal breathing. Only the health care provider assesses for a carotid pulse, taking no more than 10 seconds to palpate for the pulse. The layperson does not assess for a carotid pulse.

Circulation

Respiratory arrest is possible without cardiac arrest. Once the nurse has determined that the victim is not breathing, the nurse should assess the person's pulse. Pulselessness (cardiac arrest) indicates the need for external cardiac compressions. Performing external cardiac compressions on a victim with a pulse, however, has the potential to result in injury to the victim.

To determine pulselessness, the carotid pulse is the most reliable and accessible to the nurse. Maintain the head tilt with one hand resting on the victim's forehead while assessing for the presence of a pulse. With two or three fingers of the other hand, locate the victim's thyroid cartilage. Then gently slide the fingers into the groove between the trachea and the muscles on the side of the neck until the carotid pulse is felt. Palpate the pulse gently only on one side so as not to obliterate arterial blood flow to the brain (Fig. 16.2). The absence of a pulse confirms the presence of **cardiac arrest** (sudden cessation of functional circulation).

Performing external cardiac compressions helps blood circulate to the heart, the lungs, the brain, and the rest of the body. If external cardiac compressions are performed properly, it is possible to maintain 20% to 30% of the normal output of the heart (Jiang, 2011).

Fig. 16.2 Carotid pulse assessment.

Fig. 16.3 Proper hand placement for chest compressions.

This provides enough oxygen to the body to sustain life. Proper hand position enables as much blood to be circulated as possible. Position your hands as follows (Fig. 16.3):

1. Compress the lower half of the victim's sternum in the center (middle) of the chest, between the nipples.
2. Place the heel of one hand on the victim's sternum in the center (middle) of the chest between the nipples, and then place the heel of the second hand on top of the first so that the hands overlap and are parallel.
3. It is acceptable to extend or interlace fingers, but keep them off the chest.

Proper compression technique is important for delivering the appropriate amount of force to simulate the pumping action of the heart. Compression techniques are as follows:

1. Lock elbows in place, with arms straight and shoulders positioned over hands so that the thrusts of external cardiac compressions are in a downward motion. Some of the force of the compressions will be lost if there is a rolling or rocking motion.
2. Lean forward and push, creating pressure to depress the sternum at least 2 inches (5 cm) in an adult (see the section "Pediatric Cardiopulmonary Resuscitation: Child or Infant" for the correlated information for children). This is difficult to estimate, but some give will be felt in the sternum. The motion is smooth, never rolling or jerking. Excessive depth of chest compressions (greater than 2.4 inches, or 6 cm) should be avoided in the adult to prevent damage to surrounding tissues.
3. 2015 AHA guidelines state that it is reasonable for rescuers to avoid leaning on the chest between compressions to allow full chest wall recoil for adults in cardiac arrest. This allows blood to flow into the heart. Practice is necessary to learn how to deliver good chest compressions. (During a two-person rescue, trade off with another rescuer every few minutes to minimize fatigue, which contributes to inadequate chest compression depth and rate.) Keep the time allowed for compression to approximately equal to the time for chest recoil or relaxation. Do not pause between compressions. The proper compression rate is 100 to 120 compressions per minute.

4. Maintain hand position at all times; do not lift your hands or move them in any way. Keep hands in contact with the chest.

Complications of external chest compressions include lacerated liver, fractured ribs, and fractured sternum, as well as bruising or bleeding of the liver, the lungs, and the spleen. Do not let any concern for possible injuries from CPR interfere with its prompt and efficient application.

The sequencing of breathing to external compressions in one-rescuer and two-rescuer CPR is discussed next.

Airway

Assess the victim's airway to confirm the absence of breathing and to establish a patent airway. If there is no evidence of head or neck trauma, use the head-tilt/chin-lift maneuver to open the airway (Fig. 16.4A). Place one hand on the victim's forehead and apply firm backward pressure to tilt the head back. Place the fingers of the other hand under the jaw (avoiding the soft tissue under the chin) to lift the chin forward.

> ⚠ **Safety Alert**
>
> If a neck injury is suspected, establish the airway by using the jaw-thrust (or chin-lift) maneuver without tilting the head. To perform the jaw-thrust maneuver, grasp the angle of the victim's lower jaw with your hands on both sides of the jaw and bring the mandible forward, while keeping the neck in straight alignment and not tilting the head back (see Fig. 16.4B). Attempt again to establish whether spontaneous breathing is present once the airway is open.

Breathing

Mouth-to-mouth ventilation is the quickest method of supplying oxygen to the victim's lungs. The rescuer's exhaled air has enough oxygen to supply the victim's needs until life-support systems take over. Maintain the head-tilt/chin-lift position and an airtight seal throughout rescue breathing. If the victim has a pulse, initiate rescue breathing at a rate of one breath every 6 to 8 seconds or 8 to 10 times/min in an adult (see the section "Pediatric Cardiopulmonary Resuscitation:

Fig. 16.4 (A) Head-tilt/chin-lift maneuver. (B) Jaw-thrust maneuver.

Child or Infant"). Cardiac arrest follows if respiratory arrest continues.

To preserve the open airway, kneel by the victim's shoulders. To gently pinch the nostrils closed, use the thumb and the index finger of the same hand that he or she is using to maintain the head tilt. Take a deep breath, seal the lips around the outside of the victim's mouth (creating an airtight seal), and give two full breaths lasting 1 second each. This method is used to keep gastric distention to a minimum and decrease the potential for the victim to vomit, which sometimes results from receiving rapid breaths and excessive air volume. Allow the victim to exhale passively. When a mask is available, mouth-to-mask ventilation is performed (Fig. 16.5). Mouth-to-mask ventilation with a one-way valve prevents the transfer of microorganisms from the victim to the rescuer.

If your initial attempt to ventilate the victim is unsuccessful, reposition the head and again attempt to ventilate. Improper chin and head position is the most common reason for difficulty with ventilation. If the second attempt at ventilation is also unsuccessful, commence procedures to manage airway obstruction by a foreign body (see later discussion).

STEPS FOR ADULT ONE-RESCUER CARDIOPULMONARY RESUSCITATION

1. Determine unresponsiveness.
2. Determine breathlessness.
3. Call for help. Activate the EMS system.

Circulation
1. Determine pulselessness.
2. If pulse is present, continue rescue breathing about 8 to 10 times/min, or one breath every 6 to 8 seconds. Activate the EMS system.
3. If pulse is not present, perform 30 chest compressions at a rate of at least 100 per minute. Count "one, two, three, four, five" until you have done 30 compressions, and follow them with two slow breaths. The rescuer must be sure to provide chest compressions of the proper depth and rate to provide 100 to 120 beats/min. In order to maintain this

Fig. 16.5 Mouth-to-mask ventilation.

rate of compressions the lay person may use songs such as "Stayin' Alive" by the Bee Gees, "Crazy in Love" by Beyoncé featuring Jay-Z, "Hips Don't Lie" by Shakira, or "Walk the Line" by Johnny Cash to maintain the rate.
4. Continue with 30 compressions and two slow breaths until an AED becomes available or help arrives.

Airway
Open the victim's airway using the head-tilt/chin-lift maneuver. Gently lift the chin forward to help open the victim's airway. If the victim has a suspected neck injury, use the jaw-thrust (or chin-lift) maneuver without tilting the head.

Breathing
1. If the victim is not breathing, give two slow breaths (1 second each). Allow for exhalation between breaths.
2. If unable to give two breaths, reposition the victim's head and reattempt to ventilate.
3. If still unable to give two breaths, proceed with procedures to manage airway obstruction by a foreign body.

ADULT TWO-RESCUER CARDIOPULMONARY RESUSCITATION

Because CPR expends a great deal of energy, it is less fatiguing if two rescuers perform CPR. If the EMS system has not been activated already, direct the second rescuer to initiate CPR before starting to assist with CPR.

The rescuer at the victim's head is referred to as the "ventilator," and the rescuer at the victim's chest is referred to as the "compressor." The ventilator should determine responsiveness. If there is no response, the ventilator assesses for breathlessness for 5 to 10 seconds. The compressor or a bystander should activate the EMS and call for an AED. The ventilator should assess for pulselessness for 5 to 10 seconds. If the victim has a pulse, the ventilator should initiate rescue breathing at a rate of one breath every 6 to 8 seconds, or 8 to 10 times/min, for an adult victim. If the victim does not have a pulse, then the compressor starts compressions. The compression: ventilation ratio for two-person CPR is 30 chest compressions for every 2 breaths. Exhalation occurs during chest compressions. The compression rate for two-person CPR is at least 100 per minute. The rescuer performing chest compressions is more likely to become fatigued. The rescuers should switch positions every five cycles of 2 minutes to continue effective CPR.

The switch is initiated by the rescuer performing chest compressions at the end of a 30:2 sequence. After giving a breath, the ventilator moves to the chest and gets into position to give compressions. The compressor moves to the victim's head and checks the pulse for 5 to 10 seconds. If no pulse is felt, he or she gives the command, "Resume CPR," and compressions are restarted, followed by breaths.

PEDIATRIC CARDIOPULMONARY RESUSCITATION: CHILD OR INFANT

The basic steps of CPR and procedures to manage airway obstruction by a foreign body are the same whether the victim is an infant, a child, or an adult. For the purpose of basic life support, an *infant* is defined as anyone younger than 1 year of age, and a *child* is defined as anyone between age 1 year and puberty. First determine unresponsiveness. A child may be gently shaken, but with an infant, try gently tapping the infant's heels.

Position the victim on a firm, flat surface for the best CPR effectiveness. It is sometimes advantageous to carry a small child or infant while performing CPR, although this technique is not as effective.

Use the head-tilt/chin-lift or jaw-thrust technique to open the airway of a child while taking care not to hyperextend an infant's neck because this sometimes allows the infant's shorter trachea to become occluded. In the case of a head injury, do not tilt the head but use the jaw-thrust technique instead. Caution is necessary

with suspected neck injuries in infants and children as it is in adult cases.

After establishing that the airway is open, look for movement of the chest, listen for breath sounds, and feel for exhaled airflow. If the infant or child is not breathing, the nurse should begin the CAB sequence.

Circulation

Check for circulation by assessing the pulse on the carotid artery in a child and the brachial artery in an infant. If there is a pulse, continue rescue breathing at a rate of one breath every 6 to 8 seconds. If there is no pulse or pulse is less than 60 beats/min, begin to perform external cardiac compressions.

Airway

Use the head-tilt/chin-lift or jaw-thrust technique to open the airway of a child or infant.

Breathing

When providing breathing, give two breaths (1 second per breath). The volume of air in an infant's lungs is smaller than that in an adult's, so adjust your breaths to allow for appropriate rise and fall of the chest. A good rule of thumb is usually to use the amount of air for the infant that an adult is able to hold in the cheeks. Gastric distention is common in infants and children during CPR as a result of overinflation of the lungs.

When performing external cardiac compressions in the infant, do the following (this technique is preferred for infants when two health care providers are present):
1. Visualize an imaginary line between the nipples.
2. Use two fingers to perform chest compressions.
   a. Place two fingers about one fingerbreadth below the nipple line. Fig. 16.6A, demonstrates position of fingers for proper compression technique for one-rescuer infant CPR; Fig. 16.6B demonstrates position of fingers for proper compression technique for two-rescuer infant CPR.
3. The breastbone is compressed to a depth of at least one third the diameter of the chest, or 1.5 inches (4 cm), at a rate of at least 100 times/min. Count aloud very quickly: "One, two, three, four, five." Perform the compression-and-release action smoothly. It has been recommended to "think" the count rather than counting aloud; it is easy to lose count because the rate is so fast.
4. At the end of each compression, release pressure and allow the sternum to return to normal position without removing hands from their placement. Keep movements smooth, not jerky.
5. The sequence of compressions to ventilation is 30:2 (30 compressions to 2 breaths). If there are two health care provider rescuers, the sequence is 15:2 (15 compressions to 2 breaths).

Fig. 16.6 (A) Position of fingers for proper compression technique for one-rescuer cardiopulmonary resuscitation (CPR) in an infant. (B) Position of fingers for proper compression technique for two-rescuer CPR in an infant.

When performing cardiac compressions on a child, do the following:

1. Compress the chest with the heel of one hand at the nipple line at a depth of at least one-third the diameter of the chest, or 2 inches (5 cm), at least 100 times/min. Make sure that the fingers do not touch the ribs.
2. Keep the compressions smooth, allowing the chest to return to the natural position after each compression.
3. The sequence is 30 compressions to 2 breaths. If two health care providers are performing the rescue, the sequence is 15:2 (15 compressions to 2 ventilations).

HANDS-ONLY CARDIOPULMONARY RESUSCITATION

In their 2017 update, the AHA recommends that bystanders who are not trained in conventional CPR use only their hands without the rescue breathing in the crucial moments after they witness an out-of-hospital sudden cardiac arrest (AHA, n.d.). The AHA recommends that if a person witnesses a sudden collapse of an adult, and the victim is unresponsive, it is best to call 911 and start chest compressions "hard and fast" in the middle of the chest. Many times people nearby do not help because they are not confident in what they are doing and fear that they will hurt the victim. If the bystander is not trained in CPR or is not confident in being able to perform rescue breathing, performing hands-only CPR is the best response. Optimally, this continues until EMS arrives or an AED is made available.

Several studies have found that among people with OHCA, survival numbers were comparable between those who received chest compressions only and those who received conventional CPR (AHA, n.d.). People probably are more likely to assist with CPR if hands-only is used because they are much less likely to come into contact with microorganisms from the victim.

PROCEDURES TO MANAGE AIRWAY OBSTRUCTION BY A FOREIGN BODY

Food, particularly meat, is the most common cause of choking or airway obstruction in adults. Factors that contribute to this include large or poorly chewed

Fig. 16.7 Victims typically clutch the neck when experiencing airway obstruction.

pieces of food, talking while eating, the ingestion of alcohol, the use of sedatives, loose-fitting dentures, and neurologic deficits. In addition to food, foreign objects (e.g., marbles, balloons, beads, buttons) are the most common cause of airway obstruction in children.

If the victim can cough forcibly, the air exchange is good, although there may be wheezing between coughs. The rescuer should *not interfere* with the victim at this point. Monitor the victim closely because it is possible that air exchange may regress to a poor state.

The victim experiencing poor air exchange is likely to have a weak, ineffective cough; make a high-pitched, "crowing" noise while inhaling; exhibit increased respiratory difficulty; and develop cyanosis. With complete airway obstruction, the victim is not able to speak, breathe, or cough and sometimes clutches the neck (Fig. 16.7). This sign is a universal distress signal. To assess the inability to speak, ask the victim, "Are you choking?" Complete airway obstruction will prevent oxygen from entering the lungs and being circulated to the brain and vital organs. Unless prompt action is initiated, the victim will become unconscious, and death will result.

Fig. 16.8 Abdominal thrusts.

The following maneuver is the most effective method of removing foreign bodies that obstruct the airway.

CONSCIOUS VICTIM

Abdominal thrusts given just above the victim's navel—an emergency procedure for dislodging a bolus of food or other obstruction from the trachea to prevent asphyxiation—are recommended for relieving airway obstruction by a foreign body. These thrusts put pressure on the diaphragm, forcing air from the lungs to move and expel the foreign object. If the victim is in a sitting position, stand behind the victim and wrap your arms around the victim's waist. Then make a fist with one hand and place the thumb of the fist against the middle of the victim's abdomen, slightly above the navel and well below the tip of the xiphoid process. Wrap the other hand over the fist to provide added force. Then press the fist into the victim's abdomen with a quick upward thrust (Fig. 16.8). Repeat each thrust until the foreign body is expelled or the victim becomes unconscious. If the victim is pregnant or obese, chest thrusts are acceptable instead of abdominal thrusts. To provide chest thrusts, place your hands in the same position that is used for chest compressions during CPR.

UNCONSCIOUS VICTIM

If a victim becomes unconscious, lay him or her down in a face-up (supine) position. Blind finger sweeps are no longer recommended. Attempt to remove an object from the victim's mouth only if the object is visible. Check for the object each time you prepare to provide breaths.

Open the airway and attempt to ventilate (if the foreign body has been successfully dislodged, the victim may require artificial respirations and possibly external cardiac compressions). If ventilation is unsuccessful, perform five abdominal thrusts. To perform abdominal thrusts on an unconscious victim, kneel astride the victim's thighs and place the heel of one hand against the victim's abdomen in the midline slightly above the navel but well below the tip of the xiphoid process. Keep the second hand on top of the first hand for additional force. Press into the abdomen with a quick, upward thrust. Open the victim's mouth again and look for the foreign object. The steps should be repeated

Fig. 16.9 Clearing airway obstruction in an infant. (A) The infant is held face down and supported. Five quick, forceful blows are given with the heel of the hand. (B) In the back-lying position, two fingers are placed in the center of the infant's breastbone and five quick downward thrusts are given.

until the foreign body is dislodged and spontaneous breathing is restored. If spontaneous breathing is not restored, initiate CPR.

INFANT

Of all deaths from foreign body aspiration, many occur in infants. Aspirated materials include food, such as candies and nuts, and small objects. Infants and children experience acute respiratory distress with coughing, gagging, and stridor (harsh sound during respirations, high-pitched and resembling the blowing of wind, caused by obstruction of the air passage). The victim often becomes unconscious.

If assisting a child who has aspirated a foreign body, treat the child in a manner similar to that for an adult with performance of abdominal thrusts. However, there is a potential for injury with use of this maneuver in an infant. Use a combination of back blows and chest thrusts with an infant as follows:

1. Straddle the infant over your arm with the head lower than the trunk and the face down, and support the infant firmly at the jaw.
2. Rest the arm holding the infant on your thigh and deliver five back blows between the infant's shoulders with the heel of the hand of the other arm (Fig. 16.9A).
3. Place the free hand on the infant's back so that the victim is sandwiched between the two hands, one supporting the neck, jaw, and chest while the other supports the back.

4. While continuing to support the head and neck, turn the infant and place the infant on the thighs with the head lower than the trunk (see Fig. 16.9B).
5. Perform five chest thrusts with the hands in the same position as when performing external cardiac compressions (see Fig. 16.6).
6. Never use the blind finger-sweep technique because it is possible to cause the foreign body to become lodged within the airway. If you can see the object when the infant's mouth is open, attempt to remove it.

SHOCK

Shock is an abnormal condition of inadequate blood flow to the body's peripheral tissues (decreased tissue perfusion). The cardiovascular system fails to provide sufficient blood circulation (oxygen, nutrients, hormones, and electrolytes) to the body's tissues and major organs, and metabolic waste removal is decreased. Shock results in life-threatening cellular dysfunction, hypotension, and **oliguria** (diminished amount of urine formation, less than 500 mL of urine produced within 24 hours). To maintain circulatory homeostasis, there are several mechanisms that are necessary for the body to perform. The heart must function efficiently enough to circulate blood, and a sufficient volume of blood must be available. The vascular system must be capable of maintaining adequate circulation. The heart pumps oxygen-rich blood to the capillaries and cells. Glucose, oxygen, and essential nutrients are provided to the cells, and carbon dioxide is returned to the right side of the heart. Inability of the body to compensate for failure of one or more of these mechanisms results in shock.

CLASSIFICATION OF SHOCK

Shock is classified according to its cause. The most common causes of shock are severe loss of blood, intense pain, extensive trauma, burns, poisons, emotional stress or intense emotions, extremes of heat and cold, electrical injury, allergic reactions, and a sudden or severe illness. Box 16.3 provides several examples of types of shock.

ASSESSMENT

The signs and symptoms of shock are sometimes disguised by other signs of injury, and some often appear only in the late stages of shock. When assessing the patient for shock, monitor for the development of clinical manifestations in the following areas:

- *Level of consciousness:* The victim tends to experience changes in behavior, restlessness, anxiety, disorientation, syncope, and agitation. As the condition worsens, the victim becomes more lethargic. Coma and death are possible.
- *Skin:* The skin becomes cool and clammy. The skin and mucous membranes become pale and ashen. As shock progresses, **cyanosis** (slightly bluish, grayish,

---

| Box 16.3 | **Types of Shock** |

- *Anaphylactic shock:* Anaphylaxis (an exaggerated hypersensitivity reaction to a previously encountered antigen) results from a sudden, severe, allergic reaction to a foreign substance. Shock occurs because of the sudden decrease in the amount of circulating blood caused by the sudden release of histamine, which creates capillary hyperpermeability, which in turn causes the release of plasma through the capillary walls.
- *Cardiogenic shock:* This type results from poor heart function that results from various cardiovascular abnormalities. The heart is unable to maintain sufficient blood pressure to all body parts.
- *Hypovolemic shock* (also known as *hemorrhagic shock*): This type is caused by a decrease in fluid volume from bleeding, prolonged vomiting, or diarrhea, or by loss of fluid as a result of surgery, trauma, or burns.
- *Neurogenic shock:* This type is caused by the nervous system's failure to maintain normal contraction of the blood vessels. Common causes are spinal anesthesia, quadriplegia, or medications that cause vasodilation, which create a condition in which the blood pressure is lower because there is not enough blood to fill the dilated blood vessels.
- *Psychogenic shock syncope:* This type is caused by the nervous system's reaction to an emotional stimulus. The blood vessels dilate temporarily, decreasing blood flow to the brain, which results in unconsciousness, or syncope.
- *Septic shock:* This type results from severe infection. Toxins from the microorganisms cause loss of fluid through the blood vessel walls. This often is seen in people who have other infections such as a urinary tract infection or wound infection; in patients who recently have had surgery; in people receiving chemotherapy; or in other conditions that result in immunocompromised functioning, such as acquired immunodeficiency syndrome (AIDS).

---

slatelike, or dark purple discoloration of the skin, especially of the lips and nail beds, caused by an excess of deoxygenated hemoglobin in the blood) develops, and the victim appears dehydrated.
- *Blood pressure:* Initially the blood pressure is often normal, but as shock progresses, there is a steady decrease in blood pressure, and capillary refill time is delayed. In hypovolemic shock, hypotension is a late manifestation.
- *Pulse:* The pulse rate usually increases (**tachycardia,** abnormal rapidity of heart action, usually defined as a heart rate of more than 100 beats/min in an adult) in all types of shock. The pulse also becomes weak and thready.
- *Respirations:* The respiratory rate increases. Respirations are also frequently shallow, rapid, labored, or irregular as a result of vasoconstriction in the lungs, which causes fluid to accumulate.
- *Urinary output:* With decreased circulation of fluid volume, the patient may develop oliguria.

- *Neuromuscular system:* Decreased oxygen to the tissues results in weakness or tremors of the arms and legs. Eyelids close, and the pupils dilate.
- *Gastrointestinal system:* Because of loss of fluids and fluid shifts, the victim complains of thirst. Nausea, vomiting, and dryness of mucous membranes are also possible.

NURSING INTERVENTIONS

It is essential to treat shock immediately. Priority interventions are to establish an airway, control bleeding if present, and provide fluid replacement. Place the patient in a supine position with the legs 6 to 12 inches higher than the head as long as this does not cause the victim any increase in pain (Fig. 16.10A). This position helps improve venous flow to the right side of the heart and to the vital organs and helps increase cardiac output.

When a patient is in shock, hypotension is possible. Trendelenburg's position is not recommended. If you suspect that the patient may have head, neck, or spinal injuries, keep the victim flat and do not move him or her unless absolutely necessary to prevent further

Fig. 16.10 Body positions for shock. (A) Supine position with patient's legs elevated 6 to 12 inches. (B) Position for patients with suspected head, neck, or spinal injuries. (C) Position for patients with breathing problems.

injury (see Fig. 16.10B). If the victim is unconscious or is vomiting or bleeding around the nose and mouth, position him or her on the side to allow the airway to clear and to encourage drainage. Elevate the head and shoulders if the victim is having problems breathing (see Fig. 16.10C).

It is important to maintain the shock victim's body temperature. Wrapping the patient in blankets or other available material helps prevent heat loss. Foods and fluids are withheld in case the victim has internal injuries, which necessitate immediate surgical intervention. Provide the victim with a moistened cloth to help relieve dryness of the mouth or mucous membranes. In a clinical setting, venous access is established, usually with two large-bore intravenous catheters (ideally 14- to 16-gauge) to facilitate rapid administration of fluids and blood products if needed.

If an injury is present, pain control should be addressed. Nursing interventions include positioning, adjusting tight or uncomfortable clothing or bandages, and avoiding rough handling. Do not give analgesics or drugs unless directed by a health care provider. Victims experiencing shock are likely to be very frightened, so it is essential for the nurse to give emotional support and reassurance.

BLEEDING AND HEMORRHAGE

An average adult has approximately 5 to 6 L (8 to 12 pints) of blood circulating in the bloodstream. Blood is necessary to transport oxygen and nutrients to all parts of the body. The body may compensate for some degree of blood loss without any changes noted, but at some point, the effects of blood loss become evident. The body attempts to cause clotting of the blood to halt bleeding. Clotting usually requires 6 to 7 minutes. Bleeding, if uncontrolled, can result in shock and death.

TYPES OF BLEEDING

Bleeding from a wound may occur through one or more of the following three sources: capillaries, veins, and arteries. Capillary bleeding results from damaged or broken capillaries and is characteristic from wounds such as the oozing that occurs with minor cuts, scratches, and abrasions. This is the most common type of external hemorrhage.

Venous bleeding occurs when a vein is severed or punctured. The result is a slow, even flow of dark red blood. Besides shock from blood volume loss, a danger of venous bleeding is the entrance of air into the severed vein, which creates the risk of an **air embolism** (an abnormal circulatory condition in which air travels through the bloodstream and becomes lodged in a blood vessel) that travels to the vital organs, including the heart, lungs, and brain.

Arterial bleeding is the least common type of injury because arteries are located deep in the body and

Fig. 16.11 Applying pressure to a wound site.

usually are protected by bones, fat, and other structures. When an artery is severed or punctured, the bleeding is characterized by the heavy spurting of bright red blood in the rhythm of the heartbeat. The following arteries are the most common sites of arterial bleeding:

- Brachial (in the medial aspect of the upper arm)
- Carotid (on either side of the neck)
- Femoral (in the upper thigh and groin)
- Radial (in the medial aspect of the lower arm)

NURSING INTERVENTIONS

Direct Pressure

The most effective general treatment of bleeding is to apply direct pressure over the bleeding site. The LPN/ LVN should place a gauze dressing or the cleanest material possible over the wound and apply firm pressure with a gloved hand (Fig. 16.11). Then apply a bandage and secure it snugly over the wound to exert direct pressure. This can be accomplished by tying a knot in the bandage over the wound or by using an elasticized securing bandage. If bleeding continues after the bandage is applied, the nurse should resume pressure with a gloved hand over the bandage. Bleeding usually is controlled in 10 to 30 minutes. Do not allow anyone but a health care provider to remove the bandage while exerting direct pressure, even if it becomes saturated with blood. Instead, place an additional layer of dressing on top of the saturated bandage and continue firm pressure. Some studies advocate the practice of elevating the bleeding body part above the level of the heart, while other studies indicate this is not effective. Unless contraindicated by an injury such as a fracture, elevation is suggested if bleeding is not being controlled by applying pressure as described above.

Application of a Tourniquet to an Extremity

Bleeding is usually controlled with direct pressure. Use a tourniquet *only* when this has failed, the provider has been trained in tourniquet application, and the victim's life is in danger. Extensive damage to the affected extremity is possible because of the cessation of arterial blood flow to the area. A tourniquet also has the capacity to damage nerves and vessels directly below or under the tourniquet. An improperly, loosely applied tourniquet does not stop arterial flow but does hinder venous flow. Tourniquet use often is considered beyond the scope of first aid and of persons acting in good faith, such as a Good Samaritan, and usually is restricted to professionals such as health care providers and paramedics. Skill 16.1 provides steps to follow in applying a tourniquet.

EPISTAXIS

Epistaxis (nosebleed) is common but is seldom a serious emergency. However, profuse bleeding from the nose does have the potential to lead to shock. Epistaxis has several causes: trauma (especially a direct blow to the nose); epistaxis digitorum (self-inflicted local digital trauma from nasal picking); infections, including the common cold; snorting cocaine; overuse of nasal sprays; high blood pressure; strenuous activity; hemophilia; and low humidity in winter months. Epistaxis in an older adult may be caused by underlying conditions, such as hypertension. Always assess an adult's blood pressure if epistaxis is present.

Nursing Interventions

The victim experiencing epistaxis is kept in a quiet sitting position, leaning forward. If the victim is unable to sit up, it is best that he or she remain supine with the head and shoulders raised (if this position is not contraindicated by other injuries).

Other interventions include the following:

- Keep the victim's head tilted slightly forward so that blood will not run down the back of the throat and cause choking or vomiting.
- With the thumb and forefinger, apply steady pressure to the bridge of the nose for 10 to 15 minutes before releasing.
- Remind the victim to breathe through the mouth and to expectorate any accumulated blood.
- Apply ice compresses over the nose, which may help control bleeding.
- Look in the victim's mouth at the back of the throat to assess for bleeding from a posterior site.

If bleeding continues despite interventions, seek medical assistance because it is possible that the victim is bleeding from a posterior site, which could necessitate fluid replacement and an emergency procedure to control bleeding.

INTERNAL BLEEDING

Internal bleeding is a potentially life-threatening situation. It is difficult to diagnose and often progresses rapidly. Common causes include fractures, knife or bullet wounds, crush injuries, organ injuries, and medical conditions such as aneurysm rupture.

Skill 16.1   Applying a Tourniquet[a]

CHECK   GATHER   HELLO   ID   PRIVACY   EXPLAIN   WASH   GLOVES

NURSING ACTION *(RATIONALE)*

1. Use a strong, wide, flat piece of material, if possible (e.g., towel, necktie, wide belt). *(Never use rope or wire, which has the potential to cut the skin.)*

2. Apply a pad (piece of cloth, handkerchief, dressing) over the artery to be compressed. *(Prevents damage to the skin.)*

3. Place the tourniquet 2–4 inches proximal to the injury site and do not cross a joint. *(Prevents undue pressure on the injured site.)* Wrap the material around the limb twice, and tie a half-knot on the upper surface of the limb. *(Secures tourniquet in place.)*

4. Place a stick or rod (approximately 6 inches long) over the knot, and secure it in place. *(Enhances effect of tourniquet.)*

5. Twist the stick enough times to stop the bleeding. *(A tighter twist poses a risk for additional injury.)*

6. Secure the stick firmly with the free ends of the tourniquet. Do not cover the tourniquet. *(Tourniquet must be clearly visible to medical personnel.)*

7. Write "T" (meaning tourniquet) and the time it was applied, on the victim's forehead. Attach a note to the victim's clothing describing the time and location of the tourniquet application. *(Ensures further interventions. A tourniquet allowed to remain in place too long poses the risk of further injury.)*

8. Treat the victim for shock, and transport him or her to the nearest medical facility. Reassess the injury every 2–3 min. *(Ensures timely interventions.)*

9. Always seek medical attention once a tourniquet has been applied. *(Consistent treatment is necessary.)*

From Tactical Emergency Causality Care (TECC) Guidelines for BLS/ALS Medical Providers. March 2019. Retrieved from: http://www.c-tecc.org/images/4-2019_TECC_ALS_BLS_Guidelines_.pdf.

Assessment

All the signs and symptoms of shock are often present. Initially, some victims experience only vertigo (dizziness). Some victims expectorate blood (**hemoptysis**) or vomit blood (**hematemesis**). Dark, tarry stool (**melena**) or blood in the urine (**hematuria**) may occur. Pain, tenderness, or a dislocation at the site of a suspected injury indicates possible internal bleeding, as does bleeding from the mouth, rectum, or any other body opening.

Nursing Interventions

Internal bleeding is a priority medical emergency. Make every effort to obtain medical care immediately. Victims receiving anticoagulant therapy are likely to develop significant blood loss from minor injury. Significant blood loss also occurs in some victims with a history of alcohol abuse, as well as victims with blood dyscrasias.

The victim is placed on a flat surface with legs elevated 6 to 12 inches if this is not contraindicated by other injuries. Initiate treatment for shock. Place a cold compress or ice on the area of the suspected injury. Do not apply the ice directly to the skin because it can damage the tissue; place a towel or clean cloth between the ice and the skin. The victim's body temperature should be maintained with blankets, and the victim's vital signs should be assessed every 5 minutes. Withhold foods and fluids in case surgical intervention is necessary. Administer oxygen as ordered by the health care provider. Provide the victim with emotional support and reassurance to help decrease his or her anxiety.

WOUNDS AND TRAUMA

A *wound* is an injury to the internal or external soft tissues of the body. The basic rules for first aid treatment of wounds are as follows:

1. Stop the bleeding.
2. Treat shock.
3. Prevent infection.

CLOSED WOUNDS

Closed wounds involve the underlying tissues of the body; the top layer of skin is not broken. Examples of closed wounds are ecchymoses (discolorations of an area of the skin or mucous membrane caused by the extravasation of blood into the subcutaneous tissues; also called *bruises*), contusions (injuries that do not break the skin, caused by a blow and characterized by edema [swelling], discoloration, and pain), strains, and sprains. They most commonly occur as a result of falls, automobile accidents, or contact sports.

The following signs and symptoms are most likely to occur with a closed wound: (1) *edema* usually appears within 24 to 48 hours; (2) *discoloration* is likely to result from the formation of a hematoma (swelling containing blood): initially the discoloration is blackish blue and then turns to green or yellow within a few days; (3) *deformity* of the limbs is caused by fractures and dislocations; (4) *shock* often follows from the force of the trauma; (5) *pain* and *tenderness* at the site are possible; and (6) signs of *internal bleeding* are sometimes present.

Nursing Interventions

If the wound is small and on the patient's scalp or extremity, it may be best to apply an ice pack, along with padding, an elastic bandage, or a 4- × 4-inch abdominal dressing used for pressure. If the wound is large, monitor the patient for shock; apply cold compresses and a pressure bandage. Obtain medical assistance immediately.

OPEN WOUNDS

Open wounds are openings or breaks in the mucous membrane or skin. Regardless of the type, there is always danger of bleeding or infection. Infection is more common in wounds that do not bleed freely because active bleeding tends to flush microorganisms from the wound. There are five general types of open wounds: abrasions, punctures, incisions, lacerations, and avulsions. The following is a discussion of each of these open wound types and the appropriate nursing interventions that should be used (Fig. 16.12).

An injection of tetanus toxoid (an active immunizing agent prepared from detoxified tetanus toxin that produces an antigenic response in the body, conferring active immunity to tetanus infection) may be necessary as a general treatment for an open wound. The patient should receive the tetanus vaccine every 10 years to maintain immunity. The attending health care provider ultimately decides on administration in a given case, especially for wounds that have occurred as a result of a soiled object or are dirty.

Abrasions

Abrasions are caused by a rubbing or scraping of the outer layers of the skin. Bleeding typically is limited to oozing of blood; there is danger of infection

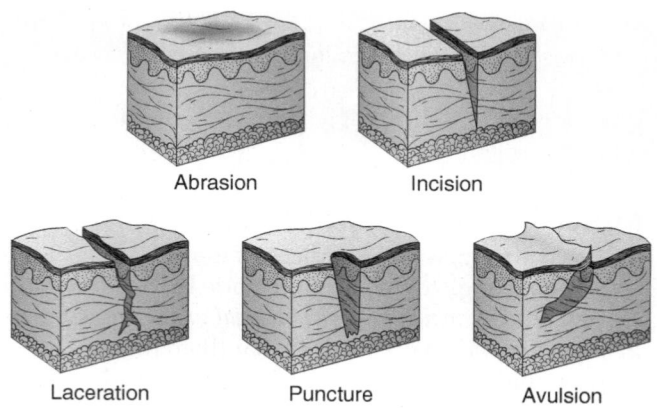

Fig. 16.12 Five types of open wounds.

from contamination with dirt and microorganisms. Examples of abrasions include rope and road burns, scratches, and scrapes of knees and elbows.

Nursing interventions. Remove all dirt, if possible. Strong antiseptics should not be used because they easily can irritate the skin. Normal saline is safe and effective, and copious irrigation with saline helps remove debris. Clean the wound from the inside out. Povidone-iodine, unless properly diluted, actually causes tissue necrosis because it is too harsh. Cover the abrasion with a sterile dressing.

Advise the victim about the signs and symptoms of infection, such as edema, erythema, pain, and purulent exudate. Instruct the victim to seek medical attention if these signs and symptoms occur.

Puncture Wounds

Puncture wounds are piercing wounds of the skin. They typically are made by knives, nails, wood, glass, or other objects that penetrate the skin. Punctures often force dirt and microorganisms deep into the tissues. If the object remains firmly in the skin, do not attempt to remove it. Leave it in place for the health care provider to remove. Removal has the potential to cause significant bleeding or other types of complications that may necessitate emergency surgical intervention.

Nursing interventions. Thoroughly irrigate all puncture wounds to remove as much debris and as many microorganisms as possible. Patients often require a tetanus booster vaccination. As with abrasions, advise the victim about signs and symptoms of infection.

Incisions

Incisions are smoothly divided wounds made by sharp instruments. Infection is not as likely to occur because blood flows freely from the wound. However, bleeding is sometimes extensive, and muscle, tendon, and nerve damage is possible. Common examples of incisional wounds include cuts from knives, broken glass, razors, or paper edges.

Nursing interventions. Carefully clean the incision and cover it with a sterile dressing. An antiseptic should be used only with a health care provider's recommendation. Typically, a butterfly bandage, Steri-Strips, or sutures are applied to hold the edges of the wound together. Help control any bleeding by applying pressure. If the incision is deep, bleeding is profuse, and function is limited, seek medical care for the patient.

Lacerations

Lacerations are wounds that are torn with jagged, irregular edges. Bleeding is often profuse, and tissue destruction and infection are possible. Auto accidents, blunt objects, and heavy machinery accidents are common causes of lacerations.

Nursing interventions. Lacerations are cleaned in a manner similar to that for abrasions and puncture wounds. Bleeding should be controlled by applying pressure (see Fig. 16.11). Use adhesive strips, Steri-Strips, or butterfly bandages to close the edges of the laceration if possible. Cover the wound with a sterile dressing, and the victim should be seen by a health care provider.

Avulsions

An avulsion is a torn piece of tissue that results in a section being completely removed or left hanging by a flap (Fig. 16.13). Avulsions are sometimes minor, with only a small amount of displaced skin, but sometimes they include large areas of tissue, with exposure of underlying bones, tendons, or muscles. Avulsions are often more difficult to heal than other types of wounds because wound edges are more difficult to approximate.

Nursing interventions. Bleeding should be controlled by direct pressure. Thoroughly cleanse the wound. Suturing is often necessary to repair an avulsion wound. Closely monitor the wound site for healing without complications.

Chest Wounds

Chest wounds are extremely dangerous and necessitate immediate medical attention. In many chest wounds, air or blood escapes into the pleural space (the potential space between the visceral and parietal layers of the pleurae). Normally this space is a vacuum created by negative pressure; therefore, air (pneumothorax) or blood (hemothorax) entering this space has the potential to cause an increase in pressure, which often results in collapse of lung tissue.

Assessment. Assess the patient for the following:
- Sharp pain at the site of the injury
- Pain associated with breathing
- Difficult and labored breathing
- Failure of one or both sides of the chest to expand normally with inspiration
- Expectoration of bright red or frothy blood (hemoptysis)

Fig. 16.13 Heel wound avulsion

- Signs and symptoms of shock: rapid, weak, thready pulse; vertigo; and hypotension
- Cyanosis of the skin and mucous membranes
- A sucking or hissing sound as air flows in and out of the chest
- Distention of the neck and arm veins
- Anxiety
- Tracheal deviation

Nursing interventions. For the first aid treatment of penetrating chest wounds, if the chest wall has been penetrated by a sharp object, do *not* remove the object; this sometimes results in further bleeding and the entrance of air into the chest wound. Instead, immobilize the object with dressings and tape. It is sometimes necessary to elevate the victim's head slightly to help facilitate breathing.

If there is a sucking chest wound (without the penetrating object in place), apply an airtight dressing. Any available material is acceptable to use: gauze, plastic wrap, clothing, or even a hand, if that is the only thing available. It is necessary for this dressing to be large enough that it is not sucked into the hole in the victim's chest and as airtight as possible. Monitor the victim for any signs and symptoms of a developing pneumothorax. Any signs of increased respiratory distress indicate the possible development of a tension pneumothorax. In that case, leave one side of the dressing untaped. Liquids should be withheld because aspiration is possible.

For the first aid treatment of crushing chest wounds, understand that the most common injury to the chest is fractured ribs. Severe blunt trauma sometimes results in flail chest (two or more ribs fractured in two or more places, resulting in instability in part of the chest wall) with associated hemothorax, pneumothorax, and

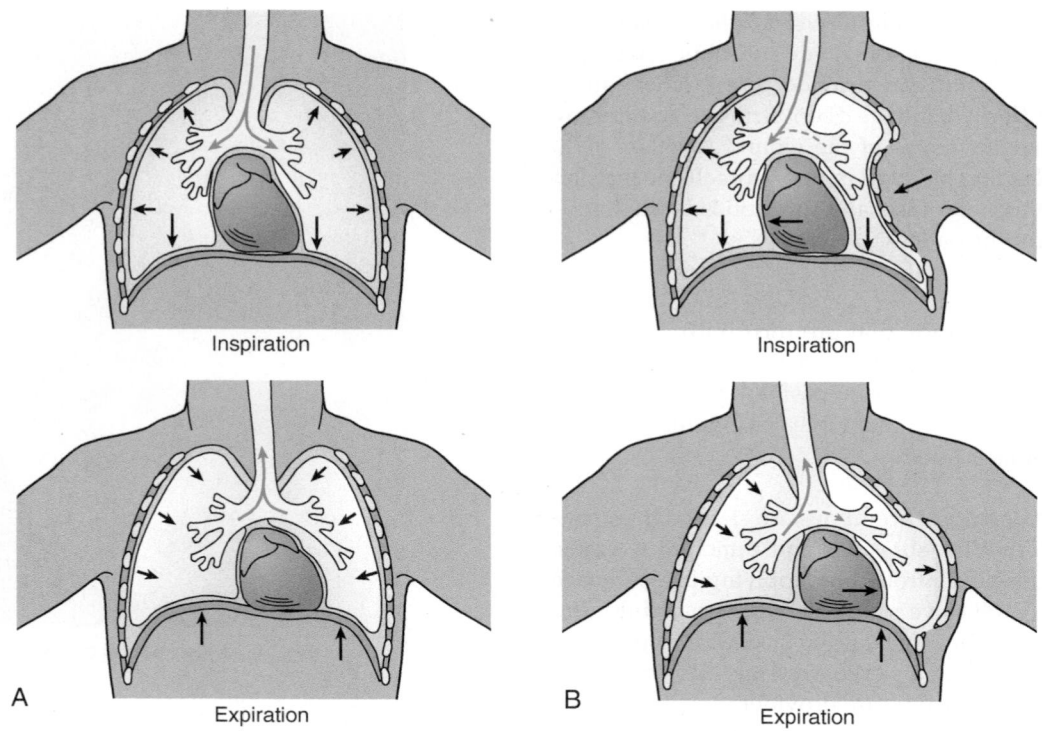

Inspiration   Inspiration

A   Expiration   B   Expiration

Fig. 16.14 (A) Normal inspiration and expiration (B) Inspiration and expiration with flail chest.

pulmonary contusion (Fig. 16.14). Paradoxic motion develops as a result of the instability this brings about in part of the chest wall, with the lung underlying the injured area contracting on inspiration and bulging on expiration. If the condition is uncorrected, respiratory distress and hypoxia result. Elevate the victim's head and shoulders to facilitate breathing if a spinal injury is not suspected. The American Heart Association currently recommends that no dressing be placed over the open chest wound during first aid care.

DRESSINGS AND BANDAGES

General Principles of Bandaging

First control bleeding before applying a sterile bandage. If sterile equipment is not available, use the cleanest material possible. The dressing should cover the entire wound and be tight enough to control bleeding but not as tight as a tourniquet. Tourniquets have the potential to cause tissue and nerve damage.

Always bandage the part in the desired alignment; do not bend a joint after it is bandaged. Tips of the fingers and the toes should be left exposed, if possible, so that the victim's circulation can be assessed. It is critical to assess for edema and adequate circulation frequently. If loose material is used for the bandage, tie it with a knot over the top of open wounds to help apply pressure and control bleeding, unless this is contraindicated.

Application of Common Types of Bandages

Bandage compress. The bandage compress is the most common type of dressing. It consists of several thicknesses of gauze covered with tape, roller gauze, or other materials. These bandages are used to control bleeding.

Triangular bandage. The triangular bandage is made of a piece of cloth that is folded diagonally and cut along the fold. Nurses use this most commonly as a sling to support injured bones. Skill 16.2 describes the application of an arm sling with a triangular bandage.

Gauze bandage. Rolls of gauze bandage are used to support an injured part, apply pressure to a dressing for control of bleeding, or secure a splint to immobilize a part (Fig. 16.15). The roll of gauze bandages is applied uniformly to ensure even pressure. The skin should be covered completely. It is best to use a greater number of evenly spaced overlapping turns rather than fewer, tighter turns of the bandage. Begin application of the gauze bandage at the point of the dressing or at the part of the limb with the smallest circumference (e.g., the wrist or the ankle). Gauze bandages are secured with either tape or a square knot. A circular or spiral roll of gauze bandages is used to cover a cylindric part. A figure-8 bandage is another option, especially if splints are necessary or when a dressing is applied to an ankle (see Chapter 22).

POISONS

Each year thousands of people die from self-inflicted or accidental poisonings. The majority of these people are children. A *poison* is any substance (solid, liquid, or gas) that even in small amounts causes damage to

Skill 16.2   Applying an Arm Sling With a Triangular (Sling and Swathe) Bandage

NURSING ACTION *(RATIONALE)*

1. Place one end of the base of the open triangle over the uninjured shoulder. *(Prevents undue pressure on injured side.)*
2. Place the apex of the triangle behind the elbow of the injured arm. *(Facilitates usefulness of sling.)*
3. Bend the arm at the elbow with the hand elevated slightly (4–5 in [10–13 cm]). *(Enables venous return from hand and forearm and facilitates drainage from edema.)*
4. Bring the forearm across the chest and over the bandage. *(Establishes position of arm in sling.)*

5. Take the lower end of the triangle and bring it over the shoulder of the injured side. Tie the bandage

on the neck at the uninjured side so that the knot is on the side of the neck. *(Prevents pressure on cervical spine.)*

6. Twist the remaining end of the bandage and tuck it in at the elbow. *(Secures sling.)*

7. Remember to keep fingertips exposed. *(Secures sling and allows for easy assessment of circulation.)*

Figures from Proehl JA: Emergency nursing procedures, ed 4, St. Louis, 2009, Saunders.

Fig. 16.15 Use of a roll of gauze bandage.

the body or interferes with the function of its systems. Poison control centers throughout the United States are equipped to give information about poisons and methods of treatment on a 24-hour-a-day, 7-day-a-week basis. Most poisons act rapidly and thus necessitate immediate first aid.

Poison control centers need the following information:

- Patient's weight
- Patient's age
- Substance ingested, inhaled, or injected
- Amount of substance taken
- Time when substance was taken
- Any medications patient has taken
- Current status of patient

GENERAL ASSESSMENT OF POISONINGS

Acute signs and symptoms of poisonings are sometimes delayed for hours. The following are possible indications of poisonings: respiratory distress; pulmonary edema; bronchospasm; severe nausea, vomiting, or diarrhea; seizures, twitching, or paralysis; decreased level of consciousness or unconsciousness;

restlessness, delirium, agitation, or panic; color changes; pale, flushed, or cyanotic skin; signs of burns or edema around the mouth or other areas of the body; pain, tenderness, or cramps on swallowing; characteristic odor on the breath; unusual urine color (red, green, bright yellow, black, bronze); slow, labored breathing or wheezing; abnormal constriction or dilation of pupils; abnormal eye movements, such as nystagmus (constant, involuntary, cyclic movement of the eyeball); skin irritation, erythema, or edema; and shock or cardiac arrest.

INGESTED POISONS

Poison ingestion by mouth is the most common type of poisoning, especially in children. Common substances include household cleaning products such as drain cleaners, oven cleaners, laundry detergents, floor or furniture polish, rat poison, cockroach sprays and baits, diaper pail deodorants, garden and garage supplies (e.g., insecticides, gasoline), drugs, medications, food, and plants, such as poinsettias. Older adults sometimes require special precautions (see the Lifespan Considerations for older adults box).

 Lifespan Considerations
Older Adults

Accidental Overdose

Older adult patients are sometimes the victims of accidental overdose for the following reasons:

- Poor eyesight potentially leads to ingesting the wrong medication. Anyone assisting with the care of an older adult should ensure that all medications and other substances are marked clearly in large lettering.
- Confusion potentially leads to repeating a medication dosage accidentally. Use of medication boxes in which medications are organized for a week at a time helps eliminate duplicate dosing.
- Older patients often are prescribed several medications. Health care providers should be sure to document a good health history, including all medications, when providing emergency treatment.

Immediate Response

The person who determines that another person has been poisoned should call the poison control center immediately (1-800-222-1222) to describe the poison ingested and to receive instructions. The poison control center will give instructions for any treatment to start in the home or recommend immediately bringing the patient to an emergency center for treatment. The poison control center number should be kept by the telephone in the home and programmed into a person's cell phone for easy access. Using syrup of ipecac is no longer recommended to induce vomiting of ingested toxins (see Chapter 10).

Treat the patient for clinical manifestations associated with shock and, if necessary, administer CPR.

Ensure that the substance's container and any vomitus are brought to the medical facility to help identify and treat the poison. No one should ever give an antidote until consulting with the poison control center.

INHALED POISONS

Poisons that can be inhaled are often present without anyone's knowledge, and thus there may be no advance warning of a problem. Once inhaled, poisons are absorbed very rapidly; therefore, prompt first aid measures are important. Common sources of inhaled poisons include carbon monoxide (from automobiles, fires, heating systems, propane engines, and paint remover), carbon dioxide (from sewers or industry), and refrigeration gases. Chlorine (used in cleaning and industry) and other spray and liquid chemicals also have the potential to give off poisonous fumes, typically when cleaning chemicals are mixed together.

Nursing Interventions

Before assisting any victim of an inhaled poison, first assess the danger. The victim should be removed from the area of exposure as soon as possible, but only if there is no danger to the nurse or any other rescuers. Loosen clothing from the victim's throat and chest, and assess the victim to determine whether CPR is necessary. The victim should be kept quiet and inactive while being transported immediately to the nearest medical facility.

ABSORBED POISONS

Poisons, caustic chemicals, and substances from poisonous plants that come in contact with the skin often are absorbed rapidly, causing burning, skin irritation, allergic responses, or severe systemic reactions. Most signs and symptoms occur within 1 to 2 hours after absorption. Signs and symptoms include nausea, vomiting, diarrhea, flushed skin, dilated pupils, cardiovascular abnormalities, and central nervous system and respiratory reactions. Poison ivy, poison oak, and poison sumac are the plants that most commonly elicit a poison response.

Nursing Interventions

First, quickly remove the source of the irritation and then wash the contacted area with soap and water. Skin preparations that are effective in the treatment of contact poisonings include baking soda, Burow's solution, and oatmeal. Calamine lotion and hydrocortisone cream (5%) are effective in relieving pruritus.

INJECTED POISONS

A person can develop an allergic reaction if the person is injected with a drug to which the person is allergic or if the person receives a venomous sting or bite from an insect, reptile, or animal. In addition, immediate follow-up treatment is recommended because bites from animals, reptiles, or rodents may lead to infection. Many health care practitioners prescribe prophylactic antibiotic treatment to prevent infection. If an animal is thought to be rabid, the person should wash the bite immediately with soap and water thoroughly and then seek emergency care for treatment of rabies (Immunization Action Coalition, n.d.). Wound cleansing is especially important in rabies prevention because, in animal studies, thorough wound cleansing alone without other postexposure prophylaxis has been shown to reduce markedly the likelihood of rabies (CDC, 2019). According to Johns Hopkins Medicine, emergency care for bites from a reptile such as a snake include the following (Johns Hopkins Medicine, n.d.):

- Restrict the movement of the affected extremity and keep it below heart level to reduce the amount of toxin flowing toward the heart and recirculating. Remove rings and any restrictive clothing in case swelling occurs. Wash the bite area thoroughly with soap and water
- Monitor the person for signs of shock and seek medical attention immediately. Note the time of the bite in order to report this information to the emergency room personnel
- If the area around the bite begins to swell or change color, it is likely that the snake was poisonous.
- Note the description of the snake to aid in identification of the type of snake, or take a picture of the snake if it is a safe distance from the victim.

Minor Reactions to Insect Bites

If a person has been stung by a bee or wasp, remove the stinger with gauze or some other clean material in a scraping motion. An attempt to grasp the barbed stinger with tweezers sometimes forces venom further into the skin. Nursing interventions include washing the area with soap and water and applying cold packs to relieve pain and slow the absorption of the poison. A paste of baking soda and water sometimes relieves pruritus at the site.

Severe Reactions to Insect Bites

Within as little as 60 minutes or up to several hours afterward, a victim of a bite or sting sometimes experiences a severe allergic reaction. Urticaria, wheezing, edema of the lips and tongue, generalized pruritus, and respiratory arrest are the most common signs and symptoms of anaphylactic shock (severe allergic reaction).

Nursing interventions. People who know that they have an allergy sometimes wear medical alert tags and carry an epinephrine pen, an anaphylaxis kit, or antihistamines such as diphenhydramine (Benadryl) to take after a bite. The patient may self-administer these types of medications. A health care provider may direct the nurse to administer such medications in this type of emergency situation.

DRUG AND ALCOHOL EMERGENCIES

Drugs (including alcohol) are chemical substances that have the potential to affect body functioning and are subject to abuse and overdose.

ALCOHOL

Alcohol is the most commonly abused drug in the world. It is a central nervous system depressant that has the capacity to cause many signs and symptoms, even death (Table 16.1).

Assessment

Signs and symptoms of *mild* intoxication include nausea, vomiting, diarrhea, lack of coordination, and poor muscle control. Flushing, erythema of the face and eyes, visual disturbances, and rapid mood swings are often present. Slurred or inappropriate speech, inappropriate behavior, and lethargy (sleepiness) are also typical.

Serious alcohol intoxication usually is caused by consuming a large quantity of alcohol over a short period of time. Signs and symptoms include drowsiness that progresses to coma; rapid, weak pulse; and depressed, labored breathing or respiratory arrest. Loss of control of urinary and bowel functions, and disorientation, restlessness, and hallucinations are possible, as are tremors that have the potential to progress to grand mal seizures, nausea, vomiting, expectoration of blood from the respiratory tract, and diarrhea. Some affected people also experience loss of memory, visual disturbances, lack of muscle coordination, and depressed reflexes.

DRUGS

Abuse of drugs is a major problem worldwide. Not only illegal drugs but also prescription and over-the-counter medications are abused. When assessing the drug abuser, observe for signs and symptoms of disorientation, hallucinations, and changes in the victim's level of consciousness; coma and death are possible results. Slurred speech, extremes in mood swings, inappropriate behavior, and anxiety are also present in some cases. Sometimes the victim has a fever and flushed skin and experiences diaphoresis (sweating). Because of lack of coordination and impaired judgment, safety is typically an issue. Depending on the drug, the pulse and blood pressure often increase or decrease, the pupils constrict or dilate, and the appetite increases or decreases. Hypodermic needle marks ("track marks") on arms, legs, hands, feet, and neck are often obvious. Many victims complain of diarrhea or pain in the abdomen, legs, or joints and experience tremors or seizures.

Nursing Interventions

Because an accurate nursing history is important, obtain as much information as possible about the substance ingested and identify any containers that contained the

Table 16.1 **Blood Alcohol Concentration and Related Effects**

BAC LEVEL	IMPAIRMENT
0.0%–0.05%	Mild Impairment • Mild speech, memory, attention, coordination, balance impairments • Perceived beneficial effects, such as relaxation • Sleepiness can begin
0.06%–0.15%	Increased Impairment • Perceived beneficial effects of alcohol, such as relaxation, give way to increasing intoxication • Increased risk of aggression in some people • Speech, memory, attention, coordination, balance further impaired • Increased risk of injury to self and others • Moderate memory impairments
0.16%–0.30%	Severe Impairment • Speech, memory, coordination, attention, reaction time, balance significantly impaired • All driving-related skills dangerously impaired • Judgment and decision-making dangerously impaired • Blackouts (amnesia) • Vomiting and other signs of alcohol overdose common • Loss of consciousness
0.31%–0.45%	Life Threatening • Loss of consciousness • Danger of life-threatening alcohol overdose • Significant risk of death in most drinkers due to suppression of vital life functions

aBAC generally is recorded in milligrams of alcohol per deciliter (mg/dL) of blood or in milligrams percentage (mg%). Percentage is used for legal definitions of intoxication. BAC is dependent on how much alcohol is consumed, how fast it is consumed, the person's weight, tolerance to alcohol, age, medication use, recent food ingestion, and gender.
BAC, Blood alcohol concentration.
From https://www.niaaa.nih.gov/publications/brochures-and-fact-sheets/understanding-dangers-of-alcohol-overdose

substance if possible. Life-threatening situations should be handled first. Establish and maintain the airway. If the victim is unconscious, the victim is turned onto his or her side. Loosen the victim's clothing to assist with ventilation. If the victim is having muscle twitching and is drowsy, do not arouse the victim because this may precipitate a seizure. If a fever is present, attempt to reduce the victim's temperature by applying cool, wet compresses. Victims must be protected from self-injury during a seizure or hallucination by removing potentially harmful objects from the patient's vicinity. Do not attempt to restrain a victim during seizure activity or place anything within the victim's mouth.

A calm, supportive, nonjudgmental approach is best when a victim is very agitated or excited. An intoxicated person should not be left alone. Frequently perform a careful assessment of the victim's mental status and vital signs. It is possible for a victim of substance abuse to go into respiratory arrest quickly. Ensure the victim is transported promptly to a medical facility.

THERMAL AND COLD EMERGENCIES

HEAT INJURIES

Heat exhaustion or heatstroke results when the body is unable to cool itself when exposed to excessive environmental heat. Normally the body reacts to heat with excessive perspiration and slowing of muscle activity. If excessive perspiration occurs without rehydration of

the body, heat exhaustion results. On the other hand, if the body is unable to cool itself, the internal body temperature rises, resulting in heatstroke. Heat exhaustion and heatstroke have different characteristics and treatment protocol.

Heat Exhaustion

Heat exhaustion is the most common type of heat injury and is the result of prolonged perspiration and the loss of large quantities of salt and water. It occurs most often in hot, humid weather when people do not adequately replace fluids (common in older adults, in whom the thirst mechanism is diminished even when they are dehydrated).

The nursing assessment of a victim of heat exhaustion includes assessing for signs and symptoms such as headache, vertigo, nausea, weakness, and diaphoresis.

Mental disorientation and brief loss of consciousness may occur. The victim has a normal body temperature with pale, cold, clammy skin. Some victims complain of abdominal cramps and loss of appetite. Breathing is typically rapid and shallow, and the pulse is weak and rapid. Blood pressure sometimes drops but usually returns to normal when the person assumes a recumbent position.

Nursing interventions. Move the victim to a cool area and cool off the victim as quickly as possible without inducing chilling and shivering. Chilling and shivering would cause the body temperature to rise. Remove as much of the victim's clothing as possible and loosen constrictive clothing to allow the circulation of air to cool the body. Cold, wet compresses are used to cool the victim, as well as a fan or air conditioner if available.

If the victim is completely conscious and alert, give the victim fluids. Water and sports drinks are recommended. If the victim is drowsy or vomiting, do not give any fluids by mouth. In the clinical setting, intravenous fluids are given. The victim should be transported to a medical facility as soon as possible.

Heatstroke

Heatstroke is a more serious heat injury; death is possible if heatstroke goes untreated. The most common cause of heatstroke is vigorous physical activity in a hot, humid environment. The body becomes overheated, but the cooling mechanism of perspiration is not helpful because of the hot, humid conditions. The body stores excessive heat because it is unable to cool itself properly. Body temperature sometimes rises to 106°F (41°C) or greater. Damage to the victim's brain and central nervous system may result.

Assessment. The signs and symptoms of heatstroke include rapidly rising body temperature; hot, dry, erythemic skin; and no visible perspiration. The pulse is rapid initially and then slows and weakens as the blood pressure falls. Breathing becomes deep and rapid. The victim complains of headache, dry mouth, and nausea and may vomit; some victims experience vertigo and decreased level of consciousness and may collapse. Muscle twitching and convulsions may occur.

Nursing interventions. It is important for the nurse to cool the victim as quickly as possible and to move him or her to a cooler area. If the victim is alert, he or she should receive 0.5 cup (120 mL) of fluid every 15 minutes. Water and sports drinks are acceptable. Assist the victim to lie down with the feet 6 to 12 inches higher than the head to avoid shock. Loosen the victim's clothing and remove excess clothing. Cool the victim's bare skin as quickly as possible with cool, wet cloths or with cool water directly on the victim's skin. Place cold packs around the neck, under the axillae, on the inguinal area, and around the ankles to cool the blood in the main arteries. Use a fan or air conditioner if available. Continue treatment until the victim's temperature falls below 100°F (37.7°C). Monitor the victim for chilling (control shivering because this will only increase the victim's body temperature) as the victim's temperature falls, and check the victim's temperature every 10 to 15 minutes to ensure that it does not rise again. Continue cooling efforts until the victim is able to obtain medical assistance.

EXPOSURE TO EXCESSIVE COLD

When the body is exposed to severe cold, body heat is lost, blood vessels constrict, and destruction of tissue sometimes results. Cold, moist air, fatigue, smoking, drugs, alcohol, dehydration, age, constricting clothing and footwear, and some diseases (such as diabetes mellitus or heart disease) accelerate the potential for injury.

Hypothermia

Hypothermia results when a person's body temperature drops lower than 95°F (35°C). The drop in body temperature affects all vital organs and body tissue because of lack of oxygenated blood perfusing tissues. Hypothermia occurs most frequently when the air is windy, cold, and moist, or when precipitation is present. Submersion in cold water is a common cause as well. Common risk factors for hypothermia include exhaustion, mental illness, medical conditions such as hypothyroidism, and medications such as narcotics and sedatives. Age is also a common risk factor. The very young and elderly are susceptible to hypothermia because of the body's decreased ability to regulate body temperature (Mayo Clinic, 2020).

Assessment. Initially, the victim is likely to shiver uncontrollably; shivering ceases when the body temperature is less than 90°F (32.2°C). Additional symptoms include lethargy and drowsiness, weakness and clumsiness, and confusion. Victims often become irritable and combative and may experience hallucinations or delirium. Symptoms may progress to seizures, stupor, and coma. Respiration and heart rate slow, and the victim may go into respiratory or cardiac arrest or both. Finally, there is a loss of all reflexes, and the victim appears to be dead. Severe problems with electrolyte disturbances create the risk of serious dysrhythmias and cardiac arrest.

Nursing interventions. Although some people who are profoundly hypothermic may appear to be dead because of the effects of the lowered metabolic rate, it is possible to revive many of these victims. Attempt to treat hypothermia by instituting first aid. Initiate CPR and continue it until the body is warmed. Place the victim in a supine position with the head lower than the feet to treat possible shock. Warm the victim *slowly* because rapid exposure to warmth tends to precipitate shock. The victim should be moved to a warm area, and all the victim's wet clothes should be removed and replaced with dry ones. Cover the victim with warm blankets. For a patient experiencing profound hypothermia (core temperature below 30°C), active internal rewarming in addition to passive external rewarming effectively will raise the core body temperature. Administration of warm, humidified oxygen per mask or per ventilator; warmed blankets; heat lamps; and heated intravenous fluids such as 5% dextrose in normal saline (D_5NS) ranging in temperatures from 104° to 113° to 149°F (40° to 45° to 65°C). The temperature of the solution should be raised gradually, dependent on the patient's condition. Patients in the final stages of hypothermia sometimes develop atrial fibrillation and therefore need continuous electrocardiographic monitoring during treatment and immediately afterward. Cardiac arrest may occur if rewarming efforts are not successful (Mayo Clinic, 2020).

If the victim is completely conscious, provide the victim with warm fluids to drink. Rescuers should *never* give alcohol to the victim because of its vasodilatory effect on the peripheral vessels, which causes the central core temperature to drop further. Obtain medical help as soon as possible.

Frostbite

Frostbite is the most common and dangerous local cold injury involving freezing and damaging of body cells. Ice crystals form in the body's interstitial and cellular fluid spaces as a result of the cold temperature leading to decreased blood flow, inhibiting sufficient heat to the body's tissues, and causing destruction of tissue integrity. Common areas affected by frostbite are the ears, nose, fingers, toes, and lips. Deep tissue frostbite can result in tissue death. Hypothermia sometimes accompanies frostbite (Zonnoor, 2020).

Assessment. Initially the frostbitten skin takes on a red flush, and the victim typically complains of numbness, tingling, or pain. The affected area becomes progressively hard and loses all sensation. The color of the affected area changes to grayish white as circulation diminishes further. If thawing occurs, the color often changes to bluish purple or black, indicating severe damage to or death of tissues. Edema often develops, followed by blisters. If frostbite damage is severe, complete loss of function of the part is possible.

Nursing interventions. If there is a possibility that the part will become refrozen after it has been thawed, it is better to leave it frozen until the victim arrives at a medical facility. Severe tissue damage is possible as a result of thawing and refreezing a frozen part. The victim may need to be treated for shock and hypothermia. It may be necessary to establish and maintain an airway. Remove any constricting clothing to encourage circulation.

If there is no risk that the part will become refrozen, warm it in the following manner: immerse the frozen part in warm water (preferably a bathtub) at 101° to 104°F (38.3° to 40°C) for approximately 30 minutes. Check the water temperature frequently and do not allow it to cool. If a tub is not available, use a very warm, moist towel or something similar. Be very careful *not* to rub the part because the friction may bruise and damage the underlying tissue. If water is not available, warm the part by placing it against a warm part of another person's body: the axilla, the abdomen, or between the legs. The frozen area should not be placed near an open flame or oven. Gentle warming is necessary to prevent burns and damage.

Once the part is warmed, the victim should be encouraged to gently move the part. If the legs or feet are involved, however, the victim should not be allowed to walk. The thawed part should be wrapped in clean towels or bulky dressing, and elevated. If toes or fingers are involved, they should be wrapped individually. Try to keep the entire body warm and offer warm fluids to drink. Keeping the victim hydrated is important. Alcohol should not be provided to the victim. The victim also should not be allowed to smoke because this will cause further vasoconstriction and more damage. A health care provider should evaluate all frostbite injuries, no matter how minor.

BONE, JOINT, AND MUSCLE INJURIES

The four major types of injuries that occur to bones, tendons, ligaments, and muscles are fractures, dislocations, sprains, and strains. Emergency care is initiated, and prompt medical care is obtained when these injuries occur.

FRACTURES

A *fracture* is a break in the continuity of a bone. Fractured bones are seldom an immediate threat to life, although they do have the potential to cause serious complications. When administering first aid to an injured victim, nurses may have to initiate CPR and treat hemorrhage. Fractures sometimes cause considerable blood loss (750 to more than 4000 mL from a fractured pelvis [Wheeless, 2016] and up to more than 1000 mL from a fractured femur [Keany, 2019]).

There are several types of common fractures (refer to *Adult Health Nursing,* Chapter 4, Fig. 4.19 for diagrams of types of fractures):

- *Closed fracture:* The skin overlying the injury is intact.
- *Open or compound fractures:* An open wound exists over the fracture site. Often the affected bone is visible as it protrudes through the skin.
- *Comminuted fracture:* The bone is shattered into two or more fragments or pieces.
- *Spiral fracture:* Results from a twisting force.
- *Impacted fracture:* Results from trauma that causes the bone ends to jam together.
- *Greenstick fracture:* An incomplete break, occurring most commonly in children because their bones are more pliable.
- *Compressed fracture:* To the vertebrae as the result of pressure.
- *Depression fracture:* Results from blunt trauma to a flat bone, causing an indentation in the bone.
- *Displaced fracture:* Fracture in which the ends of the bones are not in alignment with each other.
- *Oblique fracture:* Break runs diagonally across the bone, at approximately a 45-degree angle to the shaft of the bone.

Assessment

The health care provider, using x-ray diagnostic procedures, will determine whether a bone is fractured. Fracture is suspected if there is pain and tenderness in the area of the fracture, if pain increases during movement, and if the victim complains of an inability to adequately move the affected part. A deformity of the limb may be obvious with edema and discoloration (cyanosis, erythema) of the area. Fragments of bone sometimes protrude through the skin. If the affected part is moved, a grating sound may be heard. This is called crepitus and is caused by the broken bones scraping against each other. Sometimes victims report having heard or felt the bone snap.

Nursing Interventions

Do not move the victim unless he or she is in danger. Provide first aid and attempt to control bleeding in open fractures by cutting away the clothing around the wound and covering the wound with a large, sterile pressure dressing. No attempt should be made to reduce the fracture because this may cause further damage to the bone and tissue. The victim may need to be treated for shock.

Immobilization of the fracture is necessary, but no attempt should be made to realign the bone. Splint the body part as it was found. It is possible to change a fracture from a simple break to a comminuted or splintered one by moving it improperly. Use a lightweight but rigid splint that is long enough to extend past the joints above and beyond the fracture and is wider than the thickest part of the injury. The splint should be padded on the inner surface to prevent contact with the skin. Support the fractures while sliding the splint under the limb. Roller gauze or similar material is used to secure the limb in place (Fig. 16.16). Monitor circulation in the affected limb by assessing color, temperature, movement, and pulses below the injury; complaints of numbness and tingling; and evidence of edema. Use ice or cold packs to reduce edema.

Fig. 16.16 Immobilization of a fractured arm.

DISLOCATIONS

Dislocations occur in joints. They usually result from a blow or fall. Common sites of dislocations are the jaw, the shoulder, the elbow, the wrist, the finger, the hip, and the ankle.

Assessment

Victims usually complain of pain and edema in the area of the dislocation. Sometimes the nurse is able to observe a deformity of the part. Sometimes the part is rigid, and the victim is unable to move it.

Nursing Interventions

Never reduce dislocations, and never push dislocated joints back into place; this may further damage delicate ligaments, tendons, nerves (especially in the olecranon [elbow]), and the bone. Splint the joint in the same manner as a fracture. The splint should be large enough to support the limb in the line of the deformity. The limb should be bound to the body or supported in a sling. This is useful in dislocations of the shoulder and elbow. Apply ice or cold packs to reduce edema in surrounding tissues.

STRAINS AND SPRAINS

Strains are injuries to muscle tissue that result from stretching and tearing from overexertion. Sprains are injuries to joints resulting from stretched or torn ligaments, typically caused by twisting the joint beyond the normal range of motion. The joints most commonly affected are the knee and the ankle. Permanent damage to the tissue and joint are possible if sprains are left untreated.

Assessment

Injuries to muscle or ligaments result in the following signs and symptoms:
- *Strains:* Spasms or muscle "knots," acute pain, stiffness, and weakness on movement; back pain radiating down the leg; discoloration
- *Sprains:* Pain or tenderness around a joint; immobility of the joint; rapid and marked edema; discoloration around the joint

Nursing Interventions

Musculoskeletal injuries such as sprains and strains typically are treated initially according to the mnemonic RICE:

R *Rest* the affected extremity.

I *Ice* is applied to the part but not directly to the skin as soon as possible after the injury and for the next 48 hours, for 15 to 20 minutes, four to eight times a day. Ice should be followed with warm compresses to encourage healing by increasing the blood flow. Assess the victim's skin frequently for any evidence of burns.

C *Compression:* An elastic bandage or compression bandage is used to support the injured part.

Skill 16.3   Moving the Victim With a Suspected Spinal Cord Injury

NURSING ACTION *(RATIONALE)*

1. Carefully roll the victim, with the assistance of at least three other trained people, supporting the entire length of the body, just enough to slip a solid board underneath the victim. It is necessary for the board to extend beyond the victim's head and feet. *(Supports the entire spine.)*

2. While another person steadies the victim's head, place a towel or padding in the space underneath the victim's neck (never put the head on a pillow). *(Immobilizes the head and neck.)*

3. Place additional padding (rolled-up blankets, towels, sandbags) around the head and neck, keeping the neck in line with the body. Using a cervical collar is not currently recommended during first aid care due to an elevated risk for airway compromise and an increase in intracranial pressure. Encourage the victim to lie still. If a cervical collar is recommended following the arrival of EMS providers, then they will place it. *(Holds the head in place.)*

4. Secure the victim to the backboard with something such as bandages. Tape the head in place. *(Immobilizes the entire body.)*

5. In an emergency situation in which the victim is wearing a helmet, immobilize the victim with the helmet left in place. *(Prevents further injury.)*

E *Elevation:* The injured part should be elevated above the level of the heart to promote venous flow and reduce edema.

Some recent studies have raised the question as to whether RICE is the ideal way to treat these types of injuries. Another strategy, with the mnemonic POLICE, is being suggested by some orthopedic specialists:

P *Protection:* Protecting the injured body part. This step consists of a shorter period of rest than with RICE. Movement of the injured extremity while maintaining protection with assistive devices such as crutches is suggested with POLICE. Rest should be limited to the first few days after injury with this principle.

O, L *Optimal Loading:* Weight-bearing to be determined by the primary care provider or orthopedic specialist (this may be an orthopedic physician, nurse practitioner, or physical therapist), either with or without a boot.

The remainder is unchanged: **I** (ice), **C** (compression), **E** (elevation) (Harrison, 2014).

SPINAL CORD INJURIES

Assessment

To assess for paralysis, ask the victim whether he or she is able to move the hands and feet and whether any pain or sensation is felt. Assess for sensation by touching or gently pinching the victim's skin. Any abrasions and ecchymosis, especially on the head, shoulders, back, and abdomen, indicate possible injury to the victim's spinal cord.

Nursing Interventions

Spinal cord precautions should be taken in all cases of head trauma and multiple traumas. In patients with facial lacerations, there is a high correlation between neck injuries and spinal cord injuries. Maintain the victim's airway and ensure that the victim's head remains in a neutral position (the neck should never be hyperextended). If the victim vomits, direct several people, acting together as one unit, to help logroll the victim onto his or her side to allow drainage (see Chapter 8, Skill 8.3). When the victim is transported to a health care facility, the victim's head and neck must be kept in line with the body. Even a slight movement of the individual's head out of line with the body can potentially cause spinal damage. Do not attempt to move the victim without at least three assistants (Skill 16.3).

BURN INJURIES

Burns are a leading cause of accidental injuries; 486,000 burns per year necessitate medical treatment in the United States (American Burn Association, 2016). Burns are caused by heat from fire, hot liquids or steam, electricity from faulty wiring, chemicals such as lye, strong cleaning products, acids, solar radiation, and radioactive materials. The initial management of the patient with burns begins at the time of injury. The priority is to stop the burning process.

Burns often are classified according to their depth or the extent of the body surface area burned. The principal complications of all burns are shock from loss of fluids and electrolytes, and trauma and infection because of the loss of the skin as a barrier. The extent of burns can be calculated according to the rule of nines (Fig. 16.17).

SHALLOW PARTIAL-THICKNESS BURNS

Shallow partial-thickness burns (also classified as first-degree burns) are the least serious of all burns, involving only the outer layer of the skin. The most common first-degree burns are simple sunburns or burns from contact with hot objects. Healing usually is spontaneous

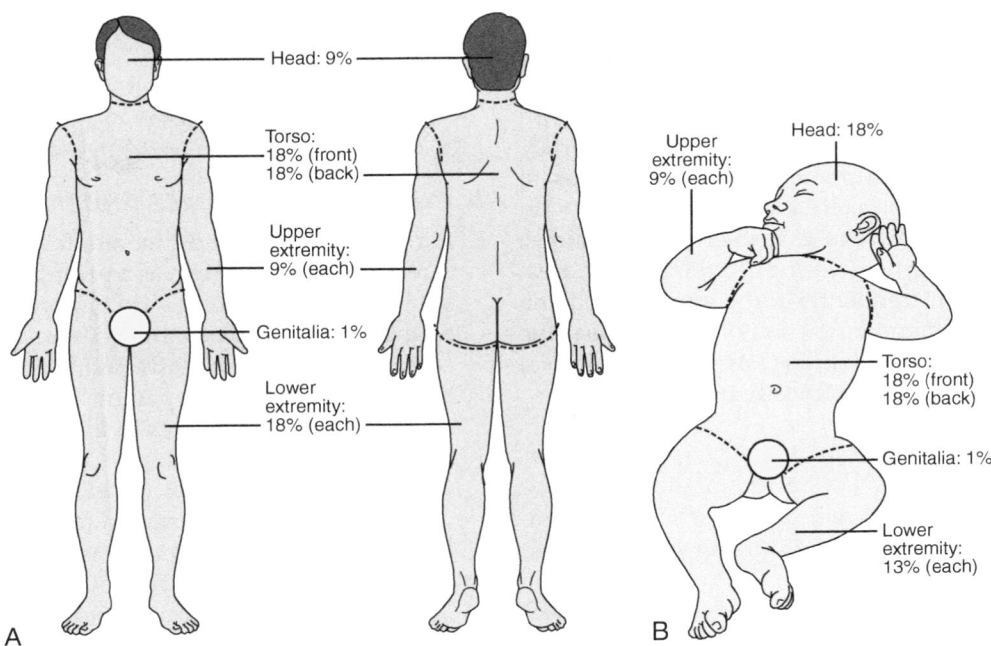

Fig. 16.17 Rule of nines. (A) Adult. (B) Child.

or occurs within 2 to 5 days and is uncomplicated. Signs and symptoms include erythema and pain.

Nursing Interventions

Cool the burn immediately by soaking the affected area in cold (not icy) water, or apply cool or cold wet compresses to the area for at least 10 minutes. Grease, butter, or salt water should not be applied to the burn. Place a sterile dressing over the burn site to help prevent infection.

DEEP PARTIAL-THICKNESS BURNS

Deep partial-thickness burns (also classified as second-degree burns) fully involve the first layer of skin (epidermis), as well as some of the underlying tissue (dermis); scarring from vesicles and infection is possible. Common causes of second-degree burns are severe sunburn, scalding liquids, direct flame, and chemical substances. Healing may take 5 to 21 days.

Assessment

Signs and symptoms include deep erythema or mottled skin with blister formation. Considerable edema often results, lasting several days. Fluid typically weeps through the skin surface (loss of plasma), and the patient complains of intense pain.

FULL-THICKNESS BURNS

Full-thickness burns (also classified as third-degree burns) involve destruction of the skin and underlying tissue, including fat, muscle, and bone. The area usually is charred, and healing is difficult. The skin is usually thick and leathery, with black or dark brown, cherry red, or dry and milky white colors. Many victims do not complain of pain because nerve endings

are damaged so severely by the burn. Capillaries become hyperpermeable, so plasma seeps into the interstitial spaces, resulting in edema and vesiculation (blistering). The larger the burned area involved, the greater the shift of fluid from the intravascular area into the interstitial area. Fluid loss causes a fluid and electrolyte imbalance. Hypovolemic shock and infection are common complications. Medical attention is urgent. Common causes of full-thickness burns are direct flame (such as ignited clothing), explosions, and gasoline and oil fires.

Nursing Interventions for Moderate to Severe Burns (Deep Partial-Thickness and Full-Thickness Burns)

It is crucial to establish an airway before edema occurs. Assess respiratory and cardiac function. CAB are the priority concerns. Remove all of the victim's clothing, as well as shoes and jewelry, which may be constricting and even smoldering. It is possible to increase the severity of the burns by leaving clothing on the victim. The victim should be kept warm, with the burned area elevated. Inspect for burns or the presence of soot around the mouth and nose, which may indicate that the patient's respiratory status has been affected. Immediately flush chemical burns with copious amounts of water.

If medical help will arrive within 15 to 30 minutes, withhold oral fluids. If medical help is delayed, it may be advisable to give oral rehydration therapy with formulations suggested by the World Health Organization (WHO) or with sports drinks to replace electrolytes (Vyas and Wong, 2013). If vomiting occurs, do not provide the victim with fluids to drink. Attempt to cool a partial-thickness burn immediately, using cool compresses. It is not appropriate to do this for other types of burns. Cool compresses or cold water sometimes cause hypothermia in victims with more extensive burns or in children. Vesicles (blisters) should not be broken intentionally; avoid touching the burn with anything except sterile dressings. It is not appropriate to apply antiseptics, ointments, sprays, or creams to the burn because they potentially may interfere with medical treatment and cause further complications. Apply loose, dry, sterile dressings to the burned area. Monitor the victim frequently to be sure that edema has not caused further constriction of the area near the burn. Honey has been identified as an antimicrobial agent that may be applied topically to burns.

❖ NURSING PROCESS

The role of the licensed practical nurse/licensed vocational nurse (LPN/LVN) in the nursing process is that the LPN/LVN will:

- Participate in planning care for patients on the basis of patient needs
- Review patient's plan of care and recommend revisions as needed
- Review and follow defined prioritization for patient care
- Use clinical pathways, care maps, or care plans to guide and review patient care

◆ ASSESSMENT

Patients requiring first aid may be suffering from a variety of injuries, not just the immediately visible problem. It is necessary to perform a complete head-to-toe assessment on all patients to determine the extent of injury. Give primary consideration to CAB. Quick and accurate assessment of the situation is vital.

In all patients who have sustained head trauma, suspect spinal injuries. Automobile accidents and falls are injuries that often result in spinal injuries. Even though no visible injury is noted, severe damage is possible in the absence of proper immobilization.

Also assess the emotional status of patients needing first aid. Even minor accidents often cause emotional distress. This is true not only for the patient but also for the patient's family and friends.

◆ PATIENT PROBLEM

Identifying patient problems provides the basis for developing a plan of care for the patient. Patients receiving emergency care often have a variety of problems that are necessary to address. The nurse is then able to plan care of the patient. Possible patient problems for first aid may include the following:

- *Anxiousness*
- *Below Normal Body Temperature*
- *Compromised Blood Flow to Tissue (cerebral, cardiopulmonary, renal, gastrointestinal, peripheral)*
- *Compromised Skin Integrity*
- *Elevated Body Temperature*
- *Inability to Clear Airway*

- *Insufficient Cardiac Output*
- *Potential for Infection*
- *Problematic Spontaneous Breathing*
- *Recent Onset of Confusion*
- *Recent Onset of Pain or Prolonged Pain*

◆ EXPECTED OUTCOMES AND PLANNING

For patients who need first aid, focus the plan on life-threatening emergencies as a priority. Specific, measurable goals and outcomes are important for preventing further injury to the patient. Be prepared to provide care quickly and efficiently and be aware of complications as they become apparent.

The plan of care relates to the specific patient problem. Examples include the following:

Goal 1: The patient will develop no infection in the open wound during stay in facility.
Outcome: No signs or symptoms of infection are noted.
Goal 2: Patient remains free of complications such as dehydration after a burn injury.
Outcome: Patient's intake and output are balanced.

◆ IMPLEMENTATION

Depending on the patient's injuries, a variety of measures is possible to implement to meet the patient's needs (Nursing Care Plan 16.1). Priorities are always to ensure that the patient has adequate circulation, has an open airway, and is breathing. Ensuring cardiac functioning sometimes involves giving cardiac compression. Severe bleeding, such as arterial spurting, is possible to control by direct pressure or a tourniquet as a last resort. Stabilization of the spine in suspected spinal injuries is possible to accomplish through the use of neck immobilizers and backboards.

Patients needing first aid care also need emotional support. Family and friends are also likely to need the nurse's understanding and comforting. Keeping the patient and family informed of procedures and the arrival of emergency aid will help them keep their anxiety levels under control. See the Cultural Considerations and Home Care Considerations boxes for additional information regarding emergency nursing interventions.

🌐 Cultural Considerations

Effect of Culture During Emergencies

- At a time of emergency, patients often fall back on their language of origin. An interpreter is able help with language barriers.
- Emergency equipment is frightening to many people. Ensure that the patient understands the rationale for any nursing interventions that are being performed and the purpose of any equipment.
- People from some cultures believe in the use of a local medicine person and are distrustful of Western health care providers. Try to work within a patient's beliefs rather than contradicting them outright. In an emergency, patients will refer to what they know best.

Home Care Considerations

Emergencies in the Home

- If ice is not available in the home, look for a bag of frozen vegetables. Peas work especially well.
- Have patients keep a list of medications, allergies, and special needs with their list of emergency numbers. This often saves time and provides valuable information for emergency medical personnel.
- Advise all patients to equip their homes with an emergency first aid kit, kept in an easily accessible place. Properly supplied kits include adhesive bandages, antiseptic, gauze dressings, tape, tweezers, scissors,

and antibiotic ointment. It is also a good idea to include directions for what to do in an emergency.
- Prevention is the key to eliminating emergencies in the home. Advise patients to "accident-proof" their homes. Advise patients to keep cleaning products and poisons, as well as medications, out of the reach of children. Handrails, nonskid surfaces, and adequate lighting help prevent falls. Advise older adults to avoid decorating with throw rugs and other objects that can cause them to trip. Keep electrical cords in good repair with no fraying.

 Nursing Care Plan 16.1   **The Patient With a Laceration**

Ms. T., 75 years of age, is living in a long-term care facility. She accidentally cuts herself with a knife during dinner. On examination, the nurse finds a 2-cm laceration in the patient's left hand that is actively bleeding.

PATIENT PROBLEM

Compromised Skin Integrity, related to trauma

Patient Goals and Expected Outcomes	Nursing Interventions	Evaluation
Bleeding wound will be controlled within 15 min Patient's wound will heal without complication within 7–10 days	Assess extent of wound, amount and type of bleeding, presence of dirt or contaminating substances. Cleanse wound, using normal saline. Apply direct pressure to control bleeding. Dress wound with sterile dressings.	Superficial 2-cm laceration to the palm of the left hand; moderate amount of bleeding noted. No visible dirt or food particles in wound. Wound irrigated with normal saline; bleeding controlled after 5 min of direct pressure. Wound dressed with a sterile 4- × 4-inch gauze secured with tape.

PATIENT PROBLEM

Potential for Infection, related to laceration

Patient Goals and Expected Outcomes	Nursing Interventions	Evaluation
Wound will heal within 7–10 days without signs of infection	Cleanse wound every shift with normal saline and apply treatment as specified by health care provider. Keep covered with sterile dressings until wound heals. Monitor the wound and patient daily for signs and symptoms of infection.	Wound edges well approximated; no bleeding, redness, swelling, or drainage from site.

CRITICAL THINKING QUESTIONS

1. Ms. T.'s wound was superficial. In contrast, what would be the nurse's actions if the wound appeared to be deep or was spurting blood?
2. What safety measures are indicated to ensure Ms. T. is not injured again?

◆ EVALUATION

Evaluation is an ongoing process. Injuries are not always visible on initial assessment. It is essential to constantly reevaluate the situation until the patient's condition is stable. The nurse will update the plan of care, depending on the evaluation. Refer to the goals and outcomes when planning care and perform procedures designed to meet those goals. Examples of goals and evaluative measures are as follows:

Goal 1: Patient will not have excessive bleeding from open wound.

Evaluative measure: No visible bleeding is noted after application of direct pressure.

Goal 2: Patient has no apparent spinal cord injury.

Evaluative measure: Patient is neurologically intact after immobilization of spine.

Get Ready for the NCLEX® Examination!

Key Points

- The goal of first aid is to preserve life until medical help arrives, not to replace medical care.
- Circulatory problems, airway problems, breathing problems, profuse bleeding, and poisonings are life-threatening situations that necessitate priority emergency care.
- Suspect shock in all situations involving traumatic injuries, diseases, and physical and emotional stress.
- Reactions to a poisonous bite often take a few minutes to several hours to appear. Take first aid measures immediately.
- Always splint a fractured part in the position it is in and never attempt to realign it.
- Take spinal cord precautions in all cases of head trauma and multiple traumas. Even a slight movement of the individual's head creates the potential for causing spinal damage.
- The dangers from burn injuries are shock, loss of fluids, and infection.
- In heat emergencies, it is important to cool the victim as soon as possible.
- Personnel trained in CPR and a rapid-response EMS system are often able to resuscitate victims of cardiac arrest or apparent sudden death.
- All health care providers need to maintain current CPR certification.
- It is necessary for rescuers to perform CPR according to the standards designated by the American Heart Association or the American Red Cross.
- There is a moral obligation to continue CPR once it has been initiated unless the rescuer is exhausted and is not able to continue, trained medical personnel take over CPR, or a licensed health care provider pronounces the victim dead.
- Circulation, airway, and breathing (CAB) are the three steps to remember in one-rescuer and two-rescuer CPR.
- If external cardiac compressions are performed accurately, it is possible to supply enough oxygen to the heart, the lungs, the brain, and the rest of the body to sustain life.
- Two fingers are used during chest compressions in an infant.
- If a victim is choking but has good air exchange (is coughing forcibly), do not interfere.
- Performing abdominal thrusts is the most effective method of removing a foreign body obstructing the airway.
- Do not use the finger-sweep technique when managing airway obstruction by a foreign body in the infant.

Additional Learning Resources

SG Go to your Study Guide for additional learning activities to help you master this chapter content.

Be sure to visit the Evolve site at http://evolve.elsevier.com/Cooper/foundations/ for additional online resources.

Review Questions for the NCLEX® Examination

1. The nurse finds a patient in a burning car. The patient is breathing with fractured arm and lacerations that are bleeding profusely. What action should the nurse take first?

   1. Splint the fractured arm.
   2. Get the patient out of the car.
   3. Give mouth-to-mouth resuscitation.
   4. Stop the bleeding.

2. A neighbor tells the nurse that her husband has been burned with scalding water. The arm is red and starting to blister. In addition to advising her to see a health care provider, what will the nurse tell the neighbor to apply to the burn?

   1. Hydrogen peroxide
   2. Petroleum jelly
   3. Cool compresses
   4. Salt water compresses

3. The nurse comes across a one-car automobile accident. The driver of the car is walking around with a dazed look on his face. He states that he was wearing his seatbelt but is unsure of what happened exactly. He has no visible injury. In checking his vital signs, the nurse finds his blood pressure is 84/56 mm Hg, his pulse is 110 beats/min, and his respirations are 32 per minute. Another bystander says that an ambulance is on the way. What is the nurse's initial action?

   1. Complete a neurologic assessment.
   2. Instruct him to get back in the car and rest.
   3. Position him on his back on the ground with legs and feet elevated 6 to 12 inches.
   4. Assess for any wounds that may be contributing to his memory loss.

4. The nurse is told in report that one of the patients has been very depressed lately. On checking the unit, the nurse finds the patient in the bathroom with one wrist bleeding profusely. The patient states that he broke a glass and used it to cut his wrist in a suicide attempt. What should the nurse do after sending someone to call for help?

   1. Attempt to find out what has been causing her depression.
   2. Apply a tourniquet above the injury.
   3. Use gauze pads and apply direct pressure.
   4. Thoroughly wash the wound.

5. A neighbor tells the nurse that her 5-year-old son has ingested one of her liquid cleaning supplies. The child is in no distress at this time. The mother shows the nurse the bottle; the nurse is unfamiliar with the ingredients. Which action by the nurse is appropriate?

   1. Give syrup of ipecac to induce vomiting.
   2. Give milk to neutralize any acids.
   3. Give water to dilute the poison.
   4. Call the poison control center.

6. The nurse comes upon a victim who is unresponsive. Place the interventions in order that the nurse should take.

   1. Administer 30 chest compressions.
   2. Give 2 mouth-to-mouth breaths.
   3. Check the carotid pulse.
   4. Activate the EMS.
   5. Open the airway.

7. The nurse is in the park and witnesses a child getting stung by a wasp. What action should the nurse implement first?

   1. Cleanse the site with soap and water.
   2. Remove the stinger using clean material using a scraping motion.
   3. Apply ice to the stung area.
   4. Determine whether the child has an allergy to wasps.

8. The nurse is assessing an adult patient who has been brought to the hospital with third-degree burns covering his head, right arm, and right leg. The nurse demonstrates accurate assessment skills by determining what to be the extent of the patient's burns?

   1. 27%
   2. 36%
   3. 45%
   4. 54%

9. A man suffers heat exhaustion while mowing the grass. The man's wife demonstrates knowledge of proper care of her husband with which action? *(Select all that apply.)*

   1. The wife calls 911 immediately.
   2. The wife encourages her husband to sit in a tub of cold water.
   3. The wife gives her husband cold water and a sports drink.
   4. The wife carefully monitors her husband while he finishes mowing.
   5. The wife loosens her husband's clothing.

10. The nurse is educating a group of hikers about how to treat frostbite. Which statement by one of the hikers indicates the need for further teaching?

    1. "I should place the frozen body part in hot water, around 110° to 114°F (43.3° to 45.6°C)."
    2. "I can wrap a frozen body part in a very warm moist towel."
    3. "I should avoid vigorously rubbing the frozen body part."
    4. "After the frozen part is warmed, I should wrap it in clean material and elevate it."

11. A patient comes to a sports medicine clinic after twisting his ankle while playing soccer. The health care provider determines he has a sprain. What discharge instructions will the nurse include in discharge summary for the patient? *(Select all that apply.)*

    1. "Apply ice to the sprained area for 1 hour, then off for 1 hour."
    2. "Wrap your ankle with an ACE bandage each morning."
    3. "Elevate your leg as much as possible to prevent further swelling."
    4. "Exercise your ankle as soon as you get home to prevent stiffness."
    5. "Use warm compresses to increase blood flow to the area after removing the ice."

12. The patient suffered a fracture of the tibia after crashing his motorcycle. He tells the nurse that his health care provider told him he shattered his tibia in three places and will need surgery. The nurse is aware that the patient has which type of fracture?

    1. Greenstick fracture
    2. Spiral fracture
    3. Comminuted fracture
    4. Compound fracture

13. Several high school teachers completed a CPR class. Which comment by one of the teachers demonstrates knowledge of proper CPR? *(Select all that apply.)*

    1. "The chest compression rate should be at least 100 per minute."
    2. "A jaw-thrust maneuver should be used on all patients when I open the airway."
    3. "The proper sequence for CPR is circulation, airway, and breathing."
    4. "I try to find the carotid pulse for no more than 10 seconds."
    5. "The adult chest should be compressed 2 to 2.4 inches during compressions."

14. When the nurse is caring for a person who has developed a nosebleed, which nursing action is appropriate?

    1. Apply steady pressure to the bridge of the nose for 5 minutes.
    2. Remind the victim to try to breathe through the nose.
    3. Avoid using ice over the nose.
    4. Keep the victim's head tilted slightly forward.

15. A nurse driving home from work one snowy night comes upon a car that's pulled over to the side of the road. A young, distraught mother pulls a limp infant from the car and, screaming, begins to wave for help. The nurse pulls over and runs to the pair, and the woman shows her an infant who seems unresponsive. "He just stopped breathing!" the mother cries. "Please help me!" "Call 911!" the nurse calls and takes the infant, kneeling with him in the headlights. As they wait for EMTs to arrive, the nurse checks the infant's airway and determines that it is open. However, the infant is not breathing.

    Identify the nursing actions below as 1—indicated (appropriate or necessary), contraindicated (could be harmful), or 3—non-essential (not necessary) for the client's care at this time. *Only one selection can be made for each nursing action.*

NURSING ACTION	INDICATED	CONTRAINDICATED	NON-ESSENTIAL
a. Gently shake the child to determine unresponsiveness.			
b. Cradle the child close and begin CPR.			
c. Use the jaw-thrust technique to open the airway.			
d. Hyperextend the neck to hold the airway open.			
e. Give two breaths (1 second per breath), delivering about what an adult can hold in the cheeks.			
f. Using two fingers, compress the breastbone of about 2.4 inches at 100 per minute			
g. Use 30 compressions to 2 breaths.			
h. Be careful not to remove the hands from their placement.			
i. Be careful not to allow the sternum to return to its initial position			

Dosage Calculation and Medication Administration

Ashley Carter

http://evolve.elsevier.com/Cooper/foundations/

Objectives

1. Demonstrate use of the most common equivalents of metric and apothecary measurement systems.
2. Correctly convert units of measurement within and between the metric, apothecary, and household measurement systems.
3. Apply mathematics skills to solve dosage calculation problems accurately.
4. Demonstrate the methods of calculating pediatric dosages.
5. Describe each phase of drug action.
6. Explain how decreased hepatic and renal functioning affect medication absorption and excretion.
7. Discuss the principles of drug actions and interactions.
8. Discuss factors that affect a patient's response to medications.
9. Identify the nurse's responsibilities regarding medication administration.
10. List the six "rights" of medication administration.
11. Describe factors to consider in choosing routes of medication administration.
12. Discuss the use of The Joint Commission's abbreviations to prevent medication errors.
13. Explain the importance of accurately transcribing medication orders.
14. Define controlled substance.
15. Discuss the three preferred sites for intramuscular injections in adults.
16. Describe the correct techniques for locating intramuscular injection sites.
17. Describe the procedures for irrigating the eye, ear, and nose.
18. Describe the correct techniques for administration of vaginal and rectal medications.

Key Terms

adverse drug reaction (ĂD-vŭrs DRŬG rē-ĂK-shŭn, p. 441)
agonist (ĂG-ŏ-nĭst, p. 440)
anaphylactic shock (ăn-ă-fĭ-LĂK-tĭk, p. 484)
antagonist (ăn-TĂG-ŏ-nĭst, p. 440)
body surface area (BŎD-ē SŬR-fĭs ĂR-ē-ŭ, p. 438)
buccal (BŬK-ŭl, p. 451)
compatibility (kŭm-păt-ŭ-BĬL-ĭ-tē, p. 440)
cumulative (kyūm-yū-lŭ-tĭv, p. 439)
denominator (dē-NŎM-ĭn-ā-tŭr, p. 431)
dimensional analysis (dĭ-MĔN-shŭn-ŭl ŭ-NĂL-ĭ-sĭs, p. 437)
drip factor (DRĬP FĂK-tŭr, p. 483)
drug interaction (DRŬG ĭn-tŭr-ĂK-shŭn, p. 440)
enteral (ĔN-tŭr-ŭl, p. 448)
enteric-coated (ĕn-TĔR-ĭk KŌT-ĭd, p. 448)
extremes (ĕk-STRĔMZ, p. 436)
gauge (GĀJ, p. 473)
graduated (GRĂD-yū-ā-tĭd, p. 452)
idiosyncratic (ĭd-ē-ō-sĭn-KRĂT-ĭk, p. 440)
intermittent venous access device (ĭn-tŭr-MĬT-ĕnt VĒ-nŭs ĂK-sĕs dĭ-VĪS, p. 480)
irrigations (ĭr-rĭ-GĀ-shŭnz, p. 429)
lumen (LŪ-mĕn, p. 473)

means (MĒNZ, p. 436)
meniscus (mĕ-NĬS-kŭs, p. 452)
metabolite (mĕ-TĂB-ŏ-līt, p. 439)
milliequivalent (mĭll-ē-ĕ-KWĬV-ă-lĕnt, p. 430)
numerator (NŪ-mŭr-ā-tŭr, p. 431)
parenteral (păr-ĔN-tŭr-ŭl, p. 448)
patient-controlled analgesia (PCA) (PĂ-shŭnt kŭn-TRŌLD ăn-ŭl-JĒ-zē-ŭ, p. 480)
percent (pŭr-SĔNT, p. 436)
percutaneous (pŭr-kyū-TĂ-nē-ŭs, p. 451)
pharmacology (făr-mŭ-KŎL-ŭ-jē, p. 439)
potentiation (pō-tĕn-shē-Ā-shŭn, p. 440)
proportion (prŭ-PŌR-shŭn, p. 436)
pulverized (PŬL-vŭr-īzd, p. 450)
ratio (RĂ-shē-ō, p. 436)
souffle cup (sū-FLĂ CŬP, p. 454)
sublingual (sŭb-LĬNG-gwŭl, p. 451)
therapeutic (thĕr-ŭ-PYŪ-tĭk, p. 439)
tolerance (TŎL-ŭr-ĭns, p. 441)
topical applications (TŎP-ĭ-kŭl ăp-lĭ-KĂ-shŭnz, p. 451)
toxicity (tŏk-SĬS-ĭ-tē, p. 440)

One of the nurse's roles is to calculate drug dosages accurately in order to administer medications safely to each patient. This chapter provides the student nurse with three measurement systems, several types of dosage calculations, and methods used to determine the appropriateness of drug orders for patients.

MATHEMATICS AND DOSAGE CALCULATION REVIEW

METRIC SYSTEM

The metric system is the preferred system of weights and measures, as it is more accurate than the imperial system in calculating dosage problems.

Like the US monetary system, which is based on the dollar, the metric system also is based on the decimal system. In the decimal system, the divisions and multiples of a unit are always in ratios of ten. For example:

1 dollar	=	10 dimes
10 dimes	=	20 nickels
20 nickels	=	100 pennies

All these units are multiples or divisions of ten.

In the metric system, the following basic units are used for volume, weight, and length:

liter (L)	volume (amount) of fluids
gram (g)	weight of solids
meter (m)	measure of length

Fractions of these units are designated by the following prefixes:

deci-	0.1 (one tenth) of the unit
centi-	0.01 (one hundredth) of the unit
milli-	0.001 (one thousandth) of the unit

Multiples of these units are designated with the following prefixes:

deca-	10 times the unit
hecto-	100 times the unit
kilo-	1000 times the unit

UNITS OF VOLUME

1 liter (L)	=	1000 milliliters (mL)
0.001 liter (L)	=	1 milliliter (mL)
1 milliliter (mL)	=	1 cubic centimeter (cc)

UNITS OF WEIGHT

1 gram (g)	=	1000 milligrams (mg)
0.001 gram (g)	=	1 milligram (mg)
1 kilogram (kg)	=	1000 grams (g)
0.001 kilogram (kg)	=	1 gram (g)

In addition to the preceding units of measurement, nurses often encounter the term *milliequivalent*, abbreviated mEq. **Milliequivalent** refers to the concentration of electrolytes in a certain volume of a solution, expressed as milliequivalents per liter (mEq/L). Potassium chloride (KCl) is an electrolyte that sometimes is ordered as an intravenous (IV) additive to a liter (1000 mL) of fluid.

EXAMPLE: The health care provider orders the following:

Add 40 mEq KCl to 1 L NS [normal saline] to infuse at 125 mL/h.

APPROXIMATE EQUIVALENTS OF THE METRIC SYSTEM

The basic unit of length in the metric system is the meter. The meter is equal to 39.37 inches, about 3½ inches longer than 1 yard (36 inches). A unit of measurement that nurses frequently use is the centimeter (cm); one inch is equivalent to 2.5 centimeters (cm). Some measurements that nurses obtain using the metric system are the following:

- Abdominal girth (obstetrics and patients with ascites and heart failure)
- Area size for topical applications
- Height, length, and head circumference (common tasks in obstetrics and pediatrics)
- Pressure injuries
- Results of intradermal skin tests (size of drug or allergen reaction on the skin)
- Wound size

0.001 meter	=	1 millimeter (mm)
0.01 meter	=	1 centimeter (cm)
0.1 meter	=	1 decimeter (dm)
10 meters	=	1 decameter (dam)
100 meters	=	1 hectometer (hm)
1000 meters	=	1 kilometer (km)

The most frequently used equivalents are the following:

1 meter (m)	=	1000 millimeters (mm)
0.001 meter (m)	=	1 millimeter (mm)
1 meter (m)	=	100 centimeters (cm)
1 centimeter (cm)	=	10 millimeters (mm)
1 millimeter (mm)	=	0.1 centimeter (cm)

APOTHECARY SYSTEM

The apothecary system is a system of measurement still used by some health care providers and hospitals. It is being replaced by the metric system. Because its use continues today, nurses may need to use the following equivalents to convert dosages from one system to another. The conversions are only approximations, but they are acceptable equivalents with which to work. Nurses need to convert from one system to another to calculate dosage problems in the same measurement units.

Volume

METRIC		APOTHECARY
30 milliliters (mL)	=	1 fluid ounce (fl oz)
500 milliliters (mL)	=	1 pint (pt)
1000 milliliters (1 L)	=	1 quart (qt)

Weight

METRIC		APOTHECARY
60 milligrams (mg)	=	1 grain (gr)
1000 milligrams (mg)	=	15 grains (gr XV)
30 grams (g)	≈	1 ounce (oz)

METRIC	APOTHECARY
0.45 kilogram (kg)	≈ 1 pound (lb)
1 kilogram (kg)	≈ 2.2 pounds (lb)

HOUSEHOLD UNITS OF MEASURE

In the clinical setting, the use of metric dosages is most common. Most medication, however, is administered in home settings, and in the home, patients may be confused by metric and apothecary units of measure. It is important for the nurse to review dosages and understand the correlation between household units of measure and metric units. Common conversions include the following:

1 teaspoon (tsp)	=	5 mL
1 tablespoon (tbsp)	=	15 mL
1 ounce	=	30 mL
1 cup	=	240 mL

BIG-TO-SMALL RULE

Whatever method is used to solve dosage problems, always convert the units of measurement in the problem to the same unit of measurement.

Some students find it difficult to convert dosages that contain decimal fractions, so this section discusses a quick and easy method called the *big-to-small rule*. It is useful in converting dosages *within the same system* (the metric system).

Because there are 1000 mL in 1 L (and 1000 mg in 1 g), this method works for converting milliliters to liters (and milligrams to grams). Likewise, liters can be converted to milliliters (and grams to milligrams) by this method.

CONVERTING LARGER UNITS OF MEASUREMENT TO SMALLER UNITS OF MEASUREMENT (GRAMS TO MILLIGRAMS; LITERS TO MILLILITERS)

RULE 1: Write down "BIG → SMALL."
RULE 2: Place the large unit under the word "BIG" and the small unit under the word "SMALL."

EXAMPLE: BIG → SMALL
                  $1.7 \, g = $ _____ mg

RULE 3: Move the decimal point three places in the direction of the arrow and then add zeros.

EXAMPLE: BIG → SMALL
                  $1.700 \, g = 1700. \, mg$

CONVERTING SMALLER UNITS OF MEASUREMENT TO LARGER UNITS OF MEASUREMENT (MILLIGRAMS TO GRAMS; MILLILITERS TO LITERS)

RULE 1: Write down the big-to-small rule formula.
    EXAMPLE: BIG → SMALL
RULE 2: Reverse the direction of the arrow.
    EXAMPLE: BIG ← SMALL
RULE 3: Place the large unit under the word "BIG" and the small unit under the word "SMALL."

EXAMPLE: BIG ← SMALL
                  $xg = 1700 \, mg$

RULE 4: Move the decimal point three places in the direction that the arrow points.

EXAMPLE: BIG ← SMALL
                  $1.7 \, g = 1700. \, mg$

ROUNDING A NUMBER

RULE 1: Round up a number that follows the decimal point if it is 5 or larger, to increase the number before it by one whole number.
    EXAMPLE 1: 7.55 is rounded up to 7.6 (rounded to the tenths place) or 8 (rounded to a whole number).
    EXAMPLE 2: 7.42 is rounded down to 7.4 (rounded to the tenths place) or 7 (rounded to a whole number).
    HINT: There are times when it is practical to round a volume of medication.
    PROBLEM: How is it possible to give 1.85 tablets?
    ANSWER: Round 1.85 to 2; give 2 tablets.

MATHEMATICS REVIEW AND PRINCIPLES

FRACTIONS

Fractions may be a challenging mathematical dilemma for some students, but it helps to understand what fractions are. A fraction is a "part" of a whole number and consists of two parts: the numerator and the denominator.

Numerator: The "top" number of a fraction
Denominator: The "bottom" number of a fraction

TYPES OF FRACTIONS

Proper fractions: The numerator is less than the denominator.

EXAMPLE: $\dfrac{1}{2}$ Numerator
                  Denominator

Improper fractions: The numerator is larger than the denominator.

EXAMPLE: $\dfrac{2}{1}$ Numerator
                  Denominator

Mixed fractions: These consist of a whole number plus a fraction.

EXAMPLE: $1\dfrac{1}{2}$, where 1 is the whole number and $\dfrac{1}{2}$ is the fraction.

CHANGING AN IMPROPER FRACTION TO A WHOLE OR MIXED NUMBER

RULE 1: Divide the denominator (bottom number) into the numerator (top number).
    EXAMPLE 1:   Change $\dfrac{10}{5}$ to a *whole* number.

                  $10 \div 5 = 2$ (a WHOLE number)

EXAMPLE 2: Change $\dfrac{40}{5}$ to a *whole* number.

$40 \div 5 = 8$ (a WHOLE number)

EXAMPLE 3: Change $\dfrac{20}{7}$ (an improper fraction) to a *mixed* number.

$$20 \div 7 = 7\overline{)20}\;\begin{array}{r}2\\\underline{14}\\6\\7\end{array} = 2\dfrac{6}{7}\text{(a MIXED number)}$$

EXAMPLE 4: Change $\dfrac{54}{5}$ to a *mixed* number.

$$54 \div 5 = 5\overline{)54}\;\begin{array}{r}10\\\underline{50}\\4\\5\end{array} = 10\dfrac{4}{5}\text{(a MIXED number)}$$

CHANGING A MIXED NUMBER TO AN IMPROPER FRACTION

RULE 1: Multiply the denominator (bottom number) by the whole number.

RULE 2: Add the numerator to the product. This sum is now the new numerator.

EXAMPLE 1: Change $2\dfrac{6}{7}$ (a mixed number) to an improper fraction.

Multiply the denominator 7 by the whole number 2.

$7 \times 2 = 14$ (The answer from numbers multiplied is called the *product*.)

EXAMPLE 2: Add the original numerator to the product.

$6 + 14 = 20$ (The answer from numbers added is called the *sum*.)

EXAMPLE 3: Place the sum, 20, over the original denominator, 7, to obtain an improper fraction: $\dfrac{20}{7}$.

The mixed number is now the improper fraction.

REDUCING FRACTIONS TO THE LOWEST TERM

Fractions commonly are reduced to the lowest term in which they can be expressed, because it is easier to work with smaller numbers.

RULE 1: Find a number that will evenly divide into the numerator *and* the denominator.

EXAMPLE: $\dfrac{2}{10}$

What number will divide into the numerator, which is 2?

2 will divide evenly into the numerator 2 one time.

2 will divide into the denominator (which is 10) five times.

$\dfrac{2}{10} = \dfrac{1}{5}$ (reduce all numbers in the fraction to their lowest terms)

DETERMINING WHICH FRACTION IS LARGER

RULE 1: If the denominators are the *same*, the fraction with the *larger numerator* is the larger fraction.

PROBLEM: Which is larger, $\dfrac{4}{6}$ or $\dfrac{2}{6}$?

ANSWER: $\dfrac{4}{6}$ is larger

RULE 2: If the denominators are *different*, as in $\dfrac{2}{5}$ and $\dfrac{1}{3}$, first find a "common denominator." Finding a common denominator means to find a number into which both denominators can be divided. Common, or equivalent, numerators will also be found.

PROBLEM: Which is larger, $\dfrac{2}{5}$ or $\dfrac{1}{3}$?

$$\dfrac{2}{5} = \dfrac{?}{15} \quad \dfrac{1}{3} = \dfrac{?}{15}$$

RULE 3: Find a common denominator. HINT: Try multiplying the denominators to get a common denominator.

$$\dfrac{2}{5} = \dfrac{?}{15} \quad \dfrac{1}{3} = \dfrac{?}{15}$$

Multiply the numerator and denominator by 3

$$\dfrac{2}{5} = \dfrac{6}{15} \quad \dfrac{1}{3} = \dfrac{5}{15}$$

OR

Find an equivalent numerator by dividing the first denominator into the equivalent denominator; multiply the answer by the first numerator.

$$\dfrac{2}{5} = \dfrac{6}{15}\,(15 \div 5 = 3\,;\,3 \times 2 = 6)$$

$$\dfrac{1}{3} = \dfrac{5}{15}\,(15 \div 3 = 5\,;\,5 \times 1 = 5)$$

RULE 4: Compare the two fractions; the one with the larger numerator is the larger fraction.

PROBLEM: Which is larger, $\dfrac{6}{15}$ or $\dfrac{5}{15}$?

ANSWER: $\dfrac{6}{15}$ is larger.

PROBLEM: Which is larger, $\dfrac{2}{3}$ or $\dfrac{6}{8}$?

$$\dfrac{2}{3} = \dfrac{16}{24} \quad \dfrac{6}{8} = \dfrac{18}{24}$$

ANSWER: $\dfrac{6}{8}$ is larger.

ADDING FRACTIONS WITH THE SAME DENOMINATOR

RULE 1: Add the numerators; place this sum of the numerators over the denominator and reduce the new fraction if possible.

$$\begin{array}{r} \frac{1}{6} \\ +\frac{1}{6} \\ \hline \frac{2}{6}=\frac{1}{3} \end{array}$$

EXAMPLE:

ADDING FRACTIONS WITH DIFFERENT DENOMINATORS

RULE 1: Find common denominators for all fractions in the problem.

EXAMPLE: $\frac{2}{4}=\frac{6}{12}$ (3 and 4 will divide into 12; 12 is the common denominator.)

ANSWER: $\frac{2}{4}=\frac{6}{12}$

RULE 2: Add the numerators.

EXAMPLE 1: $\frac{10}{12}=\frac{5}{6}$

EXAMPLE 2: $\frac{4}{18}+\frac{10}{18}=\frac{14}{18}=\frac{7}{9}$

ADDING MIXED NUMBERS

RULE 1: Add the fractions of the mixed number. Then add the sum of the fractions to the whole numbers.

EXAMPLE 1: $\begin{array}{r} 1\frac{2}{3} \\ +2\frac{1}{3} \\ \hline 3\frac{3}{3}=4 \end{array}$

EXAMPLE 2: $\begin{array}{r} 1\frac{3}{5}=1\frac{6}{10} \\ +4\frac{5}{10}=4\frac{5}{10} \\ \hline 5\frac{11}{10}=5+1\text{whole}+\frac{1}{10}, \\ \text{which}=6\frac{1}{10} \end{array}$

SUBTRACTING FRACTIONS WITH THE SAME DENOMINATOR

RULE 1: Subtract the numerators and place the answer over the denominator in the answer.

EXAMPLE 1: $\begin{array}{r} \frac{3}{5} \\ -\frac{1}{5} \\ \hline \frac{2}{5} \end{array}$ EXAMPLE 2: $\begin{array}{r} \frac{4}{7} \\ -\frac{2}{7} \\ \hline \frac{2}{7} \end{array}$

SUBTRACTING FRACTIONS WITH DIFFERENT DENOMINATORS

RULE 1: First find a common denominator, and then subtract.

EXAMPLE 1: $\begin{array}{r} \frac{3}{4}=\frac{9}{12} \\ -\frac{1}{3}=\frac{4}{12} \\ \hline \frac{5}{12} \end{array}$ EXAMPLE 2: $\begin{array}{r} \frac{2}{3}=\frac{4}{6} \\ -\frac{1}{2}=\frac{3}{6} \\ \hline \frac{1}{6} \end{array}$

SUBTRACTING MIXED NUMBERS

RULE 1: When the numerator of the top fraction is smaller than that of the bottom fraction, borrow one whole number from the whole number of the mixed fraction, and express it as a fraction.

PROBLEM: $\begin{array}{r} 3\frac{9}{15} \\ -2\frac{10}{15} \\ \hline \end{array}$

ANSWER: $3=2\frac{15}{15}$

RULE 2: Add the fraction of the original mixed number to the new fraction.

EXAMPLE: $3\frac{9}{15}=2\frac{15}{15}+\frac{9}{15}=2\frac{24}{15}$

ANSWER: 2 24/15

RULE 3: Subtract fractions and whole numbers, if any.

EXAMPLE: $2\frac{24}{15}-2\frac{10}{15}=14/15$

MULTIPLYING FRACTIONS

RULE 1: Multiply the numerators by each other; multiply the denominators by each other.

EXAMPLE 1: $\frac{1}{2}\times\frac{3}{4}=\frac{1\times3}{2\times4}=\frac{3}{8}$

EXAMPLE 2: $\frac{4}{8}\times\frac{1}{3}=\frac{4\times1}{8\times3}=\frac{4}{24}=\frac{1}{6}$

MULTIPLYING FRACTIONS AND MIXED NUMBERS

RULE 1: Change the mixed number to an improper fraction. (See the section on changing mixed numbers to improper fractions.)

PROBLEM: Multiply $3\frac{1}{2}$ by $1\frac{2}{3}$.

EXAMPLES 1 AND 2: Change $3\frac{1}{2}$ and $1\frac{2}{3}$ to improper fractions.

$$3\frac{1}{2}=\frac{7}{2}=1\frac{2}{3}=\frac{5}{3}$$

Multiply

Answer: $\dfrac{7}{2} \times \dfrac{5}{3} = \dfrac{35}{6} = 5.833$

PROBLEM: Multiply $1\dfrac{2}{3}$ by $1\dfrac{2}{3}$.

Answer: $\dfrac{5}{3} \times \dfrac{11}{4} = \dfrac{55}{12} = 4\dfrac{7}{12}$

DIVIDING FRACTIONS

RULE 1: Write the problem down correctly.
RULE 2: Invert the second fraction and multiply the two fractions; then reduce the answer to lowest terms.

PROBLEM: Divide $\dfrac{1}{2}$ by $\dfrac{3}{4}$

EXAMPLE: 1. Write the problem down *correctly*.

$\dfrac{1}{2} \div \dfrac{3}{4}$

2. Invert the second fraction, change the division sign to a multiplication sign, and multiply the two fractions.

$\dfrac{1}{2} \times \dfrac{4}{3} = \dfrac{4}{6}$

3. Reduce the answer to the lowest terms.

$\dfrac{4}{6} = \dfrac{2}{3}$

DIVIDING FRACTIONS AND WHOLE NUMBERS

RULE 1: Change the whole number to a fraction.
RULE 2: Divide as above, and then reduce to lowest terms.

PROBLEM: Divide 4 by $\dfrac{3}{5}$

EXAMPLE: 1. Change 4 to a fraction. Make 4 the numerator and use 1 as the denominator.

$\dfrac{4}{1}$

2. Invert second fraction; multiply.

$\dfrac{4 \times 5}{1 \times 3} = \dfrac{2}{3}$

3. Reduce the answer to lowest terms.

DECIMAL FRACTIONS

The decimal fraction is a type of fraction whose denominator is always some multiple of 10. The placement or position of the decimal point determines whether the denominator is 10, a multiple of 10, or a division of 10.

NAMES OF DECIMAL PLACES

0.00001	Hundred thousandths
0.0001	Ten thousandths
0.001	Thousandths
0.01	Hundredths
0.1	Tenths
1.	Unit (whole numbers)
10	Tens
100	Hundreds
1000	Thousands
10,000	Ten-thousands
100,000	Hundred-thousands

RULE 1: A decimal point found to the left of a number means that the number is a *fraction* of a whole number.

EXAMPLE: 0.1—also called "point one"—is $\dfrac{1}{10}$ of the whole number 1.

HINT: Place a zero to the left of the decimal point to prevent mistaking ".1" for "1."

Correct placement of decimal points in drug dosages is critical (see The Joint Committee's [TJC's] Official "Do No Use" list, 2019).

TJC's Official "Do Not Use" List

DO NOT USE	POTENTIAL PROBLEM	USE INSTEAD
U, u (unit)	Mistaken for "0" (zero), the number "4" (four) or "cc"	Write "unit"
IU (International Unit)	Mistaken for IV (intravenous) or the number 10 (ten)	Write "International Unit"
Q.D., QD, q.d., qd (daily)	Mistaken for each other	Write "daily"
Q.O.D., QOD, q.o.d, qod (every other day)	Period after the Q mistaken for "I" and the "O" mistaken for "I"	Write "every other day"
Trailing zero (X.0 mg)* Lack of leading zero (.X mg)	Decimal point is missed	Write X mg Write 0.X mg
MS	Can mean morphine sulfate or magnesium sulfate	Write "morphine sulfate"
MSO$_4$ and MgSO$_4$	Confused for each another	Write "magnesium sulfate"

*From The Joint Commission: Official "Do Not Use" List, 2019. Retrieved from https://www.jointcommission.org/-/media/tjc/documents/fact-sheets/do-not-use-list-fact-sheet-06-28-19.pdf?db=web&hash=043C8075920 7C3EC9616DDD3D5557113

RULE 2: A decimal point found *after* (to the right of) a number means that it is a whole number.
    EXAMPLE: 5. = 5
RULE 3: A number *without* a decimal point is understood to have an "invisible" decimal point after it.
    EXAMPLE: 2 = 2.

HINT: Do not place a zero to the right of the decimal point to prevent mistaking "2.0" for "20".

Correct placement of decimal points in drug dosages is critical. Decimal points should not be placed after a whole number.

ADDING DECIMALS

RULE 1: Align the decimal point of each decimal fraction in a column.
RULE 2: Add.
   PROBLEM: Add 3.34 and 0.6.
   EXAMPLE:

$$
\begin{array}{r}
3.34 \\
+\ 0.6 \\
\hline
3.94
\end{array}
$$
   Align decimal point in column; add

   ↑   Make sure that the decimal point is aligned properly in the answer.

SUBTRACTING DECIMALS

RULE 1: Align the decimal points of each decimal fraction in a column.
RULE 2: Subtract.
   PROBLEM: Subtract 7.45 from 15.
   EXAMPLE:

$$
\begin{array}{r}
15.00 \\
-\ 7.45 \\
\hline
7.55
\end{array}
$$
   Align decimal point in column; subtract

   ↑   Make sure that the decimal point is aligned properly in the answer.

MULTIPLYING DECIMALS

RULE 1: Multiply. You do not have to align decimal points in the problem.
RULE 2: To determine the location of the decimal point in the answer, note how many numbers are found to the right of the decimal points in all the numbers multiplied.

EXAMPLE:
$$
\begin{array}{r}
5.50 \\
\times\ \ 2.15 \\
\hline
2750 \\
550\ \ \\
1100\ \ \ \\
\hline
11.8250\ x
\end{array}
$$
(There are two numbers found after the decimal points on the top and two on the bottom.)

   $x = 11.8250$ or 12 (rounded)

NOTE: A small "x" hereafter indicates the unexpressed decimal after a whole number or a decimal point that has been moved from one place to another.

DIVIDING DECIMALS

RULE 1: Change a decimal fraction in the divisor to a whole number by moving the decimal point all the way to the right.
   PROBLEM: Divide 2.5 by 1.5.
   EXAMPLE: 1. (divisor) $1.5\overline{)2.5}$ (dividend)

   2. $1.5x\overline{)2.5}$ $15\overline{)2.5}$

RULE 2: Move the decimal point in the dividend the *same number of places moved in the divisor.*
   EXAMPLE: $1.5x\overline{)2.5x}$ The decimal point in the divisor is unexpressed after it is moved.

RULE 3: Place the decimal point in the answer directly over the decimal point in the dividend after moving the decimal point in the dividend.
   EXAMPLE: $15\overline{)25}$

RULE 4: If a decimal point is in the divisor but not in the dividend (as in $0.5\overline{)15}$), move it the same number of places as the divisor. Remember that there is an unexpressed decimal point at the right of all whole numbers.
   EXAMPLE: $0.5x\overline{)15.x}$ $5\overline{)150}$

RULE 5: If the dividend contains a decimal fraction and the divisor does not, leave the divisor as it is.
   EXAMPLE: $5\overline{)2.5}$ would remain unchanged.

CHANGING FRACTIONS TO DECIMALS

RULE 1: Divide the numerator (the top number) by the denominator (the bottom number).
   PROBLEM: Change $\dfrac{3}{4}$ to a decimal fraction.

   EXAMPLE: $\dfrac{3}{4} = 4\overline{)3.00}^{\,0.75}$

   ANSWER: 0.75

CHANGING A DECIMAL FRACTION TO A COMMON FRACTION

Decimal fractions are based on 10s, multiples of 10, and divisions by 10. The position or place of the decimal point indicates the denominator.
RULE 1: To change a decimal fraction to a common fraction, give the decimal fraction a denominator according to the position of the decimal point in the decimal fraction.
   PROBLEM: Change 0.1 to a common fraction.

   EXAMPLE: $\dfrac{0.1}{10}$ (The decimal point is in the "tens" place; 10 is the denominator.)

Now that the denominator is 10, place the 1 over it to make a common fraction.

$$\dfrac{1}{10}$$

PERCENTAGES

The word **percent** and its symbol, %, mean "hundredths." A hundredth is a fraction of a whole number; therefore, a number followed by % is a fraction, and such a fraction is called a percentage. The denominator of the fraction is understood to be 100.

EXAMPLE: 25% is the same as $\dfrac{25}{100}$.

Reduce $\dfrac{25}{100}$ to $\dfrac{1}{4}$.

CHANGING A PERCENTAGE TO A DECIMAL FRACTION

RULE 1: Remove the percent sign and move the decimal point two places to the left to indicate hundredths.
PROBLEM: Change 25% to a decimal fraction.
ANSWER: 0.25

CHANGING A FRACTION TO A PERCENTAGE

RULE 1: Change a fraction to a percentage by dividing the numerator by the denominator.
RULE 2: Multiply the answer by 100.
RULE 3: Label the answer with the percent symbol.

EXAMPLE:
$$
\begin{array}{r}
100 \\
\times 0.75 \\
\hline
500 \\
700 \\
\hline
75.00x
\end{array}
$$

(There are two decimal places in this problem; move the decimal point in the answer two places to the left)

75% Therefore $\dfrac{3}{4} = 75\%$

MULTIPLYING BY PERCENTAGE

RULE 1: Change percentage to a decimal by moving the decimal point two places to the left.
RULE 2: Multiply.

PROBLEM: Multiply 80 by 7.5%.

EXAMPLE: 7.5% is .075.

ANSWER: 6

RATIOS

Ratio is the relationship of one number or quantity to another number or quantity. Numbers of a ratio are separated by a colon. A ratio is also a fraction. The value of a ratio is not changed if both terms are multiplied or divided by the same number.
EXAMPLE: 2:4 has the same value as 1:2 or 4:8.
PROBLEM: Write numbers as ratios and express them all in the same units.
EXAMPLE: Express 1 L, 2 oz, and 30 mL all in the same way: 1000 mL:60 mL:30 mL.

PROBLEM: Write a fraction as a ratio.

EXAMPLE: $\dfrac{1}{25} = 1:25 \quad \dfrac{3}{4} = 3:4 \quad \dfrac{1}{25} = 1:25 \quad \dfrac{3}{4} = 3:4$

Ratio is an important concept that is used in the following methods of calculating dosages.

PROPORTIONS

Proportion is a relationship between two ratios of equal value.
EXAMPLE: 1 is to 2 as 4 is to 8, or 1:2 = 4:8.
Means are the inner terms of the proportion. **Extremes** are the outer terms of the proportion.

EXAMPLE:
$$
\underset{\text{means}}{1:2 = 4:8} \qquad \underset{\text{extremes}}{1:2 = 4:8}
$$

Set up the left side, or first ratio, of the proportion as the "known" side by using information that is known or given. Examples of known information are as follows:
An equivalent such as 60 milligrams = 1 grain (60 mg:1 gr)
A physician's medication or IV order, such as "give 1000 mL in 8 hr" (1000 mL:8 hr)
A drug dosage on hand or available, such as information on a drug label that reads "50 mg/mL" (50 mg:1 mL)
PROBLEM: The physician orders Demerol, 25 mg q 3–4 h, as needed (prn) for pain. On hand is a vial labeled "50 mg/1 mL."
RULE 1: Set up the known side.
EXAMPLE: 50 mg:1 mL (quantity given on the label)
RULE 2: Set up the unknown side. Use x for what the equation asks, such as "How many milliliters are needed to give 25 mg?"

EXAMPLE: **Known**   **Unknown**
50 mg:1 mL = 25 mg:x mL

RULE 3: Set up the units, such as mg and mL, in the *same position on each side* of the problem.
EXAMPLE: _____ mg:_____ mL = _____ mg:_____ mL
RULE 4: Multiply the means.

RULE 5: Multiply the extremes.

PROBLEM: 50 mg:1 mL = 25 mg:x mL

EXAMPLE: Multiply the means.
50 mg:1 mL = 25 mg:x mL

50 mg : 1 mL = 25 mg : x mL
= 25
Multiply the extremes.

50 mg : 1 mL = 25 mg : x mL
= 50x

Express the proportion.
$$50x = 25$$

RULE 6: Solve for x by dividing the number with the x into the number on the opposite side of the problem.

EXAMPLE: 50 mg : 1 mL = 25 mg : x mL

$$50x = 25 = 50\overline{)25.0}^{\,0.5}$$
$$x = 0.5$$

RULE 7: Label the answer with the unit of measurement that accompanies x in the problem.

EXAMPLE:
$$50 \text{ mg} : 1 \text{ mL} = 25 \text{ mg} : x \text{ mL}$$
$$50x = 25$$
$$x = 0.5 \text{ mL}$$

Review of Proportion Method

1. Set up problems in the *same order* on both sides.
2. Multiply the means, then multiply the extremes.
3. The number multiplied with the x is always that number with the x to the right of it.

EXAMPLE: 2 mg:1 mL = 5 mg:x mL

4. Divide the number with the x into the number on the other side of the problem.
5. Label the problem by determining which unit of measurement is associated with the x in the proportion.

$$\text{Formula Method} \quad \frac{\text{Desired dosage}}{\text{Available dose}} \times \text{Amount}$$

Many nurses use the following method of solving dosage problems:

RULE 1: Place the dose that the physician wants given over the dose that is available (on hand).

PROBLEM: The physician orders 40 mg of furosemide (Lasix). An ampule (small glass container that usually contains a single dose of a solution) of furosemide labeled "Lasix 20 mg/mL" is available.

EXAMPLE: $\dfrac{\text{(Desired dosage)}}{\text{(Available dose)}} \dfrac{40 \text{ mg}}{20 \text{ mg}} \times \dfrac{1 \text{ mL}}{1} = \dfrac{40}{20}$
$$= 40 \div 20 = 2 \text{ mL}$$

PROBLEM: The physician orders 15 mg of diazepam (Valium). Valium tablets that contain 5 mg/tablet are available.

EXAMPLE:

$\dfrac{\text{(Desired dosage)}}{\text{(Available dose)}} \dfrac{15 \text{ mg}}{15 \text{ mg}} \times \dfrac{1 \text{ tab}}{x \text{ tab}} = \dfrac{15}{5x} = x$
$$= 15 \div 5 = 3 \text{ tabs}$$

DIMENSIONAL ANALYSIS

In the dimensional analysis method (also called *factor labeling* or the *label factor method*), dosages are calculated with the use of the following three factors:

1. *Drug label factor:* The form in which the drug dose is delivered, or the vehicle *(V)*, with the equivalence in units on hand *(H)*; for example, 1 capsule *(V)* = 500 mg *(H)*.
2. *Conversion factor (C):* It helps to memorize the following common conversions (see the section on the apothecary system with its abbreviations, for a discussion of grains [gr]):

1 g = 1000 mg	1 g = 15 gr
1000 mg = 15 gr	1 gr = 60 mg

3. *Drug order factor:* The dosage desired (D).

These three factors are set up in an equation that allows the units to be canceled so you can then calculate the correct units for delivery.

$$
\begin{array}{ccc}
V = V\,(\text{vehicle}) \times & C\,(H) & \times D\,(\text{desired}) \\
H\,(\text{on hand}) \times & C\,(D) & \times \quad 1 \\
(\text{drug label}) & (\text{conversion factor}) & (\text{drug order})
\end{array}
$$

With dimensional analysis, the conversion factor is built into the equation and is included when the units of measurement of the drug order and drug container differ. If the two are of the same units of measurement, the conversion factor is eliminated from the equation.

EXAMPLE: Order calls for acetaminophen (Tylenol) gr xv, PO, prn (15 grains, by mouth, as needed)

AVAILABLE: acetaminophen (Tylenol regular strength) tablets, 325 mg each
Factors: 325 mg = 1 tablet (from drug label)
15 gr/1 (from drug order)
Conversion factor: 1000 mg = 15 gr

How many tablets should be given?

$$\text{Tab} = \frac{\text{gr}}{x} \times \frac{\text{mg}}{\text{gr}} \times \frac{\text{tab}}{\text{mg}}$$

$$\text{Tab} = \frac{15\ \cancel{\text{gr}}}{x} \times \frac{1000\ \cancel{\text{mg}}}{15\ \cancel{\text{gr}}} \times \frac{1\ \text{tab}}{325\ \cancel{\text{mg}}} = \frac{15{,}000}{4875} =$$

$$\text{Tab} = 3.07$$
$$= 3 \text{ tabs}$$

Box 17.1 lists the nurse's responsibilities in solving dosage problems accurately.

CALCULATING MEDICATIONS USING THE MILLIGRAM/KILOGRAM METHOD

Some medication dosages are based on the patient's weight. This method of calculation is used most

Box 17.1	Nursing Responsibilities in Solving Dosage Problems

- Check whether the answer is reasonable.
- Do not allow for any errors in calculating dosages.
- Recheck calculations.
- Reduce distractions while working problems.
- Work problems systematically and carefully.
- Perform dosage calculations independently, then ask another nurse to perform the same dosage calculation problem, and check answers.

commonly for dosages of medications for infants and children, but it can be used for a patient of any age. When using this method, convert the patient's weight to kilograms if the weight is measured or recorded in pounds (lb). Refer to the following example when using this method of dosage calculation.

Example: A medication order specifies administering cefazolin, 50 mg/kg, divided into four equal doses.

If the child weighs 95 lb, first convert the weight to kilograms:

95 lb/2.2 = 43.18 kg

Multiply the weight in kilograms by the milligrams:

50 mg × 43.18 kg = 2159 mg

Divide by the total number of doses to be administered:

2159 kg/4 (four equal doses) = 539.75 mg

PEDIATRIC DOSAGE CONSIDERATIONS

Administering the correct dosages of medication to children requires caution. There are various factors that the health care provider should consider when ordering medication for a child, including age, weight, body surface area, and the ability of the child to absorb, metabolize, and excrete medication. It is the health care provider's responsibility to provide medication orders and specify dosages for a pediatric patient, but the nurse must be able to recognize appropriate medication dosages and orders.

There are several different ways to determine appropriate pediatric doses, but this discussion focuses on how to use the body surface area and a nomogram.

Young's Rule

Young's rule is a method of calculating the appropriate dose of a drug for a child 2 years of age or older:

$$\frac{\text{Age of child}}{\text{Age of child} + 12} \times \frac{\text{Average}}{\text{adult dose}} = \frac{\text{Child's}}{\text{dose}}$$

This rule applies to children up to the age of 12.

Problem: The average adult dose of a medication is 50 mg. What is an appropriate dose of this medication for an 8-year-old child?

Answer: 20 mg is an appropriate dose.

Clark's Rule

Clark's rule is another method of calculating the appropriate dosage of a drug for a child. In this rule, the child's weight is used to determine dosage:

$$\frac{\text{Weight of child in pounds}}{150} \times \frac{\text{Average}}{\text{adult dose}} = \frac{\text{Child's}}{\text{dose}}$$

PROBLEM: The average adult dose of a medication is 25 mg. What is an appropriate dose of this medication for a child who weighs 40 lb?

EXAMPLE:

$$\frac{40 \text{ lb}}{150} \times 25 \text{ mg} = \frac{40}{150} \times \frac{25}{1} = \frac{1000}{150} = 150\overline{)1000.00}$$

$$= 6.7 \text{ mg or } 7 \text{ mg}$$

ANSWER: 6.7 or 7 mg is an appropriate dose.

Fried's Rule

Fried's rule is used to calculate appropriate dosages for infants younger than 2 years:

$$\frac{\text{Age in months}}{150} \times \frac{\text{Average}}{\text{adult dose}} = \frac{\text{Child's}}{\text{dose}}$$

PROBLEM: The average adult dose of a medication is 25 mg. What is an appropriate dose of this medication for a child who is 22 months of age?

EXAMPLE:

$$\frac{22}{150} \times 25 \text{ mg} = \frac{550}{150} = 150\overline{)550.00} = 3.7 \text{ or } 4 \text{ mg}$$

ANSWER: 3.7 or 4 mg is an appropriate dose.

Estimating Body Surface Area in Children

Body surface area is defined as the total area exposed to the outside environment. For pediatric patients of average size, it is acceptable to estimate body surface area with the scales shown in Fig. 17.1. Match the child's weight to the corresponding surface area. Lay a straight edge on the correct height and weight points for the pediatric patient (as on the right side of Fig. 17.1) and find the point where it intersects on the surface area scale at center.

PROBLEM: Trey, an 8-year-old, weighs 60 lb and is 51 inches tall. His body surface area (as determined with the nomogram in Fig. 17.1) is 1.0. If an adult dose is 50 mg, how many milligrams should Trey receive?

EXAMPLE: Use the following formula:

For children of normal height and weight

For other children

Fig. 17.1 Estimating body surface area *(S.A.)* in children.

$$\frac{\text{Child's body surface area}}{1.73} \times \text{Adult dose} = \text{Child's dose}$$

ANSWER: 29 mg is appropriate for a child of Trey's height and weight.

PRINCIPLES AND PRACTICE OF MEDICATION ADMINISTRATION

PHARMACOLOGY

Pharmacology is the study of drugs (medications) and their actions on the living body. Substances derived from plants and animals, vitamins and minerals, and synthetic (artificial) sources can be used as drugs in the treatment and prevention of disease. The terms *drug* and *medication* are often used interchangeably, and they are used to restore and maintain the healthy functioning of body tissues, organs, and systems and in diagnostic procedures.

The action of any drug on the body is a complicated process. This process begins with the pharmaceutical phase, or the manufacturing of the drug, until the absorption of the drug in the patient's body. Absorption occurs when the active ingredient of the drug enters the body fluids.

The pharmacokinetic phase involves the movement of the drug's active ingredients from the body fluids

| Box **17.2** | Terms Used With Dosages |

Minimal dose: The smallest amount of a drug that produces a therapeutic effect
Maximal dose: The largest amount of a drug that it is possible to give safely
Toxic dose: The amount of a drug that produces signs and symptoms of poisoning
Lethal dose: The amount of a drug that causes death

into the patient's system and to the site where the intended action of the drug takes place.

In the pharmacodynamic phase, the drug's active ingredient interacts with the intended body tissues, and the body's cells respond and change as the drug is metabolized.

The liver is the main organ that inactivates and metabolizes drugs, while the kidneys are the principal organs that eliminate the metabolites of drugs from the body. A **metabolite** is a substance produced by metabolic action, which results in the breakdown of the drug.

The nurse needs to understand the process of drug action in and elimination from the body because each patient is affected differently by prescribed medications. It is necessary to assess and consider each patient's hepatic (liver) and renal (kidney) functions, because decreased hepatic or renal function can prolong the length of time a drug stays active in the body.

Drugs that are not excreted adequately in the urine, feces, sweat, tears, breast milk (in lactating mothers), and exhaled air build up, or accumulate, in the patient's body. A drug that builds up in the body is said to have a **cumulative** (increasing by increments) effect, which sometimes leads to toxic (harmful) or even lethal (deadly) outcomes for the patient (Box 17.2).

Drug Dosage

Dosage is the schedule of administration (amount and frequency) of a drug prescribed for the patient by the health care provider. The health care provider's order includes information regarding the medication to be administered to the patient, including the drug's name, dosage, and route of administration. The order would read, "Give 100 mg Dilantin PO tid." A *dose* of medicine refers to a single administration of a drug. The dose ordered in the example is thus 100 mg. The nurse administers a 100-mg dose (one capsule) of phenytoin (Dilantin) three times a day; the total daily dosage is thus 300 mg (given in divided doses by mouth, or *per os* [PO]). It is important for the nurse to be familiar with **therapeutic** (beneficial) dosages of frequently used drugs to administer doses of medication competently to patients (Box 17.3). Always look up any unfamiliar medications in an approved resource before administering the medication.

Terms Used With Medication Orders

Stat: Medications ordered to be administered stat are those that are planned to manage an emergency patient condition. Stat orders have the highest priority ranking. They are to be completed before other orders. The time of actual administration must be documented. A stat order is a one-time-only dose.

Now: Now orders are high in priority but should be completed after stat orders.

One time only: In these orders, a medication is to be administered as a single dose.

prn (give as necessary): The patient is permitted to request prn medication, or the nurse may offer a prn medication; prn medication orders must specify a definite time interval between permitted repeat administrations.

Drug Actions and Interactions

Medications produce two general types of actions in a patient's body: local and systemic. A local action by a drug produces an effect only in the area where the drug has been placed, while a systemic action affects the entire body as the drug enters the patient's systemic circulation.

When one drug alters the action of another drug, it is called a drug interaction (a modification of the effect of a drug when administered with another drug). When two or more drugs are given together, the combined actions of the drugs sometimes produce an effect totally different from the expected action of either drug. These effects may benefit or harm the patient. When one drug increases the action or effect of another drug, it is called potentiation of the drug, or *synergism.* Drug combinations may be administered with the express purpose of boosting the action of the administered drugs. Compatibility is the quality or state of harmonious coexistence. Drug compatibility is the ability to administer medications together easily without any difficulty for the patient. Compatibility charts provide quick reference for the nurse to determine whether it is acceptable to administer one drug along with another drug in the same syringe or in an IV infusion. Always verify the compatibility of drugs with a reliable resource before mixing into the same syringe or in an IV infusion.

Some drugs should not be given together because the medications do not combine well chemically or physically. This problem is referred to as drug *incompatibility.* Suspect drug incompatibility when two drugs are mixed together and the solution changes color, becomes cloudy, or forms a precipitate (a reaction in which a new solid mass is formed). Drug interactions are more likely to occur with drugs that are especially potent, such as digitalis. Cardiotonics (drugs that slow and strengthen the heart), antihypertensives (drugs that lower blood pressure), hypoglycemic agents (oral medications that lower blood glucose level), insulin (injectable medication that lowers blood glucose level), and heparin (medication that decreases the clotting of blood) are common powerful agents; be familiar with these drugs before administering them. With drug interactions, the medication may increase or decrease the action of one or more other medications. Sometimes the medications may create an adverse reaction that is not normally associated with either drug. Drug interactions are often the result of drug incompatibilities that alter how the medication is absorbed, distributed, metabolized, or excreted. They may produce adverse effects in the patient, which may lead to reduced patient compliance and prolonged hospitalization. During the assessment of the patient, the nurse is responsible for monitoring the patient for occurrence of drug interactions and adverse reactions to medications. Assess the patient for changes in level of consciousness, slurred speech, ataxia, and changes in the patient's vital signs. Listen to what the patient says about the effects of the medication. The LPN/LVN should report any adverse reactions to the medication or possible drug interactions to the registered nurse (RN) and document these findings objectively. Health care providers depend on the ongoing nursing assessment of each patient's response to drug therapy.

The nurse must be knowledgeable about agonistic and antagonistic effects associated with medications. A drug that produces a predictable response at the intended site of action is called an agonist. An antagonist is a drug that blocks the action of another drug. Antagonistic drugs are used to counteract the effects of a previously given drug. A common antagonist prescribed is naloxone hydrochloride (Narcan), which is given when a person has received too much of an opioid medication, such as morphine sulfate. Too much morphine sulfate may produce life-threatening depression of the respiratory and central nervous systems, but naloxone blocks the action of the opioid.

Remember that each patient may respond differently to medications. Assess the patient for the development of an idiosyncratic reaction. An idiosyncratic reaction to a drug results from the individual's unique hypersensitivity to it; it is an unexpected response to a medication. For example, a patient takes a medication prescribed to help reduce anxiety, but the patient becomes more agitated and restless instead. These manifestations are consistent with an idiosyncratic reaction. It is important to monitor all patients who are receiving medication for signs of overdose, toxicity (dangerous buildup of a substance), and unexpected drug reactions.

Some patients may have had hypersensitivity reactions or allergic reactions to drugs. If possible, assess the patient's drug history before administering medication. The following questions may be helpful to ask the patient: Have you taken the drug before? Do you have any known allergies to medications? If you determine the patient has had a reaction to a prescribed medication, withhold the drug, report this information to the RN, and notify the patient's health care provider.

A reduced response to a drug over time is called drug tolerance. The patient who has developed tolerance to a drug requires a larger dose of the drug to achieve the same effect that a smaller therapeutic dose once produced. Drug tolerance is either acquired from taking increasing dosages of the drug over time or a result of genetic factors that are unique to the individual.

It is essential to monitor each patient's reaction to drug therapy, particularly when the patient receives a medication for the first time. To establish baseline information, the patient should be assessed before and after a new medication is started. Any changes in mental or physical status should be reported to the RN. Mental or physical changes that occur after administration of a medication could represent an adverse drug reaction (a harmful, unintended reaction to a drug administered at a normal dosage), drug hypersensitivity, or intolerance to the drug.

Drug administration is a tremendous nursing responsibility. The nurse should never give any unfamiliar medication to a patient without first reviewing information about the drug from an approved facility resource (such as the pharmacy department, a current drug handbook, or an online resource). Use the resource to determine the therapeutic dosage, indications for use of the drug, *contraindications* (conditions in which the drug should not be used), side effects, available formulations and routes of administration, generic and trade names, and information regarding how to manage overdoses. The following factors may affect how patients respond to medication:

- *Age:* Very young and very old people generally react more acutely to drugs than do other people. Older adults tend to have a higher ratio of fat tissue to muscle tissue, and the higher fat percentage typically affects how the fat-soluble medication is distributed and stored. Drug action is likely to be prolonged in older adults because renal and hepatic function is often diminished with age (Table 17.1). In very young children, liver and kidney function is not fully developed; as a result, metabolism or excretion of medications may be inefficient.
- *Weight:* Overweight people sometimes require more medication or higher drug dosages than do patients who are of average weight. Patients who are underweight may require lower drug dosages. Body surface area, height, and weight are often used to help determine drug dosages in children.

- *Gender:* Women tend to have a higher percentage of body fat than men. Because some drugs are fat soluble, women with a high body fat percentage tend to accumulate fat-soluble drugs in their bodies. Advise pregnant and lactating women that the substances taken during pregnancy may have the capacity to pass through the placenta and adversely affect the fetus. Some drugs may also pass to infants through breast milk.
- *Ethnicity:* There are slight differences in the responses between ethnic groups regarding the effects of certain drugs on their systems. The differences may be in part related to differences in the drug metabolism enzymes in the liver between some races. Examples include the variations in sensitivity (increased or reduced) of African Americans to certain classes of antihypertensive medications, or the increased difficulty controlling asthma in Caucasians who have certain genetic makeups (Belle and Singh, 2008; Brewster and Seedat, 2013; Ortega and Meyers, 2014).
- *Physical condition:* Disease processes may alter medication dosage requirements, particularly in patients with renal, hepatic, cardiovascular, or gastrointestinal (GI) disorders.
- *Psychological status:* Stress, emotional conflict, anxiety, and fear have the capacity to alter the patient's response to drug therapy. The nurse may help increase the patient's compliance with the medication regimen by adequately educating the patient about the medication they have been prescribed. The nurse's skill set, actions, and attitudes regarding drug administration can affect the patient's response to drug therapy as well.
- *Environmental temperature:* The patient may metabolize a drug more quickly when they are in a warm environment and may metabolize a medication more slowly when they are in a cold environment.
- *Amount of food in the stomach:* A medication taken on an empty stomach tends to reach the bloodstream faster than a medication taken on a full stomach. Irritating drugs are administered after or with meals so that they produce fewer GI side effects, such as nausea.
- *Route of administration:* The route that the medication is given influences the onset, intensity, and duration of a drug. A medication that is administered through an IV route or injected into the patient's muscle works more quickly than medications given by mouth.

Stay current regarding the basics of drug actions, how medication orders are written, how to interpret them, how the orders are received, and how they are transcribed. Always follow the basic practices and principles of safe medication administration. High personal and professional standards protect the patient and help avoid medication errors.

Table 17.1   Influence of Aging on Drug Actions in Older Adults

AGE-RELATED PHYSIOLOGIC CHANGE	EFFECT ON DRUG ACTION AND PATIENT RESPONSE	NURSING INTERVENTIONS
Gastrointestinal Tract		
Oral Cavity		
Loss of elasticity in oral mucosa, which becomes dry and easily abraded	Difficulty in swallowing tablets or capsules; sensitivity to drugs that cause dryness of mouth, which increases susceptibility to gum disease and dental caries	Have patient rinse oral cavity frequently with clear tepid water, floss daily, and brush teeth and gums gently. Recommend synthetic saliva substitute.
Esophagus		
Delayed esophageal clearance because of weakened contractions and failure of lower esophageal sphincter to relax	Difficulty in swallowing large tablets or capsules; tissue erosion caused by drugs such as aspirin and uncoated potassium chloride	Position patient upright. Administer full glass of liquid with drug. Crush tablets and mix with food (if gastric pH does not affect absorption).
Stomach		
Decrease in gastric acidity and peristalsis	Irritation from highly acidic drugs (e.g., aspirin)	Have patient drink full glass of water and take medication with nonfat snack to reduce gastric distress.
Large Intestine		
Reduced colon muscle tone; loss of defecation reflex; decreased intestinal blood flow	Slowing of drug excretion; overuse and abuse of laxatives by patient; delayed drug absorption	Provide normal fluid intake. Instruct patient to eat bulk-forming foods and to avoid use of constipating drugs.
Skin and Vascular System		
Reduced subcutaneous skinfold thickness in extremities (less body fat); reduced elasticity in skin and vascular system; increased fragility of blood vessels	Tendency for bleeding after injections	Avoid using veins in hands for intravenous (IV) injections. Apply pressure to injection sites after administration. Observe injection sites for bleeding.
Liver		
Reduced liver size; decline in hepatic blood flow	Longer biotransformation time; prolonged duration of drug action; greater risk for drug sensitivity and toxicity	Monitor for signs and symptoms of liver impairment (jaundice, pruritus, dark urine). Monitor blood chemistry values for hepatic toxicity.
Kidneys		
Reduced glomerular filtration; decreased tubular function and renal blood flow	Risk of drug accumulation and toxicity	Prevent urinary retention (keep catheters flowing freely and observe frequency of urination). Monitor for signs and symptoms of renal impairment (reduced output and difficulty in urinating). Provide normal fluid intake. Monitor blood urea nitrogen (BUN) and serum creatinine levels.

MEDICATION ORDERS

The nurse is legally and ethically responsible for ensuring that the patient receives the correct medication that has been ordered by the health care provider. Health care providers may give the nurse medication orders during patient admissions, morning and evening rounds, after surgery, or at any other time throughout the day or night as needed. As soon as possible after a health care provider writes an order it is the nurse's responsibility to read and interpret that order. Within acute care settings, the medication order is commonly shared electronically with the pharmacy department so that it may be entered accurately into the computerized system. Because of the possibility of inaccurately interpreting the handwritten medication order, more health care facilities are now requesting that health care providers enter medication orders into computers. If the nurse reads the health care provider's handwritten order and it is illegible, ask another nurse or staff member to help interpret the order. If unsure about what the order states, the nurse must contact the health care provider for clarification.

Drug Distribution Systems

There are various methods used for storing and distributing medications in health care settings. Many health care facilities have designated areas for storing

Fig. 17.2 Nurse using computer-controlled dispensing system.

medications. Medications that are stored on a patient care unit are referred to as *floor stock* because they are available on the unit and not stored solely in the pharmacy department. Areas that are used to store medications should remain locked when unattended.

In some long-term care facilities and hospitals, the unit-dose system is used to store and dispense medications. The *unit-dose system* is typically used with a portable medication cart that contains drawers. A *unit dose* is the ordered amount of medication that the patient is supposed to receive at a prescribed time. The medication cart holds the unit doses for each patient, and the nurse transports the medication cart from room to room to administer the medication at designated times. The medication cart is locked when not attended, and in some institutions, there is a locked cabinet in each patient's room where their medications are stored.

Computer-controlled dispensing systems are a combination of unit-dose and floor stock systems. These machines contain various medications that are placed in individual compartments and is commonly stocked by the pharmacy department with medications that are commonly prescribed on that unit. The nurse uses a computer to choose the medication to remove, and is assigned a security code that allows access to the medications specifically prescribed for an individual patient. The system's computer records medications removed and can be used to assist the health care facility with charging the patient for medications that were administered (Fig. 17.2).

Regardless of the type of system used to store and dispense medications, it is the nurse's responsibility to properly store medications according to the policies and procedures of the health care facility where the nurse is working. The storage instructions must be followed for each medication; the chemical properties of some medications may necessitate refrigeration or storage in cool or even reduced-lighting environments.

Medications may be referred to by several different names. The two most common names for medications are the trade name and the generic name. The trade name is the brand name given to it by the manufacturer for use especially by consumers and health care providers; on the packaging, this name is often followed by the symbol "®." The trade name is usually short, readily recognized, easy to spell, and easy to pronounce, such as "Lasix." The first letter is capitalized. The generic name is usually longer, may refer to the chemical composition of the medication, and is not capitalized; it often is written after the trade name and is listed in parentheses. Medications may be marketed under either their generic or trade names; for example, the generic name for Lasix is "furosemide" (FDA, 2009; NLM, 2017). Generic medications traditionally cost less than their more easily recognized trade (brand) names, but the generic medications have the same ingredients, potency, dosage, quality, and purity of brand-name medications. The US Food and Drug Administration requires testing for all approved medications.

Knowledge regarding suffixes (an appendage at the end of a word or phrase to form a commonality) and the category of medications associated with specific suffixes is helpful to the nurse. The suffixes provide information about the classification and uses of medications; for instance, the suffix "-semide," as in "furosemide" and "torsemide," indicates that these medications are loop diuretics.

The nurse must ensure that the medication ordered by the health care provider is administered correctly. The nurse should consult resources such as the pharmacy department, drug reference book, or online resources if they have any questions regarding a patient's medication.

The nurse must always ensure that the health care provider's order includes the following critical information to ensure the patient's safety:
- Patient's name (on the health care provider's order sheet)
- Patient's date of birth
- Date and time of the order (usually on the left side of the order sheet), written by the health care provider
- Name of drug (may be brand name, generic name, or both)
- Dosage of the drug, including size and frequency (e.g., "650 mg q 4 hr prn" [i.e., every 4 hours as needed])
- Route of administration, as prescribed by the health care provider
- Signature of the health care provider
- Any special instructions regarding any aspect of administering the drug (e.g., "650 mg q 4 hr if temperature >101°F")

Controlled Substances

Opioids, barbiturates, and other controlled medications that have a high possibility for abuse, addiction, or theft are kept in a secured area. In facilities where computerized systems are not used, special keys must be used to obtain these types of medications for patients when they are ordered. The special keys, called "narcotic keys," are kept by designated nurses each shift. The narcotic keys are used to unlock the storage container where the controlled substances are stored. The nurse usually must use a double-locking system with two separate keys. It is the nurse's responsibility to ensure that each controlled drug used during that shift is logged in a narcotic logbook. At the end of each shift, controlled drugs in the storage container are counted carefully by a designated nurse from the outgoing shift and by a nurse from the incoming shift. The number of drugs given, according to the logbook, and the actual number of medications contained in the storage container should be reviewed for accuracy. The outgoing staff should not be dismissed until the narcotic count is done and verified. If the count is incorrect and medication is missing, it is necessary to find the error or identify the issue before anyone is dismissed from the facility.

Many agencies now use computerized systems for medication access and distribution. Computerized storage has eliminated the need to perform the narcotic count at the end of each shift, as discrepancies with narcotic counts can be identified more readily with computerized systems. Counts of controlled substances are performed each time pharmacy staff members restock medications, and nurses are required to count before the removal of controlled substances from these types of computerized machines.

Medications are available in specific dosages. The dosage order may necessitate the use of only a portion of the available medication, at which time the nurse must dispose of (waste) what is remaining. When disposing of a controlled substance, the nurse must have a witness that is a licensed member of the nursing team. The witness and the nurse wasting the medication are required to document the information in accordance with the health care facility's policy and procedure (via computerized documentation or logbook) to indicate that the medication was wasted (Box 17.4).

Types of Orders

Standing orders. Standing orders are those that are already created by a health care provider for patients who are admitted to a particular unit. The nurse may enact the orders without having to contact the health care provider to request orders. The orders are accessible to the nurses on the unit via computer or on paper; the nurse must know how to locate the orders and enact the orders. Standing orders can make the admission process easier and more efficient for the patient and the nurse. The nurse is also responsible to know when to question an order because it is not applicable or appropriate for a specific patient; questions or concerns about the orders must be clarified with the health care provider before the medication may be administered.

Verbal or telephone orders. Ideally, medication orders should be written by the health care provider on the patient's order sheet. Situations may arise in which the

---

Box 17.4 · Guidelines for Safe Administration and Storage of Opioids and Other Controlled Substances

- All opioids and other controlled substances must be stored in a locked, secure cabinet, computerized medication dispenser, or secure medication storage container, per facility policy.
- Nurses must use keys to unlock secured medication storage containers or sign into a computerized medication dispenser to remove controlled substances.
- The controlled substances are counted per facility policy. In some long-term care facilities, the controlled medications may be counted at each change of shift. Other acute care agencies may require the pharmacy counts during restocking of the controlled substances within the computerized medication system. Each nurse who removes a controlled substance is required to count the remaining medication at that time.
- Discrepancies in opioid counts must be reported immediately.
- In some long-term care facilities, the paper inventory record is used to document the patient's name, birth date, room number, date, time of drug administration, name of drug, dosage, and signature of nurse dispensing the drug.
- This form provides an accurate, ongoing count of opioids and other controlled substances used and remaining.
- If only one part of a premeasured dosage of a controlled substance is given, a second nurse witnesses disposal of the unused portion and documents such on the record form or in the computer, per facility policy.

---

provider is not able to write the orders, and in this case, a verbal order may be given to the LPN/LVN or RN directly or over the phone. Follow the health care facility's policy when taking verbal or telephone orders. Verbal orders should be transcribed or entered into a computer, per facility policy. The health care provider should sign (or electronically sign) the order as soon as possible. The nurse should be careful when taking verbal orders; if anything about the order is unclear or confusing, the nurse must clarify the information with the health care provider. When receiving a verbal order, always repeat the order to the health care provider to ensure that it is correct.

SIX "RIGHTS" OF MEDICATION ADMINISTRATION

Use each step of the nursing process when carrying out responsibilities pertaining to medication administration. Medications are administered in a variety of ways. Regardless of the route by which a drug enters the body, the same practices and principles of medication administration apply.

Proper and accurate medication administration can be achieved by following the six "rights" of medication administration (Box 17.5), performing the three label checks (to be described), using standard precautions, practicing good hand hygiene, and using aseptic technique.

1. Right Medication

The Joint Commission requires nurses to reconcile the patient's medication record with the medications the patient reports in order to verify that the patient is receiving the correct medications, obtain a list of medications that the patient was taking at home and review it with the patient and/or family to make sure the information is correct, and document the information about these medications to share with the health care provider. The health care provider may wish to reorder the patient's home medications when the patient is admitted to the hospital. It is essential that the patient receives the correct medications; when the patient is transferred to another health care setting or discharged home, verify again the list of medications that the patient should take after discharge.

Make sure the drug to be given is the correct drug and perform the three label checks: checking the label on the drug's container three times—before, during, and after preparation. Take the medication to the patient's bedside in its original packaging and open the packaging immediately before administering the dose (Box 17.6).

Never give a medication that another person has prepared, and never prepare or use a medication that is not labeled. In both cases, it is impossible to know for sure which medication was prepared or which medication was in the unlabeled container.

Nurses must become familiar with generic and trade names of frequently used medications and always check the health care provider's order to verify information about a medication order. This ensures patient safety and reduces the chance for medication errors.

2. Right Dose

If there is a question regarding a medication dose, check the health care provider's order. Always check the label on the container to determine how the medication is supplied; for example, a medication may be supplied as 10 mg per 1 mL or 325 mg per tablet. Consult with another nurse or the pharmacist to check

any calculations or to clarify a dosage. Some computerized medication documentation systems require that another nurse document along with the nurse preparing and administering the dose (such as with insulin), to ensure that it is the correct dose.

The chance of an error during the process of administering medication increases when a medication is prepared from a dose formulation other than what has been ordered. Always compare the calculation of a dose with a second nurse who has calculated the dose independently. It is especially important to double-check a peer's calculation if it is an unusual or uncommonly performed calculation on that unit or if the calculation involves a dosage of a potentially toxic ("high alert") medication. Always use the correct type of measuring devices while preparing medications.

The assessment must include consideration to the appropriateness of the prescribed dose. Consider several questions: Is the dose appropriate for the age of the patient, the diagnosis of the patient's condition, and the sex of the patient? Look at the number of tablets that constitute the dose or the number of milliliters that make up the dose. Does the number of tablets or the number of milliliters in the syringe look and sound reasonable? It is important to double-check the decimal place in the dosage ordered and the calculations; a decimal in the wrong place could produce a toxic or lethal outcome.

3. Right Time

The nurse is responsible for administering the medication at the right time. Many health care facilities use a standardized schedule for medication administration; refer to the facility's policy regarding the timing of medications that are given routinely. Table 17.2 lists commonly used abbreviations.

Medications should typically be administered within 30 minutes of their scheduled time; no earlier than 30 minutes beforehand and no later than 30 minutes afterward. Follow the health care facility's policies and procedures regarding timing of medication. Some long-term care facilities allow administration as long as 60 minutes before or 60 minutes after the scheduled time. As-needed (prn) medications may not be administered before the time intervals ordered by the prescriber. The date that the order

---

Box **17.5**   Six "Rights" of Medication Administration
1. Right medication 2. Right dose 3. Right time 4. Right route 5. Right patient 6. Right documentation

Box **17.6**   Three Label Checks of Medication Administration
1. Check the label when taking the medication from where it has been stored. 2. Check the label before removing the medication from its container. 3. Check the label before discarding or replacing the medication container and before giving the medication to the patient.

Table **17.2** Commonly Used Abbreviations		
ABBREVIATION (LATIN TERM)	**MEANING**	**EXAMPLE**
bid (bis in die)	Two times a day	0900 and 1700 hr
tid (ter in die)	Three times a day	0900, 1300, and 1700 hr
qid (quater in die)	Four times a day	0800, 1200, 1600, and 2000 hr
ac (ante cibum)	Before meals	Varies with hospital or unit
pc (post cibum)	After meals	Varies with hospital or unit

was written should be reviewed to ensure that administration of the drug, the IV infusion, or the blood product is started and given on the right day and at the right time.

4. Right Route

The route chosen for administering a drug depends on the drug's properties, desired effect, and the patient's physical and mental condition. It is necessary to specify the route of administration on all prescribed medication orders, and if the route of administration is not noted on the medication order, contact the prescriber immediately. The nurse may be involved in judging the best route for a drug to be given. If an injection is prescribed, only special sterile solutions called *parenteral medications* are acceptable to use. Parenteral medications are labeled "for injectable use only." Serious complications may result if a liquid intended for oral use is injected. When the medication preparation is parenteral (intramuscular [IM], subcutaneous [subcut], intradermal [ID], or intravenous [IV]), the nurse must inject the medication into the appropriate type of body tissue.

5. Right Patient

Give the right medication to the right patient. Prevent medication errors by systematically identifying the patient before administering medication. There are several ways to do this; the nurse must always follow the facility's policy. Check the patient's identification bracelet to validate their name and date of birth, and then ask the patient to verify their name and date of birth. Some facilities employ the use of a portable cart with a laptop computer that the nurse uses to verify medications. The nurse scans a barcode located on the patient's identification bracelet to ensure that the right patient is receiving the right medication.

An unconscious or confused patient may be unable to provide self-identification. A family member or visitor may be at the bedside, but do not rely solely on others to identify the patient. Check the identification bracelet on all patients. Always review allergies before medication administration. In long-term care facilities, residents may not be required to wear identification bracelets or may be confused or unable to communicate their identity. Long-term care facility patients traditionally have numerous health concerns and as a result take large quantities of medications; this presents a unique safety challenge for the nurse who is assigned to complete the administration of medications. Follow facility policy to ensure proper identification of patients.

6. Right Documentation

Document the medication administration appropriately to help reduce medication errors (Fig. 17.3). Make a notation of the medication administration on the patient's chart or in the computer *immediately* after administering the drug. The policy of the health care facility may require that the documentation of injected (subcutaneous, intradermal, intramuscular) medications also include the site of the injection. In the medication administration record (MAR), whether a chart or in a computer, identify the drug given, the dosage, and the time the medication was actually given (not the time it was supposed to be given). In areas where immunizations are given, policy typically requires the nurse to note the lot number listed on the vial, the manufacturer of the vaccine, and the expiration date of the vaccine. The nursing assessment must include a description of any response the patient has to the medications or their administration. Examples of information to include may involve any complaints, adverse effects, and therapeutic effects. This information may have to be shared with the RN and the health care provider. The nurse should never document the administration of a medication until after the medication is given (see Box 17.8 and the Safety Alert box).

 Safety Alert

THE JOINT COMMISSION'S "DO NOT USE" LIST OF ABBREVIATIONS

Each health care facility is obliged to develop and adhere to a "Do Not Use" list of abbreviations, acronyms, and symbols, which must include those banned by The Joint Commission (2019). These abbreviations are not to be used during documentation. Each health care facility is permitted to add its own entries to the list of banned abbreviations. The Joint Commission's banned abbreviations must not appear in any documentation, including preprinted forms and computer documentation systems (see Appendix A).

If the six "rights" of medication administration are followed, it is not possible to give medication prepared by another nurse. It is impossible to assume that all the "rights" are followed unless the person who prepares the medication is the one who administers it.

To reduce the chance of making a medication error, follow the health care facility's policies and procedures and use common sense. If an error is made, the nurse must be honest when reporting the issue and perform prompt follow-up activities as directed by the RN and health care provider (Boxes 17.7 and 17.8).

IMPORTANT CONSIDERATIONS OF MEDICATION ADMINISTRATION

While handling equipment during medication administration, follow the principles of clean and sterile technique as applicable. Wash hands before and after caring for each patient, keep workspaces and equipment clean and organized, and work with the health care facility to establish practices that keep staff members and patients safe. Do not take shortcuts, and never deviate from principles that are effective. Follow these guidelines:

1. If you did not pour it, do not give it.
2. If you gave it, chart it.
3. Do not chart for someone else or have someone else chart for you.
4. Do not transport or accept a container that is not labeled.
5. Do not put down an unlabeled syringe; keep it in your hand or label it before you put it down.

6. If given a verbal order, write it down, and then repeat the order to the health care provider.
7. If you make an error, report it to the charge nurse or supervisor and health care provider immediately. An incident report also should be completed.
8. Never leave a medication tray or cart unattended or unlocked.
9. Do not leave a medication with a patient or family member. Watch the patient take and swallow all medications.
10. Monitor the patient's response to the medication.
11. Chart immediately after giving medication.
12. If a patient refuses medication even after you have performed patient education regarding the medication, do not attempt to force the patient to take it; document "Refused _____ medication because of [state reason patient refused medication]."
13. If you choose to omit a dose based on nursing judgment, request that an RN or another nurse in charge help make the decision. If the medication is omitted, the reason for the omission must be documented. Be objective and exact in charting. Report the decision to the health care provider (see the Home Care Considerations box).

🏠 Home Care Considerations

DRUG SAFETY

Instruct the patient to do the following:

- Keep each drug in its original labeled container.
- Protect drugs from exposure to heat and light, per directions from manufacturer of the medication.
- Ensure that labels are legible.
- Discard outdated medications.
- Always finish the course of a prescribed drug unless otherwise instructed, and never save a drug for future illnesses.
- The very best way to dispose of drugs is via medicine take-back programs in the community. Medications that are flushed down a sink or toilet may end up in the general drinking water. Some medications can be removed from original containers and mixed with kitty litter, coffee grounds, or another type of unpleasant substance; this would deter animals or other people who may go through the trash from taking the medications.
- Never give a family member or friend a drug prescribed for another person.
- Refrigerate drugs as directed.
- Read labels carefully and follow instructions.
- Notify health care provider of any side effects.

Fig. 17.3 (A) Medication administration record.

Fig. 17.3, cont'd (B) Computerized list of ordered medications. ([B] Courtesy Barnes-Jewish Hospital, St. Louis, Missouri. In Elkin MK, Perry AG, Potter PA: *Nursing interventions and clinical skills*, ed 4, St. Louis, 2008, Mosby.)

ROUTES OF ADMINISTRATION

Drugs enter the body through three general routes: enteral, percutaneous, and parenteral. The drugs that enter the body by these routes come in various forms, or formulations. In addition to these most common routes, medications may also be administered vaginally or through the anus.

ENTERAL ADMINISTRATION

Drugs that enter through the **enteral** routes (i.e., are absorbed within the GI tract) are given in these forms:

1. *Powders:* Often mixed with a liquid (diluent) before administration.

2. *Pills:* Round, solid drug form that must break down into solution form (dissolution) in the stomach.

3. *Tablets:* Round, spherical, or other-shaped forms that dissolve in the stomach.

   a. *Scored* tablets are indented to allow tablet to be broken in half.

   b. **Enteric-coated** tablets are encased by a coated shell that keeps the tablet from being absorbed in the stomach; absorption takes place in the intestines. *Enteric* pertains to the small intestine.

   c. *Capsules* are powders or pellets enclosed in a gelatin-like, elongated, spherical form; the medications are encapsulated because (1) the substance is bad tasting or (2) the substance is a capsule

Box 17.7 Safety Tips for Medication Administration

- *Listen to the patient.* Listening to the patient can be a mechanism for preventing medication errors. If the patient says that they do not take a certain medication when preparing to administer the medication, refer to the medication administration record to ensure an error has not been made.
- *Rely on pharmacists as a resource to prevent errors.* Pharmacists can provide information about medications, including mechanism of action, interactions, compatibility concerns, side effects, and correct dosages.
- *Unit-dose packages.* Prepare only one patient's medications at a time and leave drugs in their labeled packages. This allows for identification of the medication name before it is administered to the patient.
- *Keep calculations to a minimum.* If calculating a drug dosage, ask another nurse to independently calculate the dose and the rate, and compare answers.
- *Ask for an independent double-check of high-alert drugs before administration.* For high-risk drugs, such as insulin and heparin, a second nurse must verify the accuracy of the dose prepared.
- *Do not sacrifice safety for timeliness.* Outside of emergencies, the need to quickly administer drugs does not outweigh safe practices. Although medications are readily available from medication-dispensing systems, it is advisable to allow the pharmacist time to review medication orders.
- *Always report errors.* Incident reports for medication administration errors offer a means to track common errors and guide policies and teaching that will help prevent future errors.
- *Review the literature for error reports from other facilities.* Review of medication error literature is a common practice among quality improvement teams within a facility. A high volume of errors with similar themes may signal the need for review and modification of current medication practices.

Modified from Institute for Safe Medication Practices: www.ismp.org.

Box 17.8 Additional Safety Tips for Medication Administration

- Follow the six "rights" of medication administration (see Box 17.5).
- Be sure to read labels at least three times (comparing medication administration record with label): (1) when you remove the drug from where it has been stored, (2) before you take it to a patient's room, and (3) before you administer the drug (see Box 17.6).
- Use at least three patient identifiers when possible (e.g., name band, patient's pronouncing name, patient's verifying date of birth) whenever you administer a medication.
- Do not allow any other activity to interrupt the administration of medication to a patient.
- If the health care provider's handwriting is illegible, clarify the order with the health care provider.
- Question orders for unusually large or unusually small doses.
- Document all medications as soon as you give them.

Data from Perry AG, Potter PA, Elkin MK: *Nursing interventions and clinical skills,* ed 6, St. Louis, 2021, Mosby.

---

with time-release pellets to delay the action of the drug.

    d. *Lozenges,* or *troches,* are sweet mucilage types of tablets that dissolve in the mouth to release medication.

4. *Liquids and suspensions:* Solid particles and liquid that the nurse must shake for dispersion of solid particles throughout the liquid portion before they can be absorbed by the body.

5. *Suppositories:* Drugs mixed with a lubricated substance molded to insert into body cavities such as the rectum, vagina, or urethra; absorption occurs after substance melts at body temperature.

The following are terms used to describe how medications are administered enterally:

- *PO:* By mouth (oral)
- *Enema:* By rectum
- *Suppository:* By rectum, vagina, or urethra
- *Tubal:* By nasogastric, gastrostomy, or jejunostomy tube

Preparation of Tablets, Pills, and Capsules

Medications in tablet, pill, and capsule form enter the GI tract and are absorbed more slowly into the bloodstream than those taken by any other route. The slow absorption rate makes the PO route safer; however some PO medications are irritating to the patient's GI tract, and larger tablets may be difficult for some patients to swallow (Skill 17.1).

If the LPN/LVN makes an error in administering medication, it should be reported immediately to the RN. The facility may require the nurse to fill out an incident report to document the error. Do not hesitate to report an error, because prompt intervention may help prevent patient complications related to the error.

Preparation of Liquid Medications

Liquid medication is the formulation often chosen for children; for patients who are not able to swallow tablets, pills, or capsules; and for older adult patients. It is possible to give liquids PO or via a nasogastric, gastrostomy, or jejunostomy tube.

Never give PO liquids to unconscious patients because they could aspirate (inhale) the medication into the respiratory tract.

Some liquid medications (such as cough medicine) are not to be followed with water, and some medications (iron) tend to stain the teeth. Inspect the medication's label (Skill 17.2) for instructions before administering.

Skill 17.1   Administering Tablets, Pills, and Capsules

CHECK   GATHER   HELLO   ID   PRIVACY   EXPLAIN   WASH   GLOVES

NURSING ACTION *(RATIONALE)*

1. Follow the six "rights" of medication administration (see Box 17.5). *(Prevents medication errors.)*
2. Perform the three label checks (see Box 17.6). *(Prevents medication errors.)*
3. Follow standard precautions. *(Prevents spread of microorganisms.)*
4. Perform hand hygiene. *(Prevents spread of microorganisms.)*
5. If using a unit-dose package, place unopened medication package in medicine cup. *(Prevents medication errors.)*

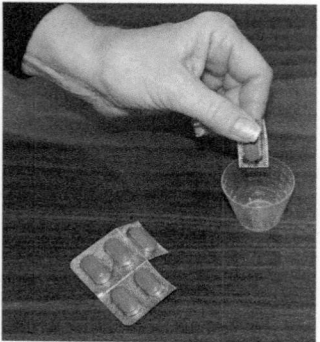

6. If using a multidose bottle, pour tablet, without touching it, into cap of bottle. *(Prevents contamination.)*
7. Pour tablet from cap into medicine cup.
8. If pouring from multidose bottle and patient is to receive several tablets, use a separate cup for medications such as digitalis, and label this cup with the name of the medication. If the patient's pulse is less than 60 bpm, withhold the medication and report this action to the RN and the health care provider. *(Placing digitalis in a separate cup marked with the medication's name allows easy identification.)*
9. If a tablet must be broken in half to administer half the dose, use gloved hands or a cutting device. Break the tablet along the scored line located at the center of the tablet. Depending on the health care facility's policy, the remainder of the tablet should either be disposed of or saved in its original container.
10. If a patient has difficulty swallowing, use a mortar and pestle or another pill-crushing device. The crushed medication is often mixed with applesauce, yogurt, or some other soft food item. Ask the patient his or her preference regarding in what to place the medication. Remember that it is not appropriate to crush drugs that are capsules, enteric coated, long acting, or slow release; these types of drugs are developed to prevent stomach irritation, or the medication may be destroyed by gastric acids. Some medications are not meant to be crushed because crushing increases the absorption rate, and the medication is meant to be released and absorbed slowly. If the medication label specifies "extended release," "sustained release," "XL," "SR," or "CD," then the medication should not be crushed.
11. Any medications dropped during the medication pass must be disposed of according to facility policy. *(Prevents contaminated medications from being administered to patient.)*
12. Transport medication to patient's room.
13. Identify patient by checking identification bracelet and per facility policy. *(Prevents medication errors.)*
14. Explain procedure to patient.
15. Document administration of medication on the medication administration record (MAR) with time, date, and name, or with computerized documentation.
16. Return at an appropriate time to assess patient's response to medication. *(Enables you to determine effectiveness of medication and any occurrence of adverse reactions. Some medication routes act more quickly than other routes.)*
17. Document side effects and therapeutic responses per facility policy.

Tubal Medications

Nasogastric (NG) tubes that are used to provide nutrition directly into the stomach are used to administer liquid medications to unconscious patients, dysphagic patients (patients who have difficulty swallowing), and those who are too ill to eat. It is also possible to use a gastrostomy tube (placed through the abdominal wall and into the stomach) or jejunostomy tube (placed through the abdominal wall and into the jejunum) in the same manner as the NG tube.

Many tubal medicines come in liquid form. Some that do not, such as those available only as solid tablets, may have to be pulverized (crushed to a powder) with the use of crushing device for some patients. Mix the crushed tablet with 30 mL of water and administer the mixture through the tube. It is also possible to open capsules, mix the contents with 30 mL of water, and administer this mixture through a tube (Skill 17.3). However, not all tablets are safe to be crushed (e.g., enteric coated), and not all capsules are safe to be opened (e.g., medications that are time released). Doing so creates the risk of toxic effects (see Skill 17.1, Step 10). Check the correct clinical pharmacology reference or the *Physician's Desk Reference* to verify the safety of pulverizing specific tablets or opening specific capsules.

OTHER METHODS OF MEDICATION ADMINISTRATION

Suppositories

A suppository is a cone-, egg-, or spindle-shaped medication made for insertion into the rectum, vagina, or urethra. Suppositories dissolve at body temperature and are absorbed directly into the bloodstream and are useful for infants, patients who cannot take oral preparations, and patients who are experiencing nausea or are vomiting (Skill 17.4).

Suppositories should be stored in a cool place so that they do not melt. They often are stored in a refrigerator. When handling a suppository, nurses should always wear gloves to prevent absorption of the medication into their skin.

Vaginal Irrigation and Medication Administration

Internal vaginal irrigation, or douching, usually is avoided medically unless as a preparation for surgery. Secretions from the vaginal membranes protect the vaginal area from infection, and so it is desirable *not* to wash these protective agents away. The health care provider orders the type of solution to use, such as saline, sterile water, or medicated solutions, and how often to perform the procedure. Commercially prepared douches are also available for one-time use, but the patient should be advised that it is not recommended to douche routinely, even at home (Skill 17.5 and the Coordinated Care box on vaginal irrigation). In addition, female patients may develop vaginal infections, which necessitate topical application of anti-infective agents.

Coordinated Care

Delegation

Vaginal Irrigation

- The task of administering a vaginal irrigation can be delegated to unlicensed assistive personnel (UAP) in some settings (check facility policy) unless the irrigation consists of medication administration. Initial patient evaluation requires the critical thinking of a nurse, and delegation of medical administration is inappropriate.
- Vaginal medications are available in foam, jelly, cream, and suppository forms. Excessive use of medicated douches can lead to irritation of the vaginal mucosa, and their use should be avoided (see Skill 17.5).

PERCUTANEOUS ADMINISTRATION

Dosage forms used with the percutaneous route (through the skin or mucous membranes) include lotions, ointments, creams, and powders.

The percutaneous routes are as follows:
1. *Topical:* applied to the skin
2. *Instillation:*
a. Applied to the mucous membranes of the mouth
   (1) **Sublingual** (under the tongue)
   (2) **Buccal** (in the cheek)
b. Applied to the mucous membranes of eye, ear, nose, and vagina
3. *Inhalation:* aerosolized liquids, gases

The percutaneous routes are routes by which medications are absorbed through the skin or the mucous membranes. Most percutaneous medications produce a local action, but some produce a systemic action.

The percutaneous routes include topical applications (applied to the skin), instillations, and inhalations. Absorption is rapid. Topical medications include ointments, creams, powders, lotions, and transdermal patches.

Ointments

An ointment is an oil-based semisolid medication; the nurse applies it to the skin or a mucous membrane. When nitroglycerin is applied topically, its effect lasts longer than that of the tablet form of nitroglycerin (which is administered sublingually).

Creams

Creams are semisolid, non-greasy emulsions that contain medication for external application. The nurse gently rubs creams into the area. Certain creams are prescription medications, and it is necessary to follow directions for application carefully to prevent overdosage.

Lotions

Lotions are generally aqueous preparations that are used as soothing agents in order to relieve pruritus (itchy skin), protect the skin, cleanse the skin, or act as astringents. Lotions contain suspended particles that are dispersed throughout the solution by gently shaking the bottle before application. Gently pat (do not rub) lotions onto the skin; they can be removed with soap and water (Skill 17.6).

Transdermal Patches (Topical Disk)

Adhesive-backed medicated patches are applied to the skin and provide sustained, continuous release of medication over several hours or days. Examples of medications used in transdermal patches are analgesics, nitroglycerin, nicotine, and estrogen. Choose a clean, dry area of the body. It should not be placed over an area where the skin is impaired, an area with body hair, or an area that is oily. If the skin is impaired, more medication may be absorbed, and if the skin has hair or is very oily, the transdermal patch does not stick well (Fig. 17.4).

Skill 17.2 Administering Liquid Medications

NURSING ACTION *(RATIONALE)*

1. Follow the six "rights" of medication administration (see Box 17.5). *(Prevents medication errors.)*
2. Perform the three label checks (see Box 17.6). *(Prevents medication errors.)*
3. Follow standard precautions. *(Prevents spread of microorganisms.)*
4. Perform hand hygiene. *(Prevents spread of microorganisms.)*
5. Remove liquid preparation from patient's drug box, bin, medication cabinet, or computerized medication dispenser.
6. Check dose/milliliter and total volume of medication in container.
7. Calculate dosage; if the dose ordered is different from the dose/milliliter stated on the label, calculate correct dose; if ordered medication is labeled according to a different measurement system, convert by using appropriate equivalent. Work calculation on paper.
8. Check calculations with another nurse. *(Helps prevent errors.)*
9. Obtain medicine cup that is **graduated** (has markings indicating marked amount; total volume of cup is 30 mL, or 1 oz) or appropriate graduated syringe. *(For accuracy.)*
10. Face label of bottle toward palm of hand *(to avoid soiling label)*; if label becomes soiled, return the bottle to the pharmacy. Do not give medication if label is unreadable. *(Maintains accuracy and prevents errors.)*
11. Place medicine cup on flat surface to pour while you watch at eye level, or hold medication cup up at eye level while you pour. *(Maintains accuracy.)*

12. Place cap of bottle with inner rim up to prevent contaminating inside of cap. *(To prevent contaminating remaining contents of bottle.)*
13. Read dosage amount at lowest level of **meniscus** (curve formed by liquid's upper surface). *(For accuracy.)* This can be achieved by holding the medicine cup or sitting it on a flat surface.

14. Transport medication to patient's room.
15. Identify patient by checking identification bracelet and per facility policy. *(Prevents medication errors.)*
16. Explain procedure to patient.
17. Document administration on medication administration record, whether on paper copy or with computer. Note time, date, and medication name.
18. Return at appropriate time to assess patient's response to medication. *(Enables you to determine effectiveness of medication and any occurrence of adverse reactions.)*
19. Document assessment findings in nursing notes.

Skill 17.3 Administering Medications Through Nasogastric Tubing

NURSING ACTION *(RATIONALE)*

1. Follow the six "rights" of medication administration (see Box 17.5). *(Prevents medication errors.)*
2. Perform the three label checks (see Box 17.6). *(Prevents medication errors.)*
3. Follow standard precautions. *(Prevents spread of microorganisms.)*
4. Perform hand hygiene. *(Prevents spread of microorganisms.)*

5. Prepare medication by using the same procedure as for liquid medications.
6. Gather equipment. *(Organizes procedure.)*
   - Disposable gloves
   - 10- to 20-mL syringe
   - One or more towels
   - Stethoscope
   - Bulb or Asepto syringe
   - Tap water

Skill 17.3 Administering Medications Through Nasogastric Tubing

7. Transport equipment and medication to patient's room.
8. Identify patient by checking identification bracelet and per facility policy. *(Prevents medication errors.)*
9. Explain procedure; answer questions that patient may have about the procedure. *(Establishes trust.)*
10. Place patient in high Fowler's position.
11. Put towel or towels over patient's chest and abdomen. *(Protects clothing and bed linens.)*
12. Don clean gloves. *(Reduces spread of microorganisms.)*
13. Check and recheck placement and patency of tube per facility policy (see also Chapter 15, Skill 15.5, Step 24). *(Ensures that tube is in the stomach and not in the respiratory tract.)* The following are several methods that may be used to check for accurate placement of a nasogastric (NG) tube:
    a. *Method A:* Verify placement of NG tube by x-ray film of chest and abdomen. Evidence suggests this is the best practice for initially verifying NG placement and before the administration of medications.

    b. *Method B:* Attach piston or Asepto syringe to end of NG tube. Pull plunger back or release suction of bulb syringe to aspirate stomach contents. If stomach contents are seen, instill 10 to 20 mL of water before medication administration to clear tube; proceed with administration of medication. Because of the difficulty in withdrawing fluid from small-bore feeding tubes, nurses often rely incorrectly on the auscultatory method to confirm NG feeding tube placement. Monitor the patient for signs and symptoms of tube displacement.
    c. *Method C:* Some facilities are using the litmus test instead of the auscultatory (air-instillation) method. Measure pH of aspirate with color-coded pH paper. The reference numbers associated with specific colors are whole

numbers and range from 1 to 11. Gastric aspirates are acidic with pH values of 5 or less.

14. Clamp enteral tube with rubber-tipped hemostats, with another clamping device, or by bending tubing in one hand, per facility policy. *(Prevents leakage of fluid from tube.)*
15. Attach syringe to end of tube (with plunger out of syringe).
16. Pour medication into syringe.

17. Unclamp tubing to allow medication to slowly flow by gravity.
18. Follow medication with 30 to 50 mL of water or per health care provider's order. *(Flushes the medication into stomach. Water is essential to enhance absorption of medication and is used to clean and maintain patency of NG tube.)*
19. Clamp tubing; secure tube after medication is given.
20. If NG tube is attached to suction, do not reconnect suction for 30 minutes or per facility policy. *(The medication will then have time to become absorbed because it will not be aspirated through tube.)*
21. Remove towel or towels from patient.
22. Remove gloves.
23. Leave patient in comfortable position.
24. Gather equipment; clean up patient and area.
25. Perform hand hygiene. *(Prevents spread of microorganisms.)*
26. Document administration of NG medication. Remember to document the amount of fluid used for medication administration as intake on the intake and output (I&O) sheet or per computerized documentation. *(Ensures accurate I&O measurement.)*
27. Return to assess patient's response to medication. *(Enables you to determine effectiveness of medication and any occurrence of adverse reactions.)*
28. Document assessment findings in nursing notes.

Continued

Skill 17.4   Administering Rectal Suppositories

1. Follow the six "rights" of medication administration (see Box 17.5). (*Prevents medication errors.*)
2. Perform the three label checks (see Box 17.6). (*Prevents medication errors.*) Ensure that the patient does not have any contraindications for giving the type of medication in a suppository form.
3. Follow standard precautions. (*Prevents spread of microorganisms.*)
4. Gather equipment. (*Organizes procedure.*)
   - Gloves
   - Lubricant
   - Suppository
   - Souffle cup
5. Perform hand hygiene. (*Prevents spread of microorganisms.*)
6. Obtain suppository from refrigerator or from patient's medication bin.
7. Place unopened suppository into medicine cup or **souffle cup** (ungraduated disposable paper cup).
8. Introduce yourself; explain procedure to patient. (*Enlists patient's cooperation and establishes trust.*)
9. Identify patient by checking identification bracelet and per facility policy. (*Prevents medication errors.*)
10. Provide privacy.
11. Don clean gloves. (*Protects you from fecal material and reduces the spread of microorganisms.*)
12. Position patient in Sims' position (on left side with upper leg flexed at knee). (*Position exposes anus and helps patient to relax external anal sphincter. Left-side positioning lessens the likelihood that the suppository or feces will be expelled.*)
13. Unwrap suppository.
14. Maintain privacy; expose patient's buttocks.
15. Assess anus externally and gently palpate rectal vault as needed. (*Enables you to determine presence of active rectal bleeding, as well as to note whether rectum contains feces, which potentially cause problems with suppository placement.*) Do not palpate a patient's rectum after rectal surgery. If a patient has hemorrhoids, always use a generous amount of a lubricating gel and gently manipulate the tissues to visualize the anus for insertion of the suppository.
16. Apply water-soluble lubricant to tapered end of suppository. (*Lubrication reduces friction as suppository enters rectal area.*)
17. Ask patient to take deep breath; insert tapered end of suppository beyond internal anal sphincter. Insert suppository as patient exhales to relax anal sphincter. (*Forcing suppository through constricted sphincter causes discomfort.*)
18. Ask patient to retain suppository as long as possible. (*This allows the medication to completely dissolve and absorb through mucous membranes of rectum into capillaries of systemic circulatory system.*) Hold the patient's buttocks together to help patient retain suppository. (*Provides sufficient time for the effects of the suppository to reach the maximum effectiveness.*)
19. Discard gloves.
20. Perform hand hygiene. (*Reduces spread of microorganisms.*)
21. Help patient assume a comfortable position.
22. Document administration of suppository per facility policy.
23. Return to assess patient's response to medication. (*Enables you to determine effectiveness of medication and any occurrence of adverse reactions.*)
24. Document assessment findings in nursing notes.

Skill 17.5   Performing a Vaginal Irrigation or Douche

NURSING ACTION (RATIONALE)

1. Refer to Standard Steps 1 to 9.
2. Assemble equipment:
   - Bath blanket
   - Bedpan and tissues
   - Clean gloves
   - Douche kit
   - Drape
   - Ordered solution (1000 to 1500 mL at body temperature or commercially prepared solutions in smaller amounts)
   - Solution container, tubing, and nozzle
   - Wash basin, washcloths, and towel (disposable washcloths are acceptable)
   - Waterproof pad

Skill 17.5   Performing a Vaginal Irrigation or Douche—cont'd

3. Assist patient to the supine position with legs abducted slightly. (*Position allows for easy access to and good exposure of vaginal orifice.*)
4. Prepare patient:
   a. Drape patient's abdomen and lower extremities with blanket. (*Minimizes patient's embarrassment.*)
   b. Position patient on bedpan with waterproof pad underneath. (*Allows hips to be higher than shoulders so that solution will reach posterior vagina and distend the vaginal wall, ensuring that solution reaches between the folds of the vagina. Bedpan collects solution, and pad protects bed linens.*)
   c. Be certain vaginal orifice is well illuminated. (*Ensures visualization of external genitalia for proper insertion.*)
5. Evaluate for the following: (*Findings provide baseline to monitor effect of therapy.*)
   a. Condition of external genitalia and vaginal canal
   b. Symptoms of pruritus, burning sensation, or discomfort
   c. Possible vaginal discharge and odor; perineal care is sometimes necessary before the douche is administered. (*A thick, white, patchy, curd-like discharge clinging to the vaginal walls is a sign of yeast infection, a common female disorder.*)
   d. Signs of inflammation, erythema, or edema in the perineal area
6. Prepare equipment. (*Organizes procedure.*) Ensure solution is at body temperature. (*Prevents burning the delicate mucosa of the vagina.*)
7. Perform hand hygiene, and don clean gloves. (*Prevents spread of microorganisms.*)
8. Allow some solution to drain down the tubing out through the nozzle into bedpan. (*Removes air from tubing and moistens nozzle.*) Gently retract labial folds and maintain position. Direct nozzle toward the sacrum, following the floor of the vagina. (*Allows correct position of nozzle.*)

9. Raise the container approximately 12 to 20 inches (30 to 50 cm) above level of vagina, and insert nozzle 3 to 4 inches (7 to 10 cm). Allow solution to flow while nozzle is inserted and rotated. Instruct patient to tighten perineal muscles as if to suppress urination and then relax. Have patient repeat this maneuver four or five times during procedure. Administer all of the solution. (*Allowing solution to flow during insertion moistens the vaginal orifice, thus reducing friction. Rotating the nozzle allows irrigation of all areas in the vagina. Periodic contracting and relaxing of perineal muscles allows solution to flow between rugae.*)
10. Withdraw nozzle, raise head of bed, and assist patient to a comfortable position while she remains on the bedpan. (The remaining solution drains by gravity. The bedpan collects solution.)
11. Refer to Standard Steps 10 to 17.
12. Allow patient to remain on bedpan for approximately 10 minutes; then don clean gloves, remove bedpan, and observe results. Dispose of returned solution in proper manner (know facility policy). Cleanse patient or allow patient to cleanse herself with basin of warm water, towel, and washcloth. Assist patient to a comfortable position. Remove gloves, discard them in proper receptacle, and perform hand hygiene. (*Reduces spread of microorganisms and provides for patient comfort.*)
13. Document the following. (*Verifies performance of procedure and ensures continuity of care.*)
    • Date and time
    • Type, amount, and temperature of solution
    • Evaluation of external genitalia and vagina. (*Documented description provides baseline to determine change in patient's condition.*)
    • Patient's response to procedure
    • Patient teaching
14. Report unusual findings.

Skills for Sensory Disorders

Eyedrops and eye ointments. Eyedrops and ointments are sterile. Ensure that the *ophthalmic* (eye) preparations are administered when at room temperature and that they remain sterile by not touching the dropper or the tube of ointment to the eye. Check the container to ensure that the medication is marked "for ophthalmic use." Eyedrops and ophthalmic ointments are prescribed for only one patient and are never meant to be shared between patients (Skill 17.7).

Eardrops. Containers of solutions to be used as eardrops are labeled *otic.* The eardrops should be at room temperature when applied. The eardrops are prescribed for only one patient and are never meant to be shared between patients (Skill 17.8).

Nose drops. Nose drops are for individual use only (Skill 17.9).

Nasal sprays. Because nasal sprays are absorbed quickly, less medication is used and wasted when the nurse administers them in this manner. Nasal sprays are for individual use only (Skill 17.10).

Skill 17.6   Applying Topical Agents

NURSING ACTION *(RATIONALE)*

1. Follow the six "rights" of medication administration (see Box 17.5). *(Prevents medication errors.)*
2. Perform the three label checks (see Box 17.6). *(Prevents medication errors.)*
3. Follow standard precautions. *(Reduces spread of microorganisms.)*
4. Gather equipment. *(Organizes procedure.)*
   - Gloves
   - Medication
   - Washing materials
5. Perform hand hygiene. *(Reduces spread of microorganisms.)*
6. Transport medication to patient's room.
7. Identify patient by checking identification bracelet and per facility policy. *(Prevents medication errors.)*
8. Introduce yourself; explain procedure to patient. *(Establishes trust.)*
9. Provide privacy; place patient in comfortable position that allows exposure of selected site.
10. Don gloves. *(Reduces spread of microorganisms and prevents absorption of topical agent into your skin.)*
11. Read prescription instructions carefully. *(For accuracy.)*
12. Prepare medicinal agent (ointments, creams, and lotions sometimes have to be squeezed or removed with a tongue blade, depending on preparation used).
13. Wash affected area, removing debris, encrustations, and previous medications. *(Removal of debris enhances penetration of topical drug through skin. Cleansing removes microorganisms resident in remaining debris.)* Area should be allowed to dry. *(Allows for better adherence to the skin.)*
14. With gloves on, apply medication lotion, ointment, or cream via paper, or apply medication patch (see Fig. 17.4) directly to skin. When using medication patches, be certain to remove old patch and remove plastic from disk of the new patch before applying to skin. Patches must be disposed of by folding it upon itself and following facility policy for disposal. *(Essential for absorption of medication. Do not massage medication into skin; this can cause a bolus of medication to be administered. Patches are folded upon themselves to prevent others from absorbing the medication. Some facilities may have special instructions for disposal of narcotic pain medication patches.)*
15. Remove gloves.
16. Leave patient in comfortable position.
17. Answer patient's questions and teach patient to perform self-applications if appropriate.
18. Clean work area.
19. Wash hands. *(Reduces spread of microorganisms.)*
20. Document administration per facility policy on paper copy of medication administration record or with computerized documentation system.
21. Return to assess patient's response to medication. *(Enables you to determine effectiveness of medication and any occurrence of adverse reactions.)*
22. Document assessment findings in nursing notes.

Patient Teaching

EYE CARE

- Use a calm, confident, soft voice when talking with patient, and reinforce the importance of the procedure.
- Remove the patient's contact lenses (if possible) before beginning irrigation or applying a compress.
- Reassure patient that the eye can be closed periodically and that no object will touch the eye.
- Ask patient to report any pain or foreign body sensation in the eye after irrigation, as well as any excessive tearing or photophobia.
- Have the patient close the eye to avoid movement, and report to the health care provider at once if any symptoms of irritation or infection occur.
- If a patient needs continuing eye irrigations at home but is unable to perform them, teach a responsible family member or caregiver.
- If the patient's field of vision is limited, the home environment should be evaluated and special safety precautions should be taken.

Fig. 17.4 Various medications are available as transdermal patches.

Skill 17.7   Administering Eyedrops and Eye Ointments

CHECK   GATHER   HELLO   ID   PRIVACY   EXPLAIN   WASH   GLOVES

NURSING ACTION *(RATIONALE)*

1. Follow the six "rights" of medication administration (see Box 17.5). *(Prevents medication errors.)*
2. Perform the three label checks (see Box 17.6). *(Prevents medication errors.)*
3. Follow standard precautions. *(Prevents spread of microorganisms.)*
4. Gather equipment. *(Organizes procedure.)*
   - Cotton ball or tissue
   - Eyedrops
   - Gloves
   - Sterile saline
5. Perform hand hygiene. *(Prevents spread of microorganisms.)*
6. Confirm medication is ophthalmic preparation. Transport medication to patient's room.
7. Identify patient by checking identification bracelet and asking patient's name and birth date. *(Prevents medication errors.)*
8. Introduce yourself; explain procedure. *(Establishes trust.)*
9. Provide privacy; position back of patient's head on pillow; direct patient's face upward toward ceiling.
10. Determine which eye is to receive the medication or whether both eyes should.
11. Don gloves. *(Reduces spread of microorganisms.)*
12. Remove exudate; clean eye as needed with sterile solution of saline or water; use cotton balls to wipe away exudate; use one cotton ball per stroke, wiping from inner canthus outward. *(Cleansing eye from inner to outer canthus avoids introducing microorganisms into lacrimal ducts. Soaking allows easy removal of dried exudate that harbors microorganisms.)*
13. To apply drops:
    a. Expose lower conjunctival sac by having patient look upward while gentle traction is applied to lower eyelid.

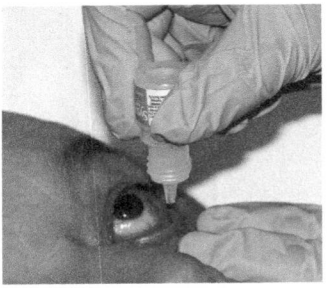

b. Put prescribed number of drops into conjunctival sac, not onto eyeball. *(Therapeutic effect of drug is obtained only when drops enter sac.)*
c. Conjunctival sac normally holds one or two drops. *(Applying drops to conjunctival sac provides even distribution of medicine across eye.)*
d. Use tissue to apply gentle pressure above bone at inner corner of eyelid for 1 to 2 minutes. *(Minimizes absorption into circulatory system.)*
e. Apply sterile dressing, if it is ordered.
14. To apply ointment:
    a. Expose lower conjunctival sac by having patient look upward while gentle traction is applied to lower eyelid.

b. Squeeze ointment into lower conjunctival sac.
c. Ask patient to close eye and move it around in circular motion. *(Spreads medication evenly.)*
d. Apply sterile dressing, if it is ordered.
15. After applying drops or ointment to an eye, leave patient in comfortable position; clean up the work area.
16. Remove gloves and wash hands. *(Reduces spread of microorganisms.)*
17. Answer patient's questions and, if appropriate, teach patient to perform self-care.
18. Record administration of medications per facility policy.
19. Return to assess patient's response to medication. *(Enables you to determine effectiveness of medication and any occurrence of adverse reactions.)*
20. Document assessment findings in nursing notes.

Skill 17.8   Administering Eardrops

CHECK   GATHER   HELLO   ID   PRIVACY   EXPLAIN   WASH   GLOVES

NURSING ACTION (RATIONALE)

1. Follow the six "rights" of medication administration (see Box 17.5). (*Prevents medication errors.*)
2. Perform the three label checks (see Box 17.6). (*Prevents medication errors.*)
3. Follow standard precautions. (*Prevents spread of microorganisms.*)
4. Gather equipment. (*Organizes procedure.*)
   - Eardrops
   - Gloves
   - Cotton ball
5. Perform hand hygiene. (*Prevents spread of microorganisms.*)
6. Confirm medication is otic preparation. Transport medication to patient's room.
7. Identify patient by checking identification bracelet and per facility policy. (*Prevents medication errors.*)
8. Introduce yourself; explain procedure. (*Establishes trust.*)
9. Provide privacy.
10. Determine which ear is to receive the medication; position patient with affected ear upward.
11. Don gloves. (*Reduces spread of microorganisms.*)
12. Remove external exudate from ear; it is necessary to obtain an order for irrigating the ear. (*Drainage harbors microorganisms and sometimes impedes distribution of medication into the canal.*)
13. Draw medication into dropper.
14. Instill drops:
    a. *For adults and for children older than 3 years:* Turn head with affected side up; pull earlobe upward and back to straighten external auditory canal; instill drops without touching ear with dropper. (*Straightening of ear canal provides direct access to deeper external structures.*)

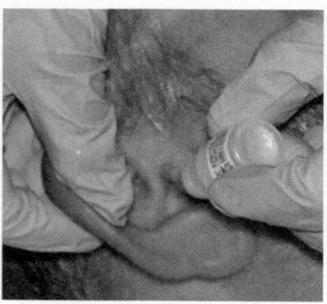

b. *For children younger than 3 years:* Turn head with affected side up; pull earlobe downward and back; instill drops without touching ear with dropper. (*Straightening of ear canal provides direct access to deeper external structures.*)

15. Tell patient to remain in same position for 5 to 10 minutes to allow medication to drain into ear by gravity. (*To promote distribution of drops in ear canal.*)
16. Place a cotton ball loosely into ear as needed. (*Prevents escape of medication when patient sits or stands.*)
17. Remove gloves.
18. Leave patient in comfortable position; clean work area.
19. Answer patient's questions and, if appropriate, teach patient self-care.
20. Perform hand hygiene. (*Reduces spread of microorganisms.*)
21. Record administration of medications per facility policy.
22. Return to assess patient's response to medication. (*Enables you to determine effectiveness of medication and any occurrence of adverse reactions.*)
23. Document assessment findings in nursing notes.

Skill 17.9   Administering Nose Drops

NURSING ACTION (RATIONALE)

1. Follow the six "rights" of medication administration (see Box 17.5). *(Prevents medication errors.)*
2. Perform the three label checks (see Box 17.6). *(Prevents medication errors.)*
3. Follow standard precautions. *(Prevents spread of microorganisms.)*
4. Gather equipment. *(Organizes procedure.)*
   - Nose drops
   - Gloves
   - Tissues
5. Perform hand hygiene. *(Prevents spread of microorganisms.)*
6. Confirm medication is nasal preparation. Transport medication to patient's room.
7. Identify patient by checking identification bracelet and per facility policy. *(Prevents medication errors.)*
8. Introduce yourself; explain procedure. *(Establishes trust.)*
9. Provide privacy.
10. Don gloves. *(Reduces spread of microorganisms.)*
11. If patient is an adult or older child, ask patient to clear nose of accumulations by blowing gently into tissue. *(Allows absorption of medication.)*
12. Determine which nostril is to receive the medication or whether both nostrils should.
13. Position patient:
    a. *Adult or older child:* Have patient lie down, hanging head backward over edge of bed (if condition permits) or with pillow under shoulders to hyperextend the neck if patient can tolerate it. *(Promotes absorption of medication.)*
    b. *Younger child:* Position child on bed with head backward and downward. *(Promotes absorption of medication.)*
    c. *Infant:* Hold infant with head backward and downward. *(Promotes absorption of medication.)*

14. After drawing medication into dropper, instill medication while holding dropper above (not touching) nostril being treated.

15. If orders specify treatment in both nostrils, repeat procedure to instill drops in other nostril.
16. Tell patient to hold position for a few minutes. *(Allows medication to remain in place.)*
17. Remove gloves.
18. Tell patient to refrain from blowing nose immediately after instillation. *(Prevents removal of medication.)*
19. Offer tissues for later use.
20. Leave patient in comfortable position; clean work area.
21. Answer patient's questions and, if appropriate, teach patient self-care.
22. Perform hand hygiene. *(Reduces spread of microorganisms.)*
23. Record administration of medications per facility policy.
24. Return to assess patient's response to medication. *(Enables you to determine effectiveness of medication and any occurrence of adverse reactions.)*
25. Document assessment findings in nursing notes.

Skill 17.10   Administering Nasal Sprays

NURSING ACTION *(RATIONALE)*

1. Follow the six "rights" of medication administration (see Box 17.5). *(Prevents medication errors.)*
2. Perform the three label checks (see Box 17.6). *(Prevents medication errors.)*
3. Follow standard precautions. *(Prevents spread of microorganisms.)*
4. Gather equipment. *(Organizes procedure.)*
   - Gloves
   - Nasal spray
   - Tissues
5. Perform hand hygiene. *(Prevents spread of microorganisms.)*
6. Confirm medication is nasal preparation. Transport medication to patient.
7. Determine which nostril is to receive the medication or whether both should.
8. Identify patient by checking identification bracelet and per facility policy. *(Prevents medication errors.)*
9. Introduce yourself; explain procedure. *(Establishes trust.)*
10. Provide privacy; position patient upright.
11. Don gloves. *(Reduces spread of microorganisms.)*
12. Have patient gently blow nose, if capable, to clear nasal passages of accumulations. *(Promotes absorption of medication.)*
13. Compress one nostril.
14. Shake bottle while holding it upright. *(To mix solution.)*
15. Insert tip of spray bottle into patient's patent nostril.
16. Instruct patient to inhale through the nose; while patient inhales, squeeze bottle.
17. If orders specify treatment in both nostrils, repeat procedure for other nostril.
18. Tell patient to refrain from blowing nose for a few minutes; offer tissues for later use. *(Promotes absorption of medication.)*
19. Answer patient's questions and, if appropriate, teach self-administration.
20. Remove gloves and wash hands. *(Reduces spread of microorganisms.)*
21. Record administration of medications per facility policy.
22. Return to assess patient's response to medication. *(Enables you to determine effectiveness of medication and any occurrence of adverse reactions.)*
23. Document assessment findings in nursing notes.

Skill 17.11   Eye Irrigation

NURSING ACTION *(RATIONALE)*

1. Refer to Standard Steps 1 to 9.
2. Assemble equipment:
   - Aseptic syringe, small bulb syringe, or plastic squeeze bottle
   - Clean gloves (mask and protective eyewear are also recommended if splashing is anticipated)
   - Cotton balls
   - Cotton-tipped applicators
   - Curved emesis basin
   - Gauze
   - Moisture-proof towel or pad
   - Sterile basin for solution
   - Warm irrigation solution as prescribed (volume depends on purpose; 200 to 500 mL)
3. Determine condition of both eyes. *(Provides baseline data to help determine change after irrigation.)*
4. Position patient with affected eye down. *(Prevents solution and contaminants from flowing into other eye.)*
5. Place moisture-proof towel or pad under patient's head. *(Prevents soiling of bed linens.)*
6. Place an emesis basin at side of face. *(Collects irrigating solution.)*
7. Don gloves. *(Reduces spread of microorganisms and protects the patient and the nurse.)*
8. Check that the irrigating solution is the correct temperature. *(Using solutions at body temperature prevents adverse reactions.)* Pour

Skill 17.11   Eye Irrigation—cont'd

a small amount of irrigating solution into sterile basin.

9. Using the thumb and index finger of the nondominant hand, separate the patient's eyelids. *(Retraction minimizes blinking and allows irrigation of conjunctiva. It also exposes eyeball and facilitates procedure.)* Never rest fingers on the eyeball but on the bone structure above and below the eye. *(Prevents placing direct pressure on the eyeball and causing damage.)*

10. Gently direct the irrigating solution along the conjunctiva from the inner to the outer canthus (see illustration). *(Follows the normal directional flow of tears and washes contaminants out of the eye.)* Use a plastic squeeze bottle unless very large amounts of solutions are needed. Sometimes a medicine dropper is sufficient or a cotton ball or a folded gauze saturated with the irrigating solution is used (depends on condition of the eye and health care provider's order).

11. Ask the patient to blink occasionally to aid in moving particles toward the conjunctival sac and out of the eye.

12. Avoid directing a forceful stream onto the eyeball. *(Reduces spread of microorganisms and decreases the risk of damage to the delicate eye structure.)*

13. Avoid touching any part of the eye with irrigation equipment. *(Prevents trauma and infection to the eye.)*

14. Gently dry the eyelids with cotton balls or a soft towel. *(Avoids force that could damage the eye structure.)*

15. Refer to Standard Steps 10 to 17.

16. Document the following. *(Verifies performance of procedure and ensures continuity of care.)*
    - Date and time of irrigation
    - Condition of eye or eyes before irrigation
    - Type of solution
    - Amount of solution
    - Duration
    - Characteristics of drainage
    - Condition of eye or eyes after irrigation
    - Patient's response
    - Patient teaching (see the Patient Teaching box on eye care)

Inner canthus

Outer canthus

© Elsevier

Irrigations

Eye irrigations. Irrigations involve a gentle washing of an area with a stream of solution delivered through a syringe. Irrigations of the eye are usually performed to relieve local inflammation of the conjunctiva, to apply antiseptic solution, or to flush out exudate or caustic or irritating solutions. In most cases, warm, normal saline and a small syringe or eyedropper are used to instill a few hundred milliliters of solution. Plain water is also acceptable, especially in an emergency situation. Always perform irrigation from the inner to the outer canthus to lessen the chances that contaminants will be absorbed through the nasolacrimal duct (Skill 17.11 and the Patient Teaching

box on eye care). Never allow the syringe tip to touch the eye. When caustic chemicals enter the eye, make sure to gently flush the eye continuously for at least 15 minutes with tap water to prevent burning of the cornea, and then refer the patient immediately to a health care provider.

Performing eye irrigation requires the skill and knowledge of a nurse. Delegation of this task to UAP is inappropriate.

In the home, a family member or the patient may perform eye irrigation with an eye cup. These cups are made of plastic or glass and are available in most drugstores. Instruct the patient about proper cleaning of the cup between uses and the need to check for chips in the glass.

Skill 17.12   Warm, Moist Eye Compresses

NURSING ACTION (RATIONALE)

1. Refer to Standard Steps 1 to 9.
2. Assemble equipment (use separate equipment for bilateral eye infections):
   - Basin of hot water
   - Prescribed solution, usually sterile water or normal saline solution
   - Sterile 4- × 4-inch gauze pads
   - Sterile basin for sterile solution
   - Sterile gloves, one pair for each eye treated
   - Sterile petroleum jelly or ophthalmic ointment and, if ordered, eye patch
   - Towels, waterproof pad, or both
3. Evaluate condition of both eyes. (*Provides baseline data to determine change after therapy.*)
4. Assist patient to a comfortable position. When applying hot compresses have the patient sit, if possible, and support patient's head with a pillow. Turn patient's head slightly to the unaffected side. (*This position helps hold the compress in place.*)
5. Place the towel or waterproof pad under patient's head. (*Protects bed linens.*)
6. Use sterile technique when infection or ulceration is present; clean technique is acceptable for all other applications. (*Reduces transmission of microorganisms.*)
7. Change gloves, dispose of in proper receptacle, and perform hand hygiene before treating each eye. (*Prevents transmission of microorganisms from one eye to the other.*)
8. Do not allow temperature of compresses to exceed 120°F (49°C). Heat solution by placing the uncapped bottle of solution in a basin of hot water. Pour the warmed solution into a sterile bowl, filling it halfway. Place sterile gauze pads in the bowl. (*Temperatures exceeding 120°F [49°C] may burn the delicate eye structures and the surrounding skin.*)

9. Take two 4- × 4-inch gauze pads from the basin. Squeeze out excess moisture. (*Prevents excess moisture from dribbling over the patient.*)
10. Instruct the patient to close the eyes. Gently apply the pads, one on top of the other, to the affected eye. Do not exert pressure on eyelids. If the patient complains that the compress is too hot, remove it immediately. (*Promotes patient's safety and prevents skin damage.*)
11. Change compress every few minutes, as necessary, for the prescribed length of time, usually 10 to 20 minutes. (*Maintains consistent temperature for the duration of therapy.*)
12. If sterility is not necessary, it is possible to apply moist heat by means of a clean washcloth. (*Clean technique is sufficient if infection or open areas are not present.*)
13. After removing each compress, check the periorbital skin for signs of redness that indicate the compress solution is too hot. (*Maintains patient's safety.*)
14. Cleanse patient's eye area and dry the skin with the remaining gauze pads. (*Promotes patient comfort.*)
15. If ordered, apply petroleum jelly or ophthalmic ointment, or eye patch. (*Petroleum jelly or ophthalmic ointment often is used on skin around the eyes to protect the skin. Promotes healing.*)
16. Refer to Standard Steps 10 to 17.
17. Document the following. (*Verifies performance of procedure and ensures continuity of care.*)
    - Date and time
    - Condition of eye or eyes before compress application
    - Type of compress
    - Temperature of solution
    - Duration of application
    - Condition of eye or eyes after treatment
    - Application of ointment, dressing, or eye patch
    - Patient's response
    - Patient teaching (see the Patient Teaching box on eye care)

If copious amounts of irrigation solution are needed, it is possible to use intravenous (IV) tubing and a bag of solution connected to a Morgan therapeutic lens for the irrigation. Connected to irrigation tubing, a Morgan lens enables continuous lavage of the eye and can be used to instill medication if needed. An adapter is used to connect the lens to the IV tubing and the solution container, and the lens is inserted into the eye.

To insert the device, ask the patient to look down as the lens is inserted under the upper eyelid. Then ask the patient to look up as the lower eyelid is retracted and released over the lens. Start the irrigation at the prescribed flow rate.

Eye compresses. Compresses (warmed, moist cloths used to reduce inflammation) are frequently used on the eyes to

Skill 17.13   Ear Irrigation

 CHECK   GATHER   HELLO   ID   PRIVACY   EXPLAIN   WASH GLOVES

NURSING ACTION *(RATIONALE)*

1. Refer to Standard Steps 1 to 9.
2. Assemble equipment:
   - Asepto or small-bulb syringe
   - Clean gloves (mask and protective eyewear are also recommended if splashing is anticipated)
   - Cotton balls
   - Cotton-tipped applicator
   - Curved emesis basin
   - Otoscope
   - Sterile basin for solution
   - Towel or moisture-proof pad
   - Warm irrigating solution prescribed (volume depends on purpose)
3. Advise patient of possible sensations involved: vertigo, fullness, and warmth. *(Prepares patient to prevent sudden movement during procedure.)*
4. Evaluate condition of external ear structures and canal for erythema, edema, and exudate.
5. Assist patient to either a side-lying or sitting position with affected ear tilted downward and position emesis basin under ear. Patient may help hold basin if able. *(Irrigating solution will flow from auditory canal into the basin. Having patient hold basin increases participation and compliance.)*

6. Place towel under patient's shoulder just under ear and emesis basin. If patient is sitting during procedure, place towel over patient's clothing. *(Prevents soiling of bed linens and of patient's clothing.)*
7. Inspect auditory canal for any accumulation of cerumen or debris. Remove what can be seen with the naked eye or the otoscope by using cotton or the applicator and solution (do not force cerumen into the canal). *(Cleanses the canal before irrigation.)*
8. Make sure irrigation solution is the proper temperature (body temperature: 98.6°F [37°C]). Test temperature of solution by sprinkling a few drops of solution on inner wrist. Fill irrigating device with appropriate volume. *(Irrigating*

solution at body temperature minimizes vertigo and discomfort and prevents damage to the ear.)*

9. Straighten auditory canal for introduction of solution. In infants, gently pull auricle (or pinna) down and back. In adults, gently pull auricle up and back. *(Facilitates entrance and flow of irrigating solution into ear canal.)*
10. With tip of syringe just above ear canal, irrigate gently by creating steady flow of solution against roof of canal. *(Flow of solution drains safely out of the canal while loosening debris.)* Do not occlude canal with tip of syringe. *(Occlusion of canal with syringe causes pressure against tympanic membrane during irrigation and could damage the tympanic membrane.)*

Stream of fluid passing behind wax or foreign body

11. Continue irrigation until all debris has been removed or all solution has been used. Check auditory canal with otoscope. *(Helps determine whether purpose of irrigation has been accomplished: to cleanse canal, instill antiseptic, or provide local heat.)*
12. Check patient for vertigo or nausea throughout procedure. Onset of symptoms may make it necessary to halt the procedure temporarily. *(Irrigating solution may cause irritation of the ear canal, which produces vertigo and nausea.)*
13. Dry auricle and apply cotton ball loosely to auditory meatus. *(Promotes comfort. Cotton ball collects drainage.)*
14. Position patient with affected ear down for 10 minutes. *(Allows solution remaining in auditory canal to drain.)*
15. Refer to Standard Steps 10 to 17.
16. Ten minutes after irrigation, return to patient to remove cotton ball and check exudate. Determine patient's level of comfort, and permit patient to resume normal level of activity when ready. *(Increase in exudate or onset of pain indicates possible injury to tympanic membrane. Aids in determining patient's tolerance of procedure.)*

Continued

Skill 17.13 Ear Irrigation—cont'd

17. Document the following. (*Verifies performance of procedure and ensures continuity of care.*)
- Date and time
- Type, temperature, and volume of solution used
- Character and amount of exudate

- Condition of the ear canal before and after irrigation
- Patient's response to irrigation
- Patient teaching (see the Patient Teaching box on ear care)

help temporarily relieve discomfort caused by irritation, inflammation, or infection. Skill 17.12 provides directions on how to apply a warm, moist eye compress safely.

Ear irrigations. Ear irrigations cleanse the external auditory canal of excess cerumen or exudate from a lesion or wound. Use a small syringe and solution at body temperature to prevent discomfort and severe vertigo in the patient. Be careful not to irritate the canal's sensitive skin lining by pulling the auricle excessively or introducing the tip of the irrigating syringe into the canal. Never occlude the auditory canal with the syringe tip; this could introduce fluid into the ear if excess pressure is applied and may cause the tympanic membrane to rupture. A slow, gentle irrigation works best (Skill 17.13 and the Patient Teaching box on ear care). Ear irrigations should not be attempted, when the obstruction is caused by a vegetable foreign body, such as a bean; vegetables tend to attract and absorb moisture and will swell, causing intense pain and complicating the removal of the object. This procedure is also contraindicated if the patient has a cold, an elevated temperature, an ear infection, or an injured or ruptured tympanic membrane.

Performing ear irrigation on the external ear requires the skill and knowledge of a nurse. Delegation of this task to UAP is inappropriate.

Nasal irrigations. Irrigation of the nasal passages is performed for several reasons. It soothes inflamed mucous membranes and washes away dried mucus, secretions, or any foreign matter present, all of which may cause obstruction of sinus drainage and airflow through the nares and may lead to development of headache, unpleasant odors, and infection. Nasal irrigation can be done with a specially designed (sometimes electronic) device, a Neti pot, or a bulb syringe. If the irrigation is meant to provide medication to the nares, the knowledge and skill of a nurse are required. If the irrigation is meant to remove dried mucus or secretions, it may be possible to delegate the task to UAP. Check facility policy.

Patients with acute or chronic nasal conditions, such as rhinitis or sinusitis, and patients who inhale allergens and toxins (e.g., coal dust, paint fumes, sawdust, pesticides) often benefit from nasal irrigations. Sometimes the health care provider orders nasal

Patient Teaching

EAR CARE
- Talk in a confident, calm voice to help the patient relax. Explain the procedure in terms that the patient will understand, and instruct the patient to inform the nurse if they feel any pain or discomfort.
- Advise the patient not to make any sudden moves in order to prevent trauma to the ear during irrigation.
- Older adults often require ongoing ear care for cerumen removal. The health care provider may recommend use of a softening agent such as slightly warmed mineral oil (0.5 to 1 mL), twice daily for several days before the irrigation.
- Older adults with large amounts of ear canal hair, those with a benign growth that narrows the ear canal, and those who habitually wear hearing aids are at higher risk for cerumen impaction.
- Instruct the patient to clean their ears with a damp washcloth wrapped around a finger. Warn the patient not to use a cotton-tipped applicator (which could rupture the eardrum).
- If patient uses a wax softener, instruct that these are softening products only and will not remove a cerumen impaction.
- Instruct patient to report the following signs and symptoms to the health care provider right away, as these may indicate a cerumen impaction:
  - Crackling noise in the ear
  - Decrease in hearing
  - Pain
  - Tinnitus (ringing in the ear)

irrigations after nasal surgery to enhance healing by removing debris and stimulating repair of the mucosal membranes.

Advanced destruction of the sinuses, foreign bodies in the nasal passages, and frequent nosebleeds are contraindications to nasal irrigation because irrigation may damage the nasal mucosa or push foreign bodies farther into the nasal cavity. Some health care providers may order nasal irrigation for such patients because they may benefit from the irrigation even if contraindications exist (Skill 17.14).

Skill 17.14   Performing a Nasal Irrigation

NURSING ACTION *(RATIONALE)*

1. Refer to Standard Steps 1 to 9.
2. Assemble equipment and supplies: *(Organizes procedure.)*
   - Apron or towels
   - Bath basin or sink
   - Bulb syringe or oral irrigation device
   - Facial tissues
   - Gloves
   - Hypertonic saline solution (500 to 1000 mL)
   - Irrigating device (prefilled kits are available at most pharmacies)
   - Plastic sheet
   - Rigid or flexible disposable irrigation tip (single use only)
3. Describe sensations that patient is likely to experience (e.g., feelings of fullness in the sinuses, warmth, and wetness). *(Helps relieve patient's anxiety and prepares patient to prevent sudden movement during procedure.)*
4. Evaluate nasal cavities and any nasal discharge. *(Provides baseline for evaluation after procedure.)*
5. Remove gloves used for evaluation of nasal cavity, dispose of appropriately, and perform hand hygiene. *(Prevents spread of microorganisms and protects patient and nurse.)*
6. Assemble and prepare equipment:
   - Warm saline solution (105°F [40.5°C]). *(A warm solution is comfortable and promotes healing. Keeping the solution at the appropriate temperature will prevent damage to the nasal cavity.)*
   - If an electrical device is to be used, plug instrument into an outlet near the patient, and run approximately 240 mL of the saline solution through the tubing. *(Facilitates procedure, rinses any residual solution from the tubing, and warms the tubing.)*
   - If a bulb syringe is to be used, fill bulb with warmed solution and then expel it. *(Rinses any residual solution from previous irrigation and warms the bulb.)*
7. Don disposable gloves. *(Reduces spread of microorganisms and protects patient and nurse.)*
8. Assist patient to sit upright close to equipment with the head bent forward over the collecting receptacle (basin or sink). The nose and the ear should be on the same plane vertically. Do not tilt the head back. *(The patient is less likely to breathe in the solution when holding the head in this position. This position will also keep solution from entering*

the eustachian tube.) Provide towels to collect any excess moisture. *(Helps keep patient dry and provides comfort.)*

9. Instruct patient to keep the mouth open and to breathe rhythmically through the mouth during the procedure. *(This causes the soft palate to seal the throat, allowing the solution to flow out the other nostril and bring any discharge with it.)*
10. Instruct patient to neither speak nor swallow during the procedure. *(This prevents forcing any infectious material into the eustachian tube or sinuses.)*
11. If the patient reports the need to sneeze or cough, remove the irrigating device tip from the patient's nares. *(Helps prevent injury to the nasal mucosa.)*
12. Perform procedure.
    a. If a commercial kit is to be used, follow directions on package.
    b. If an electrical irrigating device is to be used, insert the tip about ½ to 1 inch (1 to 3 cm) into the patient's nostril, and turn on the irrigating device. Begin with a low pressure setting, increasing pressure as needed. *(A gentle stream of solution helps prevent material in the nose from being forced into the sinuses or eustachian tube and causing an infection.)* Insert the irrigation tip far enough into the patient's nostril to ensure that the irrigating solution cleans the nasal membranes before draining out. Irrigate both nostrils.
    c. If a bulb syringe is to be used:
    (1) Fill bulb with warm saline solution, and insert tip about ½ to 1 inch (1 to 3 cm) into the patient's nostril. *(Allows the procedure to be effective without causing damage to the nasal mucosa.)*
    (2) Squeeze bulb until a gentle stream of warm solution washes through the nose. Avoid forceful squeezing. Alternate nostrils until the returned solution is clear. *(A gentle squeeze helps prevent debris from the nasal passages from being forced up into the sinuses or eustachian tube and causing an infection.)*
13. Inspect returned solution for the following. *(Indicates symptoms of infection that need to be reported to the health care provider.)*
    - Blood
    - Color
    - Necrotic material
    - Viscosity
    - Volume

Continued

Skill 17.14   Performing a Nasal Irrigation—cont'd

14. Provide the patient with tissues. (*Helps contain secretions.*) Wait a few minutes after the procedure, and then ask the patient to blow the nose gently from both nostrils at once. (*Waiting allows for more thorough cleansing of mucous membranes. Gently blowing prevents fluid or pressure buildup in the sinuses and helps loosen and expel any crusted secretions and mucus.*)

15. Clean irrigating equipment with soap and water and disinfect it according to facility policy. Rinse, dry, and properly store equipment. (*Prevents spread of microorganisms and prepares supplies for the next time the procedure is performed.*)

16. Refer to Standard Steps 10 to 17.

17. Document the following. (*Verifies performance of procedure and ensures continuity of care.*)
    - Date and time
    - Duration of procedure
    - Type of solution used (formula of ingredients used)
    - Amount and temperature of solution used
    - Appearance and amount of returned solution
    - Evaluation of patient's comfort level and ease of breathing before and after procedure
    - Patient teaching: to teach irrigations at home, include the following points:
    (a) Fill a clean 1-L plastic bottle with bottled or distilled water.
    (b) Add 1 teaspoon of non-iodized salt. (*Some health care providers also order addition of 1 tsp of baking soda.*)
    (c) Hold patient's head over the sink. Do not tilt head back.
    (d) Introduce the irrigating device approximately one finger width into the nasal cavity.

18. After irrigation, rinse equipment well to remove debris. Follow cleaning directions that accompany electrical device or equipment (*other than the bulb syringe*). Store clean equipment in a clean, dry container.

Administering Medications by Inhalation

Some drugs can be absorbed through the mucous membranes of the respiratory tract. Most often, they produce a localized effect within the respiratory tract, though they can produce a systemic effect.

Respiratory therapy departments use the inhalation route routinely to administer medications, as do anesthesiologists and nurse anesthetists.

The nurse's participation in inhalation therapy usually involves helping patients use metered-dose inhalers (MDIs) that contain bronchodilators or corticosteroids. Not all facilities employ a respiratory therapy department, so a nurse in these facilities may need to administer other types of medications via the respiratory route. Read and follow directions for use of these inhalers, because methods of use may vary among manufacturers.

Drugs administered with handheld inhalers are dispersed through an aerosol spray, mist, or powder that penetrates lung airways. The alveolar-capillary network absorbs medications rapidly. The purpose of most MDIs is to produce local effects, such as bronchodilation or reduced inflammation, but some have the capacity to create systemic side effects, such as an increased heart rate or increased blood pressure.

Many patients who routinely receive drugs by inhalation suffer from a chronic respiratory disease such as asthma, emphysema, or chronic bronchitis. Some patients have acute respiratory problems and require inhaled medications until their condition improves; medications given by inhalation help provide these patients with better air flow through their airways.

Because these patients depend on medications for disease control, they need to learn about them and how to administer them safely. Educate the patient about the importance of taking these types of medications and the correct way to administer them whenever this type of learning is needed.

An MDI delivers a measured dose of drug with each push of a canister. Approximately 5 to 10 pounds of pressure are necessary to activate the aerosol; hand strength may diminish with age and from chronic diseases that may affect an older patient, such as arthritis, chronic respiratory disease, or heart disease. A three-point or lateral hand position is effective in activating this type of canister. Some patients need to use two hands to administer the medication, or they may use an adapted inhaler device.

Proper administration of an MDI necessitates coordination during the breathing cycle. Some patients who have difficulty with this coordination do not depress the canister at the appropriate time. The medication must be administered at the beginning of an inhalation. The patient who cannot coordinate the medication with the inhalation cannot receive a full dose. A device has been created for such patients to help them receive a full dose called a *spacer* (*AeroChamber*). It fits onto the MDI and improves a patient's ability to deliver a proper dose of medication. Provide the following instructions to the patient who is using an MDI:
- Do not inhale too quickly.
- Do not hold the inhaler upside down or sideways during administration.

Skill 17.15   Administering Metered-Dose Inhaler

NURSING ACTION *(RATIONALE)*

1. Follow the six "rights" of medication administration (see Box 17.5). *(Prevents medication errors.)*
2. Perform the three label checks (see Box 17.6). *(Prevents medication errors.)*
3. Follow standard procedures. *(Prevents spread of microorganisms.)*
4. Gather equipment. *(Organizes procedure.)*
   - Canister
   - Gloves
   - Inhaler
   - Spacer device
5. Perform hand hygiene. *(Prevents spread of microorganisms.)*
6. Transport medications to patient's room.
7. Identify patient by checking identification bracelet and per facility policy. *(Prevents medication errors.)*
8. Introduce yourself; explain procedure. *(Establishes trust.)*
9. Provide privacy.
10. Don gloves. *(Reduces spread of microorganisms.)*
11. Allow patient opportunity to manipulate inhaler, canister, and spacer device (e.g., AeroChamber). Explain and demonstrate how canister fits into inhaler. *(Patient needs to be familiar with how to assemble and use equipment.)*
12. Explain what metered dose is and warn patient about overuse of inhaler, including drug side effects. *(Patient needs to know the dangers of excessive inhalations because of risk of serious side effects. If drug is received in recommended doses, side effects are minimal.)*
13. Remove mouthpiece cover from inhaler. Shake inhaler well. *(Ensures mixing of medication in canister.)*
14. Position inhaler:
    a. *Without AeroChamber (spacer):* Have patient open lips and place inhaler ½ to 1 inch (1 to 2 cm) from mouth with opening toward back of pharynx. Lips will not touch inhaler. *(Prevents rapid influx of inhaled medication and subsequent airway irritation. Positioning the mouthpiece 1 to 2 cm from the mouth is considered the best way to deliver the medication without a spacer.)*

b. *With AeroChamber (spacer):* Have patient exhale fully and then grasp mouthpiece with teeth and lips while holding inhaler with thumb at the mouthpiece and fingers at the top. *(Spacers are recommended because the device allows particles of the medication to "ride" the breath into the airways rather than hit the back of the pharynx.)*

15. Instruct patient to press down on inhaler to release medication while inhaling slowly and deeply through mouth.
16. Instruct patient to breathe in slowly for 2 to 3 seconds and to hold breath for approximately 10 seconds. *(Holding breath allows tiny drops of aerosol spray to reach deeper branches of airway.)*
17. Instruct patient to exhale through pursed lips.
18. Instruct patient to wait 2 to 5 minutes between puffs. More than one puff is usually prescribed. *(First inhalation opens airways and reduces inflammation. Second or third inhalation penetrates more deeply into airways.)*
19. If more than one type of inhaled medication is prescribed, wait 5 to 10 minutes between inhalations or as ordered by health care provider. *(Drug administration is prescribed at intervals during day to promote bronchodilation and keep side effects to a minimum.)*
20. Explain that patient will sometimes feel gagging sensation in throat caused by droplets of medication on pharynx or tongue.

Continued

Skill 17.15 Administering Metered-Dose Inhaler—cont'd

21. Instruct patient in removing medication canister and cleaning inhaler in warm water. (*To remove residue that can interfere with proper distribution of medication.*)
22. Instruct patient to rinse mouth with water and spit.
23. *Evidence-based practice for patient to determine when the metered-dose inhaler (MDI) is empty:* In the past, patients were taught to determine the remainder of medication in the canister of their MDI by floating it in water. This method was found to be inaccurate because of the variety of canister sizes and designs. Patients used different methods to try to determine whether a canister was empty and tended to use the medication canister much longer than its intended duration. Levy and colleagues (2016) recommend that when MDIs do not have built-in dose counters, it is best to instruct the patient in how to count doses still available in the canister by calculating the number of puffs used per day to calculate the number of days to expect the inhaler to last.

Skill 17.16 Administering Sublingual Medications

NURSING ACTION (*RATIONALE*)

1. Follow the six "rights" of medication administration (see Box 17.5). (*Prevents medication errors.*)
2. Perform the three label checks (see Box 17.6). (*Prevents medication errors.*)
3. Follow standard precautions. (*Prevents spread of microorganisms.*)
4. Perform hand hygiene. (*Prevents spread of microorganisms.*)
5. Transport drug to patient's room and identify patient by checking identification bracelet and per facility policy. (*Prevents medication errors.*)
6. Don gloves and place tablet under patient's tongue. (*Reduces spread of microorganisms and prevents absorption of medication into your skin.*)
7. Do not give patient water immediately afterward. (*Water reduces absorption of medication.*)
8. Instruct patient not to swallow tablet but to let it dissolve. (*Swallowing reduces absorption of medication.*)
9. Teach patient how to place medication under tongue when self-administering. Instruct patient to let it dissolve.
10. Remove gloves and wash hands. (*Reduces spread of microorganisms.*)
11. Record sublingual administration of medications per facility policy.
12. Return to assess patient's response to medication. (*Enables you to determine effectiveness of medication and any occurrence of adverse reactions.*)
13. Document assessment findings in nursing notes.

- Do not depress the canister more than once during one inhalation.
- Remain in an upright position during administration of the medicine.

Assess the patient's ability to hold and manipulate the inhaler and depress the canister (Skill 17.15).

Sublingual Administration

For sublingual administration of a drug (usually in tablet form), the tablet is placed beneath the tongue and held there until it dissolves and is absorbed into the patient's circulation. It also may be acceptable to squeeze liquid out of a capsule if it is ordered by sublingual route. Instruct the patient not to eat, drink, or smoke while the tablet is dissolving under their tongue. After dissolution, the active ingredient is absorbed rapidly into the bloodstream. Drugs given by the sublingual route bypass the liver, which reduces the time it takes for the drug to produce its desired action.

Nitroglycerin is a common type of sublingual medication. In long-term care facilities, it may be left at the bedside so that the patient is able to take it *ad lib* (as desired) if ordered this way by the health care provider. Instruct the patient to notify a nurse of any usage of nitroglycerin and its effect so that the time the medication was administered can be documented accurately and any associated effect of the drug can be noted. Follow the same procedure to prepare the administration of sublingual tablets as for solid formulations of oral medication, with the exceptions noted in Skill 17.16.

Buccal Administration

For buccal administration of a drug, a tablet is placed between the cheek and the teeth or between the cheek and the gums. It is left there until it dissolves. Absorption into the capillaries of the mucous membranes of the cheek provides rapid onset of the drug's active ingredient due to its direct entry into the systemic circulation.

Use the same procedure for buccal administration as for solid formulations of oral medication (Skill 17.17).

PARENTERAL ADMINISTRATION

The parenteral routes are those other than the digestive system route. These usually are given with a needle and syringe, and the dosage forms are liquids that are contained in the following:

- *Ampules:* Ampules are glass containers accessed by snapping off the top part of the ampule with a collar (shown in Skill 17.18, Step 10b[2]), gauze, or alcohol swab. They are intended for a single unit-dose use. Some facilities recommend the use of filter needles to prevent particles of glass from the ampule from being aspirated into the syringe barrel.
- *Vials:* Vials are glass containers sealed with a metal cap that has a rubber diaphragm in the middle. The vial may contain a single dose, or it may be used to provide multiple doses for several patients.

Large volumes of fluids meant to be infused through an IV line are placed in glass or plastic containers, such as IV fluid bags. IV fluid bags or bottles range in capacity from 50 to 1000 mL.

The parenteral routes are as follows:
- *ID:* intradermal (within the dermis)
- *IM:* intramuscular (within the muscle)
- *IV:* intravenous (within the vein)
- *Subcut:* subcutaneous (under the dermis; in fatty tissue)

Parenteral routes are used for the following reasons:
- Some medications, such as insulin, are altered or destroyed by the secretions found in the GI tract.
- Some patients, such as those who are (1) intubated, (2) severely dysphagic (unable to swallow effectively), or (3) experiencing shock, nausea, or vomiting, are unable to take medications by mouth.
- The parenteral route produces a more rapid onset of action than does the oral route.
- The duration of the action of medications that are administered through the parenteral route is commonly shorter than that of medications administered orally.
- Smaller doses of parenteral drugs can be administered, as active drug ingredients are not reduced by the action of the GI tract and liver.
- IV administration of a drug can be regulated closely; immediate entry into the bloodstream produces a very rapid response.

Always perform hand hygiene before selecting and handling syringes, needles, and other equipment. Use aseptic technique during the preparation and administration of parenteral medications; during the injection, the penetration of the skin creates a portal of entry into the body by pathogenic organisms.

Administer parenteral medication skillfully and accurately. Exact dosages are essential, as is selection of the proper site for the injection.

Equipment

Syringes. A syringe consists of a barrel, a plunger, and a tip (Fig. 17.5). The outside barrel is calibrated in milliliters, insulin units, and in some agencies, heparin units.

Skill 17.17 Administering Buccal Medications

NURSING ACTION *(RATIONALE)*

1. Follow the six "rights" of medication administration (see Box 17.5). *(Prevents medication errors.)*
2. Perform the three label checks (see Box 17.6). *(Prevents medication errors.)*
3. Follow standard precautions. *(Prevents spread of microorganisms.)*
4. Perform hand hygiene. *(Prevents spread of microorganisms.)*
5. Transport drug to patient's room and identify patient by checking identification bracelet and per facility policy. *(Prevents medication errors.)*
6. Don gloves and place medication between patient's cheek and gum. *(Prevents spread of microorganisms.)*
7. Do not give patient water immediately afterward. *(Reduces absorption of medication.)*
8. Instruct patient not to swallow tablet but to let it dissolve.
9. Teach patient how to place medication between gum and cheek when self-administering.
10. Remove gloves and wash hands. *(Reduces spread of microorganisms.)*
11. Record buccal administration of medications per facility policy.
12. Return to assess patient's response to medication. *(Enables you to determine effectiveness of medication and any occurrence of adverse reactions.)*
13. Document assessment findings in nursing notes.

Skill 17.18   Preparing Parenteral Medications

CHECK   GATHER   HELLO   ID   PRIVACY   EXPLAIN   WASH   GLOVES

NURSING ACTION *(RATIONALE)*

1. Follow the six "rights" of medication administration (see Box 17.5). *(Prevents medication errors.)*
2. Perform the three label checks (see Box 17.6). *(Prevents medication errors.)*
3. Follow standard precautions. *(Prevents spread of microorganisms.)*
4. Perform hand hygiene before handling equipment, and prepare medication in clean area. *(Prevents spread of microorganisms.)*
5. Maintain sterility of sterile parts of syringe and needle. Use aseptic technique throughout preparation. *(Prevents contamination.)*
6. Compare drug and dosage ordered with drug and dose on hand; check expiration date, dose/milliliter, and total volume of solution in vial or ampule. Look for contaminants such as solutes present in the solution or defects in vial or ampule.
7. Calculate drug dosage, and check calculations with another nurse. *(Prevents drug errors.)*
8. Check compatibility chart, consult pharmacy department, or consult facility resource if you are mixing two medications. *(It is essential that any medications mixed are compatible.)*
9. Don gloves. *(Prevents spread of microorganisms.)*
10. Prepare medication syringe:
    a. Withdrawing medication from a vial:
       (1) Remove cap from top of vial; wipe rubber stopper briskly with alcohol sponge and allow alcohol to dry. *(It is necessary to swab seals before drawing up medication, to ensure that the rubber stopper of the vial is sterile.)*
       (2) Pull plunger of syringe back to aspirate air into syringe equal to amount of drug to be withdrawn. *(It is necessary to inject air into the vial to prevent buildup of negative pressure in vial when you attempt to aspirate medication.)*
       (3) Insert needle into inverted vial; inject air and withdraw volume of solution to be given. Keep needle within solution. *(Prevents aspiration of air into syringe.)*
       (4) Push plunger gently to disperse solution to tip of needle. Remove air bubbles by gently tapping syringe.
    b. Withdrawing medication from an ampule:
       (1) Tap the top of ampule to move solution from top of ampule to bottom of ampule.

(2) Cover neck of ampule with an alcohol pad or 2- × 2-inch gauze pad; break off top of ampule; deposit top of glass ampule in sharps container. *(Prevents injury.)*

(3) Use a filter needle to aspirate medication from ampule. *(Filter or aspiration needles catch particles of glass that may be in the solution from the broken ampule.)*
(4) Insert filter needle into open neck of ampule; invert ampule to withdraw correct dose.
(5) Replace filter needle with needle appropriate for purpose and viscosity of solution.
(6) Push plunger gently until the plunger measures the correct dose.
    c. Reconstituting a powdered dosage form:
       (1) Follow instructions on manufacturer's box and drug insert. The instructions specify the type and the amount of diluent to use (e.g., the directions may direct the nurse to add 10 mL of bacteriostatic saline to prepare a solution of 500 mg/mL).
       (2) Remove the protective cap from diluent, cleanse vial top with alcohol pad, and

Skill 17.18   Preparing Parenteral Medications—cont'd

allow the alcohol to dry. Withdraw diluent by using sterile technique.

(3) Withdraw needle from diluent vial.

(4) Inject diluent into vial of powdered drug; remove syringe and needle. Gently shake and tap vial. *(Dissolves powder into solution.)*

(5) If necessary, label vial of solution with the following, if to be used for more than one dose:

(a) Date and time mixed

(b) Name of person who mixed drug and diluent

(c) Dose/milliliter obtained (concentration)

(d) Amount and type of diluent used

(6) Withdraw correct dose; facility policy may suggest to change needle and replace with a new needle of appropriate gauge and length for administering the medication to the patient. *(It is necessary to exchange the needle with the needle for injection into patient's tissue. Needles become dull as they enter the rubber stopper. Changing needles also prevents tracking of medication through patient's tissues, reducing the pain that may be associated with the injection.)*

d. Placing two medications into one syringe (insulin example used):

(1) Check compatibility of the two drugs by using compatibility chart, calling pharmacy department, or using facility-provided resource.

(2) Check and compare label of each drug ordered with label of each drug on hand.

(3) Compare each label with medication order.

(4) Roll vials of long- and intermediate-acting insulin between the palms. *(Resuspends insulin.)* Do not shake any insulin. *(Causes air bubbles.)* NOTE: Do *not* mix long-acting insulin glargine (Lantus) with any other kind of insulin. *(Lantus cannot be mixed with other kinds of insulin.)*

(5) Briskly wipe tops of both vials with separate alcohol swabs and allow to dry. *(Prevents contamination.)*

(6) Pull back plunger of syringe to amount equal to volume of longer-acting insulin to be given. *(Prevents buildup of negative pressure.)*

(7) Insert needle and inject air into vial of longer-acting insulin.

(8) Withdraw needle from vial without having removed insulin.

(9) Pull back plunger of syringe to amount equal to volume of shorter acting (regular or rapid-acting) insulin to be given.

(10) Insert needle through rubber stopper of second vial; inject air into vial.

(11) Invert vial; withdraw volume of shorter acting (regular or rapid-acting) insulin first. *(Prevents contamination of regular or rapid-acting insulin by intermediate or long-acting insulin.)*

(12) Check dosage in syringe against medication order, as well as with another nurse. *(Prevents dose error.)*

(13) Wipe rubber stopper of longer-acting insulin; insert needle of the syringe containing shorter or rapid-acting insulin and withdraw ordered dose of longer acting insulin. Check dose in syringe against medication order with second nurse. *(Prevents dose error.)*

(14) Remove needle or syringe from vial.

(15) Check labels of both vials against medication order. *(Ensures accuracy.)*

(16) Pull plunger back enough to allow space in barrel of syringe for insulin to be gently mixed. Mix by tilting syringe back and forth; remove air. Administer mixtures of insulin within 5 minutes of preparation. *(Regular insulin binds with NPH insulin and the action of regular insulin is reduced.)*

11. Identify patient by checking identification bracelet and per facility policy. *(Prevents medication errors.)*

12. Don gloves. *(Prevents spread of microorganisms.)*

13. Prepare injection site and inject according to prescribed route and method (see Skills 17.14 through 17.17).

© Elsevier

Fig. 17.5 Parts of a syringe.

Fig. 17.6 Tuberculin syringe calibration. Tuberculin syringe is marked in 0.01 increments (hundredths) for doses of less than 1 mL. (From Clayton BD, Willihnganz M: *Basic pharmacology for nurses,* ed 17, St. Louis, 2017, Elsevier.)

Fig. 17.7 Calibration of U100 insulin syringe. (From Clayton BD, Willihnganz M: *Basic pharmacology for nurses,* ed 17, St. Louis, 2017, Elsevier.)

Fig. 17.8 Reading the calibrations of a 3-mL syringe.

Barrel sizes commonly range from 0.5 to 50 mL. The outside of the barrel is not sterile, but the inside is. The tip of the barrel is either the plain slip tip or the Luer-Lock type. The needle slips directly onto the slip tip barrel tip, whereas it is necessary to turn the Luer-Lock needle to the right as the nurse attaches it onto the barrel.

The plunger that is located inside of the barrel is also sterile; avoid touching the plunger anywhere except the tip. Manipulate the plunger to draw up and inject medication with the syringe. The plunger has a rubber stopper on the end that is inside the barrel; read the volume of a medication at the area of the rubber stopper nearest the needle (see Fig. 17.5, *bottom*).

The most commonly used syringe sizes are 0.5 mL (insulin syringe), 1 mL (tuberculin syringe and insulin syringe), 3 mL, and 5 mL.

Tuberculin syringe. The tuberculin syringe (Fig. 17.6) holds a total volume of 1 mL and is used to give volumes of medication of 1 mL or less (such as for small doses of epinephrine, intradermal skin tests, and subcutaneous medication).

The tuberculin syringe is measured in milliliters. The long lines represent 0.1 (¹⁄₁₀) mL, the shorter lines represent 0.05 (⁵⁄₁₀₀) mL, and the shortest lines represent 0.01 (¹⁄₁₀₀) mL.

Insulin syringe. Use the insulin syringe only for insulin because it is calibrated in units with which insulin is measured (Fig. 17.7). Most insulin is made in the concentration of U100; the U100 syringe holds 100 units of insulin per 1 mL, and the U50 syringe holds 50 units of insulin per 0.5 mL. There is also a U30 syringe in 0.3-mL size. The unit scale on the barrel of the syringe usually differs with syringe size; the 1-mL syringe usually is marked in 2-unit increments, the 0.5-mL syringe is marked in 1-unit increments, and the 0.3-mL syringe is marked in either 1- or 0.5-unit increments (preferred for use in patients who require small doses of insulin). Check all insulin dosages with another nurse before administering the medication to the patient. Both nurses must verify and document the insulin dose to be administered to the patient.

3-mL syringe. The 3-mL syringe is chosen for giving volumes of medication of 1 to 3 mL (Fig. 17.8) and is used for most IM injections. The 3-mL syringe is calibrated in milliliters or cubic centimeters (cc), which are equivalent units. The short lines represent 0.1 mL; the longer lines represent 0.5 mL.

Select syringes based on the volume of medication to be given (Fig. 17.9A to C).

Fig. 17.9 Types of syringes. A, Insulin syringes: U-50 *(top)* and U-100 *(bottom).* B, Tuberculin syringe. C, Safety 3-mL syringe.

Safety-Glide syringes. Safety-Glide syringes are used to prevent needlesticks (see Fig. 17.9C). Many hospitals and long-term care facilities use syringes with safety glides or some sort of safety feature to protect personnel from needlestick injuries.

Disposable injection units. Disposable, single-dose, prefilled syringes are available for some medications such as morphine sulfate or enoxaparin sodium (Lovenox). Calculate the dose needed for the patient and expel any unneeded portion of the contents before administering.

The Tubex and Carpuject injection systems include reusable plastic or metal syringes that hold prefilled, disposable, sterile cartridge-needle units (Fig. 17.10). Slip the cartridge into the mechanism, secure it (per package directions), and check for air bubbles. Advance the plunger to get rid of air bubbles, obtain the correct dosage, and then inject the medication as with a regular syringe.

Needles The parts of a needle are the hub, the shaft, and the beveled tip (Fig. 17.11). The opening at the needle's beveled tip reveals the **lumen** (the inside of the hollow shaft). The diameter of the lumen determines the **gauge** (a standard or scale of measurement) of the needle (Fig. 17.12). The smaller the gauge of the needle, the larger the diameter; thus an 18-gauge needle has a much larger diameter than a 25-gauge needle. Needle gauge selection is based on the viscosity (thickness) of the medication: the thicker the medication, the smaller the gauge (the larger the lumen) required. A 20- to 22-gauge needle is usually adequate for most non-viscous IM injections. A 16- to 18-gauge needle is appropriate for blood administration, emergency IV routes, and surgical cases. A 25- to 26-gauge needle is used frequently for infants and children and for intradermal injections, and 27- to 28-gauge needles are available for subcutaneous injections. Insulin-syringe needles are typically 29- and 30-gauge.

Fig. 17.10 (A) Carpuject syringe and prefilled sterile cartridge with needle. (B) Assembling the Carpuject. (C) Cartridge slides into syringe barrel, turns, and locks at the needle end. Plunger then screws into the cartridge end.

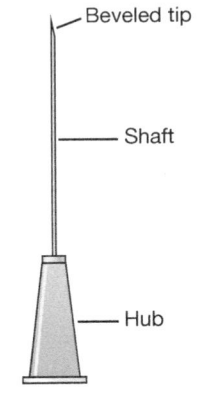

Fig. 17.11 Parts of a needle.

Needle length. Select the needle length according to the depth of the tissue into which you need to inject the medication. Intradermal injections require only ⅜ - to ⅝-inch needle length, whereas an IM injection often requires 1- to 1½-inch needle length, depending on the amount of muscle tissue the patient has. Needle length for subcutaneous injections is usually ½ to ⅝ inch, depending on the depth of the tissue where the injection is to be administered (see Fig. 17.12). Insulin-syringe needles are available in a standard ½-inch length and a ⁵⁄₁₆-inch length. The shorter needle tends to be less intimidating, and many patients with diabetes perceive it to be less painful than standard-length needles.

Intravenous needles. Two items made especially for IV use are the over-the-needle catheter and the winged-type (or butterfly) needle (Fig. 17.13A and B).

The wing-tipped (butterfly) needle is useful in administering IV fluids on a short-term basis. The nurse may use it in pediatric cases, in which veins are sometimes hard to find except in the scalp. Wing-tipped needles are easy to put in, but some health care providers prefer over-the-needle catheters. Butterfly infusion sets require that the stainless-steel needle remain in the patient's vein.

Over-the-needle catheters can be used in any situation in which an IV infusion is necessary, such as an emergency situation, surgery, and blood transfusions.

Over-the-needle catheters are plastic catheters that fit over a stainless-steel needle called a *stylet*. A stylet is a sharp, bevel-tipped metal guide used to pierce the skin and vein. Once the stylet and the catheter are in the vein, blood return occurs, and the stylet is removed. When removed from the patient's vein, the stylet can be activated or manipulated in some way to make it safer in order to reduce risk of needlesticks during IV needle insertion. The plastic catheter is left in the vein, and IV tubing or an IV lock may be attached to the catheter. The catheter is preferred over the wing-tipped needle because it is more flexible and better withstands patient movement (see Fig. 17.13A).

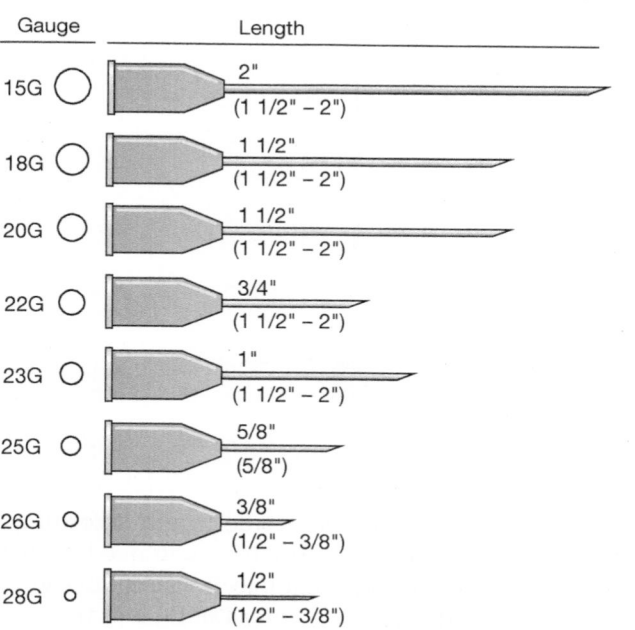

Gauge	Length
15G	2" (1 1/2" – 2")
18G	1 1/2" (1 1/2" – 2")
20G	1 1/2" (1 1/2" – 2")
22G	3/4" (1 1/2" – 2")
23G	1" (1 1/2" – 2")
25G	5/8" (5/8")
26G	3/8" (1/2" – 3/8")
28G	1/2" (1/2" – 3/8")

Fig. 17.12 Needle length and gauge.

Wing-tipped needles and over-the-needle catheters cannot be left in place indefinitely. Assess them every shift for patency, intactness, and the development of any complications. Follow the health care facility's policies regarding how long an IV catheter or needle may be left in place. If phlebitis or infiltration occurs at the IV insertion site, discontinue the infusion immediately.

A physician may insert a central line. There are several different types of central lines, and they are used for IV administration of a fluid that may be given over a long period of time, such as total parenteral nutrition, chemotherapy, or antibiotics. See Skill 17.18 for preparation of parenteral medications.

Needleless devices. Each year, many people suffer from accidental needlesticks and sharps injuries in health care settings. These injuries commonly occur when nurses attempt to recap needles, manipulate needles, or come into contact with stray needles left at a patient's bedside. The risk of exposure to bloodborne pathogens in health care workers led to the development of needleless devices, or special needle safety devices after the 1999–2000 Needlestick Safety and Prevention Act (ANA, n.d.).

Special syringes are designed with a sheath or guard that can cover the needle after it is withdrawn from the skin (see Fig. 17.9C). The safety aspect of the device is commonly required to be activated by the nurse, and the needle is covered immediately, which reduces the chance of a needlestick injury. The syringe and sheath are disposed of together in a receptacle designed for disposal of sharp items. The Centers for Disease Control and Prevention (CDC) and OSHA have mandated that health care agencies use safer medical devices (sharps disposal containers, self-sheathing needles) that eliminate or reduce exposures to bloodborne pathogens within the workplace.

IV tubing and access ports have been developed for use with Luer-Lock–tipped syringes to reduce the occurrence of injuries during medication delivery.

Intramuscular Injections

An IM injection involves inserting a needle into the muscle tissue to administer medication (Skill 17.19). Because muscle tissue has a large blood supply, IM medication is absorbed faster than medication administered subcutaneously or intradermally. The most commonly used sites are the ventrogluteal area, the vastus lateralis of the thigh, and the deltoid muscle of the arm.

When selecting an IM site, ensure that the site is free of pain, infection, necrosis, ecchymosis, and abrasions.

Fig. 17.13 (A) Over-the-needle catheter. (B) Winged-tip (butterfly) needle.

Skill 17.19   Giving an Intramuscular Injection

NURSING ACTION (RATIONALE)

1. Follow the six "rights" of medication administration (see Box 17.5). (*Prevents medication errors.*)
2. Perform the three label checks (see Box 17.6). (*Prevents medication errors.*)
3. Follow standard precautions. (*Prevents spread of microorganisms.*)
4. Perform hand hygiene. (*Prevents spread of microorganisms.*)
5. Prepare medication according to standard procedure for injectables (see Skill 17.18).
6. Don gloves. (*Prevents spread of microorganisms.*)
7. Identify patient by checking identification bracelet and per facility policy. (*Prevents medication errors.*) Explain the procedure.
8. Select and expose site (according to intramuscular [IM] site selection procedure); provide privacy.
9. Clean skin with alcohol swab (from center outward), spread skin tight with thumb and index finger; allow site to dry. (*Mechanical and chemical action removes microorganisms.*)
10. Ask patient to take a deep breath and to exhale slowly to relax muscle as needle is inserted. (*Lessens pain from injection.*)
11. Insert needle at a 90-degree angle quickly in a dartlike motion. (*Quickness reduces discomfort. A quick, dartlike insertion followed by slow injection of the medication is much less painful to the patient.*)
12. Maintain needle's position in muscle; gently aspirate (pull back plunger) to be certain needle is in muscle (and not in a vein or an artery).
    a. If blood is seen, needle is in a vein or an artery. Withdraw needle and discard medication; prepare new medication (see Skill 17.18). Select another site for new attempt and begin again from Step 8.
13. Slowly inject medication into muscle to lessen discomfort. (*A slow, steady injection rate of medication promotes comfort and minimizes tissue damage.*)
14. Withdraw needle quickly without bending or twisting it. (*Minimizes tissue injury.*)
15. Apply gentle pressure with gauze (2- × 2-inch) to stop any bleeding. (*Massaging site can cause tissue irritation.*)
16. Do not recap needle; activate safety feature of needle and discard directly into sharps container. (*Prevents needlesticks.*)
17. Remove gloves and wash hands. (*Prevents spread of microorganisms.*)
18. Record administration of medications per facility policy. Chart site used and amount and type of medication (e.g., "meperidine [Demerol], 50 mg, given IM left ventrogluteal").
19. Return to assess patient's response to medication. (*Enables you to determine effectiveness of medication and any occurrence of adverse reactions.*)
20. Document assessment findings in nursing notes.

Additional important factors to consider are the location of underlying bones, nerves, and major blood vessels, as well as the amount of solution to be injected. Each anatomic site has advantages and disadvantages; in the past, the dorsogluteal muscle site was used frequently, but because of its proximity to the sciatic nerve and superior gluteal artery, this muscle is no longer recommended as a preferred injection site. Damage to the sciatic nerve may occur as a result of accidentally hitting the nerve during the administration of an IM injection.

The ventrogluteal site is preferred for IM injections. The advantages of this site are that (1) it provides the greatest thickness of gluteal muscle, (2) fewer nerves and blood vessels penetrate this site, and (3) it has the most consistent and thinnest layer of adipose tissue covering it. Develop skill in finding the proper location for giving an IM injection by palpating anatomic landmarks correctly and being knowledgeable about the location of underlying nerves and blood vessels (Boxes 17.9 and 17.10).

Intramuscular injections for analgesia are given much less often than they were previously because of the more common use of patient-controlled analgesia (PCA) and patient-controlled epidural to help control patients' pain. IM injections are more painful than the use of PCA.

Site selection

Ventrogluteal site. The gluteal sites are the ventrogluteal and the dorsogluteal. The *ventrogluteal site* (Fig. 17.14) is located by means of three landmarks: the greater trochanter, the anterior iliac spine, and the iliac crest (the hip bone). Place the palm of your hand on the lateral portion of the patient's greater trochanter and your index (pointer) finger on the patient's anterior

Box 17.9 Characteristics of Intramuscular Sites

VASTUS LATERALIS MUSCLE
- Drug absorption at this site is rapid.
- It is the preferred site for administration of immunizations to infants younger than 12 months.[a] This site is also used for adults.
- This large, developed muscle lacks major nerves and blood vessels and is the most fully developed muscle in the newborn.

VENTROGLUTEAL MUSCLE
- This complex consists of the gluteus medius and the gluteus minimus muscles.
- It is situated deep and away from major nerves and blood vessels.
- The ventrogluteal site is preferred over other gluteal muscles because it is not associated with injuries such as fibrosis, nerve damage, abscess, tissue necrosis, muscle contraction, gangrene, or pain, as are other intramuscular sites.[a]
- It is the preferred injection site for infants, children, and adults.

DORSOGLUTEAL MUSCLE
- There is risk of striking the underlying sciatic nerve, the greater trochanter, or major blood vessels if the site is not landmarked correctly.
- Evidence-based practice no longer supports the use of this intramuscular site.[a]

DELTOID MUSCLE
- This site is easily accessible, but the muscle is not well developed in most patients.
- It is used only for small volumes (0.5 to 1 mL) of medication and is the preferred site for administration of routine immunizations in toddlers, older children, and adults.[a]
- Hepatitis B vaccine is given primarily in the deltoid.[b]
- Avoid using the deltoid muscle in infants or in children with underdeveloped muscles.

[a]Modified from Nicoll LH, Hesby A: Intramuscular injection: An integrative research review and guideline for evidence-based practice, *Appl Nurs Res* 15(3):149–162, 2002.
[b]Modified from Perry AG, Potter PA, Elkin MK: *Nursing interventions and clinical skills*, ed 6, St. Louis, 2021, Mosby.

superior iliac spine (your left hand on the patient's right hip or your right hand on the patient's left hip); then extend the middle finger toward the iliac crest. Inject medication into the V formed by the index and middle fingers. You may place the patient in a side-lying position, with muscle relaxation promoted by flexing of the upper leg.

Vastus lateralis muscle. The vastus lateralis muscle (Fig. 17.15) is the preferred site for children younger than 3 years of age because it is free of nerves and blood vessels. It is also used in adults. This muscle is located on the anterior lateral thigh. The patient may be placed in a supine or sitting position. Place one hand above the patient's knee and one hand below the greater trochanter. Give the IM injection in the area between your two hands.

Box 17.10 Locating Sites for Intramuscular Injections

VENTROGLUTEAL SITE
1. Position patient on either side, with knee of upper leg bent and upper leg slightly ahead of the bottom leg. It is also acceptable for the patient to remain supine, lie on side, or lie on abdomen. Instruct patient to relax muscles where you are placing injection.
2. Palpate the greater trochanter at the head of the femur and the anterior superior iliac spine. To locate the proper site, use your left hand when the patient lies on the left side and your right hand when the patient lies on the right side.
3. Using your right hand for the left hip and your left hand for the right hip, place the heel of your hand over the greater trochanter of the patient's hip. Point your thumb toward the patient's groin, point your index finger toward the anterior superior iliac spine, and extend your middle finger back along the iliac crest toward the buttock as far as possible (NOTE: A "V" is formed between the index and middle finger) (see Fig. 17.15).
4. The injection site is the center of the triangle formed by your index and middle fingers.
5. Spread skin taut to give injection. Use your dominant hand to give injection (see Fig. 17.15).

VASTUS LATERALIS SITE
1. Position patient lying supine or sitting with site well exposed. If patient is supine, have patient flex knee on the side where injection will be given.
2. Use the greater trochanter and the knee as landmarks for injection site. Place one hand above the knee and one hand below the greater trochanter of the femur.
3. Locate the middle third of the muscle, the midline of the anterior thigh, and the midline of the thigh's lateral (outer) side.
4. The injection site is located within a rectangle formed by these boundaries (see Fig. 17.16).

DELTOID SITE
1. Position patient sitting or lying down. Expose the upper arm and shoulder; remove any tight-fitting sleeves rather than rolling them up.
2. Ask patient to relax the arm at the side with the elbow flexed. Instruct patient to place the forearm across the abdomen or the chest.
3. Palpate the lower edge of the acromion process, which forms the base of a triangle in line with the midpoint of the lateral aspect of the upper arm (see Fig. 17.18).
4. Place four fingers across the deltoid muscle, with the top finger along the acromion process.
5. The injection site is in the center of the triangle, about 3 to 5 cm (1 to 2 inches) below the acromion process (see Fig. 17.18).

From Perry AG, Potter PA, Elkin MK: *Nursing interventions and clinical skills*, ed 6, St. Louis, 2021, Mosby.

Deltoid muscle. The deltoid muscle (Fig. 17.16) of the upper arm is a relatively small area. Position the patient in a sitting, standing, prone, or supine position, and ask them to relax his or her arm during the injection to help decrease discomfort.

Fig. 17.14 Ventrogluteal site. (A) In a child or an infant. (B) In an adult. (C) Locating ventrogluteal site for intramuscular injection.

Fig. 17.15 Vastus lateralis muscle site. (A) In a child or an infant. (B) In an adult. (C) Giving intramuscular injection in vastus lateralis site in an adult.

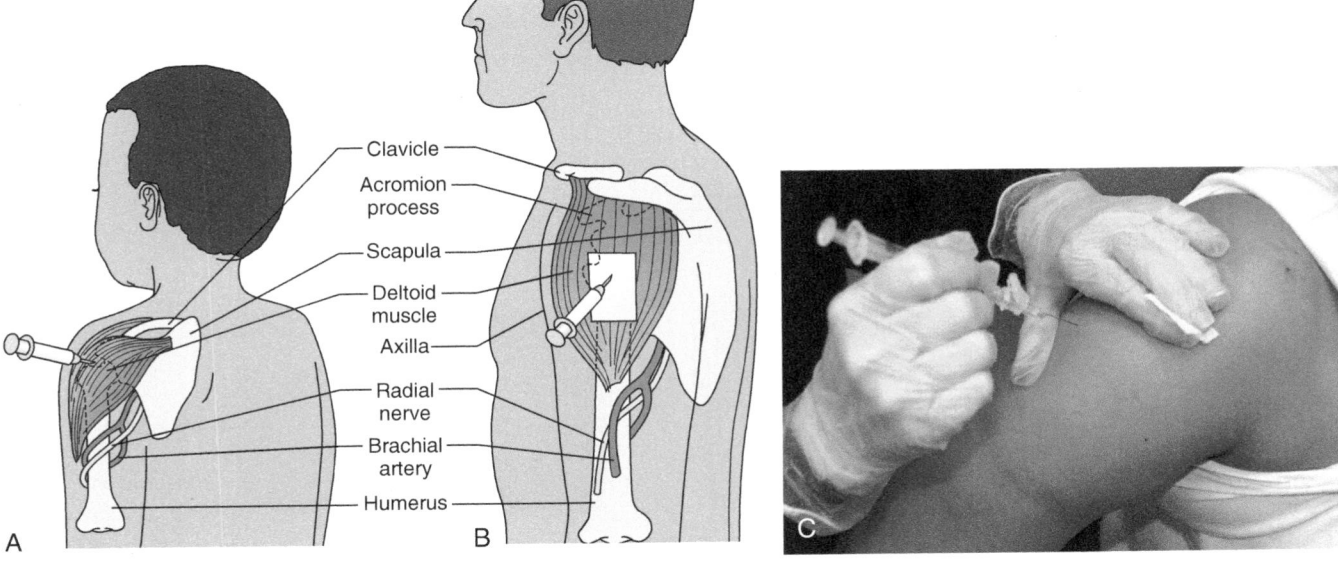

Fig. 17.16 Deltoid muscle site. (A) In a child or an infant. (B) In an adult. (C) Giving intramuscular injection in deltoid site.

The landmark for locating the proper area for this injection site is the acromion process of the scapula. Place a finger on the acromion process and move down three more fingerbreadths. The injection site is the center of the muscle, about 3 to 5 cm (1 to 2 inches) below the acromion process.

Z-track method. Use the Z-track method for injecting medications that may be irritating to the tissues. In Z-track IM administration, the medication is sealed deep within muscle tissue (see Skill 17.19). The Z-track method reduces the chance of staining or tracking of the medication back into the tissue as the needle is withdrawn, and it keeps tissue irritation to a minimum

by sealing the drug within muscle tissues (Fig. 17.17). Select an IM site in large muscles, such as those in the ventrogluteal site.

Intradermal injections

An intradermal injection is the introduction of a hypodermic needle into the dermis for the purpose of instilling a substance such as a serum, vaccine, or skin test agent (Fig. 17.18 and see Skill 17.19). Do not aspirate from the site when performing an intradermal injection.

Small volumes such as 0.1 mL are injected to form a small, bubble-like wheal just under the skin (see Skill 17.19, Step 11). Absorption in this location is slow,

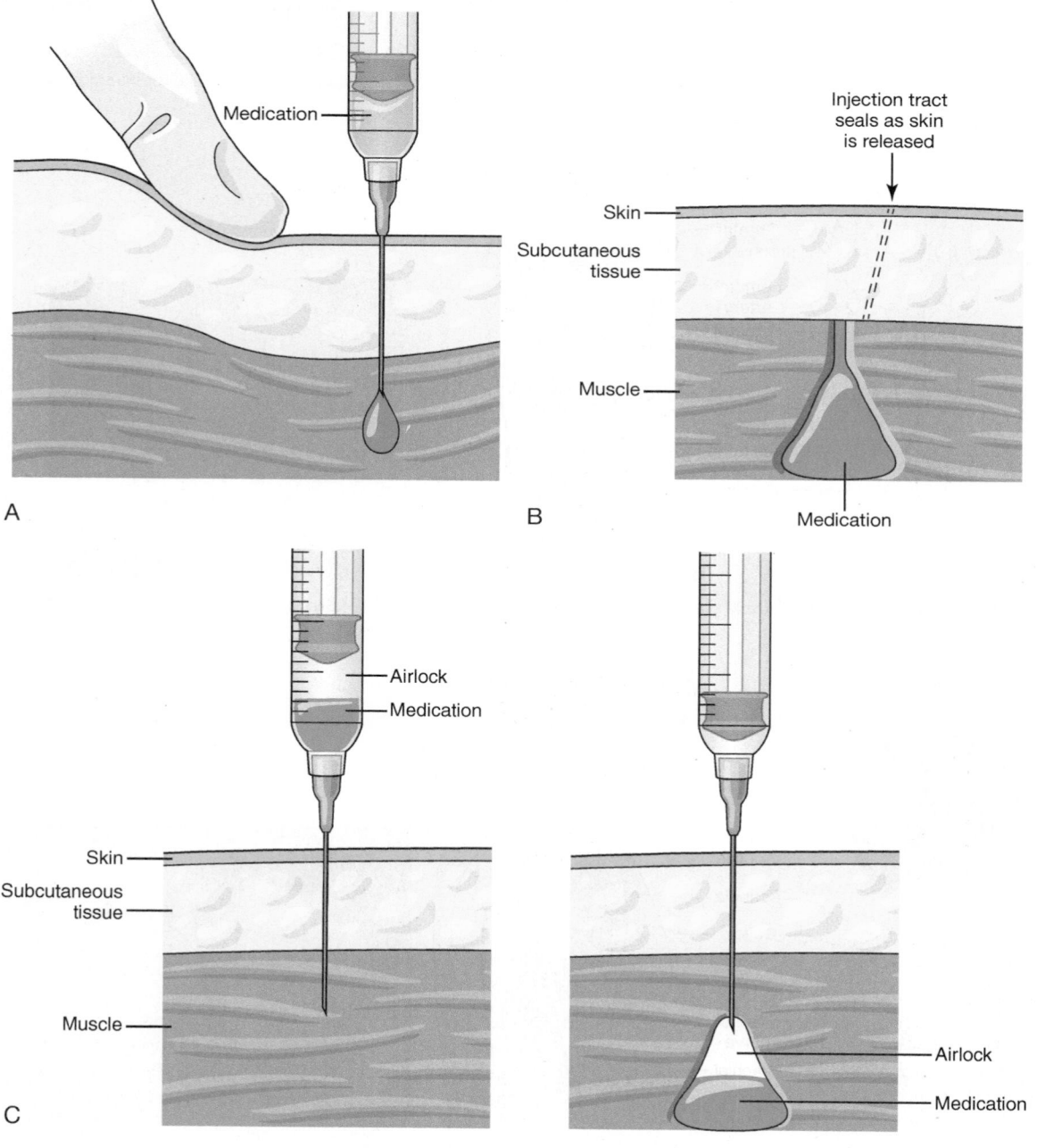

© Elsevier

Fig. 17.17 Z-track method. (A) Injection. (B) Using an air lock. (C) Administering IM injection by air lock technique.

Fig. 17.18 Angles of insertion for intramuscular (90 degrees), subcutaneous (45 degrees), and intradermal (15 degrees) injections.

Fig. 17.19 Subcutaneous injection. Angle and needle length depend on thickness of the skinfold.

which makes intradermal injection the best route for allergy sensitivity tests, tuberculin screening, desensitization injections, administration of local anesthetics, and vaccinations. Because these medications are potent, they are injected into the dermis, where the blood supply is reduced, and drug absorption occurs slowly. If the patient is allergic to the substance, a severe anaphylactic reaction is possible should the substance enter the patient's circulation too rapidly.

Use a tuberculin syringe to give intradermal injections, because the tuberculin syringe holds a maximum of 1 mL. Use a 25-gauge, ⅜- to ⅝-inch needle.

Use the upper chest, the inner aspect of the lower arm, or the scapular area for intradermal injections (see Skill 17.19).

Subcutaneous injections

Administer insulin, heparin, enoxaparin (Lovenox), dalteparin (Fragmin), epoetin alfa (Epogen), and filgrastim (Neupogen) by the subcutaneous route. Inject these types of medications into the loose connective tissue between the dermis and the muscle layer. Because subcutaneous tissue is not as richly supplied with blood as the muscles, drug absorption is slower than with IM injections. The outer aspect of the upper arms, the abdomen, the thighs, and the scapula are sites used for subcutaneous injections. Inject no more than 1 mL of solution into these sites and always carefully document the injection. With medications that must be given routinely, rotate injection sites to help prevent tissue damage.

Subcutaneous injections should be given at a 45-degree angle if the patient is thin, or at a 90-degree angle if the patient has ample subcutaneous tissue. Use your own clinical judgment in selecting sites for injection and in determining the angle of injection. Select a needle length so that the medication will be injected into subcutaneous tissue and not muscle tissue; typically, the usual needle length is ½ to ⅝ inch, and a 25-gauge needle is the one of choice (Fig. 17.19 and Skills 17.20 to 17.22).

Intravenous therapy

Advances in technology of IV equipment enable nurses and health care providers to deliver IV fluids and medications more safely. The IV route (1) provides fluid and

Fig. 17.20 Intravenous (IV) therapy. (A) IV electronic infusion pump. (B) Cleaning injection port with alcohol swab before medication administration via IV push. Injection port of IV tubing is used for drug infusion. ([A] The Alaris System images are © 2014 CareFusion Corporation; used with permission.)

electrolyte maintenance, restoration, and replacement, (2) administers medications and sterilized nutrition (such as total parenteral nutrition through a central line), (3) administers blood and blood products, (4) administers chemotherapy to patients who are being treated for cancer, (5) administers patient-controlled analgesics, and (6) keeps a vein open (KVO) for quick access.

Methods of intravenous administration

IV medications are possible to administer by several methods.

Skill 17.20 Giving a Z-Track Injection

NURSING ACTION (RATIONALE)

1. Follow the six "rights" of medication administration (see Box 17.5). (*Prevents medication errors.*)
2. Perform the three label checks (see Box 17.6). (*Prevents medication errors.*)
3. Follow standard precautions. (*Prevents spread of microorganisms.*)
4. Perform hand hygiene. (*Prevents spread of microorganisms.*)
5. Prepare medication according to standard procedure for injectables (see Skill 17.18).
6. Don gloves. (*Prevents spread of microorganisms.*)
7. Use one needle to withdraw dose from container. Use another needle (1½ to 2 inches) to inject medication so that no solution remains on the outside of needle shaft.
8. Identify patient by checking identification bracelet and per facility policy. (*Prevents medication errors.*)
9. Provide privacy. Expose and locate ventrogluteal site according to intramuscular (IM) site selection procedure.
10. Clean site with an alcohol swab and allow site to dry. (*Mechanical and chemical action removes microorganisms.*)
11. Ask the patient to take a deep breath and to slowly exhale. (*Relaxes the muscle.*) Pull skin tightly in a lateral direction (move skin at least 1 to 1½ inches laterally) to one side. Hold the skin taut with the nondominant hand. (*Z-track technique reduces discomfort and leakage of medication into tissue.*)
12. Insert needle at a 90-degree angle. (*It is necessary to insert a needle at 90-degree angle for it to enter muscle.*)
    a. inject medication at a rate of 1 mL per 10 seconds; wait 10 seconds to allow the medication to disperse slowly.
13. Withdraw needle quickly. Allow skin to return to its normal position, which leaves a zigzag path that seals the needle track wherever tissue planes slide across each other. (*The drug is not able to escape from the muscle tissue.*) (See Fig. 17.18.)
14. Place a 2- × 2-inch gauze pad or bandage on the injection site as needed.
15. Do not massage site. (*Massaging sometimes causes tissue irritation.*)
16. Do not recap needle; activate safety feature of needle and discard directly into sharps container. (*Prevents needlesticks.*)
17. Remove gloves and wash hands. (*Prevents spread of microorganisms.*)
18. Record administration of medications per facility policy. Chart site used, Z-track method used, and amount and type of medication given.
19. Return to assess patient's response to medication. (*Determines effectiveness of medication and occurrence of adverse reactions.*)
20. Document assessment findings in nursing notes.

Intravenous push. Administer the medication directly into a vein or by means of a heparin or saline lock or port of an existing IV tubing set.

Intermittent venous access device. An **intermittent venous access device** (commonly called a *saline lock,* previously called a *heparin [hep] lock*) is an IV infusion device with male adapters covered by diaphragms for the administration of intermittent infusions, and as an access site for emergency drug infusion (Fig. 17.20). Intermittent venous access devices provide ready access for IV antibiotic therapy and other IV drug therapies without causing the unnecessary pain of a re-stick with every dose. Refer to the nursing practice act in the state where you are employed to determine the role of the LPN/LVN in administering IV medication.

Intermittent venous access devices attach onto a needleless hub, and once attached, it is filled with the anticoagulant heparin or normal saline. This keeps the vein open and makes it possible to administer IV medication at intervals without the need for a continuous infusion of fluid to ensure patency.

Intermittent infusion (or piggyback). IV piggybacks are drug infusions that are given at intervals, such as every 6 hours (q 6 hr), and it is possible to connect them either to heparin or saline locks or to the injection port of the IV tubing (see Fig. 17.20B). Once the medication has been infused, remove the piggyback device from the heparin or saline lock or IV tubing and flush the lock with heparin or saline. This is a common way to administer antibiotics.

Continuous infusions. Medication is added to a bag of IV fluid and infuses with the IV fluid.

Electronic IV pumps. Pumps regulate the flow rate of IV infusions.

Patient-controlled analgesia. Patient-controlled analgesia (PCA) is a drug-delivery system that dispenses a preset IV dose of an opioid analgesic into a patient's vein when the patient pushes a button that is connected to the PCA system via a cord (Fig. 17.21). The medication is administered by a programmable pump controlled by the patient. The RN programs the pump according to the health care provider's order, which

Skill 17.21   Giving an Intradermal Injection

NURSING ACTION *(RATIONALE)*

1. Follow the six "rights" of medication administration (see Box 17.5). *(Prevents medication errors.)*
2. Perform the three label checks (see Box 17.6). *(Prevents medication errors.)*
3. Follow standard precautions. *(Prevents spread of microorganisms.)*
4. Perform hand hygiene. *(Prevents spread of microorganisms.)*
5. Prepare medication according to standard procedure for injectables (see Skill 17.18).
6. Don gloves. *(Prevents spread of microorganisms.)*
7. Identify patient by checking identification bracelet and per facility policy. *(Prevents medication errors.)*
8. Select arm and expose inner aspect of forearm.
9. Clean site gently with alcohol swab from center outward; let dry. *(Mechanical and chemical action removes microorganisms.)*
10. Two injections are made if test is for sensitivity. *(One injection is a control test with sterile water or bacteriostatic saline; the other is test substance.)* Insert a 25-gauge needle with bevel up directly under skin. Advance needle through epidermis to approximately ⅛ inch (3 mm) below the skin surface. You will be able to see the needle tip through the skin.
11. Make a small, bubble-like wheal with test solution. *(Creation of bleb shows placement of needle is correct.)* Insert needle at approximately a 15-degree angle. Do not inject into subcutaneous tissue. Inject control of saline into another site for comparison with test substance after designated time interval.
12. Do not massage site. *(Massage will most likely disperse medication into underlying tissue layers and alter test results.)*
13. Draw a circle around skin test with a marker; label area with time, date, and name of test. Another method is to make a diagram in patient's chart to indicate location of site. *(Facilitates assessment of site and reading of test results.)*
14. Remove gloves and wash hands. *(Prevents spread of microorganisms.)*
15. Record administration of medications per facility policy.
16. After the appropriate amount of time for the specific type of test has passed, note the presence of an indurated (hardened) erythematous area, measure indurated area, and record results in millimeters with metric ruler.
17. Compare control bleb with agent bleb; document results in chart.
18. Return to assess patient's response to medication. *(Enables you to determine effectiveness of medication and any occurrence of adverse reactions.)*
19. Document assessment findings in nursing notes.

A   B

specifies the amount of an opioid the patient receives per dose. The pump also controls the total amount of drug that it is possible for the patient to receive over a specific period. A lockout interval device automatically inactivates the system if a patient tries to press the button to receive another dose before the specified amount of time has passed.

Typically, RNs are responsible for programming the computerized pump and for loading medications such as morphine, fentanyl, hydromorphone hydrochloride (Dilaudid), or buprenorphine (Buprenex) into it. The LPN/LVN may perform the following activities (again, refer to the state's nursing practice act):

Skill 17.22   Giving a Subcutaneous Injection

CHECK   GATHER   HELLO   ID   PRIVACY   EXPLAIN   WASH   GLOVES

NURSING ACTION (RATIONALE)

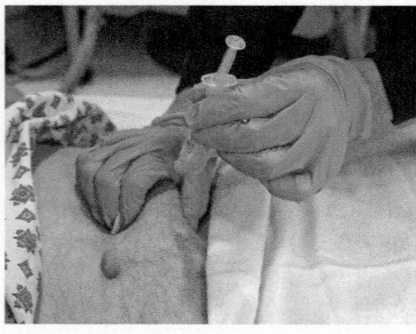

1. Follow the six "rights" of medication administration (see Box 17.5). (*Prevents medication errors.*)
2. Perform the three label checks (see Box 17.6). (*Prevents medication errors.*)
3. Follow standard precautions. (*Prevents spread of microorganisms.*)
4. Perform hand hygiene. (*Prevents spread of microorganisms.*)
5. Prepare medication according to standard procedure for injectables (see Skill 17.18).
6. Don gloves. (*Prevents spread of microorganisms.*)
7. Identify patient by checking identification bracelet and per facility policy. (*Prevents medication errors.*)
8. Select and expose site (check which site was used previously and choose a different site). The abdomen is the usual preferred site when administering heparin, enoxaparin (Lovenox), or dalteparin (Fragmin).
9. Clean site with an alcohol swab from center outward in circular motion; let dry. (*Mechanical and chemical action removes microorganisms.*)
10. Perform injection:
    a. Thin patient or child: Grasp and press together skin of selected site so that it forms roll between fingers. Insert needle at 45-degree angle. (*Angle ensures that medication reaches subcutaneous tissue rather than muscle.*) Inject medication slowly. (*Slow injection reduces pain and trauma.*)
    b. Average-size or obese patient: Grasp and press together skin of selected site so that it forms roll between fingers. Insert needle at a

90-degree angle. Inject medication slowly. (*Slow injection reduces pain and trauma.*)

11. Withdraw needle quickly and apply an antiseptic swab or a 2- × 2-inch gauze sponge. Supporting skin around injection site keeps discomfort to a minimum during withdrawal. Do not massage the site when administering insulin (*alters absorption rate*), heparin, enoxaparin (Lovenox), or dalteparin (Fragmin). (*Massage will increase local bleeding, and ecchymosis will occur.*)
12. Do not recap needle; activate safety feature of needle and discard directly into sharps container. (*Prevents needlesticks.*)
13. Remove gloves and wash hands. (*Prevents spread of microorganisms.*)
14. Record administration of medications per facility policy. Chart site used and the amount and type of medication.
15. Return to assess patient's response to medication. (*Enables the evaluation of the effectiveness of medication and any occurrence of adverse reactions.*)
16. Document assessment findings in nursing notes.

- Instruct patients to press button when analgesia is needed; ask patients to demonstrate or verbalize understanding. Reassure them that they will not receive too much medication because of the lockout mechanism.
- Maintain PCA therapy:
- Monitor number of doses received by patient.
- Monitor patient for the development of clinical manifestations that may indicate an opiate overdose.
- Monitor patient for relief of pain (if possible, use pain assessment scale).
- Document total volume infused, and remaining volume of analgesic left every shift.
- Monitor accuracy of infusion; make certain that the opioid antagonist naloxone (Narcan) is readily available in case of opiate overdose.

- Educate visitors and family members regarding the importance of allowing the patient to push the button to self-administer doses.

Two RNs are needed to verify the PCA pump settings with the order; these nurses perform the six "rights" of medication administration and program the dose volume limits, lockout interval and frequency, and 4-hour limit. The LPN/LVN should refer to the state nursing practice act and the facility policy regarding his or her responsibilities.

PCA medication infusion is considered by many patients to provide more pain relief with less medication. The patient has more control over medication administration, which often helps lessen their anxiety and pain. The PCA is an effective and efficient method for administration of analgesic medications. Special PCA

Fig. 17.21 Patient-controlled analgesia (PCA) infusion pump. The patient presses the button on a cord connected to the PCA pump. (From Lilley LL, Collins SR, Snyder JS: *Pharmacology and the Nursing Process*, ed 9, St. Louis, 2020, Elsevier.)

order sheets are used by the health care provider to specify the following:

1. Type and strength of medication
   EXAMPLE: Morphine sulfate, 1 mg/mL
2. Loading dose (an optional larger-than-usual dose to give initial pain relief)
   EXAMPLE: Range is 1 to 5 mL; usual is 1 to 2 mL
3. Maintenance dose (dose dispensed each time patient presses control button)
   EXAMPLE: Range is 0.1 to 5 mL; usual is 0.5 to 1 mL
4. Lockout interval (minimum time between doses)
   EXAMPLE: Range is 5 to 99 minutes; usual is 6 to 15 minutes
5. 4-hour limit (maximum volume delivered in 4 hours)
   EXAMPLE: Range is 5 to 30 mL in 5-mL increments; usual is 10 to 20 mL

Volumetric chambers. A volumetric chamber consists of IV tubing with a chamber that holds a prescribed amount of fluid; it is separate from the drip chamber. Medication such as oxytocin (Pitocin) or lidocaine can be added to the fluid in the chamber, and the delivery of the medication to the patient can be controlled carefully when this method is used.

Nursing responsibility. The health care provider orders the type of IV fluid, the infusion rate, and sometimes the length of time that the infusion is to run. Ensure that the ordered type and amount of fluid is started and that the fluid is regulated to be infused at the appropriate rate. The use of an electronic infusion pump eliminates the need to count drops. In the absence of an infusion pump, regulate the IV infusion by knowing the number of drops

per minute that it will take for the entire volume of fluid to infuse over the specified time ordered by the health care provider.

To find the number of drops per minute (the *drip rate*), know which type of IV tubing will be used with the infusion. Look on the IV tubing box for the **drip factor** (an apparatus that is used to deliver measured amounts of IV solutions of specific flow rates that are based on the size of drops of the solution). The box indicates whether the IV tubing is calibrated to deliver macrodrops or microdrops. To calculate IV flow rates, change milliliters to drops; for that, you need to know the drip factor. Macrodrop sets deliver 10, 15, or 20 drops per 1 mL of fluid; microdrop, or minidrop, sets deliver 60 drops per 1 mL of fluid.

EXAMPLE 1: The health care provider orders 1000 mL of 5% dextrose (D_5) in ½ normal saline (NS) with 20 mEq KCl to be infused over an 8-hour period. The nurse is using a microdrop set (60 drops per 1 mL of fluid). Use the following formula to determine how many drops will drip each minute.

First, convert number of milliliters per hour.

Then, place the information into the following formula:

$$\frac{\text{Drip rate (mL/hr)}}{60 \text{ minutes}} \times \text{drip factor} = \text{drops per minute}$$

$$\frac{125 \text{ mL/hr}}{60 \text{ minutes}} \times 60 = 124.9 \text{ drops (gtt) per minute}$$

"Drops" is also written as "gtt."
ANSWER: 125 gtt/min

EXAMPLE 2: The health care provider orders 1000 mL D_5 in ½ NS to be infused over a 4-hour period. The drip factor on the box is 10 drops per 1 mL of fluid. To get the rate of milliliters per hour, divide the amount to infuse (1000 mL) by the time (4 hours). Place the information into the formula listed above.

$$\frac{1000 \text{ mL}}{4 \text{ hours}} = 250 \text{ mL/hour}$$

$$\frac{250 \text{ mL/hour}}{60 \text{ minutes}} \times 10 = 41.66 \text{ drops (gtt)/minute}$$

ANSWER: 42 gtt/min

Infusion pumps also have the capacity to record the volume of the fluid infused. An infusion pump is designed to deliver a measured amount of fluid over a period of time (e.g., milliliters per hour). The pump has a drop sensor and an alarm that will sound if drops are not detected at the appropriate rate. There are also alarms to alert the nurse regarding increased system pressure that can occur with an infiltration (IV fluid seeping into the tissue instead of the vascular space). An accurate measurement of intake of all IV therapy is recorded.

Monitoring intravenous therapy. Check the infusion and the IV site at least every hour, or per facility policy, to ensure that the IV infusion is continuing without any difficulty. If there is a problem with the site, discontinue using it, select a new IV site, and perform another venipuncture. Refer to the state nursing practice act and the facility's policy to determine the responsibilities of the LPN/LVN regarding the IV infusion.

Monitor the IV site for the development of problems. Assess for erythema, wetness, and edema. Inflammation, erythema, warmth, and pain often signify the onset of phlebitis (inflamed vein). Edema, coolness to touch, pallor, and pain indicate a possible infiltration of fluid into the tissue. Report these conditions to the RN and discontinue the IV infusion immediately. Assess and document the degree of infiltration as evidenced by the level of discomfort, swelling, and erythema. Worsening of the site's condition requires reporting to the RN and possibly the primary care provider. In addition, report the following:

- A patient with sudden onset of chills, fever, headache, nausea, and vomiting
- An anxious, dyspneic patient with a weak and rapid pulse

These factors sometimes indicate complications of IV therapy that necessitate immediate medical intervention.

Allergic reactions are possible as a result of IV medication administration. Reactions range from a mild rash to **anaphylactic shock** (a severe, life-threatening hypersensitivity reaction). Signs and symptoms may appear suddenly or at some point after the administration of the medication. Report if any of the following occurs:

- Respiratory distress from bronchospasms, manifested by restlessness, dyspnea, wheezing, and cyanosis (bluish coloration of the skin)
- Skin reactions such as pruritus (itching) or urticaria (hives)
- Signs of circulatory collapse, such as rapidly falling blood pressure, weak and rapid (thready) pulse, or vertigo
- GI signs and symptoms such as nausea, vomiting, and diarrhea
- Change in mental status

Anaphylactic shock necessitates immediate intervention. The LPN/LVN should notify the RN immediately if the patient develops clinical manifestations of an allergic reaction.

❖ NURSING PROCESS

The role of the LPN/LVN in the nursing process as stated is that the LPN/LVN will:

- Act in accordance with the state's nurse practice act
- Act in accordance with the facility's policies and procedures
- Participate in planning care for patients based on patient needs
- Review patient's plan of care and recommend revisions as needed
- Review and follow defined prioritization for patient care
- Use clinical pathways, care maps, or care plans to guide and review patient care

◆ ASSESSMENT

The nurse assesses many factors to determine the need for and potential response to drug therapy. These factors include the patient's medical history, diet, and allergy history. Assess the patient's current physical and mental status. Poor coordination and musculoskeletal problems may sometimes interfere with the patient's ability to prepare doses and take medications correctly; consider the patient's knowledge and understanding of drug therapy. Know as much as possible about each drug given, including normal dosages, purpose, action, routes, side effects, and interactions with other drugs.

◆ PATIENT PROBLEM

Use assessment findings to determine actual or potential problems with drug therapy. Potential patient problems may include the following:

- Anxiousness
- Potential for unsafe health behaviors
- Potential for harm or damage to the body
- Insufficient knowledge (specify)
- Compromised physical mobility
- Noncooperation or nonconformity: drug regimen

◆ EXPECTED OUTCOMES AND PLANNING

The plan of care should be focused on the safe administration of drugs. Use the time during drug administration to teach patients about their medications. Collaboration with the patient's family and significant others about drug regimens after discharge is necessary.

The plan of care is likely to include the following goal and outcome:

Goal: Patient and family understand the importance of the medication and how and when to administer the medication.

Outcome: Patient and family are able to describe information about the drug, dosage, schedule, purpose, and adverse effects.

◆ IMPLEMENTATION

Identify factors that have the potential to improve or diminish a patient's health and well-being. Physical limitations, economic status, cultural beliefs, values, and habits tend to influence a patient's compliance with medication schedules. The nurse is responsible for knowing about medications and their potential adverse effects on the patient, especially if the patient has multiple prescriptions. The capabilities and limitations of older adult patients are especially important considerations (see the Lifespan Considerations box for older adults).

◆ EVALUATION

Use evaluative measures to determine whether patient outcomes were met. Always be prepared to revise the care plan based on the evaluation findings.

Goal: The patient and their family understand drug therapy.

Evaluative measure: Ask the patient or their family to describe purpose, dosage, and adverse effects of each prescribed medication.

Lifespan Considerations

Older Adults

Medications and Aging

- All phases of pharmacokinetics are affected by aging. When the nurse has an option or is required to use clinical judgment regarding a patient's dose (e.g., an order of pain medication may note that the patient may receive 1 or 2 tablets), they should give older people the lowest dosages of medication necessary to achieve the desired therapeutic results.
- Dry mouth often contributes to difficulty swallowing medications. Sipping water before attempting to swallow the medication or covering the medication with a moist food such as applesauce tends to facilitate swallowing.
- It is necessary to take more precautions when parenteral medication is administered to older adults because of a decreased amount of muscle and subcutaneous tissue. Examine sites for suitability and rotate them with each use. Carefully select needles of the proper length based on the selected site and a tissue assessment of the individual.
- Because of decreased tolerance to intravenous (IV) medications, it is necessary to carefully assess the older adult for toxicity.
- Polypharmacy (the use of excessive numbers of different medications) is a common problem for older adults. Each medication taken increases the risk of interactions or toxicity, so it is best if the older patient has only one primary health care provider who manages the patient's medications. Educate older adults to refrain from taking any medication unless it is approved by the health care provider.

- Teach the older person to keep accurate and current records of all prescription and over-the-counter medications, and to present this list each time he or she seeks medical attention.
- Because of decreased renal, cardiac, and hepatic functioning, the older adult is at greater risk of becoming adversely and even fatally affected by medications. Hospitalized older adults often have one or more chronic illnesses for which they take multiple medications.
- Monitor the patient for signs and symptoms of decreased drug excretion, cumulative effects of drugs, drug potentiation, and drug incompatibilities. Frequent assessments and careful, thoughtful monitoring of the older patient aid in the prevention of medication-related complications.
- Some older adults do not hear, see, communicate, or move about as well as younger patients. Some are disoriented, perhaps even more so at night. When administering medications to older patients, take time to carefully assess their level of consciousness before and after.
- Carefully evaluate the list of medications prescribed for each patient and ascertain whether there have been any incompatibilities or incorrect dosages, or whether any medications are possibly adversely affecting the patient.
- The prevention of drug-related problems is the combined responsibility of the nurse, the health care provider, the pharmacist, and all others who care for the patient. Effective communication between the health care team, the patient, and the patient's family is necessary to administer medication safely and effectively to the older adult.

Get Ready For The NCLEX® Examination!

Key Points

- Calculate drug dosages accurately to administer medication safely to each patient.
- To reduce the chance of making a medication error, verify the correct dosage calculation with another nurse and reduce distractions while calculating.
- The metric system is the preferred system of weights and measurements; it is more accurate and easier to use in calculating dosage problems.
- When calculating dosages, always use the same units of measurement in the problem to avoid errors; if different units are used, convert them to one type of unit.

- Age, weight, body surface area, and the ability of the body to absorb, metabolize, and excrete medication are necessary to consider when medications are administered to a child.
- Be knowledgeable about the body surface area method for calculating children's dosages.
- When preparing medications, check the medication container label against the medication administration record or computer three times.
- The six "rights" of medication administration ensure accurate preparation and administration of medication dosages.
- Administer only those medications that you prepare.

- Never administer medication without accurately identifying the patient by their name and birth date. Follow facility policy if the patient is unable to identify themselves.
- Chart medications immediately after administration.
- Never leave a prepared medication unattended.
- Failure to select injection sites by anatomic landmarks poses the risk of tissue, bone, or nerve damage.
- Nurses are ethically and legally responsible for ensuring that the patient receives the correct medication ordered by the health care provider.
- Each medication order is required to include the patient's name and date of birth, order, date, medication name, dosage, route, and frequency of administration, and health care provider's signature.
- Always have a second nurse witness the "wasting" (disposal of unused portions) of a controlled substance or medication; both nurses must sign the logbook or document via facility policy to indicate that the medication was wasted.
- Medications enter the body through oral, sublingual, buccal, parenteral, percutaneous, inhalation, and topical (skin and mucous membranes) routes.
- Irrigations of the eye are used to relieve local inflammation of the conjunctiva, to apply antiseptic solution, or to flush out exudate, caustic, or irritating solutions.
- Using a small syringe and solution at body temperature, the nurse can clean a patient's external auditory canal of excess cerumen or exudate from a lesion or inflamed area.
- Internal vaginal irrigation, or douching, should not be performed routinely as it tends to wash away protective agents.
- Medications administered parenterally are absorbed more quickly than medications administered by other routes.
- The Z-track method for intramuscular injection minimizes irritation by sealing the medication in muscle tissue.
- Intramuscular injections for analgesia are given less frequently because of the use of PCA and patient-controlled epidural pumps.
- The nurse may give intradermal injections for skin testing (e.g., tuberculin screening and allergy tests).
- Because of decreased renal, cardiac, or hepatic functioning, the older adult is at greater risk of becoming adversely and possibly fatally affected by medications.

Additional Learning Resources

SG Go to your Study Guide for additional learning activities to help you master this chapter content.

Be sure to visit the Evolve site at http://evolve.elsevier.com/Cooper/foundations/ for additional online resources.

Review Questions For The NCLEX® Examination

Work the following problems. Use the proportion method, dimensional analysis, or desired dose/available dose formula, frequently used equivalents, and the big-to-small rule.

1. The health care provider has ordered 0.5 g of ceftriaxone. The nurse has available a vial labeled "250 mg/mL." How many milliliters will the nurse give the patient?

   1. 2 mL
   2. 0.2 mL
   3. 0.05 mL
   4. 0.5 mL

2. Digoxin, 0.125 mg, is ordered. On hand is Lanoxin, 0.5 mg/mL. How many milliliters will the nurse give?

   1. 3 mL
   2. 0.25 mL
   3. 2.5 mL
   4. 0.025 mL

3. The pediatrician has requested the pediatric patient's weight in kilograms. The scales say that the patient weighs 30 lb. How many kilograms will be reported to the health care provider?

   1. 20.6 kg
   2. 15 kg
   3. 13.6 kg
   4. 66 kg

4. Ordered is 1 L of D_5 ½ NS to run over 8 hours. The drip factor stated on the IV tubing is 15 gtt/mL. How many milliliters will be infused every hour?

   1. 100 mL/h
   2. 125 mL/h
   3. 150 mL/h
   4. 175 mL/h

5. An IV infusion of 1 L of D_5 ½ NS is to run at 150 mL/h. How long will this infusion run?

   1. 6 hours
   2. 6.7 hours
   3. 7.5 hours
   4. 8 hours

6. Which injections sites are recommended for intramuscular injection? (**SELECT ALL THAT APPLY.**)

   1. Ventrogluteal site
   2. Deltoid site
   3. Vastus lateralis site
   4. Dorsogluteal site

7. The average dose of a medication is 0.4 mg (gr ⅟₁₅₀) for an adult. What is the dosage for a 12-year-old?

   1. 2 mg
   2. 0.002 mg
   3. 0.02 mg
   4. 0.2 mg

8. An adult dose of diazepam (Valium) is 5 mg. Which dose is appropriate for a child who weighs 27 kg?

   1. 2 mg
   2. 1.5 mg
   3. 3 mg
   4. 2.5 mg

9. The LPN is asked by an RN to take an unlabeled container of solution to the operating room. What is the LPN's best response?

    1. "Of course, I'll take it right away!"
    2. "What is in the container?"
    3. "I will have the orderly take it."
    4. "I am not permitted to transport an unlabeled container."

10. After a possible exposure to tuberculosis, a 25-year-old health worker receives a tuberculin skin test. What type of injection is this?

    1. Intramuscular
    2. Intradermal
    3. Subcutaneous
    4. Intravenous

11. Insulin is to be given to a 55-year-old patient with diabetes who weighs 275 lb (125 kg) and measures 72 inches (183 cm) tall. His insulin is to be given via subcutaneous injection. What angle is acceptable for the injection?

    1. 45 degrees
    2. 90 degrees
    3. 15 degrees only
    4. 72degrees only

12. The nurse is deciding on the angle used in delivering subcutaneous heparin. What factor will determine the angle to be used for the injection?

    1. The amount of solution in the syringe
    2. The gauge of the needle
    3. The amount of subcutaneous tissue of the patient
    4. The size of the bevel of the needle

13. The patient complains of nausea after having a total abdominal hysterectomy. The nurse prepares an injection of promethazine, 25 mg, for IM injection. What needle length is most appropriate for selection?

    1. ⅜ inch
    2. ⅝ inch
    3. 1 to 1½ inches
    4. 2 to 2½ inches

14. A 6-month-old is to be immunized for diphtheria, tetanus, and pertussis. Which intramuscular injection site is most appropriate for this patient?

    1. Deltoid
    2. Ventrogluteal
    3. Gluteus maximus
    4. Vastus lateralis

15. The LPN/LVN is administering 8 a.m. medications in an acute care hospital. What is the acceptable time range for the nurse to administer these medications?

    1. 0800 to 1000
    2. 0700 to 0900
    3. 0800 to 0830
    4. 0730 to 0830

16. While administering routine medications to a patient at 1200 hours, the nurse realizes they have made a medication error. What is the nurse's priority action?

    1. Notify the health care provider.
    2. Call the supervisor.
    3. Complete an incident report.
    4. Assess the patient.

17. Prescribed medications are prepared and administered during which phase of the nursing process?

    1. Assessment
    2. Planning
    3. Implementation
    4. Evaluation

18. A patient hospitalized with newly diagnosed hypertension is taking enalapril, 5 mg PO bid, to lower his blood pressure. His next dose is at 0900. When taking his vital signs, the nurse discovers the patient's blood pressure is 90/42. What action should the nurse take?

    1. Withhold the medication and inform the health care provider of the change in the patient's blood pressure.
    2. Give the medication on time (the blood pressure is within normal limits).
    3. Ask the patient how he is feeling; if he is not having adverse signs or symptoms of low blood pressure, give him the medication.
    4. Give half the dose ordered.

19. Which action would be correct when a patient's ear is irrigated?

    1. Straighten the ear canal and irrigate with a large-tipped bulb syringe.
    2. Direct the solution to the middle of the canal to avoid damaging the ear.
    3. Use a solution that is body temperature and have the patient hold a basin under the ear while the solution is directed toward the top of the canal.
    4. Repeat the irrigation with hotter water.

20. The nurse performing eye irrigation should perform which procedure?

    1. Have the patient tip her head up and run the irrigation fluid over the open eye.
    2. Direct the irrigating fluid from the inner to the outer canthus.
    3. Do not allow the patient to blink.
    4. Place the irrigating syringe directly onto the corner of the eye and allow the fluid to move across the eye.
    5. Position the patient with the effected eye down.

21. A male patient, 22, returns from an overseas mission trip and begins to develop symptoms consistent with tuberculosis (TB) infection. He is prescribed oral medications, but his symptoms continue to worsen, and it is determined that he has contracted drug-resistant TB. His health care provider prescribes streptomycin, an aminoglycoside antibiotic, to be given IM once daily for 30 to 60 days, with a gradual tapering to 3 times a week (likely for at least 9 months), with careful monitoring of treatment progression. The nurse will administer his first injection.

Highlight the *most likely* options to complete the statement below.

The **most likely** injection site for administering this patient's first dose is the **ventrogluteal** site. The site itself is centered between two fingers pointing toward the **anterior superior iliac spine** and along the **iliac crest toward the buttock**.

OPTIONS FOR 1	OPTIONS FOR 2	OPTIONS FOR 3
dorsogluteal	anterior superior iliac spine	iliac crest toward the buttock
ventrogluteal	greater trochanter of the femur	midline of the thigh's lateral side
vastus lateralis	midline of the anterior thigh	midpoint of the lateral aspect of the upper limb
deltoid muscle	lower edge of the acromion process	posterior superior iliac spine

Fluids and Electrolytes

18

Objectives

1. Discuss how very young, elderly, and obese patients are at risk for fluid volume deficit.
2. List, describe, and compare the body fluid compartments.
3. Discuss how homeostasis is maintained.
4. Describe the thirst mechanism.
5. Discuss active and passive transport processes and give an example of each.
6. Describe the cause and effect of deficits and excesses of sodium, potassium, chloride, calcium, magnesium, phosphorus, and bicarbonate.
7. Differentiate among the roles of the buffers, the lungs, and the kidneys in maintaining acid-base balance.
8. Compare and contrast the four primary types of acid-base imbalances.
9. Discuss the role of the nursing process in maintaining fluid, electrolyte, and acid-base balances.
10. Summarize the nurse's responsibilities for the patient receiving intravenous therapy and related procedures.
11. Discuss complications of intravenous therapy.
12. Explain the nurse's responsibility in the administration of blood transfusion therapy.
13. Describe the complications of blood therapy.

Key Terms

acid-base balance (ĂS-ĭd BĀS BĂL-ĭns, p. 501)
active transport (ĂK-tĭv TRĂNZ-pŏrt, p. 494)
adenosine triphosphate (ATP) (ă-DĔN-ŏ-sēn trī-FŎS-făt, p. 492)
anions (ĂN-ī-ŏnz, p. 494)
autologous blood transfusions (ăw-TŎL-ă-gŭs BLŬD trănz-FYŪ-zhŭn, p. 523)
bicarbonate (bī-KĂHR-bō-nāt, p. 501)
blood buffers (BLŬD BŬF-ŭrz, p. 503)
calcium (KĂL-sē-ŭm, p. 498)
cations (KĂT-ī-ŏnz, p. 494)
chevron (SHĔV-rŏn, p. 518)
chloride (KLŎR-īd, p. 497)
diffusion (dĭf-YŪ-zhĭn, p. 493)
electrolyte (ĕ-LĔK-trō-līt, p. 494)
extracellular (ĕks-tră-SĔL-yū-lăr, p. 490)
filtration (fĭl-TRĂ-shĭn, p. 494)
glomerular filtration rate (GFR) (glŏ-MĔR-yū-lŭr fĭl-TRĂ-shĭn RĀT, p. 492)
hemolysis (p. 525)
homeostasis (hō-mē-ō-STĀ-sĭs, p. 491)
hydrostatic pressure (hī-drō-STĂT-ĭk PRĔSH-ŭr, p. 494)

hypertonic (hī-pŭr-TŎN-ĭk, p. 494)
hypotonic (hī-pō-TŎN-ĭk, p. 494)
induration (ĭn-dū-RĀ-shŭn, p. 513)
infiltration (ĭn-fĭl-TRĂ-shŭn, p. 515)
interstitial (ĭn-tŭr-STĬSH-ăl, p. 490)
intracellular (ĭn-tră-SĔL-yū-lăr, p. 490)
intravascular (ĭn-tră-VĂS-cyū-lăr, p. 491)
intravenous (IV) (ĭn-tră-VĒ-nŭs, p. 506)
ions (Ī-ŏnz, p. 494)
isotonic (ī-sō-TŎN-ĭk, p. 494)
magnesium (măg-NĒ-zē-ŭm, p. 500)
milliequivalent (mEq) (mĭl-ē-ĕ-KWĬV-ă-lĕnt, p. 494)
orthostatic hypotension (p. 490)
osmosis (ŏz-MŌ-sĭs, p. 493)
passive transport (PĂS-ĭv TRĂNZ-pŏrt, p. 492)
patent (PĂ-tĕnt, p. 518)
peripheral (pĕ-RĬF-ŭr-ăl, p. 513)
phosphorus (FŎS-fŭ-rŭs, p. 499)
potassium (pŏ-TĂS-ē-ŭm, p. 496)
sodium (SŌ-dē-ŭm, p. 494)
venipuncture (VĔN-ĭ-pŭnk-chŭr, p. 507)

This chapter discusses fluids, electrolytes, and acid-base balance. The body's fluid, electrolyte, and acid-base balance must be maintained to keep body systems healthy and functioning properly. These are maintained by water intake and output, distribution of electrolytes in the body, and the regulation of the renal and pulmonary systems.

FLUIDS (WATER)

Water has many functions in the body. It is necessary to carry nutrients to the body cells and waste products away from the cells. Inside the cells, water provides a medium in which chemical reactions, or metabolism,

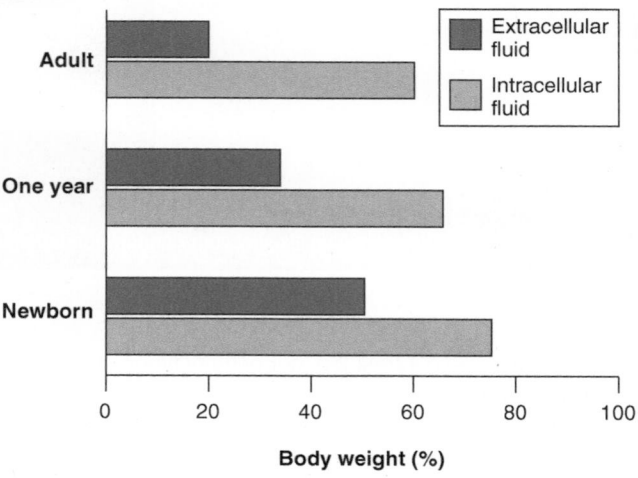

Fig. 18.1 In the newborn, more than half of total body fluid is extracellular. As the child grows, proportions gradually reach adult levels.

occur. Water also acts as a lubricant for tissues, aids in the maintenance of acid-base balance, and assists in heat regulation by evaporation.

Water is the largest component of the body. It makes up from 50% to 80% of total body weight, depending on age, sex, and body fat. This percentage depends on several factors and varies by individual. Between 70% and 80% of a newborn's body weight is water. That percentage increases in a premature infant to as high as 90%. As the infant ages, that percentage steadily decreases, and by 12 years of age, the ratio of water to body weight approaches that of an adult. The percentage of water in the adult body is 50% to 60%, and in the older adult, it drops to 45% to 55%.

In addition to age, fat also plays a role in the amount of water found in the body. Fat contains relatively little water in comparison to muscle. Women have proportionately more body fat than do men and thereby have less body fluid than do men. Individuals having more body weight, as in obesity, have smaller percentages of body water. Similarly, the more obese an individual is, the smaller the percentage of body water. Older adults and obese populations are at a greater risk for complications resulting from dehydration because of the reduced fluid reserve in their bodies (see the Lifespan Considerations box). Infants are also at higher risk for dehydration because more than half of an infant's body fluid is found outside the cells (**extracellular**) (Fig. 18.1). Extracellular fluid is lost from the body more rapidly than **intracellular** fluid (fluid inside the cells). A loss of 10% of body fluid is serious in an adult, and a 20% loss is fatal. In an infant, the percentages are even more significant: a 5% loss is serious, a 10% loss is very serious, and a 15% or more loss can be fatal.

FLUID COMPARTMENTS

Body fluids are found in two compartments in the body: inside the cells (intracellular) and outside the cells

(extracellular). However, *compartment* is an abstract term because, rather than being contained in a compartment or a specific area, the fluids are in constant motion throughout the body to carry out their functions. Although each compartment is specific in its location and functions, there is constant interaction between them.

The intracellular fluid compartment is the larger of the two compartments, making up 66% of the body's fluid. It is composed of all the fluid inside the cells within the body and contains dissolved particles, called *solutes.*

The extracellular fluid compartment contains any fluid outside of the cells. It contains large amounts of oxygen and carbon dioxide, as well as glucose, amino acids, fatty acids, sodium, calcium, chloride, and bicarbonate. The extracellular compartment is divided further into the interstitial and the intravascular fluid compartments (Fig. 18.2).

Interstitial fluid is found between the cells or in the tissues. It accounts for approximately 27% of the fluid in the body. Examples of interstitial fluid include lymph, cerebrospinal fluid, and gastrointestinal (GI) secretions.

Table 18.1   Body Fluid Distribution

COMPARTMENT	DESCRIPTION	FLUID
Intracellular	Fluid within cells	Intracellular fluid
Extracellular	Fluid outside cells	Extracellular fluid
Intravascular	Fluid within blood vessels	Plasma
Interstitial	Fluid in tissues (between cells or in body spaces)	Examples: lymph, cerebrospinal fluid, intraocular fluid, gastrointestinal secretions, urine, perspiration, exudates

Fig. 18.2 Major fluid compartments. Intracellular fluid *(ICF)* is fluid within cells. Extracellular fluid is fluid outside of cells. The extracellular fluid also includes interstitial fluid *(IF)*, which surrounds the cells, and plasma, the fluid component of blood. Fluid continually moves between the major compartments. (From Patton KT, Thibodeau GA: The human body in health and disease, ed 6, St. Louis, 2014, Mosby.)

Table 18.2   Body Fluid Distribution

COMPARTMENT	PERCENTAGE OF TOTAL BODY FLUID	FLUID VOLUME (L)
Extracellular fluid		
Interstitial fluid	27	11.2
Intravascular fluid (plasma)	7	2.8
Intracellular fluid	66	42.0

Table 18.3   Normal Fluid Intake and Output in an Adult Eating 2500 Calories Per Day (Approximate Statistics)

TYPE OF CONTENT	GAIN (ML)	ROUTE	AMOUNT OF LOSS (ML)
Water in food	1000	Skin	500
Water from oxidation	300	Lungs	350
Water as liquid	1200	Feces	150
		Kidney	1500
Total	2500	Total	2500

Intravascular fluid is the plasma within the vessels. This fluid contains serum, protein, and other substances necessary to sustain life. This fluid is usually what carries the nutrients and waste products between cells and tissues. It makes up the remaining 7% of fluid volume.

The intracellular and extracellular fluid compartments are separated by a semipermeable membrane. This membrane allows for a constant flow as nutrients are taken into the cell and waste products are carried out (Tables 18.1 and 18.2).

INTAKE AND OUTPUT

As water moves through all parts of the body, it constantly is being lost and must be replaced. Fluid leaves the body through the kidneys, the lungs, the skin, and the GI tract. **Homeostasis** is the process of keeping body fluids in balance. The body is equipped with several homeostatic mechanisms to keep the composition and volume of body fluid within narrow limits of normal. The average adult fluid intake is approximately 2200 to 2700 mL/day. Oral intake of fluids should be approximately 1100 to 1400 mL/day; solid foods contribute approximately 800 to 1000 mL/day; and fluid produced from cellular metabolism provides approximately 300 mL/day (Table 18.3). Although solid foods are not measured or counted as part of the patient's intake, they do contribute to the overall fluid intake.

Fluid intake is regulated mainly through the thirst mechanism. Receptors in the hypothalamus called *osmoreceptors* measure the concentration of the blood.

When the number of particles (solutes) in the blood is higher than normal, the sensation of thirst is present and the person drinks to satisfy that sensation. Anyone who is unable to respond to or perceive the thirst mechanism is at increased risk for dehydration and may require fluids administered by way of tube feedings, IV infusion, or total parenteral nutrition (TPN). A person may be unable to respond to perceived thirst secondary to paralysis, dementia, or injury.

Fluid loss from the body is considered either sensible (measurable) or insensible (not measurable). Sensible losses are seen in urine, feces, vomiting, and drainage from gastric tubes, chest tubes, and wounds. Insensible fluid losses include those from perspiration and expiration. Because it is difficult to measure insensible fluid losses accurately, approximations are acceptable. However, because measurement of sensible losses is possible, it is very important to keep accurate records of fluid intake and output to help determine a patient's fluid needs.

The kidneys play an extremely important role in fluid balance. If the kidneys are not functioning properly, the body has great difficulty regulating fluid balance. The nephrons are the functioning units of the kidneys and they filter blood at a rate of 125 mL/min, or about 180 L/day. This is called the glomerular filtration rate (GFR) and leads to an output of 1 to 2 L (1000 to 2000 mL) of urine per day. The kidneys are amazing organs to take 180 L per day of blood and, from that, only make 1 to 2 L of urine. The nephrons reabsorb the remaining fluid based on bodily needs. If the body loses even 1% to 2% of its fluid, the kidneys conserve fluid by reabsorbing more water from the renal filtrate, which results in less water excreted and more concentrated urine. To effectively eliminate waste products from the body, the kidneys must excrete a minimum of 30 mL/h of urine. In the presence of fluid excesses, the kidneys react by excreting more dilute urine, thus ridding the body of excess fluid and conserving electrolytes.

One simple and accurate way to determine water balance is by weighing the patient under controlled conditions: for example, at the same time of day, with the same amount of clothing, and when attached to the same equipment, such as electrodes, IV tubing, drainage devices, braces, or splints. It is important to empty all drainage bags before the patient is weighed to get an accurate measurement. One liter of fluid equals 2.2 pounds (1 kg); therefore, a weight change of 2.2 pounds reflects a loss or gain of 1 L of body fluid (Skill 18.1).

Urine-specific gravity is a measurement of urine concentration. It is also a good indicator of fluid balance. A urine-specific gravity value of more than 1.030 indicates that the urine is concentrated, as in conditions of dehydration, whereas a measurement of less than 1.003 to 1.000 indicates that the urine is dilute, as in conditions of overhydration.

MOVEMENT OF FLUID AND ELECTROLYTES

In a healthy person, body fluids are constantly in motion. This constant motion is what helps balance the fluids inside and outside the cells. The extracellular fluid transports nutrients to the cells and carries waste products away from them by way of the capillary bed. Movement of substances through the capillary bed depends on cell membrane permeability. Passage of substances across the cell membrane is accomplished in one of two ways: passive transport or active transport.

As implied by their name, active transport processes necessitate the expenditure of energy by the cell, and passive transport processes do not. The energy required for active transport processes is obtained from a chemical substance called adenosine triphosphate (ATP). ATP is produced in the mitochondria of cells from nutrients and is capable of releasing energy that enables the cell to work. For active transport processes to occur, the breakdown of ATP and the use of the related energy are required.

Two simple points to remember about active and passive transport are that (1) passive transport processes do not require cellular energy and (2) active transport processes do require cellular energy.

PASSIVE TRANSPORT

The primary passive transport processes that move substances through the cell membranes include the following:
- Diffusion
- Osmosis
- Filtration

Skill 18.1 Measuring Intake and Output

CHECK GATHER HELLO ID PRIVACY EXPLAIN WASH GLOVES

NURSING ACTION (RATIONALE)

1. Identify patient. (*Ensures accuracy.*)
2. Explain procedure. (*Enlists patient's cooperation and promotes patient participation.*)
3. Instruct patient to inform staff of all oral intake. Provide a marked I&O container. (*Facilitates accuracy of I&O measurement.*)
4. Instruct patient not to empty any output collection receptacles and to notify the nurse after elimination. (*Contributes to accuracy of I&O measurement.*)
5. Alert all staff and remind patient of need to measure I&O. (*Promotes compliance and accuracy.*)
6. Measure and record all fluids taken orally, gastric tube feedings, and all fluids administered parenterally. (*Helps ensure accurate measurement of intake.*)
7. Wash hands and don gloves. (*Prevents transmission of microorganisms.*)
8. Measure and record output in Foley drainage system, diarrhea stools, nasogastric suction, emesis, ileostomy, and surgical wound receptacles such as Davol, Jackson-Pratt, and Hemovac drains. Measure and record output from chest tube drainage in water-sealed container by marking with felt-tip pen. (*Ensures accurate measurement and proper disposal of output.*)
9. Remove gloves and wash hands. (*Prevents cross-contamination.*)
10. Compute I&O and document it on patient's record. (*Ensures accurate documentation of total I&O.*)

Table 18.4   Passive Transport Processes

PROCESS	DESCRIPTION		EXAMPLES
Diffusion	Movement of particles through a membrane from an area of high concentration to an area of low concentration—that is, down the concentration gradient		Movement of carbon dioxide out of all cells; movement of sodium ions into nerve cells as they conduct an impulse
Osmosis	Diffusion of water through a selectively permeable membrane in the presence of at least one impermeable solute		Diffusion of water molecules into and out of cells to correct imbalances in water concentration
Filtration	Movement of water and small solute particles, but not larger particles, through a filtration membrane; movement occurs from area of high pressure to area of low pressure		In the kidney, movement of water and small solutes from blood vessels but lack of movement by blood proteins and blood cells; begins the formation of urine

From Patton KT, Thibodeau GA: *Structure and function of the body*, ed 15, St. Louis, 2016, Elsevier.

DIFFUSION

Diffusion is the natural tendency of a substance to move from an area of higher concentration to one of lower concentration (Table 18.4). This eventually results in an equal distribution of solutes within the two areas. A concentration gradient is generally the stimulus for this migration or movement of molecules. A concentration gradient is the situation in which molecules become more numerous in one area of a solution. The process of diffusion occurs when the molecules move from this area of higher concentration to a less concentrated area. This results in a more even distribution of particles.

The exchange of oxygen and carbon dioxide occurs by diffusion. On inspiration, more oxygen molecules are brought into the lungs than carbon dioxide molecules. Because of this, diffusion occurs—the oxygen molecules move through the cell membranes into the capillary bed and are taken to all body tissues. At the same time, the capillary bed has more carbon dioxide molecules than oxygen molecules, and the carbon dioxide diffuses into the alveoli of the lungs to be eliminated on exhalation.

Facilitated diffusion, or carrier-mediated diffusion, is the process by which material combines with carriers to cross the cell membrane. Facilitated diffusion enables amino acids and glucose to cross the cell membrane into the cells.

OSMOSIS

Osmosis is the movement of water across a semipermeable membrane, from an area of lower concentration to an area of higher concentration (see Table 18.4). In other words, two different solutions are separated by a membrane through which they cannot pass. One side of the membrane has more particles than the other side in relationship to the water. Because of this inequality of particles, water moves through the membrane from the area of low particle concentration to the area of high particle concentration until the solutions are of equal concentration. When the solutions reach equal concentration, they are said to be *isotonic.*

The red blood cells offer an example of the osmotic process in the body; if extracellular fluid is more concentrated (has more particles) than intracellular fluid, the fluid from inside the cell moves out to the extracellular fluid, causing the red blood cell to shrink. If the fluid among the compartments is in equilibrium, fluid enters and leaves the cell at the same rate and the cell size does not change. Another example of osmosis arises when extracellular fluid is less concentrated (has fewer particles) than the fluid in the red blood cells. Fluid then moves into the cell to even out the solutions, which causes the cell to enlarge. It is possible for the cell to rupture if too much fluid moves into it.

Solutions in the body are classified according to the electrolyte (particle) concentration. Solutions that have the same concentration of electrolytes as body fluids are said to be *isotonic,* solutions that have higher concentrations of electrolytes than body fluids are considered *hypertonic,* and those with fewer electrolytes than body fluids are *hypotonic.* The concentration of the solution causes the cells of the body to react in the same way as the red blood cell does. **Hypertonic** solutions pull fluid from the cells; **isotonic** solutions expand the body's fluid volume without causing a fluid shift from one compartment to another; and **hypotonic** solutions move into the cells, causing them to enlarge. Each of these actions occurs through osmosis.

FILTRATION

Filtration is the transfer of water and dissolved substances from an area of higher pressure to an area of lower pressure. The force behind filtration is called **hydrostatic pressure,** which is the force of fluid pressing outward on a vessel wall (see Table 18.4). An example of filtration is the passage of water and electrolytes from the arterial capillary bed to the interstitial fluid. In this example, hydrostatic pressure is created by the pumping action of the heart. At the arterial end of the capillary, the hydrostatic pressure is greater than the pressure within the capillary. This forces water and electrolytes out of the capillary and into the interstitial fluid.

ACTIVE TRANSPORT

The fluid movements discussed to this point necessitate no energy expenditure by the body; they are examples of passive transport. **Active transport** is the process of moving molecules, against pressure, through a membrane with the use of "carriers" and energy from the cell. Active transport carriers are also referred to as *pumps.*

Just as with facilitated diffusion, active transport requires a carrier to move the particles from the outside of the cell to the inside. In active transport, the particles are moving against pressure and require energy to move into the cell.

The sodium-potassium pump is an example of active transport. The sodium-potassium pump is the body's way of maintaining the sodium-potassium balance. Sodium is found mostly on the outside of the cell; potassium is found mainly inside the cell. Both can flow freely through the cell membrane, and if there were no control of this flow, eventually the amount of sodium in the cell would increase and cause the cell to enlarge and burst.

To help prevent this, the sodium-potassium pump transports sodium out of the cell and pulls potassium back into the cell. Excessive sodium inside the cell can be hazardous, just as excess potassium outside the cell can be hazardous. Maintaining the proper balance is one essential component of maintaining fluid balance within the body.

ELECTROLYTES

An **electrolyte** is a substance that develops an electrical charge when it dissolves in water. These electrically charged particles are called **ions.** Ions develop either a positive or negative electrical charge. Ions with a positive charge are called **cations.** Ions with a negative charge are called *anions.*

Cations within the body include:
- Sodium (Na^+)
- Potassium (K^+)
- Calcium (Ca^{2+})
- Magnesium (Mg^{2+})

The anions found in the body are as follows:
- Chloride (Cl^-)
- Bicarbonate (HCO_3^-)
- Sulfate (SO_4^-)
- Hydrogen phosphate (HPO_4^-)

A balance exists among the electrolytes. For this balance to occur, a negatively charged anion must be present for each positively charged cation. In all fluid compartments in the body, the cations and anions combine to balance one another and keep the body in homeostasis.

Electrolytes are measured in milliequivalents. A **milliequivalent (mEq)** is a measure of the chemical activity of an ion. The chemical activity of an electrolyte is compared with the chemical activity of hydrogen. One milliequivalent of any electrolyte has the same chemical activity as 1 mEq of hydrogen. In each fluid compartment in the body, the cations and anions balance each other out with their chemical activity to maintain electrical neutrality, which again keeps the body in homeostasis.

Although the electrolytes move freely among the fluid compartments, each has a primary location. For example, sodium is the primary extracellular electrolyte, whereas potassium is the primary intracellular electrolyte. The healthy body maintains homeostasis by correcting any excesses or deficiencies of the electrolytes.

Sodium

Sodium is the most abundant electrolyte in the body. It is the major extracellular electrolyte, although a small amount is found in the intracellular fluid. Sodium has many functions in the body, one of which is to regulate the body's fluid volumes. It does this mainly through osmotic pressure because water follows the sodium throughout the body. Sodium helps regulate the contractility of muscular activity, especially in the heart, and helps maintain neuromuscular irritability to improve nerve impulse conduction. It is also necessary for maintaining acid-base balance.

The major source of all electrolytes is the diet, or oral intake; sodium is no exception. However, sodium, unlike the other electrolytes, usually is consumed in excessive amounts by most Americans. Sodium can be found in cheese, table salt, seafood, processed meat, canned vegetables, canned soups, ketchup, and snack foods, such as pretzels and potato chips.

The kidneys are the primary excretion route for sodium. Many electrolytes, such as sodium, not only pass into and out of the body but also move back and forth between several body fluids. Fig. 18.3 shows the large volumes of sodium-containing internal secretions that

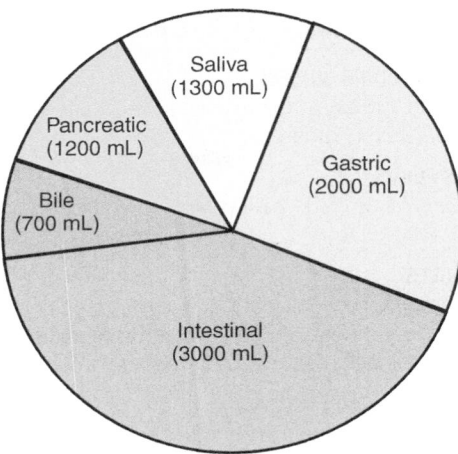

Fig. 18.3 Sodium-containing internal secretions produced every day. (Redrawn from Long BC, Phipps WJ, Cassmeyer VL: Medical-surgical nursing: A nursing process approach, ed 3, St. Louis, 1993, Mosby.)

are produced each day. During a 24-hour period, more than 8 L of fluid containing 1000 to 1300 mEq of sodium are poured into the digestive system. This sodium, along with most of that contained in the diet, is reabsorbed almost completely. The normal blood level of sodium is 135 to 145 mEq/L.

Hyponatremia. *Hyponatremia* is the state in which the concentration of sodium in the blood is less than normal. This happens when there is a sodium loss, such as with vomiting or diarrhea, or an excessive intake of water that dilutes the sodium excessively (Box 18.1). Hyponatremia occurs when the sodium level in the extracellular fluid drops to less than 135 mEq/L.

When a deficiency results from sodium loss, the body attempts to compensate by decreasing water excretion. This assists in concentrating the sodium level and allowing the sodium level to increase. The signs and symptoms of hyponatremia depend on the cause and on how rapid and severe the sodium loss is. As sodium levels decrease in the extracellular fluid, water is pulled into the cells, which causes them to become edematous. As the fluid moves into the cells, potassium is shifted out and the patient is likely to have a potassium imbalance, as well. The patient may experience weakness, anorexia, muscle cramps, confusion, fatigue, headache, edema, and seizures. Treatment for hyponatremia includes sodium replacement and water restrictions.

If the nurse remembers that sodium helps regulate muscular activity and improve nerve impulses, it is easy to associate low sodium levels with seizures (a neuromuscular condition), weakness, and muscle cramps.

Hypernatremia. *Hypernatremia* is when the concentration of sodium is greater than normal and exceeds 145 mEq/L. It is caused by an excess of sodium or a decrease in body water (Box 18.2). The body attempts to correct the imbalance by conserving water through renal reabsorption.

Box **18.1**	Hyponatremia: Causes, Signs and Symptoms, and Nursing Interventions

CAUSES
- Ascites
- Burns
- Diaphoresis
- Diarrhea
- Fistulas
- GI or biliary drainage via nasogastric tube or T tube
- Inadequate sodium intake
- Large open lesions (burns)
- Lengthy hydrotherapy
- Loss of GI fluids
- Loss through skin
- Massive edema
- Shifting of body fluids
- Small bowel obstruction
- Vomiting

SIGNS AND SYMPTOMS
- Abdominal cramps
- Apathy
- Apprehension
- Fatigue[a]
- Headache[a]
- Irritability
- Muscle weakness, muscle twitching, tremors
- Nausea and vomiting
- Postural hypotension[a]

SEVERE OR PROLONGED SODIUM DEFICIT
- Altered level of consciousness (lethargy, confusion)[b]
- Coma
- Seizures
- Shock

NURSING INTERVENTIONS
- Monitor and record vital signs, especially blood pressure and pulse.
- Monitor intake and output if patient is receiving diuretic medications.
- Monitor neurologic status frequently; report any change in level of consciousness.
- Monitor skin turgor at least every 8 h.
- Observe for abnormal fluid losses from gastrointestinal system, kidneys, or skin.
- Replace fluid loss with fluids containing sodium, not with plain water.
- Restrict fluid intake as ordered. This is the primary treatment for dilutional hyponatremia; post a sign about fluid restriction in the patient's room.
- Weigh patient daily.

[a]Most common signs and symptoms.
[b]Altered level of consciousness usually accompanies a serum sodium level lower than 125 mEq/L and indicates that the patient's condition is deteriorating.
GI, Gastrointestinal.

Hypernatremia causes fluid to shift from the cells to the interstitial spaces, which results in cellular dehydration and an interruption in cellular processes. Again, a potassium imbalance frequently occurs because potassium is excreted. Treatment for

Box 18.2 **Hypernatremia: Causes, Signs and Symptoms, and Nursing Interventions**

CAUSES
- Abnormally large intake of sodium
- Consumption of antacids containing sodium
- Dairy products in large amounts
- Loss of more water than sodium from the body
- Overuse of table salt
- Prepared foods: frozen, canned, smoked
- Taking too many salt tablets
- Too-rapid infusion of intravenous saline solution

SIGNS AND SYMPTOMS
- Dry mucous membranes with tenacious (thick) mucus
- Firm, rubbery tissue turgor
- Low urinary output
- Restlessness, agitation, confusion, flushed skin

SEVERE OR PROLONGED SODIUM EXCESS
- Death
- Manic excitement
- Tachycardia

NURSING INTERVENTIONS
- Decrease sodium intake in patient's diet.
- Monitor and record vital signs, especially blood pressure and pulse.
- Monitor for increased respiratory rate.
- Monitor intake and output.
- Monitor serum sodium level.
- Monitor water loss from fever and infection.
- Provide a safe environment for a confused or agitated patient.
- Weigh patient daily to check for body fluid loss.

Box 18.3 **Foods Rich in Potassium**

FRUITS (INCLUDING JUICES)
- Apricots, bananas, cantaloupe, dried fruits (e.g., figs, dates, raisins), grapefruit, honeydew, melon, oranges

PROTEIN FOODS
- Beef, chicken, liver, milk, nuts, peanut butter, pork, veal, turkey

VEGETABLES
- Asparagus, broccoli, cabbage, carrots, celery, dried beans, dried peas, mushrooms, potatoes (especially skins), spinach, squash, tomatoes

BEVERAGES
- Cocoa, cola drinks, fruit and vegetable juices

hypernatremia is to lower the sodium levels gradually by decreasing sodium intake or by increasing water in the body.

Potassium

Potassium (K+) is found primarily in the intracellular fluid and is the major intracellular cation. However, some potassium is present in the extracellular compartments. Of the body's potassium, 98% is inside the cells and 2% is in the extracellular fluid.

The main function of potassium is regulation of water and electrolyte content within the cell. Along with sodium and calcium, it promotes transmission of nerve impulses and skeletal muscle function. Potassium assists in the cellular metabolism of carbohydrates and proteins and helps control the hydrogen ion concentration. When potassium moves out of the cell, sodium and hydrogen ions move in. The result is the regulation of acid-base balance.

A well-balanced diet usually provides adequate potassium. Approximately 65 mEq of potassium is required each day to maintain the normal blood serum level of 3.5 to 5.0 mEq/L. Potassium is distributed in natural foods. Good sources of potassium include fruits, such as oranges, bananas, apricots, and cantaloupe; legumes; leafy vegetables; potatoes; mushrooms; tomatoes; carrots; and meat (Box 18.3).

Potassium is excreted through the kidneys (80% to 90%), as well as in the feces and perspiration (10% to 20%). In the kidneys, sodium and potassium seem to pair off against each other, and the kidneys prefer to conserve sodium, even when both electrolytes are depleted. Therefore, any condition that causes a decrease in urinary output also causes potassium retention and the potential for life-threatening consequences. Too little or too much potassium affects the heart muscle and has the potential to result in a deadly disturbance in cardiac rhythm (dysrhythmia).

Hypokalemia. *Hypokalemia* is a decrease in the body's potassium level to less than 3.5 mEq/L. Because the normal range for a serum potassium level is narrow, a slight decrease has profound consequences. The major cause of potassium loss is renal excretion (Box 18.4). The kidneys do not conserve potassium, and they excrete it even when the body needs the potassium. Intestinal fluids contain large amounts of potassium; therefore, with excessive GI losses from gastric suctioning or prolonged vomiting, potassium levels tend to become depleted. Severe diarrhea, fistulas, ileostomy, and excessive diaphoresis also can result in potassium loss, as does the use of diuretics, such as thiazides or furosemide (Lasix). Strenuous exercise and any conditions that cause injury to the cells cause the release of potassium from the cells into the interstitial spaces and, ultimately, to the kidneys. If renal function is normal, the potassium is excreted, which causes a deficiency in potassium. Hypokalemia has the capacity to affect skeletal and cardiac function. The resulting muscle weakness can cause life-threatening cardiac conduction abnormalities. Treatment of hypokalemia involves replacing the potassium orally or, possibly, with intravenous (IV) potassium supplements, as well as monitoring kidney and cardiac function until the potassium levels become normal again. It is vital to remember that potassium, when given IV or IV push (bolus of medication), must always be diluted to avoid serious cardiac dysrhythmias that may result in death.

| Box 18.4 | Hypokalemia: Causes, Signs and Symptoms, and Nursing Interventions |

CAUSES

- Conditions causing very large urine output
- Decreased potassium intake
- GI losses (vomiting, diarrhea, GI suctioning)
- Ileostomy
- Increased aldosterone activity
- Increased potassium loss
- Loss from cells, as in trauma, burns, fistulas
- Metabolic alkalosis
- Potassium shift into cells
- Potassium-losing diuretics
- Skin losses, diaphoresis
- Treatment of acidosis
- Villous adenoma (tumor of the intestine that produces potassium-containing mucus)

SIGNS AND SYMPTOMS

- Cardiac dysrhythmias; weak, irregular pulse
- Decreased bowel sounds, cramps, constipation, anorexia, nausea, vomiting[a]
- Diminished deep tendon reflexes, lethargy, confusion; paralysis involving the respiratory muscles; coma
- Electrocardiographic changes
- Orthostatic hypotension
- Paresthesia, hyporeflexia
- Polyuria
- Skeletal muscle weakness (especially in lower extremities), leg cramps[a]

SEVERE OR PROLONGED POTASSIUM DEFICIT

- Cardiac or respiratory arrest
- Flaccid paralysis
- Kidney damage
- Paralytic ileus

NURSING INTERVENTIONS

- Administer potassium chloride (KCl) supplement as prescribed by the health care provider (oral or IV).[b]
- Carefully assess patients who are taking digitalis glycosides, especially if they are also taking a diuretic. The low potassium levels could potentiate the action of the digitalis glycoside and cause digitalis toxicity.
- Encourage increased intake of foods high in potassium.
- Monitor bowel sounds.
- Monitor I&O (about 40 mEq of potassium is lost in each liter of urine; diuresis has potential to put the patient at risk for potassium loss).
- Monitor laboratory findings relating to kidney function. If renal function is impaired, there is a significant risk for hyperkalemia.
- Monitor serum potassium level.
- Monitor telemetric values.

GI, Gastrointestinal; *I&O,* intake and output; *IV,* intravenous.

Hyperkalemia. An increase in the body's serum potassium level greater than 5 mEq/L is known as *hyperkalemia.* The major cause of potassium excess is renal disease, in which potassium is not excreted adequately (Box 18.5). When tissue damage occurs, potassium is released from the cells. If kidney output also is reduced, the result is an elevation in the potassium level.

Excessive intake of foods high in potassium, especially with decreased urine output, also may cause an increase in the serum potassium level, as does excessive use of salt substitutes (most of which use potassium as a substitute for sodium); potassium supplements (oral or IV); and drugs, such as beta blockers (which inhibit potassium shifts into cells), potassium-sparing diuretics (e.g., spironolactone), chemotherapy (which causes death or lysis of cells with release of high levels of intracellular potassium into the blood), angiotensin-converting enzyme inhibitors, nonsteroidal anti-inflammatory drugs, and aminoglycosides.

Although hyperkalemia is less common than hypokalemia, it is often more dangerous because overstimulation of the cardiac muscle can cause cardiac arrest. A serum potassium level of 7 mEq/L or greater carries the risk of serious cardiac dysrhythmias. Treatment is aimed at lowering the potassium levels and correcting the underlying cause, if possible. Treatment could involve restricting potassium intake, giving IV calcium gluconate to decrease the effects of the high potassium levels on the heart, giving sodium bicarbonate or insulin in a glucose solution to shift the potassium back into the cell, or by giving sodium polystyrene sulfonate (Kayexalate) orally or rectally. Kayexalate binds with the potassium to remove it from the system by way of the GI tract.

Chloride

Chloride (Cl^-) is an extracellular anion that is rarely present alone. Chloride usually is bound to another ion, such as sodium or potassium. Chloride can diffuse quickly between the intracellular and extracellular compartments and combines easily with sodium to form sodium chloride or, less often, with potassium to form potassium chloride. The normal blood level of chloride is 96 to 106 mEq/L.

Chloride is necessary for the formation of hydrochloric acid in gastric secretions, and it is necessary in the regulation of the osmotic pressure between the body's fluid compartments. It also assists in the regulation of acid-base balance.

Foods containing sodium also contain chloride: cheese, table salt, seafood, processed meat, canned vegetables, canned soups, ketchup, and snack foods, such as pretzels and potato chips. The main route of excretion for chloride is through the kidneys.

Hypochloremia. *Hypochloremia* usually occurs when chloride levels fall below 96 mEq/L in association with sodium loss because sodium and chloride are frequently paired. Vomiting, diarrhea, gastric suctioning, and acute infections all cause a loss of both sodium and chloride. Symptoms of hypochloremia include depressed respirations, tetany, and alkalosis. Treatment involves alleviating the underlying cause and replacing the chloride with sodium chloride IV solutions.

Box 18.5 Hyperkalemia: Causes, Signs and Symptoms, and Nursing Interventions

CAUSES

- Adrenal insufficiency
- Aminoglycosides
- Angiotensin-converting enzyme inhibitors
- Beta blockers
- Entrance of potassium into the bloodstream from injured cells with extensive trauma (shift of potassium out of the cells into extracellular fluid)
- Excessive use of salt substitutes
- Infusion of large volume of blood nearing expiration date
- Metabolic acidosis
- Nonsteroidal anti-inflammatory drugs
- Potassium intake (parenteral or oral) in excess of kidney's ability to excrete
- Potassium-sparing diuretics
- Renal failure
- Tumor lysis syndrome after chemotherapy

SIGNS AND SYMPTOMS[A]

- Cardiac dysrhythmias[b]
- Diarrhea, colic[b]
- ECG changes
- Hypotension
- Irregular pulse rate
- Irritability
- Nausea, vomiting[b]
- Numbness, tingling
- Paresthesias
- Skeletal muscle weakness, especially of lower extremities

SEVERE OR PROLONGED POTASSIUM EXCESS

- Anuria
- Cardiac arrest[b] (serious dysrhythmias become especially dangerous when the serum potassium level reaches 7 mEq/L or more)
- Flaccid paralysis
- Signs and symptoms similar to those of hypokalemia (from prolonged potassium excess)

NURSING INTERVENTIONS[C]

- Administer loop diuretics.
- Administer sodium polystyrene sulfonate (Kayexalate) as prescribed by the health care provider (Kayexalate can be given orally, through a nasogastric tube, or as a retention enema); keep in mind that Kayexalate can sometimes cause serum sodium level to rise; monitor for congestive heart failure.
- Assess vital signs.
- Decrease intake of foods high in potassium.
- Decrease or stop medications associated with high potassium level.
- Monitor bowel sounds, as well as number and character of bowel movements.
- Monitor I&O (report an output of less than 30 mL/h; an inability to excrete potassium in the urine can potentially lead to dangerously high potassium level).
- Monitor serum potassium level.
- Monitor telemetric values to detect dysrhythmias.
- Monitor underlying disorders that may lead to high potassium level.

ECG, Electrocardiogram; *I&O*, intake and output.
[a]Signs and symptoms are often nonspecific; serum potassium level and ECG tracings are often the best clinical indicators.
[b]Most common signs and symptoms.
[c]Hemodialysis may be necessary for treating acute symptomatic hyperkalemia.
Note: Hyperkalemia may be the most dangerous of the electrolyte disorders.

Hyperchloremia. *Hyperchloremia* is rare; it can occur when bicarbonate levels fall and metabolic acidosis occurs. The increase in chloride anions represents an attempt to compensate and maintain equal numbers with the cations in the body fluid. Because chloride imbalances rarely occur independently of other electrolyte imbalances, there are no specific signs and symptoms to identify a chloride imbalance. However, symptoms of acidosis may indicate high chloride levels.

Calcium

Calcium (Ca^{2+}) is a positively charged ion found mainly in the bones and teeth. Of all the calcium in the body, 99% is concentrated in the bones and the teeth, where it is essentially inactive until the calcium levels in the blood fall. At that time, calcium is released from the bones to raise the serum calcium level. The remaining 1% of calcium is found in the soft tissue and the extracellular fluid. Regulation of the calcium level in the body is based on the deposition and resorption of bone, the amount of calcium absorbed from the GI tract, and the amount excreted in the urine and feces.

Vitamin D, calcitonin, and parathyroid hormone (parathormone) increase absorption and utilization of calcium; phytic acid and oxalic acid, found naturally in some plants, bind to calcium and inhibit its absorption. The normal ionized calcium level should be 4.5 to 5.6 mEq/dL. Total calcium levels may vary with the amount of albumin in the system; therefore, an ionized level is a more reliable indicator of calcium in the body. Calcium is required for the formation and maintenance of strong bones and teeth, as well as the prevention of osteoporosis. It is also necessary for normal blood clotting. Calcium has a depressing, or sedative, effect on neuromuscular irritability and, thus, promotes normal transmission of nerve impulses; it also helps regulate normal muscle contraction and relaxation. It helps hold body cells together by establishing the thickness and strength of cell membranes. One of its most important functions is to act as an enzyme activator for chemical reactions in the body.

Some of the best food sources of calcium are milk and cheese. Other sources include beans, nuts, cauliflower, lettuce, and egg yolks. Prevention of osteoporosis focuses on adequate calcium intake. Premenopausal women and postmenopausal women who are taking estrogen need at least 1000 mg of calcium per day and postmenopausal women who are not taking supplemental estrogen need about 1200 mg of calcium per day. Calcium needs in children vary, depending on their age and physiologic needs. However, during times of growth—the first year of life, puberty, and adolescence—calcium needs are increased. Calcium is removed from the body in the urine and feces.

Hypocalcemia. *Hypocalcemia* develops when the serum level of calcium falls below 4.5 mg/dL. Possible deficiencies arise from a variety of problems (Box 18.6).

Symptoms of hypocalcemia involve neuromuscular irritation and increased excitability, manifested by hyperactive deep tendon reflexes and seizures. As neuromuscular signs and symptoms increase, tetany is also possible. Tetany is a condition characterized by excessive muscle cramps, laryngeal spasms, stridor, carpal spasms (Trousseau sign), pedal spasms, and contraction of facial muscles (Chvostek sign) (Fig. 18.4). Treatment involves replacing calcium with IV calcium gluconate and 1000 mg of oral calcium supplements daily. If the low calcium level is related to decreased levels of parathyroid hormone, it is also necessary to replace that.

Hypercalcemia. *Hypercalcemia* occurs when calcium levels exceed 5.6 mEq/L. It may occur when calcium stored in the bone enters the circulation: for example, in patients who are immobilized (Box 18.7). When the bones are not being utilized for activity (such as with bedrest/immobilization), the bones give up the calcium and it enters the blood. This is why weight-bearing exercises are recommended as prevention of osteoporosis. Excessive intake of calcium or vitamin D also causes hypercalcemia. Symptoms of hypercalcemia are neuromuscular activity depression and the formation of renal calculi as a result of the excretion of high levels of calcium by the kidneys.

Phosphorus

Phosphorus is a mineral that makes up about 1% of a person's total body weight. It is present in every cell of the body, but it is found mostly in the bones and teeth, as with calcium. Phosphorus and calcium have an inverse relationship; an increase in one causes a decrease in the other. As blood calcium levels increase, a decrease in phosphorus levels is necessary, and vice versa. Most phosphorus is found combined with calcium in bones and teeth, but it also can be found in muscles and nerve tissue. Normal values range from 2.4 to 4.1 mEq/dL.

Along with calcium, phosphorus contributes to the support and maintenance of bones and teeth. It is a component of DNA and RNA, and it is an essential component of phospholipids, which are structural components of cell membranes. Phosphorous compounds are used as a buffer system to maintain the pH of the blood, and phosphorus promotes the

Box 18.6	**Hypocalcemia: Causes, Signs and Symptoms, and Nursing Interventions**

CAUSES

- Alkalosis
- Anticonvulsants, such as phenobarbital and phenytoin (Dilantin)
- Chronic renal failure
- Deficiency of parathyroid hormone or vitamin D
- Dietary deficiency of calcium and vitamin D
- Disease of small bowel; malabsorption
- Diuretics (Lasix, Edecrin)
- Draining intestinal fistulas
- Excess alcohol intake
- Excess binding of calcium ions
- Excessive nasogastric suctioning
- Increased magnesium
- Injury or disease of parathyroid gland
- Large amount of citrated blood
- Low serum albumin levels
- Pancreatic disease
- Severe burns
- Severe diarrhea
- Thyroid surgery (surgical removal of parathyroid glands, removal of parathyroid tumor)

SIGNS AND SYMPTOMS

- Anxiety, confusion, irritability
- Calcium deposits in body tissues
- Cardiac dysrhythmias, cardiac arrest
- Diarrhea[a]
- Diminished response to digitalis glycosides
- Hyperactive deep tendon reflexes
- Laryngeal spasms
- Muscle spasm of feet and hands[a]
- Nausea, vomiting[a]
- Osteoporosis, pathologic fractures
- Tetany (note positive Trousseau or Chvostek sign [see Fig. 18.4])
- Tingling sensation around nose, mouth, ears, fingers, and toes[a]
- Twitching

NURSING INTERVENTIONS

- Administer calcium and vitamin D as prescribed by the health care provider.[b]
- Encourage intake of a diet high in calcium-rich foods, vitamin D, and protein.
- For acute hypocalcemia, keep a tracheotomy tray and resuscitation bag at bedside in case of laryngeal spasms.
- Monitor electrocardiogram.
- Monitor I&O.
- Monitor pertinent laboratory values, including those of calcium, albumin, and magnesium.
- Monitor treatment of underlying causes.
- Monitor vital signs; especially monitor respiratory status, including rate, depth, and rhythm; be alert for stridor, dyspnea, or crowing (laryngeal spasms).

[a]Most common signs and symptoms.
[b]Acute hypocalcemia necessitates intravenous administration of either calcium gluconate or calcium chloride.
I&O, Intake and output.

Fig. 18.4 Tests for hypocalcemia. (A) The Chvostek sign is a contraction of facial muscles in response to a light tap over the facial nerve in front of the ear. (B) The Trousseau sign is a carpal spasm induced by inflation of a blood pressure cuff (C) above the systolic pressure for a few minutes.

Box 18.7	Hypercalcemia: Causes, Signs and Symptoms, and Nursing Interventions

CAUSES
- Movement of calcium from bone to circulation
- Immobilization
- Metastatic bone cancer
- Multiple myeloma
- Excess intake of supplemental calcium
- Excess intake of dietary calcium
- Excess intake of antacids containing calcium
- Increased absorption of calcium
- Increased levels of parathyroid hormone
- Increased levels of vitamin D

SIGNS AND SYMPTOMS
- Anorexia, nausea, vomiting
- Behavioral changes, including confusion
- Thirst, polyuria[a]
- Renal calculi
- Decreased deep tendon reflexes
- Constipation
- Paralytic ileus
- Lethargy, coma
- Cardiac dysrhythmias, cardiac arrest
- Hypertension
- Decreased muscle tone[a]
- Decreased GI motility
- Bone pain

NURSING INTERVENTIONS[b]
- Administer diuretics as ordered by the health care provider.
- Encourage patient to drink 3000–4000 L of fluids per day.
- Monitor I&O

[a]Most common signs and symptoms.
[b]In life-threatening hypercalcemia, measures to increase calcium secretion sometimes include hemodialysis or peritoneal dialysis.
GI, Gastrointestinal; *I&O,* intake and output.

effectiveness of many of the B vitamins. Phosphorus also assists in normal nerve and muscle activity and is needed in carbohydrate metabolism. Foods especially high in phosphorus include beef, pork, fish, poultry, milk products, and legumes. As with calcium, an adequate intake of vitamin D is necessary for absorption of phosphorus. The kidneys are responsible for approximately 90% of the excretion of phosphorus. The remainder is excreted in the feces.

Hypophosphatemia. Because a generous amount of phosphorus is present in many foods, a deficiency seldom occurs. However, *hypophosphatemia* is possible as a result of a dietary insufficiency, impaired kidney function, or maldistribution of phosphorus. Low phosphorus levels have been associated with muscle weakness, especially of the respiratory muscles; with bone and joint pain; and with disorientation and confusion. Treatment involves replacing the phosphorus with oral or IV supplementation and monitoring the patient.

Hyperphosphatemia. *Hyperphosphatemia,* also a rarity, occurs most commonly as a result of renal insufficiency, but can also occur with an increased intake of phosphate or vitamin D. Signs and symptoms include tetany, numbness and tingling sensation around the mouth, and muscle spasms. Restricting phosphorus intake and treating the underlying cause will bring phosphorus levels down. However, phosphate-binding gels such as aluminum hydroxide (Amphojel) and IV calcium supplementation may be needed.

Magnesium

Magnesium (Mg^{2+}) is the fourth most abundant mineral in the body and the second most abundant cation in the intracellular fluid. Only small amounts of magnesium are found in the blood, but it is important in maintaining normal body function. The majority (60%) of magnesium is found in the bone, with lesser amounts in the muscle and soft tissue; only 1% is in the extracellular fluid, mostly in the cerebrospinal fluid.

The importance of magnesium as an electrolyte was not recognized widely until recently. It is now recognized as a cofactor in the activation of many enzymes. It also promotes regulation of serum calcium, phosphate, and potassium levels and is essential for integrity of nerve tissue, skeletal muscle, and cardiac functioning. Magnesium also may enhance the effectiveness of treatment for asthma, depression, diabetes, hypertension, cardiac arrhythmias, migraine headaches, fibromyalgia, osteoporosis, and restless leg syndrome. Normal blood values are 1.5 to 2.5 mEq/L.

Magnesium is another electrolyte commonly distributed in foods. Whole grains, fruits, green vegetables, meat, fish, legumes, and dairy products are dietary sources. It is a good idea to take a multivitamin containing B-complex vitamins, along with magnesium-rich foods. The level of vitamin B_6 in the body determines how much magnesium is absorbed into the cells. The major route of magnesium excretion is through the kidneys, in which the amount of magnesium is correlated with the amount of potassium excreted. The kidneys do not conserve potassium, but they do conserve magnesium; therefore, if a magnesium deficiency develops, the body conserves magnesium at the expense of excreting potassium.

Hypomagnesemia. *Hypomagnesemia* develops when blood levels fall to less than 1.5 mEq/L. A decrease in magnesium also is associated with decreased potassium levels because the kidneys tend to conserve magnesium by excreting more potassium. Hypomagnesemia causes symptoms of increased neuromuscular irritability similar to those observed with hypocalcemia (Box 18.8): tremors, cramping, numbness, a tingling sensation in the hands and feet, disorientation, confusion, tetany, and seizures. The major causes of low magnesium levels are increased excretion by the kidneys, impaired absorption from the GI tract, and prolonged malnutrition. Oral or IV magnesium is given to treat hypomagnesemia.

Hypermagnesemia. *Hypermagnesemia* develops when magnesium blood levels exceed 2.5 mEq/L. It rarely occurs when kidney function is normal, but in the presence of impaired renal function, excess magnesium administration, and diabetic ketoacidosis with severe water loss, it may develop (Box 18.9). An excess of magnesium severely restricts nerve and muscle activity and causes respiratory depression, hypotension, and, potentially, cardiac arrest. Treatment involves decreasing the patient's intake of magnesium while supporting cardiac and respiratory function. Dialysis may be necessary to remove excess amounts from the blood.

Bicarbonate

Bicarbonate (HCO_3^-) is one of the main anions in the extracellular fluid. It is an alkaline electrolyte whose major function is the regulation of acid-base balance. Bicarbonate acts as a buffer to neutralize acids in the

---

| Box 18.8 | **Hypomagnesemia: Causes, Signs and Symptoms, and Nursing Interventions** |

CAUSES
- Alcoholism
- Conditions causing large losses of urine
- Decreased intake
- Diarrhea
- Draining intestinal fistulas
- Hypercalcemia
- Impaired absorption from GI tract
- Prolonged IV feedings without magnesium supplementation
- Prolonged malnutrition
- Starvation

SIGNS AND SYMPTOMS
- Agitation, depression, confusion
- Anorexia
- Ataxia
- Cardiac dysrhythmias
- Cramps, spasticity
- Dysphagia
- Hyperactive deep tendon reflexes
- Hypotension
- Mental changes[a]
- Nausea and vomiting
- Paresthesia[a]
- Seizures
- Tachycardia
- Tetany
- Tremors

NURSING INTERVENTIONS
- Administer magnesium supplements as prescribed by the health care provider.
- Assess dysphagia.
- Assess neuromuscular status.
- Increase patient's intake of magnesium-rich foods.
- Institute seizure precautions.
- Monitor electrocardiogram.
- Monitor I&O.
- Monitor respiratory status.
- Monitor vital signs.

[a]Most common signs and symptoms.
GI, Gastrointestinal; *I&O,* intake and output.

---

body and maintain the 20:1 ratio of bicarbonate to carbonic acid needed to keep the body in homeostasis (discussed in the next section). The normal bicarbonate level is 22 to 24 mEq/L. The kidneys selectively regulate the amount of bicarbonate retained or excreted based on need.

ACID-BASE BALANCE

Acid-base balance (also called *acid-alkaline balance*) refers to the homeostasis of the hydrogen ion (H^-) concentration in the body fluids. A solution with a high number of hydrogen ions is an acid, and a solution with a low number of hydrogen ions is an alkaline, or base. The hydrogen ion concentration is determined

| Box 18.9 | Hypermagnesemia: Causes, Signs and Symptoms, and Nursing Interventions |

CAUSES
- Diabetic ketoacidosis with severe water loss
- Renal failure

SIGNS AND SYMPTOMS
- Heat
- Hypotension[a]
- Loss of deep tendon reflexes
- Nausea and vomiting
- Respiratory depression
- Thirst
- Vasodilation[a]

PROLONGED OR SEVERE EXCESS
- Cardiac arrest
- Coma

NURSING INTERVENTIONS
- Administer diuretics as prescribed by the health care provider.
- Decrease patient's intake of foods or medications high in magnesium.
- Encourage frequent urination.
- Monitor I&O.

[a]Most common signs and symptoms.
I&O, Intake and output.

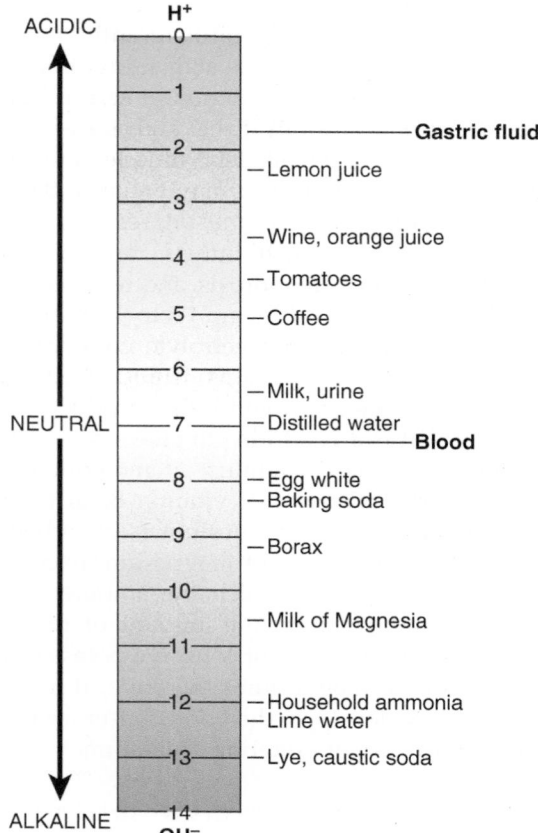

Fig. 18.5 The pH scale. A pH of 7 is considered neutral. Values toward the top (less than 7) are acidic (the lower the number, the more acidic). Values toward the bottom (greater than 7) are basic, or alkaline (the higher the number, the more basic). Representative fluids and their approximate pHs are listed at the side.

Fig. 18.6 Relationship between pH and the ratio of bicarbonate to carbonic acid. The normal plasma range is 7.35 to 7.45. A normal pH is maintained by a ratio of 1 part carbonic acid to 20 parts bicarbonate.

by the ratio of carbonic acid (H_2CO_3) to bicarbonate (HCO_3^-) in the extracellular fluid. The ratio needed for homeostasis is 1 part carbonic acid to 20 parts bicarbonate. The symbol used to indicate hydrogen ion balance is pH. A pH value is actually the hydrogen ion concentration in the body. A sample of arterial blood is used to determine the body's pH.

Arterial blood gas levels reveal whether the blood is acid, neutral, or alkaline. An inverse relationship exists between hydrogen ion concentration and the pH level; as the number of hydrogen ions increases, the acidity of the solution increases and the pH decreases. The opposite happens with alkalinity: the number of hydrogen ions decreases and the pH increases. A pH of less than 7.35 is acid. A pH of greater than 7.45 is alkaline. The normal pH of arterial blood is approximately 7.45, whereas the normal pH of venous blood and interstitial fluid is approximately 7.35. Between 7.35 and 7.45 is considered normal blood pH. A pH lower than 6.8 or higher than 7.8 is usually fatal (Fig. 18.5).

Two types of disturbances can cause a pH imbalance. One imbalance arises from an increase or decrease in the base substance bicarbonate. The other imbalance results from an increase or decrease in carbonic acid, the acid substance. The body's metabolism affects the base portion of balance, and so a bicarbonate imbalance causes metabolic acidosis or alkalosis. The body's respiratory system affects the acid side of the balance, and so a carbonic acid imbalance causes respiratory acidosis or alkalosis. Fig. 18.6 depicts the relationship between pH and the ratio of bicarbonate to carbonic acid.

The body has three systems that work to keep the pH in the narrow range of normal: the blood buffers, the respiratory system, and the kidneys. These systems are working constantly to maintain a normal pH.

BLOOD BUFFERS

Blood buffers (also called *physiologic buffers*) consist of either a weak acid and its base salt or a weak base and its acid salt. These buffers include the bicarbonate/carbonic acid buffering system, the intracellular protein buffers, and the phosphate buffers in the bone. Of these, the bicarbonate/carbonic acid system is the most important. It is responsible for buffering blood and interstitial fluid and decreasing the strength of potentially damaging acids and bases. Think of these blood buffers as chemical sponges. They circulate throughout the body in pairs, neutralizing excess acids or bases by contributing or accepting hydrogen ions. One buffer takes away a hydrogen ion if the fluid is too acid; the other adds a hydrogen ion if the solution is too alkaline. They work within a fraction of a second to prevent an excessive change in the hydrogen ion concentration. The kidneys assist the bicarbonate buffer system in regulating production of bicarbonate.

RESPIRATORY SYSTEM

Once the blood buffer systems are exhausted, the body calls on the second line of defense, the lungs, to help balance the hydrogen concentration in the body. By speeding up or slowing down respirations, the lungs have the capacity to increase or decrease the amount of carbon dioxide in the blood. Carbon dioxide is a potential acid. When it is dissolved in water, it becomes carbonic acid. Removing carbon dioxide from the blood lowers the carbonic acid level and raises the pH to make the environment more alkaline. When there is too much alkaline in the system, the respiratory system slows down and retains carbon dioxide, which results in a lower pH (acidosis). This buffering system takes 1 to 2 minutes to adjust the acid-base balance back to a normal range, whereas the blood buffers take only seconds to work. Even though the respiratory system is slower than the blood buffers, it is still just as efficient; the lungs can eliminate large amounts of acid (in the form of carbon dioxide) from the body and keep just enough carbon dioxide to maintain a normal pH level. If the pH drops suddenly, the respiratory system can return the pH to near normal within 1 minute. Chemoreceptors in the medulla of the brainstem provide the stimulus to increase respirations; however, as the hydrogen ion concentration approaches normal, the stimulus is lost and the blood buffers make the remaining adjustments needed to return the level to normal.

KIDNEYS

The third line of defense in regulating hydrogen ions is the kidneys. They regulate pH by excreting acids or bases as needed. In the state of acidosis, the kidneys excrete hydrogen in urine and retain bicarbonate. In the state of alkalosis, the kidneys excrete bicarbonate and retain hydrogen. Normal urine pH tends to be more acidic, not necessarily because the body is in a constant

Table 18.5	Acid-Base Imbalances and Compensatory Mechanisms
ACID-BASE IMBALANCE	**MODE OF COMPENSATION**
Respiratory acidosis	Kidneys retain increased amounts of HCO_3^- to increase pH
Respiratory alkalosis	Kidneys excrete increased amounts of HCO_3^- to lower pH
Metabolic acidosis	Lungs excrete CO_2 to raise pH
Metabolic alkalosis	Lungs retain CO_2 to lower pH

From Pagana K, Pagana T: *Mosby's diagnostic and laboratory test reference*, ed 11, St. Louis, 2013, Mosby.

state of acidosis and is attempting to compensate, but because the body produces excess acids in the metabolic processes and must eliminate them constantly in the urine.

The kidneys are the slowest of the systems to balance the hydrogen concentration in the body; it may take several hours or several days for the kidneys to compensate, but they are efficient enough to return the pH to exactly normal. The three systems work closely together to maintain a normal hydrogen ion concentration. The blood buffers are immediate and continuous in contributing or accepting hydrogen ions. The respiratory system has the capacity to come into play within minutes, regulating the carbon dioxide level in the blood and, thus, controlling carbonic acid. Although the kidneys work more slowly than the other two systems, they are still able to eliminate either hydrogen ions or bicarbonate ions, which means they can either increase or decrease pH.

TYPES OF ACID-BASE IMBALANCE

If the regulatory systems fail, one of four major acid-base imbalances may occur. An acid-base imbalance results in either acidosis (when blood pH is less than 7.35) or alkalosis (when blood pH is greater than 7.45). Because the lungs and the kidneys are the two major organs responsible for regulation of the acid and base substances in the body, acid-base imbalances probably are caused by an imbalance in the function of the lungs, the kidneys, or both. Many diseases create a potential for acid-base imbalances. Diseases and other conditions that predispose a patient to these imbalances include diabetes mellitus, chronic obstructive pulmonary disease, end-stage renal disease, severe vomiting, and diarrhea.

There are four primary types of acid-base imbalances: respiratory acidosis, respiratory alkalosis, metabolic acidosis, and metabolic alkalosis (Table 18.5).

RESPIRATORY ACIDOSIS

Any condition that impairs normal ventilation and prevents the respiratory system from eliminating the appropriate amount of carbon dioxide causes respiratory acidosis (Box 18.10). Carbon dioxide is retained,

Box 18.10	Respiratory Acidosis: Causes, Common Clinical Signs and Symptoms, and Laboratory Data

CAUSES
- Airway obstruction
- Atelectasis
- Barbiturate or sedative overdose
- Compromise in any of the three essential parts of breathing: ventilation, perfusion, or diffusion
- Chronic obstructive pulmonary disease (COPD)
- Cystic fibrosis
- Drowning
- Head injuries
- Obesity
- Paralysis of respiratory muscles (Guillain-Barré syndrome, poliomyelitis, myasthenia gravis)
- Pneumonia
- Respiratory failure
- Stroke (cardiovascular accident)
- Traumatic injuries to the thorax (flail chest)

COMMON CLINICAL SIGNS AND SYMPTOMS
Central Nervous System
- Coma
- Decreased deep tendon reflexes
- Decreasing level of consciousness
- Disorientation
- Dizziness
- Lethargy
- Occipital headache
- Seizures

Cardiopulmonary System
- Cardiac dysrhythmias
- Dyspnea
- Hypotension
- Tachycardia

Musculoskeletal System
- Tremors
- Weakness

LABORATORY DATA
- HCO_3^- normal in early respiratory acidosis
- K^+ <5 mEq/L
- O_2 saturation normal or <95%, depending on severity of acidosis
- $PaCO_2$ >45 mm Hg (unless the patient has COPD)
- PaO_2 normal or <80 mm Hg, depending on severity of acidosis
- pH <7.35

COPD, Chronic obstructive pulmonary disease; *$PaCO_2$,* partial pressure of arterial carbon dioxide; *PaO_2,* partial pressure of arterial oxygen.

and the level of carbonic acid in the blood increases. As pH falls and the normal 20:1 ratio of bicarbonate to carbonic acid is upset, the partial pressure of carbon dioxide (PCO_2) increases. The body then attempts to eliminate the excess carbon dioxide by increasing respirations. The activity of the central nervous system is also depressed, and the patient becomes lethargic and confused. The heart rate increases, and the patient also may experience palpitations and dizziness.

The kidneys attempt to compensate by retaining the base substance bicarbonate and eliminating hydrogen. However, because the renal system is a slow one, compensation may not occur for 24 hours or more.

Treatment for respiratory acidosis is aimed at improving ventilation. To do this, the underlying cause of the respiratory acidosis must be found and treated while support is given to the patient's respiratory efforts. Intermittent positive-pressure breathing (IPPB) or continuous positive airway pressure (CPAP) may be used to promote exhalation of carbon dioxide; antibiotics may be administered for any respiratory infection; adequate hydration (2 to 3 L/day) helps liquefy and aids in the removal of secretions; and bronchodilators may help reduce bronchial spasms. Intubation and mechanical ventilation may also be necessary.

RESPIRATORY ALKALOSIS

Respiratory alkalosis is caused most frequently by hyperventilation secondary to anxiety, pain, fear, and stress (Brinkman, 2020). Other causes include adult respiratory distress syndrome, congestive heart failure, head trauma, severe blood loss, or pneumonia (Box 18.11). Increased respiratory rate, depth, or both have the potential to cause the loss of excessive amounts of carbon dioxide, which results in a low carbonic acid level in the blood. The pH then increases because of the decrease in carbonic acid, and respiratory alkalosis results. The kidneys attempt to compensate by conserving hydrogen ions and excreting bicarbonate ions, but, as mentioned previously, the renal system is slow, and the compensation may not occur for 24 hours or more. Symptoms include lightheadedness, numbness and tingling sensation in extremities, tinnitus, blurred vision, increased heart rate, and irritability. In extreme cases, confusion, seizure activity, and loss of consciousness may occur.

Treatment for respiratory alkalosis involves treating the underlying cause. If the cause is anxiety, it helps to make the patient aware of the abnormal breathing pattern and instruct the patient to breathe slowly to retain and accumulate carbon dioxide in the body. Breathing into a paper bag may also help because the patient is inhaling some of their lost carbon dioxide. If these remedies fail, it may be necessary to sedate the patient.

METABOLIC ACIDOSIS

Metabolic acidosis occurs as a result of a gain of hydrogen ions or a loss of bicarbonate (Box 18.12). This then causes the pH of the blood to fall and acidosis to develop. Because metabolic acidosis is a problem involving the kidneys, the other compensatory system—the lungs—attempts to compensate by increasing the respiratory rate and eliminating more carbon dioxide. This results in hyperventilation. In the extracellular fluid, there is also an exchange of potassium and hydrogen. Potassium ions move out of the cell, and hydrogen ions move into the cell. This is a means to

Box 18.11	Respiratory Alkalosis: Causes, Common Clinical Signs and Symptoms, and Laboratory Data

CAUSES
- Anemia
- Asthma
- Disorders of the central nervous system (head injuries, infections)
- Drugs (aspirin overdose)
- Hypermetabolic states
- Hyperventilation (caused by hypoxia, pulmonary emboli, anxiety, fear, pain, exercise, fever)
- Inappropriate mechanical ventilator settings
- Pneumonia

COMMON CLINICAL SIGNS AND SYMPTOMS
Central Nervous System
- Anxious appearance
- Confusion
- Dizziness
- Fainting
- Irritability
- Seizures
- Tingling sensation in the extremities

Cardiopulmonary System
- Cardiac dysrhythmias
- Tachypnea

Musculoskeletal System
- Muscle weakness
- Tetany

LABORATORY DATA
- HCO_3^- levels may be normal but are more likely to be below 21 as the $PaCO_2$ levels fall.
- K^+ <3.5 mEq/L
- O_2 saturation normal
- $PaCO_2$ <35 mm Hg
- PaO_2 normal
- pH ≥7.45

PaCO₂, Partial pressure of arterial carbon dioxide; *PaO₂*, partial pressure of arterial oxygen.

Box 18.12	Metabolic Acidosis: Causes, Common Clinical Signs and Symptoms, and Laboratory Data

CAUSES
- Dehydration
- Diabetic ketoacidosis
- Drugs (methanol, ethanol, formic acid, paraldehyde, aspirin)
- Lactic acidosis
- Renal failure
- Renal tubular acidosis
- Severe diarrhea
- Shock
- Starvation

COMMON CLINICAL SIGNS AND SYMPTOMS
Central Nervous System
- Coma
- Decreasing level of consciousness
- Headache
- Lethargy

Cardiopulmonary System
- Dysrhythmias
- Kussmaul respirations (deep, rapid respirations)
- Warm, flushed skin

Gastrointestinal System
- Abdominal pain
- Anorexia
- Diarrhea
- Nausea
- Vomiting

Musculoskeletal System
- Weakness

LABORATORY DATA
- HCO_3^- <22 mEq/L
- K^+ >5 mEq/L
- O_2 saturation normal
- $PaCO_2$ normal or <35 mm Hg if lungs are compensating
- PaO_2 normal or <80 mm Hg if lungs are compensating
- pH <7.35

PaCO₂, Partial pressure of arterial carbon dioxide; *PaO₂*, partial pressure of arterial oxygen.

reduce the concentration of hydrogen in the extracellular fluid and to compensate for the acidosis that has developed. Causes of metabolic acidosis include diabetic ketoacidosis from ketone accumulation, increased levels of lactic acid (as seen in shock), starvation, severe diarrhea (dehydration), and renal failure.

Symptoms of metabolic acidosis may vary, depending on the underlying cause and severity. Common symptoms include a change in the patient's level of consciousness, headache, vomiting, diarrhea, anorexia, and cardiac dysrhythmias. Administration of sodium bicarbonate is the usual treatment for acidosis, but the underlying cause must be treated, as well. Mechanical ventilation may be necessary if the metabolic acidosis is severe and the patient is comatose.

METABOLIC ALKALOSIS

Metabolic alkalosis results when a significant amount of acid is lost from the body or if the

bicarbonate level increases (Box 18.13). The most common causes of metabolic alkalosis are vomiting gastric content (normally high in acid) and prolonged gastric suction. Metabolic alkalosis is also possible in patients who ingest excessive amounts of alkaline agents, such as bicarbonate-containing antacids. Metabolic alkalosis often develops in the presence of renal failure, as well. In this situation, the renal system is not able to correct the imbalance, and compensation is left to the respiratory system. The respiratory system responds by causing hypoventilation. Metabolic alkalosis depresses the central nervous system, which results in headaches, irritability, lethargy, changes in level of consciousness, and confusion. Changes in heart rate; slow, shallow respirations; nausea and vomiting; and numbness in the

Box 18.13	Metabolic Alkalosis: Causes, Common Clinical Signs and Symptoms, and Laboratory Data

CAUSES
- Cushing disease
- Drugs (steroids, sodium bicarbonate, diuretics); overdose of baking soda, excessive use of antacids such as Mylanta
- Electrolyte disturbance
- Excessive vomiting
- Hyperaldosteronism
- Prolonged gastric suctioning

COMMON CLINICAL SIGNS AND SYMPTOMS
Central Nervous System
- Decreases in level of consciousness
- Headache
- Irritability
- Lethargy
- Seizures

Cardiopulmonary System
- Atrial tachycardia
- Cardiac dysrhythmias (related to hypokalemia)
- Slow, shallow respirations with periods of apnea

Gastrointestinal System
- Anorexia
- Nausea
- Vomiting

Musculoskeletal System
- Hypertonicity of muscles, muscle cramps
- Numbness and tingling sensation in extremities
- Tetany
- Tremors

LABORATORY DATA
- HCO_3^- >26 mEq/L
- K^+ <3.5 mEq/L
- O_2 saturation normal
- $PaCO_2$ normal or >45 mm Hg if lungs are compensating
- PaO_2 normal
- pH >7.45

PaCO₂, Partial pressure of arterial carbon dioxide; *PaO₂,* partial pressure of arterial oxygen.

extremities may also be present. As with the other acid-base imbalances, treatment is aimed at treating the underlying cause.

INTRAVENOUS THERAPY

The body's fluid and electrolyte balance must be maintained to keep all body systems healthy and functioning properly. When there is an imbalance either in fluid intake and output or in electrolyte concentration, complications can arise. To help prevent these complications, the health care provider may order **intravenous (IV)** therapy (infusion of medication or other liquid therapeutic agents directly into the venous system).

IV therapy may be ordered for many reasons. It may be needed to maintain fluid volume if a patient is not taking in fluid or nutrients orally, or it can be used as a replacement for fluid lost through prolonged nausea or vomiting. It also can be used to give medications, blood, or blood products, and to provide the patient with nutritional support. The IV route provides faster absorption and more rapid distribution of medications, solutions, or nutrients and can be used for either long-term or short-term applications.

Each state's nurse practice act determines the legal guidelines for IV administration, and facility policy further defines the licensed practical nurse/licensed vocational nurse's (LPN/LVN's) role in the administration of IV medications, fluids, blood, or blood products. Only specially trained nurses who meet the legal qualifications and facility guidelines should be involved in IV administration (see the Coordinated Care box on IV therapy).

Coordinated Care
Collaboration

Intravenous Therapy

- The skills of basic IV needle insertion, adjusting IV flow rate, administering IV medications, and maintaining an IV site require the knowledge of a nurse. Many states include this skill in the scope of practice for LPNs/LVNs. Delegation of these tasks to unlicensed assistive personnel (UAP) is inappropriate.
- It is acceptable for UAP to inform the nurse when a fluid container is almost empty, when the patient complains of any discomfort at the IV site, and when an electronic controlling device sounds an alarm.
- In the clinical setting, the registered nurse (RN) is responsible for supervising infusion therapy and may delegate the task of IV insertion, adjusting IV flow rate, administering IV medications, and maintaining an IV site to the LPN/LVN if those tasks are within the LPN/LVN's scope of practice for that state.

The insertion of an IV catheter involves several steps (Skill 18.2 and Figs. 18.7 and 18.8). Before inserting an IV needle, always check the health care provider's order. It should indicate the solution type, as well as any medication that may have to be added to the solution, the volume to be infused, the rate of infusion, and the duration of infusion. Next, assemble and ready the equipment. Over-the-needle catheters are the most commonly used IV catheters today. They have a metal needle extending past the tip of a soft catheter. After the venipuncture, withdraw the needle and leave just the soft catheter in place (Box 18.14 and see Skill 18.2). Select a venipuncture needle and catheter according to the solution to be infused and the size and condition of the patient's veins. Choose a catheter that is smaller than the vein but large enough for the solution to flow through without clogging it. A 20-, 21-, or 22-gauge catheter is acceptable for an adult patient who is receiving only fluids or medications (or both). If administering blood, use a catheter with a larger

Skill 18.2   Initiating Intravenous Therapy

CHECK GATHER HELLO ID PRIVACY EXPLAIN WASH GLOVES

NURSING ACTION (RATIONALE)

1. Refer to Standard Steps 1–9.
2. Assemble equipment:
   - Clean gloves
   - Intravenous infusion tray or kit containing tourniquet, alcohol swab, povidone-iodine (Betadine) or chlorhexidine (follow facility policy regarding cleaning agent), angiocatheter, tubing, adhesive tape, and sterile dressing
   - Solution to be infused
3. Identify appropriate venipuncture (access of a vein with a needle for the purpose of starting an IV or withdrawing a blood sample) sites (see Fig. 18.7). (*Choosing an appropriate venipuncture site allows for patient movement and comfort. LPN/LVNs may start an IV infusion in only certain areas of the arm in some states; make sure the chosen site is in an allowable site.*)
4. Apply tourniquet, which should be tight enough to impede venous return but not occlude arterial flow (see Fig. 18.8A). (*Facilitates observation and puncture of vein.*)
5. Select venipuncture site (see Fig. 18.8A).
   a. Use the most distal site in the nondominant arm or on the nonoperative side, if possible.
   b. Avoid areas that are painful on palpation, bruised, swollen, or traumatized.
   c. In the nondominant arm, select a vein large enough for catheter placement.
   d. Choose a site that will not interfere with planned procedures or the patient's activities of daily living (ADLs).
   (1) Palpate the vein by pressing downward and noting the resistant, soft, bouncy feeling as pressure is released. (*Softness and bounciness of the vein indicate that the vein is healthy.*)
   (2) Instruct the patient to open and close the fist several times, lower the patient's arm, and rub or stroke the patient's arm. (*Promote venous distention.*)
   (3) Avoid sites distal to previous venipuncture sites, hardened cordlike veins, infiltrated sites or phlebitic vessels, and bruised areas. (*In such sites, infiltration tends to occur with new IV lines, and excessive vessel damage may result.*)

(4) Avoid vessels in an extremity with compromised circulation, as in cases of mastectomy, dialysis graft, or paralysis. (*Venous alterations increase risk of complications such as infiltration.*)
6. Release tourniquet. (*Never leave tourniquet on for longer than 1 minute to decrease the risk for vein damage.*)
7. Cleanse site with alcohol swab or other cleaning agent, using friction (see Fig. 18.8B). Cleanse in clean-to-dirty direction, starting at selected insertion site and working outward, creating concentric circles. Use alcohol first and then chlorhexidine or povidone-iodine. Allow to dry. (*Removes microorganisms from puncture site. Make sure to follow facility policy regarding cleaning agent.*)
8. Stretch skin taut and stabilize vein with nondominant hand (see Fig. 18.8C). (*Prevents vein from moving during procedure.*)
9. Insert the catheter:
   a. Using an over-the-needle catheter with safety device:
   (1) Hold the over-the-needle catheter with bevel up between index finger and thumb, and pierce skin above and slightly to side of vein at 30-degree angle (indirect method). (*Allows needle to enter smoothly through skin and approach vein wall.*)

(2) Lower angle to 10 degrees and enter vein wall. Slight resistance and "pop" sensation accompany entry into vein. (*Reduces risk of going completely through vein and enhances placement within vein.*)

Continued

Skill 18.2   Initiating Intravenous Therapy—cont'd

(3) Once the "pop" is felt, watch for blood return in flashback chamber. *(Confirms placement within vein.)*

(4) Advance catheter and stylet 3½ inches into vein, and then loosen stylet. Advance catheter over the needle into vein until hub rests at venipuncture site. Do not reinsert the stylet once it is loosened. *(Advancing the catheter and stylet ensures catheter is completely through vessel wall and into vein lumen. Threading catheter to hub reduces the risk of introducing infectious organisms along the catheter length. Reinserting the stylet has potential to cause damage to the catheter and formation of a catheter embolus.)*

(5) Release tourniquet. (Decreases potential for vein rupture and allows for venous flow.)

(6) Stabilize the catheter. Apply gentle but firm pressure with the index finger of nondominant hand 1¼ inches (3 cm) above insertion site and retract stylet from over-the-needle catheter. Do not recap the stylet. For safety, slide the catheter off the stylet while gliding the protective guard over the stylet. A click indicates that the device is locked. *(Stabilizing the catheter prevents accidental withdrawal or dislodgment. Applying gentle pressure above the insertion site decreases the flow of blood and prevents blood loss through open catheter hub. Immediately covering stylet with protective guard prevents accidental needle sticks.)*

Skill 18.2   Initiating Intravenous Therapy—cont'd

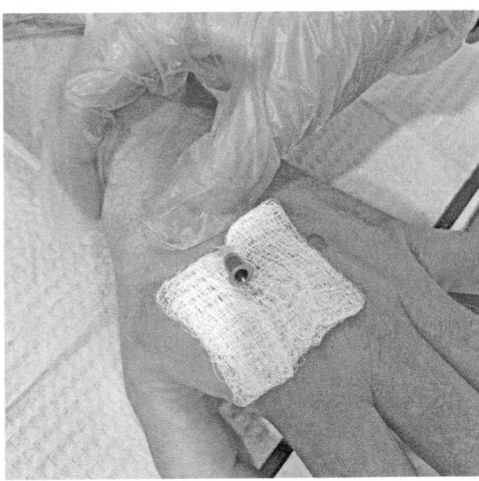

10. Attach sterile end of primed tubing to catheter hub. *(Helps prevent backflow, connects fluid source to venous access, and maintains sterility of system.)*

11. Stabilizing insertion site, slowly open roller or slide clamp to begin intravenous infusion of solution. *(Keeps catheter in place, initiates infusion, and helps prevent clotting of blood in catheter.)*

12. Secure catheter, in accordance with facility policy (see illustration). Stabilize the IV as directed by facility policy. Apply dressing recommended by facility policy. *(Prevents infection. Transparent dressings allow easier evaluation of insertion site, but facility policy should be followed.)*

13. Label site and tubing according to facility policy. *(Serves as reminder to change site and tubing at appropriate intervals.)*

14. Adjust solution flow rate according to accurate rate calculations or IV pump rate according to health care provider orders (see Chapter 17). *(Ensures patient receives appropriate amount of solution in the prescribed amount of time.)*

15. Refer to Standard Steps 10–17.

16. Document the following on appropriate facility form:
    - Date and time of insertion
    - Type of fluid
    - Insertion site
    - Size and type of catheter or needle
    - Number of attempts made
    - Flow rate
    - Patient's response
    - Patient teaching (see the Patient Teaching box and Lifespan Considerations for older adults box on intravenous therapy)

17. Immediately report to health care provider any adverse conditions or reactions, such as pulmonary congestion, shock, or thrombophlebitis.

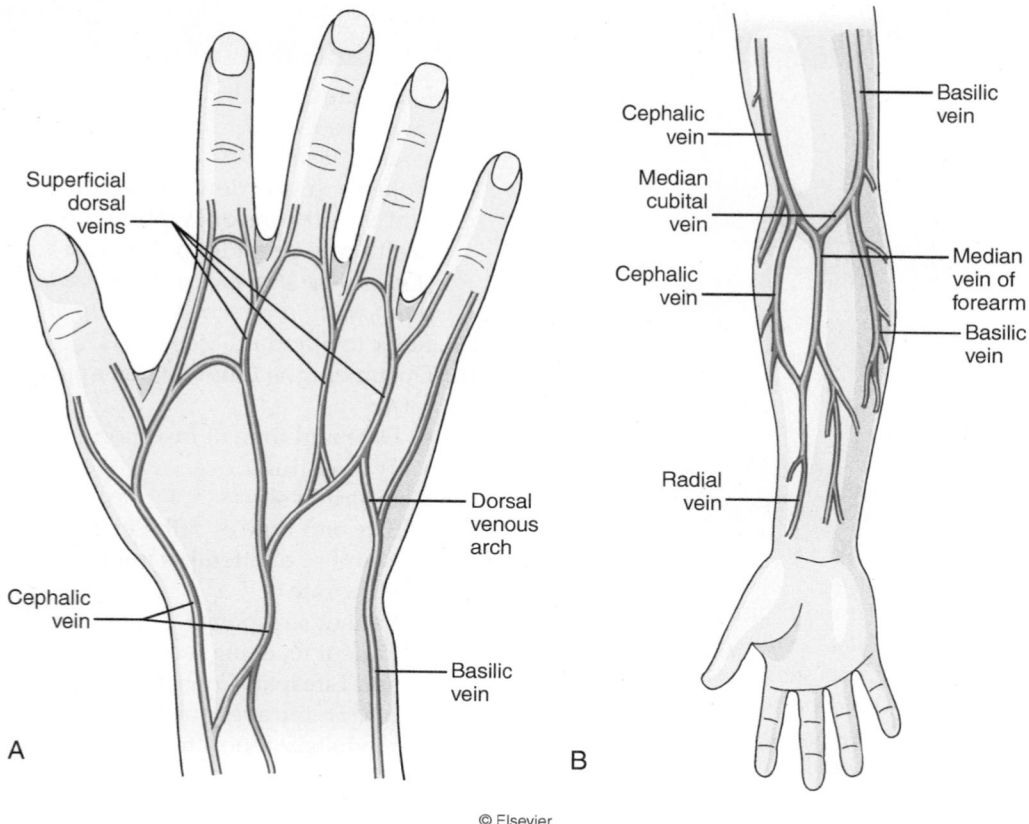

Fig. 18.7 Common intravenous sites. (A) Dorsal surface of the hand. (B) Inner arm.

Fig. 18.8 (A) Applying tourniquet and selecting site. (B) Cleansing skin for venipuncture. (C) Pulling skin taut as catheter is inserted.

| Box 18.14 | Special Considerations for Patients Receiving Intravenous Therapy |

- Very young children and older adult patients have fragile veins; avoid using sites that are easily moved or bumped.
- Venipuncture is problematic in obese patients because of difficulty in locating superficial veins.
- Avoid using any extremity with circulatory or neurologic impairment, or the dominant extremity, whenever possible.
- When the need to administer blood or blood components is anticipated or the IV is in a patient preoperatively, use a large-gauge (16- or 18-gauge) catheter that will accommodate faster infusions or thicker solutions.
- Critically ill patients at all stages of life require more frequent monitoring to check for complications related to IV therapy.
- When solution has less than 100 mL remaining, have a new bag of solution at patient's bedside so that it is readily available for changing. This reduces the risk of air entering the tubing and the patient's vein.
- In patients with fragile or engorged veins, avoid the use of tourniquets. In such patients, tourniquets increase the chance of excessive vein wall damage and hematoma formation. Consider using instead a blood pressure cuff to exert even, gentle pressure on the vessel.

- Encourage the patient to ask questions, and provide honest, forthright answers in a calm, reassuring manner.
- After all preparation is complete and immediately before you puncture the skin, inform the patient that there will be a stick. Keep reminding the patient to take slow, deep breaths to help the patient calm down. Distract the patient by talking about other subjects if necessary.
- Use a direct approach for large, easily seen veins. In the direct approach to IV insertion, the skin and the vein wall are punctured simultaneously with the catheter.
- Use an indirect approach for small, fragile, or deeper veins. In the indirect method, the skin is punctured with the IV catheter, the vein is relocated, and then the vein wall is punctured.
- If venipuncture is unsuccessful, always obtain a new catheter before you attempt a second venipuncture. Never reinsert the stylet into the catheter during insertion. This may damage the catheter and cause formation of a catheter embolism.
- If you attempt to start an IV infusion two times without success, call another nurse for assistance. The patient's anxiety level increases with multiple attempts, and this makes it more difficult to access the vein. Some facilities may have different policies regarding this. Know facility policy.

lumen (18- or 22-gauge). Many patients who require IV hydration have such low blood volume that only the smaller gauge IV catheters suffice for venipuncture.

Next, select tubing based on the patient's needs and the type of infusion to be initiated. Remove the tubing from the sterile packaging and inspect it for kinks. Ensure that the roller or slide clamp is functional and closed (Fig. 18.9A). Remove the correct solution from the sterile packaging and inspect it for expiration date, leaks, or contamination, then invert it to allow easy access to the tubing insertion port. Remove the insertion port cover (see Fig. 18.9B), remove the cover from the tubing spike, and insert the spike into the port until the plastic diaphragm covering the port is pierced (see Fig. 18.9C). Both the puncture area of the port and the tubing spike are sterile and should not be touched. Hold the fluid bag upright and gently squeeze the tubing drip chamber to fill it partially (one-third to one-half) with fluid. Open the roller or slide clamp slowly to enable the flow of the solution down the tubing. This priming prevents air from being forced through the tubing into the patient's circulatory system, which would create an air embolus and may cause death. As the fluid fills the tubing, invert injection ports to fill them with fluid, as well.

After preparing the equipment, enter the patient's room and explain the procedure to them. Allow time for the patient to ask questions and to clarify any misunderstandings. Next, evaluate the patient's veins. Select a vein in the nondominant arm, if possible. Starting low and working up the arm, look and feel for a soft, bouncy vein large enough to accommodate

the solution or medication ordered. Using alcohol, povidone-iodine, chlorhexidine, or a solution preferred by the facility, cleanse the intended puncture site. Once the site is cleaned, perform the venipuncture and secure the catheter. Begin the infusion at the prescribed infusion rate and watch the site for redness or swelling (see Skill 18.2). Because venipuncture is an invasive procedure and the pierced skin is no longer a barrier to microorganisms, follow strict aseptic technique when performing this procedure.

When the venipuncture is complete and the infusion is running, instruct the patient on limitations related to the IV infusion and the patient's responsibilities regarding the infusion (see the Patient Teaching and Lifespan Considerations for older adults boxes on IV therapy). Answer any questions that the patient may have.

CENTRAL VENOUS ACCESS DEVICES

When IV therapy is needed over a long term (several weeks or months), a central venous access device (CVAD) is inserted by the physician or advanced practice nurse. CVADs were developed to address the difficulties caused by repeated access to the venous system. CVADs provide safer access to the venous system and avoid the dangers of multiple venipunctures, such as vein sclerosis (hardening), bruising, infection, and pain. They are used primarily to administer various fluids, including chemotherapy and parenteral nutrition; to obtain blood samples on patients requiring daily laboratory tests; and for hemodialysis.

Patient Teaching

Intravenous Therapy

INTRAVENOUS THERAPY

- If intravenous (IV) apparatus is positional, instruct patient on how to position arm properly to maintain flow.
- Instruct patient to wear clothes with wide sleeves.
- Instruct patient about signs and symptoms of infiltration, phlebitis, and inflammation, such as redness, swelling, or discomfort at site.
- Instruct patient to inform the nurse if flow slows or stops, if blood is seen in the tubing, or if the site becomes red, swollen, tender, or warm.
- Instruct patient on how to ambulate with IV pole or stand.
- Instruct patient not to silence any IV pump alarms.

- Teach patient that to wash, the IV site should be securely wrapped to keep the water from the site and loosening the dressing. This can be accomplished by wrapping the IV site with a commercial product made to keep the site waterproof, or by wrapping the arm/site with plastic wrap and securing both ends with tape. After the shower, the plastic overwrap is removed and the dressing is assessed to ensure it is still in place and doesn't need changed. If the patient is taking a tub bath, the site should be wrapped as noted above and the site should not be permitted to be in the water.
- Teach the importance of not changing the flow rate, not lying on the tubing, and not allowing the tubing to kink.

 Lifespan Considerations

Older Adults

Intravenous Therapy

- Changes in cardiac and renal function related to the aging process or chronic conditions create the need for extreme accuracy in flow control and, thus, necessitate the use of electronic infusion devices (see Chapter 17).
- Fragility of veins in older adult patients increases the risk of infiltration. Monitor infusion site carefully and frequently, typically hourly.
- Fragile skin necessitates the use of nonporous tapes and skin protectant solutions.
- Older adults are more prone to fluid imbalances, and all infusions must be monitored carefully to prevent fluid volume overload.
- Visual and hearing deficits pose challenges to patient education. Face the patient and speak clearly and calmly.
- Short-term memory loss, depression, and confusion sometimes lead patients to remove the IV catheter or to change their attitude or decisions about care. An adult patient who is competent and is taught properly about the benefits and risks of IV therapy has the right to refuse it. Decisions made by competent patients to refuse treatment must be honored as legally binding.
- Because of fragility of veins, use extra care in injecting medication boluses.
- If the patient is not able to tolerate the infusion of whole blood or red blood cells in 4 hours, it may be necessary for the blood bank to split the unit into two bags. Make

sure to refrigerate the second bag during the infusion of the first.
- In older adults, use the smallest gauge catheter or needle possible (e.g., 24- to 26-gauge) for hydration fluids. This is less traumatizing to the vein and allows better blood flow to provide increased hemodilution of the IV fluids or medications. If the patient is receiving whole blood or red blood, verify the policy in regard to the size of catheter to use. Typically, a 20 gauge is the minimum size that is required for blood products.
- Avoid the back of an older adult's hand or the dominant arm for venipuncture because the resulting pain or disability at these sites greatly interferes with the patient's independence.
- If an older adult has fragile skin and veins, a tourniquet may cause rupture of veins, bruising, or both. The nurse can choose to perform the venipuncture without the use of a tourniquet or use a blood pressure cuff to provide enough pressure for vein dilation.
- When an older adult has lost subcutaneous tissue, the veins lose stability and may roll away from the needle. To stabilize the vein, apply traction to the skin below the projected insertion site.
- Using an angle of 5–15 degrees on insertion is helpful because an older adult's veins are more superficial.
- In an older person with fragile skin, prevent skin tears by minimizing the amount of tape used.

Various catheters and ports are used for patients requiring long-term IV therapy; therefore, nurses must be familiar with these devices. The three categories of CVADs currently used are tunneled central venous catheters (CVCs), percutaneous CVCs, and implanted infusion ports. Common brand names for the various catheters used include Hickman, Groshong, Raaf, and Port-a-Cath. Percutaneous CVC insertion can be performed at the patient's bedside, whereas tunneled CVCs are inserted in the operating room with the use of local or general anesthetic. Both are inserted into a large vein;

the percutaneous CVC is inserted through the cephalic or basilic veins in the arm and then advanced into the superior vena cava, and the tunneled CVC is tunneled through the subcutaneous tissue into the subclavian vein and into the superior vena cava (Fig. 18.10). The advantage of both types of CVC is that they produce less chance of irritation, inflammation, and vessel sclerosis.

Depending on the type of catheter, the device may have single, double, or triple lumens and is left in place as long as needed according to the manufacturer's guidelines (Fig. 18.11).

Fig. 18.9 (A) Closing valve. (B) Removing insertion port cover. (C) Inserting spike.

Implanted infusion ports are CVCs that are implanted surgically, with the use of local anesthetic, into the subcutaneous tissue in the area of the intraclavicular fossa. The catheter is inserted into a large vessel, as are the other CVCs, and threaded into the superior vena cava (Fig. 18.12). The body of the port is then left in the subcutaneous tissue for easy access (see Fig. 18.12B and C). The port placement is possible to palpate and is accessed with either a 90-degree angle or straight Huber needle directly through the skin (see Fig. 18.12A); to keep the port viable, it is necessary to heparinize the port every 4 weeks. The two most common complications of implanted CVCs are infection and occlusion of the catheter cannula. These complications are usually preventable by appropriate dressing changes and heparinization of the ports. It is necessary to teach patients how to care for their devices in the home setting so that they can start and discontinue infusions, heparinize their devices, and perform dressing changes appropriately.

PERIPHERALLY INSERTED CENTRAL CATHETERS

Peripherally inserted central catheters (PICCs) are an alternative to CVCs for patients requiring IV access beyond the length of time that peripheral (distal from the heart) IV lines can be maintained, usually between 7 days and 3 months. PICCs are inserted by specially trained RNs (if permitted by the state's nurse practice act) or by the health care provider. They are inserted into the cephalic or basilic vein in the upper arm and threaded into the subclavian vein. The PICC may be left in place for extended periods, as long as there are no problems with the device and complications do not occur.

PICCs pose less risk of pneumothorax, hemothorax, and air embolisms than do CVCs, are less expensive to maintain than are CVCs, and pose less risk of phlebitis and infiltration than do peripheral lines. Problems associated with PICCs include clotting, leaking from the catheter, migration of the catheter, infection, and catheter breakage.

PICCs come with single or double lumens, ranging in diameter from 16- to 24-gauge and in length from 40 to 65 cm (16 to 26 inches).

INTRAVENOUS MONITORING

To keep the IV site intact and infusing without problems, the site must be monitored frequently. Each facility specifies how often IV sites should be monitored; it may be hourly, every 2 hours, or even every 4 hours.

When monitoring an IV site, establish a routine of visualizing the entire situation, beginning at the solution container and ending at the site. Check the flow rate against the health care provider's order. Check tubing for kinks or obstructions and check the position of the patient's hand or arm. If the extremity is flexed, the vein may become occluded; remind patients to keep extremities extended. Inspect and palpate the site for edema, erythema, induration (hardness), heat, and discomfort. A burning sensation often means that the solution is irritating the vein; the infusion rate should be slowed (per provider orders), and monitoring should continue. Compare the hand or arm with the opposite hand or arm if the site seems edematous. Edema often indicates that infiltration has occurred.

If the patient is dehydrated, in shock, or critically ill, a slow infusion rate does not provide the

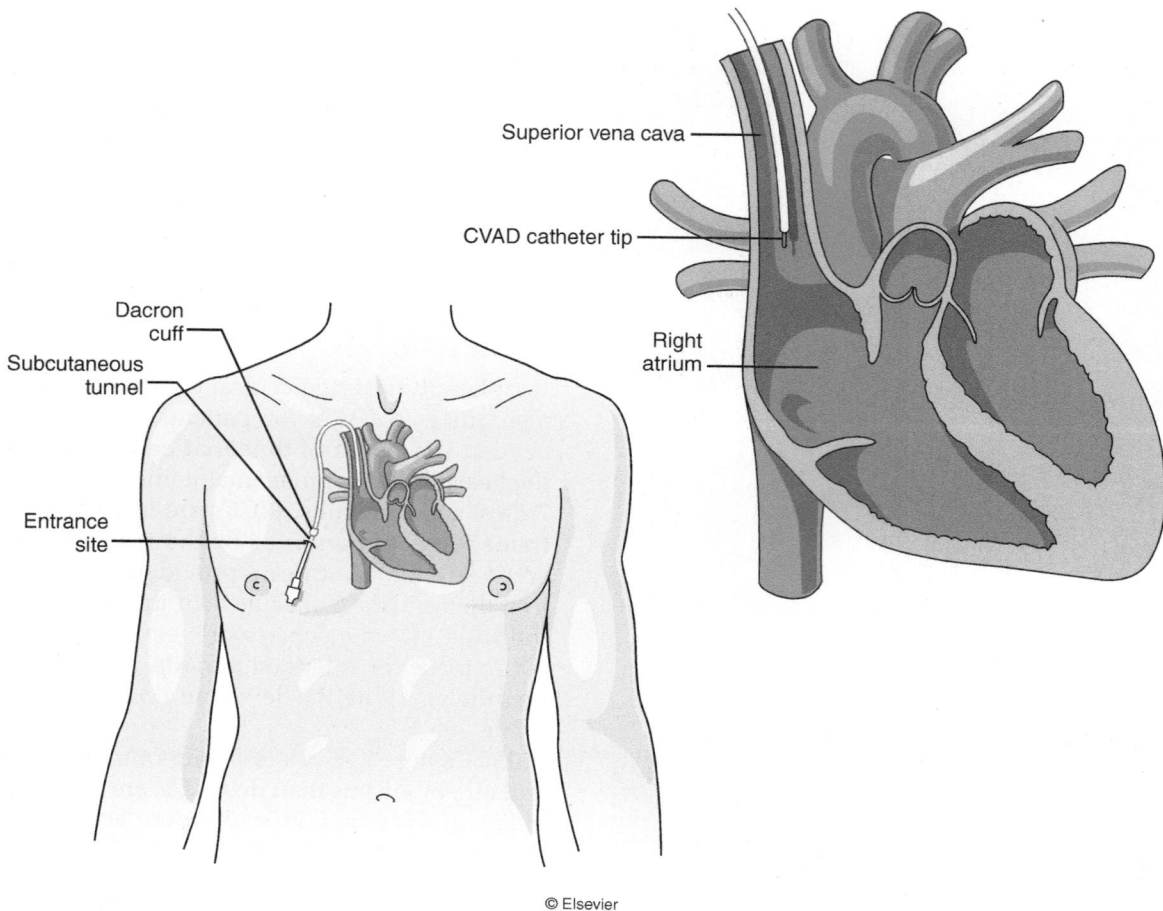

Fig. 18.10 Small-gauge tunneled catheter in its place, threaded into superior vena cava. *CVAD,* Central venous access device.

Fig. 18.11 (A) Triple-lumen central venous access device. (B) Triple-lumen central venous access device (CVAD) placed in jugular vein.

cardiovascular system with enough fluid. In contrast, an infusion rate that is too rapid may place too much fluid into the circulation and overload the cardiovascular and respiratory systems. Fluid volume overload can be fatal in certain patients. To prevent overload, monitor for symptoms such as dyspnea; a decreased oxygen saturation; a rapid, weak pulse; cough; disorientation; increased blood pressure; crackles; pitting

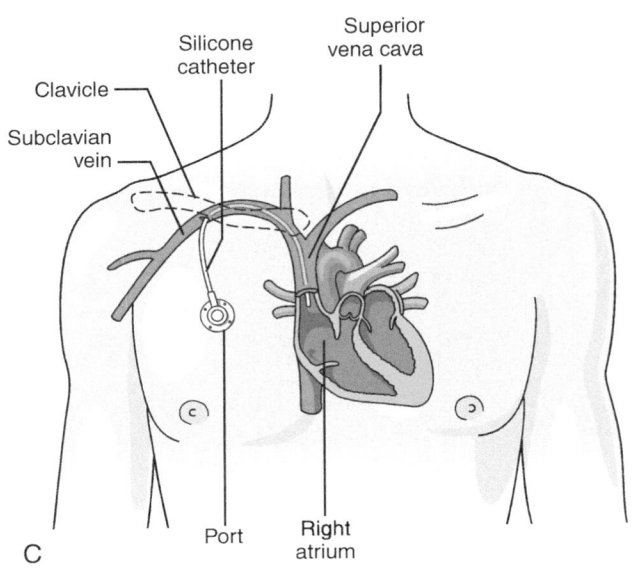

© Elsevier

Fig. 18.12 Implantation of infusion ports. (A) Infusion set with Huber needle. (B) Cross-section illustration of implantable port (C) Implanted port and catheter.

edema; and weight gain. The patient may request to "sit up" or indicate they "can't get their breath" when experiencing fluid overload. If fluid volume overload is suspected, slow the infusion rate immediately and notify the charge nurse or health care provider. Check the volume infused by comparing the bag contents with the pump readout to ensure pump accuracy.

INFILTRATION

Infiltration is the seepage of a nonirritating solution or medication into tissue surrounding the vessel. It is one of the most common complications of IV therapy and is caused by dislodgment of the IV cannula from the vein (going through vein, pulling out of vein), by phlebitis, or by excessive movement of the cannula in the vein.

If edema is detected at the insertion site, loosen the tape over the site and observe the site for a short time. Edema that does not subside generally indicates that the catheter is out of the vein and infiltration has occurred. Discomfort, burning sensation, blanching, or coolness around the site are other possible indications of infiltration. The coolness is noted because the fluid infusing will be at room temperature and the body temperature is much warmer. The room temperature fluid in the tissue will feel cool to the touch. The drip rate on gravity-flow IV lines also may decrease when an infiltration occurs. If fluid seeps into the tissue and infiltration is confirmed, discontinue the infusion and access another site to continue therapy, preferably in the opposite extremity. Monitor the site of the infiltration; fluid usually reabsorbs within 24 hours. Document the degree of infiltration (Table 18.6) and perform nursing interventions. Follow agency policy regarding care of infiltration.

PHLEBITIS

Phlebitis is an inflammation of the vein. It results from mechanical, chemical, or bacterial irritation of the vessel. The needle moving inside the vein, the low pH (acidity) of some IV solutions, highly concentrated additives, or bacteria can all cause phlebitis. Phlebitis can

Table 18.6	Infiltration Scale
GRADE	**CLINICAL CRITERIA**
0	No symptoms
1	Skin blanching Edema less than 1 inch in any direction Coolness to touch Presence or absence of pain
2	Skin blanching Edema 1–6 inches in any direction Coolness to touch Presence or absence of pain
3	Skin blanching, translucence Gross edema greater than 6 inches in any direction Coolness to touch Mild to moderate pain Possible numbness
4	Skin blanching, translucence Gross edema greater than 6 inches in any direction Deep pitting tissue edema Circulatory impairment Moderate to severe pain Infiltration of any amount of blood product, irritant, or vesicant

From Infusion Nurses Society: Infusion nursing standards of practice, *J Intraven Nurs* 34(1S):S65, 2011.

Table 18.7	Phlebitis Scale
GRADE	**CLINICAL CRITERIA**
1	Erythema at access site with or without pain
2	Pain at access site with erythema and/or edema
3	Pain at access site with erythema and/or edema Palpable venous cord
4	Pain at access site with erythema and/or edema Streak formation Palpable venous cord greater than 1 cm in length Purulent drainage

cause increased capillary permeability, which causes fluid to leak out of the vein and into the surrounding tissues. Erythema, warmth, edema, and discomfort are classic signs of phlebitis. The National Institute of Health recommends the use of a standard scale for measuring the degree of phlebitis (Urbanetto, 2016) (Table 18.7).

Prevention is the best treatment of phlebitis. To help prevent vein irritation and trauma, it is important to use large veins for hypertonic solutions, to use the smallest gauge cannula possible for the solution, to rotate IV sites every 72 hours, and to use CVCs or PICCs for long-term therapy. Some other ways to help prevent phlebitis include using aseptic technique in inserting the IV line or changing the dressing; making sure the IV catheter is secured appropriately so that it does not move; changing the IV solution, tubing, and dressings as appropriate; and decreasing the irritation of medications/solutions by diluting them or slowing the rate. Using in-line filters to remove air, bacteria, and particulate matter also aids in preventing phlebitis. If phlebitis symptoms appear, notify the health care provider, discontinue the IV infusion, and, using new IV tubing and fluids, restart it in the opposite extremity, if possible. Cold compresses applied within the first hour after phlebitis is found may help decrease complications; applying warm compresses to the inflamed area lessens discomfort. Document symptoms present, phlebitis rating, nursing interventions, and the patient's response to interventions.

SEPTICEMIA

Septicemia occurs when microorganisms enter the blood. It may occur as a result of IV therapy when poor aseptic technique or contaminated equipment is used during IV-line insertion, or when pathogens are introduced into the bloodstream. The use of sterile technique reduces the potential for introduction of pathogenic organisms. Signs and symptoms of septicemia include fever, chills, lethargy, pain, headache, nausea, vomiting, and diarrhea. If septicemia is suspected, notify the health care provider, discontinue the IV infusion, and, using new IV tubing and fluids, restart it in the opposite extremity, if possible. The discontinued IV catheter, tubing, and solution should be saved for possible culture (in accordance with the agency's policy and health care provider's orders). If an antibiotic is ordered, it should be started after cultures have been obtained. Monitor the patient closely and document symptoms present, nursing interventions, and the patient's response to interventions.

MAINTAINING AN INTRAVENOUS SITE

Complications sometimes occur with peripheral IV infusions. Infiltration of the site, phlebitis of the vessel, and local or systemic infections are possible. Appropriate management of IV sites helps prevent or minimize these complications (Skill 18.3).

Keeping the IV insertion site covered and dry helps prevent the introduction of microorganisms and reduces the possibility of infection. Most often, a gauze dressing or a transparent dressing is used to cover the insertion site. Transparent dressings make visualization of the site easier and keeps the site dry. Gauze dressings do not allow visualization of the site and can become soiled or damp; therefore, their use is limited. No matter which dressing is used, it is important to change the dressing according to facility policy, usually every 48 to 72 hours, and whenever a dressing becomes wet, soiled, or loose.

Skill 18.3   Maintaining an Intravenous Site

NURSING ACTION *(RATIONALE)*

Changing a Peripheral Intravenous Dressing

1. Refer to Standard Steps 1–9.
2. Assemble equipment:
   - Adhesive remover (optional)
   - Antiseptic swabs, alcohol, povidone-iodine, chlorhexidine
   - Arm board, hand board, or housing device (optional)
   - Clean gloves
   - Intravenous (IV) catheter stabilization device
   - Skin protectant solution (optional)
   - Strips of precut tape (if chevron method of securing IV catheter is to be used, tape should be sterile)
   - Transparent dressing or sterile 2- × 2-inch gauze pads
3. Site evaluation:
   a. Determine when the dressing was last changed by checking the dressing label. *(Labeling provides instant identification for determining status of the site.)*
   b. Observe current dressing for moisture and determine whether moisture is leakage from the puncture site or from an external source. *(Determines urgency of the dressing change. Change soiled dressing immediately.)*
   c. Observe IV system for proper functioning or complications (tubing or catheter kinks).
   d. Apply clean gloves and palpate the catheter site through the intact dressing to elicit any complaints of tenderness, pain, or burning sensation. *(These signs are indicative of phlebitis.)*
   e. Inspect catheter site for edema, erythema, drainage, or blanching. *(These signs are indicative of phlebitis or infiltration.)*
4. Remove any overlying tape. Then, remove transparent membrane dressing by picking up one corner and pulling the side laterally while holding catheter hub. Repeat for other side. *(Technique minimizes discomfort during tape removal.)*

a. Alternative is to remove gauze dressing and tape from site, one layer at a time, by pulling toward the insertion site. Tape securing catheter to skin should be left intact. *(Leaving the catheter secured prevents its accidental dislodgment and puncturing of the blood vessel.)*

5. Observe insertion site for redness, erythema, edema, exudate, pallor, or pain. If any of these is present, discontinue infusion. *(These signs are indicative of phlebitis or infiltration. Notify health care provider, and restart infusion in opposite extremity.)*
6. If IV solution is infusing properly, gently remove tape securing catheter. Leave IV stabilization device in place (if one is used) or stabilize catheter with one hand. Remove adhesive residue with adhesive remover, if necessary. *(Prevents catheter from dislodging while site is being cleaned and dressing changed.)*
7. If appropriate according to facility policy, clean insertion site with antiseptic swab. Using circular motion, start at insertion site and work outward in concentric circles. Allow antiseptic solution to dry completely. *(Allow antimicrobial solutions to air-dry completely, which effectively reduces microbial counts. If antiseptic agents are used in combination, allow each to air-dry separately.)* Option: Apply skin protectant solution (SKIN PREP Protective Barrier

Continued

Skill 18.3   Maintaining an Intravenous Site—cont'd

Wipe or 3M Cavilon No Sting Barrier Film) to the area where the tape or dressing will be applied. Allow skin protectant solution to dry.

8. Apply dressing.
   a. Transparent dressing:
   (1) Place transparent dressing over venipuncture site by smoothing dressing over IV site and catheter up to the hub (refer to manufacturer's directions). Do not completely cover the catheter hub or tubing junction with the dressing.
   b. Gauze dressing:
   (1) If IV stabilization device is not used to secure catheter, use **chevron** method (crossing the tape over the catheter) to stabilize catheter. Place single 4-inch (10-cm) strip of sterile ½-inch (1.5 cm) nonallergenic tape under peripheral catheter hub with sticky side up. Crisscross tape over catheter hub to anchor it to skin. (*Chevron method secures catheter to skin.*) Do not cover insertion site. If a second piece of sterile tape is desired, place it across catheter at hub.
   (2) Place sterile 2- × 2-inch gauze over venipuncture site and catheter hub. Secure all edges with tape. Do not cover the connection between IV tubing and catheter hub with the dressing. (*Use occlusive gauze dressings to prevent airflow. Access to catheter*

hub is needed in an emergency; therefore, when tubing is changed, hub should not be covered.)

9. Fold 2- ×2-inch gauze in half, and cover with tape 1 inch (2.5 cm) wide extending about an inch (2.5 cm) from each side of gauze. Place under the tubing and catheter hub junction. (*Placing 2- × 2-inch gauze under the catheter hub and tubing decreases skin irritation.*) When a transparent dressing is used, avoid placing tape directly over dressing. (*Tape application loosens transparent dressings.*)

10. Label the dressing with date and time of insertion, date and time of dressing change, gauge and length of catheter, and name of nurse (see illustration in Step 4). (*Allows easy recognition of type of device and time interval for site rotation.*) Option: Apply arm board, hand board, or commercial housing device if venipuncture site or dressing is affected by the motion of the elbow or wrist. (*Reduces the risk of phlebitis and infiltration from motion of the joint.*)

11. Discard used supplies, remove gloves, and perform hand hygiene.

12. Document and report the following:
   • Time dressing was changed
   • Reason for dressing change
   • Type of dressing material used
   • Condition of venipuncture site
   • Treatment of venipuncture site (if any)
   • Tubing is **patent** (tubing is open and not occluded)

13. Refer to Standard Steps 10–17.

Changing Infusion Tubing

1. Refer to Standard Steps 1–9.
2. Assemble equipment:
   a. Continuous infusion:
   • Infusion tubing as appropriate: microdrop (delivers 60 drops [gtt] per milliliter and is used for slow infusions in patients susceptible to fluid volume overload) or macrodrip (delivers 10–15 drops [gtt] per milliliter and is used for rapid infusions)
   • Filter and extension tubing if necessary (Patients sometimes require IV extension tubing to increase mobility, decrease manipulation and potential contamination at insertion site, or facilitate changes in position.)

Skill 18.3   Maintaining an Intravenous Site—cont'd

- Tubing label
b. Intermittent use saline or heparin lock:
- 5-mL syringe filled with normal saline or heparin flush solution (check facility policy)
- Clean gloves
- Injection cap or as-needed (prn) adapter
- Loop or short extension tubing (if necessary)
- Sterile 2- × 2-inch gauze pads
- Additional dressing supplies as needed if application of new IV dressing is required (see earlier Changing a Peripheral Intravenous Dressing section, Steps 4–7)

3. Evaluation of equipment:
  a. Determine when new infusion set is needed (e.g., according to facility policy or label, or after contamination or puncture of infusion tubing).
  b. Observe for occlusion in tubing such as kinking, drug or mineral precipitate, or blood. (Infusion of incompatible medication potentially leads to precipitate formation and occlusion of tubing. Blood may flow from the vein into the tubing and will adhere to tubing. Infusion of viscous blood components sometimes causes adherence to walls of tubing and results in occlusion.)
  c. Determine patient's need for continued IV infusion. (If the health care provider has discontinued the IV infusion or the nurse anticipates that the IV infusion will be discontinued, it is advisable to wait to change tubing so as not to increase costs. Call the health care provider for further orders. If the tubing has been contaminated or punctured, however, change the tubing immediately.)

4. Open new infusion set and connect add-on pieces such as filters or extension tubing. *(Use add-ons only if absolutely necessary to decrease the risk of contamination and infection.)* Keep protective covering over spike and distal adapter. *(Protective covers reduce entrance of microorganisms.)* Secure each junction with a Luer-Lok, clasping device, or threaded device. Avoid the use of tape.

5. If catheter hub is not visible, remove IV dressing as directed in Changing a Peripheral Intravenous Dressing section, Steps 3 and 4. Do not remove tape securing catheter to skin. If transparent dressing must be removed, place small piece of sterile tape across hub to temporarily anchor catheter during disconnection. *(Keeping catheter secured decreases risk of dislodging catheter.)*

6. For existing continuous infusion *(Infusion bag and tubing should be changed at the same time whenever possible to decrease risk of contamination)*:
  a. Close roller clamp on new tubing.
  b. Slow rate of infusion to keep vein open (KVO) on existing IV by regulating roller clamp on old tubing.
  c. Compress and fill drip chamber of old tubing.

7. Remove IV container from pole, invert container, and remove old tubing from solution. Carefully hold container while hanging or taping the drip chamber on IV pole 36 inches (90 cm) above IV site. *(Fluid in drip chamber will run slowly to keep catheter patent.)*

8. Place insertion spike of new tubing into old fluid container opening. Hang container on IV pole, compress and release drip chamber on new tubing, and fill drip chamber one-third to one-half full.

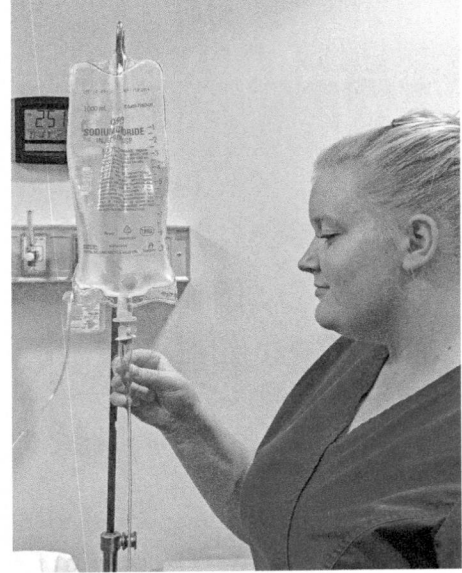

9. Slowly open roller clamp, remove protective cap from adapter (if necessary), and flush new tubing with solution. Stop infusion and replace cap. *(Slow flushing of solution into tubing reduces formation of air bubbles in tubing.)*

10. Turn roller clamp on old tubing to "off" position. Option: Place 2- × 2-inch gauze under catheter hub. *(Prevents tubing from accidentally contacting skin and collects blood that may leak from catheter hub.)*

11. Stabilize hub of catheter and apply pressure over vein just above catheter tip (at least 1½ inches above insertion site). Gently disconnect old tubing from catheter hub, and quickly insert adapter of new tubing into catheter hub. *(Minimizes loss of blood as tubing is changed.)*

Continued

Skill 18.3   Maintaining an Intravenous Site—cont'd

17. Refer to Standard Steps 10–17.

Changing Solution Container

1. Refer to Standard Steps 1–9.
2. Assemble equipment:
   - Bottle or bag of IV solution as ordered by health care provider
   - Pen
   - Time tape
3. Determine need to change solution container:
   a. Check health care provider's orders. (*Ensures that correct solution will be used and that the order is complete.*)
   b. If order is written for KVO, contact health care provider for clarification of the rate of infusion. Note date and time when solution was last changed. (*Orders for KVO do not provide complete information and have potential to result in fluid overload or deficit and in electrolyte imbalance. A KVO order is required to contain a specific infusion rate; check facility policy.*)
   c. Verify patient's identification. (*Ensures right patient receives ordered IV fluid.*)
   d. Determine the compatibility of all IV fluids and additives by consulting appropriate literature or the pharmacy. (*Precipitates caused by incompatible medications could slow infusion or occlude catheter.*)
   e. Determine patient's understanding of need for continuing IV therapy. (*Allows patient's questions to be answered and increases compliance.*)
   f. Assess patency of current IV access site. Check for blood return and free flow of infusion.
4. Prepare next solution at least 1 hour before it is needed. If it is prepared in pharmacy, be sure it has been delivered to the patient's location. Check that the solution is correct and properly labeled. (*Ensures no disruption in fluid therapy to patient.*) Check solution expiration date. Observe for precipitate and discoloration. (*Prevents infusion of contaminated or outdated solution.*)
5. Change solution when fluid remains only in neck of container or when new type of solution has been ordered. (*Prevents air in tubing and waste of solution.*)
6. Move roller clamp to stop flow rate and remove old IV fluid container from IV pole.
7. Invert old container and quickly remove spike, keeping it sterile. Remove protective cover from new fluid container. Without touching tip of spike, insert it into new bag or bottle. (*Ensures sterility of solution.*)
8. Hang new bag or bottle of solution on IV pole.
9. Check for air in tubing. If bubbles form, it is possible to remove them by closing the roller clamp, stretching the tubing downward, and tapping the tubing with the fingers (the bubbles rise in the tubing to the drip chamber). For larger amounts of air, swab port with antiseptic swab, allow to dry, and connect a syringe to

12. Open roller clamp on new tubing, allowing solution to run rapidly for 30 to 60 seconds, and then regulate IV drip according to health care provider's orders. (*Clears catheter of any blood in lumen, preventing occlusion.*)
13. Attach a piece of tape or a preprinted label with date and time of tubing change onto tubing below the drip chamber. (*Provides reference to determine next time for tubing change.*)
14. Remove and discard 2- × 2-inch gauze (if used) and old IV tubing. If necessary, apply new dressing. Dispose of gloves.
15. Form a loop of tubing and secure it to patient's arm with a strip of tape. (*Prevents accidental pulling against site and catheter movement.*)
16. Document and report the following:
    - Time tubing was changed
    - Rate of infusion

A special IV flow sheet may be used to record tubing changes. Check facility policy.

Skill 18.3   Maintaining an Intravenous Site—cont'd

an injection port below the air and aspirate the air into the syringe. *(Infusion of large amounts of air in tubing potentially results in air embolus, which is sometimes fatal.)* Reassure patient that small air bubbles are harmless.

10. Make sure drip chamber is one-third to one-half full. If drip chamber is too full, invert solution container and squeeze solution from the drip chamber back into the solution container. Replace container on IV pole. *(If chamber is completely filled, the drip rate cannot be observed.)*

11. Regulate flow to prescribed rate.
12. Place label on the side of container. Label should contain time hung, approximate time of completion, any medication added, and patient identification. If plastic bags are to be used, mark only on the label and not on the container. *(Allows accurate determination of next solution change and medication infusion.)*
13. Document and report the following:
    • Amount and type of fluid infused
    • Amount and type of new fluid
    • Patency of system
   A special IV flow sheet may be used to record parenteral fluids.
14. Refer to Standard Steps 10–17.

Discontinuing Intravenous Medications

1. Refer to Standard Steps 1–9.
2. Assemble equipment:
   • 5- or 10-mL syringe filled with normal saline, heparin flush solution, or both (depending on facility policy)
   • Antiseptic swabs
   • Clean gloves
   • Injection cap replacement (if needed)
   • Sterile cap or cover for infusion tubing

3. Evaluation:
   a. Observe fluid container for complete infusion of all medications.
   b. Review health care provider's order to determine whether blood samples are required after medication infusion. *(Monitoring of serum concentration of some IV medications is necessary to prevent reaching toxic levels. Dosage adjustment or alterations of timing for next dose are sometimes required.)*
   c. Monitor patient's response to medications. *(Enables evaluation of medication's effects.)*
4. Move roller clamp on infusion tubing to the "off" position. *(Prevents air from entering vein and prevents medication from leaking from tubing.)*
5. Disconnect medication delivery tubing from injection port and replace with a sterile cap or cover. *(Infusion tubing can be reused with next ordered medication if it is not contaminated.)*
6. If the tubing has a needle or needleless adapter on the infusion tubing, remove and discard it appropriately, and replace with a sterile cap or cover as indicated. *(If tubing is to be reused, the tubing must remain sterile. If tubing spike, connector end, fluid pathway, or fluid container is contaminated, a new tubing set or fluid container is required.)*
7. Cleanse injection port or as-needed (prn) adapter on main IV tubing with antiseptic swab. *(Ensures sterility of port.)*

8. For intermittent medication piggybacked into a continuous infusion, attach 5-mL saline-filled syringe to injection port, and flush the line gently. Regulate fluid flow of the continuous infusion as ordered. *(Saline flush prevents incompatible*

Continued

Skill 18.3 Maintaining an Intravenous Site—cont'd

medications from coming into contact in the infusion tubing. There is no way to know how much pressure is exerted inside catheter lumen. A 5-mL syringe generates less pressure than a 3-mL syringe. Do not force irrigation if resistance is felt.)

9. For intermittent medications through a saline or heparin lock, attach saline-filled 5- to 10-mL syringe to injection port and flush catheter gently, or attach syringe filled with heparin flush solution to injection port and flush gently, if necessary (check facility policy). Attach sterile injection port cover if necessary. *(Flushing with 3–10 mL of saline after each medication is crucial. Volume of flush depends on lumen size, catheter length, and medication infused.)*

   a. Approach flushing of any IV catheter carefully. If resistance is met, assess for mechanical causes (e.g., closed clamps, kinked tubing, and the position of extremity). Never force flushing. *(Fibrin formation, drug precipitates, and blood clots sometimes occlude catheter lumen. Forceful flushing against these occlusions has the potential to cause embolus formation and catheter damage.)*

10. Prepare patient for blood testing after medication infusion if necessary.

11. Document and report the following:
    • Time that medication is discontinued
    • How tubing or catheter (or both) is flushed
    • Amount and type of flush solution
    • Condition of site
    • If facility policy requires it, use special IV flow sheet to document IV interventions.

12. Refer to Standard Steps 10–17.

Discontinuing Peripheral IV Access

1. Refer to Standard Steps 1–9.

2. Assemble equipment:
    • Antiseptic swab
    • Clean gloves
    • Sterile 2- × 2-inch or 4- × 4-inch gauze pad
    • Tape

3. Site evaluation:
    a. Observe existing IV site for signs and symptoms of infection, infiltration, or phlebitis. *(Indications of need to discontinue IV infusion.)*
    b. Review health care provider's orders for discontinuation of IV therapy. *(The health care provider's order is required to discontinue IV therapy.)*
    c. Determine patient's understanding of the need for removal of peripheral IV catheter. *(Increases patient's knowledge and cooperation.)*

4. Explain procedure to patient. *(Minimizes patient's anxiety and discomfort.)*

5. Turn IV tubing roller clamp to "off" position. Remove tape securing tubing.

6. Remove IV site dressing and tape while stabilizing catheter. *(Movement of catheter will cause discomfort. Never use scissors to remove the tape or dressing because it is possible to accidentally cut the catheter.)*

7. With dry gauze held over site, apply light pressure and withdraw the catheter, using a slow steady movement, keeping the hub parallel to the skin. *(Changing the angle of the catheter inside the vein sometimes causes additional vein irritation, increasing the risk of post-infusion phlebitis.)*

8. Apply pressure to the site for 2–3 minutes, using a dry, sterile gauze pad. Secure the tape over the gauze snugly. *(Subcutaneous hematoma is a common complication. Applying tape snugly acts as a pressure dressing to stop bleeding and hematoma formation.)*

9. Inspect the catheter for intactness, noting tip integrity and length. *(Tips of catheters sometimes break off, causing an embolus, which is an emergency situation. Notify health care provider if tip is broken.)*

10. Discard used supplies.

11. Remove and discard gloves, and perform hand hygiene.

12. Instruct patient to report any erythema, pain, drainage, or edema that occurs after catheter removal. *(Post-infusion phlebitis sometimes occurs within 48–96 hours after catheter removal.)*

13. Document and record the following:
    • Time peripheral IV infusion was discontinued
    • Condition of site
    • Gauge and length of catheter
    • Whether catheter is intact

14. Refer to Standard Steps 10–17.

Box 18.15	Patient Problem Statements for the Patient Receiving Intravenous Therapy

Compromised skin integrity:
- Related to invasive procedure

Insufficient knowledge:
- Related to lack of exposure to information

Potential for inadequate fluid volume:
- Related to alterations in regulatory mechanisms of hydration
- Related to fluid and electrolyte imbalance

Potential for infection:
- Related to break in skin integrity

Potential for injury:
- Related to adverse effects of intravenous (IV) therapy
- Related to presence of IV catheter acting as a foreign body
- Related to IV medications

It is also necessary to change the IV solution container and tubing at appropriate intervals to prevent complications. There are several types of IV solution containers, including plastic and glass. These containers must be changed according to the type of solution, the type of container, and the rate at which the IV is infusing. The INS (Infusion Nurses Society, 2011) recommends changing the solution container every 24 hours or sooner if the solution has been infused completely. Most facilities follow this recommendation or have even stricter guidelines.

Most facilities recommend changing tubing every 72 to 96 hours for continuous infusions and every 24 hours for intermittent infusions or infusions through an injection or access port. Some facilities have a stricter policy and may require changing tubing on continuous infusions every 48 hours; thus, be aware of and follow facility policy.

If possible, the IV solution container, the tubing, and the dressing should be changed at the same time. This reduces the risk of introducing bacteria into the system and cuts down on infections at the site. Never disconnect the tubing when assisting with a gown or clothing change. Instead, the IV solution container and tubing should be threaded through the sleeve of the patient's garment. If the patient is allowed to shower, make sure the IV insertion site and dressing are protected with a water-resistant covering. Inspect the dressing and site after the shower and change the dressing if it becomes wet or loose. Box 18.15 lists patient problem statements for the patient receiving IV therapy.

BLOOD TRANSFUSION THERAPY

Any time a patient has a problem with the amount of blood circulating in the body or with any of the blood components, the health care provider may order a blood transfusion. Most often, a blood or blood component transfusion is ordered to replace blood volume, to preserve oxygen-carrying capacity, or to increase coagulation capabilities. It is up to the health care provider to determine the type of transfusion and how many units are to be transfused.

In some states, the initiation and administration of blood and blood components are included within the scope of practice for the LPN/LVN, and in others, the LPN/LVN may be responsible only for measuring baseline vital signs and monitoring the transfusion. Therefore, it is important to be aware of the LPN/LVN's scope of practice and facility policy when working with blood or blood component transfusions.

The fear of infection or contracting a disease leads some patients to decline transfusions of blood or blood products. The patient should receive education about the rigorous testing procedures implemented to screen donated blood. This testing has reduced the incidence of transmission of infections and blood-borne diseases, resulting in a safer supply for transfusion.

Most often, health care providers use the patient's hemoglobin level as a guideline to determine when a transfusion is necessary. Many providers do not order a transfusion for a patient until the hemoglobin level falls below 8 g/dL.

Individuals who have concerns about receiving another person's blood may donate their own blood before anticipated surgery to be infused during their hospitalization (autologous blood transfusion). Autologous blood transfusions also can be given with blood lost during surgery or after traumatic injury. Health care providers may suction a patient's lost blood into a canister, filter it, and then return it to the patient to allay fears that the patient may have regarding donated blood. The patient should discuss plans for an autologous blood transfusion with the health care provider well in advance of the planned surgery to allot time for collection and storage.

For religious reasons, some patients do not accept blood transfusions. In these situations, plasma expanders may be used instead of a blood transfusion.

INITIATING A BLOOD TRANSFUSION

Before a blood transfusion, a type and cross-matching test is done to match the donor's blood type with the recipient's blood type. A transfusion of incompatible blood can be fatal. Facilities require very strict identification and labeling procedures for transfusions.

Caring for a patient receiving a blood transfusion is the responsibility of the nurse (see the Coordinated Care box on blood transfusions). Before the initiation of a blood transfusion, the patient must be educated about the need for the transfusion, alternatives to transfusion, and risks of transfusions, as well as measures that are implemented to ensure a safe blood supply. Some facilities also require an informed consent to be signed. It is important, therefore, to know facility policy.

Coordinated Care

Collaboration

Blood Transfusions

- The skill of transfusing blood and blood products requires the critical thinking and knowledge of a nurse. In some states, the administration of blood and blood components is included within the scope of practice for the licensed practical nurse/licensed vocational nurse (LPN/LVN); in some states, it is not. Be aware of the scope of practice for the LPN/LVN, as well as facility policy.
- Tasks that may be delegated to UAP include measuring vital signs, collecting equipment, and instituting patient comfort measures. The primary responsibility for donor and recipient identification, infusing the unit within the required time, and monitoring outcomes remains with the nurse. (It is generally an RN's responsibility.)

Vital sign measurements are recorded immediately before the transfusion (to obtain a baseline) and at regular intervals throughout and after the procedure to detect or prevent transfusion reactions. Transfusion reactions are possible at any time during or even after a blood transfusion, but they usually occur within the first 15 minutes.

The health care provider's order specifies the rate of the blood infusion. Each unit of blood should be infused within 2 to 4 hours. The risk of blood cell damage and infection increases after that time. Each facility has a specific policy regarding disposal of used blood bags or any blood remaining in the bag after 4 hours. It is essential to follow the protocol for discarding or returning the container to the blood bank whenever a unit of blood is infused.

When a blood transfusion is begun, a primary IV infusion of 0.9% normal saline is started with a Y administration set (Fig. 18.13). An IV solution containing dextrose should not be used when blood is administered. Dextrose in the solution causes the blood to lyse or be destroyed. When the tubing is primed, the blood filter must be filled completely with saline solution. This prevents debris buildup within the filter and allows the blood to flow without interruption. The blood administration tubing then can be attached to a low port on an existing IV line, or it can be used with a resealable intermittent lock device.

Inspect the blood or blood product bag for signs of leakage or unusual appearance, including bubbles or purplish color. Report these signs immediately because they could indicate the presence of contamination, and the product should be returned to the laboratory or blood bank. After the donated blood and the patient have been properly identified, the blood is added to the appropriate section of the Y tubing and the rate is set according to the health care provider's order. Make sure to close the roller clamp to the normal saline before opening the roller clamp to the blood. This

Fig. 18.13 (A) Opened blood administration set and tubing primed with 0.9% normal saline. Note that the filter is filled completely with the saline. (B) Attached blood product to the 0.9% normal saline. Note that the clamp is closed on the saline and that the clamp is opened above the filter to the blood product.

prevents blood from backing up into the normal saline solution.

Remain with the patient for the first 15 to 20 minutes of the transfusion to monitor for reactions. The transfusion should be started slowly and vital signs monitored frequently, according to facility policy. Any complaint of discomfort could indicate a possible reaction and should be addressed immediately.

At the completion of the blood transfusion, the IV tubing should be flushed with the normal saline solution. If more than one unit of blood is ordered, use fresh tubing; do not reuse tubing. This prevents blood from the separate units from mixing within the tubing, and prevents clotting, as well. Always refer to agency policy for specific instructions on tubing changes for blood products.

BLOOD TRANSFUSION REACTIONS

Infusing blood that is not compatible with the patient's blood type can lead to a transfusion reaction. A transfusion reaction can be life threatening and is considered an emergency. Close monitoring is crucial to determine the patient's tolerance to the infusing blood. Patients experiencing transfusion reactions frequently say they are "not feeling right" or have a sense of impending doom. They may report or experience chills, fever, low back pain, pruritus (itching), hypotension, nausea and vomiting, decreased urine output, back pain, chest pain, wheezing, and dyspnea. If the patient is unconscious and unable to indicate symptoms, closely

| Box 18.16 | **Blood Transfusion Precautions** |

- Make sure IV catheters for blood transfusions are of appropriate size in relation to the size of the vessel.
- One unit of blood is released from the blood bank at a time. Before administration, each unit of blood and recipient information must be verified by two nurses according to facility policy.
- Completely prime blood transfusion filters with saline to prevent collection of debris in a partially primed filter. Saline reduces the viscosity of red blood cells by diluting them and, thus, flushes blood from the tubing (see Fig. 18.13A).
- In the event of a blood transfusion reaction, stop the blood infusion and remove the Y tubing from the main IV tubing or intermittent-use device. Infuse normal saline slowly through the IV line. This prevents any more of the transfusing blood from entering the patient and keeps the vein open.
- A transfusion reaction produces a hemolytic reaction that causes red blood cells to appear in the urine. Therefore, it is important that the patient voids or the catheter drainage device is emptied before the transfusion is started so that, if a reaction occurs, a fresh urine sample is available to test for red blood cells.
- An RN regulates the flow rate so that only 10–24 mL of product infuses during the first 15 min and the RN remains with the patient during this time. If a reaction occurs, only a small amount of incompatible blood product will have been administered to the patient at this slow of a rate.
- An alteration in the vital signs from baseline values indicates the possibility that a transfusion reaction has occurred.

- An RN is required to hang the blood, but an LPN/LVN is permitted to verify type with the RN in some facilities. The RN is required to sit with the patient for the first 15 to 30 minutes of transfusion.
- If the nurse believes that a transfusion reaction is occurring, the following steps should be implemented:
  1. Stop the transfusion *immediately.*
  2. Infuse 0.9% normal saline directly into the vein with new tubing to prevent any more incompatible blood from being infused into the patient.
  3. Notify the health care provider.
  4. Monitor the patient's signs and symptoms of reaction continuously and check vital signs every 5 minutes.
  5. Anticipate the health care provider's order of emergency drugs, such as antihistamines, vasopressors, IV fluids, and steroids, to counteract and treat the symptoms present.
  6. Cardiac and respiratory arrest may develop, so prepare to perform cardiopulmonary resuscitation (CPR) if necessary.
  7. Collect a urine specimen and send it to the laboratory to check for red blood cells from a hemolytic reaction.
  8. Do not discard the blood container, the tubing, the labels, or the transfusion record. These items must be sent to the laboratory, the pharmacy, or the blood bank as outlined by agency policy for review.
  9. On the appropriate forms, document the events that occurred during the transfusion reaction.

CPR, Cardiopulmonary resuscitation; *IV,* intravenous.

assess vital signs, urine output, and skin appearance. If you suspect a transfusion reaction, stop the infusion immediately. Keep the vein open with the normal saline solution and notify the health care provider and the blood bank. Keep the remaining blood product and bag and send them to the pharmacy, the laboratory, or the blood bank (depending on facility policy) so that they can be checked for infectious agents and cross-matching problems. Also, document the incident on the appropriate "blood transfusion reaction" form, and be prepared to collect blood and urine specimens from the patient. Monitor the patient's vital signs and urine output every 15 minutes; medications to treat the presenting symptoms may be necessary. Because a transfusion reaction tends to be frightening, reassure and support the patient and family.

Although a transfusion reaction normally occurs within the first 15 minutes, it is possible at any time during or after the infusion process. There are several types of blood transfusion reactions, including hemolytic, nonhemolytic, allergic, and anaphylactic reactions. Most often, these reactions occur within the first 60 to 90 minutes after the transfusion has been started and are caused by an incompatibility between the patient's blood and some component of the donated

blood. Another type of transfusion reaction is the delayed reaction, which may occur days to weeks later. This type of reaction occurs in patients who have developed antibodies to the blood from a previous transfusion and results in hemolysis (destruction or breakdown of red blood cells) of the patient's blood.

Circulatory overload is another complication of a blood transfusion and may be considered yet another form of a transfusion reaction. With circulatory overload, the patient is unable to handle the additional fluid from the transfusion and develops a cough, frothy sputum, cyanosis, and an increase in blood pressure. This can occur any time during and for several hours after the transfusion. To prevent this in susceptible patients, the rate of infusion should be slowed and the patient monitored closely for symptoms. Box 18.16 lists further precautions in giving blood transfusions.

❖ NURSING PROCESS

The role of the LPN/LVN in the nursing process involves the following:

- Participating in planning care for patients based on patient needs

- Reviewing the patient's plan of care and recommending revisions as needed
- Reviewing and following defined prioritization for patient care
- Using clinical pathways, care maps, or care plans to guide and review patient care

◆ DATA COLLECTION

When collecting data on fluid, electrolyte, and acid-base balances, know whether the patient is at risk for imbalances, be aware of the presence of any alterations, and know the extent to which body systems are involved. Data collection helps the nurse anticipate the patient's needs for nursing interventions and helps to determine the effectiveness of therapies and any adverse reactions to them.

Data collection for patients with fluid, electrolyte, or acid-base imbalances should include physical examination, including measurements of vital signs, height, weight, and neurologic function; intake and output measures; results of laboratory studies; patient's past and present medical history, with notes about renal, endocrine, or respiratory disease; and a complete medication history, including over-the-counter medications and herbal supplements.

◆ PATIENT PROBLEMS

It is particularly important that the RN choosing patient problem statements for alterations in fluid, electrolyte, and acid-base balances be skilled in critical thinking to choose appropriate patient problem statements. Some of the following patient problem statements may be appropriate for the patient with a fluid, electrolyte, or acid-base alteration:

- *Compromised Blood Flow to Tissue*
- *Compromised Oral Mucous Membrane*
- *Compromised Tissue Integrity*
- *Fluid Volume Overload*
- *Inability to Maintain Adequate Breathing Pattern*
- *Inadequate Fluid Volume*
- *Inefficient Oxygenation*
- *Insufficient Cardiac Output*
- *Insufficient Nutrition*
- *Potential for Compromised Skin Integrity*
- *Potential for Inadequate Fluid Volume*

The data collected to establish the potential for or the actual presence of a specific patient problem in these areas are often subtle. Patterns and trends emerge only when the nurse consciously looks for them because many body systems are involved. For example, relevant data for the patient problem statement of inadequate fluid volume may include the presence of insufficient oral intake, weight loss, dry skin and mucous membranes, inelastic skin turgor, decreased blood pressure, and increased heart rate. The serum sodium level may be elevated. The urine may be dark, with an elevated specific gravity. In some cases, the volume of the urine has been decreasing over a period of days.

The omission of any of these data leads the nurse to formulate an incomplete assessment of the patient's condition and perhaps results in an incorrect patient problem statement.

In addition to the accurate clustering of data, the RN must identify the related factor for the patient problem statement to plan appropriate nursing interventions. For example, for the patient problem statement of *Inadequate Fluid Volume*, the related factor is sometimes diarrhea and sometimes vomiting or difficulty swallowing. This patient problem statement is not assigned if the patient is receiving nothing by mouth (NPO) as part of the treatment regimen. If the related factor is diarrhea, administer ordered antidiarrheal medication and provide oral fluids that contain electrolytes and glucose. Teach the patient to use careful hand washing and to avoid dairy products. In contrast, if the related factor is vomiting, administer antiemetics, remove sights and odors that have the potential to induce nausea, and provide a small amount of fluids containing electrolytes. If the related factor is difficulty swallowing, attempt to ensure that the patient is fully alert; position the patient in a high-Fowler's position when possible during times of intake; provide foods and fluids with a soft, pureed, or thickened consistency; provide small amounts with each mouthful; and investigate the need for enteral or TPN.

◆ EXPECTED OUTCOMES AND PLANNING

The first step in the planning process is setting priorities. Many patient problem statements in the areas of fluid, electrolyte, and acid-base balance represent high-priority patient problems. The consequences are potentially serious, even life threatening (e.g., seizures, dysrhythmias, or coma).

During the planning process, the LPN/LVN works with the RN to formulate nursing interventions to prevent or treat fluid, electrolyte, and acid-base imbalances. It is important to collaborate with the patient and the family during this part of the planning process. The family is helpful in identifying the subtle changes in behavior associated with these imbalances, such as anxiety, confusion, or irritability. During the planning process, remember that the patient and the family need to know preventive measures, signs and symptoms to report, and measures that are possible to implement if an imbalance occurs. When medications, special diets, or oral or IV fluids are administered in the home, the patient and the family need careful teaching to be able to perform these interventions safely. Consider the patient's preferences and resources during each step of the planning process (e.g., if the patient needs to be encouraged to increase oral intake, determine the patient's favorite beverages and incorporate them into the plan of care). In the hospital, anticipate the needs of the patient and family for specific information, and initiate teaching before discharge so that they will be ready for these procedures. Inform the home health nurse of discharge preparations because the home health nurse will continue the teaching plan and evaluate the effectiveness of the home interventions.

The nurse also works closely with other members of the health care team, such as the health care provider, the dietitian, and the physical therapist. For example, when the nurse collects new data suggesting that the patient is developing a fluid, electrolyte, or acid-base imbalance, the nurse consults with the health care provider to determine the need for dietary, pharmacologic, IV fluid, or other therapy. The nurse's responsibilities also include ongoing monitoring of the patient's fluid, electrolyte, and acid-base status to determine the safety of implementing the health care provider's and nursing orders and any need for a change in the plan of care. For example, perhaps the health care provider orders an oral potassium supplement to be given to the patient three times each day. Before administering the first dose each day, the nurse must verify that the serum potassium level is normal and that the urine output is adequate. If the serum level is elevated or if the urine output has decreased, the dose of potassium must be withheld and the health care provider must be consulted.

After priority setting and collaboration with the patient, family, and health care team, the nurse should assist with the development of a care plan that is individualized according to the patient's acute or chronic fluid, electrolyte, or acid-base status.

◆ GOAL

The patient's fluid, electrolyte, and acid-base balances will be restored and maintained.

◆ OUTCOMES

- The patient's vital signs will return to baseline normal.
- The patient will have normal skin turgor.
- The patient will have moist oral mucous membranes.
- The patient's weight will be stable at baseline normal.
- The patient will have no edema.
- The patient will have clear breath sounds.
- The patient's serum and urine electrolyte and chemistry results and arterial blood gas values will be within normal limits.
- The patient's urine output will equal intake.

◆ IMPLEMENTATION

Prevention of fluid, electrolyte, and acid-base imbalances is important. When imbalances occur, remove or treat the cause of the imbalance if possible. Other nursing interventions aim to correct the imbalances.

When a patient's fluid volume is depleted, it is possible to replace fluids and electrolytes orally, with IV administration of fluids and blood components, or through TPN if the fluid deficit is caused by malnutrition. For patients with fluid volume excess, implement measures to reduce fluids, such as fluid intake restrictions, reduced sodium intake, and use of diuretics. When the patient has an electrolyte imbalance, provide an appropriate diet and administer supplements when they are ordered. For patients with acid-base imbalances, initiate such measures as reducing anxiety, improving pulmonary function, controlling the loss of GI content, or ensuring the control of conditions such as diabetes mellitus or renal failure.

◆ EVALUATION

Evaluate the interventions by comparing the patient's responses to the expected outcomes of the established goals. Be prepared to revise the plan of care based on the evaluation findings.

◆ GOAL

Patient's fluid and electrolyte balances will be restored and maintained.

◆ EVALUATIVE MEASURES

- Obtain daily weight and monitor. Be sure to weigh the patient using similar conditions as noted above.
- Obtain patient's vital signs.
- Measure all routes of intake and output.
- Auscultate for abnormal lung sounds.
- Check oral mucous membranes for dryness or moistness.
- Check tissue turgor for tenting or edema.
- Monitor serum electrolyte levels.

The patient's status and the effectiveness of the nursing care must be evaluated continuously, and the care plan must be modified as needed. If any of the measures identified have not been effective, it is important to collaborate with other health care team members to determine the changes needed to improve the patient's status.

Get Ready for the NCLEX® Examination!

Key Points

- Water is the primary fluid in the body.
- The two fluid compartments in the body are the intracellular and extracellular compartments. The extracellular compartment includes the interstitial and intravascular areas.
- Homeostasis must be maintained to maintain health.
- Fluid movement takes place by means of three passive transport systems—diffusion, osmosis, and filtration—and one active transport system in which ATP is used for energy.
- Electrolytes are chemical compounds that carry either a positive or negative charge. Positive ions are called *cations;* negative ions are called *anions.* To maintain homeostasis, it is necessary for the cations and the anions to balance each other in the body fluids.
- Sodium is the major extracellular cation in the body. Water follows sodium as it moves from one fluid compartment to another.
- Potassium is the major intracellular cation in the body. Imbalances in potassium, either high or low levels, have the potential to cause life-threatening cardiac conditions.
- Arterial blood has a normal pH range of 7.35 to 7.45. A pH lower than 7.35 is considered abnormally acidic; a pH higher than 7.45 is considered abnormally alkaline. A pH lower than 6.8 or higher than 7.8 can be fatal.
- The four types of acid-base imbalance are respiratory acidosis, respiratory alkalosis, metabolic acidosis, and metabolic alkalosis.
- Any process that interferes with normal ventilation and causes a decrease or an increase in the excretion of acids in the body poses the risk of causing respiratory acidosis or respiratory alkalosis.
- Any process that interferes with normal production or excretion of hydrogen ions poses the risk of causing metabolic acidosis or metabolic alkalosis.
- Respiratory acidosis or alkalosis results when the lungs fail to regulate the carbonic acid concentration in the blood. Metabolic acidosis or alkalosis results when the kidneys fail to regulate the bicarbonate concentration in the blood.
- If the lungs are unable to correct respiratory acidosis, the kidneys respond to correct the imbalance. If the kidneys are unable to correct metabolic acidosis, the lungs respond to correct the imbalance.
- The nurse practice act of each state legally defines the nurse's qualification for and scope of practice in administering parenteral therapy and inserting nasogastric tubes.
- Any nurse administering IV therapies must have knowledge of the complications that can occur during therapy and of the nursing interventions associated with these complications.
- IV therapy poses the risk of infiltration, phlebitis, infection at the IV site or systemic infection, fluid volume excess, and bleeding at the IV site.
- By following strict guidelines when administering blood or blood products and by being aware of the symptoms of transfusion reactions, the nurse can identify more quickly a reaction to a transfusion.

Additional Learning Resources

SG Go to your Study Guide for additional learning activities to help you master this chapter content.

Be sure to visit the Evolve site at http://evolve.elsevier.com/Cooper/foundations/ for additional online resources.

Review Questions for the NCLEX® Examination

1. An elderly patient has recently been experiencing excessive edema in their feet. The nurse discusses with the patient the dietary changes that may be causing the water retention in association with the patient's edema. Which electrolyte has the greatest influence on water balance in the body?

   1. Sodium (Na^+)
   2. Potassium (K^+)
   3. Chloride (Cl^-)
   4. Calcium (Ca^{2+})

2. Which regulatory system is the body's second line of defense in keeping the pH within normal limits?

   1. Blood buffers
   2. Respiratory system
   3. Renal system
   4. Blood pressure

3. The nurse is caring for a patient who requires additional potassium in their diet. What foods would the nurse recommend for the patient?

   1. Baked chicken, green salad, and fresh fruit plate
   2. Macaroni and cheese, cornbread, and gelatin
   3. Tacos, chips and salsa, and ice cream
   4. Seafood plate, marinated vegetables, cake

4. What is the primary route of excretion of sodium by the body?

   1. Via the skin
   2. Via the lungs
   3. Via the kidneys
   4. Via the feces

5. The movement of water from an area of lower concentration to an area of higher concentration occurs through which of the following?

   1. Diffusion
   2. Filtration
   3. Active transport
   4. Osmosis

6. What is the largest fluid compartment in the body?

   1. Intracellular
   2. Extracellular
   3. Interstitial
   4. Intravascular

7. Passive transport includes what physiologic processes? *(Select all that apply.)*

   1. Osmosis
   2. Diffusion

3. Filtration
4. Sodium-potassium pump
5. Compensatory metabolic acidosis

8. Which abbreviation is used to indicate hydrogen ion concentration in the body?

   1. mEq
   2. ATP
   3. pH
   4. mL

9. Potential causes of hypocalcemia may include which conditions? *(Select all that apply.)*

   1. Vitamin D deficiency
   2. Diuretic use
   3. Injury of the thyroid gland
   4. Severe burns
   5. Renal failure

10. The nurse is reviewing the daily weight recordings of an assigned patient who is receiving diuretic therapy. The nurse notes a weight decrease of 2 kg (4.4 lb). This will be reflected by a loss or gain of _____ body fluid.

11. When the body senses hypoxemia or hypercapnia, the chemoreceptors in the medulla of the brainstem will have what response?

    1. Slowing the respiratory rate
    2. Decreasing the heart rate
    3. Increasing the depth and rate of respirations
    4. Lowering the blood pressure

12. The nurse is caring for a patient with severe hyperkalemia. What actions should be included in the plan of care for the shift? *(Select all that apply.)*

    1. Monitor serum potassium levels.
    2. Administer Kayexalate as prescribed by the health care provider.
    3. Report a urinary output less than 30 mL/h.
    4. Monitor pulse rate every 24 hours
    5. Restrict fluid intake

13. In acute respiratory acidosis, the renal compensatory mechanisms begin to operate within how many hours?

    1. 6
    2. 12
    3. 24
    4. 48

14. Normal daily water intake and output (I&O) is approximately how many milliliters?

    1. 1500
    2. 2500
    3. 3500
    4. 6500

15. How many milliliters of urine per hour must the kidneys secrete to eliminate waste products from the body?

    1. 30
    2. 60
    3. 20
    4. 100

16. The normal pH of blood is approximately _____.

17. Which statement best describes the risk of fluid and electrolyte imbalances in the older adult?

    1. Most older adults can maintain fluid and electrolyte balance just as well as younger adults.
    2. Older adults have unlimited reserves to maintain fluid balance when abnormal losses occur.
    3. Body water increases with age, which puts the older adult at risk for fluid volume excess.
    4. Physiologic changes in the skin and mucous membranes decrease their reliability as indicators of dehydration.

18. The nurse is assigned a patient with a potassium imbalance. What assessment is most critical for this patient?

    1. Auscultate bowel sounds.
    2. Evaluate muscle strength.
    3. Monitor heart rate and rhythm.
    4. Assess reflexes.

19. The patient's potassium level is 5.2. When the nurse discusses dietary selections, the patient should be instructed to limit intake of what food items? *(Select all that apply.)*

    1. Orange juice
    2. Bananas
    3. Apples
    4. Tomatoes
    5. Red meat

20. Fluid balance is maintained in the body by which of the following systems? *(Select all that apply.)*

    1. Cardiac
    2. Respiratory
    3. Renal
    4. Hepatic
    5. Immune

21. A central line is preferred over a peripheral IV line under which conditions? *(Select all that apply.)*

    1. When irritating IV fluids are given
    2. In an infant
    3. When short-term IV therapy is required
    4. When the patient has poor peripheral veins
    5. When the patient is to receive chemotherapy

22. The nurse is assisting to prepare a nursing care plan for a patient with continuous IV infusions. What is the goal of IV therapy?

    1. Promote and maintain fluid and electrolyte balance.
    2. Promote drug blood levels when the patient is able to take liquid medication by mouth.
    3. Promote oxygen and carbon dioxide homeostasis.
    4. Balance plasma acidity levels.

23. The nurse is checking IV sites carefully for signs of infiltration. Which symptoms indicate infiltration at the IV site?

    1. Burning sensation, pain, and puffiness at the site
    2. Pain, heat, and puffiness at the site
    3. Burning sensation and numbness at the site
    4. Red streak up the arm

24. The nurse is assessing the IV site. If redness, swelling, and warmth are noted, what is the likely cause?

   1. Infiltration and air embolus
   2. Inflammation and possible phlebitis
   3. Blood loss and hemorrhage
   4. Embolus from the former catheter

25. An older adult patient is evaluated by the nurse for signs of fluid volume excess in association with IV therapy. Which symptom would indicate fluid volume excess in an elderly patient?

   1. Redness, warmth, and drainage of fluid at the IV site
   2. Decreased pulse and low urine output
   3. Complaints of shortness of breath and bounding pulse
   4. Puffiness of face, dyspnea, and decreased blood pressure

26. A patient's IV has infiltrated. When selecting a site for a new IV line, the nurse should perform which action?

   1. Choose an area proximal to the current site.
   2. Look for hard, cordlike veins.
   3. Use sites distal from the current site.
   4. Select the patient's dominant arm.

27. A patient complains of a headache, nausea, and vomiting during a blood transfusion. Which action is necessary for the nurse to take immediately?

   1. Check the vital signs.
   2. Stop the blood transfusion.
   3. Notify the health care provider and the blood bank personnel.
   4. Flush the IV line with normal saline.

28. Which nursing intervention is the most important in preventing the introduction of microorganisms to the patient when an IV infusion is initiated?

   1. Hand hygiene
   2. Checking the identification of the patient
   3. Ensuring the six rights of medication administration
   4. Carefully checking the order for the correct IV solution

29. The nurse demonstrates knowledge by choosing which needle gauge when starting a rapid transfusion of whole blood?

   1. 14- to 16-gauge
   2. 18- to 22-gauge
   3. 22- to 24-gauge
   4. 26- to 28-gauge

30. It has been 15 minutes since a blood infusion was initiated. What is most indicative that the patient is experiencing a blood transfusion reaction?

   1. The patient's blood pressure decreases.
   2. The patient feels an urgent need to void.
   3. The patient's skin is pale at the infusion site.
   4. Localized edema is noticed at the infusion site.

31. A woman, 83, does not answer her phone for 2 days, leading her son, who lives 40 miles away, to come check on her. He finds his mother a little quiet; she has trouble focusing on his questions, but otherwise she seems fine. Checking her apartment, he finds she has not done the dishes since yesterday—unusual for her— and he suspects that she hasn't eaten or had anything to drink all day. She weighs 230 lb and has hypertension, for which she keeps a blood pressure diary. She hasn't filled it out over the last 36 hours, however, so he takes her blood pressure, expecting to find it has skyrocketed, but he is shocked to find it is actually unusually low for her. She is light-headed on standing. He decides to drive her to an urgent care clinic, where her blood pressure reading is once again a bit low. Asked about her diet, she says, "I just haven't been very hungry. I'm having trouble going to the bathroom." Follow-up questions indicate that she is constipated. She has trouble producing a urine specimen, but when she does, it is a small amount and is dark, strong-smelling, and concentrated. She complains of irritated sinuses and, when asked about fluid intake, she says, "Oh, honey, I try not to drink anything after noon because, otherwise, I have to get up and pee in the night, and I hate that."

Given the symptoms observed in this patient, which steps below are most appropriate? Check all that apply.

___	A.	Assess for orthostatic hypotension and poor skin turgor.
___	B.	Assess closely for probable distended veins, especially around the neck, accompanied by decreased heart rate in response to low fluid levels.
___	C.	Monitor patient's sodium intake and teach sodium restriction.
___	D.	Monitor complete blood count for increased hematocrit in relation to hemoglobin.
___	E.	Request IV infusions that restore depleted blood serum levels of sodium and potassium.
___	F.	Teach family and caregivers the importance of skin and mucous membranes as reliable indicators of dehydration in the older adult.

Nutritional Concepts and Related Therapies

Objectives

1. Discuss the role of the nurse in promoting good nutrition.
2. Explain the use of diet planning guides in medical nutrition therapy.
3. List the six classes of essential nutrients, and identify those that provide energy.
4. List the functions and food sources of protein, carbohydrates, and fats.
5. List food sources and possible health benefits of dietary fiber.
6. Distinguish between saturated, unsaturated, and *trans* fats and cholesterol; identify current recommendations for dietary intake of fats and cholesterol.
7. Discuss key vitamins and minerals, their role in health, and their food sources.
8. Discuss changes in nutrient needs throughout the life cycle, and suggest ideas to ensure adequate nutrition during each stage of life.
9. Identify the effects of common medications on nutritional status.
10. Identify standard hospital diets and modifications for texture, consistency, and meal frequency.
11. List medical and surgical conditions that require a high-kilocalorie and high-protein diet, and suggest ways to increase kilocalories and protein in the diet.
12. Define obesity and list components of an effective weight management program.
13. Describe dietary management of type 1 and type 2 diabetes mellitus.
14. Describe fat-modified diets and list conditions requiring a fat-modified diet.
15. Identify medical and surgical conditions necessitating modifications in sodium, potassium, protein, or fluid intake, and describe the dietary adjustments necessary in these conditions.
16. Define enteral nutrition and parenteral nutrition, and list medical and surgical conditions in which nutritional support is often indicated.

Key Terms

amino acids (ă-MĒ-nō ĂS-ĭdz, p. 538)
anabolism (ă-NĂB-ŏ-lĭzm, p. 539)
basal metabolic rate (BMR) (BĀ-săl mĕt-ă-BŎL-ĭk rāt, p. 556)
body mass index (BMI) (BŎD-ē MĂS ĬN-dĕks, p. 557)
catabolism (kă-TĂB-ŏ-lĭsm, p. 539)
cholesterol (kŏ-LĔS-tŭr-ŏl, p. 538)
dietary fiber (DĪ-ĕ-tăr-ē FĪ-bŭr, p. 535)
dumping syndrome (DŬMP-ĭng SĬN-drōm, p. 561)
enteral nutrition (ĔN-tŭr-ăl nŭ-TRĪ-shŭn, p. 565)
essential nutrients (ē-SĔN-chŭl NŪ-trē-ŭnts, p. 534)
glycogen (GLĪ-kŏ-jĕn, p. 535)
hydrogenation (hī-drŏ-jĕn-Ā-shŭn, p. 537)
kilocalorie (kcal) (kĭl-ō-KĂL-ō-rē, p. 534)
lipids (LĬ-pĭdz, p. 537)
lipoproteins (lī-pō-PRŌ-tēnz, p. 538)

medical nutrition therapy (MĔD-ĭ-kŭl nŭ-TRĬSH-ŭn THĔR-ŭ-pē, p. 554)
nitrogen balance (NĪ-trŭ-jŭn BĂL-ŭns, p. 539)
nutrient (NŪ-trē-ŭnt, p. 534)
nutrient-dense foods (NŪ-trē-ŭnt–DĔNS FŪDZ, p. 548)
obesity (ō-BĒ-sĭt-ē, p. 557)
parenteral nutrition (pă-RĔN-tŭr-ăl nŭ-TRĬSH-ŭn, p. 568)
pernicious anemia (pŭr-NĬSH-ŭs ă-NĒ-mē-ă, p. 543)
residue (RĔZ-ĭ-dū, p. 555)
satiety (să-TĪ-ĕ-tē, p. 537)
therapeutic diet (thĕr-ŭ-PYŪ-tĭk DĪ-ĭt, p. 554)
total parenteral nutrition (TPN) (TŌ-tŭl pă-RĔN-tŭr-ăl nŭ-TRĬSH-ŭn, p. 538)
tube feeding (TŪB FĒD-ĭng, p. 565)
vegan (VĒ-găn, p. 539)

Nutrition is the sum of all processes involved in taking in nutrients and using them to maintain body tissue and provide energy. It is one of the foundations for life. Over the past century, tremendous progress has been made to improve the general level of health in all people, and health care providers have continued to realize that good nutrition is essential for optimal health throughout all stages of life. Eating the right kinds and amounts of food and following good dietary habits throughout one's entire life means a healthier body and mind, greater vitality and energy, and greater resistance to disease. Nurses must always consider the patient's nutritional state and evaluate the patient's nutritional history to plan quality patient care.

ROLE OF THE NURSE IN PROMOTING NUTRITION

Because the nurse spends a considerable amount of time caring for patients, patients look to the nurse as a source of health information. The licensed practical nurse (LPN/LVN) may be responsible for assisting a patient to eat, recording a patient's intake, observing a patient for signs of poor nutrition, and communicating any dietary concerns to the health care provider, dietitian, and other members of the health care team. Developing knowledge of basic nutritional principals is needed to aid patients in making appropriate nutritional choices and understanding the implications of dietary intake.

BASIC NUTRITION

DIET PLANNING GUIDES

To help people maintain optimal nutrition, most of the developed countries of the world have adopted nutrition standards. These standards are guidelines describing how good dietary habits can promote health and reduce the risk for major chronic diseases.

Over the years, these nutritional guidelines have changed in accordance with the growing knowledge of how nutrition affects health. The guidelines started as a farmers' bulletin more than 100 years ago and then evolved to the Basic Seven, the Basic Four, the Food Guide Pyramid, MyPyramid, and currently MyPlate.

MyPlate

MyPlate (Fig. 19.1) was developed in the United States by the US Department of Agriculture (USDA) and introduced in 2011. MyPlate is an image of a round plate divided into four different color sections. The colored areas show people how much they should eat from three of the four food groups: vegetables and fruits,

Fig. 19.1 MyPlate. (From the US Department of Agriculture, www.ChooseMyPlate.gov.)

grains, and proteins. A smaller circle next to the plate represents the fourth food group, dairy. Along with the image, the USDA suggests that people balance calories by reducing portions; increase intake of fruits, vegetables, and whole grains; and reduce the amount of sodium and sugary foods in the diet.

By developing this simple, visually graphic image and combining it with a few easy rules, the USDA hoped to eliminate the confusion that existed with previous guidelines and help people make better food choices (Box 19.1).

Dietary Guidelines for Americans

The US Department of Health and Human Services and the USDA have developed dietary guidelines for the US population. The *Dietary Guidelines for Americans 2015 to 2020* (USDHHS and USDA, 2015; USDHHS and USDA, n.d.) is the most current of these guidelines; it focuses on healthy eating patterns as a whole rather than on individual nutrients or foods. The recommendations are intended to help people choose an overall healthy diet. These guidelines emphasize balancing calories with activity to manage weight; consuming a variety of fruits, vegetables, and whole grains; increasing fat-free or low-fat dairy products, lean meats and seafood; and consuming less sodium, saturated fat, *trans* fat, cholesterol, added sugars, and refined grains.

The *Dietary Guidelines for Americans 2015 to 2020* (USDHHS and USDA, 2015) is used to form the US federal nutrition policy and directly affects federal nutrition programs such as food stamps, school breakfast and lunch programs, and the Special Supplemental Nutrition Program for Women, Infants, and Children (WIC).

The government developed these guidelines to address the importance of adequate nutrition, as well as the prevention of overnutrition and chronic disease. They are intended for healthy children (aged 2 years and older) and adults of any age (Box 19.2).

Dietary Reference Intakes

Dietary reference intake (DRI) refers to a set of nutrient-based values for evaluating and planning diets. The DRIs replace and expand on the recommended dietary allowances (RDAs), which have been used for more than 50 years in the United States. The DRIs are a combination of the RDAs, adequate intake, tolerable upper intake level, and the estimated average requirement of each nutrient. The purpose of DRIs is to help individuals optimize their health, prevent disease, and avoid consuming too much of a nutrient. For more information on DRIs and *Dietary Guidelines for Americans*, visit the USDA website at *www.nutrition.gov/smart-nutrition-101*.

Nutrition Facts Label

Because of heightened awareness of nutrition, Americans are learning to pick healthier foods and are

Box 19.1   **Choose MyPlate: 10 Tips to a Great Plate**

United States Department of Agriculture

10 tips
Nutrition
Education Series

Based on the
**Dietary
Guidelines
for Americans**

Build a healthy meal

Each meal is a building block in your healthy eating style. Make sure to include all the food groups throughout the day. Make fruits, vegetables, grains, dairy, and protein foods part of your daily meals and snacks. Also, limit added sugars, saturated fat, and sodium. Use the MyPlate Daily Checklist and the tips below to meet your needs throughout the day.

1 Make half your plate veggies and fruits
Vegetables and fruits are full of nutrients that support good health. Choose fruits and red, orange, and dark-green vegetables such as tomatoes, sweet potatoes, and broccoli.

2 Include whole grains
Aim to make at least half your grains whole grains. Look for the words "100% whole grain" or "100% whole wheat" on the food label. Whole grains provide more nutrients, like fiber, than refined grains.

3 Don't forget the dairy
Complete your meal with a cup of fat-free or low-fat milk. You will get the same amount of calcium and other essential nutrients as whole milk but fewer calories. Don't drink milk? Try a soy beverage (soymilk) as your drink or include low-fat yogurt in your meal or snack.

4 Add lean protein

Choose protein foods such as lean beef, pork, chicken, or turkey, and eggs, nuts, beans, or tofu. Twice a week, make seafood the protein on your plate.

5 Avoid extra fat
Using heavy gravies or sauces will add fat and calories to otherwise healthy choices. Try steamed broccoli with a sprinkling of low-fat parmesan cheese or a squeeze of lemon.

6 Get creative in the kitchen
Whether you are making a sandwich, a stir-fry, or a casserole, find ways to make them healthier. Try using less meat and cheese, which can be higher in saturated fat and sodium, and adding in more veggies that add new flavors and textures to your meals.

7 Take control of your food

Eat at home more often so you know exactly what you are eating. If you eat out, check and compare the nutrition information. Choose options that are lower in calories, saturated fat, and sodium.

8 Try new foods
Keep it interesting by picking out new foods you've never tried before, like mango, lentils, quinoa, kale, or sardines. You may find a new favorite! Trade fun and tasty recipes with friends or find them online.

9 Satisfy your sweet tooth in a healthy way
Indulge in a naturally sweet dessert dish—fruit! Serve a fresh fruit salad or a fruit parfait made with yogurt. For a hot dessert, bake apples and top with cinnamon.

10 Everything you eat and drink matters
The right mix of foods in your meals and snacks can help you be healthier now and into the future. Turn small changes in how you eat into your MyPlate, MyWins.

Center for Nutrition Policy and Promotion
USDA is an equal opportunity provider, employer, and lender.

Go to **ChooseMyPlate.gov**
for more information.

DG TipSheet No. 7
June 2011
Revised October 2016

From USDA: MyPlate. Refer to: https://health.gov/sites/default/files/2019-09/2015-2020_Dietary_Guidelines.pdf.

Box 19.2 2015–2020 Dietary Guidelines for Americans

THE GUIDELINES

1. **Follow a healthy eating pattern across the lifespan.** All food and beverage choices matter. Choose a healthy eating pattern at an appropriate calorie level to help achieve and maintain a healthy body weight, support nutrient adequacy, and reduce the risk of chronic disease.

2. **Focus on variety, nutrient density, and amount.** To meet nutrient needs within calorie limits, choose a variety of nutrient-dense foods across and within all food groups in recommended amounts.

3. **Limit calories from added sugars and saturated fats and reduce sodium intake.** Consume an eating pattern low in added sugars, saturated fats, and sodium. Cut back on foods and beverages higher in these components to amounts that fit within healthy eating patterns.

4. **Shift to healthier food and beverage choices.** Choose nutrient-dense foods and beverages across and within all food groups in place of less healthy choices. Consider cultural and personal preferences to make these shifts easier to accomplish and maintain.

5. **Support healthy eating patterns for all.** Everyone has a role in helping to create and support healthy eating patterns in multiple settings nationwide, from home to school to work to communities.

KEY RECOMMENDATIONS

Consume a healthy eating pattern that accounts for all foods and beverages within an appropriate calorie level.

A healthy eating pattern includes:

- A variety of vegetables from all of the subgroups—dark green, red and orange, legumes (beans and peas), starchy, and other
- Fruits, especially whole fruits
- Grains, at least half of which are whole grains
- Fat-free or low-fat dairy, including milk, yogurt, cheese, and/or fortified soy beverages
- A variety of protein foods, including seafood, lean meats and poultry, eggs, legumes (beans and peas), and nuts, seeds, and soy products
- Oils

A healthy eating pattern limits:

- Saturated fats and trans fats, added sugars, and sodium Key recommendations that are quantitative are provided for several components of the diet that should be limited. These components are of particular public health concern in the United States, and the specified limits can help individuals achieve healthy eating patterns within calorie limits:
- Consume less than 10% of calories per day from added sugars
- Consume less than 10% of calories per day from saturated fats
- Consume less than 2300 milligrams (mg) per day of sodium
- If alcohol is consumed, it should be consumed in moderation—up to one drink per day for women and up to two drinks per day for men—and only by adults of legal drinking age.

---

demanding that more healthy foods be made available in restaurants, vending machines, and grocery stores. To assist with this, the FDA has mandated that Nutrition Facts labels be included on all packaged foods and that restaurants make this information available to their patrons.

The FDA currently requires that the product's ingredients be listed on the label in descending order by weight. That means that there is more of the first ingredient listed on the label, based on weight, and the rest of the ingredients listed are less prevalent in the product.

The label (see Fig. 19.3) currently also must list calories from fat, total amount of fat, saturated fat, *trans* fats, and cholesterol. It also must include the amount of proteins, carbohydrates, sodium, vitamins A and C, calcium, and iron.

In 2018, the FDA set forth the Nutrition Innovation Strategy, whose goal is to reduce preventable death and disease related to poor nutrition. The initiative includes the introduction of interactive food labels, social media information and educational materials (FDA, n.d.). The FDA promotes accuracy in packaged food labels, simplified labels and updated designs (see Fig. 19.3).

ESSENTIAL NUTRIENTS

Basic Functions

A **nutrient** is a chemical compound or element necessary for good health that is found in food. **Essential** **nutrients** are nutrients that the body cannot make in the amounts essential for good health, making it necessary to obtain these nutrients through the diet or from other sources. There are six classes of essential nutrients: carbohydrates, fats, proteins, vitamins, minerals, and water. Each is necessary for life. Three major functions of nutrients include (1) providing energy, (2) building and repairing tissue, and (3) regulating body processes.

Providing energy. A **kilocalorie (kcal)** is a measurement of energy, much as a pound is a measurement of weight. If a certain food has X number of kilocalories, it provides that amount of energy. The more kilocalories a food has, the more energy it provides. Of the six essential nutrients, three provide energy: carbohydrates, fats, and proteins. Vitamins, minerals, and water do not provide energy but are nonetheless essential nutrients. Carbohydrates and protein provide approximately 4 kcal/g, whereas fat provides 9 kcal/g. Nutrition experts recommend obtaining about 45% to 65% of daily kilocalories from carbohydrates, 20% to 35% from fat, and 10% to 35% from protein. This distribution is called the *caloric distribution* of the diet.

Building and repairing tissue. Many nutrients are necessary for building and repairing tissue, but the nutrient that plays the biggest role is protein. It contains the amino acids that the body uses to build and repair tissue. Calcium and phosphorus, both minerals, are necessary nutrients in bone structure, and iron, another mineral, makes up a large part of the hemoglobin in red blood cells. Fat also plays a role in building and repairing tissues; it is found in all cell walls.

Regulating body processes. *Metabolism* is the combination of all chemical processes that take place in living organisms. It is a continuous process of building and breaking down tissues. Nutrients play various roles in metabolism and thereby help regulate certain body processes. For example, the presence of carbohydrates is required for fat to be used correctly and completely. The B vitamins are necessary for the body to derive energy from foods. Water is an integral part of almost all chemical reactions in the body. By studying how the body uses nutrients, researchers have found out two important facts: (1) individual nutrients have many functions in the body, and (2) no nutrient works alone.

Carbohydrates

Carbohydrates (CHO) are organic compounds containing carbon, hydrogen, and oxygen. The main function of carbohydrates is to provide energy. However, they also are needed in adequate amounts to keep protein from being used as an energy source. Carbohydrates are classified as either simple or complex according to the number of sugar units they contain (Table 19.1).

Simple carbohydrates. Carbohydrates are made of molecular units called *saccharides,* or sugar units. The simple carbohydrates (often called *simple sugars*) include the monosaccharides and the disaccharides. Monosaccharides have only one sugar unit. They require no digestion and are absorbed directly into the blood. Fructose, the sugar found naturally in fruits, is a monosaccharide. Another important monosaccharide is glucose. Glucose often is called "blood glucose" because it is the major form of saccharides, or sugar, in the blood.

Disaccharides are made up of two sugar units bonded together. Once taken into the body, disaccharides are reduced by hydrolysis into monosaccharides before being absorbed. Table sugar (sucrose) and the sugar found naturally in milk (lactose) are examples of disaccharides (see Table 19.1).

Simple carbohydrates are part of a healthy diet. However, in the United States, refined sugar consumption is high and is contributing to an increase in obesity. Table sugar and sweeteners such as honey and corn syrup are high in kilocalories, have low nutritive value, and contribute to dental caries (cavities). DRIs relating to carbohydrates indicate that 45% to 65% of an adult's total calorie intake should be in the form of carbohydrates and that added sugars should be limited to no more than 8% (approximately 40 g) of the total number of calories consumed daily. Simple sugars are found naturally in many nutritious foods such as milk and fruit and should not be excluded from the

diet. Encourage people to use moderation in their consumption of added sugars, sweets, and soft drinks.

Complex carbohydrates. Complex carbohydrates are termed *polysaccharides* because they are made of long chains of glucose (sugar) units. The three types of complex carbohydrates, or polysaccharides, include starch, glycogen, and dietary fiber. Starch is found in many plant foods such as grains, legumes, and vegetables, particularly starchy vegetables such as corn and potatoes. It also is found in small amounts in some fruits. All carbohydrates, including complex carbohydrates, break down into simple sugars when they are digested, but because starch is a larger, more complex molecule, it breaks down more slowly and provides energy over a longer period.

Glycogen, also called *animal starch,* is the stored form of carbohydrates. It is made from simple sugars and stored mainly in the liver and in muscles. It is used when the body's blood glucose level is low.

Dietary fiber refers to foods that humans cannot break down (digest). It is found mostly in plants and, like polysaccharides, is made of long chains of glucose units. Most of the fiber consumed eventually is

| | **Table 19.1** | **Summary of Carbohydrate Classification** |

CHEMICAL CLASS	CLASS MEMBERS	DIETARY SOURCES
Simple Carbohydrate		
Monosaccharides	Glucose	Dextrose, corn syrup
	Fructose	Fruits, honey, high-fructose corn syrup
	Galactose	Milk (only found in lactose)
Disaccharides	Sucrose	Table sugar, sugarcane, beet sugar, powdered and brown sugar, fruits
	Lactose	Milk
	Maltose	Malted grain products
Complex Carbohydrate		
Polysaccharides	Starch	Grains and grain products (e.g., cereals, breads, crackers, pasta, rice, legumes, corn, potatoes, vegetables)
	Glycogen	No significant dietary source (storage form of carbohydrate in animal tissue)
	Dietary fiber	Whole grains, legumes, fruits, vegetables, nuts, seeds

excreted in the feces and has no nutritive value. One benefit of fiber is that it provides roughage, or bulk, which is important for health maintenance. It can lower cholesterol and blood glucose levels and assist in weight loss. Dietary fiber is classified based on its ability to dissolve in water. Both types of fiber, soluble and insoluble, provide a variety of health benefits and should be included in a healthy diet.

Insoluble fiber is found in wheat bran, vegetables, whole grains, and some fibrous fruits. Insoluble fiber softens stools, speeds transit of foods through the digestive tract, and reduces pressure in the colon. Constipation and the risk of certain gastrointestinal (GI) disorders such as diverticulosis or hemorrhoids are associated to fiber intake.

Water-soluble fiber is found in fruits, oats, barley, and legumes. It binds with bile acids and cholesterol in the digestive tract to prevent their absorption. This helps lower cholesterol levels and reduces the risk of cardiovascular disease. *Soluble fiber* attracts water and turns to gel during digestion, thus slowing digestion. This provides a feeling of fullness and may aid in weight loss (Fig. 19.2).

Daily requirements. Many health organizations have recommended increasing the intake of complex carbohydrates and dietary fiber. Current DRI recommendations are that 45% to 65% of total calories should come from carbohydrates. Fiber intake should be between 25 and 38 g/day, depending on age and gender. The *Dietary Guidelines for Americans* (USDHHS and USDA, 2015; USDHHS and USDA, n.d.) and the MyPlate guide recommend increasing fruit and vegetable intake and consuming at least half of all grains as whole grains, not refined grains. Health care providers should encourage patients to choose carbohydrates and fiber closer to the whole state rather than in a refined or processed state to increase the nutritive value of the diet.

Although eating enough fiber is important in a healthy diet, there may be hazards to consuming too much fiber. Sudden increases in fiber can cause bloating, gas, and constipation. This can be avoided by slowly increasing fiber content in the diet and by adding at least 8 glasses of water a day. In addition, too much fiber can interfere with mineral absorption, which can lead to problems such as osteoporosis and anemia. It is suggested that adequate fiber be obtained by eating appropriate amounts of fruits and vegetables rather than adding fiber supplements. For more specific information concerning the fiber content of selected foods, check the Nutrition Facts label of that food (Fig. 19.3).

Digestion and metabolism of carbohydrates. Digestion of carbohydrates begins in the mouth with mechanical digestion. Chewing breaks up the food (carbohydrates) into small pieces so that it can be swallowed. In the stomach, mechanical digestion continues so that the pieces are broken down into even smaller parts and combined with gastric secretions. Once the pieces are in the small intestine, chemical digestion begins in full force. Enzymes from the intestinal wall and the pancreas aid in digesting the carbohydrates.

All carbohydrates except fiber are broken down in the digestive tract into monosaccharides (single-sugar units) before they are absorbed and eventually converted to glucose. Glucose circulates in the bloodstream and is used by the cells for energy.

When the body's energy needs are met, the extra carbohydrates are converted to glycogen, which is

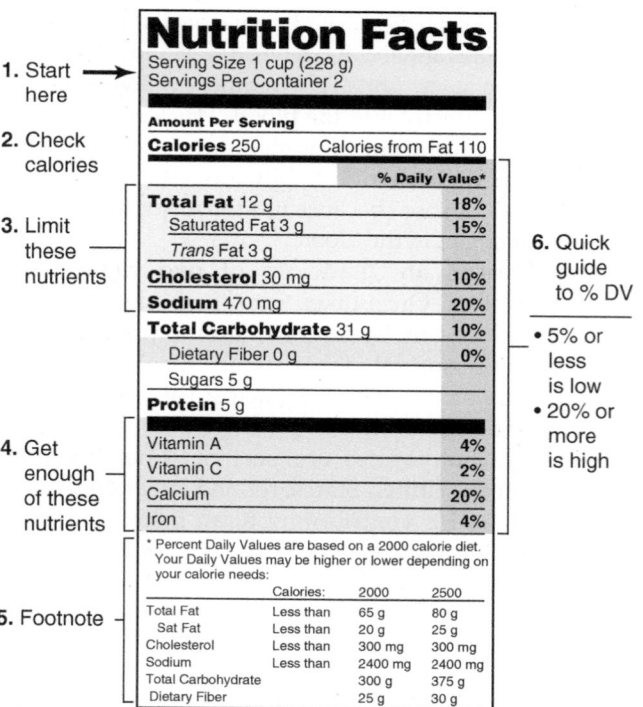

Fig. 19.3 Example of Nutrition Facts label. The food label provides a variety of information. Using the numbers listed provided a means to review and understand the information listed. (From https://www.fda.gov/Food/GuidanceRegulation/GuidanceDocumentsRegulatoryInformation/LabelingNutrition/ucm385663.htm.)

Soluble Fiber	Insoluble Fiber
Oat bran, barley, nuts, seeds, citrus, apples, strawberries, and many vegetables	Whole wheat and grains, vegetables and wheat bran

Fig. 19.2 Examples of sources of soluble and insoluble fiber.

stored in the liver and muscles until it is needed. Once glycogen stores in the liver and muscles are full, the body converts the remaining carbohydrates to fat and stores them as adipose tissue.

Fats (Lipids)

Lipids are organic substances of a fatty nature that are insoluble in water and necessary for good health. Fats and cholesterol are lipids.

Lipids perform many functions in the body. They provide the most concentrated source of energy of all the nutrients (9 kcal/g) and can be used either directly from the fat in foods or from adipose tissue, the body's stored form of fat. As *adipose tissue,* fat helps insulate the body from temperature extremes and acts as a cushion to protect organs and other tissues from being bumped or jarred. Fat is also a component of all cell membranes.

Dietary fat provides satiety, a feeling of fullness and satisfaction from food. It adds flavor and aroma to foods and provides the body with the essential fatty acids linoleic acid and linolenic acid. Dietary fat also carries the fat-soluble vitamins: A, D, E, and K.

Like carbohydrates, lipids are composed of carbon, hydrogen, and oxygen. Unlike carbohydrates, lipids contain fatty acids and glycerol. Because of this, lipids also may be called *glycerides* or, more specifically, *triglycerides* because most of the fat in the body is a combination of three fatty acids that combine with one glycerol unit.

Fatty acids, the building blocks of fat, are classified as either saturated or unsaturated. All fats and oils contain a combination of saturated and unsaturated fatty acids in various proportions.

Saturated fatty acids. A saturated fatty acid is one whose chemical bonds are filled completely, or saturated, with hydrogen. Saturated fats are generally of animal origin and are solid at room temperature. Because the chemical bond in saturated fats is so strong, they tend to take a long time to spoil, or become rancid, which allows them to have a long shelf life. Food sources of saturated fatty acids can be found in Table 19.2.

Saturated fats, although an important part of a healthy diet, tend to increase blood cholesterol levels, thus increasing the risk for atherosclerosis (the buildup of fatty deposits on the artery walls) and heart disease. In response to the effects of saturated fats the American Heart Association recommends that they be limited to only 5% to 6% of the dietary intake.

Unsaturated fatty acids. An unsaturated fatty acid has one or more places on its chemical chain in which hydrogen is missing. These are called *points of unsaturation.* A fatty acid with only one point of unsaturation is called a *monounsaturated fatty acid.* Fatty acids with two or more points of unsaturation are termed *polyunsaturated.* Most unsaturated fats are from plant sources and are liquid at

Table 19.2 Food Sources of Fatty Acids	
FATTY ACID CLASS	**FOODS CONTRIBUTING SIGNIFICANT AMOUNTS TO THE DIET**
Saturated	Coconut, palm, and palm kernel oils (tropical oils) Fat in and on meats and poultry Egg yolk Butter, cream, milk fat Cocoa butter Olive oil, olives
Monounsaturated	Canola oil Peanuts and peanut oil Most other nuts Avocados
Polyunsaturated	Safflower oil Sunflower oil Cottonseed oil Soybean oil Corn oil Most fish oil
Trans	Partially hydrogenated plant and fish oils Stick margarines, shortening Commercial fats used for frying, baking

room temperature. Sources of monounsaturated fats and polyunsaturated fats are listed in Table 19.2. Unsaturated fats, especially monounsaturated fats, are thought to lower low-density lipoprotein (LDL) cholesterol, especially when combined with lower intake of saturated fat and *trans* fat.

Hydrogenated fats. Hydrogenation is a process in which hydrogen is added to a fat of vegetable origin (unsaturated) to make it more saturated or solid. This then makes the oil more stable and less susceptible to becoming rancid. When only some of the hydrogen has been replaced, the oil is considered partially hydrogenated. Most vegetable spreads, such as corn oil margarine, have been hydrogenated to some extent.

Trans fatty acids. Trans fatty acids are unsaturated fatty acids that have been completely hydrogenated. Synthetic *trans* fatty acids are produced during hydrogenation and can be found in some deep-fried restaurant foods; packaged cookies, crackers, and other baked goods; some margarines; and shortening. Naturally occurring *trans* fatty acids are found in smaller amounts in dairy products and some meats. *Trans* fatty acids in the diet are similar to saturated fats and tend to increase blood cholesterol levels. They should be used sparingly in a healthy diet.

The American Heart Association recommends healthy individuals older than 2 years old obtain 25% to 35% of their total calories from fat, with less than 5% to 6% of total calories from saturated fats and less than 1% of total calories from *trans* fatty acids.

Cholesterol. **Cholesterol** is a lipid belonging to a class of chemical substances called *sterols*. Cholesterol is a building block for cell membranes and for hormones, such as estrogen and testosterone. It is synthesized in the liver and is found in foods of animal origin. Plant foods and oils do not contain cholesterol. In fact, plant sterols sometimes decrease cholesterol levels in the blood. The amounts of *dietary cholesterol* (the cholesterol found in foods) are highest in organ meats and egg yolks. Dietary cholesterol is also present in smaller but significant amounts in seafood, meats, poultry, and dairy products. Low-fat dairy products have less cholesterol than their higher-fat counterparts. The recommended intake of dietary cholesterol is an average of no more than 300 mg/day. Decreasing the intake of animal fats helps decrease the amount of dietary cholesterol consumed.

Digestion and metabolism of fat. For fat to be digested, it must be emulsified, or broken into smaller globules. Bile, a secretion of the liver, is necessary to emulsify fat. Bile is stored in the gallbladder and dispensed into the duodenum when fat is present. Once fats are emulsified, the body can break them down and absorb them.

After absorption, lipids are packaged as lipoproteins. **Lipoproteins** are molecules made of lipids surrounded by protein. They facilitate the transport of lipids in the bloodstream. The human body makes four types of lipoproteins: chylomicrons, high-density lipoproteins (HDLs), LDLs, and very low–density lipoproteins (VLDLs). The amounts of fat and protein in each of these lipoproteins vary. The higher the protein content of the lipoprotein, the greater the density. The type and amount of lipoproteins in the blood can protect the body from, or predispose it to, heart disease. LDLs and HDLs are important in the study of cardiovascular disease. Both of these lipoproteins carry cholesterol in the bloodstream. It appears that the cholesterol found in LDLs increases the risk of atherosclerosis by contributing to plaque buildup on the artery walls. In contrast, HDLs seem to have the opposite effect. HDLs transport cholesterol from the bloodstream to the liver to be degraded and excreted. LDLs sometimes are referred to as carrying "bad" cholesterol, whereas HDLs are referred to as carrying "good" cholesterol.

The National Institutes of Health (NIH) recommend that total serum cholesterol levels stay below 180 mg/dL. Teaching should be aimed at reducing LDL levels and increasing or maintaining HDL levels. Table 19.3 classifies the blood cholesterol values used to determine health risk. To lower cholesterol levels and maintain a healthy diet, the *Dietary Guidelines for Americans* (USDHHS and USDA, 2015; USDHHS and USDA, n.d.) recommend increasing the amount of seafood consumed to reduce the amount of cholesterol-containing meat and poultry and to replace foods containing higher solid fats with ones that contain unsaturated fats. The guidelines also recommend using oils instead of solid fats when possible.

Table 19.3 Classification of Low-Density Lipoprotein, Total, and High-Density Lipoprotein Cholesterol

LDL Cholesterol	
<100 mg/dL	Optimal
100–129 mg/dL	Near or above optimal
130–159 mg/dL	Borderline high
160–189 mg/dL	High
≥190 mg/dL	Very high
Total Cholesterol	
<200 mg/dL	Desirable
200–239 mg/dL	Borderline high
≥240 mg/dL	High
HDL Cholesterol	
<40 mg/dL for men; <50 mg/dL for women	Low

HDL, High-density lipoprotein; *LDL*, low-density lipoprotein.
Data from National Cholesterol Education Program: *ATP III executive summary*, 2001, rev. 2004; Toth PP: The "good cholesterol": High-density lipoprotein. *Circulation* 111:e89, 2005.

Protein

Protein is another nutrient vital to the human body. Proteins provide the building blocks for blood and bone, and they are a structural part of every cell. The human body contains thousands of different proteins, all of which are essential for tissue growth, repair, and wound healing. Collagen, a vital connective tissue, is made of protein. Some hormones, including thyroxine and insulin, are proteins. Enzymes are proteins produced by living cells. They cause chemical reactions within the body without being changed in the process. They are necessary for digestion and metabolism. The plasma proteins aid in fluid balance within the body. Albumin, a plasma protein, attracts water and has the capacity to pull fluid from one body compartment to another. Hemoglobin, a protein in the red blood cells, carries oxygen throughout the body. Immunoglobulins (antibodies) are also proteins, which emphasizes the role of protein in immune function.

If necessary, the body can use protein for energy. It supplies 4 kcal/g. However, if the body uses protein as an energy source, it is no longer available for any other function; thus proteins responsible for the building and repairing of tissues cannot perform their usual function.

Carbohydrates, fat, and protein contain carbon, hydrogen, and oxygen, but protein is unique in that it also contains nitrogen. All these elements—carbon, hydrogen, oxygen, and nitrogen—combine in specific ways to form amino acids. **Amino acids** are the building blocks of protein. Approximately 20 amino acids have been identified as important to the body's metabolism, but only nine of them are considered indispensable (*essential*) *amino acids*; because the body does not make them in sufficient quantity to sustain health, it is necessary to obtain them from the diet. The body can manufacture adequate amounts of the other amino acids from the indispensable (essential) amino acids.

The recommendation is for 10% to 35% of total daily calories to come from protein. The DRI for protein in healthy adults is 0.8 g/kg of body weight per day. Protein needs are increased during periods of severe illness or stress. During pregnancy the need for an increase in protein intake occurs in order to support the growth of the baby and to support changes in the body. Approximately 6 extra grams of protein per day is necessary.

Complete proteins. Food proteins are classified according to the number and kind of amino acids they contain. A complete protein is one that contains all nine essential amino acids in sufficient quantity and ratio for the body's needs. Complete proteins are generally of animal origin and are found in foods such as meat, poultry, fish, milk, cheese, eggs, and soy products.

Incomplete proteins. Incomplete proteins are those that are lacking in one or more of the essential amino acids. Incomplete proteins are of plant origin. This includes the protein in grains, legumes, nuts, and seeds. Even though the proteins in these foods are considered incomplete, these foods should not be avoided. By combining a variety of incomplete proteins in the diet, the body can obtain the necessary balance of the essential amino acids.

Vegetarian diets. For people who choose to limit their intake of animal foods, obtaining sufficient amounts of protein may be challenging. Depending on the preferences of the person following a vegetarian diet, the diet may vary, and the amount of protein may or may not be adequate to meet the body's needs. There are a variety of "vegetarian" diets, and the nurse should ask specific questions about what the patient wishes to consume and what is to be avoided. A typical vegetarian diet is made up of mainly plant foods. Some vegetarian diets include dairy products or eggs, or both, as well. Legumes play an important role in vegetarian diets. Legumes are plants that have nitrogen-fixing bacteria in their roots. These nitrogen-fixing bacteria lock nitrogen into the plant's structure, thereby increasing its protein content. Legumes contain two to three times as much protein as most vegetables. Most vegetarian diets supply sufficient protein if a variety of allowed foods are eaten throughout the day. However, the strictest vegetarian diet, the **vegan** diet, excludes all animal products, and more planning is required to obtain sufficient protein. To offset this deficit, vegans consume soybeans, soy milk, and other soy products to enhance protein intake. Strict vegetarians also need to include a reliable source of vitamin B_{12} in the diet, because vitamin B_{12} is found exclusively in animal foods.

Studies of those opting for a vegetarian diet indicate that they, because of their dietary choices, may be at lower risk for various chronic diseases such as coronary artery disease, colon cancer, obesity, and type 2 diabetes.

Digestion and metabolism of protein. Protein-containing foods are the body's only external source of nitrogen. Once a protein-containing food is eaten, the nitrogen is removed from the amino acid, and some of it is excreted as urea nitrogen in the urine. The nitrogen that is not excreted is then used to make other amino acids. **Nitrogen balance,** or nitrogen equilibrium, is achieved when the amount of nitrogen (protein) taken in is equal to the amount of nitrogen excreted in the urine. Although a healthy adult is generally in a state of nitrogen balance, under certain circumstances nitrogen balance may be either positive or negative.

Positive nitrogen balance. A positive nitrogen balance exists when more nitrogen is taken in than is excreted. In this situation, the body is building more tissue (**anabolism**) than it is breaking down. This is seen during periods of growth, such as infancy, childhood, adolescence, and pregnancy.

Negative nitrogen balance. A negative nitrogen balance exists when less nitrogen is being consumed than is being excreted. This condition occurs when insufficient protein is being taken in and the body is breaking down more tissue (**catabolism**) than it is building. Nitrogen balance is negative in states of undernutrition, illness, and trauma. Skipping protein food for one day is not likely to create a negative nitrogen balance, so noticeable physical signs are not likely to occur. In contrast, prolonged negative nitrogen balance eventually can cause atrophy of muscles, as well as poor functioning of all body systems.

When protein is consumed in amounts greater than the body needs, the amino acids are changed chemically, converted to fat, and stored as adipose tissue. Therefore more dietary protein does not necessarily make more muscle; it may create more adipose tissue.

Excess dietary protein is sometimes unhealthy. Usually high-protein diets are also high in saturated fats, which increase the risk for cardiovascular disease. High-protein diets also tend to cause excretion of more calcium, thereby increasing the risk for osteoporosis. Too much dietary protein also places an excessive burden on the kidneys, which could possibly lead to renal insufficiency or renal failure.

Protein energy malnutrition. When there is a lack of energy or protein intake, protein energy malnutrition (PEM) may result. PEM is fairly common in children and adults in developing countries, and malnutrition is associated with more than half the deaths of children younger than 5 years worldwide. In developed countries, PEM is found most often in hospital settings, usually is associated with disease, and is more common in older adults. Two types of PEM exist: marasmus and kwashiorkor.

Marasmus is a protein deficiency that affects people of all ages. It involves a deficiency of protein, as well as of all other energy-providing foods. It is a chronic condition characterized by wasting of body tissues. As the disease progresses, subcutaneous fat stores and then muscle stores are depleted, leaving the victim with a "skin-and-bones" appearance (Fig. 19.4A).

Kwashiorkor occurs as a result of severe protein restriction in the presence of other calories. It occurs most often in children in developing countries, with onset at approximately the time the child is weaned from breastfeeding. Kwashiorkor is characterized by edema in the feet, legs, and often in the face and hands (see Fig. 19.4B). There also may be swelling in the abdomen. This swelling of the abdomen is due to ascites related to hypoalbuminemia and the resulting low oncotic pressure, as well as an enlarged fatty liver. As a result of the abdominal swelling, the child sometimes appears "fat," and the parents regard the child as well fed.

PEM usually is accompanied by multiple nutrient deficiencies and can lead to stunted growth and impaired cognitive development in children, reduced mental and physical capacity, and lowered resistance to infections.

Vitamins

Vitamins are organic compounds that are essential in small quantities for normal metabolism and for growth and maintenance of the body. Organic compounds are derived from living matter and contain carbon. Vitamins themselves are not sources of energy; they work in conjunction with other nutrients in the body to regulate many processes, including energy production. Because the amount of vitamins needed by the body is so small, they sometimes are referred to as *micronutrients*.

Many compounds, including vitamins, are susceptible to destruction by heat, light, and exposure to air. Therefore some of the vitamin content may be lost when foods are prepared or stored, resulting in value of the nutrient being lessened (Box 19.3).

Vitamins have many functions in the body, and those functions are specific to each vitamin. One vitamin cannot perform the functions of another. If an insufficient amount of vitamin C is taken in, the deficiency cannot be corrected by vitamin D.

Vitamins are classified by whether they are soluble in fat or soluble in water. Vitamins A, D, E, and K are fat soluble. Fat-soluble vitamins are absorbed from the intestine in the same way as fats, and, like fats, they can be stored in the body. Because of this storage capacity, excessive intake of fat-soluble vitamins, especially A and D, can lead to toxicity and death.

The water-soluble vitamins are those that dissolve in water and include the B vitamins and vitamin C. The body is not readily able to store these vitamins because they are water soluble, and excesses generally are excreted in the urine. Daily intake of these vitamins is necessary because body reserves are minimal. Table 19.4 lists all the vitamins with their food sources, their functions, and symptoms of deficiency and toxicity.

A memory trick to recall the water-soluble vitamins is to think of the letters ADEK as sounding like the word "attic" and remembering that household items are often stored in the attic, just as fat-soluble vitamins are stored in the body. In contrast, the student could remember that "Boats and Canoes" go in water, just as the vitamins B and C are water soluble.

Fig. 19.4 Protein energy malnutrition. (A) Marasmus. (B) Kwashiorkor. (Courtesy Centers for Disease Control and Prevention.)

Antioxidant vitamins. Certain vitamins have attracted public interest and are of interest to health care professionals in the treatment of some diseases. These vitamins, E, C, and A (in the previtamin form, discussed later), have been found to delay or prevent the destruction or breakdown of cell membranes in the presence of oxygen (antioxidants) and thereby reduce the risk of developing certain cancers, inflammatory diseases, Alzheimer disease, and heart disease. The link between these vitamins and disease has led to recommendations to increase intake of foods high in vitamins. Thus a focus on eating more fruits and vegetables is the current recommendation to delay or prevent these diseases.

Vitamin C. Vitamin C, or ascorbic acid, has many functions in the body. It contributes to the healing of wounds, burns, and fractures; it serves as an antioxidant; and it is

---

Box 19.3	**Methods of Preserving the Nutrient Content of Foods**

- Avoid very high temperatures, long cooking times, and keeping foods hot for an extended time, as in a buffet line.
- Expose food to as little air as possible; keep prepared vegetables, fruits, and juices covered and airtight; cut and manipulate food as little as possible; and keep lids on pans while cooking.
- Expose food to as little water as possible; steam, microwave, stir-fry, or bake rather than boil.
- Keep and use the cooking water.
- Keep milk in opaque containers.
- Store fruits and vegetables cold.
- Use foods in whole form whenever possible.

Table 19.4   Vitamins

FOOD SOURCES	FUNCTION	SIGNS AND SYMPTOMS	
		DEFICIENCY	TOXICITY
Vitamin A[a]			
Egg yolks, liver, milk Carrots, winter squash, sweet potatoes, spinach, collards, kale, broccoli, apricots, cantaloupe	Vision, epithelial tissue integrity, growth, reproduction, embryonic development, immune function	Night blindness, xerophthalmia, increased susceptibility to infections, follicular hyperkeratosis	Fatigue, headache, nausea, vomiting, blurred vision, liver abnormalities, bone and skin change
Vitamin B$_1$ (thiamine)			
Unrefined whole grains, enriched and fortified grains and cereals, liver, pork, legumes, nuts	Carbohydrate metabolism	Beriberi: mental confusion, anorexia, muscle weakness and wasting, found in association with chronic alcoholism	None exhibited
Vitamin B$_2$ (riboflavin)			
Milk, meats, poultry, fish, enriched and fortified grains and cereals	General metabolism	Ariboflavinosis: sore throat, cheilosis (a disorder of the lips and mouth characterized by scales and fissures), glossitis, dermatitis	None exhibited
Vitamin B$_3$ (niacin)			
Meat, poultry, enriched and fortified grains and cereals (high-protein foods that contain tryptophan)	General metabolism	Pellagra: dermatitis, constipation or diarrhea, dementia, depression	Nausea, vomiting, flushing, pruritus (itching) of the skin, abnormal liver function
Vitamin B$_5$ (pantothenic acid)			
Widespread in foods; abundant in animal tissue, whole grains, and legumes	General metabolism	Listlessness and fatigue (rare)	Diarrhea and water retention
Vitamin B$_6$ (pyridoxine)			
Meat, poultry, fish, eggs, brown rice, wheat, oats, soybeans	Amino acid metabolism, general metabolism	Anemia, convulsions, dermatitis, depression, confusion	Peripheral neuropathy, irregular muscle coordination
Vitamin B$_7$ (biotin)			
Liver, egg yolks, soy flour, cereals, yeast (synthesis by intestinal bacteria)	General metabolism	Dermatitis, conjunctivitis, alopecia, depression (rare)	None exhibited
Vitamin B$_9$ (folic acid)			
Liver, green leafy vegetables, legumes, fruits, enriched grain products	Nucleic acid synthesis, amino acid metabolism	Macrocytic (large-cell) anemia, elevated homocysteine level	Sometimes masks vitamin B$_{12}$ deficiency; interferes with the anticonvulsant drug phenytoin (Dilantin)
Vitamin B$_{12}$ (cyanocobalamin)			
Animal products (meat, fish, poultry, milk, dairy products, eggs)	Synthesis of new cells, maintenance of nerve cells	Pernicious anemia: macrocytic megaloblastic anemia	None exhibited
Vitamin C (ascorbic acid)			
Citrus fruits and juices, strawberries, kiwi fruit, melons, broccoli, peppers, tomatoes, potatoes, fortified beverages	Antioxidant; wound healing, tissue growth and maintenance, proper immune function, absorption of iron	Scurvy: gingivitis, bleeding gums, easy bruising, increased infections, poor wound healing, rough skin, joint pain, muscle atrophy, fatigue	Abdominal cramps and diarrhea

Continued

Table 19.4   **Vitamins—cont'd**

FOOD SOURCES	FUNCTION	SIGNS AND SYMPTOMS	
		DEFICIENCY	**TOXICITY**
Vitamin D (calciferol)			
Fortified milk, fortified margarine, egg yolks, liver, fish oils Sunlight on skin	Maintenance of blood calcium and phosphorus balance	Rickets (children): abnormal shape and structure of bones Osteomalacia (adults): weakening and softening of bones	Calcification of soft tissues
Vitamin E (alpha-tocopherol)			
Vegetable oils, dark green, leafy vegetables, wheat germ, nuts	Antioxidant; protection of cell membranes	Peripheral neuropathy, ataxia, skeletal myopathy, retinopathy, and impairment of the immune response	Increased tendency to hemorrhage
Vitamin K			
Green, leafy vegetables, milk, dairy products, liver, meat, egg yolks, green tea (synthesis by intestinal bacteria)	Formation of blood clotting factors	Increased prothrombin time; in severe cases, hemorrhaging	None exhibited
Choline[b]			
Richest sources are liver, kidney, wheat germ, brewer's yeast, and egg yolks	Maintenance of cell membranes, memory retention, muscle control, lipid metabolism	Liver damage	Hypotension, sweating, diarrhea, fishy body odor

[a]Beta-carotene is a previtamin; it is converted to vitamin A in the body.
[b]Choline is an essential nutrient that works with folate in preventing neural tube defects and plays a role in cell functions and nerve communication.
US Department of Health and Human Services. Vitamin E Fact Sheet for Health Professionals. March 26, 2021. Retrieved from https://ods.od.nih.gov/factsheets/VitaminE-HealthProfessional.

necessary for adrenal gland function. It also enhances the absorption of iron and is needed to convert folic acid, a B vitamin, to its active form. Vitamin C supplementation has become a common practice because of claims that it helps prevent the common cold and prevents or cures cancer. Although it is true that adequate vitamin C is necessary for proper immune function, large supplemental doses of the vitamin have not been shown consistently and conclusively to be of greater value than what can be obtained solely through diet. The adult DRI for vitamin C is 90 mg/day for men and 75 mg/day for women. The National Institutes of Health's Office of Dietary Supplements suggests an additional 35 mg/day for those who smoke cigarettes because cigarette smoke increases oxidative stress. The DRI recommended a vitamin C intake upper limit of 2 g/day for adults (USDHHS, NIH, 2018g). Intakes above this level pose the risk of causing diarrhea and GI disturbances and cause the body to store too much iron, which results in tissue damage. It is easy to meet the DRI recommendations by increasing intake of citrus fruits; green, leafy, and yellow vegetables; and other foods containing vitamin C (Table 19.5). A deficiency of vitamin C can result in bleeding in the bones and joints, easy bone fracture, poor wound healing, and anemia.

B-complex vitamins. There are several different B vitamins. All are water soluble, and all are necessary for proper metabolism. Of all the B-complex vitamins, three are especially important.

Niacin. Niacin (vitamin B_3) is important in the production of energy from glucose and is involved in the repair of DNA. The body can produce some niacin if tryptophan is present. Niacin is measured in niacin equivalents. The DRI for niacin is 16 mg niacin equivalents/day for men and 14 mg niacin equivalents/day for women. This requirement is obtained easily by eating meat, poultry, fish, peanuts, or enriched whole grain breads and cereals. Niacin deficiency is rare, and there is usually no risk for toxicity except with excess vitamin supplementation.

Folate (folic acid). Folate is a water-soluble B vitamin that is the natural form found in foods such as spinach, lentils, and garbanzo beans. Folic acid is the synthetic form of the vitamin. Folic acid can be found in dietary supplements and in foods that are fortified with the vitamin. Both forms work the same in the body, but the synthetic form is easier for the body to absorb. Folic acid (vitamin B_9) is necessary for the formation of DNA and proper cell division. A deficiency can lead to megaloblastic anemia (see *Adult Health Nursing,* Chapter 7). Adequate folic acid intake before and during pregnancy has been found to reduce the risk of neural tube defects (defects of the brain, spine, or spinal cord) in the infant. The recommendation for women who are

Table 19.5   Vitamin C Content of Selected Foods

FOOD	SERVING SIZE	VITAMIN C CONTENT (mg)
Orange juice	¾ cup	93
Strawberries	½ cup	49
Red pepper	½ cup	95
Orange	1 medium	70
Grapefruit juice	¾ cup	70
Broccoli, cooked	½ cup	51
Brussels sprouts, cooked	½ cup	48
Kiwi	1 medium	64
Cantaloupe	½ cup	29
Cauliflower, raw	½ cup	26
Tomato juice	¾ cup	33
Grapefruit, pink	½ medium	39
Tomato	1 medium	17
Cabbage, cooked	½ cup	28
Potato, baked	1 medium	17
Spinach, cooked	½ cup	9

The adult recommended daily allowances (RDAs) for vitamin C are 90 mg/day for men and 75 mg/day for women.
Data from National Institutes of Health, Office of Dietary Supplements, Vitamin C. Retrieved from https://ods.od.nih.gov/factsheets/VitaminC-HealthProfessional/ March 26, 2021

capable of becoming pregnant is 400 mcg/day from fortified foods or a supplement in addition to the folic acid found in a varied diet containing green, leafy vegetables; beets; oranges; and kidney beans (USDHHS, NIH, 2018b).

Vitamin B_{12}. Cyanocobalamin (vitamin B_{12}) plays an essential part in the production of hemoglobin and myelin. To absorb vitamin B_{12}, a protein secreted by the stomach is required. This protein is called *intrinsic factor* and is produced in the lower portion of the stomach. When the intrinsic factor is missing—for example, after stomach excision or resection—vitamin B_{12} cannot be absorbed, and pernicious anemia (a progressive macrocytic megaloblastic anemia) develops. Treatment of pernicious anemia consists of vitamin B_{12} injections for a lifetime. Oral vitamin B_{12} supplementation is ineffective because of the lack of intrinsic factor. Because vitamin B_{12} is found primarily in foods of animal origin, people who follow a strict vegetarian diet (vegans) do not always receive adequate vitamin B_{12} from food and are likely to benefit from an oral supplement. People older than 50 years also tend to have difficulty absorbing vitamin B_{12} from foods because of low stomach acid secretion; therefore oral supplementation of vitamin B_{12} is recommended for them as well. It is recommended that individuals older than 50 receive most of their vitamin B_{12} from fortified foods or supplements containing vitamin B_{12} (NIH, Office of Dietary Supplements 2018f).

The DRI for vitamin B_{12} in adults is 2.4 mcg/day. This can be obtained easily from eating animal products such as lean meat, liver, seafood, eggs, and dairy products.

Vitamin A. Vitamin A, an antioxidant and a fat-soluble vitamin, is available in two forms: retinol (preformed) and carotene (provitamin). A preformed vitamin (retinol) is in a complete state when it is eaten, and it can be used immediately by the body. A provitamin (carotene) must be converted in the body to a form that can be used. Both forms of vitamin A are important for maintaining vision, as well as for skin and bone growth. The DRI for vitamin A is 700 mcg for women and 900 mcg for men (USDHHS, 2018). Most people consume vitamin A in the form of beta-carotene, found in bright yellow and orange fruits, carrots, pumpkin, and dark green, leafy vegetables. The liver contains about 90% of the body's stored vitamin A.

Vitamin D. Vitamin D promotes the absorption of calcium and phosphorus, which in turn promote bone and tooth health. It can be found in most fortified dairy products, in yeast, and in fish liver oils. The body also synthesizes vitamin D when the skin is exposed to sunlight. Because vitamin D is a fat-soluble vitamin and can be stored in the body, excess intake can cause GI upset, muscular weakness, and, in extreme cases, calcium deposits in the kidneys, lungs, brain, or heart. Vitamin D deficiency can lead to brittle bones (osteoporosis) and may be of concern for some older adult patients in long-term care facilities. A patient in long-term care who is confined indoors and does not drink milk or consume milk products is likely to be at risk for obtaining inadequate amounts of vitamin D. The DRI for vitamin D for adults up to 70 years of age is 15 mcg/day. After the age of 70, the DRI is 20 mcg/day (USDHHS, NIH, 2018h).

Vitamin K. Vitamin K plays a role in blood clotting. It is important in maintaining four of the eleven clotting factors found in the blood. There are two forms of vitamin K: one is present in green, leafy vegetables, and the other is made by intestinal bacteria. Because of the effect that vitamin K has on clotting, patients who are taking antiplatelet drugs or anticoagulants should consume consistent amounts of vitamin K from day to day. Large fluctuations in vitamin K intake have the potential to alter the effects of the anticoagulant drug. The DRI for vitamin K is 120 mcg/day for adult males and 90 mcg/day for adult females (USDHHS, NIH, 2018i).

Minerals

Minerals differ from vitamins: they are inorganic, and they are single elements rather than compounds. Minerals are also similar to vitamins: they help regulate bodily functions without providing energy and are essential to good health.

Table 19.6   Minerals

| FOOD SOURCES | FUNCTION | SIGNS AND SYMPTOMS | |
		DEFICIENCY	TOXICITY
Calcium			
Milk, cheese, milk products, green, leafy vegetables, broccoli, legumes, fish with bones, fortified cereals	Formation and maintenance of bones and teeth, blood clotting, nerve conduction, muscle contraction	Osteoporosis (adults): weak, more porous bones Stunted growth in children	Constipation; increased risk for urinary stone formation in men; reduced absorption of iron and zinc
Chloride			
Salt, processed foods, water supply	Fluid and acid-base balance	Metabolic alkalosis	None exhibited
Chromium			
Whole grains, liver, nuts, cheese	Maintenance of normal glucose metabolism	Impaired glucose tolerance, diabetes-like symptoms	None exhibited
Copper			
Organ meats, seafood, nuts, seeds, whole grains, cocoa	Necessary for utilization of iron	Anemia, vascular skeletal problems	Nausea, vomiting, liver damage
Fluoride			
Water supply, plants grown in fluoride-rich soil	Increases tooth resistance to decay, stimulates new bone formation	Increased susceptibility to tooth decay	Fluorosis: mottled tooth enamel, altered bone health
Iodine			
Iodized salt, seafood, plants grown in iodine-rich soil	Part of thyroxin, which helps regulate metabolism, growth, and development	Goiter: enlarged thyroid gland, weight gain, skin and hair changes Cretinism: mental and physical retardation of fetus	Enlarged thyroid gland
Iron			
Clams, liver, oysters, meat, poultry, fish, legumes, whole and enriched grains, fortified cereals	Part of hemoglobin and myoglobin; necessary for oxygen transport and use in the body; part of some enzymes; energy metabolism	Microcytic, hypochromic anemia: fatigue, weakness, headache, apathy, pale skin, decreased immune function Children: reduced attention span, decreased ability to learn	Tissue damage, constipation, decreased zinc absorption Accidental poisoning in children: nausea, vomiting, diarrhea, rapid heartbeat, weak pulse, dizziness, shock, disorientation
Magnesium			
Nuts, legumes, whole grains, green leafy vegetables, fortified cereals	Bone mineralization, muscle contraction and relaxation, general metabolism, blood pressure regulation	Nausea, muscle weakness, confusion, tetany (rare, usually caused by other disease states)	Diarrhea
Manganese			
Widely distributed in food; richest in whole grains, cereals, fruits, vegetables	General metabolism, formation of bone	Dermatitis, reduced bone mineralization, altered lipid and carbohydrate metabolism	Central nervous system abnormalities
Phosphorus			
Milk, meat, poultry, fish, grains, food additives; found in almost all foods	Essential component of bone, energy metabolism, acid-base balance	Rare, but sometimes occurs in patients using aluminum hydroxide antacids	Calcification of nonskeletal tissues
Potassium			
Sweet potatoes, fruits, vegetables, fresh meat, legumes, milk	Nerve conduction; muscle contraction, including the heart; fluid and acid-base balance	Severe: cardiac dysrhythmias, muscle weakness, glucose intolerance Moderate: increased blood pressure, risk of kidney stones, increased bone turnover	Cardiac arrest

Table 19.6   Minerals—cont'd

FOOD SOURCES	FUNCTION	SIGNS AND SYMPTOMS	
		DEFICIENCY	TOXICITY
Selenium			
Meat, poultry, fish, bread, grains, seeds	Antioxidant	Cardiomyopathy	Nail and hair changes, nausea, diarrhea, skin rash, garlic breath odor, fatigue
Sodium			
Salt, processed foods, small amounts in whole unprocessed foods	Fluid and acid-base balance, nerve conduction, muscle contraction	Cramps, mental confusion, apathy, appetite loss (usually secondary to diarrhea or disease)	Hypertension in susceptible individuals, increased calcium excretion
Sulfur			
All foods containing protein	Essential constituent of proteins, metabolism	None exhibited except in severe protein deficiency (problems with cartilage, tendons, and ligaments)	None exhibited
Zinc			
Red meat, liver, eggs, seafood, cereal, whole grains, legumes	Part of many enzymes involved in metabolism	Loss of appetite, growth retardation, skin changes, immune system dysfunction	Impaired immune response, impaired copper status, reduced HDL cholesterol level

HDL, High-density lipoprotein.

Minerals are classified as either major minerals or trace minerals. Major minerals are those needed in amounts greater than 100 mg/day (National Academies of Sciences, Engineering, and Medicine, n.d.). They include calcium, phosphorus, magnesium, sulfur, sodium, potassium, and chloride. The trace minerals are needed in much smaller amounts (less than 100 mg/day); they include iron, zinc, iodine, selenium, copper, manganese, fluoride, chromium, and molybdenum. Other trace minerals thought to be essential, but of which less is known, include arsenic, boron, nickel, and silicon. Table 19.6 lists the minerals with a summary of their food sources and function, as well as symptoms of deficiency and toxicity.

Calcium. Calcium has several functions in the body. It is important in the formation of bones and teeth; it plays a role in blood clotting; and it plays a role in the transmission of nerve impulses and muscle action. It is also important for metabolic reactions throughout the body. Because of these functions, calcium is necessary to protect against osteoporosis. *Osteoporosis* is an abnormal reduction in bone density that leads to bone pain, fractures, loss of stature, and deformities such as kyphosis (hunched back). In the United States, 1.5 million bone fractures are attributed to this bone disease annually. Women are affected more than men. Many hip fractures are the result of osteoporosis. Besides pain, hip fractures often result in dramatic lifestyle changes, disability, and loss of independence. An estimated 12% to 20% of people with hip fractures die from complications within 1 year of the fracture (Centers for Disease Control and Prevention, 2013).

The causes of osteoporosis are multiple. Peak bone mass is determined not only by calcium intake but also by genetic influences, gender, hormone levels, physical activity, and dietary intake of vitamin D, fluoride, and other trace minerals. In the United States, diets high in sodium and protein and low in potassium appear to contribute to osteoporosis by increasing the amount of calcium that is excreted in the urine. Growth and mineralization of bone occur from birth until early adulthood. Peak bone mass is achieved between 19 and 30 years of age. A higher peak bone mass in young adulthood lowers the risk of bone fractures later in life. In women, menopause greatly accelerates the rate of bone loss. Therefore calcium intake in childhood, adolescence, and young adulthood is important.

The recommended intakes of calcium are similar for men and women, but it varies across age groups. The requirement for older children and adolescents is set at 1300 mg/day (USDHHS, NIH, 2017). The suggested intake for adults is 1000 mg/day up to age 50 and 1200 mg/day for adults 51 years of age and older. No increases in calcium intake are recommended during pregnancy and lactation because additional dietary calcium does not appear to have any influence on the changes seen in maternal bone mass during pregnancy and lactation. The calcium recommendation for patients with osteoporosis is 1500 mg/day.

The amount of calcium recommended for good health is often difficult to achieve from diet alone, and many foods, such as orange juice and breakfast cereals, have been fortified with calcium. It is also possible to take calcium supplements, but they should never be allowed to replace calcium-rich foods in the diet. Foods provide not only calcium but also other nutrients that are beneficial in disease prevention (Table 19.7).

Calcium absorption and excretion may be affected by physiologic circumstances and dietary factors. Box 19.4 discusses factors that influence calcium absorption and excretion.

Sodium. In the body, sodium functions as an *electrolyte* (a compound that can conduct an electrical current). Sodium is needed in very small amounts for good health and is found naturally in almost all foods. Therefore dietary sodium deficiency is extremely rare in the United States. Of greater concern is that excess sodium has the potential to be detrimental to health. Salt (sodium chloride) is the largest contributor of sodium in the diet and, if eaten in large quantities, can cause hypertension and edema. Approximately 65 million, or 31%, of American adults suffer from hypertension. DRIs for sodium suggest that intake of 1500 mg/day is adequate for healthy adults younger than 50, 1300 mg is adequate for adults between 50 and 70 years of age, and 1200 mg is adequate for adults older than 70 (USDHHS and USDA, 2015). The upper limit of intake is set at 2300 mg/day. Most adults in the United States consume approximately 3400 mg of sodium per day. Because sodium may be lost with heavy sweating, diarrhea, vomiting, renal disease, and cystic fibrosis, it is important to monitor sodium levels in individuals presenting with any of these symptoms or diseases.

Potassium. Potassium, also an electrolyte, is needed for conduction of nerve impulses and the contraction of muscles, including the heart muscle. It helps maintain acid-base balance and is required for conversion of glucose to glycogen. It also plays a role in energy production and insulin release from the pancreas. A severe deficiency of potassium can lead to hypokalemia (blood potassium level less than 3.5 mmol/L), which is a life-threatening state. Individuals taking potassium-wasting diuretics and chronic laxative users also may be at risk for developing hypokalemia and need to achieve adequate potassium intake through diet or supplementation, or both. Excessive intake of potassium is also a problem and can lead to hyperkalemia (blood potassium levels above 5.0 mmol/L). This can result in renal failure, adrenal failure, and cardiac arrest.

The DRIs for potassium suggest that intake of 4700 mg/day is adequate for all adults (USDHHS, NIH, 2018d). At present, most Americans consume much less than this. Studies indicate that a moderate potassium deficiency (in the absence of hypokalemia) may lead to increased blood pressure, increased risk of kidney stones, and increased bone loss. Therefore, adequate potassium intake is necessary to prevent these health risks.

Potassium is found naturally in many foods, especially fruits, vegetables, and milk. Plant forms of potassium are water soluble; therefore much of the potassium may be lost during food processing. Processed foods usually have added salt or other sources of sodium. Therefore eating more foods in their natural states and reducing the amount of processed foods help reduce sodium intake and increase potassium intake. Potassium supplementation is not recommended, except when prescribed by a health care provider, because the risk of toxicity and cardiac arrest is high.

Iron. Iron is an essential part of hemoglobin, myoglobin, and many enzymes throughout the body. Hemoglobin is part of the red blood cell and carries oxygen to the cells. Myoglobin is similar to hemoglobin but is found in the

Table 19.7 Calcium Content of Selected Foods

FOOD	SERVING SIZE	CALCIUM CONTENT (mg)
Sardines	3 oz	371
American cheese	1 oz	348
Cheddar cheese	1 oz	306
Milk	1 cup	291–316
Yogurt	1 cup	274–415
Tofu (processed with calcium)	3 oz	225
Ice cream	1 cup	176
Salmon with bones (canned)	1 oz	167
Processed cheese	1 oz	159–199
Collard greens (cooked)	1 cup	148–357
Broccoli (cooked)	1 cup	94–177
Cottage cheese	½ cup	77

Box 19.4 Factors Affecting Calcium Absorption and Excretion

FACTORS THAT IMPROVE CALCIUM ABSORPTION FROM THE GASTROINTESTINAL TRACT
- Acidic conditions in the stomach (presence of food in the stomach increases stomach acid secretion)
- Increased physiologic need (e.g., infancy, childhood, adolescence, pregnancy)
- Small doses (less than 500 mg) of calcium are better absorbed than large doses

FACTORS THAT DECREASE CALCIUM ABSORPTION FROM THE GASTROINTESTINAL TRACT
- Calcium absorption decreases with age
- Calcium is poorly absorbed from foods rich in oxalic or phytic acids (spinach, sweet potatoes, rhubarb, beans, seeds, nuts, grains)

DIETARY FACTORS THAT INCREASE EXCRETION (LOSS) OF CALCIUM IN URINE
- Caffeine
- High-protein diets
- High-sodium diets
- Low-potassium diets

muscle tissue and is responsible for storing oxygen in the muscle. A lack of iron in the body can cause iron-deficiency anemia.

Iron-deficiency anemia seems to be the most prevalent nutritional problem in the world, and it may result not only from inadequate iron in the diet but also excessive blood loss, absorption problems, and hemoglobin production problems. A deficiency of iron limits oxygen delivery to the cells, which results in fatigue, weakness, headaches, pallor of skin and mucous membranes, poor work performance, and decreased immune function. In children, iron deficiency has been associated with a short attention span, irritability, and a reduced ability to learn.

Children aged 6 months to 4 years, adolescents, menstruating women, and pregnant women are at greatest risk for iron-deficiency anemia. Dietary requirements are higher for women than for men because of the monthly blood loss during menstruation. Iron DRIs are set at 15 mg/day for adolescent girls and 18 mg/day for premenopausal adult women (USDHHS, 2018). For postmenopausal women, men, and children, the DRI is 8 mg/day of iron. Pregnant women have an iron requirement set at 27 mg/day. Because this requirement is so high, it is almost impossible to obtain it through diet alone, and supplementation is required.

Food sources of iron include meat (especially organ meats), poultry, fish, whole grains, and soy foods, as well as fortified and enriched grain products. Dietary iron is found in two forms: heme and nonheme. Heme iron is found in animal tissues (meats, poultry, and fish) and is absorbed well. The iron in plant products and iron supplements is nonheme iron. Nonheme iron is not absorbed well from the GI tract and therefore may not be as available as heme forms of iron. Iron absorption from the GI tract may be enhanced or inhibited by certain dietary factors. For example, taking vitamin C with iron supplements may enhance the absorption, whereas consuming iron along with fiber and coffee may inhibit absorption (Box 19.5). An easy way to teach the patient is to recommend taking their iron supplement with orange juice to enhance absorption.

Even though iron is a necessary mineral, overdoses can be toxic and even fatal. Iron poisoning is seen each year in children who ingest overdoses of iron-containing vitamin and mineral supplements. Immediate medical attention is necessary if a child ingests large amounts of iron-containing supplements.

Chromium. *Chromium* is necessary for glucose metabolism and seems to work with insulin in regulating blood glucose levels. Adequate intake of chromium is thought to help patients suffering from type 2 diabetes mellitus; however, some studies have revealed that the value of chromium supplements for patients with diabetes is inconclusive and controversial and more studies are needed.

The average healthy adult (19 to 50 years old) requires only 25 mcg/day (women) to 35 mcg/day

---

Box **19.5**   Factors Affecting Iron Absorption

FACTORS THAT ENHANCE IRON ABSORPTION
- Meat, fish, and poultry (MFP) have a factor (sometimes called the *MFP factor*) that enhances iron absorption
- Vitamin C (ascorbic acid), when eaten in the same meal with iron-containing foods

FACTORS THAT INHIBIT IRON ABSORPTION
- Bran and some fibers that contain phytates bind iron in the gastrointestinal tract, so it is not absorbed
- Calcium in milk and supplement form
- Polyphenols, which are compounds found in coffee, tea, and red wine
- Some medications such as antacids
- Vegetable proteins, especially soy protein

(men), so it is possible to obtain adequate chromium through diet alone (USDHHS, NIH, 2018a). Good sources of chromium include whole grains, cheese, liver, eggs, peas, apples, and nuts.

Vitamin and mineral supplementation. Many Americans are interested in vitamin and mineral supplementation. There have been claims that these nutrients help reduce stress, prevent colds, increase sexuality, increase energy, improve physical performance, and reduce the risk for certain diseases. Many people believe that if some is good, more is better. The truth is that for most people, vitamins and minerals are obtained best from a balanced, varied diet. Except in certain cases, supplementation is not necessary. For people who like to use a supplement as "insurance" against an imperfect diet, a simple multivitamin and mineral supplement should suffice. It is best to avoid large doses, or megadoses, of nutrients and to avoid taking numerous types of supplements, except for therapeutic purposes. All medications, including vitamins and minerals, should be taken under the supervision of a health care provider.

Water

Water is the nutrient most vital to life; humans can survive longer without food than they can without water. Lack of this nutrient brings about detrimental changes in the body more rapidly than lack of any other. Water makes up approximately 60% of adult body weight and 80% of infant weight and performs many functions in the body. It provides form and structure to body tissues, acts as a solvent, and is necessary for most of the body's chemical processes. Water transports nutrients and other substances throughout the body by way of the blood, body secretions, and tissue fluids; it lubricates and protects moving parts of the body, such as joints; it aids in digestion; and it is necessary for regulating body temperature. If fluid needs are not met, in relation to inadequate intake or through abnormal losses such as vomiting, hemorrhage, burns, or an increase in perspiration or urination, dehydration results. Severe dehydration (more than 10% of body weight lost) could become a life-threatening situation. Signs of dehydration include poor skin turgor; flushed, dry skin; dry mouth; cracked, dry lips; decreased urine output; irritability; and disorientation. Dehydration in infants is evidenced by sunken fontanels, a decrease in the number of wet diapers, and no tears when the child cries.

About 80% of total water intake comes from drinking water and other beverages, and 20% comes from the water contained in foods. The need for water varies, depending on factors such as body size, age, activity level, metabolic needs, and temperature, and so it is not possible to give a specific recommendation; however, a suggested daily intake of 9 cups (women) to 13 cups (men) of fluids from drinking water and other beverages is adequate for most adults. Pregnant and lactating women have increased water needs (up to 3 L/day). Infants tend to be at greater risk for dehydration because they have a higher percentage of body water and are more susceptible to greater skin losses of water. In young infants, breast milk and formula normally provide adequate fluid, but extra fluids may be needed in warmer weather. Older adults have decreased sensitivity to thirst and are also at greater risk for dehydration. Young infants and older adults require special attention to make certain that their fluid needs are met and to avoid dehydration. Caffeinated beverages should be discouraged because caffeine is a natural diuretic and will cause addition fluid loss.

LIFE CYCLE NUTRITION

PREGNANCY AND LACTATION

Nutrient needs are greater during periods of intensive growth, such as pregnancy and infancy, than at any other time during the life cycle.

Optimal nutrition during pregnancy reduces the risk of complications, premature deliveries, and low birth weight. Even the mother's nutrition before conception plays a role in the outcome of a pregnancy. Women of childbearing age should be encouraged to consume a healthy diet and use care in the consumption of alcohol and caffeine. The focus of maternal education regarding nutrition should be expanded to include preconceptional, as well as prenatal, nutrition. Many women are unaware of their pregnancy during the first weeks after conception, and most women do not attend prenatal information classes until the later months of their pregnancy. Therefore it is important to provide information before conception or within the first few weeks of pregnancy. During these early weeks of pregnancy, adequate folic acid is thought to significantly reduce the risk of neural tube defects, such as spina bifida, in the infant. For this reason, women of childbearing age should be advised to consume adequate amounts of folate from fortified foods in addition to natural food sources.

To consume enough nutrients for mother and fetus, pregnant women should increase their caloric intake by about 300 kcal/day during the first trimester, 340 kcal/day during the second trimester, and 450 to 500 kcal/day during the third trimester of pregnancy. These additional calories should be from nutrient-dense foods (foods that contain large amounts of nutrients in relation to kilocalories). For a detailed discussion on nutrient needs during pregnancy and sample menus for pregnancy, see Tables 19.8 and 19.9.

Concerns in Pregnancy

Weight gain. Weight gain in pregnancy is important. Recommended weight gain varies based on a woman's pre-pregnancy weight. Optimal weight gain for the average woman is 25 to 35 pounds. Underweight women should gain between 28 and 40 pounds, whereas overweight women should gain only between 15 and 25 pounds. Encourage pregnant young adolescents to strive for higher weight gain to maintain their health, as well as that of the fetus.

Intentional weight loss should not be attempted during pregnancy. Mothers who do not gain adequate weight during pregnancy risk giving birth to a low–birth weight (LBW) infant (weighing less than 5.5 pounds). These babies are at greater risk for complications during and after birth.

Discomforts and complications. Many women experience discomforts during pregnancy. Common among these are nausea and vomiting, often referred to as "morning sickness." There are many ways to alleviate the nausea and vomiting associated with pregnancy. Mild nausea and vomiting, as well as other discomforts, often can be alleviated with safe and simple dietary alterations (Box 19.6). However, women should be advised to discuss any concerns they may have with their health care provider.

Occasionally, pregnancy brings about medical conditions that pose potential dangers for the mother and the fetus. Hypertensive disorders of pregnancy include chronic hypertension, preeclampsia, eclampsia, and gestational hypertension. These disorders are the second leading cause of maternal death in the United States and contribute significantly to stillbirths and neonatal complications. Proper nutrition is vital before and throughout pregnancy and may help in the management of blood pressure during pregnancy. A diet rich in fruits, vegetables, and milk products, as well as in adequate protein, and moderate sodium intake should be encouraged.

Controlling blood glucose levels during pregnancy is very difficult. Hypoglycemia is common in the first trimester because of low glucose levels, increased insulin production, and nausea and vomiting. During the latter two trimesters, insulin resistance is common, and so the woman may be more likely to experience hyperglycemia. With the incidence of diabetes on the

Table 19.8   Nutrient Needs During Pregnancy and Lactation

AMOUNT (DIETARY REFERENCE INTAKES)			REASONS FOR INCREASED NUTRIENT NEED DURING PREGNANCY	FOOD SOURCES
NONPREGNANT ADULT	PREGNANCY	LACTATION		
Protein				
46–50 g	60 g	65 g	Rapid fetal tissue growth Amniotic fluid Placental growth and development Maternal tissue growth: uterus, breasts Increased maternal circulating blood volume: • Hemoglobin increase • Plasma protein increase Maternal storage reserves for labor, delivery, and lactation	Milk, cheese, eggs, meat, grains, legumes, nuts, soy products
Calories[a]				
2200	2500	2700	Increased basal metabolic rate, energy needs Protein sparing	See individual foods
Minerals				
Calcium[b]				
1000 mg	1000 mg[b]	1000 mg[b]	Fetal skeleton formation Fetal tooth bud formation Increased maternal calcium metabolism Maternal blood pressure control	Milk, yogurt, cheese, fortified soy milk, dark green, leafy vegetables
Iron				
18 mg	27 mg	9 mg	Increased maternal circulating blood volume, increased hemoglobin Fetal liver iron storage High iron cost during pregnancy	Liver, meats, eggs, whole or enriched grain, leafy vegetables, nuts, legumes, dried fruits, fortified cereals
Iodine				
150 mcg	220 mcg	290 mcg	Increased basal metabolic rate Increased thyroxine production	Iodized salt
Magnesium				
310 mg	350 mg	310 mg	Coenzyme in energy and protein metabolism Enzyme activator Tissue growth, cell metabolism Muscle action	Nuts, soybeans, cocoa, seafood, whole grains, dried beans and peas
Vitamins				
Vitamin B$_6$ (Pyridoxine)				
1.3 mg	1.9 mg	2 mg	Coenzyme in protein metabolism Increased fetal growth requirement	Milk, wheat, corn, liver, meat
Folic Acid				
400 mcg	600 mcg	500 mcg	Increased red blood cells Prevention of macrocytic anemia Prevention of neural tube defects	Green leafy vegetables, oranges, artichokes, broccoli, asparagus, liver, fortified grain products
Vitamin C				
75 mg	85 mg	120 mg	Tissue formation and integrity Formation of connective tissue Enhanced iron absorption	Citrus fruits, strawberries, broccoli, tomatoes, raw green, leafy vegetables
Vitamin A				
700 mcg	770 mcg	1300 mcg	Vitamin content in breast milk Embryonic development Breast milk production	Milk, egg yolks, organ meats, deep orange and green fruits and vegetables

[a]Provision of adequate nonprotein calories so that protein is available for tissue synthesis and maintenance rather than used for energy needs.
[b]Calcium absorption increases during pregnancy and lactation, so no additional dietary calcium is advised.

Table 19.9	Sample Menus for Diet During Pregnancy

MENU 1	MENU 2
Breakfast	
1 cup high-fiber ready-to-eat cereal 1 slice wheat toast 1 tsp vegetable oil spread 1 banana 1 cup 1% or skim milk	2 eggs, scrambled in 1 tsp vegetable oil with ½ cup chopped onion, pepper, mushroom, tomato, 1½ oz shredded cheese 1 bran muffin 1 tbsp vegetable oil spread 6 oz orange juice
Snack	
1 apple 2 tbsp peanut butter	½ cup mixed nuts and dried fruit
Lunch	
2 oz turkey on 2 slices wheat bread 1 tsp mayonnaise 1 cup spinach salad 6 whole-grain crackers 1 cup skim or 1% milk	1 cup black bean and vegetable soup 2 slices corn bread 1 tbsp vegetable oil spread 2 tsp honey 1 cup fresh strawberries 1 cup skim or 1% milk
Snack	
½ cantaloupe with ½ cup low-fat cottage cheese	3 cups popcorn
Dinner	
Pork-vegetable stir-fry: 3 oz lean pork 1½ cups fresh vegetables 2 tsp olive oil Seasonings 1 cup steamed brown rice Water	4 oz grilled chicken breast 1 baked potato 2 tbsp sour cream and chives 1 cup steamed broccoli ½ cup pasta salad with vinegar and oil dressing 1 dinner roll 1 tsp vegetable oil spread Water
Snack	
2 oatmeal raisin cookies 1 cup 1% or skim milk	1 cup low-fat yogurt topped with ⅓ cup granola
Approximate Number of Servings Provided per Menu	
Grain group	8
Fruit group	3
Vegetable group	4
Dairy group	3
Meat group	6 oz
Fats, oils, and sweets	5–6

Box 19.6	Nutritional Suggestions to Relieve Some Discomforts of Pregnancy

NAUSEA, VOMITING, GASTRIC DISTRESS
- Allow time after eating before lying down or going to bed to prevent epigastric distress.
- Avoid high-fat or fried foods in excess.
- Avoid letting the stomach become empty.
- Consume five or six small meals that include protein each day.
- Drink plenty of fluids during the day; however, drink liquids before or after meals to avoid feeling too full.
- Limit consumption of foods with strong odors during times of nausea. Avoid odors that bother the patient.
- To reduce nausea, eat soda crackers or other dry grain products before getting out of bed.

CONSTIPATION
- Drink plenty of fluids, especially water.
- Include fiber-rich foods at each meal.
- Include moderate daily exercise.

rise in the United States, it is important to make sure all women undergo screening for gestational diabetes during pregnancy. For women with preexisting diabetes, achieving good blood glucose control before and during pregnancy is important. Gestational diabetes often is controlled through nutrition therapy and moderate exercise, but for women who are unable to achieve glycemic control, insulin therapy is often necessary.

Anemia is another common nutritional problem in pregnancy; iron-deficiency anemia and folic acid–deficiency anemia are possible. An adequate diet that includes meats, poultry, fish, vegetables (especially green, leafy vegetables), and a variety of fruits should be consumed, along with a prenatal supplement containing iron and folic acid.

Practices to avoid. During pregnancy, there are several things a woman should avoid in her diet. Alcohol, caffeine, and nicotine are three of the more important substances to avoid. Alcohol contributes to an increased risk for mental and physical disabilities in the fetus, and if the mother consumes large amounts of alcohol during pregnancy, *fetal alcohol syndrome* could develop. Fetal alcohol syndrome is characterized by physical deformities, learning disabilities, and behavioral problems. No safe level of alcohol consumption during pregnancy has been determined, and most nutrition experts favor total abstinence. The American Medical Association recommends that women of childbearing age abstain from drinking alcohol as soon as they plan to become pregnant.

High caffeine consumption may be a problem and is associated with delayed conception, increased risk of spontaneous abortion, and low birth weight. The March of Dimes recommends that women who are pregnant should not consume more than 200 mg of caffeine per day (one 12-ounce cup) to avoid decreased blood flow to the fetus and the complications that could occur (March of Dimes, 2020).

Nicotine in tobacco smoke also should be avoided during pregnancy. Studies have shown that smoking decreases blood supply to the fetus. This can cause premature birth and low birth weight. Birth defects such as cleft palate or cleft lip are also more common in babies born to mothers who have smoked during pregnancy.

Taking drugs of any kind during pregnancy should be avoided unless done under the direct supervision of a health care provider. Advise women to avoid all drugs, including over-the-counter medications and herbal or botanical supplements, until they have consulted their health care provider.

Another dietary concern for pregnant women is the intake of mercury. High mercury intake during pregnancy can cause fetal brain damage, as well as hearing and vision problems in the baby after birth. Pregnant women should be advised to avoid such foods as shark, swordfish, and king mackerel because of the high mercury content.

Lactation

During lactation, a woman should follow a diet similar to that followed during pregnancy. Kilocalorie needs and many nutrient needs are higher than during pregnancy (see Table 19.8). Lactating women should increase their caloric intake by 500 kcal/day more than their prepregnancy intake. These calories should come from foods that are going to provide the lactating woman with increased protein, calcium, phosphorus, and iron, as well as vitamins and minerals. Fluid needs are increased during lactation and should be obtained through the consumption of water, milk, juices, and other nutritious beverages. Advise moderation in any consumption of coffee, tea, and alcohol, because caffeine and alcohol can enter the breast milk and affect the infant.

During lactation, adequate fluid and nutrient intake is important to maintain the quantity and quality of breast milk. Poor kilocalorie and nutrient intake causes a decrease in the quantity of milk produced, as well as in the nutritional quality of the breast milk. Therefore it is essential for the lactating mother to be nourished properly to ensure that lactation continues and milk supply is adequate.

INFANCY

The time from birth to 1 year of age is one of rapid growth and development. The infant's birth weight doubles by 6 months and triples by 1 year of age. Nutrition plays an important part in this rapid growth.

Breast milk or iron-fortified infant formula is recommended for the entire first year of life. Breast milk contains antibodies and easily digested fats. This composition tends to lead to a lower incidence of infections in breast-fed infants and fewer episodes of GI upset. Regular cow's milk (whole, low-fat, or skim) should be avoided during the first year of life. Introduction of regular cow's milk before 1 year of age could lead to iron-deficiency anemia and increase the risk for developing milk allergies later in life. Also, the fat in cow's milk is more difficult for the infant to digest and could cause GI disturbances. The large amounts of protein, sodium, and potassium found in cow's milk also could overwhelm the infant's system and cause damage to the kidneys. Acceptable alternatives to cow's milk during the first year of life are breast milk and iron-fortified infant formula. Whole milk is acceptable after the first year, but skim and low-fat milk are inappropriate until the child is 2 years of age because the fat content is insufficient. In the first 6 months, water, juice, and other solid foods are generally unnecessary for infants. In most cases, breast milk or formula provides adequate nutrition for about the first 4 to 6 months. At approximately 4 to 6 months of age, depending on the infant's development, it is possible to introduce solid foods into the diet. Solid feedings usually are initiated with iron-fortified rice cereal, because rice cereal is less allergenic than most other foods. Infants should start with 1 to 2 teaspoons, and the amount is increased gradually. Fruits are added next, then vegetables, and then meats. Single-ingredient foods should be introduced one at a time at weekly intervals. This allows sufficient time to detect any food-related allergies. If the family has a history of food allergies, it is generally best to withhold wheat cereal, wheat products, and egg whites until the child is 1 year of age. Infants younger than 12 months of age also should never be given honey, especially wild honey, because of the potential for botulism. Wild honey is a potential source of *Clostridium botulinum* spores and easily can cause botulism in the infant.

Most commercially prepared baby foods in the United States are nutritious, safe, and of high quality. However, it is important to read labels and use foods without added salt, sugar, or honey. If baby foods are prepared at home, it is important to take care to reduce the risk of foodborne illness by having a sanitary preparation area and proper storage conditions.

There is no nutritional benefit to feeding juice to infants younger than 6 months. Offering juice before solid foods are introduced into the diet may cause the infant to prefer juice over breast milk or infant formula and tends to reduce the intake of important nutrients such as protein, fat, vitamins, and minerals.

It is important to remind parents that once the baby develops teeth, the nighttime feeding should be limited to water, and breastfeeding mothers should not allow the infant to nurse continuously throughout the night. Prolonged exposure of the teeth to formula or breast milk is a major contributing factor to dental caries.

CHILDHOOD

At approximately 1 year of age, appetite generally tapers off, and the growth rate slows. Children still need adequate nutrition, although nutrient needs relative to weight are generally less than in infancy. The website *www.ChooseMyPlate.gov* offers an appropriate guide for children's diets (see Fig. 19.1). Younger children typically need smaller serving sizes than adults, and as a child grows, serving sizes should increase. By the toddler years, the child's digestive system should be able to handle all the nutrients found in the normal family diet, and by school age, the child's taste preferences should be emerging. Most children prefer simple, plain foods and will eat what they need if they are not coaxed, nagged, bribed, rewarded, or influenced by television commercials. Childhood is a critical time for instilling good dietary habits. It is also a time for children to test their independence. Food is often a source of contention at mealtime, with the parents resorting to coaxing to get the child to eat or arguing with the child to gain compliance. Often the more pressure that is placed on the child at mealtime, the more negative the experience (see the Health Promotion box on fostering good dietary habits in children). Caregivers must supervise children's eating habits carefully and offer nutritious meals and snacks, but they also must allow the child the freedom to decide what and how much to eat.

Health Promotion

Ways to Encourage Good Dietary Habits in Children

- Encourage children to be physically active.
- Encourage children to eat meals and snacks at regular times and at the table. By having set eating times, children learn that they cannot eat and snack continually all day.
- Encourage children to help with food selection and preparation.
- Give small servings, or teach children how to serve themselves small servings. Then let them have seconds if they are still hungry.
- Keep nutritious snacks available, such as fruits, cheese, crackers, raw vegetables, and bread. Most children need to snack.
- Limit sweets, and do not use sweets and foods as rewards or bribes.
- Offer a variety of foods from all food groups, and allow children a choice of food, within reason.
- Offer new foods, but do not force children to eat foods they dislike. If the child will not eat a new food, quietly remove the food and offer it again at another time.
- Remember that physical growth and appetite come in spurts. Do not force children to eat more than they want to eat.
- Set a good example by practicing sound dietary and exercise habits.
- Try to make meals relaxed and enjoyable. Children need time to eat, and mealtimes should be a positive experience.

ADOLESCENCE

Puberty is another time in the child's life when growth is very rapid and nutrition becomes more important for proper development. Even though adolescents may understand good nutrition concepts, they may not relate this understanding to their own dietary habits. They usually react more readily to nutritional teaching if it applies to them directly. Adolescents may be more likely to practice good nutrition if they consider factors such as how nutrition helps skin (facial appearance), strength (for any athlete), and the ability to concentrate in school. Because of the accelerated growth rate and participation in sports, adolescents may need more food to supply their energy requirements. Because adolescents are seeking to establish their independence, their food choices are sometimes not wise ones and tend to be influenced by peer preference rather than by parental advice. Their diets often are filled with kilocalorie-rich and nutrient-poor snack foods. The era of fast food has given the adolescent access to high-calorie, nutritionally unbalanced meals. Too many fast food meals and too much snacking on empty calorie foods can lead to nutritional deficiencies. Common dietary inadequacies in adolescence include iron and calcium deficiencies (particularly in girls) and deficiencies in vitamins A and C and folic acid. Iron needs increase with the onset of menstruation in girls, and anemia is a common problem. When good nutritional habits have been established earlier in life, adolescent nutrition is likely to be better balanced than in cases in which nutritional teaching has been insufficient. Being part of a family that practices sound nutrition ensures that occasional lapses into sweets, fast foods, and other peer group food preferences do not create serious deficiencies.

Another nutritional factor to consider is that during adolescence, many teenagers experiment with alcohol and drugs, and these substances may have detrimental effects on their nutritional status as well.

Obesity in young people is a common problem in the United States. These years are a time of growth, and although obesity is not ideal, restrictive diets sometimes cause harm by suppressing development and can even lead to eating disorders. Adolescents should be encouraged to develop healthy eating habits and to use moderation when they consume soft drinks and sugar- and fat-laden snack foods. Adequate physical activity should be emphasized and television viewing and computer usage limited, along with other sedentary activities. Remind the adolescent that it is best to attempt weight-reduction diets only under the advice of a health care provider and with the guidance of a dietitian.

ADULTHOOD

During adulthood, nutrient needs change little in comparison with those of the adolescent. However, basal metabolic rate gradually slows, and the caloric needs decrease. At the same time, the activity level of many

Lifespan Considerations

Older Adults

Aging and Nutrition

- Aging often affects the eating process. Changes in dentition, decreased saliva production, and alterations in swallowing have the potential to affect nutrient intake. It is sometimes necessary to adjust food consistency to facilitate food intake. Chopped, ground, pureed, and liquid diets tend to be less appealing to older people; serve them in as palatable a manner as possible.
- The aroma and taste of foods sometimes are affected by normal changes of aging. In addition, many older adults are on special diets that restrict the use of salt, sugars, and fats. This could lead to inadequate nutrient intake. The use of flavorings, seasonings, and spices to enhance flavor and aroma is often helpful.
- Older adults experience changes in digestive secretions, gastrointestinal mucosa, and enzyme production. This affects how food is digested, absorbed, and excreted. Water, dietary fiber, and adequate physical activity play an important role in preventing constipation in older adults.
- Aging often leads to loss of muscle mass, thereby reducing basal metabolic rate. Kilocalorie needs may decrease approximately 5% for each decade between ages 55 and 75 and 7% for each decade after age 75 depending on the activity level.
- Older adults may have a greater need for certain nutrients, including protein, riboflavin, vitamin B_6, folic acid, vitamin B_{12}, vitamin D, and calcium. A multivitamin

and mineral supplement supplying 100% of the RDA is often beneficial for individuals with a low kilocalorie intake or during periods of poor intake. In addition, many older adults do not need as much vitamin A as do younger adults. Advise patients not to consume large doses of any nutrient unless they do so under a health care provider's supervision.
- Many older adults take numerous medications. Many medications tend to affect nutritional status. Be aware of drug-nutrient interactions and side effects that have the potential to influence dietary intake.
- Because of illness, restricted mobility, or financial limitations, or a combination of these, some older adults have difficulty obtaining and preparing nutritious food.
- Age-related social and mental changes such as forgetfulness, loneliness, and apathy are likely to affect the eating habits of older adults.
- Chronic medical conditions often necessitate the use of therapeutic diets. The most common such conditions in older adults include diabetes mellitus, cardiovascular disease, renal insufficiency, osteoporosis, diverticulosis, anemia, and lactose intolerance. Older adults who have long-standing dietary preferences and eating habits often find diet modification difficult. Always determine individual needs and situations before deciding the most appropriate nutrition therapy.

---

adults tends to decrease. The combined effects of decreased energy (caloric) needs and reduced physical activity often result in weight gain. As adults advance in years, it is important to remind them to eat nutrient-dense foods so that they can maintain adequate nutrition with fewer kilocalories and to maintain an active lifestyle.

Aging is associated with increased health concerns. Older adults suffer from conditions such as heart disease, arthritis, osteoporosis, diabetes, kidney disease, and other disorders with increased frequency. Special conditions may warrant differing nutrient needs that may vary greatly from individual to individual (see the Lifespan Considerations box for older adults). It is important to educate each patient about his or her dietary needs and explain the importance of any restrictions.

Nutritional Concerns of Adults in Long-Term Care Facilities

Malnutrition is a common problem among residents in long-term care facilities and profoundly influences physical health and quality of life. Poor nutritional status in these residents is related to several factors:

- Residents of long-term care facilities may experience cognitive or physical impairment, disease

processes, and emotional disturbances, all of which affect nutritional intake and status.
- Many residents in the long-term care environment need some assistance or encouragement with eating and drinking. All care providers within the facility must be educated and trained to ensure that residents are able to obtain the nutrients needed.
- Restricted diets may be prescribed for residents of long-term care facilities. Common modifications include sodium and fat restrictions. Diabetic features may be instituted for groups of residents. Dietary restrictions can affect the palatability of the food and thereby hinder nutritional intake.
- Inadequate fluid intake and dehydration are sometimes secondary to decreased thirst sensation, decreased independence, dysphagia (difficulty swallowing), and incontinence.
- *Pressure injuries* may occur in nonambulatory residents, increasing kilocalorie, protein, and nutrient needs.

All members of the health care team must work together to coordinate care to ensure that the nutritional needs of the facility residents are met. Concerns must be identified quickly and treatment planned to ensure that nutritional compromise does not occur.

Table **19.10**	Common Medications and Their Effect on Nutrition
DRUG TYPE	**POSSIBLE DIETARY SIGNIFICANCE**
Antacids	Reduced phosphorus, vitamin A, and iron absorption
Antibiotics	Reduced absorption as a result of vomiting, and increased excretion of multiple nutrients as a result of diarrhea Long-term therapy: may decrease vitamin K synthesis
Anticoagulants (e.g., warfarin)	Counteracted by vitamin K; consistent intake of vitamin K is essential Avoid high-dose supplements of vitamins A and E
Antihypertensives	Vitamin B_6 depletion; vitamin B_6 (hydralazine) supplementation is encouraged for patients with marginal diets
Aspirin	In long-term therapy: increased excretion of and decreased serum levels of ascorbic acid (vitamin C); with possible GI bleeding, loss of iron; vitamin K depletion Encourage diet rich in vitamin C
Diuretics (e.g., furosemide, chlorothiazide, hydrochlorothiazide)	Increased electrolyte excretion, leading to potassium, magnesium, and calcium depletion Potassium-rich diet is encouraged May necessitate potassium supplements
Diuretics (spironolactone)	Decreased potassium excretion; avoid supplements and salt substitutes
Laxatives	Decreased absorption of calcium, potassium, fat-soluble vitamins (especially vitamin D) Encourage fiber- and fluid-rich diets Encourage physical activity (may reduce the need for laxatives)

GI, Gastrointestinal.

Offering familiar foods and incorporating cultural needs within the prescribed diet is important. Long-term care facilities have begun to embrace these principles in their dietary offerings. The more liberalized diet has mild restrictions on salt, fat, and concentrated sweets but avoids severe restrictions when possible. These dietary policies promote a sense of control and independence. Liquid nutritional supplements may help increase kilocalorie, protein, and nutrient intake if the resident's intake is less than optimal; however, these supplements should not be used as a substitute for regular food.

Fluids should be offered to residents at all meals and between meals to ensure adequate intake. It is important for health care providers to watch for signs of dehydration in long-term care residents and to correct any deficits quickly.

Family involvement and socialization at mealtime may help increase residents' dietary intake; encourage it whenever possible.

Nutrient-Drug Interactions

Many older adults take many prescription medications daily to manage medical conditions or disease states. They may be taking over-the-counter medications as well and not realize the consequences to their nutritional state; many medications have the capacity to affect a person's nutritional status adversely.

Medications have the potential to either increase or decrease appetite or the ability to eat. In many instances, they also affect the absorption, metabolism, and excretion of some nutrients. Conversely, food intake and vitamin or mineral supplementation may affect the absorption, distribution, metabolism, and action of some medications (Table 19.10).

Caffeine. Caffeine is a central nervous system stimulant and a diuretic. It has potential to cause nervousness, irritability, anxiety, insomnia, and heart dysrhythmias and palpitations. It also tends to affect blood pressure, circulation, and gastric acid secretion. Caffeine tolerance may lessen with aging. Older adults should be encouraged to use moderation in their intake of caffeine, as well as to be aware of its possible effects, which may resemble an anxiety attack. Reducing caffeine intake often can alleviate the symptoms of an anxiety attack and possibly prevent the need for another drug to relieve anxiety.

MEDICAL NUTRITION THERAPY AND THERAPEUTIC DIETS

Medical nutrition therapy is the use of specific nutritional variations to build good health. It may involve simply modifying a nutritionally inadequate diet so that it becomes nutritionally adequate, or it may involve changing the texture or calorie content of the diet. A diet used as a medical treatment is called a **therapeutic diet**. Modifying a diet usually means adding or taking away specific nutrients or calories in a diet or changing the consistency of a diet, such as a pureed or soft diet. If a patient needs a special diet, the health care provider prescribes the diet, and it is up to the nurse to ensure that the patient understands and follows the diet, as well as to record how the patient reacts to it. When therapeutic diets are considered, it is important to account for the patient's cultural and religious preferences to increase compliance with the diet (see the Cultural Considerations box on nutrition).

Cultural Considerations

Culture and Nutrition

There is much to consider in dealing with patients of varied cultural, social, or religious backgrounds:

- Food habits are among the oldest and most deeply rooted aspects of many cultures.
- Food plays an important role in quality of life. The loss of culturally related foods during hospitalization or long-term care has great potential to affect the patient emotionally and physically.
- Never make assumptions. Be specific when asking questions regarding the patient's dietary preferences. Ask patients to provide a list of foods they like and dislike.
- The patient is likely to need help in marking the menu if he or she speaks another language or is unfamiliar with foods on the menu. Pictures of food are often helpful when there is a language barrier.
- Communication between the nursing staff and nutrition services is key to maintaining an adequate diet for the patient. Inform nutrition services if poor intake is noted so that the diet can be adjusted.
- Patients often have strong beliefs regarding certain foods or food combinations. Unless these beliefs are harmful to the patient, try to respect the patient's beliefs.
- In long-term care facilities, it is important to make every effort to work with the patient or family to provide special foods for observance of holidays, festivals, and other occasions.
- Occasionally, the family of a patient is permitted (with the health care provider's approval) to bring in food for the patient if the facility is unable to provide that food. Take special care to ensure food safety.

CONSISTENCY, TEXTURE, AND FREQUENCY MODIFICATIONS

The term *therapeutic diet* often is associated with nutrient-modified diets, such as low-fat or low-sodium diets. Modifications in textures, consistencies, and meal frequency, however, are also therapeutic in some cases. Most hospitals have standard diets based on consistency; these may include liquid, soft, and regular diets.

Liquid Diets

There are two types of liquid diets: clear liquid and full liquid. The clear liquid diet is nonirritating and consists of liquids that are easily digested and absorbed and leave little residue, or waste, in the GI tract. Because of that, very little stool is formed on a liquid diet. The clear liquid diet typically is used before diagnostic tests, particularly tests on the GI tract, and before surgery. It frequently is used postoperatively until peristalsis returns and sometimes is used during episodes of vomiting or diarrhea. The clear liquid diet is low in kilocalories, protein, and most nutrients. It is to be used temporarily, preferably for 2 to 3 days or less. Foods on a clear liquid diet include any type of liquid that you can see through, such as apple juice or white grape juice, fat-free broth or bouillon, plain gelatin, tea,

or black coffee. When patients are on a clear liquid diet, they usually are given small meals more frequently, usually every 2 to 3 hours (Box 19.7). It is important to note that a clear liquid diet does not mean the liquid must be colorless. Again, the term 'clear' indicates the liquid is free of pulp or solids. It may also be semi solid or solid as in gelatin or popsicles. If either of those have fruit pulp or pieces it will be classified as a full liquid product.

The full liquid diet is used as a transition diet after a clear liquid diet. It is more nutritionally complete than a clear liquid diet but still is lacking in some nutrients, such as iron, zinc, and fiber. A liquid dietary supplement, or vitamins, may be added to increase the nutritive value of the diet. This diet, too, is best used only temporarily. Examples of foods on a full liquid diet include ice cream, creamy soups, pudding, milk, and juices containing pulp.

Soft and Low-Residue Diets

Soft diets often are an intermediate step when a patient is progressing from a liquid to a regular diet. Soft diets and low-residue diets also are used for many people with conditions affecting the GI tract, such as acute diverticulitis, inflammatory bowel disease, gastritis, and esophageal varices, and during periods of indigestion or diarrhea.

A soft diet is generally low in fiber and is similar to a regular diet. It includes foods from all food groups, including meat, fish, poultry, eggs, milk, grains, fruits, and vegetables, but foods with strong spices are avoided. Mechanical soft diets often are ordered for patients who have difficulty chewing or swallowing. All meats are ground, and fruits and vegetables are cooked and pureed. This diet is nutritionally adequate, but supplements may be added.

The low-residue diet is similar to the soft diet but also includes restrictions on milk and milk products, because they leave more residue in the colon. If milk is omitted, the patient needs to get adequate calcium from other sources.

Regardless of the type of dietary restriction, the patient should be reminded why the diet has been ordered. When a patient does not understand the "why" of the restriction, compliance is difficult to ensure. Additionally, patients may perceive the provider and nurse do not care or are not concerned with their hunger (for example, on a liquid diet). These perceptions will hinder a trusting relationship with the health care team. Nurses should take the time to explain the duration and purpose of the dietary restrictions to assure the patient understands the benefit and reason.

High-Fiber Diets

The high-fiber diet is a variation of the regular diet and sometimes is used therapeutically. High-fiber diets often are used in the treatment of constipation. With adequate fluids, fiber has the capacity to

Box 19.7	Foods Included in Liquid Diets

CLEAR LIQUIDS
- Bouillon
- Fat-free broth
- Gelatin
- Ginger ale, lemon-lime soda
- Popsicles
- Tea, coffee
- White grape, apple, cranberry juice

FULL LIQUIDS
- All clear liquids
- Custard
- Fruit and vegetable juices
- Ice cream, sherbet
- Milk, milk shakes
- Puddings
- Strained cereals
- Strained soups
- Supplemental formulas

Box 19.8	Suggestions for Increasing Kilocalories and Protein

- Add cheese to casseroles, soups, and sauces.
- Add nuts and dried fruits to cereals, breads, or desserts.
- Add powdered milk or protein powder to milkshakes, beverages, soups, puddings, and cooked cereals.
- Add sugar to foods when reasonable (this adds only kilocalories).
- Encourage the patient to eat high-calorie foods first and eat the low-calorie foods if still hungry.
- Have snacks available at all times.
- Spread peanut butter on crackers, fruit, or celery.
- Use extra meat, chicken, or fish in casseroles and soups.
- Use generous amounts of calorie-dense foods such as butter, vegetable oils, mayonnaise, cream cheese, sour cream, and cream in recipes, as spreads, or as dips.

reduce constipation in young patients, as well as in older adults, which helps reduce or eliminate the need for laxatives. A high-fiber diet also is recommended for patients with diverticulosis and often helps lessen the severity of symptoms and inflammation (diverticulitis).

Patient instructions concerning high-fiber diets should include recommendations promoting higher fiber options such as whole grains. Fiber intake should be increased gradually to prevent excess gas formation. Fresh cooked or raw fruits and vegetables are preferred over processed foods, which have lesser nutritional values and contain high levels of sodium and other preservatives.

KILOCALORIE MODIFICATIONS

The body requires a specific amount of energy each day to carry out its tasks. This energy comes from the intake of food and fluids. The body uses this energy to maintain necessary, involuntary body functions, also called basal metabolic rate (BMR), to digest nutrients, or diet-induced thermogenesis, and for physical activity. When energy intake equals energy output, the body is in zero energy balance, or equilibrium. During zero energy balance, weight remains constant. If energy intake exceeds energy output, the energy balance becomes positive. Positive energy balance results in weight gain. Conversely, if energy intake is less than energy output, the energy balance becomes negative, leading to weight loss.

High-Kilocalorie and High-Protein Diets

During times of physiologic stress—such as after surgery, during sepsis, or in the presence of bone fractures, burns, or pressure injuries—the body's energy and protein needs are increased. Medical trauma has the potential to increase the BMR greatly. Therefore,

if energy needs are not met by diet, the patient loses protein stores and weight, and energy balance and nitrogen balance become negative.

In addition to the increased energy and protein needs, many patients with trauma and cancer suffer from *anorexia,* or lack of appetite. This adds to the already difficult task of maintaining adequate nutrition. High-kilocalorie and high-protein diets provide increased amounts of kilocalories and protein in small volumes and are used to help the compromised patient maintain adequate nutritional intake. Suggestions to help increase intake of kilocalories and protein are listed in Box 19.8.

When a patient is suffering from anorexia, the appearance of the food and how it is served may be the deciding factors in whether the patient eats it. Therefore it is important to maintain a positive attitude and provide encouragement when serving meals. Make meals as attractive as possible, and serve beverages, especially liquid nutritional supplements, in glasses, not cans. Make sure to serve meals promptly and at the correct temperature. Refrigerate snacks and supplements if necessary.

Obesity. The prevalence of obesity has reached epidemic proportions in the United States, and obesity is a growing health concern in developed and developing countries. In the United States, 42% of adults and more than 18% of children and adolescents are obese (CDC, 2021). Little differences are seen between genders. Obesity increases the risk for many diseases and health conditions, including hypertension, coronary heart disease, stroke, type 2 diabetes, dyslipidemias, osteoarthritis, gallbladder disease, some cancers, and sleep apnea. In addition to physical health risks, people who are obese often suffer from social prejudice and psychological issues related to their disease. Obesity dramatically affects quality of life and reduces average life expectancy.

Measurement of obesity. **Obesity** is defined as an excess of adipose tissue or body fat above the level considered healthy. **Body mass index (BMI)** is a number calculated from a person's weight and height (USDHHS, NIH, NHLBI, n.d.a). It provides an indicator of body fat and is used to screen for health problems related to weight. BMI accounts for total body weight and not just fat; some researchers say that this method is therefore not as accurate. Nonetheless, the BMI is recognized by many health care providers as the standard that defines overweight and obesity. BMI is determined by dividing body weight (in kilograms) by height (in meters squared). Fig. 19.5 lists the BMIs for various heights and weights. In general, if the BMI is below 18.5, the person is considered underweight; a BMI between 18.5 and 24.9 is considered within the "normal" range; if the BMI falls between 25 and 29.9, the person is considered overweight; and people with BMIs of 30 or greater are considered obese. To evaluate health status, it is important to consider *body composition* (the percentages of weight that comprise body fat versus lean tissue) as well as BMI. The location and amount of body fat in combination with BMI are sometimes better predictors of health risk than is BMI alone. Excess body fat in the upper body and the abdominal area in particular (central adiposity) increases the risk of cardiovascular disease and diabetes, whereas excess weight in the hips and the lower body poses a lesser risk.

Etiology of obesity. Obesity is caused by the chronic energy imbalance that results when more energy is consumed than expended. It is a complex disease, and much remains to be learned regarding its cause. Most experts agree that genetic, environmental, and behavioral factors contribute to obesity. The body has a powerful and multifaceted system that regulates energy intake and expenditure. Genetic, hormonal, and metabolic factors combine to control and regulate appetite and energy metabolism. Many obese individuals have a probable predisposition toward obesity that is precipitated by the environment in which they live and the lifestyle choices they make based on that environment.

Sedentary lifestyles are common in the United States. Only half of adults achieve the recommended amount of physical activity each day, and 25% report no leisure-time physical activity at all. Today's workforce has fewer positions requiring significant physical activity. Many workers spend their entire workday seated behind a desk. Some schools have cut physical education classes and recess time, so children are less physically active at school. Adults and children spend increasing amounts of time engaged in electronic entertainment with the television, computer, or handheld electronic devices. The typical American diet is also a factor in the cause of obesity. Because the food supply is abundant, it is easier to overeat. Food is readily available at any time of day, and it is possible to eat almost anywhere. High-fat, high-calorie prepackaged foods and sugar-laden soft drinks are readily accessible, and restaurants and supermarkets serve increasingly larger portions and package sizes. More people are consuming meals and snacks on the run, in the car, or in front of the computer or television and do not get much satiety, or satisfaction, from the food they eat.

Treatment of obesity. Obesity should be treated as a complex, chronic, relapsing disease. It is necessary to treat the obese patient with empathy and without prejudice. Effective therapy requires a lifelong commitment to healthy lifestyle behaviors and addresses the medical and the psychosocial aspects of the disease. The goal of obesity treatment should be to achieve weight management, not just weight loss. That means the person should achieve the best weight possible in the context of overall health. For many people, the ideal weight goals suggested on charts and tables are impossible to realize. Patients need to set realistic, achievable goals that they can maintain. Even a modest weight loss of 5% to 15% of body weight often reduces obesity-related health risks significantly.

A sound weight management program requires hard work and strong individual motivation. Weight management must be something the patient is able to follow; it must focus not only on reducing energy intake but also on changing the patient's dietary and exercise habits. In general, a good diet should provide no fewer than 1200 kcal/day. When the diet provides less than 1500 kcal/day, a multivitamin and mineral supplement is recommended. Caution patients against the use of very low calorie and semistarvation diets unless they are under the strict care of a health care provider.

Physical activity is an integral part of any weight loss effort and is critical for weight maintenance after initial loss. Recommend the inclusion of physical activity most days of the week for the prescribed amount of time for initial weight loss, and encourage physical activity for weight maintenance. Increasing physical activity may seem daunting to patients who have previously been inactive, but encourage a gradual increase of physical activity until the goal is achieved. It may be necessary to exert the proper amount of physical activity in shorter increments throughout the day rather than in one long session. Recreational activities such as sports and gardening count toward the physical activity total. Aerobic (oxygen-using) exercises such as brisk walking, jogging, cycling, cross-country skiing, and cross-training appear to be most helpful in decreasing body fat. Resistance training (weightlifting, calisthenics) is also beneficial to maintain lean body mass and bone density. BMR decreases when muscle mass is lost; therefore resistance training tends to help prevent a reduction of BMR. As with the diet, encourage people to find a physical activity that they enjoy and are able to continue. Exercise does not have to be extreme; in fact, moderate-intensity exercise is more sustainable and carries less risk of injury.

BMI	Normal						Overweight					Obese										Extreme Obesity															
	19	20	21	22	23	24	25	26	27	28	29	30	31	32	33	34	35	36	37	38	39	40	41	42	43	44	45	46	47	48	49	50	51	52	53	54
Height (inches)																																				
58	91	96	100	105	110	115	119	124	129	134	138	143	148	153	158	162	167	172	177	181	186	191	196	201	205	210	215	220	224	229	234	239	244	248	253	258
59	94	99	104	109	114	119	124	128	133	138	143	148	153	158	163	168	173	178	183	188	193	198	203	208	212	217	222	227	232	237	242	247	252	257	262	267
60	97	102	107	112	118	123	128	133	138	143	148	153	158	163	168	174	179	184	189	194	199	204	209	215	220	225	230	235	240	245	250	255	261	266	271	276
61	100	106	111	116	122	127	132	137	143	148	153	158	164	169	174	180	185	190	195	201	206	211	217	222	227	232	238	243	248	254	259	264	269	275	280	285
62	104	109	115	120	126	131	136	142	147	153	158	164	169	175	180	186	191	196	202	207	213	218	224	229	235	240	246	251	256	262	267	273	278	284	289	295
63	107	113	118	124	130	135	141	146	152	158	163	169	175	180	186	191	197	203	208	214	220	225	231	237	242	248	254	259	265	270	278	282	287	293	299	304
64	110	116	122	128	134	140	145	151	157	163	169	174	180	186	192	197	204	209	215	221	227	232	238	244	250	256	262	267	273	279	285	291	296	302	308	314
65	114	120	126	132	138	144	150	156	162	168	174	180	186	192	198	204	210	216	222	228	234	240	246	252	258	264	270	276	282	288	294	300	306	312	318	324
66	118	124	130	136	142	148	155	161	167	173	179	186	192	198	204	210	216	223	229	235	241	247	253	260	266	272	278	284	291	297	303	309	315	322	328	334
67	121	127	134	140	146	153	159	166	172	178	185	191	198	204	211	217	223	230	236	242	249	255	261	268	274	280	287	293	299	306	312	319	325	331	338	344
68	125	131	138	144	151	158	164	171	177	184	190	197	203	210	216	223	230	236	243	249	256	262	269	276	282	289	295	302	308	315	322	328	335	341	348	354
69	128	135	142	149	155	162	169	176	182	189	196	203	209	216	223	230	236	243	250	257	263	270	277	284	291	297	304	311	318	324	331	338	345	351	358	365
70	132	139	146	153	160	167	174	181	188	195	202	209	216	222	229	236	243	250	257	264	271	278	285	292	299	306	313	320	327	334	341	348	355	362	369	376
71	136	143	150	157	165	172	179	186	193	200	208	215	222	229	236	243	250	257	265	272	279	286	293	301	308	315	322	329	338	343	351	358	365	372	379	386
72	140	147	154	162	169	177	184	191	199	206	213	221	228	235	242	250	258	265	272	279	287	294	302	309	316	324	331	338	346	353	361	368	375	383	390	397
73	144	151	159	166	174	182	189	197	204	212	219	227	235	242	250	257	265	272	280	288	295	302	310	318	325	333	340	348	355	363	371	378	386	393	401	408
74	148	155	163	171	179	186	194	202	210	218	225	233	241	249	256	264	272	280	287	295	303	311	319	326	334	342	350	358	365	373	381	389	396	404	412	420
75	152	160	168	176	184	192	200	208	216	224	232	240	248	256	264	272	279	287	295	303	311	319	327	335	343	351	359	367	375	383	391	399	407	415	423	431
76	156	164	172	180	189	197	205	213	221	230	238	246	254	263	271	279	287	295	304	312	320	328	336	344	353	361	369	377	385	394	402	410	418	426	435	443

Body Weight (pounds)

Fig. 19.5 Body mass index. (Data from National Institutes of Health [NIH]: *Body mass index table 1*, n.d. From https://www.nhlbi.nih.gov/health/educational/lose_wt/BMI/bmi_tbl.htm.)

Effective psychological interventions in the treatment of obesity foster a healthier attitude about eating and body image. This usually includes counseling about self-esteem, body image, body acceptance, and coping with societal pressures. Patients often need to practice mindfulness and body awareness, learning to sense feelings of fullness by responding to internal rather than external cues. Through this process, many patients can reduce their focus on weight loss and food and establish a more constructive focus on life and good health. A support system—consisting of family, friends, or a support group—is also beneficial.

Bariatric surgery for the treatment of obesity has become common. Candidates for bariatric surgery are usually morbidly obese (BMI ≥40) or have a BMI of 35 or higher with other medical conditions such as cardiovascular disease or type 2 diabetes. Patients achieve substantial weight loss after bariatric surgery and, if diet and exercise recommendations are followed, do not regain the weight. Patients with weight-related disorders such as preexisting diabetes, hyperlipidemia, hypertension, or sleep apnea also may experience substantial improvement in these conditions. In addition, mortality rates among surgically treated obese patients appear to be lower than in those who receive treatment with traditional methods. For most patients, the benefits of bariatric surgery outweigh the risks; however, as with any major surgery, risks do exist and include nutrition-related complications such as nutrient deficiencies, dumping syndrome, and diarrhea. Because patients can eat only small amounts of food after bariatric surgery, the health care provider usually prescribes a multivitamin and mineral supplement, along with other nutritional supplements as needed. The most common nutritional deficiencies after bariatric surgery include those of iron, folic acid, and vitamin B_{12}. After bariatric surgery, it is important to encourage the patient to eat small portion sizes, to eat slowly, and to chew foods completely. They also should consume beverages and food at separate times and avoid foods that are poorly tolerated. It is also important to encourage adequate amounts of physical activity to help maintain the weight loss (USDHHS, NIH, NIDDK, n.d.a).

Pharmacologic therapy involves the use of prescription drugs or over-the-counter medications to treat obesity. If patients use weight-loss drugs, it is important to make these drugs part of a comprehensive program along with diet therapy and physical activity. Over-the-counter medications sometimes help suppress appetite; however, the effect is usually temporary.

CARBOHYDRATE-MODIFIED DIETS

Diabetes Mellitus

Carbohydrate-modified diets are used most often in the treatment of diabetes mellitus. Diabetes mellitus is a disease in which the body does not produce or properly use insulin. Insulin is a hormone that is needed to convert sugar, starches, and other food into the energy needed for daily life. The cause of diabetes is unknown, although genetics and environmental factors such as obesity and lack of exercise appear to play a role.

There are two major types of diabetes mellitus. Type 1 diabetes mellitus, most often diagnosed in children and young adults, is a disease in which the body does not produce any insulin (hormone produced by the pancreas needed to use glucose). People with type 1 diabetes are required to take insulin therapy for life. Type 1 diabetes accounts for approximately 5% of diabetes cases (American Diabetes Association, n.d.b). Type 2 diabetes mellitus is a metabolic disorder resulting from the body's inability to make enough or properly use insulin. It is the most common form of the disease and accounts for about 95% of diabetes cases (American Diabetes Association, n.d.a). Because of the increasing number of older Americans and a higher incidence of obesity and sedentary lifestyles, the number of people in whom type 2 diabetes is diagnosed has increased dramatically.

Nutrition therapy for diabetes mellitus. Diabetes is a disease that directly involves how well the body uses the nutrients consumed. Because of that, nutrition plays a major role in the treatment of diabetes. The goals for people with diabetes are the control and prevention of complications. Normal nutrition and dietary modification to control blood glucose and lipid levels are extremely important. Educating the patient on the proper diet is important so that the patient can make changes in food and exercise habits to improve metabolic control.

Achieving nutrition-related goals necessitates a coordinated effort by a health care team that includes the patient's health care provider, the nurse, the diabetic educator, the registered dietitian, the patient, and the patient's family. It is necessary to individualize nutrition therapy for each patient with diabetes; standardized preprinted diet sheets should be avoided. All patients with diabetes need the opportunity to develop a realistic and achievable eating plan to which they will adhere. Lifestyle, current eating and exercise patterns, caloric and nutrient needs, the presence of other diseases, and the use of insulin or oral antidiabetic medication are necessary considerations in developing an eating plan for a patient with diabetes.

Nutrition recommendations for a healthy lifestyle are important for all people; what differs for those with diabetes is the need to monitor more closely and control carbohydrate intake. The patient with newly diagnosed diabetes may erroneously want to focus on the amount of "sugar" in the diet and on food labels. It is important to educate the patient that carbohydrates are converted to glucose. So, the amount of sugar in food items is important, and it is actually the carbohydrates the patient will want to focus on.

The patient with diabetes must coordinate the timing of meals and snacks and administration of insulin or oral diabetic medications with exercise. Consistent meal timing, approximately every 4 to 5 hours, and consistent carbohydrate content are important to stress during patient teaching. Advise inclusion in the diet of foods containing carbohydrates from whole grains, fruits, vegetables, and low-fat milk. The amount of dietary carbohydrate intake should be based on individual needs as outlined in the MyPlate dietary guidelines, as well as the *Dietary Guidelines for Americans* (USDA and USDHHS, 2015; USDA and USDHHS, n.d.). The *total amount* of carbohydrate in meals and snacks is more important than the source or type of carbohydrate. Patients with diabetes should be encouraged to consume a variety of fiber-containing foods, but there is no reason to recommend a greater amount of fiber than any person in the general population would consume.

People with diabetes also should limit the amount of fat in their diet to control blood lipid levels. It is recommended that saturated fat be limited to less than 5% to 6% of calories and dietary cholesterol to less than 200 mg/day (AHA, 2017). In addition, *trans* fatty acids should be kept to a minimum. Evidence suggests that the use of monounsaturated fats in place of some carbohydrates often helps lower blood triglyceride levels and improves glycemic control as well. Two or more servings of fish per week (except commercially fried filets) are recommended (USDHHS, NIH, and NDDK, 2005).

Type 1 diabetes mellitus. Because most patients with type 1 diabetes are still in childhood or adolescence at the time of diagnosis, it is necessary for the eating plan to provide adequate kilocalories for normal growth and development and to be as flexible as possible. It is also important to balance carbohydrate intake with insulin administration and exercise. Initially, consistent timing and consistent content of meals and snacks are essential to determine insulin requirements. Patients are then able to monitor blood glucose levels and learn to adjust insulin dosages according to blood glucose patterns.

Type 2 diabetes mellitus. The primary goals of nutrition therapy for type 2 diabetes are to achieve and maintain desirable weight, normal blood cholesterol concentration, and normal blood glucose levels. Many people with type 2 diabetes are overweight and insulin resistant. Promoting changes to increase activity levels and make lifestyle changes is beneficial to reduce this resistance. Mild to moderate weight loss (5% to 7% of starting weight) has been shown to improve metabolic control, even if desirable weight is not achieved. Increased physical activity can aid in weight reduction, improve blood glucose levels, decrease insulin resistance, and reduce cardiovascular risk factors.

Meal-planning approaches. Even though patients with diabetes must monitor the carbohydrate and fat content of their diet, they do not need to buy special foods. Many meal-planning tools are available for them to use with foods normally available.

Exchange lists have been used for many years and sometimes still are used in diabetic meal planning. They are complicated and may be overwhelming for some patients. In an exchange list, foods are divided into groups based on carbohydrate, protein, and fat content. Typically, the patient receives instructions to include a certain number of servings from each food group at a particular meal or snack. By identifying correct serving sizes and the nutrient components of food groups, patients can better control their carbohydrate, fat, and kilocalorie intake throughout the day (Table 19.11).

Carbohydrate counting is a meal-planning approach that focuses on the total amount of carbohydrates eaten at meals and snacks. For some patients with diabetes, this approach is much simpler than exchange lists. It focuses on just one nutrient, and patients can see a direct correlation between carbohydrate intake and the blood glucose level, which makes it easier for them to comply with the recommended eating plan. For others, carbohydrate counting can be difficult because of the weighing and measuring of the food and the need to calculate the grams of carbohydrates consumed. Protein and fat are not counted with this type of meal planning, but the patient should be encouraged to eat the same amount of protein each day and choose foods that are low in fat.

Other nutritional considerations. If a person taking insulin fails to consume adequate carbohydrates, the blood glucose level may drop, causing hypoglycemia (low blood glucose level). Symptoms of hypoglycemia include headache, disorientation, weakness, perspiration, shallow breathing, nervousness, visual disturbances, and vertigo, and sometimes the individual may become unconscious. It is necessary to treat hypoglycemia with immediate administration of glucose or any carbohydrate that contains glucose. A good strategy for patients to practice is the 15 to 15 rule: take 15 g of carbohydrate, wait 15 minutes, and test blood glucose to see whether the response to the carbohydrate is adequate. If the patient becomes unconscious, intravenous (IV) administration of glucose is essential.

Acute illness increases the risk of diabetic ketoacidosis in patients with type 1 diabetes and increases the risk for hyperosmolar hyperglycemic nonketotic syndrome in patients with type 2 diabetes. During acute illness, it is important for the patient to continue taking insulin and carefully monitoring blood glucose levels. Encourage the patient to drink adequate amounts of fluids and to ingest carbohydrates, especially if the blood glucose level falls below normal levels. Beverages such as juices and punch, popsicles,

Table 19.11   **Example of an Exchange List**

FOOD	SERVING SIZE	FOOD	SERVING SIZE
Grains		**Vegetable**	
Bagel	¼ large bagel (1 oz)	Hominy	¾ cup
Breads		Marinara, pasta or spaghetti sauce	½ cup
White, whole-grain, French, Italian, pumpernickel, rye, sourdough, unfrosted raisin or cinnamon	1 slice (1 oz)	Mixed vegetables with corn or peas	1 cup
		Parsnips	½ cup
		Peas, green	½ cup
Reduced calorie, light	2 slices (1½ oz)	Potato	
Cornbread	1¾-inch cube (1½ oz)	Baked with skin	¼ large potato (3 oz)
Hot dog bun or hamburger bun	½ bun (¾ oz)	Boiled, all kinds	½ cup or ½ medium potato
Roll, plain	1 small roll (1 oz)	Mashed with milk and fat	½ cup
Stuffing, bread	⅓ cup	French-fried (oven baked)	1 cup (2 oz)
Crackers		Squash, winter (acorn or butternut)	1 cup
Animal	8 crackers	Yam or sweet potato, plain	½ cup (3½ oz)
Graham, 2½ inch square	3 squares	**Snacks**	
Oyster	20 crackers	Popcorn	
Round, butter-type	6 crackers	No fat added	3 cups
Saltine-type	6 crackers	With butter added	3 cups
Granola or snack bar	1 bar (¾ oz)	Pretzels	¾ oz
Matzoh, all shapes and sizes	¾ oz	Rice cakes	2 cakes (4 inches across)
Pancake	1 pancake (4 inches across, ¼ inch thick)	Snack chips	
		Baked (potato, pita)	About 8 chips (¾ oz)
Waffle	1 waffle (4-inch square or 4 inches across)	Regular (tortilla, potato)	About 13 chips (1 oz)

The Food Lists are the basis of a meal-planning system designed by a committee of the American Diabetes Association and The Academy of Nutrition and Dietetics. Although designed primarily for people with diabetes and others who must follow special diets, the Food Lists are based on principles of good nutrition that apply to everyone. Copyright 2014 by the Academy of Nutrition and Dietetics, American Diabetes Association, Inc.

flavored gelatin, crackers, puddings, and ice cream contain carbohydrates and tend to be more palatable to sick people.

For people with diabetes, the guidelines for alcohol use are the same as for the general population. If individuals choose to drink alcohol, teach them to limit intake: one drink per day for women and two drinks per day for men. Because alcohol increases the risk of hypoglycemia, consuming it with food is best.

Dumping Syndrome

Dumping syndrome is possible after surgery in which a portion or all the stomach is removed (partial or total gastrectomy) or after bariatric surgery for weight reduction. Dumping syndrome can occur when the contents of the stomach empty too quickly into the small intestine. The partially digested food draws excess fluid into the small intestine, which causes nausea, cramping, diarrhea, sweating, lightheadedness, and palpitations. These signs and symptoms usually occur shortly after meals or after the consumption of too much simple or refined sugar.

Diet therapy is aimed at slowing gastric emptying and distributing the amount of gastric contents in the bowel over time. This involves giving small, frequent meals that are higher in protein and fat and lower in carbohydrates. The patient is encouraged to avoid concentrated sweets and to drink fluids 30 to 60 minutes before or after a meal. Having the patient lie down for 30 to 60 minutes after a meal also may help slow stomach emptying. The dumping syndrome diet is, in some cases, needed only temporarily until the body adjusts to the changes caused by surgery. There are many diseases in which sitting up after a meal is recommended, but dumping syndrome is one of the few disorders in which lying down after a meal is encouraged.

Lactose Intolerance

Lactose intolerance occurs when there is a lack of the digestive enzyme *lactase*. In the absence of lactase, the GI tract is unable to break down lactose, the milk sugar. This condition is hereditary; the incidence of this disorder is increased among African Americans, Hispanics, Asian Americans, and Native Americans. Lactose intolerance is not the same condition as an allergy to cow's milk. Symptoms usually occur 30 minutes to 2 hours after ingestion of milk products and include nausea, cramps, a bloated feeling, flatulence, and diarrhea.

The diet for lactose intolerance excludes milk and milk products, such as ice cream, puddings, cheese, and powdered milk. Affected patients often need to avoid foods with milk added, such as biscuit or muffin mixes, some soups, and other prepared foods. In addition, many processed foods—such as waffles, pancakes, and processed meats—contain lactose. Dietary counseling should include alternative sources of calcium and potential recommendations for supplementation.

When there is a deficiency rather than a total absence of lactase, patients are often able to tolerate small amounts of milk products, especially yogurt and cheese. Several lactase enzyme–containing preparations are also available to take before consuming dairy products, and many grocery stores now carry lactose-free milks and milk products.

FAT-MODIFIED DIETS

Research has shown that modifying the amount of fat in the diet may reduce the risk of heart and vascular disease by about 14% and that the risk for some cancers can be reduced as well.

Low-Fat Diets

A low-fat diet has limited amounts of total fat, saturated fat, and *trans* fatty acids. This type of diet is needed for the prevention and treatment of *atherosclerosis* (a disorder characterized by buildup of cholesterol and lipids on the artery walls), heart disease, and *hyperlipidemia* (elevated levels of blood lipids).

To help Americans reduce the risk of cardiovascular disease, the American Heart Association has recommended dietary guidelines for the general population to decrease the amount of fat in the diet. The National Cholesterol Education Program has also developed the Therapeutic Lifestyle Changes (TLC) diet to help decrease the amount of fat and cholesterol ingested (Table 19.12) (USDHHS, NIH, and NIDDK, 2005).

Many patients have a difficult time complying with a low-fat diet because they think the required foods lack flavor and are not as satisfying. Even though they need to reduce saturated and *trans* fatty acids in the diet, patients are still able to choose low-fat foods from all the food groups. Encourage them to choose low-fat dairy products, lean meats, skinless poultry, and fish. Advise limiting eggs to four or fewer per week and limiting organ meats, such as liver, to one serving or less per week. Limits are also necessary on added fats, such as butter, stick margarine, mayonnaise, cream, and sour cream.

The inclusion of monounsaturated fats and omega-3 fatty acids in the diet often helps lower blood cholesterol and triglyceride levels. Patients should be encourage to substitute unsaturated fatty acids in the diet instead of saturated and *trans* fatty acids. Teach patients to identify food sources of these fats, such as fish, olive oil, canola oil, peanut oil, flaxseed oil, soy products, and nuts.

Keep in mind that fat possesses many good qualities and offers much pleasure when eaten. Many Americans tend to rebel against a low-fat diet because they believe it is necessary to eliminate all fatty foods. Choosing a low-fat and low-cholesterol diet does not mean "never eat cheese because it contains fat" or "never eat egg yolks because they contain cholesterol." It is the *total* amount of fat, saturated fat, and cholesterol that matters. Besides, foods such as cheese and egg yolks contribute nutrients necessary to the diet, and sometimes eliminating all high-fat foods compromises the diet's overall nutritional value. Therefore rather than totally eliminating high-fat foods, patients should be encouraged to use moderation. They should balance high-fat foods with other foods that contain less fat and cholesterol. By adhering to balance, variety, and moderation, patients are still able to enjoy some of their favorite foods while following a healthy, fat-controlled diet.

Fat-Controlled Diets

The fat-controlled diet is used to treat symptoms of diarrhea, steatorrhea, and flatulence or to treat diseases of the hepatobiliary tract, pancreas, intestinal mucosa, and the lymphatic system, as well as malabsorption syndromes.

These diets sometimes restrict fat to as little as 25 g/day depending on the severity of the symptoms. With this severe fat restriction, no visible fats (e.g., butter, cream, oil) are allowed. Only nonfat dairy products and lean meat, fish, and poultry (no more than 5 oz/day) are allowed. It is important to encourage adequate consumption of grains, cereals, fruits, and vegetables. Vitamin and mineral supplementation also may be necessary to offset the nutrient deficiencies caused by prolonged or excessive diarrhea or steatorrhea.

Metabolic Syndrome

Metabolic syndrome is a name for a group of metabolic risk factors that occur together and increase the risk for coronary artery disease, stroke, and type 2 diabetes. These risk factors include abdominal obesity, dyslipidemia, elevated blood pressure, and insulin resistance. The most important of these risk factors appears to be abdominal obesity (waist circumference of 40 inches or more in men and 35 inches or more in women) and insulin resistance (fasting blood glucose level of 100 mg/dL or higher). The prevalence of metabolic syndrome has increased dramatically; 50 million cases have been estimated in the United States. For affected patients without established diabetes, metabolic syndrome doubles the risk of developing atherosclerotic cardiovascular disease (ASCVD); for those with diabetes, the risk is increased fivefold. Thus the early diagnosis and treatment of metabolic syndrome is likely to help reduce the incidence of ASCVD.

The goal of treatment for metabolic syndrome is to reduce the risk for heart disease and diabetes. Lifestyle changes usually are initiated first in the treatment of metabolic syndrome. Lifestyle changes include cessation of cigarette smoking, weight loss in overweight or obese individuals, increased physical activity, and a fat-controlled diet. Depending upon the severity of

Table 19.12   Guidelines for Following the Therapeutic Lifestyle Changes (TLC) Diet

FOOD GROUPS	CHOOSE	GO EASY ON
Meat, Poultry, and Fish		
<5 oz/day; 2 servings of fish/week	• Lean fresh meats, extra-lean ground beef, and lean deli meats[a] • Poultry without the skin, ground turkey made from white meat • Fish and shellfish	• Meats with visible fat and marbling • Regular ground beef • Processed meats: sausage, bacon, frankfurters, cold cuts • Organ meats • Duck and goose • Deep-fried meats, poultry, or fish • Shellfish (some are high in cholesterol; use moderate portions)
Eggs		
<2 egg yolks/week	• Eggs (limit yolks to 2/week; substitute 2 egg whites for 1 egg in recipes)	
Dry Beans and Nuts		
	• Dry beans and peas, fat-free refried beans, tofu • Nuts[a] (in moderation)	
Milk, Yogurt, and Cheese		
2–3 servings/day	• Fat-free (skim) or 1% milk, buttermilk, soy milk • Fat-free or reduced-fat cheese[a] (3 g of fat or less per oz) • Low-fat or nonfat cottage cheese[a] • Low-fat or fat-free yogurt	• Whole or 2% milk, half-and-half • Whole-milk yogurt • Full-fat cheese with more than 3 g fat per oz
Fruits and Vegetables		
5 or more servings/day	• Fresh, frozen, canned, or dried fruits and vegetables • Add more vegetables to meat dishes, casseroles, or soups • Keep fresh fruits and vegetables readily available for snacks • Use fruit as dessert	• Vegetables with high-calorie sauces • Fruits with added sugar • Deep-fried vegetables (including French fries) • Limit juices, instead choosing whole fruits and vegetables for more fiber
Breads, Cereals, Rice, Pasta, and Other Grains		
6 or more servings/day depending on energy needs	• Breads, bread products, and cereals made from whole grains such as whole wheat, buckwheat, bulgur (cracked wheat), oats, rye, millet, quinoa, bran • Brown rice, wild rice • Whole-grain pastas • Popcorn	• White breads and products made with refined grains that are lower in fiber (check label) • Baked goods made with added fat and eggs, such as muffins, biscuits, croissants, and butter rolls
Fats and Oils		
Limited total amount; replace saturated fats with unsaturated fats; read labels to identify saturated and *trans* fat content	• Liquid vegetable oils (canola, corn, olive, peanut, safflower, sesame, soybean, and sunflower) • Margarines with liquid vegetable oils as first ingredient (soft tub, liquid, or vegetable oil spreads) • Light or nonfat mayonnaise and salad dressing • Reduced-fat sour cream, cream cheese, and whipped toppings	• Butter, lard, fatback, bacon drippings • Margarines with hydrogenated or partially hydrogenated oil as the first ingredient (read label for *trans* fat) • Solid shortening • Coconut milk; coconut, palm and palm-kernel oils • Full-fat sour cream, cream cheese, whipped cream
Sweets, Snacks, Condiments		
To be used occasionally on basis of caloric needs	• Low-fat ice cream, frozen yogurt, sorbet, sherbet, or low-fat puddings • Angel food cake; low-fat brownies • Fat-free or low-fat cookies such as animal crackers, vanilla wafers, gingersnaps, graham crackers • Whole-grain snack crackers[a]	• Regular ice cream; pudding made with whole or 2% milk • Doughnuts and pastries • Pie, regular cakes, and cookies • Snack crackers with high fat content

[a]Sometimes contain high levels of sodium.
Modified from US Department of Health and Human Services: *Lowering your cholesterol with TLC*. Retrieved from *www.nhlbi.nih.gov/health/public/heart/chol/chol_tlc.pdf*.

risk factors and the patient's response to the therapeutic lifestyle changes, more aggressive treatments or medications may be needed.

PROTEIN-, ELECTROLYTE-, AND FLUID-MODIFIED DIETS

Protein-Restricted Diets

In disease states, increased protein intake often is needed to facilitate healing. However, in the presence of defects in protein metabolism or excretion, it is best to reduce or at least control protein intake. Two such conditions, chronic renal failure and cirrhosis of the liver, sometimes necessitate protein restrictions.

In renal failure, the kidneys are unable to excrete protein waste products. These waste products build up in the bloodstream, leading to a condition known as *azotemia*. If a patient is experiencing renal failure, a modest protein restriction may delay the need for dialysis. Protein restriction in renal failure involves limiting the total amount of protein consumed and emphasizing the use of high-quality proteins. High-quality proteins are complete proteins found in eggs, meat, poultry, fish, and milk products. Incomplete proteins, those found in plant products such as dried beans and whole grains, contribute to azotemia and must be limited. Once a patient has been placed on renal dialysis, protein needs are greater than for the normal population; however, the dietary emphasis is still on complete proteins.

Cirrhosis is a chronic degenerative disease of the liver in which scar tissue develops and hinders the liver's effectiveness in removing ammonia. The ammonia then builds up in the bloodstream and, if not controlled, can lead to hepatic coma, brain damage, and death. In the presence of cirrhosis, protein intake initially should be at or above the DRI to facilitate healing and tissue regeneration. However, if blood ammonia levels become elevated, a low-protein diet is recommended. Special nutritional support formulas with modified protein content have been developed for use by patients with renal failure and cirrhosis to lower the protein content of the diet.

Sodium-Restricted Diets

Sodium-restricted diets may be used for a variety of medical conditions; however, they are used most often in the treatment of hypertension or heart failure. In 2001, the National Institutes of Health and the National Heart, Lung, and Blood Institute developed the Dietary Approaches to Stop Hypertension (DASH) diet. This diet quickly became popular among health care providers because it was shown to effectively lower blood pressure by limiting sodium intake to 1500 to 2400 mg/day. The DASH diet also emphasizes the inclusion of fruit and vegetables, as well as low-fat or nonfat milk products (Box 19.9) (USDHHS, NIH, and NHLBI, n.d.b).

Sodium-restricted diets also may be used in cases of water retention or edema, especially in the presence of heart failure. With congestive heart failure, a decrease in sodium intake is necessary to alleviate pulmonary and peripheral edema and reduce the workload of the heart. Some other conditions that may warrant a sodium-restricted diet include myocardial infarction, cirrhosis accompanied by ascites, and chronic renal failure.

Sodium-restricted diets vary in degree. The no-added-salt diet is the least restrictive, allowing 2000 to 3000 mg/day of sodium. This diet allows the use of most foods with the exception of highly salted snack foods and prepared foods. Patients following this diet must read nutrition labels to determine the sodium content of food products and then decide which foods are appropriate for their diet. Encourage patients to limit the amount of salt in cooking or at the table (Box 19.10). Other sodium-restricted diets may allow as much as 2000 mg/day or as little as 500 mg/day of sodium.

Box 19.9 Daily and Weekly DASH Eating Plan Goals for a 2000-Calorie-a-Day Diet

FOOD GROUP	DAILY SERVINGS
Grains	6–8
Meats, poultry, and fish	6 or less
Vegetables	4–5
Fruit	4–5
Low-fat or fat-free dairy products	2–3
Fats and oils	2–3
Sodium	2300 mg[a]
	WEEKLY SERVINGS
Nuts, seeds, dry beans, and peas	4–5
Sweets	5 or less

[a]1500 milligrams (mg) sodium lowers blood pressure even further than 2300 mg sodium daily.
From US Department of Health and Human Services (USDHHS), National Institutes of Health (NIH), National Heart, Lung and Blood Institute (NHLBI : DASH eating plan. Retrieved from *https://www.nhlbi.nih.gov/health-topics/dash-eating-plan*.

Box 19.10 What to Limit in Sodium-Restricted Diets

- Canned vegetables (fresh and frozen are lower in sodium)
- Commercial mixes such as pasta, stuffing, muffins, and potatoes
- Leavening agents such as baking soda and baking powder
- Processed cheeses
- Regular canned soups, broths, and bouillon
- Salt in cooking or at the table
- Salt-preserved foods such as smoked or cured meats or pickled foods
- Salty snack foods such as pretzels, popcorn, and chips
- Spices and condiments that contain sodium, such as soy sauce, barbeque sauce, Worcestershire and steak sauces, meat tenderizers, monosodium glutamate (MSG), spice salts, and salad dressings

Note: In general, the more processed or "instant" a food is, the more sodium it contains.

Potassium-Modified Diets

Potassium plays many important roles in the body, and a lack of, or an increase in the amounts of, potassium can cause a variety of problems. Increased intake of potassium may help with blood pressure control when it is in direct proportion to sodium intake. The American Heart Association and proponents of the DASH diet encourage balanced sodium/potassium intake in a diet that emphasizes fruits, vegetables, and low-fat dairy products. This diet is rich in potassium, magnesium, and calcium and helps reduce blood pressure in many cases. People taking potassium-wasting diuretics may need larger amounts of potassium in their diet or potassium supplements to offset the loss of potassium.

In end-stage renal disease and other kidney disease, it is sometimes necessary to restrict potassium intake to as little as 2000 mg/day. During renal failure, potassium is retained, which leads to a buildup of potassium in the bloodstream. If dietary intake is not controlled, blood potassium levels potentially can increase to the point of causing dysrhythmias and sudden cardiac arrest.

Fluid-Modified Diets

Fluid is a big part of the diet and can be found in many foods. Of course, all beverages add fluid to the diet, as do gelatins, ice cream, sherbet, puddings, popsicles, fruit ices, and soups. In good health, most adults need between 2 and 3 L of water a day to maintain hydration; in the presence of certain illnesses, however, the patient's water intake may be restricted.

During end-stage renal disease and other kidney disease with low urine output, fluid is restricted to 500 to 750 mL/day (approximately 2 to 3 cups) plus an amount equal to any daily urine output. Fluid restrictions are also common during congestive heart failure, directly after a myocardial infarction, in hepatic coma, or in the presence of ascites.

In the hospital, fluid restrictions often are divided between the nursing and the dietary departments. For example, if a patient has a 1000-mL fluid restriction, the dietary department sometimes can provide the patient with 600 mL/day, and the nursing department gives 400 mL/day. The amount of fluid allowed for nursing depends on the patient's IV and medication needs, as these fluids are counted into the total allotted for the day.

Although patients have fluid restrictions, they often experience excessive thirst. Some suggestions to help alleviate thirst include rinsing the mouth with cold mouthwash, putting lemon into cold water to make it more refreshing, freezing fluid so that it takes longer to consume, eating cold fruits and raw vegetables, chewing gum, sucking on breath mints or hard candies (in moderation), brushing teeth often, and limiting sodium intake (see the Patient Teaching box on fluid restrictions). Patient on a fluid restriction should be offered their choice of beverages when they are permitted to have fluids. This will alleviate some of the frustration with this type of restriction.

Patient Teaching

Fluid Restrictions

The health care provider and dietitian determine the exact fluid restriction. The nurse must teach and reinforce the fluid restriction by

- Explaining the rationale for the fluid restriction
- Indicating whether the restriction is temporary or permanent
- Identifying the various sources of fluid intake (e.g., intravenous fluids; fluid with medications; fluid in foods such as soup, ice cream, or gelatin)
- Teaching what "mL" represents and comparing it with measures with which the patient is familiar; for example, "You are allowed 1000 mL of fluid per day; this is about the same as 1 quart, or 4 cups"
- Showing patients the volume of fluid they are allowed
- Suggesting ways to alleviate thirst without drinking fluids
- Discussing the consequences of overconsumption of fluids

Increased fluid intake is a common dietary treatment for renal calculi (kidney stones) and urinary tract infection. Additional fluid helps dilute the urine and increase urinary output. Fluid needs are also higher during periods of diarrhea, vomiting, or malabsorption, as in inflammatory bowel disease. To prevent dehydration, the patient needs to replace fluids that are lost.

Patients with burn injuries lose a large amount of fluids from the wounds. Immediately after a severe burn, fluids, electrolytes, and protein are given intravenously rather than orally, because burn-injured patients experience a temporary loss of bowel function. Once bowel activity resumes, adequate fluids are a necessary part of dietary treatment. Burn-injured victims also require large amounts of protein, kilocalories, and certain vitamins and minerals.

Most conditions necessitating medical nutrition therapy involve combinations of therapeutic diets. To summarize, Table 19.13 lists different medical conditions and the diets commonly prescribed.

NUTRITIONAL SUPPORT

Occasionally a patient is unable to consume an oral diet. In these instances, alternative feeding methods are available in the form of tube feedings or IV feedings.

TUBE FEEDINGS

A tube feeding is the administration of nutritionally balanced, liquefied foods or formula through a tube inserted into the stomach, the duodenum, or the jejunum by way of a nasogastric tube or an ostomy. The feeding sometimes is referred to as enteral nutrition (administration of nutrients into the GI tract). Tube feedings typically are indicated when a patient is unable to chew or swallow, such as after oral surgery or

Table **19.13**   **Summary of Diet Modifications**

CONDITION	POSSIBLE DIET MODIFICATIONS
Acquired immunodeficiency syndrome (AIDS)	High calorie and high protein; increased fluid intake; mechanical soft diet; possible tube feeding or total parenteral nutrition (TPN)
Atherosclerosis	Low fat and cholesterol; avoid *trans* fatty acids; high fiber; increase fruits, vegetables and whole grain products; low calorie or sodium restrictions if necessary
Burns	High calorie and high protein; increased fluid intake; increased vitamins and minerals
Cancer	High calorie and high protein, depending on the type of cancer, dietary adjustments are made on the basis of symptoms; increased vitamins and minerals; increased fluids; possible tube feeding or TPN
Cirrhosis, hepatic coma	Protein restricted; possible sodium, fat, and fluid restriction; no alcohol; vitamin and mineral supplementation; mechanical soft diet
Congestive heart failure	Sodium restricted; fluid restricted; small, frequent feedings; soft diet; possible calorie restriction; avoid or limit alcohol
Constipation	High fiber; increased fluid intake; increased natural laxative fruits
Cystic fibrosis	High calorie, fat, and protein; increased sodium intake; vitamin and mineral supplementation, enzyme replacement therapy; possible tube feeding or TPN
Diabetes mellitus	Carbohydrate counting and Food Exchange System to meet individual needs; fat controlled; high fiber; planned consistent meals
Diverticular disease	Increased fiber and fluid; avoid foods that cause discomfort
Dumping syndrome	Carbohydrate restricted; no concentrated sweets; small, frequent feedings
Gallbladder disease	Low fat; when necessary, calorie-restricted; small frequent meals
Gastritis	Low fat and/or acidic foods; avoid foods that increase symptoms
Gastroesophageal reflux disease (GERD)	Calorie restrictions to decrease weight; low fat and/or acidic foods; avoid lying down after meals; don't eat within 3 h of going to bed and sleep with head of bed elevated
Hepatitis	High protein, high carbohydrate, moderate fat; tube feedings or TPN may be necessary
Hiatal hernia	Small, frequent feedings; calorie restrictions to decrease weight; avoid lying down after meals; don't eat within 3 h of going to bed and sleep with head of bed elevated
Hyperlipidemia	Low cholesterol and saturated *trans* fats; high fiber
Hypertension	Restricted calorie to decrease weight; sodium restrictions; DASH diet; vitamin/mineral supplementation esp. calcium, potassium and magnesium; increased fiber
Hypoglycemia	Carbohydrate counting and Food Exchange System to meet individual needs; fat controlled; high fiber; consistent meals
Inflammatory bowel disease	Consistent diet; avoid fructose, lactose, sorbitol, caffeine and alcohol; avoid gas forming foods; increased fiber; fluid and electrolyte replacement; vitamin and mineral supplementation
Lactose intolerance	Lactose restricted
Myocardial infarction (heart attack)	Low calorie initially then advanced to meet energy needs; small, frequent meals; soft diet; low fat and sodium; possible fluid restrictions
Nausea and vomiting	Small, frequent feedings; low fat; bland, soft, dry foods; increase fluid intake slowly
Obesity	Calorie restricted; fat controlled; high fiber
Oral disorders	
Broken jaw or oral surgery	Mechanical soft or liquid diet; small, frequent meals
Dental caries, periodontal disease, ill-fitting dentures, missing teeth	Mechanical soft diet
Dry mouth	Mechanical soft diet; increased fluid intake
Dysphagia (difficulty swallowing)	Individualize diet; mechanical soft diet; possible enteral feeding
Ulcers of mouth or gums	Mechanical soft diet; limited acidic and spicy foods
Pancreatitis	Low fat; small, frequent feedings; increased fluids; possible enteral feedings or TPN
Renal calculi (kidney stones)	Depends on type of calculi

Table 19.13	Summary of Diet Modifications—cont'd
CONDITION	**POSSIBLE DIET MODIFICATIONS**
Calcium oxalate	Low animal protein and sodium intake; increase fiber; maintain calcium intake; avoid high doses of vitamin C; increase fluid intake
Calcium phosphate	Decrease phosphorus intake; increase fluid intake
Uric acid	Low animal protein and purine intake; increase fluid intake
Cystine	Low sodium; avoid excess protein; increase fluid intake
Renal failure	
Acute	Protein restricted; high calorie; sodium and potassium controlled based on individual losses; vitamin/mineral supplementation possible; phosphate and calcium maintained based on body weight; possible fluid restrictions
Chronic	Limited protein; low sodium, potassium, phosphorus and calcium; vitamin and mineral supplementation; fluid intake balanced with output but not necessarily restricted
Underweight	High calorie; high protein; high carbohydrate; moderate fat; vitamin/mineral supplementation
Wound healing, pressure injuries	High protein, increased carbohydrate and fat intake; increased fluid intake; increased vitamins (especially vitamin C) and minerals (especially zinc and iron)

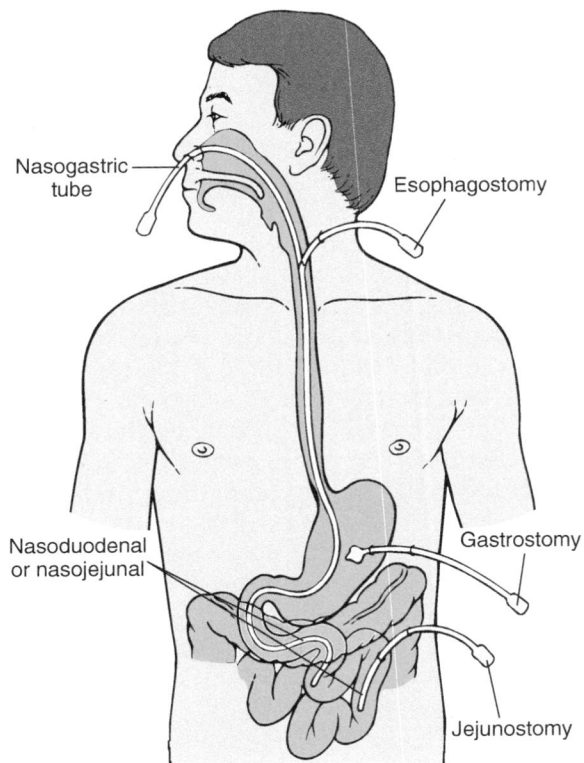

Fig. 19.6 Tube feeding sites.

facial trauma; when a patient has no appetite or refuses to eat; in times of great nutritional need, such as in the patient suffering burns or trauma; in comatose patients; or during periods of moderate malabsorption or diarrhea.

Tube feedings are used only when all or part of the GI tract is functioning. Tube feedings can be administered by way of a nasogastric tube, a tube that is passed through the nose and into the stomach (Fig. 19.6). If regurgitation is common or the amount of gastric residual is high, a nasojejunal or nasoduodenal tube (a tube that is passed through the nose and into the jejunum or the duodenum) sometimes is used to reduce the risk of aspiration.

In cases in which long-term tube feedings are necessary, as in a patient with a gastrectomy or intestinal resection or in a patient with an upper GI obstruction, feeding ostomies sometimes are employed. Feeding ostomies are surgical openings through which a feeding tube is passed. It is possible to make ostomies into the esophagus (esophagostomy), the stomach (gastrostomy), or the jejunum (jejunostomy) (see Fig. 19.6). Ostomy feedings do not have to be continuous and sometimes are given intermittently, thus permitting more freedom of movement.

Tube feedings given on a continuous basis usually are administered through a continuous-drip pump that administers the formula slowly over 16 to 24 hours. In intermittent feedings, a specific volume of formula is administered over a short time, usually about 20 to 30 minutes. This type of intermittent feeding usually is done four to six times daily. Bolus feedings (in which a 4- to 6-hour volume of formula is administered in a matter of minutes) also may be given, but most patients tolerate them poorly.

Tube feedings, although necessary in some circumstances, are not without complications, and it is necessary to monitor them closely. Distention, diarrhea, and nausea may indicate that the formula strength, volume, or rate is too great. Dumping syndrome is also possible with rapid and concentrated formula delivery. Other complications that can arise include diarrhea; contamination of formula; infection; aspiration; overhydration or dehydration; electrolyte and glucose abnormalities; and disturbances in the levels of other nutrients. The development of liver abnormalities also may occur (Table 19.14). See the Home Care Considerations box for patients receiving home enteral feeding.

Nasogastric Tube Feedings

When a nasogastric tube is used for enteral nutrition or medication administration, it is important to check for placement of the tube before administering medication or tube feedings. An improperly placed feeding tube can cause complications such as aspiration pneumonia, pneumothorax, and peritonitis, all of which can be avoided simply by checking placement of the tube before giving any medication or feeding.

The most dependable means of checking tube placement is through radiologic confirmation. Chest radiographs are considered the standard of care, especially for confirming placement of small-diameter tubes. Unfortunately, not all institutions have policies mandating this method. X-ray studies also are not performed usually for large-diameter nasogastric and nasointestinal tubes, because most clinicians believe that the tubes are less likely to enter the lung undetected. The next best method for confirming feeding tube placement is through pH measurement. By testing the pH of fluid aspirated from a newly inserted feeding tube, it is possible to make reasonable assumptions about the tube's location. Visual inspection of gastric fluid aspirated also may be implemented to verify placement.

Traditionally, the auscultatory, or "swoosh," method was used to determine nasogastric tube placement. Tube placement was determined to be accurate by pushing air through the nasogastric tube and into the stomach with a syringe and using a stethoscope to listen for a gurgling sound over the epigastric region. Air in a tube inadvertently placed in the lungs, the pharynx, or the esophagus transmits sound similar to that entering the stomach, which makes the reliability of this method questionable. Therefore it is not a good method to use solely to verify tube placement.

Many potential complications are possible with administration of tube feedings, and the cost of managing those complications or infections is high. It is important to use proper technique when administering enteral feedings and to maintain the cleanliness of the equipment. Skill 19.1 describes the administration of enteral feedings through a nasogastric tube, and Skill 19.2 describes the administration of enteral feedings via a gastrostomy or jejunostomy tube. Using good hand hygiene technique and clean equipment and hanging formula only for the recommended time to prevent spoiling are crucial steps to avoid contamination of the system and subsequent infection in the patient.

PARENTERAL NUTRITION

Parenteral nutrition, or *hyperalimentation,* is the term used to describe IV feedings. Parenteral nutrition can be given in several ways: through peripheral veins, such as those in the arms or the legs, and through a large central vein. When the nurse administers parenteral nutrition through peripheral veins, it is called *peripheral parenteral nutrition (PPN).* If it is given through a large central vein, it is called **total parenteral nutrition (TPN).**

TPN usually refers to the administration of a hypertonic solution into the superior vena cava by way of a catheter threaded through either the subclavian vein or the internal jugular vein (Fig. 19.7). TPN and PPN formulas generally are composed of glucose, amino acids, vitamins, minerals, and electrolytes in amounts individualized for the patient. Fat, in the form of triglycerides, also can be given as a supplement to the main formula, but it is administered separately through a Y-connector tube or into a peripheral vein.

Parenteral nutrition is indicated for patients with a nonfunctioning or dysfunctional GI tract, those needing 3000 kcal/day or less, those needing supplementation to an oral diet, and those requiring short-term therapy (less than 3 weeks). When IV nutrition is necessary, PPN should be considered the first choice of administration because it carries less risk of complications, necessitates less monitoring, and costs less than administration by the central venous route. TPN is indicated for patients needing a highly concentrated formula, such as those who need more kilocalories than can be administered peripherally or those requiring fluid restrictions. A concentrated formula delivers more kilocalories and nutrients in a smaller volume. Other candidates for TPN include patients who must receive IV feedings for more than 3 weeks and those with unsuitable or unavailable peripheral veins.

TPN necessitates surgical placement of a catheter in one of the central veins to establish central venous access. This imposes significant risks on the patient, including sepsis, pneumothorax, hemothorax, phlebitis, and thrombosis. It is necessary to maintain catheter site asepsis and keep feeding solutions sterile. Constant monitoring of the clinical status of the patient is essential.

Some patients receiving TPN experience fluid and electrolyte imbalances, hyperglycemia or hypoglycemia, metabolic disturbances, and bone disorders such as osteomalacia (softening of the bones). For this

Table 19.14	Common Problems and Nursing Interventions Associated With Administering Tube Feedings

PROBLEM	NURSING INTERVENTION
Abdominal distention	Abdominal distention commonly occurs when the stomach empties too slowly. Omit the nourishment if the amount aspirated from the stomach before feeding is 100–150 mL. In some instances, the health care provider orders the feedings to be stopped, at least temporarily.
Acute otitis media	Otitis media is possible when the nasogastric tube presses against the eustachian tube, which causes obstruction and edema. It is best prevented by turning the patient from side to side frequently, at least q 2 h, and by using as small a nasogastric tube as possible.
Aspiration	Aspiration is best prevented by ensuring that the tube is in the stomach before the nourishment is introduced and by keeping the head of the patient's bed elevated between 30 and 45 degrees. Suction of the mouth and throat sometimes is necessary when regurgitation and vomiting occur.
Clogged tube	Occlusion of the tube is prevented by keeping a constant flow rate when nourishment is given continuously and by flushing the tube well after single feedings. It is acceptable to gently irrigate the tube after obtaining a medical order. If irrigation does not relieve the obstruction, sometimes it is necessary to remove and replace the tube.
Diarrhea	Diarrhea commonly is caused by introducing nourishment too rapidly or using formula or nourishment that is too concentrated. The usual care is to decrease the strength of the nourishment and administer it more slowly. An antidiarrheal drug sometimes is ordered.
High electrolyte blood levels	High electrolyte blood levels are usually the result of the patient's receiving insufficient fluids. Water usually is offered through the tube at a rate of 100 mL q 4–6 h (exact amount varies according to health care provider's order).
Irritation of nasal and palate tissues	Tissue irritation occurs as a result of pressure on tissues by the nasogastric tube. Some procedures include removal of the tube a few inches every day, coating of the tube with an antibiotic ointment, and then reinsertion.
Irritation of oral mucous membranes	Oral mucous membranes often become dry and irritated when the patient is unable to take nourishment by mouth and is receiving nourishment by gavage. Frequent oral hygiene helps prevent this problem; administer it at least four times a day.
Nausea	Nausea commonly is caused by introducing nourishment too rapidly. It is also possible that the formula of the nourishment is unsatisfactory. Usual care is to administer nourishment more slowly and possibly change the formula.

reason, monitor blood chemistry values frequently and check the blood glucose level several times each day. Administration of regular insulin on a sliding scale may be necessary to maintain blood glucose levels below 200 mg/dL.

FEEDING THE PATIENT

Patients who are weak, are paralyzed, have a cast, or have some other form of physical or neurologic limitation may not be able to feed themselves or may need assistance with feeding. It may be the responsibility of the nurse or the unlicensed assistive personnel to assist these patients with meals.

In assisting patients to eat, it is necessary to create a relaxed mood so that patients do not feel rushed. It is also important to allow them time for their usual before-meal rituals. Many people pray before eating; others need to wash their hands and face. Provide the time and privacy for the patient's usual routine. This demonstrates caring and respect for the patient. Before feeding, ask the patient in which order he or she wants food and fluids offered. Also make sure the temperature of the food is not too hot to burn the patient. When feeding a patient, use a spoon because spoons are less

likely than forks to cause injury. Give the patient small bites, and allow for chewing and swallowing the food without being rushed.

Patients who are not able to feed themselves sometimes believe they are losing control over their lives and feel angry, humiliated, and embarrassed. Some of them do not like depending on others. Some may be depressed and resentful, and others may refuse to eat. Allow these patients to try to feed themselves as much as possible, offering assistance as needed. Monitor activity levels for compliance. Provide positive reinforcement and support.

Many visually impaired patients are keenly aware of food aromas. Often they can identify foods being served. Always tell a visually impaired patient what foods and fluids are on the tray and indicate their location on the tray by referring to the numbers on a clock (Fig. 19.8). When feeding a patient, announce the food that is being offered. Something simple, like "Here is another bite of mashed potatoes," allows the patient to prepare for the taste and flavor of the bite of food. Imagine being told you getting another bite of applesauce when it is actually pureed cabbage. This would make for an unpleasant eating scenario. This action is

Skill 19.1   Administering Nasogastric Tube Feedings

NURSING ACTION (RATIONALE)

1. Check health care provider's order. (*Verification of order is needed to determine formula type, rate, route, and frequency of feedings.*)
2. Introduce self. (*Decreases patient's anxiety.*)
3. Identify patient. (*Use two identifiers [name/birth date] to ensure that procedure is performed on the correct patient.*)
4. Explain procedure and reason it is being done in terms that the patient will understand. (*Decreases patient's anxiety and prepares the patient for the procedure.*)
5. Allow time for the patient to ask questions. (*May increase patient cooperation.*)
6. Determine the need for and provide patient teaching during procedure. (*Reduces patient anxiety and increases patient's knowledge of procedure. May also increase compliance.*)
7. Determine whether there is abdominal distention or tenderness. (*Absence of bowel sounds indicates inability of the GI tract to digest or absorb nutrients, and feeding should be withheld.*)
8. Listen for bowel sounds before each feeding. (*Action also provides baseline information for later comparisons.*)
9. Assemble equipment. (*Having appropriate equipment assembled may help the procedure move more smoothly and help gain patient's trust.*)
   - 30- to 60-mL syringe
   - Testing equipment. (*Some facilities require glucose testing before feedings.*)
   - Disposable feeding bag
   - Gloves
   - Infusion pump (for intestinal feedings)
   - Prescribed enteral feeding formula
   - Stethoscope and pH indicator strips
10. Wash hands and don clean gloves according to agency policy and guidelines from CDC and OSHA. (*Reduces spread of microorganisms and protects the patient and the nurse.*)
11. Close door or pull privacy curtain. (*Maintains patient's privacy.*)
12. Raise bed to comfortable working height; lower side rail on side nearest the nurse. (*Raising bed promotes proper body mechanics in the patient and prevents muscle strain in the caregiver.*)
13. Elevate head of bed (Fowler's position). (*Elevating head of bed decreases risk of aspiration during feeding.*)
14. Establish tube placement/check for residual. (*Indicates accurate tube placement and gastric emptying.*)

a. Aspirate gastric contents with syringe. (*Gastric secretions are usually green, brown, or tan.*)

b. Place drop of gastric contents on pH paper. (*Gastric contents normally have a pH range of 0–4.*)

c. If aspiration cannot be done, suspect that tube is occluded or kinked. Attempt to flush with 30 mL tap water. (*Flushing may dislodge any obstruction if present.*)
d. If flushing cannot be done, check nasal cavity or back of throat (if tube is inserted nasally). Check for kinking. (*If no kinking is seen, inability to flush may indicate tube is no longer in the correct location.*)

15. Replace gastric contents. If residual amount is greater than 150 mL, check orders for further direction. (*Prevents fluid and electrolyte imbalances.*) May need to notify health care provider of excess residual. Feeding may be withheld 1 h and then started at slower rate.
16. Prepare formula for feeding. Check expiration date to make sure formula has not expired.
   a. Before pouring from can, check expiration date, and wipe off top of can. (*Wiping off top of can prevent debris from entering the formula when it is poured.*)
   b. Before using premixed base, check date and time, as well as correct strength of formula. Check temperature. (*Some patients cannot handle full-strength formula, and it must be diluted before feeding.*) Check agency policy. Facilities

may have requirements for the temperature and storage of the solutions.

17. Administer feeding.

a. Bolus or intermittent feedings:

(1) Kink or pinch feeding tube. (*Prevents leakage and air from entering patient's stomach.*)

(2) Remove plunger from syringe and insert syringe tip into feeding tube. Release feeding tube. (*Allows formula to be poured into syringe, and allows free flow of formula through the tube.*)

(3) Fill syringe with formula. Keep syringe 18 inches or less above site. (*Keeping the syringe low prevents too rapid an infusion of formula and is better tolerated.*)

(4) Flush tube with 30–60 mL tap water (or prescribed amount/solution) when feeding is completed. (*Prevents tube from clogging with thick formula.*)

(5) Remove syringe and cap or plug tube. (*Prevents leakage of gastric contents between feedings.*)

b. Continuous drip method:

(1) Assemble gavage bag and tubing. (*Gavage bag allows larger amounts of formula to be given.*)

(2) Verify tube placement and residual. (*Ensures feeding is delivered to stomach.*)

(3) Clamp tubing, and attach gavage bag. (*Clamping prevents unwanted leakage of formula.*)

(4) Fill gavage bag with appropriate type and amount of formula. (*Verify formula type and amount before starting feeding.*)

(5) Unclamp and prime tubing, and then reclamp. (*Eliminates air from tubing and helps prevent gas formation.*)

(6) Label gavage bag with date, time, initials, formula type and strength, and amount of formula. (*Communicates essential information to all staff.*)

(7) Kink feeding tube and uncap; secure gavage tubing to feeding tube. (*Kinking tubing prevents leakage of gastric contents.*)

(8) Set rate by adjusting roller clamp on tubing. (*Set to infuse ordered amount of feeding in appropriate amount of time.*)

(9) Flush tube with 30–60 mL tap water (or prescribed amount/solution) when feeding is completed. (*Prevents clogging of the feeding tube by thick formula.*)

(10) Kink feeding tube, remove gavage tubing, and recap feeding tube. (*Prevents leakage of gastric contents between feedings.*)

(11) Place cap on end of gavage tubing. (*Protects gavage tubing from contamination between feedings.*)

c. Feeding via infusion pump:

(1) Verify feeding tube placement and residual. (*Ensures feeding is delivered to stomach and it is emptying appropriately.*)

(2) Prepare administration set with correct type and amount of formula. (*Use only enough formula for 8 h to prevent spoiling.*)

(3) Clamp gavage tubing, spike bag, unclamp and prime tubing, and reclamp tubing. (*Prevents air from entering stomach and causing gas formation.*)

(4) Label bag with date, time, initials, and formula type and strength. (*Enhances communication between caregivers.*)

(5) Hang tube feeding set on IV pole with infusion pump. Connect tubing to pump and set rate. (*Make sure to check facility policy for pump type and use.*)

(6) Kink end of feeding tube, remove cap, and attach infusion tubing. (*Kinking the feeding*

Continued

tube prevents air from entering stomach and leakage of gastric contents.)

(7) Open roller clamp on tubing, and turn on infusion pump. *(Pump will sound alarm if roller clamp is not open.)*

(8) Check residual q 4 h. *(Ensures that tubing has not been dislodged.)*

18. Flush tube with 30–60 mL water (or ordered solution) after a bolus feeding or q 4–8 h during continuous feeding. *(Prevents clogging of the*

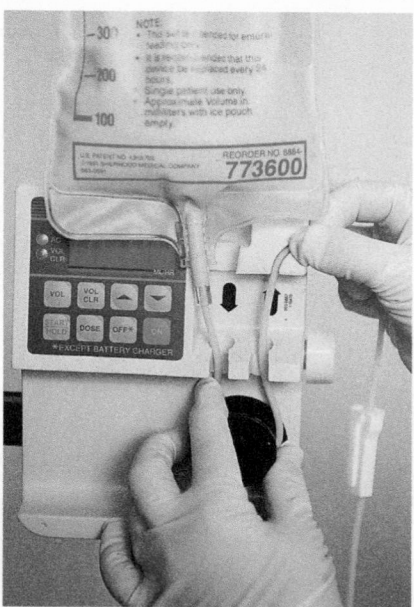

tube by thick formula or gastric secretions. Water replacement is needed to help maintain fluid volume.)*

19. Clean equipment appropriately after use. *(Helps prevent bacterial growth and allows for reuse of equipment. Most facilities require replacing equipment q 24 h.)*

20. Make sure patient is comfortable, and educate about symptoms to report. Make sure call light is within patient's reach. *(Cramping and diarrhea must be reported as this may signal the infusion is being administered too rapidly or the patient is not tolerating it.)*

21. Raise side rails and lower bed to lowest position. *(Promotes safety. Be aware of facility policy regarding side rail use.)*

22. Remove gloves, dispose of used supplies, and wash hands. *(Reduces spread of microorganisms.)*

23. Document the following. *(All treatments and patient's response must be documented.)*
    - Verification of tube placement/residual
    - Type and amount of feeding
    - Rate of feeding (if applicable)
    - How feeding tube flushed
    - Patient's tolerance of feeding
    - Any adverse effects of feeding
    - Patient education

24. Monitor weight and laboratory values daily. *(Improving laboratory values and weight gain are indications of improved nutritional status.)*

25. Observe patient for shortness of breath, low oxygenation saturation, vomiting, or color changes. *(Could indicate aspiration or intolerance of feeding.)*

CDC, Centers for Disease Control and Prevention; *GI,* gastrointestinal; *IV,* intravenous; *OSHA,* Occupational Safety and Health Administration.
Figure for Step 17c(8) from Potter PA, Perry AG: *Essentials for nursing practice,* ed 8, St. Louis, 2015, Mosby.

Skill 19.2   Administering Enteral Feedings via Gastrostomy or Jejunostomy

CHECK   GATHER   HELLO   ID   PRIVACY   EXPLAIN   WASH   GLOVES

Observe all guidelines for nasogastric tube feedings. Follow Skill 19.1 to verify tube placement; then continue with the following steps.

NURSING ACTION (*RATIONALE*)

1. Verify tube placement. (*Indicates accurate tube placement and gastric emptying.*)
   a. Gastrostomy tube:
      (1) Aspirate gastric secretions. (*Gastric secretions are usually green, brown, or tan.*)
      (2) Check appearance and pH. (*Gastric contents have a pH range of 0–4.*)
      (3) Return contents to stomach. (*Prevents fluid and electrolyte imbalances.*)
      (4) Note amount of residual. (*May need to notify health care provider if residual is excessive.*)
   b. Jejunostomy tube:
      (1) Aspirate intestinal secretions. (*Intestinal contents are medium to deep golden or bile stained.*)
      (2) Observe appearance and amount (usually 10 mL or less).
      (3) Check pH. (*Intestinal contents have a pH of 7 or greater.*)
2. Flush tube with 30 mL tap water. (*Clears tube of any remaining formula or obstructions.*)
3. Initiate feedings.
   a. Syringe feedings (*Initial feeding may be via syringe to determine patient's tolerance.*)
      (1) Pinch proximal end of tube.
      (2) Remove plunger, and attach syringe to end of tube.
      (3) Fill syringe with formula and allow it to empty gradually. (*Too rapid an infusion may cause complications.*)
      (4) Refill until appropriate amount has been delivered.
   b. Continuous drip method. (*Feedings are usually given continuously via pump to ensure proper absorption.*)
      (1) Fill feeding container with enough formula for 8 h of feeding. (*More than 8 h worth of formula may spoil.*)

    (2) Hang container on IV pole and prime tubing. (*Excess air in the GI tract can cause gas formation and patient discomfort.*)
    (3) Thread tubing on pump.
    (4) Connect tubing to end of feeding tube.
    (5) Begin infusion at prescribed rate.
4. Evaluate skin around tube exit site. (*Redness, swelling, drainage, or foul odor could indicate infection and must be reported to the health care provider.*)
5. Clean skin around tube. (*Helps prevent infection. Dressings may or may not be ordered.*)
6. Dispose of supplies. Wash hands. (*Prevents transmission of microorganisms.*)
7. Monitor fingerstick blood glucose levels q 4–6 h until maximum administration rate is reached and maintained for 24 h. (*Enteral feeding formulas may increase blood glucose levels.*)
8. Monitor intake and output q 24 h. (*Indicators of fluid balance or fluid volume excess.*)
9. Weigh patient daily until tolerance is established; then weigh three times a week. (*Weight gain is a good indicator of improved nutritional status. A sudden gain of 2 lb in 24 h may indicate fluid volume excess.*)
10. Observe return of normal laboratory values. (*Improving albumin, transferrin, and prealbumin levels indicate improved nutritional status.*)
11. Inspect tube site for signs of pressure. (*Enteral tubes may cause pressure areas on patient's skin especially if they are tucked into clothing.*)
12. Document the following. (*All treatments and patient's response must be documented.*)
    • Verification of tube placement/residual
    • Type and amount of feeding
    • Rate of feeding (if applicable)
    • How feeding tube is flushed
    • Patient's tolerance of feeding
    • Any adverse effects of feeding
    • Patient education
13. Observe patient for shortness of breath, low oxygenation saturation, vomiting, or color changes. (*Could indicate aspiration or intolerance of feeding.*)

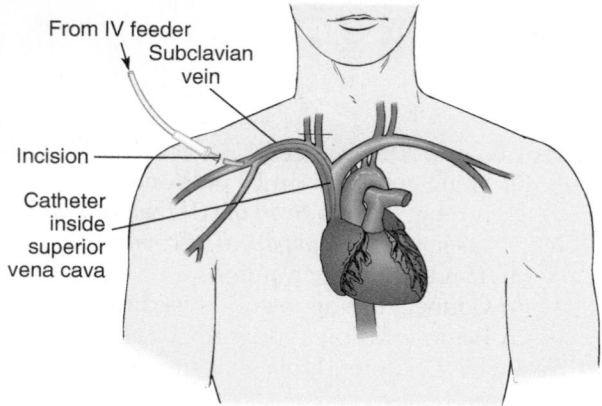

Fig. 19.7 Central venous catheter placement during administration of parenteral nutrition.

From IV feeder
Subclavian vein
Incision
Catheter inside superior vena cava

Fig. 19.8 For the visually impaired patient: "The potato is at the 12 o'clock position." (From Sorrentino SA, Remmert LN: *Mosby's textbook for nursing assistants*, ed 9, St. Louis, 2017, Mosby.)

important for the visually impaired patient, but also for any patient who is depending on another person to feed them.

Meals have always been a social activity, and many patients may not have family or friends visiting at mealtime. Eating is often a social time. Engage the patient in pleasant conversation while giving the patient enough time to chew and swallow food. Sit facing the patient. Sitting is more relaxing and demonstrates to the patient unhurried care and support from the staff. Standing communicates nonverbally that the staff does not have time and that they really are not interested in the patient. Facing the patient allows the nurse to see how well the patient is eating and

whether the patient has problems swallowing. Skill 19.3 describes techniques to use in assisting patients with eating.

Keep in mind that odors, unpleasant equipment, an uncomfortable position, the need for oral hygiene, the need to void, and the presence of pain may affect appetite. To improve a patient's appetite, remove any offensive odors or equipment and offer to help the patient void or wash before meals. Assess for pain. If needed, offer pain medication at least 30 minutes before a meal. It is also important to serve the meal as quickly as possible so that the food is at the correct temperature and more appetizing to the patient.

Skill 19.3   Assisting Patients With Eating

CHECK GATHER HELLO ID PRIVACY EXPLAIN WASH GLOVES

NURSING ACTION (RATIONALE)

1. Complete or delay care that will interfere with eating. (*It is best to serve food at its appropriate temperature.*)
2. Provide a period of rest or quiet before meals. (*A tired or excited patient is usually in no mood to eat.*)
3. Offer the patient a bedpan or urinal before mealtime. (*Having to urinate may decrease the patient's appetite.*)
4. Provide the patient with an opportunity for hand washing, and offer mouth care before the meal. (*Freshening up before a meal may increase appetite.*)
5. Remove soiled articles or clutter from room. (*An unattractive environment may decrease the desire to eat.*)
6. Make the patient comfortable for eating; give pain medication at least 30 min before a meal. (*Patients can enjoy their food more if they are comfortable.*)

7. Raise the head of the bed to a sitting position. (*Sitting or semi-sitting position makes swallowing easier.*)
8. Cover the patient's upper chest with a napkin or some form of clothing protector. (*Prevents soiling of patient's clothes or gown.*)
9. Sit beside the patient to assist with feeding. (*Sitting is more relaxing and can decrease anxiety in patients, thus encouraging them to eat better.*)
10. Encourage patients to feed themselves as much as possible. (*Encourages independence and maintains patient's dignity.*)
11. Provide a flexible straw for patients who are unable to use a cup or glass. (*Helps direct liquids into patient's mouth and allows him or her to set the pace and amount taken.*)

12. Serve manageable amounts of food in each bite. *(Too large a bite may cause choking and aspiration.)*

13. For a patient who has had a stroke, direct the food toward the side of the mouth not affected by the stroke. *(Allows for more thorough chewing and swallowing.)*

14. Serve food in the order of the patient's preference. *(Allows patients to eat in the manner in which they are accustomed.)*

15. Give the patient time to chew and swallow food. *(Allows for more relaxed atmosphere and prevents choking and aspiration.)*

16. Modify utensils and texture of food if the patient has to remain flat while eating. *(A flat position decreases the patient's ability to control food in the mouth and increases the risk of choking and aspiration.)* Use a training cup or a large syringe with flexible rubber tube. Puree or grind foods.

17. During the feeding, do not leave the patient until he or she has finished eating. Do not interrupt the meal. *(Delays or interruptions may cause food to cool or warm and become less appealing. Patients may not begin eating again if interrupted.)*

18. Carry on pleasant conversation with patient during the meal. *(Eating is a social event and should be pleasant. A pleasant atmosphere may enhance appetite.)*

19. Remove the tray from the patient's room as soon as the meal is completed. *(Having to look at or smell food that has been sitting may cause the patient to become nauseated or to vomit.)*

Get Ready for the NCLEX® Examination!

Key Points

- Nurses play an important role in promoting good nutrition.
- Nutrients are necessary for the proper functioning of all life processes in the body.
- Food planning guides are available to help plan and determine the nutritional adequacy of diets.
- Essential nutrients include protein, carbohydrates, fat, vitamins, minerals, and water.
- Deficiencies or excesses of nutrients often lead to disease or dysfunction of various body systems.
- For healthy Americans, a well-planned diet can provide adequate nutrition without supplementation.
- Nutrient needs change throughout the life cycle, and people must adjust their diet to meet those needs.
- Medications may affect nutritional status. Be aware of drug-nutrient interactions.
- Medical nutrition therapy involves using diet in the treatment of disease or injury.

- Diets often are altered in consistency or frequency when GI function precludes the use of a regular diet.
- Kilocalorie modifications are used when patients need to gain or lose weight. High-kilocalorie and high-protein diets may be necessary for weight maintenance in patients with increased metabolic needs.
- Obesity is a complex disorder; individualized treatment is necessary, and treatment involves a healthy diet combined with physical activity and psychological counseling.
- The eating disorders anorexia nervosa, bulimia nervosa, and binge eating necessitate multidisciplinary treatment efforts, including nutritional, family, and psychological therapy. Place an emphasis on the prevention of these disorders in youth by promoting good health and the value of individuality.
- Carbohydrate-controlled, fat-controlled, high-fiber diets are used in the treatment of diabetes mellitus.
- Fat-controlled and low-fat diets emphasize reduction of total fat, saturated fat, and *trans* fatty acids. They are used in the treatment of a variety of diseases, including heart

disease, atherosclerosis, obesity, diabetes, metabolic syndrome, malabsorption syndromes, and gallbladder disease.

- Sodium-restricted diets are used to treat hypertension, congestive heart failure, and renal disease. They also are used sometimes when edema is present.
- Protein- and electrolyte-modified diets are used to treat renal disease and cirrhosis.
- Fluid restrictions are necessary when urine output is decreased, when edema is present, or during heart failure. Adequate fluid is necessary to prevent dehydration, particularly in older adults.
- Nutritional support (tube feedings or parenteral nutrition) is often necessary when oral intake is impossible or inadequate. GI function usually indicates which type of feeding is appropriate.
- In feeding a patient or resident, ask about the preferred order in which to offer foods and fluids, and allow sufficient time for the patient to chew and swallow the food.
- Remove any offensive odors or equipment, offer pain medication before a meal, and then serve meals promptly to maintain appropriate temperature and increase nutritional intake.

Additional Learning Resources

SG Go to your Study Guide for additional learning activities to help you master this chapter content.

Be sure to visit the Evolve site at http://evolve.elsevier.com/Cooper/foundations/ for additional online resources.

Review Questions for the NCLEX® Examination

1. A healthy 35-year-old patient wishes to lose weight because her BMI is 27. Which suggestion would be most appropriate for her?
   1. This BMI is too low for good health; the patient needs to supplement the diet to increase weight.
   2. This is an acceptable BMI, and it is best to maintain weight at this level for continued good health.
   3. Appropriate weight loss is possible with a healthy, reduced-calorie diet and incorporating at least 30 minutes of physical activity into each day.
   4. This BMI is elevated to the point that treatments, such as surgery, are necessary.

2. A patient takes medication for hypertension and asks whether there is anything else he can do to help to reduce his blood pressure. What is the best nursing response?
   1. "A low-fat, low-cholesterol diet with only a limited amount of simple sugars will have the greatest effect on your blood pressure."
   2. "A salt-free diet will have the greatest effect on your blood pressure. Do not add salt in your cooking or at the table."
   3. "Adequate calcium and potassium intake, as well as lower sodium intake, offers some possibility of helping your blood pressure. Eat plenty of fruits, vegetables, and low-fat milk products."
   4. "Limit the use of processed foods, in your diet. That way, you will have less sodium in your diet."

3. A patient with cancer has anorexia and weight loss. Which suggestion is most likely to help him increase intake and prevent weight loss?
   1. Encourage the patient to eat double portions at each meal.
   2. Suggest that the patient snack often on high-calorie foods.
   3. Encourage the patient to eat the low-calorie foods first.
   4. Suggest to the patient that he decrease his amount of exercise.

4. Which dietary recommendation should the nurse include in the discharge instructions for a client who has been diagnosed with coronary artery disease?
   1. Limit intake of whole grains.
   2. Limit intake of tuna.
   3. Limit intake of soybean products.
   4. Limit intake of egg yolks.

5. The nurse is reviewing a patient's dietary intake. Which patient behavior reflects compliance with a 2-g sodium-restricted diet?
   1. Using only the two packets of salt found on the meal tray.
   2. Limiting milk to 1 cup per day.
   3. Avoiding use of salt in cooking.
   4. Using salt-free butter with meals.

6. A patient with iron-deficiency anemia started taking iron supplements. What recommendation can the nurse give the patient to increase iron absorption?
   1. Drink milk or take calcium supplements at the same time as eating iron-rich foods.
   2. Take iron supplements with coffee, tea, or red wine.
   3. Consume vitamin C–rich foods at the same meal with iron-containing foods.
   4. Take iron supplements with a high-fiber bran cereal.

7. The nurse determines that a hypertensive patient understands the DASH diet when the patient chooses which items from a sample menu used in dietary teaching?
   1. Caesar salad, bread sticks, and frozen yogurt.
   2. Grilled chicken sandwich, strawberries, and lettuce salad.
   3. Grilled cheese sandwich, canned pineapple, and brownie.
   4. Chicken and vegetable stir fry, rice, and egg roll.

8. A patient planning for pregnancy has heard that some experts recommend folic acid supplements for women of childbearing age. The patient understands the need for this recommendation by making which statement?
   1. "Folic acid may help prevent neural tube defects in my baby."
   2. "Folic acid provides me with extra calories to make new cells."
   3. "It is impossible for me to receive adequate amounts of folic acid in my diet."
   4. "Folic acid will help me to increase iron absorption in my diet."

9. While the nurse is completing discharge teaching for a patient with elevated cholesterol levels, the patient asks how to distinguish between an unsaturated fat and a saturated fat. Which statement is most accurate?

    1. Saturated fats are generally from plant sources and are solid at room temperature.
    2. In unsaturated fats the hydrogen bonds are full.
    3. Saturated fats are missing hydrogen at points of unsaturation.
    4. Unsaturated fats are generally from plant sources and are liquid at room temperature.

10. A nurse is caring for a patient recently diagnosed with type 2 diabetes. The patient asks the nurse to tell her about the dietary changes she will need to make. Which actions are appropriate and within the scope of practice for a nurse?

    1. Review the patient's chart and recommend a calorie and carbohydrate intake that is based on blood glucose and lipid values.
    2. Discuss the rationale for and the general principles of the diabetic diet with the patient, and then communicate the patient's concerns to the registered dietitian and health care provider.
    3. Locate the health care provider's diet order in the medical chart, and then obtain a preprinted diet sheet showing the exchange lists for meal planning and a menu pattern based on the prescribed calorie level.
    4. Decline to comment on the diet because the nurse is not a trained professional in the area of nutrition; refer all questions to a registered dietitian.

11. A middle-aged patient recently received a diagnosis of type 2 diabetes and is in the hospital for tests and is receiving a diabetic diet. The patient's spouse expresses concern because there are cookies on the patient's lunch tray. Which response by the nurse is the best?

    1. "Sugars and sweets are permitted in moderation in the diabetic diet. The important thing is that the total carbohydrate content of the meal is controlled and balanced with your spouses medication and nutrient needs."
    2. "I can understand your concern. Sugars are more rapidly absorbed and have the capacity to raise blood glucose levels more quickly than other carbohydrates. I will check with the kitchen and see if your spouse received the wrong tray."
    3. "I am sure that if the cookies were on the meal tray, they must be allowed in the diet. They are probably low in sugar. There is likely no need for concern."
    4. "Sugar is used to treat hypoglycemia or low blood sugar. Perhaps your spouse had a low blood sugar reading before breakfast, and the dietitian sent up the cookies to give extra sugar on the meal tray."

12. The health care provider has recommended that a patient increase the amount of fiber in her diet to help control her blood cholesterol levels. Which guidelines are most appropriate for increasing water-soluble fiber in the diet?

    1. Choose a daily fiber supplement that contains no artificial additives and preservatives; follow the instructions on the container, and be sure to drink plenty of water.
    2. Choose foods that are closer to their whole state rather than refined or processed, including more fruits, oats, and legumes to increase soluble fiber; and drink plenty of water.
    3. Choose more vegetables, vegetable juices, whole wheat, and whole wheat products to increase soluble fiber; and drink plenty of water.
    4. Choose more fruit juices to provide fluid and fiber, and include iron-fortified breakfast cereals to enhance the absorption of fiber from the fruit juice.

13. A patient is controlling his blood cholesterol through diet. He is familiar with food sources of saturated fat and cholesterol but is confused about *trans* fatty acids. The nurse should explain that which group of foods contributes the most *trans* fatty acids?

    1. Butter, cream, fats in meats, and tropical oils such as palm and coconut oils.
    2. Fish oils, nuts and seeds, and vegetable oils such as olive oil and canola oil.
    3. Stick margarines, shortening, deep-fried restaurant foods, and commercially prepared baked goods.
    4. Liquid margarines, vegetable oil spreads, and vegetable oils such as corn, soybean, and cottonseed.

14. A patient with a family history of osteoporosis is taking calcium supplements to help reduce her risk of developing osteoporosis. What recommendations can be made to prevent the development of reduced calcium balance? *(Select all that apply.)*

    1. Taking small doses of calcium throughout the day rather than one large dose.
    2. Choosing plenty of milk products, and avoiding excess caffeine intake.
    3. Consuming a high-protein diet.
    4. Consuming a diet that has moderate levels of sodium.
    5. Increasing potassium intake.

15. Which patient comment indicates to the nurse that more teaching is needed for the patient experiencing dumping syndrome after gastric surgery?

    1. "I should eat six small meals per day."
    2. "I should not drink fluids with my meals."
    3. "I should use honey or jelly instead of butter."
    4. "I should lie down for 30 to 60 minutes after eating."

16. An adolescent trauma patient has just been started on nasogastric tube feedings. Shortly after the formula begins, the patient complains of nausea and abdominal cramps. What is the appropriate nursing action?

    1. Check the formula rate, strength, or volume; any of these could possibly be too high.
    2. Nothing; these are normal symptoms with tube feedings.
    3. Stop the infusion immediately; these are symptoms of aspiration.
    4. Stop the infusion because the feeding tube is emptying into the lung rather than the stomach.

17. A patient in the early stages of pregnancy is experiencing some nausea and vomiting. Which suggestions would be appropriate for the nurse to recommend? *(Select all that apply.)*

   1. Limit foods with strong odors, and avoid food odors that bother you.
   2. Avoid foods with a high fat content.
   3. Try consuming five or six smaller meals each day, and include a source of protein in each meal.
   4. Try not to let your stomach get completely empty. Eat before you are overly hungry.
   5. Increase carbonated beverage intake.

18. A man, 67, is playing golf with friends when he becomes confused and begins speaking in nonsense words. At first his friends think he is joking with them about a bad swing, but then he experiences numbness in his face and legs and collapses, holding his head in pain. He is rushed to the hospital and immediately undergoes coronary angioplasty to open a blocked coronary artery. Prior to his surgery, he has had a history of diabetes and hypertension and is a 2-pack-per-day smoker. He has been taking an ACE-inhibitor for his hypertension and heart failure from atherosclerotic cardiovascular disease. He is of average weight. Within 24 hours *after* his surgery, he begins to complain of severe back pain, lower limb edema, headache, vomiting, as well as swelling around the eyes and shortness of breath. Urinalysis and blood tests reveal high serum urea and creatinine levels; glomerular filtration rate (GFR) test reveals decreased kidney function, probably caused in part by long-term effects of his ACE-inhibitor medication. He is now diagnosed with acute renal failure. After in-hospital stabilization and medication adjustments, he is referred to a dietician for nutritional support focused on his recent acute renal failure to help control and then maintain his fluid and electrolyte balance in hopes of preventing complications such as infection.

Use an X to indicate whether each potential dietary change is either indicated or not applicable for this patient's condition. All should be used and can be used only once.

DIETARY CHANGE	INDICATED	NOT APPLICABLE
Restricted protein		
Reduced calorie intake		
Mechanical soft diet		
Maintenance of phosphate based on body weight		
Increased fluid intake		
Possible fluid restriction		
Increased carbohydrate intake		

Complementary, Integrative, and Alternative Therapies

Objectives

1. Differentiate between complementary and alternative therapies.
2. Describe the practice of holistic nursing.
3. Explain why a good health history is important for a patient who is using complementary and alternative therapies.
4. Describe how herbs differ from pharmaceuticals.
5. Describe safe and unsafe herbal therapies.
6. Explain the scope of practice of chiropractic therapy.
7. Explain the difference between acupuncture and acupressure.
8. Describe the principles behind acupuncture and acupressure.
9. Identify conditions whose presence may contraindicate use of therapeutic massage.
10. Explain the use of essential oils in aromatherapy.
11. Explain the theory behind reflexology.
12. Discuss animal-assisted therapy.
13. Discuss the therapeutic results of yoga, t'ai chi, and energy field therapies.
14. Describe the purpose and principles of biofeedback.
15. Discuss the risks and benefits of marijuana used as complementary or alternative medicine.

Key Terms

acupressure (ĂK-yū-prĕsh-ŭr, p. 588)
acupuncture (ĂK-yū-pŭnk-chŭr, p. 587)
alternative therapies (ŭl-TĔR-nă-tĭv THĔR-ŭh-pēz, p. 579)
aromatherapy (ŭh-RŌM-ŭ-THĔR-ŭh-pē, p. 590)
biofeedback (bī-ō-fēd-băk, p. 594)
cannabidiol (kă-nĭ-bĭ-DĪ-ōl, p. 595)
cannabinoid (kă-NĂ-bĭ-noid, p. 595)
chiropractic therapy (kī-rō-PRĂK-tĭk, p. 585)
complementary therapies (kōm-plĭ-MĔN-tŭ-rē THĔR-ŭh-pēz, p. 579)
Efficacy (p. 580)
focusing (FŌ-kŭs-ĭng, p. 591)
herbal therapy (ĔR-bŭl THĔR-ŭh-pē, p. 581)
holistic nursing (hō-LĬS-tĭk, p. 580)

imagery (ĬM-ĭj-rē, p. 591)
integrative care (p. 580)
meridians (mĕ-RĬD-ē-ănz, p. 587)
passivity (păs-ĬV-ŭ-tē, p. 591)
Qi (CHĒ, p. 587)
receptivity (rē-sĕp-TĬV-ŭ-tē, p. 591)
reflexology (rē-flĕks-ŌL-ŭh-jē, p. 590)
Reiki (RĀ-kē, p. 588)
relaxation (rē-lăks-Ā-shŭn, p. 591)
Taiji or t'ai chi (tī JĒ, p. 593)
tetrahydrocannabinol (tĕ-trŭ-HĪ̆edrŭ-kă-NĂ-bĭ-nŭl, p. 595)
therapeutic massage (thĕr-ŭ-PYŪ-tĭk mŭ-SŌZH, p. 589)
yoga (YŌ-gŭh, p. 593)

Many patients use unconventional therapies to help restore and maintain health. This chapter discusses the use of these therapies, which are frequently referred to as either complementary, alternative, or integrative therapies.

Complementary therapies are treatments used in addition to the conventional health care regimens recommended by a person's medical doctor. As the name implies, complementary therapies do not substitute for, but rather complement the conventional treatment plan. Complementary therapies include exercise, massage, reflexology, prayer, biofeedback, creative therapies (art, music, or dance therapy), guided imagery, acupuncture, relaxation strategies, chiropractic therapy, therapeutic touch, and herbalism.

Alternative therapies, on the other hand, may include the same interventions as complementary therapies but frequently become the primary treatment modality that replaces the care provided by medical doctors. Nurses always practice under their nursing license and must be careful not to give the impression of giving medical advice or contradicting medical advice. Many of the therapies discussed in this text are given by individuals with additional training in that field. Regardless of the amount of training one receives, it is not appropriate to recommend going against the doctor's advice or to recommend discontinuation of medical care. It is appropriate to provide therapies and reinforce education that safely complements the ordered treatment.

Both complementary and alternative therapies are often provided by individuals without medical training. Providers of these treatments may have very little to extensive training in their respective modalities. These therapies tend to have a greater focus prevention of illness, rather than treatment of an existing illness.

Allopathic is a term used to describe conventional medical treatment. Allopathic doctors have medical degrees and have M.D. as part of their title. Allopathic care includes the care given by nurses, therapists, pharmacists, and medical doctors. Allopathic is also called traditional, conventional, mainstream, or Western medicine. Treatments include medication, surgery, radiation, and physical therapy. Lifestyle changes, such as smoking cessation, exercise, stress reduction, and dietary changes may be recommended as part of allopathic care. Patients may seek out complementary therapies to help them make the lifestyle changes. For example, a smoker may have been unsuccessful at quitting smoking with nicotine replacement or other pharmaceutical assistance and may choose to use acupuncture. The recommendation to quit smoking remains allopathic while the method used is complementary.

Integrative care is the assimilation of complementary therapies into conventional medical care. Earlier definitions held a strong distinction between scientifically researched conventional medicine and unconventional treatments that did not have the support of scientific research. Some therapies once seen as unconventional have since been validated by scientific research and are recommended by physicians, hospitals, and public health authorities. In the example of the patient that wants to quit smoking, the doctor may recommend the acupuncturist to assist with smoking cessation efforts. The decision to integrate complementary practices into mainstream medical care is often done after research supports safety and efficacy. **Efficacy** is the effectiveness of the therapy to produce the intended effect.

The number of patients seeking unconventional treatments is difficult to determine based on various definitions of what constitutes complementary and alternative therapies. Estimates on its use have remained high for years. For over a decade between one third to over one half of the US population reported using some form of complementary or alternative therapy.

People may turn to complementary and alternative therapies because they believe them to be less invasive and gentler than conventional medicine and perceive them to incorporate a more holistic approach. Prevention is fundamental to most of the complementary therapies. They are not usually used as an immediate cure for an illness or acute injury but provide an ongoing method of maintaining optimal health. Practitioners often recommend lifestyle changes and encourage patients to follow health practices on a daily basis, thereby improving their overall health.

Complementary and alternative therapies vary in the degree to which they are compatible with conventional medicine. Many of the complementary therapies, such as acupuncture, make use of diagnostic and therapeutic methods specific to their field, whereas others, such as guided imagery, are essentially adjunctive in nature. For example, chiropractic practitioners frequently use diagnostic terminology and methods similar to those used by allopathic practitioners. They base interventions on conventional pathophysiology, anatomy, and kinesiology but at the same time explore mind-body connections that they believe drive the physiologic condition. Some alternative therapies, however, are not supported by scientific data, and some conflict with or even contradict traditional, scientifically based medical practices.

Most patients using unconventional therapies do so in conjunction with traditional medicine. Rarely do patients choose to make the alternative health care provider the only source of health care. Patients are often hesitant to talk to the health care provider about any treatment they are receiving other than those prescribed by a provider with a medical degree.

It is important to obtain as clear a view as possible of all efforts a patient is making to improve or maintain health. Although many unconventional therapies do not interfere with therapies prescribed by a health care provider, some pose the risk of serious interactions or may result in a delay in necessary medical care. When obtaining a health history from a patient, carefully assess the patient's use of any additional therapies. Project an open, nonjudgmental attitude when obtaining a health history so that the patient feels comfortable providing all information about any therapies he or she is currently using.

Holistic nursing addresses and treats the mind-body-spirit of the patient. Nurses use holistic nursing interventions such as relaxation therapy, guided imagery, music therapy, simple touch, massage, and prayer. Such interventions affect the whole person (mind-body-spirit) and are effective, economical, noninvasive, nonpharmacologic complements to medical care. Holistic interventions can be used to augment standard treatments and to promote or maintain health. The American Holistic Nurses Association (www.ahna.org) maintains standards of holistic nursing practice, which define and establish the scope of holistic practice and describe the level of care expected from a holistic nurse.

The Office of Alternative Medicine (now the National Center for Complementary and Integrative Health [NCCIH]) was established in 1992 as part of the National Institutes of Health. *The mission of NCCIH is to define, through rigorous scientific investigation, the usefulness and safety of complementary and integrative health interventions and their roles in improving health and health* care (NCCIH, n.d.b.). The NCCIH is a leading authority and resource for health care professionals to learn about scientific research of specific complementary or integrative therapies.

The therapies discussed in this text focus on complementary and integrative therapies, rather than those therapies used as an alternative to mainstream health care. Patients may be more familiar with the older terminology of "alternative medicine", "complementary and alternative medicine", or "CAM". The distinction between the terms is academic as many patients use this terminology but continue with conventional health care and follow medical advice. As discussed, obtaining the health history with a nonjudgmental approach is essential. Many of the treatments accepted now were once labeled as "quackery". Patients that have gathered data from non-scientific sources are more prone to unscientific data, especially when it references flawed research or misrepresents the findings of actual research.

Patients that have anti-science beliefs or make decisions based on conspiracy theories are difficult to educate. Their beliefs are not based in science, so scientific evidence is unlikely to change their beliefs. Although the patient may make anti-science statements, avoid using terms such as "anti-science", "anti-intellectualism", and "conspiracy theory" while addressing the misinformation. Nurses are not immune to misinformation. The nurse should strive to maintain current knowledge and to fact check when information is conflicting or seems to be in obvious conflict with our current scientific understanding.

Media strongly influences decision making. It is often difficult to determine if media sources are reliable. Often, advertisements are disguised to promote sales, a point of view, or a cause. The spokesperson may wear a white lab coat or have medical credentials to give credibility to a claim or to increase sales. The most accurate source of information about a research study is directly from that research study. However, even experienced nurses can find research sometimes difficult to understand. Nurses as well as consumers (patients) learn about new therapies from media other than respected, peer reviewed medical and nursing journals. Because of this, it is important to know how to evaluate the credibility of the source of information. The NCCIH gives guidance to assist in determining if a media source is trustworthy. You are more likely to get correct information from a source if (1) It comes from a media source that is not trying to promote a point of view or a cause. (2) It was written by a reporter that covers medical and science topics and is trained to understand and interpret health research. (3) It includes statements from experts on the topic but were not involved in the research (NCCIH, n.d.a.).

Nurses are trusted members of society, and this may be the key to overcoming misinformation. In fact, the nursing profession has the distinction of being ranked as the most trusted profession for 18 consecutive years! The Gallup poll found that 85% of Americans rated nurses' honesty and ethical standards as "high" or "very high" (https://news.gallup.com/poll/274673/nurses-continue-rate-highest-honesty-ethics.aspx). The same poll rated doctors' and pharmacists' honesty and ethics at 65% and 64%, respectively. This is a great honor for nursing profession, but it also carries a great responsibility.

HERBAL THERAPY

The use of herbal therapy as medical treatment began thousands of years ago. Neanderthal gravesites have been found that have the remains of plants surrounding the body. Herbalists were consulted by and worked in conjunction with medical physicians until the 1930s, when the last accredited herbal schools closed. In the meantime, the number of pharmaceuticals, or drugs, was increasing and their use becoming commonplace. Nonetheless, many of those drugs, as well as medications in use today, originated in herbs. An example is digitalis, which comes from the finger-shaped foxglove herb. Used in the treatment of heart failure, it is commonly prescribed by health care providers. Interest in the use of herbs and natural supplements to treat illness and maintain health has increased among the general population.

Herbs differ from pharmaceuticals—even those that are plant based—in several ways. Herbal preparation usually includes an unpurified extract of the whole plant. One herb may be used for a variety of purposes, and its action is usually gentler than those of pharmaceuticals. Pharmaceuticals that are derived from herbs only includes the active part, and the rest of the plant is separated out and discarded; thus the pharmaceutical is likely to be more potent but may also result in more adverse effects. Herbal treatments may interact with prescribed medications. The interactions between common herbal preparations and pharmaceutical medications can be found in many drug resources. However, less common herbal preparations may or may not be listed, or even known. When considering the potential adverse effects of an herb, it may be necessary to contact a pharmacist to see if additional information is available.

Herbal medicines have not undergone the same rigorous study as have pharmaceuticals. The majority have not received approval in the United States for use as drugs. For this reason, many herbal remedies are sold as foods or food supplements in health food stores and through private companies. The Dietary Supplement Health and Education Act, passed in 1994, now allows for herbs to be sold as dietary supplements as long as no health claims are written on their labels.

Herbal products are not viewed as drugs, which reduces the level of accountability for their manufacturers compared with that required of pharmaceutical companies. Herb manufacturers are not required by law to demonstrate the safety, the efficacy, or the quality of their products. Herb manufacturing remains unregulated and is likely to continue this way. Some manufacturers voluntarily adhere to so-called "good manufacturing practices" and make every effort to produce a quality product; others do not. However, nothing guarantees that the active chemical constituents in an herbal product remain constant from manufacturer to manufacturer. Chemical analysis of samples labeled as the same herbal product but purchased from various suppliers or outlets has revealed wide variations in potency, quality, and chemical content. In contrast to prescription drugs, no standardized dosages have been established for most herbs, and few manufacturers produce the standardized preparations of

predictable and consistent strength that make an herbal regimen possible to follow.

Herbal therapy is based on a different philosophy than conventional drug therapy. The goal of herbal therapy is to restore balance within the individual by facilitating the person's self-healing capacity. Drug therapy, on the other hand, is aimed at the treatment of specific diseases or symptoms. Herbal therapy also is prescribed on an individual basis, with unique herbal concoctions tailored for each person.

Many herbs are potentially toxic if used incorrectly. Some herbs are safe and effective when used topically in the amount specified but are highly toxic if taken internally. Many of the toxic effects of herbs have yet to be determined because of insufficient research and because no law requires reporting of adverse effects from herbal products (Table 20.1). With these cautions

Table 20.1 Commonly Used Herbs

HERB	USES	CONSIDERATIONS
Asian ginseng (Panax ginseng)	Improves overall health and well-being Atherosclerosis, bleeding disorders, colitis, diabetes, depressant cancer	Do not administer to pregnant or breast-feeding patients. Do not administer to patients with cardiovascular disease, hypertension, diabetes, or concurrent therapy. Patients taking anticoagulants should avoid use because it can prolong clotting. Avoid giving to patients who are taking CNS stimulants, estrogen, furosemide, ibuprofen, caffeine, or drugs metabolized by CYP3H4. Drug and herb interactions are possible with agents that inhibit monoamine oxidase (phenelzine, St. John's wort, selegiline).
Aloe vera (Aloe ferox, Aloe barbadensis)	Burns, skin irritation Has laxative properties	Internal use produces a cathartic action and has resulted in painful cramps, electrolyte imbalance, hemorrhagic diarrhea, and kidney damage. Drug interactions exist with antidysrhythmics, cardiac glycosides (e.g., digoxin), antidiabetics, beta blockers, steroids, diuretics, and disulfiram. Herb interactions exist with licorice.
Cayenne (Capsicum sp.)	General cardiovascular health: reduces cholesterol level; topical application produces analgesia, controls bleeding	Topical application as a counterirritant produces a "heat" sensation. Repeated applications produce analgesia that results from neuronal depletion of substance P (a mediator of pain transmission between peripheral nerves and spinal cord). Burning and pruritus diminish with continued use. Drug interactions exist with ACE inhibitors, heparin, ASA, disulfiram, and theophylline. Herb interactions exist with feverfew, garlic, ginger, and ginseng.
Comfrey (Symphytum officinale)	Cell proliferant, stimulates quick healing of strains and slow-healing wounds (for external use only)	When used internally, comfrey is potentially harmful: there are reports of liver toxicity. Some preparations contain significant levels of alcohol; they should be used with caution. Monitor patients for abdominal distention, nausea, abdominal pain, and elevated liver function test results. Limit use to 4–6 wk/yr to prevent exposure to large amounts of toxic alkaloids.
Echinacea (Echinacea purpurea, E. angustifolia, E. pallida)	Stimulates immune function; excellent blood cleanser; upper respiratory infections; wound healing	Activity has been shown against influenza, herpes, and Candida infections. Adverse reactions include fever, taste disturbance, gastrointestinal disturbances, nausea and vomiting, diuresis, photosensitivity. Patients with ragweed allergies should avoid use. Prolonged use potentially leads to overstimulation of the immune system and possible immune suppression. Drug interactions are possible with protease inhibitors, disulfiram, metronidazole, immunosuppressants, cyclosporine, methotrexate, prednisone, alcohol, warfarin, digoxin, contraceptives, SSRIs, and MAOIs.

Table 20.1   Commonly Used Herbs—cont'd

HERB	USES	CONSIDERATIONS
Evening primrose oil (*Oenothera biennis*)	Premenstrual syndrome, attention-deficit hyperactivity disorder, cardiovascular problems, hot flashes, mastalgia	Use of the oil occasionally unmasks previously undiagnosed epilepsy, especially when taken with a drug that treats depression or schizophrenia. Herb should be taken with food to decrease adverse gastrointestinal reaction. Use is contraindicated in patients with an allergy to evening primrose oil and those who are pregnant or breast-feeding. Do not give to patients with a history of epilepsy or who are taking a tricyclic antidepressant, phenothiazine, or another drug that lowers the seizure threshold.
Ginger (*Zingiber officinale*)	Nausea, vomiting, motion sickness, appetite improvement, impotence, liver toxicity, burns	Overdose possibly produces CNS depression and dysrhythmias. Ginger sometimes enhances the effect of anticoagulants. Pregnant patients should not take large doses because the teratogenic potential is largely unstudied. No consensus exists regarding dosage or monitoring. Drug interactions are possible with antacids, histamine H_2 receptor blockers, proton pump inhibitors, anticoagulants, barbiturates, disulfiram, and metronidazole.
Ginkgo, maidenhair tree (*Ginkgo biloba*)	Improves memory, increases circulation to the extremities and the brain	Studies have shown that ginkgo produces arterial and venous vasoactive changes that increase tissue perfusion and cerebral blood flow. Adverse reactions include dizziness, headache, subarachnoid and subdural hemorrhage, and cardiac insufficiency. There have been reports of seizures in children and bleeding complications. Potential drug interactions exist with antiplatelet therapy, anticoagulants, anticonvulsants, bupropion, tricyclic antidepressants, disulfiram, metronidazole, MAOIs, SSRIs, and trazodone. Herb interactions include garlic.
Goldenseal (*Hydrastis canadensis*)	Antibiotic and antiseptic, especially effective on mucous membranes, urinary tract infection, diarrhea, and hemorrhoids Digestive aid and expectorant	This herb increases hypoglycemic effects in patients using insulin. Possible effects of this herb include reducing effects of anticoagulants; reducing or enhancing hypotensive effects of antihypertensives; interfering with or enhancing cardiac effects of beta blockers, calcium channel blockers, and digoxin; enhancing sedative effects of CNS depressants; and enhancing sedative effects of alcohol. Do not give to children.
Kava (kava-kava) (*Piper methysticum*)	Anxiety, stress, and restlessness, insomnia, wound healing	Kava does not appear to cause physiologic dependence. Expect enhanced sedative effects if combined with other CNS depressants (alcohol, benzodiazepines, and opioid analgesics). Heavy use sometimes causes nutritional deficiencies, skin dermopathy, blood dyscrasias, pulmonary hypertension, cirrhosis, liver failure, hepatitis, and dopamine antagonism. It is generally well tolerated except in high doses or with long-term use. Patients should not use kava when ingesting alcohol or during pregnancy and breast-feeding, and it should not be given to children younger than 12 years. Drug interactions may exist with antiplatelet medications, MAOIs, drugs metabolized in cytochrome P-450 system, hepatotoxic drugs, and levodopa.
Lavender (*Lavandula officinalis*)	Antiseptic, antidepressant, sedative, relaxation, minor cuts, psoriasis, fragrance	Lavender is used for its calming mild sedative effect. Add to warm bath water if desired to aid in relaxation. Orally it sometimes is used as a tea to calm a "nervous stomach." Monitor patient closely for oversedation because it will possibly potentiate actions of other sedative drugs. It possibly potentiates CNS depressant effects of alcohol. Avoid giving to patients who are pregnant or breast-feeding. Some patients are allergic to lavender-containing perfumes. Do not confuse true lavender oil with lavandin or spiked lavender oil; the latter two contain high enough levels of camphor to elicit neurotoxicity. Excessive inhalation of the oil sometimes leads to vertigo, nausea, and syncope. Tell patients to avoid hazardous activities until lavender's full effects are known.

Continued

Table 20.1	Commonly Used Herbs—cont'd	
HERB	**USES**	**CONSIDERATIONS**
St. John's wort (*Hypericum perforatum*)	Mild to moderate depression, anxiety, viral infection, insomnia, premenstrual syndrome, topical myalgia, inflammation	There are numerous case reports and clinical trials evaluating the efficacy and safety of St. John's wort. Most trials contain design flaws, but overall results suggest that St. John's wort is sometimes beneficial for mild to moderate depression. Adverse reactions, which are uncommon, include photosensitivity, constipation, vertigo, dry mouth, restlessness, and sleep disturbance. Patients should avoid concurrent use with MAOIs, alcoholic beverages, opioids, prescription antidepressants, sympathomimetics, and foods such as chocolate, aged cheeses, and beer. Do not give to patients who are pregnant or breast-feeding. Do not give to children. Drug interactions include amiodarone, amitriptyline, chemotherapy drugs, cyclosporine, digoxin, drugs metabolized in cytochrome P-450 system, contraceptives (oral), protease inhibitors, theophylline and warfarin, SSRIs, reserpine, and nonnucleoside reverse transcriptase inhibitors.
Tea tree oil (*Melaleuca alternifolia*)	Skin irritations, acne, athlete's foot Topical antiseptic, antifungal, inhalation for respiratory disorders	Do not give in combination with drugs that affect histamine release. Do not apply to dry skin, cracked or broken skin, open wounds, or areas affected by rash that is not fungal. It should not be used internally because of systemic toxicity. Administer externally only after dilution, especially for patients with sensitive skin. Do not apply around nose, eyes, and mouth because it sometimes causes burns or pruritus in tender areas. Use the pure oil only under close supervision by a health care provider.
Valerian (*Valeriana officinalis*)	Insomnia, hyperactivity, stress, anxiety	Valerian causes addictive effects in some patients taking barbiturates. It possibly potentiates (1) sedative effects of catnip, hops, kona, kava, and passionflower and (2) the sedative effects of alcohol. Do not give to patients who are pregnant or breast-feeding. Evidence of toxicity includes difficulty walking, hypothermia, and increased muscle relaxation. Possible adverse reactions include hepatotoxic effects upon withdrawal.

ACE, Angiotensin-converting enzyme; *ASA,* acetylsalicylic acid (aspirin); *CNS,* central nervous system; *MAOI,* monoamine oxidase inhibitor; *SSRI,* selective serotonin reuptake inhibitor.

in mind, remember that many herbs may produce beneficial effects when used as directed. Herbal medicine has yet to be subjected to the same level of scientific scrutiny as traditional medical treatments. As a result, it has not yet gained wide acceptance by mainstream medicine. Because herb use is not widely accepted or understood by mainstream medical caregivers, patients often do not disclose their use of herbs to their health care provider. Many use prescription drugs concurrently with herbal remedies and face possible health risks as a result of adverse interactions. A well-informed, nonjudgmental care provider is most likely to gain the patient's trust and obtain not only a more accurate view of the patient's herb use but also an opportunity to provide valuable information about herb safety issues (see the Patient Teaching box).

Traditional health care and prescription costs are cost prohibitive for many Americans. Many conventional prescription drugs are expensive. A portion of the cost is not often reimbursed by insurance carriers so consumers are paying more out of pocket for them. Sometimes people are interested in preventive strategies and holistic approaches to health, such as eating a nutritionally sound diet, maintaining fitness, and reducing stress. Others may view herbal treatments as a means to avoid paying for expensive prescription medications.

The nurse assists patients in making educated decisions about their health. Most patients receive information about herbs from the media and the Internet, sources whose claims do not always coincide with results of clinical studies. Teach patients that before taking any herbal product, it is best to review it with a health care provider, pharmacist, or certified herbalist.

Treatment is provided in a variety of ways. It is possible to take dried herbs orally in capsule or tablet

Patient Teaching

Using Complementary and Alternative Therapies

Herbal Preparations

- Inform your primary care provider of any drugs you use, including herbal remedies, so that all agents—whether "nutraceutical" or pharmaceutical—will be considered in the plan of care.
- Use herbal preparations according to package or health care provider's direction.
- Stop taking the herb and notify your primary care provider if adverse effects or side effects occur.
- "Natural" does not mean safe. Seek objective and scientifically based sources of information. Use caution when evaluating the claims made by herb manufacturers.
- Avoid using combinations of herbs.
- Use only products that are standardized and known to contain a specific amount of active ingredients.
- Select herbal products carefully, buying only those that list the following information on the package: herb's common and scientific names, name and address of the manufacturer, batch or lot number, expiration date, dosage and administration guidelines, potential side effects, and details of how quality is ensured.
- Avoid using herbs for at least 2 weeks before any surgery.
- Bear in mind that patients who self-prescribe medications may have serious underlying physiologic or psychological conditions that necessitate attention. Learn to devise a health regimen that best suits your needs, regardless of whether herbs are used.
- Herb-drug interactions do occur, as do herb-herb interactions, and they pose serious risks; therefore it is best to let the primary care provider determine the safety of combining herbs and drugs.
- Purchase herbal products that have been standardized: that is, products for which the effects are known for a given dosage and for which the manufacturer ensures consistency from batch to batch.

- Buy from reputable sources. Ask the primary health care provider for assistance in determining where to purchase herbs.
- Avoid herbs during pregnancy and lactation or when attempting to become pregnant.
- Neither the safety nor the efficacy of herbs has been documented conclusively in scientific literature.
- It is in your best interest to undergo a complete medical evaluation before self-medicating with supplements: whether to treat specific symptoms of an illness or as a preventive measure.
- Do not use herbs in dosages larger than recommended or for more than several weeks (unless approved by the health care provider).
- Keep all herbs out of the reach of children and pets.

Yoga and Reflexology

- Consult your health care provider before starting a yoga program, because some yoga postures are stressful to people with certain health problems (muscle injury is possible if the positions are not performed correctly or if the body is forced into certain positions).
- When practicing yoga, try different positions cautiously; few people can perform all the movements in the beginning. Yoga requires regular practice to be effective.
- Postpone reflexology treatment if your feet have cuts, boils, bruises, or other injuries.
- Check with your health care provider before trying reflexology if you have diabetes, peripheral vascular disease, or other vascular problems in the legs, such as thrombosis or phlebitis.
- Many people who claim to perform reflexology actually are performing a simple foot massage; make sure the therapist has been trained in reflexology.

---

form. Tinctures are made by placing herbs in alcohol or vinegar and allowed to sit until the liquid absorbs the properties of the herb. The liquid is then strained and used. Teas made of an infusion of herbs and hot water are consumed, or a moist compress is made from the tea and applied to the affected area. Topical application of herbs is also possible by making a salve or ointment (Table 20.2).

Thousands of herbs are available. Table 20.1 lists some of the most common herbs and their uses. Remind patients to take care to use herbs from only a reliable source. Before a patient uses any fresh herbs, it is best to obtain exact identification from a trained professional. The patient always should know exactly what any herb is and what its actions are before using it.

The nurse should be aware of herb-medication interactions. For example, the combination of valerian and barbiturates probably causes excessive sedation. Ginseng is likely to interfere with the actions of digoxin. Advise against taking St. John's wort concurrently with antidepressant medications. Screen patients carefully regarding herbal use and possible interactions with other medications.

CHIROPRACTIC THERAPY

Chiropractic therapy has been in existence since the late 1800s. Doctors of chiropractic medicine undergo extensive training in manipulation of the musculoskeletal system. Although chiropractic therapy has been criticized severely, it is currently considered an acceptable treatment for certain disorders, including back pain and headaches. Many insurance companies provide coverage for chiropractic therapy care.

This form of therapy is based on a holistic belief in the body's capacity to take care of itself. The chiropractor adjusts the joints of the body by gentle manipulation to put an area of disturbed structural integrity, usually the vertebrae, back in proper

Table 20.2   Common Essential Oils and Their Uses

ESSENTIAL OIL	USE	CONSIDERATIONS
Chamomile	Pain, gastrointestinal spasms, stress, insomnia	Chamomile oil has theoretic potential to decrease absorption of certain antispasmodic medications. Excessive anticoagulation is possible when it is used with other anticoagulants. Avoid giving to pregnant patients because of potential abortifacient and teratogenic effects. Instruct patients with atopic eczema to avoid use because of potential allergic reactions.
Eucalyptus	Respiratory problems	Eucalyptus oil sometimes causes nausea, vomiting, diarrhea, and asthma-like attacks. It may enhance the effects of hypoglycemic agents. The oil has potential to affect the action of any drug that the liver metabolizes, so monitor patients for effect and toxic reaction. It decreases blood glucose levels; monitor patients for effect. Do not use with herbs that cause hypoglycemia such as basil, glucomannan, or Queen Anne's lace. When applied to an infant's or child's face, it sometimes causes severe bronchial spasm. Do not give to patients who are pregnant or breast-feeding or to patients who have liver disease or intestinal tract inflammation.
Lavender	Insomnia, stress, depression	Lavender oil possibly causes CNS depression, confusion, vertigo, syncope, drowsiness, headache, neurotoxicity, hypotension, nausea, vomiting, constipation, and respiratory depression. It may potentiate the effects of sedative drugs, so monitor patient closely for oversedation. It also possibly potentiates CNS depressant effects of alcohol, so it should not be used with alcohol. Massaging with diluted oil is unlikely to be toxic. Do not give to pregnant or breast-feeding patients. Do not confuse true lavender oil with lavandin or spike lavender oil; the latter two contain high enough levels of camphor to elicit neurotoxicity.
Lemon	Colds and flu, mental stimulation Diuretic, antiinflammatory	Patients who are pregnant or breast-feeding should avoid oral ingestion of expressed oil. Do not give to patients who are hypersensitive to members of the citrus family. Skin reactions of photodermatotoxicity from expressed oil are possible.
Peppermint	Acne, stomach upset General stimulant	Patients with gastroesophageal reflux disease should avoid peppermint oil because it sometimes exacerbates the disease. Do not give peppermint teas and mentholated ointment to infants and small children. Menthol sometimes causes sensitization and allergic reactions. Advise patients not to apply to broken skin. Internal use of peppermint other than for flavoring is not recommended.
Rosemary	Internally: mental stimulant; alleviating stress, circulatory problems Externally: myalgias, neuralgia, pruritus, migraines	Rosemary oil promotes menstrual flow, induces abortions (do not give to pregnant patients); and relieves headache, liver, and gallbladder complaints and blood pressure problems. In high doses, it sometimes causes seizures. Asthma can result from repeated occupational exposure. The oil also sometimes causes contact dermatitis and photodermatosensitivity. Encourage patients to take precautions and use sunscreen. Avoid use with herbal products containing alcohol. Do not give to pregnant or breast-feeding patients, children, or patients with seizure disorders. Bronchospasm and glottal spasm have been reported in children.
Tea tree	Antiseptic Skin irritations, viral illness, respiratory infection	Topical applications have not shown to be toxic, but ingesting the oil possibly will produce CNS depression and gastrointestinal irritation. Its antimicrobial activity has been well documented, but only anecdotal evidence exists for its efficacy in treating skin maladies. Advise patients of various product concentrations. It is probably best for patients with propensity for contact dermatitis to avoid the use of tea tree oil.

CNS, Central nervous system.

alignment. When properly performed, this treatment does not cause pain to the patient. Often patients seek treatment from a medical physician for an acute injury or illness and use chiropractic care on a routine basis. If distress is acute, visits sometimes are recommended several times a week or daily, but monthly visits to keep the patient at a maximal level of health are typical.

Fig. 20.1 Meridians of the human body. (From Fritz S: *Mosby's fundamentals of therapeutic massage,* ed 6, St. Louis, 2017, Elsevier.)

The chiropractor often uses x-rays to assist with diagnosis. Chiropractors do not prescribe medications as part of the treatment. Other treatments, such as hot and cold packs, are sometimes used during the course of chiropractic treatment. Chiropractors often consider lifestyle changes and nutritional supplements to help keep the patient functioning well without recurrence of the injury. Various suggested exercises often play a role in treatment.

LIMITATIONS OF CHIROPRACTIC THERAPY

It is unwise to treat certain diseases or joint conditions with manipulation. Contraindications to chiropractic therapy include acute myelopathy, fractures, dislocations, rheumatoid arthritis, and osteoporosis. If a malignancy is suspected or determined through diagnostic testing, the patient is referred to a health care provider for further evaluation and treatment. Bone and joint infections also necessitate pharmaceutical or surgical intervention. Care must be taken not to compromise the structural integrity of the bone, which is possible if excessive force is used.

ACUPUNCTURE AND ACUPRESSURE

Acupuncture and acupressure are therapies that are based on the belief that there is a form of energy, or **Qi** (life force), that flows through the body along **meridians** (channels of energy). The human body has 12 meridians. These meridians can become blocked, thus causing illness or discomfort. Therapy involves stimulating the channels at specific points to open them and allow the Qi to flow freely. Pain is understood to result primarily from stagnant or blocked Qi. It is thought that opening up the dam in the flow of energy through a meridian relieves pain and increases healing (Fig. 20.1).

Acupuncture is a method of stimulating certain points (acupoints) on the body by the insertion of special needles to modify the perception of pain, normalize physiologic functions, or treat or prevent disease. Fine needles inserted at specific points open the meridians. These needles are sterile and extremely thin, much smaller than the needles used for insulin injection; each one is for one-time-use only. Acupuncturists usually insert the needles only a few millimeters. When all the needles are in place, the needles are stimulated manually, electrically, or with heat (Fig. 20.2). After the needles have been in place for about 20 minutes, the acupuncturist removes and discards them. There is usually little discomfort while the needles are inserted, and most patients state that they feel no distress at all.

Acupuncture is the primary treatment modality used by health care providers of Chinese medicine. Many Western health care providers are also being trained and certified in acupuncture. Most states require licensure to practice as an acupuncturist. There are few risks associated with acupuncture treatments provided by a licensed acupuncturist.

Acupuncture is most effective when used in patients with chronic pain. It has also been used for the

Fig. 20.2 Acupuncture uses fine needles inserted at specific points to open the meridians. (© iStock.com/tekinturkdogan.)

Fig. 20.3 Acupressure. (From Fritz S: *Clinical massage in the healthcare setting*, St. Louis, 2008, Mosby.)

prevention of tension and migraine headaches in patients that frequently suffer from them. Patients undergoing cancer treatments may find acupuncture beneficial for reducing the side effects of cancer treatment. There has not been clear evidence of benefit for smoking cessation. However, given the extensive risks of smoking and the low risk from acupuncture treatments, the patient should not be discouraged from using it.

Acupressure entails the use of gentle pressure at similar points on the body (Fig. 20.3). Pressure sometimes is applied with a finger and sometimes with a small, blunt object. Acupressure is used primarily for prevention and relief of symptoms of muscle tension. Acupressure reduces tension, increases circulation, and enables the body to relax deeply. By relieving stress, acupressure increases resistance to disease and promotes wellness. Acupressure is beneficial in situations of discomfort and promotes the ability to rest or sleep.

With acupuncture and acupressure, several treatments are usually necessary to achieve the desired results. These methods are properly performed only by a professional with appropriate training.

HEALING TOUCH, THERAPEUTIC TOUCH, AND REIKI

Energy field therapies go by many names. Healing Touch, Therapeutic Touch, and **Reiki** are probably the most popular methods taught in the United States. These therapies use the human energy field to interact with another person's energy field.

Practitioners of energy field therapies have similar general procedures. Verbal consent is established, and the person is informed he or she may end the session at any point. It is not appropriate to attempt to persuade a person who does not want the therapy to accept it. The practitioner quiets his or her own mind. Then he or she "sets the intention," which means focusing on the goal of the process. This is usually pain relief, relaxation, or healing. It may be given as part of end-of-life care to assist with a peaceful transition.

The person performing the energy field therapy often assesses the energy field. There are several methods for assessment. Often, this information is felt in the practitioner's hands while moving the hands several inches away from the body. Intuition is not only valued but also encouraged as an assessment tool. The hands are held over the body or rested gently on the body in the areas where the practitioner feels it is needed. Sometimes this is a structured sequence of positions, but intuition may direct part or all of the intervention. There is no manipulation of the physical body. Ending the session is an important part of the process. Unless there is a contraindication (situation or condition where it could be harmful), both participants benefit from increasing water intake for the day. It is believed that energy field therapies improve the flow of energy through the body. Once the session ends, the improved flow of energy through the body continues to improve the mind, the body, and the spirit.

The experience of the person receiving the energy field therapy varies. A sense of relaxation during and after the procedure is common. Physical sensations are not uncommon. The sensations may be similar to or different from those experienced by the practitioner. It is not necessary for either participant to have physical sensations or intuition for the session to be successful. Most therapies recognize the interaction does not consist of one person who "gives" and the other person who "takes." Both participants benefit from quieting the mind and allowing the energy to flow through each of them. Novice practitioners may focus on the steps and neglect humility and love as key aspects of the process. A practitioner who has excessive fatigue or discomfort after the procedure must remember the person receiving the treatment is not responsible for any unpleasant sensations experienced by the facilitator. It is the responsibility of the person offering the energy field therapy to be mindful of his or her own energy during the process.

The development of the energy field practitioner is ongoing. With practice, skills and intuition improve. It is a personal journey that may lead to a greater sense of purpose and connectedness. Just as love is not exclusive to religious beliefs, energy field therapies are not religious practices, nor are they atheistic practices. Prayer may be included to the extent that it is acceptable to the practitioner and the person receiving the treatment.

THERAPEUTIC MASSAGE

Nurses have used massage to relax patients and help prevent impairment of skin integrity in the patient confined to bed. The effects are physical and psychological (see the Lifespan Considerations for older adults box). **Therapeutic massage** is massage performed by trained professionals to manipulate the soft tissues of the body and assist with healing (Nursing Care Plan 20.1). There are various types of massage designed to heal or prevent injury. Some massage is relaxing, and other forms are energizing.

A health profile should be reviewed before the initial massage. Certain medical conditions contraindicate massage. These conditions include acute back pain, phlebitis, and thrombosis. Areas with bruises or

---

Nursing Care Plan 20.1 Using Complementary and Alternative Therapies in Treatment

Ms. L., 40 years old, underwent an abdominal hysterectomy 2 days ago. The nurse finds her awake at midnight. Ms. L. voices concern about how long she will be in the hospital because she has four children, ages 4–15 years, at home and she is worried how well her family is managing without her. She also states that she has abdominal pain at the incision site that she rates at 5 on a scale of 0–10. Her vital signs are normal. Hydrocodone, 1 or 2 tablets q 4 hr prn for pain, is ordered, but she does not want to take any more drugs. She wonders if there is anything else she can do to decrease her anxiety and pain.

PATIENT PROBLEMS

Anxiousness, level 2, related to hospitalization
Recent Onset of Pain, related to surgical procedures

Patient Goals And Expected Outcomes	Nursing Interventions	Evaluation
Patient will state that anxiety is reduced to an acceptable level Patient will state that pain rating is 1–2 on a scale of 0–10	Explain the procedure for therapeutic massage. Position the patient comfortably. Reduce noise, lighting, and distractions. Perform therapeutic massage. Make patient comfortable after procedure by proper positioning, freshening linens, darkening the room, and providing a quiet environment.	Patient states that feelings of anxiety are reduced, and pain rating is now 2 on a scale of 0–10.

Critical Thinking Questions

1. Ms. L. complains of feeling fatigued and tense. List some nonpharmacologic methods of bringing about a state of physical and mental tranquility that may be helpful. Why may each of these methods be helpful for Ms. L.?
2. Ms. L. turns on her light and is crying. She complains of feeling helpless and inadequate to assume responsibility for her children and husband when she is discharged. What are some therapeutic interventions that will promote her feelings of stability and validation of her anxiety?

Lifespan Considerations
Older Adults

Focus on Touch

- Touch is a primal need, as necessary as food, growth, or shelter. Think of touch as a nutrient transmitted through the skin. "Skin hunger," or "poverty of touch," has been described as a form of malnutrition that has reached epidemic proportions in the United States, especially among older adults.
- Older adults need touch as much as or more than any other age group. However, skin hunger is often acute among older adults. It is an unfortunate irony that older adults often have fewer family members or friends to touch them just at the time in life when there is greatest need to use simple touch to enhance communication or when other senses sometimes are reduced in acuity.
- Simple touch helps older adult patients feel more connected to and accepted by those around them and to their environment. Self-esteem and sense of worth are enhanced.
- A nurse who reacts adversely to the skin changes of older adults may find it difficult to touch an older patient. Such reluctance communicates a negative message to older adults.
- A truly holistic nursing approach to the care of older adults also includes the caregivers, who often experience poor health or have neglected their own health and find themselves challenged by their own psychosocial issues as they relate to the caregiving experience, feel the effects of multiple stressors, or feel spiritual distress.

Modified from Potter PA, Perry AG, Stockert PA, et al: *Fundamentals of nursing:*, ed 9, St. Louis: 2017, Mosby.

Fig. 20.4 Massage therapy is used to relieve tension.

Fig. 20.5 Reflexology. Foot chart shows areas that correspond to organs and systems of the body. (From Fritz S: *Mosby's fundamentals of therapeutic massage*, ed 6, St. Louis, 2017, Elsevier.)

swellings should be evaluated by a physician before massage. Infectious skin diseases are also conditions in which massage is contraindicated. Abdominal massage in pregnant women is controversial. Some practitioners receive special training in pregnancy massage. Other massage therapists do not perform massage during pregnancy. They may fear adverse effects, or they may want to avoid any suspicion that massage has contributed to unwanted outcomes.

Massage is conducted in a comfortable, relaxing atmosphere (Fig. 20.4). A session lasts approximately an hour. A whole-body massage sometimes is performed, with extra attention to the affected area. Oils or lotions are often used during the massage; ensure the patient is not allergic to them before their use.

AROMATHERAPY

Aromatherapy entails the use of pure essential oils, produced from plants, to provide health benefits. The oils are formulated for inhalation or are applied topically. Sometimes the scent is dispersed into the air using candles or oil dispersers. Aromatic oils are often used during massage. Bathing provides a good modality for aromatherapy when oil is added to the water. On occasion, essential oils are taken orally in small amounts but only when prescribed by a qualified health care professional.

Many scents are used for their psychological effects. Different scents are thought to evoke different responses in the body as well. Nurses know that certain odors in a clinical setting have the potential to cause nausea or vomiting. Aromatherapy is based on similar principles: specific scents are thought to relax or stimulate, improve digestion, increase hormone production, reduce nausea, and improve circulation or memory. Table 20.2 presents some common essences and their uses.

Patients with asthma sometimes develop exaggerated symptoms from certain aromatic essences. Do not use essential oils on the skin of a patient with atopic eczema.

REFLEXOLOGY

Reflexology is based on the premise that it is possible to exert an effect on the entire body by applying pressure to specific areas on the feet, hands, and ears with the thumbs. The theory underlying reflexology is that these areas correspond to organs and systems of the body. Reflexologists use foot charts to guide them as they apply pressure to specific areas (Fig. 20.5). The manipulation of specific reflexes removes stress, enabling the release of disharmonies by a physiologic change in the body. With stress removed and circulation improved, the body is allowed to return to a state of homeostasis.

When reflexology is performed, the patient is assisted into a comfortable position, either lying or sitting. The feet are exposed so that the practitioner is able to perform specific massage movements and techniques on the feet. Treatments typically last up to 1 hour. Most people consider treatments to be very relaxing.

Reflexologists believe that treatment has the capacity to interfere with medical or other treatments; therefore it is important that the patient informs the practitioner of any other treatments being received. Reflexology is generally considered safe for people of all ages, although very vigorous pressure may cause discomfort for some people. Lighter pressure should be used on corresponding reflex areas on people with cardiac problems, blood problems, high blood pressure, epilepsy, and diabetes. Extreme caution should be used in performing reflexology on patients with diabetes who use artificial insulin. Overstimulation of the corresponding reflexes may cause the pancreas to produce increased amounts of insulin, resulting in a decreased need of artificial insulin.

Reflexology demonstrates the following four main benefits:

1. Relaxes the body and removes stress
2. Enhances the circulation
3. Assists the body in normalizing metabolism naturally
4. Complements all other healing modalities

When the reflexes are stimulated through the process of reflexology, the body's natural electrical energy works along the nervous system pathways and meridian lines to clear any blockages along those lines and in the corresponding zones. A treatment seems to break up deposits (felt as a sandy or gritty area under the skin) that interfere with this natural flow of the body's energy. Reflexologists are not qualified to diagnose medical conditions.

MAGNET THERAPY

Early research on the use of magnets showed promise as a treatment for pain. However, larger studies failed to demonstrate a clear benefit. Magnet therapy has been marketed in a variety of products, including jewelry, shoe inserts, and mattress toppers. Most users of magnet therapy have neither beneficial nor detrimental effects. However, it is contraindicated in patients with metal devices such as defibrillators, pacemakers, cochlear implants, and insulin pumps (NCCIH, 2013).

IMAGERY

In imagery, or visualization techniques, the conscious mind is used to create mental images to evoke physical changes in the body, create a sense of improved well-being, and enhance self-awareness. Imagery is frequently combined with some form of relaxation training to facilitate the effect of the relaxation technique. Imagery is sometimes self-directed, whereby the individual creates his or her own mental images; and sometimes the process is guided, whereby a health care professional leads the individual through a particular scenario. Here is a sample scenario of guided imagery with the professional as the guide:

First direct the patient to begin slow abdominal breathing while focusing on the rhythm of breathing. Then instruct the patient to visualize ocean waves coming to shore with each inspiration and receding with each expiration. Next instruct the patient to take notice of the smells, the sounds, and the temperatures that he or she is experiencing. As the imagery session progresses, perhaps instruct the patient to visualize warmth entering the body during inspiration and tension leaving the body during expiration.

The professional works in this manner but individualizes imagery scenarios for each patient or leaves them to the patient to develop.

Imagery has the power to evoke significant psychophysiologic responses, such as alterations in immune function. Many imagery techniques involve visual imagery, but they also sometimes include the auditory, proprioceptive, gustatory, and olfactory senses. For example, visualize slicing a lemon in half and squeezing the lemon juice under your tongue. This visualization produces increased salivation as effectively as the actual event. People typically respond to the environment according to the way it is perceived. The body has a physiologic response (salivating) to the visualization of an event that did not actually happen (the lemon slicing and juice tasting). As a result, an individual learns to regulate the body's responses to environmental stimuli by appropriately regulating expectations and perceptions. Imagery has applications in a number of patient populations. Imagery has been used to visualize the destruction of cancer cells by cells of the immune system, to control or relieve pain, and to achieve calmness and serenity (University of Michigan Health System, 2020).

RELAXATION THERAPY

Relaxation is the state of a generalized decrease in cognitive, physiologic, or behavioral arousal. Relaxation also is defined as the act or process of arousal reduction. The process of relaxation elongates the muscle fibers and reduces the neural impulses sent to the brain and thus decreases the activity of the brain and other body systems. The relaxation response is characterized by decreased heart and respiratory rates, blood pressure, and oxygen consumption and increased alpha-wave brain activity and peripheral skin temperature. The relaxation response can be obtained through a variety of techniques that incorporate a repetitive mental focus and the adoption of a calm, peaceful attitude. Teaching strategies for relaxation exercises are listed in Box 20.1.

Relaxation training involves developing cognitive skills that help people reduce the negative ways in which they respond to situations and their environment. The cognitive skills include focusing (the ability to identify, differentiate, keep attention on, and return attention to simple stimuli for an extended period), passivity (the ability to stop unnecessary goal-directed and analytic activity), and receptivity (the ability to tolerate and accept experiences that are sometimes uncertain, unfamiliar, or paradoxical). In addition, the individual performs cognitive restructuring, during which he or she replaces negative thoughts with positive ones. The long-term goal of relaxation therapy is for the person to continually monitor the self for indicators of tension and to consciously let go and release the tension contained in various body parts.

ANIMAL-ASSISTED THERAPY

Animal-assisted therapy (AAT) involves the use of trained animals to enhance an individual's physical,

Box 20.1   Relaxation Strategies

RHYTHMIC BREATHING[a]
1. Provide a quiet environment.
2. Help the patient get comfortable by elevating the legs with the knees bent (relaxing the leg, back, and abdominal muscles).
3. Instruct the patient to close eyes and to breathe in and out slowly; say rhythmically, "Breathe in, 2, 3, 4; breathe out, 2, 3, 4."
4. Once rhythmic breathing is established, instruct patient to listen to your voice, and with a low and steady voice, instruct patient to do the following:
   a. Breathe in and out slowly and deeply.
   b. Try to breathe from the abdomen.
   c. Feel more relaxed with each exhalation.
   d. Try to identify your own special feeling of relaxation (e.g., light and weightless or very heavy).
   e. While you are breathing, let your imagination take you to a place you remember as peaceful and pleasant; look around, listen to the sounds, feel the air, notice the smells.
   f. When you are ready to end this relaxation exercise, count silently from 1 to 3; on 1, move your lower body; on 2, move your upper body; on 3, breathe in deeply, open your eyes, and while breathing out slowly, say silently, "I am relaxed and alert." Stretch as if just waking up.

PROGRESSIVE RELAXATION
1. Follow steps 1, 2, and 3 of rhythmic breathing.
2. Once patient is breathing slowly and comfortably, instruct patient to tighten and relax an ordered succession of muscle groups, tensing them and then relaxing them, leaving each part feeling relaxed.
3. Instruct patient to begin by tensing and then relaxing the calves, then the knees, and so on.

RELAXATION BY SENSORY PACING
1. Follow steps 1 and 2 of rhythmic breathing.
2. Instruct patient to slowly repeat and finish either in a low voice or to self each of the following sentences:
   a. "Now I am aware of seeing …"
   b. "Now I am aware of feeling …"
   c. "Now I am aware of hearing …"
3. Instruct patient to repeat and complete each sentence four times, then three times, then twice, and finally once.
4. Instruct patient to allow the eyes to close when they feel heavy.

RELAXATION BY COLOR EXCHANGE
1. Follow steps 1, 2, and 3 of rhythmic breathing.
2. Instruct patient to notice any tension, tightness, aches, or pains in the body and to give that sensation the first color that comes to mind.
3. Instruct patient to breathe in pure white light from the universe and send the light to the tense or painful place in the body, letting the white light surround the color of the discomfort.
4. Instruct patient to exhale the color of the discomfort and let the white light take its place.
5. Instruct patient to continue breathing in the white light and exhaling the color of the discomfort, allowing the white light to fill the entire body and bring about a sense of peace, well-being, and energy.

MODIFIED AUTOGENIC RELAXATION
1. Follow steps 1, 2, and 3 of rhythmic breathing.
2. Instruct patient to repeat each of the following phrases to oneself four times, saying the first part of the phrase while breathing in for 2–3 seconds, then holding the breath for 2–3 seconds, and then saying the last part of the phrase while breathing out for 2–3 seconds.

BREATHING IN	BREATHING OUT
I am	relaxed.
My arms and legs	are heavy and warm.
My heartbeat	is calm and regular.
My breathing	is free and easy.
My abdomen	is loose and warm.
My forehead	is cool.
My mind	is quiet and still.

RELAXING WITH MUSIC
1. Provide patient with an MP3 player or other listening device and headset.
2. Ask patient to select a favorite choice of slow, quiet music.
3. Instruct patient to get into a comfortable position (either sitting or lying down but with arms and legs uncrossed) and to close eyes and listen to the music through the headset.
4. Instruct patient to imagine floating or drifting with the music while listening.

[a]In conditioning a relaxation response, a "signal breath" involving deep inhalation through the nose and forceful exhalation through the mouth is the key. The signal breath precedes and follows each run through the exercise.

emotional, and social well-being (Fig. 20.6). This method improves self-esteem, reduces anxiety, and facilitates healing. AAT began in the 1940s, when an army corporal brought his Yorkshire terrier to a hospital to cheer wounded soldiers. The response was so positive that the dog continued to comfort others for 12 more years.

Research has concluded that animals have a calming effect, reducing blood pressure and anxiety. They tend to decrease loneliness and bring out positive social characteristics. Health care practitioners at many hospitals and nursing homes use AAT programs to help decrease feelings of depression and isolation in their patients, as well as stimulating mental activity through interaction with the animals.

Many different types of animals are used in AAT, from dogs and cats to horses and dolphins. Safety is always a consideration when working with any type of animal. AAT professionals and volunteer handlers must ensure that the animal has been adequately

Fig. 20.6 Animal-assisted therapy. Caring for an animal is one aspect of animal-assisted therapy.

Fig. 20.7 Yoga is useful in achieving control of the body through correct posture and breathing, control of the emotions and the mind, and meditation and contemplation.

trained and is in good health, with all necessary vaccinations. Patient allergies and autoimmunity issues necessitate consideration before implementation of AAT. Clearance by a health care provider should be obtained if there is any question regarding the patient's safety. Not all animals used in AAT are service animals. Service animals must meet specific criteria, but they are protected legally under the Americans with Disabilities Act (ADA).

AAT is a complementary intervention that is continuing to gain popularity in the medical setting. It can reduce pain, anxiety, and stress (Mayo Clinic, 2020).

YOGA

The word *yoga* means "yoke," or union of the personal self with the divine source. Yoga is a healing system of therapy and practice. It is a combination of breathing exercises, physical postures, and meditation that has been practiced for more than 5000 years. **Yoga** has emerged as a therapeutic treatment and now is being recognized by Western medical practice. As scientific research increasingly verifies the importance of the integration of the whole person in healing disease, the medical community no longer can ignore the efficacy of yoga's body-mind connection.

With consistent and earnest practice, change and personal transformation take place on numerous levels. Typically, these changes include improved health and energy, reduced stress, feelings of well-being, and the healing of disease. What perhaps started as a search for increased flexibility and stress reduction slowly enlarged to a greater understanding of the self, emotional growth, and spiritual awakening.

There are more than 100 different schools of yoga. Hatha yoga is the most familiar type in the United States. However, all systems recognize the validity of certain basic principles, including control of the body through correct posture and breathing, control of the emotions and the mind, and meditation and contemplation (Fig. 20.7).

The regular practice of yoga offers the potential to tone the muscles that balance all parts of the body, including internal organs, heart, lungs, glands, and nerves. It increases flexibility of the spine and therefore helps treat chronic back problems. It is beneficial for the nervous system, promoting deep relaxation and reduction of stress. Although the risk of injury from yoga is very small, a possibility of injury exists. Some poses may have to be modified. The participant and the instructor must be accepting of the participant's limits and present level of skill. As with most forms of exercise, the participant should not try to do too much too quickly.

Patients with glaucoma should not do inverted poses. These include downward facing dog, standing forward bend, plow, and legs up the wall. Head-down yoga poses cause a temporary, but significant, increase in pressure within the eye. The short period of time when the eye pressure is increased is not thought to be harmful to most people. However, patients with the eye disease glaucoma have a higher risk for optic nerve damage because of increases in eye pressure (Glaucoma Research Foundation, 2017).

TAIJI

Taiji (also called **t'ai chi**) originally was developed as a martial art in 17th-century China. Origins of the art are debated by proponents of various styles, but nearly all agree that the art was a fusion of existing martial arts practices with Daoist philosophical concepts, traditional Chinese medicine, and qigong theory and practice. The meaning of Taiji (Fig. 20.8) was described by Yang and colleagues (2008):

> *The word Taiji is an ancient Daoist philosophical term symbolizing the interaction of yin and yang, which are opposite manifestations of the same forces in nature. The dynamic interaction of yin and yang, underlying the relation and changing nature of all things, is epitomized in the famous "Taiji Diagram."*

A fundamental principle of Taijiquan is the relationship between seemingly opposite forces. It is helpful

Fig. 20.8 The t'ai chi diagram.

to think of yin and yang as complementary opposites: each necessarily relies upon, and "gives birth" to, the other. In Taiji practice, emphasis is placed on relaxing the body and calming and focusing the mind. Taiji form movement is performed slowly; the intention, mechanics, accuracy, and precision of the motion are accentuated. By practicing in accordance with Taiji principles of softness and slowness, the person paradoxically begins to experience a quality of hardness, strength, and efficiency of movement that are significantly different from that of ordinary natural ability (Yang, 2013).

The Taiji training system includes form movement, static and dynamic qigong exercises, and two-person balance and reaction training called "push-hands." Form movement is typically performed slowly with relaxed body and calm and focused mind and thus is referred to as a "moving meditation." Static standing and sitting meditation exercises are practiced as fundamental qigong exercises. Lying-down meditation is another qigong practice that is an effective relaxation and stretching exercise. In its complete form, Taiji is a holistic art that emphasizes mind-body integration, physical and mental balance, and spiritual development. Practice of the art is direct exercise of central and peripheral nervous system function.

Taiji practice originally was intended to improve the variables of fundamental skills, including balance, strength, flexibility, coordination, agility, reaction time, sensitivity or awareness, and confidence. Although essential for self-defense, these variables are, at the same time, fundamentally health issues. Because the intensity (e.g., range of motion and height of stance) of any Taiji form sequence is varied easily to suit the individual's physical capabilities, people of all physical abilities are able to practice Taiji. It is especially well suited as a low- to medium-intensity exercise for older adults. Those unable to learn or perform movements do well to begin with the static qigong exercises.

Other health benefits of Taiji practice have been recognized in China for a long time and are receiving more attention in Europe and the Americas. Research articles and studies are increasing as interest grows

about these concepts. Health benefits documented in these studies include significant improvements in balance, leg strength, cardiorespiratory function, range of motion and treatment of arthritic symptoms, self-efficacy, sleep quality, prevention of osteoporosis, and immune function. Other health benefits, not yet studied in Europe and the Americas but appreciated in China, include improvements in bowel function, general strengthening of the immune system, and improvements in cognitive function (attention, concentration, learning, and memory) (Harvard Health Publishing, 2019).

BIOFEEDBACK

Biofeedback is a noninvasive method that an individual can employ to learn control of the body to manage certain conditions. It may be considered when other therapies have not been successful or in conjunction with other treatments. Health concerns such as anxiety, stress, irritable bowel syndrome, and asthma may be managed through biofeedback. Monitoring equipment is used to measure vital signs and muscle tension. The messages are sent back to the individual. These responses are conveyed to the patient through auditory, visual, physical, or physiologic signals, or a combination of these (Mayo Clinic, 2021). Once the messages are sent to the patient, there is opportunity to control the body and manage the disorders. One key advantage of biofeedback is the increased awareness achieved by the patient about physiologic functions and influencing factors of these functions.

Another advantage of biofeedback is the reduction of the stress response. Biofeedback has been found to be beneficial in the treatment of disorders such as migraine headaches, pain, and urinary tract and gastrointestinal tract disorders. Commitment of the patient to the program determines a successful outcome.

Although biofeedback is considered noninvasive, precautions with the therapy are necessary in connection with repressed emotions or feelings that may surface during the relaxation or biofeedback sessions. It is important for the health care provider to be aware of these precautions so that proper psychologic support is available at the time of the sessions or proper referral is made.

MARIJUANA AND CANNABINOIDS

Cannabis (marijuana) and its chemical compounds are receiving ongoing interest as a potential treatment for a variety of health conditions. Marijuana is the common name for cannabis that can be used as a drug. Therapeutic use of marijuana remains controversial. A discussion of legal concerns must accompany a responsible discussion of marijuana. As of March of 2020, 33 states, Washington D.C., and the US territories of Puerto Rico, Guam, and the US Virgin Islands have legalized medical marijuana. Marijuana remains federally banned and is designated as a schedule I drug in the United States. Schedule I drugs are drugs designated as having no currently accepted medical use and have the highest potential for abuse. States that legalize marijuana are doing so in conflict with the current Drug Enforcement Agency's (DEA's) classification of marijuana as a schedule I drug. A petition to reschedule marijuana was denied in August of 2016. The head of the DEA, Chuck Rosenberg, told National Public Radio that "marijuana is not as dangerous as heroin, for instance…clearly not as dangerous. But this decision isn't based on danger. This decision is based on whether marijuana, as determined by the FDA, is a safe and effective medicine … and it's not." He said the DEA supports scientific research of marijuana and could change its mind based on the findings of the research. This statement was soon followed by a consensus study report by the National Academies of Sciences, Engineering, and Medicine. The study reviewed over 10,000 abstracts to outline a large body of evidence for the therapeutic uses of marijuana. They stated that "there is conclusive or substantial evidence that cannabis or cannabinoids are effective: for the treatment of chronic pain in adults." The publication also provides guidance to future researchers to fill knowledge gaps (National Academies of Sciences, Engineering, and Medicine. 2017). Later, the 2018 Farm Bill declassified hemp as a schedule I controlled substance. Since hemp is cannabis with a very low THC, this resulted in federal statements to clarify the regulation of cannabidiol (CBD). Ultimately, the 2018 Farm Bill resulted in federal legalization of CBD in all states without changing the status of THC containing cannabis as a Schedule I drug. A growing body of research shows promise for the therapeutic and medicinal use of CBD, THC, and whole plant marijuana (Russo, 2019). This evidence makes it more difficult to maintain the position that it meets the government's strict criteria of the drug as having "no currently accepted medical use" that defines a Schedule I drug.

Cannabinoids are compounds found in marijuana that attach to cannabinoid receptors in the body. There are more than 60 cannabinoids unique to marijuana. Tetrahydrocannabinol (THC) is the most well-known cannabinoid. THC is psychoactive and may cause euphoria, paranoia, drowsiness, and increased hunger. This chemical causes the "high" that is responsible for the abuse potential of the drug. Therapeutically, THC is used to treat nausea, pain, and weight loss in patients with cancer and human immunodeficiency virus (HIV). Because of breeding techniques, cannabidiol (CBD), THC, and other cannabinoids are present at highly variable levels in marijuana. CBD has no psychoactive properties and inhibits the psychoactive properties of THC. In states where marijuana is available, consumers may select varieties based on the THC to CBD content. Varieties with a high CBD content are being used for a various neurologic disorders. Parents have been using marijuana with high CBD content as a treatment for their children with life-threatening seizures that were not responsive to conventional medicine. In 2018, the FDA approved Epidiolex (cannabidiol, CBD) for the treatment of two severe forms of epilepsy. The FDA approved drug has the benefit of uniform strength and consistent delivery (FDA, 2018). Parents who have been successfully using other CBD sources may continue to do so based on the success of the treatment, cost, or convenience in obtaining it.

Three species of cannabis have been identified. *Cannabis sativa* is used for industrial purposes, therapeutic uses, and as a recreational drug. *Cannabis indica* tends to have more CBD content, but THC is present as well. Selective breeding of *C. indica* has resulted in varieties with higher CBD content. *Cannabis ruderalis* may be used as an herbal treatment but is not used as a recreational drug. Hybrids and selective breeding have led to further variation of components for therapeutic and recreational purposes.

Supporters of rescheduling marijuana point out that marijuana is a schedule I drug, like LSD and heroin. They would like to see marijuana reclassified as a schedule II drug, like narcotics used for pain control, such as morphine, hydromorphone, oxycodone, and fentanyl. Schedule II drugs have high potential for abuse but also have an accepted medical use. It is commonly accepted that marijuana is safer than opioids. Many schedule II drugs used for pain control may lead to severe respiratory depression, whereas marijuana does not. Concentrated THC preparations potentially may cause changes in blood pressure and heart rate but there is almost no risk of death. Higher concentrations of THC in products have likely contributed to more emergency room visits but have not been attributed to marijuana intoxication (NIDA, 2020).

Selective breeding may lead to new treatments for a variety of neurological conditions, such as depression, anxiety, dementia, multiple sclerosis, Parkinson disease, drug addiction, nausea, and chronic traumatic encephalopathy (Russo, 2018). Marijuana and specific cannabinoids may be used for a variety of psychological, neurologic, and inflammatory conditions. THC and synthetic THC may be used to treat the side effects of cancer treatment. Synthetic THC, dronabinol, is US Food and Drug Administration (FDA) approved for the treatment of nausea, vomiting, and anorexia in patients with cancer and AIDS. It is available in the trade names of Marinol and Syndros. They have been designated Schedule III drugs. There is ongoing research into medical uses of synthetic marijuana derivatives. These should not be confused with non–FDA-approved products marketed as "synthetic marijuana" in an effort to bypass FDA regulations. These often are sold online or in gas stations under many names, including Spice, K2, Herbal Incense, and synthetic marijuana. These have variable synthetic compounds that may or may not resemble those in marijuana. These drugs do not have FDA approval and can be lethal. Once these drugs were identified as dangerous substances, they were banned, but there have been similar drugs marketed with new names. Patients should be warned not to use over-the-counter products marketed as synthetic versions of marijuana.

There are also notable concerns regarding vaping of THC. In August 2019, the Centers for Disease Control started receiving reports of serious lung injuries in young people tied to e-cigarette use, also known as vaping. The lung injury, known as e-cigarette or vaping product use-associated lung injury (EVALI) resulted in thousands of lung injuries and over fifty deaths within a few months of the initial report. The vaping related injuries were likely to be associated with abuse rather than complementary or integrative treatments. Many of the patients with EVALI had vaped tobacco as well as THC products and additional chemicals were suspected of contributing to the development of the condition. Regardless of the intent, abuse or therapeutic use, patients considering the use of THC should be warned about the risks associated with vaping e-cigarettes (King, 2020).

This puts marijuana and cannabinoids in a unique position as potential herbal, dietary, or medicinal treatments, as well as potentially addictive substances that may necessitate treatment. Marijuana has abuse potential but is also a less addictive form of pain management than opioids. The abuse potential may be overestimated since it often based on patients that seek treatment for marijuana abuse. Over half of patients in treatment for cannabis were given the option of treatment as an alternative to incarceration. The choice for treatment is logical regardless of the need for such treatment (Russo, 2019). Marijuana may be used in place of more addictive medications or even in the treatment of addiction. The large number of cannabinoids and other natural components complicate the regulation of the drug. Although pharmaceutical companies often look at the individual components of the drug, others believe selective breeding of the whole plant has more therapeutic uses (Russo, 2019).

Most states have passed laws that permit some form of medical or recreational marijuana use. Arguments for legalization of marijuana often point out that legalization can improve state finances through tax revenue. Opponents believe that easy access to marijuana may result in increased use of more dangerous and addictive drugs. Several states have decriminalized marijuana. Decriminalizing marijuana is not the same as legalizing marijuana, but patients may be more likely to self-medicate where there are fewer consequences.

Patients that use marijuana as complementary, integrated, or alternative treatments need to stay informed of the rapidly changing state laws that restrict obtaining, cultivating, and possessing marijuana. Parents providing marijuana for their minor children may have additional legal consequences. State laws vary, and the individual is held to the law of the state they are in, regardless of residence. Even in states where marijuana is legal, employees may be terminated for obtaining a medical marijuana card or evidence of marijuana use. However, the National Conference of State Legislatures states that these same registries may also provide patients with some legal protections from criminal penalties (NCSL, 2021). With these considerations in mind, patients should be encouraged to exhaust medical options before attempting to use marijuana to treat symptoms.

Nurses must be aware of the complexities of marijuana and cannabinoid treatment. Patients may think that marijuana is safe or unsafe based on state and federal laws governing its use. The legal status of a drug does not determine its safety. Alcohol and tobacco abuse are legal, but clearly each has negative health consequences. Particularly concerning is the marketing of dangerous substances as legal alternatives to marijuana. Some state laws may require a physician to prescribe and monitor medical marijuana. However, the appropriate cannabis variety, dose, frequency, and route often are determined by providers without medical training. Plant quality, chemical components, and contamination concerns are similar to those seen with herbal treatments. Although there is no known toxic dose of marijuana, intoxication can lead to death or injury because of impaired judgment and inability to operate a vehicle safely. Concentrates of the psychoactive portion of cannabis, THC, can cause concerning changes in vital signs. Factors that may affect the response and side effects include previous marijuana use, the amount taken, the route (smoking, vaping, ingesting, applying topically or instilling eye drops), and the levels of specific cannabinoids.

The American Cannabis Nurses Association (ACNA) is a professional nursing organization that is a resource for nurses wanting to learn more about cannabinoid therapeutics. The ACNA's mission is *"to advance excellence in cannabis nursing practice through advocacy, collaboration, education, research and policy development"* (ACNA, n.d.). The Medical Cannabis Institute (TMCI) aims to *"educate a growing global community of healthcare professionals, caregivers and patients who want to learn about the science and clinical data behind medical cannabis"* (TMCI, n.d.). The ACNA and TMCI offer online curriculums for nurses and other health care professionals wanting objective, scientific information. Patients Out of Time offers conferences and resources for patients and health care providers (http://patientsoutoftime.org) (ACNA, n.d.).

From The National Organization for the Reform of Marijuana Laws—NORML, (www.norml.org/laws.), Frontiers (frontiersin.org) is an open access publisher and open science platform. They offer freely accessible research articles in this peer-reviewed journal. This platform appeals to nurses that would like to search and view full research articles as the need or interest arises.

TRENDS IN INTEGRATIVE MEDICINE AND THE NURSING ROLE

The interest in integrative therapies has increased significantly since 1990. This interest is increased not only among health care consumers but also among allopathic health care providers. Some primary health care providers do not refer their patients for unconventional treatments, because they are not familiar with the therapies and have had little, if any, education and training in them. Some health care providers may have reservations because these modalities have not been rigorously tested in clinical trials with strict controls subjects. Many studies have involved small numbers of subjects and were not well controlled, but research is improving. Continued research is needed to continue to build evidence-based practice and to validate the effectiveness of complementary and integrative therapies in different patient populations.

The NCCIH is contributing to the knowledge of complementary and integrative therapies through funding research and maintaining a database that has information for patients and health care providers. Not every research proposal can be funded so they have identified four priorities to consider when selecting which studies are funded. (1) Scientific promise. This looks at the existing research to see if the current evidence supports further research and if the proposed study fits the need for the research that is needed. (2) Amenability to rigorous scientific inquiry. This priority aims to determine if the goals of research are attainable and if the study is structured in a way to meet those goals. (3) Potential to change health practices. This aims to determine if the outcome will change patient health practices or impact health policies that will lead to changes in patient health practices. (4) Relationship to use and practice. This determines if the study can address an important need for information, for example, determining the safety or effectiveness of the therapy in the proposed research.

The integrative medicine approach is consistent with the holistic approach that nurses are taught to practice. Nurses have the potential for becoming essential participants in this type of health care model. Many nurses already offer relaxation, imagery, and massage to their patients. Nurses need a good knowledge of these therapies to make appropriate recommendations to primary

 Lifespan Considerations

Older Adults

Complementary and Integrative Therapy

- Use essential oils with caution. Older adult patients are usually more sensitive to essential oils and thus require smaller amounts and less concentrated forms of the essence.
- Advise older adult patients to take herbal treatments only under professional supervision.
- Older adults typically achieve positive results from regular exercise and weight-lifting, including increased physical strength and flexibility and improved mental status in areas such as memory and depression. It is necessary to adapt the exercise regimen to each patient's physical condition.
- In massage therapy, a lighter pressure is necessary; other modifications for body status of an older adult patient also may be needed.
- Magnet therapy has not been shown to be effective, and the use of magnets interferes with pacemaker functions.

care providers about potentially useful therapies. They should be prepared to advise patients regarding when to seek conventional therapy and when complementary therapy is appropriate (see the Patient Teaching box on using complementary and alternative therapies). For example, if a patient complains of right lower abdominal pain, nausea, and vomiting, the nurse should suspect appendicitis and recommend assessment by their primary care provider. However, if the patient has a chronic gastrointestinal disorder and irritable bowel syndrome has been diagnosed, it is possible that the patient will benefit from mind-body exercises, aimed at increasing relaxation and decreasing overactive inflammatory response. Nurses must be aware of their state's nurse practice act regarding complementary therapies and practice accordingly within the scope of these laws.

Nurses work closely with their patients and are in the unique position of becoming familiar with the patient's religious and cultural viewpoints (see the Cultural Considerations box) and existential issues. The nurse is in a good position to determine which therapies are aligned most appropriately with these beliefs and to offer recommendations accordingly.

See Chapter 6 for further discussion of cultural considerations.

Increased awareness and use of complementary and alternative therapies means that many patients whom you encounter already had experience with or are open to investigating these therapies. In making choices concerning their health care, patients tend to be receptive to holistic interventions. Therefore, be knowledgeable about the multiple options available and what is known about the safety and efficacy of the therapies. Keep abreast of the current research in this area to provide accurate information not only to patients but also to other health care providers.

🌐 Cultural Considerations

Providing Culturally Appropriate Care to patients using Complementary and Alternative Therapies

- Avoid using the term *alternative therapy;* patients may not consider their practices to be alternative at all. For some Chinese Americans, for example, treatments such as acupuncture and use of herbal preparations are grounded in their culture and passed down from generation to generation. They may consider Western medicine to be the alternative.
- Acupuncture originated in China approximately 4000–5000 years ago, but very little acupuncture was performed in the United States outside of Chinese immigrant communities until the 1970s.
- Yoga began in India more than 6000 years ago but is now one of the most popular complementary and integrative therapies in the United States.
- Members of some cultures often have more faith in an alternative or traditional care practitioner than in a conventional Western health care provider. Respect the patient's beliefs and look for ways to combine therapies when there are no contraindications.
- Regardless of your personal faith in another type of care, be sensitive to cultural differences. Question the patient appropriately and support the patient's choices as needed.
- Show respect for the cultural differences by honoring the patient's culturally based health beliefs.
- Ask permission before touching the patient. Determine the meaning of touch and which body areas are considered touchable. Acceptability of touch varies from culture to culture.
- To provide culturally appropriate care to patients using complementary therapies, remember that each individual is culturally unique and is the product of a mixture of past experiences, cultural beliefs, and cultural norms.

Get Ready for the NCLEX® Examination!

Key Points

- Complementary and alternative therapies are used to restore or maintain health.
- Patients tend to think of complementary and alternative therapies as gentler and less invasive than traditional medical treatments.
- Patients are often hesitant to tell a health care provider about unconventional therapies they are using.
- Herbs used for treatment are formulated in many ways for consumption and use: as dried herbs in capsules or tablets, tinctures, teas, compresses, salves, or ointments.
- Some herbs interfere with the actions of medications. A thorough health history is important.
- Chiropractic treatment achieves its effects through manipulation of the musculoskeletal system. Gentle manipulation puts the vertebrae in proper alignment.
- In acupuncture and acupressure, needles or pressure is applied to specific points on the body. The points correspond to meridians that flow through the body.
- Energy field therapies have benefits for the practitioner and the recipient. Energy field therapies can reduce pain and increase relaxation. Practice fosters intuition, skills, and connectedness.
- Energy field therapies do not require physical touch. Touch may be used, but there is no manipulation of the physical body.
- In its complete form, Taiji (t'ai chi) is a holistic art that emphasizes mind-body integration, physical and mental balance, and spiritual development.
- Therapeutic massage is used to promote healing and prevent injury. Contraindications include a history of phlebitis or thrombosis of the extremities.
- In aromatherapy, essential oils are used to provide health benefits. Inhalation is the most common method of using the oils.
- Pressure to the feet in the form of massage is performed in reflexology.
- Reflexology is a focused pressure technique; it is based on the premise that the feet are divided into zones or reflex areas that correspond to all organs, glands, and systems of the body.
- Regular practice of yoga potentially tones the muscles that balance all parts of the body—including internal organs, heart, lungs, glands, and nerves—and controls the emotions and mind.
- There has been an increase in state laws legalizing the use of marijuana for medicinal as well as recreational use. Marijuana remains federally banned.
- Cannabis (marijuana plant) has been bred to increase or decrease specific cannabinoids for therapeutic use.
- Patients considering self-medicating with marijuana should be encouraged to exhaust traditional medical options first.
- Although some unconventional therapies have been researched and the findings published in professional journals, others lack scientific proof. Those that lack scientific proof need not be discarded as long as they do not cause harm. Many patients report positive outcomes from these therapies.
- Patients benefit from the trusted guidance of nurses to determine the safety and efficacy of unconventional treatments. Sometimes this may include addressing anti-science beliefs and misinformation in a tactful manner.

Additional Learning Resources

SG Go to your Study Guide for additional learning activities to help you master this chapter content.

Be sure to visit the Evolve site at http://evolve.elsevier.com/Cooper/foundations/ for additional online resources.

Review Questions for the NCLEX® Examination

1. Acupressure may be most effective with which patient?

   1. A patient who is restless and anxious
   2. A patient in whom ulcerative colitis has been diagnosed
   3. A pregnant patient
   4. A patient with mental health concerns

2. The nurse is preparing a presentation on complementary therapies for a community group. Which statement should be included in the presentation?

   1. Herbal therapies are approved by the US Food and Drug Administration under the Food, Drug, and Cosmetic Act.
   2. Herbal therapies are sold as medicines in most stores because they lack major side effects.
   3. Herbal therapies may be packaged as dietary supplements if they are without health claims.
   4. Herbal therapies are consistent in their standards for concentrations of major ingredients and additives.

3. A patient asks about different herbal therapies that may promote physical endurance and reduce stress. Which herb is used to promote physical endurance and reduces stress?

   1. Ginseng
   2. Ginger
   3. Echinacea
   4. Chamomile

4. When assessing a patient's use of unconventional therapies, the nurse should ask which question?

   1. "What herbal supplements have you taken?"
   2. "Have you ever used relaxation therapy?"
   3. "What types of activities or remedies do you use when you do not feel well?"
   4. "Do you use holistic treatments?"

5. A patient questions the nurse about the use of complementary and alternative medicine. Which statement made by the nurse is correct regarding complementary and alternative medicine?

   1. One-third of the US population uses one or more forms of alternative therapy.
   2. Decreasing amounts of insurance coverage are available to meet the needs of alternative therapies.
   3. Discussion of alternative therapies is still not provided in traditional medical journals.
   4. Integration of alternative therapies is regulated by state and national agencies.

6. A patient receiving chemotherapy is implementing relaxation therapy in conjunction with medical protocol. Which benefit can this patient gain from relaxation therapy?

   1. Decreased receptivity
   2. Decreased peripheral skin temperature
   3. Decreased oxygen consumption
   4. Decreased α-wave brain activity

7. The nurse is preparing to administer medications to a patient taking several herbal preparations. Which factor makes accurate administration of precise dosages of herbs difficult?

   1. The fact that multiple clinical trials are under way
   2. Availability in many different forms
   3. Infrequent usage by consumers
   4. Excessive standardization by international organizations

8. A nurse is educating patients at a health care clinic about the use of herbs as a complementary therapy. Which instruction should be included in education about safe herbal product usage? (Select all that apply.)

   1. "Combine several herbs to maximize the benefits."
   2. "Believe all claims made by the manufacturer."
   3. "Discontinue using herbs if side effects develop."
   4. "Inform your primary care provider of all herbal products you use."
   5. "Drug interactions may exist with antiplatelet medications."

9. Patients at an integrative health care center are learning about various types of complementary health care methods. What is a method of stimulating certain points on the body by the insertion of special needles to modify the perception of pain, normalize physiologic functions, or treat or prevent disease?

   1. Acupressure
   2. Magnet therapy
   3. Acupuncture
   4. Chiropractic therapy

10. A patient has reported to the ambulatory care clinic. During the collection of data, the patient reports using reflexology on a weekly basis. What is a contraindication to the use of reflexology? (Select all that apply.)

    1. Taking chemotherapy for cancer
    2. History of hypertension
    3. Pregnancy
    4. Epilepsy
    5. History of cardiac disease

11. The patient reports a reduction in pain and spasms since taking marijuana daily for her multiple sclerosis. What side effect is the nurse most likely to assess?

    1. Decreased respiratory rate
    2. Increased appetite
    3. Nausea
    4. Rash

12. _____ (fill in the blank) nursing addresses and treats the mind, body, and spirit.

13. Which statement about complementary therapies is most correct?

    1. The patient is actively involved in the treatment.
    2. The patient becomes a total believer in what is being taught.
    3. The patient becomes increasingly submissive to the practitioner.
    4. The patient becomes less competent in his or her own care.

14. A patient is taking the herb comfrey on a daily basis for its wound-healing properties. What information is important for the nurse to tell this patient?

   1. Comfrey should be taken internally.
   2. Comfrey may cause cancer.
   3. Comfrey can be used only externally.
   4. Comfrey is a known antiseptic.

15. When the nurse reviews the patient's medical diagnoses, which condition would be a cause for concern with regard to chiropractic treatments? *(Select all that apply.)*

   1. Acute myelopathy
   2. Vertigo
   3. Osteoporosis
   4. Hypertension
   5. Rheumatoid arthritis

16. The nurse is caring for a patient on the acute care unit. The patient reports that he takes St. John's wort for mild depression. When the nurse reviews the patient's dietary selections, which choice indicates the need for further teaching? *(Select all that apply.)*

   1. Foods high in salt or sodium
   2. Milk products
   3. Anything containing barley, such as beer
   4. Aged cheese
   5. Red wine

17. A female, age 43, recently noted pain in her thighs, buttocks, and lower back, with some pain radiating along the back of the leg. She also has developed stiffness in the mornings. When her pain and stiffness increase to the point that it becomes difficult for her to walk or move around the house on rising two mornings in a row, she makes an appointment with her clinician. During the data collection it is revealed that the patient is largely sedentary and works from home sitting at a desk many hours each day. Her health care provider tells her that her thigh, hip, and back pain are from shortened, tight muscles as a result of sitting long hours at the computer. The care provider recommends ibuprofen OTC as needed for a week and gives her a sheet of stretches. After the provider leaves, the client asks the nurse about the benefits of therapeutic massage for her condition. The nurse describes both benefits and certain risks.

Use a check mark to indicate which potential issues listed in the left column may place the client at risk during therapeutic massage.

POTENTIAL ISSUES	RISK TO CLIENT
Acute back pain	
Thrombosis	
Allergies	
Bruising	
Infection	
Depression	

Pain Management, Comfort, Rest, and Sleep

21

Objectives

1. Define the key terms.
2. List 10 possible causes of discomfort.
3. Discuss McCaffery and Pasero's description of pain.
4. Describe the use of gate control theory to guide selection of nursing interventions for pain relief.
5. Identify subjective and objective data in pain assessment.
6. Discuss the concept of pain assessment as the fifth vital sign.
7. Discuss the synergistic impact of fatigue, sleep disturbance, and depression on the perception of pain.
8. Analyze several scales used to identify intensity of pain.
9. Discuss pain mechanisms affected by each analgesic group.
10. Discuss the role of the nurse in controlling pain.
11. List several methods for pain control.
12. Discuss the differences and similarities between sleep and rest.
13. Outline nursing interventions that promote rest and sleep.
14. Discuss the sleep cycle, differentiating between non–rapid eye movement (NREM) and rapid eye movement (REM) sleep.
15. List six signs and symptoms of sleep deprivation.
16. Identify two nursing diagnoses related to sleep problems.

Key Terms

abuse deterrent (p. 608)
acute pain (ă-KYŪT PĂN, p. 603)
chronic pain (KRŎN-ĭk PĂN, p. 603)
endorphins (ĕn-DŎR-fĭnz, p. 603)
gate control theory (GĂT kŏn-trŏl THĒ-ŏ-rē, p. 603)
non–rapid eye movement (NREM) (NŎN-răp-ĭd Ī MŪV-mĕnt, p. 618)
noxious (NŎK-shŭs, p. 602)

patient-controlled analgesia (PCA) (PĂ-shĕnt kŏn-TRŎLD ăn-ăl-JĒ-zē-ă, p. 610)
rapid eye movement (REM) (RĂP-ĭd Ī MŪV-mĕnt, p. 618)
referred pain (rē-FŬRD PĂN, p. 603)
synergistic (sĭn-ŭr-JĬS-tĭk, p. 603)
transcutaneous electric nerve stimulation (TENS) (trăns-kyū-TĀ-nē-ŭs ē-LĔK-trĭk NŬRV stĭm-ū-LĀ-shŭn, p. 605)
visual analog scale (VĬZH-ū-ăl ĂN-ă-lŏg SKĀL, p. 614)

One of the greatest challenges in nursing is to provide comfort to the patient. To comfort means to give strength and hope, to cheer, and to ease the grief, pain, or trouble of another. Promoting physical and psychological comfort is a vital aspect of nursing care. Many health care providers refer to pain as the fifth vital sign and recommend its assessment and management in much the same manner the traditional vital signs are regarded.

Many factors contribute to a patient's lack of comfort, which manifests in many forms, including the following:

- Anxiety
- Constipation
- Constricting edema
- Depression
- Diaphoresis
- Diarrhea
- Distention
- Dry mouth
- Dyspnea
- Fatigue
- Fear
- Flatus
- Grief
- Headache
- Hopelessness
- Hyperthermia
- Hypothermia
- Hypoxia
- Incontinence
- Muscle cramping
- Nausea
- Pain
- Powerlessness
- Pruritus
- Sadness
- Singultus
- Thirst
- Urinary retention
- Vomiting

Explore the patient's concept of what constitutes comfort. Actively listening to the patient is helpful for planning nursing interventions. Knowing the possible elements of patient discomfort allows for recognition of discomfort signals even when the patient is not able to verbalize, as in the case of a patient who is aphasic or one who is semicomatose. Be diligent in efforts and pursue all the methods to relieve patients' discomfort. If interventions are not successful, seek and apply alternative interventions.

Regardless of age, patients typically receive comfort and a sense of well-being from gentle touch and eye contact (Fig. 21.1).

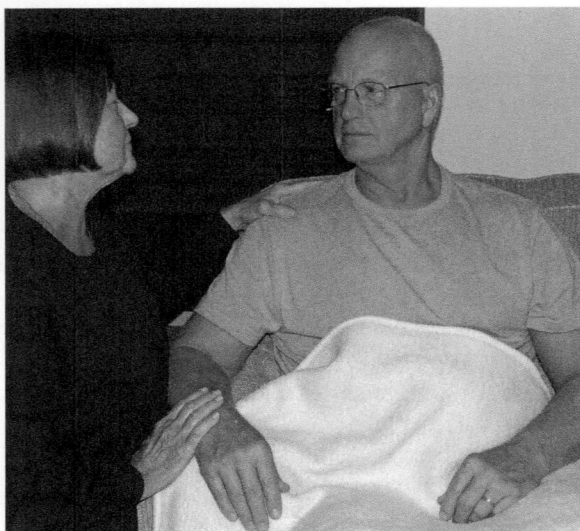

Fig. 21.1 Eye contact and gentle touch promote comfort and well-being.

PAIN

NATURE OF PAIN

Pain is a complex, abstract, personal subjective experience. It is an unpleasant sensation caused by **noxious** (injurious to physical health) stimulation of the sensory nerve endings. Pain serves as a warning to the body: it often occurs with actual or potential tissue damage. Pain is often a cardinal symptom of inflammation and is valuable in the diagnosis of many disorders and conditions. Pain also may occur when there is no tissue damage, such as the emotional pain of grief at the death of a loved one or the pain of migraine headaches. Pain causes fatigue and decreases the patient's ability to cope physically, emotionally, and mentally. Pain has the potential to be totally debilitating and is one of the most common reasons that patients seek out a health care provider.

Pain is subjective; the interpretation and significance of pain depend on an individual's learned experiences and involve psychosocial and cultural factors. The defining characteristic of pain is the verbal or nonverbal communication by the patient of the presence of pain (Box 21.1). McCaffery and Pasero's (2003) description of pain is a practical one: "Pain is whatever the experiencing person says it is, existing whenever he says it does." According to McCaffery and Pasero's description, nurses are obliged to believe every patient who says he or she has pain.

Only the person with pain, and not the health care provider, is the expert about that pain: its onset, duration, location, intensity, quality, and pattern, as well as the degree of pain relief obtained from therapy. Many patients do not recognize that health care providers are not able to tell how much pain the patients are experiencing. Individuals experiencing pain may not know how best to report their pain and its defining characteristics. Help the patient to recognize his or her expertise about the pain and to use that expertise in partnership with health care providers to obtain better pain management. Empowering the patient to be an active partner in reporting information about the pain is an important nursing skill.

DEFINITIONS OF PAIN

The most widely accepted definition of pain, adopted by the International Association for the Study of Pain and the American Pain Society, is as follows: "Pain is an unpleasant sensory and emotional experience associated with actual or potential tissue damage, or described in terms of such damage" (McCaffery and Pasero, 2003). According to this definition, pain is a phenomenon with multiple components that makes an impact on a person's psychosocial and physical functioning. It acknowledges the complexity of the pain experience. Pain is not determined by tissue damage alone. In fact, no predictable relationship exists between identifiable tissue injury and the sensation of pain. The patient's description of pain may be disproportionate to the evidence of tissue damage. In times of high stress and trauma, patients sometimes describe pain as less severe than expected. Patients with chronic nonmalignant pain often describe pain for which little or no tissue damage can be found. Such pain possibly is caused by abnormalities in the neural processing of stimuli. The inability to identify tissue damage sufficient to explain the pain is not proof that the pain is of psychological origin.

TYPES OF PAIN

There are many types of pain: mild and severe; chronic and acute; intermittent and intractable (constant); burning, dull, and sharp; precisely and poorly localized; and referred. **Referred pain** is felt at a site other than the injured or diseased organ or part of the body. An example of referred pain is the pain of coronary artery insufficiency that sometimes is felt in the left shoulder, the left arm, or the jaw.

Acute pain is intense and of short duration, usually lasting less than 6 months. In general, acute pain provides a warning to the individual of actual or potential tissue damage. It creates an autonomic response that originates within the sympathetic nervous system, flooding the body with epinephrine and commonly referred to as the *fight-or-flight response.* Anxiety usually is associated with the pain. Because the pain is of short duration, health care providers are likely to prescribe opioids and other analgesics.

Chronic pain generally is characterized as pain lasting longer than 6 months. Sometimes the pain is continuous and sometimes it is intermittent; at times, it may be as intense as acute pain. Chronic pain does not serve as a warning of tissue damage in process; rather, it signals that such damage has occurred. Chronic pain may be linked to arthritis, back injuries, fibromyalgia, accidents, or neurologic conditions. In some instances, the root cause of the pain may be elusive and unidentifiable. The pain may be the result of an active condition or from damage left to a body structure such as a joint. Because of the prolonged time involved in chronic pain, many patients develop chronic low self-esteem, change in social identity, changes in role and social interaction, fatigue, sleep disturbance, and depression. Sufferers of chronic pain are also more likely to experience comorbid psychiatric conditions.

Fatigue, sleep disturbance, and depression may act in a type of **synergistic** relationship, in which the actions of two or more substances or organs achieve an effect that cannot be achieved by an individual substance or organ. The combination of fatigue, sleep disturbance, and depression has the potential to markedly change a person's perception of pain. Depression is associated with sleep disturbance, which in turn increases the intensity of the fatigue. As the pain continues unmanaged and unchecked, the patient becomes less aware of other events and begins to focus solely on his or her own body and mind. As the focus narrows further, it entraps the individual in a vicious cycle, making the pain difficult to treat. Pain-related disability, such as inability to perform activities of daily living, contributes to low self-esteem and social problems. Depression is common in patients with chronic pain. Results of a study conducted by researchers at the University of Michigan in Ann Arbor suggested a connection between pain and an increased risk for suicide. Pain types linked most heavily to suicide were spinal pain, cancer, and arthritis (Borreli, 2018). These findings have been supported in more recent studies linking suicide and chronic pain. The study findings go further to suggest that chronic pain is a risk factor for suicide (Racine, 2018).

Because of the general differences between acute and chronic pain, some aspects of nursing interventions for these conditions often differ. Keep in mind that the patient's perception of pain, whether acute or chronic, is real, and use appropriate measures to relieve that pain.

THEORIES OF PAIN TRANSMISSION

Gate Control Theory

The **gate control theory** of pain suggests that pain impulses are regulated and even blocked by gating mechanisms located along the central nervous system (CNS). The proposed location of the gates is in the dorsal horn of the spinal cord. Pain and other sensations of the skin and muscles travel the same pathways through the large nerves in the spinal cord. If other cutaneous stimuli besides pain are transmitted, the "gate" through which the pain impulse must travel is blocked temporarily by the stimuli. The brain does not have the capacity to acknowledge the pain while it is interpreting the other stimuli. When gates are open, pain impulses flow freely (Fig. 21.2). When gates are closed, pain impulses become blocked. Partial openings sometimes occur. A bombardment of sensory impulses, such as those from the pressure of a back rub, the heat of a warm compress, or the cold from ice applications, causes the gates to close to painful stimuli. Some patients may be distracted from pain by removing the sensation of pain from their center of attention. Auditory or visual stimuli often distract patients and help make pain more tolerable.

Gating mechanisms also are subject to alteration by thoughts, feelings, and memories. The cerebral cortex and the thalamus have the capacity to influence whether pain impulses reach a person's conscious awareness. There is conscious control over how pain is perceived, and this helps explain the various ways people react and adjust to pain.

Endorphins

The body produces morphine-like substances called **endorphins** (potent polypeptides composed of many amino acids, found in the pituitary gland and other areas of the CNS). Stress and pain activate endorphins. Analgesia results when certain endorphins attach to opioid receptor sites in the brain and prevent the release of neurotransmitters, thereby inhibiting the transmission of pain impulses. People who feel less pain than do others from a similar injury have higher endorphin levels. Pain relief measures, such as transcutaneous electric nerve stimulation (TENS), acupuncture, and placebos, may cause the release of endorphins.

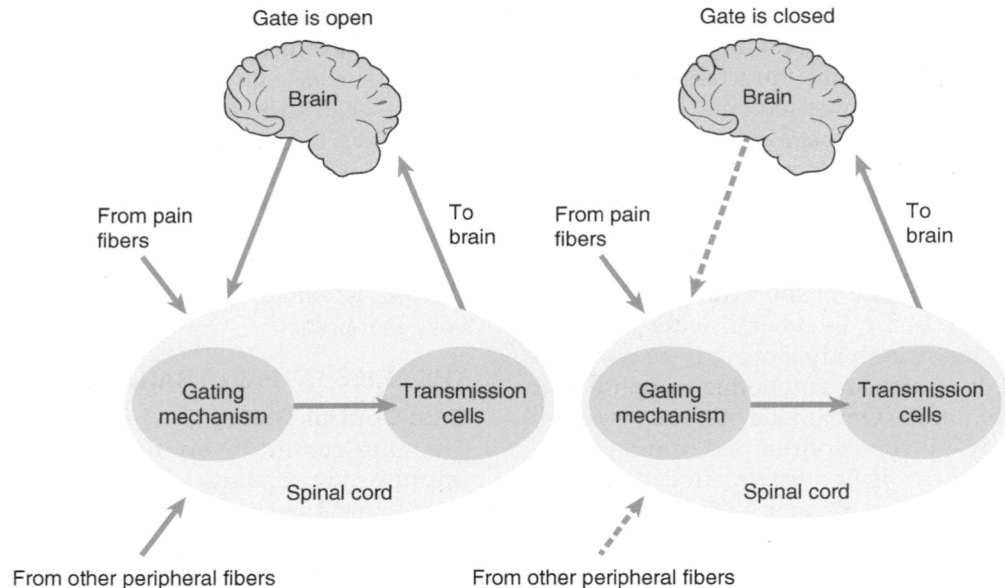

Fig. 21.2 Diagram depicting gate control theory.

CONTROLLING PAIN

Requirements of the Joint Commission for Pain Control

Assessing and managing pain have been primary nursing responsibilities for a long time. In the 1992 standards manual issued by The Joint Commission (TJC) (McCaffery and Pasero, 2003), effective pain management was stated as one of the rights of a dying patient. In 1994 TJC broadened this statement to cover all patients, stating, "The management of pain is appropriate for all patients, not just dying patients" (McCaffery and Pasero, 2003). TJC accreditation visits began to include a focus on what institutions were doing about pain management.

In 1997, under a grant from the Robert Wood Johnson Foundation, TJC began working collaboratively with institutions to create standards for pain assessment and treatment, with plans to conduct national quality improvement programs to help health care facilities meet these standards (McCaffery and Pasero, 2003). TJC now requires accredited facilities and organizations to develop policies and procedures that formalize this obligation (TJC, n.d.).

The Joint Commission standards. Under the new TJC standards, health care providers are expected to be knowledgeable about pain assessment and management, and facilities are expected to develop policies and procedures supporting the appropriate use of analgesics and other pain control therapies. The standards do NOT require or mandate the use of medications to manage the pain. These pain standards require education for practitioners on pain assessment and management; respect to the patient's right to pain management; and assessment and management of the patient's pain.

Making Pain the Fifth Vital Sign

One simple strategy to increase accountability for pain control is for an institution to make pain intensity ratings a routine part of assessment and documentation of vital signs. This makes any presence of pain known and raises awareness of the problem of unmanaged pain. Thanks to the work of pain and palliative care associations, more attention is being paid to pain management, and many institutions have included pain assessment as a vital sign.

Giving pain assessment as much attention as that of other vital signs makes it more likely the pain will be treated properly. Vital signs are monitored to detect changes or trends that signal a need for further assessment, diagnosis, and treatment. Considering pain a vital sign—along with pulse, temperature, blood pressure, and respiration—ensures regular monitoring. Use of a pain rating scale allows patients to articulate their pain clearly and makes them more likely to receive proper treatment.

The essential message about pain assessment is this: ask patients about their pain, accept and respect what they say, intervene to relieve their pain, and ask them again about their pain. It is a circle of assessment, intervention, and reassessment. Without assessment of the patient with pain, none of the pain relief measures are useful. Approximately half the people who suffer moderate to severe pain continue to suffer, primarily because nurses fail to assess pain.

Comparing the pain scale (see discussion of *pain rating scales* later in this chapter) to the thermometer is a helpful way to open a discussion about reporting pain. Explain that just as an elevation in the temperature higher than 100°F (37.8°C) would be reported to the health care provider, so would a pain rating of 4 or

Pain Assessment Guide

Tell Me About Your Pain

How does your pain feel?

aching	throbbing	shooting
stabbing	gnawing	sharp
tender	burning	exhausting
tiring	penetrating	nagging
numb	miserable	unbearable
dull	radiating	squeezing
crampy	deep	pressure

Pain in other languages

Vietnamese	Spanish	French
dau	dolor	douleur

Intensity (0-10)
If 0 is no pain and 10 is the worst pain imaginable, what is your pain now?
... in the last 24 hours?

Location
Where is your pain?

Duration
Is the pain always there?
Does the pain come and go? (Breakthrough Pain)
Do you have both types of pain?

Aggravating and Alleviating Factors
What makes the pain better?
What makes the pain worse?

How does pain affect

sleep	energy	relationships
appetite	activity	mood

Are you experiencing any other symptoms?

nausea/vomiting	itching	urinary retention
constipation	sleepiness/confusion	weakness

Things to check
vital signs, past medication history, knowledge of pain, and use of non-invasive techniques

Fig. 21.3 Pain assessment guide. (Courtesy Great Plains Regional Medical Center, North Platte, NE.)

greater on a scale of 0 to 10. As with temperature, the higher the pain score is, the more concern and urgency are warranted (Fig. 21.3).

Unrelieved pain has harmful physical effects, such as increased oxygen demand, respiratory dysfunction, decreased gastrointestinal motility, confusion, and depressed immune response. Possible emotional consequences of unrelieved pain include anxiety, depression, irritability, and an inability to enjoy life. Neglected pain erodes a patient's trust in the health care system and possibly leads to setbacks and increased costs in treatment. Conversely, appropriate pain management typically results in quicker recoveries, shorter hospital stays, fewer readmissions, and improved quality of life.

Noninvasive Pain Relief Techniques

Pain is controlled most effectively through a combination of noninvasive pain relief measures and pharmacologic therapy. The purpose of noninvasive pain relief techniques, which are sometimes helpful even when used alone, is to decrease the patient's perception of pain and to improve the patient's sense of control. Useful noninvasive approaches include cutaneous stimulation (heat, cold, massage, and TENS), the removal of painful stimuli, distraction, relaxation, guided imagery, meditation, hypnosis, and biofeedback (Table 21.1). In guided imagery, the patient is encouraged to concentrate on an image that helps relieve pain or discomfort. For the best results, help the patient choose a scene that holds especially pleasant memories. Ask the patient where he or she feels the most relaxed, such as at a lake, in a forest, or in a meadow, and then encourage the patient to use sensory memories to make the image as realistic as possible.

Regardless of whether the gate control theory explains why these techniques are successful or whether they work by decreasing anxiety, they undoubtedly have many advantages for pain control. Most are inexpensive and easy to perform, have low risk and few side effects, and frequently do not require an order by the health care provider. The greatest advantage of these techniques is patients' ability to have some control over the treatment of their pain. Having options provides comfort and assurance to the patient. Although not everyone reacts successfully to these pain relief measures, it is worthwhile to attempt any of them before advancing to more invasive techniques.

Transcutaneous electric nerve stimulation. A special pain relief system, transcutaneous electric nerve stimulation (TENS), entails the use of a pocket-sized, battery-operated device that provides a continuous, mild electric current to the skin via electrodes attached to a stimulator by flexible wires (Fig. 21.4). The electric current is adjustable. Like other forms of cutaneous stimulation, TENS is thought to work by stimulating large nerve fibers to "close the gate" in the spinal cord, thus blocking transmission of pain impulses. In addition, TENS is hypothesized to stimulate endorphin production.

TENS is used typically for patients suffering postoperative or chronic pain. It is customary to place the electrodes on or near the painful site. Be alert to the possibility that a TENS unit can interfere with the function of a cardiac pacemaker device.

Invasive Pain Relief Techniques

Invasive means anything that enters the body. Examples of invasive techniques are nerve blocks, epidural analgesics, neurosurgical procedures, and acupuncture. Certain invasive techniques offer relief for many patients with pain. However, careful patient selection and proper technique are essential because the costs and risks are potentially high.

Table 21.1   Nonpharmacologic Interventions for Pain[a]

INTERVENTIONS	COMMENTS
Physical	
Deep tissue massage	Used to reduce muscle tension and spasms. Effective for mild to moderate discomfort. May be of varying intensity.
Exercise	Physical activity can strengthen core muscles and stabilize the spine to aid in the reduction of discomfort.
Transcutaneous electric nerve stimulation (TENS)	Effective in reducing mild to moderate pain by stimulating the skin with mild electric current. Electrodes are placed over or near the site of pain. Requires special equipment.
Heat or cold application	Selection of heat versus cold varies with the type, location of the pain, and duration of the pain. Moist heat relieves stiffness of arthritis and relaxes muscles. Cold applications reduce acute pain associated with inflammation from arthritis or from acute injury.
Flotation therapy	Involves a flotation period in a chamber of water and Epsom salts (magnesium sulfate), which are absorbed through the skin. Benefits included a near zero gravity state achieved with flotation in water. Magnesium sulfate is linked to reduced musculoskeletal pain.
Acupuncture	Involves the insertion of fine, thin needles into the skin. Researchers believe it works by counteracting imbalances in the body's energy flow. This should be undertaken only by a trained professional.
Psychological and Cognitive	
Music	Music can promote relaxation and reduce anxiety. It can be used in the postoperative period to manage chronic pain and in labor and delivery. Studies have shown that postoperative pain may be reduced by 50% using music.
Biofeedback	Reduces mild to moderate pain and operative site muscle tension. Requires patient to have high level of cognitive function. Requires skilled personnel and special equipment.
Imagery	Reduces mild to moderate pain. The patient is encouraged to focus internally on positive memories or environments. Some patients may require assistance to relax and focus on attention away from the pain.
Humor	Reduces mild to moderate pain. Humor and laughter increase oxygenation and circulation. Rest and sleep also can be improved in the periods after laughter.
Education	Effective for reduction of all types of pain. Should include sensory and procedural information and instruction aimed at reducing activity-related pain.

[a]Should be used with analgesic medication.

Medication for Pain Management

Analgesics often provide effective pain relief. Members of the health care team frequently have misconceptions about the dangers and effects of analgesics. Undertreatment of pain and administration of analgesics in amounts less than what are prescribed may occur because of misunderstandings or insufficient knowledge of pharmacologic principles, concerns about addiction, and anxiety over administering too large a dose of an opioid analgesic. Because of such uncertainties, the patient's pain is only reduced, not relieved. Make sure you understand the medications available for pain relief and their effects.

Nonopioid analgesics. Acetaminophen and nonsteroidal antiinflammatory drugs (NSAIDs)—the nonopioid analgesics—are the most widely available and frequently used analgesic group. Acetaminophen may block pain impulses peripherally that occur in response to inhibition of prostaglandin synthesis, primarily in the CNS.

Nonopioid analgesics are used primarily for mild to moderate pain but sometimes also are used to relieve certain types of severe pain. Some NSAIDs are available without a prescription, such as aspirin, ibuprofen (Advil, Nuprin, Motrin), and naproxen sodium (Aleve). Aspirin blocks pain impulses in the CNS and reduces inflammation.

The maximum recommended dosage of acetaminophen is 4000 mg (4 g) in 24 hours. Its toxic side effect, a basic consideration in all analgesic regimens, is hepatotoxicity. Patient responses to NSAIDs vary, so if one is ineffective, try another. Their mechanisms of action appear to be different enough to warrant changing NSAIDs until the best one for the patient is identified. All NSAIDs pose the risk of gastrointestinal bleeding.

Opioid analgesics. Opioids such as morphine, meperidine (Demerol), hydromorphone (Dilaudid), and fentanyl (Actiq, Duragesic) act on higher centers of the brain to modify perception and reaction to pain. Opioids decrease the perception of pain by binding to pain receptor sites in the CNS.

TENS Electrode Placement

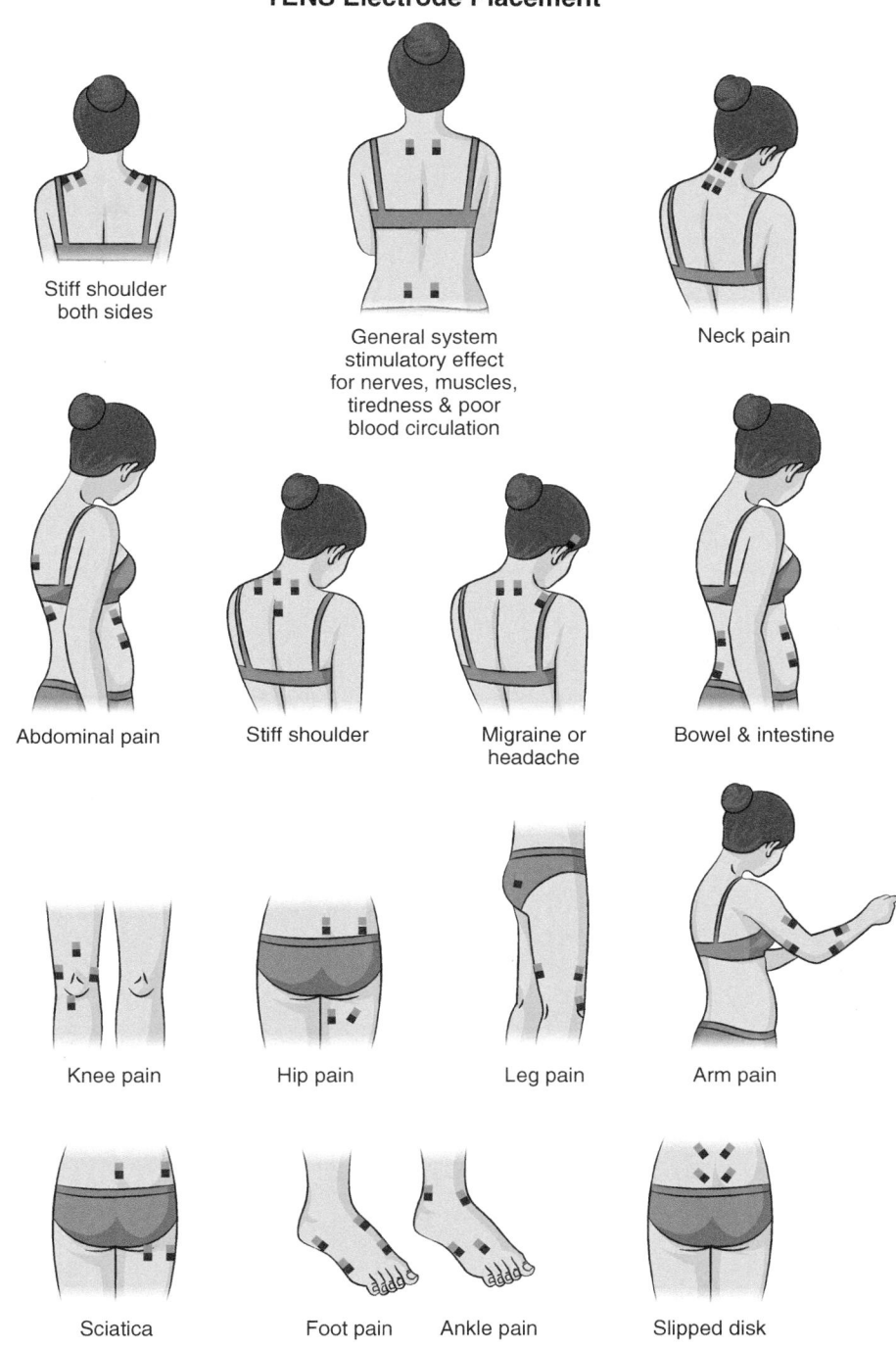

Stiff shoulder both sides

General system stimulatory effect for nerves, muscles, tiredness & poor blood circulation

Neck pain

Abdominal pain

Stiff shoulder

Migraine or headache

Bowel & intestine

Knee pain

Hip pain

Leg pain

Arm pain

Sciatica

Foot pain

Ankle pain

Slipped disk

Fig. 21.4 Transcutaneous electric nerve stimulation (TENS).

Opioid analgesics are the cornerstone for managing moderate to severe acute pain. Morphine is the standard agent in opioid therapy, but other opiates, such as hydromorphone, levorphanol, oxycodone, and fentanyl, are ordered as substitutes if the patient has an unusual reaction or allergy to morphine. Morphine is a highly effective drug; however, its use in the presence of compromised renal function must be monitored carefully.

The danger of morphine and other opioid analgesics is their potential to cause depression of vital nervous system functions. Of most significance is that opiates cause respiratory depression by depressing the respiratory center within the brainstem. The rate and regularity of respirations diminish under the influence of opiates. Instances of clinically significant or death-inducing scenarios when opiates are administered are less than 1%. However, opiate use in the unmonitored drug-addicted population is associated with less favorable outcomes. Not all opiates have the same degree of respiratory impact. In addition, the route of administration affects the influences on the respiratory system. Administering opiates via epidural or through intravenous (IV) patient-controlled analgesia (PCA, explained later in this chapter) has been shown to have fewer issues with respiratory depression. Opiates are associated with changes in sleep patterns. More time is spent in rapid eye movement (REM) sleep than in the deep sleep stage. This warrants further study to identify additional information concerning this potential complication. Predicting the potential for respiratory complications is not always possible, but a review of a patient's health history may provide insight.

Opiates may be short acting (lasting 3 to 6 hours), long acting (lasting at least 8 hours), or extended release (providing 24-hour pain relief). Short-acting medications are used best for the management of acute or breakthrough pain. Long-acting opiates traditionally are used on chronic pain.

Because of its potential for inducing seizures, meperidine (Demerol) is no longer the drug of choice for pain management. The active metabolite in meperidine, normeperidine, is a CNS stimulant and sometimes produces irritability, tremors, muscle twitching, jerking, agitation, and seizures. Because normeperidine is eliminated by the kidneys, it should not be given to patients with decreased renal function. It is a particularly poor choice in older adults and in patients with sickle cell disease because most such patients have some degree of renal insufficiency. Repeated administration increases the risk of accumulation of normeperidine, so meperidine generally is not prescribed for patients who require long-term opioid treatment, such as those with cancer or chronic nonmalignant pain. The effects of normeperidine have been observed even in young, otherwise healthy patients given sufficiently high doses of meperidine postoperatively.

Meperidine administration is contraindicated in patients receiving monoamine oxidase inhibitors and in patients with untreated hypothyroidism, Addison disease, benign prostatic hypertrophy, or urethral stricture. Meperidine is more likely than other opioid drugs to cause delirium in postoperative patients of all ages, especially if given epidurally or intravenously. The logic of using meperidine for any type of pain management, by any route of administration, is questionable. There are opioid choices that are clearly safer (see the Lifespan Considerations box on pain control in older adults).

Tolerance and addiction. In response to the rising incidence of opioid addiction the FDA is encouraging the development of analgesics that are "**abuse deterrent.**" These medications have properties that allow the management of pain but also have properties that limit their use for abusive purposes. Examples include formulations that limit the ability to crush the tablets for snorting or dissolving for injecting which are common routes of usage for addicts. It is important to recognize that these measures do not make misuse

and addiction impossible as it is still possible to take the drugs by swallowing. Examples of abuse deterrent narcotics include OxyContin, MorphaBondER, RoxyBond, Hysingla ER, and Xtampza ER. At the time of this publication there are no FDA approved generic medications identified as abuse deterrent (FDA, 2021).

Opioid tolerance and physiologic dependence are unusual with short-term postoperative use, and psychological dependence and addiction are extremely unlikely after a course of opiates for acute pain. Studies conducted over 20 years have shown uniformly that the likelihood that addiction will occur as a result of taking opioids for pain relief, even over a long period, is rare: probably less than 1%. Often the term *addiction* is applied inappropriately to a patient, and the label becomes a barrier to pain relief for that person.

Lifespan Considerations

Older Adults

Pain Control

- The effects of aging on the pain process sometimes are compounded in an older adult who has a chronic illness that affects the nervous system.
- Older adults who are well instructed in use of pain measurement tools and without diseases affecting the nervous system tend to report pain intensity similar to that reported by younger persons.
- The risk for gastric and renal toxicity from NSAIDs is increased in older adults.
- In older adults, changes in peripheral vascular function and skin, as well as decreased transmission of pain impulses, increase the risk for being unable to sense pain.
- Older age is associated with chronic health problems, increased risk for musculoskeletal pain, depression, and limitations in activities of daily living.
- Increased pain intensity has been noted in older individuals, particularly when adequate treatment is not provided for chronic and recurrent pain.
- Treatment of pain in older adults is as likely to be successful as that in younger persons.
- Because many older adults have some degree of renal insufficiency, meperidine (Demerol) is a particularly poor choice for pain control for such patients.
- Older adults sometimes become susceptible to side effects of opioids because of changes in serum proteins, liver and renal function, and a reduction in cardiac output.

Many patients will exhibit signs of physical tolerance and physical dependence after 1 to 4 weeks of regular opioid therapy. These effects are not abnormal. They should not be confused with addiction.

A helpful rule is that relief of severe pain requires a greater amount of analgesic; remembering this helps overcome any fear of overtreating patients' pain. Dosages at the upper end of normally prescribed ranges are usually safe. Administering a low dose that proves to be ineffective causes the patient to suffer until the required time interval has passed for another dose to be given.

Preventing and managing opioid-induced constipation. Opioids often delay gastric emptying, slow bowel motility, and decrease peristalsis. They also tend to reduce secretions from the colonic mucosa. The result is slow-moving, hard stool that is difficult to pass. At its worst, gastrointestinal dysfunction can result in ileus, fecal impaction, and obstruction.

Constipation is the most common side effect of opioids and the only one for which individuals do not develop tolerance. Thus it necessitates a preventive approach, regular assessment, and aggressive management. Factors contributing to constipation in patients who take opioids include advanced age, immobility, abdominal disease, and concurrent medications that also may have constipating side effects. Patients prescribed opioid analgesics also may be prescribed a stool softener with a mild peristaltic stimulant.

Instruct the patient in proper diet, fluids, and exercise, and provide for the patient's privacy and convenience. Keep in mind, however, that these aspects of bowel management are important but usually insufficient on their own to prevent opioid-induced constipation. Bulk laxatives, natural roughage, and large amounts of fluid are sometimes unpalatable and ineffective. In addition, if fluid intake is inadequate, bulk laxatives, such as psyllium (Metamucil), sometimes cause fecal impaction and obstruction. Stool softeners alone are inadequate.

Pain mechanisms affected by each analgesic group. It is useful and clinically relevant to distinguish among analgesics that relieve pain by different mechanisms. Because different analgesics relieve pain in different ways, it is sometimes logical to combine analgesics from different groups to relieve one specific type of pain or to relieve different types of pain occurring in the same patient.

Following is a brief description of selected mechanisms of action thought to be unique to each analgesic group.

- *Nonopioids* (acetylsalicylic acid [aspirin], acetaminophen, and NSAIDs). The analgesia produced by acetaminophen (Tylenol) appears to be related to the inhibition of prostaglandins that may serve as mediators of pain and fever, primarily in the CNS, but they also may block pain impulses peripherally. Aspirin blocks pain impulses in the CNS and reduces inflammation by inhibition of prostaglandin synthesis. NSAIDs such as tramadol (Ultram), ibuprofen (Motrin), naproxen (Aleve), ketorolac tromethamine (Toradol), and celecoxib (Celebrex) also work in the CNS, but their better characterized actions are peripheral (at the site of injury), where they are thought to exert analgesic effects through the inhibition of prostaglandin production. Prostaglandin is an inflammatory mediator, released when cells are damaged, that sensitizes nerves that carry information about pain. By inhibiting prostaglandin release, these drugs diminish transmission of pain stimuli.

- *Opioids.* Opioids relieve pain mainly by action in the CNS, binding to opioid receptor sites in the brain and the spinal cord. There are multiple opioid receptor sites. When a drug binds to any of these sites, pain relief occurs. When a drug attaches to these opioid receptor sites as an antagonist, pain relief and other effects are blocked. A well-known opioid antagonist is naloxone (Narcan), which antagonizes (blocks or reverses) the action of all opioids.

- *Adjuvant analgesics.* It is not possible to identify any one mechanism of action for pain relief for this analgesic group. This group is composed of diverse classes of drugs that relieve pain by a variety of mechanisms, many of which are not understood. For example, certain antidepressants appear to relieve pain by blocking the reuptake of serotonin, which results in the presence of greater amounts of serotonin. Orally formulated local anesthetics such as mexiletine (Mexitil) and certain anticonvulsants such as carbamazepine (Tegretol) are sodium channel–blocking agents, and this is perhaps part of the mechanism underlying their ability to relieve certain types of pain. Neuropathic pain is difficult to treat. Gabapentin (Neurontin), an anticonvulsant, binds to the neocortex and is used in the treatment of chronic neuropathic pain. Duloxetine (Cymbalta), an antidepressant, is used for control of the pain associated with diabetic neuropathy, as is pregabalin (Lyrica), an anticonvulsant.

Administration routes for analgesics. Learn the most effective analgesic and means of administration for the patient's specific need. It takes skill to determine the most effective method of administration.

The IV route is best for administration of opioid analgesics after major surgery. This route provides a rapid onset of pain relief and best manages escalating pain. The most appropriate opioids for pain relief for rapidly escalating, severe pain include morphine, hydromorphone, and fentanyl. For rapid onset of analgesia to treat escalating pain, these drugs should be administered via the IV route. They are suitable for bolus administration and continuous infusion, including PCA. The ability to obtain a dose when it is needed places the patient in control and eliminates the wait for medication administration.

Intramuscular (IM) administration of opioids is associated with wide fluctuations in absorption, including delayed absorption in postoperative patients making it an ineffective and potentially dangerous method of managing pain. Repeated IM injections are often painful and traumatic, which may deter patients from requesting medications for relief of pain; they also have the potential to cause fibrosis of muscle and soft tissue, as well as sterile abscesses. The use of alternative routes of analgesic administration provide opportunities. The use of IM routes should generally be avoided.

The oral route is often the optimal route, especially for chronic pain treatment, because of its convenience, its flexibility, and the relatively steady blood levels produced. However, the IV route is usually necessary when a quick onset of analgesia is desired or when the patient is unable to take oral medication. When the pain is under control, the regimen then may be changed to oral administration of the analgesic. Oral administration is convenient and inexpensive. Its use is appropriate as soon as the patient can tolerate oral intake and is the mainstay of pain management for ambulatory surgical patients.

Patient-controlled analgesia. A drug delivery system called **patient-controlled analgesia (PCA)** allows patients to self-administer analgesics whenever needed. The PCA device is a portable, computerized pump with a chamber for a syringe (Fig. 21.5). The pump delivers a small, preset dose of IV medication, usually morphine, meperidine, hydromorphone, or fentanyl. To receive a dose, the patient pushes a button on a cord attached to the pump. A timer prevents the system from delivering more than a specified number of doses every hour, to prevent overdose. Each dose may be as low as 1 mL or 1 mg of morphine every 6 to 12 minutes. It has a locked safety system that prevents tampering.

PCA is based on the idea that only the patient can feel the pain and only the patient knows how much analgesic will relieve it. By allowing patients to determine the need for doses, PCA addresses the significant variations in analgesic requirements between individuals.

Analgesia is more effective when the patient, rather than the nurse or the health care provider, is in control. PCA is similar to responsive prn dosing in that it requires patients to recognize that they are experiencing pain and to request analgesia (e.g., by pressing a button on a pump to deliver a PCA bolus). The difference between prn administration and PCA is that with PCA, the patient rather than a nurse administers the analgesic. Delays waiting for a nurse to administer analgesics are eliminated. It is important to reinforce with the patient that "staying on top of the pain" is key to achieving pain relief and preventing pain from reaching elevated levels that are difficult to control.

PCA has been used to manage all types of acute pain, although less often for cancer pain because most cancer pain is manageable with orally administered opioids. To be a candidate for PCA, a patient must be alert, oriented, and able to follow simple directions. Patient preparation and teaching are critical in the safe and effective use of PCA (see the Patient Teaching box).

Fig. 21.5 Patient-controlled analgesia (PCA) pump with syringe chamber. (Courtesy Smiths Medical ASD, Inc., St. Paul, MN.)

👥 Patient Teaching

Preparation for Patient-Controlled Analgesia

- Teach the use of patient-controlled analgesia (PCA) before surgery so that patients will know how to use it after awakening from anesthesia. (Confused and unresponsive patients, patients with neurologic disease, patients with impaired renal or pulmonary function, and those unable to press the delivery button are not candidates for PCA.)
- Instruct patients on the purpose of PCA, operating instructions, lockout intervals, expected pain relief, precautions, and potential side effects, emphasizing that the patient controls medication delivery.
- Explain that the pump prevents overdose.
- Tell family members and friends not to operate the PCA device for the patient.
- Ask the patient to demonstrate use of the PCA delivery button.

Older adult patients and those with respiratory compromise or hypovolemia are typically at high risk for respiratory complications with IV opioids of any type. They and patients with significant impairment of renal or hepatic function probably will be determined unsuitable candidates to use PCA.

If someone other than the patient pushes the button on a PCA pump, even at the patient's request, it is termed *PCA by proxy*. Proxy administration of opioids leads to possible oversedation and opioid toxicity. PCA is for patient use only, and nurses, other patients, and visitors must be reminded not to push the button.

Although patients with pain often self-administer their oral analgesics, the term *patient-controlled analgesia* is applied usually when opioids are administered by the IV and epidural routes. Typically, a special infusion pump is used to deliver PCA by these routes. In this context, PCA refers to the bolus dose that the patient controls when pressing a button on or attached to the pump. PCA is delivered by one of two modes: PCA bolus doses with a continuous infusion (also called a *basal rate*) or PCA bolus doses alone.

When caring for the patient who uses the PCA delivery system, assess the IV site and the PCA device for proper functioning and correct drug dosing. Closely monitor vital signs for signs of respiratory depression. Evaluate the patient's level of orientation for signs of oversedation. Record the amount of medication being used every shift or per agency policy.

Epidural analgesia. Another method of delivery of analgesia is the insertion of an epidural catheter and the infusion of opiates into the epidural space. Containing blood vessels, fat, and nerves, the epidural space is a "potential" space (there is no free-flowing fluid in it) between the walls of the vertebral canal and the dura mater of the spinal cord. It surrounds the spinal meninges and extends from the foramen magnum to the sacral hiatus. The epidural medication diffuses slowly from the epidural space across the dura and arachnoid membranes into the cerebrospinal fluid (Fig. 21.6). Epidural administration of opioids brings the drug close to the action site (opioid receptors); therefore, in comparison with systemic administration, relatively small doses are effective. Because of the vasculature

in the epidural space, the drug also is absorbed systemically. There are three methods of administering epidural analgesia: by bolus doses, by continuous infusion, and by patient-controlled epidural analgesia.

The epidural route of administration is an appropriate first-line route for moderate to severe acute pain expected to last for at least 24 hours. The pain relief and improvement in functional outcomes after major surgery are superior in patients who receive epidural analgesia in comparison with patients who receive traditional postoperative pain management therapies administered by IV push or intramuscularly. Epidural medications have a rapid onset: relief is experienced within 15 minutes. Drugs used for epidural analgesia are morphine, fentanyl, and hydromorphone. The epidural opioids have side effects, including urinary retention, postural hypotension, pruritus, nausea, vomiting, and respiratory depression. Epidural analgesia is beneficial for controlling acute pain during labor and for relieving chronic pain, such as that seen in patients with advanced cancer (Box 21.2).

The insertion and maintenance of the epidural catheter for the infusion are invasive techniques that are the responsibility of the anesthetist or the anesthesiologist. Nursing staff members are responsible for monitoring the patient's level of consciousness, pain intensity, respiratory rate, and the infusion rate and volume on the pump. Monitor respiratory rate, pulse, blood pressure, and oxygen saturation levels every 15 minutes during infusion. Because hypotension may occur, an IV infusion is initiated before the administration of the epidural medications. Examine the dressing site for signs of infection or leakage of medication around the catheter (Table 21.2).

There are complications associated with epidural therapies. These complications include infection, bleeding at the site, nerve damage, and seizures. Less frequently, respiratory complications may result.

Elastomeric Pumps

Elastomeric pumps or "pain balls" are used to administer local anesthetic medications (Fig. 21.7). The medication, located inside of a ball, is administered through a small catheter that has been placed beneath the skin during a surgical procedure. The medication is intended as a supplement to the regularly prescribed narcotic postoperative pain medications. Dosages of the medication may be set to provide a continuous administration, or it may allow for patient-necessitated adjustments to the dosage or even allow demand bolus administrations in the event of breakthrough pain. As the medication is dispensed, the ball gradually begins to soften and eventually appears "collapsed" or smaller. The longevity of a device varies by the size of the device employed and the dosage prescribed. The average time for a single pump to be in use is 2 to 5 days. When a device is empty, it is removed easily by the patient or a caregiver in the home. The device is small

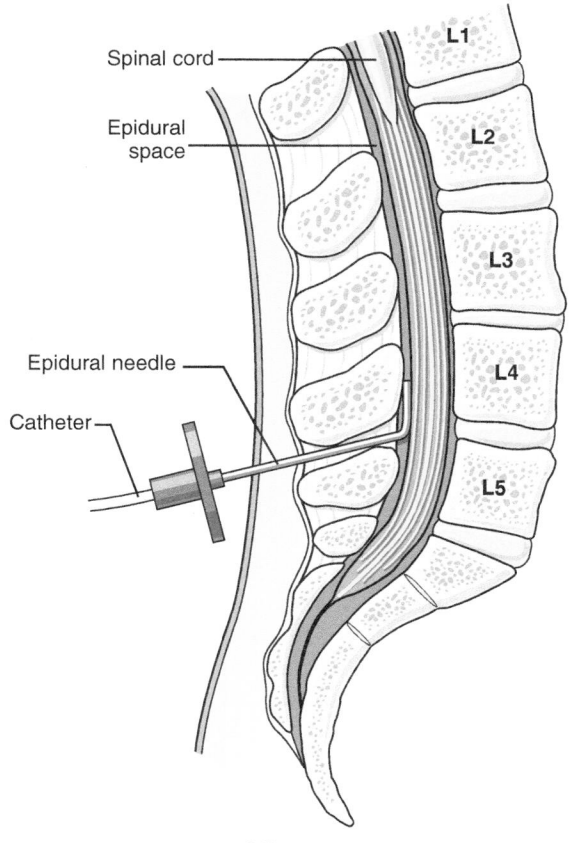

Spinal cord

Epidural space

Epidural needle

Catheter

L1

L2

L3

L4

L5

© Elsevier

Fig. 21.6 Epidural catheter placement.

Box 21.2 | **Nursing Principles for Administering Analgesics**

KNOW THE PATIENT'S PREVIOUS RESPONSE TO ANALGESICS
- Assess past history of analgesic use. Include the patient's success with the medications.
- Determine what medications have been used in the past and their degree of effectiveness.
- Determine whether the patient has allergies.

SELECT PROPER MEDICATIONS WHEN MORE THAN ONE IS ORDERED
- Use NSAIDs or milder opioids for mild to moderate pain.
- The concurrent use of opioids and NSAIDs often provides far more effective analgesia than use of an agent from either drug class alone.
- Use of NSAIDs can help reduce opioid side effects.
- In older adults, avoid combinations of opioids.
- Remember that morphine and hydromorphone are the opioids of choice for long-term management of severe pain.
- Know that injectable medications act more quickly, often relieving severe, acute pain within 1 hour, and that oral medication sometimes takes as long as 2 hours to take effect.
- For longer, more sustained relief in connection with chronic pain, give an oral drug.

KNOW THE OPTIMAL DOSAGE
- Remember that doses at the upper end of normal generally are needed for severe pain.
- Ask patient to rate pain before analgesic administration and after to determine level of effectiveness.
- Consult with members of the health care team about dosage adjustments.

DETERMINE THE RIGHT TIME AND INTERVAL FOR ADMINISTRATION
- Use an appropriate pain scale for more accurate pain assessment.
- Administer analgesics as soon as pain occurs and before it increases in severity.
- Premedicate patient if interventions or activities are planned that may cause increased discomfort.
- Do not give analgesics only on as-needed schedules. An around-the-clock administration schedule is best.
- Know the average duration of action for a drug, and time the administration so that the peak effect occurs when the pain is most intense.

CHOOSE THE RIGHT ROUTE
- Intravenous and oral routes are preferred.
- Intramuscular and subcutaneous administrations are best avoided because these routes are frequently painful and absorption is not reliable. Intramuscular injections have the potential to cause fibrosis of muscle and soft tissue and sterile abscesses.

NSAIDs, Nonsteroidal antiinflammatory drugs.

Table 21.2 | **Nursing Care for Patients With Epidural Infusions**

- Assess dressing.
- Assess catheter. Ensure the catheter remains unkinked and in place.
- Change dressing per agency policy.
- Monitor intake and output.
- Monitor vital signs and pulse oximetry.
- Monitor bowel and bladder habits.
- Assess for side effects of administration including pruritus, nausea, and vomiting. Administer medications as prescribed to manage side effects.

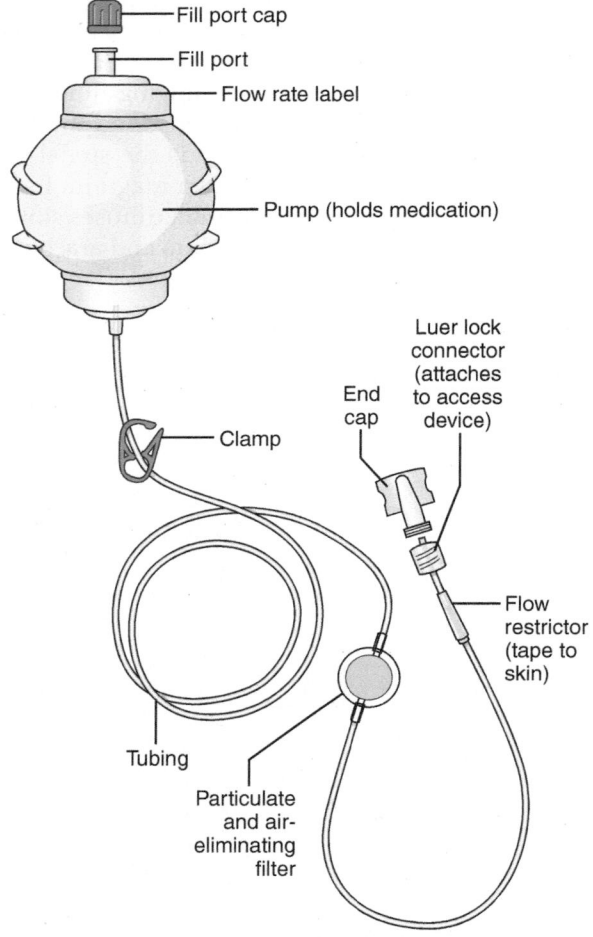

Fig. 21.7 Elastomeric pump.

Responsibility of the Nurse in Pain Control

The founding principle of effective pain management is Meinhart and McCaffery's statement that "the failure to treat pain is inhumane and constitutes professional negligence" (Meinhart and McCaffery, 1983). Every patient has the right to be free of pain; it is the nurse's responsibility to do everything possible to alleviate the patient's pain.

Assist the patient in pain relief by telling the patient, "I believe that you are in pain, and I will assist you in whatever way I can to reduce or relieve your

---

and portable and can be secured to clothing. Patients using the pumps may demonstrate a reduced intake of narcotic analgesics. If smaller doses of narcotics are used, their related side effects such as nausea, vomiting, and constipation also may be lessened.

pain." This reduces the patient's anxiety level. Patients should not be expected to convince the health care team that the pain experienced is real. Pain management interventions begin as soon as the patient states that she or he is in pain.

Encourage the patient to be an active participant in the plan of care. It is important for the patient to report pain promptly as it occurs. Teach the patient not to wait until the pain is intolerable to seek medications. Assess for nonverbal expressions of pain. If any pain-producing procedure or activity is scheduled, such as ambulating, coughing, or a dressing change, give an analgesic beforehand. Administer the medications to achieve the peak effect during the patient's most active time.

Pain control requires nurses to have a strong advocacy role. Nurses must clarify concerns, answer questions, and supply information needed by the patient. Collaboration with the health care provider is needed to ensure that the appropriate analgesics are being used. Effective patient advocacy requires time, patience, and courage. Good listening skills are essential. Ask the patient how he or she is feeling, and attentively wait to hear the answer.

The ultimate goal of pain management is to provide pain relief and enable the patient to carry on with activities of daily living in as comfortable a manner as possible. If pain is to be prevented or managed well, all members of the health care team caring for the patient must understand the pain management plan. Assessment of the patient's pain is ongoing and is documented with each assessment and reassessment. There is increasing emphasis on combining psychosocial and drug approaches in the pain treatment plan (see the Home Care Considerations box).

🏠 Home Care Considerations

Pain Management in the Home

- In current practice, nurses recognize the need to include the patient and family in planning and implementing effective pain management strategies.
- With so much care being given in clinics, physicians' offices, and patients' homes rather than in hospitals, the need for patients and families to be well informed has become even more important.
- Explain the pain management program that is likely to be used in the patient's home.
- Discuss and have the patient practice pain management techniques to use in the home.
- Home health care and hospice patients are assessed for pain at every visit. Instruct patients to notify a home health or hospice nurse at any time of unrelieved pain.

Pain management is a challenge that every nurse must face, regardless of the practice setting. In fact, the nurse's role in pain management is probably more important than that of any other member of the health care team (Nursing Care Plan 21.1).

Nursing Assessment of Pain

Collection of subjective data. Because pain is a subjective experience, you must become a well-versed and competent practitioner of the art of pain assessment. Obtaining accurate information from the patient concerning the pain, including characteristics and description of the pain, is critical. Characteristics worth noting include the site, the severity, the duration, and the location of pain. When documenting the presence of pain, describe the specific location and intensity. Charting "patient complains of pain" provides no useful information. Ask the patient what relieves the pain, what actions cause the pain to be worse, and what does not relieve the pain. Sociocultural information is beneficial. Identify normal coping mechanisms used by the patient and close family members. Determine how the pain is interpreted by those close to the patient (see the Cultural Considerations box). If medications are taken for relief of pain, the name, the dosage, the frequency, and the effect of the drugs must be determined.

Cultural Considerations

Pain Management

- The primary strategy for working with a patient in pain who is from a different culture is to establish a relationship by listening, showing respect, and allowing the patient to help develop and choose treatment options.
- To further increase cultural sensitivity, cultivate rapport with the patient and family, maintain an open attitude, and remain flexible.
- Understanding cultural background and personal characteristics aids in the accuracy of the pain assessment and its meaning to the patient.
- It may be difficult to understand some non-Western pain remedies, so it is important that the patient feels free to ask for what is needed.
- Respect the patient's attitudes and beliefs about pain, as well as preferred treatment options, even if these conflict with your personal beliefs about pain treatment.
- During the assessment process, explore how the patient feels about combining therapies so that the patient is made familiar with a range of pain treatment options.
- Traditional Latino men believe that men are supposed to endure pain without complaining and that alleviating it would be "unmanly" and demeaning in the eyes of their children.
- Chinese people may avoid eye contact, making pain assessment more difficult.
- Italian, Jewish, African American, and Spanish-speaking people often smile readily and use facial expressions and gestures to communicate pain or displeasure.
- Irish, English, and northern European people tend to show fewer facial expressions and are less responsive, especially to strangers such as professional caregivers.

Data collection is dictated largely by the patient's condition. If the patient is critically ill or in excruciating pain, limit questions to key items needed to proceed with the plan of care.

Nursing Care Plan 21.1 | **The Patient With Chronic Pain**

The nurse is caring for Mr. J., a 45-year-old male patient with a 15-year history of severe, crippling rheumatoid arthritis. He has had numerous joint replacements, has lost 40 lb (18.18 kg) in the past year, and has developed corneal ulcers from the presence of Sjögren syndrome. He is in constant chronic pain and has limited mobility. He states that he has difficulty accomplishing activities of daily living (ADLs).

PATIENT PROBLEM

Prolonged Pain, related to joint and muscle inflammation and degeneration manifested by complaints of pain, anorexia, narrow focus of interest, fatigue, guarded movement, changes in sleep pattern, and social withdrawal

Patient Goals and Expected Outcomes	Nursing Interventions	Evaluation
Patient or family (or both) will verbalize a reduction in anxiety and pain when using relaxation, massage, cutaneous stimulation, and analgesics within 1 h after initiation of pain relief measures	Encourage patient to report pain or discomfort location, intensity, and duration with the use of the pain scale. Teach relaxation exercises. Perform massage to relieve pain and to enhance communication. Administer analgesics and apply cold or heat applications as ordered. Maintain transcutaneous electric nerve stimulation (TENS) as ordered. Encourage relaxation by teaching use of guided imagery.	Patient indicates improved pain relief within 1 h of implementation of pain management techniques. Patient reports pain level reduced to 4 on a scale of 0–10.

PATIENT PROBLEM

Prolonged Low Self-Esteem, related to inability to work, carry out ADLs, and with body image changes, manifested by preoccupation with body changes, verbalization of powerlessness, expressions of guilt, and self-negating verbalizations

Patient Goals and Expected Outcomes	Nursing Interventions	Evaluation
Patient will verbalize understanding of changes in body image caused by disease process and will begin to exhibit increased confidence in dealing with self-esteem within 1 week	Encourage verbalization about fears and anxiety; listen attentively. Deal with behavioral changes, denial, powerlessness, anxiety, and dependence. Be supportive in setting goals. Encourage independence, and give praise for tasks accomplished. Modify environment, and allow time for patient to accomplish goals.	Patient states improved feeling of self-esteem within 1 week of implementation of techniques outlined.

CRITICAL THINKING QUESTIONS

1. During the morning ADLs, Mr. J. states, "I feel so useless. I can't even place the urinal for myself." What would be the nurse's most therapeutic response?
2. What would be the most useful nursing intervention to achieve the goal of reduced pain during Mr. J.'s assisted ambulation?
3. Which comfort measures could the nurse perform to ensure that the patient has several hours of restorative sleep?
4. Mr. J. complains of his eyes burning and feeling dry and the lights annoying him. What measures are most likely to help relieve his symptoms?

Try to have patients use their own words to describe the pain because the terms they use often provide clues about the cause of the pain. For example, patients who experience chest pain during a myocardial infarction frequently describe the pain as a pressure or as if someone were squeezing the chest.

Several studies have been focused on the development of tools to assess the patient's pain perception specifically. Pain is a subjective experience, and nurses face difficulty when attempting to measure and evaluate this experience for the patient. Pain rating scales aid with this assessment.

Pain rating scales. Visual analog scales and numeric scales are used commonly to qualify the intensity of the pain experience (Fig. 21.8).

With the visual analog scale, the patient marks a spot on a horizontal line to indicate pain intensity (intensity increases as the line moves from left to right). The most frequently used numeric scale is 0 to 10; the patient chooses the pain rating, with 0 being no pain and 10 being the worst pain imaginable. A visual scale with numeric ratings combines both, providing a description and facial expressions with assigned numbers from 0 to 10 (see Fig. 30.8). For clinical assessment, any of these scales is adequate and appropriate. The same scale always must be used with the same patient. All personnel in a given health care setting also must use the same scale.

A good pain scale is easy to use and not time consuming. If a patient can read and understand a scale

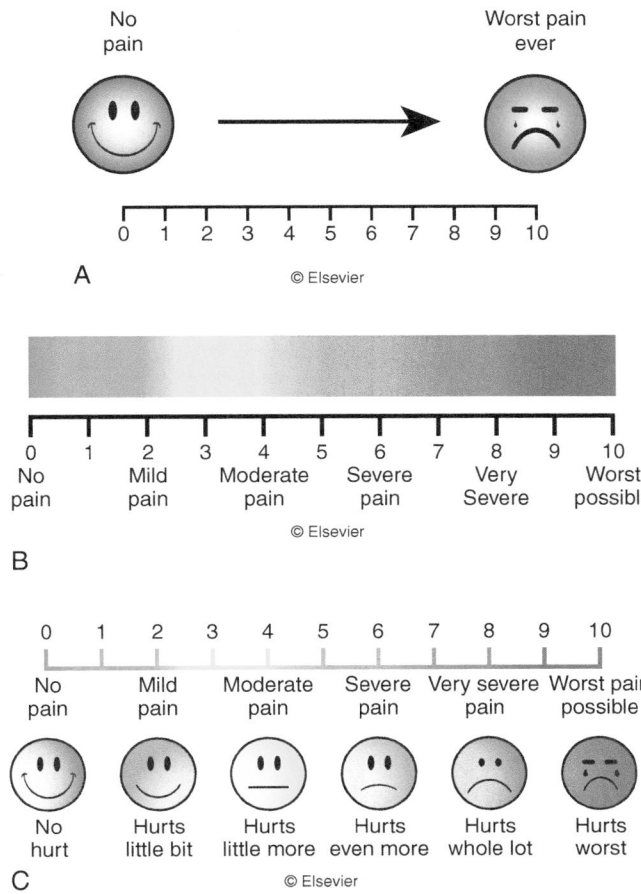

Fig. 21.8 Sample pain scales. (A) Visual analog. (B) Numeric. (C) Verbal descriptive.

Box 21.3 Objective Signs of Pain

PHYSIOLOGIC SIGNS

- *Pulse:* Increased rate
- *Respirations:* Increased depth and frequency
- *Blood pressure:* Increased systolic and diastolic
- The body seeks equilibrium. In an hour or less, vital signs usually return to what they were previously, even if the patient is still in severe pain. Continuous severe pain sometimes causes vital signs to increase again from time to time, but they rarely remain elevated.
- Diaphoresis, pallor
- Dilated pupils
- Muscle tension (face, body)
- Nausea and vomiting (if pain is severe)

BEHAVIORAL SIGNS

- Rigid body position
- Restlessness
- Frowning
- Grimacing
- Clenched teeth
- Clenched fists
- Crying
- Moaning

---

easily, the description of pain is more accurate. If the patient wears a hearing aid or glasses, be sure they are worn when the patient is answering pain assessment questions or marking a pain scale. Several pain scales have been developed to assess pain in children. Wong and Baker developed the FACES pain rating scale (see Fig. 30.8). Most patients require a pain level of 4 or less to function well.

Collection of objective data. Carefully observe the patient. Possible objective signs are tachycardia, increased rate and depth of respirations, diaphoresis, increased systolic or diastolic blood pressure, pallor, dilated pupils, and increased muscle tension. Some patients complain of nausea or weakness (Box 21.3). Other patients have a subjective complaint of pain with no observable objective signs.

If the pain is chronic or less severe, the physiologic changes are likely to be less prominent. Changes in facial expressions, such as frowning or gritting teeth, may be exhibited. Some people clench their fists and withdraw from social activities when in pain. Others complain bitterly, cry, moan, toss about in bed, assume a fetal position, or clutch at the affected body part. Pacing may be performed by some patients if their energy level allows. The amount of attention desired by a patient in pain varies; some patients in pain want someone in constant attendance, whereas others want to be left alone.

Be unbiased and nonjudgmental when gathering objective data; consider that the patient is doing the best he or she can do at the given moment. The priority intervention is to relieve or decrease the pain. Remember that pain is what the patient says it is. Do not expect the patient to behave in any set manner when in pain.

Nursing Interventions

The following measures are performed to assist in pain control and comfort (see the Health Promotion box):

- Tighten wrinkled bed linens.
- Reposition drainage tubes or other objects on which patient is lying.
- Place warm bath blankets if the patient is cold.
- Loosen constricting bandages.
- Change moist dressings.
- Check tape to prevent pulling on skin.
- Position patient in anatomic alignment.
- Check temperature of hot and cold applications, including bath water.
- Lift—do not pull—patient up in bed; handle gently.
- Position patient correctly on bedpan.
- Avoid exposing skin or mucous membranes to irritants (e.g., diarrheal stool or wound drainage).
- Prevent urinary retention by ensuring patency of Foley catheter.
- Prevent constipation by encouraging appropriate fluid intake, diet, and exercise and by administering prescribed stool softeners.

Health Promotion

Promoting Comfort

- Measures that promote a sense of well-being to minimize or avoid discomfort include warm baths, thorough personal hygiene, and adequate rest.
- Pain has the potential to disable and immobilize a person enough to impair the ability to perform self-care activities. This results in social isolation, depression, and changes in self-concept. Help patients and families learn to discuss their feelings about the loss of function and to find ways to cope with pain and the lifestyle it imposes.
- When a patient has chronic, disabling pain, instruct family members on proper positioning techniques and methods of assisting the patient with ambulation.
- Nonpharmacologic or complementary therapies used for pain relief include massage, guided imagery, music, biofeedback, meditation, hypnosis, exercise, therapeutic touch, acupuncture, and relaxation techniques.

Guidelines for individualizing pain therapy. When you provide pain relief measures, choose therapies suited to the patient's unique pain experience. McCaffery (2002) suggested the following guidelines for individualizing pain therapy:

1. *Use different types of pain relief measures.* Using more than one therapy has an additive effect in reducing pain. In addition, the character of pain often changes throughout the day, which necessitates the use of several different therapies. A combination of physical and psychological approaches (e.g., analgesics or antidepressants and relaxation) helps control all components of the pain experience.

2. *Provide pain relief measures before pain becomes severe.* It is easier to prevent severe pain than to relieve it. Giving an analgesic 30 to 40 minutes before ambulation or other care activities may help in the proactive pain management. Implement prn medications around the clock to control moderately severe to severe pain effectively. Waiting for the patient or the family to request analgesics results in delays in administration and inadequate pain control.

3. *Use measures the patient believes are effective.* The patient is the expert on the pain and probably has realistic ideas about what measures to use (e.g., rubbing lotion on an edematous finger) and when to use them.

4. *Consider the patient's ability or willingness to participate in pain relief measures.* Some patients are not able to assist actively with pain therapy because of fatigue, sedation, or altered levels of consciousness. However, some variations of pain relief measures require little effort, such as relaxation exercises in bed or listening to music as a distraction. You will not relieve pain by forcing an unwilling patient to participate in therapy. The depressed patient with chronic pain has little motivation to participate.

5. *Choose pain relief measures appropriate to the severity of the pain as reflected by the patient's behavior.* It would be poor judgment to administer a potent opioid to a patient who is displaying only mild pain. Carefully assess what the patient says before you choose pain therapy. Some patients acquire relief from severe pain after using only mild analgesics. Only the patient can determine the degree of effectiveness of a therapy.

6. *If a therapy is ineffective at first, encourage the patient to try it again before abandoning it.* Often anxiety or doubt prevents patients from obtaining relief from therapy. Some approaches, such as distraction, necessitate practice. Some measures that seem ineffective merely necessitate adjustment to become effective. For example, try increasing the dosage of an analgesic if severe pain is unrelieved initially. Be persistent and understanding in helping the patient learn to use measures that do not afford immediate relief.

7. *Keep an open mind about what has potential to relieve pain.* New ways to control pain sometimes are found. Much remains to be learned about the pain experience. Rejecting a patient's unconventional therapies leads to mistrust. Monitor therapies to ensure the patient's safety and well-being.

8. *Keep trying.* It is easy to become frustrated when efforts at pain relief fail. Do not abandon the patient when pain persists. Some patients in severe chronic pain who are ignored choose suicide as an alternative. If the patient obtains no relief, reassess the situation and consider whether alternative therapies are needed.

9. *Protect the patient.* Pain therapy that causes more distress than the pain is misguided and inappropriate. Always observe the response to therapy. Any pain relief measure poses a risk of side effects, such as fatigue, anxiety, or additional pain. The goal is to relieve pain without disabling the patient mentally, emotionally, or physically. It is important to maintain safety of the patient and environment.

SLEEP AND REST

A patient at rest feels mentally relaxed, free from worry, and physically calm. A patient at rest is free from physical or mental exertion. Everyone has his or her own method of obtaining rest and is usually able to adjust to new environments or conditions that affect the ability to rest.

Rest is important in healing the body of physical and psychological illness. Patients often are prescribed bed rest. This treatment confines patients to bed to decrease physical or psychological demands on the body. Bed rest does not necessarily mean that a patient is resting. Emotional or metabolic stressors naturally cause the patient to be restless.

Sleep is a state of rest that occurs for a sustained period. The reduced consciousness during sleep provides

| Box **21.4** | Factors Affecting Sleep |

PHYSICAL ILLNESS

- Pain and physical discomfort result in difficulty falling or staying asleep.
- Chronic pain sometimes has a circadian rhythm, including increasing in intensity at night, thus disrupting sleep.
- Illness frequently forces patients to sleep in positions to which they are unaccustomed.
- Respiratory diseases interfere with the rhythm of breathing and sometimes oblige a person to assume a certain position to be able to breathe easily. Both factors can disturb sleep.
- A patient with heart disease may be afraid to go to sleep at night.
- Hypertension causes early morning awakening and fatigue.
- Nocturia and restless legs syndrome disrupt sleep, causing the patient to awaken and have trouble going back to sleep during the night.
- Conditions that increase intracranial pressure or alter central nervous system physiology alter sleep patterns and sometimes cause excessive daytime sleepiness.

ANXIETY AND DEPRESSION

- As anxiety and depression increase, so does lack of sleep; as amount of sleep decreases, anxiety and depression increase.
- Bereaved people may experience sleep problems related to fear of intruders, loneliness, and the dreams or nightmares that occur involving the lost loved one.

DRUGS AND SUBSTANCES

- Various drugs and substances affect the pattern and the quality of sleep.
- Hypnotic medications interfere with reaching deeper sleep stages, provide only a temporary (1-week) increase in quality of sleep, and eventually cause a "hangover" feeling during the day. Hypnotic drugs often worsen sleep apnea in older adults.
- Older adults often take several drugs, the combined effects of which disrupt sleep.
- L-Tryptophan, a protein found in foods such as milk, cheese, and meats, frequently helps induce sleep.

LIFESTYLE

- Daily routines such as work shifts influence sleep patterns; changing routines, as with rotating shifts, disrupt these patterns. Only after several weeks of working a night shift does an individual's biologic clock adjust.
- Performing unaccustomed heavy work, late-night social activities, and changing evening mealtimes are activities that can disrupt sleep.

SLEEP PATTERNS

- Sleep patterns include starting time and duration of sleep. The most significant cause of daytime sleepiness is inadequate or abnormal sleep at night.
- Everyone has an increased tendency to feel sleepy from 2 a.m. to 7 a.m.
- When sleep patterns are disrupted, the natural tendency to sleep at certain times increases.
- Sleep patterns influence future attempts to fall asleep because of changes in circadian rhythm. Sleeping 1 hour later results in falling asleep 1 hour later the next night.

STRESS

- Stress resulting from personal problems or situational crises causes tension and at times causes a person to try too hard to fall asleep, to awaken frequently, or to oversleep.
- Stress causes release of corticosteroids and adrenalin, which leads to catabolism and sleeplessness.
- Patients with advanced cancer or chronic illness often are afraid to go to sleep for fear they might die.
- The stress of losses such as retirement or death of a loved one sometimes causes older adults to suffer delays in falling asleep, earlier REM (rapid eye movement) sleep, frequent awakening, increased total bedtime, and feelings of sleeping poorly.

ENVIRONMENT

- Environmental factors influence the ability to fall and remain asleep. Significant factors include ventilation, lighting, type of bed, sound level, and the presence or absence of a bed partner.
- In hospitals, unfamiliar noises and higher noise levels such as that created by wall suction, opening packages, ringing alarms, and flushing toilets can cause sleep deprivation.
- Intensive care units have high noise levels.

EXERCISE AND FATIGUE

- Exercise and fatigue in moderation usually facilitate restful sleep, but excess fatigue from exhausting or stressful work typically make falling asleep difficult.
- Performing exercise 2 hours before bedtime allows the body to cool down and promotes relaxation.

NUTRITION

- Weight gain causes longer sleep periods with fewer interruptions and later awakening.
- Weight loss sometimes causes reduction in total time spent asleep along with broken sleep and earlier awakening.

time for repair and recovery of body systems for the next period of wakefulness. The theory that sleep is associated with healing suggests that achieving optimal sleep quality is important for patients' recovery. Sleep restores a person's energy and feeling of well-being.

The routines of health care facilities easily disrupt the rest and sleep habits of patients (Box 21.4). The extent of the change depends on the gravity of the illness, as well as the environment in which the patient is placed. Remain aware of the patient's need for rest. Without it, the patient becomes fatigued and irritable and has a decreased ability to cope with stressors (see the Lifespan Considerations for Older Adults box).

Lifespan Considerations
Older Adults

Sleep

- Older adults require about the same amount of sleep as younger people but are more likely to achieve it in separate episodes; they take more daytime naps and get less sleep at night.
- The sleep of an older adult is less deep. This increases the risk of early awakening and complaints of sleep disturbance.
- Sleep is likely to be disturbed in older adults with chronic health problems such as arthritis, heart failure, and chronic obstructive pulmonary disease. Adequate pain control and positioning facilitate breathing and help promote rest and sleep.
- Many older adults take medications such as diuretics and theophylline that are likely to disturb sleep. Carefully assess time of administration and the effect on sleep, and modify the schedule when possible.
- Insufficient sleep may lead to memory and personality changes in older adults.
- Include nonpharmacologic comfort measures among nursing interventions to promote rest and sleep.

PHYSIOLOGY OF SLEEP

Sleep is a cyclic physiologic process that alternates with longer periods of wakefulness. The sleep-wake cycle influences and regulates body functions and behavioral responses. The influence of sleep is not limited to physiologic functions. Sleep and rest have an impact on memory, mood, and cognitive performance.

People experience cyclic rhythms as part of everyday life. The most familiar rhythm is the 24-hour day-night cycle known as the *diurnal* or *circadian rhythm.* All circadian rhythms, including the sleep-wake cycle, are affected by light and temperature and external factors such as social activities and environmental stressors. Each person has a biologic clock that synchronizes sleep cycles. Some people can fall asleep at 8 p.m., whereas others go to bed at midnight or early in the morning. Different people also function best at different times of the day.

The biologic rhythm of sleep frequently becomes synchronized with other body functions. Normal variations in body temperature, for example, are correlated with sleep patterns. When the sleep-wake cycle is disrupted (e.g., by working rotating shifts), other physiologic functions typically change as well.

SLEEP CYCLE

Sleep involves two phases: **rapid eye movement (REM)** and **non–rapid eye movement (NREM)** (Box 21.5). NREM sleep is further divided into four stages through which a sleeper progresses during a typical sleeping cycle. The sleeping stages are highly individualized (Fig. 21.9).

Normally an adult's routine sleep pattern begins with a presleep period, during which the person is aware only of a gradually developing drowsiness. This

Box 21.5 Stages of Sleep

NON–RAPID EYE MOVEMENT (NREM) SLEEP
Stage 1
- Lightest level of sleep
- Lasts a few minutes
- Decreased physiologic activity, beginning with a gradual fall in vital signs and metabolism
- Person is easily aroused by sensory stimuli such as noise
- If person awakes, feels as though daydreaming has occurred
- Reduction in autonomic activities (e.g., heart rate)

Stage 2
- Period of sound sleep
- Lasts 10–20 min
- Relaxation progresses
- Arousal is still easy
- Body functions are still slowing

Stage 3
- Initial stage of deep sleep
- Lasts 15–30 min
- Arousal is difficult, movement is rare
- Muscles are completely relaxed
- Vital signs decline but remain regular
- Hormonal response includes secretion of growth hormone

Stage 4
- Deepest stage of sleep
- Lasts approximately 15–30 min
- Arousal is very difficult
- If sleep loss has occurred, sleeper spends most of night in this stage
- Restores and rests the body
- Vital signs are significantly lower than during waking hours
- Sleepwalking and enuresis are possible
- Hormonal response continues

RAPID EYE MOVEMENT (REM) SLEEP
- Stage of vivid, full-color dreaming consistent with sensory experiences (less vivid dreaming sometimes occurs in other stages)
- First occurs approximately 90 min after sleep has begun, thereafter occurs at end of each NREM cycle
- Duration increasing with each cycle and averaging 20 min
- Typified by autonomic response of rapidly moving eyes, fluctuating heart and respiratory rates, and increased or fluctuating blood pressure
- Loss of skeletal muscle tone
- Responsible for mental restoration
- Stage in which sleeper is most difficult to arouse

period normally lasts 10 to 30 minutes, but if a person has difficulty falling asleep, it can last an hour or longer.

As adults fall asleep, they progress through the four stages of NREM sleep. At the end of the fourth stage, they come out of a deep sleep, go back to stage 2, and then enter a period of REM sleep. A person reaches REM sleep in about 90 minutes (average). Each person

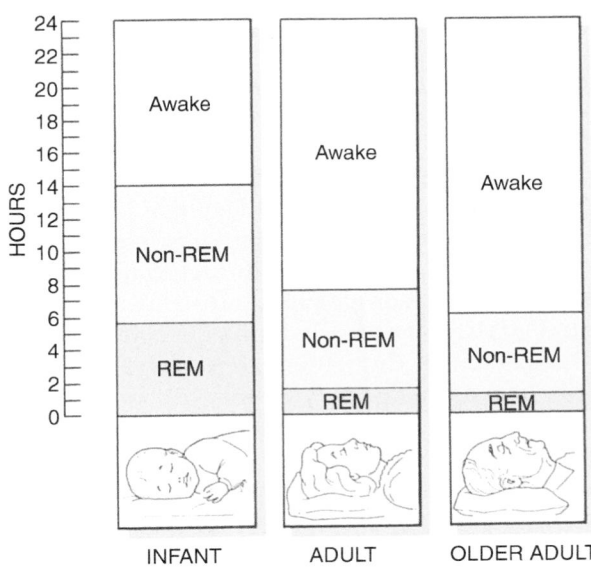

Fig. 21.9 Sleep-wake cycles across the life span. *Infants:* Approximately 40% of total sleep time is spent in rapid eye movement *(REM)* sleep. *Adults:* 20% of total sleep time is spent in REM sleep. *Older adults:* Total sleep time is slightly reduced; REM sleep continues to make up 20% of total sleep time.

differs, but a typical night's sleep consists of four to six such cycles.

Dreams occur during the NREM and REM stages. The dream of REM sleep is believed to be functionally important, more vivid, and elaborate, allowing a person to clarify emotions and prepare the mind for events of the next day.

NREM sleep provides a period of body maintenance. This stage of sleep has been attributed to wound healing, immune functions, hormone release, and muscle restoration. A person's biologic functions slow during NREM sleep. For example, a healthy adult has a heart rate of 70 to 80 beats per minute during the day; however, during sleep the heart beats at 60 beats per minute or less. Respiration rate and blood pressure also decrease during sleep. It is very difficult to arouse the sleeper in REM sleep.

REM sleep is important for brain and cognitive restoration. During REM sleep, there are changes in cerebral blood flow and increases in cortical activity, oxygen consumption, and epinephrine release, which are beneficial to memory storage and learning.

SLEEP DEPRIVATION

The amount of sleep needed varies by age and health condition. Infants need the most: 16 hours. Teens require 9 hours and adults 8 hours per night. Sleep deprivation is a problem many patients experience as a result of hospitalization. Sleep deprivation involves decreases in the amount, the quality, and the consistency of sleep. When sleep is interrupted or fragmented, changes in the normal sequence of sleep stages occur, and cycles are not completed. Cumulative deprivation

gradually develops. Sleep deprivation has been tied to hypertension, diabetes, heart disease, and stroke.

 Safety Alert

Daytime Sleepiness

- Safety precautions are important for patients and residents who awaken during the night to use the bathroom and for those with excessive daytime sleepiness.
- Set beds lower to the floor to lessen the chance that the patient or resident will fall when first standing.
- Some patients and residents who experience daytime sleepiness fall asleep while sitting up in a chair or wheelchair. Position the person so that he or she will not fall out of the chair while sleeping.

Patients with sleep deprivation experience a variety of physiologic and psychological signs and symptoms. Possible physiologic signs and symptoms include hand tremors, decreased reflexes, slowed response time, reduction in word memory, decreased reasoning and judgment, and cardiac dysrhythmias. Possible psychological signs and symptoms include mood swings, disorientation, irritability, decreased motivation, fatigue, sleepiness, and hyperexcitability.

PROMOTING REST AND SLEEP

Determine the patient's usual rest and sleep patterns, decide whether they are sufficient, and note why the patient is not getting sufficient rest. Work with the patient and the family to develop a plan to provide for more rest. A typical plan includes limiting interruptions during the night for vital sign checks and other procedures, providing a quiet environment with a comfortable room temperature, limiting the number of visitors and the duration of visits, and carrying out all procedures within a given time frame (see the Coordinated Care box).

 Coordinated Care

Supervision

Promoting Sleep

- Encourage nursing assistants to provide for patients or residents a quiet, undisturbed environment that causes the least interference with sleep.
- Instruct the nursing assistant to provide comfort measures such as toileting, a back rub, and a comfortable bed to help the patient or resident prepare for sleep.
- Communicate to the nursing assistant that it is essential to keep excessive noise from conversation or equipment to a minimum because this disturbs residents or patients who already are having difficulty sleeping.

In preparing the patient for sleep, wash the patient's back if the patient is on bed rest, gently massage it, change the linens, make certain the patient is warm enough, offer an uncaffeinated beverage such as milk (if allowed), change soiled dressings, and give the patient an opportunity to void.

Decrease environmental stimuli by dimming the lights and decreasing the noise level. Direct the patient to assume a comfortable position, and assist if needed. A night light is a necessity for promotion of safety for the older adult. Administer a sleeping medication or analgesic as ordered if the patient cannot sleep (see Box 21.4).

Patient problems and interventions for the patient with sleep disturbance include but are not limited to the following:

PATIENT PROBLEM	NURSING INTERVENTIONS
Ineffective Sleep Pattern, related to illness and psychological stress manifested by change in behavior, increased irritability, listlessness, and verbal complaints of not feeling well rested	Encourage patient to ambulate in the early evening, if permitted Provide glass of milk 30 min before patient's bedtime unless contraindicated Perform all necessary procedures before 9 p.m. to ensure uninterrupted sleep Massage patient's back, freshen linens, reduce noise, and dim lights Administer hypnotic as prescribed
Ineffective Thought Processes, related to sleep deprivation manifested by slower reaction time, altered attention span, and disorientation	Maintain periods of uninterrupted rest Provide safe environment Close door to patient room Orient patient to reality Administer analgesic or sedative (or both) about 30 min before patient's bedtime, if ordered

❖ NURSING PROCESS FOR PAIN MANAGEMENT, COMFORT, REST, AND SLEEP

The role of the licensed practical nurse/licensed vocational nurse (LPN/LVN) in the nursing process is that the LPN/LVN will:

- Participate in planning care for patients based on patient needs
- Review patient's plan of care and recommend revisions as needed
- Review and follow defined prioritization for patient care
- Use clinical pathways, care maps, or care plans to guide and review patient care

◆ ASSESSMENT

Pain assessment is one of the most frequent and difficult activities that a nurse performs. It is crucial to assess the pain experience from the patient's perspective.

Make sure patients are aware that informed reporting of pain is valuable and necessary if the health care team is to manage pain effectively.

◆ TERMINOLOGY

Specific terms are used in assessing pain. *Onset* indicates when the pain began. *Duration* is how long the pain lasts from the onset until it is resolved. Pain also is classified by location. To determine pain location, use a drawing of the body and ask the patient to mark all the areas where pain is felt. Another method is to ask the patient to point to the places where pain is felt, and you then document those places either on a body outline or descriptively in the medical record and on the care plan. Remind the patient to report new pain sites because they may signal complications.

Severity indicates whether the pain is mild, moderate, or intense. Sample pain scales are useful to assist in assessing pain (see Fig. 21.8). Terms the patient uses to describe the pain, such as "sharp," "stabbing," "dull," or "throbbing," provide more information.

Many patients experiencing acute pain exhibit a rise in pulse rate and blood pressure, diaphoresis, and dilated pupils.

◆ PATIENT PROBLEM

An accurate patient problem statement of the patient with pain enables you to plan and implement relief measures effectively. The following patient problem statements are associated directly with the care of patients with pain:

- Recent Onset of Pain
- Prolonged Pain

Other possible patient problem statements that are appropriate when pain affects other aspects of a patient's life include the following:

- Inability to Tolerate Activity
- Anxiousness
- Distorted Body Image
- Excessive Demand on Primary Caregiver
- Infrequent or Difficult Bowel Elimination
- Impaired Coping
- Impaired Family Coping
- Risk for Contractures or Muscle Atrophy
- Impaired Family Processes
- Lethargy or Malaise
- Fearfulness
- Grief
- Despair
- Insufficient Knowledge (specify)
- Compromised Physical Mobility
- Insufficient Nutrition
- Helplessness
- Impaired Role Functioning
- Inability to Bathe Self
- Inability to Toilet Self
- Impaired Sexual Function

- Deficient Sleep
- Ineffective Sleep Pattern
- Compromised Social Interaction
- Social Seclusion

The extensiveness of the list alerts you to the numerous problems that may develop because of pain.

◆ EXPECTED OUTCOMES AND PLANNING

When participating in the development of the plan of care, you establish priorities based on the patient's level of pain and its effect on the patient's condition. You and the patient set realistic expectations for pain relief and discuss the degree of pain relief to expect. Typical patient-centered goals and outcomes include the following:

Goal 1: Patient attains a sense of well-being and improved comfort within 1 hour.

Outcome: Patient nonverbally (facial expression, tone of voice) demonstrates improved relief from pain within 1 hour.

Goal 2: Patient regains ability to perform self-care independently within 24 hours.

Outcome: Patient bathes and grooms self without hesitancy or restriction within 24 hours.

◆ IMPLEMENTATION

Establish a trusting nurse-patient relationship so that the patient believes that relief measures will be beneficial. You help accomplish this when you see the patient in a holistic manner, listen attentively to concerns, attend promptly to the patient's needs, and respect any response to pain. In a successful nurse-patient relationship, the nurse understands that the patient is the expert on his or her own pain and its relief.

You probably will teach various measures to help the patient and the family deal with pain. Comfort measures sometimes avert the need for analgesics. Some measures are appropriate positioning and alignment in bed, washing and massaging the back, and ambulation, unless contraindicated.

Try teaching distraction and relaxation techniques to the patient. Sometimes distraction and relaxation do not help control the patient's pain, so it is necessary to use analgesic medications.

Nursing interventions that promote the establishment of an effective relationship with the person who is experiencing pain and with the family should include the following:

- *Believe the patient.* The patient needs to be able to trust the nurse and to recognize that the reports of pain are valid. Convey this message verbally to the patient by saying, "I know you are in pain."
- *Clarify responsibilities in pain relief.* Discuss what actions are going to be taken to manage the pain. Clarify the roles of the patient and family in the interaction.
- *Respect the patient's response to pain.* Accept the right of the patient to respond to the pain in the necessary manner. The family also needs help in this area. Sometimes the patient needs help accepting the response to the pain, if the behavior is not as expected by the patient and family.
- *Confer with the patient.* Encourage the patient to use coping techniques that have been effective in the past. Assist the patient and the family in using personal resources more effectively. Help the patient and the family to participate actively in setting goals for pain relief.
- *Explore the pain with the patient.* Find out what the pain means to the patient and the family.
- *Be with the patient often.* Act as a buffer for the patient and the family during difficult times. The physical presence of the nurse reassures or distracts the patient at times and offers comfort at others, thus relieving the pain (McCaffery and Pasero, 2003).

◆ EVALUATION

Effective communication between the nurse and the patient is essential in achieving pain control. Continuous evaluation allows you to determine whether new or revised therapies are required. Refer to the goals and outcomes identified when you plan care, and perform evaluative measures to determine whether the goals have been reached. Examples of goals and evaluative measures include the following:

Goal 1: Patient obtains a sense of well-being and improved pain relief within 1 hour.

Evaluative measure: Ask the patient to rate the pain on a scale of 0 to 10, 10 being the most severe. Observe the patient's facial expressions and body movement, noting whether there is freedom of movement.

Goal 2: Patient regains ability to perform self-care independently within 24 hours.

Evaluative measure: Observe patient performing activities of daily living.

Get Ready for the NCLEX® Examination!

Key Points

- McCaffery and Pasero (2003) provided a realistic description of pain: "Pain is whatever the experiencing person says it is, existing whenever he says it does."
- Pain is largely a subjective experience.
- Pain is often a protective mechanism that warns of tissue injury.
- A nurse's bias and misconception of pain potentially results in ineffective control of the patient's pain.
- Pain scales are used to evaluate objectively pain intensity and the effectiveness of pain therapies.
- Considering pain the fifth vital sign helps ensure that pain is monitored on a regular basis.
- Individualize pain therapy by working closely with the patient, using assessment findings, and trying a variety of therapies.
- Patient-controlled analgesic devices and epidural analgesia give pain control with low risk of overdose.
- Nursing implications for administering epidural analgesia include closely monitoring for respiratory depression.
- Appropriate pain management has the potential to bring about quicker recoveries, shorter hospital stays, fewer readmissions, and improved quality of life.
- Constipation is the most common opioid side effect and the only one for which the individual does not develop tolerance.
- Fatigue, sleep disturbance, and depression act in a type of synergistic relationship that can change a person's perception of pain markedly.
- The circadian rhythm is the 24-hour, day-night cycle known also as the diurnal rhythm.

Additional Learning Resources

SG Go to your Study Guide for additional learning activities to help you master this chapter content.

Be sure to visit the Evolve site at http://evolve.elsevier.com/Cooper/foundations/ for additional online resources.

Review Questions for the NCLEX® Examination

1. After surgery for a total knee replacement, a patient was given an epidural catheter for fentanyl epidural analgesia. What is the most important nursing intervention?

   1. Administer additional analgesic medications as needed.
   2. Change the epidural dressing every shift.
   3. Assess respiratory rate.
   4. Encourage ambulation.

2. A 52-year-old patient admitted for deep vein thrombosis of the left internal iliac vein complains of excruciating pain in his left leg. What is the most appropriate response by the nurse?

   1. "Pain is what you say it is; I will assist you in whatever way I can."
   2. "Your pain is an unpleasant sensation caused by inflammation of the vein and difficult to control."
   3. "Your pain is one of the cardinal signs of inflammation."
   4. "I know you are in pain, but it is important that we guard against possible addiction to opioids."

3. A 63-year-old patient underwent a lower anterior bowel resection yesterday. What common central nervous system analgesic is prescribed often to control pain?

   1. Aspirin
   2. Acetaminophen (Tylenol)
   3. Morphine
   4. Ibuprofen (Motrin)

4. What drug delivery system is used to control pain via a portable computerized pump with a chamber for a syringe?

   1. Patient-controlled analgesia
   2. Transcutaneous electric nerve stimulation
   3. A venous access device
   4. An intrathecal delivery system

5. The nursing student is discussing the gate control theory of pain. Which statement by the student indicates the need for further instruction? (Select all that apply.)

   1. "The gates of the pain pathways can be opened with therapeutic massage and heat treatments."
   2. "Pain has exclusive use of the pathways ahead of other stimuli, according to the theory."
   3. "Distraction is beneficial in pain management, according to the theory."
   4. "Pain is a manifestation of an intricate chain of electrochemical events."
   5. "Memories and feelings may alter gating mechanisms."

6. A patient admitted with severe cellulitis of the left breast states, "I have a severe burning pain, and it feels like my breast is on fire." She rates her pain as 7 on the 0-to-10 pain assessment scale. How would this collection of data by the nurse in assessing the patient's pain be classified?

   1. Deductive
   2. Speculative
   3. Objective
   4. Subjective

7. The nurse listens attentively while the patient describes her angina pectoris pain as radiating down her left inner arm to the little finger and upward to the jaw and the shoulder. What term is used to classify this type of pain?

   1. Precisely localized
   2. Referred
   3. Intermittent
   4. Chronic

8. The nurse is assessing the patient's description of his back pain. He states that it is "immobilizing, intense, and on a scale of 0 to 10, it is an 8." What type of pain assessment scale is the patient using?

   1. Visual analog
   2. Categorical
   3. Functional
   4. Numeric

9. The nurse is caring for two patients with similar injuries. One patient expresses severe pain, and the other reports feeling fine with low levels of pain. Which statement is most correct?

   1. The patient having more intense reports of pain has dysfunctional endorphins.
   2. The patient having lesser levels of pain has a higher level of endorphins.
   3. The patient experiencing intense pain has lower levels of endorphins.
   4. The patient having elevated levels of pain has an alteration in recognition of endorphins by the hypothalamus of the brain.

10. A patient was admitted to the orthopedic section for acute back pain. The health care provider is planning to use cutaneous stimulation management. Which is an example of this pain control method?

    1. Epidural analgesia
    2. Transcutaneous electric nerve stimulation (TENS)
    3. Nonsteroidal antiinflammatory drugs (NSAIDs)
    4. Patient-controlled analgesia

11. What statement concerning unrelieved pain is most correct?

    1. Unrelieved pain is a normal expectation after major surgery.
    2. Patients with cancer diagnoses can expect to experience unrelieved pain.
    3. Physiologic and psychological complications can result from unrelieved pain.
    4. Although unrelieved pain is stressful and annoying, it is not as important as other physical care needs.

12. What is the priority responsibility of the nurse related to pain?

    1. Leave the patient alone to rest.
    2. Help the patient appear to not be in pain.
    3. Believe what the patient says about pain.
    4. Assume responsibility for eliminating the patient's pain.

13. Research indicates that the risk of clinically significant opioid-induced respiratory depression is

    1. less than 1%.
    2. 5%.
    3. 20%.
    4. 30%.

14. Which route is most appropriate for treating rapidly escalating severe pain?

    1. Oral
    2. Intramuscular (IM)
    3. Intravenous (IV)
    4. Transdermal

15. Which opioid is no longer a drug of choice for managing pain because of its toxic complications, such as causing seizures?

    1. Codeine
    2. Morphine
    3. Meperidine
    4. Fentanyl

16. The nurse has recommended the patient consider music therapy to manage pain after an upcoming surgery. What information should be provided to the patient? *(Select all that apply.)*

    1. Music therapy works best when selections are instrumental instead of songs containing words.
    2. Music therapy is successful for at least 50% of people who try it.
    3. Music therapy promotes relaxation and takes the focus away from the pain being experienced.
    4. Music therapy is easily a self-directed means of pain management.
    5. Music therapy's success is limited to postoperative pain.

17. A patient has been prescribed acetaminophen to manage pain after a sports injury. What information can be included in the discussion about this medication with the patient? *(Select all that apply.)*

    1. This medication is limited to the management of mild pain.
    2. The dosage of acetaminophen should be limited to 4000 mg in a 24-hour period.
    3. Acetaminophen is associated with gastrointestinal upset.
    4. Excessive dosages are associated with hepatotoxicity.
    5. Acetaminophen works by blocking pain impulses.

18. A man, 64, participates every year in a number of Music & Motorcycle Festivals around the country but meets his rival in a particularly challenging open course and hill climb, in which he takes a fall. His motorcycle lands on top of him and he suffers a broken pelvis, two cracked ribs, and a punctured lung. He is put on IV hydromorphone. On transfer from the ICU to a surgical unit, he is switched to a single oral morphine. The nurse has her private doubts about this switch but says nothing. Soon after receiving the second dose of morphine tablet, the patient experiences intense pruritus. The physician is contacted and adds a medication to offset these adverse effects. He also adds a laxative as a prophylactic adjuvant. Then, the next afternoon, when his physical therapist arrives to help him practice walking the hallway on a walker, the patient's pain is at its peak, and he says, "I'm sorry. It just hurts too much this afternoon." When the physical therapist points out that he walked just fine before, he tries valiantly to stand several times, but the pain overtakes him, and he eases slowly back into his chair, rubs two fingers along his brow, and keeping his head down, quietly asks if he can be helped back into bed. After the nurse comes and helps him back into bed, observing that his face is pale and damp, another dose of oral morphine is delivered. The nurse evaluates the afternoon's disappointing outcomes. Select interventions that might have been more effective.

    ___ A. Remember that pre-medication with morphine would mean the medication will reach peak effect too soon.
    ___ B. Use NSAIDs to help reduce opioid side effects.
    ___ C. Encourage coadministration of both morphine and an NSAID for enhanced effect.
    ___ D. Give oral morphine in combination with a second opioid for maximum relief.
    ___ E. Ask to switch the patient to an injectable medication for quicker relief.
    ___ F. Time his morphine to take affect before physical activities.

Objectives

1. Discuss the classification of wounds according to the Centers for Disease Control and Prevention (CDC).
2. Discuss the body's response during each stage of wound healing.
3. Differentiate between healing by primary intention and secondary intention.
4. Discuss the role of nutrition in wound healing.
5. Discuss the factors that impair wound healing and the interventions for each type of wound.
6. Explain procedure for applying dry dressings and wet-to-dry dressings.
7. Discuss dehiscence, evisceration, and the nursing care they involve.
8. Identify the procedure for performing sterile wound irrigation.
9. Identify common complications of wound healing.
10. Identify the procedure for removing sutures and staples.
11. Discuss care of the patient with a wound drainage system: Hemovac, Davol suction, or T-tube drainage.
12. Identify the nursing interventions for the patient with vacuum-assisted closure of a wound.
13. Describe the purposes of bandages, binders, and the precautions taken when applying them.
14. List nursing diagnoses associated with wound care.

Key Terms

bandage (p. 646)
binder (p. 646)
dehiscence (dē-HĬS-ĕns, p. 652)
drainage (p. 643)
evisceration (ē-vĭs-ŭr-Ā-shŭn, p. 652)
exudate (ĔKS-ū-dāt, p. 626)
granulation (grăn-ū-LĀ-shŭn, p. 626)
incision (ĭn-SĬZH-ŭn, p. 625)
infectious process (p. 629)
inflammatory response (p. 629)
irrigation (p. 635)

primary intention (p. 626)
puncture (p. 625)
purulent (PYŪ-rū-lĕnt, p. 626)
sanguineous (săng-GWĬN-ē-ŭs, p. 629)
secondary intention (p. 626)
serosanguineous (SĒR-ō-săng-GWĬN-ē-ŭs, p. 629)
serous (SĒR-ŭs, p. 629)
tertiary intention (TŬR-shē-ăr-ē, p. 626)
T tube (p. 645)
vacuum-assisted closure (p. 645)
wound (p. 624)

The term **wound** refers to any injury to the body's tissues. Injury results in either an open or a closed wound. An open wound is one that involves a break in the skin, while in a closed wound, the trauma occurs under the surface of the skin, such as with a bruise or hematoma. Any break in the integrity of the integument results in a potential compromise to the individual's defensive barriers against outside pathogens. Prompt assessment and interventions to reduce the potentially negative impact of the skin's breech are important. Stressors to the individual affect the efficiency of wound healing. Wound healing is affected by age, nutritional status, physical well-being, and medication therapies. Social factors, including smoking, can impair wound healing. Alterations in health, including diabetes, cancer, and heart disease, slow the body's ability to heal.

During healing, any stress and strain on tissues (nausea, vomiting, abdominal distention, coughing, respiratory efforts) place tension against a surgical incision, especially an abdominal incision. During activity, the abdominal muscles contract and cause an increase in intraabdominal pressure; if the incisional area is weak, dehiscence is possible. Other factors that have the capacity to affect wound healing include preoperative skin preparation, type of surgical procedure, environment within the surgical suite, and postoperative wound care.

WOUND CLASSIFICATION

Wound classifications are determined based on a series of factors that include cause, the severity of injury, the amount of contamination, and the size. An understanding of the causative factors of a wound is vital to determination of the proper treatment plan. Obtain a complete history, including what caused the wound and any underlying disease process.

In planned surgery, the surgeon creates the wound by making an **incision** (a cut produced surgically by a sharp instrument that creates an opening into an organ or space in the body) or **puncture** (a stab wound for a drainage system); the surgical wound usually is closed or managed (e.g., a drain inserted, a stoma created) in the final stage of the procedure. By contrast, in traumatic injury (e.g., from a knife stabbing) and unplanned or emergency surgeries, the practitioner brings wound edges together to aid healing. Unless a "dirty surgery" is performed (e.g., a perforated bowel, ruptured appendix), a surgical incision is cleaner and easier to repair than a traumatic wound.

Surgical wounds are classified based on the level of contamination. The Centers for Disease Control and Prevention (CDC, 2020) has classified wounds by the level and type of contamination. Levels range from class I (clean) to class IV (dirty, infected). The Association of periOperative Registered Nurses (AORN) developed a decision tree to assist in classification of the stage of the surgical wound (Fig. 22.1).

The risk for infection in a clean surgical wound is less than 5%. The risk for other wound types increases based on the type of contamination that may be introduced. Contamination may result from the presence of gastrointestinal (GI) matter, such as feces, which contain *Escherichia coli* from the colon or from environmental conditions at the time of injury preceding the surgical intervention. Wounds that are contaminated as a result of their traumatic origin or during surgery have a significantly elevated risk of infection, nearing 39% (Carvalho, 2017).

Fig. 22.1 Surgical wound classification decision tree. (Reprinted with permission from AORN.org. Copyright 2015 AORN, Inc., 2170 Parker Road, Suite 400, Denver, CO 80231. All rights reserved.)

WOUND HEALING

The healing process begins immediately after an injury and sometimes continues for a year or longer. Although the healing process follows a consistent pattern, the type of wound and tissue, the wound's severity, and the overall condition of the patient influence the time it takes for healing to be complete. Wound healing follows four phases: hemostasis; inflammatory phase; reconstruction, also known as proliferation; and maturation, which may also be referred to as remodeling.

PHASES OF WOUND HEALING

Hemostasis (termination of bleeding) begins as soon as the injury occurs. As blood platelets adhere to the walls of the injured vessel, a clot begins to form. Fibrin in the clot begins to hold the wound together, and bleeding subsides. The inflammation phase follows.

During the inflammatory phase, there is an initial increase in the flow of blood elements (antibodies, electrolytes, plasma proteins) and water out of the blood vessel into the vascular space. The engorgement from this allows the repair cells to move toward the wound site and causes the cardinal signs and symptoms of inflammation: erythema (redness), heat, edema (swelling), pain, and tissue dysfunction. Leukocytes appear and begin to engulf bacteria, fungi, viruses, and toxic proteins. If an infection is not present, the number of leukocytes decreases. During the inflammatory phase, cells in the injured tissue migrate, divide, and form new cells within 24 to 48 hours. As the inflammatory phase ends, new cells and capillaries fill in the wound from the underlying tissue to the skin surface. This process seals the wound and protects it from contamination.

Collagen formation occurs during the reconstruction, or proliferation, phase. During this time, the wound contracts as new tissue is reconstructed. Myofibroblasts produce collagen, a gluelike protein substance that adds tensile strength to the wound and the tissue. Collagen formation increases rapidly between postoperative days 5 and 25. During this phase, the wound fills with granulation tissue and takes on the appearance of an irregular, raised, purplish, immature scar. Wound dehiscence most frequently occurs during this phase.

Approximately 3 weeks after surgery, fibroblasts begin to exit the wound. Collagen forms and cross-links, helping the tissues and skin become stronger. The wound continues to gain strength, although healing can take up to a year and healed wounds rarely return to the strength the tissue had before surgery. Although tissue heals at varying speeds, internal wounds (stomach, colon) regain strength faster than skin wounds. Occasionally, a keloid—an overgrowth of collagenous scar tissue at the site of a wound—forms during this maturation phase. The keloid's color ranges from red to pink to white. This new tissue is elevated, rounded, and firm. African Americans, dark-complexioned whites, and young women have the highest incidence of keloid formation (Xue, 2015).

PROCESS OF WOUND HEALING

The process of wound healing occurs by primary intention (primary union), secondary intention (granulation), or tertiary (third) intention (Fig. 22.2). Wounds in which skin edges are close together and little tissue is lost, such as those made surgically, heal by **primary intention**, with the result being minimal scarring. Closure can be by sutures, staples, skin glue, or Steri-Strips. Primary intention healing begins during the inflammatory phase of healing; in surgery, this is usually during closure of the wound.

Healing by **secondary intention**, when a wound must granulate during healing, occurs when skin edges are not close together (approximated) or when pus has formed. Some wounds develop a **purulent** (producing or containing pus) **exudate** (fluid, cells, or other substances that have been slowly exuded, or discharged, from cells or blood through small pores or breaks in cell membranes) when injured or diseased tissue dies. In this case, the surgeon provides a means for its release through a drainage system or by packing the wound with gauze. Slowly, the necrotized tissue decomposes and escapes, and the cavity begins to fill with **granulation** tissue, or soft, pink, fleshy projections that consist of capillaries surrounded by fibrous collagen. The amount of granulation tissue necessary to fill the wound depends on the wound's size; scarring is greater in a large wound.

In healing by **tertiary intention** (delayed primary intention), the practitioner leaves a contaminated wound open and closes it later, after the infection is controlled, by suturing two layers of granulation tissue together in the wound. This type of healing also occurs when a primary wound becomes infected, is opened, is allowed to granulate, and then is sutured. Tertiary intention healing results in a larger and deeper scar than does healing by either primary or secondary intention.

These stages provide a model for acute (as opposed to chronic) wound healing. An important concept in wound healing is that the stages of wound healing, although progressive, do not necessarily occur in a linear (strictly sequential) fashion. Some normally healing wounds are in all three stages of wound healing simultaneously.

FACTORS THAT AFFECT WOUND HEALING

To promote healing, closely monitor fluid and nutritional needs (i.e., proteins, carbohydrates, fats, vitamins) of the patient. If the patient is not able to tolerate food or fluids, provision of total parenteral nutrition or nasogastric feedings is a possibility. Patients who are unable to tolerate large meals or solid foods may need to eat small, frequent meals. Supplementation may be needed. Foods rich in protein, vitamins A and C, and zinc assist in wound repair. Sources of protein include

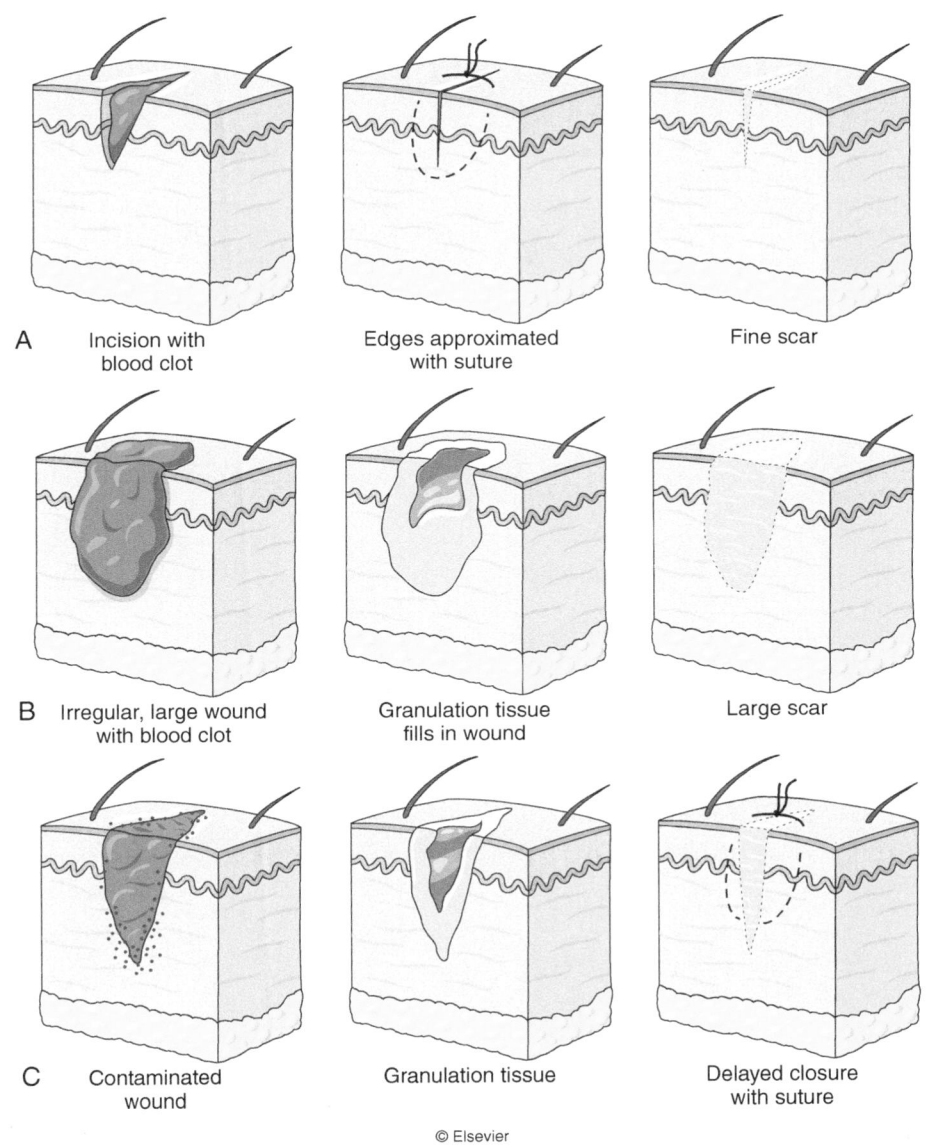

Fig. 22.2 Types of wound healing. (A) Primary intention. (B) Secondary intention. (C) Tertiary intention.

A   Incision with blood clot

Edges approximated with suture

Fine scar

B   Irregular, large wound with blood clot

Granulation tissue fills in wound

Large scar

C   Contaminated wound

Granulation tissue

Delayed closure with suture

© Elsevier

meats, peanut butter, and legumes. Dark, leafy vegetables and yellow or orange fruits and vegetables provide vitamin A. Strawberries, tomatoes, spinach, and cruciferous vegetables, including broccoli, cauliflower, and cabbage, are rich sources of vitamin C. Zinc may be obtained from fortified cereals, red meat, and seafood. Offer fluids, when tolerated, on an hourly basis. Unless contraindications exist, encourage an intake of 2000 to 2400 mL in 24 hours. As the patient progresses from clear to full liquids, provide fluids that the patient enjoys. Until the patient's hydration level is stable (usually 48 to 72 hours), monitor the patient's intake and output (I&O).

Assist the patient to achieve a balance between rest and activity. Rest helps to conserve energy that can be applied to the healing process, while activity will serve to maintain a healthy circulatory status and to decrease venous stasis. Healthy and adequate circulation is essential for delivery of oxygen and nutrients necessary for tissue reconstruction. The location and size of the incision influence the patient's movements. Take care to avoid strain on the suture line. When the patient is confined to bed, provide instruction about the best means to move in bed, moving one body section at a time—head, chest, hips, and legs. To sit up, the patient should roll to the side and, with the elbow as a lever, push to a sitting position; this reduces the stress placed on the incision. If coughing occurs, apply a pillow, rolled bath blanket, or the palms of the hands to the incisional area to lessen intraabdominal pressure; this technique is called *splinting*. Limiting of visitors sometimes may be necessary if the patient tires too easily.

Preexisting conditions, such as malnourishment, and chronic diseases (arthritis, diabetes mellitus, hypertension) add stress to the recovering body and necessitate ongoing monitoring (Table 22.1).

Table 22.1   Factors That Impair Wound Healing

PHYSIOLOGIC EFFECTS	INTERVENTIONS
Age	
Aging alters all phases of wound healing. Vascular changes impair circulation to wound site. Reduced liver function alters synthesis of clotting factors. Inflammatory response is slowed. Formation of antibodies and lymphocytes is reduced. Collagen tissue is less pliable. Scar tissue is less elastic.	Assess wound for rate of healing. Encourage diet high in vitamins A and C, protein, and zinc. Instruct patient on safety precautions to prevent injuries. Be prepared to provide wound care for longer period. Teach home caregivers wound care techniques (see the Patient Teaching box).
Malnutrition	

All phases of wound healing are impaired.
Stress from burns or severe trauma increases nutritional
   requirements.
	Provide balanced diet rich in protein, carbohydrates, lipids,
	   vitamins A and C, minerals (e.g., zinc, copper), and B
	   vitamins.
	Provide adequate amounts of calories and fluids.

Obesity	

Fatty tissue lacks adequate blood supply to resist bacterial
   infection and to deliver nutrients and cellular elements.
	Observe obese patient for signs of wound infection,
	   dehiscence, and evisceration.

Impaired Oxygenation	

Low arterial oxygen tension alters synthesis of collagen and
   formation of epithelial cells.
If local circulating blood flow is poor, tissues fail to receive
   needed oxygen.
Decreased hemoglobin (anemia) reduces arterial oxygen levels
   in capillaries and interferes with tissue repair.
	Provide diet adequate in iron, vitamin B, and folic acid.
	Monitor hematocrit and hemoglobin levels of patients with
	   wounds.

Smoking	

Smoking reduces amount of functional hemoglobin in blood,
   thus decreasing tissue oxygenation.
Smoking sometimes increases platelet aggregation and
   causes hypercoagulability.
Smoking interferes with normal cellular mechanisms that
   promote release of oxygen to tissues.
	Discourage patient from smoking by explaining its effects on
	   wound healing.

Drugs	

Steroids reduce inflammatory response.
Anti-inflammatory drugs suppress protein synthesis, wound
   contraction, epithelialization, and inflammation.
Prolonged antibiotic use increases risk of superinfection.
Chemotherapeutic drugs often depress bone marrow function,
   number of leukocytes, and inflammatory response.
	Carefully observe patient; signs of inflammation are not always
	   obvious.
	Vitamin A has the capacity to counteract effects of steroids.

Diabetes Mellitus	

Chronic disease causes small blood vessel disease that
   impairs tissue perfusion.
Diabetes causes hemoglobin to have greater affinity for
   oxygen, so it fails to release oxygen to tissues.
Hyperglycemia alters ability of leukocytes to perform
   phagocytosis and supports overgrowth of fungal and yeast
   infections.
	Instruct patient to take preventive measures to avoid cuts or
	   breaks in skin.
	Provide preventive foot care.
	Control blood sugar to reduce the physiologic changes
	   associated with diabetes.

Radiation	

Fibrosis and vascular scarring eventually develop in irradiated
   skin layers.
Tissues become fragile and poorly oxygenated.
	Closely observe patients who have had surgery for wound
	   complications.

Wound Stress	

Vomiting, abdominal distention, and respiratory effort
   sometimes stress suture line and potentially disrupt wound
   layer.
Sudden, unexpected tension on incision inhibits formation of
   endothelial cell and collagen networks.
	Control nausea with ordered antiemetics.
	Keep nasogastric tubes patent and draining to prevent
	   accumulation of secretions.
	Instruct patient to splint abdominal wound during coughing.

SURGICAL WOUND

The selection of the site for the surgical wound is based on the tissue and the organs involved, the nature of the injury or disease process, the presence of inflammation or infection, and the strength of the site. If a surgical procedure calls for a drainage system, the positioning of the drain also influences the placement of the incision. The surgeon's goal is to enter the cavity involved and repair the injured or diseased area as quickly and with the least trauma possible. To facilitate the surgery, patients often are placed in positions that add stress to the tissue. Retraction instruments often are used during procedures and compound the inflammation experienced after the surgical procedure. Pain after surgery thus results at times from strained muscles and ligaments, as well as from the surgical process.

Many options are available to the surgeon for closing the surgical incision. Common closures are sutures, staples, adhesive skin closure strips, butterfly strips, and transparent sprays and films. A binder or bandage helps to support the incision, can help secure the dressings, and makes use of adhesive materials unnecessary. A protective dressing often is used to cover the surgical wound for the first 24 hours. It is removed the day after surgery by the surgeon. After surgery, inspect the dressing hourly during the first 4 hours after the procedure. Then, inspect dressings every 2 to 4 hours for the first 24 hours. On the day of surgery, most wounds produce either sanguineous (composed of or pertaining to blood) or serosanguineous (thin and red, composed of serum and blood) exudate. Later, as the exudate subsides, it becomes serous (thin and watery, composed of the serum portion of blood) (Table 22.2). Because pressure to wounds retards bleeding, the general practice is to keep surgical wounds covered with a gauze dressing. To prevent undetected hemorrhaging, inspect the dressing or incisional area, as well as the area under the patient. Exudate follows the flow of gravity; therefore, depending on the contour of the body, the dressing sometimes remains dry even though blood or exudate is flowing away, under the body.

The extent of the inflammatory response (a tissue reaction to injury) depends on the level of injury inflicted, the size of the area involved, and the physical condition of the patient. Gradually, fluid from the cells and leukocytes collects along the vessel walls and fibrin walls of the injury and provides a matrix along which new cells form. Leukocytes perform one of their important functions, phagocytosis (a process by which certain cells engulf and dispose of microorganisms and cell debris), by surrounding, engulfing, and digesting exudate from the injured cell. The leukocyte becomes the body's vacuum cleaner by removing its debris. Evidence of leukocyte action is given through changes in the white blood cell (WBC) count. An infectious

process (a condition caused by the invasion of the body by pathogenic microorganisms) usually is evidenced by an elevated WBC count.

Table **22.2**	Types of Wound Drainage
TYPE	**APPEARANCE**
A. Serous	Watery plasma that is mostly clear, but may have some pink or yellow tinge to it
B. Purulent	Thick, yellow, green, tan, or brown
C. Serosanguineous	Pale, red, watery: mixture of serous and sanguineous
D. Sanguineous	Bright red: indicates active bleeding

STANDARD STEPS IN WOUND CARE

All nursing skills include certain basic steps to ensure the safety and well-being of both the patient and the nurse. To save space and minimize repetition, instructions for these steps are not included in the description of each skill, unless clarification of their application for that skill is necessary. Remember the following essential steps and follow them precisely to deliver appropriate and responsible nursing interventions. The rationale for the skills follows each step in parentheses.

Before performing the skill:

1. Refer to the medical record and plan of care for special interventions. *(Provides basis for care. Many nursing interventions require orders from the health care provider. Verification is ensured when the medical record is reviewed.)*

2. Provide an introduction to the patient; include name and title or role. (*Decreases patient anxiety.*)

3. Identify patients by checking armband and requesting that patients state their name and birthdate. (*Identifies correct patient for procedure.*)

4. Explain the procedure and the reason for the procedure in terms the patient is able to understand; give the patient time to ask questions. Advise the patient of any potential unpleasantness that will be experienced. (*Seeks cooperation, decreases patient's anxiety, and prepares patient. Also helps determine whether procedure is still appropriate.*)

5. Assess need for and provide patient teaching during procedure. (*Promotes patient's independence and decreases anxiety, thus improving the rate of recovery.*)

6. Assess patient. Each skill has an assessment section that includes specific data. (*Provides baseline information for later comparisons.*)

7. Perform hand hygiene and don clean gloves according to agency policy and guidelines from the CDC and the Occupational Safety and Health Administration (OSHA) (see Chapter 7). (*Reduces the spread of microorganisms.*)

8. Assemble equipment and complete necessary charges. (*Organizes procedure. Some equipment is reusable and is kept at the bedside. Some of the equipment is disposable and charged to the patient as used. Know agency policy. Specific equipment is listed for each skill.*)

9. Prepare patient for intervention:
   a. Close door or pull privacy curtain. (*Provides privacy and promotes patient's comfort.*)
   b. Raise bed to comfortable working height; lower side rail on side nearest you. (*Promotes proper body mechanics by minimizing muscle strain on caregivers and preventing injury and fatigue.*)
   c. Position and drape patient as necessary. (*Respect for privacy is basic for preserving human dignity. Patients have the right to privacy. Specific positions are included in each skill.*)

   During the skill:

10. Promote patient involvement as possible. (*Participation encourages patient motivation and cooperation.*)

11. Assess patient's tolerance, being alert for signs and symptoms of discomfort and fatigue. Inability to tolerate a procedure is described in the nursing notes. (*Patient's ability to tolerate interventions varies depending on severity of illness and disability. Nurses need to use judgment in providing the opportunity for rest and comfort measures.*)

   After completion of procedure:

12. Assist patient to a position of comfort and place needed items within easy reach. Be certain that patient has a means to call for assistance and knows how to use it. (*Promotes safety; patients who attempt to reach items that are not close risk falling or injury.*)

13. Raise the side rails and lower the bed to the lowest position. (*This reduces the risk of patients getting out of bed unattended. With use of best nursing judgment, allow alert, cooperative patients to have the side rails down during daytime hours without the risk of injury.*)

14. Remove gloves (see Skill 22.3, Step 6) and all protective barriers, such as gown, goggles, and masks, if worn. Store or remove and dispose of soiled supplies and equipment according to agency policy and guidelines from the CDC and OSHA (see Chapter 7). (*Reduces spread of microorganisms, cleans environment, and enhances patient comfort.*)

15. Perform hand hygiene after patient contact and after removing gloves (see Chapter 7). (*Wearing gloves does not eliminate the need to wash hands. Hand hygiene is the most important technique in prevention and control of the spread of microorganisms.*)

16. Document patient's response, expected or unexpected outcomes, and patient teaching. (*Timely and proper documentation records patient progress and promotes continuity of care. Recording also fulfills legal responsibility of nurse.*) Specific notes for documentation are included in each skill.

17. Report any unexpected outcomes. (*Additional therapies may be necessary.*) Specific notes for reporting are included in each skill.

CARE OF THE INCISION

Surgical wounds, because they are created under aseptic conditions, generally heal well and quickly. For prevention of trauma until epithelialization occurs, and for keeping bleeding and exposure to bacteria to a minimum, the wound usually is covered, at least initially, by a dressing. Dressings over closed wounds usually are removed by the second or third day.

Incision coverings include gauze, as well as semiocclusive and occlusive dressings (Fig. 22.3). Gauze dressings permit air to reach the wound; semiocclusive

Fig. 22.3 Types of dressings. *Clockwise, from top left:* Rolled gauze, drain dressing, Telfa non-adherent dressing, flat gauze 4 × 4, ABD.

dressings permit oxygen, but not air impurities, to pass; and occlusive dressings permit neither air nor oxygen to pass. Occlusive and semiocclusive dressings are thought to promote healing by keeping wounds moist (yet sterile), so epithelial cells are able to slide more easily over the surface of the wound during epithelialization. Tape, ties, bandages, or cloth binders sometimes may be used to secure a dressing over a wound site. The selection depends on the wound size, the location, the presence of drainage, the frequency of dressing changes, and the patient's level of activity. Montgomery straps, which remain in place around the wound while permitting the dressing over the wound to be changed, are one possibility; they reduce the need for frequent removal and reapplication of tape, which can cause considerable skin irritation (Box 22.1). The

---

Box 22.1   **How to Make Montgomery Straps**

Use of Montgomery straps to secure dressings helps prevent tape irritation of skin when dressings require frequent changing (see the figure for Step 14 in Skill 22.1). If ready-made Montgomery straps are not available, follow these steps to make them:

1. Cut several strips of 3-inch-wide (7.6 cm) hypoallergenic tape. The number of strips of tape and the length of the tape depend on the size of the dressing for the wound.
2. Fold each strip 2–3 inches (5.08–7.62 cm) back on itself (sticky sides together) to form a nonadhesive tab. Small holes should be made to allow for straps to be used to lace the Montgomery straps to secure the dressing.
3. Clean the patient's skin to prevent irritation. After the skin dries, apply skin protectant. Apply the Montgomery straps with the sticky side on the skin on either side of the dressing. Thread a separate piece of gauze tie, umbilical tape, or twill tape (about 12 inches [30.5 cm]) through each pair of holes in the straps and tie each strip similar to tying a shoelace.
4. Repeat this procedure for each of the Montgomery straps needed.
5. The straps can be left in place for several days unless they become soiled.

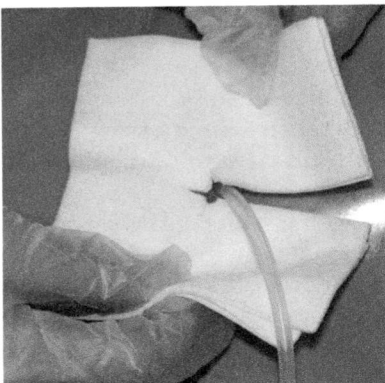

Fig. 22.4 Applying a drain dressing.

surgeon may choose to leave sutured, clean wounds undressed after surgery. This method allows atmospheric oxygen to circulate above the wound, aiding in the healing process. In some cases, if a dressing has been used for closed wounds, it is removed within 24 hours after surgery to allow air circulation. Within 24 hours, enough fibrin usually has been produced at the wound site to stop the entry of microorganisms. There are many factors that determine if this method is used, including the type of surgery, patient condition, healing process factors, and chance of infection. Refer to agency policy and the health care provider's or surgeon's preference. In many cases, the surgeon does the initial dressing change.

A dry dressing (as opposed to wet-to-dry, semiocclusive, or occlusive dressing) is often the choice for management of a wound with little exudate or drainage, such as abrasions and nondraining postoperative incisions. In addition to keeping initial bleeding to a minimum, a dry dressing protects the wound from injury, prevents introduction of bacteria, reduces discomfort, and speeds healing. A dry dressing also prevents deeper tissues from drying out by keeping the wound surface moist. The dry dressing does not debride the wound. If a dry dressing adheres to a wound, moisten the dressing with sterile normal saline solution or sterile water before removing the gauze. Moistening the dressing in this manner decreases the adherence of the dressing to the wound and reduces the risk of further trauma to the wound (Skill 22.1).

Dressing removal may be stressful to and even painful for the patient. Provide instruction about what will be experienced during the procedure. If you anticipate the dressing removal to be painful, provide analgesic at least 30 minutes before exposing a wound. If underlying drains are present, take care not to remove or displace them accidentally during dressing removal (Fig. 22.4).

Follow sterile technique whenever handling the wound or the dressing (see Chapter 7 for principles of sterile technique). *Asepsis* (absence of germs) not only protects the nurse from wound drainage, but also decreases the introduction of *pathogenic* (capable of producing disease) organisms into the wound. Use of sterile asepsis lessens the chance of the patient acquiring a health care-associated infection (Box 22.2). Use standard precautions (see Chapter 7) when handling body secretions. Good hand hygiene technique and the use of sterile aseptic procedures are essential when providing surgical wound care. Wear a gown, mask, and protective goggles if soiling or splashing of wound exudate is anticipated.

WET-TO-DRY DRESSING

The wet-to-dry dressing is a type of wound management that was used frequently in the past. Some health care providers still order wet-to-dry dressings in certain circumstances. These dressings are most appropriate for

Skill 22.1   Changing a Sterile Dry Dressing

 CHECK   GATHER   HELLO   ID   PRIVACY   EXPLAIN   WASH   GLOVES

NURSING ACTION (RATIONALE)

1. See the section "Standard Steps in Wound Care," Steps 1–9.
2. Assemble equipment:
   - Clean gloves
   - Sterile gloves
   - Refuse container
   - Dressing set
   - Sterile normal saline solution (if indicated)
   - Antiseptic swabs
   - Ointment, if ordered
   - Sterile 4 × 4 gauze squares
   - Nonadherent dressing
   - Fluff-dried or loose gauze
   - Sterile abdominal pads
   - Barrier drape (optional)
   - Tape (e.g., paper or micropore), Montgomery straps (see Box 22.1), or binder
   - Adhesive remover (optional)
   - Protective apparel (gown, goggles, mask [optional])
   - Disposable measuring device to accurately assess wound size and amount of drainage
3. Place refuse container in convenient location away from sterile field. (*Prevents need to reach across sterile field and thus prevents contamination.*)
4. Set up sterile field. (*Maintains asepsis during procedure and organizes approach to procedure.*)
   a. Open sterile dressings.
   b. Use barrier drape as needed.
   c. Open sterile gloves.
   d. Open dressing set, if needed.
   e. Prepare antiseptic swabs.
5. Loosen tape by gently removing toward incision and gently using thumb to retract skin away from tape (countertraction). (*Minimizes tissue trauma and decreases patient discomfort.*)
6. Don clean gloves, remove dressing, and discard. If drains are present, remove dressings one layer at a time. (*Prevents accidental removal of drain.*)
7. Assess status of wound and wound drainage. (*Provides evaluation of healing process and collection of data for accurate documentation.*)
8. Remove gloves; discard. Wash hands and don sterile gloves. (*Prevents spread of microorganisms and maintains surgical asepsis.*)
9. Cleanse wound and surrounding area with antiseptic swab, starting from incision and moving outward, using one stroke per swab. Discard swabs. (*Aids in removing bacteria from wound areas. Prevents contaminating previously cleaned area.*)

10. Use sterile gauze to dry in same manner or allow antiseptic to air dry. (*Drying reduces excess moisture that eventually could harbor microorganisms.*)
11. Cleanse drain site if applicable. (*Helps to remove bacteria or prevent bacteria from entering wound area.*)

12. Apply antibiotic ointment, if ordered, using same techniques as for cleansing. (*Helps reduce growth of microorganisms.*)
13. Cover wound with appropriately sized dry sterile dressing and use drain dressing, if applicable (see Fig. 22.4). (*Protects wound and skin around drain site from skin impairment.*)
14. Secure dressing with tape, Montgomery straps, or binder. Some facilities use a skin preparation at tape sites to protect skin from irritation. Consider use of Montgomery straps when dressings require frequent changing to prevent tape irritation of skin (see Box 22.1). (*Supports wound and ensures placement and stability of dressings.*)

Skill 22.1   Changing a Sterile Dry Dressing—cont'd

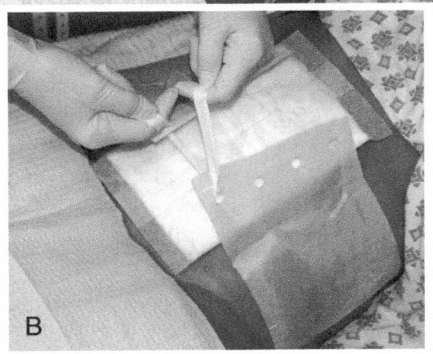

15. See the section "Standard Steps in Wound Care," Steps 10 to 17.

16. Document: *(Records patient's progress and therapy provided.)*
- Location
- Status of wound
- Description of exudate or drainage (see Table 22.2)
- Dressings applied
- Any changes
- Patient's response to procedure
- Patient teaching (see the Patient Teaching box)

17. Report to health care provider any unexpected appearance of wound or drainage or accidental removal of drain within an hour. *(Unless patient shows evidence of wound dehiscence, notification of the health care provider of unexpected findings within an hour is adequate.)*

Box 22.2	Health Care–Associated Wound Infections

- Health care–associated infections are a continual threat to patients, especially the patient after surgery.
- Virulence of the bacterial contamination and resistance of the patient are two major factors in determining whether a wound becomes infected.
- Because wound infections usually have an incubation period of 4–6 days, some patients are discharged before problems are noted.
- Patient teaching includes ongoing observations to determine whether medical treatment is necessary.
- Exudate and drainage are signs of healing, but accurate assessments sometimes provide signals of potential complications of wound healing.

wounds that do not have significant amounts of ischemic or necrotic tissue or large amounts of drainage or exudate (Skill 22.2). Traditionally, the purpose of wet-to-dry dressings was either to keep the wound bed moist or to provide mechanical debridement. Studies have called this practice into question for debridement purposes. Many health care providers no longer use this method because, during the debridement process, granulation tissue often is damaged as the dressing is removed.

Commonly used wetting agents include normal saline solution and lactated Ringer's solution, which are isotonic solutions that aid in mechanical debridement.

Acetic acid is effective against *Pseudomonas aeruginosa* but is toxic to fibroblasts in standard dilutions. Sodium hypochlorite solution (Dakin's) sometimes is used to facilitate debridement in a wound with necrotic debris and is an effective deodorizing solution. Povidone-iodine, usually one-quarter to one-half strength, is a rapid-acting antimicrobial agent for cleansing intact skin. In wounds, the solution is toxic to fibroblasts and has questionable efficacy in infected wounds. Other antibiotic solutions may be ordered, although their use is controversial. The containers of the wetting solutions should be labeled clearly with the date and time of opening. They should be discarded 24 hours after opening and replaced with fresh solution, because they can harbor microorganism growth.

ALTERNATIVES TO WET-TO-DRY DRESSING

The alternatives to wet-to-dry dressings include hydrogel gauze, hydrogel silver gauze, honey gauze, cadexomer iodine gel with high-ply gauze, hydrocolloid dressings, hydrogel dressing, and collagen dressings. The hydrocolloid dressing can be used for extra dry wound sites. This type of dressing creates an airtight bond with the skin to prevent impermeable bacteria penetration. The hydrogel dressing works with many types of wounds by providing hydration to the wound and preventing the spread of infection. The collagen dressing helps improve the movement of keratinocytes

Skill 22.2 Changing a Wet-to-Dry Dressing

CHECK | GATHER | HELLO | ID | PRIVACY | EXPLAIN | WASH | GLOVES

NURSING ACTION *(RATIONALE)*

1. See the section "Standard Steps in Wound Care," Steps 1–9.
2. Assemble equipment:
   - Barrier drape
   - Sterile dressing
   - Gauze
   - Sterile basin
   - Sterile solution
   - Antiseptic swabs
   - Instrument set, if needed
   - Clean gloves
   - Sterile gloves
   - Refuse container
   - Tape or Montgomery straps
   - Waterproof pad
3. Place waterproof pad appropriately. *(Prevents soiling of bed or linens.)*
4. Place refuse container appropriately. *(Prevents need to reach across sterile field and thus prevents contamination.)*
5. Set up sterile field. *(Maintains sterile technique during procedure and organizes approach to procedure.)*
   a. Open barrier drape.
   b. Add sterile dressing and gauze.
   c. Add sterile basin.
   d. Pour sterile solution into basin.
   e. Add instrument set, if needed.
   f. Add antiseptic swabs.
6. Loosen tape by gently removing toward incision and, using thumb, gently retracting the skin away from tape (countertraction). *(Minimizes tissue trauma. Decreases patient discomfort.)*
7. Don clean gloves. Remove dressing and discard. Do not moisten dressings to remove because this interferes with the debriding process. To be considerate of patient, provide analgesic medication at least 20–30 min before the procedure. *(Protects you from microorganisms. Prevents contamination of wound from soiled dressing and promotes patient comfort.)*
8. Assess status of wound and wound exudate or drainage on dressing (see Table 22.2). *(Provides evaluation of healing process and collection of data for accurate documentation.)*
9. Remove gloves; discard. Perform hand hygiene and don sterile gloves. *(Reduces spread of microorganisms and maintains surgical asepsis.)*

10. Cleanse wound and surrounding area with antiseptic swab, starting from incision and moving outward, using one stroke per swab. Discard swabs. *(Removes old drainage and bacteria from skin area.)*
11. Place gauze into basin. *(Wets gauze with solution.)*
12. Wring excess solution from dressing, leaving it slightly moist. *(Prevents growth of bacteria caused by dressing that is too wet.)*
13. Apply moist gauze dressing as a single layer directly onto wound surface. If wound is deep, gently pack gauze into wound with forceps until all wound surfaces are in contact with moist gauze. *(Allows solution to contact wound, which makes it effective. Moist gauze absorbs drainage and adheres to debris.)*

A

B

14. Apply dry dressing over wet gauze. *(Pulls moisture from the wound and allows for absorption of excess moisture.)*
15. Cover with additional dressing as needed. *(Protects wound from bacteria.)*
16. Secure with tape or Montgomery straps. *(Secures dressings in place.)*

Skill 22.2   Changing a Wet-to-Dry Dressing—cont'd

17. See the section "Standard Steps in Wound Care," Steps 10–17.

18. Document: (Records patient's progress and therapy provided.)
- Wound status
- Description of exudate or drainage (see Table 22.2)
- Dressings applied

- Patient's response to procedure
- Patient teaching (see the Patient Teaching box)

19. Discuss change in dressing procedure with the health care provider as wound surface becomes clean and granulation tissue is evident. (*Promotes anticipated wound healing.*)

20. Be aware this type of dressing is not widely used.

---

and fibroblasts to the wound site, which promotes healing.

TRANSPARENT DRESSINGS

Thin, self-adhesive transparent film dressings (e.g., Op-site, Tegaderm) belong in the semiocclusive or occlusive categories. As a synthetic permeable (capable of allowing the passage of fluids or substances in solution) membrane, this dressing acts as a temporary second skin. It has several advantages. It adheres to undamaged skin to contain exudate and minimize wound contamination. It also is a barrier to external fluids and bacteria, yet still allows the wound to breathe. It promotes a moist environment that speeds epithelial cell growth. This dressing type allows for wound assessment without removal of the protective film. Underlying tissue is protected against disruption caused by dressing removal. Film type dressings are beneficial for skin tears and over IV sites. Transparent dressings are available with and without adhesive borders. These dressings can stay in place up to 7 days if complete occlusion is maintained. Transparent dressings are not absorbent, so they should not be used on draining wounds.

For best results, use these dressings on clean, debrided wounds that are not bleeding actively. The film is ideal for small, superficial wounds and as a dressing over an intravenous catheter site. Apply it so that no wrinkles form, but do not stretch it over the skin. Another option in some cases is to use it over another, smaller dressing (e.g., Telfa) cut to fit the area of the wound. Impregnated gauzes are more popular. Topical medications can be applied over nonadhesive transparent dressings without disturbing the dressing. Nonadhesive transparent dressings fall off as the wound heals. Saline solution can be used to moisten dressings that may be adhering or stuck to the wound bed. Showering and bathing are permitted with the health care provider's approval.

See Skill 22.3 for applying a transparent dressing.

IRRIGATIONS

Irrigation is gentle washing of an area with a stream of solution delivered through an irrigating syringe. The benefits of wound irrigation include cleansing and medication administration. Isotonic solutions are indicated for wound irrigation. Solutions for irrigation include topical cleansers, antibiotics, antifungals, antiseptics, and anesthetics. The most common wound irrigant is normal saline solution. Principles of basic wound irrigation include the following:

1. Cleanse in a direction from the least contaminated area to the most contaminated.
2. When irrigating, be sure that all of the solution flows from the least contaminated to the most contaminated area.

Wound irrigations promote wound healing by removing debris from the wound surface, decreasing bacterial counts, and loosening and removing eschar (a black, leathery crust). Nonsurgical indications include management of pressure injuries (see Chapter 9). Meticulous hand hygiene and proper infection control procedure before and after removal of soiled dressings, coupled with proper irrigation procedures, limit the risk of health care–associated infection. Perform basic wound cleansing by applying antiseptic solutions with sterile gauze or irrigation. Skin cleansing in the area of the suture line or the drain site is indicated when an excessive amount of drainage occurs. The presence of wound exudate is an expected stage of epithelial cell growth.

When performing irrigation (Skill 22.4), be sure to provide for patient comfort; irrigation has potential to cause pain. Patients often must be medicated before the procedure is performed. Gentleness is important in performing any type of irrigation to prevent tissue damage and minimize discomfort for the patient.

Wound irrigation may be performed with various devices such as syringes, syringes with catheters attached, or syringes with needles. Gentle pressure is best in order to prevent wound trauma and reintroduction of bacteria into the wound. Use sterile technique or clean technique for wound cleansing and irrigation, depending on the type of wound. Introduce the cleansing solution directly into the wound with a syringe, syringe and catheter, shower, or whirlpool. When using a syringe, keep the tip 1 inch (2.5 cm) above the wound or area being cleansed. This prevents contamination of the syringe. Careful attention to placement of the syringe also prevents unsafe pressure of the flowing

Skill 22.3   Applying a Transparent Dressing

CHECK   GATHER   HELLO   ID   PRIVACY   EXPLAIN   WASH   GLOVES

NURSING ACTION (RATIONALE)

1. See the section "Standard Steps in Wound Care," Steps 1–9.
2. Assemble equipment:
   - Clean disposable gloves
   - Sterile gloves (optional)
   - Sterile dressing set (scissors and forceps; optional)
   - Sterile saline solution or wound cleanser (as ordered)
   - Transparent dressings (size as needed and sterile 2 × 2 gauze pad)
   - Refuse container (waterproof bag)
3. Position refuse container within easy reach of work area. (*Helps prevent spread of microorganisms.*)
4. Don clean gloves. (*Protects you from patient's body fluids.*)
5. Remove old dressings by pulling back slowly across dressing in direction of hair growth and toward the center. (*Reduces excoriation, pain, and irritation of skin after dressing removal.*)
6. Remove disposable gloves by pulling them inside out over soiled dressings and dispose of them in refuse container. (*Provides containment of soiled dressings and prevents contact of the hands with drainage.*)

7. Inspect wound for color, odor, and drainage or exudates. Measure if indicated. (*Appearance indicates status of wound healing.*)
8. Clean area gently, swabbing toward area of most exudate, or spray with cleanser; know agency policy and physician's order. (*Reduces transmission from contaminated area to cleaner site.*)
9. Reapply sterile or clean gloves as indicated. (*Prevents risk of exposure to body fluids if present.*)
10. Dry skin around wound thoroughly with sterile gauze. Be sure skin surface is dry. (*Transparent dressings with adhesive backing do not adhere to damp surface.*)
11. Apply transparent dressing according to manufacturer's direction.
    a. Remove paper backing, taking care not to allow adhesive areas to touch each other. (*Often results in wrinkles and becomes impossible to use.*) NOTE: Chevrons of tape (wrapped around the needle head) are no longer widely used because the tape is not sterile and may cause infection.
    b. Place film smoothly over wound without stretching.

c. Label with date, initials, and time, as agency policy requires. (*Communicates information to oncoming caregiver.*)

Skill 22.3   Applying a Transparent Dressing—cont'd

12. Remove gloves, discard them in refuse container, and wash hands. (*Prevents transmission of microorganisms.*)
13. See the section "Standard Steps in Wound Care," Steps 10–17.
14. Document: (*Records care given and progress of wound.*)
    - Wound status
    - Description of exudate or drainage
    - Dressing applied
    - Patient's response to procedure
    - Patient teaching
15. Report any unexpected appearance of the wound or exudates. (*Further treatment may be necessary.*)

Skill 22.4   Performing a Sterile Irrigation

CHECK   GATHER   HELLO   ID   PRIVACY   EXPLAIN   WASH   GLOVES

NURSING ACTION (RATIONALE)

1. See the section "Standard Steps in Wound Care," Steps 1–9.
2. Assemble equipment:
    - Refuse container
    - Clean gloves
    - Sterile gloves
    - Dressing set
    - Antiseptic swabs
    - Sterile basin
    - Warmed, sterile irrigation solution (200–1000 mL)
    - Irrigation syringe or spray bottle or soft catheter for deep wounds
    - Clean basin
    - Waterproof pad
    - Sterile dressings
    - Gown and goggles (optional)
    - Tape, gauze, and elastic bandage, if appropriate
    - Mask (optional)
3. Position waterproof pad appropriately. (*Protects patient and bed linens from contaminated fluids.*)
4. Place refuse container in convenient location away from sterile field. (*Prevents need to reach across sterile field and thus prevents contamination.*)
5. Set up sterile field. (*Maintains asepsis during procedure and organizes approach to procedure.*)
    a. Set up sterile basin.
    b. Add sterile, warmed irrigation solution to basin.
    c. Add antiseptic swabs.
    d. Open sterile gloves.
    e. Add dressing set (optional).
    f. Add sterile syringe and catheter if necessary.
    g. Add disposable measuring device.
6. Don gown and goggles if potential for splashing exists. (*Provides protection from body fluids.*)
7. Don clean gloves and remove dressing. Discard dressing in refuse container. (*Provides protection from pathogens and prevents wound contamination from soiled dressing.*)
8. Remove gloves, discard into proper receptacle, and wash hands. (*Reduces transmission of microorganisms.*)

Continued

Skill 22.4   Performing a Sterile Irrigation—cont'd

9. Assess status of wound and exudate or drainage on dressing (see Table 22.2). (*Provides evaluation of healing process and collection of data for accurate documentation.*)

10. Place collection basin appropriately. (*Collects contaminated solution.*)

11. Perform hand hygiene and don sterile gloves. (*Maintains asepsis.*)

12. Cleanse area around wound with antiseptic swabs. (*Removes bacteria and drainage.*)

13. Fill irrigating syringe with solution. Attach soft catheter if irrigating a deep wound with small opening. (*Allows for direct flow of solution into wound.*) Use a 19-gauge needle (or angiocatheter) with a 35-mL syringe to clean most pressure ulcers, especially deep ulcers.

14. Instill solution gently into wound, holding syringe approximately 1 inch (2.54 cm) above wound. If using catheter, gently insert into wound opening until slight resistance is met, pull back, and gently instill solution. (*Minimizes tissue trauma, irritation, and bleeding.*)

15. Allow solution to flow from clean area of wound to dirty area. Position patient to facilitate drainage. (*Prevents contamination of clean tissue by exudate.*)

16. Pinch off catheter during withdrawal from wound. (*Avoids aspiration of contaminating fluid into syringe.*)

17. Refill syringe and continue irrigation until solution returns clear. (*Thoroughly cleanses wound.*)

18. Blot wound edges with sterile gauze. (*Prevents tissue damage from excess moisture.*)

19. Dress wound again, if applicable. (*Protects wound from injury and microorganisms and provides for patient comfort.*)

20. See the section "Standard Steps in Wound Care," Steps 10–17.

21. Document: (*Records care given and progress of wound.*)
    • Status of wound
    • Performance of wound irrigation
    • Solution used
    • Character of exudate and drainage
    • Patient's response to procedure
    • Patient teaching (see the Patient Teaching box)

22. Report immediately to the health care provider any evidence of fresh bleeding, sharp increase in pain, retention of irrigant, or signs of shock. (*These are signs of tissue damage and fistula or sinus tract development. Shock phenomena sometimes indicate internal bleeding or tissue damage.*)

solution. Ensure that the flow of irrigant moves from the area being cleansed to an area that is distal to and lower than the wound area. In wound care, the area being cleansed is considered clean, and the surrounding skin surfaces are considered contaminated, without respect to whether the wound is infected. Within the wound, direct the flow from healthy tissue toward infected tissue. If the patient has a deep wound with a narrow opening, attach a soft catheter to the syringe to maintain sterile technique while permitting the fluid to enter the wound. The amount of irrigation volume is based on the wound size and level of contamination. To prevent fluid being retained in the wound, position patients on their side to encourage the irrigant to flow away from the wound. With small wounds, it is often helpful to use a 35-mL syringe with a 19-gauge needle attached to obtain optimal pressure for cleansing with

minimal risk of tissue injury. Care must be taken to not touch the wound or surrounding tissue with the needle.

If a special solution is not necessary, ambulatory or home patients are sometimes able to use a handheld shower for wound cleansing, holding the shower spray approximately 12 inches (30.48 cm) from the wound. If the force of the spray results in too much pressure for comfort, suggest that the patient tie a clean washcloth around the shower head to disperse the force. During the procedure, protect the surrounding area and assisting care providers from splashing from the wound. An alternative means of irrigating wounds in acute care areas is the shower table, frequently used for cleansing in burn and trauma wound care units. For patients who need cleansing but cannot tolerate the methods mentioned earlier, the whirlpool is useful. Physical therapists often perform or assist with performing the whirlpool procedure and then help to apply the necessary dressings.

COMPLICATIONS OF WOUND HEALING

Impaired wound healing, regardless of the cause, requires accurate observation and ongoing interventions. Because wound complications are potentially life threatening, it is vital throughout the patient's recovery phase to monitor signs and symptoms and to assess their severity (Table 22.3).

Wound bleeding potentially indicates a slipped suture, dislodged clot, coagulation problem, or trauma to blood vessels or tissue. To help detect increased drainage and color changes, inspect the wound and dressing. The dressing should be marked with the time and initials of the nurse making the observation. Initial surgical dressings may require reinforcement if they become soiled. If hemorrhage results internally, the dressing sometimes remains dry while the surrounding tissues or body cavity collect blood. Be attuned to the signs of internal bleeding, including restlessness; rapid, thready pulse; decreased blood pressure; decreased urinary output; and cool, clammy skin. Monitoring vital signs, I&O, skin condition, wound site, and overall patient response facilitates the timely identification of hemorrhage and hypovolemic shock. Internal abdominal bleeding, if allowed to continue, results in the abdomen becoming rigid and distended. If hemorrhage is not detected and stopped, hypovolemic shock occurs and can lead to collapse of the circulatory system, causing death.

When wound layers separate, resulting in dehiscence, some patients report a feeling that something has given way (refer to *Adult Health Nursing,* Chapter 2). Sometimes, this feeling is brought on by periods of sneezing, coughing, or vomiting. Evidence of serosanguineous drainage on the dressing is an important sign to assess because dehiscence sometimes is preceded by serosanguineous drainage. If the wound is not covered and dehiscence occurs, the patient remains in bed and receives nothing by mouth (NPO). If possible, encourage the patient not to cough; place a warm, moist, sterile dressing over the area until the surgeon evaluates the site; and provide reassurance. When a skin suture breaks and dehiscence occurs, the wound may be closed effectively with Steri-Strips or a butterfly strip, after which the surgeon should be notified. Dehiscence most frequently occurs between postoperative days 5 and 12. Because most patients have been discharged from the hospital by day 12, they will require patient teaching on how to recognize dehiscence and what care to provide.

If an evisceration (when internal organs protrude through opened incision) follows the dehiscence, the patient is to remain in bed in a low-Fowler's position, with the knees flexed to reduce pressure on the

Table 22.3	Terms Associated With Wound Complications
TERM	**DEFINITION**
Abscess	Cavity that contains pus and is surrounded by inflamed tissue, formed as a result of suppuration in a localized infection
Adhesion	Band of scar tissue that binds two anatomic surfaces normally separated; most commonly found in the abdomen
Cellulitis	Infection of the skin characterized by heat, pain, erythema, and edema
Dehiscence	Separation of a surgical incision or rupture of a wound closure
Evisceration	Protrusion of an internal organ through a wound or surgical incision
Extravasation	Passage or escape into the tissues; usually of blood, serum, or lymph
Hematoma	Collection of extravasated blood trapped in the tissues or in an organ that results from incomplete hemostasis after surgery or injury

Box 22.3	Responding to Wound Evisceration

If a patient's wound eviscerates, prompt action is needed to reduce further complications.
1. Remain with the patient and either notify the health care provider or ask a coworker to notify the health care provider. Wound evisceration is considered a medical emergency.
2. Place the patient into a low-Fowler's position with the knees slightly flexed. This position helps to relieve pressure on the wound. This will prevent further dehiscence of the wound edges and reduces the risk of further evisceration.
3. The protruding organ is covered with a sterile dressing moistened with sterile normal saline solution. This keeps the eviscerated organ moist and helps to prevent microorganisms from entering the wound.
4. Monitor the patient closely and assess vital signs and pulse oximetry readings to determine if the patient is exhibiting signs of shock.
5. Make sure the patient remains on NPO because the patient will need surgical correction of the evisceration.
6. Reassure the patient and family because the occurrence of a wound evisceration is often frightening.

Modified from Harkreader H, Hogan MA, Thobaben M: *Fundamentals of nursing,* ed 3, Philadelphia, 2007, Saunders.

wound. Keep the patient on NPO status, and cover the wound and contents with warm, sterile saline solution dressings. Notify the surgeon immediately (Box 22.3). Provide emotional support and explain to the patient what has happened and what can be expected in the next phase of care. Surgery is required to treat wound evisceration.

Wound infection, or wound sepsis, results when the wound becomes contaminated. The CDC labels a wound infected when it contains purulent (pus) drainage. A patient with an infected wound displays a fever, tenderness and pain at the wound site, edema, and an elevated WBC count. Purulent drainage has an odor and is brown, yellow, or green, depending on the pathogen. Culture of the exudate from an infected wound confirms the presence of the pathogenic organism, after which the appropriate medical therapy is ordered (see Chapter 23).

STAPLE AND SUTURE REMOVAL

Institutional policy determines whether only the health care provider or the health care provider and the nurse may remove sutures and staples. Always obtain the health care provider's written order before implementing either skill. The time of removal is based on the stage of incisional healing and the extent of surgery.

Sutures and staples generally are removed in 7 to 10 days after surgery if healing is adequate. Sometimes one suture or staple comes out at a time, and sometimes removal is in two phases. First, every other suture or staple is removed and replaced with a Steri-Strips. Then, the remaining sutures or staples are removed in the same fashion. The health care provider determines the timing and method and orders the removal.

Sutures are threads of wire or other material (silk, steel, cotton, linen, or nylon) used to sew body tissues together. Sutures are placed within tissue layers in deep wounds and, superficially, as the final means for wound closure. The deeper sutures usually are made of an absorbable material that disappears in several days. Many kinds of sutures are used: interrupted or separate sutures, continuous sutures, blanket sutures, and retention sutures covered with rubber tubing to provide greater strength (used primarily in obese patients who have had abdominal surgery). The cosmetic result of these latter sutures is often not as desirable as that obtained with finer suture material (Fig. 22.5).

Staples are made of stainless-steel wire, are quick to use, and provide ample strength. They are popular for skin closure of abdominal incisions and orthopedic surgery when appearance of the incision is not critical (Fig. 22.6). The time of removal is based on the stage of incisional healing and the extent of surgery. Sutures and staples are generally removed within 7 to 10 days after surgery if healing is adequate. Retention sutures are left in place longer (22 days or more). Leaving sutures in too long makes removal more difficult and increases the risk of infection. Removal of staples requires a sterile staple extractor and maintenance of aseptic technique (Skill 22.5). After the suture removal is complete, inspect the area to ensure that all of the sutures or staples have been removed.

© Elsevier

Fig. 22.5 Sutures. (A) Interrupted, or separate, sutures. (B) Continuous suture. (C) Blanket continuous suture. (D) Retention suture covered with rubber tubing to provide greater strength.

Fig. 22.6 Wound closure with staples.

Remove every other suture or staple first and replace each with an adhesive closure strip (Fig. 22.7); if the incision remains securely closed, remove the rest with the same process. If any sign of suture line separation is evident during the removal process, leave the remaining sutures in place, document a description, and report it to the health care provider. In some cases,

Skill 22.5   Removing Staples or Sutures (Applying Steri-Strips)

NURSING ACTION *(RATIONALE)*

1. See the section "Standard Steps in Wound Care," Steps 1–9.
2. Assemble equipment:
   - Refuse container
   - Clean gloves
   - Sterile gloves (optional)
   - Sterile sutures or staple removal set
   - Antiseptic swabs
   - Appropriate sterile dressings, including butterfly or adhesive Steri-Strips
   - Compound benzoin tincture or other skin protectant such as Skin Prep
3. Place refuse container in convenient location away from sterile field. *(Prevents need to reach across sterile field and thus prevents contamination.)*
4. Set up sterile field. *(Maintains asepsis during procedure and organizes approach to procedure.)*
   a. Open suture or staple set.
   b. Open sterile dressings (use sterile barrier if necessary for sterile field).
5. Remove dressing and soiled gloves. Discard into plastic refuse bag. (Use bag as needed for additional refuse.) *(Protects you from microorganisms and prevents contamination from soiled dressing.)*
6. Assess status of wound and drainage on dressing. *(Allows determination of alterations in healing process and collection of data for accurate documentation.)*
7. Perform hand hygiene and don sterile gloves. *(Allows for safe handling of sterile equipment.)*
8. Cleanse area with antiseptic swabs, starting from incision outward, using one stroke per swab. *(Removes bacteria from wound area.)*

STAPLE REMOVAL

On removal of sutures, the health care provider removes one to three sutures at a time and applies Steri-Strips in their place. This action is repeated until all sutures are removed and Steri-Strips applied.

9. Prepare patient for pulling sensation and site tenderness during removal. Place staple remover under staple while slowly closing the ends of the staple remover together. Squeeze the center of the staple with the tips, freeing the staple from the skin. *(Prevents putting excess pressure on suture line and secures removal of each staple.)*

10. Release handles and discard staple in refuse container. *(Prevents contamination of sterile field with used staple.)*
11. Repeat Steps 9 and 10 until all staples have been removed. *(Permits complete removal of all staples.)* Every other staple may be removed and Steri-Strips applied, or two or three staples removed at a time and Steri-Strips applied until all staples have been removed and Steri-Strips applied.
12. Count number of staples removed. *(Provides count for documentation.)*

SPECIAL CONSIDERATIONS FOR SUTURE AND STAPLE REMOVAL

- Wire sutures are removed by the nurse or primary care provider.
- Limit amount of dressing supplies, because either a light dressing or no dressing is needed after suture or staple removal.
- Notify health care provider immediately if inadequate wound healing is noted; discontinue removal of staples.
- It is common to see wounds closed with Steri-Strips, or sterile tape applied along both sides of a wound to keep the edges approximated and closed (see Fig. 22.7).

Continued

Skill 22.5   Removing Staples or Sutures (Applying Steri-Strips)—cont'd

INTERVENTIONS TO FOLLOW WHEN APPLYING STERI-STRIPS

13. Prepare incision for Steri-Strip application.

  a. Gently cleanse suture line with antiseptic swab. *(Removes as much surface bacteria as possible.)*

  b. Carefully inspect the incision. *(Ensures that all sutures have been removed.)*

  c. Apply tincture of benzoin to the skin on each side of suture line over an area 1½–2 inches (4–5 cm) wide and allow to dry a few minutes until tacky. *(Makes Steri-Strips adhere more securely.)*

  d. When skin is dry, cut Steri-Strips to allow strips to extend 1½–2 inches (4–5 cm) on each side of the incision. Some health care providers request that the strips be placed side by side, whereas others request they be spaced evenly and appropriately apart (see Fig. 22.6).

  e. Instruct patient to take showers rather than soak in bathtub according to health care provider's preference. During showering, the patient should be advised to engage in positions that limit direct contact by the water spray with the Steri-Strips. Steri-Strips are not removed and are allowed to loosen and peel off gradually over the course of 3–5 days. Strip edges that begin to peel away from the skin may be clipped off.

14. Assess healing status of wound. *(Determines need for butterfly or Steri-Strip skin closures.)*

  a. Cleanse area with antiseptic swabs. *(Decreases the risk of infection.)*

REMOVAL OF INTERRUPTED SUTURES (SEE FIG. 22.5A)

15. Each suture has a knot. Each interrupted suture is secured with its own knot. Knots are lined up on the same side of incision.

16. Grasp and elevate knotted end of suture with hemostat or forceps. *(Exposes the knot and ensures removal of suture and maintains skin integrity.)*

17. Snip suture at skin level on opposite side, proximal to knot. *(Releases suture.)*

18. Gently remove entire suture with forceps and discard on sterile gauze. *(Prevents contaminating sterile field with used materials.)*

19. Repeat Steps 16–18 until all sutures have been removed. *(Ensures removal of all sutures.)*

REMOVAL OF CONTINUOUS SUTURES (SEE FIG. 22.5)

20. To remove continuous sutures:

  a. Snip suture close to skin surface at end distal to knot.

  b. Snip second suture on same side.

  c. Grasp knot and gently pull with continuous smooth action, removing suture from beneath the skin. Place suture on gauze.

  d. Grasp and lift next suture, and snip with tip of scissors close to skin.

  e. Grasp suture and gently remove loop of suture. Never pull the contaminated suture through tissue.

  f. Repeat these steps until the end knot is reached. Cut the last one and remove it by grasping and pulling the knot.

REMOVAL OF BLANKET CONTINUOUS SUTURE (SEE FIG. 22.5C)

21. To remove blanket continuous sutures:

  a. Cut the suture opposite the looped blanket edge.

  b. Remove each suture by grasping at the looped end.

22. Apply sterile dressing or leave open to air as ordered. (Dressing is often needed only if patient's clothing will irritate wound area.) *(Protects wound and facilitates healing process.)*

23. See the section "Standard Steps in Wound Care," Steps 10–17.

24. Document: *(Records care given and progress of wound.)*

  • Number of staples or sutures removed

  • Condition of staple or suture line

  • Patient's response

  • Dressings applied, if necessary

  • Patient teaching (see the Patient Teaching box)

Fig. 22.7 Steri-Strips placed over incision for closure.

these sutures are left in place and removed several days to a week later.

The patient's history of wound healing, the site of the wound, the tissues involved, and the purpose of the sutures determine the selection of the suture material. For example, a patient with repeated abdominal surgeries often needs wire sutures for greater strength to promote wound closure.

EXUDATE AND DRAINAGE

Exudate is fluid, cells, or other substances that have leaked slowly from cells or blood vessels through small pores or breaks in cell membrane. Drainage is the removal of fluids from a body cavity, wound, or other source of discharge by one or more methods; it may occur passively on its own or with mechanical assistance (see the section "Drainage Systems").

Exudate and drainage are described as serous, sanguineous, or serosanguineous. Serous exudate or drainage is a clear, watery fluid that has been separated from its solid elements (e.g., the exudate from a blister). Serous fluid has the characteristics of serum, which is the clear, thin, sticky fluid portion of blood that remains after coagulation. In contrast, sanguineous exudate or drainage is fluid that contains blood. Thus, serosanguineous exudate or drainage is thin and red (usually described as pink) because it is composed of serum and blood. If the tissue is infected, exudate or drainage is likely to be purulent. The color of the purulent (pus) drainage is dependent on the causative organism and may commonly be seen as thick yellow or green exudate. Exudate or drainage from specific organs has its own color (e.g., bile from the liver and gallbladder is green or green-brown).

The type and the amount of exudate or drainage produced depend on the tissue and organs involved. Treat exudate or drainage in quantities greater than 300 mL in the first 24 hours as abnormal and report it immediately. When patients first ambulate, a slight increase of exudate or drainage sometimes occurs. If sanguineous exudate or drainage continues, small blood vessels possibly may be oozing.

Not all surgical wounds drain. If exudate or drainage does occur, accurate assessments are vital. The following exudate and drainage characteristics are important to note and chart: color, amount, consistency (thick or thin), and odor. If the exudate or drainage has a pungent or strong odor, infection is likely. Perform a wound culture (see Chapter 23). Exudate most likely is contained either in a drainage system or on a dressing. If a dressing is used, you can monitor the amount of exudate or drainage (such as from a Penrose drain) by circling and dating the drainage area and comparing the circled area with later observations, or by reporting the number and the type of dressings used and saturated over a specific interval. Until the surgeon orders a dressing change, never remove the soiled dressings, only reinforce them.

DRAINAGE SYSTEMS

Frequently, surgical procedures are performed to remove or repair organs that lie within the body (e.g., gallbladder removal, hip replacement). In these cases, the inflammatory response will result in excess fluid buildup in the cavity or tissues. The presence of this fluid can increase the pressure on the surgical area and provides an area that supports the growth of bacteria. To prevent either of these scenarios, a mechanism is needed to assist in removal of exudate from the cavity. To facilitate drainage, the surgeon makes a secondary incision, or stab wound, close to the surgical incision. The site for the stab wound is planned deliberately. The surgeon's intent is to drain exudate away from the incision, not toward it. If the exudate enters the surgical incision, contamination and infection are likely to follow.

Several methods are available to facilitate the flow of exudate away from the wound site. *Closed drainage* is a system of tubing or other apparatus attached to the body to remove fluid in an airtight circuit that prevents environmental contaminants from entering the wound or cavity. *Open drainage* passes through an open-ended tube into a receptacle or out onto the dressing. *Suction drainage* uses a pump or other mechanical device to help extract a fluid (Skill 22.6).

Gentle suction is needed in some surgeries to help gravity move the exudate. A drainage system is chosen to fit the area to be drained, according to the type of exudate and amount of drainage expected. A rubber

Skill 22.6   Maintaining Hemovac or Davol Suction and T-Tube Drainage

NURSING ACTION (RATIONALE)

1. See the section "Standard Steps in Wound Care," Steps 1–9.
2. Assemble equipment:
   - Clean gloves
   - Alcohol pads
   - Swabs
   - Calibrated drainage receptacle
   - Moisture-proof padding (optional)
3. Examine drainage system (pump and tubing) for seal, patency, and stability (see Figs. 22.8 and 22.9). If not working, notify head nurse or health care provider. (*Maintains efficiency of system.*)
4. Don goggles, if appropriate. (*Protects eyes from contaminants.*)
5. Remove Hemovac or Davol plug labeled "pouring spout." (*Permits accurate measuring of drainage.*)
   a. Empty drainage into measuring device.
   b. When emptying Hemovac, compress device by pushing top and bottom together with your hands.
6. Hold pump of Hemovac tightly compressed and reinsert plug to reestablish closed drainage system. When caring for a Davol, reestablish suction by pumping bulb until balloon is inflated completely. Recap drainage port. For Hemovac and Davol, keep plug out of drainage stream; hold the plug by stem. (*Maintains unit sterility.*)

7. Observe the drainage for color, consistency, and odor. (*Provides basis for documentation.*)
8. Measure and record amount of drainage; rinse measuring container. (*Provides basis for documentation.*)
9. Position drainage system on bed, and secure system. (*Maintains efficiency of system.*)
10. Dispose of drainage and rinse container. Remove gloves and wash hands. (*Reduces spread of microorganisms.*)
11. If specimen is ordered, send to laboratory. (If dressing change is necessary, do it at this time.) (*Provides continuity of care.*)
12. Observe Davol or Hemovac every 2–4 h. (*Ascertains integrity of suction.*) Measure drainage every 8 h or as ordered. (*Recording an accurate output of drainage is necessary so that the health care provider can determine any change in the amount or the character of wound drainage.*)
13. See the section "Standard Steps in Wound Care," Steps 10–17.
14. Document: (*Records care given and progress of wound.*)
    - Time of procedure
    - Amount of drainage
    - Characteristics of drainage
    - Patient response
    - Suction reestablished
    - Patient teaching (see the Patient Teaching box)
15. Report any abnormal characteristics of drainage (see Table 22.2).

A drainage system requires close monitoring. In addition to noting the color, the consistency, and the amount of drainage, check the tube's patency. Do not allow a tube to become kinked or occluded; if blood clots or exudate have slowed drainage, record this and report it.

or plastic drain sometimes is used to remove exudate from the wound and bring it out through the skin onto a dressing (open drainage system); sometimes, it is positioned through the surgical incision or stab wound. Although not used as frequently, the Penrose drain is an example of a drain that works by gravity. When it is inserted, a sterile safety pin is placed through the drain to keep it from sliding into the wound. When the surgeon wants a gentle vacuum, a closed drainage system can be used. The portable vacuum container (e.g., Hemovac) is an expandable unit connected by tubes to the drainage site (see Skill 22.6). As the unit creates gentle suction, exudate collects in the drainage receptacle. The Jackson-Pratt evacuator is another type of closed drainage system that uses a bulb to provide the needed vacuum (Figs. 22.8 and 22.9). Most drainage systems used today are closed systems to better control and monitor the drainage from a wound. Containment of drainage reduces the risk of infection and minimizes contact with the patient's skin, thereby reducing the risk of complications.

T-Tube Drainage System
After surgical removal of the gallbladder (via an open cholecystectomy), the bile duct often is inflamed and edematous. The health care provider frequently inserts a drainage tube into the duct to maintain a free flow of bile until edema subsides. This tube is called a **T tube**. The long end of the T tube exits through the abdominal incision or through a separate surgical wound (Fig. 22.10). The tube drains by gravity into a closed drainage system. The collection bag is emptied and measured every shift or as necessary (Box 22.4).

Wound Vacuum-Assisted Closure
Negative pressure wound therapy may be beneficial in the management of some surgical wounds. The treatment uses a machine commonly referred to as a vacuum-assisted closure device (wound VAC). The wound VAC functions by applying negative pressure to wounds. Healing of the wound is facilitated by increased blood flow, improved or increased fluid drainage, and enhanced wound closure as the pressure draws the edges of the wound together. VAC accelerates wound healing by promoting the formation of granulation tissue, collagen, fibroblasts, and inflammatory cells to close completely or improve the condition of a wound in preparation for a skin graft. The use of negative pressure removes fluid from the area surrounding the wound, thus reducing local or peripheral edema and improving circulation to the area (Fig. 22.11). In addition, after 3 or 4 days of therapy, bacterial counts in the wound drop.

Wound VAC is used to treat acute wounds (such as traumatic wounds, flaps, and grafts) and chronic wounds. The schedule for changing wound VAC dressings varies. An infected wound sometimes calls

Fig. 22.10 **T tube.** (From Parks RW, Garden OJ: *Principles and practice of surgery*, ed 7, Philadelphia, 2018, Elsevier Ltd.)

Fig. 22.8 Jackson-Pratt drains have wide, flat areas that must be brought through the stab wound with great force.

Fig. 22.9 Jackson-Pratt drainage device. (A) Drainage tubes and reservoir. (B) Emptying drainage reservoir.

Box 22.4   Care of the T-Tube Drainage System

Nursing interventions for the patient with bile drainage include the following:

- Make sure specific measures or techniques for dressing changes are in the nursing care plan to provide continuity of care.
- Assess the patency of the drainage tube frequently, preventing twists or kinks to ensure appropriate, continuous drainage.
- Keep the collection receptacle below the level of the wound or common bile duct to ensure appropriate drainage.
- Keep the receptacle compressed, and frequently monitor it to maintain a vacuum. (Many Ttube drainage systems use drainage by gravity only.)
- Protect the skin surrounding the wound from bile drainage to prevent tissue damage.
- Assess excessive bile leakage from the wound because it may indicate occlusion of drainage tube.
- Assess for normal bile drainage: amount varies from 250 to 500 mL/24 h, with color normally greenish brown, thick, and slightly blood-tinged in the first 24 hours.
- Consider the use of Montgomery straps when the dressing requires frequent changing to prevent tape from impairing skin integrity (see Box 22.1 and Skill 22.1, Step 14).
- Assess the need for patient teaching during the dressing change and wound care.
- Secure the vacuum unit to the patient's gown with a safety pin, avoiding tension on the tubing.
- Record the amount of drainage on the intake and output (I&O) sheet to provide an accurate I&O record.

Fig. 22.11 Wound VAC system uses negative pressure to remove fluid from area surrounding the wound, reducing edema and improving circulation to the area. (Courtesy Kinetic Concepts, Inc. [KCI], San Antonio, Texas.)

for a dressing change every 24 hours, whereas dressing changes three times a week suffice for a clean wound. During dressing changes, care must be taken to remove all sponges and remnants. Retained materials left on the wound may cause delays in healing and abscess formation. As the wound heals, the wound base becomes redder and granulation tissue lines its surface. The wound has a granulated appearance. Last, the surface area of the wound changes size, either increasing

or decreasing depending on wound location and the amount of drainage removed by the wound VAC system. As the wound heals, paler areas in the wound often develop. This indicates an increase in fibrous tissue. The wound has to be assessed for location, appearance, and size. This provides information regarding status of wound healing, presence of complications, and the proper type of supplies and assistance needed to apply the new transparent dressing (Skill 22.7).

Assess the patient's comfort level with use of a scale of 0 to 10. This determines effectiveness of comfort control measures before, during, and after dressing change. Determine the patient's knowledge of the purpose of the dressing change because this determines the level of support and explanation required. Focus on the expected outcomes of preventing infection, promoting healing, control of pain, and patient and family education.

BANDAGES AND BINDERS

A **bandage** is a strip or roll of cloth or other material that can be wound around a part of the body in a variety of ways for multiple purposes. Bandages are available in rolls of various widths and materials, including gauze, elasticized knit, elastic webbing, flannel, and muslin. Gauze bandages are lightweight and inexpensive, mold easily around contours of the body, and permit air circulation that helps to prevent skin maceration (the softening and breaking down of skin from prolonged exposure to moisture). Elastic bandages conform well to body parts but also can be used to exert pressure over a body part. Flannel and muslin bandages are thicker than gauze and, thus, stronger for supporting or applying pressure. A flannel bandage also insulates to provide warmth.

A **binder** is a bandage made of large pieces of material to fit a specific body part (e.g., an abdominal binder or a breast binder). Most binders are made of elastic, cotton, muslin, or flannel.

Correctly applied bandages and binders do not cause injury to underlying and nearby body parts or create discomfort for the patient (Skills 22.8 and 22.9; Table 22.4). For example, an abdominal binder must not be tight enough to restrict chest wall expansion for breathing. Before a bandage or binder is applied, the nursing responsibilities include the following (see the Coordinated Care box):

- Inspecting the skin for abrasions, edema, discoloration, or exposed wound edges
- Covering exposed wounds or open abrasions with sterile dressings
- Assessing the condition of underlying dressings and changing them if soiled
- Assessing the skin of underlying body parts and parts that will be distal to the bandage for signs of circulatory impairment (coolness, pallor or cyanosis, diminished or absent pulses, numbness, and tingling) to provide a means for comparing changes in circulation after bandage application

Skill 22.7   Wound Vacuum-Assisted Closure

NURSING ACTION *(RATIONALE)*

1. See the section "Standard Steps in Wound Care," Steps 1–9.
2. Assemble equipment:
   - VAC system (requires health care provider's order)
   - VAC foam dressing
   - Tubing for connection between VAC system and VAC dressing
   - Gloves, clean and sterile
   - Scissors (sterile)
   - SKIN-PREP or skin barrier
   - Moist washcloth
   - Plastic or waterproof refuse bag
   - Linen bag

VAC unit

Connective tubing

Absorbent foam dressing

3. Position patient comfortably and drape to expose only wound site. Instruct patient not to touch wound or sterile supplies. *(Maintaining patient comfort assists in completing skill smoothly. Draping provides access to wound while keeping exposure to a minimum.)*
4. Place disposable waterproof bag within reach of work area with top folded to make a cuff. *(Facilitates safe disposal of soiled dressings.)*
5. When VAC system is in place, begin by pushing therapy on-off button. *(Deactivates therapy and allows for proper drainage of fluid in drainage tubing.)*
   a. Keeping tube connected to VAC system, disconnect tubes from each other to drain fluids into canister.
   b. Before lowering, tighten clamp on canister tube.
6. With dressing tube unclamped, introduce 10–30 mL of normal saline solution, if ordered, into tubing to soak underneath foam. *(Facilitates loosening of foam when tissue adheres to foam.)*
7. Gently stretch transparent film horizontally and slowly pull up from the skin. *(Reduces stress on wound edges and reduces irritation and discomfort.)*

8. Remove old VAC system dressing, observing appearance and drainage on dressing. Use caution to prevent tension on any drains that are present. Discard dressing and remove gloves. Perform hand hygiene. *(Determines dressings needed for replacement. Prevents accidental removal of drains that are sometimes sutured in place and sometimes not.)*
9. Apply sterile or clean gloves. Irrigate the wound (see Skill 22.4) with normal saline solution or other solution ordered by the health care provider. Gently blot to dry. (If this is a new surgical wound, sterile technique may be ordered. Chronic wounds often require clean technique.) *(Irrigation removes wound debris.)*
10. Measure wound as ordered: at baseline, at first dressing change, weekly, and at discharge from therapy. Remove and discard gloves. (Wound cultures sometimes are ordered on a routine basis. However, when drainage looks purulent, change is seen in amount or color, or drainage has a foul odor, obtain wound cultures even when they are not scheduled for that dressing change.) *(Objectively documents wound healing process in response to negative pressure wound therapy.)*
11. Depending on the type of wound, apply sterile gloves or new clean gloves. *(Fresh sterile wounds require sterile gloves. Chronic wounds often require clean technique.)* Do not use the same gloves worn to remove old dressing. *(Cross-contamination is a possible result.)*
12. Prepare VAC foam.
   a. Select appropriate foam.
   b. With sterile scissors, cut foam to wound size. Proper size of foam dressing helps maintain negative pressure to entire wound. Dressing must be cut to fit the size and shape of the wound, including tunnels and undermined areas. *(Black polyurethane [PU] foam has larger pores and is most effective in stimulating granulation tissue and wound contraction. White polyvinyl alcohol [PVA] soft foam is denser, with smaller pores; use it when the growth of granulation tissue must be restricted.)*

A

B

Continued

Skill 22.7 Wound Vacuum-Assisted Closure—cont'd

13. Gently place foam in wound, ensuring that the foam is in contact with entire wound base, margins, and tunneled and undermined areas. *(Maintains negative pressure to entire wound. Edges of the foam dressing must be in direct contact with the patient's skin.)*

14. Apply wrinkle-free transparent dressing over foam and secure tubing to the unit. (For deep wounds, regularly reposition tubing to minimize pressure on wound edges. In addition, frequent repositioning of patients with restricted mobility or sensation is important so that they do not lie on the tubing and cause further impairment of skin integrity.) *(Connects the negative pressure from the VAC system to the wound foam.)*

A

B

15. Apply skin protectant, such as SKIN-PREP or Stomahesive to skin around the wound. *(Protects periwound skin from injury that sometimes results from the occlusive dressing.)*

16. Apply wound VAC dressing. *(Ensures that the wound is covered properly and that a negative pressure seal can be achieved.)*
    a. Cover with VAC foam, keeping margin of 1–2 inches (3–5 cm) of surrounding healthy tissue. Apply wrinkle-free transparent dressing. *(Excessive tension has the potential to compress foam dressing and impede wound healing. Excessive tension also produces a shear force on periwound area.)*
    b. Secure tubing to transparent film, aligning drainage holes to ensure an occlusive seal. **Do not apply tension to drape and tubing.**

17. Secure tubing several inches away from the dressing. *(Prevents pull on the primary dressing, which can cause leaks in the negative-pressure system.)*

18. Once wound is completely covered, connect the tubing from the dressing to the tubing from the canister and the VAC system. *(Administration of intermittent or continuous negative pressure between 5 and 200 mm Hg is acceptable, according to health care provider's order and patient comfort. The average is 125 mm Hg.)*
    a. Remove canister from sterile packaging, and push into VAC system until a click is heard. NOTE: An alarm sounds if the canister is not properly engaged.

    b. Connect the dressing tubing to the canister tubing. Be sure both clamps are open.
    c. Place VAC system on a level surface or hang from the foot of the bed. NOTE: The VAC system alarms and deactivates therapy if the unit is tilted beyond 45 degrees.
    d. Press green-lit power button, and set pressure as ordered.

19. Discard old dressing materials, remove gloves, and perform hand hygiene. *(Reduces transmission of microorganisms.)*

20. Inspect wound VAC system to verify that negative pressure is achieved. *(Negative pressure is achieved when an airtight seal is achieved.)*
    a. Verify that display screen reads "THERAPY ON."
    b. Be sure clamps are open and tubing is patent.
    c. Identify air leaks by listening with stethoscope or by moving hand around edges of wound while applying light pressure.
    d. If a leak is present, use strips of transparent film to patch the edges of the wound.

21. See the section "Standard Steps in Wound Care," Steps 10–17.

22. Document: *(Records care given and progress of wound.)*
    • Appearance of wound color; characteristics of any drainage. Compare wound with baseline wound assessment
    • Presence of wound healing augmentation such as wound VAC
    • Response to dressing change
    • Record date and time of dressing change on new dressing

23. Report immediately to the health care provider:
    • Bright, brick-red bleeding
    • Evidence of poor wound healing
    • Evisceration
    • Dehiscence
    • Possible wound infection *(These signs are abnormal and necessitate immediate interventions.)*

Figures courtesy Kinetic Concepts, Inc. (KCI), San Antonio, Texas.

Skill 22.8   Applying a Bandage

NURSING ACTION *(RATIONALE)*

1. See the section "Standard Steps in Wound Care," Steps 1–9.
2. Assemble equipment:
   - Correct width and number of bandages
   - Safety pins, fasteners, or tape
   - Gloves, if wound drainage is present
3. Ensure that skin and dressing are clean and dry. *(Allows bandages to be applied to clean, dry areas to prevent further impaired skin integrity.)*
4. Separate any adjacent skin surfaces. *(Prevents irritation and impairment of skin integrity.)*
5. Align part to be bandaged, providing slight flexion as appropriate and not contraindicated. *(Promotes comfort and functional use.)*
6. Apply bandage from distal to proximal part. *(Encourages return of venous blood flow to heart.)*

7. Apply bandage with even distribution of pressure. *(Maintains uniform bandage tension, prevents impairment of circulation.)*
   a. For the circular bandage, see Table 22.4.
   b. For the spiral bandage, see Table 22.4.
   c. For the spiral-reverse bandage, see Table 22.4.
   d. For the recurrent (stump) bandage, see Table 22.4.
   e. For the figure-of-8 bandage, see Table 22.4.
   f. Secure first bandage before applying additional rolls. Apply additional rolls without leaving any uncovered areas. *(Prevents wrinkling or loose ends.)*
8. Assess tension of bandage and circulation of extremity. *(Ensures that bandage is applied appropriately.)*
9. See the section "Standard Steps in Wound Care," Steps 10–17.
10. Document. *(Records care given and application of binder.)*

Skill 22.9   Applying a Triangular Binder (Sling), T-Binder, and Abdominal Binder

NURSING ACTION *(RATIONALE)*

1. See the section "Standard Steps in Wound Care," Steps 1–9.
2. Assemble equipment:
   - Binder
   - Safety pins
   - Washcloth
   - Towel
   - Soap
   - Water
   - Cotton or gauze pad
   - Pain medication, if indicated
   - Dressing, as necessary
3. Change dressing if appropriate; cleanse skin if needed. *(Prepares underlying skin surfaces for binder application.)*
4. Separate skin surfaces or pad bony prominences. *(Protects skin surfaces from contact, preventing irritation and impairment of skin integrity.)*
   Apply binder.
   a. Triangular binder (sling)
      (1) Have patient flex arm at approximately 80-degree angle, depending on purpose of binder. *(Allows proper angle for application.)*

(2) Place end of triangular binder over shoulder of the uninjured side, anterior to posterior. *(Places point of triangle under patient's elbow of injured arm.)*

© Elsevier

Continued

Skill 22.9 Applying a Triangular Binder (Sling), T-Binder, and Abdominal Binder—cont'd

(3) Grasp other end of binder and bring it up and over injured arm to shoulder of injured arm. (*Supports the impaired arm.*)

(4) Use square knot to tie two ends together at lateral area of neck on uninjured side. (*Prevents slippage to knot. Prevents wear on bony prominences.*)

(5) Support wrist well with binder; do not allow it to extend over end of binder. (*Maintains body alignment. Prevents circulation impairment.*)

(6) Fold third triangle end neatly around elbow and secure with safety pins. (*Secures binder. Prevents arm from slipping out.*)

b. T-binder

(1) Using appropriate binder, place the waistband smoothly under patient's waist; patient should be positioned lying supine; tails should be under patient. (*Allows use of appropriate binder; single tail for female patients and two tails for male patients.*)

(2) Secure two ends of waistband together with safety pin. (*Allows securing at the waist.*)

(3) Single tail: bring the tail up between legs to secure dressing in place. Two tails: bring tails up one on each side of penis or large dressing. (*Secures dressing, pad, or other item without causing pressure on the genitalia.*)

(4) Bring tails under and over waistband and secure with safety pins.

© Elsevier

c. Elastic abdominal binder (see illustration)

(1) Center binder smoothly under appropriate part of patient. (*Promotes effectiveness of binder.*)

(2) Close binder: pull one end of binder over center of patient's abdomen while maintaining tension on that end of binder; pull opposite end of binder over center

and secure with Velcro closure tabs, metal fasteners, or horizontally placed safety pins. (*Provides continuous wound support and comfort.*)

(3) Observe patient's respiratory status. (*Abdominal binders that are too tight often interfere with respirations.*)

© Elsevier

d. For postsurgical application of abdominal binders, proceed upward from bottom (except for a patient after cesarean delivery) to minimize pull on the suture line.

© Elsevier

6. Note comfort level of patient. Smooth out binder to prevent wrinkles. Adjust binder as necessary. (*Promotes comfort and chest expansion.*)

7. See the section "Standard Steps in Wound Care," Steps 10–17.

8. Document: (*Records care given and application of binder.*)
- Time of application
- Type of binder
- Patient's response
- Patient teaching (see the Patient Teaching box on wound care)

Table 22.4   Basic Bandage Turns

BASIC BANDAGE TURNS	USE
Circular 1. Unroll 3–4 inches (7.62–10.16 cm) of bandage from back of roll. 2. Place flat bandage surface on anterior surface of portion of body to be covered and hold end in place with thumb of nondominant hand. 3. Continue rolling bandage around same area until two overlapping layers of bandage cover part. Remove excess bandage roll. 4. Secure end of bandage with safety pin or clip if it is attached to end of bandage. If end of bandage has raw edge, fold ½–1 inch (1.27–2.54 cm) under before securing bandage. Gauze bandage is possible to secure with strip of adhesive tape.	Circular turns are used to cover small body regions such as a digit or wrist and are used to anchor bandaging materials.
Spiral 1. Anchor bandage at distal end of body part with two circular turns (note Steps 1 through 3, Circular). 2. Advance bandage on ascending angle, overlapping each preceding turn by half to two-thirds the width of bandage roll until proximal border of area is covered. 3. Secure end of bandage.	Used to cover cylindric body parts, where contour of part does not vary significantly in size (e.g., slender wrist and forearm).
Spiral-Reverse 1. Anchor bandage at distal border of area to be covered (use one to three circular turns). 2. Advance bandage on ascending angle of approximately 30 degrees. 3. Halfway through each turn fold bandage toward you and continue around part in downward stroke. Continue advancing bandage as in Steps 2 and 3 until desired proximal point is reached. Secure bandage.	Used to cover inverted cone-shaped body parts such as calf or thigh.
Figure-of-8 1. Anchor bandage at center of joint (see Steps 1 through 3, Circular). 2. Ascend obliquely around upper half of circular turn above joint followed by turn that descends obliquely below joint. 3. Continue in same manner, overlapping half of previous turn until desired immobilization is attained. 4. Be certain to cover the joint with bandage to prevent fluid shift to those tissues and subsequent impaired circulation. 5. Secure end of bandage.	Used to cover joints and provide immobilization. Outer surface of fabric is against skin during ascending application of bandage. Each reverse turn places alternate side of bandage toward skin.
Recurrent 1. Anchor bandage with two circular turns (see Steps 1 through 3, Circular) at proximal ends of body part to be covered. 2. Make reverse turn at center front, and advance fabric over distal end of the body part to center back, forming covering perpendicular to first circular turns. 3. Make reverse turn at back and bring bandage forward, overlapping one-half of perpendicular bandage on one side. Make reverse turn at front and overlap opposite side of center, continuing on to back. Repeat these steps, overlapping each previous strip of bandage until entire area is covered. 4. Anchor bandage with two circular turns. 5. Secure end of bandage.	Provides cap-like coverage for scalp or amputation stump.

Coordinated Care

Delegation

Dressing Changes

Check institutional policy and the state's nurse practice act regarding which wound care interventions can be delegated to unlicensed assistive personnel (UAP). In some states, aspects of wound care, such as emptying a drain, may be delegated. In this situation, instruct staff on what to report when a drainage container is emptied, which includes measuring the amount of drainage and reporting the amount on the patient's intake and output (I&O) record. The UAP also must know how to use clean technique to avoid cross-contamination. Assessment of wound drainage and maintenance of drains and the drainage system require the critical thinking and knowledge application unique to a nurse. All wound assessment—the care of acute new wounds and those that require sterile technique for dressing changes—remains within the domain of professional nursing practice. The assessment of the wound requires the critical thinking and knowledge application unique to a nurse, even when the dressing change is delegated to others.

The skill of suture removal requires the critical thinking and knowledge application unique to the nurse. For this skill, delegation is inappropriate.

The skills of applying a binder may be delegated to UAP, depending on the patient's condition. However, it is the responsibility of the nurse to assess the patient's ability to breathe deeply, cough effectively, and move independently before and after binder application. The nurse is also responsible for assessing the patient's skin for irritation or abrasion, the underlying wound, and the patient's level of comfort.

The skill of applying the wound vacuum-assisted closure (VAC) is inappropriate to delegate because of the unique knowledge necessary for application.

After a bandage is applied, assess, document, and immediately report changes in circulation, skin integrity, comfort level, and body function, such as ventilation or movement. When applying a bandage, loosen or readjust it as necessary. Obtain the health care provider's order before loosening or removing a bandage that the health care provider applied. Explain to the patient that any bandage or binder feels relatively firm or tight. Assess any bandage carefully to be sure it is applied properly and is providing therapeutic benefit. Replace soiled bandages. Like a damp dressing, a bandage or binder is a potential harbor for microorganisms (Box 22.5).

❖ NURSING PROCESS

The role of the licensed practical nurse/licensed vocational nurse (LPN/LVN) in the nursing process as stated is that the LPN/LVN:

- Participates in planning care for patients based on patient needs
- Reviews patient's plan of care and recommends revisions as needed
- Reviews and follows defined prioritization for patient care
- Uses clinical pathways, care maps, or care plans to guide and review patient care

◆ ASSESSMENT

Assessment consists of location, size or dimensions, exudates, wound bed or edges, tunnel or undermining, periwound characteristics, pain, and signs and symptoms of infection. Note whether wound edges are closed. A surgical incision should have clean, well-approximated edges. Crusts often form along the wound edges from exudate. A puncture wound is usually a small, circular wound with the edges coming together toward the center. If a wound is open, separate the wound edges and inspect the condition of underlying tissue such as adipose and connective tissue. Also look for complications such as **dehiscence** (separation of surgical incision or rupture of wound closure, typically an abdominal incision) and **evisceration** (the protrusion of an internal organ through a wound or surgical incision, especially in the abdominal wall). The outer edges of a wound normally appear inflamed for the first

2 to 3 days, but this slowly disappears. Within 7 to 10 days, a normally healing wound fills with epithelial cells and edges close. If infection develops, the wound edges become brightly erythematous and edematous.

If a closed wound is covered by a dressing, observe the dressing but do not change it until an order is issued. If a dressing becomes saturated with exudate before the order is given, reinforce the dressing over the incisional area by placing sterile gauze on top of the original dressing and anchoring it securely. Record and report any dressing that is reinforced. Observe and document the amount of exudate and the dressings applied.

◆ PATIENT PROBLEMS

After completing an assessment of the patient's wound, identify patient problem statements that direct supportive and preventive care. Existence of a wound clearly indicates the following patient problem:

- Compromised Skin Integrity

This patient problem statement leads to initiation of interventions that promote the healing process.

Some patients are at risk for poor wound healing because of preexisting conditions that impair healing (see Table 22.1). Thus, even though the patient's wound appears normal, it is important to identify patient problem statements that direct nursing interventions toward support of wound repair, such as the following:

- Insufficient Nutrition
- Compromised Blood Flow to Tissue

Box 22.5 Guidelines for Applying a Bandage or Binder

1. Position body part to be bandaged in comfortable position of normal anatomic alignment. Bandages cause restriction in movement. Immobilization in position of normal functioning reduces risk of deformity or injury.
2. Prevent friction between and against skin surfaces by applying gauze or cotton padding. Skin surfaces in contact with each other (e.g., between toes, under breasts) are likely to rub against each other and cause abrasion or chafing. Bandages over body prominences often rub against skin and cause impairment of skin integrity.
3. Apply bandages securely to prevent slippage during movement. Friction between bandage and skin can cause impairment of skin integrity.
4. When bandaging extremities, apply bandage first at the distal end and progress toward the trunk (heart).
5. Gradual application of pressure from the distal toward the proximal portion of the extremity promotes venous return and keeps the risk of edema or circulatory impairment to a minimum.
6. Apply bandages firmly, with equal tension exerted over each turn or layer. Avoid excess overlapping of bandage layers. (Approximately one-third to one-half of previous layer should be covered by successive layers.) Proper application prevents unequal pressure distribution over bandaged body part. Localized pressure causes circulatory impairment.
7. Position pins, knots, or ties away from wound or sensitive skin areas. These materials potentially exert localized pressure and cause irritation.
8. Remove and reapply an elastic bandage at least once every 8 h unless otherwise directed by health care provider.
9. Remove elastic bandage whenever necessary to readjust wrinkles, looseness, or tightness; because of patient discomfort; or when you note signs and symptoms of nerve or vascular impairment.
10. Apply bandages to the lower extremities before the patient sits or stands (i.e., with patient lying down).
11. Use increasingly wider bandages as size of area to be covered increases.
12. Use adhesive tape rather than loose clips or pins to fasten bandages on small child or infant. Safety pins are more effective than clips and do not fall out of bandage. Many facilities prefer tape for safety and maintenance of skin integrity.
13. Patients with tubes or drains who have binders need frequent assessment to ensure patency of tubes for drainage.

Box 22.6 Patient Problems Related to Wound Healing

- Inability to Maintain Adequate Breathing Pattern, related to:
  - Pain from abdominal or thoracic incision
  - Potential for Infection, related to:
  - Malnutrition
  - Tissue loss and increased environmental exposure
- Compromised Physical Mobility, related to:
  - Pain of surgical wound or site of surgery (e.g., joint replacement)
  - Insufficient Nutrition, related to:
  - Inability to ingest or tolerate food
  - Inability to accommodate the increased calories needed to promote wound healing
- Recent Onset of Pain, related to:
  - Surgical incision
- Impaired Self-Esteem due to Current Situation, related to:
  - Perception of scars
  - Perception of surgical drains
  - Reaction to surgically removed body part
- Compromised Skin Integrity, related to:
  - Surgical incision
  - Pressure
  - Chemical injury
  - Secretions and excretions
- Potential for Compromised Skin Integrity, related to:
  - Physical immobilization
  - Exposure to secretions

◆ EXPECTED OUTCOMES AND PLANNING

Establish a plan of care based on the patient's health care needs. These needs are identified during the assessment phase of the nursing process. Next, form the nursing diagnostic statement and devise the plan of care. Consider the patient's plan of care for discharge because patients are discharged earlier now than in the past (see the Home Care Considerations box). Incorporate patient and family teaching into the patient's plan of care (see the Patient Teaching box). Consider special needs of the older adult when performing wound care (see the Cultural Considerations and Lifespan Considerations for older adults boxes).

Goals such as the following are developed for the patient based on the patient problem. Expected outcomes are based on the goals of care.

Goal 1: Patient's wound heals without complications.

Outcome 1: Patient's wound is free of infection; edges are approximated.

Goal 2: Patient reports pain of less than 3 on a pain scale of 0 to 10.

Outcome 2: Patient reports minimal discomfort, rating 2.

◆ IMPLEMENTATION

While performing wound care, observe the wound for signs and symptoms of infection. Be certain that sterile technique is used when gloving, handling sterile equipment and dressings, performing procedures that involve care of the open wound, and caring for

The nature of a wound can cause problems unrelated to wound healing. Pain and impaired mobility can affect a patient's eventual recovery. For example, a large abdominal incision can cause enough pain to interfere with the patient's ability to turn in bed effectively (Box 22.6).

🏠 Home Care Considerations

Wound Care

- Demonstrate wound care and provide time for return demonstration.
- Explain need for specialized supplies, such as irrigating solutions and dressings, and need to maintain sterile asepsis when performing care.
- Instruct where and how to obtain additional supplies.
- Instruct about signs of improper wound healing and wound infections.
- Explain why wound is being allowed to heal by secondary intention.
- Assess understanding of need for the methods of wound care.
- Teach primary caregiver and patient how to maintain clean technique when changing dressings. Wear clean gloves and perform hand hygiene after procedure. Use of clean dressings is permitted in the home environment.
- Be certain patient knows what signs and symptoms to report to health care provider or primary caregiver, as well as when it is necessary to report them.
- Assess extent of wound or incision in relation to patient's level of activity to determine type of dressing that will achieve desired purpose.
- Assess area where procedure will be performed for adequate lighting and running water. Determine whether there is a table or cabinet on which sterile supplies may be placed with reasonable security.
- A bedroom or bathroom is usually ideal for procedure.
- Cleansing wound in the shower is acceptable if approved by health care provider.
- If drainage system is present, explain how system operates.
- Explain importance of drainage system.
- Demonstrate procedure for emptying the drainage chamber and how to reseal it without contaminating unit.
- Be sure that the drain is protected from the disoriented patient, who may pull it out.
- Teach proper application and care of binder.

👥 Patient Teaching

Wound Care

- Assist patient to accept the surgical wound by stating the progress of the wound and how healing is occurring.
- Teach importance of early ambulation after surgery.
- Teach importance of a nutritious diet in wound healing.
- Explain that dressings will perhaps be required at home and how to purchase what will be needed. Inform of home health services if needed or per health care provider's order.
- Wounds out of patient's reach and vision necessitate assistance by a family member or other caregiver.
- Explain expected wound appearance, what should be reported, and risks of improper wound care.
- After demonstrating wound care, allow the patient or the family member to perform wound care with supervision.
- Teach the importance of keeping dressings, sutures, and staples dry and clean.
- Explain the importance of washing hands before and after dressing changes.
- Teach signs and symptoms of infection.
- Instruct the patient to notify the health care provider if signs of wound infection appear.
- Follow health care provider's instructions for limiting activity.
- Provide written instructions, in addition to verbal ones.
- Allow time for patient's questions.
- If drainage system is present:
  - Explain purpose of drainage system.
  - Explain importance of measuring output.
  - Instruct to keep Hemovac or Davol tubing clipped or pinned to clothing to prevent accidental dislodgement.
  - Teach what to do if the drain accidentally comes out.
  - If binder is present, teach function of the binder.
  - Teach to report if binder is loose or causing pain or discomfort.
  - Teach to report any breathing restrictions if binder is too tight.

---

wound drainage systems. Documentation of wound care is required to include the appearance of the wound, presence of drains and drainage or exudate, medication or solutions used in wound care, type of dressings applied, and patient response to the procedure. Report any variation from normal healing. Include specific interventions or techniques of dressing changes in the nursing care plan to provide continuity of care.

◆ EVALUATION

Evaluate wound healing with each dressing change, after application of heat and cold therapies, after wound irrigation, and after stress to the wound site.

Determine whether expected outcomes have been met. Take the following evaluative measures: assess condition of the wound, ask whether patient notes discomfort during procedure, and inspect condition of dressings at least every shift. Note the following examples:

Goal 1: Patient's wound heals without complications.
Evaluative measure: Assess the wound and dressing for odor, exudate, separation, color, and edema.
Goal 2: Patient has minimal pain; rates pain at 3 or less on a scale of 0 to 10.
Evaluative measures: Compare dosage and frequency of pain medication delivered over recovery period. Request patient to rate pain on a scale of 0 to 10, with 10 being the most pain and 0 being no pain.

Cultural Considerations

Wound Care

Detection of cyanosis or pallor and other changes in skin color in patients is an important clinical skill. This detection can become a challenge in patients with dark skin. Cyanosis is defined as a slightly blue-gray, slate-like, or dark purple discoloration of the skin that results from a reduction of hemoglobin in arterial blood. Color differentiation of cyanosis or pallor varies according to skin pigmentation. The nurse needs to know the individual's baseline skin tone. Do not confuse the normal hyperpigmentation of Mongolian spots that may be seen on the sacrum of African American, Native American, and Asian American patients as cyanosis. Observe the patient's skin in daylight without glare.

Keep in mind the following points:
- Cyanosis is difficult but possible to detect in a patient with dark skin.
- Cyanosis and pallor should be assessed by examining mucus membranes, such as the conjunctiva or inside of the mouth. Nailbeds can also be assessed for pallor or cyanosis.
- Be aware of situations that produce changes in skin tone.
- Examine body sites with the least melanin for underlying color identification.
- The pigmented skin should be assessed for specific color changes in skin tone.

Lifespan Considerations

Older Adults

Wound Care

- Assess ability of the older adult to perform self-care, to reach the wound, and to manipulate the wound dressings.
- The skin of older adults is fragile and sometimes does not tolerate adhesives. Frequent dressing changes should be avoided. Assess for tape allergies. Use paper tape.
- Decrease extraneous noises as much as possible to alleviate or prevent patient anxiety.
- Increase time allowed for the skills and allow time for repetition of teaching.
- Slow the pace.
- Give small amounts of information at a time.
- Older patients learn better by doing and using multiple senses than by reading instructions.
- The increased fragility of the skin of the older adult sometimes contraindicates the use of a binder. Assess skin thoroughly before any binder application.
- Observe underlying skin of the older adult more frequently.
- The patient needs two binders because binders are washable and must be "line dried." Thus, the patient has one to wear while the other is being washed and dried.
- Older skin is frequently at higher risk for dehiscence after sutures are removed.
- Be aware that patients need additional fluid intake to prevent dehydration.
- Certain measures are sometimes necessary to prevent a confused patient from pulling out the drain.
- Compensate for any auditory, visual, or cognitive impairment that the patient has when performing a dressing change.
- A decrease in sensory receptors causes a decrease in pain sensation.

Get Ready for the NCLEX® Examination!

Key Points

- Wounds are described as open or closed. Care of the open wound is determined by the extent of the wound.
- Maintenance of sterile technique is essential when providing care for an open wound.
- Size, description of appearance, amount and type of exudate, presence of drains, integrity of wound closures, and pain level are included in a proper wound assessment.
- The wet-to-dry dressing can be used to mechanically debride a wound of necrotic tissue or wound exudate.
- Do not moisten the wet-to-dry dressing before removing it if being used for debridement. This will flush any bacteria or material that has been collected on the soiled dressing through the debridement process back into the wound and prevents removal of unwanted tissue or drainage.
- Wound drains remove secretions within tissue layers to promote wound closure.
- A drainage system requires close monitoring. In addition to noting color, consistency, and amount of drainage, checking the tube patency is important.
- After a bandage or binder is applied, assess, document, and immediately report changes in circulation, skin integrity, comfort level, and body function, such as ventilation or mobility.

- Remove dressings gently to prevent further injury to the wound. Dispose of used dressings appropriately to prevent cross-contamination.
- The type of suture securing a wound influences the method of suture removal.
- Wound care involves cleaning wounds, changing dressings, maintaining drains, irrigating, inserting packing, applying heat and cold treatments, and applying bandages and binders.
- Major types of wound exudate are serous, purulent, and sanguineous. The main complications of wound healing are hemorrhage, infection, dehiscence, and evisceration.
- Major nursing responsibilities related to wound care include preventing infection, preventing further tissue damage, preventing hemorrhage, promoting healing, and preventing skin excoriation around draining wounds.
- Wound assessment requires a description of the appearance of the wound base, the wound's size, the presence of exudates, and the periwound skin condition.
- When cleansing wounds or drain sites, clean from the least to the most contaminated area, away from the wound edges.
- Physical stress from vomiting, coughing, or sudden muscular contraction can cause separation of wound edges or dehiscence.
- Apply bandages and binders in a manner that does not impair circulation or irritate the skin.

Additional Learning Resources

SG Go to your Study Guide for additional learning activities to help you master this chapter content.

Be sure to visit the Evolve site at http://evolve.elsevier.com/Cooper/foundations/ for additional online resources.

Review Questions for the NCLEX® Examination

1. The patient has just returned from the postanesthesia care unit (PACU). During report, the nurse is told that the patient has a Jackson-Pratt drain in the left lower quadrant (LLQ). The patient asks why the drain is being used. What response by the nurse is most accurate?

   1. "The drain allows for the postoperative instillation of wound irrigation fluid in order to keep the wound clean."
   2. "The drain is used to reduce infection in the postoperative period."
   3. "Drains are used to contain and remove body fluids from the wound by mild suction."
   4. "Drains are used to minimize postoperative discomfort after a surgical procedure."

2. The nurse finds that the patient's incision has eviscerated. What action should the nurse take? (Select all that apply.)

   1. Place the patient in high-Fowler's position.
   2. Give the patient fluids to prevent shock.
   3. Do not allow the patient to get out of bed.
   4. Replace dressings with sterile fluffy pads.
   5. Apply warm, moist sterile dressings.

3. The health care provider has ordered that the patient's wound be irrigated. What is the primary rationale for this procedure?

   1. To remove debris from the wound
   2. To decrease scar formation
   3. To improve circulation from the wound
   4. To decrease irritation from wound drainage

4. What statements indicate that a wound has become infected? (Select all that apply.)

   1. Palpation of the wound reveals serosanguinous fluid under its edges.
   2. Wound cultures are positive.
   3. Purulent drainage is coming from the wound area.
   4. Upon removal, the nurse notes that the dressing is dry.
   5. Wound edges are clean and well approximated.
   6. The wound has a foul odor.

5. Which nursing entry is the most complete in its description of a wound?

   1. Wound appears to be healing well, dressing dry and intact
   2. Wound well approximated, with minimal drainage
   3. Drainage size of quarter; wound pink; 4 × 4 applied
   4. Incisional edges approximated without erythema or exudate; two 4 × 4s applied

6. Which statement is correct in regard to the use of an abdominal binder?

   1. It replaces the need for underlying dressings.
   2. It should be kept loose for patient comfort.
   3. The patient has to be sitting or standing when it is applied.
   4. The patient must have adequate ventilatory capacity.

7. What is the first step when packing a wound?

   1. Assess its size, shape, and depth.
   2. Prepare a sterile field.
   3. Select gauze packing material.
   4. Irrigate the wound.

8. What is the correct procedure for the wet-to-dry dressing method?

   1. Place dry gauze into the wound and remove it when it is wet.
   2. Medicate the patient for pain after you change the dressing.
   3. Complete this type of dressing change just once a day.
   4. Place moist gauze into the wound and remove it at prescribed intervals.

9. Which phrase best describes serous drainage?

   1. Fresh bleeding
   2. Thick and yellow
   3. Clear, watery plasma
   4. Beige to brown and foul smelling

10. The health care provider has ordered an abdominal binder placed around a surgical patient with a new abdominal wound. What is the likely indication for this intervention?

    1. Collection of wound drainage
    2. Reduction of abdominal swelling
    3. Reduction of stress on the abdominal incision
    4. Stimulation of peristalsis from direct pressure

11. What are the traditional purposes of a wet-to-dry dressing? *(Select all that apply.)*

    1. Debridement
    2. Cooling
    3. Comfort
    4. Prevention of infection
    5. Maintenance of moisture at the wound bed

12. What action should the nurse implement to reduce surgical wound infection? *(Select all that apply.)*

    1. Adhering to the principles of hand hygiene
    2. Cleansing the incision from the least contaminated to the most contaminated area
    3. Leaving the incision open to the air
    4. Changing the dressing using sterile technique
    5. Ensuring that the patient is consuming an adequate diet

13. The student nurse is changing a patient's dressing. What action indicates the need for further education? *(Select all that apply.)*

    1. Enclose the soiled dressing within a latex glove.
    2. Clean the wound in circles toward the incision.
    3. Free the tape by pulling it away from the incision.
    4. Remove the soiled dressing with sterile gloves.
    5. Apply the clean dressing with clean gloves.

14. When the drainage in a Hemovac reservoir is emptied, which nursing action is essential for reestablishing the negative pressure within this drainage device?

    1. Fill the reservoir with sterile normal saline solution.
    2. Secure the reservoir to the skin near the wound.
    3. Compress the reservoir and close the vent.
    4. Open the vent, allowing the reservoir to fill with air.

15. Which patient is more at risk for wound dehiscence?

    1. The patient who smokes
    2. The patient who is obese
    3. The patient with a history of peripheral vascular disease
    4. The patient who is immunocompromised

16. The student nurse is correct when indicating which drain is providing suction-assisted drainage?

    1. Jackson-Pratt
    2. Hemovac
    3. Penrose
    4. Wound VAC system
    5. T-tube system

17. The health care provider has ordered that all sutures on a patient with an abdominal hysterectomy be removed on the fifth postoperative day and that Steri-Strips be applied. During suture removal, the nurse notices the incision edges are slightly separating. What is the best action by the nurse?

    1. Continue removing the sutures and apply the Steri-Strips.
    2. Stop the suture removal and contact the health care provider immediately.
    3. Continue removing the sutures and applying the Steri-Strips, then cover the incision with a dry sterile dressing.
    4. Stop the suture removal, apply Steri-Strips where sutures already have been removed, and notify the health care provider.

18. When providing care to a patient with a Hemovac drain, what actions are included in the plan of care?

    1. Record the appearance of the drainage in the nursing progress notes and include the amount in the fluid output calculations.
    2. Clamp the tubing during patient ambulation and activity to prevent excess drainage during these times.
    3. Empty the bulb drainage receptacle when it is one-fourth full.
    4. Pin the bulb above the insertion site to assist in proper drainage of exudate.

19. During assessment of a patient after abdominal surgery, the nurse suspects internal hemorrhaging based on which finding?

    1. The dressing is saturated with bright red sanguineous drainage, and the patient has an increased urinary output.
    2. The dressing is dry and intact, the patient's blood pressure has decreased, and pulse and respirations have increased.
    3. The dressing is saturated with serosanguineous drainage, and the patient is diaphoretic, with a decrease in pulse and respirations.
    4. The dressing is dry and intact, and the patient reports shortness of breath and has an elevated temperature.

20. A female, 51, with COPD presents with acute cholecystitis and undergoes open cholecystectomy to remove the gallbladder after laparoscopy is ruled inappropriate. The surgeon makes a 15 cm incision and observes edema and inflammation of the bile duct. After the cholecystectomy, the surgeon makes a secondary incision near the site to insert a T tube to facilitate drainage and to prevent exudate from entering the surgical incision. The client is put on electrolytes and oral dexamethasone (a steroid). She is monitored for dehydration. On the first postsurgical night, the nurse observes serosanguineous discharge on the bandage.

Identify the nursing actions below as **Indicated** (appropriate or necessary), **Contraindicated** (could be harmful), or **Non-Essential** (not necessary) for the client's care at this time. *Only one selection can be made for each nursing action.*

NURSING ACTION	INDICATED	CONTRAINDI-CATED	NON-ESSENTIAL
a. Carefully monitor for subtle or latent signs of inflammation.			
b. Challenge any order to add vitamin A to this client's medications.			
c. Regularly measure contents of the collection bag			
d. Ensure that normal abdominal cavity drainage remains between 500 and 600 mL/24 h			
e. If bile drainage is greenish brown, thick and/or blood-tinged, immediately report this to the charge nurse and provider.			
f. Use Montgomery straps for this client's dressing.			
g. Immediately report this client's serosanguineous exudate and prep the client for anticipated emergent surgery.			
h. Report any bile duct exudate greater than 300 mL during the first 24 h.			
i. Keep the T tube collection receptacle compressed.			

Specimen Collection and Diagnostic Testing

23

Objectives

1. Describe the necessary documentation of the patient's condition before, during, and after a laboratory or diagnostic test.
2. Discuss nursing interventions necessary to properly prepare a patient who is to have a diagnostic examination.
3. Discuss patient teaching for diagnostic testing.
4. Describe the role of the nurse in procedures for specimen collection.
5. Discuss guidelines for specimen collection.
6. Explain the rationales for collection of each specimen listed.
7. State appropriate labeling for a collected specimen.
8. List the proper steps for obtaining urine specimens.
9. List the proper steps for teaching blood glucose self-monitoring.
10. Discuss the procedure for obtaining stool specimens.
11. State the correct procedures for collecting a sputum specimen.
12. Identify the procedure for performing a phlebotomy.
13. Identify the procedure for performing electrocardiography.

Key Terms

culture (KŬL-chŭr, p. 683)
cytology (sī-TŎL-ō-jē, p. 686)
electrocardiogram (ECG) (ē-lĕk-trō-KĂR-dē-ō-grăm, p. 695)
expectorate (ĕks-PĔK-tŏ-rāt, p. 683)
exudate (p. 686)
fixative (FĬKS-ŭ-tĭv, p. 671)
Hemoccult (HĒ-mō-kŭlt, p. 683)

midstream urine specimen (p. 679)
occult (ō-KŬLT, p. 683)
residual urine (p. 679)
sensitivity (SĔN-sĭ-TĬV-ĭ-tē, p. 683)
specimen (SPĔS-ĭ-mĭn, p. 678)
tourniquet (TŬR-nĭ-kĕt, p. 694)
Vacutainer (VĂC-yū-tā-nŭr, p. 692)
venipuncture (VĔN-ĭ-pŭnk-chŭr, p. 692)

DIAGNOSTIC EXAMINATION

Diagnostic examination is performed by a health care provider, sometimes at the patient's bedside and sometimes in a room specially equipped for therapeutic or diagnostic purposes. The nurse is responsible for assessing the patient's knowledge of the procedure and preparing the patient for it; assisting the health care provider with the procedure; and caring for the patient after tests are completed. The nurse's knowledge and organization of the procedure ensure that it is carried out accurately.

Patients have fundamental rights and protections during their care. One of the patient's most important rights is informed consent, which requires that the patient, parent, or guardian (or legally designated health care power of attorney if the patient is legally incompetent) fully understands what will be done during a test, surgery, or any medical procedure and understands its risks and implications *before* legally consenting to it.

Explaining a procedure, the method by which it will be performed, and its potential benefits and risks are primarily the health care provider's responsibility. Reinforcement of the health care provider's explanation is a role of the nurse. Be prepared to answer any questions the patient has and to clarify the requirements for the examination, such as whether nothing is permitted to be taken by mouth (NPO) after midnight or whether breakfast will be withheld until the examination is completed. The patient needs to know whether a special room or equipment is required for the test, as well as whether any medications are needed before or during the test. An informed patient is better prepared to participate in the testing process as required by the examination (Skill 23.1 and the Patient Teaching box). The nurse is responsible for knowing the guidelines for and the potential complications of diagnostic examinations (Boxes 23.1 and 23.2, Table 23.1).

Consent for treatment upon admission at the health care facility encompasses most diagnostic tests and

Skill 23.1 Preparing the Patient for Diagnostic Examination

NURSING ACTION *(RATIONALE)*

1. Refer to the health care provider's order.
2. Ensure that informed consent has been obtained when necessary. For most invasive diagnostic tests a signed informed consent form is required. The health care provider is ultimately responsible for disclosure, but the nurse also must be aware of agency policies regarding consent forms and ensure that informed consent is obtained before the procedure. *(Ensures that legal implications of diagnostic procedures are taken into consideration.)*
3. Assemble equipment and supplies. *(Organizes procedure.)*
4. Introduce self. *(Decreases patient's anxiety.)*
5. Identify patient. *(Ensures procedure is performed with correct patient.)*
6. Explain procedure. Assess patient's understanding of procedure and purpose. If contrast dye is to be used, assess patient for allergies (see Box 23.2). *(Promotes understanding and cooperation.)*
7. Prepare patient for procedure. *(Facilitates procedure.)*
   a. Transport patient to examining room, if necessary. Maintain safety precautions. *(Facilitates procedure; some facilities have special examination rooms, but frequently procedures are performed at the patient's bedside.)*
   b. Close door and pull curtains. *(Provides privacy.)*
   c. Raise bed or arrange examination table to convenient height. *(Promotes proper body mechanics.)*
   d. Drape patient for procedure, if necessary. *(Prevents unnecessary exposure of patient.)* (See Table 23.1.)
8. Perform hand hygiene and don clean gloves according to agency policy and guidelines from the Centers for Disease Control and Prevention (CDC) and Occupational Safety and Health

Administration (OSHA). *(Reduces spread of microorganisms.)*

9. Assist health care provider with procedure. *(Provides help to the health care provider while providing support to patient.)*
10. Answer patient's questions. *(Provides for patient's security and emotional support.)*
11. Label specimen according to agency policy (see Box 23.5): patient's name and age, room number, health care provider, date and time, type of specimen, and collector's initials. Most facility policies recommend inserting the specimen (in container) into a biohazard bag for transport to laboratory. Deliver specimen to laboratory promptly. *(Prevents loss and potential delays in obtaining results. Biohazard bag further prevents contamination from specimen.)*

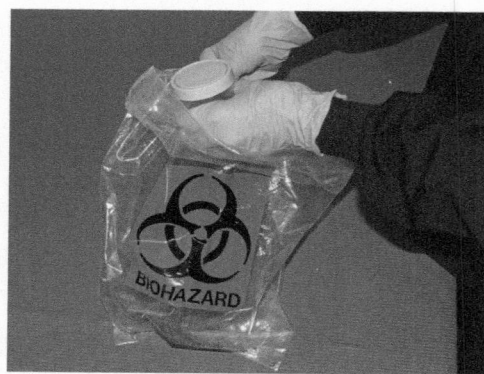

12. Document procedure. *(Communicates performed procedure and patient's response.)*
    - Type of procedure
    - Time
    - Specimen obtained
    - Sent to laboratory with requisition
    - Patient's response
13. Provide patient teaching (see the Patient Teaching box).

procedures. Some tests, however, do require the completion of additional consents. Traditionally, human immunodeficiency virus (HIV) testing and invasive procedures belong to the category requiring a more specific consent process. Written consent is not always necessary for an individual test if it is considered noninvasive; informed verbal consent is adequate in many cases. The patient retains the legal right to withdraw consent—verbal or written—at any time and for any reason and to refuse care or treatment.

Nursing responsibilities when preparing to assist with diagnostic testing and procedures includes

| Box 23.1 | General Guidelines for Diagnostic Examination |

(Rationales are provided in parentheses.)

- Know the patient's baseline vital signs. Some diagnostic tests are invasive procedures and have associated complications. *(Changes from baseline vital signs provide early physiologic data about potential complications.)*
- Assess for the presence of tattoos. Older body art may have been prepared with dyes containing metal-based components. This may present issues with CT and MRI such as burning or skin irritation. Report findings to health care provider.
- Know the patient's level of education. The nurse is required to teach the patient about diagnostic tests. *(Knowing the patient's educational background enables the development of an individualized teaching plan.)*
- Determine the patient's awareness of actual or potential medical diagnoses. *(Provides data about the patient's knowledge and perception of medical diagnoses.)*
- Perform a thorough nursing assessment, including assessment of the patient's cultural background. *(Reveals abnormal findings, which can indicate or contraindicate a diagnostic test.)*
- Determine the patient's previous experience with diagnostic testing. *(Patients who have had smooth, uncomplicated diagnostic tests are usually less anxious about a test. If a patient has had a complication from a diagnostic test, it is possible that the patient will require more pre-procedure education and support.)*
- Most agencies adhere to standard precautions; know agency policy. *(Some facilities have policies that require all specimen containers of body substances to be placed in biohazard bags for transportation to various laboratories. Attach requisitions to specimen container.)*
- Know normal values of the test being performed and causes of deviations from these normal values. (Be aware that some deviations from normal values occur as a result of medications or dietary intake.) *(Allows notification of the prescribing health care provider of end results in a timely manner.)*
- Refer to the policy manual for the facility's instructions for collection of each specimen during diagnostic examinations (see Table 23.1).
- Many factors have the potential to contribute to dysrhythmias in association with diagnostic examinations, including medications such as digitalis and quinidine, hypertrophy of cardiac muscle, alcohol, thyroid dysfunction, coffee, tea, tobacco, electrolyte imbalances, edema, acid-base imbalances, and myocardial ischemia. *(Patients with dysrhythmias are at risk for cardiac arrest. Be familiar with crash cart location, and be knowledgeable about emergency equipment, medications, and cardiopulmonary resuscitation [CPR].)*

| Box 23.2 | Patient Evaluation for Iodine Dye Allergies |

- Many types of contrast media are used in radiographic studies: for example, organic iodine and iodized oils.
- Possible allergic reactions to iodinated dye vary from mild flushing, itching, and urticaria (hives) to severe, life-threatening *anaphylaxis* (an exaggerated life-threatening hypersensitivity reaction to a previous encountered antigen; evidenced by respiratory distress, drop in blood pressure, shock, or a combination of these). In the unusual event of anaphylaxis, treatment consists of administration of drugs such as diphenhydramine (Benadryl), steroids, and epinephrine. Always have oxygen and endotracheal equipment on hand for immediate use.
- Always assess the patient for allergies to the iodine dye before its administration. Inform the radiologist if an allergy is suspected. Patients who are allergic to shellfish are likely allergic to iodine-based dyes because shellfish contain iodine. Non–iodine-based dyes often are used for these patients, or they are pretreated for the likelihood of an allergic reaction. The radiologist is likely to prescribe a diphenhydramine and steroid preparation to be administered before testing. Usually, hypoallergenic contrast media is used during the test.[a]
- After the x-ray procedure, evaluate the patient for delayed reaction to dye (dyspnea, rashes, tachycardia, urticaria). This usually occurs within 2–6 h after the test. Treat with antihistamines or steroids, according to the health care provider's order.

[a]The American College of Radiology recommends that patients who have a prior documented reaction to contrast material be given a different contrast agent in combination with a premedication regimen if it is not possible to avoid using a contrast medium.

anticipating the needs of the health care provider who performs the procedure, having the proper supplies ready, and assisting the patient through the procedure. The patient should be kept apprised of the procedural details. Certain procedures may cause discomfort. Providing support and information to these patients is key to their tolerance of the procedures. Nurses should take special care with older adults during specimen collection and diagnostic examination (see the Lifespan Considerations for Older Adults box) and be aware that sociocultural variations often affect a patient's response and willingness to participate in various diagnostic procedures (see the Cultural Considerations box).

When patients have questions about diagnostic examinations, consult the agency's procedural manual or the designated department involved. Maintain confidentiality when disclosing results from testing and diagnostic procedures. Health care agencies are required to have and to follow policies regarding confidentiality of these records.

Table 23.1	Nursing Interventions for Diagnostic Examinations

BEFORE EXAMINATION	AFTER EXAMINATION
Abdominal Scan[a]	
Order prescribed test per facility policy. Explain procedure. Obtain informed consent, if required by facility. Assess laboratory results for kidney function. If contrast medium is to be used, instruct patient to maintain NPO status for 4 h before examination. Assess patient for allergies to dye or shellfish; it is possible to perform the abdominal scan with or without the dye. Assess patient for claustrophobia. Patients who are mildly claustrophobic often benefit from premedication with antianxiety drugs. Some patients experience mild nausea from the contrast medium; provide emesis basin. Advise patient that he or she may experience a salty taste, flushing, and a sensation of warmth when dye is injected.	Evaluate patient for delayed reaction to dye (see Box 23.2). Encourage oral intake of fluids. Report results. Diarrhea is possible.
Amniocentesis	
Explain procedure. Encourage patient's verbalization of concerns. Obtain written consent from patient. Monitor fetal heart tones. No fluid or food restrictions are necessary. Monitor mother's blood pressure. Follow instructions regarding emptying the bladder, which depend on gestational age. • Before 20 weeks of gestation, it is necessary to keep the bladder full to support the uterus. • After 20 weeks, the bladder typically is emptied to minimize the chance of puncture. • After 20 weeks gestation, the health care provider may order external fetal monitoring for 30–60 min before and after the procedure. NOTE: The location of the placenta is determined by ultrasonography before the study to enable selection of a site that will help prevent placental puncture.	Monitor fetal heart tones. If patient complains of vertigo or nausea, allow her to rest on her left side for several minutes before leaving examination room; assess her vital signs. If any fluid loss or temperature elevation, abdominal pain or cramping, or fetal hyperactivity or unusual fetal lethargy occurs, instruct patient to notify her health care provider. Instruct patient to contact her health care provider to obtain results (usually after 2 weeks). For women who have Rh-negative blood and are not sensitized, administer RhoGAM because of the risk of immunization from the fetal blood. Observe puncture site for bleeding.
Arteriography	
Explain procedure. Obtain written consent. Advise patient that he or she may experience flushing and a sensation of warmth when dye is injected. Assess allergies to dye. Assess whether patient has been taking anticoagulants. Keep patient on NPO status for 2–8 h. Mark site of peripheral pulses with a pen (this enables assessment after the procedure). Document the diminished or absent peripheral pulses. Administer medications as ordered. Ensure that the appropriate coagulation studies have been done and results are within normal range. For cerebral arteriography, perform baseline neurologic assessment to compare subsequent assessment findings. Instruct patient to remove and safely store all dental prostheses and all valuables before study. Instruct patient to void before study. Inform the patient that bladder distention will possibly cause some discomfort during study.	Keep patient on bed rest for 8 h or as ordered by the health care provider. Monitor vital signs and observe for bleeding at puncture site. Assess peripheral arterial pulse at premarked site. If cerebral arteriography has been done, perform neurologic assessment. Maintain pressure at the puncture site. Perform neurovascular assessment on patient's lower extremities; compare the involved extremity with the uninvolved extremity. Administer analgesic as indicated; notify health care provider if patient has severe, continuous pain. Have patient drink fluids to prevent dehydration. Evaluate patient for delayed allergic reaction to the dye (see Box 23.2). If patient has continuous, severe pain, notify health care provider.

Table **23.1**	Nursing Interventions for Diagnostic Examinations—cont'd
BEFORE EXAMINATION	**AFTER EXAMINATION**

Barium Enema

Order prescribed test per facility policy.	Allow patient to resume regular diet as soon as examination is completed. Encourage fluid intake.
Provide needed emotional support.	Monitor stools; barium sometimes causes constipation.
Instruct patient to maintain NPO status after midnight (some facilities allow liquids for breakfast).	Administer laxative after examination per facility protocol.
Assist patient with bowel preparation, which varies among facilities. (In elderly patients, this preparation is sometimes exhausting and even causes severe dehydration in some.)	Allow time for rest.
	Be aware of dehydration and electrolyte abnormalities.
A typical day before preparation:	Inform patient that the stools will be white; when all the barium is expelled, the stool will return to normal color.
Instruct patient to have clear liquid for lunch and supper (no dairy products).	
Have patient drink one glass of water or clear liquid every hour for 8–10 h.	
Administer a cathartic as prescribed.	
Keep patient on NPO status after midnight.	
Day of examination:	
Keep patient on NPO status.	
Administer a suppository or cleansing enema as prescribed.	
Pediatric patients have specific bowel preparations.	
Patients with an ileostomy or colostomy have special preparations.	
Determine whether the bowel is cleansed adequately.	
When fecal return is similar to clear water, preparation is adequate; if large, solid fecal waste is still being evacuated, preparation is inadequate. Notify radiologist, who, in some cases, will want to extend bowel preparation.	

Barium Swallow

Order prescribed test per facility policy.	Inform the patient of the need to evacuate all the barium.
Obtain consent if required by facility or agency.	Advise patient that at first the stools are white but will return to normal color when evacuation is completed. NOTE: Laxatives sometimes are ordered to facilitate evacuation of barium.
Explain procedure.	
Instruct patient to maintain NPO status for at least 8 h (usually NPO after midnight).	
Assess patient's ability to swallow (if patient tends to aspirate, inform the radiologist).	
Accompany hospitalized patient to radiology department if vital signs are not stable and the test is to be performed.	

Blood Chemistry Test

Order prescribed test per facility policy.	Observe site for bleeding. Apply pressure as indicated.
Instruct patient to maintain NPO status (as indicated). Water is permitted.	Ensure that patient's meal is served after test is completed.
Explain procedure.	Report results.
Prohibit smoking as per agency policy.	Instruct patients with high levels regarding a low-cholesterol diet, exercise, and appropriate body weight.
Prohibit alcohol intake for 24 h before test.	
Indicate to patient that dietary intake at least 2 weeks before testing will affect results.	

Body Scan[a]

Order prescribed test per facility policy.	See specific anatomic locations for particular interventions.
Explain procedure.	
Specific anatomic locations will dictate particular interventions.	

Continued

Table **23.1**	**Nursing Interventions for Diagnostic Examinations—cont'd**
BEFORE EXAMINATION	**AFTER EXAMINATION**

Bone Marrow Aspiration

Order prescribed test per facility policy.	Apply pressure to puncture site.
Explain procedure.	Apply adhesive dressing.
Assess coagulation study results and inform health care provider of any abnormalities.	Observe the puncture site for bleeding.
Obtain written consent.	Monitor patient for signs and symptoms of shock (e.g., increased pulse rate, decreased blood pressure) and for pain.
Advise patient that the procedure may cause discomfort or a feeling of pressure, but this feeling will be brief.	Allow patient to resume normal activity 30–60 min after examination.
Assist in obtaining specimens.	Some patients need mild analgesics for tenderness at the puncture site for several days after this procedure.
Provide needed emotional support.	Instruct patient to notify health care provider if any tenderness persists or erythema occurs, because these indicate possible infection.
Obtain order for sedative, as necessary.	
Remind patient to remain very still throughout procedure.	

Bone Scan[a]

Order prescribed test per facility policy.	Because only tracer doses of radioisotopes are used, no precautions must be taken to prevent radioactive exposure of other personnel or family members.
Explain procedure.	
Instruct patient to remove dental prosthetics, jewelry, and any metal objects.	Observe injection site for erythema or edema; if hematoma forms, apply warm soaks to the area to relieve pain.
Encourage patient to drink several glasses of water.	Assure patient that the radioactive substance is usually excreted from the body within 6–24 h. (To assess for allergic reaction, see Box 23.2.)
Tell the patient the injection causes slight discomfort.	
No fasting or sedation is required.	Encourage fluid intake.
Have patient void before examination.	
Assure patient that he or she will not be exposed to large amounts of radioactivity because only tracer doses of the isotope are used.	
Tell the patient the injection causes slight discomfort; no fasting or sedation is required.	

Brain Scan[a]

Order prescribed test per facility policy.	Assess patient for iodine allergies (see Box 23.2).
Obtain informed consent.	Encourage fluid intake.
Keep patient on NPO status for 4 h before examination if contrast dye is to be used.	Report results.
Instruct patient not to wear wig, hairpins, clips, or partial denture plates.	
Observe patient for iodine allergies.	
If sedation is ordered, administer sedative.	
Inform patient that a clicking noise will be heard as the scanner moves.	

Table 23.1   Nursing Interventions for Diagnostic Examinations—cont'd

BEFORE EXAMINATION	AFTER EXAMINATION
Bronchoscopy	
Order prescribed test per facility policy. Explain procedure. Obtain informed consent before patient is premedicated. Instruct patient to maintain NPO status after midnight (4–8 h). Administer preoperative medication as ordered. Instruct patient to remove and safely store contact lenses, dentures, and glasses. Reassure patient that he or she will be able to breathe during procedure. Instruct patient to perform good mouth care to minimize risk of introducing bacteria into the lungs during procedure. Instruct patient not to swallow the local anesthetic sprayed into the throat. Provide a basin for expectoration of the lidocaine. Flexible fiberoptic bronchoscope. (Image courtesy of Olympus Corporation.)	If an anesthetic has been sprayed on the throat, do not allow the patient to eat or drink until the gag reflex returns (2–4 h). Ask patient to open mouth, and hold tongue down with tongue blade. Touch back of pharynx on each side with applicator stick. Observe any sputum for blood; small amounts are normal. Monitor vital signs frequently. Observe for impaired respirations. Observe closely until no effects of anesthesia remain. If patient complains of sore throat, provide warm saline gargles and lozenges as desired. If a tumor is suspected, collect a postbronchoscopy sputum sample for cytologic determination. Inform patient to report bronchospasms or laryngospasms immediately. Reports are available within 2–7 days.
Cardiac Catheterization	
Explain procedure. Obtain written consent. Provide needed emotional support. Instruct patient to maintain NPO status for 4–8 h. Determine whether patient has any dye allergies (see Box 23.2). Administer premedications as ordered. Prepare catheter insertion site by shaving and preparing the skin. Mark the site of the patient's peripheral pulses with a pen to facilitate postprocedure assessment. Instruct patient to void before going to the catheterization laboratory. Instruct patient to remove and safely store all valuables and dental prostheses. Obtain IV access for delivery of IV fluids and cardiac drugs, if necessary.	Monitor vital signs. Observe catheter site for bleeding; apply pressure as necessary. Encourage rest (4–8 h). Encourage fluids; monitor urinary output. Keep affected extremity extended and immobilized to decrease bleeding. Assess the patient's pulses in both extremities. Compare pulses with preprocedure marking and assessment findings. Instruct the patient that the test data will be reviewed by the cardiologist and the results will be available in 1–2 days. Perform serial neurovascular assessment on the patient's involved extremity; compare with uninvolved extremity. Instruct the patient to report any sign of numbness, tingling, pain, or loss of function in the involved extremity immediately.
Chest Radiography	
Prepare requisition form. Explain procedure; no fasting is required. Be certain that patient's gown has no snaps or pins and that the patient is not wearing a bra. Instruct patient to remove all metal objects (necklaces, pins). Tell patient that he or she will be asked to take a deep breath and to hold it while the x-ray images are taken.	Report results. NOTE: No special care is required after the procedure.

Table 23.1	Nursing Interventions for Diagnostic Examinations—cont'd

BEFORE EXAMINATION	AFTER EXAMINATION
Colonoscopy	
Order prescribed test per facility policy. Explain procedure. Obtain written consent. Assist with the bowel preparation. The bowel preparation ordered depends on the health care provider's preference. Avoid oral bowel preparation in patients with upper gastrointestinal obstruction or suspected acute diverticulitis or following recent bowel surgery. Assure patient that he or she will be draped appropriately to prevent unnecessary embarrassment. Administer appropriate preprocedure sedation as ordered. Record results from cathartics and enemas. Determine whether the bowel is cleansed adequately. When fecal return is similar to clear water, preparation is adequate; if large, solid fecal waste still is being evacuated, preparation is inadequate. Notify health care provider who will be performing the colonoscopy, who will in some cases want to extend the bowel preparation.	Observe for abdominal pain, tenderness, and bleeding or gas pains from air in the bowel. Examine stools for gross blood. Offer normal diet if no bowel perforation exists. Suggest a warm bath for relaxation. Allow time for rest. Monitor patient until the effects of the medications have diminished. Assess patient's vital signs. Watch for decrease in blood pressure with an increase in pulse rate as an indication of hemorrhage. Notify health care provider if patient develops increased pain or significant gastrointestinal bleeding. Examine abdomen for evidence of colon perforation (abdominal distention and tenderness). Encourage patient to drink a lot of fluids when intake is allowed. This will make up for the dehydration from the bowel preparation.
Complete Blood Cell (CBC) Count (See Skill 23.13)	
Order prescribed test per facility policy. Explain procedure.	Observe site for bleeding. Report results.
Computed Tomography (CT)[a]	
Explain procedure. Obtain informed consent if required. Assess for allergies to iodine (see Box 23.2). Inform patient that it is necessary to remove wigs, hairpins or clips, and dental prostheses if scan will include head. Maintain NPO status 4 h before oral contrast medium is administered, except in emergencies. See specific anatomic locations for particular interventions.	Encourage patient to drink fluids to prevent renal complications and to promote excretion of dye. See specific anatomic locations for particular interventions. 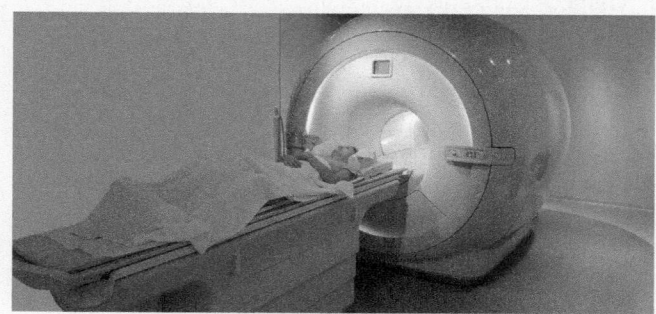 (Figure (c)iStock.com/helovi.) Machinery for computed tomography (CT).
Cystoscopy	
Explain procedure. Instruct patient to lie still during the procedure. Obtain written consent. Administer enemas as ordered, and record results. If local anesthesia is used, liquid breakfast is sometimes allowed. If general anesthesia is used, keep patient on NPO status after midnight on day of test. Administer premedications as ordered. Insert a Foley catheter if ordered.	For at least 24 h after procedure, assess patient's ability to void; urinary retention sometimes occurs secondary to edema caused by instrumentation. Record urine color; if it is bright red, report to health care provider. Suggest warm sitz baths for relaxation. Encourage fluid intake to maintain a constant flow of urine. Observe vital signs; watch for decrease in blood pressure and increase in pulse, which indicate possible hemorrhage.

Table **23.1**	Nursing Interventions for Diagnostic Examinations—cont'd
BEFORE EXAMINATION	**AFTER EXAMINATION**
	Observe for hemorrhage and for sepsis. Administer antibiotic as ordered. Instruct patient not to walk or stand alone immediately after legs have been removed from stirrups. The orthostatic hypotension that sometimes results from standing erect has the potential to cause vertigo or syncope. Mild analgesics sometimes are ordered for back pain, bladder spasms, and burning on urination. Antibiotics occasionally are ordered, to be taken 1 day before and 3 days after procedure. Encourage patient to prevent constipation. (Increases in intraabdominal pressure have the capacity to initiate severe lower urologic bleeding.) Postprocedure irrigation sometimes is ordered. If catheter remains in, provide catheter care instructions.
Echocardiography	
Order prescribed test per facility policy. Review pertinent patient history. Explain procedure; it is a painless study. Answer questions. NOTE: This procedure usually takes 45 min.	Remove the gel from the patient's chest wall with a tissue. Inform patient that the results will be available in a few hours after the health care provider has interpreted the findings.
Electrocardiography (See Skill 23.14)	
Order prescribed test per facility policy. Review all medications the patient is taking. Explain procedure. No food or fluid restriction is necessary. Expose only the patient's chest and arms. Keep the abdomen and thighs adequately covered. Assure the patient that they will not feel anything during this procedure.	Remove electrodes and gel from patient's skin with a tissue. If patient experiences chest pain during the study, indicate this on the ECG strip or request slip (it is possible that the pain will correspond to a dysrhythmia on the ECG tracing).
Electroencephalography (EEG)	
Order prescribed test per facility policy. Explain procedure. Make sure patient's hair is clean; administer shampoo as necessary; do not use any oils, sprays, or lotions. Confer with health care provider regarding the need to discontinue any medications before examination. Do not administer sedatives or hypnotics, unless ordered. Encourage food intake, but instruct patient to eliminate coffee, tea, and colas. Explain need to patient of remaining still during test; even blinking will create interference. If sleeping time is to be shortened the night before the test, instruct patient accordingly.	Assist the patient in removing the electrode paste with acetone or witch hazel. Shampoo patient's hair. Ensure safety precautions until no effects of the sedatives remain; keep side rails up. Ensure that the patient who has had sleep EEG does not have to drive home alone.
Endoscopy and Gastroscopy	
Order prescribed test per facility policy. Administer premedication, if ordered. Explain procedure. Obtain written consent before administering medication. Keep patient on NPO status after midnight. Provide emotional support.	Perform oral hygiene measures. If an anesthetic has been sprayed on the throat, do not allow the patient to eat or drink until the gag reflex returns (2–4 h). Ask patient to open mouth, and hold patient's tongue down with tongue blade. Touch back of pharynx on each side with applicator stick.

Continued

Table 23.1	Nursing Interventions for Diagnostic Examinations—cont'd

BEFORE EXAMINATION	AFTER EXAMINATION
Remove and safely store patient's dentures and eyewear.	If conscious sedation has been used, monitor patient carefully, because oversedation or adverse response to sedation has the potential to result in life-threatening complications, such as hypotension, loss of airway reflexes, inability to maintain patent airway, hypoventilation, and apnea.
Perform oral hygiene measures, because the tube will pass through the mouth.	
Reassure the patient that the procedure is not painful.	
In most of these procedures, conscious sedation is used, which is the administration of central nervous system depressant drugs or analgesics to supplement topical, local, or regional anesthesia during surgical or diagnostic procedures. It is used most often to supplement analgesia, relieve anxiety, or provide amnesia for the event. Consciousness is depressed, and some patients fall asleep but are not unconscious. Patients "wake up" in 20–30 min with no memory and no sense of the passage of time.	Explain that drinking cool fluids and gargling helps relieve some soreness.
	Observe the patient for bleeding, fever, abdominal pain, dysphagia, and dyspnea. Notify health care provider immediately if these occur.
	Monitor vital signs.
	Observe safety precautions until no effects of the sedatives remain.
If the patient's throat is to be sprayed with an anesthetic, caution patient that he or she will not be able to speak during the examination, but respiration will not be affected. Check the patient for gag reflex.	Inform patient that it is normal to have some bloating, belching, and flatulence after the procedure
Instruct the patient not to bite down on the endoscope.	

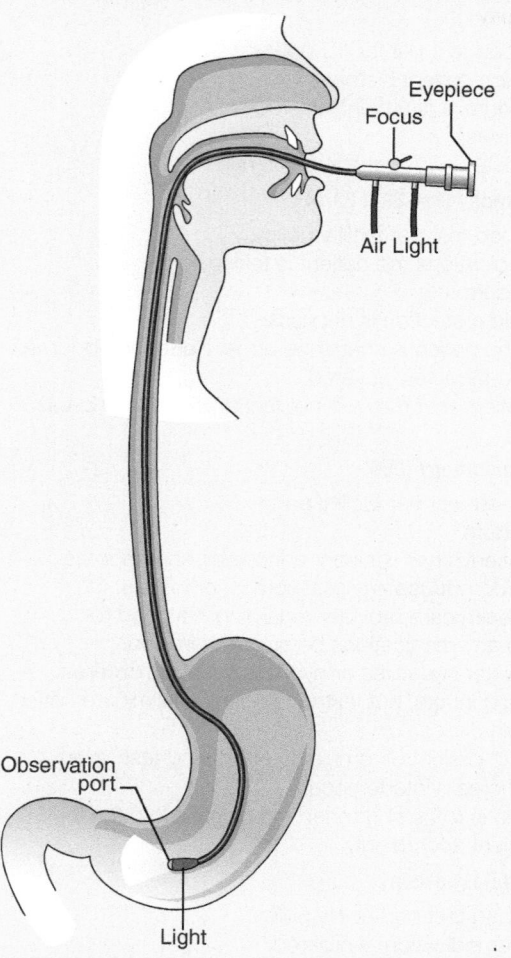

Exercise Tolerance Test (Treadmill)	
Explain procedure.	Have patient resume diet as usual.
Keep patient on NPO status for 4 h before the test, except for water, unless medications are otherwise ordered.	Have patient resume medication regimen.
	Have patient rest supine for several hours after examination.
Never withhold heart medications.	Instruct patient not to shower immediately after examination.
Instruct patient not to smoke.	Monitor and record vital signs until recordings and values return to pretest levels.
Instruct patient to wear suitable clothing; slippers are not acceptable.	Remove electrodes and paste or gel from patient's skin.

Table 23.1   Nursing Interventions for Diagnostic Examinations—cont'd

BEFORE EXAMINATION	AFTER EXAMINATION
Inform patient about the risks of the test, and obtain informed consent. Inform patient of any medications that must be discontinued before testing. Record patient's vital signs for baseline values. Apply and secure appropriate electrodes. Obtain a pretest ECG.	
Femoral Angiography (See Arteriography)	
Provide emotional support. Observe patient for allergies to iodine dye (see Box 23.2). Obtain written consent. Keep patient on NPO status after midnight.	Observe catheter insertion site for inflammation, hemorrhage, or hematoma, and observe for absence of peripheral pulses. Observe the involved extremity for numbness, tingling, pain, or loss of function. Monitor vital signs. Apply cold compresses to the puncture site as needed to reduce discomfort and edema. If patient complains of continuous, severe pain, notify health care provider.
Gallbladder Nuclear Scanning[b]	
Explain procedure. Assure patient that he or she will not be exposed to large amounts of radiation. Instruct patient to fast at least 2 h before the test. This fasting is preferred but not mandatory. Tell the patient the only discomfort associated with this procedure occurs with the IV injection of radionuclide.	Obtain a meal for the patient if indicated.
Gallbladder Series or Cholecystography	
Order prescribed test per facility policy. Explain procedure. Allow a fat-free meal the evening before examination. Assess the patient for allergy to iodine. Administer the iopanoic acid tablets (Telepaque) as ordered the day before the examination, usually early in the evening (several tablets are ordered; do not crush the tablets; have patient take them one at a time, with a 15-min interval between each tablet). Assess patient for preexisting hepatic or renal failure.	Monitor patient for side effects to the tablets, such as nausea, vomiting, diarrhea, abdominal pain, rash, and anaphylaxis. (If diarrhea develops before the examination, it is possible that the radiopaque dye will not be absorbed and, as a result, the gallbladder will not be visualized.) Instruct patient to resume usual diet as soon as series is completed. No other postprocedure care is necessary.
Glucose Tolerance Test (GTT)	

Order prescribed test per facility policy.
Explain procedure.
Consume normal intake in the days before the test.
Keep patient on NPO status for 8 h.
Collect blood and urine specimens at the same time (1 h, 3 h), and note times.[c]
The procedure is as follows:
  A laboratory assistant administers a solution containing 75 g of glucose orally.
  Instruct patient to discontinue drugs, including tobacco, that have potential to interfere with test results. Consult health care provider.
  If necessary, give patient written instructions concerning the test requirements.
  Obtain patient's weight to determine the appropriate loading dose.
	Mark on the tube the times specimens are collected.
	Send all specimens promptly to the laboratory.
	Observe venipuncture site for bleeding; apply pressure as necessary.
	Make certain patient receives meal when test is completed.
	Report results. An elevated blood glucose level at the 2-h point usually indicates some disorder of carbohydrate metabolism; depending on how elevated the blood glucose level is, glucose may be present in the urine.
	Administer insulin or oral hypoglycemic, if ordered.

Continued

Table 23.1	Nursing Interventions for Diagnostic Examinations—cont'd

BEFORE EXAMINATION	AFTER EXAMINATION
Hematest of Stools (Guaiac): Hemoccult Slide Test (See Skill 23.7)	
Explain procedure. Assist patient in obtaining specimens. There are many options for type of procedural materials (cards, tissue wipes, test paper). Tests often are permitted to be done at home with cards (Hemoccult) that can be mailed when the specimen is collected. Inform patient of the need for obtaining multiple specimens on separate days to increase test accuracy. Document specimens as sent to laboratory. Instruct patient not to eat foods that may affect the test for at least 3 days before the test. Foods include red meat, cantaloupe, uncooked broccoli, and turnips. Medications that can affect the test results include vitamin C, aspirin, and NSAID medications and should be held in the days preceding the test if approved of by the health care provider. Instruct patient not to mix urine with the stool specimen. Note on laboratory slip any anticoagulants or medications the patient is taking. Be gentle when obtaining stool by digital rectal examination. Traumatic digital examination can cause a false-positive result, especially in patients with prior anorectal disease such as hemorrhoids.	No specific follow-up care is necessary. Read results and inform patient. If test results are positive, ascertain whether the patient violated any of the preparation recommendations.
Intravenous Pyelography (IVP) or Intravenous Urography (IUG)	
Order prescribed test per facility policy. Be certain IVP is done before any barium studies. Explain procedure to patient. Check for allergies to iodine and shellfish (the intravenous dye contains iodine). Administer cathartics or laxatives as ordered (children and infants are not given cathartics or laxatives). Keep patient on NPO status after midnight (if an IV solution is infusing, ask whether health care provider wishes to decrease infusion to keep-open rate to prevent hydration; for IVP, fluid restriction is necessary for the dye to be taken up by the kidneys). Some facilities prefer abstinence from solid food for 8 h before testing; some allow a clear liquid breakfast on test day. Assess the patient's blood urea nitrogen (BUN) and creatinine levels. (Renal function that is already abnormal sometimes deteriorates further as a result of the dye injection.) Give patient an enema or suppository on the morning of study, if ordered. NOTE: Indicate specific fasting times for older adults and debilitated patients.	Observe for anaphylaxis (respiratory distress, shock, and drop in blood pressure) (see Box 23.2). Allow patient normal diet. Encourage fluid intake to help eliminate any dye left in body and counteract any fluid depletion. Encourage patient to ambulate with assistance unless contraindicated. Some patients will be weak because of the fasting and catharsis necessary for test preparation. Assess urinary output (a decreased output indicates possible renal failure).
Kidney, Ureter, and Bladder X-Ray Study (KUB, Flat Plate of the Abdomen)	
Order prescribed test per facility policy. Explain procedure; no GI contrast media will be used. No fasting or sedation is required. Schedule this study before any barium studies. Ensure all radiopaque clothing has been removed.	No specific follow-up. Report results to health care provider. Schedule IVP or gastrointestinal studies after completion of the KUB.

Table **23.1**   Nursing Interventions for Diagnostic Examinations—cont'd

BEFORE EXAMINATION	AFTER EXAMINATION
Liver Biopsy	

Explain procedure. Obtain written consent. Assess blood coagulation profile; it must be normal for study to proceed. Keep patient on NPO status after midnight before examination. Assist health care provider. Send specimens to laboratory promptly. Have specimen placed in proper **fixative** (any substance used to preserve gross or histologic specimens of tissue for later examination); usually 10% formalin is used but confirm with laboratory or pathologist. If liver specimen is for detection of lymphoma, saline solution is used. Administer any sedative medications as ordered.	Keep patient on bed rest for 24 h. Keep patient on right side for about 1–2 h immediately after the procedure. (In this position, the liver capsule is compressed against the chest wall, thereby decreasing the risk of hemorrhage or bile leak.) Observe for hemorrhage. Apply pressure dressing. Monitor vital signs frequently for evidence of hemorrhage (i.e., increased pulse and decreased blood pressure) and for peritonitis (i.e., increased temperature). Observe biopsy site. Tell patient to avoid coughing or straining, which tend to increase intraabdominal pressure. Instruct patient to avoid strenuous activities and heavy lifting for 1–2 weeks. Evaluate the rate, rhythm, and depth of respirations. Assess breath sounds. Report chest pain and signs of dyspnea, cyanosis, and restlessness (indicate possible pneumothorax).

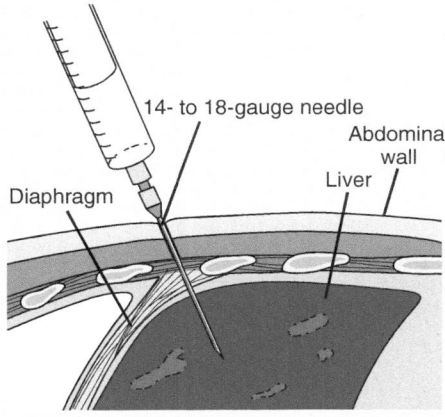

Liver biopsy: Percutaneous liver biopsy requires the patient's cooperation. The patient has to be able to lie quietly and hold his or her breath after exhaling. (From Pagana KD, Pagana TJ: *Mosby's diagnostic and laboratory test reference*, ed 12, St. Louis, 2015, Mosby.)

BEFORE EXAMINATION	AFTER EXAMINATION
Lumbar Puncture (Spinal Tap)	
Explain procedure. Obtain written consent. Have patient empty bladder and bowel. No fasting or sedation is required before procedure. Provide necessary equipment. Assist patient in assuming appropriate position. Hold manometer straight, if requested. Label and number specimen containers. Perform baseline neurologic assessment of the legs by assessing patient's strength, sensation, and movement. Explain to patient that it is necessary to lie very still throughout procedure (movement has potential to cause injury). Encourage patient to relax and take deep, slow breaths with mouth open.	Apply digital pressure and an adhesive dressing to the puncture site. Notify health care provider if any unusual findings from puncture site occur. Encourage fluids (using a drinking straw so that patient can keep head flat). Usually patient is kept in the supine position with the head of the bed elevated no more than 30 degrees until activity is changed by the health care provider to prevent discomfort from potential postpuncture spinal headache. Allow patient to turn from side to side as long as head is not raised. Transport specimens to laboratory immediately (refrigeration will alter test results). A delay between collection time and testing can result in invalid results, especially cell counts. Instruct patient to report any abnormalities such as numbness and tingling in the legs. Assess patient for numbness, tingling, and movement of the extremities; pain at the injection site; drainage of blood or CSF at the injection site; and the ability to void. Notify health care provider of any unusual findings.

Continued

Table 23.1	Nursing Interventions for Diagnostic Examinations—cont'd

BEFORE EXAMINATION	AFTER EXAMINATION

Position of patient (A) and site of needle insertion (B) for lumbar puncture.

Lung Scan[a]

Order prescribed test per facility policy.	Apply pressure to venipuncture site.
Obtain informed consent if required by facility.	Encourage fluid intake.
Explain procedure.	No radiation precautions are necessary.
Observe the patient for allergies to iodine (see Box 23.2).	Encourage patients who received dye injection to increase fluid intake because the dye causes diuresis.
Keep patient on NPO status for 4 h before test if contrast medium is administered.	
Have a recent chest radiograph available.	
Remove jewelry around the chest area.	

Magnetic Resonance Imaging (MRI), Nuclear Magnetic Resonance Imaging (NMRI)[a]

Order prescribed test per facility policy.
Explain procedure.
Obtain informed consent.
Assess the patient for any contraindications to testing (e.g., aneurysm clips, plates, pacemaker, spinal cord stimulator, and shrapnel).
Instruct patient to remove all metal objects: dentures, partial dentures, jewelry, hairpins, and belts; provide safe storage.
Inform patient of the need to remain motionless during the test.
Have patient empty bladder for comfort.
Encourage adults to read or talk to pediatric patients in scanning room.
Some patients experience claustrophobia; antianxiety medications are often helpful.
Explain that during the procedure, patient will hear a thumping sound. (Earplugs are available if the patient wishes to use them.)
There are no food or fluid restrictions.

No postprocedure care is necessary.
Patient is permitted to drive without assistance after procedure.

Assisting with magnetic resonance imaging (MRI).
(Figure from Ramsay J, Joncas J, Gilbert G, Trop I, Cheriet F, Labelle H, Parent S: Is Breast Asymmetry Present in Girls with Adolescent Idiopathic Scoliosis? *Spine Deformity* 2(5):374–379, 2014. https://doi.org/10.1016/j.jspd.2014.05.002.)

Table 23.1	Nursing Interventions for Diagnostic Examinations—cont'd
BEFORE EXAMINATION	**AFTER EXAMINATION**

Mammography

Order prescribed test per facility policy. Explain procedure. If patient is embarrassed by the procedure, ask patient to verbalize her feelings.	Explain how to obtain test results. Instruct patient on breast self-examination.
Provide emotional support. Instruct patient not to wear deodorant, powder, or lotion. Some discomfort during the examination is possible (from breast compression). This compression allows for better visualization of the breast tissue. Assure patient the breast will not be harmed. If the patient has very tender breasts, this procedure is potentially painful. No fasting is required. Patient should disrobe above the waist and put on gown.	

Myelography

Explain procedure. Obtain written consent. Assess for allergies to dye and shellfish. Obtain and assess medication history. (It is necessary to avoid some medications with the capacity to decrease seizure threshold.) Have patient empty bladder and bowel. Food and fluid restrictions vary according to the type of dye used. Check with radiologist for specific restrictions. Instruct patient to lie very still during procedure. Inform patient that he or she will be tilted into an up-and-down position on the table so that the dye can fill the spinal canal properly and provide adequate visualization in the desired area.	If necessary, assist with proper positioning, as prescribed by the health care provider. Usually, the patient is on bed rest for several hours. The head position varies with the dye used. (Examples: Elevate the head after using oil-based and water-soluble agents. After an air-contrast study, position the head lower than the rest of the body.) Observe the patient for fever, stiff neck, occipital headache, or photophobia, which are signs and symptoms of meningeal irritation. Monitor vital signs. Monitor ability to void. Encourage fluids so that patient does not get dehydrated; dehydration will result in a severe headache. Observe for seizure activity, which some types of dye potentially cause.

Paracentesis

Explain procedure. Obtain written consent. Provide emotional support. Obtain equipment. Assist health care provider. No fasting or sedation is necessary. Have patient urinate before the test (helps prevent accidental bladder trauma). Measure abdominal girth. Measure patient's weight. Measure baseline vital signs. Although local anesthetics eliminate pain at insertion site, tell patient that he or she will feel a pressure-like pain as the needle is inserted. Paracentesis. A catheter is placed through the skin and the abdominal muscle wall into the peritoneal cavity that contains free fluid.	Observe for syncope. Monitor vital signs. Encourage a period of rest after examination. Send specimen to laboratory for examination, if requested. (It is necessary to perform all laboratory tests immediately to ensure accuracy of results. Label all specimen containers appropriately.) Observe puncture site for bleeding, continued drainage, or signs of inflammation. Measure abdominal girth and weight of the patient, and compare measurements with baseline values. Observe for signs of hypotension if a large volume of fluid was removed. Record any recent antibiotic therapy on requisition slip. Monitor serum protein and electrolyte levels, especially sodium (protein content of ascitic fluid is high). Occasionally, fluid continues to leak from the needle tract. It is possible to stop this with a suture. If the suture is unsuccessful, apply a collection bag to the skin to allow for measurement of volume of fluid and treatment of fluid loss.

Continued

Table 23.1   **Nursing Interventions for Diagnostic Examinations—cont'd**

BEFORE EXAMINATION	AFTER EXAMINATION
Positron Emission Tomography (PET)	
Order prescribed test per facility policy. Obtain informed consent. Instruct patient not to have alcohol, caffeine, tobacco, sedatives, or tranquilizers for 24 h before examination; no other restrictions are necessary. Have patient empty bladder before examination. Explain procedure (because many patients have not heard of this study, they are often anxious and require emotional support). Excessive anxiety has the capacity to affect brain function evaluation. Inform patient that two IV lines probably will be inserted: one for infusion of the isotope and the other for serial blood samples. Instruct patients with diabetes to take their pretest dose of insulin at a meal 3–4 h before the test. High glucose levels potentially will decrease accuracy and invalidate results of PET scans. Inform patient that the only discomfort associated with this study is the insertion of the two IV lines. ·	Instruct patient to change position slowly from lying to standing to prevent postural hypotension. Encourage patient to drink fluids and urinate frequently to aid in removal of the radioisotope from the bladder. Report results.
Proctoscopy and Sigmoidoscopy	
Order prescribed test per facility policy. Explain procedure. Provide emotional support. Obtain written consent. Allow patient a light breakfast on day of examination. Administer enemas as ordered and record results. In most cases, two Fleet enemas are sufficient. Ensure patient is draped properly to prevent unnecessary embarrassment. Inform patient that he or she will feel discomfort and the urge to defecate as the proctoscope or sigmoidoscope is inserted. Position for proctoscopy.	Observe the patient for fever, rectal bleeding, abdominal distention, unusual complaints of pain, and increased tenderness. Inform patient that because air has been insufflated into the bowel during the procedure, he or she may have flatulence or gas pains. Ambulation often helps. If biopsy samples have been taken, slight rectal bleeding is possible. Instruct patient to report increasing abdominal pain (indicates possible bowel perforation). Fever and chills are further indications of a possible bowel perforation. Inform patient that frequent bloody bowel movements possibly indicate poor hemostasis if biopsy or polypectomy was performed. Observe for abdominal bloating and inability to pass flatus, which indicates possible colon obstruction, if a neoplasm was identified.
Renal Angiography	
Explain procedure. Answer questions. Obtain written consent. Determine whether patient has been taking anticoagulants. Assess patient for allergy to iodine dye (see Box 23.2). Keep patient on NPO status at least 2–8 h before testing. Administer cathartics as ordered. Administer premedications. Advise patient that he or she may experience flushing and a sensation of warmth when dye is injected. Mark the site of the peripheral pulses with a pen (allows for postprocedure assessment).	Observe arterial puncture site frequently; apply pressure dressings. Monitor the extremity for adequate circulation. Monitor pedal pulses and vital signs frequently. Keep patient on bed rest for about 8 h (this will allow for complete sealing of the arterial puncture site). Inform patient that cold compresses to puncture site will help reduce discomfort and edema. Encourage intake of fluids. Assess peripheral arterial pulse in the extremity used for vascular access and compare with preprocedure baseline values.

Table 23.1   Nursing Interventions for Diagnostic Examinations—cont'd

BEFORE EXAMINATION	AFTER EXAMINATION
Document abnormalities in peripheral pulses. Ensure that the appropriate coagulation studies have been performed and results are normal. Remove and safely store all valuables and dental prostheses. Have patient void (the dye sometimes acts as a diuretic). Inform patient that bladder distention sometimes causes some discomfort during the study.	Maintain pressure at the puncture site with 1- to 2-lb sandbag or IV bag. Assess extremities for signs of reduction in blood supply (i.e., absence of pulses, numbness, pallor, tingling pain, loss of sensory or motor function). Note and compare the color and temperature of the involved extremity with those of the uninvolved extremity. Notify health care provider if there is severe, continuous pain. Encourage fluids to prevent dehydration caused by diuretic action of the dye. Evaluate for delayed reaction to dye. Administer mild analgesics for minor discomfort at arterial puncture site.

Thoracentesis

Explain procedure. Obtain written consent. Obtain equipment. Assist patient in assuming the appropriate position (usually sitting). Offer emotional support. No fasting or sedation is necessary. Advise patient to keep movement or coughing to a minimum to prevent the needle from causing damage to the lung or the pleura during procedure. Administer cough suppressant if patient has troublesome cough. A radiograph or ultrasound scan often is used to assist in location of the fluid. Fluoroscopy may also be used. Inform patient that although local anesthetics eliminate pain at the insertion site, a pressure-like pain is possible when the pleura is entered and the fluid is removed	Monitor vital signs. Monitor patient for coughing or for hemoptysis, which indicates possible trauma to the lung. If patient has no complaints of dyspnea, he or she may resume normal activity in an hour. Place small dressing over needle site. Usually, you will turn patient on the unaffected side for 1 h to allow the puncture site to seal. Label specimen containers appropriately and send promptly to the laboratory. Obtain chest radiograph, if ordered, to assess for pneumothorax. Assess patient for signs and symptoms of subcutaneous emphysema or infection (e.g., tachypnea, dyspnea, diminished breath sounds, anxiety, restlessness, fever). Assess patient's lungs for diminished breath sounds, which are a sign of possible pneumothorax.

Patient positioning for thoracentesis.

Ultrasonography or Sonography[a]

Order prescribed test per facility policy. Explain procedure. If a pelvic sonogram is ordered, the patient needs a full bladder. If a gallbladder sonogram is ordered, keep patient on NPO status. For other sonograms, no fasting or sedation is needed. Obtain a signed consent form, if required.	Because this procedure is noninvasive, no specific follow-up care is needed. Patient should resume usual diet after examination. Remove the lubricant from the patient's skin. Encourage voiding.

Upper Gastrointestinal Series

Prepare requisition form. Explain procedure, and answer questions. Offer emotional support; the test will not cause discomfort. Keep patient on NPO status for at least 8 h before examination. Advise patient of potential discomfort from lying on the hard table and possible sensation of bloating or nausea during the test.	Permit patient to eat as soon as series is completed, unless food is contraindicated. Encourage intake of fluids. Administer barium liquid or per hospital protocol. Inform patient that if diatrizoate (Gastrografin) was used as contrast medium, significant diarrhea is possible. Monitor stools to make certain all of the barium has been eliminated. Initial stools will be chalky in appearance. The stools usually return to normal color after complete expulsion of the barium, which sometimes takes as long as a day and a half.

Continued

Table 23.1   Nursing Interventions for Diagnostic Examinations—cont'd

BEFORE EXAMINATION	AFTER EXAMINATION
Urinalysis (UA)	
Order prescribed test per facility policy. Explain purpose and specific method of urine collection. Wash patient's perineal area, if soiled. If patient is menstruating, note this on requisition form. Use midstream urine collection guidelines (see Skill 23.2).	Take specimen to laboratory promptly. If it is not processed immediately, refrigerate specimen. If 24-h urine collection is requested, refrigerate specimen or preserve with formalin when collected. It is necessary to perform examination for casts on fresh urine specimens.

CSF, Cerebrospinal fluid; *GI,* gastrointestinal; *IV,* intravenous; *NPO,* nothing by mouth.

[a]Showing a picture of the x-ray machine (used for scans and MRI) and encouraging the patient to verbalize concerns regarding claustrophobia help reduce anxiety. Most patients who are mildly claustrophobic are able to tolerate these studies after appropriate premedication with antianxiety medications. Most of these tests require lying still on a hard table and peripheral venipuncture, which sometimes cause mild discomfort. Mild nausea is a common sensation when contrast dye is used; have an emesis basin readily available. Some patients experience a salty taste, flushing, and a sensation of warmth during the dye injection. Encourage patients who receive dye injections to increase their fluid intake, because the dye is excreted by the kidneys and causes diuresis. Assure patients that they will be draped sufficiently to prevent unnecessary exposure.

[b]Gallbladder nuclear scanning has replaced the gallbladder series.

[c]Specific collection times depend on health care provider's orders.

 Lifespan Considerations

Older Adults

Specimen Collection and Diagnostic Tests

- Vital Signs and Monitoring
  - In older adults, slight variations in vital signs or in behavior often indicate impending problems; therefore, skilled observations are critical.
  - The use of medications (such as hypnotics and opioids) to reduce pain and anxiety during a procedure may impair respiratory and renal functioning. Monitoring vital signs and intake and output is necessary.
  - Restlessness after a procedure in an older adult possibly indicates hypoxia or pain. Assess the patient thoroughly for the cause.
- Positioning and comfort
  - Many older adults have difficulty assuming the various positions needed for specimen collection. The nurse should assess and assist as needed.
  - Because of the degree of agility necessary to collect a specimen, such as a midstream urine specimen, greater assistance from the nurse is sometimes required. Catheterization may be necessary, but other techniques and positioning (bedpans, specimen hats in toilet or commode) should be implemented before catheterization is considered.
  - If multiple procedures are necessary, schedule adequate rest time between tests.
  - Older adults often need additional clothing, slippers, and extra blankets to keep them warm in waiting rooms and examination rooms.
- Fluid Status
  - The older adult should be assessed carefully for dehydration, as the preparation for some testing requires the patient to be NPO.
- Skin integrity
  - Older adults are at greater risk for skin impairment. Assess skin integrity of a patient after he or she has been lying on the examination table.

- Vascularity
  - Decreased peripheral circulation sometimes makes it difficult to collect a specimen for blood glucose determination. Wrapping the hand in a warm, moist washcloth or massaging the hand for a few seconds may facilitate the procedure.
  - Changes in blood vessels make venipuncture more difficult in many older adults. Repeated sticks to obtain blood samples pose the risk of causing emotional and physical trauma to the older adult. Care should be taken to avoid multiple venipunctures.
  - When obtaining a specimen through venipuncture, remember that some older adults do not need a tourniquet for this procedure.
  - Older adults have fragile veins that are traumatized easily during venipuncture.
- Emotional and Educational needs
  - It is important to explain the purpose of the procedure and provide privacy during specimen collection.
  - If a patient is confused, it is helpful to have another staff member present during the testing or specimen collection to provide comfort, reassurance, and/or distraction for the patient.
  - Assessment of certain specimens involves comparing results to a color chart. Older adults may have difficulty reading the color chart.
  - Many older adult patients take multiple medications. Testing and procedures may require alteration in administration schedules. Be sure to give the patient instructions in writing if certain medications are not to be taken before or after a procedure/test.
  - When maintaining specimen collections, such as a 24-h urine specimen, older adults may benefit from a written reminder placed on the bathroom mirror or toilet to collect all urine samples during the time frame.

SPECIMEN COLLECTION

The nurse is often responsible for collecting specimens that have been ordered. Laboratory examination of specimens of urine, stool, sputum, blood, and wound drainage provides important information about body functioning and contributes to the assessment of the patient's health status. Laboratory test results often facilitate the diagnosis of health care problems, provide information about the stage and activity of a disease process, and measure the response to therapy.

Patients often experience embarrassment or discomfort when giving a sample of body excretions or secretions. Most people believe excretions should be handled discreetly; affording the patient privacy is helpful in achieving comfort during the sample collection. Anxiety also is provoked by the invasive nature of some collection procedures, as is the fear of what the test results will reveal. Patients given a clear explanation about the purpose of the specimen and how it is to be obtained will be more cooperative in its collection. With proper instruction, many patients can obtain their own specimens of urine, stool, and sputum, thus minimizing embarrassment. Often the success of specimen collection depends on cooperation.

 Cultural Considerations

Diagnostic Testing

- If the patient's language skills are inadequate for communication, assistance from interpreters, word signs, or charts may be necessary.
- A patient who is modest and self-conscious about the body will need psychological preparation before some procedures and tests.
- Patients may fear medical facilities because of language barriers, unfamiliarity with the facilities, or inadequate understanding of illness and treatment regimen. As a result, they may not comply with medical regimens.
- Be aware that diverse age groups and sociocultural groups typically use different words to describe urine and stool.
- Avoid cultural conflicts by communicating with the patient and respecting the ethnicity and individuality of each patient.

 Patient Teaching

Specimen Collection and Diagnostic Tests

- Explain importance of collecting specimens on time and in the correct amount.
- Explain the purpose of the specimen collection or diagnostic tests
- Discuss the timing for results and how the results will be communicated to the patient. For example, will the provider or nurse call the patient or will the results be emailed/mailed. Educate the patient on how long the results will take. Many facilities now have electronic patient portals that permit the patient to log in and securely review their diagnostic and specimen results. This is a convenient way for the patient to track their own health. Patient portals must be used with care. If a patient were to view alarming results from home (for example, a concerning biopsy result), they will not have immediate access to the provider to answer questions and provide clarifications of the results. Even if the results are not alarming, the patient viewing the results without the interpretation and guidance of the provider is a concern at times. For this reason, most results in a patient portal must be viewed and signed off by the provider prior to the patient being able to access these results.
- Explain appropriate hand hygiene and instruct patient to perform it before and after specimen collection.
- Explain proper procedure for obtaining each specimen and preparing for each diagnostic examination.
- Assure the patient has the correct equipment if the collection is to be done at home. For example, a specimen hat, container, gloves, and a tongue blade are needed for a stool specimen.
- Some specimen collection is completed outside the health care facility. Ensure the patient understands how to complete the collection. Ask patient to perform return demonstration of obtaining a specimen. Example: Skin puncture for measuring blood glucose level
- If dietary restrictions are required, explain importance of adhering to direction. Example: A meat-free diet often is ordered before a stool specimen for occult blood. Provide verbal and written instructions along with a phone number to call with questions.
- Explain results of test to the patient. Be sure the provider has reviewed the results and indicated the results can be shared with the patient. Results of diagnostic testing and specimen collection should always be shared with the patient but, depending on the situation, the provider may want to discuss the results formally with the patient or may permit the nurse to notify the patient and share the results.
- Explain normal laboratory values when appropriate. Example: Blood glucose levels desired
- Explain when to notify health care provider. Example: Elevated blood glucose level
- Advise patient to perform oral hygiene after sputum collection as a comfort measure.
- Explain the importance of drinking fluids to decrease thickness of mucus (this is helpful before sputum collection).
- Ensure that patient understands the importance of obtaining an uncontaminated specimen.
- Allow time for patient questions and provide answers.
- Instruct patient to check with the primary health care provider about taking, or readjusting the time schedule for, prescribed medications on the day of the test or examination.

Preventing Inaccuracy in Examination and Test Procedures

Many factors have the capacity to interfere with examinations and tests and potentially can alter the accuracy of or even nullify their results:
- Drug interactions
- Insufficient bowel cleansing
- Failure to maintain fasting requirements
- Inadequate diet preparation
- Incompleteness or absence of test requisition
- Specimen not delivered on schedule
- Inappropriate specimen amount
- Contamination of sterile specimen
- Absence of required informed consent

GUIDELINES FOR SPECIMEN COLLECTION

Laboratory tests are often expensive. Help prevent unnecessary costs by using the correct procedures for obtaining and processing specimens (Box 23.3). When a patient has questions about laboratory tests, consult the agency's procedure manual or call the laboratory.

It is the nurse's responsibility to notify the prescribing health care provider when results of laboratory and diagnostic studies deviate from the norm and intervention is necessary. Each health care facility will have policy and procedure manuals available to guide the nurse. These manuals (often in electronic form) contain routine orders for each diagnostic test. The manuals are a valuable resource that prevents the nurse from overlooking critical patient preparation information or the need to take action or notify the prescribing health care provider of results.

Regardless of the type of specimen collected, the nurse must take care to correctly label the specimen so errors in reporting are eliminated. The patient identification label should always be placed on the container and not on the lid. When the specimen is in lab, the lab personnel will remove the lid to access the specimen. If the lid is separated from the container, the lab will not have the ability to accurately report on the correct patient.

Remembering the meaning of root words, prefixes, and suffixes helps in identifying test names. Knowing the following suffixes is useful:

-ography	Procedure in which an image is produced (e.g., mammography)
-ogram	Actual image or results of a test (e.g., mammogram)
-oscopy	Procedure in which body structures are visualized (e.g., colonoscopy)
-centesis	Procedure involving puncture of a body cavity (e.g., thoracentesis)

Box 23.4 lists general guidelines for specimen collection.

General Guidelines for Specimen Collections

- Consider the patient's needs and his or her ability to participate in specimen collection procedures.
- Recognize that collection of a specimen sometimes provokes anxiety, embarrassment, or discomfort.
- Provide support for patients who are fearful about the results of a specimen examination.
- Recognize that children require a clear explanation of procedures and often benefit from the support of parents or family members.
- Obtain specimens in accordance with specific prerequisite conditions (e.g., fasting, nothing-by-mouth [NPO] status) as required.
- Wear gloves when collecting specimens of blood or other body fluids because it is not possible to identify everyone infected with bloodborne pathogens such as human immunodeficiency virus (HIV), hepatitis B, or other pathogens.
- Remove gloves, discard them in proper receptacle, and immediately perform hand hygiene; similarly cleanse other skin surfaces thoroughly if contaminated with blood or body fluids.
- Collect specimens in designated containers, at the correct time, in the appropriate amount.
- Properly label all specimens with the patient's identification; complete laboratory requisition form as necessary (see Box 23.5).
- Most specimens are transported to the laboratory in a separate biohazard bag (see illustration for Skill 23.1, Step 11).
- Deliver specimens to the laboratory within the recommended time, or ensure that they are stored properly for later transport.
- Use aseptic technique in all collections to prevent contamination, which has the potential to render test results inaccurate.
- Transport specimens under special conditions (e.g., iced specimens or special containers with preservatives) as required.

COLLECTING A MIDSTREAM URINE SPECIMEN

There are several methods for collecting a urine speci-men (a small sample of something, intended to show the nature of the whole) for urinalysis, one of the most commonly ordered diagnostic tests. Typically, the urinalysis consists of several tests, including determination of pH, specific gravity, and the presence of any protein, glucose, ketones, blood, and white blood cells (WBCs). In addition, a urine specimen sometimes is ordered for a culture and sensitivity test, which is used in the diagnosis and treatment of urinary tract infections. The nurse's responsibilities are to collect and label the urine sample, to ensure its safe and accurate delivery to the laboratory, and to assess the results. The nurse also explains the collection procedure to the patient and, if appropriate, notifies the health care provider of the results.

It is necessary that the patient is aware of the upcoming test and knows to contact the nurse before the next voiding. The nurse may instruct the patient to drink extra water to assist voiding, to avoid putting toilet tissue in the specimen container, and to prevent fecal matter from coming in contact with the urine specimen. A midstream urine specimen is collected to perform a culture and sensitivity. Urine is collected after voiding is initiated (midstream) and before voiding is completed (Skill 23.2). A midstream specimen is the cleanest part of the voided specimen and is collected in a sterile container.

COLLECTING A STERILE URINE SPECIMEN

If the provider orders a sterile urine specimen, the nurse will collect the specimen by inserting a straight catheter into the urinary bladder to remove urine or by obtaining a specimen from the port of an indwelling catheter with the use of sterile technique. Never use urine from a dependent drainage bag for a specimen. The drainage bag has been in contact with urine for an extended period of time and will be contaminated, thus making the result inaccurate. It is possible to measure residual urine (urine left in the bladder after voiding) at the time of catheterization.

Catheterization is performed within 10 minutes after the patient voids. More than 50 mL of urine remaining in the bladder is considered residual urine, and the patient may require insertion of an indwelling catheter. Most facilities will have a non-invasive bladder scanner available to determine the amount of residual urine present. However, if the nurse is catheterizing the patient for a specimen, residual urine can be obtained at that time without the use of the bladder scanner.

Prepare the patient by explaining which type of urine specimen will be collected. Relieve any anxiety by assuring the patient that there will be minimal or no discomfort if the patient remains relaxed and that he or she will experience only a sensation of mild pressure as the catheter is inserted and no discomfort or sensation when urine is collected from the catheter port. See Chapter 15 and Skill 15.1 for insertion of a sterile urinary catheter.

If a urinary catheter is already in place, a sterile urine specimen may be obtained from the port of the urinary drainage system. With this approach, the sterility of the urinary drainage system is not compromised (Skill 23.3).

COLLECTING A 24-HOUR URINE SPECIMEN

Tests of renal function and urine composition, such as measurements of levels of adrenocortical steroids, hormones, protein, and creatinine clearance, necessitate a 24-hour collection of urine. The licensed practical nurse/licensed vocational nurse (LPN/LVN) must carefully follow the procedure for ensuring accurate performance of the test. Some tests require collecting the entire volume of urine from a 24-hour period (Skill 23.4). If urine is discarded accidentally or contaminated

or if the patient is incontinent, the prescribing health care provider must order an indwelling catheter.

Care should be taken to explain the collection to the patient and, if the collection is at a facility, to the staff. Signs should be placed on the door and in the bathroom reminding the patient and staff to collect each void. Failure to collect all of the urine will result in the entire test needing to be rescheduled.

MEASURING BLOOD GLUCOSE LEVELS

Using a glucose meter to measure the blood glucose of a patient with diabetes provides more meaningful data than testing urine for the presence of glucose. The patient is able to easily perform skin puncture at home (Skill 23.5).

COLLECTING A STOOL SPECIMEN

Stool specimens are collected and examined for a variety of reasons, including the following: to determine the presence of infection or blood; to observe the amount, color, and consistency of the stool; to determine the presence of fats; or to identify parasites, ova, and bacteria. The LPN/LVN collects the feces, labels the specimen appropriately, and sends the specimen and the laboratory request to the laboratory. When stool is to be examined for parasites, it must be taken immediately to the laboratory for parasites to be examined under the microscope while they are alive. It is also possible to collect a stool specimen from a colostomy or an ileostomy.

Inform the patient that a stool specimen is needed, then carry out collection in a manner that does not cause the patient to feel hurried or embarrassed. Arrange supplies if the patient is to collect the stool. When a stool specimen is to be obtained, place the specimen hat toward the back of the toilet or commode. When a urine specimen is to be obtained, place the specimen hat toward the front (Fig. 23.1). If urine and stool specimens are to be collected, use two specimen hats: one placed at the front and one placed toward the back of the toilet or commode. A bedpan may be used to collect a stool specimen if the patient is cautioned not to void in the bedpan, which would compromise the stool specimen. The LPN/LVN must understand why the stool specimen is being collected to choose the appropriate supplies. If the stool specimen is for ova and parasites, an appropriate container with a special solution must be obtained from the laboratory (Skill 23.6).

DETERMINING THE PRESENCE OF OCCULT BLOOD IN STOOL (GUAIAC)

The presence of blood in body waste is abnormal. Bright red blood in the stool indicates that the blood is fresh and that the site of bleeding is in the lower gastrointestinal (GI) tract. In contrast, black, tarry feces indicate the presence of old blood and that the site of bleeding is higher in the GI tract. When blood

Skill 23.2   Collecting a Midstream Urine Specimen

 CHECK GATHER HELLO ID PRIVACY EXPLAIN WASH GLOVES

NURSING ACTION (*RATIONALE*)

1. Refer to the health care provider's order. (*Provides basis for care.*)
2. Assemble supplies (see illustration). (*Organizes procedure.*)
   - Antiseptic wipes
   - Sterile specimen container with label
   - Nonsterile gloves
   - Additional PPE if indicated
   - Biohazard bag
   - Requisition slip

3. Introduce self. (*Decreases patient's anxiety.*)
4. Identify patient. (*Ensures procedure is performed with correct patient.*)
5. Explain procedure. Assess patient's understanding of procedure. (*Decreases patient's anxiety, promotes patient's cooperation, and ensures accuracy.*)
6. Prepare patient for procedure. (*Facilitates procedure.*)
   a. Close door and pull curtain. (*Provides privacy.*)
   b. Varying degrees of assistance are required by patients who are seriously ill, have difficulty standing, or are disoriented. Some patients need assistance in the bathroom, whereas others require a bedpan or urinal in bed. Older patients may have difficulty maintaining balance and raising or lowering toilet seats.
7. Perform hand hygiene and don nonsterile gloves. (*Reduces spread of microorganisms.*)
8. Allow the patient to cleanse self with the antiseptic wipes if the patient is able; instruct female patients to separate the labia well and cleanse the perineum in an anterior-to-posterior direction. Instruct male patients to cleanse in a circular motion from the meatus outward; if the penis is uncircumcised, the foreskin should be retracted. If the patient is unable to cleanse the area, provide assistance. (*Provides a cleaner specimen and prevents organisms at or near the meatus from being washed into the specimen. Cleansing from anterior to posterior aspect prevents microorganisms from the anus from entering through the urinary meatus.*)
9. Guide female patients to straddle bedpan or toilet, if possible, to allow for labial spreading and to keep the labia separated during voiding. Request that patient (1) begin by voiding about 30 mL into the toilet, and then position the sterile specimen container, making sure the sides of the labia do not touch the container or each other; (2) without stopping flow, void a small amount into specimen cup; (3) remove cup and, without stopping flow, finish voiding into toilet. (*Collects midstream urine specimen appropriately. The first 30 mL, containing the organisms washed away from the meatus, is discarded.*)
10. Secure lid on container without touching the inside of the lid. (*Prevents spillage and contamination.*)
11. Remove gloves, discard them in proper receptacle, and perform hand hygiene. (*Reduces spread of microorganisms.*)
12. Cleanse and return toilet seat collector, or empty and flush bedpan or urinal if any of these are in use. (*Prepares equipment for next use.*)
13. Label specimen appropriately. Place in biohazard bag for transport to laboratory (see illustration for Skill 23.1, Step 11). (*Ensures proper identification of specimen; ensures accuracy of results; prevents loss and potential delays in obtaining results.*) Follow agency policy (see Box 23.5).
14. Ensure prompt delivery to laboratory with proper requisition slip (many facilities mandate delivery within 1 h). (*Ensures a fresh specimen for testing and prevents loss of specimen.*)
15. Document procedure. (*Provides communication of procedure and patient's response.*)
    - Time
    - Type of specimen collected
    - Sent to laboratory with requisition
    - Patient's response (if appropriate)
16. Provide patient teaching (see the Patient Teaching box on specimen collection and diagnostic tests).

PPE, Personal protective equipment.

Skill 23.3   Collecting a Sterile Urine Specimen via Catheter Port

NURSING ACTION (RATIONALE)

1. Refer to the health care provider's order. (*Provides basis for care.*)
2. Assemble supplies. (*Organizes procedure.*)
   - Nonsterile gloves
   - Sterile specimen container with label
   - Clamp or rubber band
   - Sterile syringe and needle
   - Alcohol preparation
   - Requisition slip
   - Biohazard bag
   - Additional PPE if indicated
3. Introduce self. (*Decreases patient's anxiety.*)
4. Identify patient. (*Ensures procedure is performed with correct patient.*)
5. Explain procedure. (*Promotes cooperation and decreases patient's anxiety.*)
6. Perform hand hygiene and don nonsterile gloves. (*Reduces spread of microorganisms.*)
7. Catheter port collection:
   a. Clamp just below catheter port for about 30 min. (*Allows for urine to collect for removal.*)

   b. Return in 30 min; clean port with alcohol preparation. (*Prevents needle puncture from causing contamination.*)
   c. Insert needle into port at 30-degree angle and withdraw 5–10 mL of urine for a specimen. (*Inserting needle at an angle prevents puncturing opposite side of tubing. Provides for specimen.*)
   d. Place urine in sterile specimen cup. (*Keeps specimen sterile.*)
   e. Unclamp catheter. (*Allows continuous urine flow to resume.*)
   f. Label specimen and place in biohazard bag for transport to laboratory (see illustration for Skill 23.1, Step 11, and Box 23.5) and send to laboratory with requisition. (*Ensures proper identification of specimen; ensures accuracy of results; prevents loss and potential delays in obtaining results.*)
8. Remove gloves, discard them in proper receptacle, and perform hand hygiene. (*Reduces spread of microorganisms.*)
9. Document procedure and observations (see Skill 23.2, Step 15). (*Records procedure and patient's response.*)

PPE, Personal protective equipment.

Skill 23.4   Collecting a 24-Hour Urine Specimen

NURSING ACTION (RATIONALE)

1. Refer to the health care provider's order. (*Provides basis for care.*)
2. Assemble supplies and equipment. (*Organizes procedure.*)
   - Specimen hat for bedpan, commode, or toilet; or urinal
   - Specimen container, including preservative of agency's choice, and label
   - Nonsterile gloves
   - Additional PPE if indicated
   - Requisition
3. Introduce self. (*Decreases patient's anxiety.*)
4. Identify patient. (*Ensures procedure is performed with correct patient.*)
5. Explain procedure. (*Promotes cooperation and decreases anxiety.*)
   a. Stress importance of collecting all urine for a 24-h period. (*Ensures validity of results of a 24-h kidney function test.*)

Continued

Skill 23.4   Collecting a 24-Hour Urine Specimen—cont'd

b. Instruct patient not to allow tissue or fecal material to touch specimen or enter container. *(Contaminates specimen.)*

6. Post signs on bathroom door and near patient's bed to alert staff and patient to save all urine.

7. Perform hand hygiene and don nonsterile gloves according to agency policy and guidelines from the CDC and OSHA each time a specimen is collected and transferred to the large collection container. *(Reduces spread of microorganisms.)*

8. Have patient void just before the 24-h specimen collection is to begin; discard this urine. *(This urine was formed in urinary system before the study began.)*

9. Place labeled container on ice if required. (Some agencies require refrigeration of all specimens. Others advocate that the urine container be placed on ice. For some collection procedures, refrigeration is not always necessary, or a preservative may be used in 24-h specimen collection device.) *(Keeps the specimen cool, which decreases decomposition and odor.)*

10. Save all urine for the 24-h period; place each voided specimen into the larger container. *(It is essential to save all urine; otherwise results will be altered.)*

11. Instruct patient to void a few minutes before end of 24 h; this urine is part of the 24-h specimen. *(This will empty bladder before the end of testing.)*

12. Send collection to laboratory promptly; be certain label includes date and time specimen started (see Box 23.5). If more than one container is necessary, make certain both are labeled and numbered. If patient is menstruating, be certain to note this on the requisition slip. *(Ensures proper identification of specimen; ensures accuracy of results; prevents loss and potential delays in obtaining results.)*

13. Document procedure and observations (see Skill 23.2, Step 15). *(Communicates the patient care administered.)*

14. Perform patient teaching (see the Patient Teaching box on specimen collection and diagnostic tests).

CDC, Centers for Disease Control and Prevention; *OSHA,* Occupational Safety and Health Administration; *PPE,* personal protective equipment.

Skill 23.5   Measuring Blood Glucose Levels

NURSING ACTION *(RATIONALE)*

1. Refer to the health care provider's order. *(Provides basis for care.)*

2. Assemble supplies. *(Organizes procedure.)*
   - Sterile lancet
   - Automatic lancing device
   - Alcohol swab or soap and water (see Step 10)
   - Blood glucose meter
   - Testing strips for meter
   - Cotton balls
   - Nonsterile gloves

3. Introduce self. *(Decreases patient's anxiety.)*

4. Identify patient. *(Ensures procedure is performed with correct patient.)*

5. Explain procedure to patient. *(Promotes cooperation and decreases patient's anxiety.)*

6. Perform hand hygiene and don nonsterile gloves according to agency policy and guidelines from the CDC and OSHA. *(Reduces spread of microorganisms.)*

7. Remove cap from lancet by using sterile technique. *(Maintains sterility of point.)*

8. Place lancet into automatic lancing device according to instructions in operating manual. *(Allows proper puncture of skin.)*

9. Select site on side of any fingertip (for infant, use heel). *(The side of the finger is less responsive to pain from puncture than are other sites.)*

10. Wipe selected site with alcohol swab and discard swab. *(Prepares site. Some manuals now specify washing hands with soap and water—no alcohol because it alters the test strip and dries the skin.)*

11. Ask patient to hold arm at side 30 s. *(Increases blood flow to site and allows site to dry.)*

12. Gently squeeze patient's fingertip with thumb of same hand. *(Increases blood supply to site.)*

13. Hold lancing device. *(Provides easy access to device.)*

14. Place trigger platform of lancing device on side of finger and press. *(Activates lancing mechanism.)*

Skill 23.5 Measuring Blood Glucose Levels—cont'd

15. Stroke finger with downward motion; using cotton ball, wipe off first drop of blood that appears (if recommended by glucose meter manufacturer) and continue stroking. *(Produces enough blood to cover test pad on test strip; producing and wiping first drop removes surface contaminants.)*

16. While holding strip level, touch new drop of blood on finger to test pad. Do not allow finger (skin) to touch the test pad. Apply pressure to puncture site using cotton ball. *(Causes blood to cover test pad without smearing and prevents alteration of test results.)*

17. Begin timing as recommended by glucose meter instructions. Wait for numeric readout. *(Ensures test accuracy.)*

18. Remove lancet from device and discard. *(Prevents accidental needlestick injury.)*

19. Remove gloves, discard them in proper receptacle, and perform hand hygiene. *(Reduces spread of microorganisms.)*

20. Document procedure and observations (see Skill 23.2, Step 15). *(Communicates patient care administered.)*

21. Perform patient teaching (see the Patient Teaching box on specimen collection and diagnostic tests).

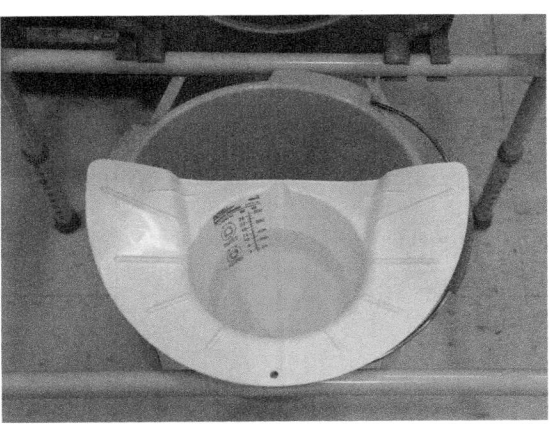

Fig. 23.1 Specimen "hat."

is present in the stool but not visible without the use of a microscope, it is referred to as **occult** (hidden). A **Hemoccult** test detects occult blood in feces (Skill 23.7).

Instruct the patient on how many stool specimens are ordered by the health care provider and how to collect a stool specimen. Then label the Hemoccult card appropriately (Box 23.5) and send it to the laboratory. Some facilities permit nursing staff to perform reagent testing without sending the Hemoccult card to the laboratory.

DETERMINING THE PRESENCE OF OCCULT BLOOD IN GASTRIC SECRETIONS OR EMESIS (GASTROCCULT TEST)

This test determines bleeding in the esophagus, the stomach, the small intestine, or the large intestine. The test confirms the suspicion of blood when gastric contents have red or black coloration or when emesis or the product of nasogastric (NG) suction has a coffee-grounds appearance (Skill 23.8) (see Chapter 15, Skill 15.5 for insertion of nasogastric tube).

COLLECTING A SPUTUM SPECIMEN

Sputum is secretion from the lungs. It contains mucus, cellular debris, microorganisms, or some combination of these, and sometimes sputum contains blood or pus. A sputum specimen must be obtained from deep in the bronchial tree. Expectoration (**expectorate**—to cough up or expel mucus or fluid from the respiratory tract) of throat and mouth secretions is not to be used as a sputum specimen, because saliva with food particles does not produce desired results. Early morning is the best time to collect a sputum specimen, because the patient has not yet cleared the respiratory passages. Many tests are possible to perform on sputum, such as **culture** (a laboratory test involving cultivation of microorganisms or cells in a special growth medium) and **sensitivity** (a laboratory method of determining

Skill 23.6   Collecting a Stool Specimen

CHECK   GATHER   HELLO   ID   PRIVACY   EXPLAIN   WASH   GLOVES

NURSING ACTION (RATIONALE)

1. Refer to the health care provider's order. (*Provides basis for care.*)
2. Assemble supplies. (*Organizes procedure.*)
   - Stool specimen cup or container
   - Nonsterile gloves
   - Additional PPE if indicated
   - Bedpan, specimen device, or commode
   - Tongue depressor
   - Specimen container label
   - Laboratory requisition
   - Biohazard bag
3. Introduce self. (*Decreases patient's anxiety.*)
4. Identify patient. (*Ensures procedure is performed with correct patient.*)
5. Explain procedure to patient; make certain patient understands what is expected. (*Promotes cooperation and decreases anxiety.*)
6. Perform hand hygiene and don nonsterile gloves according to agency policy and guidelines from the CDC and OSHA. (*Prevents transmission of microorganisms.*)
7. Assist patient to bathroom when necessary. (*Provides patient safety.*)
8. Ask patient to defecate into commode, specimen device, or bedpan, preventing urine from entering specimen. (*Prevents contamination of specimen.*)

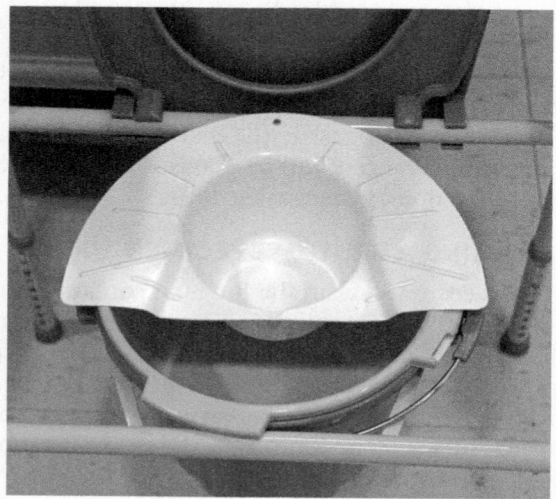

9. Transfer stool to specimen cup with use of a tongue blade, and close the lid securely. (*Protects specimen.*)

10. Remove gloves, discard them in proper receptacle, and perform hand hygiene. (*Reduces spread of microorganisms.*)
11. Attach requisition slip, enclose in a biohazard bag (see illustration for Skill 23.1, Step 11), label the bag (see Box 23.5), and send specimen to laboratory (it is necessary to take specimens for ova and parasites to the laboratory stat; it is acceptable to keep other stool specimens at room temperature). (*Ensures proper identification of specimen; ensures accuracy of results; prevents loss and potential delays in obtaining results.*)
12. Assist patient to bed. (*Provides for patient safety and comfort.*)
13. Document procedure and observations (see Skill 23.2, Step 15). (*Communicates care administered.*)
14. Perform patient teaching (see the Patient Teaching box).

CDC, Centers for Disease Control and Prevention; *OSHA,* Occupational Safety and Health Administration; *PPE,* personal protective equipment.

Skill 23.7   Determining the Presence of Occult Blood in Stool

CHECK   GATHER   HELLO   ID   PRIVACY   EXPLAIN   WASH   GLOVES

NURSING ACTION (RATIONALE)

1. Refer to the health care provider's order. (*Provides basis for care.*)
2. Assemble supplies. (*Organizes procedure.*)
   - Nonsterile gloves
   - Additional PPE if indicated
   - Clean bedpan or specimen device for commode
   - Hemoccult card
   - Wooden applicator
   - Hemoccult developer
   - Laboratory requisition
   - Biohazard bag
3. Introduce self. (*Decreases patient's anxiety.*)
4. Identify patient. (*Ensures procedure is performed with correct patient.*)
5. Explain procedure. (*Promotes cooperation and decreases patient's anxiety. It is advisable to label card before gathering specimen to prevent contamination.*)
6. Perform hand hygiene and don nonsterile gloves according to agency policy and guidelines from the CDC and OSHA. (*Reduces spread of microorganisms.*)
7. Collect stool specimen. (See Skill 23.6, Steps 8 and 9.) (*Provides stool for hemoccult test.*)
8. Follow steps on Hemoccult slide test:
   a. Open flap. (*Begins test.*)

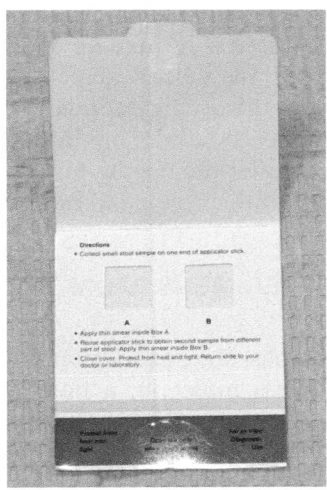

b. Use one end of tongue blade to gather stool, and smear very small amount of stool in box A. (*Prepares slide.*)

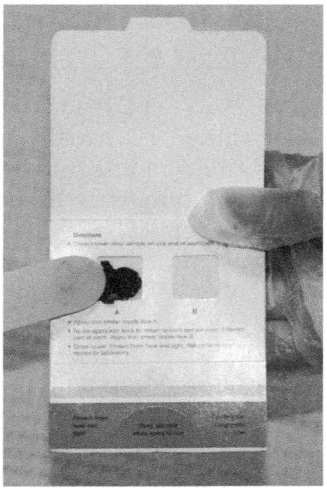

c. Use other end of tongue blade to gather from another part of stool, and smear very small amount in box B. (*Prepares second slide.*)
d. Close card and label if you have not already done so (see Box 23.5). (*Ensures accuracy in identification of specimen.*)
e. Enclose specimen in biohazard bag and send to laboratory with requisition slip. (*Ensures proper identification.*)
f. If testing is to be performed on the nursing unit, follow directions on the Hemoccult card. Document findings of occult blood in stool and results of quality control area.

9. Remove gloves, discard them in proper receptacle, and perform hand hygiene. (*Reduces spread of microorganisms.*)
10. Document procedure and observations (see Skill 23.2, Step 15). (*Communicates collection of stool specimen.*)
11. Perform patient teaching (see the Patient Teaching box).

CDC, Centers for Disease Control and Prevention; *OSHA,* Occupational Safety and Health Administration; *PPE,* personal protective equipment.

Box 23.5   Correct Labeling Information

- Patient's full name (last name, first name, and middle name or initial)
- Patient's identification number, bed number, room number, and medical record number
- Patient's age, sex (male or female)
- Health care provider's name
- Date and time of specimen collection
- Collector's name or initials
- Test ordered
- Most facilities have an electronic health record (EHR) label containing necessary information.

Fig. 23.2 Wound culture tube.

Fig. 23.3 Aerobic culture tube.

the effectiveness of antibiotics, usually performed in conjunction with culture); cytologic analysis (**cytology** is the study of cells, including their formation, origin, structure, function, biochemical activities, and pathologic processes); and examination and testing for acid-fast bacillus (the organism responsible for tuberculosis of the lung).

Collecting a Sputum Specimen by Suction

Some patients are not able to expectorate a sputum specimen, and nasotracheal suctioning is required to obtain a sputum specimen. Suctioning sometimes provokes coughing, which has potential to induce vomiting and constriction of pharyngeal, laryngeal, or bronchial muscles. In some cases, suctioning also causes direct stimulation of vagal nerve fibers, which results in cardiac dysrhythmias and increased intracranial pressure (Skill 23.9).

Closed-method collection containers, such as a Lukens specimen container, protect the nurse from contamination with body fluids. Explain the procedure and prepare the patient for the test. Provide instructions to the patient the night before the test to drink extra fluids, which helps loosen secretions and makes expectoration for the specimen easier. Instruct the patient that it is not possible to use saliva as a specimen. Saliva is clear, whereas sputum is thick, sometimes colored, and tenacious (sticky) (Skill 23.10).

OBTAINING A WOUND CULTURE

If the LPN/LVN detects purulent or suspect-looking **exudate** (drainage), the health care provider will likely order a wound culture. The patient should be assessed for fever, chills, malaise, and elevated WBC count, which indicate a possible systemic infection. It is not possible to confirm or treat infection accurately without results from a wound culture. Assess pain at the wound site with the use of a pain scale, such as a scale of 0 to 10 in which 0 indicates no pain and 10 indicates the worst pain imaginable by the patient. If a patient requires an analgesic before a dressing change, give this medication 30 minutes before the dressing change so that the analgesic effect peaks when the procedure is performed. Determine when

the dressing change is scheduled, because this is the ideal time to obtain a wound culture as part of the procedure (see Chapter 22).

A wound culture sample should not be collected from old drainage, because resident colonies of bacteria grow in exudate. Obtain the specimen from inside the wound. Aerobic organisms grow in superficial wounds exposed to the air, and anaerobic organisms tend to grow within body cavities. To collect an aerobic specimen, insert a sterile swab from the Culturette tube (Fig. 23.2) into wound secretions. Then return the swab to the Culturette tube, cap the tube, and crush the inner ampule so that the medium for organism growth coats the swab tip (Fig. 23.3). Immediately send the labeled specimen to the laboratory with a requisition slip. To collect an anaerobic specimen deep in a body cavity, use a sterile syringe tip to aspirate visible drainage from the inner wound; expel any air from the syringe and inject the syringe contents into a special vacuum container with culture medium. In some facilities, place a cork over the needle to prevent entrance of air and then send the syringe to the laboratory with a requisition slip.

COLLECTING SPECIMENS FROM THE NOSE AND THROAT

When a patient has signs and symptoms of upper respiratory or sinus infection, a nose or throat culture is a diagnostic tool often used to determine the type of infection or pathogen present. For example, a nose culture also is performed to detect methicillin-resistant *Staphylococcus aureus* (MRSA). The laboratory staff places the specimen on a culture medium to determine whether pathogenic microorganisms will grow. Regardless of what body fluids are cultured, certain principles apply. It is necessary to obtain culture specimens before antibiotic therapy is started because the antibiotics have the capacity to interrupt the

Skill 23.8   Collecting Gastric Secretions or Emesis Specimen

NURSING ACTION (RATIONALE)

1. Refer to the health care provider's order. (*Provides basis for care.*)
2. Assemble supplies. (*Organizes procedure.*)
   - Nonsterile gloves
   - Additional PPE if indicated
   - Facial tissues
   - Emesis basin
   - Wooden applicator
   - Bulb syringe (60 mL) or catheter-tip syringe
   - Gastroccult test
   - Cardboard slide
   - Gastroccult developing solution
   - Laboratory requisition
   - Biohazard bag
3. Introduce self. (*Decreases patient's anxiety.*)
4. Identify patient. (*Ensures procedure is performed with correct patient.*)
5. Explain procedure. (*Promotes cooperation and decreases patient's anxiety.*)
6. It is advisable to label card before obtaining specimen to prevent contamination.
7. Perform hand hygiene and don nonsterile gloves according to agency policy and guidelines from the CDC and OSHA. (*Prevents transmission of microorganisms.*)
8. To obtain specimen of gastric contents through nasogastric (NG) or nasoenteral tube, position patient in high Fowler's position in bed or chair. (*Keeps risk of aspiration of gastric contents to a minimum. Position relieves pressure on abdominal organs. If patient is nauseated, flat position in bed or one in which the patient is not able to sit straight sometimes causes abdominal discomfort.*)
9. Verify NG tube placement (see Chapter 15). (*Ensures aspiration of gastric contents.*)

10. Collect gastric contents via NG or nasoenteral tube (see Chapter 15). (*Only a small amount of specimen is needed for pH and occult blood testing.*)
    a. Disconnect tube from suction or gravity drainage.
    b. Attach bulb syringe or catheter-tip syringe.
    c. Aspirate 5–10 mL.
    d. Obtain sample of emesis with a 3-mL syringe or wooden applicator.
    e. Using applicator or syringe, apply 1 drop of gastric sample to test area of Gastroccult test slide. (*Sample must cover test paper for test reaction to occur.*)
    f. Follow directions on the Gastroccult card.
11. Close card and label, if you have not already done so (see Box 23.5). (*Ensures accuracy in identification of specimen.*)
12. Enclose specimen in biohazard bag and send to laboratory with requisition slip (see illustration for Skill 23.1, Step 11). (*Ensures proper identification.*)
13. Reconnect NG tube to drainage system, suction, or clamp as ordered. (*NG tube serves to decompress abdomen by promoting drainage. Clamping sometimes is ordered to determine tolerance to stomach filling.*)
14. Dispose of equipment; remove gloves and discard them in proper receptacle; and perform hand hygiene. (*Reduces spread of microorganisms.*)
15. Document procedure and observations. (*Communicates collection of specimen and completion of test.*)
16. Perform patient teaching (see the Patient Teaching box).

CDC, Centers for Disease Control and Prevention; *OSHA,* Occupational Safety and Health Administration; *PPE,* personal protective equipment.

organism's growth in the laboratory. If the patient situation or condition prevents the nurse from obtaining the specimen before an antibiotic is administered to the patient, the provider should be notified to clarify if the antibiotic should be held until the culture is collected. If the patient is already receiving antibiotic therapy, notify the laboratory and communicate specifically what antibiotics the patient is receiving.

Collection of nose and throat specimens sometimes causes the patient discomfort owing to heightened sensitivity of the mucosal membranes. Collection of a throat specimen often causes gagging, and so it is important to collect a throat culture before or at least 1

hour after mealtime to lessen the chance of inducing vomiting. To keep the patient's anxiety and discomfort to a minimum, make certain the patient clearly understands how each specimen is to be collected (Skills 23.11 and 23.12).

When collecting nose and throat specimens, perform the following:
- Assess the condition of and drainage from nasal mucosa and sinuses. (*Reveals physical signs that indicate possible infection or allergic irritation.*)
- Determine whether patient has experienced postnasal drip, sinus headache or tenderness, nasal congestion, or sore throat. (*Further clarifies nature of problem.*)

Skill 23.9 Collecting a Sputum Specimen by Suction

NURSING ACTION (RATIONALE)

1. Refer to the health care provider's order. (*Provides basis for care.*)
2. Assemble supplies. (*Organizes procedure.*)
   - Suction device (wall or portable)
   - Sterile suction catheter (size 14, 16, or 18) (*Use of a catheter that is too large causes trauma to nasal mucosa.*)
   - Sterile gloves
   - Sterile saline or container
   - In-line specimen container (sputum trap)
   - Oxygen therapy equipment, if indicated
   - Protective eyewear and other PPE as appropriate (to protect from sputum drops/particles)
   - Laboratory requisition
   - Biohazard bag
3. Introduce self. (*Decreases patient's anxiety.*)
4. Identify patient. (*Ensures procedure is performed with correct patient.*)
5. Explain procedure. Encourage patient to breathe normally to prevent hyperventilation. (*Promotes cooperation and decreases patient's anxiety.*)
6. Assess patient.
   a. Determine when patient last ate a meal. (*It is best to obtain the specimen 1–2 h after a meal or 1 h before to minimize gagging, which can cause vomiting and aspiration.*)
   b. Assess patient's respiratory status: rate, depth, pattern, lung sounds, and color. (*Changes in respirations indicate the possible presence of secretions in the tracheobronchial tree and potential need for supplementary oxygen.*)
   c. Assess patient's anxiety level. (*Procedure usually is contraindicated if patient is not able to cooperate or remain still during procedure.*)
7. Arrange equipment and prepare necessary charges. (*Facilitates procedure and facilitates proper billing.*)
8. Position patient for procedure.
   a. Close door or pull curtains. (*Provides privacy.*)
   b. The higher semi-Fowler's position is recommended. (*Promotes full lung expansion and facilitates ability to cough.*)
   c. Prepare suction machine or device and ensure that it is functioning properly. (*Adequate amount of suction is necessary to aspirate sputum.*)
   d. Drape patient as necessary. (*Prevents unnecessary exposure.*)
   e. Adjust bed to appropriate height and lower side rail. (*Promotes proper body mechanics and facilitates procedure.*)
9. Perform hand hygiene. (*Reduces spread of microorganisms.*)
10. Connect suction tube to adapter on sputum trap. (*Facilitates procedure.*)
11. Prelubricate tip of catheter with sterile water.
12. Apply sterile glove to dominant hand. (*Allows handling of suction catheter without introducing microorganisms into the tracheobronchial tree, which is a sterile body cavity.*)
13. Administer 100% oxygen to the patient for 1 min, if necessary. (*Use caution if patient has chronic obstructive pulmonary disease [COPD], because 100% oxygen has the capacity to depress respiratory effort.*)
14. Using gloved hand, connect sterile suction catheter rubber tubing on sputum trap. (*Aspirated sputum will go directly to trap instead of to suction tubing.*)
15. Gently insert tip of suction catheter prelubricated with sterile water through nasopharynx, endotracheal tube, or tracheostomy without applying suction. (*Minimizes trauma to airway as catheter is inserted. Lubrication allows for easier insertion.*)

16. Warn patient to expect to cough, and gently and quickly advance catheter into trachea. (*Triggers cough reflex.*)
17. As patient coughs, apply suction for 5–10 secs, collecting 2–10 mL of sputum. (*Suctioning longer than 10 sec risks causing hypoxia and mucosal damage.*)

Skill 23.9   Collecting a Sputum Specimen by Suction—cont'd

18. Release suction and remove catheter, and then turn off suction. (*Releasing suction prevents unnecessary trauma to mucosa as the catheter is withdrawn.*)

19. Detach catheter from specimen trap and dispose of catheter into appropriate receptacle. Connect rubber tubing on sputum trap to plastic adapter. (*Aids in keeping specimen intact.*)

20. If any sputum is present on outside of container, wash it off with disinfectant. (*Prevents spread of infection to persons handling specimen.*)

PPE, Personal protective equipment.

21. Offer patient tissues after suctioning. Dispose of tissues in emesis basin or trash container. Remove gloves, and discard them in proper receptacle. (*Reduces spread of microorganisms.*)

22. Securely attach properly completed identification label and laboratory requisition to side of specimen container (not the lid). (*Ensures proper identification of specimen; ensures accuracy of results; prevents loss and potential delays in obtaining results.*)

23. Enclose specimen in a biohazard bag (see illustration for Skill 23.1, Step 11). Send specimen immediately to laboratory. (*Bacteria multiply quickly. Prompt analysis of specimen is necessary for accurate results.*)

24. Offer patient mouth care; assist patient to a comfortable position, and place needed items within easy reach. (*Ensures patient's comfort and well-being.*)

25. Raise side rail, and lower bed to lowest position. (*Ensures patient's safety.*)

26. Store, remove, or dispose of supplies and equipment as appropriate. (*Ensures equipment is available for next use.*)

27. Document procedure. (*Provides communication that procedure was carried out and patient's response.*)
  • Method used to obtain specimen
  • Date and time collected
  • Type of test ordered and how specimen was transported to the laboratory
  • Characteristics of sputum specimen
  • Patient's oxygenation and respiratory status

28. Perform patient teaching (see the Patient Teaching box).

Skill 23.10   Collecting a Sputum Specimen by Expectoration

NURSING ACTION (RATIONALE)

1. Refer to the health care provider's order. (*Provides basis for care.*)

2. Assemble supplies. (*Organizes procedure.*)
  • Sterile sputum collector
  • Tissues
  • Label for specimen
  • Laboratory requisition
  • Nonsterile gloves
  • Additional PPE if indicated
  • Biohazard bag

3. Introduce self. (*Decreases patient's anxiety.*)

4. Identify patient. (*Ensures procedure is performed with correct patient.*)

5. Explain procedure. (*Promotes cooperation and decreases patient's anxiety.*)

6. Perform hand hygiene and don nonsterile gloves according to agency policy and guidelines from the CDC and OSHA. (*Prevents transmission of microorganisms.*)

7. Position patient in Fowler's position. (*Helps with coughing.*)

Skill 23.10   Collecting a Sputum Specimen by Expectoration—cont'd

8. Instruct patient to take three breaths and force cough into sterile container. *(Helps patient expectorate mucus.)* (Be prepared to obtain the specimen by nasotracheal suctioning if patient is not able to cough.)

9. Label specimen container (see Box 23.5). *(Ensures proper identification of specimen; ensures accuracy of results; prevents loss and potential delays in obtaining results.)*
10. Enclose specimen in biohazard bag and attach laboratory requisition. Immediately send specimen to laboratory. If any sputum is present on outside of container, wash it off with disinfectant. *(Ensures specimen is sent to the laboratory. Bacteria multiply quickly. Prompt analysis of specimens is necessary for accurate results. Removing sputum from outside of container prevents spread of infection to anyone handling specimen.)*
11. Remove gloves, discard them in proper receptacle, and perform hand hygiene. *(Reduces spread of microorganisms.)*
12. Document procedure and observations (see Skill 23.2, Step 15). *(Communicates care administered.)*
13. Perform patient teaching (see the Patient Teaching box).

CDC, Centers for Disease Control and Prevention; *OSHA,* Occupational Safety and Health Administration; *PPE,* personal protective equipment.

Skill 23.11   Obtaining a Throat Specimen

NURSING ACTION *(RATIONALE)*

1. Refer to the health care provider's order. *(Provides basis of care.)*
2. Assemble supplies. *(Organizes procedure.)*
   - Nonsterile gloves
   - Additional PPE if indicated
   - Swab and culture tube
   - Nasal speculum (optional)
   - Tongue blades
   - Penlight
   - Emesis basin or clean container (optional)
   - Facial tissues
   - Label (completed)
   - Laboratory requisition
   - Biohazard bag
3. Introduce self. *(Decreases patient's anxiety.)*
4. Identify patient. *(Ensures procedure is performed with correct patient.)*

5. Explain procedure to patient; make certain patient understands what is expected. *(Promotes cooperation and decreases anxiety.)*
6. Perform hand hygiene and don nonsterile gloves according to agency's policy and guidelines from the CDC and OSHA. *(Prevents transmission of microorganisms.)*
7. Instruct patient to tilt head backward. For patients in bed, place pillow behind shoulders. *(Facilitates visualization of pharynx.)*
8. Ask patient to open mouth and say "ah." *(Enables exposure of pharynx, relaxes throat muscles, and minimizes gag reflex.)*
9. Have swab ready for use. Loosen top of swab from culture tube for easy removal. *(Most commercially prepared tubes have a top that fits securely over end of swab, which allows touching of the outer top without contaminating swab stick.)*
10. If pharynx is not visualized, depress tongue with tongue blade and note inflamed areas of pharynx

Skill 23.11   Obtaining a Throat Specimen—cont'd

or tonsils. Depress anterior third of tongue only (illuminate with penlight as needed). *(It is necessary to visualize area to be swabbed. Placement of tongue blade along back of tongue is more likely to initiate gag reflex.)*

11. Insert swab without touching lips, teeth, tongue, or cheeks. *(Touching lips or oral mucosal structures potentially contaminates swab with resident bacteria.)*

12. Gently but quickly swab tonsillar area from side to side, making contact with inflamed or purulent sites. *(These areas contain the most microorganisms.)*

13. Carefully withdraw swab without striking oral structures. Immediately place swab securely in culture tube. Crush ampule at bottom of tube to release culture medium, and push tip of swab into liquid medium. *(Retains microorganisms within culture tube. Placing tip in culture medium maintains life of bacteria for testing.)*

14. Securely attach properly completed label and requisition slip to side of specimen container (not lid). *(Ensures proper identification of specimen;*

ensures accuracy of results; prevents loss and potential delays in obtaining results.)

15. Enclose in a biohazard bag (see illustration for Skill 23.1, Step 11). *(Complies with guidelines from the CDC and OSHA.)*

16. Send specimen immediately to laboratory or refrigerate. *(Leaving specimen at room temperature permits bacterial content to increase.)*

17. Remove gloves, discard them in a proper receptacle, and perform hand hygiene. *(Prevents spread of microorganisms.)*

18. Document procedure. *(Communicates that procedure was completed.)*
    - Date and time collected
    - Type of specimen
    - Fact that specimen sent to laboratory with requisition slip
    - Patient response (if appropriate)

19. Perform patient teaching (see the Patient Teaching box).

CDC, Centers for Disease Control and Prevention; *OSHA*, Occupational Safety and Health Administration; *PPE*, personal protective equipment.

Skill 23.12   Obtaining a Nose Culture

CHECK   GATHER   HELLO   ID   PRIVACY   EXPLAIN   WASH   GLOVES

NURSING ACTION *(RATIONALE)*

1 to 6. Refer to Steps 1–6 of Skill 23.11.

7. Ask patient to blow nose, and then check nostrils for patency with penlight. Select nostril with greatest patency. *(Clears nasal passage of mucus that contains resident bacteria.)*

8. Ask patient to tilt head back. Patients in bed should have a pillow behind the shoulders.

9. Gently insert nasal speculum in one nostril (optional). Carefully pass swab into nostril until it reaches portion of mucosa that is inflamed or contains exudate. Rotate swab quickly. **Note:** If nasopharyngeal culture is to be obtained, use a special swab on a flexible wire that is able to flex downward to reach nasopharynx. *(It is necessary that swab remain sterile until it reaches area to be cultured. Rotating swab covers all surfaces where exudate is present.)*

10. With dominant hand, remove swab without touching sides of speculum or nasal canal. *(Prevents contamination by resident bacteria.)*

11. With nondominant hand, carefully remove nasal speculum (if used) and place in basin. Offer patient facial tissue. *(Removing speculum carefully*

prevents trauma to nasal mucosa; offering patient facial tissue provides comfort.)

12. Immediately place swab securely in culture tube. *(Prevents contamination and spillage of specimen.)*

13. Crush ampule at bottom of tube to release culture medium. Push tip of swab into liquid medium. *(Placing tip in culture medium maintains life of bacteria for testing.)*

14. Discard supplies into proper receptacle. *(Prevents transmission of microorganisms.)*

15. Send culture tube to laboratory with completed requisition and attached label not attached to the lid of the container (see Box 23.5). Enclose in a biohazard bag. *(Ensures proper identification of specimen; ensures accuracy of results; prevents loss and potential delays in obtaining results.)*

16. Remove gloves, discard them in proper receptacle, and perform hand hygiene. *(Reduces spread of microorganisms.)*

17. Document procedure. *(Ensures procedure was completed.)*

18. Perform patient teaching (see the Patient Teaching box).

- Assess the condition of posterior pharynx (see Chapter 13).
- Assess for systemic indications of infection, including fever, chills, and malaise.
- Do not let the culture swab come in contact with the buccal mucosa, tongue, or teeth, because such contact contaminates the specimen.

COLLECTING A BLOOD SPECIMEN (VENIPUNCTURE) AND BLOOD FOR CULTURE

Veins are a primary source of blood for laboratory testing, as well as routes for intravenous (IV) fluids or blood replacement; therefore maintaining their integrity is essential. Acquire and maintain skill in venipuncture, if allowed by facility policy or state's nurse practice act, to prevent unnecessary injury to veins.

Venipuncture may cause discomfort and anxiety in the patient. A calm approach and skilled technique help limit anxiety. Children may benefit from being able to have access to a comforting stuffed toy or parental presence.

Blood tests, one of the most common diagnostic aids in the care and evaluation of patients, typically yield valuable information about nutritional, hematologic, metabolic, immune, and biochemical status. Tests allow health care providers to screen patients carefully for early signs of physical alterations, plot the course of existing disease, and monitor responses to therapies.

Nurses may be responsible for collecting blood specimens; however, many facilities have specially trained technicians (phlebotomists) whose sole responsibility is to draw blood. Be familiar with facility policies and procedures and the state's nurse practice act regarding guidelines for collecting blood samples.

Venipuncture, the most common method, involves inserting a hollow-bore needle into the lumen of a large vein to obtain a specimen. In some cases, a needle and syringe are used, and in others, a special **Vacutainer** tube is used to collect multiple blood samples.

Assess the patient for special conditions that will affect the test procedure or results. With some tests, certain preparations are necessary to obtain accurate measurements, such as NPO status. A variety of factors put the patient undergoing venipuncture at risk, including anticoagulant therapy, low platelet count, bleeding disorders, presence of arteriovenous shunt or fistula, and having had breast or axillary surgery performed on that side. Abnormal clotting abilities, medications, and compromised circulation tend to impair blood flow. Assess the patient's ability to cooperate with the procedure; some patients need assistance from another health care team member (e.g., children and adults who are unable to comprehend the procedure due to cognitive or emotional delay).

A health care provider's order is required for tests. Before collecting the specimen, review the order to ensure that the specimens and amount for all the tests to be performed are correct, eliminating the need for multiple blood draws. Older adults have fragile veins that are traumatized easily during venipuncture. Sometimes an application of a warm compress helps with sample collection. Using a small-bore catheter is another helpful strategy.

In the home care setting, it may be helpful to use a blood pressure cuff, rather than a tourniquet, when performing the venipuncture. Ask the patient if persistent or recurrent bleeding or expanding hematoma occurs at venipuncture site, and if so, notify the primary health care provider.

An older child should be asked if they want to help with the collecting of the specimen or to look the other way. Giving children a choice is one way to enhance cooperation. Offering the child a "special job" such as holding the adhesive bandage and to "be sure to hold it real tight and not drop it" will offer a bit of distraction and also encourage the child to be part of the experience. Children are often afraid of needles and the loss of blood. Explain the procedure and avoid phrases such as "to take blood" as children will fear losing all of their blood. When applying the tourniquet, indicate to the child the tourniquet is going to hug their arm.

Provide honest patient teaching for the pediatric patient. Fabrications and mistruths may damage the nurse-patient relationship irrevocably. Ask a parent or another staff member to hold and comfort the child. Toys or books may distract the child. Keep the needle out of the child's sight for as long as possible. Perform the venipuncture and collection of the blood quickly, and an adhesive bandage should be placed over the site.

The bloodborne pathogens standard of the Occupational Safety and Health Administration (OSHA) requires employers to protect workers from any occupational exposure that is related to bloodborne pathogens. The standard also requires that employers have a written Exposure Control Plan in place (OSHA, n.d.). As a result, phlebotomy equipment includes needle safety devices. Using standard precautions and appropriate personal protective equipment helps protect skin and mucous membranes from contact with blood; however, most barriers are penetrated easily by needles. Safety devices and features protect health care workers as follows:

- Provide a barrier between the hands and the needle after use
- Allow or require the worker's hands to remain behind the needle at all times
- Are simple to operate and necessitate little training to use effectively

A less invasive method of collecting a blood specimen is called a *capillary puncture.* It is used commonly to collect blood specimens from newborns and for glucose monitoring in all patients. The procedure usually is performed by puncturing a vascular area on a finger, toe, or heel with a lancet, although sometimes a sterile needle is used instead.

Fig. 23.4 Safety container for used needles and other sharps.

Fig. 23.5 Vacutainer method of collecting blood. (A) Parts of the Vacutainer. (B) Blood collection in a Vacutainer tube.

Even when safety needles are used, never recap needles, and always discard them carefully in puncture-resistant containers close to the patient (Fig. 23.4). A significant exposure occurs when a deep puncture is caused by a needle that has been used to collect blood. All needlestick injuries must be reported. Not all needlestick injuries are preventable; however, the use of needles with safety features has decreased substantially the risk of exposure to bloodborne pathogens for health care workers.

Blood culture, a specific blood test used to detect the presence of bacteria in the blood (bacteremia), requires a special phlebotomy technique. Specimens for cultures are drawn when the symptoms of fever and chills that often accompany bacteremia are present. It is important to draw at least two culture specimens, one each from a different site. The venipuncture sites are prepared thoroughly according to agency policy before the collection of the blood specimens. The diagnosis of bacteremia is confirmed when both cultures grow an infecting agent. If only one culture produces bacteria, the assumption is that the bacteria were skin contaminants rather than the infecting agent. Because culture specimens obtained through an IV catheter frequently are contaminated, do not perform tests on them unless catheter sepsis is suspected. Blood culture specimens always are drawn before antibiotic therapy is started, because the antibiotic usually interferes with the organism's growth in the laboratory.

Collection Methods

Several collection methods are available. Using a syringe and attached needle is one method. Another is the use of a Vacutainer. With the syringe method, blood is drawn into the barrel by pulling back on the plunger. After the blood is collected, it is transferred to a test tube.

The Vacutainer system has a needle, a holder for the needle and tube, and one or more evacuated tubes with rubber stoppers (Fig. 23.5A). In evacuated tubes, air is removed, which creates a vacuum. When a vein is punctured, blood flows into the tube (see Fig. 23.5B). After a tube fills, it is removed from the holder, and a new tube is attached without withdrawal of the needle from the vein. The Vacutainer system thus allows the collection of multiple blood specimens with one venipuncture.

Collection Tubes

Types of collection tubes. Blood collection tubes come in different sizes. The blood tests ordered determine the amount of blood needed. Some tests require additives that are added to the collection tube and mix with the blood. Some additives preserve the blood until testing; others aid in separating the blood cells from the plasma for testing. In the Vacutainer system, the tubes contain the necessary additives. The rubber stoppers are color coded. Red, lavender, blue, green, gray, and yellow are common colors. The color coding signals the type of additive, the amount of blood to collect, and the recommended blood tests to perform on the sample. Color coding sometimes varies, and so agency procedures must be followed. After the collection tubes are selected, they are placed in order of use. The order is important for preventing tube contamination. Different tubes have different additives. The additive from one tube should not be transferred inadvertently to another through use in the wrong order. Agency policy should be followed for the order in which to collect blood specimens.

Labeling collection tubes. After collection is completed and before the blood specimens are sent to the laboratory, the collection tube is labeled with the patient's identifying information (Fig. 23.6). Labeling is necessary to make sure that the right tests are done for the right patient. When wrong test results are reported for the patient, the wrong treatment will be given, and the patient is at risk for serious harm. Box 23.5 discusses a patient's identifying information. Labels generally are generated using data stored in the patient's electronic health record (EHR). Be diligent to label the tubes so the bar code (if present) is able to be scanned. Avoid applying the labels in a way that causes wrinkles or missing information.

Selecting a Venipuncture Site

The basilic and cephalic veins in the antecubital space are the most common venipuncture sites (Fig. 23.7).

Fig. 23.6 Labeling the blood collection tube.

These veins are large and near the skin surface. Hand veins offer alternative sites.

Select the arm to be used before selecting the vein. An arm on the side of a mastectomy, with a paralysis, with a hemodialysis access site, or with an IV site should not be used. An arm with existing hematomas or skin impairment also should be avoided.

A tourniquet is applied to the arm when the vein selection process begins (Fig. 23.8A). A **tourniquet** is a constricting device traditionally applied to control bleeding. It prevents arterial blood flow to the part below the tourniquet and prevents venous blood from returning to the heart. The veins fill with blood and distend, which makes them firmer and easier to see and palpate (see Fig. 23.8B); thus the tourniquet is useful for venipuncture.

The tourniquet is removed after the blood specimen is collected but before the needle is withdrawn from the vein. The tourniquet is applied 2 to 4 inches (5.08 to 10.16 cm) above the elbow. One end is crossed tightly over the other, and then the upper end is tucked under the band to form a half bow (see Fig. 23.8A). This allows for quick release.

When used for obtaining a venous specimen, tourniquets prevent venous blood flow but not arterial blood flow. Make sure the tourniquet is tight enough that the veins distend; however, the radial pulse should be palpable. If the radial pulse is not detected, release and

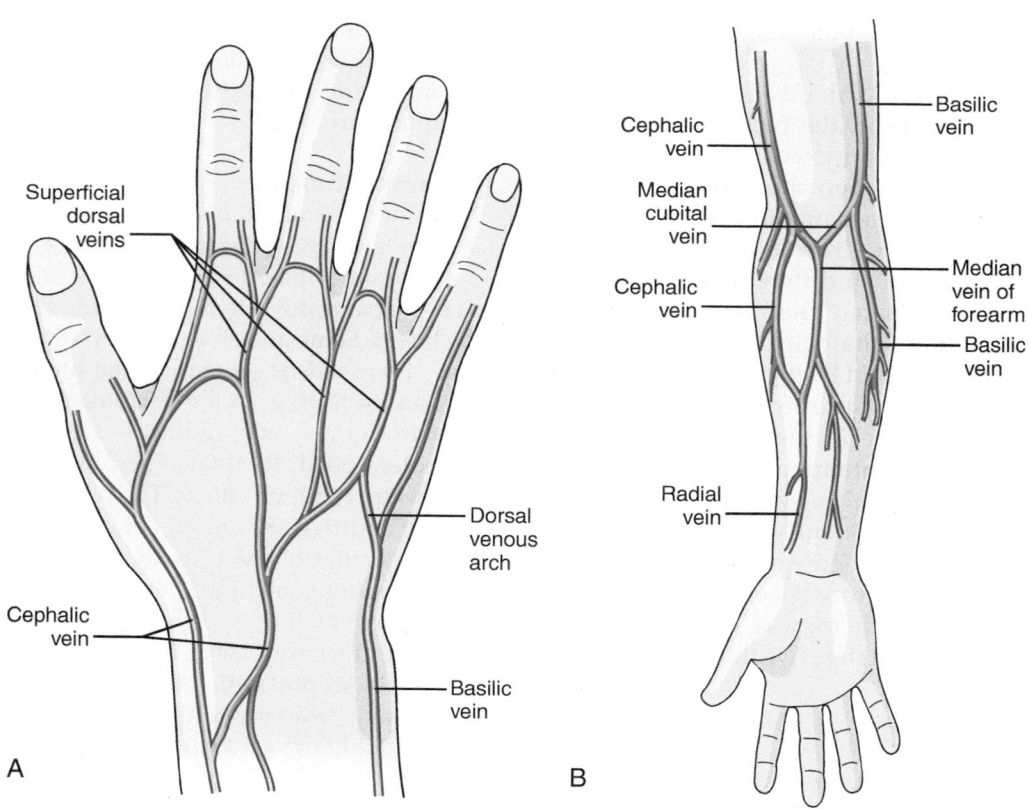

© Elsevier

Fig. 23.7 Venipuncture sites. (A) Inner arm. (B) Dorsal surface of hand.

reapply the tourniquet. The tourniquet should be in place for no longer than 1 to 2 minutes.

To select a vein in the antecubital space, a tourniquet is applied 2 to 4 inches (5.08 to 10.16 cm) above the elbow. The patient is asked to open and close the fist. While the patient's fist is closed, look and palpate for a vein. A vein that is suitable for venipuncture is straight, feels full and firm, and is elastic and springs back after palpation (see Fig. 23.8B). Veins with the following characteristics are avoided:

- Small and narrow veins are usually fragile.
- Weak veins are soft and do not rebound.
- Sclerosed veins are hard and rigid.
- Veins that are easy to roll when palpated are often difficult to pierce successfully with the needle.

Fig. 23.8 Venipuncture. (A) Applying tourniquet to select a venipuncture site. (B) Palpating a vein. (C) Pulling the skin taut over the venipuncture site. (D) Inserting a needle into the vein. E, Pulling back on the plunger to withdraw blood.

Perform the venipuncture (Skill 23.13). After the needle is withdrawn from the vein, apply pressure to the site to prevent bleeding. The patient should not bend the arm, because this may cause the formation of a hematoma.

See the Home Care Considerations and Coordinated Care boxes.

ELECTROCARDIOGRAPHY

Electrocardiography may be performed by nurses or by technicians specifically trained for this test. The electrocardiogram (ECG) is a graphic representation of electrical impulses generated by the heart during a cardiac cycle; it identifies abnormalities that interfere with electrical conduction through cardiac tissue. This procedure usually is done at the patient's bedside, but sometimes it is done in a specially equipped laboratory.

The patient is assessed for knowledge level of the procedure; ability to understand and follow directions (this procedure requires patient to follow directions closely and assume proper positioning); ability to assume proper position; and vital signs (baseline) for comparison with postprocedure vital signs.

If the patient has large amounts of hair, it is sometimes necessary to clip or shave the hair at the lead placement site. This promotes adherence of the leads (electrodes) to the chest and on the extremity. Skill 23.14 describes how the ECG is obtained.

❖ NURSING PROCESS FOR SPECIMEN COLLECTION AND DIAGNOSTIC TESTING

The role of the LPN/LVN in the nursing process is that the LPN/LVN will

- Participate in planning care for patients based on patient needs
- Review patient's plan of care and recommend revisions as needed
- Review and follow defined prioritization for patient care
- Use clinical pathways, care maps, or care plans to guide and review patient care

◆ ASSESSMENT

Do the following in regard to specimen collection and diagnostic testing:

- Assess patient's knowledge of procedure to determine level of health teaching required.
- Observe verbal and nonverbal behavior to determine patient's anxiety.
- Determine patient's ability to understand and follow directions.
- Evaluate patient's ability to assume position required for procedure and ability to remain in that position.
- Determine whether patient is allergic to antiseptics, anesthetic solutions, or any of the dyes that will possibly be used.
- Assess patient's need for preprocedure analgesic administration.

Home Care Considerations

Specimen Collection and Diagnostic Examination

SPECIMEN

Urine

- It is best to collect urine specimens for culture and sensitivity in the laboratory setting rather than at home because the chance of bacterial growth is increased by the delay in testing. If a specimen is collected at home, the patient must refrigerate the specimen until time of transport to the laboratory and must keep the specimen chilled during transport.
- When obtaining a urine testing kit, the patient needs to know that all supplies except for the specimen container are usually included in the kit.
- Urine testing at home typically is performed with reagent strips.

Stool

- Frequently, patients are instructed to obtain stool specimens at home and then bring the specimen to the laboratory setting or health care provider's office.
- If a stool specimen is obtained for occult blood testing, the patient is asked to prepare the slide at home and return the slide to the laboratory or health care provider's office for testing.
- Instruct the patient obtaining a stool specimen at home to prevent the specimen from contact with the toilet bowl by using the specimen hat provided by the health care provider.
- Many older adults need assistance with the collection of stool specimens.
- Supply the correct equipment to the patient for testing. The nurse is responsible for assuring the patient has a specimen collection hat, a collection device (tongue blade or wooden swab etc.) and a container to return the specimen.
  - If the patient is without the correct equipment, the nurse would recommend a trash bag be placed over the toilet and the seat lowered to secure it. The collection tool can be a disposable item (straw or flatware). The container should be small and disposable, such as an empty pill bottle or plastic bag. The patient will not get the collection container back after it is given to lab. After the specimen is collected, the patient can then discard the trash bag/disposable collection device.

Sputum

- Instruct patients obtaining sputum specimens at home on proper specimen collection and the importance of returning the specimen to the laboratory in a timely manner.

Wound Drainage

- Teach proper technique for obtaining a wound specimen (e.g., hand hygiene) if the specimen is obtained in the patient's home.

Venipuncture

- In the home setting, if a tourniquet is not available a blood pressure cuff can be used in place of a tourniquet for venipuncture.

Blood Glucose Testing

- Encourage patients to attend meetings of a diabetic support group.
- Various glucose meters are available for home use.
- Patient teaching should be performed on the specific glucometer model that the patient purchases.

Other Specimens and Examinations

- Driving is restricted for 24 h after procedures that necessitate moderate (conscious) sedation.
- Instruct the patient not to make any legal decisions for 24 h after procedures that necessitate conscious sedation or the use of other medications that may impair judgment.

POSTPROCEDURAL CONSIDERATIONS AT HOME

After Intravenous Pyelography (IVP)

Discharge instructions typically include the following:

- The kidneys excrete the contrast medium. Instruct the patient to drink at least 24 ounces (720 mL) of water if this is not contraindicated by a current condition.
- Delayed allergic reaction from the contrast medium is possible as much as 24 h after the procedure. Instruct patients to call the primary health care provider if they have such reactions. If the reaction is an emergency (facial swelling, especially around the eyes, lips, and mouth; difficulty breathing; difficulty swallowing; wheezing), the patient is instructed to immediately call 911 rather than calling their primary health care provider.

After Lumbar Puncture

- Provide the patient with written instructions upon discharge after a lumbar puncture. Instructions include directing the patient to get immediate medical attention if a severe headache or change in level of consciousness occurs after the procedure.

After Paracentesis

- Instruct the patient to contact the health care provider if he or she develops a fever or experiences pain, swelling, or discharge from the puncture site. The patient should rest after this procedure because he or she may feel dizzy or light-headed related to the amount of fluid removed.

After Thoracentesis

- Give patients written instructions that include signs and symptoms of complications related to perforation of the spleen, liver, or lung. Signs and symptoms to be alert to include fever, leakage of fluid from the puncture site, difficulty breathing, or chest pain. Inform the patient that sometimes these signs and symptoms do not occur until several days after the procedure.

After Bronchoscopy

- Instruct patients experiencing fever, chest pain or discomfort, or respiratory symptoms such as dyspnea, wheezing, or hemoptysis to contact the health care provider or to seek medical attention immediately.
- Inform patients that throat discomfort is common and often is relieved with throat lozenges.

Home Care Considerations—cont'd

Specimen Collection and Diagnostic Examination

After Endoscopy

- Hoarseness and sore throat sometimes occur after procedures involving endoscopes inserted through the throat; as long as the gag reflex has returned, encourage the patient to seek relief with throat lozenges or ice chips.
- After a lower GI tract endoscopy, recommend a warm tub bath to ease any rectal discomfort.

After Cardiac Catheterization

- Instruct the patient to contact the health care provider or seek immediate medical attention if any of the following occurs:

- Excessive bleeding from the puncture site (apply pressure). A small amount of dark blood may be present. Bright red blood indicates active bleeding.
- Swelling under the skin at the puncture site.
- Increase in bruising at the puncture site or movement of bruising down the extremity that was used for the procedure.
- Increased or new sensation of pain at the puncture site or in the extremity used for the procedure.
- Paleness, or if the extremity of the puncture site becomes pale or cold.
- Redness or warmth at the puncture site.

 Coordinated Care

Collaboration

Specimen Collection

- The collection of urine specimens may be performed by unlicensed assistive personnel (UAP) who are familiar with aseptic and sterile technique and if allowed by the facility policy. UAP should be informed of when to collect a specimen and proper transport of the specimen. UAP are directed to immediately notify the nurse if appearance of a specimen is abnormal (e.g., presence of blood, cloudiness, or excess sediments).
- The collection of stool and emesis for testing may be performed by UAP. However, assessing the significance of test results requires skills of critical thinking and knowledge application that are unique to a nurse. Delegation of the analysis of test results to UAP is inappropriate.
- The skills used to obtain and test gastric secretions from an NG or nasoenteral tube require the critical thinking and knowledge application unique to a nurse. Delegation of these procedures to UAP is inappropriate.
- Obtaining and testing the blood glucose level after skin puncture can be performed by UAP who are certified to perform the procedure. It is necessary to assess the patient to determine whether his or her need for glucose monitoring is appropriate for delegation. If the patient's condition changes frequently, this procedure should not be delegated to UAP.
- Phlebotomy staff, registered nurses (RNs), and licensed practical nurses/licensed vocational nurses (LPNs/ LVNs) are permitted to obtain venipuncture samples in accordance with agency policy and their state's nurse practice act. The LPN/LVN should consult agency policy to determine who is permitted to draw blood.
- The skills used to obtain throat, nasal, and nasopharyngeal cultures require the critical thinking and

knowledge application unique to a nurse. Delegation of these procedures to UAP is inappropriate.
- Collection of expectorated sputum specimens can be performed by UAP. However, the skills used to collect a sputum specimen through sterile suction require the critical thinking and knowledge application unique to a nurse. Delegation of this procedure by suction to UAP is inappropriate.
- Obtaining a wound culture requires the critical thinking and knowledge application unique to a nurse. Delegation of this procedure to UAP is inappropriate.
- UAPs are permitted to transport stable patients to the testing department. Monitoring vital signs after the procedures is possible to delegate to a UAP, but assessment is not. Monitoring during intravenous conscious sedation (IVCS) requires the critical thinking and knowledge application unique to a nurse. Delegation of this task to UAP is inappropriate.
- Diagnostic studies requiring the use of a contrast medium subject patients to potentially life-threatening complications. Direct the UAP to notify the nurse immediately of any complications (e.g., allergic reactions, bleeding, respiratory distress, or coughing up blood).
- Electrocardiography often is performed by technicians specifically trained for this test. Nurses with advanced training often monitor patient electrocardiographic patterns continuously in an intensive care setting, in the emergency department, or on units where telemetry is used. It is acceptable for UAP to monitor the vital signs of stable patients. UAPs must notify the nurse immediately of complaints of chest pain or altered vital signs.

Skill 23.13   Performing the Venipuncture

NURSING ACTION *(RATIONALE)*

1. Refer to the health care provider's order. (*A health care provider's order is necessary.*)
2. Assemble supplies. (*Organizes procedure.*)
   - Alcohol or antiseptic swab (check agency policy for specific antiseptic solution)
   - Nonsterile gloves
   - Additional PPE if indicated
   - Small pillow or folded towel
   - Rubber tourniquet
   - Sterile 2 × 2 gauze pads
   - Bandage or adhesive tape
   - Appropriate blood tubes, culture bottles
   - Identification labels
   - Laboratory requisition
   - Biohazard bag for delivery of specimen to laboratory (or container as specified by agency)
     a. Syringe method:
        (1) Sterile needles (20- to 21-gauge for adults, 23- to 25-gauge for children, 23- to 25-gauge butterfly for older adults)
        (2) Sterile syringe of appropriate size
     b. Vacuum tube method:
        (1) Vacuum tube with needle holder
        (2) Sterile double-ended needles (20- to 21-gauge for adults, 23- to 25-gauge for children)
3. Introduce self. (*Decreases patient's anxiety.*)
4. Identify patient. (*Ensures procedure is performed with correct patient.*)
5. Explain procedure, including the reason it is being done. (*Promotes patient's cooperation and decreases patient's anxiety.*)
6. Assess patient. (*To determine whether test is still appropriate.*)
7. Arrange equipment and complete necessary charges. (*Facilitates procedure and facilitates proper billing.*)
8. Prepare patient for procedure.
   a. Close door or pull curtain. (*Provides privacy.*)
   b. Assist patient into supine or semi-Fowler's position with arms extended to form straight line from shoulders to wrists. Place small pillow or towel under upper arms. (*Helps stabilize extremity. Supported position in bed reduces chance of injury to patient if fainting occurs.*)
   c. Adjust bed to appropriate height, and lower nearest side rail. (*Promotes proper body mechanics and facilitates procedure.*)
   d. Drape patient. (*Prevents unnecessary exposure.*)

9. Perform hand hygiene and don nonsterile gloves according to agency policy and guidelines from the CDC and OSHA. (*Reduces exposure to bloodborne pathogens.*)
10. Apply tourniquet 2–4 inches (5.08–10.16 cm) above puncture site (see Fig. 23.8A). (*Causes vein to distend for easier visibility.*)
11. Palpate distal pulse. If pulse is not palpable, reapply tourniquet more loosely. (*If too tight, tourniquet will impede arterial blood flow.*)
12. Keep tourniquet on patient no longer than 1–2 min. If tourniquet is left on arm too long, remove and assess other extremity or wait 60 sec before reapplying. (*Prolonged time has potential to alter test results and cause pain and venous stasis.*)
13. Ask patient to open and close fist several times, finally leaving fist clenched. Patient should avoid vigorous opening and closing of fist, which sometimes causes erroneous laboratory results. (*Facilitates distention of veins by forcing blood up from distal veins.*)
14. Quickly inspect extremity for best venipuncture site, looking for straight, prominent vein without swelling or hematoma. (*Straight and intact veins are easiest to puncture.*)
15. Palpate selected vein with fingers. Note whether vein is firm and rebounds when palpated or whether vein feels rigid and cordlike and rolls when palpated (see Fig. 23.8B). (*Patent, healthy vein is elastic and rebounds on palpation. Thrombosed vein is rigid, rolls easily, and is difficult to puncture.*)
16. Select venipuncture site (see Fig. 23.8). (*Prevents discomfort to patient and ensures accuracy of test results.*)
17. Obtain blood sample.
    a. Syringe method:
       (1) Use syringe with appropriate needle securely attached. (*Ensures needle will not dislodge from syringe during venipuncture.*)
       (2) Cleanse venipuncture site with alcohol swab, moving in circular motion outward from site for approximately 2 inches (5 cm). Allow to dry. (*Antimicrobial agent cleans skin surface of resident bacteria so that organisms do not enter puncture site. Allowing alcohol to dry reduces "sting" of venipuncture.*)
       (3) Remove needle cover, and inform patient that a "stick" lasting only a few seconds

Skill 23.13   Performing the Venipuncture—cont'd

will be felt. (Patient has better control over anxiety when prepared for what to expect.)

(4) Place thumb or forefinger of nondominant hand 1 inch (2.5 cm) below site, and pull patient's skin taut (see Fig. 23.8C). (Stabilizes vein and prevents rolling during needle insertion.)

(5) Hold syringe and needle at 15- to 30-degree angle from patient's arm with bevel up (see Fig. 23.8D). (Reduces chance of penetrating both sides of vein during insertion. Keeping bevel up reduces vein trauma.)

(6) Slowly insert needle into vein (see Fig. 23.8D). (Reduces chance of penetrating both sides of vein during insertion.)

(7) Hold syringe securely and pull back gently on plunger (see Fig. 23.8E). (Holding syringe securely prevents needle from advancing. Pulling on plunger creates vacuum needed to draw blood into syringe.)

(8) Look for blood return. (If blood flow fails to appear, needle is not well seated in vein; withdraw needle and prepare for a second attempt.) **Note:** No more than two attempts should be made by a single nurse in the same session and no more than four attempts total (Infusion Nurses Society, 2016).

(9) Obtain desired amount of blood, keeping needle stabilized. (Test results are more accurate when required amount of blood is obtained. Some tests are not possible to perform without minimal blood requirement. Movement of needle increases discomfort.)

(10) After specimen is obtained, release tourniquet. (Reduces bleeding at site when needle is withdrawn.)

(11) Apply 2 × 2 gauze pad or alcohol swab over puncture site without applying pressure, and quickly but carefully withdraw needle from vein; apply pressure with gauze after removal of needle. *(Pressure over needle causes discomfort. Careful removal of needle keeps discomfort and vein trauma to a minimum.)*

(12) Carefully transfer blood from syringe into vacuum tube.

(13) Without recapping, discard needle in proper receptacle. *(Reduces risk of needlestick injury.)*

(14) Remove gloves, discard them in proper receptacle, and perform hand hygiene. *(Reduces spread of microorganisms.)*

b. Vacuum tube method:

(1) Attach double-ended needle to vacuum tube or Vacutainer. (Long end of needle is used to puncture vein. Short end fits into blood tube.)

(2) Have proper blood specimen tube resting inside vacuum tube, but do not push onto needle and puncture rubber stopper. (Causes loss of tube's vacuum.)

(3) Cleanse venipuncture site with alcohol swab, moving in circular motion outward from site for approximately 2 inches (5 cm). *(Cleans skin surface of resident bacteria so that organisms do not enter through puncture site.)*

(4) Remove needle cover and inform patient that a "stick" lasting only a few seconds will be felt. *(Patient has better control over anxiety when prepared for what to expect.)*

(5) Place thumb or forefinger of nondominant hand 1 inch (2.5 cm) below site and pull patient's skin taut. Stretch skin down until vein is stabilized. *(Stabilizes vein and prevents rolling during needle insertion.)*

Continued

Skill 23.13 Performing the Venipuncture—cont'd

(6) Hold vacuum tube at 15- to 30-degree angle from arm with bevel up. (*Reduces chance of penetrating both sides of vein during insertion. Keeping bevel up causes less trauma to vein.*)

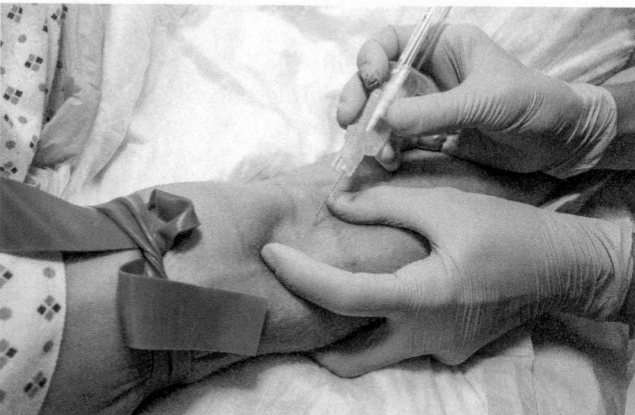

(Step 17b(1) Courtesy BD, Franklin Lakes, NJ. Step 17b(6) from Stein L, Hollen CJ: Concept-Based Clinical Nursing Skills, ed 1, St. Louis, 2021, Elsevier.)

(7) Slowly insert needle into vein (see Fig. 23.8D). (*Reduces chance of penetrating both sides of vein during insertion.*)

(8) Grasp vacuum tube securely so that you do not move it or advance needle in vein, and advance specimen tube into needle of holder. (*Pushing needle through stopper*

breaks vacuum and causes blood to flow into tube. If needle in vein advances, it is possible to puncture vein on other side.)

(9) Note flow of blood into tube (normally fairly rapid). (*Failure of blood to appear indicates that vacuum in tube is lost or needle is not well seated in vein.*)

(10) After specimen tube is filled, grasp vacuum tube firmly and remove tube without allowing needle in vein to move in or out. Insert additional specimen tubes as needed, as described in Step 8. (*Prevents needle from advancing or dislodging. It is necessary to fill tube completely to keep additives in certain tubes in proper proportion to blood volume of tube. Invert tubes with additives as soon as possible to mix.*)

(11) While last tube is filling, release tourniquet. (*Reduces bleeding at site when needle is withdrawn.*)

(12) Apply 2 × 2 gauze pad over puncture site without applying pressure, and quickly but carefully withdraw needle from vein. (*Pressure over needle causes discomfort. Careful removal of needle keeps discomfort and vein trauma to a minimum.*)

(13) Remove gloves, discard them in proper receptacle, and perform hand hygiene. (*Reduces spread of microorganisms.*)

Skill 23.13   Performing the Venipuncture—cont'd

18. For blood obtained by syringe, transfer specimen to tubes.

    a. Using one-handed technique, insert syringe needle through stopper of blood tube and allow vacuum to fill tube. Do not force blood into tube. *(Forcing blood into tube has the potential to cause hemolysis of red blood cells and invalidates test with tubes containing anticoagulants or additives. OSHA recommends one-handed technique to help prevent needlestick injury.)*

    b. Alternative method is to remove needle from syringe and stopper from each test tube. Gently inject required amount of blood into each tube. Reapply stopper. *(Blood injected too quickly sometimes causes frothing or hemolysis of red blood cells. Stopper maintains sterility of specimen.)*

19. When obtaining blood for culture (it is necessary to obtain cultures from two sites):

    a. Cleanse venipuncture sites with povidone-iodine or appropriate antiseptic. Allow to dry. (Antimicrobial agent cleans skin surface so that organisms do not enter puncture site or contaminate culture.)

    b. Clean bottle tops of vacuum tubes or culture bottles with appropriate antiseptic (check agency policy). (Ensures that specimen is sterile.)

    c. Collect 10–15 mL of venous blood by venipuncture from each venipuncture site.

    d. Discard needle on syringe; replace with new sterile needle before injecting blood sample into culture bottles. (Maintains sterile technique and prevents contamination of specimen.)

    e. If aerobic and anaerobic cultures are needed, inoculate anaerobic culture first. (Anaerobic organisms often take longer to grow.)

    f. Mix medium gently after inoculation. (Mixes medium and blood.)

    g. After venipuncture, apply 2 × 2 gauze pad over puncture site without applying pressure, and quickly but carefully withdraw needle from vein. (Pressure over needle causes discomfort. Careful removal of needle keeps discomfort and vein trauma to a minimum.)

20. For blood tubes containing additives, gently rotate tubes back and forth 8–10 times. *(It is necessary to mix additives with blood to prevent clotting. Shaking has potential to cause hemolysis of red blood cells, rendering test results inaccurate.)*

21. Inspect puncture site for bleeding and apply adhesive tape with gauze. *(Keeps puncture site clean and controls any final oozing.)*

22. Check tubes for any sign of external contamination with blood. Decontaminate with alcohol if necessary. Remove gloves, discard them in proper receptacle, and perform hand hygiene. *(Prevents cross-contamination. Reduces risk of exposure to pathogens present in blood.)*

23. Securely attach properly completed identification label to each tube, affix proper requisition, place tubes in biohazard bag, and transport to laboratory promptly. *(Ensures proper identification of specimen; ensures accuracy of results; prevents loss and potential delays in obtaining results.)*

24. Remove gloves, discard them in proper receptacle, and perform hand hygiene. *(Prevents the spread of microorganisms.)*

25. Assist patient to a comfortable position, and place needed items within easy reach. *(Ensures patient's comfort and well-being.)*

26. Raise side rail, and lower bed to lowest position. *(Promotes patient safety.)*

27. Store, remove, or dispose of supplies and equipment as appropriate. *(Ensures equipment is available for next use.)*

28. Document procedure. *(Provides communication that the procedure was carried out and patient's response.)*
    - Time
    - Test performed
    - Patient's response
    - Any adverse findings (e.g., hematoma, prolonged bleeding, unusual pain)

CDC, Centers for Disease Control and Prevention; *OSHA*, Occupational Safety and Health Administration; *PPE*, personal protective equipment.

Skill 23.14   Performing Electrocardiography

CHECK   GATHER   HELLO   ID   PRIVACY   EXPLAIN   WASH   GLOVES

NURSING ACTION (RATIONALE)

1. Refer to the health care provider's order. (*Provides basis for care.*)
2. Assemble supplies. (*Organizes procedure.*)
   - Electrocardiogram (ECG) machine
   - Electro paste (gel)
   - ECG leads or electrodes
   - Alcohol wipes
   - Razor or clippers
   - Nonsterile gloves (optional)
3. Introduce self. (*Decreases patient's anxiety.*)
4. Identify patient. (*Ensures procedure is performed with correct patient.*)
5. Explain procedure. Include the reason it is being done in terms that the patient can understand. (*Promotes cooperation and decreases patient's anxiety; ensures accuracy.*)
6. Assess patient for chest pain, pulse, and respirations. (*Enables determination of whether the test is still appropriate.*)
7. Arrange equipment and complete necessary charges. (*Facilitates procedure and proper billing.*)
8. Prepare patient for procedure.
   a. Close door or pull curtains. (*Provides privacy.*)
   b. Usually supine is the preferred position. Arrange for patient's comfort. (*Promotes accuracy of test.*)
   c. Drape patient as necessary. (*Prevents unnecessary embarrassment.*)
   d. Adjust bed to appropriate height, and lower the nearest side rail. (*Promotes proper body mechanics and facilitates procedure.*)
   e. Perform hand hygiene and don nonsterile gloves according to agency's policy and guidelines from the CDC and OSHA. (*Reduces spread of microorganisms.*)
9. Perform electrocardiography.
   a. Cleanse and prepare skin (shave or clip hair, as necessary, after obtaining consent); wipe skin with alcohol. (*Promotes adherence of leads [electrodes] to chest or extremity.*)
   b. Apply electrode paste and attach leads. (*Position of leads promotes proper display of ECG on paper.*)

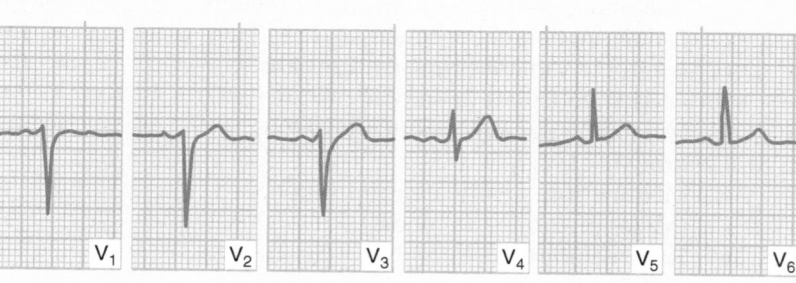

Skill 23.14   Performing Electrocardiography—cont'd

FOR 12-LEAD ELECTROCARDIOGRAPHY

(1) Chest (precordial leads)

V_1: Fourth intercostal space (ICS) at right sternal border

V_2: Fourth ICS at left sternal border

V_3: Midway between V_2 and V_4

V_4: Fifth ICS at midclavicular line

V_5: Left anterior axillary line at level of V_4 horizontally

V_6: Left midaxillary line at level of V_4 horizontally

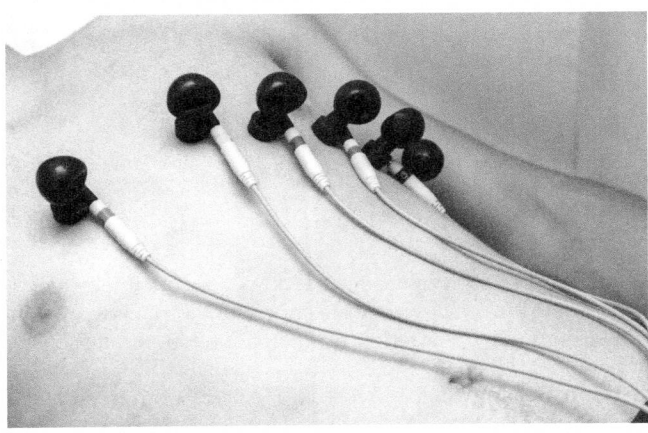

(2) Extremities: one at lower portion of each extremity:

$_aV_R$: Right wrist

$_aV_L$: Left wrist

$_aV_F$: Left ankle

c. Obtain tracing (it is possible to perform 12-lead electrocardiography without removing precordial leads). (*Transfers electrocardiac conduction on ECG tracing paper for subsequent analysis by cardiologist.*)

d. Disconnect leads; wipe excess electrode paste from patient's chest. (*Promotes comfort and hygiene.*)

e. Remove gloves, discard them in proper receptacle, and perform hand hygiene. (*Reduces spread of microorganisms.*)

f. Deliver ECG tracing to appropriate laboratory or nursing unit promptly. (*Provides for review of ECG by cardiologist.*)

10. Assist patient to a comfortable position, and place needed items within easy reach. (*Ensures patient's comfort and well-being.*)

11. Raise side rail, and lower bed to lowest position. (*Ensures patient's safety.*)

12. Store, remove, or dispose of supplies and equipment as appropriate. (*Ensures equipment is available for next use.*)

13. Document procedure. (*Provides communication that the procedure was carried out and patient's response.*)
    - Time
    - Test performed
    - Patient's response
    - Provide patient teaching (as appropriate)

CDC, Centers for Disease Control and Prevention; *OSHA*, Occupational Safety and Health Administration.
Step 9 figure (©iStock.com\portokalis.)

◆ PATIENT PROBLEM

With an accurate and thorough assessment, the LPN/LVN will be able to report patient assessment findings to the RN, who can formulate the necessary patient problem statements. Patient problems are likely to include the following:

- *Anxiousness, related to the manner in which a specimen is obtained or a procedure is performed.* Fear of the possible test results is often a factor (Nursing Care Plan 23.1).
- *Insufficient Knowledge, related to the purpose of the collection or examination and the manner in which the specimen is collected or the test is performed.*
- *Potential for Infection, related to the patient's skin or tissue impairment (broken during a diagnostic procedure).*
- *Recent Onset of Pain, related to invasive diagnostic test (when some type of instrument is inserted into a part of the body).*

Patient problems related to optimal oxygenation during diagnostic procedures involving the airway include the following:

- *Inefficient Oxygenation*
- *Inability to Maintain Adequate Breathing Pattern*
- *Potential for Aspiration Into Airway*
- *Inability to Clear Airway, related to collection of sputum specimen by sneezing and coughing or related to collection of sputum specimen by suctioning*

◆ EXPECTED OUTCOMES AND PLANNING

Identify goals and outcomes of care and set priorities for the plan of care that is likely to result in goal achievement. Expected outcomes focus on the collection of an uncontaminated specimen by the health care personnel or the patient and the patient's understanding of the purpose of the examination that requires the specimen.

All Specimens

- Patient explains procedure for specimen collection before collection is attempted.
- Patient explains purpose of specimen analysis before collection is attempted.
- Patient verbalizes lack of fear of specimen collection and test results.

Nursing Care Plan 23.1 | **Specimen Collection or Diagnostic Examination**

This care plan has been adapted for the patient who is at risk for anxiousness with regard to diagnostic tests and examinations.

PATIENT PROBLEM

Potential for Anxiousness, related to intrusive diagnostic tests and procedures

Patient Goals and Expected Outcomes	Nursing Interventions and Rationale	Evaluation
Patient describes a reduction in the level of anxiety experienced	Acknowledge awareness of patient's anxiety. (*Acknowledgment of the patient's feelings validates the feelings and communicates acceptance of these feelings.*) Stay with the patient if this appears necessary. (*The presence of a trusted person is often helpful.*) Maintain a calm manner while interacting with patient. (*The patient's feeling of stability increases in a calm and nonthreatening atmosphere.*) Orient patient to environment, new experiences, or people. (*Orientation and awareness promote comfort and may decrease anxiety.*) Use simple language and brief statements when instructing patient about diagnostic procedures. (*When experiencing moderate to severe anxiety, patients are frequently unable to comprehend anything more than simple, clear, and brief instructions.*) Encourage patient to ask questions. Assist patient in identifying factors causing anxiety. (*Patient is possibly unaware of the relationship between emotional concerns and anxiety.*)	Patient states fewer feelings of anxiety. Patient states an understanding of the upcoming examination.

CRITICAL THINKING QUESTIONS

1. The patient has been very quiet during his morning care. When you attempt a conversation, he is obviously not interested. What is a way for you to initiate a conversation to encourage him to relate his concerns over his upcoming bronchoscopy?
2. Your patient is scheduled for an intravenous pyelogram (IVP). During your preparation of this patient, he remarks he once had a reaction while eating shellfish. What will you probably do next?
3. The patient is obviously anxious about his upcoming magnetic resonance imaging (MRI) scan. He breaks out in a cold sweat and is breathing rapidly, and when assessing his pulse, you note tachycardia. How will you respond to this patient?

24-Hour Urine Collection

- All of patient's urine voided during the specified time is saved.

Urine and Stool Specimens

- Patient specimen is free of contaminants, including urine or toilet tissue in stool or toilet tissue in urine.

Sputum Specimen Obtained by Suction

- Patient maintains adequate oxygenation throughout procedure.

Wound Drainage Specimen

- Specimen is free of contaminants from skin.

Contrast Media Studies

- Patient explains the purpose and basic steps of the procedure before it begins.
- Patient assumes the correct position and remains still during the procedure.
- Patient does not experience postprocedure complications, such as flushing, pruritus, and urticaria; respiratory depression or decreased cardiovascular function; diminished or absent peripheral pulses; hypotension and tachycardia; or decreased or absent urinary output.

Nuclear Imaging Studies (Scans)

- Patient expresses fear and anxieties related to testing and results.
- Patient does not experience postprocedure complications such as hematoma, erythema, or edema at injection site.

◆ IMPLEMENTATION

Implementation includes performing preexamination and postexamination responsibilities that will assist a patient to achieve an optimal state of health (see Table 23.1).

If patient is discharged home, teach home care instructions (see the Home Care Considerations box on specimen collection and diagnostic examination).

◆ EVALUATION

Evaluation involves observing for a patient's response to determine whether goals and outcomes have been met.

1. Ask patient to state purpose and explain steps of the procedure before it is started.

2. Ask whether patient has questions or concerns about the procedure before it begins and later about test results. Assess nonverbal behaviors of anxiety before, during, and after procedure.

3. Ask patient to demonstrate body position required for procedure. Assess patient's body position throughout procedure, and assist to maintain position as necessary.

4. Ask patient to describe level of comfort during and after procedure.

5. Assess patient's respiratory status (rate, rhythm, and depth of respirations; symmetry of chest movement) during and after abdominal paracentesis, thoracentesis, and bronchoscopy.

6. Compare patient's heart rate and blood pressure during and after procedure with preprocedure baseline values. (Check hospital policy; sometimes performed as often as every 15 minutes, typically for a period of 2 hours.)

7. Inspect dressing over puncture site for drainage every hour after the procedure until patient's condition is stable.

8. Assess patient for postprocedure complications.
   a. Assess patient for a decrease in blood pressure and tachycardia (could signify hemorrhage or allergic reaction to dye [see Box 23.2]).
   b. Assess patient for flushing, itching, and urticaria (could signify allergic reaction to dye [see Box 23.2]).
   c. Assess the patient's respiratory status for sudden, severe shortness of breath (signifies possible laryngospasm and bronchospasm).
   d. Assess patient for abdominal pain, fever, and bleeding (signify possible perforation of abdominal structures).
   e. Assess patient for low oxygen saturation; rate and depth of respirations; cyanosis or mottled skin; hypotension; changes in heart rate or rhythm (usually bradycardia); decreased or nonpalpable peripheral pulses; decreased or absent reflexes; and changes in level of consciousness related to conscious sedation.

9. Ask patient to describe postprocedure positioning and activity restriction for lumbar puncture, liver biopsy, and thoracentesis.

Get Ready For The NCLEX® Examination!

Key Points

- Laboratory examinations of specimens of urine, stool, sputum, blood, and wound drainage provide important information about body functioning and contribute to the assessment of health status.
- Patients who are given a clear explanation about the purpose of the specimen and how it is obtained will be more cooperative during its collection.
- Prepare properly to ensure that the patient is ready for the test and to prevent prolonging the hospital stay because of inadequate test preparations.
- Most people prefer that excretions be handled discreetly; therefore it is important to provide the patient with as much comfort and privacy as possible.
- Health care professionals are obliged to take into consideration the patient's age and socioeconomic, cultural, and educational background when discussing and collecting laboratory specimens.
- Wear gloves when collecting specimens of blood or other body fluids to prevent spread of bloodborne pathogens such as human immunodeficiency virus (HIV), hepatitis B, and other pathogens.
- Collect specimens in proper containers at the correct time and in the appropriate amount.
- Label all specimens properly with the patient's identification, and complete laboratory requisition as necessary.
- Most invasive diagnostic tests require a signed informed consent.
- Wound cultures identify aerobic and anaerobic organisms.
- Some diagnostic tests can be performed at the patient's bedside; the nurse's responsibility in this case includes caring for the patient and assisting the health care provider.
- After diagnostic testing, provide care and teach the patient what to expect, including the outcomes or side effects of the test.

Additional Learning Resources

SG Go to your Study Guide for additional learning activities to help you master this chapter content.

Be sure to visit the Evolve site at http://evolve.elsevier.com/Cooper/foundations for additional online resources.

Review Questions for the NCLEX® Examination

1. An elderly patient who has been newly diagnosed with diabetes mellitus has been learning how to perform their own blood glucose monitoring. The patient has impaired circulation. What action would the nurse recommend to improve the specimen collection process?
   1. Use a tourniquet on the finger to be used in the specimen collection.
   2. Apply a cool, damp cloth to the finger to be used in the specimen collection.
   3. Massage the hand before performing the specimen collection.
   4. Elevate the hand above heart level before the specimen collection.

2. A sputum specimen has been ordered for a patient admitted with possible pneumonia of the right lower lobe. Which is the best method for the nurse to use with a patient who cannot expectorate sputum on their own?

   1. Pharyngeal suctioning
   2. Nasotracheal suctioning
   3. Oropharyngeal suctioning
   4. Tracheal suctioning

3. The health care provider has ordered a stool specimen for blood that it is not possible to see with the naked eye. What does this examination detect?

   1. Profuse bleeding
   2. Gross blood
   3. Obscure blood
   4. Occult blood

4. The nurse is educating a middle-aged patient who has been ordered to collect a urine sample for culture and sensitivity. What would the nurse explain is the purpose of the test?

   1. To identify the organism causing the infection
   2. To determine the presence of malignant cells
   3. To analyze the elements present in the urine
   4. To localize the site of the inflammatory process

5. Rank order the instructions that would be given to the patient who is to collect a 24-hour urine specimen.

   1. Place the collection container on ice.
   2. Discard the first voided specimen and then collect the total volume of each void.
   3. Explain the importance of collecting all voiding.
   4. Instruct the patient not to allow toilet tissue or stool to enter the collection container.
   5. Collect each void in a urine hat and add to the larger collection container.

6. A patient has an indwelling urinary catheter. A sterile urine specimen has been ordered for culture and sensitivity. Which is the best method for the nurse to collect the urine specimen?

   1. Obtain 60 mL of urine from the collection bag.
   2. Remove the current catheter, have the patient void, and then recatheterize.
   3. Disconnect the tubing from the catheter and drain 2 mL of urine.
   4. Aspirate 10 mL of urine with a sterile syringe from the tubing port after cleaning with alcohol.

7. A patient performing a fingerstick for blood glucose determination asks why the side of the fingertip is advised as the preferred site. Which is the best answer that the nurse will give to the patient?

   1. The blood supply is greater in this area.
   2. It is easier for the self-determination method.
   3. The side of the finger is less responsive to pain than other sites.
   4. It leaves more room for other site selection.

8. A patient is scheduled for a barium enema study. Which instructions will the patient be given? (Select all that apply.)

   1. Maintain NPO status after midnight before the examination.
   2. Ingest the strong laxative ordered as instructed before the procedure.
   3. Take radiographic dye tablets the evening before the examination.
   4. Monitor bowel movements after the procedure.
   5. Increase fluid intake after the procedure.

9. On evaluation of the patient after a venipuncture, the nurse recognizes which finding to be unexpected? (Select all that apply.)

   1. The patient's heart rate is 80 and regular.
   2. A large lump is noted under the skin at the venipuncture site.
   3. The patient complains of a stinging sensation when the needle is inserted.
   4. A small amount of blood is noted on the bandage over the venipuncture site.
   5. The patient reports a tingling sensation down the arm used for the venipuncture.

10. When obtaining a residual urine specimen, the nurse knows that it is important to catheterize the patient after the patient voids within which time frame?

    1. 10 minutes
    2. 30 minutes
    3. 50 minutes
    4. 90 minutes

11. The nurse has just received an order for electrocardiography. Arrange the following steps in the order that the nurse would perform them.

    1. Perform hand hygiene and don clean gloves.
    2. Obtain the tracing.
    3. Position the patient lying supine.
    4. Raise the side rail, and lower the bed to the lowest position.
    5. Shave or clip hair if necessary.
    6. Attach the leads to the patient.

12. Rank order the following instructions that the nurse would tell a female patient who needed to obtain a midstream urine specimen.

    1. Start voiding directly into the toilet.
    2. Discard the last of the stream of urine into the stool.
    3. Perform hand hygiene before obtaining the specimen.
    4. Clean the perineum by wiping from front to back.
    5. Collect a small amount of urine in the container.

13. Which nursing action is essential before a chest radiograph is obtained?

    1. Make certain the patient does not eat or drink.
    2. Remove the patient's metal necklace.
    3. Have the patient swallow contrast medium.
    4. Administer a dose of medication for pain relief.

14. A nursing student asks the nurse to explain the difference in testing between a midstream urine specimen and a urinalysis. Which explanation would answer the nursing student's question? *(Select all that apply.)*

    1. The midstream specimen is used to determine the culture and sensitivity of the urine specimen.
    2. The midstream specimen is used to measure the specific gravity of the urine.
    3. The midstream specimen is used to determine the presence of glucose and ketones in the urine.
    4. The midstream specimen is used to check the urine for the presence of white blood cells (WBCs).
    5. The midstream specimen is the cleanest portion of the urine specimen.

15. In the assessment of a patient's urine sample, what will the nurse consider an abnormal finding? *(Select all that apply.)*

    1. Clear, straw color
    2. A few mucus flecks
    3. Bloody mucus
    4. A slight aromatic odor
    5. Dark amber color with sediment

16. When is the best time to collect a sputum sample from a patient?

    1. After episodes of coughing
    2. In the morning upon awakening
    3. Immediately after respiratory treatments
    4. Before initiation of oxygen therapy

17. Because of loss of subcutaneous tissue and skin elasticity in older adults, which step of the venipuncture procedure will the nurse sometimes eliminate?

    1. Application of the tourniquet before venipuncture.
    2. Applying pressure to the venipuncture site after the procedure.
    3. Cleansing of the intended venipuncture site with a topical antiseptic.
    4. Placement of a small dressing to the venipuncture site after the procedure.

18. A male, 79, is hospitalized with suspected bladder outlet obstruction with signs of acute urinary retention. The care provider needs accurate measurements of his urinary output. The client is to be catheterized, and the provider directs the nurse to collect an initial sterile urine specimen and a measure of initial output, as well as a measure of residual urine remaining in the bladder. As a result of these tests and imaging, it was determined that the client needed to undergo bladder surgery. During recovery, the patient is restless. Which of the following nursing actions will be appropriate before, during, and after these events?

Place a check mark next to all relevant nursing actions before, during, and after these events. Check all that apply.

____ A. Perform catheterization within 20 minutes after the patient voids.

____ B. Measure residual urine at the time of catheterization.

____ C. Check carefully for residual urine in excess of 50 mL remaining in the bladder.

____ D. Collect output specimen from the closed, dependent drainage bag.

____ E. Include full patient identification information on the lid of the container to not only label securely but avoid risk of contamination.

____ F. In recovery, evaluate for hypoxia.

24 Lifespan Development

http://evolve.elsevier.com/Cooper/foundations

Objectives

1. Differentiate among the types of family patterns and their functions in society.
2. Describe different types of stresses that commonly affect today's families.
3. Describe Piaget's four stages of cognitive development.
4. Describe physical characteristics of each stage of the life cycle.
5. List psychosocial changes of the different stages of development.
6. Describe the normal age-related changes that affect the major body systems.
7. Discuss the effect of the aging process on personality, intelligence, learning, and memory.
8. Discuss Erikson's stages of psychosocial development.
9. Describe the cognitive changes that occur in the early childhood period.
10. Discuss the developmental tasks of the adolescent period.
11. List the developmental tasks for early adulthood.
12. Describe the developmental tasks for middle adulthood.
13. Define aging.
14. Discuss theories of aging.

Key Terms

adoptive family (p. 712)

ageism (ĂG-ĭzm, p. 738)

autocratic family pattern (ăw-tō-KRĂ-tĭk FĂ-mĭ-lē PĂ-tĕrn, p. 713)

blended (reconstituted) family (rē-KŎN-stĭ-tū-tĕd, p. 712)

cephalocaudal (sĕf-ă-lō-KŎ-dăl, p. 710)

chromosomes (KRŌ-mō-sōmz, p. 710)

cohabitation (kō-hăb-ĭ-TĀ-shŭn, p. 712)

conception (fertilization) (kŏn-CĔP-shŭn; fĕr-tĭ-lĭ-ZA-shŭn, p. 710)

concrete operational phase (KŎN-krēt ŏp-ĕr-Ā-shŭn-ăl FĀZ, p. 728)

democratic family pattern (dĕm-ō-KRĂ-tĭc, p. 713)

depression (dĕ-PRĔ-shŭn, p. 733)

development (dĕ-VĔL-ŏp-mĕnt, p. 710)

disengagement stage (dĭs-ĕn-GĀG-mĕnt STĀG, p. 715)

engagement or commitment stage (kŏ-MĬT-mĕnt, p. 714)

establishment stage (ĕs-TĂB-lĭsh-mĕnt, p. 714)

expectant stage (ĕks-PĔC-tănt, p. 714)

extended family (ĕks-TĔN-dĕd, p. 711)

formal operational thought stage (FŌR-măl ŏp-ĕr-Ā-shŭn-ăl THŎT, p. 731)

foster family (FŎS-tĕr, p. 713)

grandfamilies (GRĂND-fă-mĭ-lēz, p. 713)

growth (GRŌTH, p. 710)

infant mortality rate (p. 709)

life expectancy (LĪF ĕk-SPĔC-tăn-cē, p. 709)

matriarchal family pattern (mă-trē-ĂR-kăl, p. 713)

nuclear family (NŪ-clē-ăr, p. 711)

parenthood stage (PĂR-ĕnt-hūd, p. 715)

patriarchal family pattern (pă-trē-ĂR-kăl, p. 713)

preoperational thought stage (prē-ŏp-ĕr-Ā-shŭn-ăl, p. 723)

presbycusis (prĕz-bē-KYŪ-sĭs, p. 735)

presbyopia (prĕz-bē-Ō-pē-ă, p. 735)

proximodistal (prŏk-sĭ-mō-DĬS-tăl, p. 710)

schema (SKĒ-mă, p. 719)

school violence (SKŪL VĪ-ō-lĕnz, p. 730)

senescence stage (sĕ-NĔS-ăns, p. 715)

sensorimotor stage (sĕn-sŏ-rē-MŌ-tŏr, p. 719)

single-parent family (p. 712)

social contract family (SŌ-shăl KŎN-trăkt, p. 712)

surrogacy (SŬR-rŏ-gă-cē, p. 715)

teratogen (tĕ-RĂ-tō-jĕn, p. 711)

transgender family (p. 712)

zygote (ZĪ-gōt, p. 710)

Table 24.1 Healthy People 2020 Leading Health Indicators for All Ages

LEADING HEALTH INDICATORS
Increase the use of the oral health system
Reduce consumption of added sugars by people aged 2 years and older
Reduce drug overdose deaths
Reduce the number of days people are exposed to unhealthy air
Reduce homicides
Reduce household food insecurity and hunger
Increase the proportion of people who get the flu vaccine every year
Increase knowledge of HIV status
Increase the proportion of people with health insurance
Reduce the suicide rate
Substance abuse
Tobacco

From US Department of Health and Human Services: *Healthy People 2030*, Washington, DC, 2010, US Department of Health and Human Services.

The United States is in an era of increasing interest in health and well-being. Many improvements have contributed to better health and longer life. Improved sanitation, medications, immunizations, exercise, and nutrition help people stay healthy and live longer. In the coming decades, an increasing portion of the population will occupy the category of "older adult." Many factors have been identified as predictors of longevity, including health, happiness, avoidance of tobacco products, and job satisfaction. The exact number of years a person will live is not possible to predict, but estimations can be made. This estimate is referred to as the life expectancy.

Life expectancy is the number of years an individual will probably live based on the average for others with similar characteristics. Life expectancy in the United States in the beginning of the 20th century was 47.3 years, but improvements in health outcomes reflect improvements since that time. The average life expectancy for 2019 in the United States was 76.3 years for men and 81.4 years for women (Ortaliza, et. al., 2021). Unfortunately, despite the sharp increase since the early 1900s, recent mortality statistics are concerning. Since the 80s, the rate of life expectancy increases began to slow. Many countries have life expectancies greater than that of the United States. For example, life expectancy in Switzerland for men in 2019 was 82.1 years and for women it was 85.8 years; in Japan the life expectancy for men was 81.4 years and 87.5 years for women (Ortaliza, et. al., 2021).

A portion of declines in life expectancy are tied to increased death rates in young and middle-aged adults. The explosion in drug addiction statistics have resulted in lives lost too soon; drug overdoses have become too common with a rise more than five-fold (32.5 deaths/100,000). Lifestyle choices relating to dietary intake and inactivity have increased the incidence of heart attack, stroke, and diabetes. These conditions are tied not only to disease but to premature deaths

(Fleming, 2020). Within the United States, life expectancy differs between population groups as well as geographic location; for example, females outlive males by an average of 5 years. Depending on gender and race, those with household incomes of greater than $25,000 live 3 to 7 years longer than those in households with incomes of less than $10,000.

Infant mortality rate refers to the number of deaths before age 1 year. This number affects overall life expectancy statistics. The infant mortality rate for African Americans is more than double that for white infants. Education and access to preventive health care is necessary for pregnant women of all ages and races.

Other factors also influence the life expectancy for different groups, and *Healthy People 2030* has created national objectives to achieve their vision of "A society in which all people can achieve their full potential for health and well-being across the lifespan" (US Department of Health and Human Services, Office of Disease Prevention and Health Promotion, 2021). To motivate action toward change and progress, *Healthy People 2030* has organized a list of leading health indicators (LHI) (Table 24.1). These are LHIs for all ages. *Healthy People 2030* also have LHIs for specific ages.

According to *Healthy People 2030*, the five overarching goals for the population during the next 10 years are:

(1) Attain healthy, thriving lives and well-being free of preventable disease, disability, injury, and premature death; (2) Eliminate health disparities, achieve health equity, and attain health literacy to improve the health and well-being of all; (3) Create social, physical, and economic environments that promote attaining the full potential for health and well-being for all (4) Promote healthy development, healthy behaviors, and well-being across all life stages (5) Engage leadership, key constituents, and the public across multiple sectors to take action and design policies that improve the

health and well-being of all (US Department of Health and Human Services, Office of Disease Prevention and Health Promotion, 2021).

HEALTH PROMOTION ACROSS THE LIFESPAN

Development is a lifelong process that begins at conception, the beginning of pregnancy, and ends with death. Middle adulthood and late adulthood have been recognized recently as having equal importance as the earlier stages of development. Development is influenced by a series of interacting events, including personal behaviors, genetics, and the environment. An individual's experiences affect their future development. Lifespan development studies examine the changes in the life cycle of an individual and the impact of these factors on their growth and development.

Lifespan development comprises eight stages. Their approximate ages are as follows:
- Infancy: birth to 1 year
- Toddler: 1 to 3 years
- Preschool: 3 to 5 years
- School age: 6 to 12 years
- Adolescence: 13 to 19 years
- Early adulthood: 20 to 40 years
- Middle adulthood: 40 to 65 years
- Late adulthood: 65 years and over

Each stage of the lifespan is unique and has certain distinguishable features. Not all people experience the same milestones during the ages listed. Some may have delayed development or accelerated achievement of skills or behaviors. The guidelines are generalized. The goal of studying the lifespan is to enable better understanding and improved interaction and communication with individuals at various stages of development. In particular, given the significant growth of the population in the older age group, we must become more aware of the unique characteristics, needs, and problems of the older adult.

GROWTH AND DEVELOPMENT

Living beings undergo continuous changes throughout their lifespan. Some changes are physical, such as the replacement of cells, tissues, and fluids, while other changes involve cognition, communication, emotions, behavior, and feelings.

Growth refers to an increase in size and may involve the entire being or parts within. **Development** refers to function and the gradual process of change and differentiation, from simple to complex. Development proceeds as an orderly, sequential series of changes; two directional terms important to understanding growth and development are *cephalocaudal* and *proximodistal*. **Cephalocaudal** is defined as growth and development that proceeds from the head toward the feet. The infant's head is large as compared with the rest of its body; gradually the body catches up. **Proximodistal** refers to growth and development that originates in the center of the body and moves toward the outside. For example, the infant gains control of the shoulders before developing control of the hands and fingers.

The principles of growth and development can be summarized as follows:
- Growth and development proceed at a highly individualized rate that varies from person to person. Do not expect two people to react in the same manner to the same stimuli.
- Growth and development are continuous and interdependent processes characterized by spurts of growth and periods of rest.
- Growth and development proceed from the simple to the complex in a predictable sequence of progressive changes.
- Growth and development vary for specific structures at specific times. In other words, not all organs grow and develop at the same rate; for example, the ovaries in the female and the testes in the male do not mature until puberty.
- Growth and development are a total process that involves the whole person. The person grows physically, socially, mentally, and emotionally. Types of growth are interrelated.

PATTERNS OF GROWTH

Growth patterns appear to be controlled genetically. Nutrition, heredity, and environment play an important role in the patterns as well. The blueprint for all inherited traits is contained in the **chromosomes** (threadlike structures in the nucleus of a cell that function in the transmission of genetic information). At conception, the individual is endowed with a complex set of biological potential that involves characteristics such as height; skin, hair, and eye color; and talents and interests. Only identical twins have the same combinations of chromosomes (karyotype). The process of division, transmission, and mixing of chromosomes accounts for the variations in distinctive family traits or, in contrast, their continuity.

BEGINNINGS

Development begins with **conception (fertilization)**, or the union of the sperm and ovum, which combines the genetic material of both parents. This combination of genetic material and environmental influence produces a unique individual.

After fertilization, the **zygote** (the developing ovum from the time it is fertilized until, as a blastocyst, it is implanted in the uterus) contains 23 pairs of chromosomes, for a total of 46 chromosomes. One of each pair has been contributed by the mother and one by the father; the sex chromosomes (one of the chromosome pairs) determine the gender of the baby. The ovum always carries an X chromosome, whereas the sperm sometimes carries an X and sometimes a Y chromosome. The presence of a Y chromosome in the sperm that fertilizes the ovum means that the baby will be male, but if the fertilizing sperm has an X chromosome, the baby will be a female.

In some instances, environmental factors also play a role in contributing to certain diseases or defects in the unborn. A teratogen is a substance, agent, or process that interferes with normal prenatal development, causing the formation of one or more developmental abnormalities in the fetus. Drugs, alcohol, viruses, and cigarette smoke are just a few of the known harmful substances that are best avoided during pregnancy. A possible 5% to 25% of unfavorable outcomes in all pregnancies are estimated to be attributable to smoking. Smoking also may increase the incidence of low–birth weight babies.

Ethical Considerations

The transmission of certain abnormalities is determined genetically. Examples of such inherited disorders include Tay-Sachs disease, sickle cell disease, phenylketonuria, and spina bifida. Genetic testing provides prospective parents with information about whether they are carriers of genes associated with certain inherited diseases. Genetic testing may be suggested for couples based on several factors, including age, medical history, and ethnicity. Test results can provide families information to use for future decision making. Decisions may be difficult for families, and supportive services should be made available. A genetic counselor can review the test results and provide information regarding the likelihood of genes being passed on to a child.

FAMILY

The family is the basic unit of society. Families are composed of two or more individuals united by marriage, blood, adoption, emotional bonds, and social roles. The individuals of the family share emotional ties that usually persist over their entire lifetime (see the Cultural Considerations box).

🌐 Cultural Considerations

Family and Culture

- Know the patient's family and kinship.
- Understand the values, flow of authority, and decision-making patterns within the family.
- Understand different gender roles.
- Listen carefully to direct verbal and indirect nonverbal cultural cues.
- Be aware of common foods and eating rituals.
- Recognize that religious beliefs are likely to affect a person's response to health, illness, birth, and death.

Signs of several significant changes in American families are evident today, and the factors that have contributed to the changed family are listed in Box 24.1. As a result of these influences, family roles and lifestyles have changed to meet society's needs.

Box 24.1   Changes That Have Affected Modern Families

- Economic changes which resulted in an increase in the number of women in the workforce
- The feminist movement
- Postponement of marriage and childbearing
- Increase in divorce rate
  - Changes to traditional family structures
  - Increasing educational opportunities for low- and middle-income adults

TYPES OF FAMILIES

Regardless of the type of family, certain basic functions are inherent to the family unit. These basic functions include protection, nurturance, education, sustenance, and socialization. Ideally, unconditional affection, acceptance, and companionship are guaranteed to each family member. The family attempts to meet the individual's needs for growth and development, which helps support personal fulfillment and strengthen self-esteem.

The family is the first socializing agent for teaching children society's expectations and limitations. As a part of that socialization, the family is responsible for ensuring that the child receives a formal education. The family is also responsible for instilling morals, values, and ideals into the children. These roles and functions of families are not necessarily stable or constant but are vulnerable to change; for example, the birth of a baby or the death of a family member makes rearrangement of family roles and structures necessary. See Box 24.2 for types of families.

Nuclear Family

Historically, the nuclear family was considered the normal family composition. The nuclear family is a family unit that consists of parents and their biological offspring. After a rise in divorce in the 1980s, the sustainability of the traditional family unit is increasing as divorce rates decline. Nearly 70% of children live with their parents, , and 21% of children live with their mother. This supports the fact that the family dynamic is varied (Wang, 2018).

The nuclear family consists of a couple and their children living in an independent household setting. In the past, one parent (usually the father) was the primary source of income; today, these roles have been redefined in their structure and function. In many families, both parents work and share equally in the financial support, roles, and responsibilities of the family unit.

Extended Family

The extended family consists of the nuclear or traditional family as well as additional family such as grandparents, grandchildren, aunts, and uncles who live in the same household. A sharing of support, roles, and responsibilities is common to this family structure.

Box 24.2	Types of Families

NUCLEAR
- Consists of married man and woman and their children
- Lives in independent household

EXTENDED
- Consists of nuclear plus additional family members living in same household
- Provides a sharing of responsibilities

SINGLE-PARENT
- Occurs by divorce, death, separation, abandonment, or choice
- More common in recent years
- One adult performs roles of two people

BLENDED (RECONSTITUTED)
- Occurs when adults from previous marriages remarry and combine children within new household
- New children may be born from this union.

SOCIAL CONTRACT AND COHABITATION
- Made up of man and woman living together without legal commitment but sharing roles and responsibilities

LGBTQ
- Parents identifying as gay, transgender, or queer raising children
- The parents may be married, single, or cohabitating
- Adoptive
- Consists of usually traditional nuclear family members, husband, wife, and adoptive child

GRANDFAMILIES
- Children living in households headed by their grandparents
- Biological parents may or may not be involved in the child's care

FOSTER
- Responsible for care, supervision, and nurturing of children in their charge

This family type constitutes the basic family structure in many societies.

Single-Parent Family

The single-parent family exists today by choice or as the result of death, divorce, separation, or abandonment. More than 40% of single-parent families are the result of divorce. The head of the household may be male or female. This type of family unit also results when an unwed parent lives alone or a single person adopts a child. The single parent has the sole responsibility of carrying out the functions that are typically shared by two members.

Blended (Reconstituted) Family

The blended (reconstituted) family (also called the step-family) is formed when adults remarry and bring together children from previous marriages. Added to this equation is the potential addition of children to this marriage. An estimated, one in three Americans is

a part of a blended family as a stepparent or stepchild. The percentage of blended families has stayed fairly consistent over the years. This type of family potentially presents many types of stresses. Losses resulting from death or divorce sometimes cause adults and children to be fearful of love and trust; as this family type comes together, merging traditions and childrearing practices are a challenge. Children may have loyalties to one parent, which results in difficulties achieving a bond with the new stepparent, jealousies may arise as efforts are made to unite the stepchildren into a single family, and sibling rivalries may result from the children from each of the parents and toward children born of this union.

Social Contract Family and Cohabitation

The social contract family style also is referred to as cohabitation. It involves an unmarried couple living together and sharing roles and responsibilities. This family unit may or may not share children; the children in this family unit may belong to the couple or may be from previous relationships.

Lesbian, Gay, Bisexual, Gay, Transgender, Queer (LGBTQ) Families

The LGBTQ family is composed of a combination of parents who identify as lesbian, bisexual, gay, transgender or queer. In the United States, 5.6% of adults identify as members of this group. An estimated 300,000 children have parents who (Family Equality Council, 2017).are same sex partners. The specific composition of these families is not unlike those occupied by heterosexual parents. Families may consist of married, single, or cohabitating parents. Blending of families is also present. Social and political environments present challenges to these families; some report experiences of discrimination or even open hostility. Thankfully though, these families are experiencing less negativity than in the past. Those families choosing to expand their families through adoption and foster care may face legal challenges. The parenting concerns and responsibilities are consistent with other family structures.

Adoptive Family

The adoptive family is a family unit created with non-biological children. Each year, approximately 135,000 children are adopted in the United States. The road to adoption varies by family. Children may be from another country, from the foster care system, or are newborns relinquished at birth by their mothers. More than 60% of children are adopted within a month of birth. An increasing number (40%) of adoptive children are of a different race, culture, or ethnic group than the new parents.

The adoptive family will experience unique issues to this type of family creation. To reach the point of adoption, prospective parents must navigate legal and potentially expensive processes. The period from when the decision is made to adopt to completion can be time consuming and filled with anxiety. Merging cultures and addressing potential emotional concerns that may arise from feelings of abandonment by the child are common. There are also mental and physical health concerns; 54% of adoptive parents report that they have been advised that their child has a physical or mental disability that infringes on their ability to learn or engage with others. This is much higher than the 23% rate noted with biological children. The most common conditions encountered are attention deficit disorder (36%), learning disability (23%), speech impairment (16%), and developmental delay (15%). These result at a higher rate than with biological children (Zill, 2018). Families created by adoption achieve the same fulfillment associated with parenting as those families created by natural procreation.

Grandfamilies

Grandfamilies refer to families with children under the age of 18 years who live with or in the custody of grandparents. This group represents a growing demographic. Nearly 8 million children reside with their grandparents. About a third of these families also includes at least one of the biological parents (Generations United, n.d.a.). The reasons that children are removed from the care of their parents includes neglect, abuse, parental incarceration, illness, and drug use, and for some families these reasons may overlap. There is racial predominance in some groups for grandfamilies; African American children have double the likelihood of living in a grandfamily at some point in their lives (Generations United, n.d.b.). Unfortunately, 21% of these families live below the poverty line and have to deal with various other stressors, which may include their own mental health issues stemming from shame or guilt about their adult child's inability to parent or their substance abuse disorder, social isolation, and depression. Research confirms that, although it presents a challenging situation, children have more stable and safe childhoods when raised by grandparents and other relatives than when they are placed with nonrelatives.

Foster Family

The foster family results when the biological parents are unable or unwilling to provide adequate, safe care for their children. Children placed in foster care are typically placed there by the court system. The reasons for placement traditionally involve abuse, neglect, or parental drug abuse. Individual circumstances determine the amount of time for the placement; ideally, the parents can achieve stability and are again allowed to care for their children, thus protecting the parental bond. Approximately a third of children in foster care are placed with relatives. The number of US children living in foster care has decreased significantly in recent years. In 2002 more than 500,000 children were in foster care; in 2018 the number was reduced to 437,283—substantially less at fewer than 400,000 children

in foster care. The actual percentage declined by approximately 23.5% from 2002 to 2018 (Child Welfare Information Gateway, 2021). Although there has been a national decline in the number of children entering the foster care system, unfortunately many children will never return to the care of their biological parents; they face living in the foster care system until they "age out" when they reach legal adulthood.

FAMILY PATTERNS

Family patterns refer to the way in which family members relate to one another. Examples of family patterns include autocratic, patriarchal, matriarchal, and democratic patterns. Researchers have identified 12 qualities common to all functional families, listed in Box 24.3.

In the autocratic family pattern, the relationships are unequal. The parents attempt to control the children with strict rigid rules and expectations. This family pattern is least open to outside influence.

In the patriarchal family pattern, the adult male (or males) of the family assumes the dominant role. The adult male member functions in the work role, is responsible for control of finances, and makes most decisions.

In the matriarchal family pattern (also known as the matrifocal family), the adult female (or females) of the family assumes primary dominance in areas of childcare, homemaking, and financial decision making. In some families of this type, an older female relative provides childcare so that the mother is free to work outside of the home.

In the democratic family pattern, the adult members function as equals. As is often true in other types of families, children are treated with respect and recognized as individuals. This style encourages joint decision making and recognizes and supports the uniqueness of each individual member. This family pattern favors negotiation, compromise, and growth.

Box **24.3**   **Qualities of Functional Families**
• Sense of commitment toward promoting the members' well-being
• Sense of appreciation and encouragement for tasks accomplished
• Directed effort toward spending quality time with individual members
• Sense of purpose that encourages progress during good or difficult times
• Sense of harmony between members of the family
• Effective communication between individuals
• Established values, rules, and beliefs
• Variety of different coping techniques to enhance functioning
• Use of effective problem-solving measures and the use of a variety of options
• Positive outlook
• Ability to be flexible and adapt to changes
• Use of varied resources to facilitate coping skills

STAGES OF FAMILY DEVELOPMENT

Engagement or Commitment Stage

The **engagement or commitment stage** begins when the couple acknowledges to themselves and others that they are considering marriage. At this time, opposition or support is evident from friends and parents. Wedding plans are arranged. Housing, work, and furnishings are some items that require discussion and exploration.

Establishment Stage

The **establishment stage** extends from the wedding up until the birth of the first child. During this phase, one of the important tasks is the adjustment from the single, independent state to the married, interdependent state. Challenges that the newly married couple must face include learning to live with another person, together managing two-person decision making, conflict resolution, and communication. The relationship established with the couple's parents and families can enhance cohesiveness or weaken the couple's ties. To the average young adult, marriage is an important serious change that requires major adjustments. A good marriage does not just happen; both parties must work at and contribute to a marriage for success. Commitment, goals, and respect for each other require equal time and energy. Success at marriage satisfies Erikson's task of intimacy (Table 24.2 and see Psychosocial Development in the Early Adulthood section) and helps fulfill the individual's need for love and belonging (Fig. 24.1).

Expectant Stage

The **expectant stage** begins with conception and continues through pregnancy. One of the most important decisions of a person's life is that of starting a family. Many people describe becoming a parent as one of the

Fig. 24.1 Establishment stage: the newly married couple.

Table 24.2	Erickson's Stages of Psychosocial Development		
STAGE	**APPROXIMATE AGE (YEARS)**	**DEVELOPMENTAL TASK**	**OUTCOMES**
1. Infancy	Birth to 1	Basic trust vs. mistrust	Infants learn to either trust or not trust that significant others will properly care for their basic needs, including nourishment, sucking, warmth, cleanliness, and physical contact.
2. Toddler	1–3	Autonomy vs. shame and doubt	Children learn to be either self-sufficient in many activities (including toileting, feeding, walking, and talking) or doubt their own abilities.
3. Preschool	4–6	Initiative vs. guilt	Children want to undertake many adult-like activities, sometimes going beyond the limits set by parents and feeling guilty because of it.
4. School age	7–11	Industry vs. inferiority	Children eagerly learn to be competent and productive or feel inferior and unable to do any task well.
5. Adolescence	12–19	Identity vs. role confusion	Adolescents try to figure out their personal identity. They establish sexual, ethnic, and career identities, or are confused about what future roles to play.
6. Young adulthood	20–44	Intimacy vs. isolation	Young adults seek companionship and love with another person or become isolated from others.
7. Middle adulthood	45–65	Generativity vs. stagnation	Middle-aged adults are productive, performing meaningful work and raising a family, or become stagnant and inactive.
8. Late adulthood	65+	Ego integrity vs. despair	Older adults try to make sense out of their lives, either seeing life as meaningful and whole or despairing at goals never reached and questions never answered.

most challenging, and most rewarding, roles in their life. Pregnancy requires physiologic and psychological adjustments. Many important decisions must be considered during pregnancy, including childbirth methods, continuation or modification of employment, childcare, and feeding methods. The desired outcome of pregnancy is that a bond or attachment is established between the parents and the new baby.

Ethical considerations. The agreement a woman makes to be artificially inseminated, voluntarily or for a fee, to bear a child and then relinquish the parenting rights to the baby's natural father or another couple is called **surrogacy**. Presently, no national laws exist regarding surrogacy, and state laws vary. A surrogacy can cost $100,000 or more with added costs, including medical expenses and health insurance; often insurance companies do not cover surrogacy expenses.

Parenthood Stage
The parenthood stage begins at the birth or adoption of the first child. The transition to parenthood is a major event; even couples with good preparation express a great deal of anxiety associated with the onset of this new role. One of the most frequently described problems is lack of time: less free time, less sleep time, less time together, and less intimate sexual time. Compounding the lack of time is the stress of parenting and the self-doubt about ability and competency in this new role.

Disengagement stage of parenthood. The **disengagement stage** of parenthood is that period of family life when the grown children depart from the home. The role of parenting changes during this phase of the life cycle. The departure of children does not end the role of parenting. Although grown children perhaps do not live with their parents, they usually continue to need emotional guidance and some financial support. Many grown children return to living at home for financial reasons or for assistance in raising their children. Regardless, during the disengagement stage, couples or the single parent need to redefine personal roles and structure time so that there is a sense of usefulness, accomplishment, and self-fulfillment.

Senescence Stage
The senescence stage is the last stage of the life cycle and requires the individual to cope with a large range of changes. For the older adult, the family unit continues to be a major source of satisfaction and pleasure, but most older adults prefer to live independently. The greater life expectancy for women means that older women commonly outlive their spouses and continue life alone. Most older adults have regular contact with other family members. The grandparenting role requires new adaptations, such as a change in one's roles and sense of identity. In the past, grandparents often lived with their extended families because they had to,

---

Box 24.4   Common Signs of Stress in Children

- Mood swings
- Acting-out behavior
- Change in eating or sleeping patterns
- Frequent stomachaches, headaches, or other unexplained somatic symptoms
- Excessive clinging to parents
- Thumb-sucking
- Bedwetting
- Return to behavior typical of an earlier stage of development

---

not necessarily because they wanted to. Grandparents today are independent. Grandparents want close, stable, emotionally satisfying family ties. Simultaneously, they tend to want an independent life, away from kin. They want to see and love their grandchildren but not be responsible for them.

CAUSES OF FAMILY STRESS
Various stressors affect the family unit. Chronic illness, abuse, and divorce are some of the most common factors. Stress, when it occurs, affects everyone, at all ages. Like adults, children often have feelings of stress. Stress in childhood results from either internal or external pressures or from a combination of both. At very early ages, stress sometimes results when the infant's needs are not met. Toddlers often perceive stress when they are separated from their mothers. School-age children sometimes feel stress from pressures in school or from parental expectations. Even social interactions at this stage have the potential to be somewhat difficult and stressful. Parents need to observe and listen to their children and be watchful for signs of stress (Box 24.4). They must be ready to help their children deal with stress. One way to help is to anticipate what holds stress potential and to prepare children ahead of time. For example, if the child is starting a new school, the parents should talk about it before the day of the event and allow children to express their feelings. Children must know that having uneasy feelings is all right. Children need to have someone validate their feelings. Talking about what is causing the child's uneasy feelings helps minimize the child's discomfort and helps bring about possible solutions.

Chronic Illness
Chronic physical or emotional illness of the parent or the child affects all family members. Factors such as financial resources, family stability, and the adequacy of the support system determine an individual's ability to cope with a family member's chronic illness.

Working Mothers
Alternative family patterns are more common, and today's families often experience change and must adjust to new circumstances. Changes to the family's

composition and economic factors have resulted in more women in the labor force. Working mothers are considered common today. Aside from the financial rewards, many believe that working mothers create a wider range of valid role models for young children. Many working mothers compensate for the time they are not with their child by establishing quality time during their limited at-home time. Some fathers opt to assume primary childcare responsibilities. Certainly, when both parents work outside the home, caregiving arrangements must be considered. Childcare is sometimes available; some of the various forms include in-home care by a relative or paid caregiver and out-of-home care in an organized or group setting. The federal government and most states have regulations that control and regulate staff size and safety issues concerning daycare centers. Optimal qualities in a daycare center include the following: a balance of age-appropriate educational structure and an open environment, ample space with a variety of materials and activities, small class size with appropriate staff-to-child ratio, an environment that fosters active staff involvement, positive encouragement, and high-quality care in a safe and healthy environment.

Abuse

Abuse refers to physical, emotional, financial, and verbal abuse, sexual assault, and neglect. Approximately 700,000 American children are victims of child abuse each year; more than 1,700 die from abuse annually in the United States (National Children's Alliance, n.d.). Children younger than 1 year of age have the highest rate of victimization, and the abuser is most commonly a parent. Certain objective and measurable factors are related to family violence, including financial strain, social isolation, low self-esteem, and history of abuse. The presence of several of these risk factors raises the risk that an individual will resort to abuse. The following are some common characteristics of parents who abuse their children: they were abused themselves as children, they are often loners, they are harsh, strict, and punitive, they have unreasonable expectations, and they are immature, lack self-control, and have low self-esteem. Early recognition, prompt reporting, and preventive measures are called for to help detect and end all forms of abuse and neglect.

Divorce

Divorce is widespread; it continues to affect more than 1 million children annually. The effects of divorce on children are varied and complex. One of the factors is the age of the child at the time of the divorce. Younger children often feel abandoned and believe they are no longer loved by both parents. Other factors that sometimes affect the child are the bitterness and conflict surrounding the divorce, the child's prior relationship with the absent parent, the effects of the divorce on the custodial parent, and the postdivorce relationship of

---

Box 24.5	Tips for Divorcing Parents

- Encourage children to talk about their feelings
- Do not use children as pawns or "go-betweens"
- Never speak negatively about ex-spouse in front of children
- Seek professional help if children need additional support
- Reassure children that the divorce is not their fault

---

the parents. Many children have reconciliation fantasies for extended periods after the divorce is finalized. Changes in one parent's status create changes in emotional milieu, family role, finances, lifestyle, and the neighborhood to which the child has lived in prior to the divorce (Box 24.5).

STAGES OF GROWTH AND DEVELOPMENT

The following sections discuss development by age group. Fully appreciating the scope of human growth and development involves examining a few aspects of development across a larger spectrum.

PSYCHOSOCIAL DEVELOPMENT

Erik Erikson, an American psychoanalyst, viewed the life cycle as a series of developmental stages, each accompanied by a developmental task or challenge. Table 24.2 provides an overview of Erikson's stages of psychosocial development. Many of the subsections that follow include stage-appropriate characterization according to Erikson's framework.

COGNITIVE AND INTELLECTUAL DEVELOPMENT

Swiss theorist Jean Piaget's stages of cognitive development are outlined in Box 24.6.

COMMUNICATION AND LANGUAGE

Humans have an innate capacity to learn language. They are born with the mechanism and the capacity to develop speech and language skills. During infancy, the unique ability of the brain to sort out basic sounds and to extract from sentences the most meaningful elements becomes apparent. During early childhood, the brain's language-acquisition ability becomes even more sophisticated. Parents and other caregivers have an enormous potential to influence the infant's intellectual and language development. Infants do not speak spontaneously. Interaction with the environment provides a means for them to acquire these skills. Speech requires intact physiologic functioning of (1) the respiratory system; (2) the speech control centers in the cerebral cortex; and (3) the articulation and resonance structures of the mouth and nasal cavities. In addition, acquisition of language requires: (1) an intact and discriminating auditory apparatus; (2) intelligence; (3) a need to communicate; and (4) stimulation. The rate of speech development varies from child to child and is

| **Box 24.6** | **Piaget's Stages of Cognitive Development** |

SENSORIMOTOR: BIRTH TO 2 YEARS
- Uses senses and motor abilities to understand the world and coordinates sensorimotor skills; this period begins with reflexes
- Develops schema
- Begins to interact with environment
- Learns that an object still exists when it is out of sight (object permanence) and begins to remember and imagine experiences (mental representation)
- Develops thinking and goal-directed behavior

PREOPERATIONAL THOUGHT: 2–7 YEARS
- Develops egocentric thinking (understands the world from only one perspective—that of the self)
- Uses trial and error to discover new traits and characteristics
- Conceptualizes time in present terms only
- Uses symbols to represent objects
- Develops more logical, intuitive thinking
- Centers or focuses on a single aspect of an object, producing some distortion of reality
- Gains in imaginative ability
- Gradually begins to "decenter" (becomes less egocentric and understands other points of view)

CONCRETE OPERATIONAL THOUGHT: 7–11 YEARS
- Understands and applies logical operations or principles to help interpret specific experiences or perceptions
- Has more realistic views; better understands other viewpoints
- Improves use of memory
- Focuses on more than one task; develops logical, socialized thoughts
- Recognizes cause-and-effect relationships
- Learns to identify behavior outcome
- Understands basic ideas of conversation, number classification, and other concrete ideas

FORMAL OPERATIONAL THOUGHT: 12+ YEARS
- Uses a systematic, scientific problem-solving approach
- Recognizes past, present, and future
- Is able to think about abstractions and hypothetical concepts and is able to move in thought "from the real to the possible"
- Becomes more interested in ethics, politics, and all social and moral issues as ability to take a broader and more theoretic approach to experience increases

related directly to neurologic competence and intellectual development. All children go through the same sequence of stages in language and speech development in early childhood unless abnormal conditions are present (Table 24.3).

The basic sequence of language is as follows:
- *At 3 months, babbling.* When infants babble, they typically explore all the possible sounds they can make by enhancing the force of the air stream as it passes their vocal cords and by varying the positions of their tongue and mouth.

- *At 1 year, recognition of words.* Between ages 1 and 2 years, infants generally acquire the ability to produce holo phrases (one-word sentences that convey a complete message ["up"]). Infants learn to expand their holo phrases by attaching them back-to-back to other nouns or verbs. thus forming two-word sentences ("mommy milk," "daddy come"). Early speech is often referred to as telegraphic speech because, as in telegram messages, the articles, pronouns, prepositions, and conjunctions are omitted. In organizing and coding language, infants acquire an understanding of the most meaningful units of speech. No one teaches infants to use nouns and verbs first. They learn this sequence on their own.

- *At preschool age, acquisition of structure of native language.* The language explosion that occurs during the preschool years is most obvious in the growth of vocabulary, from 50 words at 18 months, to 200 words at age 2 years, to between 8000 and 14,000 words at age 6 years. From ages 2 to 6 years, the average child learns between 6 and 10 words per day. Preschoolers have an outstanding ability to learn language. Most researchers regard early childhood as a crucial period for language learning.

- *At 6 years, ability to speak and understand new words and sentences.* Even compared with the preschool years, language development from 6 years on is remarkable, albeit much more subtle, as children consciously come to understand more about the many ways language can be used. This understanding gives them greater control in their comprehension and use of language and, in turn, enhances the range of their cognitive abilities.

A common rule of thumb about the evolution of early speech acquisition is that the number of words in an average response usually corresponds to the chronologic age of the child. For example, a 2-year-old may say, "Me do," a 3-year-old may add a word, "Me do it," and a 4-year-old may say, "Let me do it."

Girls advance more rapidly in language development than do boys, firstborn children develop language earlier than do later-born children, and children of multiple births (twins, triplets) develop language later than children of single births.

INFANCY: 1 TO 12 MONTHS

Physical Characteristics

An infant's physical development happens so rapidly that size, shape, and skills seem to change daily (see Chapter 28 for discussion of the newborn). Growth, which proceeds in a cephalocaudal and proximodistal sequence, is rapid during the first 6 months of life. Infants are expected to gain about 1½ pounds (3.3 kg) per month until 5 months, and they usually double their birth weight by 4 to 6 months. By the time the baby is 1 year of age, the birth weight has tripled (average weight is 21½ pounds, or 47.3 kg). Most of the weight gain in the first months of life is in the form of

Table 24.3	Normal Language and Speech Development During Early Childhood		
AGE (YEARS)	**NORMAL LANGUAGE DEVELOPMENT**	**NORMAL SPEECH DEVELOPMENT**	**INTELLIGIBILITY**
1	Says two or three words with meaning Imitates sounds of animals	Omission of most final and some initial consonants Substitution of consonants *m, w, p, b, k, g, n, t, d,* and *h* for more difficult sounds Use of unintelligible jargon peaks at age 18 months	Usually no more than 25% intelligible to unfamiliar listener
2	Uses two-word or three-word phrases in context Has vocabulary of about 300 words and uses "I," "me," and "you"	Use of consonants *m, w, p, b, k, g, n, t, d,* and *h* with vowels, but inconsistently and with much substitution Omission of final consonants Articulation lags behind vocabulary	At age 2 years, 65% intelligible in context
3	Says four-word or five-word sentences Has vocabulary of about 900 words Uses "who," "what," and "where" in asking questions Uses plurals, pronouns, and prepositions	Mastery of *b, t, d, k,* and *g; r* and *l* may still be unclear; omission or substitution for *w* Repetitions and hesitations common	At age 3 years, 70%–80% clear
4–5	Has vocabulary of 1500–2100 words Able to use most grammatical forms correctly, such as past tense of verb with "yesterday" Uses complete sentences with nouns, verbs, prepositions, adjectives, adverbs, and conjunctions	Mastery of *f* and *v;* possible distortion of *r, l, s, z, sh, ch, y,* and *th* Little or no omission of initial or last consonant	Speech is totally intelligible, although some are still imperfect
6–7	Has vocabulary of 3000 words Comprehends "if," "because," and "why"	Mastery of *r, l,* and *th;* possible continuing distortion of *s, z, sh, ch,* and *j* (usually mastered by age 7½–8 years)	Speech is totally intelligible

fat, which provides insulation and a source of nourishment to draw on if teething or other problems decrease food intake for a few days. After 8 months, weight gain includes more bone and muscle.

Height (length) increases by about 1 inch (2.54 cm) per month for the first 6 months. By 12 months of age, the infant's birth length has increased about 50% (the typical length is 30 inches, or 75 cm).

Vital Signs. Infants are subject to wide variations in body temperature related to activity levels and state of health. Apical rates slow in infancy, while at 2 months, the average apical rate is about 120 beats/min. Count the apical pulse for a full minute, noting variations in rate, volume, and rhythm. Respiratory rates also decrease during infancy; these rates are related to activity level. Average resting respiratory rate for the 12-month-old is about 30 breaths/min. Blood pressure readings gradually increase to 90/60 mm Hg at 12 months.

Dentition. Teething begins at about 5 to 6 months of age. Signs of teething—irritability, edematous red gums, excessive drooling, and change in stooling—begin 3 to 4 weeks before the appearance of the tooth (Box 24.7).

Box 24.7	**Primary Dentition Schedule**

6	*months:*	Teething begins with eruption of two lower central incisors
7	*months:*	Eruption of upper central incisors
9	*months:*	Eruption of upper lateral incisors
11	*months:*	Eruption of lower lateral incisors
12	*months:*	Approximately 6–8 teeth present
24	*months:*	Approximately 16 teeth present
30	*months:*	Completion of primary dentition; 20 teeth present

Dental decay can begin at any time after tooth development. Oral hygiene for the young infant consists of offering sips of clear water and wiping and massaging the infant's gums. The American Academy of Pediatric Dentistry (n.d.) recommends that children have their first dental visit when the first tooth appears but no later than the child's first birthday.

Advise parents to begin toothbrushing after the first teeth appear; this element of dental hygiene is important to continue throughout the lifespan. In areas without added fluoride in the water, recommend the use of fluoride toothpaste. To prevent bottle-mouth

Fig. 24.2 Development of locomotion. (A) Infant bears full weight on feet by 7 months. (B) Infant can maneuver from sitting to kneeling position. (C) Infant can stand holding on to furniture at 9 months. (D) While standing, infant takes deliberate step at 10 months. (E) Infant crawls with abdomen on floor and pulls self forward, and then, (F) creeps on hands and knees at 9 months.

syndrome, instruct caregivers to avoid putting anything but water in the infant's night bottle. Sugar in milk, formula, and juice causes severe decay and destruction of the tooth enamel. Also, instruct all caregivers not to prop up the bottle and then leave the child alone with it, because this practice potentially leads to aspiration. Furthermore, holding the infant during feeding provides warmth, comfort, and bonding—all vital factors in providing a feeling of love and security.

Motor Development
At 2 months, the infant can hold their head up while in the prone position. By 4 months, the infant can hold their head up steadily to a 90-degree angle while in the prone position. At 6 months, most infants can balance their head well. By the end of the 7 months, infants have acquired the ability to sit up steadily without support.

Locomotion. Crawling, an early form of movement, is a motion made with the infant's abdomen touching the floor (Fig. 24.2E). A more advanced form of locomotion is creeping. The infant accomplishes this by resting the weight on the hands and knees. Infants sometimes crawl at 7 months and creep at about 9 months. Creeping appears after age 9 months in most children

(Fig. 24.2F). Standing with support and walking follow at about 8 months to 15 months (Fig. 24.2D).

Psychosocial Development
Erikson defined the task of the infant as basic trust versus mistrust. The responsiveness of others to the needs of the infant helps establish the basis of trust. Infants obtain gratification when their basic needs are fulfilled. Infants whose needs are not met develop a sense of dissatisfaction or mistrust. (See Table 24.2 for an overview of Erikson's stages of psychosocial development.)

Cognitive and Intellectual Development
During this stage, the infant uses the senses to learn about self and environment. The infant learns with exploration of objects and events and with interaction. Piaget describes the infant as being in the sensorimotor stage of cognitive development.

In the sensorimotor stage, an infant's knowledge comes about primarily through sensory impressions and motor activities. Behavior is completely reflective. The infant develops an image or schema (an innate knowledge structure that allows a child to mentally organize ways to behave in the immediate environment) and assimilates and interprets the information. Infants learn by encountering and responding to stimulation from the environment. As the infant interacts with the environment, changes occur in mental structure and in development of thinking ability. During the first 1 to 4 months, the infant follows objects visually with the eyes and auditorily with the ears. By 4 months of age, infants become notably better at using both eyes together, which makes them more astute observers. From 4 to 8 months of age, the infant begins to recognize and imitate. Reaching and grasping are improved skills.

By age 3 months, most infants respond differently to their parents or primary caregiver than they do to other people. By age 4 months, many infants can identify the voices of the most familiar people in their lives. Smiling occurs in response to different people and events; at the sight of their parents or primary caregivers, infants smile and begin to vocalize.

Studies in children ages 15 to 30 months who had good attachment relationships showed that they experienced a predictable behavior pattern after separation, known as separation anxiety. Beginning at approximately 8 months of age, infants show this anxiety when they are separated from their primary caregiver. They develop shyness and a fear of strangers. The infant may cling and protest any separation from the primary caregiver. By age 9 months, most children show alarm at the presence of a stranger.

Health Promotion

Nutrition. Human breast milk and commercially prepared formula are options that meet the nutritional needs of the infant. Although today's excellent infant formulas approximate human milk, breast milk is still almost always the best food for newborns. It has been called the "ultimate health food" because it offers so many benefits. However, infants who are fed with properly prepared formula and raised with love also grow up healthy and well adjusted. Breast milk or formula is the only food most babies need until they are 6 months of age. The American Academy of Pediatrics (n.d.b.) recommends exclusive breast-feeding for the first 6 months of a baby's life. After 6 months breastfeeding should be continued for the first year of life, or longer if desired by the mother, while foods are introduced.

Most experts agree that newborns should be fed on a demand schedule. Early in life, this practice may mean that babies are fed as often as every 2 hours. In the beginning, nursing mothers often start nursing for 10 to 15 minutes on each breast and then lengthen the feeding time as demanded by the infant. When infants suckle more slowly or appear uninterested in either the breast or the bottle, it is a good indication that they have had enough. The baby should have four to six wet diapers per day by the fourth day after birth. A baby who is breast-feeding should have at least two to three seedy stools each day. Breast milk is digested readily by the baby, which may result in a bowel movement shortly after each feeding. Signs of underfeeding include lack of satisfaction; a cranky, fussy baby; little weight gain; and persistent wrinkling of the skin. Signs of overfeeding include vomiting after feeding and frequent watery stools. Full-term infants have enough stored iron to last for at least the first 5 to 6 months of life. After this time, iron supplements or food sources are options to replenish the diminishing supply. Certain foods are best avoided in the first 6 months of life, including citrus fruits, egg whites, and wheat flour, all of which are identified frequently as allergy-producing substances.

Much controversy exists regarding the best time to introduce solid foods into the infant diet. Many physicians believe that very early introduction of solids leads to a variety of problems. A description of how to first introduce these foods into the infant diet is simpler than the decision of when to introduce solid food. The rules for solid foods include the following:

- Introduce only one new food at a time, allowing several days between new foods, which provides an opportunity to recognize allergies.
- Introduce cereals first, fruits and vegetables next, and meats last.
- Avoid mixing foods to allow the infant to develop interest in different foods and tastes.

Never leave infants alone while they are eating, because infants choke easily. Avoid giving older infants round, hard foods that can get caught in the throat easily. Foods that have high potential to cause choking include popcorn, grapes, raisins, hot dogs, and chicken nuggets.

This period is often an excellent time to look at the type of foods the whole family is eating. Limiting the amount of sodium, fats, and sugar in the family diet is best. Lifelong eating habits are established early on, in these toddler years; the entire family should be offered plenty of fresh fruits, vegetables, lean meats, and whole grains.

In warmer weather, febrile conditions, prolonged vomiting, and diarrhea place infants at higher risk for dehydration due to their small fluid volume. Infants must receive adequate breast milk or formula. Infants do not need additional fluids during the first 4 months of life. Excessive intake of water can cause water intoxication, failure to thrive, and hyponatremia in the infant. By age 8 to 9 months, most babies master eating mashed or junior foods. Self-feeding of finger foods allows the infant further opportunity for exploration. By 9 months of age, the process of weaning should begin. This is usually a gradual process, with a training cup substituted for one bottle at a time, usually starting with the lunchtime feeding.

Sleep, Play Activity, And Safety. Newborns and infants sleep 18 out of 24 hours. These sleep periods usually consist of short, nap-like periods. Infants are normally restless and make noises during these periods. Toward the end of the first 3 months, definite sleep patterns emerge, and nap and wake periods are clearly established. By the end of the first year, infants usually sleep 12 hours at night and take one nap during the day. Persistent crying during usual sleep or nap periods often signals discomfort or illness and calls for investigation.

A concern for parents of young infants is sudden infant death syndrome (SIDS). This disorder produces sudden, abrupt death with no identifiable warning signs. Formerly known as crib death, its incidence seems to peak 2 to 3 months after birth. Steps to reduce the incidence of SIDS are outlined in the Safety Alert box.

⚠ Safety Alert

Steps to Reduce the Incidence of Sudden Infant Death Syndrome

1. Back to sleep: place infants on their back to sleep.
2. Avoid exposure to cigarette smoke.
3. Avoid use of soft bedding or pillows.
4. Keep room well ventilated.
5. Breast-feed if possible.
6. Maintain regular medical checkups for infants.
7. Avoid smoking during pregnancy.
8. Consider pacifier use at night and during naps.
9. Follow the recommended vaccination schedule for infants.
10. Avoid use of bed wedges.

Play is important for learning. Play that captures the pleasures of using the senses and motor abilities is called sensorimotor play (Fig. 24.3). Early play items include turning mobiles, mirrors, colorful shapes, and toys of different textures. As hand coordination improves, other items, such as rattles and shapes, become useful play objects. Toward the end of the first year, stacking items, blocks, and puzzles encourage developing motor skills. Music is useful to soothe the infant or to stimulate awareness of sounds and rhythms. Play style during infancy is described as solitary play, which means that the infant plays alone and does not interact with or need other children to play. Allowing adequate freedom of movement helps enhance good development of muscles and bones. Young infants need room to stretch and kick, so care should be taken to prevent injury during this early stage of development. Do not push children to sit or walk before adequate muscle strength is achieved.

Accidents are the leading cause of injury and death in infants and young children. Safety precautions are essential to institute immediately at the birth of the child (Fig. 24.4). The Safety Alert box lists safety rules for infants and young children.

Infancy is also a time of daily changes. Goals for the developmental tasks of infancy are shown in Box 24.8.

Fig. 24.3 Nine-month-old infant enjoying own image in a mirror.

Fig. 24.4 Children are most likely to ingest substances that are on their level, such as cleaning agents stored under sinks, rat poison, plants, and diaper pail deodorants.

Box 24.8   Developmental Tasks of Infancy

- Establishes trusting, meaningful relationships
- Recognizes primary caregiver
- Develops attachment behavior
- Learns to recognize objects
- Develops exploration skills
- Develops communication skills by beginning vocalization, learning nonverbal communication techniques, and imitating simple vocalizations
- Develops muscular control, eye-hand coordination, and object manipulation
- Develops mobility: crawling, creeping, cruising, walking
- Establishes patterns of living: eating, sleeping, elimination habits
- Begins to develop independent living skills: self-feeding, walking, undressing, communication of needs

! Safety Alert

Safety Rules for Infants and Young Children

- Never leave an unsupervised infant on an elevated surface.
- Never leave an infant unattended in a highchair, stroller, walker, or any other device.
- Secure stairways and exits.
- Keep crib sides up and set mattress at lowest setting.
- Never leave infants or young children unattended in a bath, even for a few seconds.
- Keep windows locked and secured with child guards.
- Never use plastic bags or coverings on mattresses or near infant's playthings.
- Avoid the use of pillows with small infants.
- Infant cribs must meet US Consumer Product Safety regulations to prevent strangulation between crib bars.
- Remove wires and dangling electric cords from the crawling child's reach. Cover outlets with protective caps.
- Inspect all toys carefully for long strings and small removable parts.
- Use pacifiers that have one-piece construction.
- Do not allow children to play with balloons.
- Avoid giving infants and young children hard candies, nuts, popcorn, or other foods that are easily aspirated.
- Lock all poisons and medicines out of the reach of infants and young children (see Fig. 24.4).
- Avoid drinking hot fluids while holding an infant.
- Check temperature of foods and formula before feeding.
- Turn pot handles toward back of stove and remove burner knobs if within child's reach.

- Avoid smoking near infants and children to prevent burns and smoke inhalation.
- Keep infants and children away from hot surfaces, stoves, fireplaces, and barbecues.
- Use flame-retardant sleepwear.
- Never say that medication is candy to facilitate administration.
- Keep poison control hotline phone number accessible.
- Keep plants out of child's reach.
- Use plastic rather than glass eating and drinking utensils.
- Inspect toys and household items for sharp points.
- Inspect for chipped lead-based paint on surfaces painted before 1978 (production of lead paint for consumer use was banned in 1978).
- Keep knives and forks away from young children.
- Supervise infants and children playing around animals and pets.
- Teach children early about street dangers and supervise their play.
- Instruct children to never go anywhere with strangers.
- Teach young children the use of the telephone for emergencies.
- Instruct children that others should not touch their "private" body parts and to report happenings if they occur. Accept the child's story unless you can prove otherwise.
- Always use safety seats and restraints when transporting infants and young children.

TODDLER: 1 TO 3 YEARS

Physical Characteristics

Rate of growth in the toddler years is slower than in infancy but follows the same general principles. It is orderly, proceeding from head to foot, from the center outward, and from general to specific movements.

One of the most striking changes from infancy is the upright stance of the toddler. The chubby look of infancy is gone by 12 to 15 months. In the beginning of this stage, the toddler's body proportions result in a top-heavy appearance, but by the end of this period, rapid growth of the extremities and slowed growth in the trunk produce a more proportionate body appearance (Fig. 24.5). An exaggerated lumbar lordosis (convex lumbar curve) and protruding abdomen produce a potbelly appearance, which disappears as the abdominal muscles strengthen. By age 2½ years, all 20 deciduous teeth are present. Advise parents to begin routine dental examinations and tooth brushing during this period.

Vital Signs. During the toddler period, the pulse ranges from 90 to 120 beats/min. Blood pressure averages 80 to 100 mm Hg systolic and 64 mm Hg diastolic. Body temperature ranges between 98°F and 99°F (36.6°C and 37.2°C). Respiration slows to 20 to 30 breaths/min.

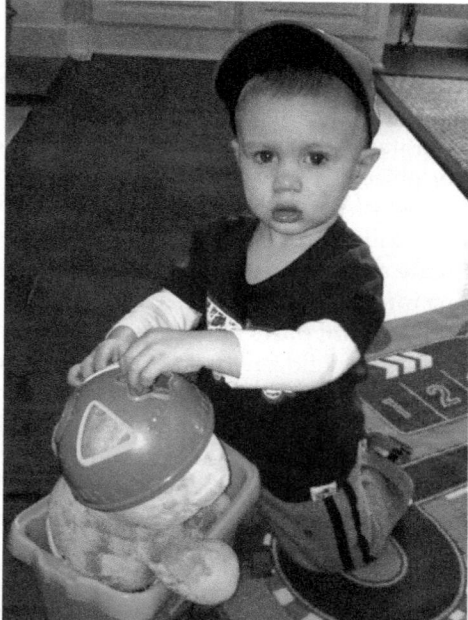

Fig. 24.5 The toddler with proportionate body appearance.

Neuromuscular Development

Many gross motor skills emerge in this period, including walking, climbing stairs (2 years), and hopping (3 years). The toddler develops running, pulling, and holding-on-tight skills, exploring the world in ways previously impossible. This time is also when the toddler begins acquiring fine motor skills, such as beginning to scribble (2 years) and copying a circle (3 years).

Toilet Training. Children do not reach the physiologic or psychological maturity necessary to begin toilet training until 18 to 24 months of age. Children need to reach maturity to have neuromuscular control, the cognitive ability to understand what is expected of them, and the language skills to express their needs. Bowel control is achieved first. Bladder control begins at the same time but takes longer to achieve. Nighttime control is usually achieved after daytime control is established. Advise parents and caregivers to expect setbacks and accidents, particularly during times of stress or illness. Deemphasize accidents; never make the child feel inadequate. Praise success and ignore accidents. If praise is given for toileting successes and accidents are cleaned up without negativism, the toddler gains a sense of self-control, inner goodness, and pride. However, if the toddler is punished and made to feel foolish, a sense of shame develops. If the toddler is kept in diapers and given no opportunities to control the urges, a sense of doubt is fostered. Feelings of shame and doubt are not healthy personality attributes.

Psychosocial Development

The toddler is an uninhibited, energetic little person who always seeks attention, approval, and achievement of personal goals. Sometimes the toddler is cuddly and loving; at other times, the toddler may bite, hit, or pinch. The toddler only slowly realizes that everything desired is not attainable and that some behaviors annoy others. The toddler tries to be independent yet becomes easily frightened and runs to the caregiver for protection, security, reassurance, and approval.

Erikson sees the toddler as struggling with autonomy (self-control) in opposition to shame and doubt. With newfound skills of independence, walking, talking, self-feeding, and beginning toilet training, the toddler is struggling to be independent. Characteristic of this search for autonomy is the toddler's use of the word "no," which gives a sense of control. The toddler possesses endless energy yet often falls asleep almost while still in motion. As toddlers struggle for independence, they frequently display possessiveness and a desire to have things go their way. Ritualistic behavior and repetitive rituals are self-consoling behaviors at this stage. Toddlers enjoy the same story, the same routine, and the same foods at each meal. Rituals decrease their anxiety by helping them know what to expect. When health care providers follow a hospitalized child's usual rituals, the toddler feels safer and more secure in the strange environment.

Temper tantrums are common and are the result of frustration. A combination of wanting things "my way," the inability to communicate feelings, and the lack of impulse control are perhaps behind outbursts

---

Box 24.9	**Basic Principles of Discipline**

- *Consistency:* Apply rules uniformly.
- *Follow-through:* Say and do what you mean.
- *Positive modeling:* Practice role model–approved behavior.
- *Promptness:* Administer any punishment in a nonhostile manner immediately after incident occurs.
- *Trust:* Express trust in the child.
- *Prevention:* Remove temptation.
- *Reinforcement:* Offer positive reinforcement for acceptable behavior.

---

of temper. This type of negativism is best ignored unless the child or others are in danger of harm.

Toddlers need many experiences of being able to choose among alternatives (to play inside or outside, to wear green pants or red pants). However, advise caregivers to make use of questions and offer alternatives for children only in situations in which either choice is acceptable. When a particular behavior is necessary (such as going to bed, holding hands to cross a street, letting go of another child's hair), it is better not to offer a choice. Erikson stressed that young children do not have the wisdom to know what behaviors are acceptable or unacceptable, healthy or unhealthy.

Discipline is a necessary means of teaching limit setting and impulse control. Basic principles of discipline are listed in Box 24.9. Toddlers seek attention, approval, and love as they struggle for independence.

Cognitive and Intellectual Development

The period from 12 to 24 months of age completes the last phase of sensorimotor development, in which the toddler's knowledge of the world comes about primarily through sensory impressions and motor activities. The period of early childhood is the **preoperational thought stage.** (When the child focuses on the use of language as a tool to meet needs, the child has the emerging ability to think.) The child uses trial and error to discover new traits and characteristics. According to Piaget, this stage extends from 2 to 7 years of age.

Toddlers are constantly absorbing new ideas, widening their cognitive world, and expanding memory. Activities can be connected to past events or memories. The toddler's concept of time is limited to the present, and the child's thinking is egocentric at this stage; toddlers are often demanding, wanting things to go their way.

Communication and Language

The cognitive and language development of toddlers makes it possible for them to express their wishes. Commonly used words at this age are "no" and "me." Toddlers use these words in an attempt to exert their will and to take on new challenges.

During the toddler period, the child identifies objects by use. At 2½ years of age, the toddler's vocabulary consists of about 450 words and two-word sentences that include a noun and verb (e.g., "Me run.").

By 3½ years of age, the child is able to answer questions and use brief sentences, and even recite television commercials. The 3-year-old's vocabulary is approximately 900 words. Regular reading to children by parents and caregivers can increase the size of the children's vocabularies greatly. This activity also promotes bonding.

Health Promotion

Nutrition. Good nutrition requires that the toddler's daily diet consist of one serving from the meat group, two or more servings of vegetables, and at least two servings of fruit, cereal, or breads. The US Department of Agriculture's guidelines (www.choosemyplate.gov) should be followed. The toddler needs two cups of food from the dairy group per day. Too few solid foods can lead to iron deficiency; many times, this is the result of consuming too much milk (more than 24 oz/day), which causes the toddler's stomach to feel full and result in a decreased appetite. Most children are more likely to eat foods with which they are familiar; therefore gradual introduction of new foods is advisable. Bite-sized pieces, finger foods, and smaller portions are generally more acceptable. Foods with a high risk for choking, such as hot dogs, grapes, carrots, and small candies, should not be given to toddlers. In the past experts suggested avoiding the early introduction of foods known to be common allergens, such as eggs, wheat, nuts, and cow's milk. Newer research is indicating that early introduction, around six months of age, actually helps prevent allergies to these foods from developing (AAP, n.d.a). There is ongoing research regarding food allergens and when to introduce these foods to children, so parents should always be referred to their pediatrician or health care provider to determine what is best for their child. Idiosyncratic eating patterns are common at this stage. Toddlers can be picky eaters and are often too busy playing to stop and eat. Parents should be encouraged to provide frequent, smaller, and nutritious meals throughout the day. Toddlers need less food per unit of body weight than they did during infancy. A general guideline for serving size is 1 tablespoon of each solid food for each year of age. Parents must be informed that during illness, brief periods of anorexia are usually not serious. Examples of nutritious finger foods that are safe and easy to eat on the run include ripe fruits such as bananas, pears, melons, and avocados; cooked vegetables including squash and sweet potatoes; shredded cheese is another good option.

Sleep, Play Activity, And Safety. Toddlers expend a high level of energy in daily growth, play, and exploration. Adequate rest and sleep are essential for maintaining optimal wellness. The toddler needs 12 hours of sleep each night plus a daytime nap. Suggestions helpful in promoting healthy sleeping patterns include limiting stimulation before sleep time, using quiet-time activities before sleep, allowing a favorite bedtime toy, telling a specified number of stories, and establishing and maintaining bedtime rituals. Box 24.10 lists guidelines for bedtime preparation.

Box 24.10	Guidelines for Bedtime Preparation

- Reduce activity level before bedtime.
- Establish a simple ritual (e.g., bathroom, story time, goodnight song).
- Make bedtime a pleasurable experience.
- Familiarize children with a nightly routine.
- Reassure children that they are not alone.
- Use a night-light.
- Expect disruptions or setbacks during and after illness and stress or after stimulating activities.

Fig. 24.6 Parallel play.

Play improves muscle coordination, balance, and muscle strength. The toddler's play style, described as parallel play (Fig. 24.6), refers to the need that toddlers have to play along with, but not directly with, their peers. Unable to share and interact with their peers at this stage, they play side by side with similar toys in similar ways, but without interacting. Toddlers thrive on activities that allow them to move. Running, jumping, and climbing activities help toddlers to develop bones and muscles. This age group's natural curiosity about how things work encourages them to explore. Play groups help encourage the shy or reluctant child to participate and try new activities. The developmental tasks of toddlers are summarized in Box 24.11.

More than half of all childhood deaths are caused by accidents, many of which are motor vehicle accidents. About 90% of the accidents that occur in the home are believed to be preventable. Prevention methods must include supervision and education.

PRESCHOOL: 3 TO 5 YEARS

Physical Characteristics

Physical development during early childhood occurs on many fronts. The most obvious are the striking

Box 24.11   Developmental Tasks of the Toddler

- Recognizes self as a separate person; tolerates separation from primary caregiver, expresses own ideas and needs
- Develops increased attention span
- Begins to develop communication skills
- Begins to develop self-control skills
- Masters toilet-training basics
- Achieves independent mobility
- Develops independent skills of daily living: feeding, dressing, toileting, and managing simple tasks

changes in size and shape, while the most important—maturation of the nervous system and mastery of motor skills—are the least obvious.

Growth during the preschool period tends to be slow and steady. The preschooler looks taller and thinner than at earlier stages, as the toddler's lordosis and protuberant abdomen are left behind (the abdominal muscles strengthen, and the child loses the potbelly appearance). Average weight gain is less than 5 pounds (11 kg) per year. Linear growth is about 2 to 2½ inches (5.08 to 6.35 cm) per year. Height of the 4-year-old is usually double the birth length. The gait of the preschooler becomes steadier. The preschooler is more capable of focusing and refining activities, and the body grows slimmer, stronger, and less top heavy. Because of these developments, gross motor skills (large body movements such as running, climbing, jumping, and throwing) improve dramatically. Tasks such as tying shoelaces, cutting food with a knife and fork, and putting together a puzzle prove more difficult because of the preschooler's undeveloped fine motor skills (skills that involve small body movements); these are much harder for them to master than gross motor skills. Development of fine motor skills is important to encourage. The scribbling of the young child is comparable with the babbling of the infant. Both are ways to obtain practice with the means to later mastery of essential communication skills. Providing pencils, crayons, markers, and paper is as important as providing things to climb, objects to throw, and places to run.

Vision in the younger preschooler is described as farsighted. Vision improves during this period, and most children achieve 20/30 visual accuracy by age 4 years. A yearly check of preschool children's vision is recommended. Sometimes amblyopia, a condition commonly known as lazy eye, is detected during a simple eye examination. Corrective measures, such as patching the good eye, usually strengthen the lazy eye and are necessary to prevent blindness.

Vital Signs. Heart rate for the preschooler ranges between 70 and 110 beats/min. Respiratory rate slows to about 23 breaths/min at rest. Blood pressure averages 110/60 mm Hg. Temperature ranges from 97°F to 99°F (36.1°C to 37.2°C), depending on the method used for measurement.

Fig. 24.7 Trying out new roles.

Fig. 24.8 Young children enjoy dressing up.

Psychosocial Development

First, children learn to function independently; they subsequently use imagination to explore new experiences creatively. Erikson describes the task of the preschooler in terms of initiative versus guilt. Preschoolers search for and create fantasies about the different kinds of people they would like to become. They pretend to be grown up and try out a variety of roles (Figs. 24.7 and 24.8). During the preschool period, the child's superego (conscience) functions as a censor of behavior. The dilemma of the preschooler, according to Erikson, is to test initiative without creating an overwhelming

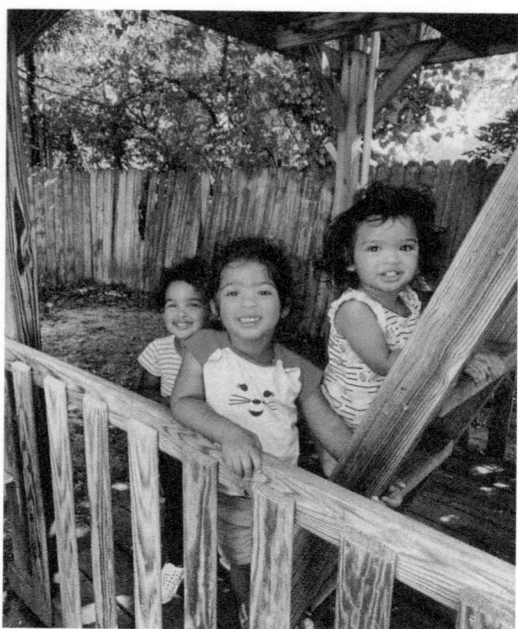

Fig. 24.9 Siblings establishing a bond.

sense of guilt. Typical development of the preschooler includes gender identification. At this time, the child commonly stereotypes roles and shows marked interest in sexual differences. Strong sibling bonding is established (Fig. 24.9).

Cognitive and Intellectual Development

According to Piaget, the preschool child is at the preoperational stage of cognitive development. Preschoolers use symbols to represent objects. They use trial and error to discover and adopt new traits and characteristics. Between ages 4 and 7 years, intuitive thinking develops, and the child begins to think logically. Children in the preoperational stage see the world from their own viewpoint; they see things as absolutes, in terms of black and white and either good or bad.

During the preschool stage, time is associated with weekly and seasonal events. Magical thoughts are typical of the child of this age, who believes that wishes have the power to make things happen. As a result, the preschool child sometimes feels powerful—and responsible—for events that occur. Because of the belief that a wish has caused serious harm or even death to a loved one, the preschooler at times feels guilty. The occasional "white lies" or untruths of this period usually reflect some of the child's fantasies. During this stage of development, the child needs trustworthy guidance to distinguish truth from fantasy. At this stage, the child is more vulnerable to certain fears, often a fallout from the typically vivid imagination. Excessive exposure to inappropriate television content and other media has the potential to further distort reality testing. Common fears that manifest at this stage include fear of thunder, lightning, the dark, pain, abandonment, and monsters.

Communication and Language

By age 3 years, children are able to carry on a conversation, but pronunciation problems continue into the school years. Language becomes more adult-like. If the child is not talking by age 3 years, evaluation by a physician for possible hearing loss or other pathologic speech disturbances is necessary. Advise parents to continue to read to their child to help expand language ability and comprehension and to continue to foster positive child-caregiver relationships.

Health Promotion

Nutrition. Because body systems and muscles are still growing steadily, the preschool child continues to need high levels of protein. Dietary calcium and phosphorus are important to toddlers and preschool children because of the increasing mineralization of their teeth and bones. Food habits, likes, dislikes, and appetites vary greatly from child to child. Some physicians recommend supplementary vitamins. Vitamins, like any other medication, are not intended to and do not have the capacity to take the place of good eating habits (see Chapter 19).

A body mass index (BMI) at or above the 85th percentile and lower than the 95th percentile for children of the same gender and age is considered overweight. A BMI at or above the 95% percentile for children of the same gender and age is considered obese (CDC, 2021a). Most cultures hold strong views regarding obesity, which results in emotional consequences for an obese child. Control of weight is an important parental concern, because it helps prevent serious health issues later in life. Overweight infants are more likely to become overweight later in life. Genetic factors may predispose individuals to obesity; additionally, children often adopt the eating habits of parents. Make suggestions to parents of ways to help with their children's weight control: model good eating behaviors, provide healthy food, and encourage physical activity.

Sleep, Play Activity, And Safety. Preschoolers often resist nap periods but still need 11 to 12 hours of sleep at night. Rest periods offered during the day enable children to reenergize and carry out the rest of their daily activities.

Play style for the preschool child becomes cooperative. The child begins to share, take turns, and interact with playmates (Fig. 24.10). Preschoolers enjoy pretending to carry out activities such as cooking, shopping, and driving. Through dramatic play, the child tries on different roles and identifies with adult models. Not only is it fun for two or more children to cooperate in creating their own scenario, but it also helps their social development to try out social roles, express their fears and fantasies, and learn to cooperate. Experiences with imaginary playmates are not uncommon in this age group. Children often feel a sense of control over what happens in their "imaginary world" and slowly learn to deal with reality through practice and experimentation.

Fig. 24.10 Playmates.

Children during the preschool period are becoming more coordinated and want to begin participating in more organized games. By age 4 to 5 years, children learn to ride a bicycle with training wheels. They need guidance because they have difficulty maneuvering the bicycle, and their judgment and awareness of safety issues is limited (see the Safety Alert box for safety and injury prevention tips for preschool children). Swimming, skating, and dancing are activities that children in this age group often begin to learn and enjoy. Activities of this nature should be fun for the child. It is not beneficial or appropriate for children to be pressured to participate in activities that they do not like or enjoy. Also advise parents and caregivers to space activities so that children are not overstressed by having too many lessons, practices, or games.

⚠ Safety Alert

Safety Tips and Injury Prevention for Preschool Children

- Use proper equipment that fits the child.
- Never leave children alone in pools of water. Teach children not to touch or go near pool drains.
- Inspect protective equipment, such as bicycle helmets, for potential hazards.
- Use protective sunscreen.

All the safety precautions described previously apply to the preschool child and the infant and toddler (see the Safety Alert box). Instruct parents and caregivers to teach preschool children their full names, addresses, and telephone numbers. Children need to know how to use the phone in case of an emergency.

Box 24.12   Steps for Discipline and Limit Setting

- Define acceptable as opposed to unacceptable behaviors.
- Set limits: "I will not let you hurt anyone."
- Be consistent: keep the same rules and enforce them reliably.
- Recognize escalating emotions and intervene: "I can see you are upset; let's go over there and sit down."
- Suggest "time out."
- Choose punishment that "fits" wrongdoing and enact it in a timely way (and in a nonhostile manner).
- Praise and reinforce positive behavior: "I like the way you…"
- Always start over with a clean slate.
- Stay calm; avoid arguing.
- Avoid putdowns: "You are acting like a bad boy."
- Remember to listen to the child.

Box 24.13   Developmental Tasks of Preschoolers

- Develops stronger sense of self; is able to express own needs, ideas, and feelings; has capacity to postpone immediate gratification
- Attains greater attention span; listens more attentively
- Develops and refines gross motor skills and fine motor skills
- Recognizes gender identification
- Begins to work and play more cooperatively with others
- Improves communication skills
- Develops self-control skills; learns socially acceptable ways of expressing anger, frustration, and disappointment; obeys simple rules; develops self-awareness and sense of self-protection
- Seeks information, asks questions, learns values and beliefs of the family

Discipline and limit setting are needed and are as important to the child as are love and security. Necessary guidance includes offering alternative ways of expressing feelings and meeting needs (Box 24.12).

The preschool period is a time of learning to function independently and exploring the imagination. Box 24.13 shows the developmental tasks of preschoolers.

SCHOOL AGE: 6 TO 12 YEARS

Physical Characteristics

During the school-age period, the growth pattern is usually gradual and subtle. The most obvious growth is in the long bones of the extremities and in the development of the facial bones. As a result of this bone growth, some children report "growing pains," particularly at night. Persistent pains call for evaluation by a physician to rule out any underlying pathologic condition. From ages 6 to 12 years, height and weight increase by about 2 inches and 4½ to 6½ pounds per year for boys and girls.

Motor skills in boys and girls develop with some differences; boys often become stronger, and girls more graceful and accurate.

The child's posture becomes straighter. The causes of poor posture range from fatigue to emotional states or even minor skeletal defects. Ensure that school-age children are screened routinely for scoliosis (abnormal lateral curvature of the spine). Muscle mass and strength gradually increase, and the body loses the "baby fat" appearance of earlier childhood. Gross motor and fine motor development continue to be refined during the school-age years.

Vision improves, and most children have 20/20 vision at this stage. Regular vision testing is advisable throughout the school years.

Vital Signs. Heart and respiratory rate steadily decrease, whereas blood pressure increases. Normal pulse rate is between 55 and 90 per minute, respiratory rate is 22 to 24 per minute, and blood pressure is 110/65 mm Hg.

Dentition. By age 6 years, the child begins to lose the deciduous teeth. Permanent teeth develop rapidly. Dental checkups should continue every 6 months throughout childhood.

Psychosocial Development

Entrance into school challenges the child and creates demands for new social and cognitive skills. The child becomes more independent and participates in a broader world of peers and new experiences. School-age children become increasingly aware of rules and socialization skills, and expectations. The beginning abilities to compromise and compete are challenges faced in this age group.

Erikson identified the task of the school-age years as industry versus inferiority. After the child realizes that "there is no workable future within the womb of his family," says Erikson, the school-age child "becomes ready to apply himself to given skills and tasks." Children develop their own goals and direct their efforts toward mastery of these goals. As children discover their talents and accomplishments, they gain self-confidence and a sense of purpose. During these years, the child learns to work and masters skills that produce satisfaction as the result of that work. Successful mastery of learning in school leads to strengthening and stabilizing the child's sense of self. According to Erikson, as children busily try to master the skills valued in their culture, they develop views of themselves as either competent or incompetent—as either industrious and productive or inferior and inadequate.

Input from the outside is a key influence on which direction the child's self-concept will take. If the environment inadequately supports a child's pursuits, the stage perhaps is set for the development of feelings of inferiority and the lack of self-confidence. A good school setting is a pleasant, comfortable environment.

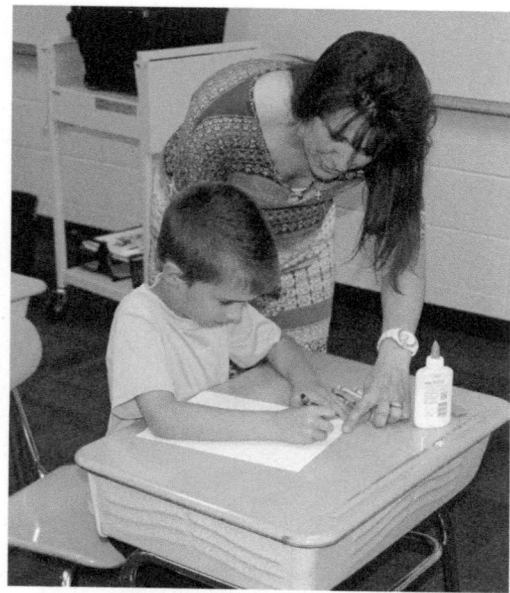

Fig. 24.11 School represents an important change in a child's life, and teachers exert a significant influence on the child.

Teachers and caregivers need to use praise, encouragement, and rewards to reinforce the school-age child's efforts positively. Teachers also must be positive role models. School helps the child learn new routines and establish important social relationships (Fig. 24.11). However, the school climate can be affected negatively by bullying. Bullying can take on many forms, including physical (hitting, tripping), verbal (name calling, teasing), relational (spreading rumors, excluding), and cyber (e-mail, text messaging). CDC defines bullying as "any unwanted aggressive behavior(s) by another youth or group of youths who are not siblings or current dating partners that involves an observed or perceived power imbalance and is repeated multiple times or is highly likely to be repeated" (CDC, 2020). In 2015, 20% of high school students reported they had been bullied on school property. Bullying can lead to physical injury as well as depression, anxiety, sleep difficulties, and even death. One way to prevent bullying is for schools to have a consistently enforced antibullying policy (CDC, 2020).

Cognitive and Intellectual Development

According to Piaget, children in the school years move into the concrete operational phase. During this phase, thoughts become increasingly logical and coherent so that the child is able to classify, sort, and organize facts while still being incapable of generalizing or dealing with abstractions. Children have the capacity to think rationally about almost any specific and concrete perception. Between ages 7 and 11 years, children usually come to understand logical principles—again, as long as the principles can be applied to concrete, specific cases. They distinguish purpose from behavior and outcome and are able to focus on more than one aspect of a task. Children in this age group have begun

| Box **24.14** | Developmental Tasks of the School-Age Child |

- Develops a sense of belonging with family and peers
- Develops work habits and learns to organize, set, and reach goals; evaluate work; and accept criticism
- Learns competence in reading, writing, calculation, grammar, and communication
- Refines fine-motor and gross-motor coordination

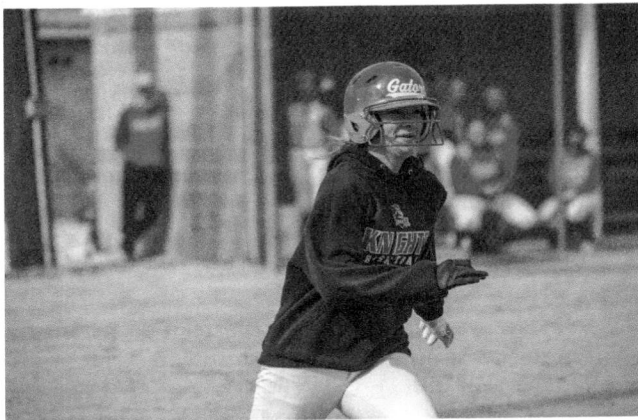

Fig. 24.12 Activities engaged in by school-age children, such as softball and football, vary according to the child's interest and opportunity.

to develop logical socialized thought. They view the world more realistically than they did at younger ages, and they are capable of understanding the views of others. Movement is away from fantasy as the child realizes that a physical cause is behind an event. The child's developing cognitive skills serve as a motivator for learning how to work. A supportive learning environment often enhances the child's approach to problem solving and helps lead to success.

The school-age child experiences gradual and subtle growth changes while learning new social and cognitive skills. Box 24.14 contains a list of the developmental tasks of the school-age child.

Communication and Language
Most 6-year-olds have a good command of sentence structure. The child's vocabulary has become more extensive and includes slang and swear words, which many children enjoy using for the effect they create. Fine motor development continues and, combined with growth in cognitive and communication skills, produces refinements in written language and musical abilities. By age 7 years, the hands of the child have become steadier. Printing becomes clearer and smaller. Between ages 8 and 10 years, the hand becomes more efficient, which enables the child to write rather than print. The 10- to 12-year-old child has the capacity to accomplish complex, intricate, fine-quality handcrafts, and sometimes begins piano, violin, or guitar lessons.

Health Promotion
Nutrition. Total metabolic needs are determined by the energy expenditure of each individual child. The sedentary, quiet child who prefers fine motor activities needs fewer calories than the child who is more oriented to athletics or is more physically active. The recommended daily intake of food is listed at the ChooseMyPlate website (www.choosemyplate.gov).

Building on toddler-age and preschool-age foundations, strong dietary habits and food preferences are established during the school-age period. Cultural influences, family habits, and peer pressure are critical factors in how a child's food habits develop. Obesity during this period is correlated closely with obesity in adult years; therefore the child's weight must be maintained within normal limits. In middle childhood, obese children are teased, picked on, and rejected. They know they are overweight, and they often hate

themselves for it. Obese children usually have fewer friends than other children. The best way to get children to lose weight is to increase their physical activity. Indeed, inactivity is possibly as responsible for childhood obesity as overeating. Diets high in saturated fat increase a child's risk for high blood cholesterol and earlier occurrence of heart disease unless steps are taken to lower these levels.

Sleep, Play Activity, and Safety. Fatigue, irritability, inattention, and poor learning are signs of inadequate sleep. The 6-year-old needs about 12 hours of sleep at night. By 12 years of age, the child usually needs about 10 hours of sleep. Some children have frequent nightmares that disrupt their sleep. Stress, violence on television, and overtiredness may contribute to a child's nightmares. Relaxation techniques such as quiet music, story time, and bathing often help the child relax before sleep.

School-age children need adequate exercise to enhance muscle development, coordination, balance, and strength. In addition, music, craft projects, board games, appropriate television, and video games are all enjoyed by the school-age child. Privacy and a place for their belongings are important at this age. The school-age child is often a willing worker and enjoys being paid for small jobs. Collection and hoarding of "treasures" among their belongings are a part of this stage of development.

Many children during the school years become involved with competitive or team sports (Fig. 24.12). Children of this age show interest and loyalty to peers of the same gender. They learn to follow the rules of games. Some may benefit from team competitiveness and use it to motivate themselves to excel. Others shy away from competition and become disinterested or develop feelings of inadequacy and disappointment.

Accidents are still the leading cause of death in this age group. Impulsiveness, poor judgment, curiosity, and incomplete control over motor coordination are some of the factors that increase the school-age child's risk of accidents.

Television often exerts a powerful influence on a child's development, and children are watching an average of 4 to 6 hours of television daily (AACAP, 2020). One concern about television today is the increased amount of violence it portrays. A common thought is that a good deal of available television content offers the child a potent model for aggressive behavior and is a significant factor in the development of aggressive behavior. Suggest ways for parents to help reduce the negative influence of television: (1) limit the amount of time children watch television; (2) screen programs for content and age appropriateness; and (3) watch programs with children and discuss the content.

Preventing school violence is another critical issue these days. **School violence** is defined as anything that physically or psychologically injures schoolchildren or damages school property. Today, school violence seems to have increased in many locations. Two factors that are possibly contributing to this increase are an increased availability of weapons and a breakdown of communication. Experts agree that children need resources to help them deal with the daily stressors that they face. Many children today spend less time with parents and more time in front of a television and on the Internet watching or playing violent shows and games (AACAP, 2014). Parents must be aware of the effects of television violence on children. Children who view violent acts are more likely to show aggression but are also fearful that something bad will happen to them. Children need to feel comfortable discussing their feelings and concerns with parents and teachers and must be able to use these discussions to learn how to recognize whether they are in danger and whether others are exhibiting signs of troubled behavior. Encourage parents to ask questions about their child's feelings and their school activities daily. If children have difficulty talking to parents or answering their questions, advise parents to seek professional help. A key responsibility of parents is to stay involved and be active participants in their child's daily affairs.

Children need to be taught constructive ways to handle their impulses; otherwise they are more likely to resort to unacceptable ways of channeling their feelings. One possibility is that they will look for revenge, which perhaps makes them feel in control and powerful. Although many children have access to weapons, most of them do not engage in violent behavior. However, we need to work to inhibit violent tendencies and to look for ways to prevent the few who do act out their feelings in violent ways from causing harm to others (see school safety tips in the Safety Alert box). The first step in preventing a tragedy is recognizing the behavioral tendencies that have the potential to lead to violence or other problem behavior. Give children the guidance and encouragement they need to recognize and report the signs of troubled behavior if they notice them in a friend or classmate without feeling that they have deceived the other person or let the other person down (Box 24.15).

Box 24.15	Common Signs of Troubled Childhood Behavior

- Problems getting along with peers
- Difficulty accepting authority and resistance to direction
- Outbursts of uncontrolled behavior
- Bullying tendencies
- Frequent victimizing or teasing
- Social isolation
- Poor school performance
- Violence to pets or other living creatures
- Preoccupation with weapons
- Verbal expression of threatening behavior or revenge

 Safety Alert

Safety in Schools

- Secure weapons in homes.
- Develop a zero-tolerance program with school officials.
- Work with a parent-teacher association (PTA) to make schools safe.
- Determine with school officials an emergency and security plan.
- Maintain open lines of communication between child, parent, and school officials.

Gun safety is necessary regardless of opinions about gun ownership. Gun enthusiasts, collectors, and law enforcement agents are obliged to ensure the safety of others. Most children and many adults have a fascination with guns. Even when children and adults are taught gun safety, some exhibit unsafe behavior when the opportunity arises. Even toy guns create the potential for dangerous situations. Parents and individuals with weapons in the home must take adequate steps to prevent accidents and injury from their weapons. Knowledge of how to handle a gun is not sufficient to protect the owner's family and others from injury. Ammunition must be removed from firearms, and guns must be locked away securely and apart from ammunition, which is kept secured in another, separate locked area. In addition, and most important, children of all ages must be taught what to do if they find a gun (see gun safety rules in the Safety Alert box).

 Safety Alert

Gun Safety Rules

FOR CHILDREN

- Stop and **DO NOT TOUCH** any gun, real or toy.
- Leave the area if a gun is found.
- Report any gun to an adult.

FOR ADULTS

- Never store ammunition with the gun.
- Keep the gun in a locked location out of reach of children.
- Lock the ammunition in a separate location from the gun.
- Lock gun-cleaning supplies, which are often poisonous.

ADOLESCENCE: 12 TO 19 YEARS

Physical Characteristics

The term *adolescence* covers the transition period from childhood to adulthood. Adolescence begins at puberty; accompanying the pubertal changes are corresponding changes in the personality. *Puberty,* the period of life at which the ability to reproduce begins, entails the maturation of the reproductive system, including all the primary and secondary sexual developmental changes. Primary changes occur in the organs related to reproduction (ovaries, breasts, uterus, testes, and penis). Secondary sexual changes occur in other parts of the body (development of pubic and facial hair, voice changes, and fat deposits). Adolescence literally means "to grow into maturity" and is generally regarded as the psychological, social, and maturational process initiated by pubertal changes.

Adolescence is characterized as the second major period of rapid growth. Females grow 2 to 8 inches (5 to 20 cm), whereas males grow 4 to 12 inches (10 to 30 cm). During this adolescent period, females gain 15 to 55 pounds (7 to 25 kg), and males gain 15 to 65 pounds (7 to 30 kg). Females develop more body fat, and males develop more muscle tissue. After puberty, men average 50% muscle and 16% fat, whereas women average 40% muscle and 27% fat. Muscle strength and muscle mass increase in the male, which causes the average male to have more muscle strength. Exercise facilitates the size, strength, and endurance of each adolescent.

In the female, menarche (the first menstrual period) signals the beginning of adolescence, while sperm production signals the beginning of adolescence in the male. Girls develop larger breasts, a narrower waist, wider hips, and a lower center of gravity. Boys develop broader shoulders, narrower hips, and larger limbs. Boys and girls experience voice changes; girls' voices become fuller and richer because of the lengthening of their vocal cords, while boys' voices become lower and louder. The deeper male voice results from enlargement of the larynx (the Adam's apple) and lengthening of the vocal cords.

Sexual interests increase markedly in vigor and intensity and usually focuses on members of the opposite sex. New problems arise as adolescents find social disapproval and prohibitions arising in their own conscience that conflict with intense sexual drives.

Vital Signs. Average pulse rate is 70 beats/min, respiratory rate averages 20 breaths/min, and blood pressure increases to 120/70 mm Hg.

Psychosocial Development

Exactly when adolescence begins is different in each person. Some enter adolescence at an early age while others develop later. Regardless of the exact age of onset, the nearing of this stage is evident by recognizing the onset of distinct behavioral changes. A mother may notice that her 11-year-old daughter has become tight-lipped about school and activities, no longer wanting her mother's opinion or listening ear. Her daughter is now spending most of her time at home in her room with the door closed. A father may delight in his son's musical talents and his band's energy and success, although the two may argue over the taste of their lyrics and the decibel level.

The period of adolescence is frequently described as difficult and involving a stormy search for oneself. Confronting every adolescent is a changing body, sexual demands, responsibilities, expectations, and questions about values and beliefs. The search for identity amid a world of social pressures creates a painful struggle.

Erikson described the developmental task of adolescence as establishing a sense of identity, and proposed the conflict of identity versus role confusion as characteristic of adolescence. The search for a sense of identity, he believed, reaches crisis proportions at this time. Not only does the adolescent need to adjust to a sexually mature body but also all previous conflicts (trust versus mistrust, autonomy versus doubt, initiative versus guilt, and industry versus inferiority) must be resolved yet again in light of the newly sensuous self. The period of adolescence requires major reorganization of the personality, resolution of childhood insecurities, and acceptance of adult responsibilities. The value of peers is usually significant to the adolescent (Fig. 24.13). Peers influence preferences of dress, speech, and leisure activities. The peer group is often the milieu to learn and test developing interpersonal skills. Many adolescents use conforming behavior to win praise and acceptance by peers. If handled properly, adolescence is often a great period of accomplishment and creativity (Box 24.16).

Cognitive Development

According to Piaget, an individual's cognitive function reaches maturity during adolescence. Piaget describes this stage as the formal operational thought stage. This is a higher process that permits abstract reasoning and systematic, scientific problem solving. Adolescents become capable of reasoning and formal logic. At this time, thoughts may be influenced more by logical principles than by personal perceptions and experiences. The adolescent thinks beyond the present. Without having to focus exclusively on the immediate situation, the adolescent can imagine the possible: a sequence of events that may occur, such as college and occupational possibilities, how things may change in the future, such as relationships with parents, and the possible consequences of actions he or she is considering, such as dropping out of school.

Moral Development

As children move through the stages of cognition and logical thinking, they also progress through stages of moral development. As with other developmental

Fig. 24.13 The peer group provides the adolescent with a sense of belonging.

Box 24.16   Parenting Tips During Adolescence

- Educate yourself and your adolescent.
- Maintain open communication.
- Choose your battles.
- Set realistic expectations.
- Set good examples for behavior.
- Honor individuality.
- Respect privacy.
- Try to remember your own experiences during this stage.
- Set appropriate rules and regulations.
- Be consistent.
- Stay involved; meet your child's friends and acquaintances.
- Be active in school and after-school activities.

processes, moral development approaches or achieves adult levels during adolescence.

In some ways, adolescence is an uncomfortable in-between phase. Old principles are challenged, but new and independent values do not emerge immediately. As a consequence, young people search for a moral code that preserves their personal integrity and guides their behavior, especially in the face of strong pressure to violate the old values. They face many decisions involving moral dilemmas; they need to gradually internalize a set of principles that provides them with the resources to evaluate the demands of a situation and to plan a course of action consistent with their ideals.

Health Promotion

Nutrition. The rate of body growth and the adolescent's increased basal metabolic rate require an increase in the individual's caloric needs. At peak growth, females may need as much as 2600 calories/day and males as much as 3600 calories/day. Many factors affect the individual's dietary habits, including cultural background, family habits, work schedules, school, concern about weight gain, peer influence, and lack of knowledge concerning correct food choices. Of particular concern are eating disorders. Anorexia nervosa and bulimia are on the rise in young women. Parents should be educated about the warning signs, because these disorders can be fatal. Protein needs are increased as a consequence of the rapid growth of this period. Advise adolescents to obtain 12% to 16% of their total daily food intake from protein.

The adolescent diet is most likely to be deficient in calcium, iron, and zinc. The need for these minerals during the period of rapid growth is increased substantially—calcium for skeletal growth; iron for expansion of muscle mass and blood volume, soft tissue growth, and the rapid growth demands of the expanding red blood cell mass; and zinc for the generation of skeletal and muscle tissue. Adolescent boys have greater muscle mass, but adolescent girls have an additional iron loss from menstruation. Consequently, the need for iron is equivalent in both sexes.

Increased amounts of milk usually are required to supplement the average diet to ensure an adequate calcium intake during this time.

The adolescent is advised to follow the guidelines at the ChooseMyPlate website (see Chapter 19).

Sleep, Play Activity, and Safety. The adolescent needs to pace activities to allow for adequate rest. The adolescent often requires increased hours of sleep to restore energy levels. During puberty and adolescence, caution must be taken to prevent injuries related to exercise and sports. Injuries sometimes occur in connection with the adolescent's growth spurt. Growth spurts cause the bones to grow more quickly than the muscles and tendons, which causes the muscles and tendons to become short and tight. Sports-related injuries may result from these factors. Teaching youngsters to perform appropriate warm-up and stretching exercises before starting any strenuous sport can lessen the risk of injury (see sports-related safety tips in the Safety Alert box). Participating in organized sports at this age helps adolescents learn to work with others, meet challenges, and set personal goals. Parents have an opportunity to encourage children to exercise by setting an example and practicing good, healthy behaviors for themselves. Having parents involved on the sidelines supporting their adolescent's efforts potentially enhances self-esteem.

! Safety Alert

Sports-Related Safety Tips

- Use safety helmets.
- Use properly fitting equipment.
- Play on properly maintained surfaces.
- Perform warm-up exercises before sports practice.
- Avoid overuse of muscles.
- Insist on adequate supervision.
- Obtain proper training.
- Treat existing injuries and prevent reinjury.

Accident prevention is vital during this stage of development. The greatest number of deaths in this age group is due to accidents. Adolescents are known to participate in more risk-taking behaviors; therefore driver's education, water safety training, education about safe sex practices, and drug education are necessary to inform adolescents of the risks and dangers inherent in these activities. The Safety Alert box lists safe sex practices that are crucial to emphasize early in adolescence, with special emphasis on abstinence.

⚠ Safety Alert

Guidelines for Practice of Safe Sex

- The safest sexual practice is abstinence.
- Be familiar with your sexual partners. Ask about their sexual lifestyle before you engage in sexual relations.
- Avoid engaging in sexual relations with intravenous drug users or with individuals who have had multiple sex partners.
- Use a latex condom as the best type of protection from infection.
- Condoms should be inspected for tears before use. Avoid lengthy storage and exposure to excessive heat.
- Fit the condom over the erect penis, leaving a small space at the end for the collection of semen.
- Hold the upper end of the condom when withdrawing from the vagina to prevent slippage.
- Avoid sexual relations with individuals who have genital lesions or unusual drainage.
- Be aware that the risk of human immunodeficiency virus (HIV) infection is increased with oral sexual practices. Anal intercourse requires additional education for safe practice.

Emotional Health. Adolescence is, as described previously, a period of maturation that covers the transition from childhood to adulthood (Box 24.17). In part as a result of the complexity of the tasks that face them, adolescents experience different moods. At times they are outgoing and gregarious and active participants in family matters. They offer their opinions and seem to ignore others. There are also times when they are moody and loners who seem not to want any part of family activities. Such mood swings generally occur at this stage. Families should recognize and distinguish normal moodiness from signs of depression. Depression is defined as a mood disturbance characterized by feelings of sadness, despair, and hopelessness. People who are depressed are often unable to improve their condition without the help of professional therapy. Teach parents, teachers, and health care workers to recognize the common signs of depression. Early detection and intervention are crucial when dealing with depression because this leads to higher success rates. Untreated depression can lead to suicide (Box 24.18). Advise parents to seek professional help if their child expresses feelings of marked depression. All threats must be taken seriously,

Box 24.17 Developmental Tasks of the Adolescent

- Recognizes individuality
- Accepts strengths and weaknesses
- Develops own value system
- Assumes responsibility for own behavior
- Develops philosophy of life
- Adapts to somatic changes (changes that affect the body)
- Acquires skills necessary for adult living
- Refines social skills
- Develops independent living skills

Box 24.18 Signs of Depression and Indicators of Suicide Risk

- Change in appetite
- Change in mood (sadness, hopelessness)
- Inability to concentrate
- Loss of interest in activities
- Change in sleep habits (either always sleeping or unable to sleep)
- Talk of suicide
- Preoccupation with death or dying
- Giving away of possessions

and it is imperative to be alert to sudden changes in behavior, such as a change from extreme sadness to manic behavior. This mood swing potentially signals a decision to carry out the person's suicide plan.

EARLY ADULTHOOD: 20 TO 40 YEARS

The transition to adulthood in the United States is marked by events such as taking on financial responsibilities, making career choices, beginning social relationships, entering marriage, and becoming a parent. All the challenges and accomplishments of the earlier developmental stages have helped prepare the individual for the responsibilities of adult maturity. Fantasies of what adulthood entails usually give way to more realistic expectations and hopes.

Early adulthood, the period of optimal physical condition, is marked by momentous changes in lifestyle. Box 24.19 contains a list of the developmental tasks of early adulthood.

Physical Characteristics

The body during early adult years is at its optimal level of functioning. The typical young adult is a fine physical specimen. During the middle 20s, most body functions are fully developed, and muscular strength, energy, and endurance are now at their peak.

Physical appearance is influenced by heredity, environment, and general state of wellness. Females usually reach their maximal height at about 16 to 17 years of age, while males continue to grow until 18 to 20 years of age. Between ages 30 and 45 years, height

Box 24.19   Developmental Tasks of Early Adulthood

- Achieves financial and social independence
- Maximizes personal worth and identity
- Develops meaningful and satisfying social relationships
- Assumes responsibilities and independent decision making
- Learns to balance personal needs and societal expectations
- Accepts self and others
- Distinguishes physical attraction from love and permanent commitment
- Decides on a marriage, career, and children

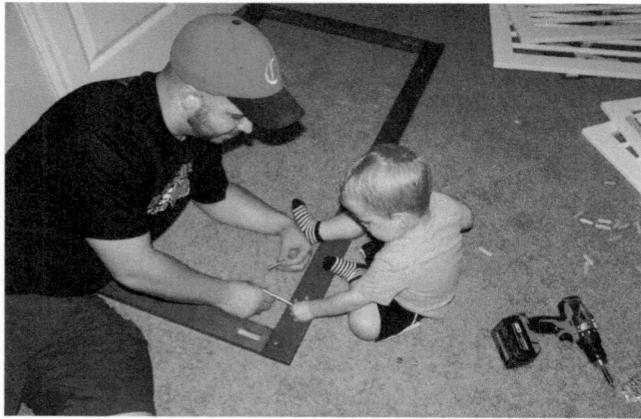

Fig. 24.14 Father and child bonding.

is stable, and then it begins to decline due to the settling of spinal disks. Often an increase in fatty tissue causes weight gain, a decrease in muscle strength, and a stabilization of reaction time. The senses are also at their sharpest during young adulthood. Visual acuity is keenest at about age 20 years and does not begin to decline until about age 40 years.

Psychosocial Development

Dual-career families have emerged based on current economic realities and women's interest in pursuing careers. The feminist movement has resulted in many positive social changes. The home and the workplace show the effects of these changes and the dual-career lifestyle.

Another important option for this age group is the decision to start a family (Fig. 24.14). If procreation is the choice, a subsequent issue is how many children to have. Further consideration is given to financial means, safety, family support, housing, the relationship to members of the extended family, and the roles and responsibilities of the nuclear family unit. Young adults who establish a family need to have open communication about self-development, which includes issues of dual careers, child-rearing practices, and domestic duties within the home.

Family development and harmony are important goals for many young adults. Although family size and structure have undergone dramatic changes in the past decades, concerns about individual members' health and safety continue to form a primary focus within the family as a unit. Family life is influenced by the characteristics of individual family members. Typically, healthy family adjustment is associated with the age of the individuals, job security, the family's and the individuals' places in the community, and healthy patterns of living (good nutrition, personal cleanliness, physical fitness). Therefore the physical and mental health of one family member affects all family members.

Erikson identified early intimacy versus isolation as the developmental task of adulthood. Intimacy is the ability to develop one's deepest hopes and concerns in connection to another person. One aspect of intimacy

is the capacity to accept the closeness of another person. Intimacy leads to commitment, sharing, and compromise. The "virtue" that develops in young adulthood is the virtue of love, or the mutuality of devotion between partners who have chosen to share their lives. As young adults resolve conflicting demands of intimacy, competitiveness, and distance, they develop an ethical sense, which Erikson considers the mark of the adult. The opposite of intimacy, the distancing of oneself from intimate relationships, is the negative resolution of the task of this life stage and leads to isolation and self-absorption.

Cognitive Development

Piaget saw adulthood as actively developing the formal operational approach to learning and problem solving. He believed that the same cognitive operations apply throughout adulthood to a larger, more expansive list of experiences. Adults tend to think in an integrative way.

Health Promotion

Nutrition. Fewer total numbers of calories are needed compared with the amount needed in adolescence because the adult has completed biophysical growth. Calories are needed to maintain body functioning for cell replacement and repair and for provision of energy. Calorie needs vary based on age, gender, size, physical activity, metabolism, and levels of stress.

Diet plays an important role, as it does throughout the developmental stages. Heart disease and cancer are major concerns in the adult years. Proper diet and exercise often have a decisive impact on the control of heart disease, which is caused by increased cholesterol deposits occluding the walls of blood vessels. Likewise, low-fat, high-fiber, and low-cholesterol diets are recommended as preventive measures against cancers of the breast, the stomach, and the intestine. Other lifestyle habits such as the use of tobacco, drugs, and alcohol affect the adult's health status (see the Health Promotion box).

Health Promotion

Recommendations for a Healthy Lifestyle

- Follow the guidelines at *www.choosemyplate.gov.*
- Drink adequate fluids.
- Avoid smoking and drugs.
- Consume little or no alcohol.
- Maintain optimal weight.
- Participate in a scheduled program of daily exercise.
- Obtain adequate restorative sleep.
- Practice stress reduction.
- Enjoy leisure activities.

Rest and Sleep. Most adults function well with 7 to 9 hours of restorative sleep. Adults commonly do not schedule daytime rest opportunities to prevent fatigue, however, they can increase their productivity by obtaining adequate rest during the day. Adequate rest is essential for the pregnant woman to ensure her health and that of her unborn baby.

Physical Activity

In the past few decades, attention to physical fitness has become more popular, with benefit to general welfare. Regular, paced exercise increases heart and lung capacity, lowers blood pressure, helps control weight, enhances body function, and improves emotional health.

By adulthood, men and women have reached their sexual maturity. Sexual drive continues for men and women throughout adulthood.

Physical and Dental Examinations. Annual physicals are recommended. A routine testicular examination for the male and an annual Papanicolaou (Pap) smear for the female are essential for early detection of cancer. The American Cancer Society recommends that women have the option to begin having mammograms between the age of 40 to 44 years. From the ages of 45 to 54 years, mammograms should be performed yearly. At age 55 and older, the health care provider and patient should determine whether to continue yearly mammograms or switch to every other year (ACS, 2021b). Beginning at age 50, men should discuss prostate cancer screening with their health care provider. Considerations should include their family history and race. African Americans or those with a father or brother who had prostate cancer before age 65 should have this talk with a health care provider starting at age 45. Testing includes a prostate-specific antigen (PSA) blood test with or without a digital rectal examination (DRE). The frequency of retesting depends on the person's PSA level (ACS, 2021a). Routine dental examinations should be scheduled for adults every 6 months. Eye examinations are necessary every 2 years unless otherwise indicated.

Safety. Accidents are the leading cause of disability and death in this age group. Injuries commonly result from work, vehicle, and sports accidents, as well as from violence.

MIDDLE ADULTHOOD: 40 TO 65 YEARS

The middle adulthood period is designated arbitrarily as occurring between 40 and 65 years of age. Most individuals of this age group enjoy a healthy body. Some changes result in a gradual shift of balance away from peak performance. The extent of these changes is related directly to diet, heredity, exercise, rest, mental outlook, stress, and disease.

Physical Characteristics

Bone mass decreases as skeletal growth cells are depleted. This bone loss leads to an increased risk of osteoporosis. Women lose calcium from bone tissue after menopause. Men also lose calcium from bones but at a more gradual rate than women, and their risk of osteoporosis is lower. Slight changes in height continue to occur as a result of the compression of the spinal vertebrae and the hardening of collagen fibers. A decrease in muscle fibers results in a reduction of muscle mass. Heredity, nutrition, and exercise patterns account for much of the individual variation commonly seen. Changes in muscle strength are perhaps related more to level of activity than to age. A redistribution of body weight leads to changes in body shape and contour. A decrease in basal metabolism and less activity often necessitate calorie reductions to prevent weight gain.

Basic neurologic functioning remains at a high level during this age period.

Noticeable changes in vision occur as a result of presbyopia (a defect in vision in advancing age that involves loss of accommodation or the recession of the near point caused by loss of elasticity of the crystalline lens and the ensuing change in close vision).

Other sensory changes may include presbycusis (a normal progressive, age-associated loss of hearing acuity, speech intelligibility, auditory threshold, and pitch). These changes usually begin around age 40 years and occur more commonly in men than in women.

One of the most noticeable changes that occurs during this period is in the appearance of the individual's skin. A decrease in the elastic fibers and a slight loss of subcutaneous tissue give skin a looser, more wrinkled appearance. Hair color often changes with age with the onset of graying. Graying usually begins at the temples. Hair growth and distribution sometimes change during the middle adult years. Scalp hair tends to become thinner.

A higher incidence of periodontal (gum) disease is seen in the middle adult years. Preventive treatment programs that include fluoride usage, regular flossing, and dental cleaning are important.

Hormonal changes include the woman's declining production of estrogen and progesterone. Menopause (female climacteric) is a gradual process that takes about 5 years to complete. A woman's perception of menopause is likely to be affected by her perceptions of her general health. The period of menopausal transition is known as perimenopause. During this process, the functions of the ovaries diminish and eventually cease. Noticeable signs and symptoms of menopause typically include irregular menstrual periods, flow changes, excess fluid retention, breast tenderness, hot flashes (feeling "hot," flushing, and blushing), palpitations, night sweats, and irritability or mood swings. Some women have very few signs or symptoms related to menopause. Some women receive small doses of estrogen aimed at relieving the complications of decreased estrogen levels. Hormone replacement therapy (HRT) is also viewed as a means to reduce osteoporosis and the risk of atherosclerosis and heart disease; however, HRT is also thought to increase the risk of stroke, endometrial cancer, and breast disease, and to raise blood pressure. The risks and the benefits of this treatment must be evaluated on an individual basis. The woman can continue to experience positive, satisfying sexuality and sexual responses throughout her middle adult years. With any fears of pregnancy now out of the picture, many women enjoy a period of enhanced sexuality.

Possible evidence of the male climacteric includes decreased libido (sex drive), loss of body hair, and delayed erection. Men do not lose the ability to reproduce during the middle adult years. Changes in male sexual function are often related more to psychological than physiologic occurrences. A man's actual capacity to function sexually often has more to do with self-perception and mental outlook, and less with the changes he experiences in body appearance, including weight gain, hair loss, and decreased muscle strength. These changes cause some men to go through what is described as a "midlife crisis." During this time, many people may engage in extramarital affairs, often leading to divorce. Many men are unaffected by the physiologic and psychological occurrences of the climacteric.

Psychosocial Development

According to Erikson, the developmental task of middle age is generativity versus stagnation, which means accepting responsibility for and offering guidance to the next generation. Generativity encompasses productivity, continuity, and creativity (Fig. 24.15). If this developmental task is not met, people become stagnant—inactive or lifeless. The middle adult years are a time for vocational, interpersonal, and personal fulfillment. The impulse to foster development of the young is not limited to guiding one's own children and does not cease with their maturation. Many middle-aged adults enjoyably express this desire through activities such as teaching and mentorship, a mutually fulfilling relationship that satisfies a younger protégé's need for guidance along with an older person's need for generativity. Resumption of education, career growth or

Fig. 24.15 According to Erikson, generativity is the developmental task of middle adulthood. Nurturing and guiding the younger generation are tasks people accomplish with their own children or with other children and adolescents in their family and community.

Box 24.20	Developmental Tasks of Middle Adulthood

- Balances goals and realities and redirects energies as necessary
- Extends caring and concern beyond immediate family (to neighborhood, community, society)
- Develops career and job satisfaction
- Adapts to physical changes
- Establishes new roles and relationships with spouse, children, grandchildren, and parents

changes, reentry into the workforce, and involvement with community activities create a multitude of possibilities for personal growth and satisfaction during the middle adult years. Box 24.20 contains a list of the developmental tasks of middle adulthood.

Family roles change during this stage. Children are sometimes present in the home. For most caregivers, a significant change in their lives occurs with the end of daily, active responsibility for children. Relationships between spouses change, and the couple often has to regain familiarity with each other. For many, this offers the opportunity for new or renewed companionship. Survival of the marriage after children leave home possibly depends on the growth, maturity, and commitment of each partner. Most women with an "empty nest" look forward to their emancipation from parenting duties, seeing it as an occasion to develop further their personal and social roles.

The role of grandparenting often begins at this developmental stage. Because it often does not have the constraints and responsibilities of childrearing, grandparenting becomes a rich and rewarding experience for many middle-aged adults. The past few decades have probably been the best time ever to be a grandparent and to experience grandparenting as a joyful experience. Grandparents now have the longest, healthiest lifespans ever recorded, the best social services, and the most independence. Many still hover just above the poverty line, and some are below it, however, many grandparents are prosperous. Many American grandparents are not involved in the upbringing and disciplining of their grandchildren, preferring a "norm of noninterference." Grandparents often refrain from giving their grown children childrearing instruction, even when they do not like something they see going on with their grandchildren. Most contemporary grandparents value their independence; many are unwilling to exchange their hard-won and long-awaited lifestyles for another round of the hard, often frustrating work of raising children.

On the other hand, most adults are not prepared for the increased responsibility of caring for aging parents. Economic stress and emotional pressure are associated with the role reversal sometimes known as "parenting the parent." Studies have indicated that a midlife daughter is most likely to be involved in elder care with her parents and her husband's parents.

Health Promotion

Nutrition. Many adult active lifestyles slow in their middle adult year, and as a result they need fewer calories than they did in their teenage years and 20s. The Centers for Disease Control and Prevention (CDC) reports that more than 40% of Americans over age 20 years are overweight or obese, which is defined as being 20% over the desirable weight for one's gender, height, and body build. The highest rate of obesity is seen in non-Hispanic black women (58.9%), followed by Hispanic men (45.7%). The lowest levels of obesity are seen in Asian men and women. The causes of obesity include the obvious factors such as excess dietary intake and inadequate physical activity. There are other factors that may be less known. Genetic predisposition has been identified as influential on body weight. Certain diseases and medications can also promote weight gain.

Positive lifestyles with regular exercise are important to maintain healthy joints and bones. Activities that are stress reducing, such as walking, swimming, golf, and tennis, also have the potential to enhance calcium utilization. Premenopausal women need to obtain about 1000 mg of dietary calcium per day, whereas postmenopausal women need 1200 mg of calcium to prevent osteoporosis if they are not taking a hormone replacement with estrogen. A good diet with supplemental vitamins and minerals combined with regular exercise often helps lessen the effects of menopause.

The diet also should be rich in phosphorus and magnesium. A diet rich in green, leafy vegetables, fresh fruits, whole-grain cereals or breads, and dairy products helps support healthy bones. A reduced intake of fat is recommended; most of it should come from unsaturated fats such as soy, sunflower, corn, or safflower oil. High blood levels of saturated fats and cholesterol contribute to atherosclerosis, coronary heart disease, and cancer.

Physical and Dental Examinations. The person in middle adulthood needs an annual physical examination and biannual dental examinations. Preventive American Cancer Society guidelines should be followed.

Sleep and Rest. During middle adulthood, sleep challenges are common. The adult in this age group sleeps less than the younger adult. Problems experienced include both difficulty falling asleep and remaining asleep. Changes to hormone levels and changes in circadian rhythms are partly to blame. In addition, during this period of life, adults may experience stressors related to health, family, and financial concerns. This may make relaxing in preparation for sleep difficult.

LATE ADULTHOOD: 65 YEARS AND OLDER

Older adults represent a rapidly growing segment of the population, and everyone should prepare for and understand the aging process (Box 24.21). There are many approaches to examining the experience of growing old. Aging is a normal condition of human existence and has been studied from sociologic, physiologic, and psychological perspectives. Throughout the lifespan, all these aspects of the human experience are interrelated. Gerontologists, who study the older adult and the aging process, note that many 70-year-olds today act and think as 50-year-olds did as recently as the 1960s.

The fact remains that everyone ages. The physiologic changes are not universal, however, or even necessarily inevitable, and the changes are often amenable to many interventions and treatments. An individual's adjustment to aging is a uniquely complex process. How an individual responds to the age-related changes visible in the mirror has much to do with the person's self-esteem. Successful aging depends on the individual's capacity to cope and ability to change. The process of aging affects the individual, the family, and society at large (see the Lifespan Considerations for Older Adults box).

The sociologically relevant issues of aging have to do with work, retirement, social security, and health care. As more and more people reach late adulthood, society must recognize and value these individuals' knowledge, skills, and contributions. Arrangements and plans for the future that are addressed and encouraged in the early adult years help prepare, support, and enhance adjustments once they are necessary. Implementation of flexible services and financial assistance programs helps people fulfill their goals.

The response to getting older is often related to lifelong health habits, diet, and exercise patterns. Family,

Lifespan Considerations
Older Adults

Effects of Aging on Older Adults

- With increased emphasis on wellness and preventive care, today's older adults are living longer, healthier lives. However, longer lifespans result in an increased presence of chronic and degenerative disorders.
- Each generation has its own central life tasks to complete. As life expectancy grows, more generations coexist, and the needs of one age group sometimes come into conflict with those of others. This increases intergenerational stress and typically causes alterations in family dynamics.
- Changes in roles and relationships present major developmental challenges to older adults.
- Health care needs of the aging population place increased demands on the health care delivery system.
- The cost of care for the older adult population is a major societal concern. This cost is likely to have a significant impact on the amount and the type of health care coverage provided by insurance companies and the government.
- Older adults are a politically active group, and as their numbers increase, they are having an impact on all aspects of society, including the entertainment, travel, and housing industries.
- Although some older adults are poor, as a group they generally have more income than younger individuals and therefore have a significant effect on the economy.

| Box 24.21 | Developmental Tasks of Late Adulthood |

- Accepts own life
- Recognizes accomplishments
- Finds satisfaction with new roles, relationships, and leisure time
- Maximizes independence and maintains high level of involvement
- Accepts own mortality and prepares for death

Fig. 24.16 According to Erikson, generativity versus stagnation is the developmental task of older adulthood. A loving relationship with a spouse is an example of a positive influence during this stage of life.

| Box 24.22 | Your Beliefs on Aging |

TRUE OR FALSE?
____ 1. All older people become senile.
____ 2. Most older people live in a nursing home or other institutional setting.
____ 3. Most older people are isolated from their families.
____ 4. Most older people have no interest in or capacity for sexual relationships.
____ 5. Older workers are less productive than younger workers.
____ 6. Intelligence declines in old age.
____ 7. Older people do better to cease exercising and just rest.
____ 8. Marked personality changes occur in the older person.
____ 9. Older people naturally become inflexible and demanding.

NOTE: All of these statements are false.

love, friendships, and intimate relationships are additional factors important to survival and well-being (Fig. 24.16). These relationships are crucial to peoples' happiness, whatever the age. Love relationships vary in intensity and meaning in adulthood. Early on, these relationships usually have an intense physical basis, which leads to intimacy, respect, and commitment. Although intense sexual drive decreases with age, sexual behavior remains an important part of many adult relationships.

Ageism

Ageism, a form of discrimination and prejudice against the older adult, is an unfortunate reality. Like racism and sexism, ageism prevents people from being as happy and productive as they otherwise can be. It is passed on from generation to generation by the process of socialization. Society must relinquish old stereotypes about the older adult and learn to affirm the positive aspects of aging. It is a mistake to view aging only as a decline; it involves growth as well. Box 24.22 provides a brief list of true-false statements that helps clarify beliefs on aging.

The number of older people has grown steadily over the past century and will continue to do so. In 2014, there were 46 million people in the United States 65 years of age or older. That number is expected to more than double by the year 2060, reaching 98 million (Mather, 2015).

Every year another group of adults reaches late adulthood. Late adulthood is defined as age 65 years and older; it can be subdivided further into "young older adult" (ages 65 to 74 years), "middle older adult" (ages 75 to 84 years), and "old older adult" (older than age 85 years). This population is changing constantly as new individuals enter the group and others leave through death. Each person has a unique personal history that reflects many influences. Box 24.23 lists keys

Keys to Successful Aging

- Practice pleasurable activities.
- View life as meaningful.
- Maintain a positive self-image.
- Accept responsibility for the past.
- Be optimistic.
- Remain motivated to maintain or expand intellectual capacity.
- Participate in a planned exercise program.

to successful aging. The fastest growing segment of the US population is the group aged 85 years and older.

Biological Theories of Aging

For centuries, humanity has been fascinated with the concept of aging. Many theories have attempted to define the causes of aging and to develop measures to halt or postpone the aging process. One of the earliest theories of aging, generated by Hippocrates, speculated that aging was an irreversible natural event caused by a decrease in body heat. Later, Galen supported this concept and claimed that aging was a lifelong process rather than an event that occurred at the end of the lifespan. Leonardo da Vinci, among the first to attempt to identify the physical changes associated with aging, performed autopsies to compare old men and young children. In the period after 1900, only a few scientists focused on aging as their main interest. Finally, in the past 30 years, we have begun to see a renewed interest in researching the causes of the aging process. Recent theories focus on the roles of autoimmunity, free radicals (compounds with an extra electron or protein), wear and tear, and biological programming, among others. The only definitive conclusion, however, is that aging is a slow, continuous, complex process that probably involves intrinsic and extrinsic factors.

Autoimmunity Theory. The autoimmunity theory states that with aging, the body becomes less able to recognize or tolerate the "self." As a result, the immune system produces antibodies that act against the self. This theory is supported by the increased accumulation of lymphocytes (plasma cells found in the tissues of healthy older people).

The primary organs of the immune system (thymus and bone marrow) are believed to be affected by the aging process. With aging, the thymus decreases in size and weight and becomes less able to produce T cells. The bone marrow stem cells also show reduced efficiency in performing certain functions. As immune system function decreases, the risk of development of infection and cancer increases.

Free radical Theory. Free radicals are highly reactive cellular components derived from unstable atoms or molecules. Free radicals have a reduced cellular efficiency and cause cellular waste to accumulate. Some free radicals are produced by radiation, heat, and oxidation. The presence of free radicals possibly accelerates aging and results in the death of an organism. Lipofuscin is a pigmented material that accumulates in many organs as a part of aging. This accumulation interferes with the diffusion and transportation of essential metabolites and perhaps also contributes to the aging process.

Wear-and-Tear Theory. According to the wear-and-tear theory, age is not based on chronologic age but is determined by the amount of wear and tear experienced. Many believe that the structural and functional changes associated with growing old are accelerated by abuse of the body.

Genetic Theory. Similar life expectancies within families lend support to the idea of a hereditary basis for aging. After all, our hair color and height are determined by our genes, so it could be that our lifespan is also determined by our genes. Scientists have been studying short-lived animals to identify longevity genes and manipulate them to study how those changes affect the animal's lifespan. Studying the genetics of aging is complex and requires much more research to fully understand; however, it is not expected that one gene solely determines the lifespan for a human, but rather several genes affect the process of aging (Stibich, 2020).

Psychological Theories of Aging

Disengagement Theory. According to supporters of the disengagement theory of aging, a natural withdrawal, or disengagement, between the individual and society is best. This withdrawal is initiated either by the individual or by others in society. Adherents to this belief suggest that such withdrawal prevents older adults from experiencing frustration when they can no longer function adequately and allows a younger member of society to fulfill the now-empty role. They characterize this process as a normal, inevitable, universal process. Two major criticisms of the disengagement theory are as follows:

- It does not allow for the many active, functional older adults.
- The process is not seen in all cultural groups; it is therefore not universal.

Activity Theory. According to this theory, the older person who is more active socially is more likely to adjust well to aging. Older adults with more social involvement have higher morale and better life satisfaction and personal adjustment. The number and the quality of the activities are important. People who give up activities or roles should be advised to find replacements. Meaningful activities that involve close personal contact with others are extremely important. Activities of this nature reinforce self-concept, which in turn is associated with a higher life satisfaction.

Continuity Theory. Supporters of this theory suggest that the critical factors in adjustment to old age are the coping abilities developed previously in life and an ability to maintain previous roles and activities. Knowledge and understanding of a person's personality type are often useful in predicting response to the aging process. People who were never highly involved in society are likely to maintain the same mild level of involvement in old age; on the other hand, individuals who were highly involved and actively engaged with society need to remain active and involved with similar intensity. Supporters of the continuity theory contend that adjustment to the aging process is eased by maintaining roles and interests similar to those developed earlier in life.

Physical Characteristics

Aging is a complex process that affects cells, tissues, and organs. Like growth and development, aging occurs at a highly individualized rate. A gradual reduction in the number of aging cells and a change in the composition of aging cells occur. A slow increase in body weight is usually seen until 45 to 50 years of age, and then a gradual decline begins. Body fat content and distribution differ in men and women. The accumulation of adipose tissue in females is typically found over the chest, the waist, the hips, and the thighs. Adipose

tissue in the male is deposited mostly in the waist, the chest, and the lower abdomen.

Loss of height begins after age 50 years. Most of the noticeable decrease in trunk length is a result of the increase in spinal curvature caused by a slight thinning of the intervertebral disks. In addition to the shortening of the spine, certain abnormal postures and contours are noted. Kyphosis, an exaggeration of the thoracic curvature, may increase with aging. This sometimes leads to a barrel-chest appearance, which possibly affects the position of the diaphragm and reduces the effectiveness of inspiration. These and other postural changes have the potential to affect body posture, mobility, gait, and respiratory efficiency.

Common age-related changes specific to each body system are listed in Table 24.4, along with suggested nursing interventions to minimize the effect of these changes.

Psychosocial Development

Years of living along with successes, failures, strengths, weaknesses, and all the early experiences influence the emotional stability of older adults. Despite the physiologic changes associated with the aging process, the

Table 24.4   Common Age-Related Changes

SYSTEM	NORMAL CHANGES	SUGGESTED NURSING INTERVENTIONS
Musculoskeletal System		
Bones, muscles, joints, and connective tissue	Mineral salts move from bones to blood, making bones more porous; tendons, ligaments less elastic; increase in joint stiffness with less range of motion; varying degrees of increase of flexion at wrists, hips, knees, producing less joint mobility, agility, and endurance; thinning of vertebral disks	Maintain mobility. Encourage exercise (with physician's guidance). Encourage passive and active exercises. Avoid fatigue. Use assistive aids when indicated.
Nervous System		
	Fewer, smaller neurons (nerve cells), slowed reaction time, decrease in tactile sensitivity, decrease in pain perception, altered motor coordination	Allow adequate time to complete activities. Be alert to danger of and prevent burning and chilling related to diminished sensitivity. Encourage position changes; inspect skin daily.
Special Senses		
Taste and smell	Decline in taste and smell perception	Use smoke detectors. Serve attractive, colorful food.
Vision	Decreased tear production, increase in lens density; presbyopia (farsightedness; loss of elasticity of lens); yellowing of lens; slowing of accommodation (reaction to changes in light and distance); narrowing of visual field; decrease in depth perception	Encourage annual eye examinations. Use more diffuse lighting. Use bright colors (red, yellow). Place articles within visual field. Use night-lights.
Hearing	Presbycusis (increased difficulty hearing high-pitched sounds); increase in degenerative changes within ear structure; increase in buildup of wax production	Speak slowly, clearly. Face individual. Do not shout. Speak in lower tones. Control background noise. Encourage use of hearing aids if available.
Respiratory System		
Ribcage	Increase in calcification of thorax; respiratory muscles weaken, producing diminished respiratory efficiency; maximum breathing capacity reduced; more susceptible to respiratory infection; easily fatigued	Allow for rest periods. Encourage coughing and deep breathing.

Table **24.4**	Common Age-Related Changes—cont'd	

SYSTEM	NORMAL CHANGES	SUGGESTED NURSING INTERVENTIONS
Lungs	Alveoli (air sacs) thinner, smaller, with decreased alveolar surface for gaseous exchange; decreased cough reflex action; decreased ciliary action, reduced maximum breathing capacity	Maintain adequate exercise and nutrition. Encourage regular physical examinations. Avoid overexertion and allow for rest between activities. Discourage smoking. Obtain streptococcal pneumonia (pneumococcal) vaccine.
Cardiovascular System		
	Fewer blood cells produced; loss of elasticity and narrowing of blood vessels, with an increase in blood pressure; valves thicker, more rigid; heart needs more time to return to resting state; decreased cardiac output	Encourage regular, paced exercise with adequate rest periods. Maintain low-fat, low-sodium diet. Obtain regular physician examinations.
Integumentary System		
Skin	Paler, thinner, irregularly pigmented; decrease in moisture; decrease in sweat and sebaceous gland activity; less elastic, more wrinkling; loss of subcutaneous fat; skin more fragile and prone to injury	Inspect skin for impairment or signs of pressure. Change position frequently. Wash with water and mild soap as needed. Rinse thoroughly and pat skin dry. Use lotions to replenish moisture. To maintain body warmth, provide adequate clothing.
Reproductive System		
Female	Fallopian tubes atrophy and shorten; ovaries smaller, thinner; uterus, cervix smaller; vagina less elastic, more alkaline, drier; reproductive capacity ceases	Suggest use of vaginal lubricants if indicated. Instruct person to have annual mammogram and vaginal examination with Papanicolaou test.
Male	Increased size of prostate; decreased testosterone levels; decreased circulation, and decreased rate and force of ejaculation	Instruct person to have annual prostate examination and prostate-specific antigen (PSA) test.
Endocrine System		
	Slowing of thyroid gland activity; decreased basal metabolic rate; decreased hormone production that affects other systems	Recommend annual physical examination with thyroid function testing.
Urinary System		
	Fewer cells in kidney, decreased renal blood flow; less effective filtration; decreased bladder elasticity and capacity; need for more frequent voiding	Observe for signs of urinary tract infections. Observe closely for adverse drug reactions. Observe male for signs of benign prostatic hypertrophy causing impairment of urinary flow.
Hair		
	Increase in graying; balding and changes in thickness of hair occur; changes in distribution of body hair	
Nails		
	More fragile, brittle; appear dull, opaque yellow or gray in color; toenails thicken	Have toenails trimmed by podiatrist as indicated.
Gastrointestinal System		
	Decreased saliva production; decreased chewing efficiency; decreased esophageal motility; total capacity of stomach reduced; decreased gastric enzyme secretion; liver smaller; less absorption of nutrients; slowing of peristalsis	Ensure adequate fluid intake. Encourage annual dental checkups. Offer five or six small daily meals, rather than three large ones. Assess for indigestion. Encourage regular toileting habits.

Fig. 24.17 Many older people continue to work and learn after the traditional retirement age.

older years should be viewed as a time of satisfaction and pleasure. Many older adults choose to work after age 65 years. These activities provide interest, intellectual stimulation, and added income (Fig. 24.17). Older people need to recognize their changing capabilities and begin a process of adjustment.

Erikson described the challenge of late adulthood as ego integrity versus a sense of despair. The task here is to evaluate one's life and accomplishments and find satisfaction and meaning. The process of reminiscing with others often further validates the meaning and importance of the individual's life. Those who can believe that their lives have been well spent and are satisfied with their decisions and achievements have mastered this task of integrity. This allows the person to continue life with a sense of dignity and peacefulness. Adults who are dissatisfied with their accomplishments often experience conflict and despair. Dissatisfaction contributes to a feeling of restlessness and a sense of panic that time is "running out." Often the individual feels the need for more time and a chance to do things over again differently.

Many other factors also affect the older adult's adjustment to this stage of life. Retirement is a major adjustment for the older adult. Health and financial resources are critical elements in determination of life satisfaction after retirement. Generally speaking, society is relatively unprepared for the phenomenon known as retirement. Retirement creates many changes—some welcome, some not. Examples are changes in roles, self-esteem, support systems, life patterns, and leisure time. Individuals need to plan and discuss their hopes and expectations for the retirement period. Planning for retirement helps identify activities that will be meaningful and promote self-esteem and a sense of usefulness to oneself and society.

Family Roles

For many individuals, the older years become a time to explore feelings about parenting and grandparenting. Grandparenting today, as discussed previously, is often very different from the role of grandparenting three or four decades ago. Today's grandparent often works and remains highly active. For some grandparents, caring for grandchildren has become a full-time responsibility that leads to multiple stresses. Raising grandchildren has the potential to create financial stress, cause a decrease in living space, and limit roles. Events that affect children such as divorce, abandonment, unemployment, death or illness, and incarceration are some of the factors that have contributed to the increased numbers of grandparents raising grandchildren on a full-time basis. Support groups, community resources, and other organizations are some of the resources that assist grandparents in their grandparenting roles.

During this stage, couples may need to adjust to increased time together; couples often enjoy the increase in companionship and closeness. Maintaining old friendships and exploring ways to form new ones, along with continuing strong family ties, are means to help soften the losses that are frequently experienced during this period.

The death of a spouse is traumatic at any age. In the older years, widowhood is more common for women than men. Children and a strong social network often play important roles in supporting the surviving spouse. The experience of being widowed goes beyond ending a partnership. Role changes, changes in lifestyle, and access to fewer financial resources are just some of the adjustments that are called for when a spouse dies. Some older people find remarriage or new partnerships to be a solution to the challenge of being widowed, and through this they discover the companionship, love, and security they seek.

Cognitive and Intellectual Development

A common misconception about aging relates to the loss of cognition. Evidence suggests that older adults in good health and in nurturing environments have the capacity to maintain or increase their level of functioning, particularly in their areas of interest or specialization. Factors important to continued cognitive functioning include reduction or limitations of stress, maintaining health, engaging in mentally stimulating activities, and engaging in activities to promote memory and cognition. Language skills are preserved with aging. Problem solving skills and overall intelligence remain intact. There may be problems when multiple stimuli are vying for attention. This is managed by encouraging the older adult to manage one task at a time. The speed of cognitive processing may be reduced with aging. This does not mean there is a lack of capability, but that it takes longer (Murman, 2015).

Memory. Some older adults notice changes in memory. Such benign forgetfulness is far more common than the forgetfulness associated with Alzheimer's disease. As adults advance in years, there appears to be a greater loss of recent memory over remote memory. An older individual perhaps forgets what was served for breakfast 2 hours earlier and yet may remember in great detail the events of a wedding many decades ago. Older people are slower than younger people but are often more accurate in what they remember and do. There are tools to help promote improved memory in the older adult. Remaining socially engaged with others is beneficial. Continuing to remain mentally engaged in activities such as puzzles, reading, and hobbies such as gardening or cooking will provide mental stimulation.

Health Promotion
Health promotion rests on the belief that individuals can have a strong influence on their health status. Environment, social patterns, diet, exercise, and personal habits are factors that determine a person's state of health. Health care workers must clarify the common misconceptions about health and aging. It is essential to emphasize that people of all ages can benefit from living a healthy lifestyle, even in the later years (see the Health Promotion box on the benefits of exercise).

Health Promotion
Benefits of Exercise in the Older Adult
- Maintains or improves cardiovascular fitness.
- Prevents or reduces intensity of chronic diseases, such as coronary artery disease, congestive heart failure, hypertension, osteoarthritis, osteoporosis, diabetes, obesity, and chronic obstructive lung disease.
- Prevents many falls and fractures.
- Improves muscle strength, flexibility, and balance.
- Enhances self-care abilities and promotes independent activities.
- Encourages social contact.
- Decreases anxiety, depression, and insomnia.

Advise older adults to receive pneumococcal and influenza vaccines yearly. Individuals who have compromised immune systems, who have a history of an allergy to eggs or egg products, or who have had a severe reaction to a previous vaccine should check with their physician before immunization.

Nutrition. Adequate nutrition plays a significant role in health maintenance and contributes to the older person's quality of life. Activities related to food and diet include transportation for food purchase, meal planning, and meal preparation. The task of providing older individuals with assistance for these activities often falls to family members. Older adults need a diet of foods of higher quality and lower quantity that provide the basic necessary nutrients. Although caloric needs are individualized, older adults are generally less active and have more adipose tissue and less body mass and therefore often need less daily caloric intake. Diets that are low in saturated fats and carbohydrates and high in fiber are usually recommended. Common threats to the adequacy of the older adult's diet are poor oral health, lack of appetite, food intolerances, and constipation. Proper nutritional assessment and counseling help identify problems and useful

interventions. To ensure dietary compliance, take long-standing habits and cultural influences into consideration when introducing any dietary changes.

Various psychosocial factors also have the potential to affect the older person's diet. The choice of foods purchased and included in the diet is sometimes the result of economic factors. Loneliness also contributes to inadequate dietary intake for some people. If people are not able to shop for and prepare meals, their diets are likely to become less than desirable. Another crucial component in the older person's diet is adequate fluid intake. Advise older adults to maintain a minimum daily intake of 1500 mL/day. Often an older person avoids fluids out of a fear of incontinence and a lack of thirst.

Activity. Throughout the lifespan, evenly paced, satisfying exercise is crucial to general well-being. Exercise has benefits for cardiovascular functioning, lowering blood pressure while enhancing oxygen utilization, and maintaining joint mobility. Exercise to the point of exhaustion is misguided; always recommend a rest period after exercise to recuperate and restore the body to its maximum level of functioning (see the Health Promotion box for benefits of exercise).

Sleep. Older individuals need more rest but less actual sleep. The incidence of accidents that occur during nighttime awakenings is increased, and safety concerns must be handled. Use of night-lights and reduced excess furniture and clutter are some methods of decreasing the risk of nighttime injury. Sleep for the older person often is affected by medications, alcohol, caffeine, stress, and environmental noise and temperature.

Safety. Most accidents are preventable (see safety tips for the older adult in the Safety Alert box). The key to prevention is knowledge and recognition of and attention to the factors that contribute to the increased risk for accident or injury. Diminished sight and changes in posture or balance sometimes expose the older person to the risk of falls. A single fall has the potential to produce an injury that necessitates a long period of immobilization, thus diminishing the person's independence and self-esteem.

Safety Alert
Safety Tips for the Older Adult
- Minimize clutter and excess furniture in rooms and hallways.
- Remove scatter rugs.
- Use handrails on stairs.
- Install grab bars in showers and bathrooms.
- Use night-lights.
- Get up slowly from a lying-flat position.
- Use caution in going from well-lit areas to darkened areas or vice versa.
- If self-medicating, use dispensing aids to decrease the risk of error.
- Wear properly fitting shoes and clothing.
- Allow enough time; do not rush or hurry.

Get Ready For The NCLEX® Examination!

Key Points

- Development is a lifelong process that begins at conception and ends at death.
- All types of families serve similar basic functions: protection, nurturance, education, sustenance, and socialization of their members.
- Growth patterns suggest rapid growth during infancy, continued growth during toddler and preschool years, and slowed but steady growth during the school years, followed by a rapid surge of growth during puberty and adolescence.
- Erikson identified a central task that must be resolved at each stage of the lifespan: infancy, toddler, preschool, school age, adolescence, early adulthood, middle adulthood, and late adulthood.
- Piaget focused on the concept of cognitive development beginning in infancy and continuing throughout the childhood years.
- Accidental injuries are a major cause of death during infancy, childhood, and adolescence.
- Consistent discipline and supervision are needed throughout childhood.
- Peer relationships become significant at school age.
- Adolescence is the transitional period between childhood and adulthood.
- Adulthood is marked by significant events: career decisions, marriage, new social relationships, and financial concerns.
- Certain physical changes become evident during middle age, including graying of hair and vision changes.
- Menopause and hormonal changes characterize the reproductive changes of the middle-age female.
- Roles undergo change during middle adulthood, including nuclear family roles, relationships with grown children, grandparenting, and possibly career changes.
- Late adulthood is marked by a gradual slowing of the body's functioning.
- Several significant physical changes become evident in the older adult.
- Family changes and an increased awareness of one's mortality are common adjustments called for by the aging process.
- Life review and acceptance of one's strengths and weaknesses are necessary aspects of the aging process.
- Several theories attempt to explain aging, however, no one theory is accepted universally.
- Aging, like growth, is a highly individualized process.

Additional Learning Resources

SG Go to your Study Guide for additional learning activities to help you master this chapter content.

Be sure to visit the Evolve site at http://evolve.elsevier.com/Cooper/foundations/ for additional online resources.

Review Questions for the NCLEX® Examination

1. The nurse is aware that the first socializing agent for the child is:
   1. daycare
   2. family
   3. school
   4. play groups

2. The nurse is educating a group of preschool teachers about psychosocial development for their population. The nurse is correct when stating a 4-year-old child is working on achieving which of Erikson's developmental tasks?
   1. Trust versus mistrust
   2. Industry versus inferiority
   3. Autonomy versus shame and doubt
   4. Initiative versus guilt

3. The student nurse is preparing for a clinical day at a local long-term care facility. The student has a correct understanding of the theories of aging when she/he makes which statement? *(Select all that apply.)*
   1. "Free radicals improve cellular efficiency and delay the aging process."
   2. "With aging, the body becomes less able to recognize itself and produces antibodies that act against the self."
   3. "Free radicals cause an accumulation of cellular waste that may accelerate the aging process."
   4. "Abuse of the body can accelerate functional and structural changes associated with growing old."
   5. "The immune system function increases, reducing the risk for infection as people age."

4. An 8-year-old loves to draw and do craft projects. The nurse understands that the child's need for praise and encouragement for the work efforts demonstrates the development of which of Erikson's tasks?
   1. Autonomy
   2. Initiative
   3. Industry
   4. Identity

5. The school nurse is preparing a presentation for the high school football team. The nurse should include that peak physical strength and endurance occurs during what period of life?
   1. Adolescence
   2. Early adulthood
   3. Middle adulthood
   4. Late adulthood

6. The nurse is completing the assessment of an 8-month-old infant at a well child visit. The nurse notes that the child has good head control and can now sit up unsupported. What term accurately describes this sequence of growth and development?

   1. Integrated
   2. Proximodistal
   3. Cephalocaudal
   4. Differential

7. The nurse is discussing stressors that are common for children when their parents remarry after a divorce. Which statement by the nurse indicates a need for further teaching? *(Select all that apply.)*

   1. Losses from a previous divorce can cause children to be fearful of love and trust.
   2. Children may have loyalties to the other parent.
   3. Jealousies may arise from the unity of stepchildren.
   4. There are no stressors to consider because the new marriage only concerns the parents, not the children.

8. A 5-year-old child is brought to the doctor's office for an annual well child visit by his grandmother. The student nurse knows which of the following is true regarding grandfamilies?

   1. Children have more stable childhoods when placed with nonrelative foster families.
   2. Finances are never a concern for grandfamilies.
   3. The number of children in foster care being raised by relatives because of substance abuse is increasing.
   4. If the grandparent is the primary caregiver for a child, the biological parents are not involved in the child's life.
   5. As long as counseling is sought before a new marriage occurs the children will not experience any difficulties.

9. The parents of a 1-week-old infant are concerned that they are going to "spoil" their baby if they hold him too much. The nurse understands that according to Erikson, when infants are cuddled, fed, and loved, they develop which characteristic?

   1. Autonomy
   2. Trust
   3. Industry
   4. Identity

10. The nurse is observing a group of preschool children playing. What type of play is most common with this age group?

    1. Parallel play
    2. Imaginary play
    3. Organized, team play
    4. Cognitive play

11. The nurse understands that characteristics of the cognitive development for a 10-year-old child include which concepts? *(Select all that apply.)*

    1. Better understands other viewpoints
    2. Recognizes cause-and-effect relationships
    3. Uses a systematic, scientific problem-solving approach
    4. Is able to think about abstractions and hypothetical concepts
    5. Understands basic ideas of conversation and number classification

12. The young adult struggles with which of Erikson's developmental tasks?

    1. Trust versus mistrust
    2. Identity versus confusion
    3. Generativity versus stagnation
    4. Intimacy versus isolation

13. A mother asks the nurse why her toddler always says "no" and has a negative attitude. The nurse assures the mother that such behavior is common in toddlers and helps the child meet which developmental task?

    1. Discipline
    2. Trust
    3. Independence
    4. Love

14. The nurse is explaining Piaget's preoperational thought stage of development to a mother. Which statements by the mother indicate that the teaching was effective? *(Select all that apply.)*

    1. "This stage of development will last from ages 2 through 7 years."
    2. "My child's thinking will be focused mainly on himself during this time."
    3. "My child will be able to use his imagination."
    4. "My child will use trial and error to discover new things."
    5. "My child will begin to show behaviors that embrace the feelings and needs of others."

15. A father is concerned that his 8-year-old son does not seem to be growing very quickly. The nurse reassures the father that growth during the school-age period can best be described in what manner?

    1. Irregular and slow
    2. Steady and slow
    3. Regular and fast
    4. Irregular and fast

16. The nurse is caring for a hospitalized 2-year-old child. What interventions are appropriate for inclusion in the plan of care? *(Select all that apply.)*

    1. Establish a routine.
    2. Offer choices when possible.
    3. Provide detailed explanations for care activities.
    4. Encourage parental involvement.
    5. Encourage play interaction with other older children also hospitalized on the care unit.

17. A 60-year-old female is being seen for her annual physical. She conveys to the nurse that she is concerned about losing her memory and intelligence as she enters her late adult years. Which statement by the nurse indicates a need for further teaching? *(Select all that apply.)*

    1. "Older adults have a greater loss of recent memory, rather than remote memory."
    2. "Benign forgetfulness is uncommon in older adults and indicates a need for further examination."
    3. "Older adults may be slower to recall past memories but are more accurate in what they recall."
    4. "Older adults in good health have the capacity to maintain or increase their cognitive function."
    5. "The older adult often confuses recent memories and past memories."

18. Which statement by the older adult indicates that nutritional counseling was effective?

    1. "I need to eat more fats and proteins."
    2. "I need to eat less fiber."
    3. "I need to eat less saturated fats and carbohydrates."
    4. "I can take a supplement for all my nutritional needs."

19. The nurse is reviewing the assigned patients for the shift. One assigned patient is a 45-year-old man. When considering the needs of the patient, the nurse should recognize that the patient is in which developmental stage?

    1. Intimacy versus isolation
    2. Generativity versus stagnation
    3. Ego integrity versus despair
    4. Initiative versus guilt

20. Which developmental skill commonly is accomplished by the fourth month of life?

    1. Sitting up unsupported
    2. Holding head up at 90-degree angle
    3. Creeping
    4. Transferring objects from one hand to the other

21. A new parent asks how to introduce solid foods to the infant. Which statement indicates that teaching was effective?

    1. "I will introduce several foods at once to see what food my baby likes best."
    2. "I will start feeding my baby my favorite foods first."
    3. "I will introduce one new food at a time."
    4. "I will mix foods together to cover up tastes that he might not like."

22. When teaching a parenting class, the nurse explains that nighttime bottles should be avoided to help prevent which occurrence?

    1. Dental caries
    2. Dental malocclusion
    3. Otitis media
    4. Lactose intolerance

23. The father of 17-year-old boy is concerned because his son is questioning all of the family's morals and values. Which is true regarding the developmental tasks of an adolescent?

    1. Adolescents should achieve independence from their parents financially and socially.
    2. Adolescents learn to accept their own mortality and prepare for death.
    3. Adolescents question their own values and beliefs as they search for their own identity.
    4. Adolescents continue to deny responsibility for their behavior.

24. A couple, Joe and Terry, are in their 30's and have no children. They have attended classes for fostering children and have just learned that they have been approved to foster an 8-year-old boy named Ayden. They learned in their classes that establishing discipline and setting limits are important to effectively parent children. Which statements confirm that the couple understand how to best establish discipline and set limits with their new foster child?

Choose the *most likely* options for the information missing from the statements below by selecting from the list of options provided.

Joe and Terry tell Ayden that they are _____ of the way he cleans his room.
Joe and Terry tell Ayden that bedtime will be _____ time each night and they will _____ maintain 8pm as his bedtime.
Joe and Terry use a _____ when Ayden is acting out.
Joe and Terry remain _____ when Ayden is angry and talk to him in a normal tone of voice.

OPTIONS
Disappointed
Whatever
Proud
Inconsistently
The same
Calm approach
Time out
Consistently
Loud voice

25

Loss, Grief, Dying, and Death

Charlotte Connerton

http://evolve.elsevier.com/Cooper/foundations

Objectives

1. Explain the role of loss in the grief reaction.
2. Describe the stages of dying.
3. Explain the concepts of euthanasia, do-not-resuscitate (DNR) orders, organ donations, fraudulent methods of treatment, and the Dying Person's Bill of Rights.
4. Describe techniques in assisting the dying patient to say goodbye.
5. Discuss the principles of palliative care.
6. Discuss nursing interventions for the dying patient.
7. List nursing interventions that may facilitate grieving in special circumstances (perinatal, pediatric, older adult, and suicide).
8. Identify the unique physical signs and symptoms of the patient who is near death.
9. Describe nursing responsibilities in care of the body after death.
10. Identify needs and discuss support for the grieving family.
11. Discuss support for the nurse who experiences grief after the loss of a patient.

Key Terms

advance directives (p. 763)
allow natural death (p. 763)
anticipatory grief (ăn-TĬS-ĭ-pă-TŌ-rē, p. 750)
autopsy (ĂW-tŏp-sē, p. 769)
bereavement (bĭ-RĒV-mĕnt, p. 749)
bereavement overload (p. 751)
complicated grieving (p. 752)
death (p. 763)
do-not-resuscitate (DNR) (p. 763)
durable powers of attorney (p. 763)
dysfunctional grieving (p. 752)
euthanasia (yū-thĕ-NĂ-zhă, p. 762)
grief (p. 747)
grief therapy (p. 748)

grief work (p. 747)
inquest (ĬN-kwĕst, p. 769)
living will (p. 747)
loss (p. 747)
maturational loss (măch-ŭ-RĂ-shŭn-ăl, p. 749)
morbidity (mōr-BĬ-dĭ-tē, p. 749)
mortality (mōr-TĂ-lĭ-tē, p. 748)
mortician (mōr-TĬ-shŭn, p. 769)
mourning (p. 749)
palliative care (PĂL-ē-ă-tĭv, p. 765)
postmortem care (pōst-MŌR-tĕm, p. 769)
situational loss (p. 749)
thanatology (thăn-ă-TŎL-ŏ-jē, p. 752)
unresolved grief (p. 752)

Life is a series of losses and gains. When any aspect of self is no longer available to a person, that person suffers a loss. Loss and death (cessation of life) are universal in the human experience, but they are unique events to the individual. Coping mechanisms determine a person's ability to face and accept loss. Grief is a pattern of physical and emotional responses to bereavement, separation, or loss. It is a natural response to loss. All losses have the possibility of triggering the grief process. The severity of the loss may vary, but the grief that accompanies it is real nonetheless.

Illness and hospitalization frequently cause loss, and nurses work with many patients who experience losses of different types. The nurse helps them understand and accept loss so that life can continue. The process of adapting to and mourning a loss is called grief work. After a loss, serious emotional, mental, and social problems may occur if a patient does not perform grief work.

Humans can anticipate death. This anticipation causes a variety of possible responses: anxiety, planning, denial, love, loneliness, achievement, or lack of achievement. Death affects dying patients and their families, significant others, friends, and caregivers. It can be an overwhelming experience. A person's style of dying reflects that person's style of living, and attitudes about death depend on a person's beliefs and emotional strengths.

Care of dying patients and their families can be one of the most challenging aspects of nursing care. Dying is the final stage of human growth and development which requires nurses be as knowledgeable about the process of dying as they are about the process of birth. Because health care usually emphasizes the cure of disease and the promotion of health, health care providers often perceive the death of a patient as a form of failure. Health care personnel who care for dying patients often withdraw from patients emotionally while providing adequate physical care.

When nurses deal with grieving families and dying patients, they are confronted with their own **mortality** (the condition of being subject to death) and other distressing issues that accompany loss. Nurses can deliver quality of care to patients and families experiencing death if they understand the stages of the grief process and the task of dying.

CHANGES IN HEALTH CARE RELATED TO DYING AND DEATH

Before the 1950s, patients commonly died at home in their own beds with assistance only from their family. From the 1950s to the 1980s, the health care system became highly mechanized, and dying occurred mostly in institutions, often with sophisticated equipment attached to the dying individual to prolong life. When diagnosis-related groups (DRGs) came into play in the early 1980s, the trend changed again. Today, in general, the only patients placed in hospital beds are those who are considered at risk for medical complications or who need hospital recovery time after surgery or special procedures. This type of bed is often also used in the home. Many recuperating or terminally ill patients are discharged to home, a convalescent center, or a nursing home. Nurses who provide care to the terminally ill patient in the home health care setting have felt the impact of this development. At home, these patients receive intravenous infusions and other technical and mechanical assistance. Nurses in health care facilities and homes are the health care providers most often available to the grieving family during the crisis of death.

During pandemics or other illness outbreaks such as influenza season, health care facilities may restrict the number of visitors for patients. The severity of the communicable disease may lead to death. The restrictions on the number of visitors for patients may interfere with the grieving process of the patient, family, and care givers. The nurse needs to take this into consideration while providing care to the patient and family.

HISTORICAL OVERVIEW

Discussions of the dynamics that surround grief, dying, and death are not new. In the 1960s, pioneers in death and dying theory, such as Kübler-Ross and Glasser and Strauss, produced works that stimulated the health care industry. Dying and death became topics of research and seminars. In the 1970s, hospices in the United States became recognized as health care delivery systems (see Chapter 40). **Grief therapy** (mental health treatment aimed at helping a patient deal with the pain of loss; a program that assists the bereaved

to cope with a loss) continues to evolve as various theories on grief and loss are developed. Grief therapy helps the nurse meet the needs and plan the care for the dying patient.

The US Supreme court did find in 1990 that patients have the right to refuse or withdraw from treatment to hasten their deaths. A limited number of states have "Death with Dignity" legislation allowing health care providers to assist with the ending of life. The construction of these state laws varies. They are limited to patients 18 years or older. Most also mandate the patient make the request to the physician twice 15 days apart. On October 27, 1997, Oregon enacted the Death With Dignity Act, which allows terminally ill Oregonians to end their lives through the voluntary self-administration of lethal medications, expressly prescribed by a physician for that purpose. The Oregon Death With Dignity Act required the Oregon Health Authority to collect information about the patients and physicians who participate in the Act and publish an annual statistical report (The Oregon Death With Dignity Act, 1997). Since that time, similar acts have been enacted in other states. At the date of this publication, states that have such acts include Washington (*Washington Death with Dignity Act*, 2008), Vermont (*Patient Choice and Control at the End of Life Act*, 2013), California (*End of Life Option Act*, 2015/2016), Colorado (*End of Life Options Act*, 2016), District of Columbia (*D.C. Death with Dignity Act*, 2016/2017), Hawaii (*Our Care, Our Choice Act*, 2018/2019), Maine (*Death with Dignity Act*, 2019), and New Jersey (*Aid in Dying for the Terminally Ill Act*, 2019). The state of Montana does not actually have an act that supports physician-assisted suicide, but in 2009 the state's supreme court did not rule against any physician who has prescribed medication that allows voluntary self-administration of lethal medications (Death With Dignity, n.d.).

Care providers have been learning to assist patients and families to exercise more control over their care. Individuals become involved by determining treatment options and choosing the setting, circumstances, and management of the dying process. Advance directives are upheld as legal documents in courts of law, and terminal health care is shifting away from hospital settings. Because of such developments, nurses continue to play a primary role in the care of the dying person at home and of the family experiencing loss.

When viewing death as a natural process, the nurse helps the patient die comfortably and with dignity. The eight domains established by the National Consensus Project for Quality Palliative Care (2018) are structure and processes of care; physical aspects of care; psychological and psychiatric aspects of care; social aspects of care; spiritual, religious, and existential aspects of care; cultural aspects of care; care of patient nearing the end of life; and ethical and legal aspects of care. The structure and processes of care involve a comprehensive interdisciplinary assessment that is used as a baseline to develop a comprehensive, individualized care plan carried out through the nursing process. This individual plan of care involves coordination of care across settings with high-quality of communication between health care providers and the patient/family unit. The physical aspects of care focus on pain and symptom control and relief of suffering to improve or maintain functioning and quality of life. The psychological and psychiatric aspects of care focus on stress, coping strategies, grieving processes, and treatment of psychiatric conditions. Nurses can provide support and education on the dying process, the grieving process, and the decision-making process by including the benefits and burdens of treatment. Social aspects of care focus on the patient and family structure of culture, values, beliefs, and strengths, which drives the patient's goals and treatment preferences. Restriction of visitors during flu season and a pandemic can interfere with the function of family processes for end-of-life care.

Spiritual, religious, and existential aspects of care focus on those practices and rituals that bring the patient and family hope, meaning, purpose, comfort, and closure to the dying process. Cultural aspects of care convey a respect of the patient's and family's perceptions, preferences, and practices and tailor communication to the patient's and family's literacy level. Care of the patient nearing the end of life focuses on promoting care that will help the patient incorporate perceptions, preferences, and practices of spiritual, religious, and cultural needs to achieve a peaceful, dignified, and respectful death. Ethical and legal aspects of care can be followed by practicing within one's guidelines established by the governing board's code of ethics.

Not all losses are obvious or immediate. Obvious losses are such events as the death of a loved one, divorce, breakup of a relationship, or loss of a job. Not as obvious are the losses precipitated by illness, aging, birth of a child with defects, and changes in schools, jobs, or neighborhoods.

Some losses are actual, and some are perceived. An actual loss is identified easily, such as a woman who has a mastectomy. A perceived loss, such as the loss of confidence or when a woman who hopes to give birth to a female child delivers a male child instead, is less obvious. Perceived losses are overlooked or misunderstood easily, yet the associated process of grief follows the same sequence as with losses that are considered "real."

Another way to look at loss is to classify it as maturational, situational, or both. **Maturational loss** is a loss that results from normal life transitions. Examples include the loss of childhood dreams, the loss felt by an adolescent when a romance fails, and the loss felt when leaving the family home for college or marriage and establishing a home of one's own. Later, as individuals age, they may experience losses such as menopause and loss of hair, teeth, hearing, sight, and "youth." Situational loss is defined as a loss that occurs suddenly in response to a specific external event, such as the sudden death of a loved one. Loss of a job can lead to

a loss of self-esteem. Such changes promote emotional growth and the development of coping skills. People use these skills later to cope with even more significant losses. Early experiences with loss can prepare the individual to deal with loss throughout the life cycle. Each person experiences loss as it individually affects him or her. Each loss is followed by a time of grieving.

Personal loss is any significant loss that necessitates adaptation through the grieving process. When something or someone can no longer be seen, felt, heard, known, or experienced, a sense of loss occurs. The type of loss influences the degree of stress it causes. For example, the loss of an object may not generate the same stress as the loss of a significant other. On the other hand, individuals respond to loss differently. In general, people expect the death of a family member to cause more stress than the loss of a pet. For an older person living alone, however, the death of a pet that has been a constant companion can cause more emotional stress than that of a cousin who had not been seen in years.

Therefore, recognize how highly individualized each person's interpretation of a loss is, whatever type of loss it may be. Loss is a complex phenomenon influenced by many factors (Box 25.1). It threatens self-concept, self-esteem, security, and sense of worth. Recognize the meaning of each loss to a patient and its impact on physical and psychological functioning.

GRIEF

Grief is the subjective response to actual or anticipated loss. It is a natural, normal, and universal part of human experience. **Bereavement** is defined as a common depressed reaction to the death of a loved one. Mourning (reaction activated by a person to assist in overcoming a great personal loss) refers to culturally defined patterns for the expression of grief. Mourning patterns include funerals, wakes, memorials, black dress, and defined time of social withdrawal.

Grief involves thoughts, feelings, and behaviors. Many examples of increased morbidity (an illness or

| Box 25.1 | Factors That Influence the Experience of Loss |

- Childhood experiences
- Significance assigned to the loss
- Physical and emotional state
- Accumulated loss experience
- View of loss as crisis
- Duration and timing
- Abruptness or suddenness
- Financial impact
- Availability of resources
- Cultural factors
- Personal attributes
- Coping mechanisms
- Relationship with the lost person or object

an abnormal condition), physical and mental, are seen after significant losses. For example, an increase in the breakup of marriages and other significant relationships after the loss of a child or when one partner suffers a loss of a body part or function is observed.

When allowed to operate normally, grief has a useful function. Grief is not an episode. It is a process, sometimes one that goes on forever (e.g., parents grieving for a child). On the other hand, the grieving process can lead to resolution of the hurt and the reestablishment of one's life. Still, the emotional pain involved in grief comes and goes with a person's life experiences. Many years after a loss, something reminds the person of the loss and the associated feelings return. The reminder may be an encounter with smells, places, foods, dates, holidays, clothing, or other people.

The grieving person may try a variety of strategies to cope. The following tasks facilitate the passage from grief to closure:

- Accepting the reality of the loss
- Experiencing the pain of grief
- Adjusting to an environment that no longer includes the lost person, object, or aspect of self
- Reinvesting emotional energy into new relationships

The successful completion of these tasks leads to healthy adjustment to loss. These tasks are not sequential. In fact, grieving people often work on all four tasks simultaneously or place priority on only one or two. One of the nurse's roles is to assist patients and families in working through these tasks. Unresolved grief can result if the tasks are not completed and can lead to incomplete relationships and health problems.

In the past, society discouraged the open display of emotions such as grief. Unhappy children were told not to cry when playmates moved away, awkward adolescents were told not to be embarrassed about sudden growth spurts, and dying people were told to remain calm and dignified. Changes in attitudes, beliefs, and values have promoted more open expressions of grief. For example, nurses learn to seek support from peers and to express their concerns about dealing with terminally ill patients. Similarly, family members seek support from caregivers to express anger over loss. Grieving leads to new understandings that promote growth if a person can be open and obtains encouragement and adequate support from others.

Sometimes losses such as physical disfigurement or the death of close friends stimulate behaviors and feelings associated with the grieving process. These behaviors and feelings also occur when individuals face their own death. A patient who is dying is undergoing loss and the impact of the family's grief. Some patients feel that their families do not need any other problems and cannot cope with additional concerns. The dying patient in this situation sometimes depends extensively on the nurse, and identification of sources of support becomes a major task (Fig. 25.1).

Fig. 25.1 Nurses assist family members in finding resources to help with the grieving process.

Loss, through death or otherwise, is somewhat easier to cope with if it is expected. Sometimes the diagnosis of terminal illness allows a period of **anticipatory grief** (to expect, await, or prepare for the loss of a family member or significant other) when the dying person and the mourners can cry together and enjoy their mutual affection. Time for anticipation does not ease the pain of loss necessarily because attachment often is strengthened during the period of anticipatory grief. However, sometimes the emotions expressed at this time make the loss less conflicted than when such exchanges never occur. When individuals achieve an awareness of mortality, this maturity often leads them to anticipate eventual grief. They make a special effort to express affection and appreciation of their older adult relatives, even without evidence of impending death.

The sudden death of someone who is not "supposed to" die (sometimes referred to as "out-of-sequence" death) is the most difficult grief to bear. The clearest example is the death of a child, especially one who has lived long enough to have a distinct personality and position in the family. If the death is a violent and sudden one, the loss is particularly devastating. Parents and siblings often are wracked by powerful and personal emotions of guilt, denial, and anger, as well as sorrow. One protective impulse is to blame someone—perhaps oneself for not having been more careful or more loving, perhaps a spouse, and perhaps even the dead child.

Blame and guilt may destroy a family just when family members need one another most. The Compassionate Friends, a national self-help support organization that assists families after the death of a child, finds that many couples are driven apart by their separate reactions to the death. Perhaps one parent needs to talk about the death, whereas the other cannot bear to hear the child's name. Siblings suffer, too—partly because parents are so involved in their own grief that the surviving children are deprived of attention, and partly because a child's grief may follow a different course from that of adults. Denial and regression are common at first, with sorrow and acceptance coming much later than for adults. Each family member should try to understand and accept the many possible individual forms and paces of mourning that may be exhibited by others. Children, in particular, need to know that all questions and feelings are acceptable.

SENSE OF PRESENCE

Individuals who have experienced a loss sometimes have a nonthreatening, comforting perception that the deceased is present. Such perceptions, known as *sense of presence,* vary from general feelings of the deceased's presence to actual sensory experiences. Sometimes these sensory experiences manifest as dreams or conversations; sometimes they involve the senses and include visions, hallucinations, or the perception of voices, smells, or touch. This is a part of the mourning process that occurs because of the bond that continues between the bereaved loved ones and the deceased. Searching allows the individual to see the deceased as safe, comfortable, and at peace. Sense of presence is known to occur during the grief process and beyond.

GRIEF ATTACKS

The involuntary and unexpected reappearance of emotions and behaviors associated with grief is known as a *grief attack.* These attacks can occur in response to a variety of triggers. Eating at a restaurant or eating a certain food that triggers a memory of the deceased loved one may cause a grief attack. At other times a memory about the deceased may enter the loved one's mind and cause an attack for no particular reason. Hearing about the death of someone or reading a book that depicts a similar death as the loved one could also trigger a grief attack.

When a loved one dies, the hurt of their loss does not typically ever disappear. Time does seem to help most people with coping with the loss in a way that does not bring sadness as frequently as it once did. Generally, after some time, the sadness is replaced with fond memories of the loved one except during special occasions such as birthdays or holidays.

NURSES' GRIEF

The universality of the loss experience often leads nurses who work with the terminally ill and the bereaved to develop a heightened empathy for their patients. Identifying with patients and sharing the impact of the loss are likely to help the nurse prepare for the death experience. On the other hand, the nurse's role in supporting grieving patients and families can become complicated when nurses experience grief themselves, especially when working with dying patients. Nurses should not allow their grief to overshadow the care of patients and families. Nurses who are not aware of their own grief issues have more difficulty relating to patients as unique individuals. An example is a dying patient who reminds the nurse of a beloved grandparent, and the nurse becomes too emotionally involved. Other tasks and abilities that may be useful to the nurse working with dying patients include coming to grips with and understanding the grief process, appreciating the experience of the dying patient, using effective listening skills, acknowledging personal limits, and knowing when there is a need to get away and take care of one's self. Recognizing the need to grieve assists the nurse in moving through this process.

Nurses who experience multiple losses during work and fail to process them adequately run the risk of **bereavement overload** (before an initial loss is resolved, it is compounded by an additional loss). Frustration, anger, guilt, sadness, helplessness, anxiety, depression, and feelings of being overwhelmed are common. Self-care is critical to survival. Practice self-care and take the time to work through the grief process and mourn losses (Box 25.2). Unrelieved grief and stress can lead to diminished well-being and inability to care for others (Fig. 25.2).

Box 25.2   Survival Strategies for Nurses

- Identify personal spiritual beliefs.
- Take regular breaks or "time-outs" from the patient care area; consider rotating out of high-stress areas.
- Identify specific patients who are the most stressful so that stress can be anticipated.
- Trade patients or ask for special assistance in working in stressful situations.
- Acknowledge physical needs as key factors in stress reduction.
- Integrate decompression routines into daily life (e.g., before leaving the work area and going home, take a moment to review the day and set it aside).
- Engage in life-affirming activities (e.g., spend time with loved ones and friends).
- View losses as an opportunity to reevaluate and grow.
- Avoid the "rescuer" or "savior" complex; recognize limits.
- Recognize the need for support and do not hesitate to ask for it.
- Say "I choose" rather than "I should."
- Develop the skills of setting limits and feeling OK about saying no.
- Laugh and play in the face of tragedy without guilt.
- Seek consultation on a regular basis.

Fig. 25.2 Nurses benefit from support of colleagues during their time of loss.

Develop an ongoing personal support system when working in areas where a high number of deaths occur. Opportunities for energy renewal and mutual support foster a sense of closure for each experience. When the stresses of the job exceed its rewards and the support of peers is lacking, the result is burnout. (See Chapter 41 for further discussion of burnout.)

The nurse, who is always giving, eventually realizes that receiving is also necessary to be effective. Nursing is a job with increasingly high demands. Nurses need the ability to modify their role, acquire new ones compatible with new trends in health care delivery, and permit ethical decision making about allocation of resources. Understanding the impact of work allows improved use of problem-solving techniques to guide choices and prevent dysfunctional responses to loss.

Being informed and current, practicing within the legal parameters of professional responsibilities, and using current trends in health care promote competence in many fields, including the expertise of caring for the dying patient.

STAGES OF GRIEF AND DYING

There is no right or wrong way to grieve. The concepts and theories of grief are only tools for the nurse to use to anticipate potential needs of patients and families and to plan interventions to help patients understand their grief while trying to deal with it. It is a mistake, and possibly harmful, to expect patients to progress in some specific manner over a specified time. The nurse's role is to assess grieving behaviors, recognize the influence of grief on behavior, and provide empathic support.

Thanatology (the study of dying and death) has sparked much interest since the 1970s. See Box 25.3 for more information on theories of grief and mourning.

Table 25.1 describes some of the concepts of death and dying typically held by specific age groups. With knowledge of these developmental stages, the nurse can better understand a patient's responses to a life-threatening situation and the grief responses of individuals after a loss.

COMPLICATED GRIEF

Bereavement is a state of great risk physically, emotionally, and socially. For this reason, the importance of grief work cannot be overstated.

Various theorists have described behaviors indicative of unresolved grief. As the term indicates, unresolved grief signifies some disturbance of the normal progression toward resolution. Complicated grieving (unresolved grief or complicated mourning; also called dysfunctional grieving) is a delayed or exaggerated response to a perceived, actual, or potential loss. Complicated

---

Box **25.3**	Theories of Grief and Mourning

KÜBLER-ROSS'S STAGES OF DYING

A behavior-oriented theory that includes five stages:

- *Denial:* Individual acts as though nothing has happened and may refuse to believe or understand loss has occurred.
- *Anger:* Individual resists the loss and may strike out at everyone and everything.
- *Bargaining:* Individual postpones awareness of reality of the loss and may try to deal in a subtle or overt way as though the loss can be prevented.
- *Depression:* Individual feels overwhelmingly lonely and withdraws from interpersonal interaction.
- *Acceptance:* Individual accepts the loss and looks to the future.

BOWLBY'S PHASES OF MOURNING

A behavioral theory that includes four phases:

- *Numbing:* Individual describes phase as feeling "stunned" or "unreal." It is a period of intense emotion that serves to protect the body from consequences of loss and lasts from a few hours to a week or more.
- *Yearning and searching:* Phase arouses acute distress in most people. Painful phase is characterized by physical symptoms such as tightness in the chest and throat, shortness of breath, a feeling of weakness, and lethargy, insomnia, and anorexia. Phase may last for months or years.
- *Disorganization and despair:* Individual endlessly examines how and why the loss occurred. It is a

common time for person to express anger. Gradually phase gives way to an acceptance that loss is permanent.

- *Reorganization:* Individual begins to accept unaccustomed roles, acquire new skills, and build new relationships. Phase may last a year or more. Individual needs support to unlink self from the lost relationships.

WORDEN'S TASKS OF MOURNING

A behavioral theory that indicates four tasks:

- *Accept reality of loss:* There is always some period of disbelief and surprise over a loss. This task involves processes needed to accept that the person or object is gone and will not return.
- *Work through pain and grief:* Emotional pain comes as a natural part of loss. Individuals who deny or shut off the pain prolong their grief.
- *Adjust to environment in which the deceased is missing:* Individual does not realize full impact of loss for at least 3 months. At this point, friends and associates stop calling, and the person is left prey to loneliness. Often the individual must take on roles formerly filled by the deceased.
- *To find an enduring connection with the deceased while embarking on a new life:* Individual does not forget the deceased or give up the relationship with the deceased. The deceased, however, must take a new, less prominent, place in a person's emotional life. People dealing with this task fear they will forget their loved one.

From Perry A, Potter P, Ostendorf W: *Clinical nursing skills and techniques,* ed 9, St. Louis, 2018, Elsevier.

Table **25.1**   Age-Related Influences on the Concept of Death

Infancy to 5 years	• Does not understand concept of death • Infant's sense of separation forms basis for later understanding of loss and death • Believes death is reversible, a temporary departure, or sleep
5–9 years	• Understands that death is final • Believes own death can be avoided • Associates death with aggression or violence • Believes wishes or unrelated actions can be responsible for death
9–12 years	• Understands death as the inevitable end of life • Begins to understand own mortality • Concept of death expressed as interest in afterlife or as fear of death
12–18 years	• Fears a lingering death • May fantasize that death can be defied, acting out defiance through reckless behaviors (e.g., dangerous driving, substance abuse) • Seldom thinks about death, but views it in religious and philosophic terms • May seem to reach "adult" perception of death but is emotionally unable to accept it
18–45 years	• Has attitude toward death influenced by religious and cultural beliefs
45–65 years	• Accepts own mortality • Encounters death of parents and some peers • Experiences peaks of death anxiety • Death anxiety diminishes with emotional well-being
65+ years	• Fears prolonged illness • Encounters death of family members and peers • Sees death as having multiple meanings (e.g., freedom from pain, reunion with already deceased family members)

Box **25.4**   Complicated Grief

When a person has difficulty progressing through the normal stages of grieving, bereavement becomes complicated. In these cases, bereavement appears to "go wrong," and loss never resolves, which threatens a person's relationships with others. Complicated grief includes four types:
- *Chronic grief:* Active acute mourning characterized by normal grief reactions that do not decrease but persist over long periods. People verbalize an inability to "get past" the grief.
- *Delayed grief:* Characterized by normal grief reactions that are suppressed or postponed. The survivor consciously or unconsciously avoids the pain of the loss. Active grieving is held back, only to resurface later, usually in response to a trivial loss or upset. For example, a wife only grieves a few weeks after the death of her spouse, only to become hysterical and sad a year later when she loses her car keys. The extreme sadness is a delayed response to the death of her husband.
- *Exaggerated grief:* People become overwhelmed by grief, and they cannot function. This is reflected in the form of severe phobias or self-destructive behaviors such as alcoholism, substance abuse, or suicide.
- *Masked grief:* Survivors are not aware that behaviors that interfere with normal functioning are a result of their loss. For example, a person who has lost a pet has changes in sleeping or eating patterns develop.

From Perry A, Potter P, Ostendorf W: *Clinical nursing skills and techniques,* ed 9, St. Louis, 2018, Elsevier.

grieving occurs when individuals: (1) get "stuck" in the grief process and become depressed; (2) are unable to express feelings; (3) cannot find anyone in their daily life who acts as the listener they need; (4) suffer a loss that stirs up other, unresolved losses and causes them to explore long-standing feelings or emotional concerns; or (5) lack the reassurance and support to trust the grief process and fail to believe that they can work through the loss. A surviving spouse who seeks additional support for many years after the loss of a significant other (Box 25.4) provides one example. The more signs, symptoms, and behaviors the mourner has, the stronger the likelihood of unresolved grief (see Nursing Care Plan 25.1). These individuals must be recognized and referred for appropriate counseling or treatment (see Fig. 25.1).

SUPPORTIVE CARE DURING THE DYING AND GRIEVING PROCESS

Assessment

To give compassionate nursing care and support to the family and the patient during the grieving and dying process, consider the five aspects of human functioning: physical, emotional, intellectual, sociocultural, and spiritual. Assess each area, using the nursing process, to fully understand the patient's needs and provide appropriate interventions.

Physical assessment. While interviewing and observing the patient, assess such areas as sleeping patterns, body

Nursing Care Plan 25.1 | **The Patient Experiencing Complicated Grieving (Unresolved Grief)**

Ms. S. is 78 years old and is being admitted for weakness, chronic fatigue, anorexia, and weight loss. Her nursing history reveals that Ms. S. refuses to care for herself, has stopped participating in her church activities, and is unable to discuss the deceased without crying. The social history of Ms. S. reveals that her only child, a daughter, died unexpectedly at age 47. Her husband of 50 years died 1 year later. Ms. S. is accompanied by her grandchildren, who offer support and concern. The nursing assessment reveals that Ms. S. lacks resolution of previous grieving response and is experiencing bereavement overload.

PATIENT PROBLEM
Complex Grief, related to bereavement overload, as a result of death of daughter and husband, manifested by refusing to care for self, abstaining from participation in church activities, the inability to discuss the deceased without crying, alterations in eating habits, and interference with performance of activities of daily living (ADLs).

Patient Goals And Expected Outcomes	Nursing Interventions
Patient will establish new and meaningful relationships and interests Patient will engage in constructive, meaningful lifestyle (precrisis level of functioning)Patient will relate realistically to the pleasures and the disappointments of the lost relationships Patient will participate in decision making and cooperate with recommended treatment within 2 weeks	Establish trust and positive regard by creating an atmosphere of sharing.Offer privacy and security. Identify significance of multiple losses. Promote resolution of the grieving process. Discuss ambivalence. Assess stage of grief and support patient's expressions of grief. Use active listening. Facilitate discussion of positive and negative aspects of loss. Provide opportunities for social interaction, especially with those who have coped with similar losses. Teach patient and significant others about the grieving process. Assure patient that feelings are normal. Expect patient to meet responsibilities and give positive reinforcement. Help patient identify ways to adapt lifestyle to accommodate loss. Explore ways to assist patient to make new emotional investments. If you become uncomfortable with your unresolved feelings of loss, contact another nurse to counsel the patient.

CRITICAL THINKING QUESTIONS
1. Ms. S. is admitted to the medical unit for severe weakness, weight loss, and chronic depression. She is reluctant to get out of bed to dress and have meals. How can the nurse facilitate progression through the grieving process?
2. Ms. S. appears thin, with poor tissue turgor. How can the nurse and dietitian encourage improvement of her nutritional status?
3. The nursing assessment for Ms. S. revealed a flat affect, little verbalization, and poor personal hygiene. Which therapeutic nursing interventions can help achieve patient goals and expected outcomes?

From Moorhead S, Johnson M, Maas M, Swanson E: *Nursing outcome classification (NOC)*, ed 6, St. Louis, 2018, Elsevier.

 Nursing Care Plan 25.2 | **The Patient Facing Death**

Ms. B. is 68 years old and has been admitted to the hospital for weakness and debilitation caused by widespread metastatic cancer of the colon. She reports pain and is anxious to return home. Ms. B. and her family are aware of her terminal prognosis. The nursing history identified that Ms. B.: (1) is unable to care for herself because of severe weakness; (2) has chronic pain; (3) has a decreased appetite; (4) appears anxious and wants to be home with her family; and (5) is grieving the loss of her health and expresses fears regarding her death.

PATIENT PROBLEM
Prolonged Pain, related to disease progression.

Nursing Care Plan 25.2   The Patient Facing Death—cont'd

Patient Goals And Expected Outcomes	Nursing Interventions	Evaluation
Patient will verbalize moderate comfort and decreased pain while receiving analgesics and other comfort measures	Position patient comfortably; change position gradually and unhurriedly. Provide pain-relief measures patient prefers (e.g., relaxation therapy, diversion, and distraction). Give analgesics as ordered. Evaluate pain for intensity and quality. Know that pain is what patient says it is. Observe patient's freedom of movement. Ask patient to rate pain on a scale of 1–10 and compare with baseline data. Use after nursing therapies are administered. Use combinations of analgesics or other therapies as patient's needs change. Provide frequent rest periods in a quiet environment. Time and pace nursing activities to conserve patient's energy. Minimize irritants through skin care, including daily baths, lubrication of skin, frequent repositioning, and dry, clean bed linens.	Patient states pain is relieved or decreased in intensity within 30 min to 1 h after administration of medication 75% of the time.

PATIENT PROBLEM

Inability to bathe self, dress self, toilet self, or feed self, related to weakness and advanced disease.

Patient Goals And Expected Outcomes	Nursing Interventions	Evaluation
Patient will carry out ADLs at highest ability with nurse's assistance as necessary	Assist with ADLs but allow patient and family to assist when able. Provide sufficient time for ADLs. Include patient in determining care routine. Provide frequent oral care q 2–4 h. Use soft toothbrushes or foam swabs for frequent mouth care. Apply a light film of petroleum jelly to lips and tongue. Remove crusts from eyelid margins and provide eye care. Reduce corneal drying with artificial tears. Protect skin from irritation and breakdown using absorbent pads and clean linen. Cluster hygiene activities to conserve strength	Patient indicates satisfaction with level of personal hygiene achieved.

PATIENT PROBLEM

Insufficient Nutrition, related to disease progression

Patient Goals And Expected Outcomes	Nursing Interventions	Evaluation
The patient will be able to consume 50% of her meals	Maintain and document food intake. Confer with dietitian to increase kilocalories and protein intake and discuss patient's nutritional needs. Assist with frequent oral hygiene. Assist with environmental control (temperature, appearance, odors). Identify food preferences and provide the preferences as often as possible. Suggest that smaller portions may be more palatable. Allow home-cooked meals, as preferred by patient (gives family a chance to participate). Provide relief of thirst by using ice chips, sips of fluids, or moist cloth to lips.	Patient has maintained weight for 2 weeks.

CRITICAL THINKING QUESTIONS

1. Ms. B. reports severe bone pain and nausea. She appears cachexic and extremely weak. What are some nursing interventions to decrease Ms. B.'s symptoms?
2. Ms. B. says, "I want to go home to die. I don't want to stay in the hospital. All I want to do is go home and be with my family." How can the hospice team most beneficially assist Ms. B.?
3. When the nurse enters Ms. B.'s room to begin ADLs, she notes the patient's extreme fatigue and lethargy. What are some nursing interventions to conserve Ms. B.'s strength?

From Moorhead S, Johnson M, Maas M, Swanson E: *Nursing outcome classification (NOC)*, ed 6, St. Louis, 2018, Elsevier.

image, activities of daily living (ADLs), mobility, general health, medication use, and pain. Additional areas of concern include the basic needs of nutrition, elimination, oxygenation, activity, rest, sleep, and safety (see Nursing Care Plan 25.2).

Interventions should target: (1) energy conservation; (2) pain-reduction techniques; (3) comfort measures; (4) promotion of sleep and rest; and (5) increasing self-esteem through body image acceptance.

Emotional assessment. Preparation for death is an endeavor filled with anxiety and fear for most people. Assess the patient's and the family's level of anxiety, guilt, anger, and acceptance. Major fears of the dying patient include fears of abandonment (fear of dying alone), loss of control, pain and discomfort, and the unknown.

Nurses intervene appropriately when they can accept the patient's and the family's feelings, whatever they may be. Offer encouragement and support and give the patient "permission to die" by assisting the patient in saying goodbye.

Intellectual assessment. Intellectual assessment includes an evaluation of the patient's and the family's educational level, their knowledge and abilities, and the expectations they have in regard to how and when death will occur. Some aspects of functioning in the intellectual dimension frequently are altered during the dying process because of physiologic changes, medications, the patient's emotional state, and the disease process. Remaining alert to these changes allows for the avoidance of problems if the patient's memory or sensations are decreased.

In most cases, interventions are directed toward patient and family education and support. Keeping everyone informed of procedures, changes in the patient's condition, and hospital policies can allow the patient and family to make well-informed and satisfactory decisions.

Sociocultural assessment. The assessment of the patient's and the family's support systems is valuable. Assessment helps to ascertain whether family members want to assist in the patient's daily care. Not only does this lessen the family's sense of loss of control but it also helps clarify what tasks the family will do and what will be done by nursing staff. If these needs and desires are not clear, distrust and hostility between family and nursing staff can result. Each family and each member in that family are unique in what they wish to do. Never assume that families want to deliver daily care. Many do, but others do not, and they need the opportunity to make that choice (Box 25.5).

Family members need support to get through the dying and death of their loved one. It is also beneficial for family members and loved ones to provide support for one another; encourage this mutual support. Recognize the value of family members as resources and assist them in working with the dying person.

Box 25.5   **Suggestions for Involving the Family in the Care of the Dying Patient**

- The thanatologic philosophy dictates that family members are free to choose if and when they wish to be with the patient who is dying. Do not raise a barrier because of "visitation hours."
- Allow young children to visit a dying patient when the patient is able to communicate.
- Be willing to listen to family members' complaints about the patient's care and to their feelings about the patient.
- Help family members learn to interact with the dying patient (e.g., using attentive listening, avoiding false reassurances, conducting conversations about normal family activities or problems).
- Allow family members to help with as much or as little patient care as they desire.
- When the family becomes fatigued with care activities, relieve them from their duties so that they can get the rest and support they need. Refer them to resources for meals and lodging.
- Support the act of shared grieving among patient and family. Provide privacy when preferred. Do not discourage open expression of grief between family and patient.
- As the time of death approaches, assist family members to stay in communication with the dying patient through short visits, caring silence, touch, and telling the patient of their love for him or her.
- After death, assist the family with decision making, such as selection of a mortician, transportation of family members, and collection of the patient's belongings.

In the home, the family becomes closely involved in the patient's care (see Chapters 37 and 40). A terminal illness places heavy demands on the social and financial resources. The emotional strain often disrupts normal communication channels. The family may become increasingly afraid to interact with the patient.

When families choose to take the patient home for care, be sure that they are well prepared before discharge for what they need to know. Arrange for hospice services to assist the family, if they are receptive. Emphasize continuity of care and constant availability for when the patient has an emotional or physical crisis and needs ongoing support.

During the social assessment, learn whom the patient considers to be the most supportive person in his or her life. It may be a friend, coworker, or fellow church member. Help this person to become a part of the patient's supportive network and be included in planning the patient's care. Encourage these social support people to become involved, and at the same time, maintain and promote the patient's independence whenever possible.

Spiritual assessment. Assess the spiritual dimension by gaining insight into the patient's philosophy of life, spirituality, and religious resources. Find out what significance the rituals of the particular faith group have for the patient in dealing with death. It is imperative for the nurse to self-assess feelings related to death and dying experiences. It is equally important to avoid judging others and avoid attempting to interpret and analyze the spiritual aspect of death and dying. Create an atmosphere of openness to discuss the patient's spiritual concerns.

Therapeutic interventions related to topics of death and dying involve an interaction between the members of the intradisciplinary care team, clergy, friends and family. Support of the patient's and the family's belief systems and values is important (see Chapter 6).

One aspect of this belief system is hope. Hope can take many forms. The challenge is to assist the patient and the family to identify those hopes that are most important to them to help them to cope.

Hope can be considered a life force that is multidimensional (taking many forms) and fluid. Hope is the common thread identified in all stages of grief. It is characterized by confidence, even though the hopeful individual does not necessarily expect to achieve a specific goal. Hope does not comprise a single act but is a complex series of changing thoughts, feelings, and actions. Many sources report a significant relationship between the level of hope and the level of coping. In addition, the strength of religious connections and the performance of family role responsibilities are related significantly to the variables of hope and coping.

Hope is difficult to maintain during the dying process. As the patient's condition deteriorates, the nurse's challenge becomes one of assisting the patient and family in translating their hope for a cure into realistic hopes that are focused on short-term, achievable goals. These may be the hope for a comfortable and pain-free life or the desire to live long enough to participate in some important family event, such as the wedding of a child. A total lack of hope exhausts the human spirit. When hope is relinquished, death follows rapidly.

Shock and Denial

Shock and denial are common reactions that occur during the grieving process. Nurses can be a great source of support during the time of experiencing these reactions. Nursing responsibilities often include providing guidance and understanding and answering questions that loved ones have when in shock or denial. The nurse frequently spends time with the family while dealing with shock and denial and may offer further support through counselors, clergy, or various support groups. See Box 25.6 for tips on breaking bad news to the family or patient.

❖ NURSING PROCESS IN LOSS AND GRIEF

The role of the licensed practical nurse/licensed vocational nurse (LPN/LVN) in the nursing process as stated is that the LPN/LVN will:

| Box 25.6 | Breaking Bad News |

Generally, the health care provider delivers any unexpected bad news, but occasionally, nurses must give families the news of a death or participate in the delivery of the bad news. Accompany the health care provider who is approaching a family with unexpected or traumatic news, especially when it involves a death, and remain with the family after the health care provider leaves. When you must deliver bad news, use the following guidelines:

- Deliver the news in a private location.
  - Have a self awareness that delivering this information may cause feelings of sadness and helplessness.
  - Provide tissues
  - Provide an introduction of the health care members who will be meeting with the family and their roles.
  - Plan what information will be shared with the family members.
- Review the relationship of the audience to the deceased. Determine the role they fill for the deceased.
- Assess the family dynamic to ensure that the information is provided to the appropriate person.
- Allow time for questions.
- Provide resources for support after the news is delivered.
  - Allow time for questions to be asked. Provide the information clearly. Avoid using potentially difficult to understand medical or technical terms.
- If needed be prepared to remain with the family members after the information is provided.
  - Determine if the family wants to have time with the deceased.
  - Ensure the family members are feeling able to safely leave the health care facility.
- Bring in clergy who can support and remain with families after the formal discussion of facts has concluded, if the family desires. Seek nursing supervisor assistance when needed to further assist family members as indicated (see Fig. 25.1).

- Participate in planning care for patients based on patient needs.
- Review the patient's plan of care and recommend revisions as needed.
- Review and follow defined prioritization for patient care.
- Use clinical pathways, care maps, or care plans to guide and review patient care.

By completing the assessment, diagnosis, planning, outcomes identification, implementation, and evaluation, the LPN/LVN can develop a nursing care plan.

◆ ASSESSMENT

Begin care of the grieving patient by collecting subjective and objective data about the meaning of loss to the patient and family or significant others. Interview the patient and family, observing their responses and behavior. Do not try to assess how the patient *should be* reacting but rather how the patient *is* reacting. Some behaviors or phases occur in sequence. In contrast, sometimes behaviors or phases in the death and dying process may be skipped, omitted, or experienced in a different order. Many variables affect grief. Assessment of these variables gives the nurse a broad database with which to individualize care. When nurses provide care to patients from other backgrounds, they should perform the assessment attentively and listen for clues to beliefs and practices regarding health and illness.

Interpretation of a loss varies greatly with a person's cultural and ethnic background. Many sources note that ethnicity is related strongly to attitudes toward life-sustaining treatments during terminal illness. The form the expression of grief takes generally is linked to cultural background and family practices. Culturally determined traditions often dictate how a family support system is to behave. For example, in the Western tradition, the grieving process is usually personal and private, with individuals showing emotional restraint. The ceremonies that surround a person's death offer time and a means for grief resolution and reminiscing. In Eastern nations, respect for the dead may be shown with louder verbal expression and physical demonstration of grief for a specified period. Despite these general tendencies, however, members of the same ethnocultural background often respond differently to loss and death.

◆ PATIENT PROBLEM

After thorough and thoughtful data collection, identify patient problems related to the patient's clinical situation. Formulate an individualized patient problem statement by noting and analyzing any clustering of patient or family behaviors, actual or potential losses, and data involving the loss (Box 25.7).

The mere presence of one or two defining characteristics is usually insufficient to identify a patient problem accurately. Be vigilant and do not overlook competing patient problems. For example, if a patient who is dying manifests an increase in crying or tearfulness, displays of anger, and frequent nightmares, consider several possible patient problem statements, because these characteristics are common to more than one patient problem. Among the choices are *Recent Onset of Pain, Impaired Coping,* and *Impaired Belief System.* Until you examine all the available data and inquire about the presence of other behaviors and symptoms, you are unable to determine a correct patient problem with any accuracy.

For selection of appropriate interventions for the patient's care, identification of the relevant context, or the related factor, is also necessary. For example, *Grief* that results from the loss of a job greatly differs than the interventions for *Grief* experienced from the loss of health and wellbeing.

For the patient who is seriously ill, several patient problems are possible. Addressing all of these complex problems simultaneously is impossible. On any given

---

Box 25.7	**Patient Problem Statements Related to Grieving**

Grief, related to:
- Potential loss of significant other
- Potential loss of physiopsychosocial well-being

Complex grief or potential for complex grief, related to:
- Actual or potential object loss
- Absence of anticipatory grieving
- Lack of resolution of previous grieving response
- Loss of significant other
- Thwarted grieving response to a loss

Fear of dying/death, related to:
- Anticipation of pain, suffering, and impact of death on others
- Confronting the reality of terminal disease
- Discussions on the topic of death
- Uncertainty about the after-life following death

Insufficient nutrition, related to:
- Depressed grief response
- Loss of significant other
- Change in social status
- Situational transition or crisis

Side effects of medication therapies
  Impaired family processes related to:
  - Situational transition or crisis
  Despair, related to:
  - Failing or deteriorating physiologic condition

Impaired belief system or potential for impaired belief system, related to:
- Separation from religious and cultural ties
- Situational transition or crisis

Potential for Impaired Human Dignity, related to:
- Compromised maintenance of health
- Impaired decision-making ability

---

day or at any one time, two or three problem areas demand the nurse's attention. These priorities shift according to the patient's condition, so reevaluate and restate priorities constantly.

In addition to a patient problem related directly to grief, other health problems common to grieving are also likely to be diagnosed, such as *Anxiousness* or *Insufficient Nutrition.* In these situations, focus the interventions on supporting or resolving grief before attempting to solve the other problems. For example, if the patient continues to have loss of appetite related to severe anxiousness, simply improving the nutritional value and variety of available foods has little impact on nutritional status.

◆ EXPECTED OUTCOMES AND PLANNING

Nursing interventions should be planned to meet the physiologic, emotional, developmental, and spiritual needs of the grieving patient. Draw on resources among the patient's friends and family, clergy, support groups, and legal consultants and focus on achieving specific goals and outcomes that relate to the identified patient problem statement.

The following are examples of possible goals and outcomes:

Goal 1: Patient will actively participate in grief work.

Outcome: Patient expresses thoughts and feelings related to loss.

Goal 2: Patient will verbalize finding meaning in life.

Outcome: Patient verbalizes future goals and plans.

In developing a comprehensive plan to help patients deal with loss and grief, include other professionals within the health care team and in the greater community as resources. Suggesting consultation with other professionals or providing resources contributes to the patient's well-being. These external resources should be incorporated into the plan of care. Patients may have concerns about financial matters or the making or revising of a will; the best intervention for them may be referral to legal aid or to a private attorney. Also remember to treat each patient and family as unique, and recognize that their needs, fears, hopes, expectations, and concerns change throughout the illness.

◆ IMPLEMENTATION

Nursing care of the terminally ill patient is often demanding and stressful. It is important to recognize the value of family members as resources and assist them in working with the dying patient (see Box 25.5 and the Patient Teaching box on the dying patient and family). Also, consider any special needs of the older adult (see the Lifespan Considerations for Older Adults box).

 Patient Teaching

DYING PATIENT AND FAMILY

- Describe and demonstrate feeding techniques and selection of foods to facilitate ease of chewing and swallowing.
- Demonstrate bathing, mouth care, and other hygiene measures and allow the family to perform a return demonstration.
- Show a video on simple transfer techniques to prevent injury to themselves and the patient; help family members practice.
- Teach the family to recognize the signs and symptoms to expect as the patient's condition worsens and provide information on whom to call in an emergency.
- Discuss ways to support the dying person and listen to needs and fears.
- Solicit questions from the family and provide information as needed.
- Provide teaching, information, and encouragement in the use of creative outlets for expressing feelings and communicating with others. Encourage the use of tape-recorded messages, drawings, writings, imagery, music, and poetry. (This also assists patients and families in creating memories that can be comforting later.)
- Inform the patient and family of relaxation techniques.
- Observe the family and patient interacting with effective communication skills.

 Lifespan Considerations

Older Adults

Dying And Death

- Many older adults have long-standing religious beliefs that are likely to influence their response to death and dying. Be sure spiritual counselors are available.
- Despite their age, older adults may still struggle to accept impending death.
- Encourage open communication between the older adult and their family support system.
- Respect patients who are not comfortable talking about death and dying.
- Attitudes of older adults about death vary greatly. Some will accept it others continue to avoid discussions about it.
- Some older adults feel free to discuss death; others avoid this topic. Encourage patients to discuss their feelings by giving permission and making yourself available to the bereaved.
- With aging comes increasing experiences with death and loss. Losses may include friends, family, significant other/spouse,
- The loss of independence can be as significant as the loss of a friend or family member.
- The older adult often needs emotional support to cope with grief.
  Open communication by the dying patient is key to ensuring their wishes are carried out.
- Loss of a partner/spouse in older adulthood is may also result in relocation. This increases the stress level of an already grieving older person and the risk of new health problems or an exacerbation of existing illness.
- Increasing number of older adults have advance directive.
- Older adults have the right to a dignified death.
- When caring for an older patient who is dying, it is important to prevent feelings of loneliness and abandonment and to maintain the patient's self-esteem. This can be achieved by ensuring that attentive care is given: speak directly to the patient, ensure that pain control measures are effective, and keep the room environment pleasant.
- The older adult often feels a loss of control; therefore, the nurse should offer choices to the patient regarding care. Family members are often unaware that the dying older adult seeks their permission to die. Educate family members about this need and allow family members to be with the dying patient at any time.
- Comorbidity (more than one disease process) is common among older adults.
- Uncertainty of the prognosis of chronic illnesses can make treatment decisions difficult.
- Geriatric pharmacology and awareness of multiple drug interactions is vital.
- The most frequent symptoms experienced by the dying older adult are pain, respiratory distress, and confusion.

A return to full functioning is not an expected outcome for a terminally ill patient or even a person who experiences significant disability or other loss of function. Always have the goal of enabling the patient to return to optimal physical and emotional functioning.

This does not mean that the patient and family do not experience sadness or other disturbing emotions but that they adapt and cope effectively with the stressors in their life. Use a variety of techniques and interventions to assist patients to function optimally under severe stress; to make effective decisions regarding their care; and to cope with disappointment, frustration, and other emotions caused by their illness.

◆ EVALUATION

Refer to the goals and outcomes identified when planning care, and perform measures designed to evaluate the achievement of those goals.

Goal 1: Patient will actively participate in grief work.
Evaluative measures:
- Patient observed discussing loss with significant other.
- Patient demonstrates progress in dealing with stages of grief at his or her own pace.
- Patient participates in self-care, ADLs, and family conversations.

Goal 2: Patient will verbalize finding meaning in life.
Evaluative measures:
- Patient indicates to the health care team or family that he or she finds "peace" in meditation.
- Patient verbalizes goals and plans.
- Patient verbalizes progress in resolution of grief.

The patient expects individualization of care, including comfort, dignity, and cooperation, to maximize quality of life. The success of the evaluation depends partially on the bond you form with the patient. Unless the patient can trust you fully, he or she is not likely to share personal desires. Once you establish rapport, be ever vigilant to avoid problems that threaten it.

The following questions validate the achievement of the nursing interventions:
- "Am I meeting your expectations while providing your care?"
- "Would you like me to assist you in a different manner?"
- "Do you have a specific request that I can use in your care at this time?"
- "Is there another problem that we are overlooking or that you feel is of higher priority?"
- "Are we dealing with your problems in a timely manner?"

Through communication and assessment, continue to evaluate whether the outcome criteria have been satisfied. Use this process to judge the extent to which the goals that were chosen initially have been accomplished. Often evaluation of how well the patient's needs have been met is easy, but ascertaining the same for the family may prove to be more difficult.

SPECIAL SUPPORTIVE CARE

Often death occurs outside the realm of serious illness, injury, or aging. Perinatal, pediatric, suicidal, and older adult deaths are some examples that warrant special consideration.

PERINATAL DEATH

The death of a child is often viewed as one of the most devastating losses that can occur in a family. If the death of the child occurs before, during, or shortly after birth, it is called perinatal death.

Give special consideration to permitting the parents and family to grieve adequately. Loved ones will be left with few or no memories about the child to hold on to. "Acting as though it never happened" places parents in jeopardy of living with unresolved grief. When possible, enable the parents to see, touch, and hold the infant so that they can face the reality of the situation and resolve their grief. Listen attentively, and allow the parents to express their feelings over their loss. Refer to the baby as "your baby," "your son," or "your daughter," or use the given name, to reinforce that the baby was a unique individual who was loved and will be missed. Support the usual cultural rituals after death for the baby, such as a funeral or memorial service.

Some agencies give a lock of the baby's hair, a blanket the baby was wrapped in, or an identification bracelet to the parents. Photographs and footprints may be made to provide additional mementos to the parents. Hospitals often have policies to retain such items for a later date in case the parents initially refuse them. Agencies also often acknowledge the first-year anniversary of the infant's death.

Other agencies provide angel boxes, which are decorated or painted memorial boxes containing some mementos for the bereaved parents. Suggested items for the angel boxes are booklets on loss and coping with a loss, a wooden angel, a crocheted angel that was touched by the newborn or used during the pictures, a quilt or crocheted blanket, a lock of hair of the newborn if the hair is long enough, footprints and handprints, a clay imprint of the foot, seeds to plant in remembrance of the infant, and the digital camera card with pictures of the infant.

The Angel Gown program provides comfort to the bereaved families through the gift of a beautiful custom-made gown or vest for final photos and for burial services along with support resources and mentoring programs for the family (NICU Helping Hands, n.d.). The custom-made gown or vest is made from wedding and pastel bridesmaid dresses that were donated to the organization. "Now I Lay Me Down to Sleep" provides a specially trained photographer to take pictures of the infant and family for free (Now I Lay Me Down to Sleep, n.d.). Each agency handles the death of an infant in a specific way; please check with your facility for the nursing practices being used.

PEDIATRIC DEATH

The nurse caring for children faced with death needs special skills. Be aware of how children view or understand death, their own and that of others. These

Lifespan Considerations

Infants and Children

A Child's Understanding Of Death

A child's reaction to and understanding of death and dying depends on the developmental stage of the child and parental values and beliefs, culture, and religious orientation. The first way to help children develop a positive attitude toward death is to counsel parents. Parents need to understand a child's age-specific understanding of death and the normal reactions of a child to death. Parents may use "small deaths"—of a pet, for example—to help children become familiar and comfortable with a loss.

When death occurs in a family, parents often try to shield children from the loss. They fear the child will not be able to cope with the grief. However, allowing children to feel emotions appropriate to events prepares them for more traumatic experiences later in life. The child's developmental level determines the proper amount and type of detailed information to discuss with the child.

When a child is dying, parents and siblings often feel considerable anger and resentment. The death of a child usually is seen as unfair. Some parents' inclination is to withhold information about the illness from the dying child. Even young children, however, often perceive that something is wrong with them because of the changes in behavior they see in parents. Work together with parents to plan their child's care, and determine the level of participation they desire. Do not attempt to assume a parental role or relinquish important nursing responsibilities. Parents and children need to know specifics about the plan of therapy and the normalcy of their reaction to the loss. Friends and relatives commonly avoid contact with the dying child and family because of fear over the child's illness. Parents must decide whether they wish to maintain contact with significant others. Such a resource frequently proves valuable.

The following are basic guidelines to follow while providing care for a child who is dying or experiencing the death of a loved one:

- Allow young children to visit a dying parent or grandparent if all parties consent. (Some dying patients have strong feelings about possibly traumatizing children during this transition.)
- Ascertain the child's understanding and experience of death. Developmental theories regarding children's concepts of death are based on cognitive stage of development.
- Respect the family's wishes for how and what to tell children about serious illness, dying, and death. If the parents wish to be honest with the child, straightforward, yet caring, explanations are important.
- Use of play therapy or drawing may help a child express emotions, fears, and understanding about death.
- Answer parents' questions with specific details, taking into consideration the family's cultural background and knowledge level.
- Parents should be allowed to stay with the child at any time of day or night.
- Explain signs and symptoms of approaching death.
- Reassure parents that everything possible was done for the child.
- When possible, the topic of organ donation should be approached with the family before the death of the child. Many families appreciate this topic being brought to their attention because they would not think of it on their own. Many find it comforting to know they can help others.
- Make every effort to arrange for family members, especially parents, to be with the child at the time of death, if they wish to be present. For many, viewing the body is a sign of closure, an opportunity to finish their goodbyes.
- Treat the family and child as a unit. Encourage parents to stay with the child and participate in care as much as desired or possible.
- Understand that decisions to end treatment can be more difficult when children are involved.

Data from Perry A, Potter P, Ostendorf W: *Clinical nursing skills and techniques,* ed 9, St. Louis, 2018, Elsevier; and Hockenberry M, Wilson D, Rogers C: *Wong's essentials of pediatric nursing,* ed 10, St. Louis, 2017, Elsevier.

---

children are usually aware that they are going to die. They often try to protect their parents. They need to be told the truth in language they can understand and be allowed to share fears, feelings, and opinions (see the Lifespan Considerations for Infants and Children box).

Most of all, children, like adults, need reassurance from their nurse, health care provider, and family that they will not suffer or be abandoned and left alone. A letter written by a 13-year-old boy who died of leukemia beautifully summarizes the needs of the dying child. This letter was written to the editor of a newspaper in the 1970s and published in a column written by Saul Kapel, MD (1974):

I am a 13-year-old boy. I am dying. I write this to you who are and will become nurses and doctors in the hope that by sharing my feelings with you, you may someday be better able to help those who share my experience.

But no one likes to talk about such things. In fact, no one likes to talk much at all. Doctoring and nursing must be advancing, but I wish it would hurry. The dying person is not yet seen as a person and thus cannot be communicated with as such. He is a symbol of what every human fears and what we each know….

But for me, fear is today and dying now. You slip in and out of my room, give me medication and check my blood pressure. Is it because you are insecure or just a human being that I sense your fright? Why are you afraid?

I am the one who is dying. I know you feel insecure, don't know what to say, don't know what to do. But please believe me, if you care, you can't go wrong. Just admit that you care. This is really what we search for.

We may ask for whys and wherefores, but we really don't want answers.

Don't run away. Wait. All I want to know is that there will be someone to hold my hand when I need it. I'm afraid. Death may be routine to you, but it is new to me. You may not see me as unique, but I've never died before. To me once is unique.

You whisper about my youth, but when one is dying, is he really so young anymore? I have lots I wish we could talk about. It really would not take much of your time, because you are in here quite a bit anyway.

If only we could be honest—both admit of our fears, touch one another. If you really care, would you lose so much of your professionalism if you even cried with me just person to person? Then it might not be so hard to die in a hospital with friends and relatives close by.

This heartrending essay describes the need of a child for honest and caring communication. Parents and loved ones have much difficulty in accepting the reality of a child's impending death. The death of a child is an "out-of-sequence" death and therefore is often more difficult to accept. Parents often harbor extreme guilt. They may express hostility and anger toward health care providers, God, or the world in general. Grandparents suffer a double grief—for themselves and for their son or daughter. Siblings also are affected extremely and need much support at this time. During the dying process and after a child's death, survivors often can derive benefit from supportive group therapy.

SUICIDE

There were 47,511 suicides according to 2019 statistics in the United States, an average of 130 each day. Suicide was the tenth leading cause of death for all ages (CDC, 2021). Survivors of someone who has committed suicide suffer grief in its many forms, in addition to profound guilt or shame. Sometimes they become obsessed with their failure to "see the signs." Rejection and lack of social and religious support is something survivors fear and, unfortunately, often experience. Suicide sometimes is not considered acceptable; many families of suicide victims are not given the same support from the church, community, or workplace as those whose loved ones have died from other causes. Because of the family's anger, fear, and shame, others may avoid reaching out to help. The grief of survivors is complicated and intense. Survivors may be at an increased risk for suicide themselves, and a grief counselor is frequently helpful.

GERONTOLOGIC DEATH

Older adults often are assumed to have some understanding and acceptance of the death process. This is not always true. Treat the older patient as an individual and assess the patient's needs in the same way as those of any individual facing a terminal illness (see the Lifespan Considerations for Older Adults box earlier in the chapter). The older person must be included in self-care and in decisions to undergo or refuse extensive therapeutic or resuscitative measures. Even when aggressive technological options are rejected, patients still need intensive nursing interventions and pain control measures. Sometimes families who suffer the loss of an older person accept the death, but they must experience the grieving process nonetheless.

Factors that influence grief in older adults include the following:
- Physical changes that accompany aging
- Loss of employment
- Loss of social respect
- Loss of relationships
- Loss of self-care capabilities
- Fear of loss of control
- Sense of fulfillment and contributions made
- Personality traits
- Feelings of self-worth
- Degree to which functional ability is retained

SUDDEN OR UNEXPECTED DEATH

Coping with a sudden, unexpected, or violent death, such as through accident, homicide, or sudden illness (e.g., myocardial infarction), is often difficult. Families experiencing this type of loss require a great deal of support. Often there is preoccupation with the final hours or minutes before death. There is "unfinished business," such as things left unsaid or undone. There are usually guilt feelings (e.g., "If only I had not let him go to the party, he would still be alive"). There may be involvement of law authorities, such as the police or coroner. Sometimes there is an obsessive need to understand or know why this has happened. Grief therapy and referral to support groups can be beneficial to those who are left behind from the death of a loved one.

ISSUES RELATED TO DYING AND DEATH

EUTHANASIA

Euthanasia (Greek for "easy death") is sometimes active, a deliberate action taken with the purpose of shortening life to end suffering or to carry out the wishes of a terminally ill patient. Passive euthanasia is permitting the death of a patient by withholding treatment that may extend life, such as medication, life-support systems, or feeding tubes. Active euthanasia is assisting in such a death.

Euthanasia raises many moral and ethical questions for society and for patients and their families. Technologies that can keep patients alive indefinitely after the brain has, for all practical purposes, stopped functioning are largely responsible for the change in attitudes in the past 25 years.

A 2017 Gallop Poll on values and beliefs asked the following two questions: When a person has a disease that cannot be cured, do you think doctors should be allowed by law to end the patient's life by some painless means if the patient and his or her family request it? When a person has a disease that cannot be cured and is living in severe pain, do you think doctors should or should not be allowed by law to assist the patient to commit suicide if the patient requests it? A total of 73% of 518 people answered yes to the first question and 67% of 518 people answered yes to the second question (ProCon.org, 2017).

DO-NOT-RESUSCITATE ORDER

It is proper for patients and families to retain control over decisions about withholding or withdrawing treatment. Death with dignity remains a concern for all. A joint decision for a do-not-resuscitate (DNR) decision made by the patient, the family, and the health care providers is best. Be sure the patient and family obtain an explanation of all facts regarding the patient's condition and all treatment options. DNR means only not to resuscitate. It does not mean to withhold any other care, such as hygiene, nutrition, fluids, or medications. The health care provider writes a "no code" or "do not resuscitate" order once a health care provider has documented in the progress notes the deterioration of the patient's condition and the decision by the health care provider and the patient not to administer cardiopulmonary resuscitation. Often the instructions regarding lifesaving treatment are written in the patient's living will or durable power of attorney. Check that the no-code or DNR order is written, not given verbally. In optimal circumstances, the health care provider regularly reviews DNR orders because of changes in the patient's condition. The nurse must be familiar with the institution's policies and procedures concerning DNR orders. Health care providers can list all specifics of DNR orders as a follow-up to the patient's living will. The patient may choose to allow some parts of resuscitative efforts, such as medication administration, but specifically prohibit chest compression or intubation for cardiac dysrhythmias or respiratory arrest. Thoroughly document in the patient's chart all DNR orders and the associated discussion with the patient and family.

With pediatric populations, the term allow natural death is more acceptable to parents. "Allow a natural death" acknowledges that one is going to die and forgoes aggressive treatment. Resources that can help patients and families decide what type of care they want to receive are "My Wishes" for children and "Five Wishes" for adults (Aging with Dignity, n.d.). PartingWishes.com is a website where individuals can write wills, living wills, powers of attorney, funerals, and memorials.

ADVANCE DIRECTIVES

The two basic types of advance directives are living wills and durable powers of attorney for health care. Many patients have instituted one or both. Advance directives are signed and witnessed documents that provide specific instructions for health care treatment if a person is unable to make these decisions personally at the time they are needed. For more information on advance directives, see Chapter 2.

ORGAN DONATIONS

Legally competent people are free to donate their bodies or organs for medical use. Consent forms are available for this purpose. In many states, adults can request organ donation by signing the back of their driver's license. State laws determine whether a nurse is allowed to serve as a witness when individuals wish to give consent for the donation of organs, tissue, or the body. Be aware of the policies and procedures of your employing institution.

In most states (National Organ Transplantation Act, Public Law 98-507, 10-14, 1984), required request laws stipulate that at the time of a person's death, a qualified health care provider must ask family members to consider organ or tissue donation. Required request laws are the result of the shortage of suitable organs for transplant.

The Uniform Anatomical Gifts Act addresses many problems of organ donation and stipulates that the health care provider who certifies death shall not be involved in removal or transplantation of the organs. The National Organ Transplantation Act, which governs this area of medical and nursing practice, prohibits selling or purchasing organs. Organ and tissue donations remain voluntary.

Donations can include the following:
- Vital organs
  - Kidney
  - Heart
  - Lung
  - Liver
  - Pancreas
  - Small intestine
- Nonvital tissues
  - Cornea
  - Long bones
  - Skin
  - Middle ear bones
  - Saphenous and femoral veins
  - Heart valves
  - Tendons
  - Hands and face

Vital organs are recovered after a patient is pronounced clinically dead or brain dead; circulatory and ventilatory support is maintained to perfuse the organs before removal. Additional information about organ and tissue donation can be found at https://www.giftofhope.org/faq/

RIGHTS OF DYING PATIENTS

Death with dignity is the goal in caring for the dying patient. The Dying Person's Bill of Rights (Box 25.8) is honored at hospitals and other health care agencies and is posted in prominent areas.

The Dying Person's Bill of Rights

- I have the right to be treated as a living human being until I die.
- I have the right to maintain a sense of hopefulness, however changing its focus may be.
- I have the right to be cared for by those who can maintain a sense of hopefulness, however changing this might be.
- I have the right to express my feelings and emotions about my approaching death in my own way.
- I have the right to participate in decisions concerning my care.
- I have the right to expect continuing medical and nursing attention, even though "cure" goals must be changed to "comfort" goals.
- I have the right not to die alone.
- I have the right to be free from pain.
- I have the right to have my questions answered honestly.
- I have the right not to be deceived.
- I have the right to have help from and for my family in accepting my death.
- I have the right to die in peace and dignity.
- I have the right to retain my individuality and not be judged for my decisions that may be contrary to beliefs of others.
- I have the right to discuss and enlarge my religious and/or spiritual experiences, whatever these may mean to others.
- I have the right to expect that the sanctity of the human body will be respected after death.
- I have the right to be cared for by caring, sensitive, knowledgeable people who will attempt to understand my needs and will be able to gain some satisfaction in helping me face my death.

From Barbus A: The dying patient's bill of rights, *Am J Nurs* 75:99, 1975.

FRAUDULENT METHODS OF TREATMENT

Often, the patient and family seek unconventional methods of treatment to prolong the patient's life. Such treatments may include special diets, enemas, unproven drugs, and machines or devices. The nurse may be asked to help patients and families sort out which treatments are real and which are fraudulent. Fraudulent treatments are those that are misrepresented, whether by concealment or nondisclosure of facts, for the purpose of inducing another to use them. View with suspicion any treatment that does not offer the patient informed consent after providing information regarding options, results, and approvals from federal agencies.

DYING PATIENT

COMMUNICATING WITH THE DYING PATIENT

Express respect for the patient, offer realistic hope, and impart appropriate reassurance and support when using therapeutic communication. Supportive words without an accompanying supportive attitude are empty in meaning and fail to provide comfort. Verbal and nonverbal communication should be equivalent in message. Reassurance that is unrealistic or given merely to calm a patient does not work. Stating that "everything will be just fine" when this is untrue or uncertain only increases the patient's anxiety and violates trust in the nurse. Do not offer false reassurance. Limited reassurance that is consistent with the facts is far better.

Therapeutic communication also requires paying careful attention to what the patient expresses verbally and nonverbally. Always verify with the patient any interpretations or summaries of the patient's thoughts and feelings to ensure they are accurate and effective.

If patients prefer not to communicate at a particular time, accept and respect their wishes. Indicate a willingness to return at another time when the patient is feeling more comfortable. Be available to listen actively, without judgment, and with acceptance. Allow the patient to express emotions and feelings without fear.

Behavior that indicates listening to the patient is called "attending behavior." It includes appropriate eye contact, attentive body language, and verbally acknowledging that the nurse is listening by using terms such as "uh huh," "I understand what you are saying," or "go on." Demonstrate attentiveness in nonverbal and verbal ways. For instance, sit in a chair close to the patient's bed to reduce the physical distance and the emotional distance it implies. When appropriately used, touching is a highly effective means of communication. Later in the illness, when strength for or interest in verbal communication has dwindled, a patient derives benefit from being touched. Holding a hand, patting an arm, or gently wiping away a tear indicates attending behavior and concern and care.

Remember that you cannot "solve" the problem of dying, but you can have a positive impact on the dying patient's feelings and fears. Communicate openly and sensitively with the patient. This facilitates the expression of emotion and affirms that the patient is a living human who has your support and compassion.

One of the most important tasks of the bedside nurse is to empower patients and families to participate in the final act of living. Communicate reassurance, confidence, and support for the vulnerable patient and family by sustaining nursing assessment practices, continuing to communicate, and providing skilled physical care. The seasoned hand of a skilled professional supporting and guiding the patient can change the journey through dying and death from a frightening process to one of peace and comfort.

Other resources to summon during management of the dying patient depend on the patient's needs and wishes. Patients sometimes desire greater focus on spiritual needs; many request a visit by a clergyman or clergywoman or the performance of a religious ritual. You may be asked to assist in religious rituals such as prayer or reading of scripture. If you are uncomfortable with this task, ask another nurse who is comfortable assisting with the patient's needs or contact chaplain services. Other patients seek answers in nutritional approaches, miracles, and other sources of hope, although these often come with a high price tag. Support nontraditional therapies if they give the patient hope and do no harm (see Chapter 20). The nurse's primary role in the care of the dying patient is to explain realistic options without destroying hope. The attitude of the nurse and the patient makes the difference between the perceived success or failure of a dying experience.

ASSISTING THE PATIENT IN SAYING GOODBYE

One of the most difficult tasks a terminally ill patient faces is leaving loved ones behind. The patient who is aware of dying must say goodbye, whether in a verbal, nonverbal, concrete, or symbolic way. For their part, family members also must work through the process of acknowledging the impending parting. Goodbyes help them move toward the completion of unfinished business with the patient that otherwise could complicate their transition through the grieving process. The nurse's assistance in this area is important to the dying person and the family (see the Communication box).

 Communication

Counseling a Family Member

Family member: I can't go back in that room. He just lies there and stares. I don't know what to do or say.

Nurse: Being near someone who is dying can be uncomfortable.

Family member: It makes me so sad to see him like that. Do you think he knows I'm there?

Nurse: It's very possible that he does. Would you like me to go in with you?

Family member: Yes, please. I wonder if he can hear me?

Nurse: It must be very difficult for you not to be certain that he is hearing you. The last sense to go is hearing. If there is something you want to say to him, get close, take his hand, and speak directly to him. Most people in his condition can hear but are very weak and may not have the strength to respond.

Family member: I just feel like I am not able to do anything for him anymore.

Nurse: Just being there is letting him know that you care. That's something very important to any person.

Family member: I suppose you're right. I guess I'm ready to go in now.

Nurse: I'll be right here by your side.

First, provide a private, comfortable environment. Sometimes emotional expression becomes overwhelming for the patient, the family, or both; offer to remain present or nearby to help support the family member or loved one and the patient. Various ways are available to assist patients in saying their goodbyes, such as role playing, letter writing, or making audio or video recordings. Help patients focus on what they want to say. One way to facilitate this is to ask them to talk to

their loved ones as if they were going to be separated for a long time. Encourage them to express those feelings and thoughts they most want their loved ones to know in their absence. Help the dying person to formulate appropriate letters or tape recordings by asking, "What would you want to say to your 6-year-old when the child is 12?" Often dying patients become depressed because they do not have a purpose in life. Working on tasks such as poems, letters, and recordings affords patients feelings of control and productivity in their last days.

PALLIATIVE CARE

People who face life-threatening illnesses can take advantage of many medical and technological advances to reverse the course of their disease or to prolong their lives. For patients with life-limiting illness, finding ways to help them approach their end of life becomes important. Such is the goal of palliative care: the prevention, relief, reduction, or soothing of symptoms of disease or disorders without affecting a cure. Palliative care allows patients to make more informed choices, achieve better alleviation of symptoms, and have more opportunity to work on issues of life closure. According to the World Health Organization (n.d.), when delivering palliative care, the nurse does the following:

- Provides relief from pain and other distressing symptoms
- Affirms life and regards dying as a normal process
- Intends neither to hasten or postpone death
- Integrates the psychological and spiritual aspects of patient care
- Offers a support system to help patients live as actively as possible until death
- Offers a support system to help families cope during the patient's illness and their own bereavement
- Uses a team approach to address the needs of patients and their families, including bereavement counseling, if indicated
- Will enhance quality of life, and may also positively influence the course of illness
- Is applicable early in the course of illness, in conjunction with other therapies that are intended to prolong life, such as chemotherapy or radiation therapy, and includes those investigations needed to better understand and manage distressing clinical complications.

Palliative care is a philosophy of total care. Palliative care is appropriate to deliver at any time and to patients of any age, with any diagnosis. Although it has particular relevance to the care of the terminally ill, it is not reserved for only the last few months of life. The approach to care usually involves an interdisciplinary team of health care providers, nurses, social workers, pastoral care professionals, physical and occupational therapists, and pharmacists. Massage therapists or music or art therapists who provide alternative therapies are also a part of the team. In the context of end of life,

Box 25.9   Long-Term Care Considerations

- In settings outside of the hospital there may be less physician involvement which gives nurses the vital role in assessing and managing pain and symptom control.
- Challenges include providing privacy and autonomy for the patient and family, involving the family as much as possible or desired, individualizing care, keeping family members informed of changes, and making the environment as homelike as possible.
- The goal of a nursing facility is to provide a caring environment for those who are dying. However, many facilities sorely lack appropriate supportive care. Compassionate care allows family members to be present whenever they choose, day or night, and involves aggressive and appropriate symptom management.
- Nighttime is a time of least attention and a time of loneliness and pain. Night is also a time when people fear they will die alone and no one will know. If a friend or relative cannot stay with the patient, a mature sitter is an option. A volunteer from hospice may provide the same support. For those older adults who have developed a lifestyle around aloneness, solitude may be preferred. Be sensitive to the patient's preference.

Data from Perry A, Potter P, Ostendorf W: *Clinical nursing skills and techniques,* ed 9, St. Louis, 2018, Elsevier.

a palliative care approach ensures that a patient experiences a "good death," free of avoidable pain and suffering in accord with the patient's and family's wishes and reasonably consistent with clinical, cultural, and ethical standards.

One of the most important tasks for a nurse providing palliative care is to establish a caring relationship with patient and family. Furthermore, the symptom-control measures the nurse provides are important to help maintain the patient's dignity and self-esteem, prevent abandonment or isolation, and establish a comfortable and peaceful environment for death to occur (Box 25.9).

PHYSICAL CARE

The nurse has an important responsibility in assisting patients to meet their physical needs. Providing adequate nutrition and maintaining elimination patterns are priorities for the dying patient (see Chapter 40). Keep the patient clean, dry, well groomed, odor free, and comfortable to decrease the chances of skin impairment and provide the patient with feelings of self-esteem and self-worth (see Chapter 9). Sometimes nurses provide care in a facility (see the Coordinated Care box) and sometimes in the patient's home (see the Home Care Considerations box).

Adjusting the environment to increase comfort and safety is paramount. Use side rails for safety and, when possible, to assist weak patients to adjust their own positions.

 Coordinated Care

Collaboration

Caring For The Dying Patient

A multidisciplinary team is needed to appropriately care for the dying patient. Nurses are educated to assess the psychosocial needs of patients and family who are experiencing impending death. Support of these families is the role of the nurse. Determining the need for referrals and consultations is a role of the nurse. The assistive personnel's roles include:

- Ask assistive personnel to inform the nurse when the patient expresses behaviors of grief (e.g., crying, anger, loss of appetite).
- Communicate the reports of patient/family needs to the nurse.
- Monitor visitors

A professional nurse is responsible for assessment of patient symptoms and a determination of which symptoms can be managed independently and which symptoms necessitate medical intervention. Certain symptom therapies can be delegated to assistive personnel, such as positioning and environmental controls, hygiene approaches, and hydration. Therapies such as administration of opioids, anxiolytics, and antidepressants require a nurse's intervention. The nurse provides assistive personnel with instruction and assistance regarding the following:

- When to notify the nurse if the patient's symptoms worsen or change in nature
- Potential adverse effects of pharmacologic agents and what to report to the nurse
- The need to maintain communication with dying patients who still retain the sense of hearing

Certain aspects of care of the body after death can be delegated to assistive personnel. Also, care after death can, in fact, begin before the actual death so that patients and families can preserve cultural practices. Check agency policy regarding which staff members are permitted to remove invasive tubes or lines. At the time of death, it may be best for the nurse and assistive personnel to work together in preparing the body (see Skill 25.1).

- Inform other care providers of any preference the family may have because of cultural, religious, or ethnic beliefs that influence the routine procedures of caring for the patient's body.
- Reinforce the importance of handling the body with respect.

Modified from Perry A, Potter P, Ostendorf W: *Clinical nursing skills and techniques,* ed 9, St. Louis, 2018, Elsevier.

ASSESSMENTS AND INTERVENTIONS

Care of the dying patient has many facets. Of all the needs of the dying patient, the three most crucial are the need for love and affection, for the control of pain, and for the preservation of dignity and self-worth.

As death approaches the body is in an increasing state of weakness and deterioration. Nursing assessment and care remain important. One of the nurse's goals in end-of-life nursing goes beyond merely allaying the physical suffering of patients to the greatest extent possible. Ideally, the nurse also helps patients

Skill 25.1   Care of the Body After Death

NURSING ACTION (RATIONALE)

1. Gather equipment. (Organizes procedure.)
   - Disposable gloves, gown, and other protective clothing
   - Plastic bag for hazardous waste disposal
   - Washbasin, washcloth, warm water, bath towel
   - Clean gown or disposable gown for body
   - Absorbent pads
   - Body bag or shroud kit (know agency policy)
   - Paper tape and gauze dressing
   - Suitable receptacle for patient's belongings and other items to be returned to family
   - Valuables envelope
   - Identification tags, as required by agency policy
2. Wash hands. (Reduces spread of microorganisms.)
3. Don clean gloves. (Protects nurse from contamination.)
4. Close patient's eyes and mouth if needed. (Provides a more normal appearance.) A rolled towel placed under the chin is helpful to keep the mouth closed.
5. Remove all tubing and other devices from patient's body.[a] (Makes patient look more peaceful.)
6. Place patient in supine position. (Allows access for procedures.) Elevate the head. (Prevents discoloration.) Do not place one hand on top of the other. (This can lead to discoloration.)
7. Replace soiled dressings with clean ones. *(Prevents odor.)*
8. Bathe patient as necessary. *(Reduces odor.)*
9. Brush or comb hair. *(Gives more normal appearance.)*
10. Apply clean gown. (Prepares body for viewing.)
11. Care for valuables and personal belongings. (For legal considerations.) If wedding band is to remain on the deceased, secure ring to finger with a small strip of tape over ring. (Prevents loss and protects jewelry.)
12. Allow family to view body and remain in room for as much time as needed. (Provide emotional support if family wishes.) A sheet or light blanket placed over the body with only the head and upper shoulders exposed maintains dignity and respect for the deceased. Remove unneeded equipment from the room. Provide soft lighting and offer chairs. (Demonstrates respect for significant others.)
13. After the family has left the room, attach identification per hospital policy. Attach special label if patient had a contagious disease. (Protects those who handle the body.)
14. Close door to room. (Prevents exposure to patients and visitors.)
15. Await arrival of ambulance or transfer to morgue. (Out of respect for patient.) (Some agencies use a shroud to enclose the body before transfer to the morgue.)

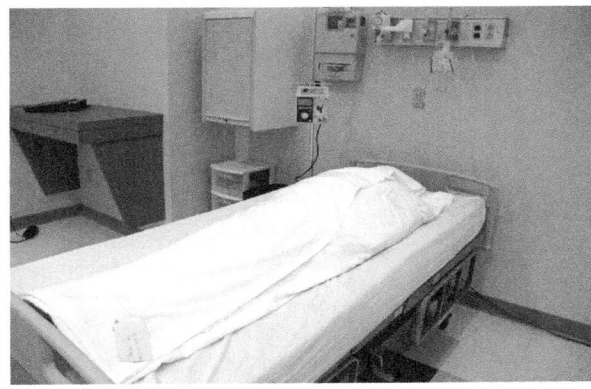

16. Document procedure and disposition of patient's body and of belongings and valuables. *(For legal purposes.)*

[a]Some situations require that all tubing remain in the body (e.g., when an autopsy is scheduled). Know agency policy.

recognize and accept death as a reality of life so that they can undertake their last task in life with self-esteem and dignity. Work to prevent the abandonment by family, friends, and caregivers that is sometimes a part of the dying patient's experience. Ensuring support by others can help prevent a patient from being left to die alone. Be aware of the availability of the *No One Dies Alone program* in your employing institute. *No One Dies Alone* is a national volunteer program that will allow compassionate companions to sit with the dying patient so that the patient will not die alone. During the dying process the compassionate companion can talk to the patient, hold the patient's hand, or just be a loving presence in the room (Eskanazi Health, 2016).

Assess the patient for impending death. Patients may appear comatose, unconscious, or unresponsive. Such appearance is often a result of extreme fatigue, and patients may be aware of activities that occur around them. Decreased oxygenation may cause the patient to become restless. They may pick and pull at the bed linens. Discoloration of arms and legs is a result of impaired circulation. Table 25.2 shows signs of

Home Care Considerations

The Dying Patient

- At least 50% of Americans will die in their home while in the care of hospice.
  - Terminally ill patients may have trepidation about dying at home because they fear causing a burden to their families.

Home care resources are key to patients feeling comfortable dying at home.

- The family members need to have information about who to call in the event there are significant condition changes.
- Family members assume primary care responsibility, necessitating ongoing teaching and support. Educate family members about symptom management approaches and when to seek help.
- Volunteers may be needed to give family respite time.

approaching death as expressed in patient needs and the appropriate interventions.

Changes in vital signs are observed, including (1) slow, weak, and thready pulse; (2) lowered blood pressure; and (3) rapid, shallow, irregular, or abnormally slow respirations. Mouth breathing occurs, which leads to dry oral mucous membranes. The patient often has a detached look in the eyes. Diminished sensory and motor function is seen in the lower extremities, which progresses to the upper extremities. Touch sensation diminishes while pressure and pain sensations may remain intact. As death becomes imminent, the pupils become dilated and fixed, Cheyne-Stokes respirations occur, the pulse becomes increasingly weaker and more rapid, and the blood pressure continues to fall. Peripheral circulation diminishes. The skin is cool and clammy; profuse diaphoresis may occur. If mucus collects in the patient's

Table 25.2   Needs and Interventions for the Patient Near Death

PATIENT NEEDS	INTERVENTIONS
Discomfort	Provide thorough skin care, including daily baths, lubrication of skin, and dry clean bed linens to reduce irritants. Provide oral care at least q 2–4 h. Use soft toothbrushes or foam swabs for frequent mouth care. Apply a light film of water-soluble lubricant or lip balm to lips and tongue. Eye care removes crusts from eyelid margins. Artificial tears reduce corneal drying.
Fatigue	Help patient to identify values or desired tasks; then help patient to conserve energy for only those tasks. Promote frequent rest periods in a quiet environment. Time and pace nursing care activities.
Nausea	Administer antiemetics; provide oral care at least q 2–4 h; offer clear liquid diet and ice chips; avoid liquids that increase stomach acidity such as coffee, milk, and juices with citric acid; and uncover food outside of the room to reduce strong odors.
Constipation	Give preventive care, which is most effective: increase fluid intake; include bran, whole-grain products, and fresh vegetables in diet; and encourage exercise. Administer prophylactic stool softeners. Assess for fecal impaction.
Diarrhea	Confer with health care provider to change medication, or get order for antidiarrheal medication, if possible. Provide low-residue diet.
Urinary incontinence	Protect skin from irritation or breakdown. Indwelling urinary catheter or condom catheters may be used.
Inadequate nutrition	Serve smaller portions and bland foods, which may be more palatable. Allow home-cooked meals, which may be preferred by patient and gives the family a chance to participate.
Dehydration	Remove factors that cause decreased intake; give antiemetics, and apply topical analgesics to oral lesions. Reduce discomfort from dehydration; give mouth care at least q 2–4 h; and offer ice chips or moist cloth to lips.
Dyspnea, shortness of breath	Treat or control underlying cause. Maximize patient's oxygenation (e.g., position patient upright, provide supplemental oxygen, maintain a patent airway, and reduce anxiety or fear). Administer medications such as bronchodilators, inhaled steroids, or narcotics to suppress cough and ease breathing and apprehension.

From Potter PA, Perry AG, Stockert P, et al: *Fundamentals of nursing*, ed 9, St. Louis, 2017, Elsevier.

throat, noisy respirations are heard. This sound is referred to as the *death rattle*. A period of peace may immediately precede the moment of death. The clinical signs of death are given in the following list:

1. Unreceptivity and unresponsiveness
2. No movement or breathing
3. No reflexes
4. Flat encephalogram
5. Absence of apical pulse
6. Cessation of respirations

INQUEST

An inquest is a legal inquiry into the cause or the manner of a death. When a death is the result of an accident, for example, an inquest is held into the circumstances of the accident to determine any blame. The inquest is conducted under the jurisdiction of a coroner or medical examiner. A *coroner* is a public official, not necessarily a health care provider appointed or elected to inquire into cause of death. A *medical examiner* is a trained health care provider and usually has advanced education in pathology or forensic medicine. Agency policy dictates who is responsible for reporting deaths to the coroner or medical examiner.

POSTMORTEM CARE

In most states, the health care provider is responsible for certifying a death in the medical record. The health care provider notes time of death and records a description of therapies or actions taken in the medical record. The health care provider may request permission from the family for the autopsy (examination performed after a person's death to confirm or determine the cause of death). Autopsies are required in circumstances of unusual death (e.g., violent trauma or unexpected death in the home).

Because of the therapeutic nurse-patient relationship, the nurse may be the best person to provide postmortem care (care for the patient's body after death). Keep in mind the need to care for the patient's body with dignity and sensitivity. Provide postmortem care as soon as possible after death to prevent tissue damage or disfigurement. If the family has requested organ donation, take immediate measures as appropriate. Know the state laws and the policies and procedures of the employing institution.

Prepare the body and the room to keep the stress of the experience to a minimum, after the patient has been pronounced dead by a health care provider or professional nurse and before the family views the body. Remove supplies and equipment from sight. Remove, clamp, or cut tubes that remain in the body to within 1 inch (2.5 cm) of the skin, and tape them in place. Care of tubes and specimens depends on agency policy and whether an autopsy will be performed. Never, however, remove tubes, dressings, drains, and other equipment that is in place on or in the patient when an autopsy is to be performed. Clear away soiled linen and other clutter. Use spray deodorizer to help eliminate unpleasant odors.

Prepare the body by making it look as natural and comfortable as possible. Place the body in the supine position with arms at the sides, palms down or across the abdomen (but not one hand over the other); this helps the mortician (person trained in the care of the dead) better prepare it for interment. Discoloration of the face can result if blood is allowed to pool; to prevent this, place a small pillow or folded towel under the head. The eyelids usually remain closed if gently held down for a few seconds. If not, a moistened cotton ball can hold them in place. Insert the patient's dentures to maintain normal facial features. A rolled-up towel under the chin keeps the mouth closed (see Skill 25.1). The Cultural Considerations box on care of the

 Cultural Considerations

Care of the Body After Death*

African Americans: Most families prefer that members of the health care team clean and prepare the loved one's body. Some may have misgivings about organ donation but may agree to an autopsy. Historically the African American community has not embraced cremation after death but this form of after life management is growing in popularity.

Chinese Americans: Some families may prefer to bathe the deceased themselves. Often, they feel the body should remain intact; organ donation and autopsy are uncommon.

Filipino Americans: Some families may prefer to wash the body themselves and are likely to want time for all family members to say goodbye. The family may not permit organ donation or autopsy.

Hispanics or Latino Americans: Family members may want to help with care of the body and are likely to want to say goodbye. Organ donation and autopsy are uncommon.

Jews: The dying person may want to make a deathbed confession or desire prayers. Observant Jews usually oppose autopsies but may consider organ donation. The body must not be left unattended until burial; a family member may remain present while the body is prepared by nursing staff, during transport to and while in the morgue, and then to the funeral home.

Roman Catholics: The dying person may desire to receive the sacraments of Reconciliation and Anointing of the Sick within 30 days before death. The religion does not oppose autopsies or organ donation.

Muslims: When close to death, a devout Muslim may wish to recite the Islamic Creed with help from others. After death, the person's eyes and mouth should be closed and the limbs should be straightened. Fully clothe the deceased. It is preferred that the deceased by handled by members of the same gender wearing gloves.

Hindus: The dying person should be in a peaceful room if not at home. The patient or someone else should recite the Gita. Family members may prefer to wash the body and may feel that organ donation is an individual choice.

Buddhists: An ordained monk or nun should care for the dying person. After death, the body should be covered with a cotton sheet. Keep the body as still as possible during movement. The eyes and the mouth should not be closed. No noise, talking, or crying is allowed. Buddhists consider organ donation to be an individual choice.

*These are common practices; not all practices listed are the beliefs of members in a culture.

body after death presents culturally related attitudes toward preparation of the body. It should be noted that these are only common attitudes of the cultural groups listed. These are not necessarily the beliefs or practices of all members of these cultural groups.

At the time of death, make a notation of any valuables, such as watch, rings, or money, and secure these articles so that they may be delivered to the family according to agency policy. Documentation of all valuables and their disposition in the patient's medical record is required (Box 25.10).

Offer the family the opportunity to view the body and opportunity to say goodbye to their loved one, especially if they were not present at the time of death. If the family hesitates to view the body, let them think about it. If they decide not to view the body, accept their decision without judgment. If the family decides to view the body, assure them that they will not be alone if they prefer the nurse be present. Offer to accompany them, or ask to call on someone else to be present if they would like. Spend as much time as possible assisting the grieving family, and offer to contact other support services, such as social services and the spiritual adviser. (Many health care facilities employ a full-time chaplain who may be summoned in the event of death.) The family now becomes the patient.

DOCUMENTATION

Document the care given to the dying patient objectively, completely, legibly, and accurately. As death approaches, make frequent documentation, and include the signs of impending death as they occur. Recording who was present at the time of the patient's death is important. Continue documentation until the last entry, which states where and to whom the body was transferred (see Box 25.10).

GRIEVING FAMILY

SUPPORT

The needs of the grieving family and significant others deserve the nurse's caring, compassionate attention. Make every attempt to contact someone—family, clergy, or friends—to be with the grieving survivor if he or she is alone at the time of the loved one's death. Express words that convey sympathy. If appropriate, use a spontaneous touch, such as a hand on the arm or an embrace, as a comforting gesture. Answer any questions the family may have, and encourage them to view, touch, and talk to the deceased family member. Remain nonjudgmental as the family expresses feelings of anger, guilt, or unfairness. Help with the notification of the mortician and any individuals involved in the procurement of donated organs.

Informing others can be a major emotional step for family members. The nurse's presence and assistance in this area is very supportive. Direct family members to support groups and other referral agencies

---

| Box **25.10** | Documentation of End-of-Life Care |

Documentation includes the following:
- Time of death and actions taken to prevent the death if applicable
- Who pronounced the death of the patient
- Any special preparation and type of donation, including time, staff, and company
- Who was called and who came to the hospital: donor organization, morgue, funeral home, chaplain, or individual family members making any decisions
- Personal articles left on the body and taped to skin or tubes left in
- Personal items given to the family and specific names and description of items
- Time of discharge and destination of the body
- Location of name tags on the body
- Special requests by the family
- Any other personal statements that may be needed to clarify the situation

---

(churches, therapists, social workers); such connections expand the family's social network, foster relatedness, and decrease isolation.

The restriction of visitors during a pandemic will disrupt the family process of being at the bedside during the dying process and being able to say goodbye to a loved one. This action could have an impact on the grieving process.

Grief work helps an individual cope with the loss of a loved one. The use of counseling techniques in order to address symptoms related to suffering a loss is one way grief work can be achieved. Grief work includes:
- Adapting to life without their loved one
- Realizing the reality of the loss of the loved one
- Reinvesting in life while maintaining a healthy bond with the deceased loved one
- Dealing effectively with the emotional pain of the loss (Worden, 2009)

RESOLUTION OF GRIEF

Resolution of grief has begun when, after the loss, the grieving person or family can complete the following tasks:
- Have positive interactions with others
- Participate in support groups with others who are similarly bereaved to articulate loss together and offer companionship
- Establish goals, and work to achieve them
- Discuss the meaning of the loss and its effect on the survivor's life

People need support and understanding to deal with the grief that comes with the loss of a loved one. Months or years may elapse before an individual can complete grief work and begin the full process of resolution. The grief experienced by an individual depends on the energy expended in the relationship. Many believe that about a year must pass before the bereaved can begin to think of the deceased without feeling intense emotional pain.

Get Ready for the NCLEX® Examination!

Key Points

- Care of the dying patient has moved from the home to hospitals and back again in the past 50 years.
- Dr. Elizabeth Kübler-Ross has been instrumental in identifying the five stages of death and dying: denial, anger, bargaining, depression, and acceptance.
- Losses occur throughout the life cycle, provide the individual experience with loss, and promote emotional growth and development of coping skills.
- The effect a loss has on a person is individualized: duration, abruptness, extent, time required for treatment or replacement, and financial impact affect the sense of loss.
- Grief is not an episode but a process—an active, not a passive, process. It takes work and emotional energy. The grief experienced by an individual depends on the energy expended in the relationship.
- When people do not do "grief work" after any significant loss, they are at risk for emotional, mental, and social problems.
- The grief theory demonstrates that the normal grief process includes an onset, active grief work, and a resolution or reorganization of the survivors' lives after the loss.
- Nurses experience all the emotions of grief in response to not only their own losses but also the death of their patients.
- Assessment of whether family members are willing to be involved in a dying patient's care is mandatory before they are used as resources.
- The major concerns of the dying patient are (1) fear of abandonment (fear of dying alone); (2) fear of loss of control; (3) fear of pain and discomfort; and (4) fear of the unknown.
- Euthanasia is an ethical and legal issue faced by nurses. Oregon, Washington, Vermont, California, Colorado, District of Columbia, Hawaii, Maine, and New Jersey have a form of Death with Dignity Acts at the time of this publication.
- A do-not-resuscitate (DNR) order or allow natural death order means only that. It does not mean to withhold hygiene, hydration, nutrition, or medications.
- Patients who decide ahead of time what kind of care they want and communicate these decisions to others help to ensure they receive the extent of care they desire. These communications, called advance directives, most often involve the living will and the durable power of attorney.
- The Dying Person's Bill of Rights includes the elements characteristic of dying with dignity.
- Assisting a dying patient in saying goodbye is an intervention nurses can initiate.
- The physical care requirements of the dying patient are primarily nursing interventions. Providing adequate nutrition, elimination, hygiene, safety, and comfort is a nursing priority.
- Continuing to speak to and include patients in their care is essential, because as death approaches, the dying patient becomes weaker. Patients may appear comatose yet be aware of activities around them.
- Signs of impending death are (1) slow, thready, and weaker pulse; (2) lowered blood pressure; (3) rapid, shallow, irregular, or abnormally slow respirations; and (4) mottling of lower extremities.
- Postmortem care is the care administered to the body after death. Follow procedures including cleansing, positioning, and labeling the body.

Additional Learning Resources

SG Go to your Study Guide for additional learning activities to help you master this chapter content.

Be sure to visit the Evolve site at http://evolve.elsevier.com/ Cooper/foundations/ for additional online resources.

Review Questions For The NCLEX® Examination

1. **A 77-year-old patient has been admitted with pneumonia. Her husband asks the nurse about the living will. Which statement is correct about living wills?**

   1. Living wills allow the courts to decide when care can be given.
   2. Living wills allow individuals to express their wishes regarding care.
   3. Living wills are legally binding in all states.
   4. Living wills allow health care workers to withhold fluids and medications.

2. **The patient's daughter remained at the bedside of her dying mother throughout the night. When her mother died the following morning, the daughter cried out angrily at the nurse and the physician. Which is the most appropriate action by the nurse?**

   1. Explain that everything possible was done for her mother.
   2. Remain with the daughter and listen to what she is saying.
   3. Leave the daughter in privacy and allow her to work through her grief.
   4. Notify a clergyman and call other family members.

3. **A newly licensed nurse is assigned to his first dying patient. When he is caring for a dying patient, what best prepares the nurse?**

   1. Having completed a course dealing with death and dying
   2. Being able to control his own emotions about death
   3. Having experienced the death of a loved one
   4. Being aware of his own thoughts and feelings toward death

4. **A nurse is assigned to a patient who recently was diagnosed with a terminal illness. While the nurse was assisting her with morning care, the patient asked about organ donation. Which nursing action is most appropriate?**

   1. Assist her in obtaining the necessary information to make this decision.
   2. Have the patient first discuss the subject with her family.
   3. Suggest she delay making a decision at this time.
   4. Contact the physician so that consent can be obtained from the family.

5. Which statement describes a person experiencing anticipatory grief?

   1. A person faces the possibility of losing a loved one.
   2. A person has placed the death of a loved one in perspective.
   3. A person displays grief responses after a loved one's death.
   4. A person has difficulty making decisions after a loved one's death.

6. When talking with a patient what would be considered a therapeutic communication technique? *(Select all that apply.)*

   1. Stating, "I know just how you feel"
   2. Saying, "Her death was for the best"
   3. Never crying in front of family members
   4. Encouraging family members to share their feelings
   5. Sitting at the same level of the patient when conversing with them.

7. Which of the following helps family members make difficult decisions?

   1. Discussing autopsy and organ donation at the time of the loved one's death
   2. Addressing one matter at a time, giving them adequate time to discuss each issue
   3. Publicly discussing issues with other hospital staff
   4. Addressing all of the issues at once

8. Which comment is most likely to help grieving family members express themselves more easily? *(Select all that apply.)*

   1. "Tell me how you're feeling."
   2. "I know just how you feel."
   3. "Things will get better."
   4. "Time heals all wounds."
   5. "I hear you saying that you miss your loved one very much."

9. Which of the following is most therapeutic when talking with family members with an unresolved issue?

   1. Explain that they are simply experiencing normal anticipatory grief.
   2. Explain that they missed their chance to make amends and now it is too late.
   3. Encourage them to verbalize their thoughts and feelings to the loved one.
   4. Tell them not to worry, and explain that they are just going through the searching and yearning phase of bereavement.

10. Nurses care for all types of patients with various conditions, including those with a terminal illness. Which statement is true about terminal illnesses?

    1. Death from terminal illness is sudden and unexpected.
    2. Physicians know when death will occur.
    3. An illness is terminal when no reasonable hope of recovery exists.
    4. All severe injuries result in death.

11. After the death of a patient, the nurse leaves the room quickly; she is found sobbing in the utility room. Which action is the most supportive to the nurse?

    1. Sending the nurse home for the rest of the shift
    2. Reassigning the nurse to an area where it is unlikely a patient will die
    3. Sitting with her and allowing her to express herself
    4. Insisting that she perform postmortem care for the patient

12. What type of care allows a patient to make more informed choices, achieve better alleviation of symptoms, and have more opportunity to work on issues such as closure?

    1. Acute care
    2. Mourning care
    3. Palliative care
    4. Terminal care

13. A healthy 25-year-old who sustained a head injury during a motor vehicle accident is in the emergency department. The patient has no brain activity and is on life support. The family has expressed an interest in organ donation. What should the nurse know about organ donations?

    1. Organ donations can occur only if the patient has given prior consent.
    2. Vital organs, such as the heart and pancreas, must be harvested while the patient remains on the ventilator.
    3. Brain death can be reversed, so the family should be informed to take more time in making their decision.
    4. The attending physician must be present in the operating room during harvesting of the organs.

14. A bereaved widow of 3 months tells the nurse she has smelled her deceased husband's aftershave scent clearly as she sat in church recently. She questions if she might be "going crazy." What is the widow experiencing?

    1. Intrusive memories
    2. Dysfunctional or complicated grief
    3. Sense of presence
    4. Grief attacks

15. The adult children of a dying patient, who is alert and oriented, disagree on the patient's choice of a do-not-resuscitate order. The children ask the opinion of the nurse, who has cared for this patient over an extended period. How should the nurse respond to this question about the patient's dying request?

    1. Encourage the children to speak with the physician regarding their concerns.
    2. Remind the children that this is the wish of their parent.
    3. Ask the patient to speak with the children regarding their concerns.
    4. Listen to the children's concerns and encourage them to talk to their parent.

16. A nurse is preparing to care for a dying patient, and several family members are at the bedside. Select the therapeutic techniques that the nurse uses when communicating with the family. *(Select all that apply.)*

    1. Be honest and truthful and let the patient and family know that the nurse will not abandon them.
    2. Explain everything that is happening to all family members.
    3. Encourage expression of feelings, concerns, and fears.
    4. Extend touch and hold the patient's or family member's hand if appropriate.
    5. Make the decisions for the family.
    6. Discourage reminiscing.

17. The nurse is providing postmortem care for a patient. Which interventions are appropriate before allowing the family to visit? *(Select all that apply.)*

    1. Prepare the body to look as clean and natural as possible.
    2. Wear sterile gloves to provide postmortem care.
    3. Keep the sheet cover over the patient's face until the family is comfortably seated in the room.
    4. Remove the external tubes and drains if there is no autopsy required.
    5. Call the health care provider to obtain an order to release the body to the mortician.

18. The nurse is caring for a dying patient. What are clinical signs of death? *(Select all that apply.)*

    1. Slow, thready pulse
    2. Absence of apical pulse
    3. Cessation of respirations
    4. Cessation of bowel sounds
    5. Flat encephalogram

19. The nurse is conducting an assessment on the dying patient. Which statement by the patient would indicate the patient is experiencing the stage of acceptance by Kübler-Ross?

    1. "I am helping my spouse plan my obituary and funeral."
    2. "I can do anything I want. I plan to live forever."
    3. "I promise I will do better for my family if I just could live a few more weeks."
    4. "This cannot be happening. I did not do anything to deserve this condition."

20. A young mother has just given birth to a boy born with severe birth defects. She states, "I feel so sad, I wanted a normal child. I do not want to see the baby." Which type of loss is the mother experiencing?

    1. Anticipatory loss
    2. Complicated loss
    3. Maturational loss
    4. Situational loss

21. The community hospice nurse is conducting a follow-up visit with the family 3 months after the death of a loved one. Which statement by the family member indicates that she is experiencing grief?

    1. "I really miss Charlie; it is hard to accept that he is gone."
    2. "I realize that Charlie is gone; I am adjusting to sleeping alone."
    3. "I was able to go on a date with a friend I met a couple of weeks ago."
    4. "I believe that Charlie would want me to move on with my life and meet new people."

22. The dying patient asks the nurse to assist him to say goodbye to his son, who is 4 years old. Which suggestion by the nurse is age appropriate for the 4-year-old?

    1. We could do a role play.
    2. You could read him a poem.
    3. Tell him you are going on a trip to heaven.
    4. You could write him a letter that he can read when he gets older.

23. A teenager brought by ambulance to the Emergency Room from the scene of a motor vehicular accident is pronounced dead upon arrival. The family is notified of the death and request to see their child before the funeral home picks up the body. Which actions by the nurse are most respectful when caring for the patient and family during a sudden death? *(Select all that apply.)*

    1. Preparing the body to look as clean and natural as possible
    2. Encouraging the parents to discuss what caused the accident
    3. Allowing the parents to spend as much time as possible with the body
    4. Leaving the body uncovered while it is being transferred to a quiet room
    5. Rushing the parents to say goodbye because it's almost time for a shift change
    6. Offering to call the pastor of the family's church while the family is viewing the body

24. A male patient, 87, is dying of lung cancer. He lives alone and at his request, he is moved into a hospice facility. The patient is conscious and communicates but no longer desires food. He has cachexia, dehydration, dry mouth, anorexia, and fatigue. He expresses acceptance of his own death but wants closure with his family. His only son is deceased, but his granddaughter, her husband, and two small grandchildren live 20 minutes away. The granddaughter is anxious about leaving her grandfather alone in a new place but is equally anxious about spending time alone with him. She says she has always had tension with her grandfather—they used to argue bitterly about politics a lot when she was a teenager—but she loves him and wants to be of help. Her own children, ages seven and ten, are another story. They adore their great-grandfather and have asked to see him. He is in favor of it and says, "Can you make sure I'm not in any pain when they come?" His daughter asks the nurse's advice about this. She also asks, "How do I talk to my grandpa while he is dying? Being alone with him terrifies me. I'm afraid I might make him cry." The nurse counsels the granddaughter and the patient's anxiolytic and pain control are timed for optimal comfort during the visit.

Given what you know about this patient, what are the most effective actions to take? *(Select all that apply.)*

ACTIONS	EFFECTIVE
a. Assure the daughter that it is okay for children to visit a dying patient in hospice.	
b. Gently discourage the patient's hopes of a reconciliation in case it cannot be achieved, causing more grief.	
c. Teach the daughter to reassure her grandfather that he is not dying and that there is always hope of recovery.	
d. Provide oral care at least every 2–4 h.	
e. Remind support staff that only a nurse can position a patient who has trouble breathing.	
f. Remind staff that only the nurse can administer this patient's medications.	

Health Promotion and Pregnancy

Objectives

1. Explain the physiology of conception.
2. Discuss the anatomic and physiologic alterations that occur during pregnancy.
3. Identify the components of antepartal assessment.
4. Differentiate among the presumptive, possible, and positive signs of pregnancy.
5. List the danger signs that might occur during pregnancy.
6. Describe nutritional requirements during pregnancy.
7. Discuss the common discomforts of pregnancy.
8. Discuss cultural practices and beliefs that may affect ongoing health care during pregnancy.
9. Identify nursing diagnoses relevant to care of the prenatal patient.

Key Terms

abortion (ă-BŎR-shĕn, p. 776)
amniocentesis (ăm-nē-ō-sĕn-TĒ-sĭs, p. 789)
antepartal (ăn-tē-PĂR-tăl, p. 791)
ballottement (bă-LŎT-mĕnt, p. 792)
blastocyst (BLĂS-tō-sĭst, p. 776)
chorionic villi (kō-rē-ŎN-ĭk VĬL-ī, p. 776)
chorionic villus sampling (p. 788)
crown-rump length (p. 787)
ectoderm (ĔK-tō-dĕrm, p. 776)
ectopic pregnancy (ĕk-TŎP-ĭk PRĔG-năn-sē, p. 776)
endoderm (ĔN-dō-dĕrm, p. 776)
flagellation (flăj-ĕ-LĀ-shŭn, p. 776)
fundus (fŭn-dŭs, p. 785)
Goodell's sign (p. 792)
gravida (GRĂV-ĭ-dă, p. 794)
Hëgar's sign (p. 792)
implantation (p. 776)

intrapartal (p. 791)
lanugo (lă-NŪ-gō, p. 777)
mesoderm (MĔZ-ō-dĕrm, p. 775)
morula (MŎR-ū-lă, p. 776)
nuchal translucency screening (p. 788)
para (p. 794)
perinatal (p. 791)
postpartal (p. 791)
prenatal (p. 791)
relaxin (p. 798)
teratogenic agents (tĕr-ă-tō-JĔN-ĭk Ā-gĕnts, p. 775)
trimesters (p. 791)
ultrasonography (ŭl-tră-sŏ-NŎG-ră-fē, p. 785)
villi (VĬL-ī, p. 776)
Wharton's jelly (p. 777)
zygote (ZĪ-gōt, p. 776)

Few experiences in life are as exciting and as challenging as childbearing. Profound and dramatic changes occur in a relatively short time. Childbearing is a challenge to the new mother, to the newly developing or changing family unit, to society, and to the nurse who assists in the childbearing process. The maternity nurse is in a unique position of providing care to the unborn.

The goal of maternity care is a healthy pregnancy with a physically safe and emotionally satisfying outcome for mother and infant. Consistent health supervision and surveillance are paramount. Many pregnant women and their families are unfamiliar with the changes that accompany pregnancy. The knowledgeable maternity nurse can help a pregnant woman recognize the relationship between her physical status and her care plan. Sharing information encourages the pregnant woman to participate in her own care, depending on her interest, need to know, and readiness to learn.

PHYSIOLOGY OF PREGNANCY

Understanding the physiologic changes of pregnancy begins with understanding the normal anatomy and physiology of the male and female reproductive systems. A review of the menstrual cycle and related hormonal activity is particularly important. Also important is recognition that specific cells (ova in the female and sperm in the male) carry genetic messages to their offspring. These cells are united to form a new individual with a unique genetic makeup.

FERTILIZATION

During sexual intercourse, sperm carried in the male's ejaculatory semen enter the female's vagina. By flagellation (whiplike movement), the sperm travel through the mucus of the cervical canal (if the mucus is receptive), enter the uterine chamber, and move into the ampulla—the outer third of the fallopian tube. If the timing is right, an ovum has been produced and is also within the ampulla of the tube; in such cases, fertilization may occur. Fertilization (also called *conception*) takes place when the sperm joins or fuses with the ovum. The fusion of the sperm into the ovum requires approximately 24 hours. Once fertilization has occurred, the new cell is referred to as a zygote (cell formed by the union of two reproductive cells) or a fertilized ovum. This cell carries 46 chromosomes (44 autosomes and 2 sex chromosomes). At the moment of fertilization, the sex of the zygote and all other genetic characteristics are determined and do not change.

IMPLANTATION

The zygote moves through the uterine tube via ciliary action and some irregular peristaltic activity. It takes 3 or 4 days to enter the uterine cavity. During this time, the zygote is in a phase of rapid cell division called *mitosis*. Further changes result in formation of a structure called the morula (developmental stage of the fertilized ovum in which a solid mass of cells resembles a mulberry), which develops into the blastocyst (the embryonic form; a spherical mass of cells with a central fluid-filled cavity surrounded by two layers of cells). Stem cells are derived from the inner cell mass of the blastocyst. After the blastocyst is free in the uterine cavity for 1 or 2 days, the exposed cell walls of the blastocyst (called the *trophoblast*) secrete enzymes that can break down protein and penetrate cell membranes. These enzymes allow the blastocyst to enter the endometrium and implant. The action of the enzymes normally stops short of the myometrium, but may cause slight bleeding in some individuals. This is called *implantation bleeding*. Although this bleeding is rarely more than spotting, it may confuse some women, who think that they had a very light and short menstrual cycle, when actually they are pregnant.

The condition of the uterine lining is critical for implantation (embedding of the fertilized ovum in the uterine mucosa) of the zygote. During the secretory phase of the menstrual cycle, the endometrium has an enriched vascular bed with enlarged blood vessels and an increased store of glycogen, which support development of the embryo if implantation occurs. Implantation usually occurs in the fundus of the uterus on either the anterior or the posterior surfaces. If uterine conditions are not suitable, implantation is unlikely to occur. If intrauterine vascular or hormonal conditions cannot sustain the implanted embryo, a spontaneous abortion occurs. Abortion is the medical term used to refer to the loss of a pregnancy before 20 weeks' gestation. Most spontaneous abortions occur during the first 8 weeks of pregnancy for these reasons. Ectopic pregnancy is a serious condition that refers to the implantation of the fertilized egg outside of the uterine cavity. These conditions are discussed further in Chapter 29.

During the first few weeks after implantation, primary villi (short vascular processes or protrusions that grow on certain membranous surfaces) appear. These villi use maternal blood vessels as a source of nourishment and oxygen for the developing embryo. The villi nourish the embryo from the time of implantation (about 2 weeks after conception) until the seventh or eighth week. Also during these first few weeks, the first stages of the chorionic villi (tiny vascular protrusions on the chorionic surface that project into the maternal blood sinuses of the uterus and help form the placenta) occur. Chorionic villi secrete human chorionic gonadotropin (hCG), a hormone that stimulates the continued production of progesterone and estrogen by the corpus luteum, which is the reason ovulation and menstruation cease during pregnancy. Primary villi also synthesize protein and glucose for approximately 12 weeks, until the fetus is developed adequately to meet its own needs. The chorionic villi become the fetal portion of the placenta.

EMBRYONIC AND FETAL DEVELOPMENT

Until the time of implantation (the germinal phase), the cell mass is referred to as the zygote. During this period, the fertilized ovum develops from the two original cells into a many-celled organism. When the growing mass of cells reaches about 32 cells, it is referred to as a morula. As the cells continue to divide, they separate into an inner and outer group of cells. This stage is referred to as the blastocyst. The inner cells become the embryo. The zygote develops two separate and distinct cavities: the amniotic cavity and the yolk sac. The amniotic cavity has walls lined with the ectoderm (outer layer of embryonic tissue that gives rise to skin, nails, and hair) and is filled with amniotic fluid. The yolk sac is lined with the endoderm (the innermost of the cell layers, which develop into the lining of cavities, passages of the body, and the covering of most internal organs). The yolk sac supplies nourishment until implantation. A third layer of primary cells, the mesoderm (embryonic middle layer of germ cells that gives rise to all types of muscles, connective tissue, bone marrow, blood, lymphoid tissue, and all epithelial tissue), is located between the two cavities. The embryo develops at the point at which these three layers meet, called the *trilaminar embryonic disk*.

The embryonic stage begins with implantation and encompasses approximately the first 8 weeks of pregnancy. During the embryonic stage, the three primary cell layers differentiate into tissue and layers, which form the placenta, embryonic membranes, and the embryo. Cell growth is rapid. A simple heart begins beating, and rudimentary (basic, initial, or primary) forms of all the major organs and systems develop. By the end of this stage, the embryo has acquired a human appearance. Starting with the ninth week, the embryo is referred to as the *fetus,* and the fetal stage begins. (See Chapter 32 and Fig. 32.1 for fetal circulation.)

Many structures develop simultaneously in the embryo; therefore, when an infant is born with one birth defect or abnormality, the physician checks for others that may be associated with the identified defect. During the early weeks of pregnancy, often before a woman even knows that she is pregnant, teratogenic agents (any drug, virus, or substance that can cause malformation of the fetus) can cause serious harm. For example, rubella, or German measles, is a known *teratogen* (a nongenetic factor that causes malformations and disease syndromes in utero). Although rubella is usually a mild childhood disease, at this stage of pregnancy, the virus can affect all of the germ layers and cause serious anomalies, such as cardiac defects, deafness, and cognitive impairment.

The prenatal calendar (Table 26.1) describes fetal development and maternal changes throughout pregnancy.

EMBRYONIC AND FETAL PHYSIOLOGY

Placenta

The *placenta* (Greek, "flat plate") is a disklike organ made up of about 20 sections called *cotyledons.* It is a unique structure, present only during pregnancy. The placenta becomes fully functioning by week 12. At full term, the placenta looks like a large red disk with a diameter of 8 inches (20 cm) and a thickness of 1 inch (2.5 cm). It normally weighs between 1 lb and 1 lb, 5 oz (450 and 600 g). The bulk of the placenta is fetal in origin. The side attached to the uterine wall ("Dirty Duncan") appears dark red and has a rough surface; the cotyledons are apparent as distinct lobes, with clefts or divisions between each lobe. Presentation of the Duncan side after delivery is associated with blood expulsion with the placenta. The fetal side is smooth and shiny ("Shiny Schultze"). It consists of the membranes of the amniotic sac that encases the fetus. A small gush of blood precedes the placenta when the Schultze side is presenting. On delivery, the placenta is assessed and the presenting side determined; then, the placenta is examined for intactness. The findings are documented.

As mentioned, the placenta functions as an endocrine gland that secretes hCG and the steroidal hormones estrogen and progesterone, which maintain the pregnancy. In addition, the placenta is the site of the exchange of nutrients, oxygen, and waste products between the fetus and the maternal circulation. The placenta allows transfer of oxygen and nutrients through such processes as diffusion and active transport, and it also blocks the transfer of certain substances. This is called the placental barrier. Some viruses can cross the placental barrier, but most bacteria are too large to cross. Some drugs do not cross the placenta, but most do and can cause serious harm to the growing embryo or fetus. After delivery, the placenta is of no further use and is expelled.

Fetal Membranes

The amniotic sac is composed of two layers, both of which originate in the zygote. The outer layer, the *chorion,* attaches to the fetal portion of the placenta. The inner layer, the *amnion,* blends with the fetal umbilical cord. These membranes appear fragile, but in fact, they are strong enough to contain the fetus and amniotic fluid even at full term.

Umbilical Cord

The umbilical cord joins the embryo to the placenta. It originates in the fetal portion of the placenta and normally is attached near the center. The cord is typically 20 to 22 inches (50 to 55 cm) long and less than 1 inch (2.5 cm) in diameter at the time of delivery. Umbilical cords can vary widely in appearance. The major part of the cord is a pale, white, gelatinous-mucoid substance called Wharton's jelly (a gelatinous tissue that remains when the embryonic body stalk blends with the yolk sac within the umbilical cord). This substance prevents compression of the blood vessels and aids in insulating the vessels within the umbilical cord. The normal umbilical cord has two arteries and one vein that may give the cord a ropelike appearance. On occasion, the cord has only two vessels—one artery and one vein. This phenomenon is seen in less than 3% of deliveries. It may be associated with fetal anomalies and requires follow-up. The vein carries oxygenated blood to the fetus; the arteries carry deoxygenated blood back to the placenta. The cord has no pain receptors, so cutting at the time of delivery does not cause pain.

Amniotic Fluid

Amniotic fluid surrounds the fetus in utero. It begins production early in the pregnancy and is present in increasing amounts. Approximately 30 mL (1 oz) are present at 10 to 12 weeks' gestation. The peak volume is noted around 34 weeks' gestation at approximately 800 to 1000 mL. The amniotic fluid has several important functions for the fetus. It acts as a cushion against mechanical injury; helps regulate fetal temperature; allows the developing embryo or fetus room for growth, which promotes musculoskeletal development; and provides for fetal lung development. The fluid is clear yellow with a slightly alkaline pH. Amniotic fluid contains albumin, urea, uric acid, creatinine, bilirubin, *lecithin* (phospholipids for fat metabolism), *sphingomyelin* (a compound of lipids and sphingosine, found in high concentrations in the brain and other tissues of the nervous system), fructose, fat, leukocytes, proteins, epithelial cells, enzymes, and strands of lanugo (downy, fine hair found on the fetus from 20 weeks' gestation until birth). Amniocentesis (discussed subsequently) can be done after the first trimester of pregnancy to aid in determination of fetal development, maturity, health, and gender.

Table 26.1   Fetal Development and Maternal Events During Pregnancy and Drug Substances to Avoid

	WEEK 1	WEEK 2	WEEK 3	WEEK 4	WEEK 5	WEEK 6	WEEK 7	WEEK 8
Embryonic Development	The ovum becomes fertilized, divides, and burrows into the uterus.	The embryonic disk (ectoderm, endoderm, mesoderm) is formed. These three primitive germ layers generate every organ and tissue in the infant's body.	The first body segments appear; they eventually form the primitive spine, brain, and spinal cord.	Heart, blood circulation, and digestive tract take shape. The embryo is now 0.2 inch long; the head is a third of its total length.	The heart starts to pump blood; limb buds appear. Major divisions of the brain can now be discerned.	Eyes begin to take shape; external ears develop from skin folds.	Development proceeds rapidly. The face is now complete, with eyes, nose, lips, and tongue—even primitive milk teeth. Tiny bones and muscles appear beneath the thin skin.	The embryo is now a little more than 1 inch long.
Maternal Events	Ovaries increase production of the pregnancy-maintaining hormone, progesterone.	The first period is missed.	Placenta grows to cover 1/15 of the uterine interior. Breasts may begin to feel tender. There is no weight gain.			Exchange of fetal and maternal metabolites across the placenta begins, yet the two circulations are completely separate.	No noticeable weight gain occurs.	The placenta now covers about one-third of the uterine lining.

Common Maternal Discomforts | **Remedies**

- Morning sickness occurs because increased hormonal activity slows down the digestive system, apparently to enhance the absorption of nutrients for the baby. | Eat a few dry crackers before rising. Eat frequent, small, low-fat meals during the day. Drink liquids.

- Fatigue is thought to be caused by a change in ovarian hormone production (progesterone and relaxin), the purpose of which is to relax pelvic ligaments, stimulate breast growth, and soften the cervix. | Exercise regularly and get plenty of sleep with frequent naps during the day.

- Urinary frequency is caused by the uterus compressing the bladder against the pelvic bones, thus reducing its capacity, and by hormonal changes that affect the water balance in the body. | Decrease pressure on the bladder at night by sleeping on the side.

Drug Substances to Avoid | **Acceptable Alternatives**

- Antiemetics: Most traditionally used antiemetic medications are avoided during pregnancy. | Doxylamine succinate (Diclegis) a prescribed medication to manage nausea and vomiting in pregnancy.

- Stimulants: amphetamines, excessive caffeine. *(Avoid throughout pregnancy.)*

WEEK 9	WEEK 10	WEEK 11	WEEK 12	WEEK 13	WEEK 14	WEEK 15	WEEK 16
Embryonic and Fetal Development							
Genitalia are now well defined; the baby's sex is determined. Eyelids finish forming and seal shut. The embryo becomes a fetus.	The fetus assumes a more human shape as the lower body rapidly develops. Blood and bone cells form. The first movements begin.	Organs begin to function. The pancreas produces insulin; the kidneys produce urine.	The lungs have taken shape; primitive breathing motions begin. The swallowing reflex has been mastered as the fetus sucks its thumb while floating weightlessly in the amniotic fluid.		The musculoskeletal system has matured. The nervous system begins to exercise some control over the body; blood vessels rapidly develop.	With hands ready to grasp, the fetus, now weighing about 7 oz, kicks against the amniotic sac.	All organs and structures have been formed, and a period of growth begins.

Continued

Table 26.1   Fetal Development and Maternal Events During Pregnancy and Drug Substances to Avoid—cont'd

	WEEK 1	WEEK 2	WEEK 3	WEEK 4	WEEK 5	WEEK 6	WEEK 7	WEEK 8
Maternal Events								
	Maternal blood volume has increased 30%–40%.	Some women describe the sensation of these first movements as if something were blowing bubbles through a straw in their stomachs.	There is a 2- to 3-lb weight gain and a possible increase in perspiration.	The placenta has reached complete functional maturity, acting as the baby's lungs, kidneys, liver, and digestive and immune systems.		There is a 3- to 4-lb weight gain, and her belly begins to show.		Placenta begins producing the estrogen hormone.

Common Maternal Discomforts

	Remedies
• Sleeplessness may result from the discomfort or anxieties of pregnancy.	Take warm shower before sleeping. Support body parts with pillows.
• Vaginal secretions are the result of an increased supply of blood and glucose to the vaginal mucosa. Severe pruritus, irritation, and malodor suggest infection. If infection is suspected, consult a professional.	Cleanse daily with warm water, keeping the area dry to prevent chafing. Apply yogurt for vulvar pruritus.
• Headaches may occur while her body adjusts to changes in blood volume and vascular tone. Emotional tension may also be a factor.	Change body positions slowly. Resting with a damp cloth on the forehead may help. Drink milk or eat a small snack to obtain some relief.

Drug Substances to Avoid

	Acceptable Alternatives
• Tranquilizers, narcotics, antihistamines, alcohol, barbiturates *(Avoid throughout pregnancy.)*	None
• Vaginal antiinfectives may be employed in pregnancy but options such as metronidazole are avoided.	Nystatin, miconazole, and clortrimazole
• Avoid x-rays.	None
• Analgesics: salicylates (aspirin), phenacetin-caffeine, indomethacin (Indocin), tranquilizers. *(Avoid throughout pregnancy.)*	Acetaminophen

	WEEK 17	WEEK 18	WEEK 19	WEEK 20	WEEK 21	WEEK 22	WEEK 23	WEEK 24
Fetal Development		An oily coating protects the fetus. Fine hair covers the body and keeps the oil on the skin.	Eyebrows, eyelashes, and head hair develop.	The fetus is now following a regular schedule of sleeping, turning, sucking, and kicking and has settled on a favorite position in the uterus.		The skeleton is developing rapidly as the bone-forming cells increase their activity.	Eyelids begin to open and close.	The fetus now weighs about 27 oz.
Maternal Events		There is a 3- to 4-lb weight gain. The fetal heartbeat can now be heard with an amplified stethoscope.	Breasts begin secreting colostrum in preparation for nursing.	Placenta reaches its largest size relative to fetus, covering half the uterine lining. The amniotic sac contains 400 mL of fluid.		There is a 3- to 4-lb weight gain.		The placenta becomes thicker rather than wider. Mother can now sense when baby is awake.

Continued

Table 26.1 Fetal Development and Maternal Events During Pregnancy and Drug Substances to Avoid—cont'd

WEEK 1	WEEK 2	WEEK 3	WEEK 4	WEEK 5	WEEK 6	WEEK 7	WEEK 8

Common Maternal Discomforts

Remedies

- Faintness or dizziness occurs when standing suddenly, caused by reduced blood flow to the brain as the body adjusts to new circulatory patterns. Shortness of breath may occur.

  Try to sit with feet up when possible; rise slowly and support yourself. Smelling salts, aromatic spirits of ammonia.

- Varicose veins are often the result of rising blood pressure in the lower extremities. This is caused by the enlarged uterus cutting off blood flow back from the legs to the heart.

  When sitting, rest legs on footstool with feet elevated; avoid pressure on lower thighs. Many women find support stockings helpful.

- Allergies, such as hay fever, are a common problem.

  Use air conditioning (with a clean filter) and wear a pollen mask to screen out allergens.

- Skin changes such as darkened nipples, stretch marks, splotches on cheeks and forehead, acne, and redness on palms and soles are the result of increased hormone levels in the blood.

  Be patient. Virtually all of these effects subside soon after childbirth. If nipples or abdomen itch, a lanolin-based cream or baby oil can provide relief.

- Epistaxis sometimes occurs because of increased blood volume and nasal congestion.

  Apply a little petroleum jelly in each nostril, which should stop the bleeding. Use a humidifier. Do not irritate nasal mucosa.

Drug Substances to Avoid

Acceptable Alternatives

- Tranquilizers, alcohol (Avoid throughout pregnancy.)

  None

- Traditionally antihistamines have been largely avoided in pregnancy.

  Chlorpheniramine for congestion; pseudoephedrine or nasal spray for stuffy nose may be used occasionally, if necessary; calamine lotion for rashes.

- Tetracycline (for acne) (Avoid throughout pregnancy.)

  A mild soap can remove the excessive facial oil produced by acne.

WEEK 25	WEEK 26	WEEK 27	WEEK 28	WEEK 29	WEEK 30	WEEK 31	WEEK 32

Fetal Development

To a certain extent, the fetus can now breathe, swallow, and regulate its body temperature, but it still depends greatly on maternal support.

A substance called surfactant forms in the lungs, preparing them to function independently after birth.

Fetus is two-thirds grown.

Fat deposits are building up beneath the skin to insulate the fetus against the abrupt change in temperature at birth.

The digestive tract and the lungs are now nearly fully matured, and the skin becomes less red and wrinkled.

The fetus has grown to about 14 inches.

Maternal Events

- There is a 3- to 4-lb weight gain.
- Respiratory movements can be detected with ultrasound scan. Mother sometimes feels baby's breathing as "hiccups."
- The volume of amniotic fluid decreases to make room for growing fetus.
- There is a 3- to 5-lb weight gain.

Common Maternal Discomforts

Common Maternal Discomforts	Remedies
Leg and muscle cramps may be caused by fatigue, pressure exerted on the nerves by the uterus, or too little calcium or too much phosphorus in the diet.	Exercise regularly, especially walking. Elevate legs and flex toes when resting. Increase milk consumption.
Pyrosis (heartburn) often occurs because the stomach emptying time is delayed, causing a burning sensation in the throat.	Drink milk between small, frequent meals. This problem disappears soon after the baby's birth.
Edema of ankles occurs. The pressure of the uterus on the large veins returning blood to the heart may induce water retention.	Elevate legs, once or twice a day for an hour or so, level with the hips. Sleep on the left side.
Constipation is another result of the decelerated digestive process. As food moves slowly through the intestines, more water is extracted, leaving the stool drier and harder.	Eat foods that contain roughage, such as raw fruits, vegetables, and cereals with bran. Drink liquids and exercise frequently.
Mother may have trouble sleeping because of baby's activity.	Soak in a warm bath or sit on soft pillows to soothe the symptoms.
Hemorrhoids may develop.	Dibucaine (Nupercainal) suppositories or cream, hydrocortisone (Anusol), benzocaine (Medicone)

Drug Substances to Avoid

Drug Substances to Avoid	Acceptable Alternatives
Salicylates (aspirin), tranquilizers (Avoid throughout pregnancy.)	Calcium supplements with little or no phosphorus
Antacids: calcium carbonate, magnesium trisilicate (Gaviscon), sodium bicarbonate (baking soda), cimetidine (Tagamet) (Avoid throughout pregnancy.)	Maalox, Mylanta (also for "gas")
Most diuretics ("water pills") (Avoid throughout pregnancy.)	
Laxatives: mineral oil, castor oil (Avoid throughout pregnancy.)	Metamucil, Senokot, teaspoon of Milk of Magnesia at bedtime

Continued

Table 26.1	Fetal Development and Maternal Events During Pregnancy and Drug Substances to Avoid—cont'd

WEEK 33

Fetal Development

TO TERM

Virtually the entire uterus is now occupied by the fetus, and its activity is restricted.

Maternal antibodies against measles, mumps, rubella, whooping cough, and scarlet fever are transferred to the baby, providing protection for about 6 mo until the infant's own immune system can take over.

In 9 mo, the miracle is complete; a single, microscopic, fertilized cell has transformed into a 6 trillion–celled human.

Maternal Events

The placenta is nearly four times as thick as it was 20 weeks before and weighs about 20 oz.

Preparing for birth, the fetus descends deeper into the mother's pelvis. There is a 3- to 5-lb weight gain.

Common Maternal Discomforts

Remedies

- Backaches are often caused by muscles and ligaments relaxing in preparation for the stretching required in delivery and by the added off-center weight of the enlarged uterus.

Do back exercises, such as the "pelvic tilt," which can help strengthen back and abdominal muscles. Wear low-heeled shoes or flats; avoid heavy lifting.

- Urinary frequency is caused (for the second time in pregnancy) by the uterus compressing the bladder against the pelvic bones, thus reducing its capacity.

Decrease pressure on the bladder at night by sleeping on your side. Urinate frequently.

- Uterine contractions become perceptible as the cervix and lower uterine segment prepare for labor.

Drug Substances to Avoid

Acceptable Alternatives

- Analgesics: salicylates (aspirin), propoxyphene (Darvon), phenacetin-caffeine, indomethacin (Indocin), codeine *(Avoid throughout pregnancy.)*

Tylenol brand acetaminophen (occasional use)

ASSESSMENT OF FETAL WELL-BEING

A variety of technological and assessment tools can be used in evaluation of fetal well-being. These tools are used to evaluate maternal and fetal health problems, fetal congenital anomalies, and fetal growth and maturity (Table 26.2).

Fetal Heart Tones

The fetal heart shows activity by the seventh week of gestation. Practitioners can auscultate fetal heart tones (FHTs) between 10 and 12 weeks with a Doppler scan (see Fig. 26.1). To hear the FHTs, place the instrument in the midline, just above the symphysis pubis, and apply firm pressure. Some difficulty may be encountered in locating FHTs in obese women during the early stages. Offer the woman and her family the opportunity to listen to the FHTs, which are to be assessed for a full minute. The rate and characteristics of the tones should be evaluated. FHTs are assessed at each of the expectant mother's visits for the remainder of the pregnancy.

Fundal Height

During the second trimester, the growing uterus rises from the pelvic cavity and becomes an abdominal organ. The top portion of the uterus is referred to as the fundus. The fundal height, or measurement of the height of the uterus above the symphysis pubis, is one indicator of fetal growth. McDonald's method is used commonly. The measurement also provides a gross estimate of the duration of pregnancy. When the fundal height is measured, the woman should be lying flat. Her bladder should be emptied. A paper tape measure or a pelvimeter may be used to measure fundal height. For increased reliability of the measurement, the same person should examine the pregnant woman at each of her prenatal visits. Often, this is not possible, so a protocol should be established that specifies the measurement technique, including the woman's position on the examining table, the measuring device, and the method of measurement used (Fig. 26.2).

During the second and third trimesters (weeks 18 to 30), the height of the fundus in centimeters is approximately the same as the number of weeks of gestation. Some maternal characteristics may affect the accuracy of the measurement (Box 26.1). The measurement of fundal height may aid in identification of high-risk factors. A decreased fundal height may indicate intrauterine growth restriction (IUGR) or an inadequate level of amniotic fluid (oligohydramnios); an excessive increase could indicate multifetal gestation or hydramnios (excessive amniotic fluid).

Human Chorionic Gonadotropin Levels

hCG is the hormone assessed in pregnancy tests. This hormone can be detected in urine and blood. Testing for hCG can be quantitative or qualitative. Quantitative

Fig. 26.1 Detecting fetal heartbeat. (A) Fetoscope (18–20 weeks). (B) Doppler ultrasound stethoscope (12 weeks). (A, From McKinney ES, James SR, Murray SS: *Maternal-child nursing*, ed 4, St. Louis, 2013, Saunders.)

testing considers the level or amount of the hormone in the specimen. Quantitative results are obtained from a blood specimen. Qualitative testing simply determines the presence or absence of a substance. Qualitative testing for hCG may be performed on the blood and the urine. During pregnancy, the levels of HCG may be used to assess the viability and gestation of the pregnancy. hCG levels that are less than anticipated for a specific point in gestation may signal a pregnancy that is no longer viable. Quantitative hCG levels may be reported every few days to determine whether they are rising, as in a normally developing pregnancy, or whether they are declining in a manner consistent with miscarriage.

Ultrasound Scan

During ultrasonography, high-frequency sound waves are used to visualize the fetus. Because soft tissue is visualized, this noninvasive tool can be used to determine gestational age, monitor fetal growth, determine the number of fetuses and the location of the placenta, estimate the volume of amniotic fluid, and detect anomalies. It also can be used in conjunction with invasive tests such as amniocentesis. The gestational

Table 26.2   Assessment Tools to Evaluate Fetal Well-Being

DIAGNOSTIC TEST OR ASSESSMENT TOOL	DESCRIPTION AND PURPOSE	GESTATIONAL AGE
Transvaginal ultrasound	High-frequency sound waves visualize fetus to help confirm pregnancy, determine gestational age, visualize number of fetuses and location of placenta, estimate volume of amniotic fluid, note presence of anomalies.	Performed up to the 12th week of pregnancy.
Abdominal ultrasound	High-frequency sound waves to visualize the fetus. Uses: • Confirmation of pregnancy • Assess viability of pregnancy • Assessment and estimation of gestational age • Confirmation of number of fetal numbers, presentation and position • Assessment of placental position • Confirm pregnancy, assess viability • Assessment of amniotic fluid volume • Assistance with other diagnostic tests in pregnancy such as chorionic villus sampling and amniocentesis	Performed throughout the pregnancy.
Maternal serum alpha-fetoprotein (AFP) screening	Provides probability for the presence of neural tube defects or chromosomal disorders such as Down syndrome or	Performed between 16 and 18 weeks' gestation.
Chorionic villus sampling (CVS)	Aspiration of small amount of tissue from the villi of the placenta. It may be performed transabdominally or transcervically. Assesses for genetic or chromosomal disorders in the fetus.	Performed between 10 and 12 weeks' gestation.
Amniocentesis	Aspiration of small amount of amniotic fluid. Used to determine the presence of chromosomal abnormalities, health status, gender and fetal lung maturity. May be used to reduce amniotic fluid levels in the gravid woman with severe hydramnios.	May be performed as early as the 15th week of gestation and onward.
Nuchal translucency testing	Employs an ultrasound to assess the nuchal thickness of the fetus. Thicknesses greater than 2.5 mm are suspicious and may signal Down syndrome.	Performed between 11 and 14 weeks' gestation.
Nonstress test (NST)	Fetal movement and fetal heart rate recorded with external fetal monitors to evaluate the response of the fetal heart rate to fetal movement. The mother notes when movements are felt. This is reviewed in correlation to the fetal heart rates.	Performed from 28 weeks' gestation onward.
Contraction stress test (CST)	Contractions are simulated by nipple stimulation or the administration of oxytocin. The fetal heart rate is reviewed in relation to the contractions. Declines in heart rate at the midpoint or after of the contraction indicate the need for follow-up.	Performed after 34th week of pregnancy with stimulation of uterine contractions.
Magnetic resonance imaging (MRI)	Noninvasive tool provides images of soft tissue. Vascular structures within the body may be seen without the use of iodinated contrast medium, without biological risk. Interference from skeletal, fatty, or gas-filled structures is not a problem as it is in ultrasound scan.	May be performed throughout the pregnancy.
Biophysical profile (BPP)	Assesses the adequacy of the uterine environment to support the pregnancy. It applies a score to fetal breathing movements, fetal muscle tone, fetal movements, amniotic fluid volume, and an evaluation of the NST.	Normally performed after 32 weeks' gestation but can be considered as early as 24 weeks' gestation if fetal compromise is suggested.
Daily fetal movement count (DFMC; kick count)	Measurement of fetal movement as an indicator of fetal health. Advantages of the test include that it is simple, low cost, noninvasive, and fast. Instruct woman to count fetal movements for 1 h two or three times daily. No exact number of movements has been identified as a "failing test." However, fewer than three fetal movements in a 1-h period or the absence of fetal movements for 12 h is an indication for further evaluation (see the Patient Teaching box on guidelines for counting fetal movements).	Daily fetal movement count can be done to evaluate the fetus in high-risk pregnancies for complications related to reduced oxygenation.

age often determines the type of ultrasound scan performed. When used to determine the gestational age, the health care provider performs a series of measurements. In the first trimester (13 weeks 6/7 days), the fetal crown-rump length is used. **Crown-rump length** is the measurement from the top of the fetal head to the buttocks. This recording is correct within 5 to 7 days. As the pregnancy progresses and the fetal positioning changes, this becomes an ineffective means to measure gestational age. In the second trimester, the examiner measures fetal head circumference, biparietal diameter, and femur length to calculate gestational age. The degree of accuracy is 7 to 14 days. Estimation of fetal age in the third trimester is even less accurate because of a variety of interrelated factors that include genetics, gender differences, and maternal-related concerns. In the third trimester, the discrepancy may be as great as 21 days. During the first trimester, the transvaginal ultrasound scan may be used. The small distance between the probe, which is inserted vaginally, and the uterus makes the transvaginal ultrasound scan a prime tool for assessment of the early pregnancy to confirm the presence and viability of the pregnancy (American College of Obstetricians and Gynecologists' Committee on Obstetric Practice, 2017).

After the first trimester, the abdominal ultrasound scan is preferred. It may be used singularly or in conjunction with other methods of maternal fetal assessment. Early in pregnancy, the mother is required to drink a quart of water and not void. This allows for the bladder to elevate the uterus for better viewing with the technology.

A growing number of nurses perform ultrasound scans and biophysical profiles (BPPs; a system of estimating current fetal status by analyzing five variables via ultrasound scan and nonstress testing). However, most nurses are involved primarily in counseling and educating women about the procedure (see the Patient Teaching box on ultrasound scan examination).

Patient Teaching

Preparing for Ultrasound Scan Examination

Abdominal ultrasounds completed in the first and second trimester will require a full bladder. This will allow for improved imaging of the fetus. Position the patient comfortably, with pillows under her head and knees, while the test is conducted. A small back roll may be needed to ensure that the patient is not lying flat on her back. Apply ultrasonic gel to the abdomen and pass the scanner over it while images are reproduced. The woman and her partner can watch if they wish. The woman should not feel any discomfort.

For a transvaginal ultrasound scan, tell the woman that she may either be in a lithotomy position or have her pelvis elevated. These positions are optimal for imaging the pelvic structures. Introduce a transducer with a protective sheath covering into the vagina. If the patient has a latex allergy, ensure that the probe covering in use will not be latex. If the woman wants to insert it herself, allow her to do so. The angle of the probe or the tilt of the table may be altered during the examination, but the procedure should not be painful.

Maternal Serum Alpha-Fetoprotein Screening (Quadruple Marker Screening)

Maternal serum alpha-fetoprotein screening is referred to commonly as the quadruple marker screening. The assessment is a screening with results that provide a prediction for the occurrence of certain birth defects. The results do not provide a definitive diagnosis or presence of a disorder. Screening of the levels may be

Fig. 26.2 (A) Measurement of fundal height. (B) McDonald's method.

Box 26.1	Factors That Influence Fundal Height Measurement

- Maternal position
- Maternal stature
- Maternal obesity
- Presence of uterine fibroids
- Elevations in amniotic fluid volume

Data from Davidson M, London M, Ladewig P: *Olds' maternal-newborn nursing and women's health across the lifespan*, ed 9, Upper Saddle River, NJ, 2010, Pearson.

performed to identify the presence of chromosomal abnormalities, such as Down syndrome, or birth defects, such as neural tube defects. The factors assessed with the screening are alpha-fetoprotein, estriol levels, hCG, and inhibin A. Alpha-fetoprotein is a protein produced by the fetal yoke sac and liver. Serum testing should be done between 16 and 18 weeks of gestation. Elevated levels are suggestive of neural tube defects, whereas low levels may suggest a fetus with Down syndrome (trisomy 21). Screening results may be influenced by maternal age and weight, gestational age, and the presence of more than one fetus.

There are factors that may affect the reliability of the results. These include the maternal age, the presence of a multifetal pregnancy, and an incorrect recording of gestational age. Abnormal findings result in additional testing. Ultrasound scan may be performed to assess fetal structures. The ultrasound scan provides no definitive means to rule out the presence of chromosomal defects, which makes an amniocentesis an option for consideration by the mother and her health care provider.

Nuchal Translucency Testing

Nuchal translucency screening is a test that has grown in popularity since the late 1990s. It is a diagnostic procedure used to assess the back of the neck for characteristics consistent with Down syndrome. Fetuses with larger nuchal folds (thickness at the back of the neck) have a greater incidence of Down syndrome (Fig. 26.3). The examination uses an ultrasound scan to measure the nuchal folds. At this point in the pregnancy the patient is asked to drink and not void before the ultrasound. This provides better visualization when the urinary bladder raises the uterus. The test typically is performed between 10 and 13 weeks' gestation. Normal findings for a fetus at this point in development would be up to 2 mm. A finding of excessive nuchal folds is not a definitive diagnosis for Down syndrome, but indicates the need for additional testing, such as an amniocentesis (American College of Obstetricians and Gynecologists [ACOG], n.d.). Other conditions should be considered if findings show an excess in the nuchal region. They include trisomy 13, trisomy 18, Turner syndrome, or congenital heart disorders (National Library of Medicine (NLM), 2020a).

Chorionic Villus Sampling

Chorionic villus sampling (CVS) is a test to detect genetic disorders of the fetus. It usually is performed between 10 and 12 weeks of gestation and requires aspiration of a small amount of tissue from the chorion of the placenta. A primary advantage of the test is the ability to perform it at an early point in the pregnancy, which allows for preparation of the mother in the event of fetal abnormalities. The test may be performed vaginally or abdominally. There are minimal risks with the procedure, including Rh sensitization, infection, and miscarriage. At about 7%, the rate of pregnancy loss with CVS is slightly higher than with the amniocentesis.

Fig. 26.3 Nuchal translucency testing. (Courtesy Dr. Greggory R. DeVore, Fetal Diagnostic Center, Pasadena, California. Reprinted with permission.)

© Elsevier

Fig. 26.4 Transabdominal amniocentesis.

Amniocentesis

Amniocentesis involves removal of a small amount of amniotic fluid with a needle passed through the abdominal wall (Fig. 26.4). This procedure is conducted in conjunction with an abdominal ultrasound scan, which enables the physician to visualize the location of the fetus, the placenta, and a pocket of amniotic fluid. Laboratory examination of the amniotic fluid can reveal valuable information regarding genetic factors such as sex and chromosomal abnormalities, health status, and maturity of the fetus.

Early amniocentesis is performed at approximately the 15th week of pregnancy and is used to detect biochemical or chromosomal abnormalities. This is the earliest point at which there is adequate amniotic fluid for testing. Testing at this time allows the mother to consider termination of the pregnancy before the legal point of viability is reached. The fetus's ability to survive outside the uterus is known as *viability*. In the past several decades, the age of viability has decreased as a result of technological advances. A fetus as young as 22 to 25 weeks' gestation may survive outside of the mother's womb. Later in pregnancy, amniocentesis is used primarily to determine fetal lung maturity. It also may be performed to detect intrauterine infection and fetal distress, and to assess fetal laboratory values.

Nonstress Test

The nonstress test (NST) is done to evaluate how the fetal heart rate responds to periods of fetal movement. It is indicated when a risk exists for placental insufficiency, such as pregnancy-induced hypertension, diabetes,

postmaturity, maternal smoking, or inadequate maternal nutrition. It also may be done as a preventive screening tool for women who have had a past stillbirth. The test can be completed starting at 28 weeks' gestation. It may be ordered as a single test or repeated weekly or biweekly, depending on the mother's individual health history. With a baseline fetal heart rate of 120 to 160 beats/min, the fetal heart rate normally accelerates at least 15 beats/min for at least 15 seconds with fetal movement. Testing is done with external fetal monitors (see Chapter 27), with the tocotransducer recording fetal movement and the ultrasound transducer recording the fetal heart rate. A reactive result indicates a healthy fetus, with findings of at least two fetal movements accompanied by two increases of 15 beats/min in a 20-minute period. A nonreactive NST results when the fetal heart rate does not increase with fetal movements. This may indicate a compromised fetus and requires further evaluation with another NST, a BPP, or a contraction stress test (CST).

Nursing responsibilities include explaining the procedure to the patient, assuring the patient that no discomfort is associated with the NST, encouraging the patient to verbalize her fears, ensuring that the patient eats before the test to elevate serum glucose levels, requesting that the patient empty her bladder and then assume a Sims position, applying the external fetal monitors to the patient's abdomen, observing for an increase in fetal heart rate with fetal movement, and stimulating fetal activity with external methods if the fetus remains quiet for more than 20 minutes.

Contraction Stress Test

The CST, or oxytocin stress test, uses external fetal monitoring and stimulation of contractions to evaluate how the fetal heart rate responds to the decreased oxygen supply during uterine contractions. The test is usually completed 34 weeks' gestation and beyond. Administering the test prior to this point in the pregnancy is not recommended as it can result in the onset of preterm labor. Additional contraindications include undiagnosed vaginal bleeding, preterm rupture of membranes, and placenta previa. The test is commonly used after unsuccessful BPPs, postterm pregnancies, or other complications encountered in the later weeks of pregnancy. Contractions are elicited with the administration of oxytocin or nipple stimulation. The desired response is termed negative, which means that the fetal heart rate increases with the contractions. A positive test is noted when late decelerations are noted in 50% or more of the contractions. A drop in fetal heart rate indicates placental insufficiency and fetal hypoxia. Declines in fetal heart rates are identified by where in the cycle of the contraction they occur. Declines in the heart rate at or after the midpoint of the contraction are referred to as late decelerations. Late decelerations are considered an ominous sign. The fetus may be at risk during labor and need delivery via cesarean section. Equivocal findings result when there are late decelerations, but they occur in less than 50% of the contractions. This result is still concerning and does warrant further assessment. Tests that do not achieve the needed number of contractions or contractions that are inadequate in strength or duration are termed unsatisfactory.

Magnetic Resonance Imaging

Magnetic resonance imaging (MRI) is a noninvasive tool that can be used for obstetric and gynecologic diagnosis. As with computed tomographic (CT) scan, MRI provides excellent pictures of soft tissue. Unlike CT scan, ionizing radiation is not used; thus, vascular structures within the body can be evaluated without injection of an iodinated contrast medium, thereby eliminating any known biological risk. As with sonography, MRI is noninvasive and can provide images in multiple planes, but interference from skeletal, fatty, or gas-filled structures is not a problem. Also, imaging of deep pelvic structures does not depend on a full bladder. Although this procedure has many advantages, its complete safety has not been determined.

Biophysical Profile

The BPP assesses fetal status with evaluation of several factors (Table 26.3). These include the NST, fetal breathing movements, fetal muscle tone, fetal movements, and amniotic fluid volume. Each category is given a score of 0 or 2. A total score of 8 or more is reassuring; lower scores may warrant interruption of the pregnancy.

MATERNAL PHYSIOLOGY

HORMONAL CHANGES

During pregnancy, hormonal changes help to prepare the woman's body to accommodate the advancing pregnancy. Most pregnancy-related hormones initially are produced by the corpus luteum until the placenta begins to function adequately. Pregnancy-related hormones include the following:

- *hCG:* Initially secreted by the trophoplast in the developing pregnancy. It is responsible for stimulation of the corpus luteum to promote production of estrogen and progesterone until the placenta is functioning. hCG is the hormone assessed with a pregnancy test.
- *Human placental lactogen (HPL), also called human chorionic somatomammotropin:* This hormone promotes insulin resistance by the maternal cells, resulting in elevations in serum glucose levels. It affects maternal metabolism, resulting in the maintenance of energy sources for the fetus.
- *Estrogen:* This primary hormone of pregnancy is secreted by the corpus luteum and, later, the placenta. It is responsible for the increased vascularity needed in the developing pregnancy.
- *Progesterone:* This important hormone of pregnancy is secreted by the corpus luteum and, later, the placenta. It often is referred to as the maintenance hormone of pregnancy. This hormone has properties that enable it to relax the organs. It frequently is referred to as the maintenance hormone of pregnancy because it is responsible for the normal contractility

Table 26.3 Interpretation of Biophysical Profile Score Variables

FETAL VARIABLE	NORMAL BEHAVIOR (SCORE = 2)	ABNORMAL BEHAVIOR (SCORE = 0)
Fetal breathing movements (FBMs)	Intermittent multiple episodes of more than 30-s duration, within 30-min BPS time frame. Hiccups count. With continuous FBM for 30 min, exclude fetal acidosis.	Continuous breathing without cessation. Completely absent breathing or no sustained episodes.
Body or limb movements	At least four discrete body movements in 30 min. Continuous active movement episodes count as a single movement. Includes fine motor movements, rolling movements, and so on, but not REM or mouthing movements.	Three or fewer body or limb movements in a 30-min observation period.
Fetal tone and posture	Demonstration of active extension with rapid return to flexion of fetal limbs and brisk repositioning or trunk rotation. Opening and closing of hand, mouth, kicking, and so on.	Low-velocity movement only. Incomplete flexion, flaccid extremity positions, abnormal fetal posture. Must score 0 when FM completely absent.
Cardiotocogram (CTG)	Normal mean variation (computerized FHR interpretation), accelerations associated with maternal palpation of FM (accelerations graded for gestation), 20-min CTG.	Fetal movement and accelerations not coupled. Insufficient accelerations, absent accelerations, or decelerated trace. Mean variation <20 on numeric analysis of CTG.
Amniotic fluid evaluation	At least one pocket >3 cm with no umbilical cord.	No cord-free pocket >2 cm or elements of subjectively reduced amniotic fluid volume deficit.

BPS, Biophysical profile score; *FHR,* fetal heart rate; *FM,* fetal movement; *REM,* rapid eye movement.
From Harman CR: Assessment of fetal health. In Creasy RK, Resnik R, Iams JD, editors: *Maternal-fetal medicine: principles and practice,* ed 6, Philadelphia, 2008, Saunders.

of the uterus being halted, which enables implantation to take place without interruption.

- *Relaxin:* This hormone is secreted by the corpus luteum and, later, the decidua of the uterine lining and the placenta. Relaxin is linked to the softening of the cervix and pubic symphysis in preparation for labor and delivery.

UTERUS

The uterus enlarges during pregnancy as a result of hormonal stimulus, which causes an increase in vascularity, hyperplasia (new muscle fiber and tissue), and hypertrophy (enlargement of existing fiber and tissue). The nonpregnant uterus is pear shaped and weighs approximately 2 oz (50 g). By the third trimester (the last 3 months of a 9-month pregnancy), it is egg shaped and has increased in weight to 2.2 lb (1000 g). At term, it can hold a fetus, a placenta, and amniotic fluid, totaling more than 8.5 lb (4000 g).

The consistency of the tissue changes also. Changes in the cervix and fundus, along with an altered position in the pelvis, are early signs of pregnancy. The uterus, which, in a nonpregnant state, is a pelvic organ, rises to the base of the rib cage. The superior aspect of the uterus (the fundus) is located at the level of the xiphoid process by the end of the third trimester.

BREASTS

Changes in the breasts during pregnancy are caused by hormonal stimulation. The changes include hypertrophy of the mammary glandular tissue and increased vascularization, pigmentation, size, and prominence of nipples and areolae. During the second trimester, the breasts begin to produce colostrum, often referred to as "premilk." The colostrum is produced actively from the second trimester to after delivery until the mother's milk comes in. This fluid is low in fat but high in carbohydrates and protein. It also contains valuable antibodies to provide protection to the newborn. The first newborn stool, meconium, is aided in passage by the laxative-like effects of the colostrum.

CYCLES OF PREGNANCY AND CHILDBIRTH

The maternity cycle, which is discussed in this and successive chapters, is divided into three distinct periods. The first portion of the cycle is called the antepartal period, (from Latin root *ante,* "before," and *parere,* "to bring to bear") or prenatal period (from Latin root *pre-,* "before," and *natal,* "birth"). The antepartal period begins with conception and ends with the onset of labor.

The next portion of the cycle is referred to as the intrapartal period (from Latin *intra,* "within," and *parere,* "to bring to bear"). This period begins with the onset of labor and ends with delivery of the placenta. The same period sometimes is called the perinatal portion (from Latin *peri,* "around," and *natal,* "birth").

The final stage of the cycle is the postpartal period (from Latin *post,* "after," and *parere,* "to bring to bear").

This period starts after the delivery of the placenta and lasts for approximately 6 weeks or until the reproductive organs return to the prepregnancy state.

Pregnancy spans 9 months, approximately 40 weeks. Pregnancy is also divided into 3-month periods, or trimesters. The first trimester covers weeks 1 through 13; the second, weeks 14 through 26; and the third, weeks 27 through term gestation (38 to 40 weeks).

ANTEPARTAL ASSESSMENT

GENERAL PHYSICAL ASSESSMENT

Prenatal care and assessment should begin when pregnancy is planned or as soon as the first menstrual period is missed. Ideally, the woman has been receiving regular medical attention and already is known by the health care provider. Unfortunately, because of cost or frequent changes of residence, many people do not receive regular, routine health care. Some women seek the attention of a specialist, an obstetrician, a nurse practitioner, or a midwife during pregnancy.

The first visit is the most in-depth. Demographic information about the patient is recorded. This will include data such as age, occupation, and marital status. Insurance information will also be investigated. Referrals to programs to assist with prenatal care expenses may be made if needed. Risk factors will also be identified. This may include age, lifestyle, socioeconomic status, and education level.

A basic family and personal medical history are obtained. To anticipate any problems, the practitioner must be aware of any genetic diseases in either the mother's or the father's family. The mother's personal health history will also be included. If serious genetic problems are known, couples may seek genetic counseling before they consider having children.

GENETIC COUNSELING

An assessment of potential risks to a fetus is discussed during genetic counseling. The process can be initiated prior to or during pregnancy. The genetic counseling team may be multidisciplinary and include physicians and nurses. The motivation for genetic counseling may begin with the desire to further investigate repeated pregnancy losses or it may be the result of a known familial condition. The need for genetic screening may be identified during the initial prenatal data collection. Genetic counseling is not needed for all families. It should, however, be considered for mothers over the age of 35 years, families who have a child with a birth defect or genetic disorder, and in response to concerning results of prenatal testing from the CVS, amniocentesis, or nuchal translucency test.

Assessment begins with a personal medical history and a review of systems. Information is obtained about chronic diseases such as cardiac problems, hypertension, diabetes mellitus, and infectious diseases (e.g., rubella, acquired immunodeficiency syndrome [AIDS],

Box 26.2	Basic Prenatal Physical Examination

- Measurement of vital signs, height, and weight
- Assessment of heart, lungs, and reflexes
- General physical inspection of skin and mobility
- Laboratory studies (hemoglobin; hematocrit; serology tests for detection of syphilis, human immunodeficiency virus, and hepatitis virus; ABO and Rh factor; rubella titer)
- Routine urinalysis for glucose, protein, and ketones
- Pregnancy test if pregnancy has not been confirmed already

Box 26.3	Gynecologic Examination

- Palpation and auscultation of the abdomen
- Visualization of the cervix and vagina
- Evaluation of the bony pelvis
- Palpation of the uterus externally or bimanually
- Examination of the vulva, the perineum, the anus, and the rectum
- Pap smear (done at the beginning of the examination)

or other sexually transmitted infections [STIs]). Any history of accidents or previous surgeries is documented. Significant findings in these areas may indicate the potential for problems and the need for early medical and nursing interventions. High-risk pregnancies are discussed in Chapter 29.

Assessment is made of lifestyle patterns, including recreational activities; nutrition and eating habits; use of prescription medications, street drugs, alcohol, or tobacco; and work exposure to hazardous conditions. Early detection and correction of problem situations can reduce hazards to the woman and prevent detrimental effects on the fetus.

A basic physical examination is completed (Box 26.2). These tests increase the data available and enable the primary care practitioner to plan comprehensive care.

OBSTETRIC ASSESSMENT

When collecting health information on the pregnant woman, it is important to pay close attention to her gynecologic, menstrual, and obstetric history. This includes the use of contraceptives and the regularity of the menstrual period, including frequency, duration, amount of flow, presence of pain, and any other significant comments. A review is made of any history of gynecologic surgery, vaginal discharge, or STIs.

The number of pregnancies the patient has had and their outcomes are discussed. This includes the course of the pregnancy, with special attention to any complications; the type of delivery (vaginal or cesarean); any complications during delivery; the use of forceps or other medical assistance; the type of anesthetic used; the condition of the newborn; and any complications of the postpartal period.

GYNECOLOGIC EXAMINATION

The gynecologic examination is also performed at this time. The nurse is often called on to prepare the necessary equipment, assist in the examination, and to provide explanations and emotional support to the patient (Box 26.3).

DETERMINATION OF PREGNANCY

The woman may report to the physician after having suspected pregnancy and then taking a home

pregnancy test to confirm suspicions. During the first prenatal care visit, another test may be performed to confirm the pregnancy. The test results, history, and physical examination will provide the physician the needed information to confirm the pregnancy and establish gestational age.

PRESUMPTIVE SIGNS

The presumptive signs are indicators that a woman may be pregnant. They are subjective. These signs are those frequently attributed to pregnancy, but they may also indicate other conditions not related to pregnancy:

- Amenorrhea: Absence of menstruation
- Nausea and vomiting
- Frequent urination
- Breast changes: Swelling, tingling, and tenderness of the breasts are common during pregnancy, along with changes in pigmentation of the areolae. The sebaceous material secreted from the ducts of the glands to the skin of each areola lubricates and protects the breasts from infection and trauma during breastfeeding.
- Change in the shape of the abdomen
- Quickening: The subjective sensation of fetal movement first occurs at about 16 to 18 weeks of gestation in multigravida women. First-time mothers may not report these sensations until 18 to 20 weeks' gestation.
- Skin changes: Pigment changes, including darkening of some areas of the body such as the areolae, may occur. Some women may experience chloasma (melasma).

PROBABLE SIGNS

The probable signs indicate a high likelihood that the woman is pregnant. These findings are objective and can be confirmed by an examiner. Still, these signs are not 100% reliable indicators:

- *Changes in the reproductive organs:* The uterus begins to grow early in the pregnancy. Enlargement of the uterus indicates a high probability of pregnancy, particularly if accompanied by changes in the consistency of the isthmus of the uterus (the segment between the fundus and the cervix). A softening of this segment is called **Hëgar's sign** (Fig. 26.5). This change and a softening or increased pliability of the cervix called **Goodell's sign** are seen most commonly in pregnancy. **Ballottement**, which may be used at approximately 16 to 18 weeks of gestation, is a technique that involves palpating the uterus in such a way that the examiner feels the rebound of the floating fetus (Fig. 26.6). During the pelvic examination, the physician may note that the vagina, the cervix, and sometimes the vulva have a violet or purplish discoloration. This is referred to as Chadwick's sign and this change in color is the result of increased vascularity to the area. Ladin's sign refers to softening in the center of the uterus.

- *Positive pregnancy test result:* Assessment of pregnancy may be done with either serum or urine testing. These tests measure the presence and/or levels of hCG. A positive pregnancy test is not a definitive determination of pregnancy because other conditions may result in positive test results. Urine tests are readily available over the counter in stores. Reliability of these products depends on the technique used in collecting the urine specimen and performing the test. Tests administered by the primary care practitioner have a high level of reliability, between 95% and 99%. The greatest advantages of pregnancy tests are that they can be administered early in pregnancy and are reasonably inexpensive. If the test results are positive and other indicators such as uterine changes are abnormal, the primary care provider may suspect complications such as an ectopic (outside the uterus) pregnancy or hydatidiform mole (abnormal growth of a fertilized ovum in which a large vascular mass, but no fetus, develops). Hydatidiform mole frequently results in a highly reactive pregnancy test, and the test may continue to indicate positive results even after surgical removal.

POSITIVE SIGNS

Positive signs are those that occur only with pregnancy and cannot be attributed to other physiologic occurrences. Positive signs definitively identify the presence of the fetus. The signs include palpation of the fetal outline, visualization of the pregnancy with ultrasound scan, and presence of a fetal heartbeat (Box 26.4).

© Elsevier

Fig. 26.5 Hëgar's sign. Bimanual examination for assessment of compressibility and softening of isthmus (lower uterine segment) while the cervix is still firm.

© Elsevier

Fig. 26.6 Internal ballottement (18 weeks).

Box 26.4	Positive Signs of Pregnancy

- *Visualization:* The fetal skeleton seen on x-ray examination is a positive sign of pregnancy, but radiation is generally limited during pregnancy because of possible danger to the fetus. Ultrasound tracing of the fetus is also a positive indication of pregnancy.
- *Fetal movement:* Fetal movement may be detected by a trained observer (the primary care practitioner).
- *Auscultation of fetal heart tone:* Fetal heart activity can be detected with ultrasound scan at 6 weeks; tones are heard with Doppler at 10–12 weeks and with stethoscope at approximately 18–20 weeks.

Box 26.5	Defining Parity

FIVE-DIGIT SYSTEM: GTPAL
G: Gravidity
T: Term births
P: Preterm births
A: Abortions
L: Living children

FOUR-DIGIT SYSTEM: TPAL
T: Term births (also may be noted as F)
P: Preterm births
A: Abortions
L: Living children

DETERMINATION OF THE ESTIMATED DATE OF BIRTH

Normal human pregnancy, counting from the first day of the last menstrual period, is about 280 days, 40 weeks, 10 lunar months (28 days each), or slightly more than 9 calendar months.

The estimated date of delivery (EDD), often known as the "due date," involves calculations based on the woman's menstrual cycle. In the past, this date was referred to as the estimated date of confinement, or EDC. The term confinement is not used commonly today, because pregnancy and childbirth are seen as highly anticipated wellness-related experiences. The most common method is called *Nägele's rule.* To calculate, start with the first day of the woman's last normal menstrual period and count back 3 months, then add 7 days. For example, if the first day of the last menstrual period was June 14, counting back 3 months to March 14 and then adding 7 days would yield an EDB of March 21. Studies reveal that only a small percentage of infants actually are born on the date predicted; most deliveries, however, do occur within 10 days before or after the EDB.

If the woman is unaware of her last menstrual period or has an irregular cycle, the calculation of the EDB may be more difficult. The health care provider must then rely on observations such as quickening, fundal height measurement, measurement of fetal size with ultrasonography. If it is essential for the primary care practitioner to know the level of fetal maturity, specialized tests can be performed later in the pregnancy.

OBSTETRIC TERMINOLOGY

Specific terms are used in obstetrics to describe the number of times a woman has been pregnant and has given birth. **Gravida** (from the Latin root *gravidus,* "heavy") indicates a pregnant woman. Latin numeric fixes are added to this term to indicate the number of pregnancies, such as *primigravida* (one), *nulligravida* (none), and *multigravida* (multiple). Similarly, prefixes are added to the Latin root **para** ("to bring forth") to indicate the number of births, such as *nullipara* (none), *primipara* (one), and *multipara* (multiple). Shorthand for noting the patient's overall obstetric status is "GP," with the correct numerals included.

A four-point or five-point description may be used to provide obstetric history. The four-part description, referred to as TPAL or FPAL, sometimes is used, as well (Box 26.5). The first digit represents the total number of term pregnancies (or, in the FPAL notation, full-term), including the present one. A *term pregnancy* is one that results in delivery after conclusion of the 37th week of gestation through the 42nd week of gestation. The second digit indicates the number of preterm deliveries. A *preterm delivery* is one that takes place from the 20th week of gestation through the end of the 37th week of gestation. The third notation indicates the number of abortions. The abortion may be spontaneous, as in a miscarriage, or an elective procedure. Multifetal pregnancies are recorded as singular events when calculating the number of abortions and preterm and term pregnancies. The last number indicates the number of living children. In one case, if a woman has experienced normal pregnancies and deliveries, but all of her children have died in a fire, the last number is 0. For example, a descriptive number such as 3-1-0-3 indicates that a woman has delivered three term pregnancies, had one preterm pregnancy and no abortions, and has three living children. The more detailed five-point method includes information about the total number of pregnancies a woman has had. It is denoted as GTPAL. In the case of a multifetal pregnancy, the gravida notion, as well as the information about the delivery, are counted as one.

ANTEPARTAL CARE

HEALTH PROMOTION

Most pregnant women want to learn more about pregnancy, childbirth, and motherhood. Pregnancy is a time in life when most women see the importance of regular medical supervision and are willing to make changes in their habits. Most will begin to think of their baby first and do everything that is best for the infant.

A checklist for antepartal needs throughout pregnancy is a valuable teaching tool. It provides the team of care providers with a communication tool to prevent gaps and to identify areas of repeated concerns for patients. Sharing the checklist with patients reassures them that other pregnant women and their

Box 26.6	Trimester Checklist

- Schedule and events of visits
- Counseling for self-care
- Adaptations and discomforts
  - Dyspnea
  - Insomnia
  - Psychosocial responses and family dynamics
  - Gingivitis
  - Urinary frequency
  - Perineal discomfort and pressure
  - Braxton Hicks contractions
  - Leg cramps
  - Ankle edema
- Safety (balance)
- Exercise and rest
- Relaxation
- Nutrition
- Sexuality
- Personal hygiene
- Danger signs, general
- Danger signs, preterm labor
- Fetal growth and development
- Preparation for baby
  - Feeding method
  - Nipple preparation
- Preparation for labor
  - Recognition: false versus true
  - Prenatal classes
  - Control of discomfort
  - Hospital tour
  - Provision for other family members
- Preparation for homecoming
- Diagnostic tests (specify)
- Other

Box 26.7	US Food and Drug Administration Drug Categories

The rational use of any medication requires a risk-versus-benefit assessment. Among the many risk factors that complicate assessment, pregnancy is one of the most perplexing. The US Food and Drug Administration (FDA) has established five categories to indicate the potential of a systemically absorbed drug for causing birth defects. The key differences among the categories are the degree (reliability) of evidence and the risk:benefit ratio. Pregnancy category X is particularly notable; it is assigned to a drug if any data indicate that the drug is a teratogen and the risk:benefit ratio does not support use of the drug. Category X drugs are contraindicated during pregnancy.

PREGNANCY CATEGORY AND DEFINITION

A: Adequate studies in pregnant women have not demonstrated a risk to the fetus in the first trimester of pregnancy, and no evidence of risk is found in later trimesters.

B: Animal studies have not demonstrated a risk to the fetus, but no adequate studies are found in pregnant women; or animal studies have shown an adverse effect, but adequate studies in pregnant women have not demonstrated a risk to the fetus during the first trimester of pregnancy, and no evidence of risk is found in later trimesters.

C: Animal studies have shown an adverse effect on the fetus, but no adequate studies are found in humans; the benefits from the use of the drug in pregnant women may be acceptable despite its potential risks; or no animal reproduction studies and no adequate studies in humans are found.

D: Evidence is seen of human fetal risk, but the potential benefits from the use of the drug in pregnant women may be acceptable despite its potential risks.

X: Studies in animals or humans demonstrate fetal abnormalities, or adverse reaction reports indicate evidence of fetal risk. The risk of use in a pregnant woman clearly outweighs any possible benefit.

NR: Not rated.

Regardless of the designated pregnancy category or presumed safety, no drug should be administered during pregnancy unless it is clearly needed and potential benefits outweigh potential risks. Modified from Skidmore-Roth L: *Mosby's 2013 nursing drug reference*, ed 26, St. Louis, 2013, Mosby.

families face the same issues. Reading the checklist also reminds patients of information they may otherwise forget (Box 26.6).

Once pregnancy is determined, prenatal care is instituted. Nursing interventions follow the nursing process: assessment, analysis, identification of patient problems, planning, implementation, and evaluation.

Pregnancy is an excellent time to establish good general health practices. Until they become pregnant, many women do not have regular physical examinations or Papanicolaou (Pap) smears and do not do home screening tests such as breast self-examination (BSE). The high motivation level makes this a good time to teach patients about health maintenance practices.

Early in pregnancy, the woman often begins to seek information and make choices regarding how and where she wishes to give birth. Information should be provided regarding the available options in her community (see Chapter 27).

Routine care during pregnancy begins with the initial examination and history, as previously described. Appointments are recommended once a month through the seventh month, once every 2 weeks for the next month, and then, once every week until delivery. If any problems occur or the health care provider suspects anything unusual, such as a multiple pregnancy, the schedule of visits may be altered. Dental care should continue during pregnancy. Any major dental work, such as oral surgery or extractions, is usually delayed until after delivery, however.

Smoking during pregnancy can be dangerous to the developing fetus. Oxygen deprivation can lead to decreased intrauterine growth and low birth weight. Preterm delivery is also linked to maternal smoking. Drinking of alcoholic beverages during pregnancy is contraindicated, as well. Fetal alcohol syndrome is discussed in Chapter 29.

Ideally, women should avoid taking any medication or drugs during pregnancy. The use of over-the-counter drugs and prescription medications must be reviewed with the health care provider (see Box 26.7). Most drugs can cross the placenta and are transmitted to the fetus. Street drugs, such as marijuana and cocaine, are dangerous to mother and fetus and must be avoided. Although complementary and alternative therapies may be used safely before pregnancy, certain elements may be dangerous to the developing fetus. To ensure safety, the nurse must be vigilant in assessing for their use and in subsequent reporting to the primary health care provider (Box 26.8).

Embryonic and fetal development is vulnerable to environmental teratogens. Many potentially dangerous chemicals are present in the home, yard, and workplace, including cleaning agents, paints, sprays, herbicides, and pesticides. The soil and water supply may be unsafe. Therefore, the woman should: (1) read all labels for ingredients and proper use of product; (2) ensure adequate ventilation with clean air; (3) dispose of wastes appropriately; (4) wear gloves when handling chemicals and gardening; and (5) change job assignments or workplace as necessary.

Today, many women continue to work throughout pregnancy. The work environment must be checked for chemicals and other hazards. The Occupational Safety and Health Administration (OSHA) has numerous guidelines for hazards in the workplace. Address working conditions, such as lifting and standing or sitting for long periods. Encourage the woman to take frequent rest periods.

DANGER SIGNS DURING PREGNANCY

Although pregnancy involves many changes and normal discomforts, certain conditions signal the need for immediate medical attention (Box 26.9). Teach the pregnant woman these danger signs and how to monitor fetal movements (see the Patient Teaching box for guidelines for counting fetal movements). Stress the importance of contacting the primary care practitioner promptly if any of these signs are present.

Patient Teaching

Guidelines for Counting Fetal Movements (Kick Counts)

- Kick count monitoring should begin at 28 weeks' gestation.
- The expectant mother should pick a time of day when she can sit or lie quietly. If deciding to lie down, a left side-lying position should be selected.
- Each fetal movement or kick should be counted. The goal is to experience 10 to 12 movements/kicks in a 1- to 2-h period.

If an inadequate number of movements is felt, the health care provider should be notified.

Box 26.8   Complementary and Alternative Therapies Used in Pregnancy

NAUSEA AND VOMITING IN PREGNANCY
- Acupuncture
- Acupressure discs (Sea Bands)
- Hypnotherapy
- Shiatzu
- Aromatherapy Peppermint
- Lavender
- Herbal remedies[a]
  - Lemon balm
  - Spearmint
  - Ginger root
  - Raspberry leaf
  - Fennel
  - Chamomile
  - Hops
  - Meadowsweet
  - Wild yam root

RELAXATION AND MUSCLE ACHE RELIEF
- Yoga
- Biofeedback
- Reflexology
- Therapeutic touch
- Massage

[a]Some herbs can cause miscarriage, preterm labor, or fetal or maternal injury. Pregnant women should discuss use in pregnancy and during lactation with the health care provider.

Box 26.9   Danger Signs and Symptoms During Pregnancy

- Visual disturbances: diplopia (double vision), blurring, or spots
- Headaches: severe, sudden, or continuous
- Edema: swelling of the face, presacral area, or fingers
- Rapid weight gain in excess of normal gain for gestation
- Pain: severe abdominal or epigastric pain
- Signs of infection: fever, chills, diarrhea, changes in vaginal drainage, pain or burning with urination
- Vaginal bleeding (no matter how slight)
- Vaginal drainage (aside from normal mucus)
- Persistent vomiting
- Muscular irritability or convulsions
- Absence or decrease in fetal movement once felt

NUTRITIONAL AND METABOLIC HEALTH PATTERN

See Chapter 19 for information about basic nutrition and nutritional therapy for the life cycle, stages of pregnancy, and lactation.

Pica

Pica refers to craving and eating substances that are not normally considered edible. Pica may be associated by nutrient deficits such as iron or zinc. Some report the craving is due to a smell or need to experience a certain texture in their mouths (NLM, 2020b). It is seen more in lower socioeconomic groups and linked to certain cultural groups. Substances ingested may include clay, laundry starch, dirt, and chalk. Although the substances are not considered toxic, complications are associated with pica. Patients may experience constipation or other gastrointestinal ailments from the ingestion of the nonfood substances. Eating the craved items may reduce quality nutritional intake, resulting in deficiencies. Problems that may occur as a result of pica include interference with iron absorption, constipation, and loss of important nutrients when normal caloric intake is replaced with the pica-related substances.

Common Discomforts

Many pregnant women experience some discomforts of the gastrointestinal tract during pregnancy. Some women have excessive salivation (ptyalism), presumably in response to the high levels of estrogen during pregnancy. Although it may be uncomfortable and awkward at times, ptyalism causes no serious problems and disappears late in pregnancy or after delivery. Teach the patient to try using astringent mouthwash, chewing gum, or sucking on hard candy to provide relief.

Nausea is common in the early stages of pregnancy. It typically occurs when the woman awakens in the morning, hence the name "morning sickness." However, it can occur at any time of the day. Nausea is thought to be caused by increased HCG levels and changes in carbohydrate metabolism. Mild nausea usually can be controlled by slowly eating a few soda crackers or dry toast before rising from bed. Other suggestions are eating smaller, more frequent meals and avoiding spicy or greasy food. Morning sickness rarely lasts beyond the fourth month. If it lasts longer, if it is more severe, and, particularly, if it involves vomiting, the health care provider should be contacted. The most severe form is called *hyperemesis gravidarum*. Its cause is not clear, but if left untreated, it can lead to dehydration, fluid and electrolyte imbalance, acid-base imbalance, altered kidney and cardiac function, and even fetal death. Hospitalization with close medical supervision, including intravenous therapy, may be necessary (see Chapter 29).

Pyrosis (heartburn) from gastric reflux into the esophagus can be caused by the increasing size of the fetus in the abdominal cavity, which displaces the stomach. Increased progesterone levels cause relaxation of the cardiac sphincter. Decreased gastric mobility, which results in delayed stomach-emptying time, also may contribute to the problem. Smaller, more frequent meals; decreased fat intake; low-sodium antacids; and avoidance of lying down after meals often give relief.

Skin Changes

Changes in pigmentation often occur during pregnancy as a result of increased amounts of melanocyte-stimulating hormone. The changes occur primarily in areas that already have greater pigmentation, such as the areolae, nipples, vulva, and perineal area. A darkening of a line from the midline of the abdomen from the pubis to the umbilicus may result and is called the *linea nigra*.

Chloasma, the mask of pregnancy, is an irregular darkening of the cheeks, forehead, and nose. These changes are often more obvious in women with darker hair and skin and may be worsened with sun exposure. This generally disappears or fades significantly soon after delivery.

Striae gravidarum, or stretch marks, are reddish, wavy streaks that can appear on the thighs, the abdomen, and the breasts. They are more common with distention, but may occur even in relatively thin women. They usually fade after delivery. Because integumentary system changes vary greatly among women of different racial backgrounds, the color of a woman's skin, along with any changes that may be attributed to pregnancy, should be noted in the physical assessment.

Spider nevi (a branched growth of dilated capillaries on the skin) and *palmar erythema* (reddened palms) sometimes are seen. These conditions are caused by increased blood flow that results from high estrogen levels. Both usually disappear when the pregnancy ends.

Hair and nail growth frequently are accelerated during pregnancy, with *hirsutism* (excessive body hair in a masculine distribution pattern as a result of heredity, hormonal dysfunction, or medication) commonly reported. Oily skin and acne may occur in some women, whereas others report a clearing of their skin. This is usually temporary unless other physiologic problems are active.

Occasionally, decreased emptying of the gallbladder may result in subclinical jaundice, which causes generalized pruritus (itching). This and other concerns are noted in Table 26.4.

Changes in the Cardiovascular System

Maternal adjustments to pregnancy involve extensive anatomic and physiologic changes in the cardiovascular system. Changes can result in episodes of orthostatic hypotension. An increase of platelets and fibrinogen increases the woman's risk for blood clots. Cardiovascular adaptations protect the woman's normal physiologic functioning, meet the metabolic demands of pregnancy, and provide for fetal development and growth (Table 26.5).

Changes in the Respiratory System

Structural and ventilatory adaptations during pregnancy provide for maternal and fetal needs. Maternal oxygen requirements increase in response to the accelerated metabolic rate and the need to add to the tissue mass in the uterus and breasts. In addition, the fetus needs oxygen and a way to eliminate carbon dioxide. Elevation of estrogen causes the ligaments of the rib cage to relax, permitting increased chest expansion (Table 26.6).

Table 26.4	Discomforts and Concerns Related to Maternal Adaptations During the Third Trimester	
DISCOMFORT	**PHYSIOLOGY**	**TEACHING FOR SELF-CARE**
Shortness of breath and dyspnea in 60% of pregnant women	Expansion of diaphragm limited by enlarging uterus; diaphragm elevated approximately 1.5 inches (4 cm); some relief after lightening (when the fetus settles lower in the true pelvis, leaving more space in the upper abdomen)	Good posture; sleep with extra pillow; avoid overloading stomach; stop smoking; refer to physician if symptoms worsen to rule out anemia, emphysema, and asthma
Insomnia (later weeks of pregnancy)	Fetal movements, muscular cramping, urinary frequency, shortness of breath, or other discomforts	Reassurance; conscious relaxation; back massage or effleurage (deep or gentle stroking); support of body parts with pillows; warm milk or shower before retiring
Psychosocial responses: mood swings, mixed feelings, increased anxiety	Hormonal and metabolic adaptations; feelings about impending labor, delivery, and parenthood	Reassurance and support from significant other and nurse; improved communication with partner, family, and others
Return of urinary frequency and urgency	Vascular engorgement and altered bladder function caused by hormones; bladder capacity reduced by enlarging uterus and fetal presenting part; lightening	Kegel exercises (see the Patient Teaching box on Kegel exercises); limit fluid intake before bedtime; reassurance; wear perineal pad; refer to health care provider for pain or burning sensation
Perineal discomfort and pressure	Pressure from enlarging uterus, especially when standing or walking; multifetal gestation	Rest, conscious relaxation, and good posture; maternity girdle; refer to physician for assessment and treatment if pain is present; rule out labor
Braxton Hicks contractions	Intensification of uterine contractions in preparation for the onset of true labor	Reassurance; rest; change of position; practice breathing techniques when contractions are bothersome; effleurage; rule out labor
Leg cramps (gastrocnemius spasm), especially when reclining	Compression of nerves supplying lower extremities because of enlarging uterus; reduced level of diffusible serum calcium or elevation of serum phosphorus; aggravating factors: fatigue, poor peripheral circulation, pointing toes when stretching legs or when walking, drinking >1 quart (1 L) of milk per day; cause unclear	Assess lower extremities for redness, warmth, tenderness, or swelling; some facilities may use the Homan's sign; this assessment is presently under review by many medical professionals because it is not considered completely reliable, and concerns exist about the safety of the practice Heat may be used over affected muscle; stretch affected muscle until spasm relaxes
Ankle edema (nonpitting) to lower extremities	Edema aggravated by prolonged standing, sitting, poor posture, lack of exercise, constrictive clothing (e.g., garters), or hot weather	Ample fluid intake for "natural" diuretic effect; put on support stockings before rising; rest periodically with legs and hips elevated; exercise moderately; refer to physician if generalized edema develops (diuretics are contraindicated)

Changes in the Musculoskeletal System

The gradually changing body and increasing weight of the pregnant woman cause noticeable alterations in her posture (Fig. 26.7) and the way she walks late in pregnancy. The great abdominal distention that gives the pelvis a forward tilt, decreased abdominal muscle tone, and increased weight bearing create a realignment of the spinal curvature. The woman's center of gravity shifts forward. Lordosis (an increase in the normal lumbosacral curve) develops. An increased curvature in the cervicodorsal region also is seen. The expectant mother may be noted with an exaggerated anterior flexion of the head, as well. This is done to promote balance. As the pregnancy advances, common symptoms include muscle aches and numbness. Enlarging breasts and a stoop-shouldered stance

further accentuate the lumbar and dorsal curves. Walking is more difficult, and the pregnant woman's waddling gait is well known. The ligamentous and muscular structures of the middle and lower spine may be severely stressed. Pregnant women who gain excessive weight or who carry more than one fetus may experience overdistention. This excessive stress on the abdominal wall muscles may cause a separation (diastasis recti abdominis). Management of this condition is typically conservative, but severe cases may necessitate surgical repair.

Slight relaxation and increased mobility of the pelvic joints are normal during pregnancy. They are a result of the exaggerated elasticity and softening of the connective tissue caused by increased circulating steroid sex hormones, especially estrogen. **Relaxin**, an ovarian

Table **26.5**   Cardiovascular Changes in Pregnancy

PARAMETER	CHANGE
Heart rate	Increases 10–15 beats/min
Blood pressure	Blood pressure declines from the prepregnancy baseline in the first and second trimesters. Blood pressure returns to normal in the third trimester.
Blood volume	40%–50% above prepregnancy level Changes begin in the first trimester and peak at 34 weeks gestation
Red blood cell mass	Increases 18%
Hemoglobin	Physiologic anemia of pregnancy results as plasma levels increase earlier in gestation than the cells.
Hematocrit	Non pregnant levels are 35%-44%. Levels decline throughout the pregnancy as a result of the excess fluid volume. In the first trimester levels range from 31% to 41% and reach the lowest level in the third trimester (28%–40%). (Perinatology.com, 2010)
White blood cell count	Non pregnant values 5,000–10,000 mcL. Values increase in pregnancy due to the physiological stress and immune response of the maternal system. Changes during in pregnancy begin in first trimester (5.7–13.6 mcL) and reach their highest point in the first 24 h of the post partum period (20,000–30,000 mcL). (Perinatology.com, 2010; Moldenhauer, 2020)
Cardiac output	Increases 40%–50%
Cardiac Murmur	Seen in nearly 90% of pregnant women. It is the result of positional changes of the heart in response to the growing uterus. This is a benign condition and resolves after delivery.

Table **26.6**   Respiratory Changes in Pregnancy

PARAMETER	CHANGE
Respiratory rate	Unchanged or slightly increased
Tidal volume	Increased 30%–40%
Vital capacity	Unchanged
Inspiratory capacity	Increased
Expiratory volume	Decreased
Total lung capacity	Unchanged to slightly decreased
Oxygen consumption	Increased 20%–40%

From Lowdermilk DL, Perry SE, Cashion K, et al: *Maternal and women's health care*, ed 10, St. Louis, 2012, Mosby.

hormone, assists in the relaxation and softening. These adaptations permit enlargement of pelvic dimensions to facilitate labor and birth. The degree of relaxation varies, but considerable separation of the symphysis pubis and the instability of the sacroiliac joints may cause pain and difficulty in walking. Obesity and multifetal pregnancy tend to increase the pelvic instability.

Hygiene Practices

Bathing or showering during pregnancy should continue as part of routine hygiene. Increased perspiration is common, and good personal hygiene is important to prevent body odor. Tub bathing may become difficult in the later months of pregnancy because of changes in mobility and balance. Some primary care practitioners restrict tub baths in the last month because the cervix may have begun to dilate.

Most primary care practitioners recommend that women avoid hot tubs, sauna baths, and spas during pregnancy, because maternal hyperthermia during the first trimester may result in central nervous system defects of the fetus or pregnancy loss. Because a woman may not be aware she is pregnant early in the first trimester, those women who are not taking measures to prevent pregnancy are well advised to also avoid hyperthermic baths.

Pregnant women experience increased vaginal discharge. Douching is not recommended. Vaginal drainage that causes pruritus or other symptoms should be reported to the primary care practitioner.

Pregnant women do not have to buy special clothing but should choose garments that are comfortable and do not restrict movement. Circulation-restricting clothing, such as garters and socks with tight elastic bands, should be avoided. Larger bras may be necessary as breasts enlarge; a bra that is too tight may interfere with breathing.

ELIMINATION

Gastrointestinal System

Slowing of intestinal peristalsis can result in abdominal distention, flatulence, and constipation. Constipation also may be linked to iron supplements the woman is taking.

Hemorrhoids can result from straining as a result of constipation. They can also be caused by the enlarged uterus putting pressure on the pelvic blood vessels, slowing venous return from the lower extremities. Women with a history of cholelithiasis may experience problems with this as a result of an increased cholesterol level, which is common during pregnancy. Adequate fluid intake, dietary roughage, and exercise may help reduce problems related to constipation.

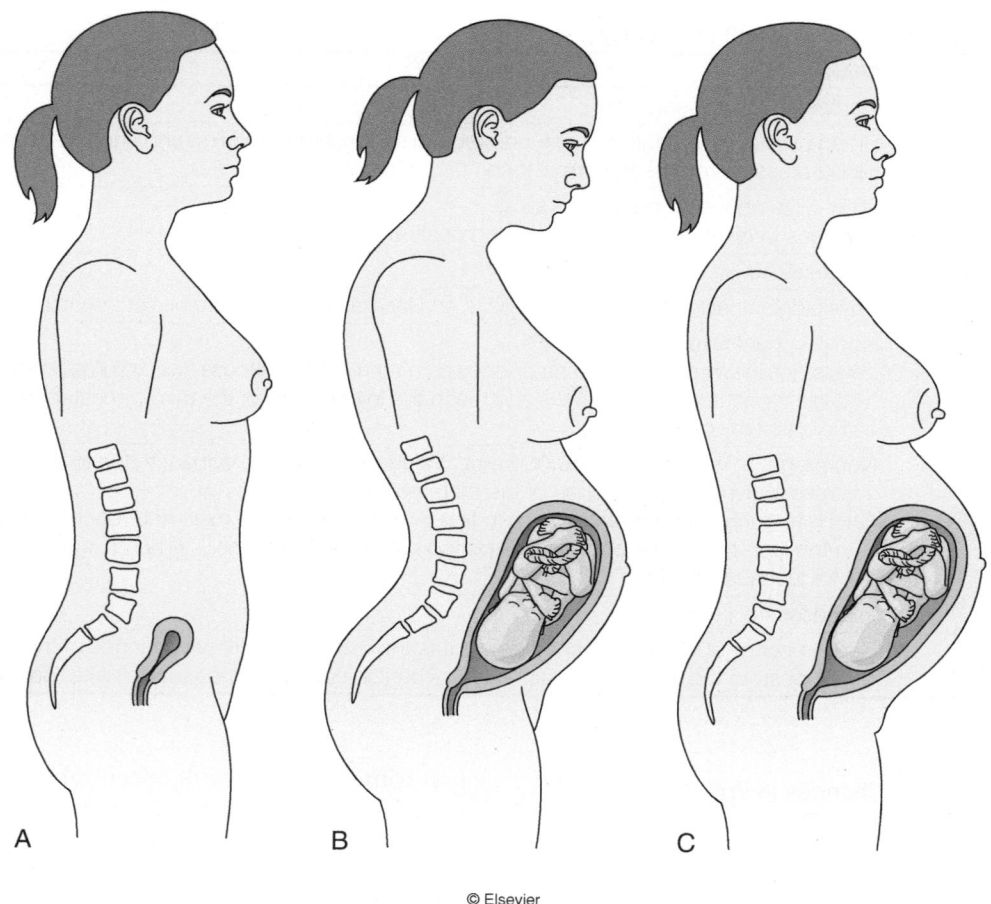

© Elsevier

Fig. 26.7 Postural changes during pregnancy. (A) Nonpregnant. (B) Incorrect posture during pregnancy. (C) Correct posture during pregnancy.

Urinary System

Frequency of urination is a common symptom of pregnancy. In the first trimester, this results from the enlarging uterus putting pressure on the bladder. Later, during the third trimester, the uterus moves back into the pelvic cavity in preparation for labor and delivery, again placing pressure on the urinary bladder. The increase in circulating blood volume results in increases in glomerular filtration rate (GFR). This causes an increase in urinary output. The stressors placed on the kidneys during pregnancy may result in protein and glucose to be detected in the urine samples. During the prenatal care period, the woman's urine is evaluated with a dipstick test to assess for the presence of glucose or protein. The patient can be taught Kegel exercises to help tone the muscles of the perineum and prevent stress incontinence (see the Patient Teaching box on Kegel exercises).

The ureter and kidneys may become dilated, particularly on the right side, as a result of placental progesterone and pressure from the enlarging uterus. Restricted circulation in the pelvis as the uterus enlarges increases the risk of bladder trauma and urinary tract infection.

ACTIVITY AND EXERCISE

Patients should continue normal activity throughout an uncomplicated pregnancy. If a woman regularly participates in a fitness program or sport, she probably can continue with most activities. This should be discussed with the health care provider. High-risk activities or those that require a great deal of balance and coordination are discouraged. Common sense is the best guide.

Changes in balance and posture occur as the fetus increases in size. To compensate for the shifting center of gravity, the lumbodorsal curve increases (lordosis), which may result in low backaches. Hormonal influence on pelvic bones, which results in joint relaxation, can lead to a waddling gait. Wearing footwear with low heels and using good body mechanics help reduce discomfort.

Leg cramps are common, perhaps related to pressure on the pelvic blood vessels and nerves or altered calcium and phosphorus balance. Dorsiflexion of the foot may help reduce these cramps. Dependent edema and varicose veins also may result from increasing intraabdominal pressure. Many women wear support hose to reduce edema; resting with legs elevated is also helpful.

Patient Teaching

Kegel Exercises

- The muscles that stop the flow of urine are the pubococcygeal muscles. These muscles support the pelvic floor, the bladder, and the urethra. Attempts to stop the flow of urine or forestall the expulsion of gas aid the woman in targeting the involved muscles. Doing Kegel exercises during urination helps the woman know whether she is doing them correctly. If she can stop the stream of urine, her tone is good.
- After a woman has located the targeted muscles, she can do Kegel exercises in the following ways:
  - *Slow:* Tighten the muscle, hold it for a count of 3, and relax it.
  - *Quick:* Tighten the muscle and relax it as rapidly as possible.
  - *Push out, pull in:* Pull up the entire pelvic floor as though trying to suck up water into the vagina. Then, bear down as if trying to push the imaginary water out. This also uses abdominal muscles.

PRACTICE

- Kegel exercises must be practiced several times a day to be effective. They must be done every day for the rest of the woman's life.
- These exercises can be done 10 times in a row at least 3 times or more per day. Although some people recommend doing this as many as 100 times in a row, this only fatigues the pelvic floor muscles.
- A good time to practice is during trips to the bathroom, but additional practice at other times is even more beneficial.

Fatigue is reported commonly during pregnancy. The woman must pace herself and not overdo tiring activities.

Round ligament pain or tenderness in the lower abdomen is a result of stretching of the ligaments by the enlarging uterus. There is no way to prevent this but use of good body mechanics reduces the discomfort.

Dyspnea (shortness of breath) may be experienced as the uterus enlarges and pushes the diaphragm upward, decreasing the size of the chest cavity. Avoiding large meals, which distend the stomach, and maintaining good posture help relieve this problem. Exercises often are recommended to help reduce discomfort and prepare for childbirth (Box 26.10).

REST AND SLEEP

Early in pregnancy, women experience increased fatigue. Napping is encouraged during this time. Left side-lying positioning is recommended to promote oxygenation. As the pregnancy progresses and the abdomen grows larger, the pregnant woman may have difficulty finding a position of comfort, particularly if she prefers to sleep in the prone position. The supine position is not recommended because the enlarged uterus may place excessive pressure on the aorta and vena cava. The pressure can result in vena cava syndrome (supine hypotensive syndrome). The woman

may experience syncope and vertigo. The supine position also may result in decreased circulation for the fetus. A side-lying position is recommended (Fig. 26.8).

Encourage rest periods during the day, with feet elevated. Placing pillows under the legs and abdomen promotes good body alignment and rest. Naps at intervals during the day can be helpful, but these are not always possible with busy lifestyles.

SEXUALITY AND REPRODUCTIVE SYSTEM

Breast Changes

Breast changes begin early in pregnancy. Many women report tingling and a feeling of fullness. Increased sensitivity is also common. Generally, the breasts grow in preparation for lactation. Nipples and areolae darken. Colostrum may be secreted by the nipples in the second half of pregnancy. Supportive bras are recommended. If colostrum leakage is problematic, the woman should be encouraged to use breast pads.

Sexual Activity

Sexual desire is normal during pregnancy. The pregnant woman can have sexual relations unless contraindicated by other conditions. Complications during pregnancy, such as premature labor, bleeding, or rupture of membranes, necessitate that sexual activity be halted. Many factors have a strong influence on the frequency and type of sexual activity, including cultural, religious, and psychological influences. Partners must communicate their fears, concerns, and needs to each other. Many women experience a decrease in desire as a result of hormonal changes and discomfort. Change in body shape and body image also may cause concern. Discussion of various coital positions and sexual activity that does not include intercourse is appropriate. The health care provider may promote this discussion by introducing the topic during routine prenatal care.

Increased vaginal secretions are common during pregnancy. *Leukorrhea,* an increase in vaginal mucus, results from hormonal changes. If the discharge changes in color or odor, the physician should be informed at once.

Vaginal Bleeding

Vaginal bleeding at any time during pregnancy should be reported to the physician at once. Sexual activity should cease until the cause of the bleeding is determined and should be resumed only when the physician determines that no danger exists.

COPING AND STRESS TOLERANCE

Pregnancy is a developmental milestone. As with other significant developmental changes, anxiety is normal. All the physical and hormonal changes of pregnancy place additional stress on the woman. The woman and her partner normally have fears. They are concerned with the ability to cope with the pregnancy, the potential pain related to labor and delivery, and the health and well-being of the baby. Mood swings and ambivalence

| Box 26.10 | Exercise Tips for Pregnant Women |

- Consult your health care provider when you know or suspect you are pregnant. Discuss your medical and obstetric history, your current regimen, and the exercises you would like to continue throughout pregnancy.
- Seek help in determining an exercise routine that is well within your limit of tolerance, especially if you have not been exercising regularly.
- Consider decreasing weight-bearing exercises (jogging, running), and concentrate on non-weight-bearing activities such as swimming, cycling, or stretching. If you are a runner, you may wish to walk instead, starting in your 7th month.
- Avoid risky activities, such as surfing, mountain climbing, sky diving, and racquetball. Activities that require precise balance and coordination may be dangerous.
- Exercise regularly at least three times a week, as long as you are healthy, to improve muscle tone and increase or maintain your stamina. Sporadic exercises may put undue strain on your muscles.
- Limit activity to shorter intervals. Exercise for 10–15 min, rest for 2–3 min, then exercise for another 10–15 min.
- Decrease your exercise level as your pregnancy progresses. The normal alterations of advancing pregnancy, such as decreased cardiac reserve and increased respiratory effort, may produce physiologic stress if you exercise strenuously for a long time.
- Take your pulse every 10–15 min while you are exercising. If it is more than 140 beats/min, slow down until it returns to a maximum of 90 beats/min.
- Avoid becoming overheated for extended periods. It is best not to exercise for more than 35 min, especially in hot, humid weather. As your body temperature rises, the heat is transmitted to your fetus. Prolonged or repeated fetal temperature elevation may result in birth defects, especially during the first 3 months.
- Warm-up and stretching exercises prepare your joints for more strenuous exercise and lessen the likelihood of strain or injury to your joints.
- A cool-down period of mild activity after exercising helps bring your respiratory, heart, and metabolic rates back to normal and avoid pooling of blood in the exercise muscles.
- Rest for 10 min after exercising, lying on your left side. As the uterus grows, it puts pressure on a major vein carrying blood to your heart on the right side of your abdomen. Lying on your left side takes the pressure off and promotes return circulation from your extremities and muscles to your heart, increasing blood flow to your placenta and fetus.
- Drink two or three 8-oz glasses of water after you exercise to replace the body fluids you lost through perspiration. While exercising, drink water whenever you feel the need.
- Increase your caloric intake to replace the calories burned during exercise. Choose such high-protein foods as fish, cheese, eggs, or meat.
- Take your time. This is not the time to be competitive or train for activities that require long endurance.
- Wear a supportive bra. Your increased breast weight may cause changes in posture and put pressure on the ulnar nerve.
- Wear supportive shoes. As your uterus grows, your center of gravity shifts and you compensate by arching your back. These natural changes may make you feel off balance and more likely to fall.
- Stop exercising immediately if you experience shortness of breath, dizziness, numbness, tingling, abdominal pain, or vaginal bleeding, and consult your health care provider.

(conflicting emotions) are common as the woman works through her fears and comes to grips with the reality of pregnancy and how it will affect her life. During the early part of the pregnancy, the sudden hormonal changes combined with fatigue, nausea, and vomiting affect her concerns and ability to cope. As the pregnancy progresses, she will likely feel better and become increasingly able to adapt to the changes she experiences.

Women use problem-solving skills and methods of coping that worked in the past to adjust to this new situation. Provide support as this problem solving occurs and help the woman work through her unique situation. Explain the normal physiologic changes and discomforts. Listening and allowing the woman adequate time to verbalize her fears also may help reduce anxieties.

Roles, Relationships, and Adaptation

The expectant woman has generally held several roles in her life, such as child, student, employee, and wife. Pregnancy introduces a totally new role, that of mother. The woman often looks to her own life for role models and tends to seek guidance from family and friends. Culture has much to do with how she defines her role (Box 26.11).

Dynamics also change between the woman and the baby's father, particularly with the first pregnancy. The mother is no longer just a wife or girlfriend; she is also a mother. While she is coping with the role change to mother, he is coping with the role change to father (Box 26.12).

SELF-PERCEPTION AND SELF-CONCEPT

The rapid changes in body shape and size can lead to changes in self-image. Many women feel unattractive when they are pregnant. They also may feel a loss of control related to the changes taking place. They are no longer free to do as they please because all of their actions may affect the growing fetus.

COGNITIVE AND PERCEPTUAL CHANGES

Although sensory changes are uncommon with pregnancy, blurred vision or diplopia (double vision) may indicate problems with a hypertensive condition of pregnancy (see Chapter 28).

PREPARATION FOR CHILDBIRTH

Prenatal education is important. Most primary care practitioners give explanations during routine visits,

© Elsevier

Fig. 26.8 During the third trimester, pillows that support the abdomen and back provide a comfortable position for rest.

but the time available is too brief to meet all of the average woman's needs. The nurse plays an important role in prenatal education. Provide pamphlets and referrals to community-based resources whenever possible. Libraries and bookstores also have many good books on prenatal care. Another source of information the expectant mother may consider are the special classes provided by hospitals and public health agencies to help the childbearing family understand and prepare for the demands of pregnancy, labor, the newborn, and parenthood. An increasing number of women seek information from internet resources. Address the selection of reliable and safe online sites for obtaining information.

CHILDBIRTH PREPARATION CLASSES

Communities often have a variety of courses that complement one another and meet the differing needs of specific segments of the population (Fig. 26.9). Some classes are general, whereas others are targeted toward specific groups such as adolescents, those having cesarean or vaginal birth after cesarean delivery, siblings, or grandparents (Box 26.13).

Common methods of prepared childbirth include Dick-Read, which focuses on progressive relaxation techniques and avoidance of analgesics; Bradley, which stresses control of environmental factors, such as lighting, temperature, and noise, to provide a calm, supportive environment for childbirth; Leboyer, which

Patient Teaching

Safety During Pregnancy

Changes in the body as a result of pregnancy include relaxation of joints, alteration of the center of gravity, faintness, and discomfort. Problems with coordination and balance are common. Therefore, the woman should follow these guidelines:
- Use good body mechanics.
- Use safety features on tools or vehicles (safety seatbelts, shoulder harnesses, headrests, goggles, helmets) as specified.
- Avoid activities that require coordination, balance, and concentration.
- Take rest periods; reschedule daily activities to meet rest and relaxation needs.

uses a warm water bath to reduce the trauma of birth; and Lamaze, which uses breathing, distraction, and focusing techniques to control pain mentally and requires disciplined training throughout the pregnancy. The Patient Teaching box on safety during pregnancy provides activity and environmental guidelines.

CULTURAL VARIATIONS IN PRENATAL CARE

The practitioner must determine and explore cultural practices and beliefs with the patient (see the Cultural Considerations box; see Chapter 6 for further discussion of the cultural aspects of nursing).

❖ NURSING PROCESS FOR NORMAL PREGNANCY

The role of the licensed practical nurse/licensed vocational nurse (LPN/LVN) in the nursing process as stated is that the LPN/LVN will:
- Participate in planning care for patients based on patient needs.
- Review the patient's plan of care and recommend revisions as needed.
- Review and follow defined prioritization for patient care.
- Use clinical pathways, care maps, or care plans to guide and review patient care.

◆ ASSESSMENT

Assessment begins when the woman visits the physician's office or clinic during the early part of her pregnancy. The first visit includes obtaining demographic data, taking a health history, and performing a general physical assessment, as well as an obstetric assessment. The general assessment includes lifestyle patterns, body system examination, and laboratory screening of blood and urine. Also explore the woman's perceptions of her condition, cultural and ethnic influences, experiences with other caregivers, lifestyle, and patterns of coping. A symptom diary, in which the woman records emotions, behaviors, physical symptoms, diet, and exercise and rest patterns, is a useful diagnostic tool. The obstetric assessment includes a gynecologic

| Box 26.11 | **Maternal Adaptation** |

Adaptation to the maternal role involves a complex social and cognitive learning process. Pregnancy functions as a rite of passage and indicates that physiologic maturity has been reached. Reva Rubin began studying maternal role adaptation in the 1960s. She described the developing tasks of pregnancy as accepting the pregnancy, identifying the role of mother, reordering the relationships between her mother and herself and between herself and her partner, establishing a relationship with the unborn child, and preparing for the birth experience.

Women who are prepared to accept a pregnancy seek medical validation early. When pregnancy is confirmed, a woman's emotional responses may range from delight to shock, disbelief, and despair. A general state of well-being predominates, but emotional lability is common. These rapid mood changes include increased irritability, explosions of tears and anger, and feelings of great joy and cheerfulness. Such changes are often attributed to hormonal changes.

Rubin describes changes in pregnancy as follows. The subjective experience of time and space changes during pregnancy; early in pregnancy, nothing seems to be happening, and the woman spends much time sleeping. With quickening (feelings of fetal movement) in the second trimester, there is a reduction of time and space, both geographic and social, as the woman turns her attention inward to her pregnancy. She examines or fosters relationships with her mother and other women who have been or are pregnant. With the third trimester, there is a slower pace and a sense that time is running out as the woman's activities are curtailed. A mother's positive reaction to her daughter's pregnancy signifies her acceptance of the grandchild and of her daughter. If the mother is supportive, the daughter has an opportunity to discuss pregnancy and labor and her feelings of joy or ambivalence with a knowledgeable and accepting woman.

The partner's emotional support is an important factor in successfully accomplishing the developmental tasks of pregnancy. Pregnant women express two major needs concerning their partner: feeling loved and valued and having the child accepted. The addition of a child changes forever the nature of the bond between partners. The partner can be a stabilizing influence, a good listener to expressions of doubts and fears, and a source of physical and emotional reassurance. The partner can also feel jealous of the unborn baby. Lesbian and unpartnered women have received little attention in the literature. Some suggest that a woman partner may be better able to understand and nurture her partner. An unpartnered woman may seek out her mother or other women friends to meet her dependence needs.

From Hockenberry MJ, Lowdermilk DL, et al: *Wong's maternal-child nursing care,* ed 8, St. Louis, 2007, Mosby.

🌐 Cultural Considerations

Pregnancy

- Many cultures and religions have customs that affect pregnant women. It is important not to generalize when giving care. Not all members of a cultural group behave in exactly the same way. Discuss beliefs with each individual to determine her unique cultural practices. If the practices do not cause harm, include them in planning care.
- Because of cultural and other factors—such as lack of money, lack of transportation, and poor communication on the part of health care providers—many women do not receive adequate prenatal care. Do not misinterpret the woman's behavior as uncaring, lazy, or ignorant.
- A concern for modesty can be a deterrent for prenatal care. Exposure of one's genitalia, especially to a male practitioner, is a significant breach of modesty. Thus, many women prefer a midwife instead of a male practitioner. Health care providers frequently assume that women lose this sense of modesty during pregnancy and labor. Most women value and appreciate efforts to maintain their modesty.
- Almost all cultures advocate a socially harmonious and agreeable environment during pregnancy. Stressful relationships can hinder a successful outcome for the mother and baby.
- Extended family members may wish to accompany the pregnant woman to her prenatal care visits and during labor. To avoid discord, the nurse and other staff members must accommodate the situation in culturally prescribed ways.
- Some belief systems include magical thinking about events that may occur during pregnancy. Among some Hispanics, it traditionally is thought that witnessing an eclipse of the moon may cause a cleft palate in the infant, or that exposure to an earthquake may result in preterm delivery, miscarriage, or a breech presentation if the earthquake was exceptionally strong. Some African Americans may warn a pregnant woman not to ridicule someone with an affliction or her child may be born with the same handicap. A widely held folk belief persists that raising one's arm above one's head or tying knots may cause the umbilical cord to wrap around the baby's neck and become knotted.
- Native people from some cultures of the American Southwest may wear amulets (charm, talisman, fetish, lucky piece), spirit medals, and beads to ward off evil.
- Pregnant Filipino women may be cautioned that any activity is dangerous, and others willingly take over their work. For those holding this belief, inactivity is considered to be a protection for the mother and baby, and the mother is encouraged to simply produce the succeeding generation. This behavior should not be misinterpreted as laziness or noncompliance.

and obstetric history, as well as a gynecologic examination with Pap smear, if needed.

◆ PATIENT PROBLEM

Nursing assessment helps identify the needs of the pregnant patient. Care can then be based on these needs. Possible patient problems for a normal pregnancy include the following:

- *Deficient Sleep*
- *Distorted Body Image*
- *Fearfulness*
- *Impaired Family Processes*
- *Inability to Control Urination due to Physical Stress*
- *Inability to Tolerate Activity*
- *Infrequent or Difficult Bowel Elimination*
- *Insufficient Knowledge*

Box **26.12**	Paternal Adaptation

A man's emotional response to becoming a father, his concerns, and his informational needs change during the pregnancy. Men can experience three styles of involvement and one style of relative noninvolvement during pregnancy (May, 1982). Men may be relatively uninvolved in pregnancy as observers, avoiding direct involvement in activities such as parent education classes and decisions about breastfeeding. Others are more involved and expressive, displaying a strong emotional response to pregnancy and a desire to be a full partner in the project. Some expectant fathers experience *couvade syndrome* and have pregnancy-like symptoms such as nausea, other gastrointestinal issues, and fatigue (couvade is a custom in some non-Western cultures in which a husband goes through mock pregnancy and labor). Some fathers adopt the instrumental style, performing tasks in their role as manager of the pregnancy. They feel responsible for the outcome of the pregnancy and are protective and supportive of their partners.

The father's beliefs and feelings about the ideal mother and father and his cultural expectation of appropriate behavior during pregnancy affect his response to his partner's need for him. One man may engage in nurturing behavior; another may feel lonely and alienated as the woman becomes physically and emotionally engrossed in the unborn child. The man may seek comfort and understanding outside the home or become interested in a new hobby or involved with his work. Some men view pregnancy as a proof of their masculinity and their dominant role. To others, pregnancy has no meaning in terms of responsibility to either mother or child. However, for most men, pregnancy is a time of preparation for the parental role, of fantasy or great pleasure, and of intense learning.

Perry S, Hockenberry M, Lowdermilk D, et al: *Maternal-child nursing care,* ed 5, St. Louis, 2014, Mosby.

- *Insufficient Nutrition*
- *Lethargy or Malaise*
- *Potential for Compromised Parenting Skills*
- *Potential for Injury*

◆ EXPECTED OUTCOMES AND PLANNING

The care plan should focus on the pregnant patient's needs and the nurse's ability to address those needs effectively (Nursing Care Plan 26.1). Each patient has different needs, and care must be individualized accordingly.

The care plan focuses on goals and outcomes specific to the patient problem. Examples include the following:

Goal 1: Patient will use self-care behaviors to maintain optimal levels of wellness for herself and the fetus.

Outcome: Patient keeps all prenatal appointments, does not smoke or drink alcoholic beverages, and does not use other drugs unless prescribed by her physician.

Goal 2: Patient will become knowledgeable about needs and concerns experienced during each trimester.

Outcome: Patient keeps a symptom diary and discusses it on each visit to the primary caregiver. Patient attends prenatal classes regularly.

Fig. 26.9 Entire family participating in a childbirth preparation course.

Box **26.13**	Topics Typically Discussed in Childbirth Preparation Classes

- A review of reproductive anatomy and physiology
- Physical and emotional changes commonly observed during pregnancy
- Fetal growth and development
- Nutrition
- Routine aspects of prenatal hygiene and exercise
- Danger signs during pregnancy
- Birth process, vaginal and cesarean
- Analgesia and anesthesia during labor and delivery
- Care of the newborn infant
- Selection of infant feeding methods
- Sibling preparation
- Changing family dynamics
- Postpartal exercises

◆ IMPLEMENTATION

Nursing interventions during the prenatal period may include the following:

- Identify factors that may interfere with health maintenance.
- Provide information to the patient to promote health maintenance.
- Assess and counsel on nutritional habits and weight gain.
- Stress safety issues regarding risk of injury as the pregnancy progresses.
- Teach the importance of pacing activities.
- Review the importance of adequate fluid intake.
- Review patterns of elimination and any changes that have occurred.

Nursing Care Plan 26.1   The Patient With a Normal Pregnancy

Ms. P. is a 23-year-old gravida 1, para 0 at 30 weeks of gestation. She has gained 12 lb since the beginning of her pregnancy. She has a full-time job at an insurance company and plays tennis twice a week. She considers herself a vegan but reports she does eat some fish. She takes prenatal vitamins daily. She reports some constipation, although her bowel habits were normal before her pregnancy.

PATIENT PROBLEM

Insufficient Nutrition, related to dietary habits

Patient Goals and Expected Outcomes	Nursing Interventions	Evaluation
Patient will meet nutritional needs Patient will know about additional nutritional needs during pregnancy and how to fulfill them	Assess weight at regular intervals. Review the ChooseMyPlate guide. Provide information related to nutritional needs during pregnancy. Have patient keep dietary diary. Encourage patient to drink 6–8 glasses of water daily to aid in bowel regularity.	Patient meets her nutritional needs as evidenced by recommended weight gain. Patient displays knowledge of additional nutritional needs by eating a well-balanced diet as evidenced by dietary diary and appropriate weight gain. Patient reports water intake of 6–8 glasses daily.

PATIENT PROBLEM

Potential for Compromised Parenting Skills or Ineffective Attachment, related to developmental stressors of pregnancy and to lack of knowledge and skill

Patient Goals and Expected Outcomes	Nursing Interventions	Evaluation
Patient will follow a lifestyle that is conducive to a positive pregnancy outcome	Discuss measures that promote a healthy pregnancy outcome, including nutrition, physical activity, rest, stress reduction, and lifestyle changes. Encourage patient to ask questions and express concerns.	The patient makes necessary lifestyle changes to promote a positive pregnancy outcome. Patient uses effective coping strategies regarding stressors of pregnancy.
Patient will express ability to cope with the changes and stressors of pregnancy	Provide encouragement for effective coping strategies used. Encourage patient to keep a symptom diary and bring it with her to each prenatal visit. Inform parents of community resources to assist and support them as needed. Help parents develop realistic expectations of newborn behaviors and demands. Assess parents' plans to incorporate the newborn into the family circle. Offer opportunity for demonstration of infant care skills, with return demonstration.	Patient keeps symptom diary and brings it to each prenatal visit; feels free to discuss concerns. Parents complete infant bathing, diapering, cord care, and feeding appropriately in return demonstration.

CRITICAL THINKING QUESTIONS

1. How should the nurse respond to Ms. P. if she expresses concern about her dietary practices and their effects on her baby? What suggestions can the nurse give her to ensure that her diet is adequate to support the pregnancy?
2. Ms. P. states that she is concerned about having to reduce her activity schedule, particularly tennis, which she enjoys. She is worried that she will begin to resent her baby because of the need to alter her activities. How should the nurse respond to her concerns? What suggestions should the nurse give her?

- Teach ways to position body for sleep promotion and rest.
- Provide information on prenatal classes.
- Explain discomforts and danger signs.
- Encourage verbalization of fears and concerns.
- Incorporate patient's cultural values into the care plan.

See the Health Promotion box for self-care prenatal health maintenance measures.

◆ EVALUATION

Continually evaluate the success of the interventions. As the pregnancy progresses, the focus and interventions change. Refer to the goals and outcomes to determine whether the care plan was successful and the outcomes were met. Be assured that care has been effective when the woman reports improvements in the quality of her life, skill in self-care, and a positive self-concept and body image.

Health Promotion

Prenatal Health Maintenance Measures

Health maintenance is an important aspect of prenatal care. Patient participation in their own care ensures prompt reporting of problematic responses to pregnancy. Patient responsibility for health maintenance is strengthened by a readiness to learn and by the nurse's understanding of maternal adaptations to the growth of the unborn child.

The expectant mother needs information about many topics. Be observant, listen, and know the typical concerns of expectant parents to anticipate what questions will be asked and to prompt mothers and their partners to discuss what is on their minds. Provide printed literature to supplement the individualized teaching; women often avidly read books and pamphlets related to their own experience. Read the literature before distributing them and point out areas that may not correspond to local health care practices. Patients who receive conflicting advice or instruction may grow frustrated with members of the health care team and the care provided.

Topics to discuss with pregnant women may include the following:

EMPLOYMENT
- Employment of pregnant women usually has no adverse effects on pregnancy outcomes. Job discrimination that is based solely on pregnancy is illegal. However, some job environments pose a potential risk to the fetus (e.g., dry-cleaning plants, chemical laboratories, and parking garages).
- Discourage activities that require a good sense of balance, especially during the last half of pregnancy.
- Commonly, excessive fatigue is the deciding factor in the termination of employment.
- Women in sedentary jobs need to walk around at intervals and should neither sit nor stand in one position for long periods. Activity counters sluggish leg circulation, which can cause varices and thrombophlebitis. Women also should avoid crossing their legs at the knees because this fosters such conditions. Standing for long periods increases the risk of preterm labor.
- The pregnant woman's chair should provide adequate back support. Use of a footstool can prevent pressure on veins, relieve strain on varicosities, and reduce swelling of feet.

CLOTHING
- Comfortable, loose clothing is best. Washable fabrics (e.g., absorbent cottons) often are preferred. Maternity clothes may be purchased new or found in good condition at thrift shops or garage sales. Tight bras and belts, stretch pants, garters, tight-top knee socks, panty girdles, and other constrictive clothing should be avoided, because tight clothing over the perineum encourages vaginitis, and impaired circulation in the legs can cause varices.
- Maternity bras are constructed to accommodate the increased breast weight. These bras have drop-flaps over the nipples to facilitate breastfeeding. A good bra can help prevent neck and back discomfort.
- Elastic hosiery is comfortable and promotes greater venous emptying in women with large varicose veins. Ideally, the supportive hose should be worn during waking hours.
- Comfortable shoes that provide firm support and promote good posture and balance are advisable. Tall high heels and platform shoes are not recommended because of the woman's changed center of gravity, which can cause her to lose balance. In addition, the woman's pelvis tilts forward in the third trimester, increasing her lumbar curve. The resulting leg aches and cramps are aggravated by shoes that do not provide good support.

TRAVEL
- Travel is not contraindicated for pregnant women at low risk, but those with high-risk pregnancies are advised to avoid long-distance travel after fetal viability has been reached. This is to avoid the economic and psychological consequences of delivering a preterm infant far from home.
- The second trimester is the ideal time for travel.
- Travel to areas where medical care is poor, water is untreated, and malaria is prevalent should be avoided if possible.
- Women who contemplate foreign travel should be aware that many health insurance carriers do not cover birth in a foreign setting or even hospitalization for preterm labor.
- Pregnant women who travel long distances should schedule periods of activity and rest. While sitting, women can practice deep breathing, foot circling, and alternately contracting and relaxing different muscle groups. They should avoid becoming fatigued.
- Although travel is not a cause of adverse outcomes, such as miscarriage or preterm labor, certain precautions are recommended while traveling in a car. The woman always should use automobile restraints—generally a combination lap belt and shoulder harness. The lap belt is worn low across the hip bones and as snug as is comfortable. The shoulder belt is worn above the pregnant uterus and below the neck to avoid chafing. The pregnant woman should sit upright and use the headrest to avoid a whiplash injury.
- Maternal death as a result of injury is the most common cause of fetal death. The next most common cause is placental separation. This occurs because body contours change in reaction to the force of a collision. The uterus as a muscular organ can adapt its shape to that of the body, but the placenta lacks the resiliency to change. At the impact of collision, placental separation can occur.
- Airline travel in large commercial jets usually poses little risk to the pregnant woman, but policies vary from airline to airline. The pregnant woman is advised to inquire about restrictions or recommendations from her carrier. Magnetometers (metal detectors) used at airport security checkpoints are not harmful to the fetus. Cabins of commercial airlines are maintained at 8% humidity, which may result in some water loss; hydration (with water) should be maintained under these conditions. Sitting in a cramped seat of an airliner for prolonged periods may increase the risk of superficial and deep thrombophlebitis. A pregnant woman is encouraged to take a 15-min walk around the aircraft cabin during each hour of travel to minimize this risk.

Get Ready for the NCLEX® Examination!

Key Points

- Pregnancy is a normal process that involves many complex physiologic changes in the mother.
- Over a period of 280 days, two initial cells join and develop into a unique, viable human.
- Structures such as the placenta, membranes, the umbilical cord, and amniotic fluid protect and support the developing fetus. These structures are unique to pregnancy.
- All aspects of the mother's lifestyle potentially can affect her developing fetus.
- Many drugs and viruses can cross the placenta and present serious hazards to the developing embryo, particularly during the first trimester of pregnancy.
- Sophisticated diagnostic tests often are performed to identify genetic or developmental problems during pregnancy. Early identification of problems may influence a woman's decisions regarding a pregnancy.
- Although pregnancy is a normal process, regular and ongoing health care is important throughout pregnancy.
- At present, the best means of reducing the number of children born with genetic defects is for health professionals to provide families with genetic information and services.
- Many signs and symptoms of pregnancy are similar to those that are characteristic of other medical conditions. The positive signs of pregnancy are visualization of the fetus, fetal motion detected by a trained observer, and auscultation of fetal heart sounds.
- Every pregnant woman should be aware of the danger signs during pregnancy and contact her physician if any of them are present.
- The rational use of any medication requires a risk-versus-benefit assessment. Among the many risk factors that complicate assessment, pregnancy is one of the most perplexing.
- Nutritional needs change during pregnancy. To support normal growth and development of the fetus, the woman needs increased calories, minerals, and vitamins.
- Many discomforts may occur during pregnancy. Be aware of measures that can reduce these discomforts without harming the mother or the fetus.
- Pregnancy is a time of role adjustment for both prospective parents. All family members are affected by the addition of a new member.
- Adequate preparation enables the woman to become a knowledgeable participant in the entire childbearing process. Be aware of classes available in the community and the materials covered in these classes.
- The nurse and the patient are influenced by cultural and personal values and beliefs during the patient's pregnancy. Careful assessment is imperative.

Additional Learning Resources

SG Go to your Study Guide for additional learning activities to help you master this chapter content.

Be sure to visit the Evolve site at http://evolve.elsevier.com/Cooper/foundations/ for additional online resources.

Review Questions for the NCLEX® Examination

1. A 25-year-old woman comes to the clinic and says she thinks she is pregnant. Her last period was July 20. Based on this fact, what is the expected date of delivery (EDD)?

   1. April 13
   2. April 27
   3. May 20
   4. March 27

2. The patient reports experiencing nausea, vomiting, and breast tenderness, along with missing her period. These symptoms are considered to be what type of signs of pregnancy?

   1. Probable
   2. Positive
   3. Presumptive
   4. Possible

3. A pregnant patient is seen during her second trimester at the health care provider's office. She asks the nurse, "What can I do when my leg goes into a cramp?" The patient demonstrates understanding of the nurse's instruction regarding relief of leg cramps if she takes which action?

   1. Wiggles and points her toes during the cramp
   2. Applies cold compresses to the affected leg
   3. Extends her leg and dorsiflexes her foot during the cramp
   4. Avoids weight bearing on the affected leg during the cramp

4. A woman who is in her first trimester is talking with the nurse. The patient has inquired about the feelings she will have when she first feels her baby move. What information can be provided by the nurse?

   1. The movement will feel like cramps.
   2. The movement is rhythmic and called Goodell's sign.
   3. The movement is flutter-like and is called quickening.
   4. The movement is like a thud and is called Hëgar's sign.

5. While giving a health history to the nurse, the patient reports that she usually has a glass of wine with dinner. What is the safe level of alcohol intake for her during her pregnancy?

   1. No alcohol
   2. Wine only; one or two glasses daily with meals
   3. Up to 4 oz daily
   4. Beer or wine only after the first trimester

6. The nurse explains to the patient that she should contact her health care provider if she experiences any of the danger signs of pregnancy. Which symptoms are a danger sign during pregnancy? (Select all that apply.)

   1. Urinary frequency
   2. Severe headaches
   3. Dyspepsia
   4. Heartburn
   5. Diplopia
   6. Abdominal cramping
   7. Vaginal spotting

7. A test that may be done in late pregnancy to determine fetal well-being is the nonstress test. This test is based on which phenomenon?

   1. Fetal heart rate increases in connection with fetal movement.
   2. Braxton Hicks contractions cause an increase in fetal heart rate.
   3. Fetal heart rate slows in response to contractions.
   4. Fetal movement causes an increase in maternal heart rate.

8. Constipation is a frequent symptom as a pregnancy progresses. Which measures should be recommended to the gravid woman? *(Select all that apply.)*

   1. Drink six to eight glasses of water daily.
   2. Take an over-the-counter laxative.
   3. Take an iron supplement only every other day.
   4. Take mineral oil at bedtime.
   5. Increase dietary fiber intake.

9. At one of her prenatal visits, the patient is scheduled for a sonogram. Sonography can be used to assess which of the following? *(Select all that apply.)*

   1. Number of fetuses
   2. Gestational age of fetus
   3. Down syndrome
   4. Congenital anomalies
   5. Placement of the placenta
   6. Gender of fetus
   7. Quantity of amniotic fluid

10. Which symptom is considered a first-trimester warning sign and should be reported immediately to the health care provider?

    1. Nausea with occasional vomiting
    2. Fatigue
    3. Urinary frequency
    4. Vaginal bleeding

11. A pregnant woman at 10 weeks of gestation jogs three or four times per week. She is concerned about the effect of exercise on the fetus. What information can be provided by the nurse?

    1. "You do not need to modify your exercising at any time during your pregnancy."
    2. "Stop exercising because it will harm the fetus."
    3. "You may find that you need to modify your exercising to walking later in your pregnancy, around the seventh month."
    4. "Jogging is too hard on your body; switch to walking now."

12. A woman at 23 weeks of gestation calls to tell the nurse she thinks she is leaking fluid from her vagina. What information should be included in the nurse's response to the patient?

    1. "As long as the baby is still moving around, there is nothing to worry about."
    2. "Come to the office right away."
    3. "Call me back in 2 hours and tell me if there is any change in the leakage."
    4. "We can wait until your next appointment to check you."

13. A woman admitted in labor has an obstetric history that indicates that she has had four pregnancies and has three living children. One was born at 39 weeks of gestation, another at 34 of weeks of gestation, and another at 35 weeks of gestation. She had a miscarriage at 16 weeks gestation. What are her gravidity and parity with the TPAL system?

    1. 1-2-1-3
    2. 1-2-0-3
    3. 3-0-3-0
    4. 2-2-0-3

14. The nurse teaches a pregnant woman about the presumptive, probable, and positive signs of pregnancy. Which are positive signs of pregnancy? *(Select all that apply.)*

    1. A positive pregnancy test
    2. Fetal movement palpated by the primary caregiver
    3. Braxton Hicks contractions
    4. Nausea and vomiting
    5. Presence of fetal heart tones

15. A patient is scheduled for an ultrasound scan. She is at 22 weeks' gestation. The patient asks how they will be able to tell the gestational age of her fetus. When planning the response, the nurse correctly recognizes that which measurements will be used in this determination? *(Select all that apply.)*

    1. Abdominal circumference
    2. Biparietal diameter
    3. Quantity of amniotic fluid
    4. Femur length
    5. Crown rump length

16. An expectant father confides to the nurse that his pregnant wife (10 weeks of gestation) is driving him crazy. "One minute, she seems happy, and the next minute, she seems unhappy, and the next, she is crying over nothing at all. Is there something wrong with her?" What is the most appropriate response by the nurse?

    1. "This is normal behavior and should begin to subside by the second trimester."
    2. "She may be having difficulty relating to the pregnancy. I will refer her to a counselor I know."
    3. "This is called emotional lability and is related to hormone changes and anxiety during pregnancy. The mood swings will subside as she adjusts to being pregnant."
    4. "You seem impatient with her. Perhaps this is precipitating her behavior."

17. When planning a diet with a pregnant woman, what should the nurse's initial action be?

    1. Review the woman's dietary intake.
    2. Teach the woman about the ChooseMyPlate guide.
    3. Caution the woman to avoid large doses of vitamins, especially those that are fat soluble.
    4. Instruct the woman to limit the intake of fatty foods.

18. A pregnant woman at 32 weeks of gestation reports feeling dizzy and lightheaded while her fundal height is being measured. Her skin is pale and moist. What should the nurse's initial action be?

    1. Assess the woman's blood pressure and pulse.
    2. Have the woman breathe into a paper bag.
    3. Raise the woman's legs.
    4. Turn the woman on her side.

19. When obtaining a reproductive health history from a female patient, what should the nurse do?

    1. Limit the time spent on exploration of intimate topics.
    2. Explain the purpose of questions asked and how they will be used.
    3. Avoid asking questions that may embarrass the patient.
    4. Use only acceptable medical terminology when referring to body parts and functions.

20. After admitting a new patient to the maternity unit, the nurse writes a care plan. This process of determining outcomes and interventions is which stage of the nursing process?

    1. Assessment
    2. Planning
    3. Implementation
    4. Evaluation

Fill in the Blank
Fill in the blank with the correct medical term.

21. _____ Woman who is pregnant

22. _____ Woman who is pregnant for the first time

23. _____ Woman who has had two or more pregnancies

24. _____ Capacity to live outside the uterus

Labor and Delivery

Objectives

1. Discuss birth planning.
2. Discuss birth setting choices.
3. Discuss the signs and symptoms of impending labor.
4. Distinguish between true and false labor.
5. Explain the five factors that affect the labor process.
6. Discuss cephalopelvic disproportion.
7. Describe the "powers" involved in labor and delivery.
8. Identify the mechanisms of labor.
9. Identify the stages of labor.
10. Describe the assessment for labor and delivery.
11. Identify nursing diagnoses relevant to the woman in labor.
12. Discuss nursing interventions related to labor and delivery.
13. Outline medical interventions related to labor and delivery.

Key Terms

amniotomy (ăm-nē-ŎT-ŏ-mē, p. 843)
attitude (p. 816)
Braxton Hicks contractions (p. 813)
cardinal movements of labor (p. 821)
cephalopelvic disproportion (sĕf-ă-lō-PĔL-vĭk dĭs-prō-PŌR-shŭn, p. 844)
descent (p. 822)
effacement (ĕ-FĀS-mĕnt, p. 813)
engagement (ĕn-GĀJ-mĕnt, p. 822)
episiotomy (ĕ-pĭs-ē-ŎT-ŏ-mē, p. 826)
expulsion (p. 826)
extension (p. 823)
external rotation (p. 823)

fetal lie (p. 816)
fetal position (p. 816)
fetal presentation (p. 816)
flexion (FLĔK-shŭn, p. 816)
hypoxia (hī-PŎK-sē-ă, p. 831)
internal rotation (p. 823)
lightening (p. 812)
meconium (mĕ-KŌ-nē-ŭm, p. 831)
oligohydramnios (ŏl-ĭ-gō-hī-DRĂM-nē-ŏs, p. 834)
oxytocin (ŏks-ē-TŌ-sĭn, p. 826)
restitution (p. 823)
surfactant (sŭr-FĂK-tănt, p. 831)
uterine inertia (YŪ-tĕr-ĭn ĭn-ĔR-shă, p. 843)

BIRTH PLANNING

Preparation of the mother and her partner for the birth of the baby ideally begins early in the pregnancy. Beginning teaching in the first trimester allows the family time to ask questions and retain information provided. The education provided should include information about the pregnancy-related changes the mother will experience, fetal development, labor, delivery, and the postpartum periods. Some health care providers and mothers initiate a birth plan. The plan begins as an outline of the options available for the mother and her baby for the labor, delivery, and postpartum periods. The mother is then encouraged to select preferred options, but must recognize that some desires for the plan cannot be satisfied. Inability to achieve all the preferences may result from concern for the health and well-being of the mother and her baby or from facility policies.

BIRTH SETTING CHOICES

The expectant mother should consider the location in which to give birth. Choices may be limited by the community of residence, the medical privileges and preferences of the selected practitioner, and the health of the mother and baby. The three primary options to consider are the hospital, birthing center, or home.

Hospitals

In previous generations, home deliveries were considered commonplace. Technological advances, anesthesia options, and desires for the convenience of birthing in a facility have resulted in the movement of births to hospital settings. Today, the majority of births take place in medical facilities. Only 1.4% of births occur outside of a hospital (CDC, 2015). In 2013, more than 56,000 births occurred outside of the hospital. More than 60% of those deliveries took place in the home. The remaining deliveries were in a free-standing birthing center.

Birthing in a hospital has many advantages. The greatest is the availability of trained personnel in the event that complications occur. Within the hospital facility, a variety of rooming options are available. Some facilities offer single-room LDRP (labor, delivery, recovery, postpartum) units. This type of arrangement allows for the labor, delivery, and birth to take place in a single location. After delivery, the new mother and her baby continue to be cared for in the same room by a single team of nurses. Some facilities have more traditional arrangements with LDR (labor, delivery, recovery) units. In the LDR setting, the mother is admitted to the labor suite and remains there for a specified time after birth. Then she is transferred to a postpartum care unit. The baby either is transferred to a nursery or remains with the mother.

Birthing Centers

A birthing center is a care facility focused on childbirth. These facilities allow the mother to experience labor and delivery in a more homelike setting. An emphasis is placed on the wishes of the woman and her partner. Typical birthing center rooms are LDRP units. The center may be privately held or affiliated with an acute care hospital. A relationship with a hospital provides a degree of security should a complication arise requiring more invasive care. Although still limited, the use of birthing centers has increased. Presently, less than 1% of births take place in birthing centers. Birthing centers are family focused and are considered ideal only for those with low-risk pregnancies. Complications of pregnancy or necessary cesarean sections would discourage the woman's use of a birthing center.

Home

Home births were common in the United States until the early 1900s. (In the early decades of the 20th century, a shift toward hospital births took place.) Currently, women who want to have more control over their birth experience and desire reduced technology have led a renewed interest in home births. Despite the renewed interest, this is still an option only undertaken by less than 1% of the nearly 4 million births annually. Giving birth at home is not an option for all women. It is intended for the healthy pregnant woman and fetus who have not experienced complications during the gestational period. For those women choosing to deliver at home, this is not a risk-free option. Women who have experienced complications in previous pregnancies or have a history of cesarean section are also not likely candidates for home births. Unexpected complications such as failure of the labor to naturally progress may result in a needed transfer to a hospital facility. The rates of cesarean section, augmentation, induction, and complication are lower than those found in hospital deliveries. Although most home births are attended by midwives, they also may be managed by a variety of medical professionals, including a physician, nurse, or physician's assistant.

NORMAL LABOR

ONSET

In most pregnancies, the uterus begins the process of labor once the fetus is matured and ready for birth. Although this process has been occurring throughout human history, researchers still are trying to discover the exact cause for the onset of labor. The theories fall into two main categories: those based on mechanical changes and those based on hormonal changes.

One mechanical theory involves uterine stretching. It is based on the principle that once a hollow-body organ reaches a certain state of distention, it spontaneously contracts and empties. For example, a full bladder empties by incontinence and a distended stomach empties by vomiting. The hypothesis is that when the uterus stretches to a certain size, it empties spontaneously. However, the wide variation of uterine size between different pregnancies in the same woman makes this a weak theory. For example, a woman may have one pregnancy in which she delivers a 6-pound baby at term. In her next pregnancy, she may again reach term but deliver twins, each weighing 6 pounds.

Hormonal theories for the onset of labor are based on either an increase or a decrease in hormones. In some theories, the source of the hormones is the mother; in other theories, it is the fetus. Some of the more common (but still unproven) theories relating to hormones are (1) oxytocin stimulation; (2) progesterone withdrawal; (3) estrogen stimulation; and (4) fetal cortisol.

SIGNS OF IMPENDING LABOR

A series of signs may occur as labor is about to begin. Approximately 2 weeks before the onset of labor, the woman may notice that the fetus seems to have settled, or "dropped," into the pelvis. This is called lightening and is seen most often in nulliparas. Once lightening has occurred, the woman often notices that urinary frequency returns. She may be able to breathe more normally because the abdominal cavity holds more space. Multiparas may not experience this change until they are in active labor.

The gravid woman may experience a slight leakage or even a larger flow of fluid vaginally. Although urine does not seep from the vagina, the close proximity of the urinary meatus may cause the woman to believe that it is amniotic fluid. Evaluation should be performed to determine what the fluid is. A simple test with nitrazine paper can distinguish between fluids (Box 27.1). The paper is moistened with discharge from

Box **27.1**	Nitrazine Test for Rupture of Membranes

- Explain the procedure to the woman or the couple.
- Perform the procedure.
- Wash hands.
- Put on sterile gloves.
- Use nitrazine test paper, a dye-impregnated test paper for determination of pH (differentiates amniotic fluid, which is slightly alkaline, from urine and purulent material [pus], which are acidic).
- While wearing a sterile glove lubricated with water, place a piece of test paper on the cervical opening.

or

- With a sterile, cotton-tipped applicator, dip deep into the vagina to pick up fluid; touch applicator to test paper. (Procedure may be done during speculum examination.)
- Read results:
- Membranes probably intact: identifies vaginal and most body fluids that are acidic:
  Yellow, pH 5.0
  Olive-yellow, pH 5.5
  Olive-green, pH 6.0
- Membranes probably ruptured: identifies amniotic fluid that is alkaline:
  Blue-green, pH 6.5
  Blue-gray, pH 7.0
  Deep blue, pH 7.5
- False test results are possible because of presence of bloody show, insufficient amniotic fluid, or semen.
- Provide pericare as needed.
- Remove gloves and wash hands.
- Document results (positive or negative).

Table **27.1**	Comparison of True and False Labor	
TRUE LABOR	**FALSE LABOR**
Contractions follow a regular pattern.	Contractions rarely follow a pattern.
Contractions come closer together, are stronger, and tend to last longer.	Contractions vary in length and intensity.
Contractions get stronger with ambulation.	Contractions frequently stop with ambulation or position change.
Contractions seem to start in the lower back and then travel to the lower abdomen.	Contractions may be felt in the back but are noticed most often in the fundus.
Contractions usually are not stopped with controlled breathing, sedation, or other relaxation interventions.	Contractions eventually stop with relaxation interventions.
The cervix softens, effaces, and dilates.	The cervix may soften, but with little or no change in effacement or dilation.
The fetus continues descent into the pelvis.	No significant change in the fetal position occurs.

the unwashed area. If the paper reacts (turns blue), the discharge is likely amniotic fluid. If the test is nonreactive, the discharge is urine and the membranes are more likely intact. The amniotic sac generally ruptures after labor has begun. If it ruptures before labor starts, medical attention is essential. If labor does not occur within a few hours of the rupture of the membranes, the physician usually will attempt to induce (initiate) labor with administration of medication. Delivery should occur within 24 hours after membranes rupture. Prolonged rupture of membranes puts the woman and her fetus at risk for infection. Inability of delivery to take place within the specified time likely results in birth via cesarean section.

The amount of vaginal drainage typically increases as term approaches, and a blood-tinged mucus called *bloody show* may be observed. This mucus occludes the cervical os (the opening of the cervix) during pregnancy (mucous plug). The health care provider will likely perform a vaginal examination during the last weeks of the pregnancy. Findings that the cervix has begun to soften, efface (thin), and open (dilate) are normal. Backache and contractions of the uterus, called **Braxton Hicks contractions** (irregular tightening of the pregnant uterus that begins in the first trimester and

increases in frequency, duration, and intensity as pregnancy progresses), are common as the pregnancy approaches term. The severity of these contractions varies from mild to moderate. They remain irregular and do not dilate the cervix.

Some women notice a slight loss of weight (1 to 3 pounds) a few days before labor. Reports of nausea and diarrhea are not uncommon during this period. An energy burst often is experienced. Expectant mothers report cooking, cleaning, and preparing for the baby's arrival with renewed energy; this can be compared with the nesting behaviors noted in pregnant animals.

True labor is marked by the onset of regular, rhythmic contractions that cause progressive cervical dilation and **effacement** (thinning and shortening or obliteration of the cervix that occurs during late pregnancy, labor, or both).

FALSE LABOR VERSUS TRUE LABOR

Before the onset of true labor, many women may experience false labor. The discomforts of false labor do not promote the needed fetal descent and cervical changes that accompany true labor. The contractions experienced during this time often convince the woman that labor has begun. Fear of going to the hospital at the wrong time is common in expectant women. Explain how true and false labors differ (Table 27.1). The information should include an emphasis on the importance of seeking medical attention when any doubt exists.

LABOR AND DELIVERY

STANDARD PRECAUTIONS DURING CHILDBIRTH

During birth, nurses and other health care providers are exposed to a great deal of maternal and newborn blood and body fluids. Use standard precautions to avoid transmission of infection through contact with body fluids. The standard precautions applicable to childbirth include the following:

- Wash hands before donning gloves and after performing procedures and removing gloves.
- Wear gloves (clean or sterile, as appropriate) when performing procedures that require contact with the woman's genitalia and body fluids, including bloody show (e.g., during vaginal examination, amniotomy, hygienic care of the perineum, insertion of an internal scalp electrode and intrauterine pressure monitor, and catheterization).
- When assisting with a birth, wear a cover gown and a mask with a shield or protective eyewear. Cap and shoe covers are worn for cesarean birth but are optional for vaginal birth in a birthing room. The primary health care provider who is attending the birth should wear a sterile gown with a waterproof front and sleeves.
- Drape the woman with sterile towels and sheets as appropriate. Explain to the woman what can and cannot be touched.
- Help the woman's partner put on appropriate coverings for the type of birth, such as cap, mask, gown, and shoe covers. Show the partner where to stand and what can and cannot be touched.
- Wear gloves and gown when handling the newborn immediately after birth.
- Use an appropriate method to suction the newborn's airway, such as a bulb syringe, mechanical wall suction, or DeLee oral suction device.

PROCESS OF LABOR AND DELIVERY

To understand the complex process of labor and delivery, examine each of the factors involved. These factors are frequently called the five *P*s:

- *Passageway:* The pelvis and soft tissues
- *Passenger:* The fetus
- *Powers:* Contractions
- *Position of mother:* Standing, walking, side lying, squatting, or on hands and knees
- *Psyche:* Psychological response

Passageway

Pelvis. The superior portion of the pelvis (iliac segment of the innominate bones) supports the uterus and fetus during the late months of pregnancy. These bones aid in directing the fetus into the inferior (lower) portion of the pelvis, which is called the *true pelvis.* The two sections are divided by an imaginary line called the *linea terminalis,* or pelvic inlet.

The size and shape of the true pelvis are more important than those of the false pelvis because the fetal head must be able to pass through this section of the pelvis for vaginal delivery to occur. Four different types of pelvises are recognized, each with a unique shape and characteristics (Table 27.2).

The true pelvis is divided further into three segments: the inlet, the cavity (midpelvis), and the outlet (Fig. 27.1). The primary care practitioner can use several methods for evaluation of the size of the true pelvis:

Table 27.2 Comparison of Pelvic Types

CHARACTERISTIC	GYNECOID	ANDROID	ANTHROPOID	PLATYPELLOID
Percent of women	50%	23%	24%	3%
Brim	Slightly ovoid or transversely rounded	Heart-shaped, angulated	Oval, wider anteroposteriorly	Flattened anteroposteriorly, wide transversely
Shape of opening	Round	Heart	Oval	Flat
Depth	Moderate	Deep	Deep	Shallow
Side walls	Straight	Convergent	Straight	Straight
Ischial spines	Blunt, somewhat widely separated	Prominent, narrow interspinous diameter	Prominent, often with narrow interspinous diameter	Blunted, widely separated
Sacrum	Deep, curved	Slightly curved, terminal portion often beaked	Slightly curved	Slightly curved
Subpubic arch	Wide	Narrow	Narrow	Wide
Usual mode of delivery	Vaginal • Spontaneous • Occiput anterior position	Cesarean, Vaginal • Difficult, with forceps	Vaginal • With forceps or spontaneous • Occiput posterior or occiput anterior position	Vaginal • Spontaneous

- *Palpation:* Externally, the health care provider can use a pelvimeter to determine the distance between the ischial tuberosities. This measurement helps estimate the distance between the ischial spines, which otherwise can be obtained only with pelvic x-ray examination. Internally, additional bony prominences are evaluated to determine pelvic adequacy.
- *Pelvimetry:* With x-ray films from different views, the health care provider can measure accurately the bony prominences. This type of assessment may be done for a woman who is not currently pregnant but is seeking preconception care. The diagnostic measurement may be performed for women who have had an injury or known developmental problem, such as rickets.
- *Ultrasound scan:* Sound waves above the range of human hearing also can be used to estimate pelvic adequacy. Because ultrasound scanning does not involve the use of radiation, it generally is regarded as safe for the fetus. An ultrasound scan can show soft tissue and helps gather information regarding fetal growth, multiple pregnancy, placental location, and abnormal presentation that may complicate delivery.

Understand that adequacy of the pelvis is relative. For each delivery, a determination must be made whether the pelvis is adequate to allow passage of the fetus. Although certain measurements are considered "normal," the size and position of the fetus make each situation unique.

Soft tissues. During labor, the uterus, the cervix, the vagina, and the muscles of the perineum change in consistency and shape to allow passage of the fetus in the following ways:

- *Uterine tissues:* During labor, the walls of the upper section of the uterus have a thickened musculature that provides the force of contractions. The muscle walls of the lower section become thinner and act as a passive tube. Located between the two sections is a band of tissue: the physiologic retraction ring.
- *Cervical tissues:* As contractions of the muscular upper segment apply downward pressure, the uterine contents (fetal presenting part) efface and dilate the cervix.
- *Vagina:* In response to hormonal changes during pregnancy, the vagina undergoes many changes. Increased blood supply (vascularity) and thickness of the mucosa, loosening of the connective tissue, and enlargement (hypertrophy) of smooth muscle cells make the vagina capable of stretching (dilating) to allow passage of the fetus.
- *Perineum:* The muscles of the pelvic floor are stretched and thinned by the pressure of the presenting part. The anus may appear dilated and bulging.

Passenger

Fetus. To be born, the fetus must be able to exit through the bony passageway just described. The fetal head is the largest part of the body. Delivery of the head is of the highest concern.

The bones of the fetal skull are not rigidly fused (joined), which allows the bony plates to move and overlap as they progress through the maternal pelvis. This reshaping of the skull bones in response to pressure against the maternal pelvis is called *molding.*

The major bones of the skull are the two frontal bones, the two parietal bones, the two temporal bones, and the occiput. They are joined by membranous spaces called *sutures.* Sutures meet at larger membranous

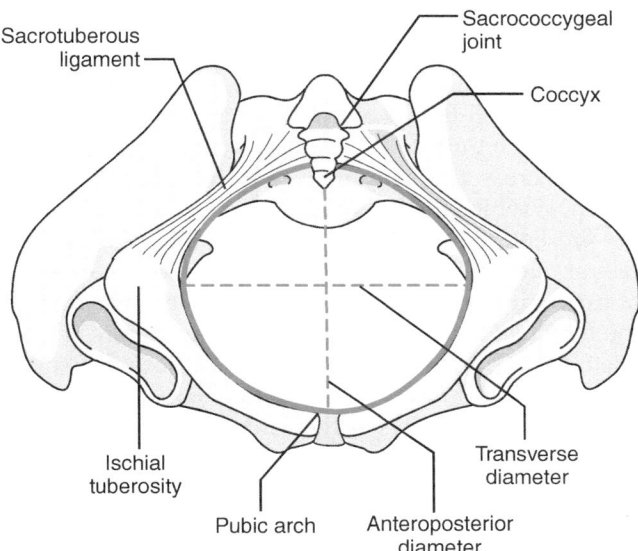

Fig. 27.1 Female pelvis. (A) Pelvic brim (inlet, linea terminalis, or iliopectineal line) from above. (B) Pelvic outlet from below.

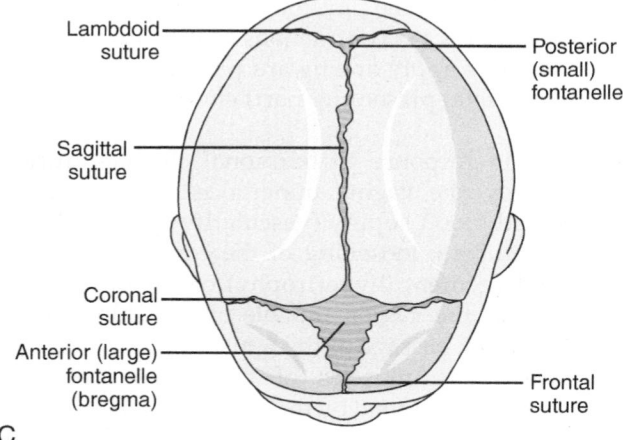

Fig. 27.2 Fetal head at term. (A) Bones. (B) Fontanelles. (C) Sutures.

areas called *fontanelles* (Fig. 27.2). The anterior fontanel (bregma) is formed by four bones and thus tends to be larger and diamond shaped. The posterior fontanel is formed by three bones and is smaller and triangular. With palpation of the sutures and fontanelles through the dilated cervix, the primary care practitioner can determine the presentation of the fetus during labor. The largest transverse diameter of the skull is the biparietal measurement. If this is too large, the skull may not be able to enter the mother's pelvis.

Fetal attitude. The relationship of fetal body parts to one another is called **attitude**. At term, the ideal attitude for

the fetal body is **flexion**. The back is bowed outward, the chin is touching the sternum, the arms are crossed over the chest, and the thighs are flexed on the abdomen. This is called the **fetal position** (the relationship of the occiput, sacrum, chin, or scapula of the fetus to the front, back, or sides of the mother's pelvis). This attitude takes up minimal space and allows the best angle of approach to the pelvis. **Fetal lie** is the relationship of the cephalocaudal (head-to-buttocks) axis of the fetus to the cephalocaudal axis of the mother. If the spine of the fetus is parallel to the spine of the mother, the lie is called *longitudinal.* The presentation could be cephalic (head down) or breech (buttocks down). The lie is longitudinal in 99% of deliveries. If the spine of the fetus is perpendicular to that of the mother, it is called *transverse lie.* Only 1% of deliveries involve a transverse lie. This lie is most common in women who have had many pregnancies (resulting in weakened abdominal walls), maternal pelvic contracture, or placenta previa (see Chapter 28). Early in gestation, the fetus will change positions frequently. As the pregnancy progresses and the fetus grows, position changes become less frequent as space is limited.

Fetal presentation. **Fetal presentation** (that part of the fetus [head, face, buttocks, feet, or shoulders] that first enters the pelvis and lies over the inlet) describes the part that will be in contact with the cervix and is determined by attitude and lie. In about 96% of deliveries, the presentation is cephalic. In cephalic presentation, some part of the fetal head is in contact with the cervix. Cephalic presentation is divided into four types: vertex (region between the fontanelles), brow, face, and mentum (chin). The portion of the head that enters the birth canal first greatly impacts the labor progression and outcome. Each of the cephalic presentations has a differing presenting diameter.

In about 3% of deliveries, the presentation is breech. Either the buttocks or legs are in contact with the cervix. Three types of breech presentation are possible: complete breech, in which the buttocks present and the thighs are well-flexed on the abdomen; frank breech, in which the buttocks present and the thighs are extended across the abdomen and chest; and footling breech, in which there is no flexion and one foot or two feet present. Breech presentations are more difficult to deliver vaginally. Attempts to deliver a breech presentation vaginally may result in fetal head entrapment. The fetal head is larger than the torso and may be unable to pass through the birth canal without difficulty. To decrease risks to the fetus, most breech births are delivered surgically (see the later section "Cesarean Delivery"). Vaginal deliveries of breech infants may be allowed under controlled circumstances if the fetus is preterm or the mother is multiparous.

In about 1% of deliveries, some other body part presents. These presentations occur when the fetus has been in a transverse lie. The shoulder, hand, elbow, and iliac crest are possible presenting parts. These cases also necessitate a cesarean birth.

Fig. 27.3 Leopold's maneuvers. (From Lowdermilk DL, Perry SE, Cashion K, et al: *Maternity and women's health care*, ed 10, St. Louis, 2012, Mosby.)

ROP
Right
occipitoposterior

LOP
Left
occipitoposterior

POSTERIOR

ROT
Right
occipito-
transverse

LOT
Left
occipito-
transverse

RIGHT   *LEFT*

ANTERIOR

ROA
Right
occipitoanterior

LOA
Left
occipitoanterior

Lie: Longitudinal or vertical   **Reference point:** Occiput
Presentation: Vertex   **Attitude:** General flexion

Fig. 27.4 Cephalic positions. Examples of fetal vertex (occiput) presentation in relation to front, back, and side of maternal pelvis.

Fetal position. Position is the relationship of the presenting fetal part to a quadrant of the maternal pelvis. Fetal position can be determined with abdominal inspection and palpation (Leopold's maneuvers) (Fig. 27.3), vaginal or rectal examination, auscultation of fetal heart tones, or ultrasound scan or x-ray examination. Positions are expressed in abbreviated form—for example, the most common position for delivery is left occiput anterior (LOA), in which the occiput of the fetus points toward the left anterior segment of the maternal pelvis. The right occiput anterior (ROA) position is the next most common position. Many combinations are possible (Figs. 27.4 and 27.5).

Fig. 27.5 Various presentations and positions. *LMT*, Left mentotransverse; *LSA*, left sacroanterior; *LSP*, left sacroposterior; *RADA*, right acromio-dorsoanterior; *RSA*, right sacroanterior; *RScA*, right scapuloanterior; *RSP*, right sacroposterior.

A longitudinal lie, well-flexed attitude, and vertex presentation is the ideal. This position best enables the fetal skull bones to mold as they progress through the maternal pelvis. The fetal skull also provides a smooth, round surface, which is most effective in effacing and dilating the cervix. The smooth, regular shape also fills the cervix and prevents the umbilical cord from prolapsing, or coming before the fetus. Cord prolapse is dangerous because pressure on the vessels in the cord can restrict blood flow to the fetus.

If a part other than the vertex presents, labor is generally longer, more tiring to the mother, and more likely to necessitate surgical intervention.

Prompt recognition of a prolapsed umbilical cord is important because fetal hypoxia from prolonged cord compression (occlusion of blood flow to and from the fetus for more than 5 minutes) usually results in central nervous system damage or death of the fetus. The examiner can relieve pressure on the cord by putting a sterile gloved hand into the vagina and holding the presenting part off of the umbilical cord (Figs. 27.6A and B). The woman is assisted into a position such as a modified Sims (Fig. 27.6C), Trendelenburg, or knee-chest (Fig. 27.6D) position so that gravity keeps the pressure of the presenting part off of the cord. If the cervix is fully dilated, forceps- or vacuum-assisted delivery can be performed for the fetus in a

cephalic presentation; otherwise, a cesarean birth is likely. Nonreassuring fetal status, inadequate uterine relaxation, and bleeding also can occur as a result of a prolapsed umbilical cord.

Placenta. The placenta is also referred to as a passenger. After the fetus is delivered with strong uterine contractions, the placental attachment site is significantly smaller. This reduced size causes the placenta to separate from its attachment. Normally, the first few strong contractions 5 to 7 minutes after the birth of the baby disrupt the placenta from its base. A placenta is not freed easily from a flaccid (relaxed) uterus because the placental attachment site is not reduced in size.

Placental separation is indicated by the following signs (Fig. 27.7):
- A firmly contracting fundus
- A change in the uterus from discoid (disklike) to globular ovoid (egg-shaped) as the placenta moves to the lower segment
- A sudden gush of dark blood from the introitus (the entrance into the vagina)
- Apparent lengthening of the umbilical cord as the placenta gets closer to the introitus
- A vaginal fullness (the placenta) noted on vaginal or rectal examination or fetal membranes seen at the introitus

Fig. 27.6 *Arrows* indicate direction of pressure against presenting part to relieve compression of prolapsed umbilical cord. Pressure exerted by examiner's fingers in: (A) vertex presentation and (B) breech presentation. (C) Gravity relieves pressure when woman is in modified Sims position with hips elevated as high as possible without pillows. (D) Knee-chest position.

Whether the placenta shows its shiny fetal surface ("Shiny Schultze") or its dark, roughened maternal surface ("Dirty Duncan") first is of no clinical significance. The delivery of the placenta completes the third stage of labor. This stage lasts 15 to 30 minutes, or longer if the health care provider waits for the mother to express the placenta. When the delivery of the placenta is managed actively, it can take less than 5 minutes (Fig. 27.7 B).

After the placenta (with its membranes) emerges, it is examined for intactness to be certain that no portion of it remains in the uterine cavity. The goal of this stage of labor is the prompt separation and expulsion of the placenta, achieved in the easiest and safest manner. If the fundus is not firm, stimulate the uterine muscle to regain tone and to expel any clots before measuring the distance from the umbilicus. Palpate the uterus gently only until it is firm; overstimulation causes uterine muscle fatigue and results in atonia (relaxation).

The uterus can contract only if it is free of intra-uterine clots. Take care to avoid inversion of the uterus during expulsion of clots. To expel clots, place the hands as shown in Fig. 27.8, supporting the uterus from below with one hand. With the upper hand, apply firm pressure downward toward the vagina while observing the perineum for the number and size of expelled clots. While performing these assessments, teach the patient the rationale for the assessment and how to maintain uterine tone with self-palpation.

Powers

Involuntary and voluntary contractions combine to aid the fetus in movement through the birth canal and expulsion from the mother. They are also responsible for delivery of the placenta. Involuntary uterine contractions, called primary powers, signal the beginning of labor. Once the cervix has dilated, the woman's voluntary bearing-down efforts, called secondary powers, augment the force of the involuntary contractions.

A

B

Fig. 27.7 Third stage of labor – Steps of placental delivery. *(A)* Placenta begins to separate in central portion accompanied by retroplacental bleeding. Uterus changes from discoid to globular shape. *(B)* Placenta completes separation and enters lower uterine segment. Uterus is globular shaped. *(C)* Placenta enters vagina, cord is seen to lengthen, and bleeding may increase. *(D)* Expulsion (delivery) of placenta and completion of third stage. (B) The placenta after delivery.

Fig. 27.8 Palpating fundus of uterus during first hour after delivery.

0%   50%   100%

Fig. 27.9 Cervical effacement.

Primary powers. The involuntary contractions originate at certain pacemaker points in the thickened muscle layers of the upper uterine segment. From the pacemaker points, contractions move downward over the uterus in waves, separated by short rest periods.

The primary powers are responsible for the effacement and dilation of the cervix and the descent of the fetus. Effacement is the shortening and thinning of the cervix during the first stage of labor. The cervix, normally 2 to 3 cm long and about 1 cm thick, is obliterated or "taken up" by shortening of the uterine muscle bundles in advancing labor. Only a thin edge of the cervix can be palpated when effacement is complete. In a first pregnancy, effacement generally occurs at term before significant dilation occurs. In subsequent pregnancies, effacement and dilation of the cervix tend to progress together. Degree of

effacement is expressed in percentages from 0% to 100% (e.g., a cervix 50% effaced) (Fig. 27.9).

Dilation of the cervix is the enlargement of the cervical opening and the cervical canal that occurs once labor has begun. The diameter of the cervix increases from less than 1 cm to approximately 10 cm (full dilation) to allow birth of a term fetus. When the cervix is dilated fully (and completely retracted), it can no longer be palpated. Full cervical dilation marks the end of the first stage of labor.

Dilation of the cervix occurs with the drawing upward of the musculofibrous components of the cervix as a result of strong uterine contractions. Pressure from the amniotic fluid while the membranes are intact and the force applied by the presenting part also promote cervical dilation. Scarring of the cervix from prior infection or surgery may slow cervical dilation.

In the first and second stages of labor, increased intrauterine pressure caused by contractions places pressure on the descending fetus and the cervix. When the presenting part of the fetus reaches the perineal floor, mechanical stretching of the cervix occurs. Stretch receptors in the posterior vagina cause release of exogenous oxytocin, which triggers the maternal urge to bear down, or Ferguson's reflex.

Uterine contractions are involuntary and usually independent from external forces. For example, laboring women who are paraplegic have normal uterine contractions. Uterine contractions may temporarily become less frequent and intense when the woman receives narcotic analgesic medication or epidural analgesia early in labor. The relationship between prolonged labor and epidural analgesia is still under investigation.

Secondary powers. As soon as the presenting part reaches the pelvic floor, the contractions change in character and become expulsive. The woman experiences an involuntary urge to push. She uses secondary powers (bearing-down efforts) as she contracts her diaphragm and abdominal muscles and pushes. These bearing-down efforts result in increased intraabdominal pressure that compresses the uterus on all sides and strengthens the expulsive forces.

The secondary powers have no effect on cervical dilation, but they are important in expelling the infant from the uterus and vagina after the cervix is dilated fully. Pushing in the second stage is more effective, and the woman is less fatigued when she begins to push only after she has the urge to do so, rather than when she is fully dilated but does not yet have the urge to push. The woman should not push before complete dilation. This can result in swelling or tearing of the cervix and ultimately may slow the birthing process.

The way a woman pushes in the second stage is much debated. Spontaneous bearing-down efforts, Valsalva's maneuver (closed glottis and prolonged bearing down), pushing, open glottis pushing, "mini" pushing, and forced methods of pushing have been investigated. Although no significant differences in length of second-stage labor have been found among these methods, fetal hypoxia and acidosis are associated with directed pushing. Continued study is needed to determine the effectiveness and safety of various pushing techniques in relation to maternal and fetal outcomes.

Position of the Woman in Labor

Maternal position affects the woman's anatomic and physiologic adaptations to labor. Frequent changes in position relieve fatigue, increase comfort, and improve circulation. Encourage a woman in labor to find the positions that are most comfortable for her (Fig. 27.10).

An upright position (e.g., walking, sitting, kneeling, or squatting) offers many advantages. Gravity can promote the descent of the fetus. Uterine contractions are generally stronger and more efficient in effacing and dilating the cervix, which results in shorter labor. An upright position is also beneficial for the mother's cardiac output, which normally increases during labor as uterine contractions return blood to the vascular bed. Increased cardiac output improves blood flow to the uteroplacental unit and the maternal kidneys. An upright position also helps reduce pressure on the descending aorta and ascending vena cava and prevents their compression. Compression of these vessels can compromise cardiac output and lead to supine hypotension and decreased placental perfusion. If the woman wishes to lie down, a lateral position is suggested.

The "all fours" position (on hands and knees) may be used to relieve backache if the fetus is in an occipitoposterior position. It also may assist in anterior rotation of the fetus.

The woman's preference may determine positioning for second-stage labor, but the decision is also affected by the condition of the woman or fetus, the environment, and the health care provider's confidence in assisting a birth in a specific position. For physician-attended births in the United States, the lithotomy position is predominant. Alternative positions and position changes are practiced most commonly by nurse-midwives.

A woman in a semirecumbent position needs adequate body support to push effectively because her weight is on her sacrum, which moves the coccyx forward and causes a reduction in the pelvic outlet. In a sitting or squatting position, abdominal muscles work in greater synchrony with uterine contractions during bearing-down effort. Kneeling or squatting moves the uterus forward, straightens the long axis of the birth canal, and can facilitate the second stage of labor by increasing the pelvic outlet.

Women can use the lateral position to help rotate a fetus that is in a posterior position. This position also may be used when less force is needed during bearing down, such as when the woman needs to control the speed of a precipitous birth.

In addition to position changes, the use of birthing devices such as the birthing ball are helpful. These balls are similar to devices used in workouts but are larger. Made of rubber or PVC materials, they are strong and not subject to puncture. The balls allow the laboring woman to site astride and engage in gentle rocking movements. Engaging with the ball in this manner allows the woman to achieve levels of comfort in her hips, back, and perineal regions. Proponents of the birthing ball believe that it promotes dilation as the woman sits and gently rocks. Women experiencing posterior positions which are associated with "back labor" report it is beneficial.

No evidence shows that any of these positions for second-stage labor increases the need for operative techniques (e.g., forceps- or vacuum-assisted birth, cesarean birth, and episiotomy) or causes perineal trauma. Also, no evidence shows that use of any of these positions adversely affects the newborn.

Psyche

The fifth "*P*" involves the psyche, or psychological response, which is a crucial part of childbirth. Anxiety, fear, and fatigue decrease the woman's ability to cope with pain and the stressors of childbirth. Provision of information and support to the mother and her partner is imperative to her success.

MECHANISMS OF LABOR

As the fetus moves through the maternal pelvis, several maneuvers are necessary. These turns and adjustments are called the cardinal movements of labor. The mechanisms of labor in the vertex position are as follows.

Hands and knees

Sitting/leaning

Tailor sitting

Semirecumbent

Walking

Standing

Squatting

Kneeling and leaning forward with support

A

Lithotomy

Lateral recumbent

Semirecumbent

Squatting

B

Fig. 27.10 (A) Positions for labor. (B) Positions for birth.

Engagement occurs when the biparietal diameter of the fetal head crosses the pelvic inlet; the head is said to be fixed or engaged in the pelvis. In nulliparous women, this tends to occur early, often several days or weeks before labor begins. Multiparous women may not experience engagement until labor has started.

Descent is the downward progress of the presenting part. The amount of progress is measured by comparing the lowest point of the presenting part with the ischial spines. This is referred to as the *station* and is measured in centimeters above or below the level of the spines. For example, if the presenting part is even with the ischial spines, the station is 0; if the presenting part is 2 cm above the spines, the station is −2; if the presenting part is 2 cm below the ischial spines, the station is +2 (Fig. 27.11).

Internal rotation enables the fetal head to progress through the maternal pelvis. The largest diameter of the fetal head aligns with the largest diameter of the pelvis.

Extension occurs when the occiput passes under the symphysis pubis. This bony structure acts as a stable point and provides leverage, which enables the head to leave the pelvis. The actual delivery of the head is done by extension. As soon as the head is delivered, it moves to realign with the body and shoulders, referred to as **restitution** (Fig. 27.12).

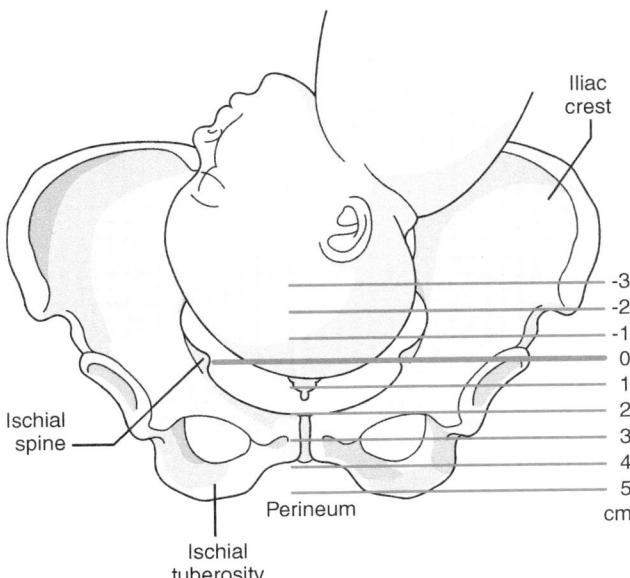

Fig. 27.11 Stations of presenting part, or degree of engagement. The station represents the location of the presenting part in relation to the level of ischial spines and indicates degree of advancement of the presenting part through the pelvis. Stations are expressed in centimeters above (minus) and below (plus) the level of the ischial spines.

External rotation occurs as the shoulders and body move through the birth canal, with the same maneuvers as the head. The shoulders are delivered similarly to the head, with the anterior shoulder pressing under the symphysis pubis, which again acts as a leverage point and assists in delivering the posterior shoulder. After the shoulders are delivered, the delivery ends with **expulsion**, in which the body of the infant leaves the pelvis. Delivery of the body occurs rapidly once the shoulders have been delivered (Fig. 27.13).

STAGES OF LABOR AND DELIVERY

First Stage: Dilation
The first stage begins with the onset of regular contractions and ends with complete dilation of the cervix (Fig. 27.14). This stage is generally the longest stage of labor; it averages 10 to 12 hours in nulliparas and 6 to 8 hours in multiparas. This stage often is divided into the following three phases:

1. *Latent phase* (0 to 3 cm dilation): Contractions occur 5 to 8 minutes apart and last 20 to 35 seconds. Dilation at this point is about the size of a penny. The woman generally is alert and talkative. The nulliparous woman may feel anxious about childbirth. This phase is ideal for teaching and establishing rapport. The nurse or a significant other may be the coach, reviewing techniques learned in prenatal classes. Pain tends to be mild and easily controlled. Backache is common. Many women, particularly multiparas, prefer to remain home during this stage. If the bag of waters has not ruptured, many women walk during this stage. Women should be advised that if the membranes rupture, they should seek care to be evaluated.

Fig. 27.12 Normal vaginal birth. (A) Anteroposterior slit. Vertex visible during contraction. (B) Oval opening. Vertex presenting. (C) Crowning. (D) Nurse-midwife using the Ritgen maneuver as head is born via extension. (E) After nurse-midwife checks for nuchal cord, she supports the head during external rotation and restitution.

Continued

Fig. 27.12, cont'd (F) Note the use of bulb syringe to suction mucus. (G) Birth of posterior shoulder. (H) Birth of newborn via slow expulsion. (I and J) Second stage complete. Note that newborn is not completely pink yet. (K) Note increased bleeding as placenta separates. (L) Expulsion of placenta. (M), Expulsion is complete, marking the end of the third stage. (N) Newborn awaiting assessment. Note that color is almost completely pink. (O) Newborn assessment under radiant warmer. (P) Parents admiring their newborn. (Courtesy Michael S. Clement in Lowdermilk DL, Perry SE, Cashion K, et al: *Maternity and women's health care*, ed 10, St. Louis, 2012, Mosby.)

Fig. 27.13 Cardinal movements of labor in left occipitoanterior (LOA) presentation. (A) Engagement and descent. (B) Flexion. (C) Internal rotation to OA. (D) Extension. € Restitution. (F) External rotation.

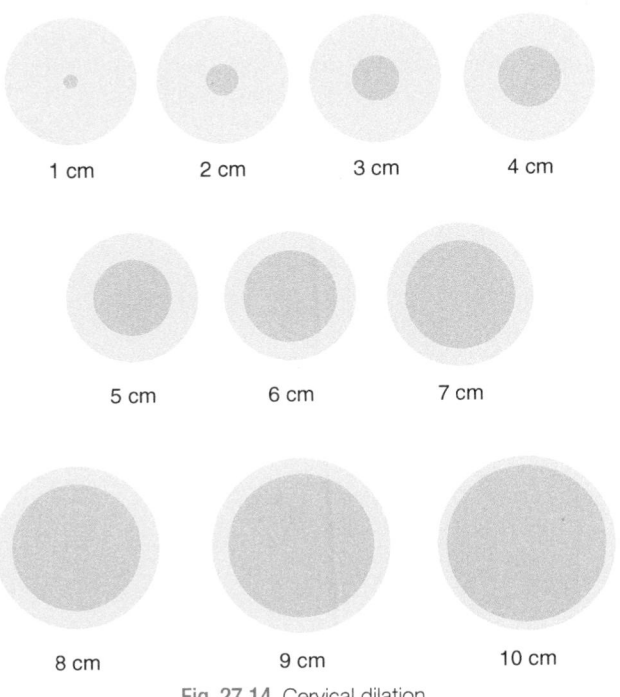

Fig. 27.14 Cervical dilation.

2. *Active phase* (4 to 7 cm dilation): Contractions occur at 3- to 5-minute intervals and last 40 to 60 seconds. The woman becomes less talkative and focuses on breathing techniques learned during prenatal classes. During this period, the woman may worry that she will not be capable of achieving the birth experience she may have imagined. If she has not learned breathing techniques already, teach them to her during labor. The intensity of the pain increases but still may be manageable without medication.

3. *Transitional phase* (8 to 10 cm dilation): Contractions occur at 2- to 3-minute intervals and last up to 90 seconds. The woman is focused deeply and may not wish to communicate with the nurse or significant other. She may be irritated easily by distractions. If the woman has not requested pain medication earlier, she may desire it at this time. Nausea is common.

Second Stage: Delivery of the Fetus

The second stage of labor begins with complete dilation at 10 cm and ends with the birth of the baby. This stage lasts an average of 30 minutes to 2 hours in nulliparas and 20 minutes to 90 minutes in multiparas. Contractions continue to last 80 to 90 seconds or slightly shorter.

Once the cervix is completely dilated, the woman usually feels the urge to push and is anxious to do so. Pushing is hard work, and the woman needs ongoing encouragement from the coach and the nurse. Resting between contractions, if possible, is important to conserve energy.

During this stage, the primary care practitioner may provide anesthesia and perform an episiotomy.

The **episiotomy** is a surgical incision of the perineum performed at the end of the second stage of labor (see Fig. 27.15). Episiotomies were once considered almost standard in vaginal births. The goal of the procedure was to reduce bleeding, minimize tearing, and aid in the prevention of future bowel and bladder complications. Episiotomy use soared in the 1970s with an incidence rate over 60%. In 2006, The American Academy of Obstetricians and Gynecologists recommended against the use of "routine" episiotomies. In the years that followed, their use declined. By 2012, episiotomy use was just below 12%. The change in the use of the procedure has been tied to research demonstrating that the complications it was used to prevent were not associated significantly with vaginal births. Today, the incision is used for the delivery of macrosomic infants, in rapid deliveries, to aid in the management of shoulder dystocia, to facilitate delivery when the fetal heart rates (FHRs) indicate immediate delivery is warranted, and abnormal presentations.

The most common type of episiotomy is a midline, or median, incision that separates the tissues of the perineum at an anatomic junction. Advantages of the midline episiotomy include greater ease in completing the procedure, speed of healing, and comfort over the mediolateral incision. Unfortunately, this type does have a higher risk for further extension and tearing. If the perineum is too small or the fetus is anticipated to be large, a mediolateral incision, which involves cutting the muscle, is performed. This is generally more uncomfortable and is done only when necessary. Complications of an episiotomy include infection, blood loss, pain, and painful sexual intercourse.

Immediately after delivery, the baby's airway is established (see the section "Response of the Newborn to Birth") and the umbilical cord is clamped with two clamps and then severed between the two. If there are no complications, show the baby to the parents. Then either give the infant to the mother to hold or position the infant in a warming unit that allows for close observation and care. If any problems occur with the infant, administer care immediately. This emergency care may have to be performed in the delivery area. Remain calm and supportive to the parents. Be aware that the parents may be alarmed and need support and explanations to allay their fears for the newborn.

Third Stage: Delivery of the Placenta

The third stage begins with the delivery of the infant and ends with the delivery of the placenta. The average for primiparas and multiparas is 5 to 20 minutes.

When the placenta detaches from the uterine wall, blood suddenly pours out of the vagina. The cord protruding from the vagina lengthens, and the uterus becomes firmer and more rounded. The woman may again experience contractions. The size and consistency of the placenta usually permit delivery with one or two pushes. During this time, the primary care practitioner repairs the episiotomy if one was performed. Women who do not have an episiotomy will still often have lacerations or tears that occur during the birth process. These soft tissue injuries will need to be repaired. Those stitches will absorb and not require removal. They will be checked closely during the postpartum period (see Fig. 27.16). Total blood loss is normally 200 to 300 mL; more than 500 mL of blood lost during delivery is considered excessive. An oxytocic medication, such as oxytocin (Pitocin) or methylergonovine maleate (Methergine), is administered commonly during this stage (Table 27.3). An *oxytocic* (**oxytocin** is a hormone produced by the pituitary gland) is a drug that stimulates uterine contractions and works to prevent postdelivery hemorrhage. These medications cause the uterus to contract firmly, compressing blood vessels inside the uterus and keeping blood loss to a minimum.

Fig 27.16 Repair of perineal/vaginal tears and lacerations.

Mediolateral

Median
(or midline)

Fig. 27.15 Types of episiotomies.

Table **27.3**   **Medications for Normal Labor and Delivery**

GENERIC NAME (BRAND NAME)	ACTION	SIDE EFFECTS	NURSING IMPLICATIONS
butorphanol	Synthetic, centrally acting analgesic; provides relief of moderate to severe pain during labor	Drowsiness, sedation, headache, vertigo, dizziness, weakness, confusion, insomnia, nervousness, respiratory depression, change in blood pressure, palpitations, bradycardia, nausea, clammy skin, tingling, flushing and warmth, diaphoresis, skin rash, pruritus, increased urinary output Neonatal: respiratory depression, disorganized infant behavior, tendency for frequent crying	Monitor for respiratory depression; do not give if respiratory rate is <15 breaths/min; monitor vital signs; observe neonate for respiratory depression; observe safety precautions because of sedation and dizziness.
carboprost tromethamine (Hemabate)	Produces strong, prompt contractions of uterine smooth muscle; used in postpartum hemorrhage from uterine atony not managed with conventional methods	Headache, anxiety, weakness, arrhythmias, eye pain, nausea, vomiting, uterine rupture, backache, leg cramps, wheezing, fever, chills	It is used only by trained personnel in a hospital setting and may be injected into the uterus.
fentanyl citrate (Sublimaze): epidural	Binds with opiate receptors in the central nervous system, altering perception of and emotional response to pain through an unknown mechanism	Sedation, euphoria, vertigo, headache, confusion, anxiety, depression, seizures, blood pressure deviations, nausea, vomiting, respiratory depression	It is used occasionally. Monitor circulatory and respiratory status and urinary function. Monitor arterial oxygen saturation.
hydroxyzine (Vistaril)	Antianxiety antepartum and postpartum adjunctive therapy	Drowsiness, dry mouth, marked discomfort at IM injection site	It is used less frequently. Aspirate IM injection carefully to prevent inadvertent IV injection. Inject deeply into a large muscle mass. Observe for sedation.
magnesium sulfate	Decreases acetylcholine in motor nerve terminals, which is responsible for seizure prevention in preeclampsia and eclampsia	Diarrhea; side effects are related to magnesium levels: with >3 mg/dL, depressed central nervous system, blocked neuromuscular transmission that leads to anticonvulsant effects; with >5 mg/dL, depressed deep tendon reflexes; with >12.5 mg/dL, respiratory paralysis	Obtain vital signs q 15 min after IV dose; do not exceed 150 mg/min; monitor cardiac function; time contractions and monitor fetal heart rate; monitor intake and output (should remain ≥30 mL/h). When given in close proximity to delivery may contribute to uterine atony. Monitor maternal lochia.
meperidine (Demerol)	Synthetic morphine-like compound that produces comparable analgesic effects and provides relief of moderate to severe pain	Pruritus, dizziness, sedation, weakness, euphoria, respiratory depression, hypotension, palpitations, bradycardia or tachycardia, dry mouth, nausea, constipation, oliguria, urinary retention Neonatal: respiratory depression	It is used less and less frequently. Monitor vital signs closely, especially respiratory rate, depth, and rhythm; encourage deep breathing and coughing to overcome respiratory depressant effects; assess patient's need for medication as needed; give IM or IV as ordered in smallest effective dose.
methylergonovine maleate (Methergine)	Stimulates uterine contraction, decreases bleeding	Headache, dizziness, nausea, vomiting, chest pain, palpitations, hypertension, tinnitus, sweating, rash	Monitor blood pressure, pulse, character, and amount of vaginal bleeding; monitor respiratory rate; give IM in deep muscle mass and IV only in emergency.

Continued

Table 27.3   Medications for Normal Labor and Delivery—cont'd

GENERIC NAME (BRAND NAME)	ACTION	SIDE EFFECTS	NURSING IMPLICATIONS
misoprostol (synthetic prostaglandin E; Cytotec)	Used most widely to prevent nonsteroidal anti-inflammatory drug–induced gastric ulcer in patients at high risk	Headache, nausea, dyspepsia, vomiting, constipation, flatulence	Some physicians use it to induce labor, especially in the event of fetal death, administered vaginally in the posterior fornix. It is easier on the mother because labor and delivery can be over in as little as 45 min. To induce labor when fetal death has not occurred, administered vaginally into the posterior fornix.
nalbuphine hydrochloride	Binds with opiate receptors in the central nervous system, altering perception of and emotional response to pain through an unknown mechanism	Headache, sedation, vertigo, syncope, restlessness, crying, confusion, blood pressure variations, bradycardia, blurred vision, nausea and vomiting, urinary urgency, respiratory depression, asthma; Neonatal: disorganized infant behavior, fussiness, refusal to nurse	Usually administer one or two doses and then begin an epidural. Monitor circulatory and respiratory status and bladder and bowel function; withhold dose and notify physician if respirations become shallow or fall below 12 breaths/min. Stool softeners may be ordered.
naloxone hydrochloride (Narcan)	Thought to displace previously administered narcotic-opioid analgesics from their receptors (competitive antagonism); indicated for use in known or suspected narcotic-induced respiratory depression in neonates (asphyxia neonatorum)	Tremors, seizures, blood pressure variations, nausea, vomiting; Can cause seizure when used with street drugs (of which the health care worker is sometimes unaware)	It is not used as often as it once was. Respiratory rate increases within 1–2 min. Monitor respiratory depth and rate. Be prepared to provide oxygen, ventilation, and other resuscitation measures. Administer IV into umbilical vein. May be repeated q 2–3 min.
oxytocin (Pitocin)	Acts directly on myofibrils, producing uterine contractions; stimulates milk ejection by breasts	Anaphylaxis, postpartum hemorrhage, cardiac arrhythmias, nausea, vomiting, premature ventricular contractions, hypertension, convulsions; Fetal: bradycardia, arrhythmias, jaundice, hypoxia, intracranial hemorrhage	Monitor intake and output ratio, contractions, fetal heart rate, blood pressure, pulse, and respirations.
promethazine hydrochloride	Prevents but does not reverse histamine-mediated responses; at high dosage, exhibits local anesthetic effects; used as adjunct to analgesics	Sedation, blood pressure deviations, blurred vision, nausea, vomiting, urine retention, seizures	It is used most of the time for postoperative cesarean delivery. Inject deep into large muscle mass. Often used as an adjunct to analgesics. It may be mixed with meperidine in the same syringe.
prostaglandin E (dinoprostone [Prepidil, Cervidil])	Stimulates uterine contractions like those seen in normal labor	Uterine contractile abnormalities, nausea, vomiting, diarrhea, back pain, warm feeling in vagina, fever; Fetal: heart rate abnormalities, bradycardia	Use caution to prevent contact with skin; wash thoroughly after administration; bring to room temperature before administering; do not force warming process; have patient remain supine for 15–30 min after insertion.
ritodrine hydrochloride	Uterine beta$_2$-adrenergic receptor–stimulating effect, which reduces uterine contractions	Erythema, rash, dyspnea, hyperglycemia, headache, restlessness, anxiety, chills, tremor, nausea, vomiting, diarrhea, constipation, altered maternal and fetal heart rates	It is used less and less frequently. Monitor maternal and fetal heart tones during infusion; watch intensity and length of uterine contractions; monitor fluid intake to prevent overload; monitor blood glucose level in patients with diabetes.

IM, Intramuscularly, intramuscular; *IV,* intravenously, intravenous.

Box 27.2   **Changes in Fetal Health Rate**

NORMAL BASELINE RATE
- 120–160 bpm

TACHYCARDIA
- Moderate increase to 160–180 bpm
- Marked increase greater than 180 bpm; significant if variability is absent and late or variable decelerations (decreases in the speed or velocity of an object or reaction) are present

CAUSES
Maternal thyroid disease
Maternal fever
Maternal dehydration
Early fetal hypoxia
Maternal anemia
Fetal anemia
Fetal prematurity
Nursing Interventions[a]
- Interventions depend on the cause.
- Reduce maternal fever with cooling measures and antipyretics as ordered.
- Oxygen at 8–10 L/min per face mask may be of some value.
- Carry out health care provider's orders to alleviate cause.

BRADYCARDIA
- Moderate decrease to 100–120 bpm
- Marked decrease to fewer than 100 bpm; significant if variability is decreased or absent or if late or variable decelerations are present

CAUSES
Maternal hypotension
Prolonged fetal hypoxia
Maternal narcotic use
Placental abruption
Uterine hyperstimulation

Nursing Interventions[a]
- Interventions depend on the cause.
- Intervention is not warranted in fetus with heart block diagnosed with electrocardiogram.
- Oxygen at 8–10 L/min per face mask may be of some value.
- Carry out health care provider's orders to alleviate cause.
- Scalp stimulation may be performed to determine whether the fetus is able to compensate physiologically for stress (fetal heart rate [FHR] accelerates).

VARIABILITY
- Measures the normal fluctuation of the FHR from the baseline.
- Absent or minimal variability possibly indicative of fetal distress.
- Variability classified as long-term variability (LTV) or short-term variability (STV).

DECELERATIONS
- Periodic decreases in the FHR in response to contractions; classified as early, late, or variable (Fig. 27.16).
- Early decelerations: caused by pressure on fetal skull; tend to be uniform; onset, shape, and recovery correspond to contractions.
- Late decelerations: caused by decreased oxygen and blood flow to fetus through the placenta; noted at or after the peak of the contraction; may indicate fetal distress, particularly if associated with changes in baseline FHR and absence of variability.
- Variable decelerations: caused by compression on the umbilical cord; occur randomly and onset may be sudden; FHR decreases below normal range.

Nursing Interventions[a]
- Notify the primary caregiver immediately and initiate appropriate treatment when patient has a prolonged deceleration.

[a]See Box 27.3 for care of the woman being monitored electronically for fetal status during labor.

Fourth Stage: Stabilization

The time immediately after delivery is critical as the mother's body attempts to recover from the efforts of labor. Usually, the mother is monitored closely for 2 to 4 hours after delivery in the birthing room or in a recovery room. Some women, particularly those who have had a long or difficult labor and delivery, are exhausted and wish only to rest. Others seem euphoric and wish to talk about the experience or spend time with the baby and their significant other.

Monitor physiologic changes closely during the fourth stage. Assess vital signs, uterine tone, vaginal drainage, and the perineal tissue. During the first hour, perform assessments every 15 minutes. If observations are within normal limits, assessments are done every 30 minutes for the next hour. If all observations remain normal, the woman is transferred to a patient room for the remainder of her hospitalization (unless she is in a birthing center or in a facility that has an LDRP room configuration, where she may remain until discharge).

MONITORING FETAL STATUS

The process of labor is stressful to the fetus, and continuous monitoring of the fetus is important during this time. FHR is a good indicator of the fetus's condition. The normal FHR range is 120 to 160 bpm. An increase or decrease of 30 bpm may indicate fetal distress and should be reported immediately (Box 27.2).

Auscultate the FHR with a fetoscope or a Doppler instrument every 15 to 30 minutes during the first stage of labor and every 5 minutes during the second stage. Also assess the FHR immediately after rupture of the membranes, particularly if the head is not engaged (i.e., not firmly settled into the pelvis).

Electronic Fetal Monitoring

Frequently, continuous electronic monitors, either internal or external, are applied for electronic fetal monitoring (EFM). Monitors can detect subtle changes of condition before they can be recognized with auscultation. The external, or indirect, mode uses external transducers on the maternal abdominal wall to assess FHR and uterine activity. An ultrasound transducer uses high-frequency sound waves to reflect movement of the fetal heart ventricles. A tocotransducer monitors uterine activity and records frequency and duration of contractions. A strip chart prints out FHR (upper part of the strip) and uterine activity (lower part of the strip) (Fig. 27.18A). External monitoring can be used in the antepartal and intrapartal periods. It does not require rupture of membranes or cervical dilation; however, the tocotransducer cannot assess the intensity of contractions (see Fig. 27.17). Maternal position can affect the accuracy of the recordings.

Internal monitoring uses a spiral electrode applied to the presenting part to monitor the FHR (Fig. 27.19). An intrauterine catheter is used to monitor frequency, duration, intensity, and resting tone of uterine contractions. This catheter is compressed during contractions, which places pressure on a strain gauge or pressure transducer. FHR and uterine pressure are reflected on a strip chart (see Fig. 27.18B). Internal monitoring can be used only during the intrapartal period, because membranes must be ruptured and the cervix dilated 2 to 3 cm. Display of FHR and uterine activity is accurate regardless of maternal position. Box 27.3 lists guidelines for care of the woman being monitored electronically for fetal status during labor.

FHR is monitored in relation to the contractions. A decrease in FHR occurs in response to the contractions and is called a *deceleration.* Decelerations can be early, late, or variable (Fig. 27.20 and see Box 27.2).

In the United States, electronic monitoring is used routinely for both low-risk and high-risk labor.

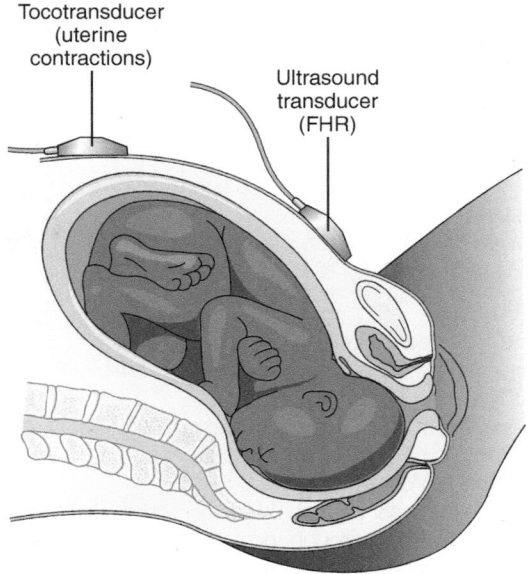

Fig. 27.17 Diagram of external noninvasive fetal monitoring with tocotransducer and ultrasound transducer, with ultrasound transducer placed below umbilicus and tocotransducer placed on uterine fundus position. *FHR,* Fetal heart rate.

Fig. 27.18 Display of fetal heart rate *(FHR)* and uterine activity *(UA)* on chart paper. (A) External mode with ultrasound transducer and tocotransducer as signal sources. (B) Internal mode with spiral electrode and intrauterine catheter as signal sources.

Fig. 27.19 Diagram of internal invasive fetal monitoring with intrauterine catheter and spiral electrode in place (membranes ruptured and cervix dilated). *FHR,* Fetal heart rate.

Fetal Distress

Fetal distress from hypoxia (insufficient availability of oxygen to meet metabolic needs) is indicated with nonreassuring FHR patterns. These patterns can include a progressive increase or decrease in the baseline FHR, progressive decrease in baseline variability, tachycardia (more than 160 bpm), severe bradycardia (less than 100 bpm), persistent late decelerations, and severe variable decelerations with slow return to baseline. Another indication of fetal distress is greenish-stained amniotic fluid in a cephalic presentation. The color is a result of meconium (the infant's first stool, a viscid, sticky, dark greenish-brown (almost black), sterile, odorless stool) being released from the fetal rectum in response to hypoxia (which increases intestinal activity and relaxes the anal sphincter). This color is referred to often as *meconium staining.* Table 27.4 describes characteristics of amniotic fluid.

Nurses who care for women during childbirth are legally responsible for correctly interpreting the FHR pattern, indicating appropriate nursing interventions based on that pattern, and documenting the outcome of those interventions. Notify the primary caregiver in a timely manner if an abnormal FHR pattern is detected. Initiate the institutional chain of command if health care providers disagree on the interpretation of the FHR pattern and the intervention necessitated.

RESPONSE OF THE NEWBORN TO BIRTH

The process of delivery is stressful to the newborn. Rapid adaptation from the intrauterine climate to that of extrauterine life is essential if the newborn is to survive.

The infant's physical condition is evaluated at birth. Most facilities use an evaluation guide called the *Apgar score* (Table 27.5). This scoring is done at 1 and 5 minutes of age. The score can range from 0 to 10, with 8 to 10 considered optimal. The criteria used include heart rate, respiratory effort, muscle tone, reflex irritability, and skin color. A low score indicates serious problems that may necessitate resuscitation. A high score indicates good condition, necessitating only routine care.

In utero, the fetus's need for oxygen was met by the mother. Once the umbilical cord is severed, the newborn must breathe to obtain oxygen. Fetal lungs must be mature enough that the alveoli can expand adequately. As the infant lungs begin to mature, they begin to produce increasing amounts of a substance called surfactant, which decreases surface tension within the alveoli and permits inflation. At the time of delivery, a combination of chemical, thermal, tactile, and mechanical changes initiates the first breath.

The airway must be cleared of fluids that are in the lungs. Some fluids are forced from the lungs as the thorax passes through the pelvis during delivery. Use a bulb syringe to remove excess fluid from the mouth and nasopharynx (Box 27.4). Positioning of the infant is also important (Fig. 27.21).

Warmth is necessary to prevent a rapid drop in body temperature. The environment in utero is approximately 99°F (37.2°C); the external environment in the delivery room is usually about 70°F (21.1°C). To prevent hypothermia, immediately dry the infant to help reduce heat loss from evaporation. Then place the baby in contact with the mother's skin, especially if she wishes to breastfeed, or transfer the baby to a radiant warming unit.

If no complications occur, the infant remains in the mother's view until her care is completed. Place identification bracelets on mother and baby before they leave the delivery room. In many institutions a bracelet is also worn by the baby's father or other person designated by the mother. These are used to verify infant identification and match it with that of the mother until discharge. Footprinting the infant is another method of identification; this may be done in the delivery area or in the nursery. Additional security devices that may be used by a birthing unit include microchips placed in the cord clamp or bracelets.

NURSING ASSESSMENT AND INTERVENTIONS

HEALTH PERCEPTION AND HEALTH MANAGEMENT

Find out what the woman has done to prepare for childbirth. The woman who has attended classes and practiced breathing techniques needs a different level of explanation and support than one who has had no preparation. If a hospital delivery is planned, admission generally is prearranged and much of the paperwork completed ahead of time to minimize delays. If

Box 27.3   Care of the Woman With Electronic Fetal Monitoring

The following guidelines relate to patient teaching and the functioning of the monitor.

- Explain that fetal status can be assessed continuously with electronic fetal monitoring (EFM), even during contractions.
- Explain that the lower tracing on the monitor strip paper shows uterine activity; the upper tracing shows the fetal heart rate (FHR).
- Reassure woman and partner that prepared childbirth techniques can be implemented without difficulty.
- Explain that during external monitoring, effleurage can be performed on sides of abdomen or upper portion of thighs.
- Explain that breathing patterns based on the time and the intensity of contractions can be enhanced by the observation of uterine activity on the monitor strip paper, which shows the onset of contractions.
- Note peak of contraction; knowledge that a contraction will not get stronger and is half over usually is helpful.
- Note diminishing intensity.
- Coordinate with appropriate breathing and relaxation techniques.
- Reassure woman and partner that the use of internal monitoring does not restrict movement, although she is confined to bed.[a]
- Explain that use of external monitoring usually requires the woman's cooperation during positioning and movement.
- Reassure woman and partner that use of monitoring does not imply fetal jeopardy.
- Reassure woman that the equipment is removed periodically to permit the applicator site to be washed and other care to be given.

EXTERNAL MONITORING
Ultrasound Transducer
Function
Monitors FHR with high-frequency sound waves.
Nursing Care
- Tap transducer before use to ensure sound transmission.
- Apply ultrasound transmission gel to transducer, clean abdomen and transducer, and reapply gel every 2 h and as needed.
- Massage reddened skin areas gently and reposition belt or adhesive device every 2 h and as needed.
- Auscultate FHR with stethoscope or fetoscope if in doubt as to validity or tracing.
- Position and reposition transducer as needed to ensure receipt of clean, interpretable FHR data.

Tocotransducer
Function
Monitors uterine activity via a pressure-sensing device placed on the maternal abdomen.
Nursing Care
- Position and reposition every 2 h and as needed on the fundus, the area of least maternal tissue.
- Keep abdominal strap snug but comfortable for the laboring woman.
- Adjust pen-set between contractions to print between 10 and 20 mm Hg on the monitor strip paper.
- Palpate fundus every 30–60 min to assess strength of contraction; only frequency and duration of contractions can be assessed with tocotransducer.
- Do not determine woman's need for analgesia based on uterine activity displayed on monitor strip.
- Gently massage reddened areas under transducer and belt every hour and as needed.

INTERNAL MONITORING
Spiral Electrode
Function
Obtains fetal electrocardiogram from presenting part and converts it into FHR.
Nursing Care
- Ensure that wires are appropriately attached to leg plate.
- Reapply electrode paste to leg plate if needed.
- Observe FHR tracing on monitor strip for variability.
- Turn electrode counterclockwise to remove; never pull straight out from presenting part.
- Administer perineal care after the woman voids during labor and as needed.

Intrauterine Catheter
Function
Catheter (solid- or fluid-filled) that monitors intraamniotic pressure internally.
Nursing Care
- Flush open system catheter with sterile water before insertion and as needed.
- Ensure that the length line on catheter is visible at introitus.
- For closed-system catheters, turn off stopcock to woman; then, with pressure valve of strain gauge released, flush strain gauge, remove syringe, and set stylus to 0 line of chart paper; test further according to manufacturer's instructions every 3–4 h and as needed.
- Check proper functioning by tapping catheter, asking woman to cough, or applying fundal pressure; observe appropriate inflection on strip chart.
- Keep catheter taped to woman's leg to prevent dislodgement.

[a]Portable telemetry monitors allow the FHR and uterine contraction patterns to be observed on centrally located electronic display stations. These portable units pvermit ambulation during electronic monitoring.

---

home delivery is anticipated, the primary care practitioner gives instructions to the family.

When hospitalization is anticipated, it is a good idea for the prospective parents to prepare a suitcase with necessary items well in advance of the date of delivery. A trial run to the hospital also can reduce fears of not getting to the hospital on time. If children are at home, parents should make plans for their care. Advise the

parents-to-be to anticipate as many problems as possible and make several alternate plans. On admission, begin the assessment (Box 27.5).

NUTRITIONAL AND METABOLIC PATTERN

Gastrointestinal motility and absorption decrease during labor and delivery. Food eaten before labor may remain in the digestive tract and lead to symptoms of

Fig. 27.20 Summary of periodic changes. *FHR*, Fetal heart rate.

nausea and vomiting. Once active labor begins, solid foods generally are withheld. Find out when food was consumed last in case administration of a general anesthetic becomes necessary. In addition, assess fluid intake. Increased physical exertion and mouth breathing are common during labor. When these factors are combined with restricted oral intake, a fluid deficit may result. Some primary care practitioners allow small amounts of ice chips or clear beverages during labor. Orders for intravenous (IV) fluids, such as a 5% dextrose solution, to prevent fluid imbalance are common.

ELIMINATION

Depending on the amount of fluid intake, urinary output may be normal or decreased. Voiding every 2 hours is desirable. *A full bladder can interfere with the progress of labor.* When membranes are intact, use of the toilet is permitted. Once membranes are ruptured, the bedpan is preferred. If the presenting part is compressing the urethra, catheterization may be ordered.

Assess bowel elimination. Some women experience diarrhea with the onset of labor. Careful hygiene

Table 27.4   Assessment of Amniotic Fluid Characteristics

CHARACTERISTIC OF FLUID	NORMAL FINDING	DEVIATION FROM NORMAL FINDING	CAUSE OF DEVIATION FROM NORMAL
Color	Pale, straw-colored; may contain white flecks of vernix caseosa, lanugo, scalp hair	Pea green or brown fluid	Episodes of fetal distress resulting in hypoxia may cause the fetus to pass meconium, which will present into the amniotic fluid. A fetus in a breech presentation may pass meconium in the absence of distress because of abdominal wall pressure in the descent into the birth canal.
		Yellow-stained fluid	Fetal hypoxia ≥36 h before rupture of membranes; fetal hemolytic disease; intrauterine infection
		Port-wine color	Bleeding associated with premature separation of the placenta (abruptio placentae)
Viscosity and odor	Watery; no strong odor	Thick, cloudy, foul-smelling	Intrauterine infection Large amount of meconium makes fluid thick
Amount (normally varies with gestational age)	400 mL (20 weeks of gestation)	>2000 mL (32–36 weeks of gestation)	Hydramnios (excessive amount of amniotic fluid): associated with congenital anomalies of the fetus when fetus cannot drink or fluid is trapped in the body (e.g., fetal gastrointestinal obstruction or atresias); increased risk with maternal pregestational or gestational diabetes mellitus
	1000 mL (36–38 weeks of gestation)	<500 mL (32–36 weeks of gestation)	**Oligohydramnios** (a condition in which the volume of amniotic fluid is <300 mL in the third trimester): associated with incomplete or absent kidney; obstruction of urethra; fetus cannot secrete or excrete urine

Modified from Lowdermilk DL, Perry SE: *Maternity and women's health care,* ed 9, St. Louis, 2007, Mosby.

Table 27.5   Apgar Scoring Chart

SIGN	0 POINTS	1 POINT	2 POINTS
Heart rate	Absent	Slow, <100 bpm	>100 bpm
Respiratory effort	Absent	Slow, irregular	Good crying
Muscle tone	Flaccid, limp	Some flexion of extremities	Active motion
Reflex irritability	No response	Grimace	Vigorous cry, cough, or sneeze
Color[a]	Pale blue	Body pink, extremities blue	Completely pink

[a]Skin color or its absence may not be a reliable guide in nonwhite infants, although melanin (the pigment that gives color to the skin) is less apparent at birth than later.

technique is important to reduce the possibility of contamination. Enemas once were administered routinely to empty the colon and maximize space in the pelvic cavity; today they are given only when specifically ordered. *Enemas should not be given if vaginal bleeding or premature labor is present, if the presenting part is not engaged, or if the presentation is not vertex.* If membranes are ruptured, the enema should be expelled into a bedpan.

The urge to defecate during labor may indicate the start of the second stage. Before the woman attempts to have a bowel movement, inspect the perineum and assess dilation for progress of labor.

ACTIVITY AND EXERCISE

Encourage ambulation as long as the membranes have not ruptured. Ambulation also may be permitted if the membranes have ruptured and the presenting part is fully engaged. Walking provides distraction and tends to strengthen the effectiveness of labor. If ambulation becomes too uncomfortable, or if the mother has been given analgesics, she usually is advised to rest. Positioning becomes important; encourage the woman to assume the position most comfortable for her. Some women prefer sitting or semiseated positions. Low back pain is common. A side-lying position is frequently more comfortable than a supine position. Changing

Box 27.4   Suctioning With a Bulb Syringe

- Suction the mouth first to prevent the infant from inhaling pharyngeal secretions by gasping as the nares are touched. This is necessary because the neonate is an obligatory nose breather.
- Compress the bulb (see illustration) and insert it into one side of the mouth. Avoid the center of the infant's mouth, which could stimulate the gag reflex.
- Suction the nasal passages one nostril at a time.
- When the infant's cry does not sound as though it is through mucus or a bubble, stop suctioning. The bulb syringe should be kept in an easily accessible place.
- Give the parents demonstrations on how to use the bulb syringe and ask them to perform a return demonstration.

Box 27.5   Admission Assessment

- *Review the prenatal record,* including general medical history, obstetric history, and history of the current pregnancy. This record should include information about allergies and any current health problems, such as respiratory tract or other types of infection.
- *Interview the patient* for signs and symptoms of the onset of labor, such as the nature and frequency of contractions, the level of discomfort, and the presence of vaginal discharge, such as bloody show or loss of amniotic fluid. If these data indicate that the woman is in labor, obtain information regarding the type of preparation for childbirth, support person present, special cultural practices or expectations, type of anesthesia planned, method of infant feeding desired, and name of pediatrician.
- *Perform the physical examination,* including a complete set of vital signs and fetal heart tones. These data function as a baseline for further assessment. Auscultate heart and lung sounds. Inspect the face, the hands, the legs, and the sacrum for signs of edema. Palpate the abdomen to determine the fetal lie and presentation. Assess the status of the membranes. If any question exists regarding ruptured membranes, perform a nitrazine test (see Box 27.1) before the vaginal examination because solutions used may make the test results unreliable. Time contractions to determine frequency, regularity, duration, and intensity. A vaginal examination is performed to determine the progress of labor, including position, dilation, effacement, and station.
- *Perform diagnostic tests,* including a urinalysis to check for glucose, protein, or ketones, which may indicate potential complications. If blood analyses were not performed during pregnancy, they should be done at this time. Information about hemoglobin and hematocrit levels, blood type and Rh factor, and antibody titer and screening for sexually transmitted infections help in assessment of actual or potential problems.

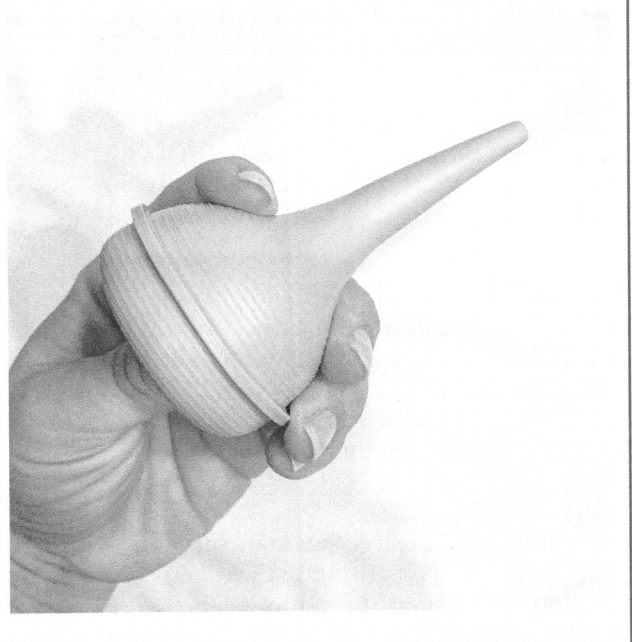

Fig. 27.21 Infant is turned to right side and supported in this position to facilitate drainage from the mouth and to promote emptying of stomach contents into the small intestine.

position may help reduce discomfort. If the patient is allowed to be up, a warm shower provides much relief for low back pain during labor. Side-lying positions reduce pressure on the vena cava. The left side is recommended if the FHR shows late deceleration or if the woman experiences hypotension (Fig. 27.22). If a prolapsed cord is suspected, special positioning is necessary (see Fig. 27.6).

VAGINAL EXAMINATION

Continue assessment of vaginal drainage throughout labor. If not observed sooner, bloody show may be seen. Moderate amounts of discharge are common; a linen change provides comfort. Report any bright red bleeding immediately.

Vaginal examination to assess the progress of labor continues through the first stage of labor. Monitor contractions for frequency, duration, and intensity.

Fig. 27.22 Supine hypotension. Note relationship of gravid uterus to ascending vena cava in standing posture (A) and in supine posture (B). (C) Compression of aorta and inferior vena cava with woman in supine position. (D) Relieved with use of a wedge pillow placed under woman's right side.

PSYCHOSOCIAL ASSESSMENT

Coping and Stress Tolerance

During labor and delivery, many women, particularly primigravidas, express fears. They may have unrealistic expectations and believe that they should be able to control their labor. Controlled breathing techniques help, but the involuntary nature of labor troubles many women. Encouragement and support in breathing exercises along with explanations regarding the progress of labor are helpful. Fatigue and pain lower the woman's ability to cope. Understanding the cultural and religious background of each woman is important, because these factors may strongly influence behavior.

Nursing observations also should include the mother's support team. The woman's partner may feel fear and anxiety. Questions should be answered in an effort to relieve concerns. At times, fathers express guilt about their role, either in not being able to help enough or in being responsible for the pregnancy. Tell the father that he is an important participant, not an unwanted guest, in the process of childbirth. Encourage him to help make the woman comfortable and provide the companionship and caring needed.

Roles and Relationships

Many women want their spouse or a significant other to be with them during labor and delivery. Most childbirth education programs include this individual in the preparation. Often this person works as the "coach" to remind the woman of breathing techniques and provide encouragement.

In some situations, however, the woman faces labor and delivery alone. This may be at her request, or it may be a matter of circumstances. If she is alone, the nursing staff must provide extra support. Many other individuals, such as grandparents, siblings, and extended family, may be interested in the progress of labor. Depending on the situation, try to pay attention to the needs of these family members.

Doulas

The term doula means "woman servant." The term today refers to the continuous presence of a trained, experienced woman throughout labor and delivery. Women who are cared for by a trained doula are less likely to require pain medication, receive Pitocin, or deliver via cesarean section. The birth experience reported by women laboring with a doula is more favorable than those women who do not have a doula (DONA International, n.d.). In addition, women often demonstrate increased maternal-infant bonding and ability to care for their new baby. The doula is trained in the care of the laboring family. Her role is to provide physical support using therapeutic touch, counterpressure, and assistance with breathing patterns. The doula provides emotional support to the laboring woman and her partner. It is not the role of the doula to administer medications or to insert herself into the dynamic that exists between the patient and her primary care provider. Doulas may be assigned upon arrival to a birthing center/hospital, or this relationship may be established early in the pregnancy. The financial model used to compensate the doula varies. Doulas may be employees of the birthing center/hospital, or they may be independently hired by the pregnant woman.

Father or Partner During Labor

The support partner during labor is usually the baby's father, although a family member or friend of any gender may perform this role. (This discussion refers to the partner as the father.) No matter who the support partner is, include that person in the circle of communication while caring for the woman in labor. They often can provide comfort measures and touch that the laboring woman needs. When the woman becomes focused on her pain, sometimes the father can persuade her to try nonpharmacologic variations of comfort measures. He usually can interpret her needs and desires to staff members. He may be focused and involved with the woman, or he may be more passive because of cultural norms or fear. Assess his level of comfort in asking questions and in being present and involved during the second-stage labor and birth. This helps determine what level of support to provide to the couple.

The father is exposed to many sights and smells that he may never have experienced before. Tell him what to expect and make him comfortable about leaving the room to gather his composure should something shock him. First, arrange for someone else to support the mother during his absence. Tell the father that his presence is helpful and encourage his involvement in the care of his partner to the extent of his comfort level. This is especially important when his partner has become angry and told him to go away. Reassure the father that this is normal behavior for a woman in transition and that if he reenters after a few minutes, the woman may ask him why he was gone so long.

When the father is active and supportive, the mother turns to him. The primary care practitioner remains the medical-surgical expert without taking on the significant other-surrogate role as well. The couple's future relationship and their relationship with the child may be influenced positively.

Supporting the father as well as the mother during labor elevates the nurse's role from custodial care to a therapeutic role. Support of the father reflects the nurse's commitment to the person, the family, and the community. Therapeutic nursing actions convey to the father several important concepts: (1) he is of value and competent as a person, (2) he can learn to be a partner in the mother's care, and (3) childbearing is a partnership. The nurse can support the father in various ways (Box 27.6). Fewer women had postdelivery emotional upsets when their partners received support and assistance from parent education classes, physicians, midwives, and nurses throughout the childbearing cycle.

Self-Perception

The prepared mother generally feels more able to deal with labor and delivery than the unprepared one. Multigravidas generally have more confidence because they have previous experience on which to draw. Women who have experienced problems during

---

Box 27.6   Supporting the Father

- Regardless of the degree of involvement desired, orient the father to the maternity unit, including the woman's labor room, the cafeteria, the waiting room, the nursery, and names and functions of personnel present.
- Respect decisions as to the father's degree of involvement, whether the decision is active participation in the delivery room or just information updates. When appropriate, provide information on which decisions can be based; offer choice as opposed to coercion. This is the parents' experience and baby.
- Let the father know when his presence has been helpful and continue to reinforce this throughout labor.
- Offer to teach the father comfort measures to the degree he wants to know them. Reassure him that he is not assuming the responsibility for observation and management of his partner's labor but supporting her as she progresses.
- Communicate with the father frequently regarding the mother's progress, procedures to be performed, what to expect from procedures, and what is expected of him.
- Prepare the father for changes in the mother's behavior and physical appearance.
- Remind the father to eat; offer snacks and fluids if possible.
- Relieve the father as necessary; offer blankets and a pillow if he is to sleep in a chair by the bedside. Acknowledge the stress of the situation on each partner and identify normal responses. The nonjudgmental attitudes of staff members help the father and the mother accept their own and the other person's behavior.
- Try to modify or eliminate unsettling stimuli (e.g., extra noise, extra light, chatter).

---

pregnancy or in past labors and deliveries may need reassurance that they can be successful. Even an unprepared woman can participate in simple breathing exercises with coaching from the nurse.

Women With a History of Sexual Abuse

Memories of sexual abuse can be triggered during labor with intrusive procedures, such as vaginal examination; loss of control; confinement to bed and "restraint" by monitors, IV lines, and epidurals; observation by students; and intense sensations in the uterus and genital area, especially while pushing the baby out. Women who are survivors of abuse may fight the labor process by reacting in panic or anger toward care providers, may take control of everyone and everything related to their childbirth, may surrender by being submissive and dependent, or may retreat by mentally dissociating themselves from the sensations of labor and birth.

Help these women associate the sensations they are experiencing with the process of childbirth and not their past abuse. Maintain the woman's sense of control by explaining all procedures and why they are needed,

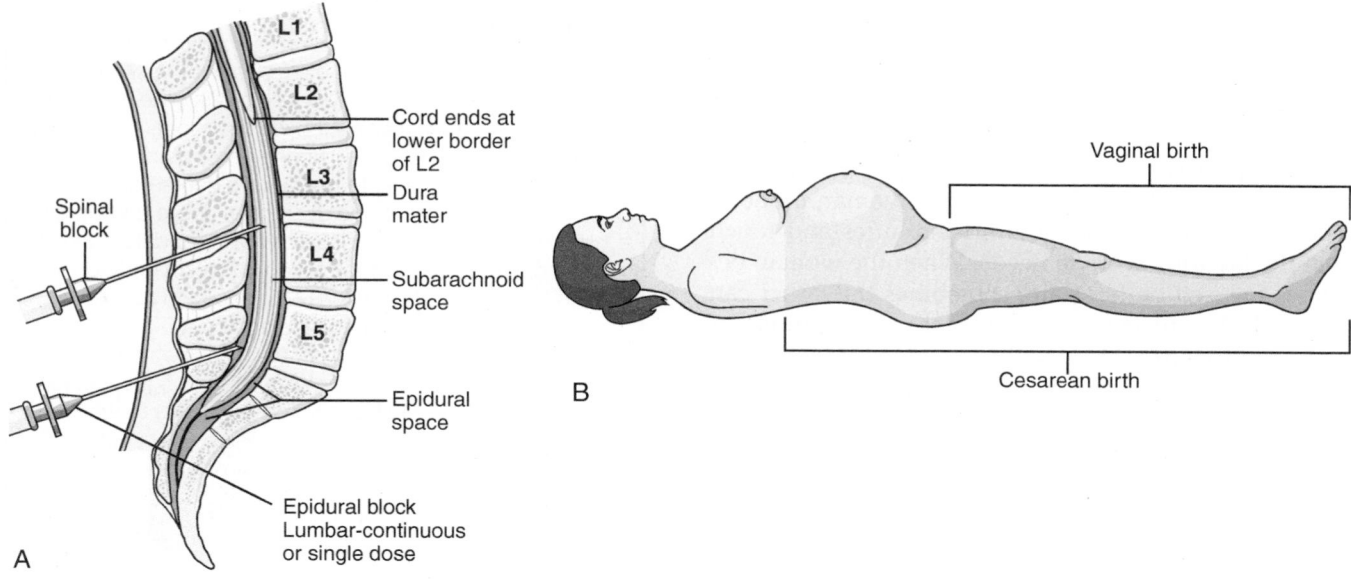

Fig. 27.23 (A) Regional anesthesia in obstetrics. (B) Level of anesthesia necessary for cesarean delivery and vaginal delivery.

validating her needs and paying close attention to her requests, proceeding at the woman's pace by waiting for her permission to touch her, accepting her reactions to labor, and protecting her privacy by limiting the exposure of her body and the number of people involved in her care. All laboring women should be cared for in this manner because they may have chosen not to reveal a history of sexual abuse.

Cognitive and Perceptual Issues

Pain is a major concern during labor and delivery. Breathing exercises help reduce discomfort, but as the intensity of labor increases, most women need some form of analgesia or anesthesia. The physician prescribes these medications with caution because they pass through the placenta and affect the fetus. Timing is critical to prevent diminished or depressed respiratory effort at the time of birth. Carefully assess the condition of mother and fetus before and after medication administration.

The most commonly used analgesics are meperidine hydrochloride (Demerol) and butorphanol tartrate, which may be given intramuscularly or intravenously. Antianxiety medications such as hydroxyzine (Vistaril) and diazepam (Valium) may be administered to reduce apprehension and anxiety. These medications also potentiate the effects of narcotics. Occasionally, sedative-hypnotics such as pentobarbital (Nembutal sodium) and secobarbital (Seconal sodium) are given in early labor to promote relaxation and rest.

The form of anesthesia used depends on the patient's wishes and the primary care practitioner's assessment of maternal and fetal needs. Anesthetics are classified as general, regional, and local. Most vaginal deliveries today include a form of regional anesthetic (Fig. 27.23). Regional anesthetics include paracervical, epidural, spinal, and pudendal blocks (Table 27.6 and Figs. 27.24 and 27.25).

GENERAL ANESTHESIA

General anesthesia is systemic pain control that involves loss of consciousness. It rarely is used for vaginal births, but still has a place in cesarean deliveries. Some women need surgery but either refuse or are not good candidates for epidural or spinal block. Occasionally, a planned epidural or spinal block proves inadequate for surgical anesthesia, or a cesarean birth may need to be performed so quickly that no time is available to establish either type of regional block. General anesthesia may be required for emergency procedures at any stage of pregnancy in the event that surgery is necessary.

Technique

Before induction of anesthesia, the woman breathes oxygen for 3 to 5 minutes or takes four deep breaths to increase her and her fetus's oxygen stores for the short period of apnea during anesthesia induction. A wedge is placed under the woman's right side (or the operating table is tilted toward her left side) to displace the uterus from the aorta and inferior vena cava, which promotes placental blood flow.

Adverse Effects of General Anesthesia

Major adverse effects are possible with the use of general anesthesia. *Maternal aspiration of gastric contents* can occur. Regurgitation with aspiration of acidic gastric contents is a potentially fatal complication. Aspiration of food particles may result in airway obstruction. Aspiration of acidic secretions causes chemical injury to the airways (aspiration pneumonitis). Infection often occurs after the initial lung injury. For purposes

Table 27.6 Anesthesia for Labor and Delivery

TYPE OF ANESTHESIA	ADMINISTRATION	AREA ANESTHETIZED OR EFFECTS	POSSIBLE SIDE EFFECTS		NURSING INTERVENTIONS AFTER ADMINISTRATION
			MOTHER	FETUS	
Regional					
Paracervical block	Injection, either side of cervix at 4-cm dilation	Cervix and uterus	Can slow labor	30% incidence rate of temporary slowing of fetal heart rate	Closely monitor fetal heart tones and maternal vital signs and contractions.
Pudendal block (see Figs. 27.24 and 27.25)	Injection into area of pudendal nerves for birth	Perineum	None unless allergy to drug	None	Provide reassurance and explanation; monitor fetal heart tones and maternal vital signs closely.
Caudal and lumbar epidural (see Figs. 27.24 and 27.25)	Caudal canal Epidural space at 4-cm dilation	Pelvic region	Hypotension; cannot "push" for delivery; may slow labor if started too early	Slowing of fetal heart and fetal heart deceleration	Monitor fetal heart tones and maternal vital signs closely; use excellent aseptic techniques.
Saddle block (low spinal)	Injection under dura of spinal cord for birth	Pelvic region	Postspinal headache, hypotension	None	Intravenous injection and oxygen are usually used.
General Inhalation					
Nitrous oxide	Inhaled through mask	Complete body	Aspiration possible with vomiting	Respiratory depression; hypoxia	Be alert and prepared for vomiting (with aspiration of food) and excessive uterine bleeding as a result of uterine relaxation.

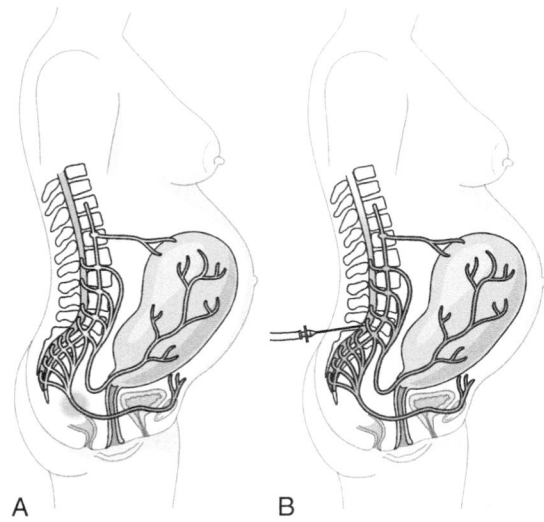

Fig. 27.24 Pain pathways and sites of pharmacologic nerve blocks. (A) Pudendal block: suitable during second and third stages of labor and for repair of episiotomy or lacerations. (B) Epidural block: suitable for all stages of labor and for repair of episiotomy or lacerations.

Fig. 27.25 Pudendal block. Use of needle guide (Iowa trumpet) and Luer-Lok syringe to inject medication.

of general anesthesia, anesthesia providers assume a pregnant woman has a full stomach.

Respiratory depression may occur in either the mother or the infant but is more likely in the infant if delivery is delayed after anesthesia is started.

Uterine relaxation can occur with some inhalational anesthetics. This characteristic is desirable for treatment of some complications, such as replacing an inverted uterus. However, postpartum hemorrhage may occur if the uterus relaxes after birth.

Methods to Minimize Adverse Effects
Measures to reduce the risk of maternal aspiration (or of lung injury, if aspiration occurs) include the following:
- Restrict intake to clear fluids or maintain nothing-by-mouth status if surgery is expected, such as with a scheduled cesarean birth.
- Administer drugs to raise the gastric pH and make secretions less acidic, such as sodium citrate and

citric acid (Bicitra), ranitidine (Zantac), cimetidine (Tagamet), or famotidine (Pepcid).
- Administer drugs to reduce secretions, such as glycopyrrolate (Robinul).

Avert neonatal respiratory depression by (1) reducing the time from induction of anesthesia to clamping of the umbilical cord and (2) keeping use of sedating drugs and anesthetics to a minimum until the cord is clamped.

To reduce the time from induction of anesthesia to cord clamping, prepare and drape the woman and alert the physicians before anesthesia is begun. Before cord clamping, the anesthesia is so light that the woman may move on the operating table as the incision is made, but she rarely remembers the experience or does not recall it as painful. The anesthesia level is deepened after the cord is clamped.

Values and Beliefs

Cultural beliefs and practices have implications for labor and delivery, as they do in all aspects of life. Respect the values and beliefs of women in labor. Seek information about specific cultural practices, values, and beliefs and incorporate these into the care plan.

Non–English-Speaking Women in Labor

A woman's level of anxiety in labor rises when she does not understand what is happening or what is said. English-speaking women may feel some stress from a misunderstanding, but the effect on a non–English-speaking woman is more dramatic, because she may feel a complete loss of control over her situation if no health care providers speak her language. She can panic and withdraw or become physically abusive when someone tries to do something she perceives may harm her or her baby.

Sometimes a support person can be a translator, although ideally a bilingual nurse cares for the woman. Alternatively, contact an employee or volunteer translator for assistance. If no one in the hospital can translate, call a translation service to translate over the telephone. For some women, a female translator may be more acceptable. If no translator is available, the labor and birth unit staff can prepare a set of cards with graphic depictions that illustrate common situations. Even when the nurse has limited ability to communicate verbally with the woman, in most instances, efforts to communicate are meaningful and appreciated by the woman.

Precipitous Labor and Emergency Birth

Precipitous labor is defined as labor that lasts less than 3 hours from the onset of contractions to the time of birth. Precipitous labor may result from hypertonic uterine contractions that are tetanic-like in intensity. In addition, lower resistance than normal in the maternal soft tissues may promote a rapid fetal descent through the birth canal. Maternal and fetal complications can

result. Maternal complications include uterine rupture, lacerations of the birth canal, amniotic fluid embolism, and postpartum hemorrhage. Fetal complications include hypoxia from decreased periods of uterine relaxation between contractions and intracranial hemorrhage related to rapid birth. As a result of the rapid descent and related fetal distress, meconium staining and aspiration may result. The neonate also may have lower Apgar scores.

Women who experience precipitous labor often describe feelings of disbelief, alarm, panic, and finally relief when they arrive at the hospital. They express frustration when nurses do not believe that they are ready to push. Some women have difficulty remembering the details of their labor and birth and need others, including caregivers, to help them fill in the gaps in their memory. If the baby is responsive, placing the child at the mother's breast to nurse is a positive intervention because it stimulates the uterus to contract.

❖ NURSING PROCESS FOR NORMAL LABOR

The role of the licensed practical/vocational nurse (LPN/LVN) in the nursing process as stated is that the LPN/LVN will:
- Participate in planning care for patients based on patient needs.
- Review patients' care plans and recommend revisions as needed.
- Review and follow defined prioritization for patient care.
- Use clinical pathways, care maps, or care plans to guide and review patient care.

◆ ASSESSMENT

Assessment begins with admission of the patient to the labor and delivery unit. Take a nursing history, including current labor, birth plan, current pregnancy and complications, previous pregnancies and complications, general medical history, and support system. Assess uterine contractions for frequency, duration, intensity, and resting tone. Frequency refers to the time from the beginning of one contraction to the beginning of the next. Duration is the time from the onset of the contraction to its completion. Intensity refers to the strength of the contraction. It may be measured definitively with an intrauterine pressure catheter. If the membranes are intact, the intensity is evaluated by palpating the firmness of the maternal abdomen during the contraction. Resting tone is the period between contractions. Assess FHR for baseline and decelerations. Assess cervical changes, condition of the membranes, and vaginal discharge. Also assess the patient's general physical status, including degree of pain or discomfort, and her psychosocial reaction to labor. The assessments, except for the history, are ongoing, with findings changing as the labor progresses.

Nursing Care Plan 27.1   **The Patient With Spontaneous Rupture of Membranes**

Ms. G. is a 27-year-old gravida 2, para 1 at 39½ weeks of gestation who appears on the labor and delivery unit with spontaneous rupture of membranes and regular contractions every 3 min. She has had a normal pregnancy without complications and has an insignificant medical history. Her first pregnancy ended with a vaginal delivery of a 7-lb, 8-oz boy after a 10-h labor.

PATIENT PROBLEM

Recent Onset of Pain, related to the process of labor and birth

Patient Goals and Expected Outcomes	Nursing Interventions	Evaluation
Patient will use techniques learned in prenatal classes to cope with pain of labor and birth Patient will have reduced pain with use of relief measures	Provide comfort measures to reduce anxiety, enhance relaxation, and increase the effectiveness of pain relief measures (see Table 27.3): • Back massage with sacral counter pressure • Cold, moist cloth to forehead • Frequent change of position • Hygienic care: sponge bath, perineal care • Use alternative measures for pain relief: • Effleurage • Relaxation, guided imagery, focal points • Breathing • Administer analgesics safely. • Encourage use of techniques and provide positive reinforcement.	Patient performs breathing techniques during contractions. Patient uses techniques and expresses their effectiveness. Patient expresses pain reduction with use of analgesics and other pain relief measures.

Patient Problem

Anxiousness, related to the childbirth experience

Patient Goals and Expected Outcomes	Nursing Interventions	Evaluation
Patient's level of anxiety will be maintained at a mild to moderate level Patient will participate in anxiety-reducing activities	Encourage use of childbirth relaxation techniques (see Box 27.7). Review birth plan with patient and coach. Use comfort measures to facilitate relaxation (see Box 27.7). Use calm, confident, caring approach. Encourage expression of feelings. Inform patient and coach of progress and procedures. Maintain privacy. Administer medications as necessary.	Patient's anxiety is reduced through breathing techniques and guided imagery with assistance of coach. Patient dozes between contractions.

CRITICAL THINKING QUESTIONS

1. Ms. G.'s labor is progressing normally with continuous monitoring. Suddenly the fetal heart rate drops to 90 bpm with late decelerations with each contraction. What should the nurse do? Explain the reason for these actions.
2. Ms. G. and her coach have been working well together to manage her labor, using a focal point, breathing techniques, and guided imagery. Suddenly she becomes irritable and tells her coach, "Don't touch me!" Her coach is bewildered by this change in behavior. How should the nurse explain Ms. G.'s behavior to her coach? How can the nurse help the coach continue to be effective during this time?

◆ **PATIENT PROBLEM**

Nursing assessment helps identify the needs of the laboring patient. Care can then be based on these needs (Nursing Care Plan 27.1). Possible problems for a laboring patient include but are not limited to the following:

• *Alteration in Urinary Elimination*
• *Anxiousness*
• *Compromised Blood Flow to Tissue (Maternal)*
• *Fearfulness*
• *Impaired Coping*
• *Insufficient Knowledge*
• *Lethargy or Malaise*
• *Potential for Inadequate Fluid Volume*

• *Potential for Infection*
• *Potential for Injury*
• *Recent Onset of Pain*

◆ **EXPECTED OUTCOMES AND PLANNING**

The care plan focuses on the needs of the laboring patient and the nurse's ability to meet those needs effectively. Each patient has differing needs, and care must be individualized accordingly. The care plan focuses on goals and outcomes specific to the patient problem. Examples include the following:

Goal 1: Patient will use techniques learned in prenatal childbirth classes to cope with pain during labor.

Box 27.7	**Nurse's Role in Relaxation and Breathing Techniques**

FIRST STAGE

Goal: Promote Relaxation of Abdominal Muscles

- Provide support during contractions: coach breathing, give back rubs, provide cool cloths.
- Provide distracting activities: guided imagery, focal point, effleurage (rhythmic stroking of abdomen by woman), progressive muscle relaxation, breathing techniques, music.
- Provide support and reminders for previously learned breathing techniques. If no specific method has been learned, encourage the following pattern:
  - Early, or latent, phase: slow, deep chest or abdominal breathing, six to nine breaths/min; inhalations through nose and out through pursed lips.
  - Middle, or active, phase: Slow acceleration, then deceleration of breaths through contraction; breaths shallow; approximately 16–20 breaths/min.
  - Transitional phase: four to six pants followed by a blow for duration of contraction.
- Remind patient to use breathing techniques only during contractions and normal breathing patterns between contractions.
- Remind patient to take deep, cleansing breath before and after contraction to increase oxygen intake.
- Remind patient to avoid rapid breathing, which leads to hyperventilation, because this can result in decreased oxygenation to fetus and symptoms for the mother.

SECOND STAGE

Goal: Increase Abdominal Pressure and Assist in Expelling Fetus

- Assist patient with natural bearing-down effort (BDE) or urge to push.
- Help patient into a position that facilitates BDE during contractions: upright (squatting on bed), semirecumbent with shoulders curved and knees bent, or lateral (raise and support upper leg during BDE).
- Assist patient with breathing during BDE:
  - Two deep, cleansing breaths at contraction onset; patient takes a breath, holds a few seconds, then pushes while exhaling in short (7-s) periods.
  - Two deep, cleansing breaths at contraction end.
- Help patient into a position of comfort between contractions.
- Provide encouragement for effort and encourage relaxation techniques between contractions.
- Remind patient to pant during contraction if BDE is to be avoided.

Outcome: Patient demonstrates ability to relax between contractions and effectively perform breathing techniques during contractions.

Goal 2: Patient's level of anxiety will remain mild to moderate as labor progresses.

Outcome: Patient participates in anxiety-reducing activities and dozes between contractions.

◆ IMPLEMENTATION

Nursing interventions during labor include the following:

- Provide emotional support to both the patient and her coach or significant other.
- Maintain a supportive environment.
- Give physical care to provide comfort to the patient.
- Explain all procedures performed.
- Identify any factors that may indicate interference with labor.
- Provide encouragement throughout the labor process.
- Encourage verbalization of fears and concerns.
- Continually monitor the progress of the labor to ensure the safety and well-being of the mother and fetus.

◆ EVALUATION

Continually evaluate the effectiveness of the interventions. As the labor progresses, the focus and interventions change. Refer to the goals and outcomes to determine whether the care plan was effective and the outcomes met. Examples include the following:

Goal 1: Patient will use techniques learned in prenatal childbirth classes to cope with pain during labor.

Evaluative measure: Observe the patient correctly performing breathing techniques during contractions.

Goal 2: Patient's level of anxiety will remain mild to moderate as labor progresses.

Evaluative measure: Ask patient to demonstrate relaxation techniques used to reduce anxiety (Box 27.7).

MEDICAL INTERVENTIONS

Although labor and delivery are normal processes, sometimes complications arise. At times, the physician must intervene to protect the mother or fetus.

INDUCTION

Induction is an attempt to start labor at a chosen time rather than waiting for it to begin spontaneously. It may be indicated for either maternal or fetal factors. Maternal factors include rupture of membranes greater than 24 hours, hypertensive disorders, diabetes mellitus, and history of stillbirth or fetal demise (death). Fetal indications may include intrauterine growth restriction (IUGR), nonreassuring fetal status, and oligohydramnios. Occasionally an elective induction is scheduled when the woman has a history of precipitous labor (under 3 hours). This is done to prevent an emergency out-of-hospital delivery. Contraindications for induction of labor include active herpes simplex infection, placenta previa (placenta covers the cervical os), and cord prolapse.

The health care provider assesses the woman to determine whether she and the fetus are good candidates for the induction. Bishop scoring is a tool used

Fig. 27.26 (A) Amnihook. (B) Finger cot amnihook. (A, From McKinney ES, James SR, Murray SS, et al: Maternal-child nursing, ed 4, St. Louis, 2013, Saunders. B, Image provided by Utah Medical Products, Inc. [UTMD].)

Fig. 27.27 Amniotomy.

to evaluate the readiness of the expectant mother for induction of labor. Factors that are evaluated with this tool include cervical dilation, effacement, cervical position, station, and cervical consistency. The medically approved methods of inducing labor include amniotomy, prostaglandin gel application, and oxytocin administration.

Amniotomy

If the amniotic membranes have not ruptured, the primary care practitioner may use a sterile hook-shaped instrument to open the sac and allow the fluid to drain; this procedure is called an amniotomy (or artificial rupture of the fetal membrane) (Figs. 27.25 and 27.26). An amniotomy has the advantage of facilitating contractions much like those in natural labor. In addition, once the membranes are ruptured, internal monitoring can be implemented. Minimal cervical dilation (−2 cm) must be present for rupture of the membranes. Caution is used when performing an amniotomy in the presence of hydramnios or if the fetal presenting part is not engaged. Assess FHR for a full minute immediately before and after this procedure. Assess the amount and color of amniotic fluid. Once an amniotomy has been performed, the woman traditionally is allowed 24 hours to deliver. Prolonged rupture of membranes carries the risk of infection.

Prostaglandin Gel Application

Successful induction of labor requires cervical dilation. The cervix begins to soften in the last weeks of pregnancy. In the event the consistency of the cervix is not favorable, prostaglandins may be used to ripen the cervix. Before administration of the prostaglandin, the patient must be assessed. Fetal heart tones are recorded to establish a baseline. The mother is placed on continuous monitoring. After assessment of the mother and fetus, the primary care practitioner applies prostaglandin E (PGE) gel intracervically with a plastic catheter (see Table 27.3). Contractions normally begin within an hour of instillation of the gel. Assessment during the ripening procedure includes close monitoring of vital signs, FHR, and contractions. Uterine

hyperstimulation is a possible side effect of prostaglandin administration. An amniotomy is performed in conjunction with the gel application. An internal fetal monitor also is applied routinely when PGE gel is used. In most facilities, the LPN/LVN does not apply this gel, but does monitor vital signs, FHR, and labor progress.

Oxytocin Stimulation

Use of oxytocin is indicated to induce labor or to augment (stimulate) a labor that is not making adequate progress because of uterine inertia (absence or weakness of uterine contractions). A primary IV line is initiated. Oxytocin (Pitocin) is administered intravenously with a piggyback procedure (see Table 27.3). The medication levels are titrated based on the characteristics of the contraction elicited. After induction, monitor the progress of labor. Because the contractions that result from oxytocin can be very strong, monitor the FHR and contractions carefully and document care. Stop the infusion and contact the primary care practitioner if signs or symptoms of complications appear, such as changes in FHR, bradycardia, tachycardia, arrhythmias, or excessive frequency, duration, or pressure of contractions. In addition, if hypertonic labor patterns result, administer oxygen.

FORCEPS DELIVERY

Forceps are spoonlike devices that fit around the fetal head to aid in expulsion. They most commonly are used to assist in the presence of a prolonged second stage or when intervention is necessary to speed the second stage of labor in the presence of actual or anticipated fetal compromise (Fig. 27.28). As with induction, certain criteria must be met before use. Membranes must be ruptured. Complete cervical dilation must be achieved. The precise location and positioning of the head must be known. The head must be engaged.

A

B

Fig. 27.28 (Forceps (A) and vacuum (B) extraction.)

The nurse assisting in the delivery is responsible for providing the type of forceps requested by the primary care practitioner. Closely monitor the FHR before and during the forceps maneuvers. Also explain to the mother that these actions help the baby. The newborn with a forceps-assisted delivery may have ecchymosis (bruising) or edema. Maternal complications may include lacerations, episiotomy extension, hematomas, and increased bleeding.

VACUUM EXTRACTION

An alternative to forceps delivery is vacuum extraction, which involves attaching a vacuum cup to the fetal head and applying negative pressure. Criteria for this procedure include vertex presentation, ruptured membranes, complete dilation of the cervix, and lack of cephalopelvic disproportion. During this procedure, assess the FHR frequently and encourage the mother to remain active in the birth process by pushing with contractions. The most common neonatal findings after this procedure are caput succedaneum, edema of the scalp, and circular bruising of the

scalp. Reassure the parents that these conditions are temporary.

CESAREAN DELIVERY

Cesarean birth is delivery through an abdominal and uterine incision. This type of delivery may be scheduled or may be performed in cases of emergency. The number of cesarean deliveries has increased greatly over the past 30 years. Cesarean sections total nearly a third of all births at 31.9%. Although the outcomes for most operative births are positive, it should not be forgotten that they are a major operative procedure. Potential complications include infection, hemorrhage, and injury to the bladder, bowel, and the uterus. In early 2020, Joint Commission announced plans to report hospitals with consistently elevated cesarean section rates.

Indications for cesarean birth can be maternal or fetal. The major maternal indications for cesarean delivery are:

1. **Cephalopelvic disproportion** (the head of the fetus is larger than the pelvic outlet), so that the fetus is unable to pass through the maternal pelvis
2. Previous cesarean delivery
3. Breech presentation
4. Medical conditions that endanger the mother's health, such as cardiac complications
5. Abnormal conditions of the placenta, such as placenta previa
6. Infections of the vaginal canal
7. Pelvic abnormalities
   The major fetal indicators are:
1. Fetal oxygen deprivation (hypoxia)
2. Prolapse of the umbilical cord
3. Breech presentation
4. Malpresentations, such as transverse
5. Congenital anomalies
   These conditions are discussed in greater depth in Chapter 28.

In past years, women who gave birth via cesarean section would be expected to deliver any future children in the same operative manner. This gave birth to the adage, "Once a C-section, always a C-section." The ability of a woman to experience a vaginal birth after cesarean (VBAC) is potentially possible. Factors such as the reason for the initial cesarean section and type of operative incisions performed will determine the feasibility of a VBAC. After a review of the woman's medical history, the nature of the current pregnancy, and the reason for the earlier cesarean, the primary care practitioner may permit a trial labor. In these cases, the woman must be monitored carefully, and the facility must be prepared to perform an emergency cesarean if complications arise (Box 27.8).

To perform a cesarean delivery, the primary care practitioner makes incisions in the abdominal and the uterine walls. Depending on the technique, several different incision types may be used.

Box 27.8   Vaginal Birth After Cesarean Birth

Approximately 60%–80% of women with one low transverse uterine incision from a cesarean birth have successful vaginal births. Women who had their prior cesarean for a nonrecurring reason (e.g., breech presentation) are more likely to have a successful vaginal birth after cesarean birth (VBAC) than women who had their prior cesarean for dystocia. Women who had a vaginal birth before or since the prior cesarean birth are more likely to have successful VBAC.

Candidates for VBAC include the following:

- A woman with one or two low transverse uterine scars but none from removal of fibroid tumors or uterine rupture.
- A woman whose pelvis is adequate for estimated fetal size.

Management of women who plan VBAC includes the following considerations:

- External cephalic version may be as successful for women with a prior cesarean as for women with an unscarred uterus.
- Epidural analgesia and anesthesia may be used.
- Induction and augmentation of labor with oxytocin may be done. Use of prostaglandin gel appears to be safe. Misoprostol (Cytotec) currently is contraindicated.
- Most authorities recommend electronic fetal monitoring.
- A physician, anesthesia, and personnel must be immediately available during active labor in case an emergency cesarean is needed.

Data from American Academy of Pediatrics (AAP) and American College of Obstetricians and Gynecologists (ACOG): *Guidelines for perinatal care,* ed 6, Elk Grove Village, IL, and Washington, DC, 2007, Author; ACOG: *Vaginal birth after previous cesarean delivery (ACOG practice bulletin no. 54),* Washington, DC, 2006, Author; ACOG: *Induction of labor with misoprostol (ACOG committee opinion no. 228),* Washington, DC, 2006, Author.

Patient problems and interventions for the patient delivering by cesarean section include but are not limited to the following:

PATIENT PROBLEM	NURSING INTERVENTIONS
Potential for Infection, related to a surgical procedure	Monitor and document vital signs and fetal heart rate
	Maintain good aseptic technique during vaginal examinations, catheterization, and preoperative skin preparation
	Monitor blood loss and white blood cell count
	Administer antibiotics as ordered
	Monitor and encourage fluid intake
Impaired Self-Esteem due to Current Situation, related to change in birth plan	Discuss changes in birth plan, including the reasons for the changes
	Encourage patient to verbalize feelings about cesarean birth
	Provide positive reassurance
	Involve patient in decision making
	Accept patient's own pace in working through grief or crisis situations

Get Ready for the NCLEX® Examination!

Key Points

- Although various theories have been proposed, the process that starts labor has not yet been determined.
- True labor and false labor can be confusing to the patient and health care personnel; even knowledgeable individuals can be mistaken.
- The birth process can occur in a variety of settings. The most important concern is protecting the welfare of the mother and the newborn.
- Vaginal delivery involves a complex interrelationship of the passageway, the passengers, and the powers.
- The first stage of labor is usually the longest. Mother and fetus face significant risks during this time and must be assessed carefully and continually.
- Fetal monitoring, internal or external, helps the nurse monitor labor and recognize signs of fetal distress.
- Many women learn specific breathing techniques to reduce pain and facilitate control of the birthing process. Be prepared to assist with these.

- The fourth stage of labor, the time of stabilization, requires careful nursing assessment of the mother. Assess vital signs and perform fundal checks to detect excessive blood loss.
- Episiotomies may be performed and lacerations may occur even during "normal" childbirth. Their appropriate and prompt repair is essential.
- The Apgar scoring system is used 1 and 5 minutes after birth to assess the newborn's condition.
- Modification of functional health patterns occurs during labor and delivery. Assess all areas to detect problems quickly and report them promptly.
- In some cases, the practitioner may have to intervene in the process of labor and delivery and use forceps or surgical means to deliver a healthy newborn.
- Facilitate mother-infant attachment by meeting the new mother's physical, support, and teaching needs.
- Anticipate an immediate birth if any laboring woman states, "The baby is coming!"

Review Questions for the NCLEX® Examination

1. A 23-year-old primigravida arrives at the labor unit in early labor. Which assessment finding indicates that labor has begun?

   1. Decreased vaginal secretions
   2. Weight gain of 1 to 3 lb
   3. Cervical dilation
   4. Increased fetal movement

2. To determine fetal lie, presentation, and position, the caregiver uses which assessment technique?

   1. Abdominal ultrasound scan
   2. Fetal heart tone auscultation
   3. Palpation of contractions
   4. Leopold's maneuvers

3. The fetal position is ROA. Where is the fetal presenting part in relation to the maternal pelvis?

   1. The occiput is facing the right side and the front of the maternal pelvis.
   2. The mentum is facing the right side and the front of the maternal pelvis.
   3. The occiput is facing the left side and the back of the maternal pelvis.
   4. The sacrum is facing the right side and the front of the maternal pelvis.

4. To assess the frequency of regular labor contractions, what should the nurse record?

   1. The interval between the peaks of the contractions
   2. The interval from the start of one contraction to the start of the next
   3. The interval from the end of one contraction to the start of the next
   4. How many contractions she has in 15 minutes

5. A pregnant woman is attending childbirth classes. She asks the nurse teaching the class when she can have an internal fetal monitor applied. What is the best nursing response?

   1. "Because you have had a low-risk pregnancy, you are not considered a candidate for internal monitoring."
   2. "Your health care provider decides when to apply the internal monitor."
   3. "Your cervix must be 2 to 3 cm dilated and your membranes ruptured before an internal monitor can be applied."
   4. "We can apply the internal monitor at any time after your membranes rupture."

6. A woman tells the nurse she thinks her membranes have ruptured. What action by the nurse best validates rupture of membranes?

   1. Feeling the draw sheet for wetness
   2. Performing a nitrazine test
   3. Inserting a Foley catheter into the bladder
   4. Performing an ultrasound

7. A woman has progressed through her labor without difficulty. However, the fetal heart rate has been decreasing with each contraction for the past 15 minutes. The rate decreases from 150 to 125 bpm after the peak of the contraction and returns to 150 bpm 15 seconds after the contraction is finished. What phenomena do the clinical manifestations most support?

   1. Variable decelerations
   2. Early decelerations
   3. Late decelerations
   4. Combination decelerations

8. When the woman enters the transition phase to active labor, which behaviors should the nurse expect to see?

   1. A desire for personal contact and touch
   2. Sleepiness and quietness, with a desire for touch
   3. Responsiveness to teaching
   4. Irritability, resistance to touch, and withdrawal

9. As the woman's labor progresses, which assessment finding indicates that the second stage of labor has begun?

   1. Passage of a mucous plug
   2. Bearing-down reflex
   3. Dilation of the cervix to 7 cm
   4. Change in shape of the uterus

10. The nurse has just reviewed the fetal heart rate on an assigned laboring patient. What finding indicates the need to notify the charge nurse?

    1. Accelerations
    2. Early decelerations
    3. Average fetal heart rate (FHR) of 126 bpm
    4. Late decelerations

11. Which maternal cardiovascular finding is expected during labor?

    1. Increased cardiac output
    2. Increased pulse rate
    3. Decreased white blood cell count
    4. Decreased blood pressure

12. The nurse notes heart rate accelerations with fetal movement. The nurse correctly recognizes that heart accelerations most commonly:

    1. are reassuring.
    2. are caused by umbilical cord compression.
    3. warrant close observation.
    4. are caused by uteroplacental insufficiency.

13. The patient delivers an 8-lb, 1-oz boy. Ten minutes later, there is a sudden gush of blood from her vagina. At the same time, the woman's uterus becomes globular in shape and the umbilical cord lengthens. What do these findings most likely indicate?

    1. Separation of the placenta
    2. Uterine hemorrhage
    3. Cervical or vaginal laceration
    4. Uterine involution

14. A woman pregnant for the first time is dilated 3 cm, with contractions every 5 minutes. She is groaning and perspiring excessively and states that she did not attend childbirth classes. What is the most important nursing action?

    1. Notify the woman's health care provider.
    2. Administer the prescribed narcotic analgesic.
    3. Ensure that her labor will be overseen.
    4. Give simple breathing and relaxation instructions.

15. When planning care for a woman whose membranes have ruptured, the nurse recognizes that the woman's risk for what has increased?

    1. Intrauterine infection
    2. Hemorrhage
    3. Precipitous labor
    4. Supine hypotension

16. The nurse is caring for a patient in labor who has had meperidine (Demerol) for pain relief. Which side effects are commonly associated with this drug? *(Select all that apply.)*

    1. Dry mouth
    2. Hypotension
    3. Bradycardia
    4. Pruritus
    5. Tachypnea

17. The nurse is preparing a patient for a scheduled cesarean section. The nurse will administer medications to reduce gastric acidity. Which medications may be used? *(Select all that apply.)*

    1. Sodium citrate (Bicitra)
    2. Ranitidine (Zantac)
    3. Cimetidine (Tagamet)
    4. Famotidine (Pepcid)
    5. Glycopyrrolate (Robinul)

18. When caring for a patient who gave birth via cesarean section, her ability to deliver vaginally will be determined by _____ and the _____ used.

19. The fetus is noted to be experiencing tachycardia. What are potential causes? *(Select all that apply.)*

    1. Fetal anemia
    2. Maternal anemia
    3. Maternal dehydration
    4. Prolonged cord compression
    5. Administration of meperidine to the mother
    6. Uterine hyperstimulation
    7. Maternal hypotension
    8. Maternal hyperthyroidism
    9. Maternal infection
    10. Early fetal distress

Objectives

1. Describe the postpartum assessment of the mother.
2. Identify the physiologic changes that occur in the postpartum period.
3. Discuss the nursing responsibilities during the postpartum period.
4. Recognize complications in the postpartum period.
5. Explain the importance of teaching personal and infant care.
6. Discuss the psychosocial adaptations that occur after birth.
7. Discuss interventions for the prevention of infant abductions.
8. Describe the assessment of the healthy newborn.
9. Identify the physical characteristics of the healthy newborn.
10. Identify normal findings and common variations observed in the newborn.
11. Describe the behavioral characteristics of the newborn.
12. Discuss nursing interventions for the circumcised newborn.
13. Explain parent-child attachment (bonding).
14. Discuss nutritional needs and feeding of the newborn.
15. Discuss quieting techniques for the fussy newborn.

Key Terms

acrocyanosis (ăk-rō-sī-ă-NŌ-sĭs, p. 875)
autolysis (ăw-TŎL-ĭ-sĭs, p. 849)
circumcision (p. 877)
colostrum (kō-LŌS-trŭm, p. 882)
cryptorchidism (krĭp-TŎR-kĭ-dĭz-ĕm, p. 877)
diaphoresis (dī-ă-fŏ-RĒ-sĭs, p. 852)
diuresis (dī-ŭr-RĒ-sĭs, p. 852)
engorgement (ĕn-GŎRJ-mĕnt, p. 866)
fontanelles (FŎN-tă-nĕlz, p. 875)
gynecomastia (jĭn-ĕ-kō-MĂS-tē-ă, p. 877)
harlequin sign (HĂR-lĕ-kwĭn, p. 875)
involution (p. 849)

lactation (p. 851)
lanugo (p. 875)
latch-on (p. 867)
lochia (LŌ-kē-ă, p. 849)
meconium (p. 884)
parent-child attachment (bonding) (p. 886)
polydactyly (pŏl-ē-DĂK-tĕ-lē, p. 878)
prolactin (p. 851)
pseudomenstruation (sū-dō-mĕn-strū-Ā-shŭn, p. 877)
puerperium (pū-ĕr-PĔR-ē-ŭm, p. 848)
syndactyly (sĭn-DĂK-tĕ-lē, p. 877)
vernix caseosa (VĔR-nĭks kăs-ē-Ō-să, p. 875)

The postpartum period, also called the puerperium, lasts from the time the woman delivers the placenta until the reproductive organs return to approximately the nonpregnant size and position. The puerperium lasts about 3 to 6 weeks and consists of two stages. The immediate postpartum period, which lasts up to 6 hours after delivery, sometimes is called the *fourth stage of labor,* or the recovery stage. The new mother needs emotional support and close assessment after giving birth. This is a time for close observation and assessment to ensure that no problems occur. The later postpartum stage follows the stage of recovery and lasts until about 6 weeks after delivery.

During the postpartum period, the mother's body makes rapid physiologic adaptations. The anatomic and physiologic changes that took place over 9 months begin a reversal within 6 short weeks. Many psychological changes also occur as the woman and her family adjust to expansion of the family.

ANATOMIC AND PHYSIOLOGIC CHANGES OF THE MOTHER

REPRODUCTIVE ORGANS
Uterus
After the birth of the baby and the delivery of the placenta, the uterus contracts in response to *oxytocin* (a hormone produced by the posterior pituitary gland that stimulates uterine contractions and release of milk in the mammary glands [let-down reflex]). This contraction compresses blood vessels at the site where the placenta separated from the uterine wall. This site, an area 3 to 4 inches (8 to 10 cm) in diameter, has open venous sinuses. If the uterus does not contract adequately,

there will be increased blood loss. The placental site heals through exfoliation, in which necrotic tissue is sloughed from the uterine lining, leaving a fresh layer of endometrial tissue free from scars. This process is necessary for successive pregnancies to occur.

Immediately after delivery, the uterine fundus is about midway between the umbilicus and the symphysis pubis or slightly higher. It weighs approximately 2 lb (907 g). During the first 12 hours after birth, it rises to the level of the umbilicus at midline. In the following 24 to 48 hours, the uterus begins a gradual descent. It moves approximately one fingerbreadth per day; within a week, it is barely palpable at the level of the symphysis pubis and weighs 1 lb (453 g). Within 6 to 8 weeks, the uterus again is a pelvic organ, approximately the nonpregnant size of 2 oz (57 g) and no longer palpable. This decrease in size is called involution (Fig. 28.1). Complications during the recovery process related to the uterus are termed subinvolution.

Involution is carried out by a process called autolysis. **Autolysis** (the self-dissolution or self-digestion that occurs in tissues or cells by enzymes in the cells themselves) is a result of the sudden withdrawal of estrogen and progesterone, which releases proteolytic enzymes into the endometrium. These enzymes cause the cells to lose protein materials and thereby shrink. The number of muscle cells remains the same, but the size of each cell changes dramatically.

After delivery, the uterine lining is shed. This bloody discharge is termed lochia. It consists of blood, tissue, and mucus. As the uterine lining is shed, the necrotic tissue, blood, and mucus leave the body through the vagina. Lochia has a fleshy odor similar to that of menstrual discharge. For the first day or two after delivery, the lochia is made up mostly of blood, which results in a bright red drainage called *lochia rubra.* Some small clots may be passed during this phase. As the placental site heals, the discharge thins and becomes pink to

Fig. 28.1 Assessment of involution of uterus after delivery. (A) The progress of involution. (B) Fundal assessment. Size and position of uterus 2 hours after delivery. (C) Two days after delivery. (D) Four days after delivery.

Table 28.1	Lochia and Non-lochia Bleeding
LOCHIA	**NONLOCHIA BLEEDING**
Lochia usually trickles from the vaginal opening. The steady flow is greater as the uterus contracts.	If the blood discharge spurts from the vagina, cervical or vaginal tears may exist in addition to the normal lochia.
A gush of lochia may result as the uterus is massaged. If it is dark in color, it has been pooled in the relaxed vagina, and the amount soon lessens to a trickle of bright red lochia (in the early puerperium).	If the amount of bleeding continues to be excessive and bright red, a tear may be the source.

brown; this is called *lochia serosa*. After the seventh day, the drainage is slightly yellow to white and is called *lochia alba*. This drainage continues for another 10 days to 2 weeks. If fragments of the placenta are retained in the uterus, the uterus is not able to contract and seal blood vessels adequately, which can result in excessive blood loss and may necessitate surgical intervention (Table 28.1). See Box 28.1 for signs and symptoms of hypovolemic shock and nursing interventions.

Cervix, Vagina, and Perineum
The cervix appears edematous, with bruising. The external cervical os has a ragged, slit-like appearance instead of a round shape as seen in the nulliparous woman. The vaginal walls are thin and dry, with an absence of rugae. Vaginal mucus production returns with the return of estrogen production. Rugae reappear in 4 weeks.

Bruising and edema of the perineum is common. The episiotomy (if present) should be free of erythema, with the edges well approximated and without discharge. It should heal in 2 to 3 weeks. Sutures that are used are absorbed by the woman's body. Lacerations of the perineum are classified from first to fourth degree, depending on depth of involvement. The repaired laceration also should have well-approximated edges and no drainage (Fig. 28.2). Healing time depends on laceration depth. Return of these areas to the nonpregnant state should be complete in 6 to 8 weeks.

Lacerations of the genital tract. Lacerations of the cervix, the vagina, and the perineum are also causes of postpartum hemorrhage. Hemorrhage related to lacerations should be suspected if bleeding continues despite a firm, contracted uterine fundus. This bleeding can be a slow trickle, an oozing, or frank hemorrhage.

Factors that can lead to obstetric lacerations of the lower genital tract include operative birth, precipitous birth, congenital abnormalities of the maternal soft parts (vulva perineum), and a contracted pelvis. Other causes include size, abnormal presentation, and position of the fetus; relative size of the presenting part to

Box 28.1	Hypovolemic Shock

SIGNS AND SYMPTOMS
- Woman has persistent significant bleeding (perineal pad soaked within 15 min); this bleeding may not be accompanied by a change in vital signs or maternal color or behavior.
- Woman states she feels weak, lightheaded, "funny," or "sick to my stomach" or she "sees stars."
- Woman begins to act anxious or exhibits air hunger.
- Skin turns ashen or grayish.
- Skin feels cool and clammy.
- Pulse rate increases.
- Blood pressure declines.

INTERVENTIONS
- Notify primary health care provider.
- If uterus is atonic, massage gently and expel clots to cause uterus to contract; compress uterus manually, as needed, with two hands. Add oxytocic agent to IV drip, as ordered.
- Give oxygen via face mask or nasal prongs at 8–10 L/min.
- Tilt the woman to her side or elevate the right hip; elevate her legs to at least a 30-degree angle.
- Provide additional or maintain existing IV infusion of lactated Ringer's solution or normal saline solution to restore circulatory volume.
- Administer blood or blood products, as ordered.
- Monitor vital signs.
- Insert an indwelling urinary catheter to monitor perfusion of kidneys.
- Administer emergency drugs, as ordered.
- Prepare for possible surgery or other emergency treatments or procedures.
- Chart incident, medical and nursing interventions instituted, and results of treatments.

the size of the birth canal; scarring from prior vaginal infections, injury, or surgery; and vulvar, perineal, and vaginal varicosities. Extreme vascularity in the labia and periclitoral area often results in profuse bleeding if laceration occurs. Pelvic hematomas (i.e., a collection of blood in the connective tissue) may be vulvar, vaginal, or retroperitoneal in origin. Vulvar hematomas are the most common. They usually are visible and painful. Vaginal hematomas typically are associated with a forceps-assisted birth, episiotomy, or primigravidity. Retroperitoneal hematomas are the least common, but they are life threatening. They are caused by laceration of one of the vessels attached to the hypogastric artery, usually because of the rupture of a cesarean scar during labor.

Most acute injuries and lacerations of the perineum, the vagina, the uterus, and their support tissues occur during childbirth. Ideally, injuries are repaired at the time of delivery, which facilitates healing, limits residual damage, and reduces the incidence of infection. Future gynecologic problems, including pelvic relaxation, uterine prolapse, cystocele, and rectocele, may be attributed to childbirth.

Fig 28.2 The perineal region may appear bruised and swollen.

The tendency to sustain lacerations varies with each woman; in some women, the soft tissue may be less distensible. Heredity may be a factor. For example, the tissue of light-skinned women, especially those with reddish hair, is not as readily distensible as that of darker-skinned women, and healing may be less efficient.

Perineal lacerations. Perineal lacerations are the most common of all injuries in the lower genital tract. They usually occur when the fetal head is being born. The extent of the laceration is defined in terms of its depth (Fig. 28.3):
- *First-degree:* Laceration extends through the skin and structures superficial to muscles.
- *Second-degree:* Laceration extends through muscles of perineal body.
- *Third-degree:* Laceration continues through the sphincter muscle.
- *Fourth-degree:* Laceration also involves the anterior rectal wall.

Perineal injury often is accompanied by small lacerations on the medial surfaces of the labia minora below the pubic rami and to the sides of the urethra and the clitoris. Lacerations in this vascular area often result in profuse bleeding and necessitate repair with absorbable sutures.

When caring for the woman with a third-degree or fourth-degree laceration, assess the bowel habits. Include assessment of fecal continence. The initial stool after delivery may be uncomfortable, and measures to promote soft stools should be implemented.

Some health care providers may prescribe stool softeners. Additional measures include promoting fluid intake and encouraging increased dietary fiber and activity such as walking. Rectal treatments such as enemas or suppositories are contraindicated for women who have third-degree or fourth-degree lacerations. Antimicrobial therapy may be used in some cases.

Vaginal and urethral lacerations. Vaginal lacerations often occur in conjunction with perineal lacerations. Vaginal lacerations tend to extend up the lateral walls (sulci) and, if deep enough, involve the levator ani muscle. Additional injury may occur high in the vaginal vault near the level of the ischial spines. Vaginal vault lacerations may be circular and may result from forceps rotation, especially in cases of cephalopelvic disproportion, rapid fetal descent, and precipitous birth. Lacerations also can occur around the urethra (periurethral) and in the area of the clitoris.

Cervical injuries. Cervical injuries occur when the cervix retracts over the advancing fetal head. These cervical lacerations occur at the lateral angles of the external os; most are shallow, and bleeding is minimal. Larger lacerations may extend to the vaginal vault or beyond the vault into the lower uterine segment; serious bleeding may occur. Extensive lacerations may follow if the woman is allowed to push before full cervical dilation is achieved. Injuries to the cervix can affect pregnancies and childbirths.

Nursing interventions for episiotomy, lacerations, and hemorrhoids are listed in Box 28.2.

Breasts

Breast changes begin early in pregnancy. Increased amounts of estrogen stimulate enlargement of breast size by increasing adipose tissue and fluid retention. Estrogen also stimulates the growth of the milk ducts to prepare for lactation (function of secreting milk or period during which milk is secreted).

The first secretion produced by the breast is colostrum. This precursor to milk is thin, watery, and slightly yellow. It is rich in protein, calories, antibodies, and lymphocytes. Colostrum production begins in the second trimester. Expectant mothers begin to leak colostrum in the later weeks of the third trimester. Its production continues for about 2 days after delivery, when true milk production begins.

Lactation is a combination of hormonal, neurologic, and psychological responses. After delivery, estrogen and progesterone levels diminish rapidly. As they drop, the level of prolactin increases. Prolactin, a hormone secreted by the anterior pituitary gland, is responsible for stimulating milk production in the mammary alveolar cells. Stimulation of the nipples, particularly by the infant's sucking, causes the release of oxytocin from the posterior pituitary gland. Oxytocin stimulates contraction of the mammary ducts, and milk is ejected from the breast. This cycle is called the *let-down reflex.*

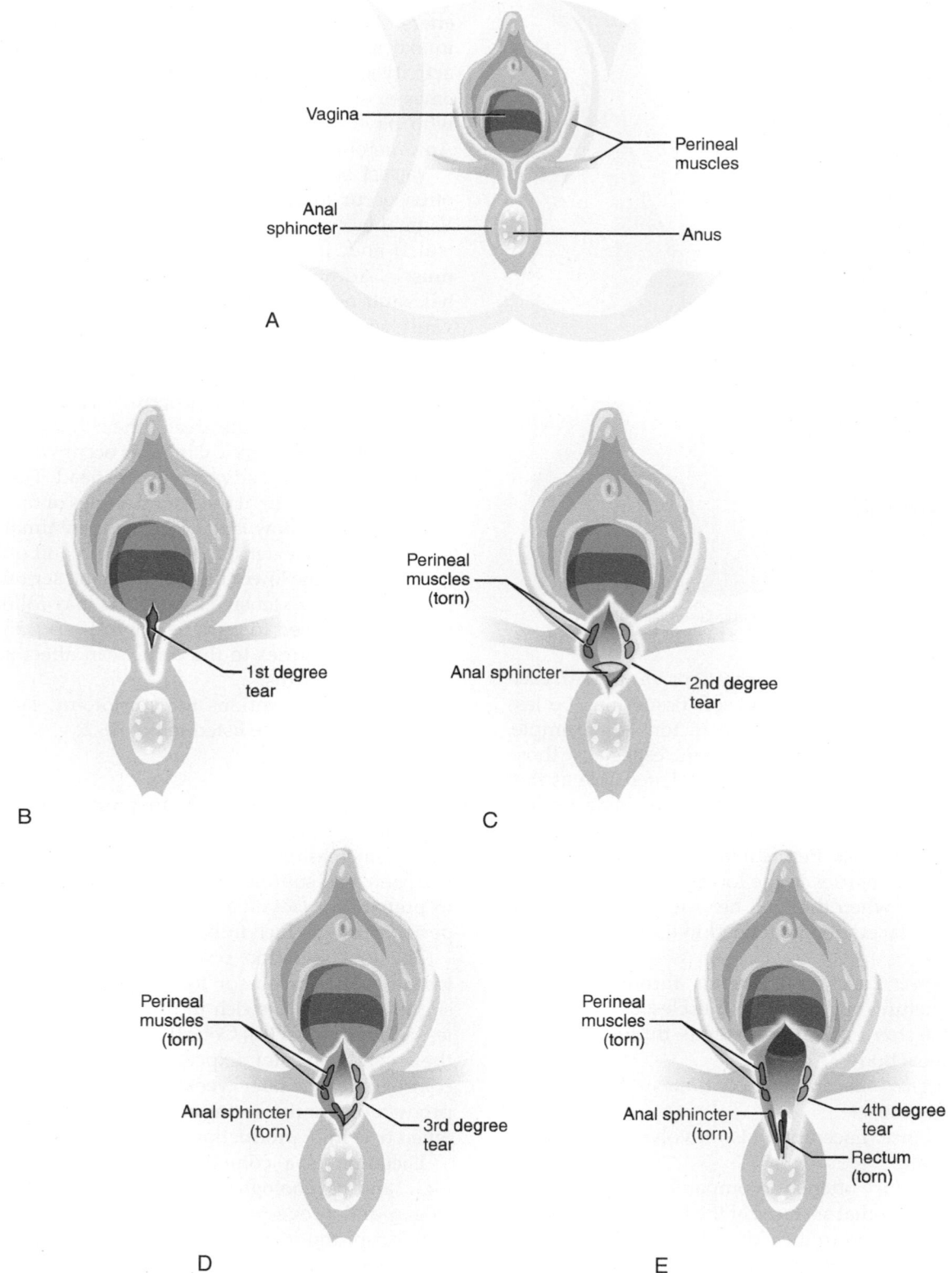

Fig. 28.3 Vaginal lacerations. (A) normal perineum (B) 1ˢᵗ degree laceration (C) 2ⁿᵈ degree laceration (D) 3ʳᵈ degree laceration (E) 4ᵗʰ degree laceration

OTHER BODY SYSTEMS

Cardiovascular

Blood volume is reduced to nonpregnant levels by 2 to 4 weeks after delivery. Diuresis (the increased formation and secretion of urine) and diaphoresis (the secretion of sweat, especially when profuse) account for most of the fluid loss. Blood loss during delivery accounts for an additional 300 to 500 mL (600 to 800 mL

Box 28.2 Interventions for Episiotomy, Lacerations, and Hemorrhoids

CLEANSING
- Wash hands before and after cleaning perineum and changing pads.
- Explain procedure.
- Wash perineum with mild soap and warm water at least once daily.
- Cleanse from symphysis pubis to anal area.
- Apply peripad from front to back, protecting inner surface of pad from contamination.
- Wrap soiled pad and place in covered waste container.
- Change pad with each void or defecation or at least four times per day.
- Assess amount and character of lochia with each pad change.

ICE PACK
- Apply a covered ice pack to perineum from front to back:
  - During first 2 h after the birth, to decrease edema formation and increase comfort
  - After the first 2 h, to provide anesthetic effect

SQUEEZE BOTTLE
- Demonstrate for and assist woman; explain rationale.
- Fill bottle with tap water warmed to approximately 100.4°F (38°C; comfortably warm on the wrist).
- Instruct woman to position nozzle between her legs so that squirts of water reach perineum as she sits on toilet.
- Explain that it takes a whole bottle of water to cleanse perineum.
- Remind her to blot dry with toilet paper or clean wipes.
- Remind her to avoid contamination from anal area.
- Apply clean pad.

SITZ BATH
Built-in Type
- Prepare bath by thoroughly scrubbing with cleaning agent and rinsing. Pad with towel before filling.
- Explain procedure.

- Fill one-half to one-third with water of correct temperature (100.4°F–105°F [38°C–40.6°C]). Some women prefer cool sitz baths; add ice to lower the temperature to a comfortable level.
- Encourage woman to use at least twice a day for 20 min.
- Place call bell within easy reach.
- Teach woman to enter bath by tightening gluteal muscles and keeping them tightened and then relaxing them after she is in the bath.
- Place dry towels within reach.
- Ensure privacy.
- Check on woman in 15 min; assess pulse as needed.

Disposable Type
- Clamp tubing and fill bag with warm water.
- Raise toilet seat, place bath in bowl with overflow opening directed toward back of toilet.
- Place container above toilet bowl.
- Attach tube into groove at front of bath.
- Loosen tube clamp to regulate rate of flow; fill bath to half full; continue as previously described for built-in sitz bath.

DRY HEAT
- Inspect lamp for defects.
- Cover lamp with towels.
- Position lamp 50 cm from perineum; use three times a day for 20-min periods.
- Provide draping over woman.
- If same lamp is used by several women, clean it carefully between uses.
- Teach woman regarding use of 40-watt bulb at home.

TOPICAL APPLICATIONS
- Apply anesthetic cream or spray; use sparingly three or four times a day.
- Offer witch hazel pads (Tucks) after voiding or defecating; woman pats perineum dry from front to back, then applies witch hazel pads. Explain rationale.

---

with cesarean delivery). Cardiac output also declines rapidly. The patient is at risk for thrombus formation as a result of elevation of platelets in the early postpartum period.

Urinary

After childbirth, as a result of trauma, increased bladder capacity, and the effects of conduction anesthesia, women have a decreased urge to void. In addition, pelvic soreness and edema caused by forceps used during labor, vaginal lacerations, or the episiotomy reduce or alter the voiding reflex. Decreased voiding combined with postpartum diuresis may result in bladder distention. Immediately after giving birth, the woman may bleed excessively if the bladder becomes distended because it pushes the uterus up and to the side and prevents the uterus from firmly contracting. Later in the puerperium, overdistention can make the bladder more susceptible to infection and delay the return of

normal voiding. With adequate emptying of the bladder, bladder tone usually is restored 5 to 7 days after childbirth, with daily urinary output of up to 3 L common.

Neurologic

Neurologic changes during the puerperium result from a reversal of maternal adaptations to pregnancy or from trauma during labor and childbirth. Pregnancy-induced neurologic discomforts abate after birth. Through diuresis, edema is eliminated, which relieves carpal tunnel syndrome by easing compression of the medial nerve. The periodic numbness and tingling of fingers that affect 5% of pregnant women usually disappear after birth, unless lifting and carrying the baby aggravate the condition.

Headache requires careful assessment. Postpartum headaches may be caused by various conditions, including gestational hypertension, stress, and leakage of cerebrospinal fluid into the extradural space during placement of the needle for epidural or spinal anesthesia. Depending on the cause and the effectiveness of the treatment, the headaches can last from 1 to 3 days to several weeks.

Gastrointestinal

Appetite generally returns to normal immediately after delivery. Gastric motility, however, may continue to decline, leading to constipation. Normal bowel elimination should resume within 2 or 3 days after delivery. Decreased abdominal tone and tenderness from the episiotomy or hemorrhoids may make the patient reluctant to strain for a bowel movement.

Endocrine

Placental hormone levels rapidly fall after delivery and are soon undetectable or at their nonpregnant values. Estrogen and progesterone levels drop markedly after expulsion of the placenta and reach their lowest levels 1 week into the postpartum period. Decreased estrogen levels are associated with breast engorgement and with the diuresis of excess extracellular fluid that has accumulated during pregnancy. The estrogen levels in nonlactating women begin to rise by 2 weeks after birth and are higher by postpartum day 17 than in women who breast-feed. The anterior pituitary secretes prolactin, but only in response to nipple stimulation. Other endocrine glands (thyroid, adrenal, and pancreas) return to prepregnant size and function.

Musculoskeletal

Abdominal muscle tone returns, and joint stabilization occurs over a 6- to 8-week period after delivery. The return of muscle tone depends on previous tone, proper exercise, and the amount of adipose tissue. Some pelvic joints may never return fully to their prepregnant position. Patients may feel discomfort in the joints immediately after delivery because of secretion of the hormone relaxin. However, even when all other joints return to their normal pregnant state, those of the parous woman's feet do not. The new mother may notice a permanent increase in shoe size.

Integumentary

Chloasma of pregnancy usually disappears at the end of pregnancy. Hyperpigmentation of the areola (the area encircling the nipple) and linea nigra (a dark line on the abdomen of a pregnant woman, usually extending from the symphysis pubis midline to the umbilicus) may not disappear completely after childbirth. Some women have permanent darker pigmentation of those areas. Striae gravidarum (stretch marks) on the breasts, the abdomen, and the thighs may fade but usually do not disappear.

Vascular abnormalities such as spider angiomas (nevi), palmar erythema, and epulis generally regress as estrogen rapidly declines after the end of pregnancy. For some women, spider nevi persist indefinitely.

The abundance of fine hair seen during pregnancy usually disappears after birth; however, any coarse or bristly hair that appears during pregnancy usually remains. Fingernails return to their prepregnancy consistency and strength.

Profuse diaphoresis in the immediate postpartum period is the most noticeable change in the integumentary system. This is common, especially at night, during the first week postpartum.

Immune

No significant changes in the maternal immune system occur during the postpartum period. Whether the mother needs a rubella vaccination or $Rh_o(D)$ immune globulin (RhoGAM) for prevention of Rh isoimmunization should be determined. Pregnant women are screened routinely for immunity to rubella early in the prenatal period. Women who are not immune are immunized early in the postpartum period before discharge. Patients who are Rh negative are screened in pregnancy for isoimmunization. If they are not found to be sensitized and give birth to infants who are Rh positive, they must receive RhoGAM within 72 hours of delivery.

TRANSFER FROM THE RECOVERY AREA

After the initial recovery period of 1 to 2 hours, the woman may be transferred to a postpartum room in the same or another nursing unit. In labor, delivery, recovery, postpartum (LDRP) room settings, the nurse who provided care during the recovery period usually continues to care for the woman. In the labor, delivery, recovery (LDR) room or a traditional setting, the woman is transferred to a separate unit where the postpartum nursing staff provide her care. In some settings, the baby remains with the mother wherever she goes. In other facilities, the baby is taken to the nursery for several hours of observation during the mother's initial recovery period.

The move to another area of the maternity unit requires the nurse to prepare a transfer report. The information to be provided to the nurse accepting the patient must be accurate and concise. Sources of information include the admission record, the birth record, and the recovery record. The postpartum nurse should be advised about the name of the primary care provider; gravidity and parity; age; anesthetic used; medications given; duration of labor and time of rupture of membranes; oxytocin induction or augmentation; type of birth and repair; blood type and Rh status; rubella immunity status; syphilis and hepatitis serology test results; intravenous (IV) infusion of any fluids; physiologic status since birth; description of fundus, lochia, bladder, and perineum; infant's gender and weight; time of birth; pediatrician; chosen method of feeding;

Box 28.3 Postpartum Maternal Danger Signs

- Fever with or without chills
- Malodorous vaginal discharge
- Excessive amount of vaginal discharge
- Bright red vaginal bleeding after it has changed to pink or rust
- Edema; erythematous or painful area on the legs
- Pain or burning sensation with urination or an inability to void
- Breast changes, such as localized pain, heat, edema, or malodorous drainage
- Pain in the perineal or pelvic area

Box 28.4 Assessment of Attachment Behaviors

- When the infant is brought to the parents, do they reach out for the infant and call the infant by name? (Recognize that in some cultures parents may not name the infant in the early newborn period.)
- Do the parents speak about the infant in terms of identification, such as who the infant looks like, what appears special about their infant compared with other infants?
- When parents are holding the infant, what kind of body contact is there? Do parents feel at ease changing the infant's position? Do they use fingertips or whole hands? Are there parts of the body they avoid touching or parts of the body they investigate and scrutinize?
- When the infant is awake, what kinds of stimulation do the parents provide? Do they talk to the infant, to each other, or to no one? How do they look at the infant? With direct visual contact, avoidance of eye contact, or looking at other people or objects?
- How comfortable do the parents appear in terms of caring for the infant? Do they express any concern regarding their ability or disgust for certain activities, such as changing diapers?
- What type of affection do they demonstrate to the newborn, such as smiling, stroking, kissing, or rocking?
- If the infant is fussy, what kinds of comforting techniques do the parents use, such as rocking, swaddling, talking, or stroking?

any abnormalities noted; and assessment of initial parent-infant interaction.

Most of this information is also documented for the nursing staff in the newborn nursery. In addition, specific information should be provided on the infant's Apgar scores: weight, voiding, and feeding since birth. Also, nursing interventions that have been completed (e.g., prophylaxis, vitamin K injection) should be recorded.

NURSING ASSESSMENT OF AND INTERVENTIONS FOR THE MOTHER

HEALTH MANAGEMENT AND HEALTH PERCEPTION

In the early 1980s, the average length of stay after childbirth was 4 days for a vaginal delivery and 1 to 2 days longer for a cesarean birth. During the early 1990s, discharge time shrunk. The movement was largely the result of changes in insurance coverage. Resistance to the progressively shorter stays was swift and vocal. Many states began enacting legislation to restrict facilities, health care practitioners, and insurance companies from requiring women be discharged in less than 48 hours after a vaginal delivery or 96 hours after a cesarean. Most women are stable and can be discharged within 48 (vaginal birth) and 72 (cesarean section) hours. Women who have uneventful, uncomplicated deliveries may opt to stay 24 hours or less. Regardless of the timing of the discharge, the woman's ability to meet her needs and those of her infant must be assessed. The assessment must include physiological and psychological parameters.

Discuss the home situation. If any aspect of the home situation appears unsafe or questionable, confer with the health care provider and discuss a referral to social services before discharge. Self-care concerns, including postpartum danger signs (Box 28.3), the importance of medical follow-up, infant care, and family planning should be incorporated.

Parent-Newborn Relationships

The nursing assessment must include the mother's reaction to the sight of her newborn. Some new mothers may appear excited, laughing, talking, and even crying; some exhibit apparent apathy. Occasionally, the mother appears angry or indifferent, turns away from the baby, concentrates on her own pain, or makes hostile comments. These varying reactions can arise from pleasure, exhaustion, or deep disappointment. Whatever the reaction and cause may be, the mother needs continuing acceptance and support from all the staff. Consider the woman's age, placement within Erikson's stages of growth and development, and unique circumstances surrounding the pregnancy. For example, a teen mother may be more self-absorbed and less able to focus on the needs of her infant. A woman who has given birth to an unwanted pregnancy may have impaired bonding. Documentation in the nurse's notes concerning bonding behaviors is needed. Observations should include verbal and nonverbal behaviors of the parents (Box 28.4).

Childbearing practices and rituals of other cultures may be different from standard practices associated with bonding in the Anglo-American culture. For example, Chinese families traditionally use extended family members to care for the newborn so that the mother can rest and recover, especially after a cesarean birth. In some cultures, women do not initiate breastfeeding until their breast milk comes in. In other cultures, families do not name their babies until after the confinement month. The amount of eye contact also varies among cultures.

Box 28.5	Postpartum Danger Signs for Parent-Newborn Relationships

- Passive reaction, either verbal or nonverbal. (Parents do not touch, hold, or examine baby or talk in affectionate terms or tones about baby.)
- Hostile reaction, either verbal or nonverbal. (Parents make inappropriate verbalization, glances, or disparaging remarks about child's physical characteristics.)
- Disappointment over gender of baby.
- Lack of eye contact.
- Non-supportive interaction between parents. (If interaction seems questionable, talk to nurse and physician involved with delivery for further information.)

Become knowledgeable about the childbearing beliefs and practices of diverse cultural and ethnic groups. Because individual cultural variations exist within groups, clarify with the patient and family members or friends what cultural norms the patient follows. Incorrect judgments may be made about mother-infant bonding if culturally sensitive care is not practiced.

Some warning signs of possible difficulties in parent-child relationships, apparent immediately after delivery, are listed in Box 28.5.

Maternal Self-Image

An important assessment concerns the woman's self-concept, body image, and sexuality. How a new mother feels about herself and her body during the puerperium may affect her behavior, adaptation to parenting, and sexuality.

Feelings related to sexual adjustment after childbirth often cause concern for new parents. Women who recently have given birth may be reluctant to resume sexual intercourse for fear of pain or damage to healing perineal tissue. Because many new parents are anxious for information but reluctant to bring up the subject, postpartum nurses should include the topic of postpartum sexuality in a matter-of-fact manner. This may be addressed during the routine physical assessment and reinforced during the discharge teaching period (Box 28.6). This approach assures the woman and her partner that resuming sexual activity is a legitimate concern for new parents and indicates the nurse's willingness to answer questions.

Promoting Parenting Skills

Parents are responsive to praise of their newborn. Many need reassurance that the baby's blue appearance after delivery is normal until respirations are well established. Review the reason for the molding of the baby's head. Repeat information about the hospital's routine for future parent-child contacts. Encourage siblings to get acquainted with the new family member (Fig. 28.4). The hospital staff, with their interest and their concern, can do much to make this experience satisfying for parents, family, and significant others.

Box 28.6	Resumption of Sexual Intercourse

- A woman can resume sexual intercourse safely when bleeding has stopped and the episiotomy has healed. The mother should be scheduled to see her primary care provider at 6 weeks postpartum. At that time, the woman's perineum and cervix are assessed for readiness for sexual intercourse. For the first 6 weeks to 6 months postpartum, the vagina does not lubricate well.
- The physiologic reactions to sexual stimulation for the first 3 months after birth are slower and less intense. The strength of the orgasm is reduced.
- A water-soluble gel, cocoa butter, or a contraceptive cream or jelly may be used for lubrication. If some vaginal tenderness is present, the partner can insert one or more clean lubricated fingers into the vagina and rotate them within the vagina to help relax it and to identify possible areas of discomfort. A position in which the woman has control of the depth of the insertion of the penis also is useful. The side-by-side or female-on-top position may be more comfortable.
- The presence of the baby influences post-birth lovemaking. Parents hear every sound made by the baby; conversely, they may be concerned that the baby hears every sound they make. In either case, any phase of the sexual response cycle may be interrupted by hearing the baby cry or move, leaving both partners frustrated and unsatisfied. In addition, the amount of psychological energy expended in childcare activities may lead to fatigue.
- Some women report feeling sexual stimulation and orgasms when breast-feeding their babies.
- Instruct the woman to correctly perform Kegel exercises to strengthen the pubococcygeal muscle. This muscle is associated with bowel and bladder function and with vaginal feeling during intercourse.

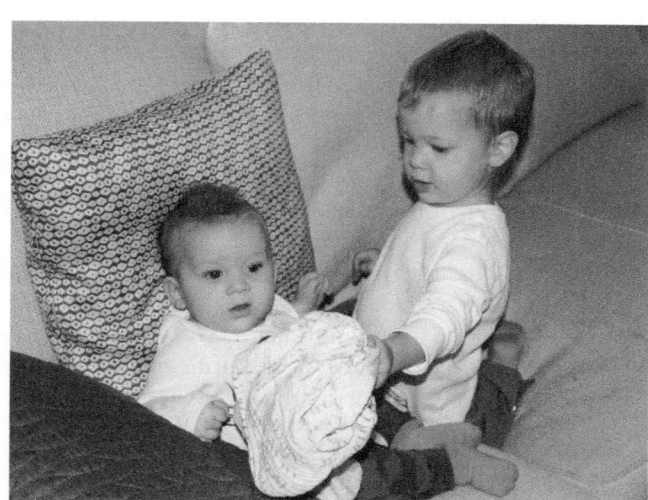

Fig. 28.4 Sibling involvement.

| Box 28.7 | Postpartum Maternal Teaching Summary |

FUNDUS (HEIGHT, MASSAGE)

- Fundus height shrinks one fingerbreadth a day.
- It is back into pelvis in 10 days.
- It feels firm, like a softball.
- Report bogginess to primary care practitioner immediately.
- Cramping may occur with nursing.

LOCHIA (AMOUNT, CHANGES, WARNING SIGNS)

- For the first 3 days, lochia is dark red, like menstrual flow; 2 or 3 days after this, it is pinkish brown.
- Moderate flow consists of four to eight lightly saturated pads a day.
- Flow continues for 3–4 weeks.
- In the last couple of weeks, lochia is a yellowish color with a musty, stale odor.
- Report any foul-smelling or bright red discharge or large clots.
- Flow may increase with overactivity. Rest; if flow does not subside, notify primary care practitioner.

PERINEUM (EPISIOTOMY CARE, CLEANSING, HEALING, DOUCHING, TAMPONS)

- Take sitz baths two or three times daily with vaginal delivery.
- Cleanse from front to back.
- Use perineal spray water bottle after voiding.
- Change pad frequently—after each voiding and when soiled.
- Do not douche or use tampons until after first office visit when primary care practitioner says it is okay.
- Continue using witch hazel (Tucks pads) for discomfort and to aid in healing.
- Episiotomy heals in approximately 3 weeks (when the lochia has stopped).

BREASTS

- Breast-feeding (nipple care, engorgement, feeding techniques, breast pump)
  - Air dry; use proper technique to break infant's suction to the nipple; wear a good supportive bra.
  - Pregnancy can occur while nursing; use a contraceptive.
  - For engorgement, apply heat, warm shower; may pump to enable baby to latch on.
  - Feeding techniques: demonstrate proper use; advise where to purchase materials; demonstrate manual expression; expressed milk may be frozen in plastic bottles or bags for up to 2 weeks.
  - May take a mild analgesic 1 h before nursing.
- Dry breasts (engorgement, fluid intake)
  - Wear supportive, well-fitting bra.
  - Avoid breast stimulation (warm showers).
  - Apply ice bags for 20 min four times a day.
  - Suppression of lactation takes about 5 days.
  - Do not drink excessive amounts of fluids (normal: six to eight 8-ounce glasses).

NUTRITION (NURSING, DIETING)

- Continue prenatal vitamins until gone.
- Nursing: need 500 kcal more than prepregnant diet; need increased protein, 400 mg calcium each day, 8–10 glasses of fluid each day; avoid onions, cabbage, chocolate, spices, and foods that may distress infant; no dieting during breast-feeding.

SEXUALITY (SEXUAL ACTIVITY)

(See Box 28.6)

- 45% of nonnursing mothers resume menses by sixth week.
- Breast-feeding does not protect against pregnancy.
- Avoid sexual activity until after first post-birth office visit and approval by primary care practitioner.
- If episiotomy is not healed and sexual activity is resumed, there is increased discomfort and chance of infection.

EXERCISE (WHEN, HOW MUCH)

- Increased lochia or pain means you need to reevaluate activity.
- Do not resume strenuous exercises until primary care practitioner approves.
- Gradually increase activity.

EMOTIONS (BONDING, "BABY BLUES")

- Parent-child attachment (bonding): schedule time to enjoy baby; use eye contact, cuddling, and caressing; enjoy infant feedings.
- Postpartum depression:
  - Mother may be tearful or anorexic and have difficulty sleeping.
  - Hormonal factors and fatigue are often responsible.
  - Notify primary care practitioner if prolonged, increased, or unmanageable.

CESAREAN BIRTH (INCISION, ACTIVITY)

- Notify primary care practitioner of any redness, drainage, separation of incision, temperature greater than 100.4°F (38°C).
- Do not lift anything heavier than baby, gradually increase activity.
- Take pain medications as ordered and needed.

REPORT TO PRIMARY CAREGIVER

- Temperature greater than 100.4°F (38°C)
- Chills
- Change in lochia: foul odor, return to bright red, excessive amount
- Calf pain, tenderness, or swelling
- Evidence of mastitis: breast tenderness, cracking, redness, or a feeling of discomfort or uneasiness
- Urinary urgency, burning, or frequency
- Severe or incapacitating depression

SAFETY (CAR SEAT SAFETY VIDEO, CAR SEAT DEMONSTRATION)

- Review infant safety from baby discharge sheet.
- Review car seat safety video if available.
- Volunteers have car seats to rent.
- Demonstrate proper use of car seat.

New parents may feel anxious about their abilities to care for their child. They may demonstrate uncertainty when attempting to perform care. Educate new parents about the needs of the baby and reassure them. Parents first become acquainted with their new baby as the nurse performs a physical examination and describes any normal variations. Nurses act as role models by providing compassionate, attentive care (Boxes 28.7 and 28.8). As one nurse described it:

I found the mother crying and distraught as she wrapped and unwrapped her baby. She said, "I don't seem to be

doing anything right." I took the baby from her and talked to him, "What are you doing to your mother? You have her all upset!" The baby alerted to my voice and looked at me. Then, I said to the mother, "Now you talk to him." She said, "You're a big, lovely boy; don't cry so much." The baby, hearing her voice, promptly turned his head to look at her. I said, "You see, he knows his mother's voice and prefers it to mine." The mother was surprised and seemed very pleased and excited. We then reviewed how to wrap a baby snugly.

Box 28.8   Newborn Teaching Summary

SECURITY
- Know the caregiver. Check references.
- Ask others who are trusted to babysit.
- Do not leave baby alone on flat surface because the baby could roll over and fall off the surface.
- Do not lay baby on abdomen; place on the side or back to prevent sudden infant death syndrome (SIDS).
- Car seat safety and the law:
  - Use until age 4 years or 40 lb.
  - Infant in car seat should be secured in back seat, facing the rear of the car.
  - These are the laws in most states; if you are stopped, you could be fined.

BATH DEMONSTRATION AND NORMAL SKIN CONDITIONS
- Skin should be soft, pinkish, and dry.
- Clean perineum from front to back to prevent urinary tract infections.
- Use hypoallergenic soap. Most babies need bathing only every other day.
- Keep diaper area as clean as possible. (Use no talc.)
- Keep head clean, rinsing well after each shampoo to prevent cradle cap.

UMBILICAL CORD CARE
- Use alcohol on cord stump daily. (Be careful to prevent alcohol from dripping down to perineal area.)
- Keep area dry; fold diaper down with plastic side on outside to prevent moisture retention.
- Sponge bathe for 7–10 days until umbilical cord comes off. (Do not soak in bath water.)
- Report any redness, drainage, or foul odor coming from umbilical area.

CIRCUMCISION CARE
- If a Gomco or Mogen clamp was used, apply petroleum jelly-covered gauze to penis after every diaper change. Keep area clean to prevent infection; cleanse penis carefully with warm water at least every 4 h.
- If a Plastibell is used, the plastic rim remains in place for about a week while healing takes place, after which the Plastibell falls off. Petroleum gauze is not necessary.
- Do not allow pressure on circumcised area. Loose diapering is necessary.
- Do not be alarmed when a yellowish crust forms; this is part of the normal healing process. Do not attempt to

remove this crust; it lasts only 2 or 3 days. Fanfold the diaper so that it does not press on the area.

EYE CARE
- Wash with water from inner to outer corner with a different area of the washcloth for each eye.
- Note that a special treatment was administered to baby's eyes on delivery. This may cause some swelling and redness. Do not be alarmed; this is normal.

DIAPER AREA CARE
- Change diaper as soon as possible.
- Wash from front to back, especially on girls, to prevent urinary tract infection.
- Cleanse with warm water and mild soap; dry well.
- If rash persists, call the health care provider.
- Use no powder. Air out diaper area when possible.

FEEDING METHOD
Breast
- Position: Entire body of infant should face the breast.
- Feed baby before he or she gets frantic and very hungry.
- Lightly brush the infant's lips with the nipple to start the rooting reflex.
- Alternate breasts with each feeding.
- Direct the nipple into infant's mouth with as much of the areola tissue as possible in the baby's mouth and over the tongue.
- Gently hold breast away from baby's nostrils; babies are nose breathers.
- To break suction, place finger between the baby's lips and the breast; do not pull breast away from baby.
- Mothers who have cesarean births need to support infant so that he or she does not rest on the abdomen for long periods.
- Burping baby:
  - Burp between breasts, over the shoulder, sitting up supported by your hands, or lying across your lap.
- Length of time to nurse:
  - Feed for 10–15 min from each breast.
  - Emptying both breasts is important because an empty breast signals the woman's body to produce more milk.
- Supplement: You may pump your breasts while away from baby; keep breast milk cold during transport.
- Breast milk can be safely stored in a refrigerator for 24–48 h.

Box 28.8   **Newborn Teaching Summary—cont'd**

- If breast milk will not be used within 48 h, it should be frozen immediately after being expressed. Breast milk may be frozen for 2 weeks.
- To thaw, gently shake container under warm tap water or place breast milk in a container of warm water. Thawed breast milk should be used immediately. It should not be refrozen. Do not use a microwave to thaw or heat breast milk.
- After the milk supply is established, an occasional bottle does not affect lactation or breast-feeding.
- Stooling pattern: Stools of breast-fed babies are loose. Some infants have a stool with each feeding.

Bottle
- Positions:
  - Never prop the bottle.
  - Hold the bottle so that fluid fills the nipple and none of the air in the bottle is allowed to enter the nipple.
  - Avoid overfeeding; be alert to infant cues that enough formula has been taken (e.g., falls asleep, turns head to side, or ceases to suck).
- Burping baby:
  - Burp baby every 0.5–1 oz of milk.
  - Position baby over the shoulder, sitting up supported by your hands, or lying across your lap.
- Preparing bottles:
  - Purchase formula in ready-to-use powder or in liquid concentrate to be mixed with water.
  - Many helpful pamphlets on formula preparations are available.
  - Prepare formulas with scrupulous cleanliness; if home conditions or the water supply is unsafe (such as from a private well), then water should be boiled for 15 min.
  - Give formula at room temperature; test formula temperature on inner wrist or back of hand.
  - Opened container of ready-to-feed or concentrated formula should be discarded after 24 h; date the opened container.
- After feeding, position baby on right side to discourage regurgitation.

CLOTHING
- Dress infant for the season.
- Dress infant in soft, comfortable clothing.
- Dress infant as you are dressed.

VAGINAL AND BREAST SECRETIONS
- As the maternal hormones clear the infant's bloodstream,

the infant may have a mucus-like, bloody vaginal discharge.
- Girl and boy babies may have a swelling of the breast tissue, and sometimes a thin discharge may be seen; this subsides as the mother's hormones are eliminated from infant's body.

BULB SYRINGE
- Squeeze out air to establish suction by compressing the bulb and holding it in.
- Gently insert tip of syringe into the side of infant's mouth and release; then suction the nares.
- Clean well after each use.

INFANT CARDIOPULMONARY RESUSCITATION
- Be sure to see video before dismissal if available.
- Teaching:
  - Give fingertip compressions (5–1).
  - Give puffs for breaths (1–5).
  - Cover baby's nose with cheek as you cover mouth.
  - Avoid stretching back too far in the head-tilt/chin-lift.

PHENYLKETONURIA, BIOTINIDASE, AND THYROID TESTING
- These tests should be performed on all newborns.
- Undetected abnormalities could lead to brain damage or death. With early detection and proper treatment, these are preventable.

AFTER DISCHARGE
- Keep, read, and refer to pamphlets if you have any questions.
- Use medication prescribed only by a physician. (Do not use nose drops because aspiration may result in lung complications.)

WHEN TO CALL PHYSICIAN
- If baby has sudden fever, rash, excessive vomiting, diarrhea, distended abdomen, or bleeding from circumcision, call the physician.
- Normal body temperature ranges from 97.6°F–99°F (36.4°C–37.2°C) when taken via the axillary route. This method is recommended until age 6 years.

NUTRITIONAL AND METABOLIC ISSUES

Recovery Stage

After the time and exertion involved in labor and delivery, the mother is often hungry. Most women do not have dietary restrictions after vaginal childbirth. After a cesarean section, women often have restrictions that limit oral intake to ice or liquids for the first day with a gradual reintroduction to normal diet. Fluids are important during the recovery phase to replace the fluids and blood lost during delivery; offer a variety of fluids such as water and juices. If the physician orders IV fluids, administer them promptly. When a general anesthetic has been used, such as during a cesarean delivery, verify the *presence of bowel sounds* before giving solid food.

If the woman used mouth-breathing techniques during labor, she may have dry mucous membranes, cracked lips, and noticeable breath odor. Good oral hygiene relieves these symptoms and reduces discomfort. A complete sponge bath or a shower with assistance enhances well-being and comfort by removing perspiration and other waste products from the skin.

Later Postpartum Stage

Diet remains an important concern postpartum. Many women are concerned about the weight gained during pregnancy and wish to lose the excess as soon as possible. Dieting must not deprive the woman of necessary nutrition. If the woman has not gained excessive weight during pregnancy, she usually returns to her prepregnant weight in 6 to 8 weeks without significant dietary restrictions. Most physicians do not recommend any weight-loss diets until after this time. Women who are not breast-feeding should continue to eat a well-balanced diet that follows MyPlate suggestions. Women who are breast-feeding generally continue the diet recommended during pregnancy because the body needs extra calories, vitamins, and minerals for lactation. The breast-feeding mother should maintain the increased caloric intake of 300 to 500 kcal/day as part of a well-balanced diet and should maintain a daily fluid intake of 2 to 3 L.

HYGIENE

During the postpartum stage, excessive perspiration is normal. The lochia has a characteristic musty odor. It should not have a foul or decaying smell. Encourage regular bathing (showers are preferred) to minimize odors and promote comfort. Most women are permitted to be up as tolerated within hours of giving birth, but they may experience vertigo as a result of vascular shifts related to the heat of the shower. If this occurs while the woman is standing in the shower, she may experience syncope and injure herself. The first time the newly delivered woman takes a shower, provide for safety by instructing her on the use of the emergency call signal and the length of shower time

recommended, and by placing a chair in the shower room. Also, check the patient frequently during her first shower to verify she is safe. Tub baths are not recommended until after the postpartum examination at 6 weeks so that no water that has been contaminated with bodily waste enters the vaginal canal or uterus until healing is completed.

Sitz baths, peri bottles, and witch hazel pads may be used to provide cleansing, reduce discomfort, and promote healing of the perineum. Peri bottles are filled with warm water and used every time the new mother urinates or has a bowel movement. The mother sits on the toilet and sprays the warm water over the perineum. Witch hazel contains chemicals that help reduce swelling. Sitz baths and peri bottles cause vasodilation from the warm the water, which helps reduce edema and speed tissue repair. Instruct the patient about water temperature and length of time. Most facilities use a personal, portable sitz bath that the patient can take home at discharge (Fig. 28.5).

If the woman has delivered via cesarean section, she has an abdominal incision with sutures or staples. Assess this incision in the same manner as any other surgical incision. It should remain approximated with no erythema, little exudate, and no malodor (foul odor). Traditionally, the patient has a dressing covering the incision the day of surgery. This usually is removed the next day by the surgeon. The incision likely is left open to the air. Those patients with staples closing their wounds have them removed in approximately 3 days. Adhesive strips may be applied after their removal and remain on for the next 5 to 7 days. Care should be taken so that clothing does not irritate the incision. The patient may shower with the incision

Fig. 28.5 Perineal care items. (A) Peri bottle. (B) Witch hazel pads. (C) Portable sitz bath.

that contains sutures or staples. Wounds with adhesive strips must be protected from the direct flow of water during a shower.

ELIMINATION

Recovery Stage

Diuresis and diaphoresis are common immediately after delivery. If the woman received IV fluids, urinary output may be increased. Support the bladder above the symphysis pubis and palpate it to check for fullness. Encourage voiding because a full bladder may interfere with complete contraction of the uterus, potentially causing hemorrhage.

The initial voiding should occur within 4 to 6 hours after delivery. Tissue edema from the delivery may cause difficulty with voiding. In addition, some women may have reduced sensitivity and are unaware that the bladder is full. Some agencies have a policy to assess voiding three times in measurable amounts of 300 mL or more after delivery to determine urinary elimination. Try measures to stimulate voiding. If the patient is unsuccessful voiding a sufficient quantity, catheterization may be necessary. If repeated catheterization is needed, a Foley catheter may be inserted. An indwelling catheter is inserted routinely before cesarean delivery and may remain in place for 1 or 2 days after delivery.

Later Postpartum Stage

Women may not have a strong sense of urgency when the bladder is full. The perineum also may be sore, resulting in a reluctance to regularly void. Encourage the woman to void at regular intervals of 2 to 4 hours. Urinary retention should be considered if a woman is voiding small amounts (less than 100 mL) frequently. The assessment of voiding patterns should include inquiries about symptom urgency and frequency or dysuria. Incomplete emptying of the bladder prevents the uterus from contracting normally and predisposes the patient to urinary tract infections.

Review proper cleansing technique after delivery. Instruct the woman to cleanse gently and pat dry from the anterior to posterior of the perineum. This method of cleansing prevents microorganisms from the rectal area being transported to the cleaner urinary or vaginal areas. A peri bottle may be used after each urination or bowel movement. Water should be warm (100°F [37.7°C]). Cleansing with toilet tissue is discouraged until the episiotomy or laceration is healed.

The shortened length of hospitalization after childbirth may result in the woman being discharged before she has a bowel movement. Health care providers differ on requirements that the new mother have a bowel movement before discharge. Fear of discomfort from the episiotomy, lacerations, or hemorrhoids may result in the woman resisting the urge to defecate. Bowel peristalsis may continue to be slow. Constipation may result when these factors are combined with a decrease in activity and loss of abdominal tone. Stool softeners may be prescribed. Promote good bowel habits by encouraging activity, fluid intake, and increased fiber in the diet. Occasionally, suppositories or fleet enemas are administered to promote bowel evacuation. Enemas and suppositories are contraindicated for women who have experienced third-degree or fourth-degree lacerations or extensions to their episiotomies. Sitz baths can also soothe the perineum and promote bowel elimination.

Patients with cesarean births, particularly those who received general anesthesia, are likely to develop problems with bowel function. The combination of general anesthesia and loss of abdominal tone increases the risk of ileus, so pay close attention to bowel function and report any abnormal observations promptly. To promote bowel function, assist with and encourage the patient to ambulate periodically throughout the day.

Perineal pads, worn to absorb vaginal drainage, should be changed after each urination or defecation. Teach the woman the importance of correct application and changing of the pad. Pads should be applied and removed from anterior to posterior and secured so as not to move about. If they are not worn correctly, contaminated areas could touch cleaner areas of the perineum and increase the risk of infection. Stress correct and scrupulous handwashing before and after changing to prevent cross contamination.

MAINTENANCE OF SAFETY

ACTIVITY AND EXERCISE

Recovery Stage

Monitor vital signs every 15 minutes for the first hour and then hourly for the next 4 hours during the recovery stage (Table 28.2). Ensure the mother is settled comfortably in bed. A patient who has just given birth may need to remain in bed for a time to allow her body systems to adjust to fluid volume changes. Early ambulation is key in the prevention of complications. Consider the baseline blood pressure, amount of blood lost, type and amount of analgesic or anesthetic medications administered during labor and birth, and level of pain when preparing to assist the woman to ambulate for the first time. The rapid decrease in intraabdominal pressure after birth results in a dilation of the blood vessels that supply the intestines (known as splanchnic engorgement), which causes blood to pool in the viscera. This contributes to orthostatic hypotension; when a woman who has recently given birth stands up, she may faint or feel lightheaded.

Instruct the patient to use her call bell to summon help before she attempts to get out of bed. Assess her color, pulse, and level of consciousness (LOC) in response to conversation and then assist her in ambulating to the bathroom. Once the woman has reached the bathroom, remain close with frequent inquiries as to her well-being. Have a wheelchair available in the

Table 28.2   **Vital Signs and Blood Pressure After Delivery**

NORMAL FINDINGS	DEVIATIONS FROM NORMAL FINDINGS AND PROBABLE CAUSES
Temperature	
During first 24 h, temperature may rise to 100.4°F (38°C) as a result of dehydrating effects of labor. After 24 h, the woman should be afebrile.	A diagnosis of puerperal sepsis is suggested if a rise in maternal temperature to 100.4°F (38°C) is noted after the first 24 h after delivery and recurs or persists for 2 days. Other possibilities are mastitis, endometritis, urinary tract infection, and other systemic infections.
Pulse	
Bradycardia is common for the first 6–8 days after delivery. It is caused by increased cardiac output and stroke volume. The pulse returns to nonpregnant levels within 3 months of delivery. A pulse rate between 50 and 70 beats/min is considered normal.	A rapid or increasing pulse rate or one that is increasing may indicate hypovolemia
Respirations	
Respirations should fall to within the woman's normal predelivery range.	Hypoventilation may follow an unusually high subarachnoid (spinal) block.
Blood Pressure	
Blood pressure is altered slightly, if at all. Orthostatic hypotension, as indicated by feelings of vertigo or syncope immediately after standing up, can develop in the first 48 h as a result of the splanchnic engorgement (the excessive filling or pooling of blood within the visceral vasculature after removal of pressure from the abdomen) that may occur after delivery.	Low or falling blood pressure may reflect hypovolemia as a result of hemorrhage. However, it is a late sign, and other symptoms of hemorrhage usually alert the staff. An increased reading may result from excessive use of vasopressor or oxytocic medications. Because gestational hypertension can persist into or begin in the postpartum period, routinely evaluate blood pressure. If a woman reports headache, rule out hypertension as a cause before administering analgesics. If the blood pressure is elevated, confine the woman to bed and notify the physician.

room or just outside in case the woman is too weak to walk back to bed. Encourage her to rest after the ambulation so that she can regain her strength. Keep aromatic ammonia ampules on hand; these can be broken if necessary to revive the patient who is ambulating for the first time.

The patient who had epidural anesthesia is kept in bed until she can fully move, feels sensation in her legs, and has blood pressure and pulse within normal limits. Assess her ability to communicate, her LOC, and her vital signs for stability (within normal limits) before allowing her to get out of bed. The patient should wear slippers when ambulating to prevent slipping or sliding.

The patient who has received analgesics must be observed closely until she has recovered fully from the medication (i.e., vital signs are stable within her normal range, and she is fully awake).

During the first 24 hours after giving birth, the woman's temperature may be elevated slightly if she is dehydrated. Elevations noted after the first 24 hours may signal the onset of an infection, and temperatures higher than 100.4°F (38°C) are significant and should be reported. Many women feel chilled after giving birth and appreciate an extra blanket or one that has been warmed. Sometimes a beverage such as hot tea or warm milk provides comfort. Tell the patient this chilling is a normal reaction to the stress of labor.

Slight bradycardia, 50 to 70 beats/min, is sometimes observed and is not considered abnormal if the other vital signs are within normal limits. Tachycardia may also occur in response to increased blood loss or physical exertion.

Blood pressure may be slightly elevated from exertion, excitement, and possibly the oxytocic medications. If the blood pressure is consistently elevated, or if the patient also reports headache or visual disturbances, complications related to gestational hypertension could be occurring. These often persist even after delivery. Notify the physician immediately. A decrease in blood pressure could be caused by altered intraabdominal pressure or hemorrhage. Watch changes closely and report them.

Later Postpartum Stage

Vital signs normally stabilize within the first 2 hours after delivery; report immediately any abnormality that persists longer than this. If vital signs have not stabilized within this time, continue to monitor them every 15 minutes to 1 hour and report significant changes.

A temperature of 100.4°F (38°C) or higher on 2 successive days during the first 10 days after delivery (not including the first 24 hours) is considered indicative of puerperal infection. Closely monitor any signs and symptoms of infection during the postpartum stage. Use good aseptic technique when caring for the postpartum patient. Review the signs and symptoms of infection with the new mother before discharge, and stress the importance of contacting the physician promptly if any of these occur (see Box 28.3).

Also assess pulse and blood pressure. Bradycardia may persist up to 10 days after delivery. Elevated blood pressure readings or a continued decrease in blood pressure may be significant and should be reported promptly.

Thrombophlebitis is a potential complication of the postpartum period. Early and frequent ambulation is the key to preventing this problem. Encourage new mothers to get out of bed and move about in the room. If the baby is kept in a nursery away from the mother's room, this is a good target for ambulation. If the perineum is uncomfortable, teach the woman to stand using the muscles of the legs while squeezing the buttocks together. This technique also helps when she attempts to sit. If she appears unsteady, accompany her when she ambulates. Ambulation is important for women who delivered via cesarean birth and may be initiated as early as the same day of surgery. Remember that inactivity predisposes patients to development of thrombophlebitis.

The flow of lochia may increase suddenly when the patient gets out of bed; secretions that pooled in the vagina drain out of the body when she stands. Once the lochia has changed to *serosa* or *alba,* excessive exercise or activity may result in the lochia changing back to *rubra.* This is a sign to slow down and increase activity gradually.

The physician indicates when postpartum exercises are suitable for the new mother, whether she delivered vaginally or via cesarean. The woman should begin gradually and avoid vigorous exercise until after the examination at 6 weeks, when the physician releases her to do so. Teach her isometric exercises that help with toning without causing undue exertion.

REST AND SLEEP

Rest and sleep are important through the postpartum period. After the difficulties most women encounter at the end of pregnancy, it is a pleasure to sleep in any position desired. Many women report that the night after delivery they get the best sleep they have experienced in weeks.

Hospital noises interrupt the sleep of many new mothers. Keeping environmental noise to a minimum to promote rest and sleep is helpful. Do not disturb the patient's sleep unless it is necessary to protect her well-being.

If she is breast-feeding, the new mother nurses her baby at 2- to 3-hour intervals during the night. This interrupted sleep pattern may persist for weeks until the infant is capable of sleeping for 5 or 6 hours without a feeding. Encourage the patient to take advantage of periods during the day when the baby is sleeping to rest and nap to compensate for lost sleep. If sleep

deprivation is prolonged, it may interfere with milk production and the let-down reflex.

REPRODUCTIVE ISSUES

Recovery Stage

Check the fundus and lochia every 15 minutes for the first 1 or 2 hours after delivery. The fundus should remain contracted, firm, and midline. This is critical because severe bleeding may occur if the uterus does not tightly constrict the placental site. A full bladder can displace the uterus and prevent its contraction. Encourage the patient to empty her bladder before checking the fundus. Palpate the uterus by placing one hand over the lower segment of the uterus near the pubic bone. Use the side of the other hand to feel the location and consistency of the uterus (see Fig. 28.1B).

If the fundus is not firm, it may be difficult to locate. An atonic uterus, one that has lost muscle tone, feels soft or boggy. Gently massage the fundus to increase contractility. Small clots are frequently expressed during this maneuver, and the uterus regains good contracted tone. If this does not result in contraction, the primary care provider should be notified. Oxytocic medications may be prescribed. Examples include oxytocin (Pitocin) and methylergonovine maleate (Methergine). These are usually administered intravenously to obtain prompt response. Methylergonovine may be administered intramuscularly or orally. Monitor vital signs closely if these medications are given because they may cause elevated blood pressure, bradycardia, nausea, headache, vertigo, and other side effects (Table 28.3).

While palpating the uterus, observe the amount of lochia. If the uterus is contracting well, small to moderate amounts of drainage are observed. If tone is poor, the amount of lochia is increased. Learn what amount is considered scant, light, moderate, and heavy. This is usually determined by the number of absorbent pads saturated in a period, such as pads per hour (Fig. 28.6). The time factor is important when assessing lochia. One pad saturated in 30 minutes is more serious than one pad saturated in 4 hours. Pay attention to the patient who has a small but steady trickle of lochia; the blood loss may be significantly greater than in those who seem to bleed larger amounts (see Table 28.1). Also, be sure to check under the buttocks of the patient who remains in the supine position; often, gravity causes drainage to miss the pad and pool under the patient.

Later Postpartum Stage

Perform daily assessments of the breasts, the fundus, lochia, the perineum, the rectum, and the vascular condition of the legs.

As done in the recovery stage, assess the location and consistency of the uterine fundus for the normal signs of involution. It is normally located at the level of the umbilicus on the day of delivery. The first day

Table 28.3   **Medications for the Mother and Newborn**

GENERIC NAME	ACTION	SIDE EFFECTS	NURSING IMPLICATIONS
benzocaine	Local anesthetic that inhibits conduction of nerve impulses from sensory nerves, temporarily reducing perception of local discomfort	Urticaria, edema, contact dermatitis	Cleanse area with clear, warm water after each trip to the toilet. Hold spray 6–12 inches from affected area and spray liberally. Use up to four times a day.
codeine (with acetaminophen oxycodone terephthalate	Pain reliever, narcotic	Drowsiness, sedation, nausea, vomiting, constipation, respiratory depression, urinary retention, allergic reactions, rash, urticaria	Avoid concomitant use of alcohol or other central nervous system-depressant drugs; tell patient to avoid driving or other hazardous tasks while taking these medications; warn patient that extended use may result in dependency; avoid overdosing mother on acetaminophen.
dibucaine ointment	Topical anesthetic	Allergic reactions, burning, stinging	Instruct mother that it is for external use only (application to severely denuded tissue may result in systemic absorption).
erythromycin ophthalmic ointment or drops	Ophthalmic antibiotic agent	Irritation of eye that lasts 24–48 h Vision may be blurred temporarily	Apply to conjunctival sacs of baby. Wear gloves. Cleanse eye first, if necessary. Spread the ointment from the inner canthus to the outer canthus on lower lid. Do not touch the tube to the eye. After 1 min, wipe off excess ointment. Observe eyes for irritation.
ibuprofen	Nonsteroidal antiinflammatory with antipyretic and analgesic properties	Heartburn, nausea, pruritus, lightheadedness, gastrointestinal bleeding	Give 1 h before or 2 h after meals; with gastrointestinal intolerance, give with meals; instruct patient to avoid taking aspirin or acetaminophen concurrently; teach patient to avoid alcohol intake and to report gastrointestinal distress or bleeding.
methylergonovine maleate	Oxytocic agent, stimulates uterine contraction, used to control postpartum bleeding	Headache, dizziness, nausea, chest pain, tachycardia, hypertension	Contraindicated in patients sensitive to ergot derivatives. Monitor blood pressure and heart rate after administration
oxytocin	Oxytocic agent, stimulates uterine contractions	*Mother:* nausea, vomiting, uterine spasm or rupture, water intoxication, seizures, cardiac arrhythmias, hypotension *Fetus:* cardiac arrhythmias, central nervous system or brain damage	Carefully monitor intake and output; fetal heart tones; and length, duration, and force of uterine contractions.
purified lanolin cream	Retains the skin's natural moisture and protects the mother's nipple from further abrasions	None; does not need to be washed off for the next feeding	Applied to the mother's nipple. Mothers with a history of wool allergy should not use lanolin before a skin test can be done.
Rh_o(D) immune globulin	Gamma globulin solution containing immunoglobulins (IgG); provides passive immunity by suppressing antibody response and formation of anti-Rh(D) in Rh-negative individual exposed to Rh-positive blood	Injection site irritation; slight fever and lethargy	Check lot number, administer IM only to mother, using deltoid muscle within 72 h of pregnancy termination.

Table 28.3	Medications for the Mother and Newborn—cont'd		
GENERIC NAME	**ACTION**	**SIDE EFFECTS**	**NURSING IMPLICATIONS**
rubella vaccine	Live virus vaccine	Rash, joint pain, pain at site Does not harm breast-feeding mothers	Administer IM in deltoid muscle during postpartum period; warn patient to avoid pregnancy for at least 3 months. Obtain informed consent.
simethicone	Antiflatulent	None	Instruct patient to chew tablet thoroughly before swallowing; give after meals.
vitamin K	Antidote for inadequate absorption and synthesis of vitamin K in neonate	With a large dose: hyperbilirubinemia, hemolytic anemia, kernicterus	Administer IM in the middle third of the infant's vastus lateralis muscle of thigh after delivery. Stabilize leg firmly.
vitamin, prenatal	Vitamin supplement	Nausea, vomiting	Tell patient it is important that pregnant women take prenatal vitamins and not regular vitamin supplements and that prenatal vitamins contain extra folic acid, which is needed for normal fetal development.
witch hazel	Astringent	Local irritation	Instruct mother that it is for external use only; use for relief of perineal discomfort.

Note: Hepatitis B vaccine is no longer given at birth while the patient is still in the hospital but in the physician's office, as determined by the health care provider.
IgG, Immunoglobulin G; *IM*, intramuscularly.

Fig. 28.6 Suggested guidelines for assessment of lochia volume. The pad may also be weighed and compared with the weight of a clean dry pad (1 g of weight equals 1 mL). (A) Scant, less than 1 inch (2.5 cm). (B) Light, less than 4 inches (10 cm). (C) Moderate, less than 6 inches (15 cm). (D) Heavy, pad saturated within 1 hour.

postpartum it may be one fingerbreadth above or at the level of the umbilicus; after that, it normally descends at the rate of one fingerbreadth per day (see Fig. 28.1A). When assessing the fundus of a woman who delivered via cesarean, carefully palpate the sides of the incision to determine uterine tone and position.

As during the early recovery stage, the fundus should remain firmly contracted. Manage any atony as described. If massage does not result in adequate contraction, notify the physician. Lochia may begin to change within the first 2 days from the rubra to the serosa form. Assess the amount of drainage. Frequently, less lochia is observed after cesarean deliveries because the uterine cavity is suctioned as part of the surgical procedure. The odor of the lochia should remain fleshy. If a fetid odor is detected, infection may be present; report this promptly.

Inspect the perineum and the rectum by having the woman assume a lateral position with the upper leg drawn toward the chest. The perineum should be approximated. If an episiotomy was performed, the tissue may appear edematous. Erythema is common. Ecchymosis is also common, particularly after a difficult delivery. Many physicians order some form of topical anesthetic, such as witch hazel (Tucks pads), to soothe the perineum (see Table 28.3). This should be applied to the perineum with a clean, lint-free tissue, not the fingers.

If localized edema, discoloration, and intense pain are observed in the perineal area, a hematoma may be present. This hematoma is caused by excessive bleeding into the tissue. A hematoma is most common after deliveries in which forceps were used. Hematomas may be obvious or may be concealed in the vaginal canal. If the woman reports persistent perineal pain or fullness in the vagina, notify the physician. This problem necessitates medical attention and perhaps surgical intervention.

Although the rectum and legs are not part of the reproductive system, these areas typically are included in postpartum assessments. Hemorrhoids (varicosities of the rectum) usually disappear quickly after delivery if there is no longstanding history of this problem. Use topical anesthetics to relieve pain if ordered by the physician. Sitz baths also provide relief and should be offered if the physician has ordered them. Suppositories may be ordered for hemorrhoid treatment.

Examine the patient's legs closely for warmth and redness. Question the patient about the sensation of pain in the legs. Early ambulation is the leading means of prevention of this potential complication.

The postpartum assessment can be organized as a head-to-toe assessment with the eight-letter mnemonic BUBBLE-HE (Box 28.9).

Box 28.9   Postpartum Assessment: BUBBLE-HE

Breast: For assessment of the breast, have the patient lie down and remove her bra. Palpate both breasts for engorgement or nodules. Inspect nipples for pressure, soreness, cracks, or fissures.

Uterus: The top of the uterus, the fundus, should remain very firm. If it becomes soft, the uterine muscles probably are not contracting properly, or the uterus has retained placental fragments. Both conditions predispose the patient to hemorrhage. Gently massage the uterus to help the muscles contract and expel placental fragments.

Bladder: The new mother may urinate frequently the first few days after giving birth. Be alert for signs and symptoms of infection. Also note any dysuria or urinary retention.

Bowel: Because of early discharge from the hospital, many women leave without having had a bowel movement. Assess for bowel sounds, encourage activity with rest periods, and encourage adequate fluid intake.

Lochia: Lochia has a definite fleshy scent, but if it has a fetid odor, it may indicate infection. Assess carefully.

Episiotomy: Most new mothers have an episiotomy and, in some cases, a laceration. (NOTE: There is movement away from doing an episiotomy on the side—either left or right—and possibly even away from doing episiotomies at all, but midline is the site of choice. For a lateral episiotomy, use the following procedures.) Position the patient on her affected side. Instruct her to flex her top leg at the knee and draw it up toward her waist. Use a flashlight and wear gloves. Stand behind the patient and gently lift her top buttock to expose the perineum. Also assess for hemorrhoids.

Homans' sign: For patient assessment, position the legs flat on the bed while she reclines in the supine position. Dorsiflex her foot toward the ankle. Assess both extremities. If she reports calf pain, Homans' sign is positive; further assessment is needed because a blood clot in a vessel in the leg is indicated.

Emotional status: Consider the three phases most new mothers pass through:
1. The first is "taking in," the time immediately after birth. She sleeps, depends on others for nurturing and food, and relives the events surrounding the birth.
2. Over the next few days, she is "taking hold." She is preoccupied with the present and concerned about her health and her baby's condition. She cares for herself and wants to learn to care for her newborn.
3. The next phase, "letting go," comes later in the postpartum period. She reestablishes relationships with other people.

Monitor the patient's emotional status, noting how she interacts with her family, her level of independence, sleep and rest patterns, mood swings, irritability, or crying.

Modified from Ferguson H: Planning letter-perfect postpartum care, *Nursing* 17(5):50, 1987.

Lactation and breast-feeding. All new mothers should be encouraged to wear a bra regardless of breast size. The bra should be comfortable and fitted to provide support. Non-nursing mothers need a bra that provides adequate compression to inhibit lactation without being uncomfortable.

With the bra removed, inspect and palpate the breasts. Observe for erythema, heat, edema, and engorgement. Visually assess the nipples for cracking and blisters.

Engorgement is an uncomfortable fullness of the breasts that occurs when the milk supply initially comes in. Three interrelated factors—congestion, increased vascularity, and the accumulation of breast milk—are the underlying causes. Filling of the breast with milk usually begins in the axillary region, so palpate the body and the tail of the breast. The condition may range from feelings of fullness to hard, painful breast tissues. In severe cases, women may even experience numbness and tingling of the arms and hands. Engorgement usually is observed around the third day postpartum and resolves in about 48 hours but may continue for up to a week. Because most patients are home by the time engorgement occurs, teach the new mother the symptoms of engorgement and methods of obtaining relief. If the patient is breast-feeding, interventions such as manual expression of milk and application of warm, moist heat are most useful. If the patient is not breast-feeding, compression of the breasts with a firm bra, wrapped ice packs, and analgesics are recommended most often. The use of cabbage leaves has been shown in some research studies to provide relief and reduction of engorgement (Gagandeep, 2013). Lactation experts recommend the placement of clean cabbage leaves inside the bra over the breasts. Some recommend the use of room temperature leaves and others suggest refrigerated, cooled leaves.

Inspect the nipples for inflammation, fissures, or tenderness. The nipples generally do not cause problems for nonlactating mothers; however, if the patient is breast-feeding, the nipples should be kept soft and supple. Most physicians recommend avoiding soap or other chemicals because they dry the skin and may be ingested by the infant. Plain water and air drying may prevent problems. Some physicians recommend allowing the nipples to dry after feeding without removing the milk residue. If additional moisturizer is needed, small amounts of unscented lanolin or a nipple cream may be used to soften and soothe dry, tender nipples. Modifications in the positioning of the baby may be needed if tender or cracked nipples continue to be a problem.

In addition to assessing the breasts, help the breast-feeding mother succeed in establishing lactation. To establish the lactation response, the breast must be stimulated adequately so that prolactin can be released by the anterior pituitary. Once the milk supply is established, prolactin production decreases, and oxytocin, released as the baby suckles, primarily maintains the supply of milk.

The mother may feel a tingling or prickling sensation, known as the *let-down reflex*, when feeding time

Fig. 28.7 Positioning the baby for breast-feeding. (A) Football hold. (B) Cradling. (C) Lying down. (D) Across the lap.

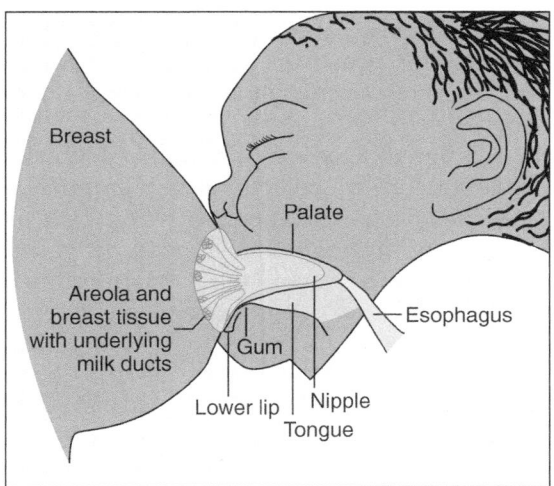

Fig. 28.8 Correct attachment (latch-on) of infant at breast. (From Lowdermilk DL, Perry SE: *Maternity and women's health care*, ed 9, St. Louis, 2007, Mosby.)

approaches. If the mother nurses the baby at regular, frequent intervals and empties the breasts, the supply of milk increases in response to the baby's demands. If the breast is not stimulated adequately, the lactation response may not be established. This can happen when the baby has a weak suck or is not put to breast often enough. If the breast is not emptied adequately, the pressure of the milk in the alveoli can also suppress milk production. Incorrect placement at the breast may also lead to problems. If the baby's mouth grasps only the nipple and does not apply pressure on the lactiferous glands (mammary glands or Montgomery's glands, consisting of 20 to 24 glands in the areolae of the nipples), milk is not released and the needed stimulation does not occur. This may also lead to nipple trauma and soreness.

Become knowledgeable about correct breast-feeding techniques to accurately instruct the breast-feeding mother. These techniques include correct position and placement of the nipple and areola in the baby's mouth, stimulation of the infant to enable correct **latch-on** (attachment of the infant to the breast for feeding), frequency and length of nursing, and care of the breasts. Also assist the mother's efforts by providing support and encouragement. Lactation consultants, teaching videos, and support groups, such as La Leche League, are excellent resources that supplement and reinforce teaching by the nurse (Figs. 28.7 and 28.8).

Manual pumping of the breasts may be necessary in some cases. The mother whose infant is unable to suckle at the breast at birth may pump to establish

| Box 28.10 | Advantages of Breast-Feeding |

- *Antiinfective properties:* Immunoglobulins, lymphocytes, and other immune components that are present in breast milk protect the infant against infection. The bifidus factor in breast milk encourages growth of normal bacterial flora in the infant's gastrointestinal tract.
- *Nutrition:* Breast milk is specifically made for the human infant. Its protein, carbohydrate, and fat ratios are thought to be ideal for growth and development. It is well digested and readily absorbed.
- *Growth and development:* Breast-feeding promotes better tooth and jaw alignment. It may be less likely to produce obesity in the child, and it may favor optimal bonding between mother and infant.
- *Allergy:* Breast-feeding may reduce the incidence of allergies in infants at high risk for allergic conditions.
- *Maternal benefits:* Hormones produced in breast-feeding help contract and shrink the uterus. Breast-feeding requires no formula preparation or bottle sterilization and is more economical than formula feeding.

lactation and provide milk that can be fed to her baby by alternate means. The mother who must spend an extended time away from her infant—going to work, for example—may pump to maintain lactation and provide breast milk for her baby during her absence.

Breast-feeding has many benefits for the mother (Box 28.10). The release of oxytocin during breast-feeding stimulates contraction of the uterus, so it undergoes more rapid involution. A lower incidence of breast cancer is found in women who have nursed for at least 3 months. Also, many women who breast-feed report a special closeness to their infants because they provide important nourishment. Human milk provides many factors that are suited uniquely to the infant and enhance growth and development. Human milk has antibacterial and antiviral properties, immunoglobulin, and antiallergy factors that protect the infant against many infections and diseases. Mother's milk also contains growth factors, digestive enzymes, and proteins that foster the maturation process begun in utero.

Patient problems and interventions for the breast-feeding patient include but are not limited to the following:

PATIENT PROBLEM	NURSING INTERVENTIONS
Insufficient Nutrition, related to nutritional demands during lactation	Review dietary choices
	Instruct patient to continue diet recommended during pregnancy
	Arrange consultation with a dietitian
	Inform patient of Women, Infants, and Children (WIC) supplemental food program

PATIENT PROBLEM	NURSING INTERVENTIONS
Anxiousness, related to initiating feedings as a result of inexperience	Evaluate patient's readiness to initiate feedings
	Initiate feedings as soon as possible
	Position mother and infant for comfort
	Initiate correct latch-on and position correctly
	Support and encourage mother in breast-feeding attempts

Bottle feeding is another choice for the new mother. If the mother chooses not to breast-feed, lactation must be suppressed. This can be accomplished by mechanical means, starting before milk production begins. The woman wears a supportive bra within 4 to 6 hours after delivery. Ice to the breasts also decreases the discomfort that may result from engorgement. She should avoid any form of breast stimulation, such as pumping the breasts, and avoid applying heat to the breasts, such as facing the hot water when showering. Do not restrict maternal fluid intake.

PSYCHOSOCIAL ASSESSMENT

COPING AND STRESS TOLERANCE

Many new mothers feel overwhelmed by the responsibility of motherhood. They may be intimidated by the nurses' capability and skill with the newborn. They often feel inept and may not wish to ask questions that may be viewed as unintelligent. Establishing rapport, listening, and anticipating fears and anxieties are important nursing measures. False reassurances are not helpful; thorough teaching and encouragement are far more beneficial.

Often, women experience a period of depression after delivery that is triggered by rapid hormonal shifts. This so-called postpartum depression, or "baby blues," may be mild or severe. It often appears between 2 and 7 days postpartum. Prepare the woman for the possibility of this and plan a course of action if it occurs.

SIGNS OF POTENTIAL PROBLEMS

No assessment of psychosocial needs is complete without an assessment for signs of potential problems. Not all potential psychosocial problems are identified easily. However, some signs may indicate a need for further evaluation by a caregiver skilled in that area (Box 28.11). The presence of one or more of these signs does not prove that a problem exists but may indicate a need for further assessment (see Chapter 29).

Roles and Relationships

The addition of a new family member has a major effect on roles and relationships. These changes are most obvious when the first child is born, but

Box 28.11   Signs of Potential Psychosocial Problems

- Inability or refusal to discuss labor and birth experience
- Refusal to interact with or care for baby (e.g., does not name baby, does not want to hold or feed baby)
- Refusal to attend infant care (including breast-feeding) classes
- Refusal to discuss contraception
- References to self as ugly and useless
- Excessive preoccupation with self (body image)
- Marked depression
- Lack of support system
- Partner or other family members reacting negatively to baby
- Expression of disappointment over baby's sex
- View of baby as messy or unattractive
- Baby reminding mother of family member or friend she does not like

Table 28.4   Transition to Fatherhood: A Three-Stage Process

STAGE	CHARACTERISTICS
Stage 1: Expectations	Father has preconceptions about what life will be like after baby comes home.
Stage 2: Reality	Father realizes that expectations are not always based on fact. Common feelings experienced are sadness, ambivalence, jealousy, and frustration. Father has overwhelming desire to be more involved. Some fathers are pleasantly surprised at ease and fun of parenting.
Stage 3: Transition to mastery	Father makes conscious decision to take control and become more actively involved with infant.

adjustments take place whenever another child joins a family. Time, money, and environmental and emotional resources must be divided to include the new member.

In our society, the mother still fills the role of the child's primary caregiver and faces the greatest number of changes. The responsibility of this role, 24 hours a day, 7 days a week, is overwhelming to many women. Today, because many women are independent wage earners, the loss of freedom is a difficult adjustment. The transition to motherhood can lead to feelings of guilt and confusion. Be sensitive to the mother's concerns.

The responsibilities of fatherhood often become a reality when the father sees his child for the first time. The realization that a totally dependent individual needs him is frightening to many men. The financial concerns of feeding, clothing, and sheltering his family take on new significance. A formerly two-income family may have only one income, the father's wages, at least temporarily. Even if the mother returns to work, there are new expenses for childcare. Both parents find that the child's needs take priority over their own needs or wishes. Freedom and spontaneity give way to a life circumscribed by feeding schedules, diaper bags, and babysitters.

Some men have little knowledge or experience in caring for infants; simple things, such as feeding, changing diapers, or even carrying a baby, may be intimidating. Help alleviate these fears by including the father in teaching whenever possible and by allowing him to verbalize his fears and concerns. Fathers go through a predictable three-stage process during the first 3 weeks of their transition to parenthood (Table 28.4).

Additional role adjustments relate to friends and the extended family. Friendships and socialization may take lower priority. Siblings assume a new position in the family order. Parents now become grandparents, and in-laws share grandchildren. These situations are all dynamic, and each family makes a variety of accommodations in incorporating their new roles.

SELF-PERCEPTION

The new mother commonly wishes to discuss her perception of the labor and delivery. She may spend considerable time with friends or in telephone conversation relaying her experiences of labor and delivery. Allow time for her to verbalize and work through her experiences. Reality may differ greatly from her expectations. She may need explanations to clarify things in her mind.

The new mother may be passive for the first day or two. This is called the taking-in stage (see Box 28.9). During this time, the mother needs supportive care. Her primary focus may be on herself and on personal needs such as sleep, food, and attention. She may defer to the nurses and let others care for the baby. This is followed by the taking-hold stage, when the woman is ready to assume greater authority and responsibility for herself and her baby.

Mood swings are common early in the postpartum period, related to recent stresses, fatigue, and rapid hormonal changes. Explain this to the new mother so that she does not become unduly concerned.

New mothers, particularly primiparas, commonly expect that they will regain their prepregnancy figures quickly after delivery. Many bring clothes that they hoped to wear home, only to be sadly disappointed. Be supportive and explain that it takes time for the body to regain the prepregnancy tone and shape.

COGNITIVE AND PERCEPTUAL ISSUES

Control of discomfort during the postpartum period is necessary for the woman to resume a normal activity level and get adequate rest. The most common discomforts experienced are perineal pain from the episiotomy and *afterbirth pains*. Afterbirth pains are cramping sensations that result from the contraction of the uterus. They are more common and may be more severe in multiparas and breast-feeding mothers.

Most physicians prescribe analgesics for these discomforts. Acetaminophen is commonly used, with or without codeine. Codeine is generally effective but is a controlled substance and has side effects, such as constipation and vertigo, which may be undesirable in the postpartum patient (see Table 28.3). Salicylates, such as aspirin, are usually avoided because they may interfere with clotting mechanisms. Recently, ibuprofen (Motrin) has been popular. Ibuprofen is an analgesic, an anti-inflammatory, and a prostaglandin inhibitor. It is often effective in reducing the severity of the cramping without altering the contraction of the uterine muscle. CAUTION: Ibuprofen is to be used with caution in people with kidney or heart disease or those taking diuretics.

Another major challenge of the postpartum period for the mother involves learning how to care for herself and the newborn. This can be overwhelming for the first-time mother. The nurse has limited time to teach all the necessary information. Most hospitals have teaching lists and printed handouts or booklets that cover all the key areas (see Box 28.7). To prevent the woman from becoming overwhelmed, pace teaching throughout the hospital stay, rather than leaving it until discharge. Be sure to document teaching about newborn care (see Box 28.8).

❖ NURSING PROCESS FOR THE POSTPARTUM MOTHER

The role of the licensed practical nurse/licensed vocational nurse (LPN/LVN) in the nursing process as stated is that the LPN/LVN will:
* Participate in planning care for patients based on patient needs.
* Review patient's care plan and recommend revisions as needed.
* Review and follow defined prioritization for patient care.
* Use clinical pathways, care maps, or care plans to guide and review patient care.

◆ ASSESSMENT

Assessment begins with admission of the patient to the postpartum unit from the labor and delivery unit. Review the prenatal history for obstetric history, prenatal care, and health status during the pregnancy. Also review the events of labor, delivery, and recovery, including the onset of labor, the mother's physical and emotional status during labor, progress of labor, status of fetus, birth, and status of neonate. A physical and psychosocial assessment should follow. Areas assessed should include the reproductive system, cardiovascular status, nutrition, elimination, activity and rest, maternal self-concept, knowledge level, parenting role,

attachment, home environment, and support system. Physical and psychosocial assessments are ongoing during the postpartum stay.

◆ PATIENT PROBLEM

Nursing assessment helps identify the needs of the postpartum patient. Care can then be based on these needs. Possible problems for the postpartum patient include, but are not limited to, the following:
* *Alteration in Family Processes*
* *Alteration in Urinary Elimination*
* *Anxiousness*
* *Compromised Parenting Skills*
* *Compromised Tissue Integrity*
* *Impaired Self-Esteem due to Current Situation*
* *Ineffective Sleep Pattern*
* *Infrequent or Difficult Bowel Elimination*
* *Insufficient Knowledge*
* *Insufficient Nutrition*
* *Potential for Compromised Parenting Skills*
* *Potential for Inadequate Fluid Volume*
* *Potential for Infection*
* *Recent Onset of Pain*

◆ EXPECTED OUTCOMES AND PLANNING

The care plan focuses on the needs of the postpartum patient and the nurse's ability to meet those needs effectively (Nursing Care Plan 28.1). Each patient has differing needs; care must be individualized accordingly.

The care plan focuses on goals and outcomes specific to the patient problem. Examples include the following:

Goal 1: Patient will experience relief of pain at episiotomy site.

Outcome: Patient uses appropriate pain relief measures, such as a sitz bath, topical anesthetic spray, and medication, as necessary.

Goal 2: Patient will provide appropriate safe care to infant.

Outcome: Patient demonstrates competence in bathing, feeding, diapering, and comforting infant.

◆ IMPLEMENTATION

Nursing interventions during the postpartum period include the following:
* Assess progress of involution by monitoring vital signs, breasts, fundus, lochia, and episiotomy.
* Administer oxytocics, analgesics, and stool softeners as ordered.
* Use aseptic techniques, good handwashing, and standard precautions when caring for patient and baby.
* Teach or demonstrate the following (see Boxes 28.7 and 28.8):
  * Breast care measures
  * Signs and symptoms of infection; prevention measures

Nursing Care Plan 28.1 | **The Mother With a Newborn**

Baby Caleb is a 39-week-gestation male neonate, 7 lb, 3 oz, and 21 inches long, born today to Philip and Anne P. Caleb was born via vaginal delivery after a 7-h labor. Ms. P. had epidural anesthesia. Her pregnancy and medical history were unremarkable. Caleb is Philip and Anne's first child, and Ms. P. has begun breast-feeding. Caleb will be circumcised tomorrow. He has been nursing every 3 h for approximately 20 min with a strong suck. At the initial assessment of Caleb 1 h after birth, findings were all within normal limits. He was given 0.5 mL vitamin K (AquaMEPHYTON) in the left anterolateral thigh, and erythromycin (Ilotycin) was placed in both eyes. His temperature on admission to the nursery was 97.5°F (36.4°C) axillary. After he spent an hour under the radiant warmer, his temperature was 98.6°F (37°C) axillary, and he was given his initial bath. Caleb currently is rooming with his mother, who is asking numerous questions about his care.

INFANT PATIENT PROBLEM

Potential for inability to regulate body temperature, related to exposure to cool environment.

Patient Goals and Expected Outcomes	Nursing Interventions	Evaluation
Stable infant temperature will be established and maintained	Dry infant immediately after birth. Wrap infant in warm blanket. Place infant under radiant warmer on admission to nursery. Place cap on infant's head. Keep infant away from drafts, exterior walls, and windows. Keep infant off cold surfaces. Monitor temperature q 30 min until normal, then q 4 h. Delay bath until temperature is above 97.7°F (36.5°C) axillary.	Infant's temperature remains greater than 97.7°F (36.5°C) axillary. Infant is placed under radiant warmer on admission to nursery. Infant is properly dressed. Infant shows no signs of cold stress.

MATERNAL PATIENT PROBLEM

Insufficient knowledge, maternal, related to being a first-time parent.

Patient Goals and Expected Outcomes	Nursing Interventions	Evaluation
Mother will verbalize understanding of infant care Mother will demonstrate infant bath and diaper change Mother will verbalize correct safety practices Mother will use correct breast-feeding techniques	Demonstrate and encourage return demonstration of infant bath, including umbilical cord care, circumcision care, and dressing. Demonstrate diaper change and cleaning of genital area. Teach correct positioning of infant. Teach techniques for breast-feeding. Teach methods to maintain infant's temperature.	Mother correctly bathes and diapers infant. Mother practices safe technique when handling infant. Mother successfully breast-feeds infant with correct techniques.

CRITICAL THINKING QUESTIONS

1. Even though Caleb is nursing well at each feeding, Ms. P. is anxious about her ability to successfully breast-feed. She asks how she will know whether Caleb is getting enough breast milk and whether she should supplement with formula, juice, or cereal. How should the nurse answer her?
2. A Gomco circumcision is performed on Caleb. After the procedure is completed, Caleb is returned to his mother's room. What should the nurse tell Ms. P. in response to her questions regarding diaper changes and care of the circumcision? How should the nurse describe the expected appearance of the circumcised penis?

- Nutritional and dietary requirements for healing and lactation
- Postpartum exercises
- Infant care techniques
- Provide comfort and pain-relief measures.
- Encourage patient and family to express feelings.
- Make referrals to community agencies as appropriate.

Implementation of nursing care involves putting into practice specific activities that should result in the expected outcomes planned for each individual patient.

◆ **EVALUATION**

Continually evaluate the success of the interventions. As the postpartum period progresses, the goals and interventions may change. Refer to the goals and outcomes to determine whether the plan was successful and the outcomes met. Examples include the following:

Goal 1: Patient will experience relief of pain at episiotomy site.

Evaluative measures: Patient uses sitz bath twice a day, applies topical anesthetic spray with each peripad change, and requests analgesics for episiotomy pain.

Goal 2: Patient will provide appropriate safe care to infant.

Evaluative measures: Patient demonstrates appropriate infant bathing techniques, use of infant car seat, and feeding techniques.

VALUES AND BELIEFS

Cultural beliefs and practices are important determinants of parenting behaviors. They influence the interactions with the infant and the parent's or family's caregiving style. For example, Asian mothers may remain at home with the baby for at least 30 days after birth and are not supposed to engage in household chores, including care of the infant. Many times, the grandmother takes over the baby's care immediately, even before discharge from the hospital. Similarly, a Jordanian mother may have a 40-day lying-in after birth, during which her mother or sisters care for the baby. Hispanics may practice a 40-day period after birth during which the mother is expected to recuperate and get acquainted with her infant. Traditionally this involves many restrictions concerning food (spicy or cold foods, fish, pork, and citrus are avoided; tortillas and chicken soup are encouraged), exercise, and activities, including sexual intercourse. Abdominal binding is a traditional practice, and many grown women avoid tub bathing and washing their hair. A traditional Hispanic husband may not expect to see his wife or infant until both have been cleaned and dressed after birth.

People in all cultures desire and value children. In Asian families, children are valued as a source of family strength and stability, are perceived as wealth, and are objects of parental love and affection. In the Yup'ik culture of the Alaskan Eskimos, where sharing traditionally has been necessary for survival, children are looked on as security. There is no concept of illegitimacy; every child is welcomed and loved. Adoption is common and is usually within the extended family.

Differing cultural values can influence parents' interactions with health care professionals. Because all members of a cultural group do not necessarily adhere to traditional practices, validate which cultural practices are important to individual parents. Knowledge of cultural beliefs can help with accurate assessments and diagnoses of observed parenting behaviors. For example, nurses may become concerned when they observe cultural practices that appear to reflect poor maternal-infant bonding.

Traditionally, Asians are taught to be humble and obedient. They are often brought up to not question authority figures (such as a nurse) and to avoid confrontation and respect the yin-yang balance in nature.

Because of these learned values, an Asian mother may not confront the nurse about the length of time before she receives the medication requested for her episiotomy pain. A mother may nod and say "Yes" in response to the nurse's directions for using an iced sitz bath but then not use the bath. The "Yes," in this case, is a courtesy, meaning "I'm listening," rather than an indication of agreement. The mother does not use the iced sitz bath because of her traditional avoidance of bathing and cold in the puerperium.

An Algerian mother may not unwrap and explore her infant as part of the acquaintance process, because in Algeria babies are wrapped tightly in swaddling clothes to protect them physically and psychologically. A Vietnamese woman may care for her infant but refuse to cuddle or further interact with her child. This apparent lack of interest in the newborn is this cultural group's attempt to ward off "evil spirits" and actually reflects an intense love and concern for the child. An Asian mother may be criticized for almost immediately relinquishing care of her infant to grandmothers and not even attempting to hold her baby when he or she is brought to the room. Family members show their support for a new mother's rest and recuperation by assisting with the care of the baby. Contrary to the guidance given to mothers in the United States about "nipple confusion," a mix of breast-feeding and bottle feeding is standard practice for Japanese mothers. This is out of concern for the mother's rest during the first 2 to 3 months and does not interfere with lactation; breast-feeding is widespread among Japanese women.

In helping new families adjust to parenthood, follow principles that facilitate nursing practice within transcultural situations (see the Cultural Considerations box).

PREVENTING INFANT ABDUCTION

An essential nursing role is protecting the infant from abduction (kidnapping). Precautions include teaching parents how to recognize the picture identification badge worn by birth facility personnel; this may be done by providing parents with written and oral information, including a picture of staff identification badges, and cautioning parents to never give their infant to anyone who does not have proper identification.

Staff members who are working temporarily on the unit are assigned special identification badges that are monitored carefully so that they cannot be removed from the premises without alerting the staff. In some agencies, an electronic sensor is attached to each infant with a bracelet or tag. The sensor activates an alarm if it goes near an exit or if it is cut or removed from the infant. With some systems, all exits lock automatically if an alarm is activated.

Entrances to the maternity unit should be in areas where staff can watch people enter and leave. Unit doors may be locked at all times. Entrance requires knocking, pressing a call signal, or using a card key

Cultural Considerations

Postpartum Period

- Many cultures emphasize certain postpartum rituals for mother and baby. In some cultures, including Chinese, Mexican, Korean, and Southeast Asian, these rituals may include bathing, activity, and dietary restrictions designed to restore the hot-cold (yin-yang) balance of the body. Please be aware that not all members of a culture follow the same practices. The following are only examples of some common cultural practices:
    - The mother may observe a long period of seclusion and rest with avoidance of physical activity. Household responsibilities and infant care are provided by other female family members. The period of seclusion may last from 2 weeks to 40 days.
    - These cultures avoid cold and maintain increased body warmth; avoid bathing, hair washing, exercise, and exposure to wind for 7–30 days after childbirth; and add extra heat (cover with blankets).
    - The woman may avoid cold and raw foods and water. She may eat only warm foods and drink hot beverages to replace blood loss and to restore the balance of hot and cold in her body. Traditional foods of culture are encouraged.
- The woman may wear an abdominal binder. She may prefer not to give her baby colostrum.
- In other cultures, breast-feeding practices are not established until after milk comes in because of belief that colostrum is "bad" for the baby.
- A low-income mother may need to contend with stressors that distract her from developing a relationship with her baby. Inability to pay for infant supplies or childcare, chaotic home situations, and worry over eligibility for social and health care services deplete the woman's mental and physical energy.
- An Arabic woman may eat special meals designed to restore her energy. She is expected to stay at home for 40 days after delivery to avoid illness from exposure to the outside air.
- A Haitian woman may request to take the placenta home to bury or burn.

Box 28.12   Precautions to Prevent Infant Abductions

- All personnel must wear appropriate identification that is easily visible at all times. No one without appropriate identification should handle or transport infants.
- Enlist parents' help in preventing kidnapping. Teach them to allow only hospital staff with proper identification to take their infant from them.
- Teach parents and staff to transport infants only in their cribs and never by carrying them. Question anyone walking in the hallway carrying an infant.
- Investigate anyone with a newborn near an exit or in an unusual part of the facility.
- Be suspicious of anyone who does not seem to be visiting a specific mother or who asks detailed questions about nursery or discharge routine.
- Be suspicious of unknown people carrying large bags or packages that could contain an infant.
- Respond immediately when an alarm sounds signaling that a remote exit has been opened or an infant has been taken to an unauthorized area.
- Never leave infants unattended at any time. Teach parents that their infant must be observed at all times. If no family members are present, the mother can take her infant into the bathroom with her, or send the infant back to the nursery if she wishes to nap.
- Take infants to mothers one at a time. Never leave an infant in the hallway unsupervised.
- When an infant is left in a mother's room, place the crib away from the doorway.
- If entrances to the maternity unit or nurseries are equipped with locks that open to codes or card keys, protect them from others.
- When a parent or a family member comes to the nursery to take an infant, always match the infant and adult identification bracelet numbers. Never give an infant to anyone without the correct identification bracelet or other proper identification.
- Alert hospital security immediately of any suspicious activity.
- Suggest that parents not place announcements in the newspaper or signs in their yard that may alert an abductor that a new baby is in the home.

or a code on the lock. Visitors to maternity units may be required to check in with security guards or other staff members and wear special visitor identification tags. Remote exits are locked and often equipped with video cameras and alarms. Staff must respond quickly whenever a door alarm sounds.

Newborns usually are abducted by women who are familiar with the birth facility and its routines. They are likely of childbearing age, are often overweight, and may live near the birth facility. They usually visit several times to learn the routines so that they can impersonate birth facility staff to gain access to a newborn. They often know the layout of the facility and the locations of exits well. The woman may have had a previous pregnancy loss or be unable to get pregnant. She may want an infant to solidify her relationship with her husband or boyfriend.

Although the woman plans the kidnapping scheme, she waits for an appropriate opportunity to take an infant (Box 28.12).

DISCHARGE: BEFORE 24 HOURS AND AFTER 48 HOURS

Early postpartum discharge, shortened hospital stays, and *1-day maternity stays* are all terms for the length of hospital stays of a mother and her baby after a low-risk birth. The trend of shortened hospital stays is based largely on efforts to reduce health care costs, coupled with consumer demands to have less medical intervention and more family-focused experiences.

Laws Relating to Discharge

Health care providers have expressed concern with shortened stays because some medical problems do not show up in the first 24 hours after birth. New mothers do not have sufficient time to learn how to care for their newborns and identify problems, such as jaundice and dehydration related to breast-feeding difficulties.

The concern for the potential increase in adverse maternal-infant outcomes from hospital early discharge practices led the American College of Obstetricians and Gynecologists, the American Academy of Pediatrics (AAP), and other professional health care organizations to promote the enactment of federal and state maternity length-of-stay bills to ensure adequate care for the mother and the newborn. The Newborns' and Mothers' Health Protection Act of 1996 provides minimum federal standards for health plan coverage for mothers and their newborns. The act requires all health plans to allow the new mother and the newborn to remain in the hospital for a minimum of 48 hours after a normal vaginal birth and 96 hours after a cesarean birth, unless the attending provider, in consultation with the mother, decides on early discharge.

MATERNAL FOLLOW-UP CARE

After delivery, the woman is instructed to make a follow-up appointment with her health care provider in 6 weeks. Some birthing units require this appointment be made before discharge. If the nurse schedules the appointment, the patient needs prompt notification of the date and time of the appointment. Women with complications may be seen sooner.

WELL BABY FOLLOW-UP CARE

Healthy infants are seen by the physician at 2 weeks of age. Babies who are discharged before 48 hours of age traditionally are seen by the health care provider within 3 to 5 days after discharge. The purpose of this appointment is to review nutritional status, elimination, and the presence of jaundice. The schedule of appointments for a well baby is every 2 to 3 months until age 18 months. Milestone visits are planned for ages 2 and 3 years and then every 2 years. These visits focus on preventive care such as health education, nutritional assessments, review of growth and development, and routine immunizations (see Chapter 30).

ANATOMY AND PHYSIOLOGY OF THE HEALTHY NEWBORN

ASSESSMENT IMMEDIATELY AFTER DELIVERY

In addition to Apgar scoring (see Chapter 27), which is done immediately after delivery, other assessments are performed to establish the newborn's gestational age. Gestational age is the actual number of weeks since conception. This age is important because many problems observed in newborns are age related. Because many women are unsure of the exact date of conception, calendar-based gestational age is unreliable. Physical and neurologic assessments based on established criteria are more reliable. Evaluate physical characteristics

within the first few hours of life. Neurologic assessment is done 24 hours later, after the nervous system has had the opportunity to stabilize from the trauma of delivery.

CHARACTERISTICS

Body Size and Shape

The newborn's head is disproportionately large for the body. The abdomen is prominent, with a smaller chest and narrow hips. The body usually is held in a moderately flexed position. A wide variation of size is seen in healthy newborns. The average newborn weighs 7 lb, 8 oz (3400 g) and is approximately 20 inches (50 cm) long. Charts are available for plotting height and weight. The head circumference averages 13 to 14 inches (33 to 35.5 cm) and is generally about 1 inch (2.5 cm) larger than the chest circumference, which averages 12 to 13 inches (30.5 to 33 cm).

Vital Signs

Respiratory rate averages from 30 to 60 breaths/min with brief periods of apnea. Breathing is diaphragmatic and should be effortless, without evidence of respiratory distress. Rate and rhythm vary with activity. Pulse rate averages 120 to 160 beats/min, with higher and lower variations depending on activity.

The heartbeat should have a regular rate and rhythm. Auscultate the apical beat between the fourth and fifth intercostal spaces. This is best done when the infant is asleep. Murmurs are common in the newborn and the physician determines whether they are significant. The blood pressure averages 60 to 80/40 to 50 mm Hg and should be approximately the same in all four extremities. A drop in systolic blood pressure (about 15 mm Hg) in the first hour after birth is common. Crying and moving usually cause increases in systolic blood pressure. The axillary temperature of the newborn should be between 97.6°F and 98.6°F (36.4°C and 37°C), with stabilization of temperature occurring within 8 to 10 hours after birth.

Skin

The infant's skin can exhibit a wide range of rashes and color changes (Box 28.13). Most are not significant and disappear within a few days. However, parents may be concerned until the changes are explained.

Color. The white newborn is usually pink to slightly reddish in appearance. The black newborn may appear pinkish or yellowish brown. Newborns of Spanish descent may have an olive tint or a slight yellow cast to the skin. Newborns of Asian descent may be a rosy or yellowish tan. The color of Native American newborns depends on the tribe and can vary from a light pink to a dark, reddish brown. By the second or third day, the skin turns to its more natural tone and is drier and flakier. The ruddiness results from normally elevated red blood cell concentration.

| Box 28.13 | Common Skin Observations in the Newborn |

- *Milia* are small white spots usually seen on the nose and chin. They are a result of occluded sebaceous glands and disappear spontaneously within a few weeks.
- *Newborn rash*, or erythema toxicum neonatorum, is an elevated, hivelike rash that may result in small white vesicles. It is not contagious and, like milia, disappears without treatment.
- *Telangiectatic nevi*, "stork bites," are flat pink or red marks often seen on the eyelids, nose, or nape of the neck. These are dilated capillaries that become more vivid when the infant cries. They are not significant to the health of the infant and disappear at 1–2 years of age.
- *Mongolian spots* are areas of increased pigmentation. The lumbar dorsal area is the most common location. The area may appear bluish black. These are most often seen in darker-skinned people.
- *Nevus flammeus*, port-wine stain, is a reddish-purple discoloration often seen on the face. This is a capillary angioma below the epidermis. Unfortunately, these do not disappear spontaneously. Medical techniques have been developed that reduce or remove port-wine birthmarks.
- *Strawberry birthmarks*, nevus vasculosus, are capillary hemangiomas. These may continue to increase in size for several months. Normally, they then begin to shrink spontaneously and usually disappear early in childhood.

The hands and feet may appear slightly blue; this is called **acrocyanosis** and is caused by poor peripheral circulation. Acrocyanosis can last for 7 to 10 days. It is observed most commonly when the infant becomes cold. Mottling, a lacy pattern with dilated vessels on pale skin, is also common. Another normal variation is called the **harlequin sign**; half of the newborn's body appears deep red, and the other half appears pale, as a result of vasomotor disturbance, with some vessels constricting while others dilate. When the infant is placed on one side, the dependent half is noticeably pinker than the superior half. This may last for up to 20 minutes. Although disturbing to view, it is not harmful.

The newborn's hemoglobin and hematocrit levels frequently are elevated; hemoglobin may range from 14 to 24 g/dL, and hematocrit from 44% to 64%. These elevated levels are needed by the fetus to assist with oxygen transport. After delivery, the neonate does not require these same levels. As the infant's body begins to manage this elevation and cells are broken down, jaundice results. *Jaundice,* a yellow discoloration caused by deposits of bile pigments and known as *icterus neonatorum,* is detected first over bony prominences on the face and the mucous membranes. Normally occurring jaundice results approximately 48 hours after birth and is termed physiologic jaundice. It gradually disappears by the 7th to 10th day. Jaundice that occurs sooner than 48 hours after birth is termed pathologic jaundice. This type of jaundice is not normal and may be the result of a maternal-fetal blood incompatibility. Further assessment of jaundice is necessary. The physician may order laboratory and diagnostic tests to determine the nature of the problem and begin treatment to prevent complications. Causes of jaundice are discussed further in Chapter 29.

Appearance. At birth, the skin is covered with a yellowish white, cream cheese-like substance called **vernix caseosa**. This substance protects the infant's skin from the amniotic fluid. When the vernix caseosa is removed, the skin may appear dry and may crack, flake, and peel. Another common finding is **lanugo** (downy, fine hair characteristic of the fetus between 20 weeks of gestation and birth). Lanugo is most noticeable over the shoulders, forehead, and cheeks, but it is found on nearly all parts of the body, except the palms, soles, and scalp.

Good turgor and tissue elasticity are normally observed. Desquamation of the skin of the term infant does not occur until a few days after birth. Its presence at birth is an indication of postmaturity.

Head

The **fontanelles** (broad area or soft spot that consists of a strong band of connective tissue contiguous with [touching] cranial bones and located at the junction of the bones) should be palpable. The *anterior fontanelle* is normally large and diamond shaped and closes at approximately 18 months of age. The *posterior fontanelle* is smaller and triangular and normally closes at 2 months of age. The sagittal suture may be felt by running the fingers between the two fontanelles (see Chapter 27, Fig. 27.2).

The newborn's head may manifest many variations. Most of these are a result of the birth process and disappear without treatment shortly after the delivery.
- *Molding* is overlapping of the bones of the skull. The head may appear elongated and misshapen; this condition is a result of compression during delivery and normally disappears within a day or two.
- *Caput succedaneum* is commonly seen with molding. It is the result of edema in the soft tissue of the scalp. The tissue feels spongy and may be felt over suture lines. This also disappears without treatment (Fig. 28.9A).
- *Cephalhematoma* is caused by bleeding within the periosteum of a cranial bone. It is confined to a particular bone and does not cross suture lines. This is usually a result of difficult labor. Cephalhematomas generally appear 1 or 2 days after birth. These normally absorb without treatment. Large hematomas may lead to anemia and jaundice, which necessitate medical intervention (see Fig. 28.9B).

Face. The newborn's chin is receding, and the nose is relatively flat. Fat pads make the cheeks appear full and

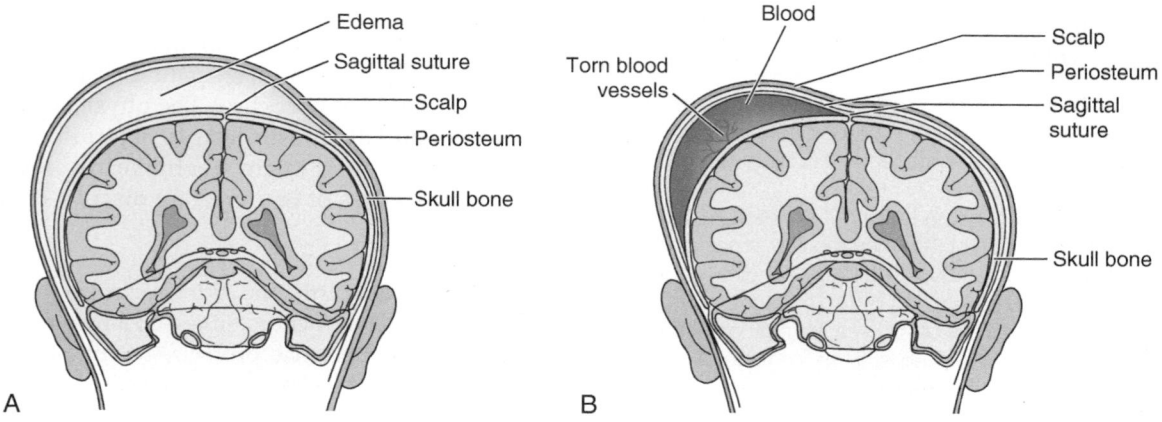

Fig. 28.9 Differences between caput succedaneum and cephalhematoma. (A) Caput succedaneum: edema of scalp noted at birth; crosses suture line. (B) Cephalhematoma: bleeding between periosteum and skull bone that appears within first 2 days; does not cross suture lines.

Fig. 28.10 External genitalia. (A) Genitalia in female term infant. (B) Genitalia in male infant. Uncircumcised penis. Rugae cover scrotum, indicating term gestation.

round. Movements of the face should be symmetric. The mouth should open freely, and the oral cavity should be intact with a closed palate. Small white nodules called *Epstein's pearls* may be observed on the hard palate. These are a result of epithelial cells and disappear spontaneously within a few weeks. Rarely, an infant is born with teeth; these teeth should be watched closely, because they may become loose and be aspirated. The oral cavity should be clean and free from lesions. A fungal infection may be acquired during passage through the birth canal if the mother is infected with *Candida albicans*. This results in thrush, a white, patchy coating of the mucous membranes that cannot be wiped off. Treatment with antifungal medications such as nystatin or gentian violet is necessary.

Eyes. The eyelids may appear edematous because of prophylactic antibiotic medication that was applied to the eyes after birth to prevent *ophthalmia neonatorum* (infection in the neonate's eyes, usually resulting from gonorrheal or other infection contracted when the fetus passes through the birth canal [vagina]). The eyes appear wide set. *Strabismus* (crossed eyes) and *nystagmus* (abnormal motion of the eyes) are commonly seen as a result of the newborn's immature nervous system. Most white infants have slate-gray to blue irises at birth; in darker skinned infants, the irises may appear darker. The newborn does not produce tears because the lacrimal structures have not fully matured. Tears may not be present during crying for the first few months of life. Vision has been found to be more acute than previously believed. Newborns are nearsighted and can see objects best at 8 to 10 inches; most prefer simple patterns in black and white and human faces. Make certain the parents know this, because eye contact with the baby is an important part of bonding.

Ears. The ears are normally positioned with the upper insertion of the pinna located even with the outer canthus of the eye. Low-set ears may indicate a chromosomal disorder. Newborns are most attentive to high-pitched sounds and the mother's voice. The fetus becomes familiar with the mother's voice in utero.

Fig. 28.11 The cord clamp is removed when the end of the cord is dry and crisp. The clamp is cut (A) and separated (B). NOTE: No triple dye was used; the diaper is folded down away from the cord area.

Umbilical Cord

The umbilical cord is whitish blue-gray with three vessels (one vein and two arteries) and contains a gelatinous tissue called Wharton's jelly. Inspect the cord for the number of vessels, because a two-vessel cord may indicate congenital anomalies. In Fig. 28.10, note the cord stump in *A* and the cord stump in *B* (triple dye gives it the purplish color).

Providing cord care. Check the cord for bleeding or oozing during the early hours after birth. The cord clamp must be fastened securely with no skin caught in it. Purulent drainage, redness, or edema at the base indicates infection. The cord becomes brownish black within 2 or 3 days and falls off in about 10 to 14 days.

Care of the cord varies in different agencies. It may be treated with a bactericidal substance, such as triple-dye solution (see Fig. 28.10B), antibiotic ointment, or alcohol, three times a day or allowed to dry naturally. None of the commonly used treatments are better at keeping the cord clean and dry than the others. When soiled, the cord should be cleaned with water. This natural treatment of cords may shorten the time to cord separation and does not lead to increased infections. The diaper is folded below the cord to keep the cord dry and free from contamination with urine.

Remove the cord clamp about 24 hours after birth if the end of the cord is dry (Fig. 28.11). Although the base of the cord is still moist, it does not bleed if the end is dry and crisp.

Reflexes

Healthy newborns exhibit a wide variety of reflexes (Table 28.5). Some are protective reflexes, such as the rooting, sucking, gag, swallow, blink, burp, hiccup, and sneeze reflexes. Other reflexes, such as the Babinski's, Moro, tonic neck, and stepping reflexes, are related to the immature nervous system. Many are present for a limited time and then disappear.

Genitalia

The genitalia in female newborns may be edematous (see Fig. 28.10A). Discharge of blood-tinged mucus from the vagina, called **pseudomenstruation**, may occur in response to maternal hormones. Either gender may have enlarged breasts. This is called **gynecomastia** and is also a result of maternal hormones. The labia majora cover the minora in term infants (see Fig. 28.10A). The scrotum in the male may be enlarged and edematous, which indicates a hydrocele. The testicles are normally descended in term infants (see Fig. 28.10B); in preterm infants, they may not be descended (**cryptorchidism**). If the testicles are not descended, the condition is monitored until they do descend. In the event they have not by the age of 18 months to 2 years, surgical intervention is necessary. Inspect the penis for position of the urethral meatus. Abnormal placement may result in problems with voiding. **Circumcision** (the surgical removal of the foreskin) normally is not done if there is any malplacement, because the foreskin may be used as part of the surgical correction.

Spine

The spine should be straight without curves. The normal cervical and lumbar curves develop once the infant begins to stand. Also, examine the spine for dimples, tufts of hair, and masses that may indicate abnormalities of spinal column development.

Extremities

The arms and hands generally are flexed against the body. Both arms should move evenly. Trauma during delivery may result in fracture of the clavicle or in brachial palsy. Both hands should be free from webbing (**syndactyly**, malformation of digits, commonly seen as webbing or fusion of two or more digits to form one structure) or extra digits **(polydactyly)**. A single crease in the palm of the hand, a simian line, may indicate chromosomal disorders such as *Down syndrome* (mongolism or trisomy 21, caused by an extra chromosome 21 in the G group) (see Chapter 31). Nails often extend beyond the fingertips. Legs should be equal in length. If one leg appears longer or if the gluteal or popliteal folds are *asymmetric* (unequal in size or shape), congenital hip dysplasia may be suspected. The hips should move freely.

Also assess the feet for syndactyly or polydactyly. Creases should cover at least the anterior two-thirds of the sole. The feet may appear to be turned abnormally, often the result of the newborn's position in utero.

NURSING ASSESSMENT AND INTERVENTIONS FOR THE NEWBORN

HEALTH MANAGEMENT AND HEALTH PERCEPTION

Each time the baby is given to the mother, the identification must be checked to prevent giving the wrong baby to the wrong mother.

Instruct the mother about hand hygiene when caring for the baby to prevent the spread of microorganisms.

Table 28.5	Assessment of Reflexes in the Healthy Newborn

EXPECTED BEHAVIORAL RESPONSE	COMMENTS	
Moro (Startle) Reflex		
Sudden jarring or change in equilibrium causes extension and abduction of extremities and fanning of fingers, with index finger and thumb forming a C shape, followed by flexion and adduction of extremities; legs may weakly flex; infant may cry.	Elicit reflex by holding the infant above the examining table in a supine position with one hand beneath the sacrum and the other supporting the upper back and head; then allow the infant's head to suddenly fall about 30 degrees. Disappears after 3–4 months; usually strongest during first 2 months.	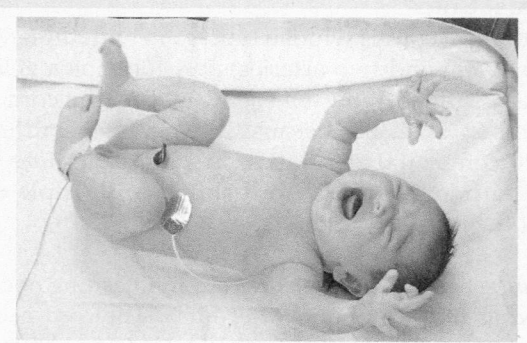
Tonic Neck Reflex		
When infant's head is quickly turned to one side, arm and leg extend on that side, and opposite arm and leg flex; posture resembles a fencing position.	Disappears by 3–4 months of age, to be replaced by symmetric positioning of both sides of body.	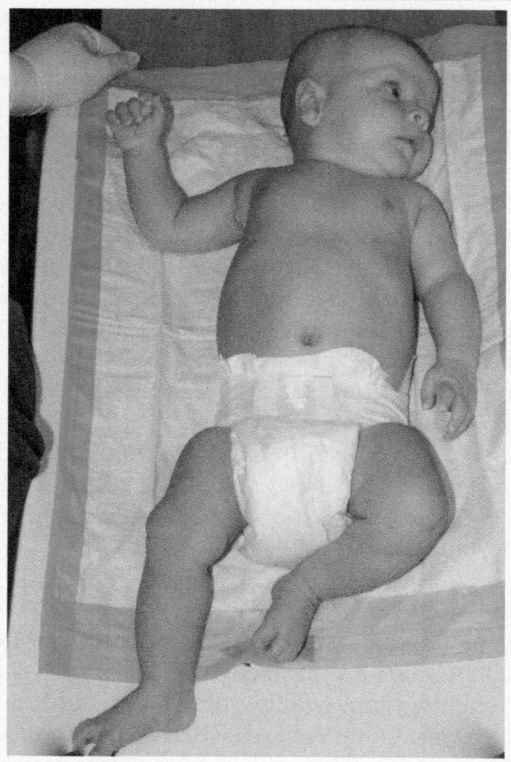

Table 28.5   Assessment of Reflexes in the Healthy Newborn—cont'd

EXPECTED BEHAVIORAL RESPONSE	COMMENTS	
Dance or Stepping Reflex		
If infant is held so that sole of foot touches a hard surface, there is a reciprocal flexion and extension of the leg, simulating walking.	Disappears after 3–4 weeks, to be replaced by deliberate movement.	
Babinski's Reflex		
When the sole of the foot is stroked along side of sole beginning at heel and then moving across ball of foot to big toe, toes fan out with dorsiflexion of big toe.	Disappears by 1 year. Absence laterally indicates central nervous system damage.	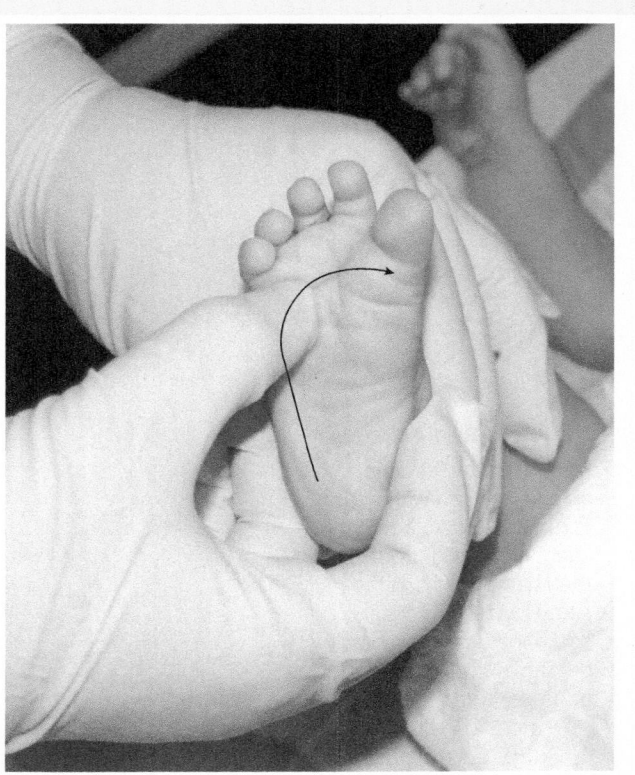

Continued

Table **28.5** **Assessment of Reflexes in the Healthy Newborn—cont'd**

EXPECTED BEHAVIORAL RESPONSE	COMMENTS
Grasp Reflex	
Palmar. Place finger in the palm of the hand. Infant's fingers curl around examiner's fingers.	
Plantar. Place fingers at the base of the toes. Toes curl downward.	
Pull to Sit (Traction) Reflex	
Pull infant up by the wrist from supine position with head in midline. Head lags until infant is in upright position, then head is held in the same place with chest and shoulder momentarily before falling forward; infant attempts to right head.	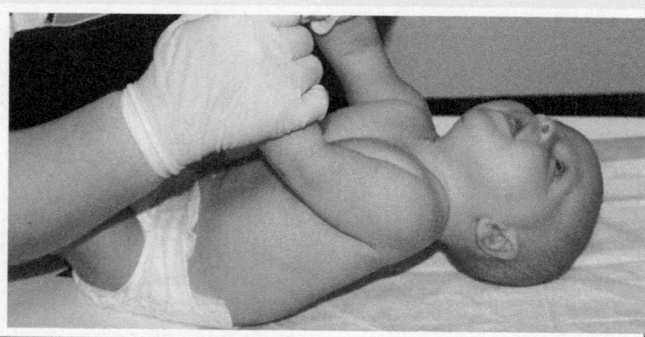

Moro reflex image from McKinney ES, James SR, Murray SS, et al: *Maternal-child nursing,* ed 4, St. Louis, 2013, Saunders.

Fig. 28.12 Holding baby securely with support for head. (A) Holding newborn while moving from one place to another. (B) Holding newborn upright in burping position. (C) Football hold. (D) Cradle hold.

Stress the importance of hand hygiene after performing personal care and before caring for the infant.

Instruct the new mother in safety practices to reduce the likelihood of injury to the infant. Education should include positions that provide head support to the infant during handling (Fig. 28.12). The mother must recognize the safety hazards of leaving the baby unattended in unsafe locations, such as the bed or changing table. To reduce the incidence of sudden infant death syndrome (SIDS), instruct parents to place babies on their back for sleeping. Include discussions concerning the risk to the infant from secondhand smoke. Babies exposed to smoke are more likely to die of SIDS. To prevent aspiration, the infant should not be placed immediately in the prone position after feeding (CDC, 2020). The environment should be kept free of hazards, such as pins or other sharp objects. Demonstrate bathing techniques and temperature taking. Bottles should never be propped for feeding because this may lead to choking or aspiration. All 50 states have legislation mandating the use of car seats for infants (Governors Highway Safety Association, n.d.).

NUTRITIONAL AND METABOLIC ISSUES

Each state has laws requiring that newborn screening testing be completed. The laws vary by state. These tests are done to detect conditions that result in serious complications, such as neurologic disorders and cognitive impairment. With early detection and proper treatment, many complications can be eliminated or reduced. Most of the diseases being tested for involve inborn errors of metabolism in which the newborn is unable to metabolize various nutrients. Some of the more common tests are done to detect phenylketonuria, maple sugar urine disease, galactosemia, and hypothyroidism. These tests involve either blood or urine samples. For accurate results, the newborn must have consumed an adequate amount of nutrition (human milk or commercial infant formula preparation). This period is traditionally after 48 hours of age. Infants discharged before this period have an initial screening completed and are required to return for the remaining screening during 2 to 5 days of age. The parents must understand the importance of the tests and when the newborn is to be tested (Table 28.6).

Newborns have low prothrombin levels at birth and are at risk for hemorrhage. Because they are not able to synthesize vitamin K in the colon until they have adequate intestinal flora, a vitamin K injection (AquaMEPHYTON) is administered routinely. Injections are best administered in the vastus lateralis

Table 28.6	Standard Laboratory Results for a Full-Term Infant
PARAMETER	**VALUE**
Hematocrit	14–24 g/dL
Glucose	40–60 mg/dL
Bilirubin, direct	0–1 mg/dL
Hemoglobin	14–24 g/dL

Heel-stick capillary blood.

muscle because it is more developed than the newborn's other muscles.

Monitor weight daily. A newborn normally loses up to 10% of body weight in the first week of life, from a combination of factors. More weight is lost through the passing of meconium and urine than is taken in by the newborn. This is particularly true in breast-fed babies. Most newborns regain their birth weight within the second week.

Nutritional Requirements

The healthy newborn needs approximately 120 kcal/kg of body weight each day. This includes proteins, carbohydrates, fats, vitamins, and minerals. Breast milk and prepared formulas are balanced to meet the newborn's needs. Because newborns cannot concentrate urine efficiently, fluid intake needs are high; 140 to 160 mL/kg/day is necessary (1 kg = 2.2 lb).

With the improved formulas available today, the infant's fluid and nutritional needs can be met with either breast-feeding or bottle feeding. The mother can choose the method she prefers. Provide support and instructions appropriate to the mother's chosen method.

Breast milk is produced in three stages. **Colostrum**, the first substance produced, is thin, watery, and slightly yellow. It is rich in protein and calories in addition to antibodies and lymphocytes. It also contains high levels of immunoglobulins, which transfer some immunity to the newborn. The mother begins producing colostrum in the last trimester of pregnancy and continues for 2 to 4 days after delivery; she then produces transitional milk for about 1 week. This milk may appear thinner and more watery but is high in fats, lactose, and water-soluble vitamins and contains more calories than colostrum. Mature milk generally is established by 2 weeks after delivery. This milk may appear very thin and watery. It provides 20 kcal/oz and contains lactose, proteins, minerals, and vitamins. If the mother is eating properly, only supplemental vitamin D may be needed; the primary care provider should be consulted.

Because human milk is uniquely designed to meet the needs of the human infant, it is used as the standard for all infant feedings. Infants who are not breast-fed should be given commercial formulas. Low-income families should be referred to WIC to determine their eligibility for services through the program, which provides iron-fortified infant formula.

Bovine milk (cow's milk) is the basis of most formulas. Infants with an allergic reaction to cow's milk formula may experience diarrhea, rash, colic, vomiting, and, in extreme cases, failure to thrive. Soy milk formula is acceptable for some of these infants, but others are allergic to soy protein. If hypersensitivity to cow's milk protein is suspected, a hydrolyzed casein formula may be effective; however, these special formulas are expensive.

Formulas are produced by modifying cow's milk to make it more similar to human milk. It appears thicker and richer but also contains 20 kcal/oz. Formulas are available in ready-to-feed, powdered, and concentrated forms. Instruct the mother in proper preparation and storage to prevent nutritional or digestive problems in her infant.

In bottle-fed infants, the first feeding is normally 15 to 30 mL of sterile water. This must be given with caution to verify that the infant is able to swallow normally and has no anomalies of the digestive tract. If the infant takes the water without difficulty, begin bottle feeding. Breast-fed newborns can be put to breast to nurse immediately after birth, without a sterile water feeding.

Regurgitation of mucus after the first few feedings is normal for infants. Food intake is necessary to prevent hypoglycemia, which is stressful to the newborn. Some facilities have a policy that requires a blood glucose determination test. Excessive maternal glucose results in fetal hyperglycemia and fetal hyperinsulinism. After birth, the neonate's high levels of insulin deplete the glucose stores, and hypoglycemia results. If the infant's blood glucose level is 40 mg/dL or less, sterile glucose water is given in the first hours after birth.

The frequency of feeding depends on the type of feeding. Breast-fed babies tend to do best on an "on demand" schedule, generally nursing at 2- to 3-hour intervals. Bottle-fed babies tend to eat less frequently, usually every 2 to 4 hours, because formula is digested more slowly. Each baby establishes a pattern over time. It is important not to overfeed, particularly with bottle-fed babies, because this can lead to regurgitation. Breast-fed infants are not normally given glucose water supplements because doing so may interfere with the process of establishing lactation; the neonate may not be adequately hungry when put to breast, so exceptions may be made in cases in which the newborn's blood glucose is low.

Bottle-fed and breast-fed babies need to be burped at intervals. While sucking, the baby normally swallows air; if this air is not cleared from the stomach, the infant may feel satisfied and stop eating. When the air clears the stomach, the infant may again appear hungry.

Before starting, the mother should choose a feeding position that is comfortable and that facilitates the flow of milk into the infant's stomach. Many different positions are suitable for breast-feeding or bottle feeding (see Fig. 28.7).

Hypothermia

Maintenance of body temperature is a major concern in the care of newborns. Prolonged exposure to a cold environment can result in increased oxygen consumption and depleted glycogen reserves. Newborns have a relatively large surface area and a limited amount of protective adipose tissue. They lose heat through radiation, evaporation, conduction, and convection. Be aware of this and take precautions to reduce the losses (Table 28.7).

Monitor temperature with a skin sensor or thermometer. Verify that the anus is patent. The rectal method of temperature assessment is used rarely because of the chance of rectal irritation or perforation. Most facilities use the axillary route because it is considered safest. The normal axillary temperature is 97.6°F to 98.6°F (36.4°C to 37°C). Mercury thermometers are used rarely in health care settings today, although they may still be used in the home.

Hygiene

Inspection and bathing of the neonate take place after the body temperature has stabilized. The frequency and type of baths depend on facility policies. Bathing serves a number of purposes: complete cleansing, observation of the infant's condition, comfort, and parent-child socialization.

Gather all bathing articles and the infant's change of clothing before bathing. The room temperature should be 75°F (24°C), and the bathing area should be free of drafts to prevent heat loss. The bath water should be approximately 100°F (38°C). Heat loss in the infant is greater than heat loss in the adult because of the relatively large ratio of the skin surface to body mass in the newborn. To conserve the infant's energy, control heat loss by bathing the infant quickly, padding cold surfaces, exposing only a portion of the body at a time, and thoroughly drying the infant. Until the initial bath is completed, wear gloves when handling the newborn.

The Centers for Disease Control and Prevention regulations related to standard precautions against human immunodeficiency virus and other bloodborne pathogens have increased the use of soap solutions for bathing newborn infants. Use a nonmedicated mild soap for the initial bath. Shampoo the hair and use a brush or a comb to remove dried blood and vernix caseosa. Use cotton balls, not gauze, to cleanse the nostrils and ears. Careful drying reduces the heat lost during bathing. The order of the bath is essentially the same as for an adult, beginning with the eyes, the face, and the head and ending with the anal region. Do not vigorously remove vernix caseosa (the white material that looks like cold cream), because it is attached to the upper, protective layer of the skin. Vernix caseosa may be left on for 48 hours; if it persists beyond that time, wash it off gently. Some nurses advocate massaging the vernix caseosa gently into the skin. No studies have confirmed the benefits or disadvantages of this technique.

Reassess the temperature 30 minutes after completion of the bath.

After the initial bath, washing with warm water is sufficient for the first week. Full submersion into a tub of water should not be done until the cord has fallen off. The infant's skin is thin and delicate. The infant's fragile skin can be injured by vigorous cleansing. Daily bathing is not needed; however, the perineal area should be washed carefully with nonmedicated mild soap and warm water and carefully dried with each diaper change. Parents may make personal decisions about the brand and type of cleaning agents used. Recommendations are that oils and scented products should be avoided. After the bath, talc use should be limited because it may cause aspiration if it comes too close to the nose and mouth.

Discuss the choice of cloth or disposable diapers with parents. Cloth diapers today are different from those used years ago with plastic or rubber pants. Exclusive use of disposable diapers is the most expensive and most popular method. Over 1 or 2 years, the cost can be considerable, particularly if more than one child is wearing diapers. However, some disposable diapers may help prevent diaper dermatitis.

Pay special attention to care of the umbilical area. At delivery, the cord is moist. Over the next few days, a drying process called *mummification* (producing a dry, hard mass) begins. Avoid getting the cord wet during bathing. Most facilities have a routine to promote

Table 28.7	Precautions to Minimize Heat Loss in Infants
TYPES OF HEAT LOSS	**NURSING INTERVENTIONS TO PREVENT HEAT LOSS**
Radiation: Loss that occurs when heat transfers from the body to cooler surfaces and objects not in contact with the body	Keep body well wrapped to prevent radiant loss. Work quickly to avoid excessive time with skin exposed. Use radiant warmer to minimize loss. Locate crib away from outside wall.
Evaporation: Loss when water is converted into a vapor	Dry infant thoroughly after delivery and promptly when bathing.
Conduction: Loss of heat to a cooler surface via direct skin contact	Pad surfaces under infant, including tables and scales. Warm other equipment, such as stethoscopes, before use.
Convection: Loss of heat to cooler air currents	Reduce drafts from open doors, windows, or air conditioning; wrap newborn to protect from cold.

drying with use of alcohol or other substances (triple dye) that inhibit microbial growth. Odor or exudate from the cord is abnormal and should be reported promptly. Delay tub bathing until the fully dried cord drops off at about 10 days of age.

Give the mother a demonstration of temperature taking and bathing the newborn. If possible, encourage her to bathe the infant while you observe. This helps her gain confidence and provides an opportunity to answer questions about care. It is also a good time to demonstrate safe methods of holding and positioning the infant.

Circumcision refers to the surgical removal of the foreskin. Many parents elect to have the procedure performed on their newborn infant. A review of the procedure's rates for 1997 to 2010 showed an overall decline. The national rate in 1997 was 64.5% and in 2010 it was 58.3%. There are regional differences across the country. Rates of circumcision are highest in the southern and midwestern states and lowest in the west. The reasons parents opt to have their sons circumcised are varied. Some parents choose circumcision to follow family tradition, and others out of concern for their son's reproductive health. The Jewish faith promotes the circumcision of infant boys. Jewish families who follow the time-honored ritual of their faith opt to have the circumcision performed 7 days after birth. The procedure is performed in a religious ceremony by a religious figure. The AAP reported in 1999 that acknowledged health benefits were associated with circumcision but that these benefits were not significant enough to warrant a recommendation to mandate this procedure for all male infants. In 2012 the AAP again reaffirmed this position (American Academy of Pediatrics, 2012). The AAP further states that analgesia should be used if a circumcision is performed; a consent form for both is required.

If circumcision is performed, keep the area clean and assess it for bleeding every hour for the first 12 hours after surgery. Apply gentle pressure to the bleeding area with a folded gauze pad. Sterile petroleum gauze usually is applied to the penis after a Gomco or Mogen circumcision and is left in place for 24 hours; it is replaced if it becomes dislodged prematurely. If a Plastibell circumcision is performed, the petroleum gauze is not needed because the plastic bell that covers the glans does not stick to the diaper.

Wash the penis gently at diaper changes to remove urine and feces, and reapply fresh sterile petroleum gauze. Do not attempt to remove the dried yellow exudate that forms in 24 hours and persists for 2 to 3 days; this is part of the normal healing process. Some practitioners may recommend the use of cloth diapers during the first week to promote healing. Loose diapering is necessary. If bleeding is not controlled, continue application of intermittent pressure, notify the physician, and prepare for blood vessel ligation. If the infant has undergone this procedure without anesthesia, he

should be comforted until he is quieted and then returned to his crib. These infants usually are fussy for about 2 to 3 hours and may refuse a feeding.

Teach the parents appropriate home care before discharge of the newborn. Teaching should include measures to promote hygiene and thus reduce the risks of infection. Educate the parents to immediately report any unusual signs and symptoms such as edema; purulent, malodorous discharge; elevated temperature; and delayed healing.

ELIMINATION

The newborn should urinate within 24 hours of delivery. If this does not occur, notify the physician. The average newborn voids small amounts of poorly concentrated urine; it is normally clear and odorless. Occasionally, a small pink or brownish discharge may be observed as a result of uric acid crystals that were formed in the bladder in utero. As fluid intake increases and kidney function improves, urination becomes more frequent and assumes the normal color.

Bowel elimination should occur within 24 hours of birth. The newborn's initial stools are odorless, black-green, and sticky. This is called meconium and is made up of vernix, strands of lanugo, mucus, and other substances from the amniotic fluid. Occasionally, the first stool is encased in mucus and called a *meconium plug*. If no stool is observed, notify the physician so that an examination can be performed to determine the problem. Once the infant begins to take nourishment, the stool changes. Transitional stools, which occur on about the second day, tend to be greenish and loose. These are seen until about the fourth day, when the milk stool is seen. Breast-fed babies tend to pass stool frequently, sometimes with every feeding. The stool is pale yellow and sweet smelling. Small curds may be observed. Babies who are bottle fed tend to have fewer stools, usually two or three per day after the first 2 weeks. These are bright yellow and pasty in consistency; the odor may be slightly stronger than that of breast-fed babies. This type of stool continues until solid food is introduced. Very watery stools, green stools (after the transition), or stools expelled with force may indicate gastrointestinal irritation or infection and should be reported promptly (Fig. 28.13). Newborns can lose a great deal of fluid rapidly and become dehydrated (see Box 28.14 for stooling patterns of newborns). (Note that newborns normally give the impression of straining with a stool because their muscles are underdeveloped. This can cause parents undue concern if they are not advised about it. The straining subsides as growth and maturity continue.)

The skin of the perineum and buttocks can become irritated if waste products are left in contact for too long. Teach the parents to wash the skin, wiping from anterior to posterior, after each voiding or stool, and to change diapers promptly. Recommend minimal use of

Fig. 28.13 Infant stool. (A) Breast-fed. (B) Formula fed.

| Box 28.14 | **Change in Stooling of Newborns** |

MECONIUM
- Infant's first stool is composed of amniotic fluid and its constituents, intestinal secretions, shed mucosal cells, and possibly blood (ingested maternal blood or minor bleeding of alimentary tract vessels).
- Passage of meconium should occur within the first 24–48 h, although it may be delayed up to 7 days in very low-birth-weight infants.
- Colostrum has a laxative effect that aids the infant to expel the meconium.

TRANSITIONAL STOOLS
- Transitional stools usually appear by the third day after initiation of feeding.
- They are greenish brown to yellowish brown, thin, and less sticky than meconium; they may contain some milk curds.

MILK STOOL
- Milk stools usually appear by the fourth day.
- In *breast-fed* infants, stools are yellow to golden, are pasty in consistency, and have an odor similar to that of sour milk.
- In *formula-fed* infants, stools are pale yellow to light brown, are firmer in consistency, and have a more offensive odor.

---

creams, which can irritate the skin. Disposable or cloth diapers may be chosen.

REST AND SLEEP

Most newborns spend 16 to 20 hours per day sleeping. They may be observed to startle and make sucking motions during sleep. Breathing may be regular and even or irregular, depending on the sleep state. The time awake is spent crying, eating, or in quiet alertness. Each infant establishes a unique pattern, which may be erratic but stabilizes over time as the nervous and digestive systems mature. Most infants do not exceed 5 continuous hours of sleep for some months, which can be disruptive to the sleep of others in the household.

ACTIVITY AND EXERCISE

Maintenance of a clear airway is critical. Many infants need suctioning to remove mucus from the nose and mouth. Newborns are obligate (necessary or required) nose breathers; they must be able to breathe through the nose while suckling. The nasal passageway must be kept open and free from mucus. A small bulb syringe is commonly used. Compress it before insertion and then gently release it to suction secretions. Explain to parents the use of the bulb syringe before the first feeding. For the first few days, a bulb syringe always should be kept with the newborn, particularly during feeding.

Crying is the newborn's only means of communication. The cry can indicate hunger, pain, the need for attention, or fussiness. The newborn's cry should be strong, vigorous, and of medium pitch. As mother and infant become more adept at interpreting each other's behavior, some mothers can distinguish the reason for crying. The following report indicates that mother and baby are communicating effectively:

I can tell when she's hungry. Crying starts in a plaintive [sorrowful, sad] way and then becomes more and more demanding. When she is hurt, she lets out a startled yell as though she couldn't believe it was happening to her. Sometimes when she is put down to sleep, she starts a kind of talking cry, jerky and demanding; it gets louder, and if nothing happens, fades away in little spurts. The fussy cry is the hardest to take—nothing seems to work; like a complaining that goes on and on.

A high-pitched cry may indicate neurologic problems and should be observed further and evaluated by a physician. See the Patient Teaching box for infant quieting techniques.

👥 Patient Teaching

Infant Quieting Techniques

- Many newborns feel insecure in the center of a large crib. They prefer a small, warm, soft space that reminds them of intrauterine life. Try a smaller bed, such as a bassinet, portable crib, buggy, or cradle, or use a rolled-up blanket to turn a corner of the big crib into a smaller place.
- Carry baby in a front pack or backpack.
- Swaddle newborn snugly in a receiving blanket. Swaddling keeps the newborn's arms and legs close to his or her body, similar to the intrauterine position. It makes the newborn feel more secure. Swaddling should never be used when a baby is not placed on the back to sleep. Swaddling is viewed as safe for the first 2 months of life (AAP, 2020).
- Prewarm the crib sheets with a hot water bottle or heating pad that is removed before putting the baby to bed. Some babies startle when placed on a cold sheet.
- Some newborns need extra sucking to soothe themselves to sleep. Breast-feeding mothers may prefer to let their infant suckle at the breast as a soothing technique. Other mothers choose to use a pacifier. Stroke the pacifier against the roof of the baby's mouth to encourage him or her to suck it during the first 2 weeks. Around age 3 months, infants can find and suck their thumbs as a way of self-consoling.
- A rhythmic, monotonous noise that simulates the intrauterine sounds of the maternal heartbeat and blood flow may help the infant settle down. Some parents have found it helpful to put a fussy baby in a portable crib beside the dishwasher or washing machine.
- Movement often helps quiet a baby. Take the baby for a ride in the car or an outing in a stroller or carriage. Rock the baby in a rocking chair or cradle.
- Place the baby on his or her stomach across the lap; pat and rub the back while gently bouncing legs or swaying them from left to right.
- Babies enjoy skin-to-skin contact. A combination of this and warm water often helps soothe a fussy baby. Fill the tub with warm water. Get in and let the baby lie on the chest so that the baby is immersed in the water up to his or her neck. Cuddle the baby.
- Let the baby see your face. Talk in a soothing voice.
- The baby may simply need more stimulation. Bring him or her into the room where the family is gathered. Change the baby's position; many babies like to be upright, such as being held up on the shoulder.

Fig. 28.14 Parents and sibling interacting with a newborn.

Fig. 28.15 The infant is quiet and alert during the initial sensitive period. The newborn gazes at the mother and responds to her voice and touch.

PARENT-CHILD ATTACHMENT

The human infant is born defenseless and could not survive without a caregiver. The parents are responsible for the infant's physical and psychological development.

Parenting is not instinctive; a new parent must bond with the baby first. **Parent-child attachment (bonding)** is defined as the initial phase in a relationship characterized by strong attraction and a desire to interact (Fig. 28.14). Without bonding, parents find the energy needed to meet the newborn's needs difficult to maintain. The nurse cannot make bonding occur but can facilitate its development.

Early contact with the infant is important to establish bonding. A new mother normally wishes to touch and explore her baby. Holding the infant close and looking eye to eye (the en face position) helps bonding occur (Fig. 28.15). It is normal for a new mother to talk in high-pitched tones to the baby. Encourage early and frequent interaction between the newborn and the parents (Fig. 28.16). Attachment increases when the infant begins to respond.

Fig. 28.16 The behavior of fathers at initial contact with their infant often corresponds to maternal behaviors. The intense fascination that fathers exhibit is called engrossment. Note eye-to-eye contact between father and infant.

The newborn has amazing capabilities. The infant is a socially responsive human who can probably learn better on the first day of life than ever again. Immediately after birth, the baby stares intently at the parents' faces and sees them. In fact, the newborn prefers looking at the mother's face, especially the eyes, to looking at other objects. The newborn also can recognize an approaching object as a threat and turns away to avoid it. He or she reaches for an object and usually comes close to touching it. The newborn imitates another person's facial expressions, such as sticking out the tongue, opening the mouth, and pursing the lips. Newborn babies are active stimulus seekers where repetition and the level of stimulation are important. The baby can shut out stimuli and may even turn his or her head at the sound of the mother's voice.

Indeed, babies are not passive and unresponsive creatures to be hurried off to the hospital nursery after birth. The affectionate bond between parents and child begins at the moment of birth (see Figs. 28.14 and 28.16). As long as the newborn is responding normally, immediate skin-to-skin contact with the parents is important in bonding. The newborn has difficulty opening the eyes under bright spotlights but looks around if the lights are dimmed. (If necessary, dim the main lights in the delivery area and keep a light focused over the perineum for episiotomy repair or other procedures.) Shielding the infant's face with a hand or a blanket also provides enough protection from the light to encourage the baby to open the eyes. Objects are in clearest range for the newborn at about 8 to 10 inches. Newborns prefer faces over other patterns. Refraining from using prophylactic eye drops and weighing and measuring the baby for 30 minutes to 1 hour after birth allows the parents time alone with their baby so that the attachment process can proceed without interruption. The mother may wish to breast-feed in the first hour after birth; the nurse or the father can assist her.

Periods of quiet alertness are best for interaction. Explain the different levels of alertness to the parents so that they can recognize them. Time care so that the mother is available to enjoy quiet moments with her newborn.

Patient problems for the newborn infant may include the following:
- Inability to maintain adequate breathing pattern
- Inability to regulate body temperature
- Potential for infection
- Potential for injury
- Potential for inability to clear airway
- Recent onset of pain

Get Ready for the NCLEX® Examination!

Key Points

- During the 6 weeks after delivery, the reproductive organs return to approximately the prepregnant size and location.
- The new mother should avoid dieting and excessive activity during the early postpartum period.
- Postpartum fatigue and depression are common as a result of hormonal and physiologic changes.
- Complications can occur during the postpartum period. Each woman must be assessed carefully.
- Before discharge, provide instruction concerning the danger signs of the postpartum period and verify that the woman knows when and how to contact her physician.
- Hormonal changes enable the woman to produce enough milk to meet the nutritional needs of the growing infant. Nutritional needs of the lactating woman are similar to those during pregnancy.
- Motherhood is a learned skill. The new mother needs extensive teaching and encouragement about parenting skills.
- Early discharge necessitates that the nurse provides essential teaching in a brief period. Be careful to document teaching.
- Supplement teaching with written materials so that the new mother has something to refer to when at home.

- Conduct assessment of the newborn in a head-to-toe format. Thoroughly review each body system.
- Newborns exhibit a wide range of normal variation. Verify any questionable observations with another nurse or physician.
- Hypothermia and infection are two major areas of concern in care of the newborn.
- Circumcision is an elective surgical procedure.
- The newborn has social and physical needs.
- Injuries to the cervix can have adverse effects on future pregnancies. Repair should be immediate.
- In preparing the transfer report, the recovery nurse uses information from the admission record, the birth record, and the recovery record.
- In helping new families adjust to parenthood, provide culturally sensitive care following principles that facilitate nursing practice within transcultural situations.
- Infant abduction from hospitals in the United States has been on the increase. Parents and nurses must work together to ensure the safety of newborns in the hospital environment.
- Provide demonstration and instruction to educate the mother about the newborn's hygiene needs.
- Whether or not this is the couple's first baby, parents appreciate anticipatory guidance in the care of their child.
- Parent-child attachment (bonding) is the process by which parent and child come to love and accept each other.

Additional Learning Resources

SG Go to your Study Guide for additional learning activities to help you master this chapter content.

Be sure to visit the Evolve site at http://evolve.elsevier.com/Cooper/foundations for additional online resources.

Review Questions For The NCLEX® Examination

1. **A primigravida has delivered a baby vaginally after 6 hours of labor. She had an uneventful pregnancy and is in good general health. She is transferred from the recovery room to the postpartum unit. What interventions are included in routine postpartum care?** *(Select all that apply.)*

    1. Assessment of intake and output until the patient is voiding in sufficient quantities
    2. Insertion of a catheter to assess residual urine after the initial voiding
    3. Firm massage of the fundus every 15 minutes
    4. Assessment of the emotional status of the new mother
    5. Checking of breasts for engorgement and cracking of nipples

2. **The nurse is performing a routine postpartum assessment. Which action is indicated before the fundal height is measured?**

    1. Massage the uterus.
    2. Apply pressure to the fundus to check for clots.
    3. Elevate the head of the bed.
    4. Ask the patient to empty her bladder.

3. **The nurse finds bright red bleeding on a patient's peripad. The stain is about 6 inches long. What is the correct description of the character and amount of lochia?**

    1. Lochia rubra, moderate
    2. Lochia serosa, heavy
    3. Lochia rubra, heavy
    4. Lochia serosa, light

4. **The nurse is teaching breast care for the lactating woman. What information should be included?** *(Select all that apply.)*

    1. Expose the nipples to air for 20 to 30 minutes daily.
    2. Wear a supportive bra 24 hours a day for the first few weeks.
    3. Wash breasts and nipples with soap and water before each feeding.
    4. Use plastic liners in bras.
    5. Use ice packs every 4 hours as needed for discomfort associated with engorgement.

5. **A woman asks the nurse how she will know her baby is getting enough milk. The nurse's response is based on understanding that which is the best determinant?**

    1. The baby awakens every 4 to 6 hours to eat.
    2. The baby stops nursing when full.
    3. The baby has 6 to 10 wet diapers per day.
    4. The baby cries when hungry.

6. **In evaluating maternal adjustment, which behavior leads the nurse to believe that the patient is still in the taking-in phase?** *(Select all that apply.)*

    1. The mother states she is "starving" and can't wait to eat.
    2. The majority of the mother's time is spent talking about her delivery experience.
    3. The mother takes a shower and washes her hair.
    4. The mother asks the nurse to teach her how to give her baby a bath.
    5. The mother reports she feels as if she needs to get more rest.

7. **A baby boy is 1 hour old when admitted to the newborn nursery. He weighs 7 lb, 3 oz; is 21 inches long; has irregular respirations of 42 breaths/min with adequate chest movement, a heart rate of 145 beats/min, and a temperature of 35.6°C, axillary; and is acrocyanotic. What is an appropriate goal for this baby within the next 2 hours, based on these findings?**

    1. Color will remain unchanged.
    2. Respirations will slow.
    3. Temperature will stabilize at 36.5°C to 37°C.
    4. Heart rate will decrease to 100 beats/min.

8. **When teaching parents how to bathe their baby, which point should the nurse stress?**

    1. Avoid immersing the baby in water until after the umbilical cord has fallen off.
    2. Use only mild medicated or scented soap.
    3. Apply baby powder after the bath to keep the skin dry.
    4. Apply baby oil after the bath to keep the skin soft and smooth.

9. When providing education to parents about care of the umbilical cord, what information should be included? *(Select all that apply.)*

   1. Cleaning the cord with an alcohol swab
   2. Keeping the diaper folded below the cord
   3. Applying triple dye to the cord
   4. Keeping the cord moist to promote healing
   5. Oiling the cord to facilitate it falling off

10. A baby has a Gomco circumcision. What instruction should the nurse give his parents for care of the circumcised penis?

    1. Soak the penis in warm water daily.
    2. Cover the glans with a petroleum gauze dressing.
    3. Clean the glans with alcohol to promote healing.
    4. Remove any yellowish exudate that forms within 24 hours.

11. On examining a woman who gave birth 5 hours previously, the nurse finds that the woman has saturated a perineal pad within 15 minutes. What action is the nurse's first priority?

    1. Increase the drip rate of an IV infusion of Ringer's lactate solution.
    2. Assess the patient's vital signs.
    3. Call the patient's primary health care provider.
    4. Palpate the woman's fundus.

12. A woman gave birth 48 hours ago to a healthy baby girl. She has decided to bottle feed. During the assessment, the nurse notices that both breasts are swollen, warm, and tender on palpation. The patient should be advised that this is best treated with which action?

    1. Running warm water over her breasts during a shower
    2. Applying ice to the breasts for comfort
    3. Expressing small amounts of milk from the breasts to relieve pressure
    4. Wearing a loose-fitting bra to prevent nipple irritation
    5. Wearing a snug bra

13. A first-time mother is to be discharged from the hospital tomorrow with her baby girl. Which maternal behavior indicates a need for further intervention by the nurse before she can be discharged?

    1. The mother leaves the baby on her bed while she takes a shower.
    2. The mother continues to hold and cuddle her baby after she has fed her.
    3. The mother reads a magazine while her baby sleeps.
    4. The mother changes her baby's diaper, then shows the nurse the contents of the diaper.

14. The nurse observes several interactions between a postpartum woman and her new son. Which behavior, if exhibited by this woman, does the nurse identify as maladaptive regarding parent-infant attachment?

    1. The mother talks and coos to her son.
    2. The mother seldom makes eye contact with her son.
    3. The mother cuddles her son close to her.
    4. The mother tells visitors how well her son is feeding.

15. The nurse can help a father in his transition to parenthood with what action?

    1. Pointing out that the infant turned to his voice
    2. Encouraging him to go home to get some sleep
    3. Taping the baby's diaper a different way
    4. Suggesting that he let the baby sleep in the bassinet

16. A breast-feeding mother reports to the nurse that her breasts are very firm and tender. What information should be included in the response by the nurse? *(Select all that apply.)*

    1. "Avoiding breast-feeding for several hours will be helpful."
    2. "Let's try to apply lettuce leaves to your breasts."
    3. "This is known as engorgement."
    4. "More frequent breast-feeding will be helpful in managing this condition."
    5. "Let's take off your bra for a few hours."
    6. "Bottle feeding will prevent you from having this problem."
    7. "There isn't much we can do to help this. It just takes time."
    8. "We have a medication we can give you to help dry up the milk."
    9. "Ice works very well to help prevent these symptoms."

17. During the vaginal delivery there was tearing of the perineal region. The tearing extended into the lumen of the rectum. When planning care and teaching for the postpartum patient, what should be included? Select all that apply.

    1. Administer a suppository to promote a bowel movement if one does not naturally occur within 48 hours.
    2. Administer a fleet enema after 72 hours.
    3. Encourage fluid intake.
    4. Encourage the woman attempt to avoid a bowel movement for the first 24 to 48 hours post-delivery to allow healing to start.
    5. Encourage frequent ambulation.
    6. Recommend protein increases in the diet to promote stool elimination.

18. The nurse helps the breast-feeding woman change her newborn's diaper after the baby's first bowel movement. The mother expresses concern because of a large amount of sticky, dark green—almost black—stool. She asks the nurse if something is wrong. What information should be included in the nurse's response?

    1. Tell the woman not to worry because all breast-fed babies have this type of stool.
    2. Explain that this type of stool is called meconium and is expected for the first few bowel movements of all newborns.
    3. Ask the woman what she ate at her last meal before giving birth.
    4. Suggest that the mother ask her pediatrician to explain newborn stool patterns.

Care of the High-Risk Mother, Newborn, and Family With Special Needs

Objectives

1. List conditions that increase maternal and fetal risk.
2. Compare and contrast abruptio placentae and placenta previa, noting signs and symptoms, complications, and nursing and medical management.
3. Identify diagnostic tests used to determine high-risk situations.
4. Compare and contrast hypertensive disorders experienced during pregnancy.
5. Identify preexisting maternal health conditions that influence pregnancy.
6. List the infectious diseases most likely to cause serious complications.
7. Discuss the care of the pregnant adolescent.
8. Discuss the problems created by alcohol and drug abuse.
9. Identify concerns related to preterm infants.
10. Explain the hemolytic diseases of the newborn.
11. Discuss patient problems related to high-risk conditions of the mother and the newborn.
12. Identify nursing interventions for the pregnant woman with a cardiac disorder.
13. Explain the care of a pregnant woman with a pulmonary disorder.

Key Terms

anasarca (ăn-ă-SĂR-kă, p. 906)
atony (ĂT-ŏ-nē, p. 904)
brown fat (p. 923)
cerclage (sĕr-KLĂHZH, p. 899)
direct Coombs' test (p. 928)
dizygotic (dī-zī-GŎT-ĭk, p. 894)
eclampsia (ĕ-KLĂMP-sē-ă, p. 905)
erythroblastosis fetalis (ĕ-rĭth-rō-blăs-TŌ-sĭs fĕ-TĂL-ĭs, p. 927)
gestational diabetes mellitus (GDM) (jĕs-TĀ-shŭn-ăl dī-ă-BĒ-tēz MĔL-ĭ-tŭs, p. 913)
gestational hypertension (GH) (jĕs-TĀ-shŭn-ăl hī-pĕr-TĔN-shŭn, p. 905)
glycosylated hemoglobin (glī-KŌ-sĭ-lāt-ĕd HĒ-mō-glō-bĭn, p. 914)
high-risk pregnancy (p. 892)

hydramnios (hī-DRĂM-nē-ŏs, p. 892)
hyperbilirubinemia (hī-pĕr-bĭl-ĭ-rū-bĭ-NĒ-mē-ă, p. 927)
incompetent cervix (p. 899)
indirect Coombs' test (p. 928)
infant mortality (p. 890)
kernicterus (kĕr-NĬK-tĕr-ŭs, p. 927)
kick counting (p. 907)
monozygotic (mŏn-ō-zī-GŎT-ĭk, p. 894)
morbidity (p. 892)
phototherapy (p. 928)
placental barrier (plă-SĔN-tăl, p. 927)
preeclampsia (prē-ĕ-KLĂMP-sē-ă, p. 905)
severe preeclampsia (p. 906)
TORCH (p. 910)

One of the indicators considered in the health of the nation is the rate of infant mortality (the number of infants who die within the first year of life, expressed as the number per thousand live births). The infant mortality rate is higher in the United States than in many other countries in the world such as Canada, Japan, and the United Kingdom (Kamal, 2019). Approximately 4 million babies are born in the United States each year. After making slight strides to reduce the rates in the last decade, the rate is still nearly 5.8. per 1000 live births. This number is troubling in a nation considered a super power. For those babies who do not survive their first year of life, the factors primarily associated with mortality rates are prematurity and low birth weight, chromosomal defects, congenital malformations, maternal complications, sudden infant death syndrome, and injuries. A staggering 40% of these deaths take place within in the first day of life. Prevention of morbidity and mortality among mothers and infants depends on identification of the risk, along with appropriate and timely intervention during the perinatal period.

With the changing demographics in the United States, more women and families are at risk for complications because of nonphysiologic factors. The influences of socioeconomic and lifestyle factors are seen in the increasing numbers of homeless and uninsured women of childbearing age, single, and uninsured pregnant women with limited access to prenatal care during any stage of pregnancy. The nation's highly publicized drug addictions are contributing factors to maternal illness and fetal mortality (Box 29.1).

Although most pregnancies proceed normally, complications and high-risk situations can occur at any stage of the childbearing process. Women from all demographics can face complications. Awareness of risk factors and condition changes will facilitate timely action and care. The importance of early and consistent prenatal care is key to the promotion of positive outcomes for the mother and her baby. Despite resources available, only 77.1% of women who gave birth in 2016 initiated prenatal care in the first trimester. In the second trimester, 4.6% sought care for their pregnancy. Seeking care in the third trimester was pursued by 1.6% of women.

Box 29.1   Classification of High-Risk Factors of Pregnancy

BIOPHYSICAL
- *Genetic considerations:* Genetic factors may interfere with normal fetal or neonatal development, result in congenital anomalies, or create difficulties for the mother.
- *Nutritional status:* Adequate nutrition, without which fetal growth and development cannot proceed normally, is one of the most important determinants of pregnancy outcome.
- *Medical and obstetric disorders:* Complications of current and past pregnancies, obstetric-related illnesses, and pregnancy losses put the patient at risk.

PSYCHOSOCIAL
- *Smoking:* A strong, consistent, causal relationship has been established between maternal smoking and reduced birth weight.
- *Caffeine:* Birth defects in humans have not been related to caffeine consumption. High intake (three or more cups of coffee per day) has been related to a slight decrease in birth weight.
- *Alcohol:* Alcohol exerts adverse effects on the fetus, resulting in fetal alcohol syndrome, fetal alcohol effects, learning disabilities, and hyperactivity.
- *Drugs:* The developing fetus may be affected adversely by drugs through several mechanisms. Drugs can cause metabolic disturbances, produce chemical effects, or depress or alter central nervous system function. This category includes medications prescribed by a health care provider or bought over the counter, and commonly abused drugs such as heroin, cocaine, and marijuana.
- *Psychological status:* Childbearing triggers profound and complex physiologic, psychological, and social changes, with evidence to suggest a relationship between emotional distress and birth complications. This risk factor includes conditions such as specific intrapsychic disturbances and addictive lifestyles.

SOCIODEMOGRAPHIC
- *Low income:* Poverty underlies many other risk factors and leads to inadequate financial resources for food and prenatal care, poor general health, increased risk of medical complications of pregnancy, and greater prevalence of adverse environmental influences.
- *Lack of prenatal care:* Failure to diagnose and treat complications early is a major risk factor that arises from financial barriers or lack of access to care; cultural beliefs that do not support this need; and fear of the health care system and its providers.
- *Age:* Women at both ends of the childbearing age spectrum have a higher incidence of poor outcomes; however, age may not be a risk factor in all cases.

- *Adolescents:* More complications are seen in young mothers (less than 15 years old), who have a 60% higher mortality rate than those over age 20 years, and in pregnancies that occur less than 3 years after menarche. Complications include anemia, preeclampsia, gestational hypertension (GH), prolonged labor, and contracted pelvis and cephalopelvic disproportion. Long-term social implications of early motherhood are lower educational status, lower income, increased dependence on government support programs, higher divorce rates, and higher parity.
- *Geriatric pregnancies:* The risks to mothers over 35 years old are not from age alone but from other considerations, such as number and spacing of previous pregnancies, genetic disposition of the parents, medical history, lifestyle, nutrition, and prenatal care. Medical conditions more likely to be experienced by mature women include hypertension and GH, diabetes, extended labor, cesarean birth, placenta previa, abruptio placentae, and death. Her fetus is at greater risk for low birth weight.
- *Parity:* The number of previous pregnancies is a risk factor that is associated with age and includes all first pregnancies, especially a first pregnancy at either end of the childbearing age spectrum. The incidence of GH and dystocia is higher with a first birth.
- *Marital status:* The increased mortality and morbidity rates for unmarried women, including a greater risk for GH, often are related to inadequate prenatal care and a younger childbearing age.
- *Residence:* The availability and quality of prenatal care varies widely with geographic residence. Women in metropolitan areas have more prenatal visits than those in rural areas, who have fewer opportunities for specialized care and consequently a higher incidence of maternal mortality.
- *Ethnicity:* Although ethnicity is not a major risk factor, race is an indicator of other sociodemographic risk factors. Nonwhite women are more than three times as likely as white women to die of pregnancy-related causes. Black babies have the highest rates of prematurity and low birth weight, with an infant mortality rate more than double that for whites.

ENVIRONMENTAL
- Various environmental substances can affect fertility and fetal development, the chance of a live birth, and the child's subsequent mental and physical development. Environmental influences include infections; radiation; chemicals such as pesticides, therapeutic drugs, illicit drugs, industrial pollutants, and cigarette smoke; stress; and diet.
- Paternal exposure to mutagenic agents in the workplace has been associated with an increased risk of spontaneous abortion.

This leaves more than 15% of women who navigated through their pregnancies without care (Osterman, 2018). When pregnant women are tardy or fail to seek prenatal care, the reasons may include a lack of awareness of available resources, cultural barriers, and financial limitations (Jones, 2020). Absent or delayed care will hinder access to testing, and assessment which allow for the development of a comprehensive plan of care for the mother and her baby (see the Cultural Considerations box on high-risk pregnancies).

COMPLICATIONS OF PREGNANCY

The care team for the pregnant woman and her baby is multidisciplinary. Members collaborate closely to care for the patient at high risk. A high-risk pregnancy is one in which the life or health of the mother or the infant is jeopardized by a health concern. The condition may be preexisting (pregestational onset), or it may be the result of pregnancy (gestational onset). For the mother, the high-risk status extends (based on medical judgment) through the puerperium (6 weeks after delivery). Postdelivery maternal complications usually are resolved within a month, but perinatal morbidity (state of having disease) may continue for months or years.

A better understanding of human reproduction has greatly reduced morbidity and mortality (quality or state of being subject to death). Knowledge about fetal and neonatal disorders has increased However, less significant improvements have occurred in perinatal morbidity and mortality rates when only high-risk pregnancies are considered. Infant mortality rates vary by racial and ethnic groups, maternal age, and geography, with the highest rate among infants born to non-Hispanic black mothers followed closely by Native Hawaiian or other pacific islander, and Native American (CDC, 2021). Understanding the high-risk patient allows individualized therapeutic nursing interventions. Nurses can be instrumental in educating the public about the importance of obtaining early and regular care during pregnancy. See Box 29.2 for factors that place the postpartum woman and neonate at high risk.

Cultural Considerations

High-Risk Pregnancies

- Providers must consider culturally based differences that could affect the treatment of diverse groups of women, and women must share practices and beliefs that could affect their nursing care or their willingness to comply. Health care providers are obligated to respect their patients' various sources of information and beliefs about sickness and health.
- Beliefs that pregnancy is a period of wellness may contribute to the plan to seek care later in pregnancy.
- Recognize that many women may be reluctant to disrobe and may avoid physical examination unless absolutely necessary.
- Gender of the care provider may be concerning to some groups if limited numbers of female health care physicians are available.
- Consider who in the family traditionally makes the "major" decisions. In some families, the husband may be charged with these decisions, including those that affect the woman's health.
- Religious beliefs may dictate a care plan (e.g., with birth control measures or blood transfusions).
- Folk medicine, homeopathy, prayer, or a combination of these may be preferred to traditional Western medicine. Even the perceived effectiveness of medications may be affected by route of administration or color of pills.

Box 29.2   **Factors That Place the Postpartum Patient and the Newborn at Risk**

MOTHER
- Hemorrhage
- Traumatic labor or birth
- Infection
- Psychosocial factors
- Abnormal vital signs
- Previous medical conditions (e.g., diabetes, cardiovascular disease)

INFANT (FACTORS FOR ADMISSION TO NEONATAL INTENSIVE CARE UNIT)
High-Risk Category
- Continuing or developing signs of respiratory distress syndrome
- Asphyxiation (Apgar score, 6 at 5 min); resuscitation necessary at birth
- Preterm infants
- Cyanosis or suspected cardiovascular disease; persistent cyanosis
- Major congenital malformations that necessitate surgery; chromosomal anomalies
- Convulsions, sepsis, hemorrhagic diathesis (constitutional predisposition to certain disease conditions), or shock
- Meconium aspiration syndrome
- Central nervous system depression for longer than 24 h
- Hypoglycemia
- Hypocalcemia
- Hyperbilirubinemia

MODERATE-RISK CATEGORY
- Dysmaturity (premature weight between 2000 and 2500 g)
- Apgar score of less than 5 at 1 min
- Feeding problems
- Multifetal birth
- Transient tachypnea
- Hypomagnesemia or hypermagnesemia
- Hypoparathyroidism
- Jitteriness or hyperactivity
- Cardiac anomalies that do not necessitate immediate catheterization
- Heart murmur
- Anemia
- Central nervous system depression for less than 24 h

HYPEREMESIS GRAVIDARUM

Etiology

Mild nausea and vomiting occurring during the first trimester of pregnancy are common and, to some extent, normal symptoms known as morning sickness. Prolonged and severe nausea and vomiting may result in electrolyte, metabolic, and nutritional imbalances. This condition, termed hyperemesis gravidarum, is a serious complication.

There is no diagnostic test to confirm the condition. The presentation of symptoms will provide the needed affirmation of the disorder. Hyperemesis criteria include a weight loss exceeding 5% of the prepregnant weight. The resulting dehydration and hypovolemia will lead to electrolyte imbalances, chiefly hypokalemia. When the gravid woman does not receive adequate nutrition, her body may begin to break down fats for energy, resulting in ketones in the urine. Short-term hepatic dysfunction with elevated liver enzymes may occur. Vitamin and mineral deficiencies may result. Thiamine deficiency can cause encephalopathy.

The exact cause of this condition is not known. The disorder is more common with conditions that involve high levels of HCG, such as gestational trophoblastic disease (hydatidiform mole) or multifetal pregnancies. Women who have experienced the disorder in past pregnancies are at higher risk. Primigravidas also have a higher risk for developing the condition. Psychogenic factors also may play a role. Hyperemesis gravidarum is one of the most common nutrition-related discomforts of pregnancy.

Clinical Manifestations

The mother with hyperemesis gravidarum experiences nausea, vomiting and retching far worse than the usual morning sickness. The nausea and vomiting are not limited to the morning hours. Women may border on starvation and become severely dehydrated. The result may be various serious complications that endanger the mother and the fetus. Acid-base imbalance related to the loss of excessive amounts of hydrochloric acid or intestinal juices may result in alkalosis or acidosis. Potassium may become depleted, leading to cardiac arrhythmias. Vitamin deficiencies can lead to jaundice, hemorrhage, and neurological complications.

Assessment

Assess, record, and report the frequency, amount, and character of emesis. Carefully measure fluid intake and output (I&O). Obtaining the patient's daily weight for comparison purposes also is recommended. Assess the patient's skin turgor and mucous membranes. Psychosocial assessment includes asking the woman about anxiety, fears, and concerns related to her own health and the effects on her pregnancy. Assess family members' anxiety and their role in supporting the woman.

Assessment of the status of the fetus is also important. Monitor fetal heart rate (FHR) regularly and immediately report any significant changes (see Chapter 26).

Medical Management

Medical treatment is directed at rehydration, meeting nutritional needs, the prevention of additional complications, and emotional support. An electrolyte profile should be obtained to determine the impact of the vomiting. Oral intake is restricted until the vomiting ceases. Once oral intake is resumed, it may be increased gradually, beginning with clear liquids and advancing the diet as tolerated. Intravenous (IV) fluid replacement is initiated. Fluids used in the replacement often include normal saline, lactated Ringer's solution, and dextrose solutions. Additives in the fluids administered often include multivitamins, magnesium, potassium chloride, pyridoxine, and thiamine.

Complications may result if the woman is not hydrated adequately, and electrolyte imbalances result. Observe the patient for any signs of complications, such as metabolic acidosis, jaundice, premature labor, and hemorrhage. Alert the physician if these occur.

Nursing Interventions and Patient Teaching

Ideally, the woman who experiences nausea and vomiting can maintain adequate hydration and nutritional intake. Consuming small, frequent meals is helpful. Avoidance of greasy or spicy foods is encouraged. High-protein snacks and intake of carbonated beverages may be beneficial. Ingesting dry crackers before getting out of bed is encouraged.

The patient who requires hospitalization will be given parenteral fluids. The IV fluids will include potassium chloride and vitamins. They may also be placed on NPO. Then, once the vomiting has eased, there can be a gradual reintroduction of oral intake. Oral hygiene is essential because the mouth may be irritated by the vomitus. Weigh the woman daily during acute illness. Test the urine for ketones. Weight loss and ketones in the urine suggest that fat stores and protein are being metabolized to meet energy needs. A consultation with a dietitian is recommended (see Chapter 19 for further diet modification suggestions). Take steps to reduce the mother's emotional distress. Provide emotional support and explanations. Include the family in the care plan whenever possible. Their participation may help alleviate some of the emotional stress associated with hospitalization. Complementary therapies may be included in the management of the condition. Acupuncture, Sea-Bands, and aromatherapy may be used.

More severe cases of hyperemesis may require pharmacologic intervention. Currently doxylamine-pyridoxine (Diclegis) is the only medication listed with FDA approval to treat vomiting in pregnancy. Other medications may be prescribed as deemed appropriate by the physician (see Table 29.3).

After treatment in the hospital, most women return home with nourishment by mouth. A few women continue to experience intractable nausea and vomiting throughout pregnancy. If the woman remains unable to achieve adequate nutrition orally, she may require enteral, parenteral, or total parenteral nutrition to provide the needed nutrients to sustain both herself and the fetus.

Patient problems and interventions for the patient with hyperemesis gravidarum include but are not limited to the following:

PATIENT PROBLEM	NURSING INTERVENTIONS
Insufficient Nutrition, related to nausea and persistent vomiting secondary to pregnancy	Monitor food intake; caloric record may be desirable
	Offer dry crackers and bland food as tolerated
	Provide a pleasant atmosphere at mealtimes
	Administer antiemetics as prescribed
	Measure and record intake and output (I&O)
	Weigh daily
	Encourage oral fluids, slowly increasing amount as tolerated
	Maintain a calm, compassionate, and sympathetic manner
	Encourage patient to discuss concerns
	Encourage family participation
Fearfulness, related to concern for self and fetus	Convey acceptance of patient's perception of fear
	Help patient identify personal strengths and previous coping mechanisms
	Help patient identify sources of support
	Provide opportunities to verbalize fears
	Provide continuity of care; refer to social worker as indicated

Patient teaching includes: (1) arranging for dietary consultation; (2) educating patient regarding condition, including signs of improvement or deterioration, and treatment measures; (3) teaching patient how to assist with her own treatment (e.g., eating small, frequent meals with high carbohydrate content); and (4) providing referrals for follow-up treatment, such as psychological counseling, or for support from a social worker.

Prognosis

In most instances, hyperemesis gravidarum responds to therapy, and the prognosis is good. If untreated, hyperemesis gravidarum can result in maternal and fetal death.

MULTIFETAL PREGNANCY

Etiology

Pregnancy involving twins occurs in approximately 32.6 in 1000 live births in the United States. Triplets and higher order multiples occur in 93 per 100,000 live births (CDC, 2021). Pregnancies that involve more than three fetuses are even rarer. Between 2014 and 2018 the rate of twin births declined. Women who become pregnant with multiple fetuses most often are nonwhite, have a family history of multifetal pregnancies, or have taken fertility treatments.

Twins are classified as monozygotic (identical) or dizygotic (fraternal). **Monozygotic** twins begin with one fertilized ovum; the embryonic disk divides, causing identical twins. Because the genetic message is identical, the twins are of the same sex and carry an identical genetic code. They sometimes share a placenta or amniotic sac, but each has a separate umbilical cord. **Dizygotic** twins are the result of two separate ova being fertilized at the same time. These twins almost always have separate placentas. Gender may differ; genetic makeup varies as they are no more closely related than siblings born at different times (Fig. 29.1). Dizygotic twinning may be hereditary in some families, presumably because the woman inherited a tendency to release more than one ovum per cycle.

A   Monochorionic/monoamniotic

Monochorionic/diamniotic

Identical twins

Dichorionic/diamniotic

B   Fraternal twins

Fig. 29.1 Multiple pregnancies. (A) Monozygotic (identical) twins develop from one ovum and one sperm. (B) Dizygotic (fraternal) twins develop from two ova and two sperm.

Pathophysiology

Maternal and fetal risks increase during a multiple pregnancy. Spontaneous abortions, maternal anemia, gestational hypertension (GH), hydramnios, and bleeding from placenta previa or abruptio placentae are more common in women with twins. The elevations in HCG levels promote increased incidence of nausea and vomiting. The fetuses are more likely to have congenital anomalies, problems with entangled cords, and growth problems. An incomplete separation of the embryonic disk can result in conjoined twins.

Labor may be complicated by the loss of uterine tone that results from overstretching of the musculature, abnormal presentations, and preterm labor. Many twin pregnancies and almost all with more than two fetuses require a cesarean delivery.

Because of overdistention of the uterus, twins usually deliver before term and may have extended hospital stays. Additional referrals may be needed if the nursing assessment reveals the parents do not have the needed resources to care for multiple newborns.

Clinical Manifestations

A multiple pregnancy is suspected when uterine enlargement exceeds the anticipated rate for growth, excess nausea and vomiting occurs, or levels of HCG are significantly elevated. Abdominal palpation with Leopold maneuvers, auscultation of two distinct heart tones, and ultrasound scan reveal the presence of multiple fetuses.

GESTATIONAL TROPHOBLASTIC PREGNANCY (HYDATIDIFORM MOLE OR MOLAR PREGNANCY)

Gestational Trophoblastic Pregnancy (Hydatidiform Mole) is a gestational trophoblastic disease. Hydatidiform moles come in two distinct types: complete (or classic) mole and partial mole.

Etiology

These pregnancies result 1 of every 1000 pregnancies in the United States and Europe (Johns Hopkins Medicine, n.d.). The cause is unknown, although an ovular defect may occur. Risk factors include maternal age (under 20 or over 35 years), history of miscarriage, family or personal history of past gestational trophoblastic disease (American Cancer Society [ACS], n.d.). The risk of a second mole is 1% to 2%.

Pathophysiology

The complete mole results from fertilization of an egg whose nucleus has been lost or inactivated. The nucleus of a sperm (23X) duplicates itself (resulting in the diploid number 46XX), because the ovum has no genetic material or the material is inactive. The developing cells resemble a cluster of grapes. The fluid-filled vesicles grow rapidly, causing the uterus to be larger than expected for the duration of the pregnancy. Usually the complete mole contains no fetus, placenta, amniotic membranes, or fluid. With no placenta to receive maternal blood, hemorrhage into the uterine cavity and vaginal bleeding occur. While rare, the development of choriocarcinoma is tied to women having a history of a molar pregnancy (National Library of Medicine [NLM], 2020).

Clinical Manifestations

The signs and symptoms of a complete hydatidiform mole in the early stage cannot be distinguished from those of normal pregnancy. There are the traditional symptoms associated with early pregnancy. The pregnancy is confirmed with a serum or urine HCG test. Early in pregnancy, the uterus in approximately half of affected women is significantly larger than expected based on the date of the last menstrual period. The percentage of women with an excessively enlarged uterus increases as the pregnancy advances. Approximately 25% of affected women have a uterus smaller than would be expected from menstrual dates. Findings that result in suspicion that the patient may have a gestational trophoblast include the inability to locate fetal heart tones on a routine care visit.

Later, vaginal bleeding occurs in almost 95% of cases. The vaginal discharge may be dark brown (resembling prune juice) or bright red and either scant or profuse. It may continue for a few days or off and on for weeks.

Anemia resulting from blood loss, excessive nausea and vomiting (hyperemesis gravidarum), and abdominal cramps caused by uterine distention are relatively common findings. Preeclampsia occurs in about 15% of cases, usually between 9 and 12 weeks of gestation, but any symptoms of GH before 20 weeks of gestation may suggest hydatidiform mole. Hyperthyroidism and pulmonary embolization of trophoblastic elements occur infrequently but are serious complications of hydatidiform mole. Partial moles cause few of these symptoms and may be mistaken for an incomplete or missed abortion.

Passages of vesicles (grapelike clusters) may occur around 16 weeks of gestation. There is no fetal movement, FHR, or palpable fetal parts. Some women have signs and symptoms of hyperthyroidism.

Diagnostic Measures

Diagnosis can be made with ultrasound scan, amniography, and measurement of HCG level in the blood. The ultrasound shows an enlarged uterus with no identifiable fetal parts. The uterine trophoblastic cells will be visualized. In most cases, the mole is discovered when abortion is threatened or in progress.

Medical Management

The molar pregnancy traditionally is managed with a suction curettage. After this is completed, the woman's medical management includes the assessment of serum HCG levels. The levels are assessed weekly until they are negative. Once the levels are negative, the

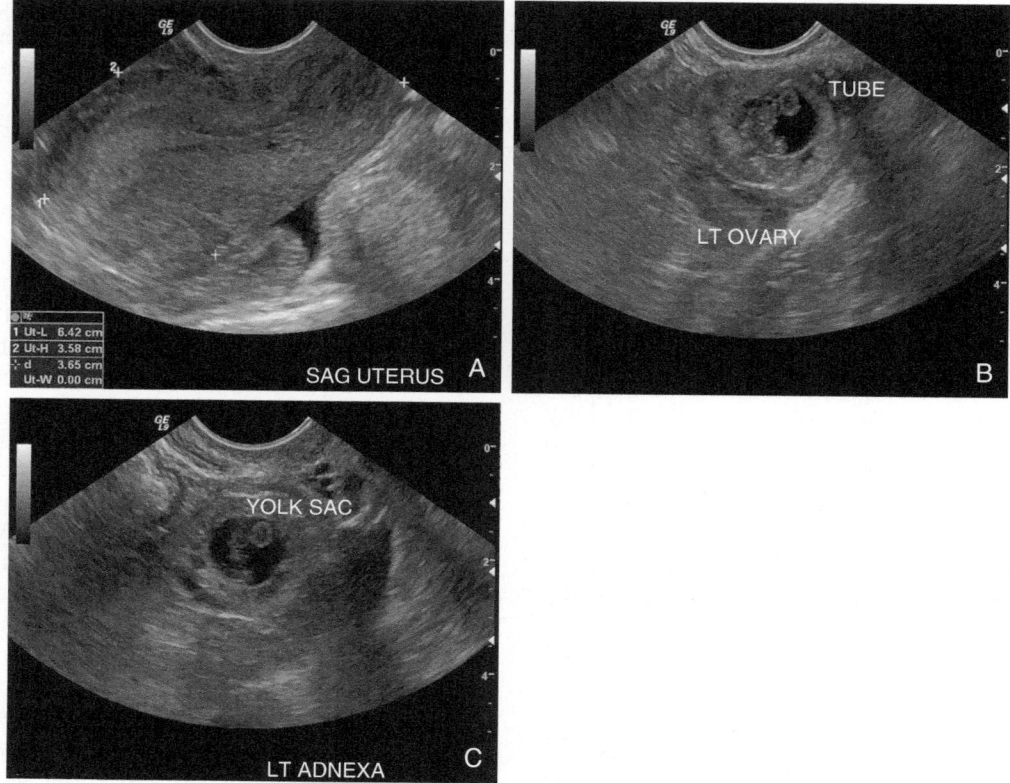

Fig. 29.2 Ectopic pregnancy, abdominal.

monitoring is repeated monthly. A return to positive findings may signal the presence of carcinoma. Rho(D) immune globulin is administered to women who are Rh negative to prevent isoimmunization. Women who have experienced a molar pregnancy must avoid becoming pregnant for a year. Even with removal of the products of conception, cells may remain behind and develop into a malignancy.

Nursing Interventions and Patient Teaching

The woman and her family need information about the disease process, the necessity for a long course of follow-up, and the possible consequences of the disease. Help the woman understand and cope with pregnancy loss and recognize that the pregnancy was abnormal. Encourage the woman and her family to express their feelings and provide information about support groups or counseling resources if needed. Explain the need to postpone a subsequent pregnancy the next year, and provide contraception counseling to emphasize the importance of consistent, reliable use of the method chosen.

ECTOPIC PREGNANCY

Etiology

In ectopic pregnancy, implantation occurs somewhere other than within the uterus, most commonly the fallopian tube (Fig. 29.2). An estimated 1% to 2% of reported pregnancies are ectopic. About 95% of all ectopic pregnancies occur in the fallopian tube. Other sites include

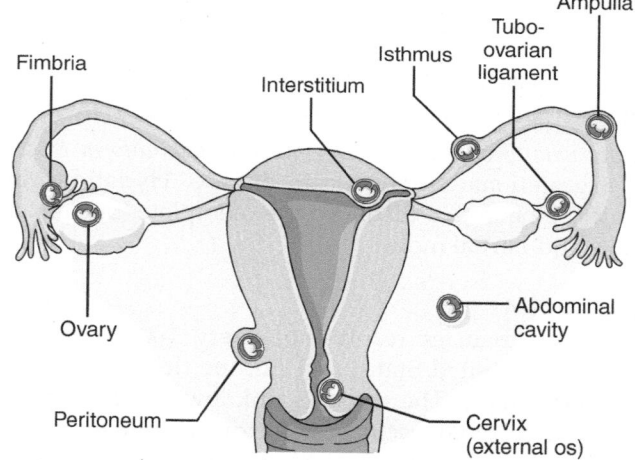

Fig. 29.3 Sites of implantation of ectopic pregnancies in order of frequency of occurrence: ampulla, isthmus, interstitium, fimbria, tuboovarian ligament, ovary, abdominal cavity, and cervix (external os).

the abdominal cavity, an ovary, ligaments, and the cervix (Fig. 29.3). Rarely is the ectopic pregnancy located in the abdomen (1% of ectopic pregnancies); in this case, the pregnancy may have a minimal chance to achieve viability. Tubal pregnancy occurs when the progress of the fertilized ovum through the fallopian tube is slowed or obstructed. The incidence of ectopic pregnancy has increased dramatically throughout the world in the past 20 years. Ectopic pregnancy rates are higher in nonwhite and older women, particularly those over age 35. Risk factors for the development include history of pelvic inflammatory disease, tubal structural defects, endometriosis, history of surgery to the reproductive organs, smoking, the use of assistive reproductive techniques, and elevated progesterone levels.

Pathophysiology

Once the fertilized ovum implants, it begins to grow and develop. It becomes too large to be contained. This results in pain. If the pregnancy is not aborted, it ultimately results in rupture of the tube and bleeding into the abdominal cavity. At least three-fourths of ectopic pregnancies become symptomatic and are diagnosed during the first trimester. Ectopic pregnancy is a significant cause of maternal morbidity and mortality, even in developed countries.

Clinical Manifestations

The woman already may have had pregnancy confirmed with an HCG test. She may have experienced symptoms associated with pregnancy such as amenorrhea, nausea and vomiting, and breast tenderness. Uterine examination reveals enlargement in 25% of cases. These normal symptoms associated with pregnancy are the result of the hormonal changes of the pregnancy.

The initial symptom signaling there is a concern is lower abdominal pain. The pain may be one-sided or across the entire abdomen. Vaginal bleeding may be present. If the fallopian tube has ruptured, she may have vaginal bleeding, referred shoulder pain, and abdominal rigidity. The shoulder pain will be the result of nerve irritation from the bleeding. The risk for hypovolemic shock is present.

Diagnosis, Medical Management and Nursing Interventions

The initial management includes confirmation of the condition. HCG testing is performed, and levels are traditionally lower than normal for the stage of gestation. An ultrasound is completed to determine the location of the pregnancy. A vaginal examination also is performed. The vaginal exam may cause discomfort.

Management of the ectopic pregnancy may be done surgically or pharmacologically. Surgical treatment, a laparotomy, requires removal of the pregnancy and related damaged tissue. It may necessitate removal of the fallopian tube (salpingectomy) or repair of the damaged tube (salpingostomy). If the fallopian tube is ruptured and significant bleeding occurs, blood transfusions may be necessary.

Pharmacologic therapy, when applicable, may allow for preservation of the tube and help to improve the chances of future pregnancies. Single or multiple doses of methotrexate may be prescribed for treatment of the unruptured ectopic pregnancy. Methotrexate is a folic acid antagonist that has been used for years to treat actively proliferating trophoblastic disease. It destroys the rapidly dividing cells. Not all women are candidates for the use of methotrexate. The fallopian tube must be unruptured and the size of the pregnancy less than 3.5 cm. The woman must be free of blood, liver, or kidney disorders. The medication may be administered once or twice if needed. Patient education concerning signs and symptoms to report include increased abdominal pain and vaginal bleeding. These may signal fallopian tube rupture. Patients are advised to avoid alcohol ingestion, vitamins containing folic acid, NSAID pain relievers and penicillin. Administration of Rho(D) immune globulin (RhoGAM) is indicated for those women who are Rh negative.

The woman and her family often need support to resolve emotions that may include anger, grief, guilt, and self-blame. The woman also may be anxious about her ability to become pregnant. Unfortunately, conditions that led to the ectopic pregnancy may exist in the other tube, placing the woman at increased risk for a repeated ectopic pregnancy. Additionally, the population who experience an ectopic pregnancy may have a history of risk factors associated with infertility. This can heighten the sense of loss and grief. The family experiencing an ectopic pregnancy may experience an acute sense of loss similar to that of women suffering a miscarriage. Ensure that the mother and family understand what has happened to the pregnancy and the reasons for the care options selected.

Prognosis

The prognosis varies. Accounting for less than 2.5% of pregnancies, ectopic pregnancies are the leading cause of maternal mortality in the first trimester of pregnancy (Stremick, 2019). The rates of maternal morbidity and secondary surgery are high, however, principally because of inaccurate or delayed diagnosis. When a potential ectopic pregnancy presents, other conditions that share similar manifestations must be considered. This may include threatened abortion, ruptured corpus luteum cyst, appendicitis, salpingitis, ovarian cysts, torsion of the ovary, and urinary tract infection. The perinatal mortality rate in ectopic pregnancy is virtually 100%. Ectopic pregnancy recurs in approximately 10% of women, but more than 50% of women who have had an ectopic pregnancy achieve at least one normal pregnancy thereafter. The diagnosis and management of this condition are changing rapidly with technological advances.

SPONTANEOUS ABORTION

Etiology

Abortion is the termination of pregnancy before the age of viability—or 20 weeks of gestation in the United States. The two types of abortion are (1) spontaneous abortion, which results from natural causes, and (2) therapeutic abortion (including elective abortion), which is the interruption of the pregnancy for medical or personal reasons. Spontaneous abortion is referred to generally as a miscarriage. Most spontaneous abortions occur during the first trimester of pregnancy. Estimates are that as many as 10% to 15% of all pregnancies end in first-trimester spontaneous abortion. Many of these go unrecognized, with the woman merely thinking that her menstrual period was delayed.

More than half of all spontaneous abortions are caused by abnormal embryonic development, chromosomal defects, and inheritable disorders. Maternal causes linked to spontaneous abortions include advancing maternal age and parity, chronic infections, chronic debilitating diseases, poor nutrition, and recreational drug use.

Pathophysiology

The pathophysiology depends on the specific cause.

Clinical Manifestations

The main presenting symptom is bleeding, which may or may not be accompanied by cramps or backache. Spontaneous abortions are classified as follows:

- *Threatened:* Unexplained bleeding and cramping occur. The fetus may or may not be alive. Membranes remain intact, and the cervical os remains closed.
- *Inevitable:* Bleeding increases, and the cervical os begins to dilate. Membranes may rupture.
- *Complete:* All products of conception are expelled from the uterus. The cervica os may be slightly opened or closed.
- *Incomplete:* Some, but not all, of the products of conception are expelled.
- *Missed:* The fetus dies and growth ceases, but the fetus remains in utero. Amenorrhea continues, but no uterine growth is measurable. The patient may report the decline or absence of pregnancy related symptoms.
- *Septic:* Malodorous bleeding, elevated temperature, and cramping may be present; cervical os is opened; and abdominal tenderness is typical.
- *Habitual:* This often is referred to as recurrent spontaneous abortion, when the woman has aborted spontaneously in three or more consecutive pregnancies; emotional trauma is increased, especially with subsequent pregnancies.

Diagnosis and Medical Management

When a woman presents with symptomology consistent with an actual or potential spontaneous abortion, the first step is to confirm diagnosis. Diagnostic confirmation will involve an assessment of HCG levels. Although the products of conception may no longer be viable, HCG testing may reveal positive levels. These levels, while positive, may not be at the value of a pregnancy at the gestation in question. Repeated (serial) testing may be performed to determine if levels decline over a period of days. An ultrasound to assess fetal viability is completed.

When a spontaneous abortion occurs, administer IV fluids and replace blood loss with transfusions, as

Box 29.3	Types of Spontaneous Abortion and Therapeutic Management

- *Threatened:* Decreased activity, sedation, and avoidance of stress and orgasm are recommended. Further treatment depends on patient's course.
- *Inevitable, incomplete:* Prompt termination of pregnancy is accomplished, usually by dilation and evacuation (D&E).
- *Complete:* No further intervention may be needed if uterine contractions are adequate to prevent hemorrhage and if there is no infection.
- *Missed:* If spontaneous evacuation of the uterus does not occur, pregnancy is terminated with method appropriate to duration of pregnancy. Blood clotting factors are monitored until uterus is empty. Disseminated intravascular coagulation (DIC) and incoagulability of blood with uncontrolled hemorrhage may develop in cases of fetal death after 12th week if products of conception are retained for longer than 5 weeks (see discussion of DIC).
- *Septic:* Pregnancy is terminated immediately with method appropriate to duration of pregnancy. Cervical culture and sensitivity studies are done, and broad-spectrum antibiotic therapy (e.g., ampicillin) is started. Treatment for septic shock is initiated if necessary. If signs of uterine infection are seen, such as an elevated temperature, vaginal discharge with a foul odor, or abdominal pain, evacuation of the uterus is delayed until antibiotic therapy is initiated.

ordered. A dilation and curettage (D&C) or dilation and evacuation (suction; D&E) may be indicated to remove retained placental tissue (Box 29.3). If significant blood loss occurred, iron supplementation may be ordered. Rh-negative women need the administration of RhoGAM.

Patient Teaching

Patient teaching should include the need for rest (see the Patient Teaching box on spontaneous abortion).

Patient Teaching

Spontaneous Abortion

- Refer patient to appropriate support groups, clergy, or professional counseling.
- Advise patient to report any heavy, profuse, or bright red bleeding to physician.
- Reassure patient that a scant, dark discharge may persist for 1–2 weeks.
- Instruct patient not to use tampons or douches until bleeding has stopped.
- Instruct patient to avoid sexual intercourse until bleeding has stopped.
- Acknowledge that patient has experienced a loss and that time is needed for recovery. She may experience mood swings and depression.
- Advise patient that attempts to become pregnant are not recommended for at least 2 months or as recommended by the healthcare provider to allow the body to recover.

INCOMPETENT CERVIX

Late abortion and preterm delivery may be associated with incompetent cervix. This condition traditionally was defined as the passive and painless dilation of the cervix during the second trimester. A more recent idea is that cervical competence is variable and is determined in part by cervical length. Other related factors include composition of the cervical tissue and the individual circumstances associated with the pregnancy, such as maternal stress and lifestyle. Women who have a history of delivering at an earlier point in gestation with subsequent pregnancies should be evaluated for cervical competence issues.

Etiology

Etiologic factors include a history of cervical lacerations during childbirth, excessive cervical dilation for curettage or biopsy, and the patient's mother's ingestion of diethylstilbestrol during pregnancy with the patient. Other instances may result from a congenitally short cervix or cervical or uterine anomalies. Reduced cervical competence is a clinical diagnosis, based on a history of short labors and recurring loss of the pregnancy at progressively earlier gestational ages. Ultrasound scan is used to diagnose this condition objectively. A short cervix (less than 20 mm long) is indicative of reduced cervical competence. Often, but not always, the short cervix is accompanied by effacement of the internal cervical os.

Medical Management

Women with a history of painless cervical dilation and effacement in a previous pregnancy or with a previous second-trimester loss in which short cervix and effacement were documented with ultrasound scan are candidates for prophylactic cerclage, a technique that uses suture material to constrict the internal os of the cervix (Fig. 29.4). Prophylactic cerclage is placed at 10 to 14 weeks of gestation. It is typically an outpatient procedure. After the placement of the cerclage, the woman is observed for approximately 1 to 2 hours. The observation will require the gravid woman to be placed on a monitor. Uterine activity and fetal heart tones will be assessed. Discharge teaching provided includes instructions to refrain from intercourse and to avoid prolonged standing and heavy lifting. The signs of premature labor and preterm rupture of membranes must be reviewed with the patient. Signs and symptoms to report include ramping, bleeding, rupture of membranes, or elevated temperatures. During the remainder of the pregnancy, assess for cervical shortening and effacement. The cerclage is removed electively (usually with an office or clinic procedure) when the woman reaches 37 weeks of gestation, or it may be left in place and a cesarean birth performed. Approximately 80% to 90% of pregnancies treated with cerclage result in live, viable births. If removed, the cerclage must be replaced with each successive pregnancy.

A woman whose reduced cervical competence is diagnosed during the current pregnancy may undergo emergency cerclage placement. Risks of the procedure include premature rupture of membranes, preterm labor, and *chorioamnionitis* (an inflammatory reaction in fetal membranes to bacteria or viruses in amniotic fluid). Because of these risks and because bed rest and *tocolytic therapy* (drugs used to relax the uterus) can be used to prolong the pregnancy, cerclage rarely is performed after 26 weeks of gestation.

Because the diagnosis of reduced cervical competence usually is not made until the woman has lost one or two pregnancies, there may be feelings of guilt or self-blame for this impending loss; therefore, assess the patient for previous reactions to stress and appropriateness of coping responses. Emotional support for the gravid woman and her family are indicated. If management is unsuccessful and the fetus is born before viability, provide appropriate grief support. If the fetus is born prematurely, appropriate anticipatory guidance and support are necessary.

Prognosis

Prognosis for the fetus in the woman who has an incompetent cervix is based on early recognition and prompt medical management. The woman with the incompetent cervix likely will continue to face spontaneous abortions and premature labor if not managed with each pregnancy. Complications beyond pregnancy are very limited.

BLEEDING DISORDERS

Vaginal bleeding during pregnancy warrants investigation. Instruct the patient to contact her physician if any bleeding occurs. Depending on the stage of pregnancy, several different conditions may cause the bleeding.

PLACENTA PREVIA

Etiology

Placenta previa occurs when the placenta implants in the lower uterine segment. Placenta previa is described by the degree to which the placenta covers the internal cervical os: complete with total coverage; partial with incomplete coverage; and marginal, which indicates that only an edge of the placenta approaches the internal os (Fig. 29.5). The term *low implantation* is used when the placenta is situated in the lower uterine segment away from the internal os. In the second trimester, approximately 45% of all placentas are implanted in the lower uterine segment. As the lower uterine segment lengthens (stretches), the placenta seems to migrate upward.

Placenta previa occurs in 1 in 200 pregnancies. The cause is unknown. Risk factors include cesarean birth, possibly related to endometrial scarring; multiple gestation (because of the larger placental area);

Fig. 29.4 (A) Cerclage correction of recurrent premature dilation of cervix. (B) Cross section of closed internal os. (From Shiland BJ: *Mastering healthcare terminology*, ed 6, St. Louis, 2019, Elsevier.)

closely spaced pregnancies; and advanced maternal age (older than 35 years).

Pathophysiology

In the last trimester of pregnancy, uterine size increases, and the cervix begins to dilate and efface. As the placenta separates from the uterus at the internal os of the cervix, sinuses at the site begin to bleed. The amount of bleeding depends on the amount of separation that occurs.

Clinical Manifestations

The main presenting symptom of placenta previa is painless, bright red, vaginal bleeding that occurs after 20 weeks of gestation. The bright red bleeding may be intermittent, may occur in gushes, or more rarely, may be continuous. It may start while the patient is resting or during any activity.

Abdominal examination usually reveals a soft (relaxed), nontender uterus of normal tone.

Fig. 29.5 Types of placenta previa after onset of labor. (A) Incomplete, or partial. (B) Complete, or total. (C) Marginal, or low lying.

Diagnostic Testing

Obstetric ultrasound scan is the diagnostic method of choice. Vaginal examinations are restricted in the pregnant woman with undiagnosed vaginal bleeding as the manipulation may result in additional bleeding. When deemed necessary, the vaginal examination is performed by the primary care provider. The vaginal examination is performed in a care environment that allows for a *double setup*. This allows for the availability of a staffed operating room, with trained personnel and equipment available to manage an immediate vaginal or cesarean birth. Manipulation of the lower uterine segment or cervix may result in profound hemorrhage; preparation for immediate delivery is necessary.

Medical Management

Medical care of the patient with placenta previa is traditionally conservative. Laboratory testing includes blood typing and cross-match. Close observation of the patient's hemoglobin and hematocrit levels is completed. The patient is monitored with hopes of prolonging the pregnancy to promote fetal lung maturity. Those placentas that are implanted low, near the cervical os, may be delivered vaginally if they "migrate upward" as the pregnancy continues. Placentas that cover the cervical os partially or completely are delivered via cesarean section. The common practice is to schedule the cesarean birth at 36 weeks of gestation. If bleeding cannot be controlled or labor begins, delivery is indicated. If labor onset occurs prior to the scheduled cesarean delivery, the patient must have prompt treatment to surgically deliver the fetus. Fluid volume replacement may be indicated. Blood transfusions may be indicated to manage large volumes of blood loss or low hemoglobin levels. Betamethasone, a steroid, may be administered to promote fetal lung maturity in preparation for a potential preterm delivery.

Nursing Management

Patients with stable conditions often can be managed from home. Activity is limited to bed rest with bathroom privileges. The patient with placenta previa requires education about the condition. Instruct the patient about the signs and symptoms to report, such as increases in vaginal bleeding, the onset of labor, or rupture of membranes. Discuss the use of kick counts daily. Sexual intercourse is not permitted for the patient diagnosed with placenta previa. Emotional support related to the diagnosis, potential compromise to the fetus, and related management strategies is indicated.

Blood loss may cease with delivery of the infant and placenta. However, the interlacing muscle bundles that contract around open vessels so characteristic of the upper part of the uterus are absent in the lower part of the uterus. The patient has an elevated risk for postpartum hemorrhage (PPH). During emergency preparations, constantly provide reassurance to reduce the woman's anxiety and that of her family.

Prognosis

Maternal mortality rate in placenta previa is low, about 0.6%. Fetal outcomes are related directly to the level of bleeding and the gestational age of the fetus at the time of delivery.

ABRUPTIO PLACENTAE

Etiology

Abruptio placentae is premature separation of the normally implanted placenta from the uterine wall. This generally occurs late in pregnancy, frequently during labor. Abruptio placentae occurs in about 1% of all pregnancies. The cause is unknown. Predisposing factors include history of abruption in a past pregnancy

Table 29.1	Classification of Placental Abruption
TYPE	**SEVERITY**
Grade I (mild, 1)	The woman has vaginal bleeding, perhaps with uterine tenderness and mild tetany (extremely prolonged uterine contraction), but neither mother nor baby is in distress. Approximately 10%–20% of placental surface is detached.
Grade II (moderate, 2)	The woman has uterine tenderness and tetany, with or without external evidence of bleeding. The mother is not in shock, but there is fetal distress. Approximately 20%–50% of the total surface is detached.
Grade III (severe, 3)	Uterine atony is severe, the woman is in shock (although the bleeding may not be obvious), and the fetus is dead. Often the woman has coagulopathy (defect in blood-clotting mechanisms). More than 50% of the placental surface area is detached.

not caused by trauma, trauma, hypertension and advancing maternal age. Abruptio placentae is three times more likely to occur in women with gravidity of more than five. Smoking and cocaine use in pregnancy significantly increases the risk of premature separation of the placenta. Blunt external abdominal trauma, usually the result of motor vehicle accidents or maternal battering, is an increasingly significant cause of placental abruption.

Pathophysiology

When the placenta separates from the uterine wall, bleeding from uterine sinuses occurs, as in placenta previa. The most common classification of placental abruption is according to type and severity (Table 29.1).

Clinical Manifestations

The major symptoms of abruptio placentae are sudden, severe pain accompanied by uterine rigidity. The uterus also may increase in size because of the hemorrhage. The first sign during labor may be strong and constant contractions (tetany). Symptoms vary with the degree of separation. The presence of vaginal bleeding is determined by the location of the abruption. If the placenta has torn, and the blood is trapped in the uterus, little to no vaginal bleeding will be noted.

Assessment

When any vaginal bleeding occurs during pregnancy, assess the following:

- *Duration, amount, color, and characteristics of the bleeding:* This includes assessment of: (1) the time since the onset of bleeding; (2) what, if any, activity preceded the bleeding episode; (3) the number of pads saturated per

hour; and (4) the color of the bleeding (bright red, dark red, or brown). If a clot or tissue is passed, save it for examination by the health care provider.

- *Vital signs:* Depending on the origin and severity of the bleeding, signs of shock may be present. In addition to pulse and blood pressure, observe for pallor; diaphoresis; cool, clammy skin; and dyspnea. These physical signs seem out of proportion to the amount of bleeding if the hemorrhage is concealed, as in central abruptio placentae.

- *Pain:* Note the presence, location, nature, and duration of pain.

- *FHR:* Depending on the stage of pregnancy, measure FHR with a fetoscope or Doppler amplifier. If pregnancy is in the early stages, fetal heart sounds may not be heard. In labor, when there is uteroplacental insufficiency, the fetus, in its struggle to obtain more oxygen, may be restless and active. The FHR either accelerates greatly or slows.

- *Emotional response:* In addition to a physical assessment, address the emotional response of the expectant mother and her partner. Common feelings include anxiety, fear and confusion. The care team and their interactions may feel overwhelming. Concerns about the viability of the pregnancy will also be present.

Diagnostic Tests

The most common laboratory tests include measurement of hemoglobin and hematocrit levels to determine the amount of blood lost. Blood typing and cross-matching are ordered in case blood replacement is necessary. Ultrasound scans may be performed to determine placental location and fetal life. Vaginal examinations are avoided because they may increase the bleeding.

Medical Management

Abruptio placentae constitutes an obstetric emergency. The treatment often includes delivery via cesarean birth and blood replacement.

A modified side-lying position with a wedge placed under the patient's right hip facilitates uterine-placental perfusion. Carefully monitor blood and fluid replacement therapy. Insert a retention catheter to monitor urinary output. The fetus is monitored and delivered when indicated. If signs of fetal compromise such as hypoxia are present, or if the expectant mother exhibits signs of excessive bleeding, either obvious or concealed, the fetus is delivered immediately. Intensive monitoring of the woman and the fetus is essential because rapid deterioration in the condition of either can occur.

A woman undergoing immediate cesarean delivery may feel powerless as the health care team hurriedly prepares her for surgery. If possible, explain anticipated procedures to the woman and her family to reduce their fear and anxiety.

Nursing Interventions

Nursing measures are structured to support and promote optimal physical and psychological functioning.

Oxygen should be available. If blood loss is significant, oxygen-carrying capability is decreased; oxygen may be ordered to prevent maternal or fetal hypoxia.

IV or blood replacement therapy may be necessary, so be prepared for this. Possible loss of the pregnancy is a crisis. Be supportive of the patient's and family's emotional needs. Remain with the woman as much as possible, listen to her concerns, give clear explanations about medical treatment, and prepare her for the possible loss.

Patient problems and interventions for the patient with abruptio placentae include but are not limited to the following:

PATIENT PROBLEM	NURSING INTERVENTIONS
Insufficient Cardiac Output, related to excessive bleeding secondary to abruptio placentae	Monitor and record vital signs q 15 min until stable, then q h as indicated Measure and record I&O Weigh daily Assess skin turgor and mucous membranes Help patient ambulate Monitor blood replacement therapy
Potential for Grief, related to possible loss of pregnancy	Allow time for patient to verbalize concerns about loss Assist with grieving processes Encourage contact with support system Encourage session with spiritual advisor if patient desires Foster active participation of significant other

Prognosis

Premature separation of the placenta is a serious disorder and accounts for about 15% of all perinatal deaths. Maternal mortality rate approaches 1% in abruptio placentae; this condition remains a leading cause of maternal death. The mother's prognosis depends on the extent of placental detachment, overall blood loss, degree of disseminated intravascular coagulation (DIC), and time between the placental separation and delivery.

Approximately one-third of infants of women with premature separation of the placenta die. More than 50% die as a result of preterm delivery, and many others die of intrauterine hypoxia.

DISSEMINATED INTRAVASCULAR COAGULATION

Etiology

Disseminated intravascular coagulation is a potentially life-threatening disorder that results from alterations in the normal clotting mechanism. DIC is always a secondary diagnosis. It may be seen with abruptio placentae, incomplete abortion, hypertensive disease, or infectious process. It may occur with a postterm delivery.

Pathophysiology

In DIC, the body's attempts to prevent excessive blood loss put stress on the coagulation processes. The body produces excessive amounts of thrombin, stimulating the conversion of fibrinogen to fibrin. Elevated fibrin levels result in multiple small clots forming in small blood vessels, which may lead to obstruction of vessels, ischemia, and damage to vital organs. This clot formation also traps platelets and can result in generalized hemorrhage.

Clinical Manifestations

The onset of symptoms is sudden. The patient may report chest pain or dyspnea and become extremely restless and cyanotic, occasionally expectorating frothy, blood-tinged mucus. Profound circulatory shock from hemorrhage may occur rapidly. Fetal and maternal death may result.

Assessment

All women with complications that may result in DIC should be observed closely for signs of bleeding, such as epistaxis (nosebleeds), bleeding gums, or petechiae, particularly around the blood pressure cuff on the patient's arm. Excessive bleeding may occur from a site of slight trauma, such as venipuncture sites, intramuscular or subcutaneous injection sites, nicks from shaving of perineum or abdomen, and injury from insertion of urinary catheter. Continue to monitor the maternal and fetal conditions with assessment of vital signs, FHR, and I&O and with general careful assessment.

Diagnostic Tests

Blood testing includes determination of hemoglobin and hematocrit levels. Clotting factor studies, such as fibrinogen levels, platelet counts, prothrombin time (PT), and partial thromboplastin time (PTT), typically are ordered for the patient. Laboratory tests may reveal various degrees of anemia and decreased fibrinogen and platelet counts. Prolonged PT and PTT are also typical.

Medical Management

Emergency care for DIC includes IV administration of fibrinogen, blood, and other substances that help restore normal clotting mechanisms. Paradoxically, DIC therapy may include heparin via continuous infusion pump (although its use is controversial) and oxygen therapy with a tight-fitting mask at 10 to 12 L/min. If the fetus is not yet born, delivery should occur as soon as possible. Carefully monitor urinary output (it must be maintained at more than 30 mL/h) because renal failure is one consequence of DIC.

If the woman is still pregnant, position her in a side-lying tilt to maximize blood flow to the uterus.

Nursing Interventions

Nursing interventions are directed at supporting medical treatment. Report signs and symptoms promptly. Use caution when providing care to minimize the risk of additional trauma to tissue, which may lead to further bleeding. Recognize and support the emotional needs of the patient and the family.

Prognosis

DIC is a life-threatening disorder. The prognosis depends on the degree and extent of the underlying disorder and the response of the woman to prompt and proper treatment.

POSTPARTUM HEMORRHAGE

Etiology

PPH is classified as early or late. Early PPH is blood loss greater than 500 mL after vaginal childbirth or 1000 mL after cesarean birth. Estimating blood loss may be difficult if the blood loss is rapid or concealed. Hemorrhage is one of the leading causes of maternal morbidity and mortality in the first 24 hours after delivery; late PPH occurs after the first 24 hours. At least 5% of women experience PPH. Studies have shown that women who have an extended second stage of labor, instrument-assisted delivery, large-for-gestational-age newborn, or induction or augmentation of labor, or who are obese have an increased incidence of PPH.

The most common causes of early hemorrhage are uterine atony, *retained placental fragments,* and *perineal lacerations. Uterine atony* (lack of normal tone or strength) has several potential causes, including excessive distention of the uterus from multiple pregnancy, hydramnios (excessive amount of amniotic fluid), or a large infant. Atony is also more prevalent in grand multiparas or when labor is prolonged or traumatic. Pharmacologic therapies also may be linked to PPH. Magnesium sulfate and nifedipine are associated with PPH. Placental disorders, including implantation in the lower uterine segment and failure of the placenta to detach as in placenta accrete, are implicated as well. Infection is another contributing factor to PPH. The most common cause of late PPH is retained placental fragments.

Pathophysiology

Contraction of the uterus seals the uterine sinuses, aiding in the prevention of PPH. Hemorrhage results when loss of tone or tissue remaining in the cavity prevents adequate uterine contraction. In addition, hemorrhage may result when there is unchecked bleeding from lacerations or tears. These tears may be uterine, perineal, or cervical.

Assessment

Nursing assessment of uterine contraction and lochia is part of routine postpartum assessment. If the uterus is boggy (soft, uncontracted) or the flow of lochia is heavy, suspect hemorrhage. Bleeding accompanied by a boggy uterus is consistent with atony. Bleeding that occurs in the presence of a firm, contracted uterus should be investigated because potential causes include lacerations or tears. Vital sign changes such as tachycardia and hypotension are reflective of excessive blood loss. Compare findings with the patient's baseline values.

PPH can progress rapidly to shock. Symptoms consistent with advancing PPH include oliguria, lethargy or restlessness, air hunger, and ultimately collapse. Review the history for factors that predispose to PPH.

For the first 24 hours after childbirth, the uterus should feel like a firmly contracted ball roughly the size of a large grapefruit. It should be located easily at about the level of the umbilicus. Lochia should be dark red and moderate in amount. Saturation of more than one peripad per hour is considered a large amount, and saturation of more than one peripad in 15 minutes is excessive. Significant blood loss may also happen with a constant trickle or dribble.

Assess the bleeding color, amount, and, if possible, source. Note the time of the last pad change. If the pad is loose, blood may pool under the patient, so assessment must include checking under the patient.

Vital signs may not be reliable indicators of shock in the immediate postpartum period because of physiologic adaptations of this stage. Data should include assessment for bladder distention because a full bladder lifts and displaces the uterus and prevents effective contraction of the uterine muscles. Help the mother urinate or catheterize her as necessary.

Medical Management

Medical management begins with determination of the cause of bleeding. Diagnostic studies include a complete blood count, type, and cross-match. The presenting hemoglobin and hematocrit levels are compared with baseline studies. IV fluid replacement is initiated. Transfusion with packed red blood cells (RBCs) may be performed. Treatment is based on the underlying case of the bleeding. Retained placental fragments are managed with a D&E to remove the tissue surgically. Lacerations are identified and repaired.

The management for uterine atony includes fundal massage, with the bladder kept empty. Fluid replacement is initiated with IV therapy. Oxytocic agents such as Methergine and Pitocin are administered. Failure to control bleeding may necessitate a hysterectomy.

Nursing Interventions

Nursing interventions are directed at the early identification of excess blood loss and the prevention of hemorrhage. If the uterus is boggy, massage is initiated. If the uterus remains atonic, the primary care provider may prescribe an oxytocic. If a D&E is necessary, preparation of the patient for surgery is completed by the nurse. Provide emotional support. Other surgical preparations include obtaining signed consent forms; verifying that laboratory data are on the chart, the patient has had nothing by mouth, and identification and allergy bands are in place; completing skin preparations as ordered; having the patient empty her bladder or inserting an indwelling catheter; removing jewelry, contact lenses, and dentures; obtaining vital signs; administering preoperative medication as scheduled; monitoring safety with side rails up; and documenting all preoperative care.

Trauma. If the fundus is firm, but bleeding is excessive, the cause may be a laceration of the cervix or birth canal. Inspect the perineum for a laceration in that area. Lacerations of the cervix or vagina are not visible, but bleeding when the uterus is contracted suggests a laceration. This sign warrants examination of the vaginal walls and the cervix by the health care provider (see Chapter 28 and Box 28.2).

If the mother reports deep, severe pelvic or rectal pain, or if vital signs or skin changes suggest hemorrhage, but excessive bleeding is not obvious, the cause may be concealed bleeding and the formation of a hematoma. Examine the vulva for a bulging mass or skin discoloration. A hematoma in the vagina or in the retroperitoneal area is not obvious. Notify the health care provider.

Keep the woman on bed rest to increase venous return and maintain cardiac output. The Trendelenburg position may interfere with cardiac function and is not advised. Continue assessments; call for assistance; and save all pads, linen savers, and linen so that blood loss can be estimated accurately. Assistance is necessary so that one nurse can continue to massage the uncontracted uterus and perform and record assessments while the other notifies the health care provider of the mother's condition.

The unusual activity of the hospital staff may make the mother and her family anxious. Keeping the family informed is one of the most effective ways of reducing anxiety.

Patient problems and interventions for the patient with PPH include but are not limited to the following:

PATIENT PROBLEM	NURSING INTERVENTIONS
Insufficient Knowledge related to signs of hemorrhage	Select teaching strategies appropriate to patient's need and willingness to learn
	Demonstrate postpartum checks of fundus and lochia
	Observe patient performing self-check
	Review importance of contacting the health care provider if signs are abnormal or questionable
Inadequate Fluid Volume, related to hypovolemia secondary to excessive blood loss	Perform fundal massage until firm
	Monitor vital signs and intake and output closely
	Assess blood loss by pad saturation
	Monitor fluid replacement therapy
	Monitor for signs and symptoms of infection
	Teach patient fundal massage
	Encourage fluids by mouth unless contraindicated

Patient Teaching

Patient education includes the importance and purpose of the fundal assessment. Teach them how to palpate their fundus. Observation of lochia and the normal parameters is discussed. Late PPH, which typically occurs without warning 7 to 14 days after delivery, can be dangerous for the unsuspecting mother. Alert her to call the physician if bleeding is excessive or persistent beyond expectations.

Prognosis

In the United States, 700 women will lose their lives as a result of pregnancy-related issues. This represents 17.4 women per 100,000 live births in the United States (CDC, 2020). Similar to the infant mortality statistics the largest population impacted will be non-Hispanic black women. The leading causes are cardiovascular conditions, infection, and hemorrhage.

HYPERTENSIVE CONDITIONS IN PREGNANCY

Etiology

Vascular resistance is reduced during pregnancy. Rising progesterone levels are responsible for this physiological change. In response, the blood pressure levels are normally reduced during the first and second trimesters. The blood pressure levels gradually return to the prepregnancy baseline levels by the later weeks of the second trimester or early in the third trimester. Pregnancy may cause blood pressure elevations. The timing and associated factors determine the type of disorder.

Chronic hypertension: Elevation of blood pressure 140/90 or greater occurring before pregnancy or prior to 20 weeks gestation. There is no proteinuria. When a patient experiences chronic hypertension, the likelihood of preeclampsia is heightened.

Gestational hypertension (GH): Formerly referred to as pregnancy-induced hypertension (PIH), GH is a disease encountered during pregnancy or early in the puerperium, characterized by increasing hypertension. The condition begins after 20 weeks' gestation. Unlike preeclampsia, it is not accompanied by proteinuria. As the pregnancy continues, the condition may progress to preeclampsia.

Preeclampsia *and eclampsia:* Blood pressure increases of 140/90 or higher, taken twice 6 hours or more apart, occurring after 20 weeks' gestation and accompanied by mild proteinuria and edema is indicative of preeclampsia. If the blood pressure increases to 160/110 or greater and is accompanied by moderate proteinuria, the condition is termed severe. Additional symptoms of the condition include headache, visual disturbances, and epigastric pain. These symptoms may signal worsening of the condition.

Risk factors for the condition include maternal age (under 18 or over 40 years of age), first pregnancy, African American, history of chronic or GH, obesity, family history of preeclampsia, diabetes, multifetal pregnancy, and gestational trophoblastic disease.

Mild preeclampsia. Early preeclampsia has few clinical symptoms. Change in the blood pressure readings (an increase of 30 mm Hg systolic and 15 mm Hg diastolic, or a reading of 140/90 mm Hg in a woman whose blood pressure has been normal) indicates a problem. The blood pressure readings are reflective of hypertension when taken two times 6 hours apart. Generalized edema may be evident in the face, the hands, and the ankles. Periorbital edema may be a more ominous finding. Weight may increase as much as 3 pounds (1.4 kg) per month in the second trimester and 1 pound (0.5 kg) per week in the third trimester. Urine testing frequently shows 1+ to 2+ protein level readings. The urinary output is at least 500 mL/24 h.

Severe preeclampsia. The symptoms of severe preeclampsia may appear suddenly. Blood pressure readings increase; readings of 160/110 mm Hg or higher on two separate occasions 6 hours apart with the pregnant woman on bed rest are common. The presence and location of edema were once considered key criteria for the diagnosis of preeclampsia. Currently, edema is monitored but it does not determine the severity of the condition. Edema becomes increasingly obvious and may be observed in the face, the hands, the sacral area, the abdomen, and throughout the lower extremities. Weight increases dramatically. The woman may gain as much as 2 pounds (0.9 kg) in a matter of a few days or a week. Urine testing for albumin shows 3+ to 4+ readings. The urinary output is less than 500 mL/24 hours. The patient often reports headache, blurred vision, and epigastric discomfort. The assessment reveals hyperreflexia. Clonus is noted with pending seizure activity. Increasing headache, visual changes and hyperreflexia signal worsening neurological involvement.

Eclampsia. Eclampsia is the most severe form of preeclampsia. The most dramatic characteristic is seizure activity. The patient exhibits tonic (pertaining to or characterized by muscular tension) and clonic (spasmodic alteration of muscular contractions) phases. This generally is followed by a coma that lasts from minutes to hours. Other signs are elevated blood pressure, proteinuria, and oliguria. If untreated, this sequence of seizure-coma may repeat, and death may follow.

Assessment

During each prenatal care visit, blood pressure assessment is completed. Hypertensive conditions can begin at any point in the prenatal period through the postpartum period. Weight gain patterns should be reviewed. Excessive or rapid weight gain, particularly when accompanied by edema, may signal complication onset. The presence and location of edema is recorded (see Fig. 8.16 in *Adult Health Nursing*). Edema typically is described with a scale of 1+ to 4+:

1+ Minimal edema on pedal and pretibial area
2+ Obvious edema of lower extremities
3+ Edema of face, hands, sacrum, and abdomen
4+ Massive, generalized edema (anasarca)

Test urine for protein with each prenatal appointment. If rupture of membranes has occurred, the readings may be inaccurate. Certain symptoms, such as continuous headache, drowsiness, or mental confusion,

indicate poor cerebral perfusion and may be precursors of convulsions. Visual disturbances, such as blurred or double vision or spots before the eyes, indicate arterial spasms and edema in the retina. Some symptoms such as epigastric pain or "upset stomach" are particularly ominous, because they indicate distention of the hepatic capsule and often warn that a convulsion is imminent. Decreased urinary output indicates poor perfusion of the kidneys and may precede acute renal failure.

If the patient is hospitalized for GH, monitor deep tendon reflexes (Table 29.2 and Fig. 29.6) and urinary output; also electronically monitor FHR.

Diagnostic Tests

Serum laboratory tests include blood urea nitrogen, complete blood cell count, clotting studies, liver enzymes, type and screen, and possible cross-match. Urine screenings, such as specific gravity and protein, and a 24-hour urine collection are obtained to measure creatinine and protein clearance. Electrolyte panels commonly are drawn. If symptoms indicate severe preeclampsia or eclampsia, liver function and platelet count evaluations also are performed. If the health care provider is considering induction of labor before term, gestation tests to establish fetal maturity are indicated. These tests include amniocentesis and ultrasound scan. Nonstress tests, contraction stress tests, and biophysical profiles may be performed to assess fetal well-being.

Medical Management

The level of severity will determine if the patient is managed at home or hospitalized. Management strategies may include activity modification, maternal and fetal monitoring, and medication administration. While the goal is to maintain the pregnancy as long as possible to help ensure fetal lung maturity, ultimately, delivery is the only means to interrupt the condition. Activity is restricted, with rest periods encouraged. Severe symptoms necessitate hospitalization. Bed rest typically is ordered, preferably in the left lateral recumbent position, to reduce pressure on the inferior vena cava and promote venous return. A well-balanced diet with adequate protein is important. Moderate sodium intake is allowed, but high-sodium foods should be avoided. Patients with GH and preeclampsia do not face restricted-sodium diets. Instead, balance is the

Table 29.2 Assessment of Deep Tendon Reflexes	
DEGREE	**GRADING**
Hyperactive response (brisk with intermittent or transient clonus)	4+
More than normal (brisk), slightly hyperactive	3+
Normal, active, expected response	2+
Sluggish or diminished	1+
No response	0

Fig. 29.6 Location of tendons for evaluation of deep tendon reflexes. (A) Triceps. (B) Biceps. (C) Brachioradial. (D) Patellar. (E) Achilles. (F) Evaluation of ankle tonus.

goal. IV access is needed to provide a line if emergency medications are to be administered. The infant's fetal heart tones are monitored in conjunction with prenatal testing. Non stress testing or biophysical profiles may be ordered periodically to assess fetal condition.

Medication therapies to manage severe preeclampsia or eclampsia include the administration of magnesium sulfate or antihypertensive medications. Magnesium sulfate ($MgSO_4$) is not an antihypertensive agent. It acts as a relaxant that works to reduce blood pressure. It is administered intravenously and may be prescribed parenterally to prevent seizure activity. Antihypertensive medications are not used routinely for the patient with mild preeclampsia or GH. Antihypertensive medications are prescribed for blood pressure readings that exceed 160/100 mm Hg. The administration of medications in less severe conditions may impair perfusion to the fetus.

Nursing Interventions

Nursing care for the woman with elevations of blood pressure during pregnancy focuses on assessment of the expectant woman, monitoring of the fetus, administration of prescribed medications, and emotional support. Subtle changes in blood pressure should be noted and reported. The assessment of the woman's mental status and any noteworthy changes necessitates consultation with the health care provider.

In mild cases, monitor routine I&O; in severe cases, it may be necessary to insert an indwelling catheter and record hourly urinary output. Record the patient's daily weight. Evaluate daily weight changes in conjunction with I&O to determine levels of fluid retention.

Monitor fetal condition carefully. In mild cases, routine auscultation of FHR is adequate. Severe cases necessitate continuous fetal monitoring. **Kick counting** is encouraged if the mother has reached 28 weeks gestation. The mother is asked to spend an hour noting the amount of movement felt in a one hour period of time during a period of maternal rest and relaxation. Fetal activity of less than three kicks per hour is considered serious and must be reported. Fetal activity decreases in the presence of hypoxia.

Monitor blood pressure every 4 hours or more frequently if condition indicates. Encouraging compliance with treatment can help prevent the patient from convulsing. Because stress may exacerbate this condition, keep the environment quiet and stress-free. Maintaining a stress-free environment is difficult, however, because enforced bed rest may last for several weeks. Enforced bed rest or hospitalization can be highly disruptive for the patient and her family; there are financial implications, and the woman's condition can affect family dynamics. Explain the necessity of treatment and the care and the treatment that will be given (Box 29.4).

Box 29.4	Eclamptic Seizure Precautions and Interventions

- Keep the environment quiet and nonstimulating, with subdued lighting. Limit visitation.
- For seizure precautions, use padded side rails.
- Suction and oxygen administration equipment and airway kept at bedside.
- Keep the call button within easy reach.
- Emergency medication tray is immediately accessible.
- If magnesium sulfate is administered, keep calcium gluconate readily available.
- Cluster nursing assessments and care to promote periods of rest.

The complications of the pregnancy and fear of the unknown will be challenging for the patient and her family. Emotional and psychological support are essential in helping the woman and her family cope. Their perception of the disease process, the reasons for it, and the care received affects their compliance with and participation in therapy. A care plan designed for the woman with preeclampsia must be integrated with the nursing care all women need during labor and birth.

Protecting the woman and fetus during a convulsion.
The nurse's primary responsibilities to protect the woman and the fetus during a convulsion include the following:

- Remain with the woman and press the call light for assistance.
- If she is not on her side already, attempt to turn the woman onto her side when the tonic phase begins. The left side-lying position permits greater circulation through the placenta, and it may help prevent aspiration.
- Note the time and sequence of the convulsion.
- Insert an airway after the convulsion, and suction the woman's mouth and nose to clear secretions and prevent aspiration. Provide oxygen by mask at 8 to 10 L/min to increase oxygenation of the placenta and all maternal body organs.
- Observe fetal monitor patterns for nonreassuring signs, such as bradycardia, tachycardia, or decreased variability. These usually resolve within a few minutes as maternal oxygenation is restored.
- Notify the physician that a convulsion has occurred. Administer medications and prepare for additional medical interventions as directed by the physician.

Providing information and support for the family.
Explain to the family what has happened without minimizing the seriousness of the situation. A convulsion is frightening for anyone who witnesses it, and the family often is reassured when the nurse explains that the convulsion lasts only a few minutes and that the woman probably will not be conscious for some time afterward. Acknowledge that the convulsion indicates worsening of the condition and that the physician needs to determine future management; this may include delivery of the infant as soon as possible. Vaginal birth is preferred if the maternal and fetal conditions permit because of abnormalities in coagulation and other body systems.

Patient problems and interventions for the patient with GH include but are not limited to the following:

PATIENT PROBLEM	NURSING INTERVENTIONS
Insufficient Diversional Activity, related to environmental lack of stimulation	Find out about hobbies or interests that the woman can perform while resting
	Involve patient in conversation while performing care
	Encourage family to visit and bring books or other recreational items
	Encourage relaxation techniques
	Encourage listening to music
	Gentle exercise such as range of motion, stretching, Kegel exercises, pelvic tilt (important in maintaining muscle tone, blood flow, regularity of bowel function, and a sense of well-being)
Potential for Injury, related to elevated blood pressure and central nervous system irritability	Determine prepregnant baseline vital sign values
	Monitor blood pressure q 4 h (or more frequently as necessary) in supine and lateral recumbent positions
	Assess for headache and visual disturbances
	Weigh patient daily
	Monitor intake and output
	Assess deep tendon reflexes and for the presence of clonus
	Monitor urine for protein
	Observe for pitting edema of upper extremities, periorbital area, and face. Monitor laboratory values
	Maintain bed rest as needed

Patient Teaching

Teach all pregnant women the danger signs of complications in pregnancy and the importance of regular medical supervision. Many of the symptoms of GH, particularly the mild, early symptoms, are detected only with regular physician contact. If GH is diagnosed, explain the consequences of failure to comply.

Encourage high-quality protein, vitamin, and mineral intake. Salt restriction below the normal dietary levels (4 to 6 g/24 hours) usually is not recommended.

Be certain that the patient understands that bed rest is vital because it slows metabolism and relieves dependent edema.

Prognosis

Delivery of the baby is the only cure for preeclampsia and GH. The condition remains a cause for concern for 6 weeks during the postpartum period. Potential complications associated with the condition include bleeding problems, placental abruption, liver rupture, stroke, and death. Immediate and continuous care by the obstetric team is mandatory to prevent maternal and fetal morbidity and mortality.

HELLP SYNDROME

The *HELLP syndrome (H,* hemolysis; *EL,* elevated liver enzymes; *LP,* low platelet count) represents an extension of the pathology of severe preeclampsia and eclampsia. The initial symptoms of the HELLP syndrome usually appear early in the third trimester, although they may appear in the early postpartum period.

For a woman to be diagnosed with the HELLP syndrome, her platelet count must be less than 100,000/mm^3, her liver enzyme levels (aspartate aminotransferase and alanine aminotransferase) must be elevated, and some evidence for intravascular hemolysis must be present. The hemolysis accounts for the large drop in the hematocrit value, out of proportion to blood loss, that occurs in most new mothers with HELLP syndrome during the postpartum period. A unique form of coagulopathy (not DIC) occurs with the HELLP syndrome.

Recognition of the clinical and laboratory findings of the HELLP syndrome is essential to initiate early, aggressive therapy and prevent maternal and fetal mortality.

The prominent symptom of the HELLP syndrome is pain in the right upper quadrant, the lower chest, or the epigastric area. The woman may have tenderness from liver distention. Additional signs and symptoms include nausea, vomiting, and severe edema. Avoid traumatizing the liver with abdominal palpation and use care in transporting the woman. A sudden increase in intraabdominal pressure, including a seizure, could lead to rupture of a subcapsular hematoma, resulting in internal bleeding and hypovolemic shock (see Chapter 28 and Box 28.1).

Women with HELLP syndrome should be managed in a setting with full intensive care facilities available. Their treatment is the same as for preeclampsia or eclampsia. After delivery, most women begin recovering within 72 hours.

Intrapartum nursing care of the woman with severe preeclampsia or HELLP syndrome involves continuous monitoring of maternal and fetal status as labor progresses. Continue the assessment and prevention of tissue hypoxia and hemorrhage, both of which can lead to permanent compromise of vital organs throughout the intrapartum and postpartum period.

An unfavorable (uneffaced and undilated) cervix and the aggressive nature of this disorder support the need for cesarean birth. Prolonged induction of labor could increase maternal morbidity. Fresh-frozen plasma may be needed if bleeding occurs and persists. The major laboratory manifestations of the disease, however, may not appear until the early postpartum period (48 to 72 hours). Delayed transfusion of packed RBCs and platelets often is necessary because of the continued hemolysis. Attempt to lower the blood pressure if the diastolic pressure is consistently greater than 110 mm Hg. However, blood pressure may be normal or slightly elevated; thus, it is not an adequate indicator of the severity of the disease. Hypoglycemia may be present in the woman with HELLP syndrome and, when the blood glucose is less than 40 mg/dL, is associated with a high maternal mortality rate.

COMPLICATIONS RELATED TO INFECTION

Mother and fetus must be considered in the assessment of maternal infection. In some diseases, such as tuberculosis, the fetus usually is spared, even though the mother may be dying. With other infections, such as rubella, the fetus may be critically compromised, while the mother is only slightly ill.

Pregnancy generally is regarded as an immunosuppressed condition. Hormonal changes provide protection to the fetus by reducing the chance it will be expelled. Altered immune responses during pregnancy may decrease the maternal ability to fight infection. In addition, genital tract changes may affect susceptibility. As pregnancy advances, vaginal walls engorge, the cervix enlarges, and vaginal pH decreases, contributing to susceptibility.

Some consequences of maternal infection, such as infertility and sterility, last a lifetime. Psychosocial problems as a result of maternal infections may include altered interpersonal relationships and lowered self-esteem. Other conditions, such as a congenitally acquired infection, often affect the length and quality of a child's life.

Education and counseling are important in the prevention of maternal infections. Adolescent mothers are at risk because of earlier onset of intercourse and increased likelihood of multiple partners. The recent trend of exchanging sex for drugs is contributing to a rise in infection rates, especially among urban, poor, and minority women.

The prevention of disease and reduction of maternal and neonatal complications continue to be enormous challenges. Many microorganisms can increase maternal and fetal risk. Mortality and morbidity rates are increased when infection is present; thus, it is important to prevent infection or at least to recognize and treat it promptly.

GROUP B STREPTOCOCCUS

Group B Streptococcus is a bacteria pathogen. It usually resides in the genitourinary and gastrointestinal systems. Normally the virus is benign, and the host carries no adverse symptoms or damage. The virus, however, can cause damage in the fetus. The illnesses caused may include pneumonia, meningitis and sepsis. The transmission takes place during the birth process. Testing for Group B Streptococcus is routinely completed between 35- and 37-weeks' gestation. The diagnostic test consists of both a vaginal and a rectal swab. Treatment of the disease is initiated during the labor process. At that time antibiotics are administered intravenously. Treating the patient prior to labor is not sufficient. Treating after delivery does not prevent transmission of the infection. When a patient has not had prenatal care, or they have not yet completed the Group B Streptococcus testing, the medication will be administered prophylactically.

MASTITIS

Mastitis is an infection of the lactating breast. Although it occurs most commonly during the first 3 weeks after childbirth, it can occur at any time. It usually affects in only one breast.

Mastitis often is caused by *Staphylococcus aureus*. The bacteria typically are carried on the hands of the mother or agency staff or in the newborn's mouth. The organism may enter through an injured area of the nipple, such as a crack or blister, although there may be no sign of injury. Nipple soreness may result in insufficient emptying of the breast.

Engorgement and stasis of milk frequently precede mastitis, often when a feeding is skipped, when the infant begins sleeping through the night, or when breastfeeding is stopped suddenly. Constriction of the breasts from a tight bra may interfere with emptying all of the ducts and may lead to infection. The mother who is fatigued or stressed or who has other health problems that compromise her immune system is at increased risk for mastitis.

Initial symptoms may be flulike, with fatigue and aching muscles. Symptoms progress to include fever of 101.1°F (38.3°C) or higher, chills, malaise, and headache. Mastitis is characterized by a localized area of redness and inflammation.

Antibiotic therapy, antiinfective agents (antimicrobial agents), and continued emptying of the breast with breastfeeding or breast pump constitute the first line of treatment. With early antibiotic treatment, mastitis usually resolves in 24 to 48 hours. Approximately 5% of women with mastitis develop a breast abscess, which is treated with surgical drainage and antibiotics.

Supportive measures include application of heat or ice packs, breast support, and analgesics. The mother should continue to breastfeed from both breasts. If the affected breast is too sore, she can use a breast pump. Regular emptying of the breast helps prevent abscess formation. If an abscess forms and ruptures into the breast ducts, breast-feeding on that side should be discontinued and a breast pump used to empty the breast temporarily. Milk obtained should be discarded.

Nursing Interventions and Patient Teaching

Mastitis rarely occurs before discharge from the birth facility, making the provision of information about condition prevention and recognition important. Breastfeeding behaviors are key to preventing mastitis. Nipple trauma and milk stasis can be limited by positioning the infant during breast feeding to ensure there is a good latch onto the nipple during nursing. Breast-fed babies feed on a demand schedule. The new mother should seek to feed her baby every 2 to 3 hours. Babies who are "sleepy" or lethargic should be encouraged to nurse. Avoidance of supplemental formula and water will prevent the baby from filling up on another non-breast source of nutrition. When the baby is provided nonbreast sources of nutrition, the amount of milk produced by the mother will be reduced. Nipple shields should be avoided as they can promote chafing of the nipple and surrounding skin. Change nursing pads when they are damp.

Once mastitis occurs, nursing measures are aimed at increasing comfort and helping the mother maintain lactation. Moist heat promotes comfort and increases circulation. A shower or warm compresses should be used before feeding or pumping the breasts. Cold packs can be used between feedings to reduce edema. The woman should complete the entire course of antibiotic therapy to prevent recurrence or a breast abscess.

The woman should empty the breast completely at each feeding to prevent stasis of milk, which can result in an abscess. If she is too sore to breastfeed on the affected side, or if she is taking medications that are contraindicated during lactation, instruct her to express the milk or use a pump to empty the breasts. Starting the feeding on the unaffected side causes the milk-ejection reflex to occur in the painful breast and makes the process more efficient. Massaging over the affected area before and during the feeding helps ensure complete emptying. Unless contraindicated, fluid intake should be 3000 mL/day. Analgesics may be needed to relieve discomfort.

The mother with mastitis is likely to be discouraged and may decide to stop breastfeeding because of the discomfort involved. Weaning during an episode of mastitis may increase engorgement and stasis, leading to abscess formation or recurrent infection.

TORCH INFECTIONS AND HUMAN IMMUNODEFICIENCY VIRUS

TORCH infections—or *T*oxoplasmosis, *O*ther infections such as hepatitis, *R*ubella virus, *C*ytomegalovirus, and *H*erpes simplex viruses—are a group of organisms capable of crossing the placenta and adversely affecting the development of the fetus (Box 29.5).

Transmission of human immunodeficiency virus (HIV), a retrovirus, occurs primarily through the exchange of body fluids. Severe depression of the cellular immune system characterizes acquired immunodeficiency syndrome (AIDS) (Box 29.6). Although the

Box 29.5   TORCH Infections

T: TOXOPLASMOSIS

- Toxoplasmosis is caused by a protozoan, *Toxoplasma gondii,* which can be contracted by eating raw contaminated meats, drinking contaminated water or having contact with and ingestion of contaminated feces or soil (due to poor or absent handwashing). Toxoplasmosis is one of the common accompanying opportunistic infections of acquired immunodeficiency syndrome (AIDS). The mother may be free of symptoms or may have development of myalgia, enlarged posterior cervical lymph nodes, malaise, and rash that disappear in a matter of days. Acute infection in pregnancy produces flulike symptoms and lymphadenopathy.
- Diagnosis is confirmed with blood studies, and women in at-risk groups should have toxoplasmosis titer evaluated.
- The effects on the fetus can be profound: spontaneous abortion, stillbirth, neonatal death, blindness, retardation, and a wide range of congenital anomalies.
- Teach all pregnant women to avoid undercooked meats and potentially contaminated water sources.
- If cats are present in the woman's environment, she should wear gloves whenever chance of contact with feces exists.
- Medications used include pyrimethamine (when contracted after 18 weeks gestation) and spiramycin (when contracted before 18 weeks gestation).

O: OTHER

- The primary infection in this category is hepatitis. Hepatitis A is a virus spread by droplets or hands and is associated with poor handwashing after defecation.
- Pregnancy effects include spontaneous abortion and flulike signs and symptoms: fever, malaise, and nausea. If the fetus is exposed in the first trimester and is untreated, possible effects include fetal anomalies, preterm birth, fetal or neonatal hepatitis, and intrauterine death. Gamma globulin vaccination is given to mothers and newborns for prophylaxis.
- Hepatitis B is a virus transmitted in a manner similar to that of human immunodeficiency virus (HIV). Routes of transmission include contaminated needles, syringes, or blood products; sexual intercourse; and body fluid exchange.
- During pregnancy, common signs and symptoms include fever, rash, anorexia, malaise, myalgias, and jaundice if the liver is affected acutely. Fetal and newborn effects are the same as those listed for hepatitis A. Vaccination during pregnancy is not thought to pose a risk to the fetus. Hepatitis B vaccine is recommended for all mothers and neonates.
- The "other" group includes other miscellaneous infections that may affect the mother or fetus (or both). Varicella zoster and mumps are included in this listing.
- Urinary tract and vaginal infections can cause fever, chills, dysuria, pain, malaise, and changes in vaginal drainage. Report any of these symptoms promptly to the physician. Culture and sensitivity tests usually reveal the specific organism. Treatment is based on the causative organism and the severity of the problem. Treatment must be done cautiously because of the possibility of teratogenic effects from the antibiotics.
- Sexually transmitted infections (STIs) are also a serious concern. Syphilis can cross the placental barrier and infect the fetus. Chlamydia may cause pneumonia or eye infections in the newborn. Gonorrhea can cause pelvic inflammatory disease in the mother and eye infections in the newborn.

- Human immunodeficiency virus (HIV) is an infection that has potentially lethal implications for both the mother and fetus. See Box 29.6.

R: RUBELLA, GERMAN MEASLES, OR 3-DAY MEASLES

- Rubella is a viral infection transmitted by droplets. Fever, rash, and mild lymphedema usually are seen in the affected mother. If contracted during the first trimester, rubella can cause a wide range of congenital defects, including congenital heart disease, mental retardation, and cataracts. Congenital infection is the leading cause of deafness.
- Serologic testing for rubella is completed at the initial prenatal health check.
- As a live virus immunization is not possible during pregnancy, if a pregnant woman does not have immunity, caution her to avoid risk of exposure to the disease.
- Nonimmune women will receive vaccination prior to discharge after childbirth.
- Further caution the woman to avoid becoming pregnant for 2–3 months after vaccination because the attenuated virus used for immunization may still be present.

C: CYTOMEGALOVIRUS

- Cytomegalovirus (CMV) belongs to the herpesvirus group.
- CMV is a common infection that can be spread by close contact, breast-feeding, sexual relations, and kissing.
- More than half of all adults have antibodies to the virus by the age of 40. Nearly a third of children have been infected by the age of 3.
- This virus is capable of crossing the placental barrier and causing serious damage to the fetus, including cognitive impairment, hearing problems, and congenital anomalies. It is unusual in that the mother may be totally asymptomatic, and it does not always cause fetal complications.
- Antiviral therapies can be administered but will not reverse damages that may be experienced by the fetus.

H: HERPES SIMPLEX

- Herpes simplex causes painful lesions on the external genitalia and also can involve the cervix.
- Intrauterine infection of the fetus can occur if the membranes rupture or vaginal delivery takes place when active lesions are present. If the virus is not treated, the neonatal mortality rate is extremely high.
- Mothers who have herpes simplex prior to pregnancy have a lower risk of transmission to their fetus than those who contract herpes simplex for the first-time during pregnancy.
- Diagnosis is made based on maternal symptoms and a culture of the lesions.
- Women with active herpes infection should deliver via cesarean birth. Women who are inactive at the time of labor onset, may choose a vaginal delivery after consultation with their physician.
- The pregnancy effects of primary genital herpes infection include spontaneous abortion, preterm labor, and intrauterine growth restriction.
- Health care providers with herpes simplex virus (HSV) infections should take precautions. Anyone with oral HSV lesions should wear a mask if in close contact with newborns, and anyone with skin lesions should not give direct care until lesions are dried and crusted. Scrupulous handwashing is essential.

| Box 29.6 | Acquired Immunodeficiency Syndrome |

- Acquired immunodeficiency syndrome (AIDS) is a substantial health concern. It has had a significant effect on all areas of health care, including maternal nursing.
- The causative organism is the human immunodeficiency virus (HIV), which enters the body through blood, blood products, or sexual contact. It is capable of crossing the placental barrier and infecting the fetus in utero, causing congenital defects such as microcephaly (abnormal smallness of the head) and facial deformities.
- Because of the long incubation period, infants born to HIV-seropositive mothers may show no indication at birth but develop signs of the infection later. These signs include failure to thrive, recurrent infection, interstitial pneumonia, and neurologic abnormalities.
- Early in the pregnancy HIV testing is discussed with the patient.
- Studies place the risk of perinatal transmission at 20%–50%. Most children diagnosed with AIDS die within the first few years of life. The use of antiviral medications by the gravid woman can reduce neonatal transmission to 2% or less.
- All pregnant women diagnosed with HIV benefit from antiretroviral therapy. Most mother-to-fetus transmissions occur in the final weeks of pregnancy.
- Rapid HIV testing is available for women who come in for delivery without having had prenatal care. Results are rapidly available and allow for safer management of mother and baby.
- Vaginal birth is strongly discouraged, and cesarean delivery is advisable. Cesarean births have been shown to reduce contact with maternal virus.

populations at high risk have been well documented, assess all women for the possibility of HIV exposure. HIV infection in women commonly is reported at a later stage in the disease; patients usually enter the hospital for initiation of treatment when the illness is more severe. The delay may be due in part to the fact that the symptoms are different from those in men. Chronic vaginitis and candidiasis are common presenting problems.

Obstetric risk in people with HIV infection is difficult to determine because so many other factors are often present. Many women who are HIV positive also have drug and alcohol addiction, poor nutrition, limited access to prenatal care, or concurrent sexually transmitted infections (STIs). Women who are HIV positive are at a higher risk for preterm labor and birth, premature rupture of membranes, intrauterine growth restriction (IUGR), perinatal mortality, and postpartum endometritis (see Chapter 16 in *Adult Health Nursing*).

Etiology

Numerous infectious diseases may cause complications during pregnancy. Some are airborne or ingested, but most are spread via direct contact, usually through sexual transmission. Others are contracted with use of contaminated needles or blood transfusions.

Nursing Interventions

The presence of infection is not always evident. Because of the increased incidence of serious infectious diseases, the Centers for Disease Control and Prevention recommends use of standard precautions with all patients. These precautions are most important when dealing with blood and body fluids. Those caring for mothers and newborns frequently are exposed to blood and body fluids and must be particularly alert. Wear gloves, masks, gowns, and glasses during procedures that involve splashing of body fluids, such as amniotomy. Use gloves when cleaning or assessing the breasts or perineal area. Also use gloves when performing the initial newborn bath or changing diapers. Thorough handwashing, as always, is essential. Suction or resuscitate the infant with use of mechanical barriers or equipment such as mouth shields, suction devices, and ventilators. Take care when handling needles and syringes; dispose of these in special containers without breaking or recapping.

During the birthing process, every effort should be made to decrease the neonate's exposure to infected maternal blood and secretions. If feasible, the membranes should be left intact until the birth. Women who give birth within 4 hours after membrane rupture are less likely to transmit the virus to their neonates than women who experience a longer interval between rupture and birth. Avoid fetal scalp electrodes and scalp pH sampling because these procedures may result in inoculation of the virus into the fetus. Likewise, avoid the use of forceps and a vacuum extractor when possible. Episiotomy and cesarean birth do not seem to influence the infection rate greatly.

Breastfeeding is discouraged because of possible HIV transmission in breast milk. (The World Health Organization has not discouraged breastfeeding in nonindustrialized nations because of the decreased availability of infant formula and hygiene risks in the preparation of formula but may be changing its recommendation.) After discharge, the woman and her infant are referred to physicians who are experienced in the treatment of AIDS and associated conditions.

Psychological support is important to the patient with an infectious disease. Because many of these diseases are life threatening to the mother, the fetus, or the newborn, fear and anxiety are common. If the infection results in fetal mortality or defects, the mother may express guilt. Nurses also must cope with their own feelings about these serious infectious diseases. Caring for mothers and newborns with AIDS and other such diseases can create judgmental feelings in nurses that they must resolve.

Patient Teaching

Education on prevention of infection should start long before pregnancy. Infections acquired by a woman before she becomes pregnant can seriously affect the outcome of pregnancy. Immunization for rubella before childbearing years is essential; stress to all new

Box 29.7	**Comfort Measures for the Pregnant Woman With a Vaginal Infection**

- Pour warm water over the urethra and vulva.
- Take warm sitz baths for 15 min three to five times daily.
- Avoid strong deodorant soaps, creams, and ointments.
- Dry the genital area with a blow dryer. (To prevent burning, beware of high temperatures.)
- Wear 100% cotton underwear.
- Do not wear tight-fitting jeans.
- Do not wear nylon panties or panties with nylon inserts.
- Obtain early and regular Papanicolaou (Pap) smears.
- Avoid any sexual contact during outbreaks.

mothers the importance of having children routinely immunized. Review hygiene practices such as careful hand washing and proper storage and preparation of meats. Discuss safer sex practices, including use of condoms, with individuals at risk, and stress the importance of regular medical care and treatment.

Counseling the pregnant woman with a vaginal infection also should include measures to deal with the discomfort (Box 29.7).

Prognosis

The success of the prevention measures depends on the conscientious effort of the health care worker in carrying out all recommended procedures carefully and the patient's willingness to comply with preventive measures or prescribed therapy.

COMPLICATIONS RELATED TO EXISTING MEDICAL CONDITIONS

DIABETES MELLITUS
Etiology

Diabetes mellitus is an endocrine disorder that affects metabolism and the utilization of glucose. This disease is not curable and is often difficult to control. In pregnancy, hormonal changes and stresses placed on all the maternal body systems result in even more complex medical and nursing management.

Pathophysiology

In diabetes mellitus, the pancreas does not produce adequate amounts of insulin to metabolize glucose normally. Because glucose does not enter the cells without adequate insulin, blood glucose levels remain high. The cells release stored fat and protein for energy, leading to ketosis and a negative nitrogen balance.

Diabetes is classified into various forms. Type 1 (formerly called insulin-dependent diabetes mellitus) requires regular administration of insulin for control. Type 2 (formerly called non–insulin-dependent diabetes mellitus) is controlled most often with diet or oral hypoglycemic medications. *Pregestational diabetes*

mellitus is the label sometimes given to type 1 or type 2 diabetes that exists before pregnancy.

Gestational diabetes mellitus (GDM) is the inability to produce enough insulin to maintain normal glucose levels during pregnancy. Increased dietary glucose needs, along with insulin resistance from placental hormones, cortisol, and insulinase, result in hyperglycemia and GDM. The patient with GDM usually is diagnosed in the middle of the pregnancy and may have sustained hyperglycemia in the early months of the pregnancy. Risk factors for gestational diabetes includes older than age 25 years at the time of pregnancy, family history of diabetes, history of gestational diabetes, nonwhite race, obesity, a history of large for gestational age babies, a history of unexplained fetal loss, and hypertension.

Improved control of this disease process has reduced the risk to mother and fetus; however, the incidence of complications is still significant. Maternal complications include infections (urinary tract and vaginal), difficult labor related to increased fetal size (which frequently results in cesarean birth), vascular complications (including retinopathy), azotemia, ketoacidosis, hypertensive disorders such as preeclampsia, and cesarean birth. Fetal complications include stillbirth, spontaneous abortion, hydramnios (excessive amniotic fluid), large placenta, alteration in size for gestational age (macrosomia), congenital anomalies, neonatal hypoglycemia, neonatal hyperbilirubinemia, respiratory distress syndrome, and fetal or neonatal death.

Clinical Manifestations

Alteration in blood glucose levels is the major manifestation of the disease. Blood glucose levels greater than 120 mg/dL significantly increase the risk of complications. When blood glucose levels are elevated, the classic symptoms of diabetes—polyuria, polydipsia, and polyphagia—may be observed (Box 29.8).

Assessment

Perform urine testing at all prenatal visits. If testing indicates the presence of glucose, additional testing is necessary. For the patient with known diabetes, assess diet, activity, and medication compliance. Assess the vascular system regularly for possible complications and watch the patient closely for signs of infection. Also assess the condition of the fetus with serial ultrasound scans and other medical measures.

Diagnostic Tests

A 1-hour, 50-g diabetes screening test or glucose tolerance test is scheduled routinely between 24 and 28 weeks' gestation. Women with a history of gestational diabetes or who present with risk factors for development of the condition are tested earlier in the pregnancy. Results that indicate hyperglycemia in the fasting

Box 29.8	Signs and Symptoms of Maternal Hypoglycemia and Hyperglycemia

HYPOGLYCEMIA
- Shakiness (tremors)
- Sweating
- Pallor; cold, clammy skin
- Disorientation, irritability
- Headache
- Hunger
- Blurred vision

HYPERGLYCEMIA
- Fatigue
- Flushed, hot skin
- Dry mouth, excessive thirst
- Frequent urination
- Rapid, deep respirations; odor of acetone on breath
- Drowsiness, headache
- Depressed reflexes

portion of the test (blood sugar [BS], >92 mg/dL) or the 1-hour reading (180 mg/dL) result in an order for the woman to undergo the 3-hour glucose tolerance test. The results from the 3-hour test are used to confirm the diagnosis. Any two results of displaying elevations establish the diagnosis (Davidson et al., 2012).

- Fasting, 95 mg/dL
- 1 hour, 180 mg/dL
- 2 hours, 155 mg/dL
- 3 hours, 140 mg/dL

Glycosylated hemoglobin (Hgb A_{1C}) may be used in the first trimester to assess a woman's history of hyperglycemia for the preceding 3 months. After the second trimester, it is not used. Diagnostic techniques for fetal surveillance often performed during pregnancy are complicated by diabetes mellitus. Tests to evaluate fetal well-being include alpha-fetoprotein screening, nonstress test, contraction stress test, and biophysical profile. An ultrasound may be completed to assess fetal growth and development. The frequency of the biophysical profile, nonstress test and contraction stress test may be repeated at intervals to ensure the fetus continues to have adequate perfusion. The patient who is diagnosed with gestational diabetes or who has been diagnosed with diabetes mellitus before pregnancy often has labor induced before the due date in an effort to avoid complications. Determination of the estimated due date (EDD) and assessments as the pregnancy progresses to determine fetal lung maturity are performed. Try to determine the estimated date of birth. A baseline ultrasound scan is done to assess the fetus's gestational age. Follow-up ultrasound examinations are performed as often as every 4 to 6 weeks to monitor fetal growth and development and to assess for congenital abnormalities. Biochemical analysis of amniotic fluid is performed to ascertain fetal lung maturity, typically in the third trimester.

Nursing Interventions

Nursing care is directed at maintaining the patient in a euglycemic (normal blood glucose) status. The patient's insulin requirements change significantly throughout pregnancy, labor, and delivery. Assess the patient carefully at each visit, complete all blood glucose level evaluations as ordered, and report any abnormalities to the health care provider promptly. Because of possible teratogenic effects, patients with type 2 diabetes mellitus have oral hypoglycemic medications discontinued and insulin prescribed. The initial plan of action for patients diagnosed with gestational diabetes is control of the condition with dietary interventions. In the event this is not successful, insulin therapy is prescribed. Regular and intermediate-acting insulin are most often administered. Blood glucose monitoring is recommended at fasting and then 1 to 2 hours after meals.

A patient problem and interventions for the patient with GDM include but are not limited to the following:

PATIENT PROBLEM	NURSING INTERVENTIONS
Impaired Health Maintenance, related to deficient knowledge of the effects of pregnancy on diabetes control	Review pathophysiology of the disease
	Assist the patient in formulating questions for the physician
	Clarify misconceptions
	Teach home monitoring of blood glucose levels
	Review effects of diabetes on the pregnant patient
	Explain in simple terms the advantages to the fetus of maintaining a normal maternal blood glucose level; advantages include an optimal pattern of growth, the increased likelihood that the baby will be born near term, and fewer complications associated with prematurity
	Teach danger signs of diabetes and whom to notify (provide written as well as oral instructions)
	Stress importance of weekly prenatal visits during second half of pregnancy
	Refer patient to community diabetic support groups

Patient Teaching

The need for teaching differs with the classification of the disease and the patient's willingness to learn. A woman who has been diagnosed before pregnancy needs reinforcement of diet, medication, and health practices. Also explain the effects pregnancy has on diabetes throughout the course of pregnancy, labor, delivery, and the postpartum period.

Table 29.3 **Medications for the Mother and Newborn at Risk**

GENERIC NAME (TRADE NAME)	ACTION	SIDE EFFECTS	NURSING IMPLICATIONS
Metoclopramide	Antiemetic	Headache, weakness, fatigue	IV administration deliver dosage over 15 min.
Betamethasone	Steroid administered to promote fetal lung maturity.	Weakness, fatigue, increased serum glucose levels	IV administration. May administer a single dose or 2 over the course of a 24-h period.
doxylamine-pyridoxine (Diclegis)	Antiemetic	Drowsiness, headache, constipation	Take on an empty stomach with water. Do not crush or chew pill. This medication is not a prn medication. Consult with physician before discontinuing.
Methotrexate	Antimetabolite compound that interferes with DNA synthesis	Nausea, vomiting, photosensitivity, skin redness	Administer intramuscularly. Review lab records to ensure patient is hemodynamically stable. Instruct patient of signs and symptoms to report.
valacyclovir (converts to acyclovir; Valtrex)	Antiviral	Topical: Stinging, burning, rash, pruritus; Systemic: Headache, seizures, renal toxicity, phlebitis at intravenous site	Topical: Use glove to apply, cover lesion completely. Adequate hydration to prevent crystallization in kidneys; give IV dose for 1 h.
Hepatitis B immune globulin (HBIG)	Series provides immunity to hepatitis B	Pain, redness and itching at site of injection. Headache, fatigue and fever	Provide education on scheduling of subsequent injections in the series.
hydralazine	Arterial vasodilator	Headache, flushing, tachycardia	Assess for tachycardia, hypotension, urinary output; maintain bed rest.
Lung surfactant: colfosceril palmitate (Exosurf [synthetic]) beractant (Survanta [natural lung surfactant])	Replaces natural lung surfactant that maintains lung inflation and prevents lung collapse; used to treat and prevent respiratory distress syndrome in premature neonates	Synthetic: Apnea, pulmonary hemorrhage, pulmonary air leak; Natural: Transient bradycardia, oxygen desaturation, hypotension, apnea	Administer endotracheally only; suction before administration (drug may reflux into endotracheal tube during administration); slow or stop administration until tube is clear.
Magnesium sulfate (MgSO$_4$)	See Chapter 26.		
oxytocin (Pitocin)	See Chapter 27.		
Rh$_o$(D) immune globulin (RhoGAM)	See Chapter 27.		
ritodrine	See Chapter 26.		
Rubella vaccine	See Chapter 27.		
naloxone hydrochloride (Narcan)	Reverses central nervous system and respiratory depression caused by narcotics (opiates) Competes with narcotics at receptor sites	If given to an infant of a mother addicted to drugs, causes withdrawal and may cause seizures	Prepare the syringe before birth by drawing up more than is needed. After birth, remove excess from the syringe and give the amount according to the estimate of the infant's weight. Inject rapidly. Monitor for response and be prepared to give repeated doses if necessary. Use resuscitation measures as necessary.

Continued

Table 29.3   Medications for the Mother and Newborn at Risk—cont'd

GENERIC NAME (TRADE NAME)	ACTION	SIDE EFFECTS	NURSING IMPLICATIONS
terbutaline[a]	Stimulates beta-adrenergic receptors of the sympathetic nervous system Results primarily in bronchodilation and inhibition of uterine muscle activity Increases pulse rate and widens pulse pressure	Maternal and fetal tachycardia, palpitations, cardiac arrhythmias, chest pain, wide pulse pressure, dyspnea, tremors, weakness, dizziness, headache, hyperglycemia, nausea, vomiting, skin flushing, and diaphoresis	Explain common side effects, which usually are well tolerated. Assess FHR, usually with continuous fetal monitoring. Assess maternal pulse, respirations and blood pressure by the same schedule as for FHR. Maintain adequate hydration. Encourage patient to urinate every 2 h. Report any significant or unacceptable side effects. Repeat continuing or recurrent uterine activity. Teach signs and symptoms of recurrent preterm labor and follow-up medical care after discharge.
nifedipine (Procardia)	Relaxes smooth muscles (tocolytic) Inhibits uterine contractions in preterm labor Not approved by the FDA for inhibiting uterine activity, although it is widely used for this purpose	Dizziness, headache, palpitations, weaknesses, shortness of breath, feelings of warmth, and tightness in chest	See nursing implications for terbutaline.
penicillin	Used for group B streptococcus Administered after culture and sensitivity is completed	Interferes with contraception usage	Assess for allergies; hypersensitivity reaction may be delayed. Assess respiratory system for abnormalities such as rate, status, character, any tightness in chest.

FDA, US Food and Drug Administration; *FHR,* fetal heart rate; *IV,* intravenous.
[a]Not approved by the FDA for inhibiting uterine activity, although it is widely used for this purpose; research has been mixed regarding the drug effects of terbutaline for this purpose, but its lower risk for adverse side effects, combined with some efficacy, has encouraged its use.

The patient with newly diagnosed gestational diabetes needs significant education. It is important to stress the necessity of good control of the disease. The training normally provided to a patient with newly diagnosed diabetes mellitus also may be helpful.

Be an active listener and allow time for the woman and her family to express concerns and feelings. Convey acceptance of expressed feelings whether they are negative or positive. Sharing emotions helps the woman cope with her anxiety and frustration and thus promotes her active participation in her care.

Prognosis

Maintenance of glycemic control promotes improved outcomes. Potential complications for the mother include increased risk for operative birth and tissue trauma resulting from vaginal delivery of a large-for-gestational-age infant. Complications in the infant include risk for preterm delivery, IUGR, and macrosomia. Although the baby born to the diabetic woman is often large for gestational age, or macrosomic, they may also exhibit signs of IUGR. This can result from circulatory

impairments that can result from diabetes. Insulin does not cross the placental barrier (placental tissue limits passage of certain substances); consequently, control of the mother's diabetes is vital to the health of the fetus. Most women benefit from praise when diabetic control is well maintained. They feel competent and trusted by the health care team and motivated to continue.

CARDIAC DISEASE

Pregnancy increases the demands on the cardiovascular system. This is not a problem for the normal, healthy heart, which is able to adapt to the increased demands. However, women who have preexisting cardiac disease face increased risk when cardiac function is challenged by pregnancy. About 1% of pregnancies are complicated by heart disease. The degree of disability is often more important than the type of cardiovascular disease in the treatment and prognosis during pregnancy.

Etiology

The most common cardiac problems of maternity patients result from rheumatic heart disease, congenital heart defects, and mitral valve prolapse. Occasionally, a condition called *peripartum cardiomyopathy* (disease of the myocardium, especially as a result of primary diseases of the heart muscle) is observed in pregnant patients who have no history of cardiac problems. This may be seen in the last month of pregnancy or during the postpartum period. The symptoms are similar to those of congestive heart failure.

With successful treatment of congenital cardiac anomalies or mitral stenosis from rheumatic heart disease, many girls are now reaching childbearing age and bearing children. Rheumatic heart disease, a complication of streptococcal infection, is not common in the United States but may be found in recent immigrants. Hypertensive heart disease, often a secondary effect of obesity, can be expected to affect more childbearing women because of the growing incidence in the general population. Cardiomyopathy is a disorder of the muscle structure of the heart that may have any of several causes. Congestive heart failure may result from underlying heart disease or from treatment for other conditions.

Pathophysiology

During pregnancy, increased blood volume, heart rate, and cardiac output are normal. In the woman with existing cardiac problems, the muscle, the valves, or the vessels are overly stressed by these changes. Symptoms of the underlying pathologic condition are exacerbated, which results in cardiac decompensation, congestive failure, and other medical problems.

Clinical Manifestations

The symptoms depend on the underlying pathologic condition. Edema, cyanosis, tachycardia, palpitations, arrhythmias, chest pain, dyspnea, and fatigue may occur. Physical exertion may increase the severity of the symptoms. Clinical findings are those of heart failure (left ventricular failure). The patient has decreased cardiac output and pulmonary congestion, with fluid collecting in the lungs. Pulmonary edema and pleural effusion also occur, and pulmonary crackles, hemoptysis, and cough may be present.

Assessment

At each prenatal visit, measure the patient's vital signs and evaluate her ability to participate in activities. Unusual fatigue with activity may reveal problems. Monitor for edema, weight gain, murmurs, cough, dyspnea, and abnormal lung sounds. Compare these data with normal changes during pregnancy. The patient with preexisting heart disease also should be followed by her cardiologist during her pregnancy.

The pregnant woman with cardiac disease needs detailed assessment to determine the potential for optimal maternal health and a viable fetus throughout the peripartum period. If she chooses to continue the pregnancy, assess the condition of the woman with a high-risk pregnancy as often as weekly.

Diagnostic Tests

Chest x-ray evaluation, electrocardiograms, echocardiograms, and auscultation are used to determine the type and severity of the cardiac problem. Blood gas analysis may be performed if severe decompensation is observed. A woman's sudden inability to perform activities that she previously was comfortable doing may indicate cardiovascular decompensation.

Nursing Interventions

Nursing care is directed at helping the woman maintain normal physical and psychosocial function. During pregnancy, teach the importance of diet, medications, paced activity, and adequate rest. This includes education about the specific disease and its management. Iron intake must be adequate to prevent anemia, which further stresses the heart. Sodium may be restricted to control the fluid volume and decrease cardiac stress. If cardiac palpations are being experienced, caffeine limitations will be helpful. Stool softeners may be prescribed to decrease use of the Valsalva maneuver (holding the breath while bearing down) when defecating. The activity level is dictated by the severity of the cardiac problem. Be aware of the medical recommendations and help the woman incorporate these into her daily life. Patients with more severe cardiac problems need the greatest adjustments. Be highly sensitive to personal and family needs.

If cardiopulmonary arrest occurs during pregnancy, cardiopulmonary resuscitation may be performed within certain guidelines.

During labor, the semi-Fowler's or side-lying position with the head elevated enhances respiratory effort and improves circulation. During every contraction, 300 to 500 mL of blood shifts from the uterus and placenta into the central circulation. This extra fluid causes a sharp rise in cardiac workload. The efforts of labor may necessitate oxygen administration to increase the blood oxygen saturation, which is monitored with pulse oximetry. Administer medications such as cardiotonics, diuretics, prophylactic antibiotics, sedatives, and analgesics as directed by the physician. Reduce discomfort to a minimum. Also try to eliminate unnecessary activity by the patient during labor. Resting between contractions and using shorter, open-glottis pushing are recommended to conserve energy. Closely monitor fetal condition for any signs of distress; use a fetal monitor for continuous assessment. Calmly explain everything to decrease anxiety.

A vaginal delivery is recommended for a woman with heart disease unless there are specific indications for a cesarean birth. Vacuum extraction or outlet forceps often are used to minimize the mother's use of the Valsalva maneuver when pushing during the second stage.

Postpartum care varies according to the severity of the cardiac problem. Explore methods of incorporating care of the infant into the mother's activities. Because extravascular fluid returns to the bloodstream after delivery, the mother is at risk for development of cardiac decompression during the 48 hours after the birth.

To promote normal parent-child attachment, establish contact as early as possible. Discuss breastfeeding with the physician because the physical effort may be excessive for the mother, and the transfer of medications in the breast milk may be harmful to the infant. As in all other areas of nursing, continue to assess the patient's status and give explanations for all care.

Amnioinfusion. Amnioinfusion, an infusion of fluids directly into the amniotic sac, may be performed during pregnancy to treat patients with *oligohydramnios,* a deficit in the level of amniotic fluid. During labor, amnioinfusion may be performed with saline or lactated Ringer's solution to manage women with cord compression resulting in variable decelerations. Amniotic fluid provides buoyancy to the fetus, preventing cord compression and promoting musculoskeletal development.

Prognosis

In cardiac complications, the maternal mortality rate has been estimated in the range of 30% to 60%; the infant mortality rate is approximately 10%. The prognosis is good if cardiomegaly is not persistent after 6 months. The prognosis for women whose hearts remain enlarged is not as favorable. Future pregnancies usually result in some cardiac failure (50% to 88%). The mortality rate may be as high as 60%. Oral contraceptives are contraindicated because of the risk of thromboembolism.

COMPLICATIONS RELATED TO AGE

ADOLESCENTS

Adolescent patients present the nurse with a unique challenge. A significant number are sexually active and in need of contraceptive counseling; many become pregnant. The pregnant adolescent, her family, and her partner need sensitive, competent nursing interventions. The young woman may choose to terminate the pregnancy or carry it to term. She may place the infant up for adoption or elect to keep the baby. The nurse plays a vital role in helping the patient make informed decisions and in supporting her, physically and emotionally, in carrying out her chosen option. Never recommend a choice.

Growth and Development

The period of adolescence is divided into three stages: early, middle, and late. The higher the developmental level, the greater the readiness to accept responsibility for self and others.

Adolescent development is characterized by physical, cognitive, and behavioral development that approximates chronologic age. Adolescents are characteristically egocentric, concrete thinkers, and have feelings of invincibility, which lead to risky behaviors, such as smoking, drug and alcohol abuse, and unprotected sex with multiple partners.

Before children can become mature adults, they must accomplish the developmental tasks of adolescence, including acceptance of body image, acceptance of sexual identity, development of a personal value system, preparation for making a living, independence from parents, development of decision-making skills, and development of an adult identity. These tasks vary from culture to culture and with individual adolescents and their goals.

Pregnancy interrupts the process of identifying formation and developmental tasks. Attempting to accomplish developmental tasks of pregnancy and of normal adolescence simultaneously may be overwhelming. The psychological burden may lead to depression and to postponement in attaining an adult identity. The pregnant adolescent faces further developmental tasks of parenthood. These tasks are as important to the new adolescent parents as they organize ways to behave in their environment as they are for the adult (see lifespan discussion in Chapter 24).

Although the number of adolescent pregnancies in the United States has not increased in the past 5 to 10 years, pregnancies have increased significantly among very young adolescents (ages 10 to 14 years). This trend is attributed to many sociologic factors, including breakdown of the traditional family and changes in social mores that result in earlier sexual activity. Teenagers account for an increasingly large percentage of births and abortions. Physiologic immaturity, incomplete education, and unresolved developmental tasks are complicating factors.

Several physiologic concerns are associated with the young pregnant adolescent. These include an increased risk for GH, cephalopelvic disproportion that results in cesarean birth, abruptio placentae, low birth weight, IUGR, anemia, infection, preterm delivery, and perinatal death. Pregnant teenagers also commonly fear or deny the pregnancy and go without medical attention until late in pregnancy. Lack of prenatal care increases the risk to the pregnant teenager and her infant.

Sociocultural concerns are seen in educational and economic arenas. The pregnancy frequently ends the adolescent's formal education, which leads to reduced job opportunities because of lack of training. This results in an increased poverty risk with potentially prolonged dependence on public assistance.

Assessment

Assessment of all health patterns for each adolescent is essential. When prenatal care is initiated early and consistently, and confounding variables (e.g., socioeconomic factors) are controlled, very young pregnant adolescents are at no greater risk (nor are their infants) for an adverse outcome than older pregnant women. The nurse's role in reducing the risks and consequences of adolescent pregnancy is twofold: to encourage early and continued prenatal care, and to refer the adolescent, if necessary, for appropriate social support services, which can help reverse the effects of a negative socioeconomic environment.

Nursing Interventions

When caring for the pregnant adolescent, be aware of the patient's unique nature and incorporate physical and psychological interventions into the care plan. An understanding of adolescent growth and development is necessary to successfully relate to and care for this patient.

Patient problems and interventions for the pregnant adolescent patient include but are not limited to the following:

PATIENT PROBLEM	NURSING INTERVENTIONS
Insufficient Knowledge, related to choices regarding pregnancy, childbirth experiences, and parenthood	Examine own views regarding sexuality to be able to maintain nonjudgmental approach
	Listen and give honest answers
	Create a safe and stable environment that engenders trust
	Evaluate which stage of development the adolescent is experiencing
	Teach the adolescent about pregnancy choices, childbirth, and parenthood
	Encourage questions and verbalization of fears and concerns
	Compliment teens on the questions asked and efforts made to learn about issues
	Encourage support personnel to attend and participate in prenatal care
	Refer to childbirth and parenthood class and community support and information groups
Imbalanced Nutrition, related to inadequate diet	Perform 24-h diet recall to establish dietary habits
	Assess height and weight and compare with norms for age
	Assess for frequent dieting, eating disorders, smoking, alcohol use, and substance abuse
	Assess fat content of diet
	Assess fluid intake for caffeine levels
	Explain fetal need for weight gain
	Refer to dietitian for nutrition counseling
	Provide sample menus, including increased vitamins, minerals, and calories
	Refer to the Women, Infants, and Children (WIC) program for dietary supplements

Labor and birth. The very young adolescent may be frightened of needles, pelvic examinations, noises from other women in labor or from equipment, and birth rooms. Provide a single, private room when possible. Ensure the patient has the support of a knowledgeable coach, whether husband, friend, parent, or nurse. Many teenagers come to labor lacking preparation; they are frightened and often alone. If they are admitted early in the first stage, teach about relaxation with contractions, ambulation, side-lying positions, and comfort measures. The adolescent is more concerned with how the baby will get out than with fetal well-being.

Pregnant young adolescents often are still growing, so there is an increased chance of cephalopelvic disproportion and cesarean birth. This provides an additional fear for the laboring adolescent. Be prepared to provide the necessary support and encouragement. Always provide anticipatory guidance and explain procedures. Many adolescents keep their infants and are responsive to staff members who share their delight. For these young parents, efforts to promote parent-child attachment are particularly important.

Postpartum care. Physically, the adolescent mother needs the same care as any woman who has given birth. Provide explicit directions for self-care and infant care. Most adolescents view the care of the infant as their primary area of concern. Continue to assess the new mother's parenting abilities during the postpartum period. In addition, continue to support the patient by involving grandparents or other family members, making home visits, and referring to group sessions for discussion of infant care and parenting problems. Outreach programs concerned with self-care, parent-child interactions, child injuries, and failure to thrive, and those that provide prompt and effective intervention prevent more serious problems.

Postpartum contraception education is a high priority for the adolescent. The risk of repeat pregnancy in adolescence is high, and all the accompanying risks of adolescent pregnancy increase with each subsequent pregnancy. Almost universally, postpartum adolescents say that they will never have sex again and therefore need no birth control. This attitude is not realistic. Adolescents need to leave the hospital with a plan for contraception. The decision must be based on the adolescent and her life situation with consideration of her emotional and cognitive developmental status. Cultural values and practices also should be considered. Barrier methods (foam and condoms) and the knowledge of how and when to use them should be considered. Some health care providers send adolescents home on a regimen of oral contraceptives. This practice is controversial because of the increased risk of thromboembolic disease in the immediate postpartum period (first 4 weeks). Medroxyprogesterone (Depo-Provera) because of the longevity of the method may be considered and can potentially be initiated prior to discharge.

Adolescent males must be considered and included in any interventions in sexuality education, family planning, and parent education.

The adolescent mother needs support if she is considering adoption for her child. Avoid use of phrases that give negative connotations to the adoption process. Phrases such as "put up for adoption" and "give up for adoption" imply the biological parents are uncaring. Neither should the terms "real parents" or "natural parents" be used exclusively for genetic parents. The adoptive parents are the "real parents," because they care for the child. Neutral language, such as "arranging for an adoption," "biological parent" or "birth mother," and "adoptive parent," is preferred. Give the mother the option of either remaining on the postpartum floor or transferring to another unit. Assure her that she will have as much access to the baby as she desires.

Grief results from actual or perceived loss. The adolescent may experience grief from thoughts about adoption, the birth of a preterm infant who may be in intensive care, or the infant's death. Help the patient move through the grieving process. The adolescent who gives birth to a preterm infant or one who is small for gestational age may find it difficult to reconcile a tiny infant with images she may have imagined about the "perfect baby." She may be afraid of caring for the child introduced to her in the intensive care unit. The confidence in her abilities gained during the prenatal period may be replaced by feelings of being overwhelmed and incompetent. Intensive teaching and continual support programs are essential to keep the young mother and her vulnerable infant from becoming estranged.

Many young mothers pattern their parenting on what they experienced. It is important to assess the level of support available to the young mother. Referrals may be needed to address identified needs. The adolescent may have conflict with dependence versus independence issues as she performs her mothering role within the framework of her family of origin. The adolescent's family also may need help adapting to their new roles.

Adolescent father. The adolescent father also faces immediate developmental crises: completing the developmental tasks of adolescence and making a transition to parenthood and, sometimes, to marriage. These transitions can be stressful. Begin interacting with the adolescent father by asking his pregnant partner to bring him to the clinic with her so that he may participate in the birth. With the pregnant teen's agreement, the father also may be contacted directly.

To include the young father in all aspects of the care, assess four areas: (1) the couple's relationship; (2) levels of stress, concern, and coping; (3) educational and vocational goals; and (4) level of health care knowledge. Like all fathers, adolescent fathers need support to discuss their emotional responses to the pregnancy. The nurse's nonjudgmental attitude is essential for open communication. Recognize the father's feelings of guilt, powerlessness, or bravado and their negative consequences for parents and child. Counseling must be reality oriented. Discuss topics such as finances, child care, parenting skills, and the father's role in the birth experience. Teenage fathers also need knowledge of reproductive physiology and birth control options.

The adolescent mother's partner and family affect how she deals with her pregnancy, labor, birth, and subsequent parenthood. The adolescent father may continue to be involved with the young mother. In many instances, he plays an important role in the decisions she faces in pregnancy, including whether to continue the pregnancy, have an abortion, keep the child, or arrange for adoption.

Support the young father by helping him develop realistic perceptions of his role as "father of a child." Encourage his use of coping mechanisms that are not detrimental to his, his partner's, or his child's well-being. Enlist support systems, parents, and professional agencies on his behalf. Encourage mutual responsibility for birth control.

Patient Teaching

Education of the pregnant adolescent is essential. To work effectively with adolescents, be sensitive, nonjudgmental, and knowledgeable about the stages of adolescence. Because no two adolescents are alike, use a wide range of skills to reach each individual (see the Patient Teaching box on adolescent parents). Patient teaching may have to be directed toward the adolescent mother, who is often the primary caregiver. Efforts should be made to keep the adolescent in school. Many high schools have programs to assist adolescent parents in their educational endeavors.

Patient Teaching

Adolescent Parents

- Nutrition is a major area of concern for the teenager. The teen often is still growing, and her nutritional intake must meet her own needs and those of the fetus. Fad diets and food idiosyncrasies are common in teenagers; take this into account when teaching nutrition. Body image disturbance is a problem even for a mature woman. The teenager, particularly one who has not yet accepted the fact of pregnancy, may limit food intake to avoid gaining weight. This can be exceedingly dangerous to mother and infant.

- Preparation for labor and delivery is also essential. Many adolescents have little knowledge of human anatomy and have fears and misconceptions about the process of childbirth. They may have heard stories from friends that increase their anxiety. Be factual without being harsh when describing the birth process.

- Most adolescents plan to keep and raise their infants. Instruction should include child care, growth, and development. Refer the women to community agencies that provide ongoing support.

- Involve the adolescent father. Consider the effect of pregnancy on him, particularly if he remains meaningfully involved with the teenage mother. Counseling is important for both because the physical, financial, and emotional consequences of the pregnancy will affect both of them for the rest of their lives.

OLDER PREGNANT WOMAN

At the other end of the reproductive cycle are women who have their first child after they are 35 years of age. These pregnancies are termed "geriatric pregnancies." There is an increased risk of maternal and fetal complications. Issues and concerns related to the over-35 age group have become increasingly prominent in the past decade. Some women have always borne children at a later age, either by choice or because of lack or failure of contraception during the perimenopausal years. Today this group also includes women who have postponed pregnancy because of careers or other reasons and women with infertility problems who become pregnant through technological advances that have expanded alternatives for couples desiring children.

Many women become aware of the so-called biological clock as menopause approaches and wish to have a child while they are still able to do so. The potential for infertility increases with age. Although most women who wait until later in life are well educated and have decided to become pregnant, conception and pregnancy are not always easy. The incidence of ectopic pregnancy, placenta previa, and various medical conditions such as diabetes or hypertension increases with age. If the woman does become pregnant, each year after age 35 increases the risk of conceiving a child with Down syndrome or other chromosomal anomalies. Amniocentesis, chorionic villus sampling and the maternal serum alphafeto protein screenings are performed commonly to detect genetic problems. Detection of genetic disorders can raise ethical dilemmas regarding aborting or raising a disabled child.

Older women who are without medical problems have a much lower risk for problems than previously thought. Those who do have some complications often can have a successful pregnancy with good medical and nursing care. As women maintain better overall health and fitness, increased age appears to be less of an impediment to a normal pregnancy. Most first-time mothers older than 35 have waited and chosen this specific time for pregnancy; this choice is influenced by their awareness of the increasing possibility of infertility or of genetic defects in the infants of older women. Many women seek information about pregnancy from books and friends. They actively try to prevent fetal disorders and are careful in searching for the best possible maternity care. They identify sources of stress in their lives. They are concerned about having enough energy and stamina to meet the demands of parenting and their new roles and relationships.

Psychosocial adjustment to parenthood at this time of life depends greatly on the individual and her situation. Changes in income, lifestyle, and work routines can present challenges that are stressful, even if the pregnancy is desired.

Peer support may be less available for the mature primigravida. Many friends have teenage children and do not relate to the concerns of a new mother. Younger mothers have some of the same concerns, but they often do not share the perspective of older mothers. Family support may also be limited due to the potential age of the grandparents.

Mature gravidas also worry about complications that may affect the fetus or their own health. They are aware that they may not have another opportunity for pregnancy because of their age. They may be concerned about their ability to balance their career with increased family responsibilities.

Emphasize measures to assist the mother in regaining strength and muscle tone (e.g., prenatal and postnatal exercises). Some older mothers may find that the care of the newborn infant exhausts their physical capabilities. Many women may benefit from referral to supportive resources in the community.

ADOPTION

Some women carry the pregnancy to term and then give up the newborn to the care of another family for adoption. The decision to place the infant for adoption is a painful one that can produce long-lasting feelings of ambivalence and sorrow. On one hand, the birth mother may be satisfied that the infant is going into a stable home where a child is wanted and will receive excellent care. On the other hand, the social pressures and personal feelings against giving up one's child are often intense.

The relationship between the birth mother and the adoptive parents varies greatly. The adoptive parents may be unknown to the birth mother, or she may have chosen them. Some adoptive mothers participate in the birth. The birth mother may never see the infant again or may keep in contact and participate in the child's life.

Nurses are sometimes unsure of how to communicate with the woman who is giving up her infant. The nursing staff who come into contact with the woman must be informed of her decision to place the infant for adoption. Information prevents inadvertent comments that could cause distress. Second, remember that adoption is an act of love, not one of abandonment, as the woman gives the newborn to a family who is better able to provide financial and emotional support.

Also be prepared to respect any special wishes that the mother may have about the birth. For instance, most birth mothers want to know all about the infant. They may want to see and hold the newborn and give the child a name. Many take photographs or save the crib card. Such actions provide memories of the infant and help the mother through the grieving process that may accompany adoption of the child.

Try to establish rapport and a trusting relationship with the mother. Acknowledgment of the situation at the initial contact with the woman is helpful: "Hello, my name is Claire, and I'll be your nurse today. I understand the adoptive family is coming this morning. What can I do to help you get ready?" This communication is more helpful than ignoring the event that is of primary concern to the mother. It also provides an opening for her to express feelings such as attachment to the infant, ambivalence about her decision, and profound sadness.

Nurses also teach adoptive families how to care for the newborn and what to expect in growth and development. Teaching requires adequate time and a private place. This family benefits from all the teaching provided to other new parents. They may be anxious, and demonstrations and return demonstrations are appropriate.

CONTRACEPTION

Contraception refers to actions taken to avoid becoming pregnant. Women and men actively engage in family planning and determine when to attempt to conceive a child or avoid pregnancy. A wide variety of birth control products are available. Selection of one involves a review of personal preferences and consideration of the woman's medical history and age. The assessment should include methods of interest and lifestyle concerns with the goal of pairing the best option for the couple. Provide information about the use, effectiveness in preventing pregnancy, cost, potential protection from STIs, and pros and cons of the method selected. A visit with her primary care provider or health care professional also is advised. Also consider cultural values and practices (see the Cultural Considerations box on contraception).

POSTPARTUM THROMBOPHLEBITIS

Development of a blood clot in the interior of a blood vessel that results from inflammation or obstruction of a vessel is known as a *thrombosis*. The postpartum period may be affected by three types of thrombosis:

- *Superficial venous thrombosis:* Venous inflammation just below the skin's surface
- *Deep vein thrombosis:* A blood clot in a vein deep within the body, usually in the lower extremities
- *Pulmonary embolism:* Occlusion of the pulmonary artery by a blood clot traveling from elsewhere in the body

Incidence and Etiology

Thromboembolic disease is seen in less than 1% of postpartum women. Early ambulation after childbirth helps reduce the incidence. Risk factors for thromboembolic disease are increasing age, obesity, surgery, multiparity, and immobility.

Clinical Manifestations

Pain and tenderness in the lower extremities, along with warmth, redness, and hardening over the involved vessel, are common manifestations of superficial venous thrombosis.

During pregnancy, calf tenderness or leg pain and swelling may indicate deep vein thrombosis. The positive Homans' sign is not considered a definitive test, because it may be associated with other conditions. Be alert for the respiratory changes of dyspnea and tachycardia, which may signal pulmonary embolism.

Diagnosis is not based solely on the physical examination. Doppler ultrasound scan provides a noninvasive means to confirm the presence of thromboembolic disease. Compression ultrasound or magnetic resonance imaging also may be used.

Medical Management

A conservative approach is used to manage superficial venous thrombosis. Pharmacologic management includes the use of nonsteroidal anti-inflammatory medications. Administer pain medications as needed and limit activity. The goal is to rest the affected extremity in an elevated position. Heat applications and elastic stockings also are recommended.

The acute phase of treatment for deep venous thrombosis includes IV anticoagulant therapy, activity restriction, leg elevation, and pain management. Once the symptoms have eased, elastic stockings are applied, and the woman is able to ambulate. Begin administration of oral anticoagulant medications during this phase. Oral therapy can be anticipated for 3 months.

Management of a pulmonary embolism involves IV heparin therapy. Warfarin is contraindicated in pregnancy. After the acute phase of the illness, the patient takes subcutaneous heparin or oral anticoagulant therapies for 6 months. The use of aspirin is contraindicated in patients taking anticoagulant medications because of the increased risk for bleeding.

Nursing Interventions

To assess the woman with a thrombosis, observe and gently palpate the affected area, palpate peripheral pulses, measure the circumference of the leg for comparison, observe for signs of bleeding, and determine the presence of crackles or respiratory distress.

Evaluate the effectiveness of anticoagulant therapy in part with laboratory values. The PT or PTT is drawn and reviewed throughout the therapy. Report to the physician any laboratory values that fall outside the recommended therapeutic range.

During the acute phase of the illness, the patient requires emotional support and education to ensure her compliance with the treatment regimen. Assistance with self-care may be needed. Provide instruction about positions to avoid in the bed such as crossing the legs. Encourage leg elevation. Instruct her to change positions frequently.

Nursing care of a woman experiencing a thrombosis involves patient and family education and ongoing assessment. Teach the patient about the diagnosis and treatment plans. Activity limitations may be difficult, so educate the patient about the risks associated with noncompliance. Massage of the thrombus is contraindicated because it may cause the clot to break free and travel to vital body organs.

Discharge teaching also should include information about the prescribed medication regimen and follow-up appointments with the laboratory and the physician. Medication education includes scheduling, dosages, potential side effects, and problems to report. Laboratory monitoring is needed throughout the therapy. The risk for injury is increased as a result of the anticoagulant therapy, so advise her to use a soft toothbrush and electric razor. Warfarin is associated with birth defects, so have a frank discussion about the need for contraception.

COMPLICATIONS RELATED TO THE NEWBORN

NEWBORNS AT RISK

Many maternal conditions can place the newborn in increased danger of illness or death. Identify any maternal risk factors as soon as possible to decrease the risk to the fetus or the newborn. Once these risks are identified, all medical and nursing measures possible should be undertaken to minimize the consequences to the mother and the newborn.

When risk factors are identified early, care providers can prepare to meet the needs of the newborn at risk. New equipment, such as fetal monitors and more sensitive diagnostic tests, has made problems during labor and delivery easier to recognize. Despite all progress, however, many infants still are born in need of special attention.

Assess the newborn at the time of delivery. The Apgar score gives important information about the newborn's status at 1 and 5 minutes after delivery (see Chapter 27). This is followed by a more detailed assessment of size related to gestational age. Distinguish between infants who are preterm and those who are small for gestational age. Although both groups are at risk, the problems they present are different.

GESTATIONAL AGE

Gestational age is a significant factor in neonatal mortality and morbidity (Figs. 29.7 and 29.8). Preterm and postterm infants are at risk. Gestational age is classified as follows:

- *Preterm:* 20 to 37 completed weeks' gestation
- *Term:* 38 to 41 completed weeks' gestation
- *Postterm:* 42 weeks' gestation

Physical assessment procedures to determine gestational age are based on the method devised by Lilly and Victor Dubowitz, South African physicians. Their method is based on 21 strictly defined physical and neurologic signs and provides the correct gestational age ±2 weeks in 95% of infants. Most birthing facilities use this scale or one similar for determination of gestational age. Ideally the tests are performed between 2 and 8 hours of age. For the first hour, the infant is recovering from the stress of birth, and this is reflected in muscle movements; for example, the arm recoil is slower in a fatigued infant. After 48 hours, some responses change significantly. The plantar creases on the soles of the feet appear to increase in number and become visible as the skin loses fluid and dries. Fig. 29.8 shows newborn maturity ratings and classification.

PRETERM INFANT

Etiology and Pathophysiology

The exact causes of preterm labor are unknown. In some cases, it is related to maternal or placental problems, but in other cases, the cause cannot be determined. Fetal size does not negate the complications that may arise when the fetus is born prematurely. The prematurity may also be combined with maternal conditions that promoted less than ideal intrauterine conditions. This can further hinder the path to a positive end outcome.

The preterm infant is developmentally immature. The lungs do not produce enough surfactant to allow adequate oxygenation. Circulation may not have adapted from fetal to neonatal as it usually does in a term infant, which leads to oxygenation problems.

Problems with heat conservation stem from lack of subcutaneous fat, a large surface area relative to body weight, and poor reserves of glucose and brown fat (a source of heat unique to neonates that is capable of greater thermogenic [heat-producing] activity than ordinary fat; deposits are found around the adrenals, the kidneys, and the neck; between scapulae; and behind the sternum for several weeks after birth). The digestive system is formed, but problems with absorption of nutrients are common. The renal system is immature and ineffective. Fluid and acid-base imbalance frequently is observed. The infant is also neurologically immature; the gag, suck, and swallow reflexes may be weak or absent, and other normal reflexes may be absent or atypical.

The preterm infant is at risk because of immaturity of organ systems and lack of reserves. The morbidity and mortality rate for preterm infants is three to four times higher than that of older infants of comparable weight. The potential problems and care needs of the preterm infant of 2000 g differ from those of the term, postterm, or postmature infant of equal weight.

Fig. 29.7 (A) Three babies of the same gestational age, with weights of 600, 1400, and 2750 g, respectively, from *left* to *right.* Their weights are plotted in B at points *A, B,* and *C.* (B) Intrauterine growth status for gestational age and according to appropriateness of growth. (A, From *Perinatal assessment of maturation,* National Audiovisual Center, Washington, DC. B, Modified from Battaglia FC, Lubchenco LO: A practical classification of newborn infants by weight and gestational age. J Pediatr 1967;71[2]:59–63.)

Preterm infants are at a disadvantage when they face the transition from intrauterine to extrauterine life. The degree of disadvantage depends primarily on their level of maturity. Physiologic disorders and anomalous malformations affect their response to treatment as well. In general, the closer they are to the normal term infant in gestational age and birth weight, the easier is their adjustment to the external environment.

Clinical Manifestations

The preterm newborn's posture is froglike or flaccid. The color is usually ruddy, and cyanosis may be present immediately after birth and for the first few hours of life. The head appears large in proportion to the body, and the bones of the skull are pliable with large, flat fontanelles. The skin is thin and translucent with obvious blood vessels and little subcutaneous fat. A layer of fine hair (lanugo) may coat large areas of the body. Cartilage in the ears is pliable, and the ears can be easily folded. The genitalia in boys are small, and frequently the testes are undescended. In girls, the labia majora are small and less prominent than the labia minora. The cry is weak, and reflexes are immature or absent.

NEUROMUSCULAR MATURITY

	−1	0	1	2	3	4	5
Posture							
Square Window (wrist)	> 90°	90°	60°	45°	30°	0°	
Arm Recoil		180°	140° - 180°	110° - 140°	90° - 110°	< 90°	
Popliteal Angle	180°	160°	140°	120°	100°	90°	< 90°
Scarf Sign							
Heel to Ear							

PHYSICAL MATURITY

Skin	sticky friable transparent	gelatinous red, translucent	smooth pink, visible veins	superficial peeling or rash, few veins	cracking pale areas rare veins	parchment deep cracking no vessels	leathery cracked wrinkled
Lanugo	none	sparse	abundant	thinning	bald areas	mostly bald	
Plantar Surface	heel-toe 40-50 mm: -1 <40 mm: -2	>50 mm no crease	faint red marks	anterior transverse crease only	creases ant. 2/3	creases over entire sole	
Breast	imperceptible	barely perceptible	flat areola no bud	stippled areola 1-2 mm bud	raised areola 3-4 mm bud	full areola 5-10 mm bud	
Eye/Ear	lids fused loosely: -1 tightly: -2	lids open pinna flat stays folded	sl. curved pinna; soft; slow recoil	well-curved pinna; soft but ready recoil	formed & firm instant recoil	thick cartilage ear stiff	
Genitals (male)	scrotum flat, smooth	scrotum empty faint rugae	testes in upper canal rare rugae	testes descending few rugae	testes down good rugae	testes pendulous deep rugae	
Genitals (female)	clitoris prominent labia flat	prominent clitoris small labia minora	prominent clitoris enlarging minora	majora & minora equally prominent	majora large minora small	majora cover clitoris & minora	

MATURITY RATING

score	weeks
-10	20
-5	22
0	24
5	26
10	28
15	30
20	32
25	34
30	36
35	38
40	40
45	42
50	44

Fig. 29.8 Estimation of gestational age. New Ballard scale for newborn maturity rating. Expanded scale includes extremely premature infants and has been refined to improve accuracy in more mature infants. (From Ballard JL, Khoury JC, Wedig K, et al: New Ballard score, expanded to include extremely premature infants. *J Pediatr* 1991;119[3]:417–423.)

Assessment

Assess all systems of the preterm newborn carefully and continually; changes occur rapidly and necessitate continuous monitoring. Preterm infants typically are placed in an intensive care nursery and receive care from nurses specially trained to meet their needs.

The preterm infant's greatest potential problem is respiratory distress syndrome, which results from an immature respiratory system (see Chapter 31). The first symptom of respiratory distress is usually grunting on expiration, followed by nasal flaring, circumoral cyanosis, substernal retractions, and tachypnea. It is treated with oxygen therapy and artificial surfactant. Providing periods of rest and maintaining body temperature are important components of treatment.

An accurate assessment of gestational age is a good indicator of the problems a preterm newborn is likely to experience. Follow a systematic approach in assessment. The preterm infant's response to extrauterine life is different from that of the term infant. Knowledge of the physiologic basis of these differences helps in assessment of these infants, understanding of their responses, and determination of which potential problems are most likely to occur.

Diagnostic Tests

A wide range of diagnostic tests may be performed based on the newborn's specific needs.

Nursing Interventions

The specifics of care of the preterm newborn are beyond the scope of this text. The main goals include maintaining and stabilizing the conditions of preterm newborns until they mature adequately. Respiratory regulation, thermoregulation, fluid and electrolyte regulation, sensory stimulation, and promotion of bonding with the parents are major areas of concern for the nurse.

Patient problems and interventions for the preterm infant include but are not limited to the following:

PATIENT PROBLEM	NURSING INTERVENTIONS
Potential for Inability to Regulate Body Temperature, related to immature temperature regulation center, large body surface in relation to body weight, and minimal brown fat stores	Use skin probe to measure skin temperature and take steps to maintain it at 97–98°F (36.1–36.7°C)
	Monitor heart rate and rhythm
	Keep infant well covered and wrapped in blankets
	Pad cold surfaces
	Use radiant warmer if infant is uncovered for extended periods
	Keep skin dry
	Avoid drafts
	Keep crib, warmer, or Isolette away from windows and cold external walls
	Monitor for signs and symptoms of cold stress: decreased temperature, lethargy, and pallor (cold stress increases oxygen requirements)
	Avoid taking rectal temperature
	Obtain axillary temperatures and compare with registered skin probe temperature every 30 min for 2 h and until stable
Potential for Anxiousness (parental), related to preterm birth, separation, and breastfeeding	Encourage parents to stay with baby in the neonatal intensive care unit
	Encourage parents to actively participate in all aspects of care, if possible
	Encourage parents to hold baby and engage in en face positions (allowing mutual gazing at each other's face). This promotes eye contact and bonding.
	Encourage mother to breastfeed
	Explain the use of all equipment being used
	Discuss baby's behavioral cues and physical characteristics
	Encourage parents to express their feelings about the pregnancy, the labor, and the birth
	Discuss parents' feeding decisions
	Facilitate milk expression and storage by providing equipment or referral for lactation consultation

POSTTERM INFANT

The postterm infant may show signs of placental insufficiency because the aging placenta was not fully functioning. Fetal malnutrition may occur as a result of deteriorating metabolic exchanges in the aging placenta. The infant also may be at increased risk for perinatal mortality from intrauterine hypoxia during labor and birth. This infant is at risk for asphyxia, respiratory distress, and hypoglycemia.

GESTATIONAL SIZE

Newborns are also classified according to their weight at any given gestational age. An infant may be as follows:

- *Small for gestational age (SGA):* Weight is less than the 10th percentile for age.
- *Appropriate for gestational age (AGA):* Weight is between the 10th and 90th percentiles.
- *Large for gestational age (LGA):* Weight is greater than the 90th percentile.
- *Low birth weight:* Weight is 2500 g or less at birth.

An SGA infant may be preterm, term, or postterm; an AGA infant may be preterm, term, or postterm; and an LGA infant may be preterm, term, or postterm.

The SGA infant may be small because of problems in the first trimester, such as infections or chromosomal abnormalities, or a later reduction in the fetal oxygen supply and fetal nutrition as a result of smoking, maternal hypertension, or malnutrition. Problems seen with SGA infants include asphyxia, meconium aspiration syndrome, hypoglycemia, and hypothermia. LGA infants often have hypoglycemia, respiratory distress, birth injuries, and asphyxia.

INFANT OF A MOTHER WITH DIABETES

The infant of a mother with diabetes, whether preterm, term, or postterm, is at risk. This infant frequently exhibits macrosomia (excessive size and stature), hypoglycemia, perinatal asphyxia, hypocalcemia, respiratory difficulties, and hyperbilirubinemia. The infant of the mother with gestational diabetes also may have congenital anomalies resulting from the uncontrolled maternal blood glucose levels in early pregnancy. The infant born to a woman with long-term and poorly controlled diabetes mellitus may be small for gestational age as a result of poor perfusion to the placenta and fetus.

HEMOLYTIC DISEASES

Etiology

Hemolysis may result from basic incompatibility of blood groups, such as ABO or Rh incompatibility, or from a transfer of antibodies through the placenta.

Pathophysiology

The term *Rh negative* indicates that an individual's RBCs do not have a specific antigen on their surface. The majority of people are classified as being Rh positive as they do have the blood protein on the surface of

⚠	Rh– Red blood cell (RBC) of mother
⚠	Rh+ RBC of fetus with Rh antigen on surface
Ⓐ⚡	Anti–Rh antibody made against Rh+ RBC
⚡	Hemolysis of Rh+ RBC

Fig. 29.9 Mechanisms of erythroblastosis fetalis, which is caused by Rh incompatibility. (A) Rh-positive fetus is carried by Rh-negative mother. Rh protein crosses placental barrier and invades mother's bloodstream. (B) Mother's system manufactures antibodies to destroy foreign Rh protein. (C) Antibodies cross back over placenta and destroy fetus's blood cells, which are associated intimately with Rh protein. (From Herlihy B: *The human body in health and illness,* ed 4, St. Louis, 2011, Saunders.)

their RBCs. Being Rh negative is a benign matter and of limited relevance except during pregnancy.

If a Rh-negative woman is exposed to Rh-positive blood cells, she may become sensitized (isoimmunization). If the woman is sensitized (i.e., exposed to the antigen), she produces antibodies. Exposure can occur through blood transfusion of incompatible blood or during pregnancy when some fetal blood cells enter the maternal circulation. This transfer of antigen may occur in cases of abortion or abruption or at the time of delivery. Once the mother develops Rh antibodies, they remain in her blood, as do other antibodies.

When the woman becomes pregnant, maternal antibodies may cross the **placental barrier** (the boundary provided by placental tissue between the fetal and maternal circulations; small substances, excluding blood cells, may cross this barrier). If the fetal RBCs contain the Rh antigen, the maternal Rh antibodies cause hemolysis (destruction) of the fetal RBCs. The higher the level of maternal antibodies, the greater the destruction of fetal RBCs. This destruction of fetal RBCs results in pathologic jaundice, which occurs within the first 24 hours after birth.

Because sensitization most often occurs at delivery, the firstborn fetus generally has no signs of hemolysis; successive fetuses are most likely to be affected. Today, serious problems related to Rh incompatibility, such as **erythroblastosis fetalis** (a type of hemolytic anemia that occurs in newborns as a result of maternal-fetal blood group incompatibility, especially involving the Rh factor and ABO blood groups), usually are prevented (see Fig. 29.9).

ABO incompatibility is also an antigen-antibody process. Type O blood naturally contains anti-A and anti-B antibodies. These antibodies cross the placenta and cause hemolysis if the fetus has blood type A or B. Incompatibility is also possible if the mother is A, and the infant is B, or if the mother is B, and the infant is A. No sensitization is necessary, and it may affect the first and all successive pregnancies.

Clinical Manifestations

The mother shows no clinical symptoms. Hemolysis may occur in utero, and detection must be made with diagnostic tests on amniotic fluid, suspected by changes in fetal condition or maternal diagnostic tests. Jaundice present at birth or in the first 24 hours of life is considered an indicator of a pathologic condition. **Kernicterus** (an abnormal toxic accumulation of bilirubin in central nervous system tissues caused by **hyperbilirubinemia** [an excess of bilirubin in the blood of the newborn]) may result in neurologic damage or death. Anemia caused by RBC destruction is also possible.

Assessment

Determine the maternal blood type and Rh factor during pregnancy. If the mother is Rh negative, find out the father's blood type. If he is also Rh negative, no Rh-based problem will occur. If the father is Rh positive, problems are possible. Also assess the woman's history for any events that may have caused sensitization, such as previous pregnancy, birth, abortion, or amniocentesis and transfusion with Rh-positive blood,

Box 29.9	**Home Phototherapy With a portable blanket device—Biliblanket**

Information for parents:

- As much of the infant's skin as possible should be in direct contact with the lighted section of the pad. The infant's back or chest should be placed directly on the pad, with the tip of the pad at the shoulder and the cable at the feet.
- Follow the equipment supplier's instructions regarding safety and use of the phototherapy unit.
- Phototherapy can be discontinued for brief periods without harming your baby.
- Temperature instability may occur when starting and stopping phototherapy and when collecting laboratory specimens.
- Effects of phototherapy may include changes in frequency and color of the infant's stools and rash from an increase in the number of loose stools.

Notify your child's health care provider if:

- A notable change is seen in activity level.
- The infant's temperature is not maintained at 97° or 100°F (33.3° to 37.7°C).
- The infant is feeding poorly.
- The infant is not voiding six times per day or does not void within a 6-h period.
- Infant vomits two or more feedings.

Notify your home care agency if:

- Phototherapy is discontinued.
- An equipment malfunction occurs.

Modified From University of California San Francisco Home Health Care: Guidelines for home therapy, San Francisco, 2001, University of California. In Lowdermilk DL, Perry SE, editors: *Maternity and women's health care*, ed 9, St. Louis, 2007, Mosby.

which causes immediate sensitization. Even premature separation of the placenta and trauma may cause sensitization.

Diagnostic Tests

An indirect Coombs' test is completed on Rh-negative women with their initial prenatal lab studies. The purpose of the test is to determine if there has been exposure to Rh-positive cells and thus becoming sensitized. After delivery, a direct Coombs' test is performed on infant blood to determine the presence of antibody-coated RBCs. Bilirubin levels of infant blood indicate the extent of RBC destruction.

Nursing Interventions

Maternal. If the results of an Rh-negative mother's indirect Coombs' test are negative, the mother is given an intramuscular injection of RhoGAM. This currently is recommended at 28 weeks of pregnancy and again within 72 hours of delivery. RhoGAM provides passive antibodies and prevents development of naturally occurring maternal antibodies. RhoGAM also should be given to an Rh-negative mother in cases of abortion, ectopic pregnancy, and amniocentesis. Give the mother an identification card with vital information, including date of last injection of RhoGAM. She should carry this card with her always. If

the indirect Coombs' is positive there will be close observation of the pregnancy for potential complications. This will include antibody titer testing to monitor the level of sensitization throughout the pregnancy. The fetus will be monitored by ultrasound. The medical plan will be to deliver the fetus once the there is adequate lung maturity. To provide this information an amniocentesis will be completed.

Newborn. Carefully observe the newborn affected by a hemolytic process; jaundice and anemia may become severe and lead to other complications. Monitor the bilirubin, hemoglobin, and hematocrit levels and notify the physician of any abnormal results. The infant with severe jaundice may be treated with phototherapy or may need transfusion. Phototherapy usually is begun when the bilirubin levels reach 12 to 15 mg/dL.

Phototherapy requires several precautions. Phototherapy involves exposure of the skin to fluorescent lights, which converts the bilirubin to a water-soluble form that can be excreted in the urine. Maintain body temperature and protect the infant's eyes during this treatment. Phototherapy may be carried out at home with the use of a biliblanket (Box 29.9).

Eye patches should be removed and lights turned off during feedings and bathing to allow infant stimulation and face-to-face interaction with the mother or other caregiver. Stools may be loose, and the urine contains excessive waste products, so it is important to maintain skin integrity with careful cleansing and frequent diaper changes. Because fluid loss is increased, adequate fluids are important to maintain necessary hydration.

Patient problems and interventions for the patient with hemolytic disease include but are not limited to the following:

PATIENT PROBLEM	NURSING INTERVENTIONS
Potential for Inadequate Fluid Volume, related to insensible weight loss and dehydration	Do not clothe infant; diapering is questionable
	Maintain thermoneutral phototherapy environment
	Maintain axillary temperature at 97.7°F (36.5°C)
	Assess axillary temperature at least q 2 h and as needed
	Avoid exposure of skin temperature probe to phototherapy lights
	Weigh infant daily unclothed at the same time on the same scale before feeding
	Measure accurate intake and output
	Check urine specific gravity every shift
	Test strength of bililight according to hospital's and manufacturer's policy

PATIENT PROBLEM	NURSING INTERVENTIONS
Potential for Compromised Parenting Skills, related to disruption of parent-infant interaction secondary to phototherapy	Explain need to provide adequate fluid intake, including water between feedings Discuss signs and symptoms to report to physician, such as recurrence of jaundice or persistent diarrhea Emphasize importance of having laboratory tests done as ordered Emphasize importance of follow-up care Encourage parent participation in infant care activities such as feeding, bathing, and cuddling Review care of infant with hyperbilirubinemia as necessary with parents Permit siblings to visit according to hospital policy When parents visit, turn off lights and remove eye shields for the time period ordered by physician Reinforce explanation of phototherapy, reasons for particular interventions, and care plan

Patient Teaching

Rh-negative women should be aware of the process involved in Rh sensitization. Answer all questions that the woman or her partner may have. Phototherapy can be disturbing to the parents. They may voice concerns about not being able to hold their child as much as desired and thus interrupt the bonding. Explain the reasons for treatment and provide opportunities for maternal-infant interaction. Today many newborns are sent home receiving this form of therapy. Many insurance companies recognize the therapeutic value of phototherapy at home and include phototherapy in their policies. Teach the parents correct use of the equipment and the special care needed by the infant.

SUBSTANCE ABUSE

The use of legal substances, such as alcohol and tobacco, or illicit drugs, such as cocaine and marijuana, increases the risk for medical complications in the mother and poor birth outcomes in the infant. Approximately 1 in 10 infants is exposed to one or more mood-altering drugs during pregnancy. Although tobacco, alcohol, and marijuana are the most commonly abused drugs, the use of cocaine and heroin has had a major effect on health care for pregnant women and their offspring.

When the pregnant woman takes a substance, the fetus experiences the same systemic effects as the expectant mother but often more severely. The damage incurred by the fetus related to maternal substance abuse cannot be reversed. For instance, cocaine raises the blood pressure of the woman and the fetus and puts both at risk for intracranial bleeding. The quantity or frequency of alcohol ingestion to cause an adverse impact on the fetus varies. A drug that causes intoxication in the woman causes it for prolonged periods in the fetus. The fetus cannot metabolize drugs efficiently and experiences the effects long after they have disappeared in the woman. Maternal, fetal, and neonatal effects of commonly abused substances are summarized in Table 29.4. It is important to note that the damage may not be readily evident at birth. Learning disabilities and behavioral problems may not be evident until the child is school age. This sharply limits the ability for condition improvement.

Nursing Interventions

Nursing care relating to substance abuse in pregnancy ideally begins early in prenatal care. The nursing assessment includes inquiries about the use of tobacco, alcohol, and drugs. It is important to ensure that this data collection is comprehensive. When a gravid woman reports use of potentially damaging substances, work toward providing education to the woman about the dangers faced by her fetus. The need to assist the woman withdrawing from their use is a priority.

In some cases, the substance abuse may not be noted until after delivery. The policies in individual states may indicate meconium screening for newborns suspected of being born to women who are using drugs during pregnancy or for infants who are born prematurely. Infants of known drug and alcohol users generally are placed in a neonatal intensive care unit. Physical care includes careful temperature regulation and monitoring of vital signs. Observe the newborn to detect increasing instability. Provide small feedings, and observe the infant for diarrhea, regurgitation, and vomiting. Positioning on the right side helps prevent aspiration. IV therapy may be necessary. Administer medications as ordered to prevent the most serious withdrawal symptoms. Reduce stimuli that may aggravate seizures. These infants are often inconsolable, which makes caring for them difficult and stressful.

Include the newborn's parents in care whenever possible. Depending on the severity of the problems encountered, the infant may remain in the hospital, be discharged to the parent, or be placed in the custody of social services. Establishing a therapeutic relationship with the chemically dependent parent is a significant challenge. Consult with social welfare or other departments that are best able to protect the newborn and help the parent obtain the treatment needed to overcome an addiction.

Table 29.4	Maternal and Fetal or Neonatal Effects of Commonly Abused Substances	
SUBSTANCE	**MATERNAL EFFECTS**	**FETAL OR NEONATAL EFFECTS**
Caffeine (coffee, tea, cola, chocolate, cold remedies, analgesics)	Stimulation of CNS and cardiac function, vasoconstriction, mild diuresis; half-life triples during pregnancy Limit ingestion to 200 mg/day	Crosses placental barrier and stimulates fetus; teratogenic effects are undocumented High usage when breastfeeding may cause the baby to be fussy.
Tobacco	Decreased placental perfusion, anemia, PROM, preterm labor, spontaneous abortion, placental abruption	Prematurity, LBW, fetal demise, developmental delays, increased incidence of SIDS, pneumonia
Alcohol (beer, wine, mixed drinks, after-dinner drinks)	Spontaneous abortion	Fetal demise, IUGR, FAS (facial and cranial anomalies, developmental delay, mental retardation, short attention span), fetal alcohol effects (milder form of FAS)
Cocaine ("crack")	Hyperarousal state, generalized vasoconstriction, hypertension, increased incidence of spontaneous abortion, abruptio placentae, preterm labor, cardiovascular complications (stroke, heart attack), seizures, increased STIs	Tachycardia; stillbirth; prematurity; LBW; tremors; IUGR; irritability; decreased ability to interact with environmental stimuli; poor feeding reflexes; nausea, vomiting, diarrhea; decreased intellectual development; distended, flabby, creased abdomen (prune-belly syndrome) caused by absence of abdominal muscles
Narcotics (heroin, methadone, morphine)	Spontaneous abortion, PROM, preterm labor, increased incidence of STIs, HIV exposure, hepatitis, malnutrition	IUGR, perinatal asphyxia, intellectual impairment, neonatal abstinence syndrome, neonatal infections, fetal or neonatal death (SIDS, child abuse, and neglect)
Sedatives (barbiturates, tranquilizers)	Lethargy, drowsiness, CNS depression	Neonatal abstinence syndrome, seizures, delayed lung maturity, possible teratogenic effect
Amphetamines ("speed," "crystal," or "ice" when processed in crystals to smoke)	Malnutrition, tachycardia, withdrawal symptoms (lethargy, depression)	Increased risk for IUGR, prematurity, cardiac anomalies, cleft palate, abruptio placentae, hypoglycemia, sweating, poor visual tracing, "glassy-eyed" look, lethargy, feeding problems
Marijuana ("pot" or "grass")	Often used with other drugs (alcohol, cocaine, tobacco), increased incidence of anemia and inadequate weight gain	Unclear, more study needed; believed related to prematurity, IUGR, tremors, sensitivity to light

Modified from CNS, Central nervous system; *FAS,* fetal alcohol syndrome; *HIV,* human immunodeficiency virus; *IUGR,* intrauterine growth restriction; *LBW,* low birth weight; *PROM,* premature rupture of membranes; *SIDS,* sudden infant death syndrome; *STIs,* sexually transmitted infections.
From McKinney ES, James SR, Murray SS, et al: *Maternal-child nursing,* ed 2, St. Louis, 2005, Saunders.

COMPLICATIONS RELATED TO POSTPARTUM MENTAL HEALTH DISORDERS

Mental health disorders have implications for the mother, the newborn, and the entire family. Such conditions can interfere with attachment to the newborn and family integration, and some may threaten the safety and well-being of the mother, the newborn, and other children. Because birth usually is thought to be a happy event, a new mother's emotional distress may confuse family and friends and leave them unable to act. At a time when she most needs the caring attention of loved ones, they may either criticize or withdraw because of their own anxiety.

MOOD DISORDERS

Mood disorders are the predominant mental health disorder in the postpartum period, typically occurring within 4 weeks of childbirth. Feelings of mild

depression or "baby blues" is common. An estimated 70% to 80% of new mothers are impacted. Women with a history of depression or other mood disorders are at an increased risk (Langdon, n.d.). The stressors associated with childbirth contribute to these feelings. The postpartum patient undergoes a rapid change in hormones with the birth of the baby. Taking home an infant who requires total care and relies on the mother for survival is overwhelming. Preparing or accessing nutritious meals during the early postpartum period may be difficult with so many other responsibilities. When combined with sleep alterations encountered when faced with feeding and caring for an infant around the clock. feeling "blue" or down is understandable. The blues present intermittently. The individual may be happy and contented and then with little warning, feel tearful and sad. In most cases this "moodiness" self resolves. Nurses can help by suggesting new mothers accept help from friends and family members. This will also help to prevent feelings of isolation. Promoting rest by encouraging she rest when the baby rests will also be beneficial.

More serious depression eventually can incapacitate them to the point of being unable to care for themselves or their babies. Postpartum depression (PPD) can lead to a disturbance in the interaction of mothers and infants. Postpartum psychosis is a rare condition in which the mother becomes very disturbed and is unable to care for herself or her infant. She may feel directed to harm herself or her infant.

Nurses are positioned strategically to offer anticipatory guidance, to assess the mental health of new mothers, to offer therapeutic interventions, and to provide referrals when necessary. Failure to do so may have tragic consequences. Many women feel guilty about being depressed at a time when they believe they should be happy. They may be reluctant to discuss their symptoms or their negative feelings toward the child or this time in their life.

Medical Management

The depth or duration of sadness and depression may require medical intervention. Women experiencing PPD may require short term pharmacologic therapy with antidepressants and counseling. Women experiencing severe PPD or postpartum psychosis, a multifaceted approach involving antidepressants, anxiolytic agents (a sedative or minor tranquilizer), and electroconvulsive therapy. Psychotherapy focuses on the mother's fears and concerns regarding her new responsibilities and roles and monitoring for suicidal or homicidal thoughts. For some women, hospitalization is necessary.

❖ NURSING PROCESS FOR THE MOTHER AND NEWBORN AT RISK

The role of the licensed practical nurse/licensed vocational nurse (LPN/LVN) in the nursing process as stated is that the LPN/LVN will:

- Participate in planning care for patients based on patient needs.
- Review patient's care plan and recommend revisions as needed.
- Review and follow defined prioritization for patient care.
- Use clinical pathways, care maps, or care plans to guide and review patient care.

◆ ASSESSMENT

Nursing process for the patient at risk begins with assessment, which focuses on the history of the pregnancy and the patient's symptoms. Assessment includes physical and psychological arenas. Specific assessment items depend on the patient's disorder. Assessment also should include medical history, obstetric history, and social history.

◆ PATIENT PROBLEM

Nursing assessment helps identify the needs of the patient at high risk. Care then can be based on these needs. Patient problems depend on the high-risk condition and symptoms observed (see patient problem statements throughout the chapter).

◆ EXPECTED OUTCOMES AND PLANNING

The care plan focuses on the needs of the patient at high risk and the nurse's ability to meet those needs effectively. Each patient has different needs, and care is individualized accordingly. The care plan focuses on goals and outcomes specific to the patient problem. Examples include the following:

Goal 1: The patient with hyperemesis gravidarum will maintain caloric intake adequate to provide for fetal health and growth.

Outcome: Patient eats and retains 1800 kcal/day and drinks 2000 mL of fluid per day.

Goal 2: The preterm neonate will maintain skin temperature of 97.5° to 98.6°F (36.4° to 37°C) axillary while in an open crib.

Outcome: Neonate's temperature is 97.8° to 98.6°F (36.6° to 37°C) axillary on three successive occasions 4 hours apart.

◆ IMPLEMENTATION

Nursing interventions for the patient at high risk are determined by the patient problem and goals for the specific condition being treated.

◆ EVALUATION

Continually evaluate the success of the interventions. As the high-risk patient's situation changes, so too may the goals and interventions. Refer to the goals and outcomes to determine whether the plan was successful and the outcomes met. For example:

Goal 1: The patient with hyperemesis gravidarum will maintain caloric intake adequate to provide for fetal health and growth.

Evaluative measures: Patient ate six small meals totaling 1500 kcal with one emesis of 200 mL. Fluid intake of water and tea was 1200 mL.

Goal 2: The preterm neonate will maintain skin temperature of 97.5° to 98.6°F (36.4° to 37°C) axillary while in an open crib.

Evaluative measure: Neonate's temperature was 98.6°F (37°C) axillary at 0600, 98.2°F (36.8°C) axillary at 1000, and 98.9°F (37.2°C) axillary at 1400.

Get Ready for the NCLEX® Examination!

Key Points

- Complications can occur during any stage of the childbearing process.
- Continually assess pregnant women and newborns for any signs of complications.
- Educate all pregnant women about danger signs that indicate complications, stressing the importance of prompt medical attention.
- Hemorrhage is a danger sign during pregnancy and after delivery.
- Bleeding disorders of pregnancy are medical emergencies that demand expert teamwork from health care professionals.
- Premature separation, or placental abruption, is characterized by painful vaginal bleeding. A concealed bleed is possible depending on the location of the separation. Concealed bleeding is associated with abdominal rigidity.
- Placenta previa results from an abnormal location of implantation of the placenta, completely or partially covering the cervical os. This is associated with third trimester and painless vaginal bleeding.
- The type of spontaneous abortion determines the management.
- The cause of GH is unknown, and no known reliable tests are available for predicting women at risk for preeclampsia.
- Magnesium sulfate, the anticonvulsant agent of choice for prevention of eclampsia, necessitates careful monitoring of reflexes, respirations, and urinary output; its antidote, calcium gluconate, should be at the bedside.
- A wide range of infectious diseases present a threat to the mother and the newborn.
- The Rh-negative mother may need special interventions to prevent sensitization, which may affect future pregnancies.
- Preexisting health conditions, such as cardiac problems or diabetes mellitus, increase the risks of childbearing.
- Routine screening for GDM is performed for most women during the second trimester. Women with increased risk factors or those who are suspected of having diabetes-related issues may be tested earlier in gestation.
- The mother's age is significant in childbearing. The very young and the older mother are at increased risk.
- Adolescents can develop trusting relationships with helping professionals whom they respect.
- Drug and alcohol use have a serious impact on the developing fetus.
- Approximately 80% to 90% of pregnancies treated with cerclage result in live, viable births.
- The woman who is addicted to narcotics may have infections that compound the risk to the infant, including hepatitis; septicemia; and STIs, including AIDS.
- Newborns born to drug-abusing or alcohol-abusing mothers may manifest a variety of anatomic and neurologic defects.
- Infants born preterm or postterm and SGA or LGA are at greater risk for complications.
- Preterm infants are physiologically immature and at risk for respiratory distress syndrome, hypoglycemia, hyperbilirubinemia, and thermoregulation problems.

Additional Learning Resources

SG Go to your Study Guide for additional learning activities to help you master this chapter content.

Be sure to visit the Evolve site at http://evolve.elsevier.com/Cooper/foundations/ for additional online resources.

Review Questions for the NCLEX® Examination

1. The nurse is reviewing the plan of care for a patient being treated for acute deep vein thrombosis. Which can be anticipated to be included in the plan of care at this time? Select all that apply.

   1. Frequent ambulation
   2. Extremity elevation
   3. Intravenous anticoagulant therapies
   4. Oral anticoagulant therapies
   5. Activity restriction

2. A patient is admitted to the hospital with a diagnosis of suspected ectopic pregnancy. Which findings in the patient's history and assessment would be supportive of this diagnosis? *(Select all that apply.)*

   1. History of genital herpes simplex
   2. History of pelvic inflammatory disease
   3. Positive serum HCG test results
   4. Uterine enlargement
   5. Abdominal pain
   6. History of endometriosis
   7. Shoulder pain
   8. Vaginal spotting
   9. Positive urine HCG test results
   10. Chadwick's sign noted during the pelvic examination

3. A patient has been diagnosed with placenta previa. Which symptom is considered the classic diagnostic criterion for placenta previa?

   1. Painful vaginal bleeding
   2. Uterine irritability
   3. Elevation of temperature
   4. Painless vaginal bleeding

4. A patient is in labor and suddenly reports sharp fundal pain. She begins to have vaginal bleeding as well. What is the most likely cause of her symptoms?

   1. Preterm labor
   2. Abruptio placentae
   3. Pelvic inflammatory disease
   4. Placenta previa

5. A patient is diagnosed with an inevitable abortion. Which assessment finding distinguishes an inevitable abortion from a threatened abortion?

   1. Uterine cramping
   2. Vaginal bleeding
   3. Cervical dilation
   4. History of previous abortions

6. A patient is suspected of having gestational hypertension. Which assessments are likely to be included in the nursing assessment? *(Select all that apply.)*

   1. Deep tendon reflexes
   2. Determination of when she last ate
   3. Daily weight
   4. Intake and output
   5. Nitrazine testing

7. What is the most common cause of postpartum hemorrhage?

   1. Cervical lacerations
   2. Uterine atony
   3. Cesarean birth
   4. Disseminated intravascular coagulation

8. A baby boy was born at 38 weeks of gestation to a mother with type 1 diabetes. Into which category does this infant most likely fall?

   1. Premature
   2. Average for gestational age
   3. Intrauterine growth restriction
   4. Large for gestational age

9. A baby girl was born at 34 weeks of gestation. At 3 hours old, she is diagnosed with respiratory distress. What is an early symptom of respiratory distress?

   1. Nasal flaring
   2. Expiratory grunting
   3. Cyanosis
   4. Substernal retractions

10. A patient is Rh negative and delivers an infant with Rh-positive blood. RhoGAM is prescribed. What is the rationale for the use of this medication?

    1. To stimulate formation of maternal blood antigens
    2. To stimulate production of maternal blood antibodies
    3. To prevent production of maternal blood antibodies
    4. To prevent production of fetal blood antigens

11. After giving birth to a healthy baby boy, a primiparous woman, age 16 years, is admitted to the postpartum unit. An appropriate patient problem statement for her at this time is *Potential for Compromised Parenting Skills, related to deficient knowledge of newborn care.* In planning for the woman's discharge, the nurse should include what in the care plan?

    1. Tell the woman how to feed and bathe her baby.
    2. Give the woman written information on bathing her baby.
    3. Advise the woman that all mothers instinctively know how to care for their babies.
    4. Provide time for the woman to bathe her baby after she views a baby bath demonstration.

12. A newborn is jaundiced and receiving phototherapy. What is an appropriate nursing intervention when caring for an infant with hyperbilirubinemia who is receiving phototherapy? *(Select all that apply.)*

    1. Apply an oil-based lotion to the newborn's skin to prevent drying and cracking.
    2. Lay the baby down with the back directly on the biliblanket.
    3. Place eye shields over the newborn's eyes.
    4. Place the cord of the device near the head of the bed.
    5. Change the newborn's position every 3 to 4 hours.

13. A 26-year-old pregnant woman, gravida 2, para 1, is 28 weeks pregnant when she experiences bright red, painless vaginal bleeding. On her arrival at the hospital, what is an expected diagnostic procedure?

    1. Amniocentesis for fetal lung maturity
    2. Ultrasound scan for placental location
    3. Contraction stress test
    4. Internal fetal monitoring

14. In planning care of a 30-year-old woman with pregestational diabetes, what is the most important factor that affects pregnancy outcome?

    1. Mother's age
    2. Number of years since diabetes was diagnosed
    3. Amount of insulin required prenatally
    4. Degree of blood glucose control during pregnancy

15. When caring for a pregnant woman with cardiac problems, the nurse should be alert for what signs and symptoms that suggest cardiac decompensation? *(Select all that apply.)*

    1. Hypotension
    2. Hypertension
    3. Bradycardia
    4. Tachycardia
    5. Shortness of breath

16. The gravid woman is suspected of having mild preeclampsia when a blood pressure of _____ or higher on _____ occasions, twice, _____ hours apart.

Objectives

1. List three benefits of regular physical activity in children.
2. Identify barriers to health promotion and maintenance for the pediatric population.
3. State the American Academy of Pediatrics' recommendations for immunization administration in healthy infants and children.
4. State three strategies to promote dental health.
5. State the causes and prevention of accidental poisonings.
6. Describe four strategies to prevent aspiration of a foreign body.
7. Discuss the proper use of infant safety seats in motor vehicles.
8. List safety precautions important in educating parents to prevent environmental injuries to children.
9. Identify health risks for adolescents and interventions to reduce them.
10. Discuss the impact of social media on children.

key terms

anticipatory guidance (p. 934)
botulism (BŎT-ū-lĭzm, p. 943)
nursing bottle caries (p. 943)

The focus of health promotion is to assist individuals to realize their full potential. Active participation by patients and family is needed to develop and maintain a lifestyle that optimizes wellness. Traditionally, the primary care of children has fostered health promotion through health supervision and health maintenance visits, immunizations, screenings and surveillance, and anticipatory guidance (psychological preparation, based on developmental stage of a person for an event expected to be stressful, as in preparing a child for surgery by explaining what will happen and what it will feel like; also used to prepare parents for normal growth and development of their children). Health promotion activities are essential in identifying risks and encouraging healthy behaviors in children and their families. Ideally, these undertakings begin before the birth of the baby as the parents are prepared for the needs of their growing family. This lays a foundation for a continued health promotion in subsequent years.

One of the major roles in nursing is promoting wellness and disease prevention. Pediatric nursing provides many unique opportunities to participate in this role. The pediatric population offers several challenges not found in the adult population. Pediatric nurses need to use a multidisciplinary approach to meet the demands related to the promotion of wellness and disease prevention concerning the pediatric population.

To assist a population in the achievement of optimal states of health and wellness it is necessary to understand the barriers standing in the way of these initiatives. Obstacles for care can be grouped as financial and nonfinancial. Financial barriers include available monetary resources to pay for the care or items that are not covered readily by any existing insurance. Families having insurance also may experience problems locating a desired provider who will accept their insurance. Families who do not have insurance face the problem of having to balance health care related costs and the costs for necessities such as food and shelter. Children are not the decision makers in the family unit and are only to access care when deemed appropriate by their parents or guardians. Other non-financial barriers include physical access to care as a result of the availability of medical practitioners in the area or transportation. Working parents may face problems seeking care due to their work schedules. Psychosocial barriers also, may play a role in accessing health services. Language and cultural beliefs may affect ability and willingness to use care resources. Finally, an understanding and belief in the importance of health promotion affect a family's willingness to participate in care services (Unite for Sight, n.d.). Nurses have a key role in the identification of real and perceived barriers. Once these have been highlighted, the nurse, in conjunction with the other members of the health care team, can initiate a plan to assist families in the achievement of health promotion and maintenance.

This chapter identifies health promotion and disease prevention factors unique to the pediatric population. The primary focus of this chapter is the indicators identified in *Healthy People 2030* US Department of Health and Human Services, 2021) and dental health, poisoning, aspiration, and burn injuries related to children.

KEY HEALTH PROMOTION TOPICS FOR CHILDREN

The health and wellness of children is not limited to the hopes of their experiencing a well childhood. It is an investment. The prevention of illness and the establishment of health promotion activities for children provide a means to imbed behaviors in children in hopes of avoiding disease and chronic health concerns.

ACCESS TO HEALTH CARE

Health promotion and the care and treatment of disease are affected most by the access the family has to health care. The inability to engage in health care services can result in the absence or delay in receiving education about healthful practices. It can cause delays in the diagnosis and treatment of diseases. Millions of American children do not have any type of health care insurance. There are racial and socioeconomic divides regarding the coverage of children with health insurance. An estimated 4.3 million children under the age of 19 years do not have health insurance. An estimated 10% of Hispanic children do not have insurance in comparison with 4% for white non-Hispanic and black non-Hispanic children. The rates pertaining to how the coverage is provided is also racially significant: the majority of white non-Hispanic children (68%) are privately insured; black non-Hispanic (34%) and Hispanic children (31%) are privately insured at a much-lower rate (Berchick, 2019). This creates a somewhat impassable obstacle for people seeking health care services.

Other common barriers associated with access to health care in addition to the financial one include, lack of primary care providers, cultural and spiritual differences, language barriers, discrimination, and concerns about confidentiality. All health care providers have a responsibility to improve health care access for all people.

NUTRITION, PHYSICAL ACTIVITY, AND OBESITY

Physical activity and a balanced diet are for the healthy growth and development of children and adolescents. Diet and exercise lay a foundation to maintain health throughout the lifetime. Diet and exercise aid in the prevention of diseases such as hypertension, cancer, and heart disease. Unfortunately, many American children do not follow the recommended

dietary guidelines. Fewer than 1 in 3 children eat the recommended daily intake of vegetables. Exercise is also a concern, with more than 80% of adolescents not achieving the recommended level of physical activity.

Diet and exercise are intertwined with obesity in children. The number of overweight children in the United States is increasing and seems to be approaching an epidemic status. In economically developed countries, the most common disease seen in childhood and adolescence is now obesity. An estimated 19.3% of American children are overweight (CDC, 2021a). This number reflects a slight increase over the past decade from 14.94% noted in 2010 (CDC, 2017a). Children with a body mass index (BMI) between the 85th and 95th percentiles are considered overweight, and obesity is defined as a BMI greater than the 95th percentile. Children in the 99th percentile are considered extremely obese. Racial differences are noted: non-Hispanic blacks (24.2%) and Hispanics (25.6%) have higher rates of obesity than non-Hispanic whites. The rates of obesity increase with age. In children ages 2 to 5 years the rate of obesity is 13.4%. The most concerning rate of increase was in children ages 6 to 11. Since 2010 their rate more than doubled from 7.5% to 20.3%. Teens ages 12 to 19 years of age saw no significant changes (CDC, 2021a).

Regular physical activity lowers death rates in adults and reduces the risk for development of heart disease, high blood pressure, diabetes mellitus, and colon cancer. In children, regular physical activity increases bone and muscle strength and helps decrease body fat. Psychological benefits of regular physical activity include improvement in self-esteem and reduction in stress and depression (Fig. 30.1). The establishment of health-seeking behaviors in childhood affects the long-range health status of those same individuals as they reach adulthood.

Nurses have the opportunity to promote physical activity in the pediatric population by educating parents, teachers, school administrators, and daycare providers. Physical activity in children is often reflective of the adults within their environment. Positive role modeling is another way to promote healthy living. Programs geared toward combining healthy eating and activity are most effective (Table 30.1).

Physical risks associated with excess weight include high blood pressure, high cholesterol, type 2 diabetes mellitus, fatty liver disease, heart disease, stroke, gallbladder disease, arthritis, sleep apnea, and problems breathing. Psychological risks associated with excess weight include discrimination, social stigmatization, lowered self-esteem, social isolation, and feelings of depression and rejection.

Many factors contribute to the excess weight carried by children. Some of the most common factors are lack of physical activity, increased fast food consumption, working mothers, and poverty. Although not all of these factors are possible to eliminate, many of them are amenable to significant improvement.

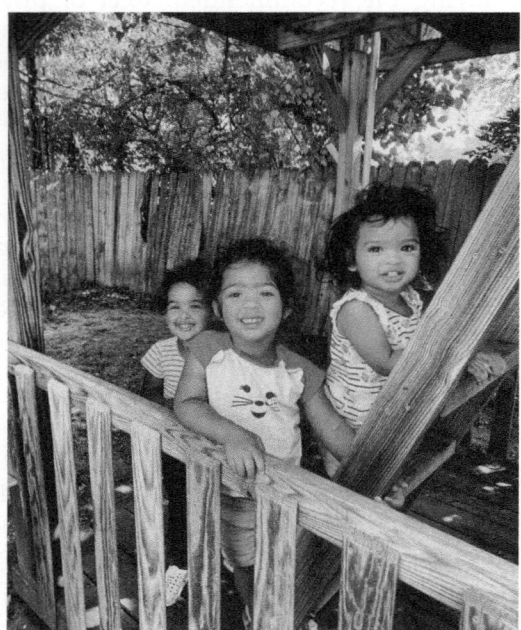

Fig. 30.1 Children engaging in physical activity.

Nutrition

Families today often are pressed for time. The convenience of fast food combined with the increase in families with two working parents has contributed to poor eating habits for many children. Only 2% of children meet the daily nutritional recommendations of the USDA. This is reflective of diets that have excessive amounts of fats, sodium and added sugar. Children often prefer foods laden with fat and empty calories. The intake of fast food is elevated as well. More than 20% of the calories taken in by adolescents ages 12 to 18 come from fast foods (Casslbury, 2018). This is a definite cause for concern about the dietary intake of children. Children's diets contain an estimated 11% to 15% of calories from saturated fat instead of the American Heart Association's recommendation of a maximum of 7%. Children tend to consume high-calorie, poorer-quality diets that do not meet federal dietary recommendations for healthy growth and development. Childhood obesity results from a diet high in calories from saturated fat and lack of exercise.

In contrast, the *Dietary Guidelines for Americans* (USDHHS & USDA, 2015), written jointly by the US Department of Health and Human Services, and the US Department of Agriculture, recommends that children ages 2 years and older consume a diet of an assortment

Table 30.1 **National Resources for Childhood Physical Activity and Dietary Intake**

RESOURCE	WEBSITE	MAJOR RECOMMENDATIONS
Physical Activity		
Physical Activity Guidelines for Americans	https://health.gov/our-work/nutrition-physical-activity/physical-activity-guidelines/current-guidelines	60 min or more of physical activity daily
		Most activity should be of moderate or vigorous intensity[a]
		Muscle-strengthening activity at least 3 days/week[b]
		Bone-strengthening activity at least 3 days/week[c]
Dietary		
Dietary Guidelines for Americans	https://www.dietaryguidelines.gov/sites/default/files/2020-12/DGA_2020-2025_ExecutiveSummary_English.pdf	Follow a healthy dietary pattern
		Cut back on foods high in solid fats, added sugars, and salt and limit alcohol intake
		Eat nutrient dense food and drinks to meet personal preferences
		Stay within personal calorie limits while meeting food group needs
Combined		
5-2-1-0 Let's Go!	http://www.letsgo.org	Five or more fruits and vegetables daily
		Two hours or less of screen time daily
		One hour or more of physical activity daily
		More water and low-fat milk, no sugary drinks
Let's Move!	https://letsmove.obamawhitehouse.archives.gov	Children: have fun being active and eating healthy
		Parents: get on track to eat well and stay fit
		Schools: add healthy living to the lesson plan
		Community leaders: empower families to make healthy decisions
		Health care professionals: educate and support patients in living healthier

[a]Examples of aerobic activity: running, biking, swimming, and dancing.
[b]Examples of muscle-strengthening activity: playing on playground equipment, climbing trees, and lifting weights.
[c]Examples of bone-strengthening activity: running, jumping rope, and basketball.
Modified from United States Department of Health and Human Services: Physical Activity Guidelines for Americans, ed 2 (https://health.gov/our-work/physical-activity/current-guidelines); United States Department of Agriculture: Dietary Guidelines (https://www.dietaryguidelines.gov/sites/default/files/2020-12/DGA_2020-2025.); MaineHealth: Let's Go (https://mainehealth.org/lets-go); Let's Move! America's Move to Raise a Healthier Generation of Kids (https://letsmove.obamawhitehouse.archives.gov/).

Health Promotion

Encouraging Healthy Behaviors in the Infant, Toddler and Child, and Adolescent

INFANT
- Encourage parental bonding.
- Monitor growth and development through well-baby clinic appointments.
- Encourage breast-feeding, if appropriate.
- Use prescribed baby formula to provide necessary nutrients and vitamins.
- Introduce baby foods as recommended. Begin with rice cereal and introduce one new food per week to monitor for allergic reactions.
- Monitor transitioning stools as the gastrointestinal system matures.
- Provide age-appropriate play to encourage physical and mental development.
- Transport infant in child carrier that faces the rear of the car (birth to 20 pounds).
- Maintain immunization schedule as recommended.

TODDLER AND CHILD
- Encourage a healthy diet to include high-nutrient foods such as fruits, vegetables, whole grains, and low-fat dairy and protein products (child and adolescent).
- Continue to provide health care, including immunizations and dental care.
- Encourage developmentally appropriate play.
- Remember that autonomy and initiative are paramount and offer toddler and child choice of nutritionally dense foods.
- Teach parents and child appropriate methods for good hygiene, such as handwashing and covering mouth when coughing or sneezing.
- Mandate use of seatbelts while riding in vehicle:
  - Toddler, 20 to 40 pounds: Front-facing safety seat secured in rear seat

- Child, more than 40 pounds: Secured in booster seat with lap and shoulder belt
- Children should wear protective helmets when riding tricycles and bicycles.
- Maintain immunization schedule as recommended.

ADOLESCENTS
- Instruct parents to monitor adolescent for use of drugs or alcohol by noting changes in behavior.
- Adolescents should wear protective helmets when riding bikes or motorcycles, or when skateboarding.
- Provide nutritionally dense foods and snacks to support this period of growth.
- Allow privacy in telephone use and interactions with friends.
- Allow the child to establish an identity even if it is different from that of the parents.
- Insist on mandatory use of seatbelts when in vehicle.
- Maintain immunization schedule as recommended.
- Encourage dental care.
- Encourage safe sun practices:
  - Teach that the long-term effects of sun exposure, such as tanning, include premature aging of the skin, increased risk of skin cancer, and in susceptible individuals, phototoxic reactions.
  - Teach that the long-term effects of tanning machines are similar to those of the sun; dermatologists do not recommend sun tanning by this means.
  - Provide education that the use of sunscreens, including hypoallergenic products, with a sun protective factor (SPF) of at least 15 and a non-alcohol base without lanolin or fragrance is important.

---

of foods that include fruits, vegetables, grains (especially whole grains), fish, lean meats, poultry, and beans. Fat restriction is not appropriate for toddlers; 30% of their calories optimally come from fat. Children under the age of 2 years should drink whole milk or 2% milk. Children who are at risk for obesity or who have a family history of heart disease or high cholesterol may be moved to a lower-fat option after 12 months of age (Riley, 2018). It is acceptable for the child and the adolescent to consume low-fat or fat-free milk products.

The patterns in the dietary intake of children shape their future health report card. Overweight children are at an increased risk for developing health conditions such as diabetes and heart diseases, which are largely considered health disorders of adults. Obese children are at an increased risk for obesity in adulthood. This makes the need for change imperative.

Promoting Lifestyle Changes
The nurse's most important role in relation to overweight and obese children is in education. Education of children and parents concerning dietary choices is

essential. Children and adolescents ages 6 to 17 years get at least 60 minutes of physical activity per day. It is recommended that children under 5 years just need to be active throughout the day (CDC, 2021b). Teaching about the optimal types and amounts of physical activity is important. Many parents do not realize the magnitude of this problem; however, simply by acquiring an awareness of the need, many parents are motivated to make significant lifestyle changes for their children.

TOBACCO USE
Cigarette smoking continues to be the single most preventable cause of death and disease in the United States. Fortunately, the use of tobacco products among teens has been steadily declining. Despite these improvements, nearly 4.6% of high schoolers and 1.6% of students in middle school report having smoked a cigarette in the past 30 days. Since 2014, smokeless tobacco products have outpaced cigarette use in teens. Nearly 20% of high school teens report having used an e-cigarette product in the past month (CDC, 2020b). Behaviors associated with teen smoking were use and

approval of smoking by peers or siblings, smoking parents, accessibility of tobacco products, low self-esteem, and exposure to advertising for tobacco products. Many states have implemented laws that restrict the sale of tobacco products to minors. Cigarettes are considered to be a gateway drug, and teenagers who smoke are more likely to use illicit drugs.

Other forms of tobacco exposure that also arouse concern include, smokeless tobacco, cigar smoking, and environmental tobacco smoke (ETS), commonly referred to as *"secondhand smoke."* Adolescents rarely understand the risks involved in smokeless tobacco. These risks include lip, gum, throat, and stomach cancers. There is also a heightened risk for heart disease and hypertension. There is also an impact on pregnancy, with stillbirths increasing due to the use of smokeless tobacco (CDC, 2020c). Cigar smoking has been showing increasing popularity. Cigar bar establishments, embracement by pop culture icons has lent to the mystique. Use by male high school students (9%) exceeds that of female students (6.7%). ETS results in an increased risk for heart and lung diseases, particularly asthma and bronchitis in children. Parents often point out that they do not smoke in front of their child; however, the damaging smoke is often trapped in clothing, drapes, and household furnishings.

New pastimes related to smoking involve ENDS (electronic nicotine delivery systems). ENDS include hookahs, e-cigarettes, and vaping (Fig. 30.2). Initially ENDS were not under the purview of the FDA; however, in 2016 they became regulated by the FDA. Forty states have regulations prohibiting the sale of ENDS to minors. Hookah uses water and a special type of tobacco, which often is flavored. In a study, 23 high school seniors had participated in hookah smoking in the past year. Some who enjoy hookah-smoking activities feel it is a safer alternative. The practice still allows exposure to nicotine and other toxins of tobacco. Hookah smoking traditionally takes place in a hookah establishment, where many others are engaged in the practice. When the hookah is smoked, a repetitive puffing and inhalation pattern is used. This may increase the concentration of the toxin exposure. The Centers for Disease Control and Prevention report, "A typical 1-hour-long hookah smoking session involves 200 puffs, whereas an average cigarette is 20 puffs. The amount of smoke inhaled during a typical hookah session is about 90,000 milliliters, compared with 500 to 600 milliliters inhaled when smoking a cigarette" Hookah smoking is associated with the same health risks as cigarettes (Box 30.1) (CDC, 2021c).

Box **30.1**   **Electronic Nicotine Delivery Systems**
• More than 3 million middle and high school students were current users of e-cigarettes in 2015, up from an estimated 2.46 million in 2014.
• 16% of high school and 5.3% of middle school students were current users of e-cigarettes in 2015, making e-cigarettes the most commonly used tobacco product among youth for the second consecutive year.
• During 2011–2015, e-cigarette use rose from 1.5% to 16.0% among high school students and from 0.6% to 5.3% among middle school students.
• In 2013–2014, 81% of current youth e-cigarette users cited the availability of appealing flavors as the primary reason for use.

From US Food and Drug Administration (FDA): Vaporizers, e-cigarettes, and other electronic nicotine delivery systems (ENDS), 2020. Retrieved from: https://www.fda.gov/tobacco-products/products-ingredients-components/vaporizers-e-cigarettes-and-other-electronic-nicotine-delivery-systems-ends.

Fig. 30.2 Electronic nicotine delivery systems (ENDS). (From http://www.fda.gov/TobaccoProducts/Labeling/ProductsIngredientsComponents/ucm456610.htm.)

Electronic cigarettes and vaping are increasing in popularity. Many incorrectly feel they are not a danger and are much safer than traditional cigarettes. These provide an aerosolized nicotine to the user. There are concerns they carry the same risks as their paper and tobacco predecessor (CDC, 2020a).

The American Cancer Society (ACS) and many other organizations offer excellent programs and resource materials aimed at educating children and adolescents concerning the dangers involved in tobacco use. These programs are available at no cost to schools, civic organizations, and health care professionals. Some teens volunteer with these programs to discourage tobacco use. Knowledge of available resources and the ability to promote their use are part of every pediatric nurse's toolbox and professional responsibility.

SUBSTANCE ABUSE

Statistics highlight the use of drugs by teens; 23.9% of teens ages 12 to 17 years reported they have tried an illicit drug. The rates are higher in males (24.5%) in comparison to only 4% of females. The racial differences in use are also striking. Drug use in high school is highest among white, non-Hispanics (24%) followed by Asians and mixed-race youths at 7%. The lowest rates were reported in black and Hispanic youths at 2%. These rates increase with age, showing a rapid increase as students reach high school. Studies indicate that the early age onset for use of alcohol and drugs is a large determining factor in dependency on them later in life. *Healthy People 2030* seeks to reduce this statistic. Substance abuse is associated with many social problems found in the United States. These problems include domestic violence, sexually transmitted infections (STIs), teen pregnancy, school failure, motor vehicle accidents (MVAs), increased health care costs, decreased worker productivity, and increased homelessness. Teens who engage in alcohol and drug use are less likely to participate in healthy relationships with their peers and face more problems related to discipline and school truancy (Juergen, 2021). Adolescents experiment with marijuana, cocaine, crack, heroin, lysergic acid diethylamide (LSD), inhalants, methamphetamines, ecstasy, other street drugs and the misuse of prescription drugs. Recently, abuse of prescription and synthetic drugs has become a concern for professionals who work with children and adolescents. In addition, health professionals are concerned about the use of alcohol and volatile substances (such as gasoline, spray paint, antifreeze, and organic solvents) that are inhaled to achieve altered sensorium. The good news is, generally, drug use in teens has been declining with the exception of marijuana (Paresky, 2017). However, an increase has been seen in children ages 12 and 13 years who are experimenting with drugs. This is of particular concern because the younger a person is when drug use (abuse) becomes habitual, the stronger the addiction, and the more difficult the task of breaking it.

The reasons teens initially try drugs can vary. Some of the leading reasons include boredom, a desire to "fit in," curiosity and peer pressure. Encourage parents to talk with their children about the risks of substance abuse and to plan appropriate child care and supervision. Children who are left unattended are more likely to experiment with drugs. After-school programs are available in many areas. Also, help educate parents regarding the signs of potential drug use in their children.

TELEVISION, VIDEO GAMES, AND THE INTERNET

The meaning of screen time extends beyond television. Today's youth have more options for media engagement. Children mark screen time with television, cell phones and video games. Parents and child development specialists are concerned about the influence these platforms have on child development and behavior. Electronic media time and television viewing are largely sedentary activities. Inactivity is tied to health problems such as diabetes and obesity.

The majority of teens have a cell phone. Most of these phones are "smart phones" which provide access to a variety of applications such as social media, video streaming and gaming. Teens spend more than 7 hours/day on their phones. Children ages 8 to 12 years spend close to 5 hours daily (Paresky, 2017). Many spend an equal number of additional hours using the computer. Time spent using these services reduces time available for other activities such as family, school, and friends. The volume of time spent engaged in cell phone use raises the question about why children are so tied to these devices. One study of teens found that feelings of loneliness and anxiety were associated with being apart from their phones (Schaeffer, 2019).

Children in the United States spend more than 3 hours/day watching television (Medline, 2019).

Children with televisions in their bedrooms spend more time watching than those who do not. The average American home has three or more televisions. Teens who watched more television were more overweight than those who watched less (Harvard T.H. Chan School of Public Health, n.d.). Although television is capable of producing positive learning outcomes, the values and attitudes represented on television are often not realistic, and at times, they clash with the values that the child has been taught. Television seldom represents the actual daily experiences that a child faces. The American Academy of Pediatrics reports that violent television and video games increase aggressive thoughts and angry feelings, which in turn cause an increase in aggressive behavior. Violent media also leads to youths being desensitized to violent acts. This causes them to not be empathetic to the pain and suffering of others (Anderson, et al., 2017). Parental control of television viewing is beneficial to ensure the appropriateness of programming selected.

Violence on television and other screen time has shown increased difficulty sleeping at night for children. In addition, problems with attentiveness, anxiety and depression are a result of increased screen time (Anderson, et. al., 2017).

There are critics and supporters of children and adolescents' exposure to video games. Critics argue that video games have detrimental effects, which include preventing children from completion of their homework, producing tension and violence, and causing sleeplessness. Critics also suggest video games have potentially negative physical and psychological results. Adverse physical effects possibly include triggering of epileptic seizures (AACAP, 2015). However, some believe that video games possibly may have a positive influence on children. Supporters believe video games can have positive effects, depending on the type of video games being played. Some can offer increased socialization with others as well as increased physical activity (Halbrook, et. al., 2019).

More than 80% of teens use a social media site (Herold, 2018). On average nearly 3 hours/day is spent on social media. For 20% of children, this figure is a whopping 5 hours/day or more (Vaughn, 2019). The increasing popularity of social media sites has brought some benefits but also challenges for children. As of 2018, an estimated 90% of teens ages 12 to 17 have a personal cellphone. Ready access to social media can promote socialization and communication (Box 30.2). There also is easily obtained health information online. Concerns related to social media use in children include cyberbullying and online harassment, privacy violations, sexting, and Facebook depression. Some early research between social media usage and depression appeared to support a tie to depression as a possible cause (News Medical Life Sciences, 2012). Recent studies, however, have linked the two together in a different manner. Teens, especially females, report turning to social media during periods of depression. It is suggested that teen girls may reach out for the connections felt from social media when feeling depressed (Engeln, 2019). Regardless of the causation, depression is a condition that can leave a teen vulnerable to potential dangers found on social media sites.

In the United States, 71% of families who have children ages 8 to 17 years have computers. Computers and the Internet provide valuable educational and recreational information, but just as in television programming, there are many dangers. Children sometimes are exposed to dangerous or illegal material and negative contact with others through e-mail or in chat rooms. Sharing of personal data or meeting with strangers puts the child and the family at financial and physical risk. Parents and children need to be educated about the potential risks involved in accessing the Internet, and the child always needs adult supervision.

Parents and teachers can provide safeguards by limiting the amount of time that children are

Box 30.2	Social Media Use

Top Social Media Platforms for Teens
% of all teens 13 to 17 who use:

Facebook	71%
Instagram	52%
Snapchat	11%
Twitter	6%
Google+	5%

Source: Ballard J: Teens use these social media platforms the most. October 25, 2019. YouGovAmerica. Retrieved from: https://today.yougov.com/topics/lifestyle/articles-reports/2019/10/25/teens-social-media-use-online-survey-poll-youth.

allowed to watch television, play video games, or be online. Advise them to monitor content and to increase access to educational alternatives. The goal is balance with activities using electronic devices and media with time dedicated toward friends, family, and school.

RESPONSIBLE SEXUAL BEHAVIOR

Teens are waiting longer to engage in sexual activity than in they did in past decades. Statistics from 2016 show that the average age for the onset of sexual activity is 17 (Guttmacher Institute, 2019). Between 2006 and 2008, approximately 11% of females and 15% of males reported having sexual intercourse before age 15 years. In 1995 this number was 19% and 21%, respectively. Although this is a positive change, sexual activity in teens continues to be a concern. The major risks associated with irresponsible sexual behavior include unintended pregnancy, STIs, and human immunodeficiency virus and acquired immunodeficiency syndrome (HIV/AIDS). Approximately one half of all new HIV cases in the United States occur among people younger than 25 years of age.

Although abstinence is the only protection that is 100%, effective, proper use of condoms helps prevent unintended pregnancies and transmission of STIs. This topic always has been a controversial issue with parents, school officials, and health care professionals. The rate of contraceptive use has increased to 80% (CDC, 2017b). The lack of either full compliance with the use of contraception or total abstinence indicates that education still is needed. It does not matter who provides the education. The bottom line is the necessity of teaching adolescents about responsible sexual behavior, because it is often a matter of life and death.

MENTAL HEALTH

Healthy People 2030 cites target areas related to adolescents and mental health. The initiatives have identified the following areas for improvement for children (USDHHS, ODPHP, 2021):

- Reduce suicide attempts by adolescents
- Increase the proportion of children and adolescents with mental health problems who get treatment
- Increase the proportion of children and adolescents who get appropriate treatment for behavior problems
- Increase the proportion of children and adolescents who get preventive mental health care in schools
- The teenage years are among the most difficult times of a person's life. Teenagers want to fit in. They need to belong. They want to look and act like others their age. Parents often forget how difficult this time is for the adolescent.

Mental health issues often are considered less important than physical illnesses. Nurses who feel confident to help with physical symptoms all too commonly feel powerless when confronting matters concerning mental health.

Pediatric nurses are obliged to treat patients holistically, which means addressing physical and mental health. Nurses often underestimate the effect they can have on their patients' mental health. Keep these mental health issues in mind in the practice of pediatric nursing: depression, suicide, eating disorders, and substance abuse.

INJURY AND VIOLENCE

Injuries historically have been a problem in the pediatric population. Common injuries found in children and adolescents involve MVAs, accidental poisoning, suffocation, drowning, falls, aspiration of foreign bodies, and burns. Accidental firearm injuries continue to occur in the pediatric population. Premeditated intentional shootings also occur more frequently among today's adolescents.

The target goals related to injury and violence involving children and adolescents include a reduction in pediatric deaths caused by MVAs and homicides. The nurse contributes to these goals by encouraging proper use of child safety restraints and seatbelts. Advise parents of the following guidelines:

- Use infant car seats designed according to federal safety guidelines:
  - Birth to 20 pounds: Rear-facing safety seats secured in the rear seat (Fig. 30.3)
  - Toddlers 20 to 40 pounds: Front-facing safety seats secured in the rear seat
  - Children more than 40 pounds: Secured in booster seats with lap and shoulder belts. The properly fitted shoulder belt lies across the chest, and the lap belt sits below the hip bones to prevent internal injuries in the event of a vehicular accident.
- Teach the child pedestrian safety: "Stop, Look, Listen" at crosswalks; use sidewalks; wear light-colored clothing at night.
- Supervise children when playing outdoors—no playing at the curb or behind parked cars.

Fig. 30.3 Toddler in rear-facing safety seat, secured in the rear seat.

Fig. 30.4 Proper use of a safety helmet begins at an early age.

- Insist that the child wear an approved helmet when riding tricycles, bicycles, scooters, mopeds, and skateboards (Fig. 30.4). Protective wrist, elbow, and kneepads are necessary during play involving skateboards and while roller-skating or in-line skating.
- Reinforce the danger of using drugs or alcohol when driving, and insist that no child ride in a car with a person who has been drinking alcohol or using drugs.
- Emphasize rules for safe driving with the adolescent driver.

The role in pediatric nursing in the reduction of pediatric deaths by homicide includes assessment for potential violent behaviors and mental health disorders. Encourage parents to monitor their children's activities. Parents need to be aware of where their children are going and with whom. Encourage teachers, parents, and students to report strange behavior or threats made by other students.

Other significant injury prevention concepts call for awareness and concern. Poisoning, aspiration, and burn injuries in children are addressed subsequently in this chapter.

"Unwanted aggressive behavior(s) by another youth or group of youths, who are not siblings or current dating partners, that involves an observed or perceived power imbalance, and is repeated multiple times or is highly likely to be repeated" (CDC, 2020). In the United States, an estimated 28% of students in grades 6 to 12 reported being the victim of a bully. The risk factors for being bullied include the following:

- Have a history of depression
- Are viewed by others as not "fitting in"
- Are overweight or have some other physical characteristic that makes them stand apart from the rest of the peer group

Bullies also have some characteristics placing them at risk for the behavior, including the following:

- Display aggression
- Have friends who bully others
- Have limited parental involvement
- Are experiencing problems at home
- Have difficulty following rules

The methods used vary and can be combined by the attacker (Stopbullying.gov, n.d.). Some assaults are by cyber methods. In this case, the bullying may involve sending threatening messages, texts, or photographs. Emotional attacks may include spreading rumors with the intent to harm the reputation of the victimized individual. Physical attacks may include hitting, tripping, or other types of violence. The verbal attack is just as powerful and may involve shaming, name calling, or rude comments. The impact of bullying can result in physical injuries and long- and short-term emotional harm. It can cause feelings of isolation, depression, or despair. When providing care for at-risk youth, include an assessment for bullying in the data collected. Make certain that the child is aware that bullying behaviors are not acceptable. Determine what reporting may be necessary.

ENVIRONMENTAL QUALITY

Environmental quality concerns specific to children and adolescents include, exposure to ETS, ozone (outdoor) standards, and (for infants and young children) exposure to lead-based paint. Make sure parents are aware of potential exposure to lead-based paint in older housing and possibly furniture, such as cribs. They need additional education regarding proper testing for lead levels in children, who are in some circumstances at risk for lead poisoning.

See the previous section on tobacco for a discussion of exposure to ETS and the potential problems related to it. Nursing responsibilities regarding ozone standards include awareness of any dangers in the area and of possible measures to take for prevention or avoidance and sharing of this information with others.

IMMUNIZATION

Immunizations are an excellent way to prevent the occurrence and spread of certain infectious diseases. More than 70% of all children in the United States have received a full schedule of recommended immunizations (CDC, 2019). Although these statistics show a strong compliance rate, those children who do not have their immunizations completed not only face personal risk but also can endanger medically fragile individuals by exposing them to communicable infections. Healthy People 2030 continues to have as goal to increase immunizations for children in the United States. Immunization standards offer a challenge for the pediatric nurse because these standards often change. With modern advances in medical research, new immunizations are being developed. The most recent recommended childhood immunization schedule for the United States, valid as of February 2018, was approved by the Advisory Committee on Immunization Practices (ACIP), the American Academy of Pediatrics (AAP), and the American Academy of Family Physicians (AAFP). It can be reviewed at www.cdc.gov/vaccines/schedules/hcp/child-adolescent.html. Children who are vaccinated according to the recommended immunization schedule are protected against 10 vaccine-preventable childhood diseases by age 2 years.

It should be noted that lower levels of compliance with immunization is noted for the vaccines to prevent human papillomavirus (HPV), the main cause of genital warts and cervical cancer. The rates for this immunization are less than 50%. Gardasil (Human Papillomavirus Quadrivalent [Types 6, 11, 16, 18] Vaccine) offers coverage against HPV types 6, 11, 16, and 18 (FDA, 2019b); Cervarix (Human Papillomavirus Bivalent [Types 16 and 18] Vaccine, Recombinant) is effective against HPV types 16 and 18 (FDA, 2019a). It is recommended that both boys and girls between the ages of 11 to 12 years. The vaccine can be given to older children and young adults as long as they are not sexually active. These vaccines are not effective after exposure to HPV (CDC, 2020d).

Barriers to proper immunization include lack of insurance and funding, lack of transportation, lack of education about the importance of immunizations, and personal and cultural beliefs. Vaccination assistance programs provide vaccinations to children whose parents are unable to pay. Know the current recommended immunization schedule and be able to answer parents' questions regarding immunizations.

DENTAL HEALTH

A multidisciplinary approach to all aspects of pediatric health promotion is fundamental to safeguarding the physical and emotional health of all children. Dental health promotion, an aspect of proper health care, is best to begin with the eruption of the primary teeth, usually at about 6 months of age; advise parents to begin it no later than when the child has reached 2½ years of age, the average age when deciduous dentition is complete. Although the incidence of dental

Fig. 30.5 Nursing bottle caries. (From Swartz MH: *Textbook of physical diagnosis: History and examination*, ed 4, Philadelphia, 2005, Saunders.)

caries has decreased considerably since the introduction of fluorides and increased dental health education and promotion, nursing bottle caries continues to be a significant concern for infants and toddlers. **Nursing bottle caries** is tooth decay that is the result of prolonged drinking from a bottle after the infant has been put to bed, when the milk, juice, or other fluid is allowed to bathe the teeth, thus providing sugar to oral bacteria for growth. During sleep, decreased salivary flow prevents clearance of the liquid from the mouth, and the liquid pools on the teeth (Fig. 30.5). The nurse is in a unique position to prevent these and other problems by promoting good dental health through counseling and education.

STRATEGIES TO PROMOTE DENTAL HEALTH

Make early institution of good dental hygiene and practices to prevent dental caries a part of the anticipatory guidance for all children and their parents. Help children and parents by teaching them to use the following strategies:

- Begin cleansing of the oral cavity in infancy by wiping the teeth and gums with a damp washcloth (Fig. 30.6). A toothbrush usually is too harsh for an infant's tender gums. As an infant gets more teeth, use a small soft-bristled toothbrush with plain water to cleanse the teeth and gums. Avoid use of toothpaste during this age, especially if fluoridated, because swallowing by the infant leads to ingestion of excessive amounts of fluoride.
- Initiate fluoride supplementation at 6 months of age if the water in the infant's residential area is not fluoridated. Fluoride supplementation no longer is recommended for infants under 6 months of age.
- Encourage proper nutrition during infancy and childhood to promote good dental health. Avoid, or use sparingly, food with concentrated sugars. In addition, advise against use of honey during the first year of life because some cases of infant **botulism** (an often-fatal form of food poisoning caused by an endotoxin produced by the bacillus *Clostridium*

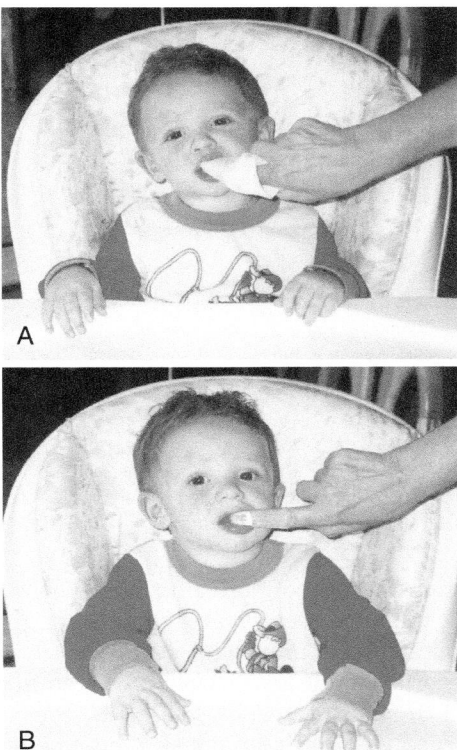

Fig. 30.6 For the infant, wipe the oral cavity and teeth with a damp washcloth. (A) Cleansing with a damp washcloth. (B) Cleansing with a finger cot toothbrush.

botulinum) have been associated with it. Other foods associated with an increased incidence of dental caries include molasses, corn syrup, and dried fruits such as raisins.

Specific interventions are possible to prevent nursing bottle caries. Give the last bottle *before* bedtime, with proper cleansing of the teeth and gums *before* putting the child down to sleep. Use water in the bedtime bottle instead of juice or milk. Do not use sugar-coated or honey-coated pacifiers. Offer juice in cups, which the child drinks from and then sets down, rather than in bottles.

After infancy, dental hygiene and health care needs to continue through the various stages of development.

- For preschool children, when the eruption of the deciduous teeth is complete, continuous good dental hygiene is important. Parental assistance and supervision is necessary with brushing; also teach parents to perform flossing (Fig. 30.7). Promote continuation of professional dental care and fluoride supplementation. Encourage proper nutrition (see Chapter 19).
- Eruption of permanent teeth begins during the school-age years. Good dental hygiene and professional dental supervision are especially important during this period. Screening for malocclusion problems that result from abnormal eruption of permanent teeth is also important. Teach or reinforce correct brushing and flossing techniques. Have children brush teeth after meals and snacks and at bedtime. Encourage the child to decrease the ingestion of sugary food.

Fig. 30.7 Young children can participate in tooth brushing, but parents need to brush all the child's teeth thoroughly.

- Although the rate of caries formation slows down during the adolescent years, continuing good dental practice is still important. Adolescence is a stage where orthodontic appliances are often applied to correct malocclusions. Adolescents are typically concerned with body image and must be reminded often of the temporary nature of these devices and their proper use and care.

INJURY PREVENTION

Injuries in children are associated with age, developmental level, and the physical and cognitive skills of the child. The inexperience of infants with the environment and their immature motor skills make them vulnerable to falls and suffocation. Toddlers and preschoolers are at increased risk of injuries from water-related accidents, poisoning, and burns as they acquire new skills. School-age children become more competitive in their activities and sometimes suffer injuries from bicycle accidents, MVAs, and skating accidents. In their struggle to gain independence and freedom, adolescents become more vulnerable to injuries and death from MVAs and accidents that involve firearms, alcohol, and illegal drugs. *Anticipatory guidance* education has been the most widely used approach to educate parents in accident prevention. Use every opportunity to educate parents about injury prevention (see the Safety Alert box).

POISONING

The ingestion of harmful or poisonous substances is a common cause of morbidity and mortality in children younger than the age of 5 years. Children in the 1 to 2 years age group are at an increased risk because of their natural curiosity to explore their environment once they become mobile. The Poison Prevention Packaging Act of 1970, which requires childproof packaging of medications, has reduced greatly the incidence of poisoning; however, continued strategies

and educational efforts are needed to reduce the morbidity and mortality of this preventable cause. Children are vulnerable to becoming poisoned from a variety of substances including, pharmaceuticals (especially acetaminophen, cough and cold preparations, iron, vitamins, and oral contraceptives) and non-pharmaceuticals (cleaning products, lead, plants, insecticides and pesticides, mouthwashes, and cosmetics).

Prevention

All parents must be educated to prevent accidental poisoning. Despite parents' best efforts, children are still at risk, especially when visiting the homes of relatives or friends. Parents must know the number of the poison control center (PCC) in their area. Advise parents to place the PCC telephone number close to each telephone in the home and program it into their cell phones. The PCC hotline number usually is found in the front of the telephone directory. The US Poison Control Center no longer recommends syrup of ipecac for routine treatment of poisoning. Help parents institute prevention strategies by instructing them to do the following:

- Never refer to medicines as candy; medicines are drugs. Store them with childproof caps, and keep them out of reach or in a locked cabinet.
- Place cleaning supplies and other toxic substances, including batteries, up high and out of reach of curious youngsters or in a locked cabinet.
- Do not keep large quantities of toxic agents (e.g., pesticides, cleaning fluids, drugs) in the home.
- Inspect the home for possible sources of lead contamination, including lead-based paint on windowsills, stair rails, and door moldings and peeling wall paint.
- Keep toxic plants out of reach of small hands.
- Remember that many grandparents take medications, and they, too, need to keep them in a locked cabinet or up high and out of the reach of children. Keep purses out of the child's reach.
- Educate older children and adolescents about the dangers of drugs and alcohol.

A patient problem and interventions for the patient with poisoning include, but are not limited to the following:

PATIENT PROBLEM	NURSING INTERVENTIONS
Potential for Injury, related to lack of knowledge of safeguarding child's environment from harmful, poisonous substances	Counsel parents to store medicines with childproof caps
	Teach parents to store harmful substances out of child's reach and in a locked cabinet
	Educate parents to contact health care facility and poison control center immediately if suspected ingestion of harmful substance is noted

Safety Alert

Infant, Toddler and Child, and Adolescent

INFANT

- Keep your hands on the infant at all times when the crib rail is down.
- Use an infant car safety seat restraint that has been federally approved.
- Children should remain in the size appropriate car safety seat facing the rear until they are 2 years of age.
- Children should remain seated in the back seat of the vehicle until they are 12 years of age.
- Leave no gaps between the crib side and mattress.
- Place infants on the back to sleep. The risk of sudden infant death syndrome (SIDS) is increased in infants placed on side-lying or prone position.
- Check all toys for small parts to reduce risk of choking or wounds.
- Support head and shield head from injury.
- Do not prop bottle.
- Place infant in upright position when feeding solid foods.
- Use clean bowl and spoon to feed and do not feed directly from jar: this prevents contamination of food.
- *Never* leave infant unattended in or near water.
- *Never,* under any circumstances, leave infant unsupervised in a bathtub.
- Apply a sunscreen when infant is exposed to sunlight (year round).

TODDLER AND CHILD

- Use a toddler car safety seat restraint that has been federally approved.
- Use car booster seats also known as belt-positioning devices for children less than 4 feet 9 inches tall and weighing more than 40 pounds, typically between 4 and 8 years.
- *Never* leave toddler unattended in a vehicle or shopping cart.
- Protect from falls, burns, and collisions with objects that result from running and climbing.
- Use washable toys without small parts or sharp edges.
- Supervise closely when near any source of water.
- *Never* leave a toddler unsupervised in a bathtub.
- Cover electrical outlets with protective plastic caps.
- Do not allow toddler or child to play on a curb or behind a parked car.
- Supervise tricycle and bicycle riding; have child wear a helmet.
- Teach child to obey pedestrian safety rules.
- Never leave infant or toddler unattended in high chair.
- Supervise at playgrounds; select safe play areas.
- Apply a sunscreen when toddler or child is exposed to sunlight (year round).

- Stress on the dangers of open flames.
- Always check the bath water temperature; adjust water temperature to 120°F (48.9°C) or cooler (infants, toddlers, children).
- Place all potentially toxic agents out of reach or in a locked cabinet.
- Discard all unused refrigerators, ovens, and other appliances; if storing an old appliance, remove the door.
- Keep venetian blind cords out of reach of a toddler or child.
- Teach child never to go with strangers.
- Teach child to tell parents if anyone makes him or her feel uncomfortable in any way.

ADOLESCENT

- Adolescents feel indestructible and tend to be more prone to deliberate (suicide) or non-deliberate accidents such as in the use of guns, drugs, or motor vehicles.
- Emphasize and encourage safe pedestrian behavior.
- At night, walk with a friend.
- Do not walk in a secluded area; take well-traveled walkways.
- Provide competent driving education; encourage the judicious use of a vehicle; discourage drag racing, "playing chicken"; teach how to maintain vehicle in proper condition (e.g., brakes, tires).
- Teach and promote safety and maintenance of two-wheeled vehicles.
- Promote use of seatbelts.
- Promote and encourage wearing of safety apparel, such as helmet or long pants when skateboarding and bike riding.
- Reinforce the dangers of using drugs, including alcohol, when operating a motor vehicle.
- Teach a nonswimmer how to swim.
- Teach basic rules of water safety; stress the need to make sure water is of sufficient depth for diving.
- Reinforce proper behavior in areas that involve contact with burn hazards (gasoline, electrical wires, fires).
- Advise regarding excessive exposure to natural or artificial sunlight (ultraviolet burn); encourage use of sunscreen.
- Discourage use of all tobacco products.
- Educate in hazards of drug use, including alcohol.
- Promote acquisition of proper instruction in sports and use of sports equipment.
- Instruct in safe use of and respect for firearms and other devices with potential danger (e.g., power tools, fireworks).

ASPIRATION OF A FOREIGN BODY

In children younger than 1 year of age, the leading cause of fatal injury is asphyxiation by aspiration of foreign materials into the respiratory tract. Although all children younger than age 3 years are at risk, the older infant 6 months to 1 year of age is at greatest risk because of the normal hand-to-mouth activities

common in this age group. The severity of respiratory tract obstruction depends on the location and the type of material aspirated. Foods that pose the greatest danger include hot dogs, round candy, nuts, grapes, popcorn, peanuts, cookies or biscuits, other meats, carrots, apples, peanut butter, and beans. Common objects that are aspirated easily include buttons on clothing

Box 30.3	Foreign Body Aspiration Prevention Strategies

- Keep small objects and toys away from infants and young children who are developmentally unable to obey restrictions. Small children may place small objects in the nose or the ear, causing obstruction.
- Inform parents of the dangers of round foods to children too young to chew these foods properly; they are acceptable to introduce when the child is older.
- When administering medications via syringe, stress to parents the need to remove the cap first.
- Encourage parents to choose one-piece pacifiers that do not come apart and cause aspiration. Have the parents check the pacifier frequently by pulling on the nipple. If it becomes separated from the shield, it is to be discarded.

or toys, beads, coins, balloons, pins, and barrettes. Toys with small or loosely attached parts and pacifier nipples that become detached from the shield are also dangerous. More recently, the caps of medication syringes also have been implicated when caretakers forget to remove them before administering medication to a child.

Families need to be cognizant of choking hazards for small children. Counsel families about prevention strategies. Box 30.3 summarizes areas to discuss with parents during routine health supervision visits.

BURN INJURIES

Burns are the result of thermal damage to skin and tissues. Severity is related to the temperature and length of time the skin is exposed to the heat source. Burns occur because of flames, chemicals, hot objects, radiation, or electricity. Burns are the third leading cause of accidental death in children 1 to 4 years of age, the second in children 5 to 9 years of age, and the third in children 10 to 14 years of age. Up to 75% of all burn injuries occur in the home; children younger than age 2 years experience more scald burns, and children older than 5 years frequently have flame burns.

Prevention

As infants and children acquire new motor skills, they are more vulnerable to accidental burns and other injuries. The nurse has a unique opportunity to educate parents to avoid risks and provide a safe environment for their children. Teach the following safety precautions:

- Keep the hot water heater set at no more than 120°F (49°C).
- Turn all pot handles on the stove toward the back of the stove.
- Keep hot objects, such as cigarettes, coffee pots, and hot liquids or foods, out of the reach of small hands.
- Remove hanging tablecloths and electrical cords especially around children who crawl or walk.
- Teach older children safe cooking methods and emphasize that it is never acceptable to wear loose clothing near the stove or other heat source (e.g., fireplace, wood-burning stove).
- Use guardrails or guards around fireplaces, space heaters, and other heating sources.
- Use and maintain smoke detectors in the home.
- Keep electrical wires hidden and out of the reach of children.
- Use plastic caps to cover electrical outlets.
- Keep small, hot appliances such as curling irons and steam irons out of the reach of children.
- Keep a fire extinguisher in the home and know how to operate it.
- Use a cool mist rather than a hot mist vaporizer.
- Use a hat and sunscreen on children when outdoors, especially during peak sun hours.
- Teach older children the potential of burn hazards, such as gasoline, matches, barbecue grills, candles, and fireworks (e.g., Roman candles).
- Have parents map out an escape route in the home and practice fire drills with family members.
- Keep the telephone numbers of the fire and rescue squads near the telephone (911 in most areas). Teach small children "nine-one-one" (911), because how to dial nine-eleven is not necessarily a concept they are able to grasp.

Get Ready for the NCLEX® Examination!

Key Points

- Anticipatory guidance is education of parents to prepare them for normal growth and development of their children. It is also psychological preparation of a person for an event expected to be stressful, as in preparation of a child for surgery by explaining what will happen and what it will feel like.
- *Healthy People 2030* identified 13 leading health indicators for health promotion and disease prevention.
- Initiate fluoride supplementation at 6 months of age if the water in the infant's residential area is not fluoridated.
- The development of immunizations against communicable diseases has significantly reduced the morbidity and mortality associated with many diseases.
- Injuries in children are associated with age, developmental level, and the physical and cognitive skills of the child.
- Use infant safety seats designed according to federal safety guidelines: birth to 20 pounds, rear-facing safety seats secured in the rear seat; toddlers 20 to 40 pounds,

front-facing safety seats secured in the rear seat; children over 40 pounds, secured in booster seats with lap and shoulder belts per federal safety protocol.

- The use of electronic media is a strong presence in the lives of children. The healthful balance of the media and other activities is needed.

Additional Learning Resources

SG Go to your Study Guide for additional learning activities to help you master this chapter content.

Be sure to visit the Evolve site at http://evolve.elsevier.com/Co oper/foundations/ for additional online resources.

Review Questions for the NCLEX® Examination

1. When counseling the parents of a 6-month-old about dental health, the nurse includes which statement(s)? *(Select all that apply.)*

    1. "Begin cleansing the oral cavity by wiping teeth and gums with a damp washcloth."
    2. "Avoid toothpaste at this age, especially if it is fluoridated."
    3. "Initiate fluoride supplementation at 6 months of age if infant's home water supply is not fluoridated."
    4. "It is acceptable to prop a bottle with juice or milk for the infant if limited to nighttime periods."
    5. "Dilute fluids made with tap water if fluoridation is present."

2. The nurse is planning a program for parents and adolescents in the community related to obesity. What information is most appropriate for inclusion in the information that will be provided?

    1. Because more mothers work outside the home, children and adolescents eat only fast foods.
    2. Obese children always become obese adults.
    3. Being overweight or obese sometimes results in major physical and psychological health problems.
    4. It is best for families to have more meals at home.

3. Responsible sexual behavior among young people most importantly should include what characteristic?

    1. Having sexual activity only with someone you know
    2. Abstaining from sexual activity or properly using condoms
    3. Having sexual activity only once a month
    4. Requiring sexual partners to be tested for HIV

4. A 15-year-old male patient states that he does not smoke. Further assessment reveals he uses chewing tobacco. What information should the nurse provide to the patient about smokeless tobacco?

    1. The use of smokeless tobacco carries a similar risk for the development of lung cancer.
    2. Individuals using smokeless tobacco have an increased risk for the development of lip, gum, and throat cancer.
    3. People using smokeless tobacco are at an elevated risk for becoming a smoker later in life.
    4. The use of the tobacco must stop immediately.

    5. Heart disease risk is increased by the use of smokeless tobacco.

5. The parents of a 10-month-old are concerned about motor vehicle safety. What education should be provided from the nurse to the parents?

    1. Children who weigh more than 35 pounds must be secured with a lap and shoulder belt.
    2. Infants from birth to age 2 years must be in a rear-facing safety seat.
    3. When using a lap and shoulder belt, have the lap belt rest above the hip bones.
    4. When using a lap and shoulder belt, have the shoulder belt fit across the upper abdomen.

6. Proper counseling of the parent of a 1-year-old regarding safety includes which instruction(s)? *(Select all that apply.)*

    1. Fence pools with a self-locking gate.
    2. Keep drapery cords out of children's reach.
    3. Place infant on back to sleep.
    4. Do not tie pacifiers on a string around the infant's neck.
    5. Limit bottle-feeding to the periods before bedtime.

7. Human papillomavirus (HPV) vaccine is recommended for what population?

    1. Carriers of the disease
    2. Women with sexual partners who are carriers of the virus
    3. Boys or girls between the ages of 11 to 12 who are not sexually active
    4. Girls who have been sexually active for less than 12 months

8. HPV infection is associated with what health complication?

    1. Infertility in women
    2. Menorrhagia
    3. Pelvic inflammatory disease
    4. Cervical cancer

9. The nurse is discussing dietary intake with the mother of an 18-month-old child. What statement(s) by the mother indicate(s) the need for further instruction? *(Select all that apply.)*

    1. "Whole milk is not a good option for my child."
    2. "I need to begin to decrease the amount of milk my child is allowed to drink."
    3. "2% milk is a good alternative to whole milk for my child."
    4. "Until my child is 3 years of age, whole milk is recommended."
    5. "I can continue to provide 2% milk for my child to drink."

10. The parents of a 13-year-old boy report their son spends several hours on the Internet and social media sites each day before and after school. What information should be provided by the nurse? *(Select all that apply.)*

    1. As long as the child's school grades are good, this is a safe practice.
    2. Excessive hours on social media can result in an imbalance between the rest of the social activities of the child.
    3. Social media use may result in mental health concerns.

4. Social media has some benefits including improved communication with others.

5. The Internet can provide educational benefits.

11. **A 16-year-old teen reports he uses smokeless tobacco. Which statements by the teen indicate the need for further instruction?**

1. "Smokeless tobacco is safer for me than a cigarette."
2. "As long as I brush my teeth after use I am going to be OK."
3. "My breath may have a foul odor from smokeless tobacco."
4. "I can become sterile from smokeless tobacco use."
5. "I am at increased risk for heart disease from using this product."

12. **When preparing snacks for an 18-month-old child, which would be appropriate?** *(Select all that apply.)*

1. Apple sauce
2. Peanuts
3. Grapes
4. Orange segments
5. Crackers
6. Hot dogs
7. Marshmallows
8. Sliced strawberries
9. Mashed bananas
10. Cottage cheese

13. **The nurse is discussing planned well child appointments with the mother of a toddler who frequently misses them. What actions should be taken by the nurse?** *(Select all that apply.)*

1. Assess the parent's beliefs on the importance of the health promotion activities.
2. Determine if the family has transportation for the appointments.
3. Seek family input on the dates and times for scheduling the appointments.
4. Report the family to Child Protective Services.
5. Review the family's ability to pay for health care.

14. Burns are the _____ leading cause of accidental death in children 1 to _____ years of age.

Basic Pediatric Nursing Care

Objectives

1. Identify events that were significant to the health care of children in the United States in the 20th century.
2. Discuss the works of Abraham Jacobi and Lillian Wald.
3. Describe the purposes and outcomes of the White House Conferences on Children between 1909 and the 1980s.
4. Discuss the personal characteristics and professional skills of a successful pediatric nurse.
5. Identify key elements of family-centered care.
6. Describe areas in which the pediatric nurse uses principles of growth and development.
7. Discuss how to use the head-to-toe method for the physical assessment of a child.
8. Describe metabolism in the child and its relationship with nutrition.
9. List general strategies to consider when talking with children.
10. Describe the three categories of child abuse.
11. Outline several approaches for making the hospitalization of children a positive experience for them and their families.
12. Discuss pain management in infants and children.
13. Explain the needs of parents during their child's hospitalization.
14. Discuss common pediatric procedures.
15. Discuss administration of pediatric medications.
16. Discuss hazards and accident prevention in the pediatric population.

Key Terms

anterior fontanelle (fŏn-tă-NĔL, p. 976)

anticipatory guidance (p. 954)

birth defects (congenital anomalies) (kŏn-JĔN-ĭ-tăl ă-NŎM-ă-lēz, p. 951)

body surface area (BSA) (p. 983)

children with special needs (p. 952)

cognitive impairment (p. 953)

en face position (ăhn FĂS, p. 959)

family-centered care (p. 952)

morbidity (mŏr-BĬD-ĭ-tē, p. 987)

mortality (mŏr-TĂL-ĭ-tē, p. 949)

primary (deciduous) teeth (dĕ-SĬD-ū-ŭs, p. 961)

sex trafficking (p. 966)

vastus lateralis muscle (VĂS-tŭs lăt-ŭŭ-Ă-lĭs, p. 985)

weaning (p. 964)

HISTORY OF CHILD CARE: THEN AND NOW

In today's society, children are recognized as individuals with unique medical needs that are different than those of adults. The care of children has not always been viewed as an important stage of life. For centuries, children were considered miniature adults.

In colonial America, children had to assume adult responsibilities as soon as they were capable. The value of children was related directly to the work they could perform. Infant and childhood mortality (or death) rates were high. Epidemic diseases were common, and there was no control over or treatment for such diseases as smallpox, diphtheria, measles, dysentery, mumps, chickenpox, yellow fever, cholera, or whooping cough. Farm accidents and burns from open fireplaces and gunpowder also contributed to high mortality rates.

Industrialization in America resulted in a population shift from rural to urban settings, where people lived in overcrowded and unsanitary conditions. Often unsanitary conditions were caused by lack of knowledge about how disease occurs. For instance, milk was not refrigerated and contained hundreds of millions of bacteria, which contributed to the development of diarrhea and tuberculosis. In addition to poor living conditions, children were treated as adults, working in factories for 12 to 14 hours a day. With no legal rights for children and no workplace laws, family life was sacrificed to focus on survival.

Children's health care needs were not considered different from those of adults until 1860, when Abraham Jacobi, a New York physician referred to as the "father of pediatrics," first lectured to medical students on the special diseases and health problems of children. With several other physicians, Dr. Jacobi pioneered the scientific and clinical investigation of childhood diseases. One outstanding achievement during Dr. Jacobi's era was the establishment of "milk stations" in 1893, in partnership with New York merchant Nathan Straus. At these free stations, infants were weighed and mothers were taught how to prepare milk before giving it to their babies. Mothers also had access to nurses who taught them the benefits of fresh air, clean water, and adequate clothing and how to satisfy the recreational needs of children. The crusade for pure milk resulted in improved sanitation, the advent of pasteurization of milk, and increased interest in infant care. Despite a remarkable decline in the infant mortality rate, 20% of children still died before their second birthday, and 50% died before age 21 (CDC, 1999).

During the late 1800s, increasing concern developed for the social welfare of children, especially those who were poor, homeless, immigrants, tenement residents, or employed as factory laborers. Reformer Lillian Wald (1867–1940) founded the Henry Street Settlement in New York City, which provided nursing services, social work, and an organized program of social, cultural, and educational activities. She is regarded as the founder of public health or community nursing. Wald believed that public health nurses should treat social and economic problems for the entire neighborhood. Her work had far-reaching effects on child health and nursing.

As medical and scientific advances revealed more causes of disease, emphasis was placed on isolation and asepsis. In the early 1900s children with contagious disease were isolated from adult patients. Parents were prohibited from visiting because of the possibility of transmitting disease to and from home. The works of Spitz (1945, 1946) and Robertson (1990) on institutionalized children helped health care professionals recognize how isolation and maternal deprivation affected children. The growing interest in the psychological health of children resulted in changes for hospitalized children, such as rooming in, prehospitalization, parent education, and hospital schooling.

Influenced by social reformers such as Lillian Wald, national leaders began to take action to improve children's living conditions. In 1909 President Theodore Roosevelt called the first White House Conference on Children. The conference focused on such issues as child labor, dependent children, and infant care. In 1912 the US Children's Bureau was established as a direct result of that conference. Its charge was to investigate all aspects of child care, including infant mortality, child labor laws, conditions of social agencies, and the country's birthrate.

The second White House Conference on Children convened in 1919, after World War I. This conference addressed the socioeconomic situation of mothers and children and resulted in the first federally supported health programs for mothers and children. The Great Depression of 1929 paralyzed the United States and resulted in devastating social and economic conditions. A White House Conference on Children was called in 1930 to study the economic effects of the Great Depression on the health and well-being of children.

Thereafter a conference was held at the beginning of each decade until the 1980s. These conferences have been responsible over the years for many changes in child health and welfare, including funding for essential programs, legislation, and shifting the focus from treatment of diseases to preventive health care. Attendees were professionals who worked with children, representatives of federal and state agencies and volunteer organizations, and members of various citizen groups. Although the group did not have legislative powers, together its members raised the consciousness of public officials and private citizens regarding the status of children and families.

The United States did not recover from the Great Depression for many years. In the interim, the Children's Bureau was able to propose legislation to assist children. Some of the most remarkable pieces of legislation were those authorized by the Social Security Act of 1937, which was signed by President Franklin D. Roosevelt. The health care needs of children were incorporated into the provisions of Title V, Maternal and Child Health Services, which, among other accomplishments, recognized for the first time the needs of disabled children. Another important milestone was the Women, Infants, and Children (WIC) program, which opened its first distribution site in 1974. WIC offers assistance with food and nutrition counseling for low-income pregnant, breast-feeding, and non–breast-feeding postpartum women and infants and children under the age of 5 years.

Today the Office of Child Development, established in 1967, oversees children's programs. It houses the Children's Bureau and the Bureau of Child Development Services, which operates such programs as Head Start. The Secretary of Health and Human Services is the cabinet officer responsible for all their activities. In December 1987, the United States Congress and President Ronald Reagan created the National Commission on Children to serve as a forum on behalf of the children of the nation. In May 1991, after 2½ years of intensive investigation and deliberation, the 34-member commission concluded that the United States was failing many of its children. For example, the proportion of children who were not immunized adequately for preventable childhood diseases had increased dramatically since the early 1980s. Lack of immunization resulted in 26,500 cases of measles and 60 deaths from measles in 1990. The commission's final report listed numerous recommendations for addressing pressing children's issues, such as the need to ensure income security, improve health, increase educational achievement, prepare adolescents for adulthood, strengthen and support families, and protect vulnerable children and their families.

Children are the focus of many of our century's reform initiatives, and solutions are sure to emphasize collaboration between various disciplines. For example, violence, once considered solely a criminal justice problem, now is acknowledged as a preventable public health problem. The most effective solutions for this and other multifaceted problems require the expertise of health care professionals, and law enforcement and criminal justice officials, social workers, economists, and educators.

PEDIATRIC NURSING

The nursing of infants and children is consistent with the revised definition of nursing proposed by the Social Policy Task Force of the American Nurses Association (ANA) in 2003. The definition states that "nursing is the protection, promotion, and optimization of health and abilities; prevention of illness and injury; alleviation of suffering through the diagnosis and treatment of human response; and advocacy in the care of individuals, families, communities, and populations" (ANA, n.d.). This definition incorporates the four essential features of nursing practice:

1. *Human responses* of individuals to actual or potential health problems of concern to nurses, including any observable need, concern, condition, or fact of interest that may be the target of evidence-based nursing practice.
2. *Theory application* is built on understanding theories of nursing and other disciplines as a basis for evidence-based nursing actions.
3. *Nursing actions* are theoretically derived and evidence based and require well-developed intellectual competencies to prevent illness and injury, to alleviate suffering, and to advocate for all populations.
4. *Outcomes of nursing actions* produce beneficial results in relation to identified human responses. Evaluation of those actions determines whether they have been effective. Findings from nursing research provide rigorous scientific evidence of beneficial outcomes of specific nursing actions.

According to Hockenberry and Wilson (2015), "The major goal of pediatric nursing is to improve the quality of health care for children and their families." This can be attained by mechanisms such as improvements with immunization rates, nutrition counseling, teen pregnancy prevention, and improved oral health.

CHARACTERISTICS OF A PEDIATRIC NURSE

Pediatric nursing is different from other clinical specialties. First, the nurse must enjoy working with children of all ages and have enhanced growth and development knowledge. Second, when a child has a health problem, the child, family, and the disease become a nursing focus, and none of the three components can be separated from the other two during care consideration. Pediatric nursing is family-centered nursing in its truest sense. It is important for the family to be totally involved and have a feeling of control over the decision making concerning their child's health care. The nurse must provide care to the child while also identifying family stressors and caring for other members of the family. Working with pediatric patients requires the nurse to have specialized skills, including excellent assessment skills; the ability to establish trust; teaching ability; and the ability to serve as a patient advocate.

By watching children play or perform certain tasks, a nurse should be able to assess their developmental ages. Not all birth defects are diagnosed in the neonatal period. Sometimes nurses identify a problem as a result of a careful nursing assessment. Birth defects, also known as congenital anomalies, are any abnormality present at birth, particularly a structural one that could be inherited in genes from one or both parents, developed during the gestational period, or acquired during the process of giving birth. When children are very ill, minor changes in their physical status sometimes result in a variety of complications; therefore, any changes must be noted as early as possible.

Often the nurse is involved in supporting children through a difficult procedure or serious illness. Such an endeavor not only includes preparation for the event but also requires a level of trust that permits children to express their fear, apprehension, and anxiety. To establish a trusting relationship, convey respect to children, talk with them at a level they can understand, and, most importantly, be honest.

Teaching is ongoing in pediatrics and can be direct or indirect. Innumerable opportunities are available to help children and parents adapt to a chronic illness or disorder through direct teaching, but these require a nurse's knowledge of community resources or volunteer agencies. Be aware of the indirect teaching that occurs through example. A pediatric nurse serves as a role model for children by demonstrating appropriate health promotion and prevention behaviors, such as maintaining good nutrition, a healthy lifestyle, and personal hygiene, and for parents by exhibiting age-appropriate responses to children.

Another role the nurse fills is that of child and family advocate, whether the situation involves ethical decision making or the quality of care given. Sometimes this takes the form of coordinating the activities of a health team and collaborating with members of different disciplines to provide a child with the expert care that is necessary. The nurse often is the intermediary person between the child, family, and other health care providers, providing information, encouragement, clarification, and support.

To enjoy a career and continue working in pediatrics, the nurse needs the ability to recognize and appreciate the uniqueness that each child or adolescent brings to the nurse-patient relationship. It is that special quality—uniqueness—that anyone who provides care for children must understand, respect, and cherish.

CHILDREN WITH SPECIAL NEEDS

Medical advances over the past two decades have resulted in significant changes in the pediatric population. Fragile or premature infants and children with severe injuries or disabilities are now surviving, unlike in the past. With the aid of technology, babies born long before their due dates live into childhood and beyond, but they may face lifelong chronic or debilitating conditions. The term children with special needs refers to infants and children with congenital abnormalities; chronic physical conditions, such as malignant disease, gastrointestinal (GI) disease, or central nervous system (CNS) anomalies; and chronic developmental, behavioral, and emotional conditions. Many of these children need specialized care throughout childhood and into other developmental stages as they age.

Although children with special needs make up a large percentage of the hospitalized children, many forms of technology previously found only in hospital settings have been adapted for home use. With appropriate services and support, even children with severe disabilities can live at home with their family and attend school with their peers.

FAMILY-CENTERED CARE

Family-centered care is a philosophy of care that recognizes the family as the constant in the child's life and holds that systems and personnel are called on to support, respect, encourage, and enhance the strengths and competence of the family (Box 31.1). Nurses and others in the community support families in their natural caregiving and decision-making roles by building on existing unique strengths and acknowledging their expertise in caring for their children within and outside the hospital setting.

Two basic concepts in family-centered care are enabling and empowering. Professionals *enable* families by creating opportunities for all family members to make use of their abilities and competencies and to acquire new ones that are necessary to meet the needs of the child and the family. Professionals *empower*

Box 31.1 Key Elements of Family-Centered Care

- Identify and mobilize internal and external strengths.
- Access appropriate resources in the extended family and community.
- Recognize and enhance positive communication patterns.
- Decide on a consistent discipline approach and access parenting programs if needed.
- Maintain comforting cultural and religious traditions and sources of healing.
- Engage in joint problem solving.
- Acquire new knowledge by providing information about a specific health problem or issue.
- Become empowered.
- Allocate sufficient privacy, space, and time for leisure activities.
- Promote health for all family members during times of crisis.

From James SR, Nelson KA, Ashwill JW: *Nursing care of children: Principles and practice*, ed 4, St. Louis, 2013, Saunders.

families to establish or confirm a sense of control over their lives. Empowerment frees families to foster their own strengths, abilities, and actions and thus enables them to make positive changes in their lives.

The *parent-professional partnership* is a powerful mechanism for enabling and empowering families. Parents serve as respected equals with professionals and have the right to decide what is important for themselves and their family. The professional supports strengthen the family's ability to nurture and promote family development. In a parent-professional partnership, all persons involved in the care of the patient work together and share their talents and resources to provide the best care possible for the patient. The pediatric nurse should assist family members with identifying their strengths and needs and encourage family members to contribute to the plan of care. Last, all professionals involved in the care of the patient also must work together as a team to benefit the child(ren) and family.

Mutual respect is the foundation for effective partnerships with parents. Parents know their child better than anyone else and are able to provide the nurse with important information that cannot be obtained in any other way. Parents of a child with special needs also often become experts on their child's condition. The tradition of the authoritarian nurse has been replaced by a system in which nurses are consultants to the parents and share their unique knowledge and decision-making responsibility (Box 31.2).

Children are vulnerable to the major stressors inherent in hospitalization, such as separation from family and familiar environment, loss of control, bodily trauma, and pain. Many factors, including the child's age, available family support, coping skills, and diagnosis influence the child's response to the illness and hospitalization. Family-centered care is better understood with a comparison of the typical handling of child hospitalization or care needs in the past with today's family-centered approach to care. In the past, parents usually were denied access to their child's medical records or hospital chart. With a family-centered care approach, parents have the same access to information about their child as do all other members of the child's health care team. Other changes, such as hospitals welcoming parents 24 hours a day, reflect increased acknowledgment of the importance of family to the child and of family well-being to members of the family unit. A family-centered approach to care is an important concept in the nursing care of all children. However, it is crucial for optimum care of children with special needs, who are likely to experience repeated contact with the health care system throughout their life.

FUTURE CHALLENGES FOR THE PEDIATRIC NURSE

The present shift in focus from treatment of disease to promotion of health is likely to expand nurses' roles further in ambulatory and outpatient care, with

Box 31.2 Implementation of Family-Centered Care

Although professionals readily accept the concept of family-centered care, they have been slow to implement practices that embody "the family as the patient." This lag has occurred in part because family-centered care requires a shift in orientation regarding the provision of services. The philosophy behind family-centered care requires stretching beyond clinical practices that have become traditional because of their convenience to the institution and personnel.

- Common examples of *system-based care* are exclusionary policies, such as not allowing family members to stay with their children during a procedure and restricting visiting hours and the number and the age of visitors.
- Family-centered care means putting families at the center of the caregiving process, with their input serving as the major determinant of the interventions provided. For example, exclusionary policies are replaced with *family-based care,* such as parental and child *choice* regarding separation during procedures, open visiting hours, and no limitations on the age or the number of visitors, except per family request. In fact, the question arises: Are we misusing the word *visitor* altogether? Family members certainly are not visitors to their child; nurses and other staff are.
- Even *child-based care* is not synonymous with family-based care. For example, often the hospital dietary service provides selections for children but fails to provide inexpensive meals for parents or consider family cultural and religious traditions. Primary nurses at times focus on the child's needs but place little emphasis on the family's concerns.
  - In your practice, what policies can be considered system-based, child-based, or family-based care? How can those that are not family-based be changed? What reasons do staff give for preferring system-based care?
- Compare your agency's policies with its mission statement and purpose. Fortunately, models of family-centered care do exist and have documented benefits:
  - Families experience greater feelings of confidence and competence and less stress in caring for their children.
  - The dependence of families on professional caregivers decreases.
  - Costs of care decrease.
  - Professionals experience greater job satisfaction.
  - Parents and providers are empowered to develop new skills and expertise.

an emphasis on prevention and health teaching. Childhood diseases such as obesity and diabetes will continue to be a major challenge in the years ahead. The need for home care and community health services will make it imperative for nurses to become more independent and acquire skills well beyond those needed in traditional care settings.

Of the 73.4 million children in America, 65% live in a home with two married parents. Although the number of total children in America is on the decline, the number of minority children has increased slightly. Of the children ages 5 to 17 years, 22.6% speak a language other than English at home; 14.4% of children live in poverty; and an estimated 5% of children are without health care insurance (Forum on Child and Family Statistics, 2019). This results in limitations in access to affordable care. The provision of family-centered care to these children and their family is the challenge presented to the pediatric nurse.

NURSING IMPLICATIONS OF GROWTH AND DEVELOPMENT

The nurse must know the basic principles of normal growth and development to understand what can be expected from infants and children, what their needs are, and why they behave as they do. Although each child is unique, groups of children of the same age are more alike than they are different. For example, significant differences are found among the babies in a newborn nursery, but a number of general statements can be made about them. In knowing their similarities, the nurse is better able to perform assessments, develop interventions, identify problems, and promote healthy development (see the Health Promotion box).

Growth and development are complex processes that occur in stages as the body grows, the mind develops, and the personality unfolds. The newborn moves through infancy, toddlerhood, preschool, school age, and adolescence, and each stage consists of predictable, orderly events. Knowledge of the normal milestones of a 6-year-old, for example, makes for easier identification of a developmental delay in a 6-year-old who has not mastered the expected developmental milestones. Differences occur in the rate or the timing with which a child accomplishes a particular task. One infant may sit up at 5 months of age, perhaps, and another at 7 months. However, most infants do so by 6 months of age. Illness or a lack of stimulation interferes with normal development. Other variables that affect development include a baby's genetic makeup and a host of factors such as ethnic background, religion, family size, socioeconomic bracket, and education of the parents.

Growth and development is an important aspect of pediatric nursing. One of the nurse's primary responsibilities is to identify an infant or child who is demonstrating cognitive impairment (the preferred term for mental retardation). The earlier intervention takes place, the greater the likelihood of improvement or remediation. The pediatric nurse also has the opportunity to play a significant role in other types of interventions. For example, the nurse may caution expectant mothers on the hazards of consuming alcohol or smoking while pregnant, refer children with suspected delays to early interventionists, teach parents therapeutic activities and exercises to use with their children, and become knowledgeable about resources in the community that serve children and their families.

Health Promotion

Characteristics of the Infant, Toddler, Child, and Adolescent: Encouraging Healthy Behaviors at Each Stage

INFANT

- Weight doubles by 6 months and triples by 1 year.
- Vision at birth is approximately 20/400; by 12 months, vision is 20/100.
- Play requires stimulation activities that involve motor skills, language, and social skills.
- Infants like toys that bang, shake, or can be pulled and enjoy playing "peek-a-boo."
- Infants like verbal praise and encouragement.

GUIDANCE

- Encourage parents to not use baby talk but to instead pronounce words correctly.
- Sleep usually is established by the spacing of feedings. Encourage parents to give care during awake times either before or after feedings.

TODDLER AND CHILD

- Weight gain from 1 to 3 years is about 5 pounds per year. The weight is usually four times the birth weight by 3 years of age.
- This period consists of intense activity and exploration.
- The toddler or child takes 1 or 2 naps a day and sleeps up to 9 to 12 hours a night.
- Bowel and bladder control usually are achieved by 3 years of age.
- The toddler or child practices parallel play.
- Cognition regarding thinking and reasoning is based on magical or egocentric processes.
- The toddler or child experiences physiologic anorexia, which causes the child to either binge or be picky depending on individual growth spurts and plateaus.

GUIDANCE

- Recommend milk as a drink of choice because of increased needs for calcium. Milk should be fat free or low fat to avoid a large number of "empty calories." Lactose-free milk and soymilk are available for those who are lactose intolerant.

ADOLESCENT

- Adolescents need to be more independent and vacillate between independent and dependent roles, which may be reflected in mood swings.
- Concern about body image, looks, and clothes increases.
- Interest in the opposite sex is heightened.
- Adolescents exhibit logical thought and reasoning and often question the values of parents.
- Adolescents prefer being with peers to establish identity, spending less time with parents and more time with friends.

GUIDANCE

- Adolescence is a time of transition from childhood to becoming a young adult and making one's own choices. Adolescents struggle for greater independence yet are prone to risk taking behavior. Encourage parents to assist with problem solving by having the teen discuss their choices and potential outcomes of those choices.
- Allow the adolescent the freedom to make some unwise choices and do not rescue them from the consequences. For example, they may be saving money for a larger purchase, but spend the money on going to the movies. If the child must wait until they have the money for the larger purchase, they have learned about choices and consequences.
- Sex education and pregnancy prevention education needs to begin before the adolescent is sexually active. Schools may offer some sex education, but there are large differences in what is taught from one school to another. Consequently, parents should not rely on schools as the only source of sex and health education.
- The adolescent diet is prone to deficiencies from eating quick, cheap junk foods. Dietary teaching needs to focus on maintaining a balanced diet and healthy snacks rather than weight or appearance. Be observant for indications of an eating disorder, which may require treatment with a mental health professional.

Knowledge of child development allows the nurse to use a developmental rather than a chronologic approach to pediatric nursing care. A developmental approach emphasizes the child's abilities and strengths rather than disabilities and weaknesses. It considers children's individuality and personalities and builds on what they *can* do rather than concentrating on what they *cannot* do.

An understanding of normal growth and development enables the nurse to select age-appropriate toys for the infant or young toddler and devise activities that appeal to the school-age child or adolescent. Children learn through every opportunity made available to them. For example, observe a 2-year-old playing with a large box, which demonstrates a child's curiosity and creativity.

Age and developmental level influence the ways in which children perceive and make sense of experiences

such as illness or disability and therefore, make an impact on their ability to cope. Knowledge of these levels prepares nurses to develop appropriate nursing plans of care. Some generalizations are possible to make regarding children's concept of illness at different stages of development (Box 31.3). Keep in mind that children, particularly very young ones, sometimes change very rapidly physically and developmentally. Therefore, be sure to reassess and modify nursing care plans continually to reflect these changes.

Knowledge of growth and development is also the basis for anticipatory guidance with parents. Anticipatory guidance (psychological preparation) is preparation for what is likely to occur in the coming weeks and months so that it is possible to lay the groundwork now to protect and promote the child's well-being at that time. For example, parents learn that their 9-month-old or 10-month-old will begin to crawl

INFANTS
Perceive illness as generalized discomfort and pain.

PRESCHOOLERS
Conceive of illness as a punishment for bad thoughts or behavior; believe that adults have the power to magically cure the illness if they want.

SCHOOL-AGE CHILDREN
Sometimes perceive illness as a result of bad or indiscreet behavior; sometimes have an accurate awareness of the location of body parts and a beginning understanding of body processes and functions.

ADOLESCENTS
Focus on discrete symptoms rather than overall effect of illness; often intellectually question and deal with information about illness; at times use denial of illness or overcompensate in areas not affected.

from one place to another. It is normal, it is expected, and it must be allowed. However, parents must remove any harmful objects from the child's reach.

Once a child becomes mobile, the environment should be made "childproof" so that it is safe for the curious crawler. Play is the work of childhood. It is best done in a safe environment, with toys that are safe. The nurse plays an important role in assisting parents to understand the physical and behavioral changes that occur rapidly in the developing infant or toddler. These principles also are useful in working with school-age children, who are exposed to many new experiences once they start school, and preadolescents, who need to be ready to manage the hormonal and growth changes they will experience. The parents of the adolescent are usually as confused and perplexed as the youngster is about changes and behavior at this stage of development. Nurses play an important role in supporting and guiding parent and adolescent through this trying time of life.

PHYSICAL ASSESSMENT OF THE PEDIATRIC PATIENT

Children's rate of growth, level of understanding, and means of communicating differ from adults'. Each stage of childhood is unique. The challenges that children present are constant, exciting, and satisfying. Different assessment skills must be used with children of different age groups.

As in the adult, the sequence of assessment of a child follows a head-to-toe direction. Sometimes you must alter the sequence to accommodate the child's developmental needs, but the findings are documented in the traditional way.

To prepare a child for a physical assessment, use developmental and chronologic age as the main criteria

for the choice of method to assess each body system (Boxes 31.4 and 31.5).

GROWTH MEASUREMENTS

Measurement of physical growth is a key element in evaluation of the health status of children. The growth parameters include weight, height, and head circumference and sometimes skinfold thickness and arm circumference. Plot the child's measurements with percentiles on growth charts and compare them with those of the general pediatric population to determine deviations from the norm. Evaluation of growth trends demonstrated by the child is imperative because growth is a continuous but uneven process, and therefore the most reliable evaluation lies in comparison of growth measurements of each child over a prolonged time (Table 31.1).

The most commonly used growth charts in the United States are from the National Center for Health Statistics (NCHS). The growth charts include 3rd and 97th smoothed percentiles for all charts, and the 85th percentile for the weight-for-stature and BMI-for-age charts.

Children whose growth necessitates further investigation include the following:

- Children whose height and weight percentiles are widely disparate (e.g., height in the 10th percentile and weight in the 90th percentile, especially with above-average skinfold thickness).
- Children who fail to show the expected growth rates in height and weight, especially during the rapid growth periods of infancy and adolescence.
- Children who show a sudden increase, except during puberty, or a decrease in a previously steady growth pattern.

Common Measurements

Head circumference is measured in children up to 36 months. Head circumference usually is measured above the eyebrows and pinna of the ears and around the occipital prominence at the back of the skull (Fig. 31.1).

Length refers to measurements taken when children are supine. Until children are 2 years old, recumbent length is measured. Request assistance in holding the child's head in midline while you extend the child's legs to take a measurement.

Height refers to a measurement when a child stands upright.

Weight

A child's weight reflects fluid loss and inadequate calories, especially in the infant and the toddler. Because of the information that the child's weight conveys, consider the following:

- Use the same scale and weigh the child at the same time every day.
- Perform weight measurements in a warm room.
- What children wear and what is attached to them affects weight.

Box 31.4   Guidelines for Pediatric Physical Assessment

- Perform examination in appropriate, nonthreatening area:
  - Have room well lit and decorated with neutral colors.
  - Have room temperature comfortably warm.
  - Place all strange and potentially frightening equipment out of sight.
  - Have some toys, dolls, stuffed animals, and games available for child.
  - If possible, have rooms decorated and equipped for children of different ages.
- Provide privacy, especially for school-age children and adolescents.
- Provide time for play and becoming acquainted.
- Look for behaviors that signal child's readiness to cooperate:
  - Talking to nurse
  - Making eye contact
  - Accepting offered equipment
  - Allowing physical touching
  - Choosing to sit on examining table rather than parent's lap
- If you observe no signs of readiness, use the following techniques:
  - Talk to patient; gradually focus on a favorite object, such as a doll.
  - Make complimentary remarks about child, such as appearance, dress, or a favorite object.
  - Tell a funny story or play a simple magic trick.
  - Have a nonthreatening "friend" available, such as a hand puppet, to "talk" to child for the nurse.
- If child refuses to cooperate, use the following techniques:
  - Assess reason for uncooperative behavior; consider that a child who is unduly afraid has perhaps had a previous experience that was traumatic.
  - Try to involve child and parent in process.
  - Avoid prolonged explanations about examining procedure.
  - Use a firm, direct approach regarding expected behavior.

- Perform examination as quickly as possible.
- Have attendant gently restrain child.
- Minimize any disruptions or stimulations: limit number of people in room; use isolated room; use quiet, calm, confident voice.
- Begin examination in a nonthreatening manner for young children or children who are fearful:
  - Use approaches such as "Simon says" to encourage child to make a face, squeeze a hand, stand on one foot, and so on.
- Use "paper-doll" technique:
  1. Lay child supine on an examining table or floor that is covered with a large sheet of paper.
  2. Trace around child's body.
  3. Use body outline to demonstrate what will be examined, such as drawing a heart and listening with the stethoscope before performing the activity on child.
- Involve child in examination process:
  - Provide choices, such as sitting on the bed or the chair.
  - Allow child to handle or hold equipment.
  - Encourage child to use equipment on a doll, family member, or examiner.
  - Explain each step of the procedure in simple language.
  - Examine child in a comfortable and secure position: sitting in parent's lap; sitting upright if in respiratory distress.
- Proceed to examine the body in an organized sequence (usually head-to-toe) with the following exceptions: examine painful areas last; in emergency situation, examine vital functions (airway, breathing, and circulation) and injured area first.
- Reassure child throughout examination, especially about bodily concerns that arise during puberty.
- Discuss findings with family at end of examination.
- Praise child for cooperation during examination; give reward such as small toy, stickers, or sucker.

Box 31.5   Assessment of Body Systems

Use of developmental and chronologic age as the main criteria for the choice of method to assess each body system accomplishes several goals:
- It minimizes stress and anxiety associated with assessment of various body parts.
- It fosters a trusting nurse-child-parent relationship.
- It allows for maximum preparation of the child.
- It preserves the essential security of the parent-child relationship, especially with young children.
- It maximizes the accuracy and reliability of assessment findings.

Table 31.1   Expected Growth Rates at Various Ages

AGE	EXPECTED GROWTH RATE PER YEAR	
	cm	inches
1–6 months	18–22	7.2–8.8
6–12 months	14–18	5.6–7.2
Second year	11	4.4
Third year	8	3.2
Fourth year	7	2.8
Fifth to tenth years	5–6	2–2.4

- If equipment has been added or removed, document this on the graphic sheet.
- Usually older children are weighed with underpants or a light gown (Fig. 31.2).
- Respect the privacy of all children.

Skinfold Thickness and Arm Circumference
Skinfold thickness is determined at one site, with at least two measurements taken for the greatest reliability (Box 31.6).

Arm circumference measures muscle mass. The same procedure is followed as for skinfold thickness, except the measurement is made with a tape measure rather than calipers.

VITAL SIGNS

Key elements in evaluation of physical status are vital signs: temperature, pulse, respiration, and blood pressure. (For best results taking vital signs of an infant, count respirations first, before the infant is disturbed; take pulse second, and temperature last.)

Temperature

Body temperature, which also reflects metabolism, is fairly stable from infancy through adulthood. After the unstable regulatory ability in the neonatal period, heat production steadily declines as the infant grows into childhood. In an air-conditioned delivery room, the newborn's temperature sometimes drops to 97°F (36.1°C) or lower, which accounts for the use of radiant warmers for newborns after delivery. Newborns also tend to have difficulty dissipating heat in an overheated environment, which increases the risk of hyperthermia.

Despite the ability to regulate their temperature, infants and toddlers are prone to wide variations, especially after crying for extended periods or after active play. Temperature elevations also occur rapidly in young children when infections are present.

Crown-to-heel recumbent length

Fig. 31.1 Measurement of head, chest, and abdominal circumference and crown-to-heel measurement (recumbent length).

Box **31.6**	**Measurement of Triceps Skinfold Thickness**

- With child's right arm flexed 90 degrees at elbow, mark midpoint between acromion and olecranon on posterior aspect of arm.
- With arm hanging freely, grasp a fold of skin between thumb and forefinger 1 cm above midpoint.
- Gently pull fold away from underlying muscle and continue to hold through the remaining steps until measurement is completed.
- Place caliper jaws over skinfold at midpoint mark; if a plastic catheter (e.g., Ross Adipometer) is used, apply pressure with thumb to align lines on caliper; follow directions for use of other calipers.
- Estimate reading to nearest millimeter, 2 or 3 s after applying pressure.
- Take measurements until you obtain two readings that agree within 1 mm.

Fig. 31.2 (A) Infant on scale. (B) Toddler on scale.

Table 31.2   Normal Temperature in Children

| AGE | TEMPERATURE | |
	°F	°C
3 months	99.4	37.5
6 months	99.5	37.5
1 year	99.7	37.7
3 years	99.0	37.2
5 years	98.6	37.0
7 years	98.3	36.8
9 years	98.1	36.7
11 years	98.0	36.7
13 years	97.8	36.6

Table 31.3   Vital Signs (Averages)

AGE	HEART RATE (beats/min)	RESPIRATIONS (breaths/min)	BLOOD PRESSURE (mm Hg)
Newborn	120	35	70/50
1–11 months	120	30	90/60
2 years	110	25	96/68
4 years	100	23	100/70
6 years	100	21	105/70
10 years	90	20	108/70
12 years	88	20	110/70
16 years	70	20	120/70

Beginning at approximately 12 years of age, girls display a temperature that remains relatively stable, whereas the temperature in boys continues to fall for a few years longer. Females maintain a temperature slightly above that of males throughout life (for normal temperature in children, see Table 31.2).

The primary purpose of body temperature measurement is detection of abnormal values. In patients with febrile conditions, the chief concern is the temperature of the brain, because very high temperatures have the capacity to cause neural damage. Thus, the best sites for measurement of temperature are those closest to the brain, which reflect central, or core, body heat. Other core sites are the esophagus and the bladder. However, these sites involve invasive thermometry and are impractical for routine temperature measurement.

The oral and axillary sites are used commonly in clinical practice. Other sites that also are used for temperature measurement are the tympanic membrane and temporal artery (temporal artery thermometry). Historically, the temperatures of infants and young children were taken rectally. Safety concerns and the availability of safer and more reliable methods have made this practice rare today. In infants and young children, tympanic or axillary temperatures often are preferred. Oral temperatures are acceptable when children are old enough to be cooperative and understand directions, typically around 5 or 6 years old.

Many facilities now use tympanic temperatures for all ages. The ear's proximity to the hypothalamus, the body's temperature-regulating center, makes it a desirable area for reflecting true core temperature. In comparisons with rectal, oral, or axillary temperature assessments in children, tympanic membrane measurements are fairly insensitive in detecting fevers and should be used with caution for children younger than 3 years of age. The size of the probe has the potential to influence the reading. Many ear probes are too large to be placed correctly in the pediatric ear canal. Use of correctly sized pediatric materials and supplies is

important. Technique is another important factor. For the sensor to detect heat from the drum, instead of from the cooler canals, straighten the ear canal. When the ear is pulled back and down and the probe tip points at the midpoint between the eyebrow and the sideburn on the opposite side of the face, the most accurate temperature readings are obtained.

In considering all the findings for and against different sites of temperature measurement, think critically about why the temperature is needed, how clinically significant a small difference in temperature between routes really is, and how much the procedure upsets the child and the caregiver. Finally, in deciding which route to use, consider which method will be the least traumatic to the child. Children are less upset having their temperature measured via the ear route than via the rectal route. Parents also sometimes have objections to the rectal route.

Heart Rate or Pulse

Variations exist in the heart rates of children. Although an average apical beat of a newborn is around 120 per minute, the heart rate gradually slows to an average of 70 beats/min by adolescence (Table 31.3). The presence of infection increases the heart rate, as does physical activity. During sleep, a child's pulse is at its slowest rate.

In assessment of the heart rate, note the rhythm and any irregularities. Count the pulse rate for 1 full minute. An apical pulse measurement, heard at the apex of the heart (located at the fifth intercostal space on the left side), is more reliable if taken while the patient is asleep. For assessment for murmurs of the heart, listen at the second intercostal space. Whereas an apical pulse is taken in infants and young children, with children 5 years of age and older, a radial pulse often is taken.

Respiration

Respirations are counted in the pediatric patient in the same manner as in the adult. Newborns are obligate nasal breathers, meaning they breathe only through their noses; they do not breathe through the mouth until they reach 3 or 4 weeks of age. The infant's respirations are primarily diaphragmatic; the abdominal movements should be observed when respirations are counted. In children younger than 7 years of age, respiratory movements are abdominal or diaphragmatic. In older children, respirations are chiefly thoracic. The respiratory rate also slows as a child progresses from infancy to adolescence.

A newborn's respiratory rate is extremely erratic, so for accuracy, count it for 1 full minute to notice any irregularities. Assess the rate, the depth, and the quality of respirations. The rate in the newborn sometimes is as rapid as 40 to 50 breaths/min, gradually slowing to 25 to 32 per minute by 36 hours of age (see Table 31.3 for normal respiratory rate in children).

Blood Pressure

Blood pressure typically is not measured until a child reaches 3 years of age (Box 31.7). Children with symptoms of hypertension, and those in intensive care, at high risk, and in emergency departments, need to have their blood pressure measured.

Blood pressure is low in a newborn. Gradually it rises, so by the end of adolescence it is about 120/78 mm Hg (see Table 31.3).

To ensure accuracy with a blood pressure reading, use the correct cuff size. Be sure the cuff covers two-thirds of the length of the upper arm or leg (Box 31.8).

See sites for measuring children's blood pressure in Fig. 31.3.

The technique for measuring blood pressure in children is the same as that for an adult. Because children are upset easily by unfamiliar procedures, an explanation of each step is helpful. For preschool and early school-age children, explain how the cuff will feel, such as "tight feeling," "arm hug," or "I want to feel your muscle." Use an explanation such as, "I want to see how strong your muscle is."

Because results are best when the child is quiet and relaxed during the procedure, measure blood pressure before performing any anxiety-producing procedures. Infants and small children are often quieter if the blood pressure is taken while they are sitting on the parent's lap. Never place the blood pressure cuff on any limb with an intravenous site.

HEAD-TO-TOE ASSESSMENT

Skin

Genetic factors influence assessment of skin color, as do physiologic factors. Edema decreases intensity of skin color, sometimes producing false pallor. Pallor is a sign of potential anemia, chronic disease, edema, or shock. Compare pallor or cyanosis (bluish tone) against the color change normally produced by blanching, with use of the nonpigmented nail: press down on the free

---

Box 31.7	Calculation of Normal Blood Pressure

Use the following quick formula to calculate normal systolic blood pressure:
- *1–7 years:* Age in years + 90 mm Hg
- *8–18 years:* (2 × Age in years) + 83 mm Hg
  Use the following quick formula to calculate normal diastolic blood pressure:
- 1–5 years: 56 mm Hg
- 6–8 years: Age in years + 52 mm Hg

Box 31.8	Correct Blood Pressure Cuff Size

- In choosing cuffs, use an appropriately sized one.
- A cuff of proper size covers two-thirds of the length of the upper arm or leg.
- If a cuff of the correct size is not available, use an oversized cuff rather than an undersized one, or use another site that more appropriately fits the cuff size.
- Do not choose a cuff based on the name of the cuff (e.g., an "infant" cuff is too small for some infants).

---

edge of the nail and observe return blood flow. Apply pressure to the lips or gums of dark-skinned individuals to observe color change. A yellow tint may indicate jaundice.

Erythema usually is the result of increased temperature, local inflammation, or infection. Normal skin texture in the young child is smooth, soft, and slightly dry to the touch.

Accessory Structures

Scalp hair is usually lustrous, silky, and elastic. Genetic factors influence the appearance of hair. Tufts of hair anywhere along the spine, especially the sacrum, are significant because they sometimes mark the site of spina bifida occulta.

Healthy nails are pink, convex, smooth, and hard but flexible, not brittle. Dark-skinned individuals sometimes have more deeply pigmented nail beds. Variation in color, such as blueness, suggests cyanosis.

Each person has a distinct set of handprints and footprints. The palm normally shows three flexion creases. If grossly abnormal lines or folds are observed, a specialist may investigate further. Note that the skin and accessory structures change with the aging process of an individual.

Eyes

The eyes of a newborn undergo many changes before vision is comparable with that of an adult. The baby achieves clear vision only at very close range. At birth, visual acuity is normally around 20/400, which makes it important for the adult holding a baby to assume an **en face position** (position in which the adult's face and the infant's face are approximately 8 inches apart and on the same plane, as when the mother holds the infant up in front of her face or

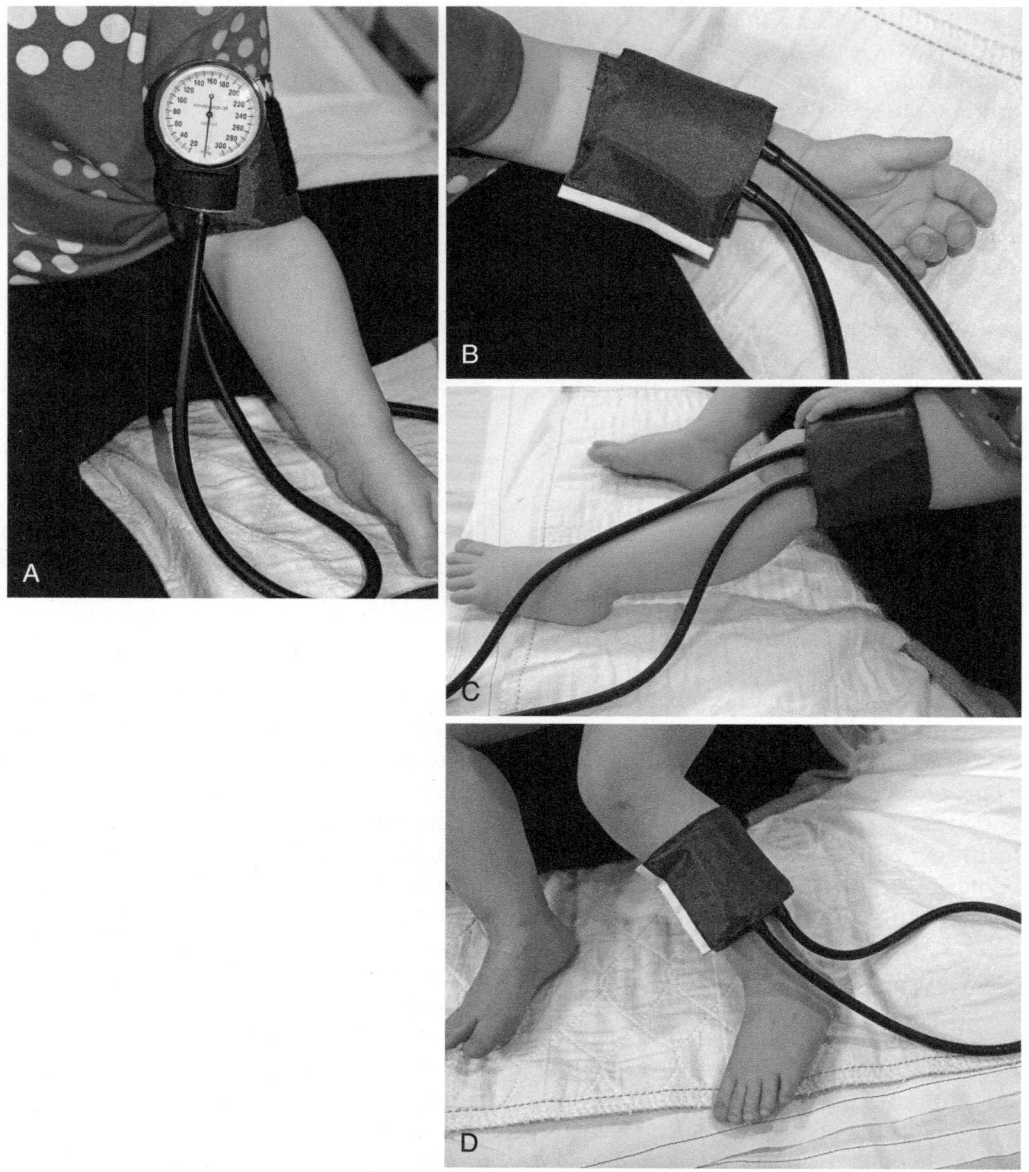

Fig. 31.3 Sites for measuring blood pressure. (A) Upper arm. (B) Lower arm or forearm. (C) Thigh. (D) Calf or ankle.

when she nurses the infant) (Fig. 31.4). Teach parents to hold the baby comfortably so that they can make eye contact and the newborn can gaze on the face of the holder. Although tears are absent immediately after birth, by the second week of life, tear glands begin to function. Newborns develop the ability to follow bright, colorful objects by the second or third week of life.

Although visual acuity is typically 20/200 by the fourth or fifth month, depth perception does not develop before the ninth or tenth month. One-year-olds, who enjoy playing with large objects (blocks, toys, and boxes), often bump into obstacles because their vision is only about 20/100. Vision improves to 20/30 to 20/22 by age 2 to 3 years. When a child starts school, *accommodation* (changes in ciliary muscle and the lens in bringing light rays from various distances to focus

on the retina) and *refraction* (the production by the normal eye of the proper image of the object on the retina) also are present. Almost 6 years of continual development are needed for the parts of the eyes to function as they do in an adult.

Ears
The tops of the ears, or pinnae, are generally on a horizontal line with the outer canthus of the eye. The pinna should be flexible with cartilage present. Low-set ears may be indicative of some congenital anomalies, and additional investigation may be necessary to determine the difference between signaling a significant anomaly or only as a familial trait (dad's ears). The ears should be inspected for general hygiene. If the ear canal appears free of *cerumen* (a waxy substance produced by the ceruminous gland in the outer

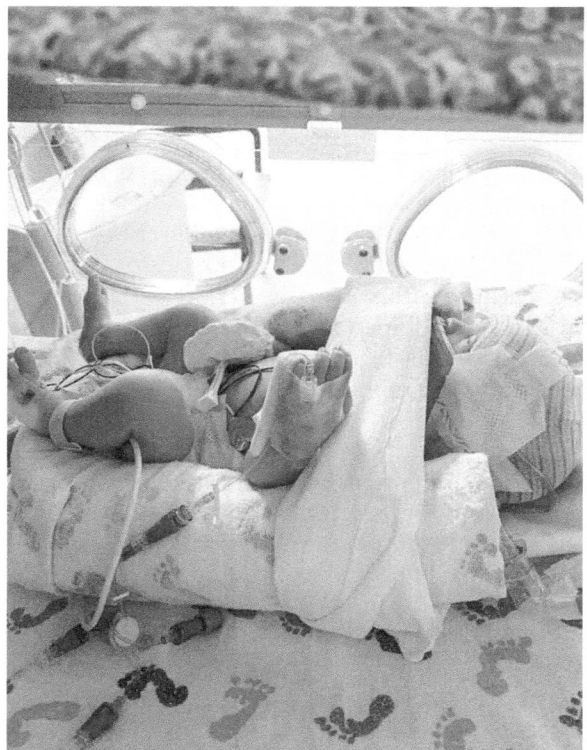

Fig. 31.4 Promoting bonding may require the mother overcome a physical barrier to achieve the en face position.

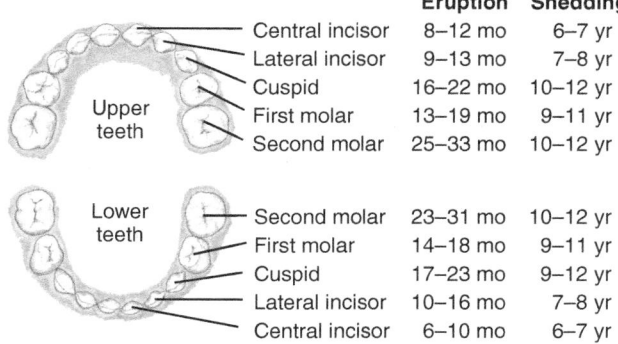

		Eruption	Shedding
Upper teeth	Central incisor	8–12 mo	6–7 yr
	Lateral incisor	9–13 mo	7–8 yr
	Cuspid	16–22 mo	10–12 yr
	First molar	13–19 mo	9–11 yr
	Second molar	25–33 mo	10–12 yr
Lower teeth	Second molar	23–31 mo	10–12 yr
	First molar	14–18 mo	9–11 yr
	Cuspid	17–23 mo	9–12 yr
	Lateral incisor	10–16 mo	7–8 yr
	Central incisor	6–10 mo	6–7 yr

Fig. 31.5 Sequence of eruption of primary teeth. (Modified from James SR, Nelson KA, Ashwill JW: *Nursing care of children: Principles and practice,* ed 4, St. Louis, 2013, Saunders.)

portion of the canal), ask about ear-cleaning methods. It is best to question the parent and child about ear cleaning by remarking on how clean the ears are and asking how they remove wax. This approach is more likely to yield an honest answer. Advise parents and children to clean the ears with a washcloth and to gently wipe only the outer portion of the external canal. Also advise that they can soften any cerumen that is hard by instilling 2 or 3 drops of mineral oil into the ear for a few days and then rinsing the external canal with an ear syringe. Discourage the use of cotton swabs in the ear canal.

Nose, Mouth, and Throat

The nose normally lies from the center point between the eyes to the notch of the upper lip. No discharge usually is emitted from the nose. Inspect the lining of the mouth. Ask the child to open the mouth wide, to move the tongue in different directions, and to say "Ahh," which depresses the tongue for full view of the mouth.

Infants and toddlers, however, usually resist and do not open their mouth. Place the tongue blade along the side of the tongue, not the center where the gag reflex is elicited. Frequently, a protrusion of the tongue is seen in children with cognitive impairment.

The number of teeth is also important to check. The **primary (deciduous) teeth** (the set of 20 teeth that normally appear during infancy) begin to descend between the sixth and ninth months of life. The central incisors are normally the first teeth to appear. By a child's third birthday, all 20 primary teeth are typically present. The exact mechanisms responsible for the eruption of teeth are not fully understood. The eruption of teeth is distressing to most babies, whose gums become erythematous and edematous. The fussiness demonstrated sometimes results in a refusal to eat. A cold teething ring and numbing (locally anesthetizing) agents provide some relief to painful gums. See Fig. 31.5 for the sequence of eruption of primary teeth.

Permanent teeth begin to appear at about 6 years, and most are present by 12 years.

Good dental hygiene should begin as soon as the primary teeth erupt. The first dental visit should be conducted by age 1 year. The promotion of dental health is important in the lives of children (American Academy of Pediatric Dentists [AAPD], n.d.). Dental caries are the leading chronic disease in children in the United States. Fluoride is a mineral that protects against tooth decay. Almost all water contains naturally occurring fluoride, but at levels that are not high enough to prevent tooth decay. Fluoride often is added to community drinking water and toothpaste to provide tooth protection benefits. The positive outcomes prompted a goal to increase adequately fluoridated community water to 80% by 2020 (Centers for Disease Control [CDC], 2020).

Lungs

Guidelines for effective auscultation of lung sounds in children are seen in Box 31.9 and Fig. 31.6.

Chest

During infancy, the chest appears circular. As the child grows, the chest size normally increases symmetrically. Asymmetry in the chest indicates the possibility of serious underlying problems such as cardiac enlargement (bulging on left side of ribcage) or pulmonary dysfunction. In an older child, a barrel-shaped chest sometimes indicates chronic obstructive pulmonary disease such as cystic fibrosis or asthma.

| Box **31.9** | Guidelines for Effective Auscultation of Lungs |

- Be sure the child is relaxed and not crying, talking, or laughing. Record if the child is crying.
- Check that the room is comfortable and quiet.
- Warm the stethoscope before placing it against the skin.
- Apply firm pressure on the chest piece but not enough to prevent vibrations and transmission of sound.
- Avoid placing the stethoscope over hair or clothing, moving it against the skin, breathing on the tubing, or sliding fingers over the chest piece, all of which often cause sounds that falsely resemble pathologic findings.
- Use a symmetric and orderly approach to compare sounds.
- Ask the child to "blow out" the light on an otoscope or pocket flashlight; discreetly turn off the light on the last try so that the child feels successful (see Fig. 31.6).
- Place a cotton ball in the child's palm; ask the child to blow the ball into the air, and have the parent catch it.
- Place a small tissue on the top of a pencil and ask the child to blow off the tissue.
- Have child blow a pinwheel, a party horn, or bubbles.

Fig. 31.6 Auscultation of lungs while child "blows out" otoscope light.

Back

The back of a newborn is C-shaped (Fig. 31.7A). As growth occurs, the typical S-shaped curve is seen in the older child and the adult. Marked curvature in posture is abnormal. Symmetry of the spine in the adolescent may be a sign of *scoliosis* (lateral curvature of the spine) (Fig. 31.7C). Scoliosis is an important childhood problem that is more common in females.

Abdomen

Examination of the abdomen involves the following:

- *Inspection:* Done while the child is erect and supine. Normally in infants and young children, the abdomen appears slightly rounded. In the supine position, the abdomen appears flat.

- *Auscultation:* Heart or lung sounds can be heard with a stethoscope placed gently on the skin, but the diaphragm of the stethoscope must be pressed firmly against the abdominal surface to hear bowel sounds.

The most important sound to listen for is peristalsis, which you may possibly hear every 10 to 30 seconds. Normal peristalsis sounds like metallic clicks and gurgles. Report the absence of bowel sounds or hyperperistalsis, because either usually denotes an abdominal disorder. The abdomen should be auscultated among all four quadrants for a full 3 minutes before absent bowel sounds are reported.

Extremities

Examine the extremities at birth for symmetry, range of motion, and signs of malformation. Count fingers and toes to be certain of normal numbers. As a toddler begins to walk, the legs are usually bowlegged until lower body and leg muscles develop. The infant and the toddler also must be observed for arch development and correct gait. By school age, the walking posture is more graceful and balanced. During puberty, adolescents sometimes experience awkward posture that results from rapid growth of extremities.

Renal Function

All structural components are present in the renal system of a newborn, but functional deficiency is found in the kidneys' abilities to concentrate urine and to cope with conditions of fluid and electrolyte fluctuation, such as dehydration or fluid overload. Infants are more prone to fluid volume fluctuations because glomerular filtration and absorption are low as a result of the immature kidney function. The kidneys in children are not protected by padding and are consequently susceptible to injury.

Urine output varies and depends on the size of the infant or child. Table 31.4 identifies average volumes excreted at given ages. The urine is colorless and odorless and has a specific gravity of approximately 1.020.

Anus

Assess history of bowel movements for diarrhea, constipation, or rectal bleeding. Different stooling patterns are noted by feeding method and age. The stool of a baby who is breast-fed exclusively is typically light mustard color, grainy in texture, and runny in consistency. The stool of a formula-fed baby is usually tan, yellow, or light brown in color and firmer than that of the breast-fed baby. The presence of lesions or skin irritations near the anus necessitates further investigation. Reports of itching may signal parasitic infections.

Genitalia

Genitalia examination is usually uneventful for infants. It can be anxiety producing for toddlers, older preschoolers, school-age children, and adolescents.

Fig. 31.7 (A) Newborn showing normal "C" spinal curvature. (B) Normal spine. © Scoliosis.

Table **31.4**	Kidney Function and Urine Output
AGE	**VOLUME OF URINE OUTPUT**
Preterm newborn	1–3 mL/kg/h
Full-term newborn	3–4 mL/kg/h
6 months	12 mL/h
1 year	22 mL/h
5 years	28 mL/h
12 years	33–35 mL/h

The genital examination is an excellent time for eliciting questions concerning body functions or sexual activity. It provides an opportunity to increase or reinforce the child's knowledge of reproductive anatomy and explain its function.

During the male genital examination, assess the external appearance of the glans and the shaft of the penis, the prepuce, the urethral meatus, and the scrotum. Edema, skin lesions, inflammation, or other irregularities are possible signs of underlying disorders, especially sexually transmitted infections (STIs). The examination of the female genitalia usually is limited to the inspection and palpation of external structures.

FACTORS THAT INFLUENCE GROWTH AND DEVELOPMENT

NUTRITION

A holistic look at the child requires an assessment of current family nutrition. Nutrition is probably the single most important influence on growth. During infancy and childhood, the demand for calories is great because of rapid increase in height and weight. Growth is uneven during infancy and adolescence. A child's appetite fluctuates in response to growth spurts. Good nutrition begins before conception and is related closely to good health throughout life.

Infants begin life outside the womb nursing at the breast or ingesting formula or breast milk by bottle or tube. Human milk is the most desirable complete diet for the infant for the first 6 months of life. The American Academy of Pediatrics (2012) recommends breast-feeding exclusively until the infant reaches 6 months of age. Exclusive breast-feeding means that the infant receives only breast milk and no additional foods (except vitamin D) or fluids unless recommended by the primary health care provider (National Institute of Child Health and Human Development [NICHD], n.d.). Whole cow's milk should be advised against until the child passes the 12-month mark because cow's milk contains high amounts of protein and minerals, which can stress an infant's immature kidneys. Skim or low-fat milk is not recommended because the essential fatty acids are inadequate and the solute concentration of protein and electrolytes, such as sodium, is too high. An allergy to protein in milk can cause the infant to be fussy and irritable.

Most infants are given solid foods at 4 to 6 months of age when they begin to need more iron in the diet and their teeth begin to erupt. Iron-fortified cereal is the first solid food most parents give to a baby. Rice cereal is digested easily and has low allergenic potential, so it is a common choice. However, oatmeal and barley are high-protein cereals and also make good options. After several months of breast milk or formula, the addition of solid foods to an infant's diet is a significant developmental step.

Although the order of introduction of foods other than cereal is arbitrary, the usual sequence is strained fruits, fruit juices, strained vegetables, and strained meats. As more teeth erupt, suggest offering finger food, such as zwieback (teething biscuit). This helps infants develop a hand-to-mouth cycle, which is basic to feeding themselves.

Each new food must be introduced at weekly intervals to allow recognition of any food allergies (an allergic response sometimes takes several days to appear). Development of a rash, wheezing, or diarrhea is a common sign that indicates the presence of an allergy to a food.

By 9 months, several teeth have erupted, and junior foods can be offered, which are of much coarser texture. These fruits, vegetables, and meats taste different, and their different texture encourages the infant to chew. Good choices of finger foods to give at this time include small pieces of fruit (excluding grapes, which could choke the infant) and cooked vegetables.

The cost of baby foods is significant; therefore, as the infant acquires more teeth and does not experience difficulty eating solids, encourage parents to prepare these foods at home. Canned foods, other than those prepared for infants, often contain excessive sodium or sugar. If sweetening is needed, refined sugar is acceptable to use, but advise against using honey and corn syrup because of the risk of infant botulism. Encourage cooking fresh or frozen foods and using a blender or food processor. By 12 to 15 months, toddlers usually are eating table food prepared for the family. Although use of a spoon is messy, typical toddlers become angry and frustrated when they are "ready" to feed themselves and parents continue to feed them.

Weaning (gradually eliminating breast-feeding or bottle feeding and instituting cup and table feedings) is a major accomplishment of toddlerhood. The earlier method of feeding has provided the child with a great deal of pleasure and satisfaction. Giving it up is sometimes difficult for child and parent. Breast-feeding should be continued until 12 months of age. After 12 months, the American Academy of Pediatrics (2012) states that the discontinuation of breast-feeding is a personal choice. The American Academy of Pediatrics (2012) recommends weaning bottle-fed infants by 15 months of age. Solid foods also are pleasing to the taste buds, but when toddlers feed themselves with a spoon, they may turn it upside down as they navigate the utensil toward their mouth, and they lose much of the food. The same occurs with a cup. A plastic cup with a spout decreases the amount of milk or juice that is spilled. Most 9-month-old or 10-month-old infants who can sit in a high chair begin to demonstrate a readiness to wean. They become much more active and squirm when they are held for feedings. In addition, they observe siblings and adults drinking from cups or glasses and desire to do the same. Gradually, parents replace bottle feedings or breast-feeding with the cup. Usually the bedtime feeding is the last one parents discontinue. A parent should never allow a child to take a bottle of milk or any sweetened liquids to bed and should never prop a bottle, because this is a major cause of dental caries in deciduous teeth. If the child needs a bottle at bedtime, the parent should give water.

Ideally, concentrated sugars and high-carbohydrate snacks are absent from the young child's diet. The form of sugar in foods is important. Cariogenic (promoting or producing tooth decay) foods are those that are sticky and hard and remain in the mouth longer (e.g., lollipops). Help parents plan meals and snacks that include foods less damaging to teeth.

As children move through toddler and preschool stages, they often develop fads with strong preferences. Teach the school-age child and the parent the value of a diet balanced to promote growth. Adolescent problems include dietary imbalance and excesses. Excess intake of calories, sugar, fat, cholesterol, and sodium are common. Inadequate intake of certain vitamins is evident among teens. These dietary patterns can contribute to an increased risk of such chronic illnesses as heart disease and osteoporosis and some types of cancer later in life. The American Academy of Pediatrics recommends cholesterol testing for children whose parents or grandparents have total cholesterol levels of 240 mg/dL or higher and for children whose parents or grandparents have had heart attacks or have been diagnosed with blocked arteries at age 55 or earlier in men or age 65 or earlier in women. For children in these categories, the first cholesterol test should be after 2 years of age but no later than 10 years of age (Healthychildren.org, 2020).

Approximately 18.8 per 1000 females between the ages of 15 and 19 give birth. Although the rate of pregnancy in this demographic has been slightly declining in recent years, it remains higher than the rates in similarly developed countries (Office of Population Affairs, n.d.). The pregnant teen exhibits food preferences, eating behaviors, and lifestyle habits similar to nonpregnant peers. Frequent snacking on foods high in fat and sugar and low in essential nutrients (calcium, iron, zinc, folate, and vitamins B_6, A, and C) causes special dietary concerns during pregnancy. Nurses play a central role in meeting the needs of pregnant teenagers. The nurse is frequently the one the young girl turns to for help and guidance in her dilemma and the one she relies on for support and reassurance. The nutritional assessment focuses on the dietary adequacy of iron, calcium, and multivitamins with folic acid.

METABOLISM

Metabolic needs vary among individuals. The rate of metabolism is highest in the newborn infant because the ratio of total body surface area to body weight is much greater in the infant than it is in the adult. This proportion decreases as the child grows and matures. The basal metabolic rate (BMR) is a measure of metabolism when the body is at rest; it changes dramatically as the body increases in size. Newborns double their birth weight by 5 to 6 months and triple it by about 1 year of age, which demonstrates the rapid rate at which metabolism occurs in very young children.

The body uses energy provided by foods. Whereas the energy requirements for an infant are highest during the first 6 months of life, they are fairly constant from 4 to 10 years and vary in adolescence, depending on the teen's physical development (Table 31.5).

Table **31.5**	Daily Caloric Needs of Infants, Children, and Adolescents

AGE GROUP	CALORIC NEEDS
Infants	
Birth to 6 months	108 kcal/kg
6–12 months	94.4 kcal/kg
Children	
1–3 years	100 kcal/kg
4–6 years	90 kcal/kg
7–10 years	71.4 kcal/kg
Adolescents	
Males	
11–14 years	55.6 kcal/kg
15–18 years	45.5 kcal/kg
Females	
11–14 years	47.8 kcal/kg
15–18 years	40 kcal/kg

Modified from *https://www.merckmanuals.com/professional/nutritional-disorders/nutrition-general-considerations/overview-of-nutrition#v881783*, 2019.

Because metabolism is so high in infants and children, their ability to recover from surgery or a fractured bone is swift compared with that of an adult. With the accelerated rate of all bodily functions, healing occurs quickly, provided all necessary nutritional components are in place. For example, a fractured femur at birth is united in 3 weeks, but an 8-year-old with the same type of fracture needs 8 weeks for union, and a 20-year-old takes 20 weeks to heal.

SLEEP AND REST

Children spend less total time sleeping as they mature. The newborn sleeps much of the time not occupied with feeding and other aspects of care. Most babies sleep through the night by the latter part of their first year and take one or two naps a day. Most 12- to 18-month-olds usually nap once a day. The 3-year-old child usually has given up all daytime naps.

The best way to prevent sleep problems with the infant and child is to establish bedtime rituals that do not foster problematic patterns. One of the most constructive ways is to place infants awake in their own crib or bed. Advise using the bed for sleeping only, not as a playpen.

SPEECH AND COMMUNICATION

Crying at birth is the earliest evidence of speech, wordless though it is. Infants use this method of communication when they are hungry or in pain or need to be changed. Crying is followed gradually by other sounds, such as cooing, laughing, or babbling. By 9 months, infants practice the noises they can make and painstakingly repeat them. Infants enjoy the sounds of their own voice. While they begin to express themselves, they also begin to imitate the vocal sounds of an adult. It is possible to have an actual conversation with the infant. Although no formal words are exchanged, it is a pleasant experience. The adult speaks, the infant responds, the adult answers, and so on. As the infant begins to enjoy experimenting with these sounds, encouragement of these vocalizations is important; it is positive reinforcement for oral communication.

A 1-year-old has a three-word or four-word vocabulary. It usually includes *mama* and *dada*. In toddlerhood, more words are understood than expressed. Children usually know 25 to 50 words by 18 months, but by 2 years, they often know more than 250 words. Speech develops rapidly at this stage, as children practice and learn new words and their meanings. Soon they are able to say a two-word or three-word sentence. Preschoolers have a fairly extensive vocabulary to convey their wants, needs, and desires.

Speech ability is determined by the child's stage of development, the amount of stimulation or encouragement received from adults, the child's health status, and many other factors. In addition, the development of language does not occur in isolation; it is related to the physiologic, neurologic, and psychosocial progress that is occurring simultaneously. Children learn the complex symbol system of language with astonishing speed.

It is important to know what typifies speech at each stage of childhood for identification of problems. For example, the lack of babbling or the inability of a 9-month-old to imitate sounds is a possible indication of deafness or hearing impairment. All babies make verbal sounds until 6 or 7 months of age, but then the child who is unable to hear decreases these verbalizations in favor of gesturing or some expression of body language (or nonverbal communication).

Verbal communication is used in a variety of ways in nursing practice. Talking softly to infants while cuddling them is an important part of establishing trust in a relationship with babies. Although the toddler is leery of strangers, if the nurse talks with a parent first, the 2-year-old senses the trusting attitude of the adult and begins to participate in the conversation. As a result of improving verbal skills, preschoolers and school-age children understand more and share their concerns more easily. Teaching 8- to 10-year-olds is particularly satisfying because they are eager to learn. On the other hand, adolescents who have refined their verbal abilities communicate a significant amount of information nonverbally through body language, gestures, and facial expressions. General strategies to consider when talking with children include the following:

- Use a calm, unhurried, and confident voice.
- Speak clearly, be specific, and use as few words as possible. As a general guide, use sentences whose sum of words is equal to the child's age in years plus one.

- State directions and suggestions in a positive way; for example, say, "You need to stay very still," rather than, "Don't move."
- Because children see things only in relation to themselves and from their viewpoint, focus communication on them.
- After greeting the child, continue to talk to the child and the parent while pursuing activities that do not involve the child directly.
- Use play as a strategy for getting to know the child. For example, if the child has a doll or a stuffed animal, begin by speaking to the toy. Then, initiate conversation with the child by asking simple questions about the toy.
- Listen to and observe the child at play. Often children express important information, such as complicated or difficult feelings, through this familiar medium.
- Look for opportunities to offer the child choices but offer them only when they really exist. (Children are confused by choices being offered when there actually are none.) For example, when a child needs to change into a gown, a statement such as, "I need your dress off so that I can listen to your chest. Shall I help you take it off?" gives the child an explanation, a choice, and some control.
- Be honest with children. However, be careful about creating overly scary impressions. Instead of saying, "This will hurt" before a procedure, it is better to prepare the child with a statement such as, "Children tell me different things about how this feels. Some say it feels like a cat or dog scratching. Afterward, will you tell me what it felt like for you?"
- Use direct and concrete communication with young children because they are unable to work with abstractions or to separate fact from fantasy. For example, they attach literal meanings to such common phrases as "a frog in the throat" or "hold your horses."
- Avoid use of a phrase that is open to a young child's misinterpretation. For example, the statement, "Let's see how warm your body is," is preferred to "Let's take your temperature," because young children may wonder what you are going to do with their temperature once you have it and whether you are planning to give it back. Words such as "shot" are frightening if a child envisions a shot from a gun. Instead substitute "putting some medicine under the skin."
- Children between 5 and 8 years want concrete explanations and reasons for everything because they rely more on what they know than what they see when faced with new problems. Continue to use relatively simple explanations, remembering that their expanding vocabulary facilitates communication.

One of the most important points to remember is to speak with a child according to the child's stage of development. A conversation with a 2-year-old differs greatly from a conversation with a 12-year-old. To be successful in establishing relationships with children and to be effective in teaching or sharing information, be sure to communicate with them at the appropriate level.

Nonverbal Communication

Young children become very adept at understanding nonverbal communication. They sense anxiety or fear by the rise in pitch of the parent's voice. Nodding of the head, using direct eye contact, tapping finger or foot, avoiding eye contact, and using sign language are nonverbal symbols. Sometimes nonverbal behaviors are necessary to receive confirmation from the children in return. Children are very sensitive to nonverbal cues.

CHILD MALTREATMENT

The maltreatment of children is a complicated and prevalent problem in today's society. The problem of maltreatment is not confined to one specific race, religion, or socioeconomic level. Although certain groups have higher reported rates of abuse, this problem occurs in every level of society. *Child maltreatment* is a broad term used to describe physical and emotional neglect and physical, emotional, and sexual abuse of children. In recent years, the rates of reported cases of child maltreatment has increased dramatically. The 2018 statistics from the US Department of Health and Human Services' (DHHS) Children's Bureau showed that nearly 678,000 children were abused or neglected. The leading age of the victims was from birth to one year of age. The rates of abuse were slightly higher for girls, but deaths from abuse were higher in boys. Unfortunately, many cases of child maltreatment are insidious and go undetected and unreported. Most reports of maltreatment are made by professionals, such as nurses. Nurses need to be aware that the suspicion of abuse (not the confirmation of abuse) requires reporting through appropriate channels. This is part of the role of the nurse.

Recently, the DHHS began collecting data for a newly identified type of maltreatment, sex trafficking. **Sex trafficking** is "a type of maltreatment that refers to the recruitment, harboring, transportation, provision, or obtaining of a person for the purpose of a commercial sex act" (DHHS, 2020).

CHILD NEGLECT

Neglect can be divided into two broad categories: physical neglect and emotional neglect. *Physical neglect* is the failure of a parent or caretaker to supply a child with adequate food, clothing, shelter, education, or health care despite being financially able to do so or offered financial or other means to do so. *Emotional neglect,* in contrast, is the failure by a parent or caretaker to meet a child's needs for emotional nurturance, affection, and attention.

CHILD ABUSE

Child abuse can be divided into three broad categories: physical, emotional, and sexual. *Physical abuse* is the intentional infliction of physical injury on a child, usually by the child's caregiver. *Emotional abuse* is the intentional attempt by a parent or caretaker to impair or destroy the mental or emotional state of a child. *Sexual abuse* is defined as commission of a sexual offense by a person responsible for the child's care, such as a parent, relative, acquaintance of the family, or babysitter, against a child who is dependent or developmentally immature, for the purpose of the perpetrator's own sexual stimulation or gratification.

Sadly, statistics show that in 2018, 15.5% of abused children experienced more than one type of maltreatment. Of the remaining children experiencing abuse, the most common single form of maltreatment was neglect (DHHS, 2020).

SEX TRAFFICKING

In 2015 a bill was introduced to address the problems of sex trafficking, The Justice for Victims of Trafficking Act of 2015. When it became a federal law, it updated criminal penalties for offenses, provided for care and services for victims, and outlined requirements for states to report data. The law also redefined the Victims of Child Abuse Act of 1990 to include child pornography and human trafficking within the definition of "child abuse." Child Protective Services (CPS) is the agency that investigates the caregivers in abuse cases. In the context of sex trafficking, the perpetrator usually does not have a family or custodial relationship with the victim. Repeated, deliberate relocation of the victim is used to perpetuate the crime. This law encourages states to involve CPS, even though the victimizer is generally not the caregiver. It also allows for an expanded definition of "child abuse" to include older victims if it is before their 24th birthday.

The earliest data became available in 2018. Not all states participated, some provided incomplete data, and they may have only had a few months to report. Despite these severe limitations in data reporting, 741 victims of child sex trafficking were identified. Although the majority of sex trafficking victims are female, over 10% of the victims identified were male. Unlike the other types of child maltreatment, older children are at a greater risk. Racial demographics of the victims were mostly white (41.6%), black (23.5%), or Hispanic (19.3%). It will take years to get a clearer picture of the scope of the problem, how to prevent sex trafficking, and how to best meet the needs of victims (DHHS, 2020). In the meantime, nurses can continue to play a key role as reporters of suspected sex trafficking, including the expanded definition of a child in this type of abuse.

Etiology

Many factors contribute to the cause of child maltreatment, including parental, child, and situational factors. Parental factors include the parent's culture (see the Cultural Considerations box); socialization history and history of abuse as a child; the parent's age and developmental level; attitudes toward the child and child rearing; knowledge of normal child behavior and development; and the parent's psychological state. Characteristics of the child sometimes place the child at risk for maltreatment. Many factors—including temperament, age, exceptional physical needs, disabilities, and health or behavior problems—have the potential to increase the potential for maltreatment by a parent or caretaker. Situational factors include sources of stress and support within the family's environment. Other factors sometimes present include marital problems, financial difficulties, drug or alcohol abuse, lack of social support or the inability of the parent or caretaker to ask for support, poor social network, and poor relationships with extended families. These factors have the power to increase the potential for an abusive reaction by adding stress to an environment in which a parent or caretaker is already lacking resources.

Child maltreatment in the form of sex trafficking needs additional data to determine the etiology. Sex trafficking is different from other types of maltreatment because the perpetrator of the abuse is generally not a parent or other person designated to care for the child. The victims are primarily older children. It is generally accepted that internet contact, grooming, and initial recruitment of children play a role in the entry into sex trafficking. Frequent relocation and isolation are key in maintaining the abusive situation. Ultimately, the etiology of sex trafficking is the traffickers themselves as they exploit and increase the vulnerabilities of their victims.

 Cultural Considerations

Child Abuse

Uninformed health professionals run the risk of mistaking many cultural practices for evidence of child abuse. An understanding of these practices is important, yet the family should be informed that the practices are possibly harmful and may place them in jeopardy with Child Protective Services. Examples of such practices include coining (repeatedly rubbing the edge of a coin on a child's skin, producing welts, to rid the body of a disease) and moxibustion (practice of burning small areas of the skin to treat temper tantrums and enuresis).

Clinical Manifestations

Children who have been abused or neglected often manifest certain physical or behavioral indicators that suggest maltreatment. Table 31.6 summarizes these manifestations.

Nursing Interventions

The most important role for any health care provider, especially nurses, is the identification of a child who is

Table 31.6   Clinical Manifestations of Possible Child Maltreatment

BEHAVIORAL INDICATORS	PHYSICAL INDICATORS
Physical Neglect	
Begging or stealing food Extended stays at school Fatigue or listlessness at school Delinquency Alcohol or drug abuse	Failure to thrive (the abnormal retardation of growth and development of the infant resulting from conditions that interfere with normal metabolism, appetite, and activity) Lag in growth and development Consistent hunger Poor personal hygiene Inappropriate dress for season Unattended medical needs Abandonment
Physical Abuse	
Frequent injuries explained as accidents Conflicting stories about the "accident" or injury from the parents or others Wary of contacts with parents or other adults Apprehension when other children cry Fear of parents or going home Concealing clothing worn to hide injuries Low self-esteem Suicide attempts	Ecchymosis, welts, and bite marks Ecchymosis reflecting the shape of object used to inflict injury (electrical cord, belt buckle, iron, radiator, or a hand) Evidence of human bites Lacerations or abrasions Burns that are symmetric and have no "splash marks" Cigar or cigarette burns on soles, palms, back, or buttocks Fractures: • To skull, nose, or face • Multiple or spiral • Various stages of healing • Discovered during examination, not reported by caretaker
Sexual Abuse	
Nonspecific symptoms such as sleep disturbances or abdominal pain noted by provider Promiscuous behavior Unwillingness to change for gym Withdrawal, fantasy, or infantile behavior Age-inappropriate sexual knowledge Poor peer relationships Delinquency Prostitution Forcing of sexual acts on other children Fear of being touched Suicide attempts Low self-esteem Excessive or public masturbation Declining school performance	Difficulty in walking or sitting Torn, stained, or bloody underclothing Pain or pruritus in genital area Ecchymosis or bleeding in external genitalia, vaginal, or anal areas Ecchymosis to the hard or soft palate Sexually transmitted diseases in preteens Adolescent pregnancy Enuresis or encopresis Vaginal or penile discharge Foreign bodies in vagina or rectum Presence of semen Recurrent urinary tract infections
Emotional Neglect and Abuse	
Stranger anxiety Emotional withdrawal Inappropriate fearfulness Delinquency Lag in emotional and intellectual development Language difficulties Suicide attempts	Failure to thrive Feeding difficulties Enuresis or encopresis Sleep disturbances

being maltreated. Often the nurse is the first person to interact with the child and the parent. A thorough history and physical examination are the most effective diagnostic tools in recognizing a child who has been abused or neglected. A behavioral or physical indicator of maltreatment should be a cue to investigate further because these indicators rarely appear as single factors. Carefully document any manifestations of

abuse in the medical record, along with the caretaker's explanation for these findings. When documenting, use direct quotes, and report only objective findings. Pay special attention to injuries that are unexplained or inconsistent with the parent's or caretaker's explanation of how the injury was incurred.

If abuse is suspected, the child and the parent must be questioned separately. A child rarely betrays a parent and admits the abuse. Even the most battered of children remain loyal to the *perpetrators* (those guilty of committing the act). The use of drawings, play, diagrams, and anatomically correct dolls sometimes help a child to express what has happened.

All states have regulations for the mandatory reporting of child maltreatment when a health professional has reason to suspect that child abuse or neglect has occurred or is occurring. The professional does not need to be certain or prove that a child has been maltreated; it is enough for the reporter to distrust or doubt the caretaker's explanation of what has been observed in the child. Many states have a toll-free number where reports are taken by a state central registry and then referred to the social services office in the locality where the child resides. All health care providers are obliged to be alert to, assess, and report any abusive situations to proper authorities.

If the child needs hospitalization as a result of the abuse, a nonjudgmental attitude must be maintained toward the parents or caretakers. Establishing a rapport with the family promotes a trusting and open relationship between you and the parents. The hospitalization provides a unique opportunity to demonstrate positive caretaking activities and offer education through role modeling. Consistency in the caregivers assigned to the child is important. Explain all procedures and treatment to the child to prevent the child from misinterpreting invasive or painful events. If the child is to return to the parents' care, integrate their participation into the daily routine. In this situation, document interactions between the child and the parents in an objective and factual manner.

Prevention of child maltreatment is an area in which the nurse can play an active role. During the prenatal period, identify any families at risk for abuse and refer them for intervention. During the child's health care visits, identify families at risk when you observe behaviors indicating a lack of understanding of the child's care requirements or when the support systems available to the family in stress are assessed. Encourage parents to search for and make use of resources that provide supportive services. Reinforcement of positive caretaking behaviors is an effective way of affirming positive parenting practices.

HOSPITALIZATION OF A CHILD

Hospitalization is an anxiety-producing experience for children and their families, primarily because of a basic fear of not knowing what will occur. It creates an interruption in the child's normal development. Every member of the family is affected by the hospitalization because of the disruption it brings about in routines. Hospitalization is often the first crisis children face. How a child deals with this crisis is influenced by developmental age, previous illness experience, separation coping skills, seriousness of the illness, and support of parents and staff. An experience sometimes can be made less traumatic with *anticipatory guidance,* explanations and preparation to help relieve fear and anxiety. However, infants and toddlers are not able to understand; therefore, separation is especially painful for them. Preparation for a scheduled admission is possible; however, emergencies arise, and unplanned hospitalizations occur. In those instances, always give explanations whenever possible and as soon as feasible to avoid aggravating an already traumatic situation.

Adequate preparation makes the transition from the security of a home to the unfamiliar atmosphere of a hospital less difficult. When it is best to begin preparation and how much information is right to give varies. The age of the child has a significant influence. A physician provides a family with details about a treatment plan, the length of stay, and expected results or outcomes. Parents then can reinforce the information by providing explanations to the child, using simple, age-appropriate terms. Usually time and opportunity are available before the actual admission for the child to talk about what will occur.

PREADMISSION PROGRAMS

Many hospitals have orientation programs for children who are to be admitted. In some hospitals, nurses conduct preadmission programs; other hospitals use *child life specialists* (health care professionals with extensive knowledge of child growth and development and the special emotional needs of children who are hospitalized).

The programs are based on the child's level of understanding and stage of development, with the purpose of familiarizing the child with hospital surroundings. These programs help to dismiss the child's fantasies and correct misconceptions. The programs include tours and audiovisual aids, such as movies, videos, and puppet shows. The child is given simple explanations of equipment used during surgery and hospitalization.

It is helpful for children to handle some of the items they will see while hospitalized, such as masks and gowns, stethoscopes, anesthesia masks, and syringes (without the needles attached). Be sure time is allowed for questions. Encourage children to talk about what they have seen or heard so that you can identify problem areas or areas of concern. Some hospitals distribute coloring books or storybooks that focus on the information covered in the orientation program. This material reinforces information and helps parents answer their child's questions. Many programs send the parents away with a brochure that describes hospital routines and lists items the hospital permits children to bring with them to the hospital. Keep written information simple, clear, and at an understandable level.

Timing of the orientation is important. Enough advance time must be allowed for the child to be able

Communication

Developmental Considerations: Communicating Effectively With Young Children

INFANTS

- Consider your body language, such as gestures and posture, and the pitch, intonation, and intensity of your voice.
- Nonverbal approaches work especially well for infants, with cuddling, patting, or some other form of gentle physical contact often quieting them.
- Maintain a calm voice and avoid sudden, loud noises. The actual words spoken are not as important as the way they are spoken.
- Because infants often begin fearing strangers at ages as young as 6 months, holding out the hands and asking the older infant to "come over" is seldom successful. If handling is necessary, the best approach is to pick up the infant firmly without using gestures.
- Infants are usually more at ease when upright and in visual contact with and proximity to their parents.

PRESCHOOL AND YOUNG SCHOOL-AGE CHILDREN

- Avoid quick approaches with preschool and young school-age children. Let them make the first move whenever possible.
- Broad smiles and other facial contortions sometimes have a threatening appearance.
- Avoid extended eye contact until after the child is comfortable.
- Position yourself at the child's eye level. You appear less threatening to the child, and you deemphasize the child's smallness.
- Children are often more responsive when they remain close to the parent, such as when they sit on the parent's lap.
- New or intimidating situations, such as hospitalization, are potentially stressful; thus, children have even more difficulty grasping the new words they encounter in this environment, even simple words that express unfamiliar ideas. Avoid use of expressions with dual meanings, such as "put to sleep."
- Substitute words that have potentially threatening interpretations with words that are less emotionally charged, such as replacing "stick" with "gently slide," or "hurt" with "feel uncomfortable."

OLDER SCHOOL-AGE CHILDREN

- Give children an opportunity to express their thoughts, concerns, and feelings. Listen and respond to underlying messages rather than just verbal content. Be attentive, try not to interrupt, and avoid making comments that convey disapproval or surprise.
- Avoid prying, asking embarrassing questions, and lecturing when giving advice.

ADOLESCENTS

- Be prepared to deal with a wide range of emotions and behaviors with adolescents. Give concrete explanations that focus on the teenager's concerns. Recognize that the adolescent's capacity to think in abstract terms increases with age.
- Fluency in teen jargon is not necessary, but ask for clarification when necessary.
- To enhance communication, exchange information without using questions that back the teenager into a corner. Initially confine discussions to less-threatening topics to allow time for trust to develop.
- Ask broad, open-ended questions before specific questions, such as "How's school?" before asking, "What is the best (or worst) thing about school?"

to assimilate the information after the program, but not so much time that the child forgets the information. Generally, the younger the child, the shorter the period between when the child is told about pending hospitalization and the actual admission date. Usually, a toddler is told only days before. However, school-age children have a better understanding of time and the future; therefore, they can be told that they are going to the hospital "in 2 weeks." Tell adolescents as far in advance as possible to allow them time to inform peers and solicit their support.

Children must be allowed to prepare for this new experience in their own way. This preparation involves telling friends and selecting pictures of family members, toys, or clothes they wish to take, if they are permitted. Packing a bag with these items reinforces the event's reality.

Parents also benefit from such orientation programs. They receive information that is helpful in answering a child's questions at home. Printed materials provide parents a reference guide for reviewing what the child has been told.

Emergency Admission

An emergency admission, in contrast to a well-planned and well-prepared-for admission, thrusts the child into an unknown environment with strange equipment, frightening sounds, and many unfamiliar adults. The incident that results in the hospitalization usually is sudden, serious, and possibly painful. The speed with which a health team responds to the emergency is critical, and little time is available for explanations. Whenever possible, explain to the child and family what is happening. This can prevent an escalating crisis situation. When the child is stable and awake, assess the child's perception of what happened, correct any misconceptions, and provide information not given initially.

ADMISSION

Confidentiality is important while interviewing the hospitalized pediatric patient and is particularly important with adolescents when they have concerns related to issues such as substance use or sexual behaviors.

Adolescents are more likely to participate in health care services when caring, respectful professionals are the ones providing them. Characteristics of good providers include compassion, warmth, understanding, an ability to communicate with the adolescent, a willingness to be straightforward and honest, and competency.

Pediatric units are usually bright, colorful, and cheery areas with cartoon figures on the walls (or ceilings of treatment rooms), many pictures, and large photographs of sports figures and popular singers. Often the unit or room is decorated to reflect the age group admitted there. For example, an infant and toddler unit usually has many age-appropriate toys, high chairs, playpens, and strollers. A typical adolescent area has a lounge with a television, video games, DVD player, CD player, and computers with age-appropriate software and Internet access. To decrease anxiety, most hospitals try to make the pediatric environment different from adult units and include many items that are found in the child's normal home or school environment.

First impressions are important and have the potential to color the child's entire hospital stay. Therefore, be sure to greet children warmly and welcome them by name when they arrive on the unit. After they see their room and meet their roommate(s), give them a tour of the unit. Two important locations to point out are the area in which snacks or liquid refreshments are available and the playroom (or activity room when speaking to adolescents), where they will spend time when allowed out of bed. The play area is a safe, secure place for children. It contains an assortment of toys, games, and crafts for diversional activities. Newly admitted children also need explanations about when meals are served, how to operate the bed, and how to communicate with nurses by using a call bell or intercommunication system.

Sometimes anxiety levels about a hospital admission are high. Perhaps heart surgery is scheduled or a brain tumor is suspected. In those instances, a tour or an in-depth orientation may be postponed. The development of a therapeutic relationship with the family very possibly seems more important because it has the potential to affect the entire course of a hospitalization. Inform parents that a tour and further orientation are available and that the timing of such events is the parent's choice.

After the child is admitted, obtain a nursing history. An identification bracelet, usually worn on the wrist, is important to verify identity when medications are given, or procedures are done. Often these bands are placed on the ankles of infants and toddlers because they are curious about items on their wrists. When applying the band, allow enough space for one finger to fit between the band and the skin. Be sure the band is not constrictive and check the skin underneath for its integrity.

Assess vital signs, including blood pressure. Measure and record the height (or length for infants) and weight. These are important baseline data. The height and weight are used in calculating a child's body surface area, especially when treating a child with burns or in calculating fluid and electrolyte requirements. Most medical centers use body weight in kilograms to compute drug dosages. An important nursing responsibility is identifying the scale used to weigh a child, if more than one is available, so that all staff use the same scale for subsequent weighings.

A laboratory technician draws routine blood samples on all newly admitted infants and children. Some hospitals make efforts to reduce the number of "sticks" a child receives by coordinating various physician requests whenever possible. A urine specimen also typically is collected. The laboratory values provide a physician with baseline information and are sometimes diagnostic. The physician orders additional x-ray examinations or procedures as appropriate to the child's specific health problem.

HOSPITAL POLICIES

Changes in hospitals' policies over recent years reflect their changed attitude toward parents. Most hospitals no longer consider parents "visitors" and welcome their presence throughout the child's hospitalization. Many hospitals have developed a system of family-centered care. This philosophy of care validates the integral role of the family in a child's life and acknowledges the family as an essential part of the child's care and illness experience. In this kind of system, the family becomes a partner in the care of the child.

Hospitalization is especially traumatic to very young children, and the presence of supportive parents increases their feelings of security. The typical fear and apprehension children experience when they are isolated from their parents and family is known as *separation anxiety* and causes major stress for the hospitalized child, especially between ages 15 and 30 months. Many hospitals have facilities that allow one parent to live in or room in, which means a parent can stay 24 hours a day. Make parents aware that beds, meals, and shower facilities are available for their use. Allowing parents or other family members to stay with the pediatric patient alleviates stress and is therapeutic for the patient.

Parents who are involved in care have a sense of contributing to the child's recovery, which is an important consideration. The presence of a parent increases the available teaching opportunities. It also enables the nurse to assess a family's strengths, needs, and potential problem areas. However, parents need time to relax and to get away from the child's bedside periodically. Rooming-in is sometimes an exhausting experience. Parents need breaks and relief to remain effective in supporting the child. Hospitals with a family-centered philosophy set aside a room or other specified area on the nursing unit for parents where they have the chance to socialize, support each other, and share their thoughts. Note that the presence of parents does not mean that nurses give up their responsibilities in caring for these children.

Some hospitals allow children to wear their own clothes, which is especially important for a hospitalized adolescent. However, if a child is scheduled for surgery or needs an IV line, hospital gowns usually are required.

DEVELOPMENTAL SUPPORT FOR THE CHILD

Hospitalization not only interrupts children's normal routines but also threatens their normal developmental process. Children often regress when hospitalized. For instance, some young school-age children resume the practice of thumb sucking. Often regression persists for several months after a child is discharged.

Some of the traumatic effects of hospitalization on a child's normal development can be alleviated or even eliminated in several ways. A child's developmental level influences his or her understanding and response to hospitalization. Strategies for supporting children are likely to be more effective when developmental concerns and needs are considered (Table 31.7).

Take particular care to meet the psychosocial needs of children with special needs who are hospitalized. Because of the nature of their conditions, these children are even more likely to experience invasive and traumatic procedures during frequent and lengthy hospital stays. These factors result in a group of children more vulnerable to the emotional and developmental consequences of hospitalization.

PAIN MANAGEMENT

Health care professionals, including nurses, tend to underestimate pain in children. Some people falsely believe that infants or young children are not able to feel pain. Another explanation for this tendency is a misconception of what playing, reading, or any other activity means about a child's comfort level. Anything that is painful to adults should be assumed to be painful to infants and children. Children, like adults, engage in activities for distraction, as a method of coping with pain. These behaviors do not signal the absence of pain.

Pain is known commonly as the fifth vital sign, and it must be documented during each shift assessment. A critical component in management of pain is its assessment. However, pain assessment, especially for

Table 31.7	Age-Related Concerns and Needs of Children Who Are Hospitalized	
CONCERNS	**POSSIBLE RESPONSES**	**POSITIVE PARENT AND NURSE RESPONSES**
Infancy		
Anxiety is common during this age because of separation from the parent(s).	Bonding is often an issue as well as distrust; skills may be delayed because of anxiety experienced by the infant.	Encourage rooming in of parent(s); teach parents procedures they are capable of being taught to perform; assign the same nurse when possible to maintain consistency.
Toddler/Preschool		
Separation from parents is a major issue because of stranger fear and separation anxiety. The toddler fears bodily injury and pain.	It is common for the hospitalized toddler to be uncooperative, throw temper tantrums, and show regression in behavior.	Praise for appropriate behavior (e.g., dressing or feeding self); set appropriate limits on negative behavior and encourage parents to do so; encourage home routines and rituals, such as bedtime stories.
School-Age		
The school-age child is concerned with bodily injury related to medical procedures. In addition to anxiety resulting from separation from parents, the school-age child also is anxious from separation from friends and school, and other family members.	The school-age child may show some level of regression. In addition, anger, acts of aggression, boredom, isolation, and withdraw from family may occur.	Encourage friends and family to visit and/or encourage talking to them on the phone if visits are not possible; ensure homework is obtained for child if condition permits; include the child in decision making.
Adolescence		
Adolescence is a time for establishment of identity. Inability to interact with peers is especially difficult during this time. Loss of control and fear of the unknown are paramount during this phase.	Rejection of the parents is a common reaction as well as being uncooperative and regression in regard to coping behaviors. Fear and anxiousness are typical reactions.	Always include the adolescent in decisions; encourage visits from peers or talking to them on the phone; in some situations the adolescent does not want the parent to be present as much as with previous ages.

Data modified from *http://www.austincc.edu/adnlev3/ol_hosp_child/care_plans_psychosocial_need.htm*.

MY PAIN RATING SCALE*

Please keep a record of how well your child's pain medicines are working. Rate your child's pain before and after pain medicine is given.

0	1	2	3	4	5
No Hurt	Hurts Little Bit	Hurts Little More	Hurts Even More	Hurts Whole Lot	Hurts Worst

Explain to your child that each face is for a person who has no hurt (pain) or some or a lot of hurt (pain). Point to each face and say the words under the face. Ask the child to pick the face that best describes how much hurt he (or she) has. Record the number of that face in the Pain Rating column. If your child's pain is above 2, or if you have other concerns with pain, let your nurse or physician know.

Date and time	Pain rating	Medicine I took	Side effects, such as drowsiness or upset stomach

Fig. 31.8 Wong-Baker FACES Pain Rating Scale. Explain to the patient that each face is for a person who feels happy because he has no pain (hurt) or sad because he has some or a lot of pain. Face 0 is very happy because he does not hurt at all. Face 1 hurts just a little bit. Face 2 hurts a little more. Face 3 hurts even more. Face 4 hurts a whole lot. Face 5 hurts as much as you can imagine, although you do not have to be crying to feel this bad. Ask the patient to choose the face that best describes now how he or she is feeling. Recommended for children ages 3 years or older. (From Wong-Baker FACES Foundation (2020). Wong-Baker FACES® Pain Rating Scale. Retrieved January 27, 2021, with permission from www.WongBakerFACES.org . Originally published in Whaley & Wong's Nursing Care of Infants and Children. © Elsevier Inc.)

children who have limited cognitive and language skills, continues to be a challenge for health care providers. The pain that occurs in a child and the intensity of the pain are often difficult to ascertain. Infants are not able to verbalize that they are in pain or the pain's location. Rely on physiologic variables and behavioral variables, such as vocalization, facial expressions, and body movements. Pain assessment tools such as the Wong-Baker FACES Pain Rating Scale (Fig. 31.8) are helpful in the assessment of pain in children. Remember that some children are reluctant to let you know they are experiencing pain for fear of getting pain medication via injection. Advocate for IV analgesic administration, particularly when IV lines are already in place, and promote oral analgesic administration as soon as possible.

Reasons other than inaccurate pain assessment also lead to undertreatment of pain in children. Fear of respiratory depression or addiction sometimes means that a child does not receive an adequate amount of analgesic, does not receive it often enough, or is not considered a candidate for certain opioids. Although respiratory depression is a possible side effect with opioids in children older than 3 months of age (and possibly younger), opioids cause no greater respiratory depression than in adults. As for addiction, nothing indicates that children are at any increased risk of physiologic or psychological dependence from the use of opioids for pain management.

In addition to learning to assess pain accurately in children and advocating for and administering adequate analgesics, encourage parental presence and use sensitive care practices to lessen children's pain. Try integrating soothing talk or musical tapes into care practices. Infants often derive benefit from pacifiers, swaddling, rocking, or simply being held. Take care, whenever possible, to let the child's needs determine the timing of care routines, procedures, and tests. Also take appropriate action to reduce noise and other disturbing sensations to create a soothing and calming environment for the child in pain.

SURGERY

Undergoing a surgical procedure tends to be an especially stressful event for children and their families. Children who face surgery without information and preparation often develop misconceptions about the surgical event or any of the series of events that led up to or occur after surgery. Fantasies built on misconceptions typically lead to fears, which in turn often lead to negative reactions and long-term consequences, such as behavioral problems or an inability to trust others.

Table 31.8	Age-Related Fears Associated With Surgery	

AGE	PRIMARY CONCERNS	INTERVENTION
Younger than 5 years	What will happen when I wake up? Where will I be? Who will be with me?	Show recovery room, if possible. Tell when parents will visit after surgery. Encourage parents to be with child as soon as possible.
School-age	Anesthesia	Show mask.
Younger	That I might wake up during surgery	Explain "gas" or "medicine" and how it works.
Older	How doctor knows when, or if doctor knows how, to awaken me	Stress concept of "special sleep." Explain that it is a special person's job to control the sleep.
	Same as above plus the following: • Operation • Mutilation • Possible death	Same as above. Provide knowledge about procedure.
Adolescent	Same as above plus the following: • Special anxiety for change in body image • Loss of control while under anesthesia (in terms of behavior and for body integrity) • Peer reaction to scars • Effect on sexuality • Effect on adolescent mode of dress	Same as above. Reassure that only what is supposed to be done will be performed. Introduce to peer with similar surgery.

Preparing a child for surgery entails providing information to parents and child about what will happen and what the child will experience. Addressing the events surrounding surgery that are most difficult for children is a good place to begin. Six stress points are common for children undergoing surgery: (1) admission; (2) blood tests; (3) the afternoon of the day before surgery; (4) injection of preoperative medication; (5) the moments before and during transport to the operating room; and (6) return from the postanesthesia care unit (PACU). Think through each stress point from the child's perspective and develop an individualized preparation plan. Explain the hospital system to the parents and inform them of the operation's progress.

Age influences the types of fears and concerns a child is likely to experience regarding surgery. Table 31.8 lists common age-related fears and effective interventions. Use of children's ages as a guide increases the likelihood that children are prepared adequately for surgery and all the surrounding events.

PARENT PARTICIPATION

An effective working relationship with parents must be established as soon as possible. Parents are the most significant individuals to a child. Also, they know their child better than anyone else and often play an important role in assessing the child's responses. Therefore, take care to project a positive attitude toward parents: give them a warm greeting, smile, and establish eye contact. Gain the trust of the parents by: (1) reviewing and interpreting information from the physician as needed; (2) asking the parents whether they have any questions; (3) conveying concern for the parents' well-being; (4) listening and being available; and (5) respecting them as experts on their child and soliciting their

input. These activities are time consuming, and yet for a nurse who works with families, they are some of the most satisfying.

When obtaining a nursing history, select a quiet place on the unit to listen to parents' responses and to provide them with opportunities to ask questions. Even if the physician sees the reason for hospitalization as minor, in some cases a parent perceives it as very serious. Parents experience fear and anxiety because of the seriousness of the illness, the procedures involved, or the pain the child will experience. Their apprehension then is transmitted to the child. Therefore, convey interest and concern and try to decrease their anxieties.

Parents experience a series of reactions when a child is hospitalized. They too are in an unfamiliar environment, meeting different groups of people who ask many questions and give them much information. Perhaps the tests or procedures mentioned are unknown to them. They may become frustrated because they do not understand much of what is being told to them. Parents often do not know hospital rules and regulations and what is expected of them. They lose control in this setting and feel powerless. To this point, they alone have cared for their son or daughter. Now a nurse assumes control over the child's care. If an accident is the cause for hospitalization, parents sometimes blame themselves and feel guilty.

On admission, parents need specific information on routines, hospital policies that affect them, any limitations that exist, and what is expected of them. When parents receive information that they can apply immediately, their anxiety levels decrease and they feel more comfortable. When the emotional needs of a parent are met, that parent is better able to support the child (Box 31.10).

| Box 31.10 | Factors That Affect Parents' Reactions to Their Child's Illness |

- Seriousness of the threat to the child
- Previous experience with illness or hospitalization
- Medical procedures involved in diagnosis and treatment
- Available support systems
- Personal ego strengths
- Previous coping abilities
- Additional stresses on the family system
- Cultural and religious beliefs
- Communication patterns among family members

Later, be sure to explain to the parents any diagnostic tests, medications, or procedures that the physician plans. Keep in mind that anxiety and the sheer volume of information they have to absorb sometimes results in parents becoming confused or forgetting what they have heard. Any change in plans has the potential to generate anxiety and result in a parent being unable to process the information. Be sure to explain the tests and treatments thoroughly. Offer information several times to the parents, if necessary, to be certain they fully comprehend it.

As the parents' comfort increases, they become more involved in meeting their child's physical needs. Mothers tend to spend more time with their hospitalized children and participate early in providing care. Fathers are often more reluctant, so encourage them to become involved. When parents participate, they contribute to the child's recovery. Another strategy is to ask for parents' assistance in establishing goals or revising a care plan.

The equipment that surrounds a child is often overwhelming, with the strange-sounding alarms or with electrodes placed on different parts of the child's body (Fig. 31.9). When the function of a monitor or some other device is explained, it often becomes less threatening. However, use terms the parent can understand.

Initially parents watch the nurse perform a procedure for their child. When the nurse describes what is being done and why, parents become more interested. Information exchange, demonstrations, and teaching motivate parents to perform the procedure and improve their overall confidence in caregiving activities. Parents often become skillful in performing a variety of technical skills if taught in a patient, nonthreatening manner. Some activities in which parents become involved include gastrostomy tube feedings, tracheostomy suctioning, and subcutaneous injections.

Be sure parents are confident and knowledgeable in their ability to perform given tasks in their child's care and encourage them to participate only in as many activities as they feel comfortable performing. Generally, the extent of parental involvement is a good measure of the nurse's effectiveness as a teacher.

Fig. 31.9 A parent can easily feel overwhelmed by the equipment that surrounds an infant.

The last phase of adaptation for parents of a child who is hospitalized relates to discharge. Do not postpone teaching until the time of discharge. Teaching begins at admission and is an ongoing process throughout the hospitalization. The child often has some activity restrictions, care requirements, or ongoing follow-up after discharge, but after you have instructed them and ascertained their competence, parents usually are able to provide any nursing interventions that are needed at home.

COMMON PEDIATRIC PROCEDURES

Some of the following procedures are for general care of children and procedures that healthy children experience in the home. Others take place primarily in health care settings. Many events that are common in health care settings are sometimes frightening for children. As is appropriate to the child's age, prepare children and their parents for all procedures, even those that you consider insignificant. Preparing children for procedures increases their cooperation, helps them cope, and promotes a sense of self-esteem and mastery.

A sensation-based approach is the most effective method of preparation. Provide information about what the child is likely to feel, see, smell, hear, or taste, along with emotions commonly experienced. For example, children scheduled for x-ray examinations or computed tomographic (CT) scans perhaps feel frightened, anxious, guilty ("Am I being punished for being bad?"), powerless, or curious. The sights they see probably include a "big machine" or "camera" over them and a lead shield or apron on themselves, the x-ray technician, and a parent if present. They hear noises of the machine "buzzing" and the sliding of x-ray plates. The room and the table most likely feel cold, and the lead shield heavy.

Timing is important in preparing the child. Young children are usually best to prepare close to the time of the procedure. Older children may be prepared further in advance. Preparation just before less-complicated procedures, such as injections, finger sticks, or vital sign assessments, is acceptable for children of all ages.

BATHING

Bathing the child provides the nurse with the opportunity to do a complete skin assessment. When giving a bath, protect the infant from drafts and chilling. Usually the best time to bathe the infant is before a feeding to avoid stimulating regurgitation or vomiting. Check the water temperature. If the umbilical cord is still attached, give a sponge bath. Clean the cord and keep it dry. Some providers may recommend cleaning the area around it with alcohol, which may help to dry the cord and prevent infection.

Use only water to clean areas around the eyes. Use a mild soap on the rest of the body; start with the face and move downward. Expose, wash, rinse, and dry one section of the body thoroughly before bathing another area. A baby's creases need special attention. Babies have very short necks; if they are not cleaned and dried thoroughly, skin impairment is possible.

If a sponge bath is given at the bedside, place the infant across the width of the bed facing you. This practice allows greater control of any movement by the baby and decreases the likelihood of the baby rolling out of the crib. Never use cotton-tipped applicators to clean the ear canal because injuries are possible; a washcloth is adequate. Give special care to the genitalia. In females, separate the labia and wash them in the anterior-to-posterior direction. Wash the penis and the scrotum of a circumcised male. In an uncircumcised male, daily external washing and rinsing are all that is necessary. It is best not to attempt to retract the foreskin because it is almost always attached to the glans. Forcing the foreskin back risks harm to the penis, causing pain, bleeding, and possibly adhesions. No ointments or powders usually are advised.

Infants enjoy being placed in basins or bathtub seats for baths. After washing the baby's face, lather the trunk and extremities. When placing the infant in the basin, use dry hands to pick up the infant more securely. The head needs the support of one hand; use the other hand to rinse the infant. Allow the baby to play and splash the water, which encourages

development. After the infant is removed from the basin, wrap the infant in a towel and dry the infant thoroughly.

Hold the infant "football style" when washing the infant's head. In this position, the infant's hip rests on your hip. Your hand supports the baby's head, and the baby's back rests on your forearm. This position allows the infant to look at your face while the hair is washed. After the hair is lathered well, rinse the head over the basin at the bedside. Sometimes parents ask about the baby's soft spot (anterior fontanelle) (a space, roughly diamond-shaped, covered by tough membranes between the bones of an infant's cranium; the posterior fontanelle is triangular). Assure them that the area is not injured by shampooing.

Most toddlers love to be placed in a tub for their baths. Provide toys for the child to use in splashing, water play, and bathing. For most young children, 15 to 30 minutes is enough time to allow them to enjoy themselves in a tub. Remember that water is fascinating to a toddler because it has no shape or form. Safety is an issue: never leave a child in a tub without supervision.

The school-age child sometimes is reluctant to bathe, and many children are not accustomed to a daily bath. With encouragement, children who are feeling fairly well usually participate in their daily care. Use judgment of the child's physical and mental condition and advice from the child's parents to determine how much supervision a particular child needs.

Most adolescents become accustomed to bathing or showering as part of their daily routine. The need for an underarm deodorant usually becomes evident during puberty. Privacy when bathing and dressing is paramount during the teenage years.

FEEDINGS

Breast-Feeding

Breast milk is the preferred nutrition for the full-term infant, and a mother should be encouraged to continue breast-feeding her baby who is ill or hospitalized. Assist the mother by providing a quiet environment and a comfortable chair for her to sit in when nursing her baby. Some mothers are unable to be present for every feeding, or the baby is unable to take milk directly from the breast. Encourage the mother in this case to use a breast pump and provide a private place for this activity. Bottles of breast milk may be frozen and given later by bottle or tube feeding.

Bottle Feeding

The correct position for feeding an infant is one that is comfortable for adult and infant. The caregiver holds the infant securely. Place a table or stand within arm's reach so that it is possible to set the bottle aside while *burping* (inducing belching or eructation) the baby. If a burp is not elicited by one position, try another.

Hold the bottle so that formula fills the nipple entirely to decrease the amount of air the baby swallows in the course of the feeding. Infants are not able to push the bottle voluntarily away when finished, so feed them only as much as they actively consume to prevent overfeeding. During the feeding, remove the bottle and burp the infant periodically. Newborns need burping more often than older babies.

Burping and Finishing a Feeding

There are three common methods of burping an infant. One way is to place the infant in a sitting position on the lap. With one hand over the infant's chin and chest supporting the body as the infant leans forward, use the other to gently pat or rub the infant's back from the waist to the shoulders. The infant also may be placed flat across the lap, face down, with one hand used to rub or pat the back and the other hand used to secure the body. The third position is with the baby upright against the body, looking backward over the shoulder. One arm holds the baby, and the other hand is free to rub the infant's back from the waist to the shoulders. Once the baby has released any trapped air, resume the feeding if the baby has not yet finished. Repeat this process until the infant has consumed the desired amount, ending with burping.

After feeding, position the infant on the right side to permit the feeding to flow toward the lower end of the stomach and allow any swallowed air to rise above the fluid and through the esophagus. Place infants only on their back to sleep; this measure helps prevent sudden infant death syndrome (SIDS). The Academy of Pediatrics (2017) has recommended the use of a pacifier at naptime and bedtime as a protective mechanism against the incidence of SIDS during the first year of life.

Solids

When the infant starts solid food, assist the parent to learn the proper feeding position. The parent feeds the infant in an infant seat. Always secure the safety strap. In an infant seat, the baby can focus the eyes on the adult, and both hands of an adult are free to introduce solids to the infant. Once an infant achieves control, caregivers can hold the baby in their arms. Older infants (8 or 9 months old) can sit in a high chair with a safety strap in place. Additional support is sometimes necessary. Try rolling up baby blankets and placing them on either side of the infant's trunk.

Gavage

Some infants and children need gavage feedings. Gavage involves passing of a feeding tube through the nose or mouth, down the esophagus, and into the stomach. Although in many health care settings, nurses are required to have additional training before performing this function, the nurse usually assists with the tube placement and is permitted to perform the actual tube feedings.

To measure the tube before placing it, a qualified staff member uses one of the following procedures: (1) measure from the nose to the distal area of the earlobe and then to the end of the xiphoid process or (2) measure from the nose to the earlobe and then to a point midway between the xiphoid process and the umbilicus.

Some restraint of infant activity is likely to be necessary when passing the tube. Pulling up the bottom of the shirt over both arms is often all that is needed to restrain the newborn. Some infants may need to be wrapped in a mummy type of safety reminder device (SRD) before proceeding. (See the description of the mummy SRD in a later section.) In the unlikely event that a premature infant needs restraint, a small towel folded across the chest and secured beneath the shoulders is usually sufficient; take care not to compromise breathing.

Because infants are nose breathers, the mouth is the preferred route for tube insertion. The tube often is passed through the nose for older infants and children. Ask children who are able to understand to swallow while the tube is being inserted. A tube that will be indwelling is inserted almost always through the nose; to prevent irritation, use alternate nostrils for reinsertion. Once the tube is inserted, tape it in place. If the tube is inserted through a nostril, tape the tube to the cheek, not to the forehead, to prevent possible structural and cosmetic damage to the nostril.

Before feedings, check tube placement by (1) aspirating for stomach contents and (2) injecting a small amount of air (0.5 to 1 mL in premature or very small infants to 5 mL in larger children) through the syringe into the tube while simultaneously listening with a stethoscope over the stomach area for sounds of gurgling or growling. If any doubt exists about tube placement, do not proceed with feeding, and consult the practitioner. Sometimes radiographic data are necessary to confirm proper tube placement (see Chapters 15 and 19).

Whenever possible, hold the infant during the feeding. If this is impossible, position the infant or child on his or her back or toward the right side with the head and chest elevated. Give infants a pacifier during feedings to encourage sucking and help them associate sucking with satisfying hunger. Warm the formula to room temperature and, after a gentle push with the plunger, allow it to flow into the stomach via gravity. To prevent nausea and regurgitation, use rates of no more than 5 mL every 5 to 10 minutes in premature and very small infants and 10 mL per minute in older infants and children. At the completion of the feeding, flush the tube with sterile water (using from 1 or 2 mL for small tubes to 5 mL or more for large ones). Clamp or cap indwelling tubes after feeding. If the tube is to be removed, pinch it firmly to prevent escape of fluid and withdraw it quickly. Keep the child positioned on the right side for at least 1 hour to keep the possibility of regurgitation and aspiration to a minimum. Burp the infant if the medical condition permits. Record the type and the amount of feeding given and the child's response.

Gastrostomy

A gastrostomy tube (G tube) often is used in children in whom a nasogastric tube is contraindicated or in children who need tube feeding over an extended period. The physician places the tube during surgery when the child is under general anesthesia, or percutaneously with an endoscope with the child under local anesthesia. The practitioner inserts the tube through the abdominal wall into the stomach and secures it with a purse-string suture and anchors the stomach to the peritoneum at the operative site. Feeding is carried out in the same manner and rate as in gavage feeding. After feedings, place the child on the right side or in Fowler's position. The tube is left open and suspended or clamped between feedings, depending on the child's condition.

Total Parenteral Nutrition

When feeding by way of the GI tract is impossible, inadequate, or hazardous, total parenteral nutrition (TPN; also called IV alimentation or hyperalimentation) is an option. A highly concentrated solution of protein, glucose, and other nutrients is passed intravenously through conventional tubing with a special filter attached to remove particulate matter and microorganisms. Wide-diameter vessels, such as the subclavian vein, are the usual sites of infusion. In most health care settings, the nurse is required to have additional training before assisting with TPN. Nursing responsibilities include control of sepsis, monitoring of the infusion rate, and continuous observations. **Never** confuse this method of feeding with the use of "kangaroo" feedings, in which a mechanical pump is used to regulate the volume and rate of continuous gastric feedings per gastrostomy tube.

SAFETY REMINDER DEVICES

For safety reasons, children sometimes must be restrained after surgery or during a procedure or examination. SRDs are used only as a last resort. The SRD is used to ensure that safe care is given to the patient. The following clinical situations allow for the use of SRDs:

- Maintenance of oxygen therapy without interruption
- Protection from harm if child has an indwelling catheter, IV tubes, pacemaker wire, or sutures
- Patients who are confused, agitated, or unable to comprehend instructions (Leifer, 2019)

Make sure to apply the SRD correctly, and closely monitor circulation and skin integrity. Remove the

SRD every 2 hours to permit exercise of the body area. If you need to restrain the extremities, release them one at a time so that the child cannot pull out an IV or NG tube. Attach the ties of all SRDs to bed frames only, not to side rails.

Elbow Safety Reminder Devices

Elbow SRDs prevent flexion or bending of elbows. They allow an infant or toddler to move the upper extremities but prevent them from touching the head and neck area; thus, for example, they protect the newly repaired cleft lip or palate or scalp vein infusion site. Slip clean tongue blades into the parallel pockets of a wraparound SRD. Pull the shirt or pajama sleeve down to the wrist and place the elbow in the center of this SRD. Wrap the SRD around the arm and tie it securely. Cuff the sleeve over the bottom of the SRD to protect the skin. Check the axilla and the wrist routinely for skin impairment.

Mummy Safety Reminder Device

A mummy SRD is used when it is necessary to immobilize head, neck, trunk, and upper and lower extremities. A jugular venipuncture or the insertion of an NG tube sometimes calls for this type of SRD. Place a square baby blanket on a crib, and fold over one corner. Place the infant on his or her back on the blanket so that the shoulders are at the level of the fold and arms are at the sides. Wrap one corner of the blanket over the right arm and tuck it under the infant's left side. Place the opposite corner over the left arm and place it securely under the right side of the body (Fig. 31.10). A commercially prepared mummy SRD is also available.

A modified version sometimes is needed so that it is possible to expose the chest. While you place one corner of the blanket around the right arm and tuck it under the baby's body, encircle the left arm with the opposite corner and secure it too. Bring the corner beneath the feet up to the abdomen and pin it, thereby leaving the chest exposed.

Clove-Hitch Safety Reminder Device

This type of four-point SRD is for use on all extremities of a child. Rolls of Kerlix, roller bandage, or strips of muslin can be used. Pad the wrists and ankles with gauze squares or other soft material. A clove hitch is not a square knot. Make a figure-8 with the material, slip it over the padded wrist or ankle, and tighten it gently (see Chapter 10). Check each SRD frequently to be sure that circulation is not affected and pressure is not excessive. Use a slip knot to tie the ends of this SRD to the bed frame.

Jacket Safety Reminder Device

Sometimes a jacket SRD is needed to keep an extremely active older infant or toddler safely in bed or in a high

Fig. 31.10 Mummy restraint. (A) Fold material over the right arm, and then tuck the corner under the left side. (B) Fold the bottom up and the opposite corner over the infant's left arm. (C) Tuck it under the right side to secure it.

Table **31.9**   Advantages and Disadvantages of Various Oxygen-Delivery Systems

SYSTEM	ADVANTAGES	DISADVANTAGES
Oxygen mask	Delivers a more precise concentration of oxygen than the nasal cannula (most precise mask is the Venturi mask). Oxygen delivery is achieved even if child is a nose breather.	Patient unable to eat. Talking is muffled. Mask may be irritating to the face. Depending on the age of the child the mask may increase the chance of aspiration if patient vomits.
Nasal cannula	The child can eat and talk normally. Child is typically more compliant with nasal cannula than a mask because it is less intrusive.	Less precise concentration of oxygen delivered. Skin irritation is more likely along cheeks and over ears from tubing. May insert prongs in wrong direction, thus decreasing amount of oxygen received.
Oxygen tent	Child can eat and talk normally. Humidification easily achieved. Less intrusive than other devices.	Delivery of oxygen is interrupted when tent is open. May cause child to feel cold from moisture. Child may feel isolated in tent.
Oxygen hood, face tent	Less intrusive than a tent. Can administer higher concentration of oxygen than with a nasal cannula.	Child is unable to eat with hood or face tent. Excess moisture.

chair. It resembles a vest and has ties in the back. Pull the child's arms through the jacket and tie the jacket in the back. Attach the long ties to a bed frame or under the seat of a high chair. Although children are able to move all body parts, they cannot climb out of beds or high chairs.

OXYGEN THERAPY

Supplemental oxygen helps improve the child's respiratory status by increasing the amount of oxygen in the blood. It also is used in children who have cardiac or neurologic disorders. When administering oxygen to a newborn or infant, remember the harmful effects of oxygen on the developing pulmonary system. Oxygen is forced through sterile water to humidify it to counteract its drying effect. Check oxygen levels frequently (every 2 hours).

Monitor infants and children receiving oxygen with an oximeter, a flexible noninvasive photoelectric device with adhesive backing that is placed on the foot or the hand of an infant or the finger of an adolescent.

The monitoring screen gives an instant reading of the oxygen saturation of blood. Correlation is high between this measurement and the arterial oxygenation. Table 31.9 presents advantages and disadvantages of various oxygen delivery systems.

Hood and Incubator

Oxygen often is delivered to small infants through a plastic hood that fits over the baby's head. It is an efficient method of providing oxygen at well-controlled levels. More important, the body is accessible for starting an IV line or performing a procedure.

A less-efficient method of delivering oxygen to an infant is use of a closed incubator. Incubators have imperfectly fitted lids, uncovered vents, and portholes that must be opened to perform an activity on the infant, all of which contribute to fluctuations in oxygen levels. Maintenance of a constant temperature within the incubator is a problem as well. As an infant's metabolism increases in an effort to maintain body temperature, larger amounts of oxygen are needed.

Mist Tents

The purpose of a mist tent is to improve a child's respiratory status by liquefying pulmonary secretions. The child is observed easily through the plastic canopy. All of the device's working parts are outside of the tent, which is a distinct advantage when a toddler needs this form of therapy. Compressed air or oxygen runs through sterile water to form the therapeutic mist. A disadvantage is that the canopy must be opened for the treatments and procedures, which lowers the concentration of the mist.

Organize all activities and thus limit the number of times the tent is opened, to make maintenance of desired concentrations possible and to give the child longer rest periods. Tuck the tent under the mattress of a crib to maintain humidity levels. If the tent is functioning efficiently, dampness within it is significant, and frequent (every 3 to 4 hours) linen and clothing changes often are necessary.

Nasal Cannula

Delivery of oxygen to newborns and all ages of children is possible by means of a nasal cannula. This mode of delivery is used commonly with infants with conditions such as bronchopulmonary dysplasia (abnormal development of the bronchi and the lungs), respiratory syncytial (sin-SISH-uhl) virus (RSV), and bronchiolitis (inflammation and congestion of the bronchioles). Maintenance of the cannula's placement is often problematic in the infant, whose random head and hand movements disturb its position. Clear plastic tape or special adhesive anchoring devices that are less harmful to the delicate skin (Fig. 31.11) is placed around the oxygen tubing and over the nose and cheek and helps prevent this. Adjusting the device at the back of an infant's head allows the tubing to be fitted to the child and hooking it over the pinnae helps stabilize it. In older children, keep the nasal cannula in place by using the adjustable elastic straps on the child's head.

SUCTIONING

Patent airway maintenance sometimes necessitates suctioning. Air passages in children become occluded more commonly because of the small size of their respiratory tract structures. Signs that a child possibly needs suctioning include pallor; restlessness or anxiety; increased pulse, respiration, and temperature; dyspnea; bubbling (copious amounts of thin secretions); rattling (thick, tenacious secretions); drooling; mouth breathing; nasal flaring; grunting; gasping; retractions; cyanosis; and erythema (flushed face). Infants often have an anxious look in their eyes or fidget constantly. An older child perhaps constantly seeks attention with no explanation, tosses and turns in bed, or fingers the edge of a blanket.

Use suctioning when secretions are audible in the airway or when signs of airway obstruction or

Fig. 31.11 Oxygen is administered to an infant by means of a nasal cannula.

oxygen deficit are present. Various devices can be used to suction children, such as a bulb syringe or a straight suction catheter of the proper size for the child. In nonemergency situations, demonstrate how the suction machine operates by suctioning some water from a cup. Reassure the small child that the machine is only suctioning excess fluid from the mouth or nose, not body contents. Recommended pressures for airway suctioning with wall suction range from 50 to 95 mm Hg for infants to 95 to 110 mm Hg for children.

The use of artificial airways has become a routine life-sustaining measure in the pediatric and neonatal population. Depth, timing, and frequency are important considerations when suctioning a tracheostomy or endotracheal tube:

- *Depth:* Approximately ¼ to ½ inch beyond the tip of the artificial airway; determine placement by placing an appropriately sized suction catheter into an artificial airway of the same size, insert the catheter to the appropriate depth, mark with tape, and keep at the bedside as a reference.
- *Timing:* Limit suctioning to not more than 5 seconds.
- *Frequency:* Allow 30 seconds between suctioning attempts (two or three attempts at most).

INTAKE AND OUTPUT

Many health disorders necessitate accurate monitoring of the amount of solids and liquids taken in and the amount excreted. For example, measuring and recording intake and output (I&O) is extremely important in infants with diarrhea, toddlers with burns, or adolescents with renal disorders. Infants who are hospitalized because they fail to thrive or to grow as expected are placed on "calorie counts," which call for the careful recording of all food ingested and liquids given. This intake is recorded at the bedside, and a nutritionist calculates the calories the child actually consumes. It is helpful in determining whether the cause is organic or the result of an inadequate intake. These causes are ruled out before a maternal-infant problem is considered.

All fluids given to a child are documented on a record kept at the bedside. Adolescents are usually able to assume this responsibility after an explanation.

Many fluids are acceptable for encouraging fluid intake in the hospital and at home. They include diluted fruit juices, liquid or solid gelatin, sweetened tea, flavored ice pops, and sports electrolyte replacement drinks and infant solution (e.g., Pedialyte).

Persuading a reluctant child to drink fluids is often a nursing challenge. Offer fluids in small amounts at frequent intervals to prevent dehydration. Do not force them, and do not awaken the child from rest for this purpose.

When teaching parents about fluid management, determination of whether they understand the concept of clear liquids is always wise. Emphasize that milk is not a liquid because it forms curds when it comes in contact with the stomach lining. Caution parents about broths because most are high in sodium.

Encourage parents to relax any pressure on a child to eat during an acute illness. They need to understand that liquids can provide the necessary fluid and calories.

Infants and children who are unable or not permitted to take fluids by mouth face obligatory parenteral fluid therapy. Before an IV infusion is started, prepare the child and the family for this stressful procedure.

An understanding of the child's feeding habits often helps increase consumption after the child is able to step up the diet from fluids to solids. Once the child feels better, appetite begins to improve. Take advantage of any hungry period by serving high-quality foods and snacks. With the permission of the health care provider, encourage parents to bring in food items from home. This is especially important if the family's cultural eating habits differ from what hospital food services provide. The importance of recording all intake is key to preventing complications.

Measure all urine voided before discarding it. Remind older children to save all urine. Measuring urine output in the infant or toddler who is not toilet trained is sometimes a challenge. Most hospitals require routine weighing of diapers (before and after voiding) of all children who are not toilet trained. Subtract the weight of a dry disposable diaper from the

Fig. 31.12 Suprapubic bladder aspiration.

weight of the wet diaper. The difference in the weight in grams equals the milliliters voided: 1 g equals 1 mL of urine.

SPECIMEN COLLECTION

Urine Collection

Collection of a urine specimen when the child is not toilet trained is sometimes a major problem in pediatrics. It is often a routine part of the admission procedure and provides important information. In addition, kidney infections are common, so urine must be collected and examined often.

Qualified personnel sometimes perform suprapubic bladder aspiration on newborns and infants (Fig. 31.12). Contamination is a minimal concern with this method. Place an infant in a froglike position for the procedure, similar to the position described subsequently for femoral venipuncture. A qualified health care provider prepares the skin above the bladder and inserts a 20-gauge or 21-gauge needle into the bladder and removes several milliliters of urine. Gently prevent the legs from excessive movement, which has the potential to cause injury at the insertion site, by holding the infant's legs in a froglike position. Usually the best time for the procedure is 30 to 60 minutes after voiding.

Plastic urine collection bags sometimes are used for specimen collection. They must be applied correctly. Application of skin preparation to the area increases the adhesiveness of these bags (Fig. 31.13). In girls, give special attention to the narrow area between the vagina and the rectum. If the adhesive backing is not attached securely to this area, the anus is covered, and stool may contaminate the specimen.

When the bag is in place, cut a slit into the disposable diaper before it is placed on the child. This makes it possible to pull the urine bag through to the outside so that you can monitor it. As soon as the child voids, remove the bag, so there is less chance of losing the urine specimen.

Fig. 31.13 Application of a urine collection bag. (A) On male infant, apply adhesive portion to exposed and dried perineum first. (B) Bag adheres firmly around perineal area to prevent urine leakage.

Catheterizations are done occasionally. Because of the high possibility of contamination, especially in regard to introducing organisms into the urinary system, practitioners use this procedure as little as possible.

Venipunctures to Obtain Blood Specimens

In infants and young children, the physician sometimes uses a jugular or femoral vein to obtain a blood specimen. The nurse prepares, positions, and restrains the child. Holding the head or lower extremities absolutely immobile is critical.

When a jugular vein is used, place the child in a mummy SRD beforehand. Place the child's body on the examining table so that the shoulders are at the edge of the table. Turning the infant's head 45 degrees provides the best angle for successful entry (Fig. 31.14). For a femoral venipuncture, place the infant on the back with both legs in a froglike position (Fig. 31.15).

Gentle pressure to both knees is necessary to restrict movement. Once the needle has been removed from the vein, apply pressure to the site to prevent the formation of a hematoma.

Sometimes the chosen site for venipuncture is one of the veins of the extremities, especially the arm and the

Fig. 31.14 Correct position for jugular venipuncture procedure.

Fig. 31.15 Position for femoral venipuncture procedure.

hand. Older children, with appropriate explanation, preparation, and support, usually need only minimal, if any, restraint. One way of restraining younger children is to have the technician on one side of the child's bed and the nurse on the other. Lean across the child's upper body to prevent movement and immobilize the venipuncture site with an arm.

Lumbar Puncture

Lumbar punctures are often frightening for children and parents. Explain the procedure to the parents and the child, if old enough to understand, and answer any questions they have. Application of EMLA (eutectic mixture of local anesthetics), a local anesthetic cream, to the lumbar area usually is permitted. However, the EMLA cream should be applied at least 1 hour before the procedure.

This procedure requires positioning the child at the edge of the examining table or bed, on the side, facing you. Often the infant is placed in a sitting position.

Fig. 31.16 (A) Modified side-lying position for lumbar puncture. (B) Older child in side-lying position.

Gently flex the neck and the legs, as shown in Fig. 31.16. This angle increases the spinal curvature and helps the physician gain entry into the subarachnoid space of the lumbar spinal canal. The child must be observed for any signs of difficulty. The toddler's legs may have to be wrapped in a blanket to decrease activity. Hold the child gently and securely in that position until the physician completes the spinal tap. Label the spinal fluid specimen immediately, and send it to the laboratory for analysis.

Normal spinal fluid pressure ranges from 60 to 180 mm Hg; the lower end of the range is typical in infants. Help adolescents avoid headache after a lumbar puncture by advising them to lie flat for several hours; young children usually do not have headaches, and quiet play after the procedure is generally appropriate.

MEDICATION ADMINISTRATION

A critical responsibility of a pediatric nurse is the administration of pediatric medications. For safety reasons, have a second nurse check all computed dosages. Do not forget the "six rights" of medication administration discussed in Chapter 17: Give the *right* medication and the *right* amount of the *right* medication to the *right* child at the *right* time and by the *right* route with the *right* documentation. Also remember to assess and document the child's response to the drug. Factors related to growth and maturation alter the child's capacity to metabolize and excrete drugs (see the Safety Alert box).

Immaturity or defects in all or part of the process of absorption, distribution, or excretion have the potential to alter the effect of a drug. Newborn and young children are more susceptible than adults to the toxic effects of certain medications because of their immature organ system's limited ability to detoxify or eliminate drugs. The side effects and toxic signs and symptoms are difficult to evaluate in a preverbal child.

Unit doses are not used in pediatrics because children are of various ages and weights. Methods of calculating dosages for children consider age, body weight, and body surface area (BSA) (total area exposed to the outside environment).

Also, see Chapter 17 for a detailed explanation of pediatric considerations in medication administration.

Oral Medications

When administering liquids, take care to prevent aspiration. With the infant held in a semireclining position, place the medicine in the mouth using a spoon, plastic cup, plastic dropper, or plastic syringe (without the needle). Place the dropper or syringe along the side of the infant's tongue and administer the liquid slowly, waiting for the infant to swallow between deposits. Another option is to use an empty nipple to deposit liquid medication. Remove the nipple as soon as the infant consumes all of the medication. Young children who refuse to cooperate or who resist despite explanation will need mild physical coercion at times. If this is necessary, carry it out quickly, kindly, and carefully. Remember the possibility that a crying child will aspirate medication when lying on his or her back.

To encourage the child's acceptance of oral medications:

- Give the child an ice pop or small ice cube to suck to numb the tongue before giving the drug.
- Mix the drug with a small amount (about 1 tsp) of a sweet-tasting substance, such as honey (except in infants because of the risk of botulism), flavored syrups, jam, fruit purées, or ice cream; avoid using essential food items because the child may later refuse to eat them.
- Give a "chaser" of water, juice, a soft drink, or an ice pop or frozen juice bar after the drug.
- If nausea is a problem, give a carbonated beverage poured over finely crushed ice before or immediately after the medication.
- When medication has an unpleasant taste, have the child pinch the nose and drink the medicine through a straw. Much of what we taste is associated with smell.

Many pediatric medications are given via drops or dropper. A misunderstanding of these terms on parents' part creates a risk of overdose. In addition, many droppers that come with medications are marked in

Safety Alert

Administering Medication to the Infant, Toddler and Child, and Adolescent

INFANT

- The health care provider is responsible for prescribing drugs in the correct dosage to achieve the desired effect without endangering the health of the child.
- The nurse must understand the safe dosage of medications being administered to children, and of the expected action, possible side effects, and signs of toxicity.
- Calculate dosage for all medications using the method desired by the facility. Any small differences in dosage have the potential to result in toxemia.
- A second nurse must check all computed dosages.
- When an ordered dose is outside the usual range or some question exists regarding the preparation or the route of administration, always check with the prescribing practitioner before proceeding with the administration of the drug. The nurse is legally liable for any drug administered.
- The vastus lateralis muscle is an acceptable injection site because it is the most developed and not located close to any major circulatory or nerve structures.
- The ventrogluteal muscle is situated away from major nerves and blood vessels and is identified easily by a prominent bony landmark. It is the preferred injection site for children of all ages.
- Administer oral medications with a disposable plastic syringe (without a needle), releasing them slowly into buccal pouch; medication also can be placed in an empty nipple and the infant allowed to suck.

TODDLER AND CHILD

- Usually 1 mL is the maximal volume that is acceptable to administer parenterally (intramuscular [IM] or subcutaneous [SQ]) in a single site to small children.

- The ventrogluteal site is relatively free of major nerves and blood vessels, is a relatively large muscle, and is a safe injection site for young children.
- Allow toddler or child choices of drink to consume with oral medications.
- If possible, allow child to choose chewable or liquid medication if available.
- Never mix oral medications with essential foods, liquids, or honey (because of risk of botulism); use nonessential foods like applesauce or pudding.
- Use childproof tops on all medications for safety.
- Provide for sufficient help in restraining young child before giving IM or SQ injections; children are often unable to cooperate, and their behavior is usually unpredictable.
- Apply EMLA (eutectic mixture of local anesthetics, a topical anesthetic) over IM site if time permits (at least 60 minutes before giving injection). Applying LMX cream (lidocaine) is possible if time interval must be shorter.

ADOLESCENT

- The adolescent is capable of logical thought and reasoning and needs an explanation of hospital routine and purpose of treatments and medications.
- Older children and adolescents usually pose few problems in selecting a suitable site for IM injections.
- When administering medications to an adolescent, follow the same protocol as for an adult.
- The ventrogluteal site is the preferred site for IM injections for the adolescent.

---

tenths of cubic centimeters. If parents use a syringe instead, which is marked in cubic centimeters, they run the risk of administering 4 cc instead of 0.4 cc. Parents also do not realize that cubic centimeters (cc) and milliliters (mL) are considered the same. If the prescription is written in cubic centimeters, parents often do not know what to do when droppers are in milliliters. Provide education to parents on correct methods for measuring and giving medication. Demonstrate the technique.

Intradermal, Subcutaneous, and Intramuscular Medications

Injections are a source of discomfort and fear for children, so drugs usually are given via injection only when other routes cannot be used. Table 31.10 lists recommendations for injection sites and needles. The primary site for IM injections are the vastus lateralis muscle (Fig. 31.17) and the ventrogluteal muscle (Fig. 31.18). The deltoid muscle is possible to use in children who are 18 months or older as a site for intramuscular injections and in infants who are receiving their hepatitis B vaccine (Leifer, 2019) (Fig. 31.19). If time permits, apply EMLA, a local anesthetic cream, to the injection site at least 1 hour before the injection.

Table 31.10	Needle and Site Recommendations for Selected Injections
NEEDLE	**SITE**
Intradermal (ID)	
⅜-inch to ½-inch 25-gauge to 27-gauge	Primary: ventral forearm
Subcutaneous (SQ)	
⅜-inch to ⅝-inch 24-gauge to 26-gauge	Primary: upper outer aspect of arm; lower abdomen; anterior thigh
Intramuscular (IM)	
⅝-inch to 1-inch	Primary: 0–2 years, vastus lateralis, ventrogluteal
20-gauge to 25-gauge	2–12 years: vastus lateralis; ventrogluteal; deltoid

Wearing gloves prevents anesthesia from affecting the nurse's fingers.

Injections administered with care seldom produce trauma to the child. Repeated use of a single site has been associated with fibrosis of the muscle and subsequent muscle contracture. Most children are unpredictable, and few cooperate totally when receiving an

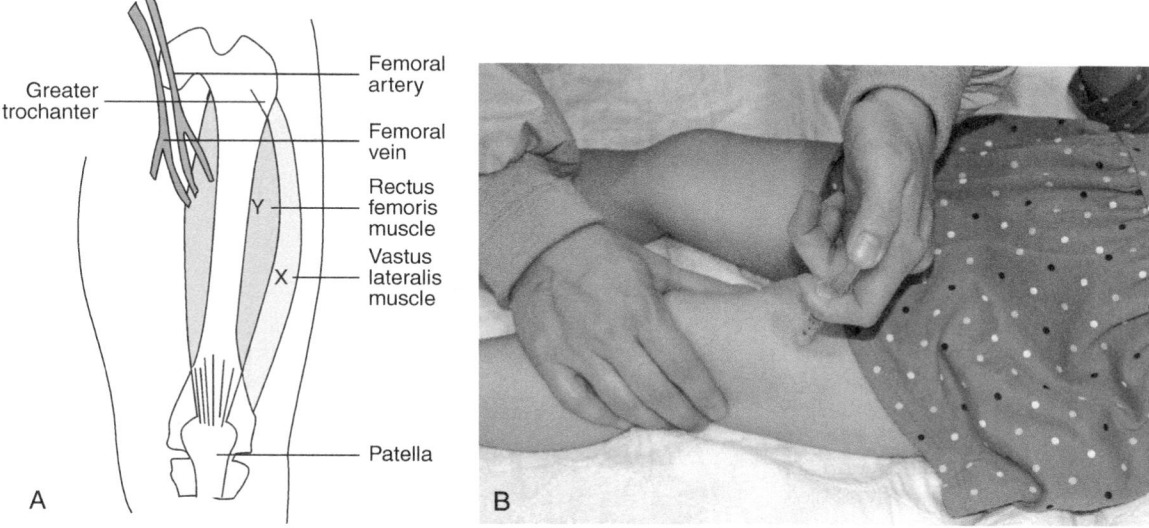

Fig. 31.17 Intramuscular injection sites. (A) The middle third of the vastus lateralis muscle is the primary site for intramuscular injections in the thigh. (B) Infant's leg is stabilized for intramuscular injection. The needle penetrates the midlateral thigh on a front-to-back course.

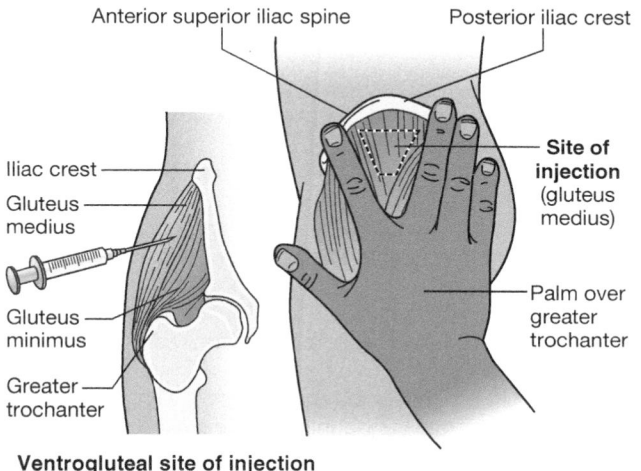

Ventrogluteal site of injection

Fig. 31.18 Ventrogluteal site for intramuscular injection.

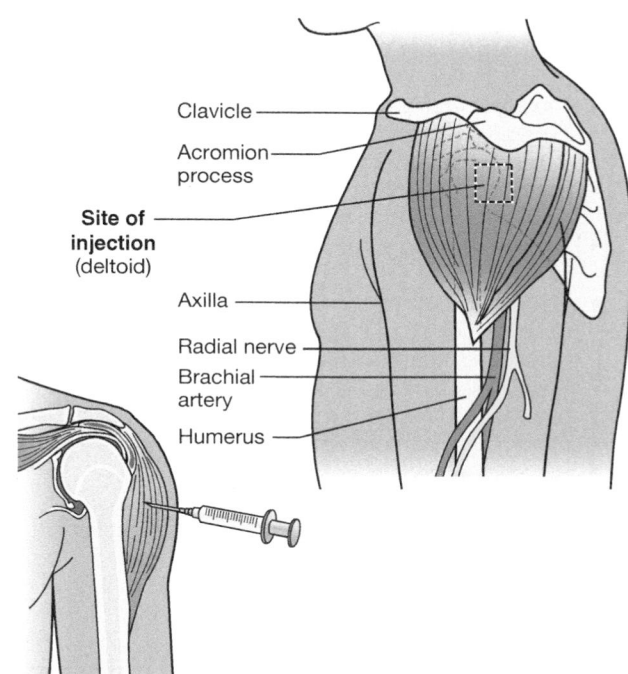

Fig. 31.19 Deltoid site for intramuscular injection.

injection. It is advisable to have someone available to help gently restrain the child.

To estimate the needle length for IM injections, first grasp the **vastus lateralis muscle** (the largest of the four muscles of the quadriceps femoris, situated on the lateral side of the thigh; see Fig. 31.17A) or the deltoid muscle (see Fig. 31.19), and choose a needle length that is approximately half the distance between the thumb and index finger. With the ventrogluteal site, grasp only subcutaneous tissue, so choose a needle length that is slightly more than half the distance (see Fig. 31.18). Needle length should allow for a small portion of the needle to be exposed at the skin surface as a precaution if the needle breaks off from the hub.

Factors to consider when selecting a site for IM injection on an infant or child include the following (Box 31.11):

- The amount and character of the medication to be injected
- The amount and the general condition of the muscle mass
- The frequency or number of injections to be given during treatment
- The type of medication being given
- Factors that will possibly impede access to or cause contamination of the site
- The ability of the child to assume the required position safely

Box 31.11	Guidelines for Intramuscular Administration of Medication in Infants and Children

1. Use all usual safety precautions in administering medication (e.g., check child's identification). Apply EMLA cream (eutectic mixture of local anesthetics, a topical anesthetic) over site if time permits.
2. Prepare medication.
   - Select needle and syringe appropriate to the following:
   - Amount of fluid to be administered (syringe size)
   - Viscosity of fluid to be administered (needle gauge)
   - Amount of tissue to be penetrated (needle length)
   - Maximal volume to be administered in a single site is 1 mL for older infants and small children.
3. Determine the site of injection, and be certain muscle is large enough to accommodate volume and type of medication.
   - Older children: select site as with adult patient; allow child some choice of site, if feasible.
   - Vastus lateralis muscle and ventrogluteal muscle are acceptable sites for infants and small or debilitated children.
   - Dorsogluteal muscle is insufficiently developed to be a safe site for infants and small children. **The dorsogluteal muscle is not used for infants or children of any age.**
4. Administer medication.
   - Provide for sufficient help in restraining child; children are often uncooperative, and their behavior is usually unpredictable.
   - Explain briefly what is to be done and, if appropriate, what child can do to help.
   - Expose injection area for unobstructed view of landmarks.
   - Select a site where skin is free of irritation and danger of infection; palpate for and avoid sensitive or hardened areas. With multiple injections, rotate sites.
   - Place child in a lying or sitting position; child is not allowed to stand for the following reasons:
   - Landmarks are more difficult to assess.
   - Restraint is more difficult.
   - The child could faint and fall.
   - Use a new, sharp needle with smallest diameter that permits free flow of the medication.
   - Grasp muscle firmly between thumb and fingers to isolate and stabilize muscle for deposition of drug in its deepest part; in obese children, spread skin with

thumb and index finger to displace subcutaneous tissue, and grasp muscle deeply on each side.
   - Allow skin preparation to dry completely before penetrating skin.
   - Have medication at room temperature.
5. Decrease perception of pain:
   - Distract child with conversation.
   - Give child something on which to concentrate (e.g., squeezing a hand or bed rail, pinching own nose, humming, counting).
   - Place a cold compress or wrapped ice cube on site about a minute before injection or apply cold to contralateral site.
   - Say to child, "If you feel this, tell me to take it out, please."
   - Have child hold a small bandage and place it on puncture site after intramuscular (IM) injection is given.
6. Insert needle quickly, using a dartlike motion.
7. Avoid tracking any medication through superficial tissues:
   - If withdrawing medication from an ampule, use a needle equipped with a filter that removes glass particles; then use a new, nonfilter needle for injection.
   - Use the Z-track technique as indicated.
   - Do not depress the plunger at all during insertion of the needle.
8. Inject medication slowly (over 20 seconds) or as indicated.
9. Remove needle quickly; hold gauze sponge firmly against skin near needle when removing it to avoid pulling on tissue.
10. Apply pressure to site after injection; massage site to hasten absorption unless contraindicated, as with irritating drugs.
11. Place a small bandage on puncture site; with young children, decorate bandage by drawing a smiling face or other symbol of acceptance.
12. Hold and cuddle young child and encourage parents to comfort child; praise older child.
13. Allow expression of feelings.
14. Discard syringe and uncapped needle in puncture-resistant container located near site of use.
15. Record time of injection, drug, dose, and injection site.

Intravenous Medications

The IV route of administering a medication often is selected for the following reasons:

- Medication is distributed almost immediately to tissues, and prompt physiologic action occurs.
- With consecutive doses, predictable drug levels and maintenance of therapeutic effects are possible.
- After initial insertion, IV administration is more comfortable for the child than other types of parenteral injections.
- The IV sites in children differ from those of adults. A superficial scalp vein is used commonly in infants younger than 9 months of age, because these

veins have no valves, so it is possible to insert a needle in either direction. In addition, the child can move the head from side to side without dislodging the needle. Any accessible vein is acceptable to use in older children. The use of peripheral lines in a child's lower extremities impedes ambulation.

- An infusion line may be converted to a saline lock when a child does not need additional IV fluids but still needs additional medications, such as antibiotics or pain medication. With a saline lock, a child can move about except for those brief periods when drugs are infused. Irrigate the tube regularly to keep the line open as per agency policy.

OCULAR, OTIC, AND NASAL ADMINISTRATION

A few differences are found in administering eye, ear, and nose medication to children or adults. Gaining children's cooperation is necessary for these procedures, and the child may need to be restrained.

Instilling eye drops in infants can be difficult because infants often clench their lids together. One approach is to place drops in the nasal corner where the lids meet. When the child opens the lids, medication flows into the conjunctiva. For younger children, playing a game tends to be helpful. If eye ointment and eye drops are ordered, give drops first, wait 3 minutes, and then apply the ointment to allow each drug to work. When possible, administer eye ointments before bedtime or naptime because the child's vision will be blurred for a while.

Instill eardrops with the child restrained. For children 3 years of age and younger, straighten the external auditory canal by pulling the pinna downward and back. For children older than 3 years of age, pull the pinna upward and back. After instillation, have the child remain lying on the opposite side for a few minutes. Gentle massage of the area in front of the ear usually facilitates entry of the drops. Sterile cotton may be placed loosely in the ear to prevent infected material from being forced into the mastoid area.

For nasal administration, position the child with the head hyperextended to prevent the strangling sensations caused by medication trickling into the pharynx rather than up into the nasal passages.

RECTAL ADMINISTRATION

The rectal route is less reliable but sometimes is used when the oral route is difficult or contraindicated. Lubricate the suppository with water-soluble jelly or warm water and insert it quickly and gently into the rectum beyond the rectal sphincters. Then hold the buttocks together firmly to relieve pressure on the anal sphincter until the urge to expel the suppository has passed (5 to 10 minutes).

Enema

The procedure for an enema for a child does not differ essentially from that for an adult (Table 31.11). Use an

Table **31.11**	Guidelines for Administration of Enemas to Children	
AGE	**AMOUNT**	**INSERTION DISTANCE**
Infant	120–240 mL	1 inch
2–4 years	240–360 mL	2 inches
4–10 years	360–480 mL	3 inches
11 years	480–720 mL	4 inches

isotonic solution in children. Do not use plain water, because it is hypertonic and has the potential to cause rapid fluid shift and overload.

Proper insertion of the catheter tip, especially in infants, is essential to prevent rectal damage and perforation. If insertion of the enema tip causes discomfort, remove the tip and notify the physician.

SAFETY

Protecting a child from harm is paramount in pediatrics. Anticipatory guidance for parents of infants and toddlers and health teaching for school-age children and adolescents are two methods of preventing accidents. However, hazards and dangers are everywhere—in the home, at the playground, at school, and in the hospital.

Injuries cause more deaths and disabilities in children than all causes of disease combined. The risk-taking activities of adolescents also contribute to the morbidity (an illness or an abnormal condition or quality) and mortality of adolescence. Table 31.12 identifies common developmental characteristics, potential hazards, and preventive measures that help decrease the incidence of accidents and injuries.

Parents and children need to talk and listen to each other to prevent many accidents. Maintaining open communication between and among all members of a family is one method of prevention. The adult who is a role model, who thinks about safety, and who identifies potential dangers in the environment or a particular activity has immense power to influence a child.

Table 31.12	Prevention of Accidents	
BEHAVIOR OR AGE-RELATED FACTOR	**ACCIDENT OR HAZARD**	**PREVENTION**
Newborn		
Sleeping Poor head control Somewhat capable of moving body around	Suffocation	Do not tuck blankets in. Do not use pillows. Do not use plastic bags in crib. Avoid soft, moldable mattresses. Place healthy infants in supine or side-lying positions for sleep.
	Accidents	Use an approved car seat and follow manufacturer's instructions. Check crib slats; have them no more than 2⅜ inches apart.
	Burns	Test bath water temperature. Never smoke or drink hot liquids while holding baby.
	Falls	Never leave baby alone or unattended on bed, sofa, or counter. Always have one hand on baby. Carry newborn with two hands.
	Lead poisoning	Eliminate or reduce the child's exposure to any surfaces or substances that contain lead.[a]
1–6 Months		
Head control improving	Suffocation	Keep crib free of plastic bags. Do not use pillows.
Placing objects in mouth	Foreign body aspiration Injury from toys: loose parts or sharp edges	Inspect all toys; remove button eyes or detach small wheels. Do not offer foods that pose risk of choking, such as grapes, nuts, potato chips, and raisins. Remove open safety pins, needles, and nails from baby's reach.
Moving body from one place to another	Falls	Do not leave baby unattended on bed, sofa, or counter.
Beginning to pull self to sitting position	Burns	Test bath water; hold infant securely. Keep hot liquids in cups away from child's grasp.
7–12 Months		
Sitting up	Falls, drownings	Never leave infant unattended in high chair, on bed, or in tub.
Crawling	Accidents	Use gates at bottom and top of stairs. Place guards around fireplaces; never leave infant alone near space heater.
	Suffocation	Do not leave plastic bags or balloons in crib or playpen or within infant's reach.
Feeding self	Aspiration, ingestion	Do not offer foods on which child is likely to choke, such as popcorn; small, hard candies; gum; or hot dogs. Lock up all medications and poisonous household substances. Purchase medicines and household cleaners in childproof containers. Keep number of local poison control center by telephone. Childproof the entire house, including placing poisonous houseplants out of reach.
1–2 Years		
Holding on or walking	Falls, lacerations, abrasions	Keep furniture with sharp edges and glass tabletops out of child's way or protect with special corner protectors. Keep sharp kitchen utensils and garden equipment out of reach or locked up.
Exploring environment	Electrical injuries	Always know where the toddler is playing. Supervise all outdoor play activities.

Table 31.12   Prevention of Accidents—cont'd

BEHAVIOR OR AGE-RELATED FACTOR	ACCIDENT OR HAZARD	PREVENTION
Running		Do not allow child to run with objects in mouth. Begin teaching safety outdoors, including dangers of traffic, climbing, and walking in front of swings at playgrounds.
	Motor vehicle accidents	Always use an approved car seat and follow manufacturer's instructions. Keep toddler in fenced area. Install childproof locks on car doors. Teach child to cross street holding an adult's hand. Keep car doors locked in garage or driveway. Do not allow play in driver's seat without adult present.
	Ingestion, inhalation	Keep insecticides, medications, and all harmful cleaners locked up.
	Suffocation	Supervise play with balloons. Do not allow plastic bags in play. Remove doors of refrigerators or chain shut before discarding.
	Drowning	Keep bath water level low in tub. Never leave child alone in tub or wading pool; empty wading pool after use. Supervise child closely at beach. Never allow child near water without an adult. Fence around swimming pool. Enroll toddler in swimming class.
	Burns	Remove matches and lighters from reach. Teach fire safety. Keep handles of pots toward center of stove when cooking. Keep child away from stove while preparing meals. Keep child away from charcoal fires.
3–5 Years		
Climbing Running Exploring environment outside the home Improving motor skills	Falls, lacerations, and abrasions	Check yard, playground, and daycare center for potential hazards. Begin teaching: safety in using playground equipment; dangers of pushing and shoving playmates; and avoiding strangers. Supervise child using scissors, tricycles, and Big Wheels. Discourage approaching animals without an adult present. Teach child his or her own name, address, and telephone number.
	Drowning	Supervise action-related activities, such as swimming. Never leave child alone in bathtub or wading pool. Never allow child near water without an adult.
	Motor vehicle and pedestrian accidents	Use car seat or safety belts in car according to Department of Transportation (DOT) standards. Review acceptable behavior in a moving car. Review crossing street at corner, watching lights and flow of traffic.
	Assault, abuse	Teach child to keep parent informed of whereabouts. Confine play to yard; do not allow child to play in street.
	Burns	Practice fire drills in the home. Implement other practices similar to those for 1- to 2-year-olds.
	Firearms	Never keep loaded guns or rifles in house or garage. Keep service guns locked. Instruct child never to touch gun or bullets.

Continued

Table 31.12   **Prevention of Accidents—cont'd**

BEHAVIOR OR AGE-RELATED FACTOR	ACCIDENT OR HAZARD	PREVENTION
6–11 Years		
Motor skills continuing to improve Enjoying large muscle activities Becoming increasingly independent Engaging in competitive sports, unsupervised activities	Motor vehicle and pedestrian accidents, injuries, fractures	Review traffic safety. Use safety belts. Teach skateboard safety: control speed; refrain from jumping; use helmet, knee, and elbow pads. Teach bicycle safety: rules of the road, use of reflectors, proper signaling, use of helmets. Review safety regarding use of lawn mowers, farm equipment, and tools. Teach child not to hide in or play near cars.
	Assault, abuse	Caution child about playing in vacant buildings, quarries, or sand pits. Teach proper use of protective gear in competitive sports. Teach child not to throw objects at people or moving vehicles. Teach child how to call fire department, police, and emergency medical assistance.
	Drownings	Review swimming and boating safety. Do not allow ice skating on pond unless its safety has been determined. Never allow the child to swim or skate alone.
	Inhalation, ingestions	Evaluate health education programs at school. Emphasize the hazards of glue sniffing and drug or alcohol use. Encourage family discussions about substance abuse.
12–18 Years		
Rapid growth spurt Demonstrating risk-taking behaviors Demonstrating increased independence Engaging in extracurricular activities Reacting to peer group influence Driving a car	Motor vehicle, motorcycle, and bicycle injuries and fractures	Evaluate the high school's safety and health education programs. Review bicycle and motorcycle safety, including use of helmets. Enroll child in driver education classes. Establish limits regarding care, use, and consequences of drinking alcohol and driving.
	Sporting injuries	Encourage group participation in outdoor activities, such as running or jogging. Supervise competitive sports activities. Encourage enrolling in first aid classes. Maintain a physical conditioning program.
	Drownings	Review water safety in seasonal activities. Discourage risk-taking behaviors at pool or beach. Discuss dangers of swimming and skating alone.
	Firearms	Keep guns empty and locked up. Teach proper care of firearms. Supervise target practice in isolated areas.

ªContinued attention to this precaution is necessary throughout childhood.

Get Ready for the NCLEX® Examination!

Key Points

- Knowledge of basic principles of normal growth and development is important to understand what infants and children are like, what is possible to expect from them, what their needs are, and why they behave as they do.
- Knowledge of physical assessment with the systematic (head-to-toe) method is important for accurate documentation.
- Metabolism is highest in the newborn.
- Nutrition is probably the single most important influence on growth and is closely related to good health throughout life.
- Children are at risk of maltreatment in the form of abuse and neglect.
- Neglect is the most common form of maltreatment.
- The youngest children are most susceptible to all types of maltreatment, except sex trafficking.
- Sex traffickers exploit the vulnerabilities of children then isolate them from their caregivers and victimize them for commercial sex use.
- Nurses are required to report suspected maltreatment of children through appropriate channels.
- By understanding that hospitalization is an anxiety-producing experience for the child and the family, the nurse is better able to address the needs of both.
- The goal of the pediatric nurse is to promote the highest state of health in each child.
- Family-centered care is a philosophy of care that recognizes the family as the constant in the child's life and holds that systems and personnel are called on to support, respect, encourage, and enhance the strengths and competence of the family.
- By understanding parents' responses to hospitalization of a child, the nurse is better able to address the parents' needs.
- Children in different age categories show varying concerns and needs while hospitalized.
- One way to decrease the traumatic effects of a child's hospitalization is to have the child and the parents attend a preadmission orientation program.
- Rooming-in facilities allow a parent to become as involved as desired and provide the child with the security of an adult who is known, trusted, and loved.
- Preparing children for pediatric procedures increases their cooperation, helps them cope, and promotes a sense of self-esteem and mastery.
- Always provide explanations to children at an age-appropriate level so that the child is able to understand them. Age and developmental level influence the ways in which children perceive and make sense of experiences such as illness or disability and therefore make an impact on their ability to cope.
- The administration of pediatric medications is a serious responsibility.
- The preparation of medication for a child requires precise computation of dosage.
- Accidents are a leading cause of death in children and adolescents, and identification and avoidance of potential hazards is necessary.

Additional Learning Resources

SG Go to your Study Guide for additional learning activities to help you master this chapter content.

Be sure to visit the Evolve site at *http://evolve.elsevier.com/Cooper/foundations/* for additional online resources.

Review Questions for the NCLEX® Examination

1. **The nursing student is reviewing what he/she knows about the development of pediatrics as a discipline. The nursing student recognizes which of the following individuals as being credited with being the "father of pediatrics"?**

   1. Hippocrates
   2. Abraham Jacobi
   3. James Mott
   4. R.E. Behrman

2. **Lillian Ward, founder of the Henry Street Settlement in New York City, focused on which of the following?** *(Select all that apply.)*

   1. Nursing services
   2. Social work
   3. Recreational sports
   4. Educational activities

3. **The first White House Conference on Children focused on issues of child labor, dependent children, and infant care. As a result, what was established in 1987 on behalf of children?**

   1. US Children's Bureau
   2. Office of Child Development
   3. National Commission on Children
   4. Women, Infants, and Children program

4. **A 4-year-old child is to be hospitalized for the first time, and the parents voice anxiety about his condition and hospitalization. Which action by the nurse best addresses the concerns of the child's parents?**

   1. Provide only necessary information.
   2. Provide an orientation to the child before hospitalization.
   3. Provide a tour of the entire hospital.
   4. Provide anticipatory guidance and explain all procedures.

5. **Which method is the most effective when preparing a child for a pediatric procedure?**

   1. Problem-solving approach
   2. Sensation-based approach
   3. Symbol-based approach
   4. Autonomy-based approach

6. **A 16-month-old child is admitted to the pediatric floor after surgery to repair a cleft palate. The child's mother asks why her child is restrained. The nurse explains that the elbow safety reminder device (SRD) is being used to:**

   1. monitor pressure to the suture line.
   2. prevent excessive movement in bed.
   3. help to prevent injury to the operative site.
   4. reduce the likelihood your baby will fall out of the bed.

7. Which statement by the new pediatric nurse indicates an understanding of medication administration to children? *(Select all that apply.)*

   1. "Children and adults are susceptible to toxic effects of medication at the same rate."
   2. "There are unit doses for children."
   3. "BSA is a reliable method of calculating children's medication dosage."
   4. "The route of choice is always the rectal route."
   5. The six rights of medication must be followed when administering medication.

8. A 7-year-old is about to have a finger-stick blood draw. Which statement by the nurse is most effective?

   1. "It will hurt, but you are a big girl, so you can just grin and bear it."
   2. "It will hurt a lot, and you can cry if you want to."
   3. "Some children say that they feel a little pinch."
   4. "Close your eyes, and don't look; it will be over in a minute."

9. An 18-month-old is hospitalized for surgery in the morning. Which intervention is most helpful in relieving the child's stress?

   1. Maintaining a normal routine
   2. Providing opportunities for play
   3. Encouraging parental presence and rooming-in
   4. Encouraging self-care activities

10. The mother of a 6-month-old is worried because the child's grandmother is concerned that the child is "slow" because she is not yet crawling. What action by the nurse is most appropriate?

    1. Assure the parent that grandmothers are often overly concerned when it comes to grandchildren.
    2. Ask the mother at what age her other children began crawling.
    3. Refer the mother for additional evaluation because most children do crawl by 6 months of age.
    4. Assure the mother that children develop at their own rate, but most children do not crawl at age 6 months.

11. An accurate apical heart rate measurement is assessed at the _____ intercostal space.

12. A nurse is meeting a new 4-year-old patient for the first time. Which intervention is most effective when entering the patient's room for the first time?

    1. Speak only to the parents because the child will be very scared.
    2. Explain all procedures in detail because the child will want to know what is going on.
    3. Be careful not to use words that may be misinterpreted by the child, such as "take your temperature."
    4. Tell the parents they must leave the room until the physical assessment is complete.

13. The nurse is providing postoperative care instructions to parents of a 5-month-old who is recovering from surgery. Which statement indicates that the teaching was effective? *(Select all that apply.)*

    1. "The baby will perhaps be comforted by sucking on a pacifier, being swaddled, or being rocked."
    2. "Analgesics are best given only if the child will not stop crying."
    3. "At 5 months of age, the baby has immature pain receptors and therefore will not need analgesics."
    4. "The baby will have less pain if left alone in the bed for all activities."
    5. "I can continue to breast feed as soon as my child is able to eat."

14. What is true regarding the child's nutrition? *(Select all that apply.)*

    1. The toddler needs to eat twice as much as a 6-month-old infant.
    2. Infants can begin solid foods at 4 to 6 months of age.
    3. The toddler is too busy to eat, so give finger foods such as hot dogs, grapes, and nuts.
    4. The toddler has no risk of food allergies.
    5. Solid foods should be introduced one at a time and a new one each week.

15. What is the most accurate method to measure urine output in an infant?

    1. Weigh the diaper before and after the infant voids.
    2. Weigh the infant after each wet diaper.
    3. Have the parents try to catch the urine in a plastic cup.
    4. Insert a Foley catheter for all infants who are not potty trained.

16. What is true of intramuscular injections in children younger than 2 years old? *(Select all that apply.)*

    1. Not possible to give because of poor muscular development.
    2. Possible to give in the vastus lateralis muscle.
    3. Possible to give in the ventrogluteal muscle.
    4. Possible to give in the deltoid muscle.
    5. Apply EMLA cream 15 minutes before injection.
    6. Possible to give in the dorsogluteal muscle.
    7. Help should be obtained to restrain the child.

17. The most common asymmetry with lateral curvature of the spine in the adolescent is known as _____.

18. What is the appropriate method to examine a 6-month-old's ear with an otoscope?

    1. Pull the ear up and back.
    2. Pull the ear down and forward.
    3. Pull the ear up and forward.
    4. Pull the ear down and back.

19. A female, 16, gives birth to a low birthweight (LBW) baby girl, estimated gestational age 32 weeks. The young mother surrenders the infant at birth for adoption. The infant weighs 3 lb, 12 oz (1.7 kg) and is 16.5 in (42 cm) long. Her head circumference is 11.4 in (29 cm). Heart rate is 150 bpm and blood pressure is 65/41. Respiratory rate is 63 breaths/min. Her 1-minute Apgar score is 6, with a 5-minute score of 8. The infant is jaundiced. Babinski reflex is downgoing bilaterally. Sucking reflex is absent, and there is some immaturity of bowel function. The infant is moved into the NICU where, initially, bottle feeding is encouraged. However, with the absence of a sucking reflex, these efforts soon cause significant fatigue and agitation in the infant, and a decision is made to temporarily initiate gavage while the staff continues to encourage development of the sucking reflex and attend intestinal development and function.

Choose the *most likely* options to complete the statement below.

For this patient, before each feeding the nurse should _____1_____ and then _____2_____; then after feeding, the nurse should _____3_____.

OPTIONS FOR 1	OPTIONS FOR 2	OPTIONS FOR 3
Position the infant on her left side	Cool the formula slightly.	Wrap her in a mummy type safety reminder device
Ensure that the tube is inserted through and secured to her right nostril	Apply a steady, gentle push with the plunger for continuous feeding	Ensure that she remains prone for 30 min
Inject 2.0–5.5 mL of air into the tube to clear it	Administer 5 mL formula every 5–10 min	Inject 2.0–5.5 mL of air into the tube to clear it
Flush the tube with 1–2 mL sterile water	Administer 10 mL formula per minute	Flush the tube with 1–2 mL sterile water
Give the infant a pacifier to suck during procedure	Aspirate periodically for air	Aspirate periodically for air

Objectives

1. Describe the etiology and pathophysiology, types, clinical manifestations, diagnostic tests, and medical management of and nursing interventions, patient teaching, and prognosis for children affected by the following:
   - Congenital heart defects
   - Iron-deficiency anemia, sickle cell anemia, and aplastic anemia
   - Hemophilia and idiopathic thrombocytopenia purpura
   - Leukemia
   - Acquired immunodeficiency syndrome (AIDS)
   - Juvenile rheumatoid arthritis
   - Disorders of the respiratory system, including respiratory distress syndrome, bronchopulmonary dysplasia, pneumonia, sudden infant death syndrome, upper respiratory tract infections, tonsillitis, croup, bronchitis, respiratory syncytial virus, pulmonary tuberculosis, cystic fibrosis, and bronchial asthma
   - Disorders of the gastrointestinal system, including cleft lip and cleft palate, dehydration, diarrhea, gastroenteritis, constipation, gastroesophageal reflux, hypertrophic pyloric stenosis, intussusception, and Hirschsprung disease
   - Disorders of the genitourinary system, including nephrotic syndrome, acute glomerulonephritis, and Wilms tumor
   - Disorders of the endocrine system, including hypothyroidism, hyperthyroidism, and diabetes mellitus
   - Disorders of the musculoskeletal system, including hip dysplasia, Legg-Calvé-Perthes disease, osteomyelitis, talipes, Duchenne muscular dystrophy, and septic arthritis
   - Disorders of the nervous system, including meningitis, encephalitis, hydrocephalus, cerebral palsy, seizures, spina bifida, neonatal abstinence syndrome, and neuroblastoma
   - Lead poisoning
   - Disorders of the integumentary system, including contact dermatitis, diaper dermatitis, eczema, seborrheic dermatitis, acne vulgaris, herpes simplex virus type I, tinea infections, candidiasis, and parasitic infections
   - Disorders of the sensory system, including otitis media, refractive errors (myopia, hyperopia), strabismus, periorbital cellulitis, and allergic rhinitis
2. Discuss the parent teaching necessary to assist in prevention of urinary tract infection in infants and children.
3. Identify six possible causes of cognitive impairment.
4. Describe the clinical manifestations of Down syndrome.
5. Discuss the appropriate nursing interventions in caring for a child with autism.
6. Demonstrate an understanding of the medical management and nursing interventions for a child with a learning disability.
7. Describe four nursing interventions for a child with attention deficit/hyperactivity disorder.
8. Identify six clinical manifestations of depression in children.
9. Discuss three nursing interventions for the child who is suicidal.

Key Terms

acquired heart disorders (ŭ-KWĪRD HŌRT dĭs-ŌR-dŭrz, p. 995)

alpha-fetoprotein (ĂL-fŭ fē-tō-PRŌ-tēn, p. 1051)

amblyopia (ăm-blē-Ō-pē-ă, p. 1066)

attention deficit/hyperactivity disorder (ADHD) (ŭ-TĔN-shŭn DĔF-ĭ-sĭt hī-pŭr-ăk-TĬV-ĭ-tē dĭs-ŌR-dŭr, p. 1072)

autism (AW-tĭz-ŭm, p. 1070)

chelation therapy (kĕ-LĀ-shŭn THĔR-ŭ-pē, p. 1053)

cognitive impairment (KŎG-nĭ-tĭv ĭm-PĀR-mŭnt, p. 1067)

congenital heart disease (CHD) (kŏn-JĔN-ĭ-tŭl HŌRT dĭz-ĒZ, p. 995)

"currant jelly" stools (KŬR-ŭnt JĔL-ē STŪLZ, p. 1028)

Down syndrome (DOUN SĬN-drōm, p. 1068)

glomerulonephritis (glō-mĕr-ŭ-lō-nĕf-RĪ-tĭs, p. 1032)

Gowers sign (GOU-ŭrz SĬN, p. 1043)

intelligence quotient (IQ) (ĭn-TĔL-ĭ-jŭns KWŌ-shŭnt, p. 1067)

Legg-Calvé-Perthes disease (LĔG kăl-VĀ PĔR-tēz dĭz-ĒZ, p. 1039)

lichenification (lī-kĕn-ĭ-fĭ-KĀ-shŭn, p. 1056)

neural tube (NŪ-rŭl TŪB, p. 1050)

Nissen fundoplication (NĬS-ĕn fŭn-dō-plĭ-KĀ-shŭn, p. 1026)

nuchal rigidity (NŪ-kŭl rĭj-ĬD-ĭ-tē, p. 1044)

pica (PĪ-kŭ, p. 1053)

pneumothorax (nū-mō-THŌ-răks, p. 1012)

priapism (prī-ŭ-PĬZ-ŭm, p. 1003)

prodromal (prō-DRŌ-mǎl, p. 1061)

psychogenic (sī-kō-JĔN-ĭk, p. 1074)

school avoidance (SKŪL ŭ-VOYD-ŭns, p. 1071)

sickled cell (SĬK-ŭld sĕl, p. 1002)

somatization disorders (sō-mǎt-ŭ-ZĀ-shŭn dĭs-ŌR-dŭrz, p. 1073)

subluxation (sŭb-lŭk-SĀ-shŭn, p. 1039)

Many of the health problems that affect children differ from those of adults, and management of these problems also can be different. Nurses must be aware of the unique way they provide care to children and their families. When providing nursing interventions to children, include parents as much as possible, delegating to them any interventions that are appropriate. It is also necessary to provide them with resources within their community so that they can provide for the continued health of their child after hospital discharge.

This chapter provides the reader with an understanding of the physical, mental, and cognitive (the process of knowing) disorders affecting children. Although it is dedicated to the understanding of the most prevalent health issues affecting children, it is beyond the scope of this chapter to address all disorders that may affect children.

PHYSICAL DISORDERS

DISORDERS OF CARDIOVASCULAR FUNCTION

Many cardiovascular disorders in children are the result of congenital heart disease (CHD), an abnormality or anomaly of the heart that is present at birth. Consequences of many of these defects include heart failure, predisposition to infection, hypoxia, and alterations in growth. Another group of cardiovascular disorders, acquired heart disorders, comprises abnormalities occurring after birth that compromise the heart's function.

Any type of cardiovascular disorder tends to be frightening to the child and parents. It is important to educate and prepare them regarding the disorder and its management.

Congenital Heart Disease

It is estimated that 5% to 10% of full-term newborns have CHD. The rate is even higher among infants born prematurely.

Etiology And Pathophysiology. The causes of many congenital heart defects are unknown, although genetics and maternal medication use may play a role. There are several probable environmental and genetic risk factors for the various types of defects. Environmental factors include intrauterine rubella exposure, maternal alcoholism, diabetes mellitus, advanced maternal age, and maternal drug ingestion (e.g., lithium, thalidomide, or phenytoin [Dilantin]). Genetic risk factors include the presence of a sibling or parent with a CHD, chromosomal anomalies (trisomy G [trisomy 21, Down syndrome]; trisomy D [trisomies 13, Patau syndrome; 14; and 15]; and monosomy X [Turner syndrome]), and the presence of other noncardiac congenital anomalies (Mayo Clinic, 2018b).

Principles of Fetal And Postnatal Circulation. During fetal development, the placenta is the source of oxygen and nutrients. Oxygenated blood is brought to the fetus by the umbilical vein and enters the fetal heart via the inferior vena cava. The fetal lungs, which are collapsed and full of fluid, pose a strong resistance to the right side of the heart, increasing the pressures in the right atrium and the right ventricle. Because of the increased pressure in the right side of the heart, blood entering the heart from the inferior vena cava is directed across the right atrium through the foramen ovale to the left atrium. This blood is then ejected from the left ventricle into the aorta. Thus, the blood richest in oxygen is pumped through the aorta to the coronary arteries, the brain, and the upper extremities. Venous blood returning from this region returns to the right atrium through the superior vena cava and is directed downward through the tricuspid valve into the right ventricle. From there it is pumped into the pulmonary artery, where the majority of the blood is shunted to the descending aorta through the ductus arteriosus and perfuses the lower body (Fig. 32.1). Only a small amount enters the fetal lungs for structure development, owing to high pulmonary resistance (Fig. 32.2A).

At delivery, with the first breath, the newborn's lungs expand, and the fluid within them is absorbed into the pulmonary circulation. As a result, pulmonary and right-sided heart pressures fall and, with the removal of the placenta, systemic pressures rise. The foramen ovale closes as the pressure in the left atrium exceeds the pressure in the right atrium. The ductus arteriosus closes with the increased oxygen content of the newborn's blood (see Fig. 32.2B).

Types of Defects. In the past, diagnoses were based on a classification into two basic categories of CHD: disorders related to symptoms of color (cyanotic or acyanotic) and disorders related to the direction of blood flow (left-to-right shunt or right-to-left shunt). These categories sometimes have been difficult to understand because it was not possible to classify all disorders by these criteria.

A new classification system of CHD has emerged. The most current CHD categories are related to four physiologic characteristics: increased pulmonary blood flow, decreased pulmonary blood flow, obstruction to systemic blood flow, and mixed blood flow.

Fig. 32.3 illustrates hemodynamics related to the first three categories. The figure does not illustrate mixed blood flow, which includes many possible combinations of the mixing of oxygenated and unoxygenated blood in the heart or great vessels.

In this chapter, several of the major CHDs, clinical manifestations, and medical management are discussed. They also are described in the nursing care plans and critical thinking activities.

Clinical Manifestations. Children with suspected cardiac dysfunction may exhibit cyanosis, pallor, cardiomegaly, pericardial rubs, murmurs, additional heart sounds (S_3 or S_4), discrepancies between apical and radial pulses, tachypnea, dyspnea, grunting, digital clubbing, hepatomegaly, splenomegaly, discrepancies between upper and

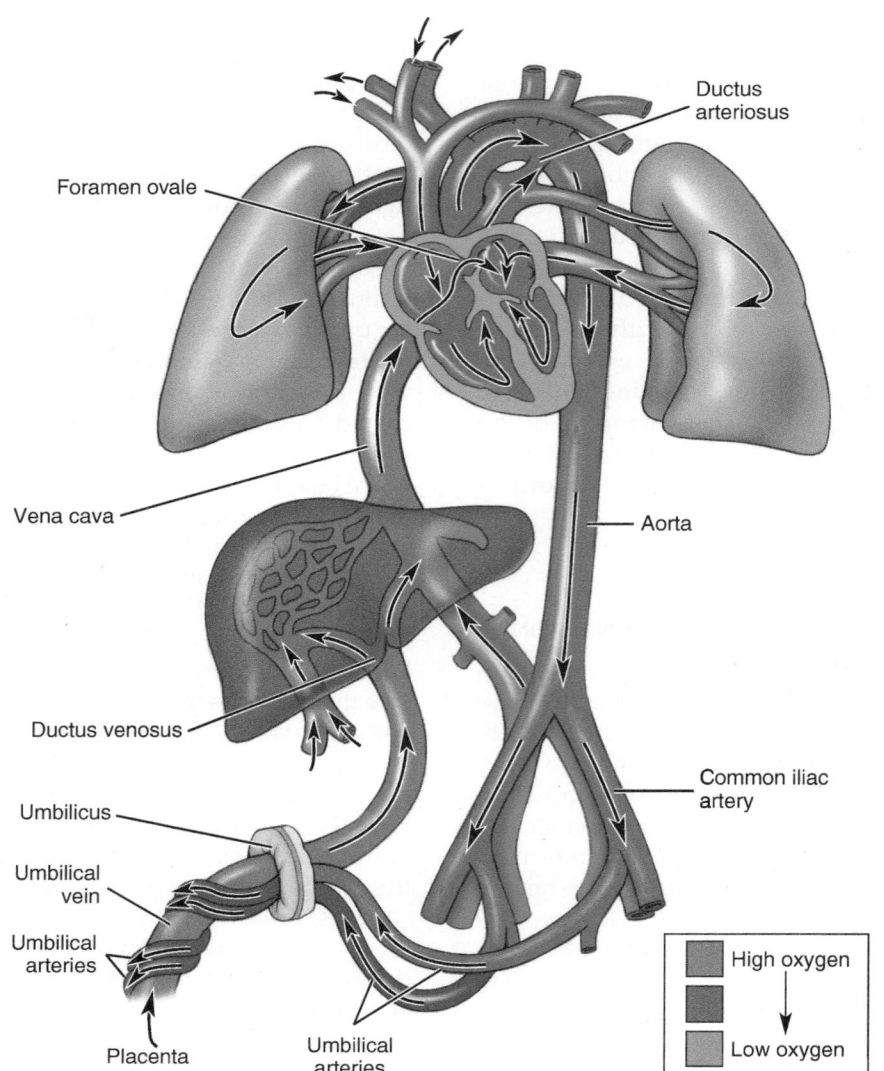

Fig. 32.1 Fetal circulation. (From Herlihy B: *The human body in health and illness*, ed 4, St. Louis, 2011, Saunders.)

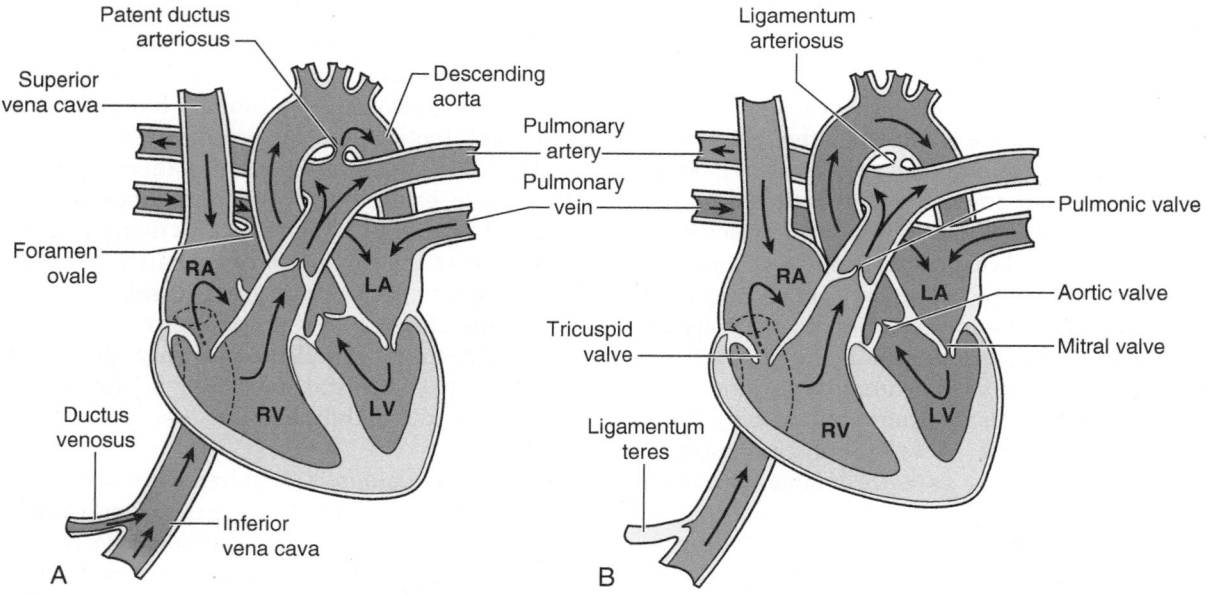

Fig. 32.2 Changes in circulation at birth. (A) Prenatal circulation. (B) Postnatal circulation. *Arrows* indicate direction of blood flow. *LA,* Left atrium; *LV,* left ventricle; *RA,* right atrium; *RV,* right ventricle.

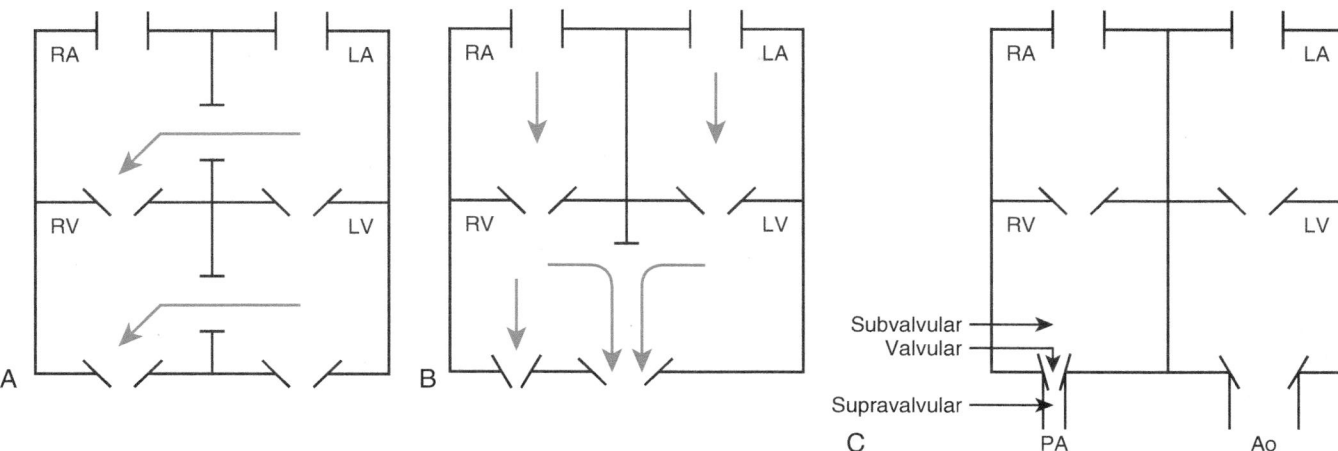

Fig. 32.3 Hemodynamics in congenital heart disease. (A) Increased pulmonary blood flow. (B) Decreased pulmonary blood flow. (C) Obstruction to systemic blood flow. *Ao,* Aorta; *LA,* left atrium; *LV,* left ventricle; *RA,* right atrium; *RV,* right ventricle.

lower extremity blood pressures, crackles, and wheezing. (See the discussions of specific clinical manifestations of common congenital heart defects throughout this chapter.)

Diagnostic Tests. Many invasive and noninvasive tests are available to diagnose cardiovascular disorders. The choice of studies the health care provider orders will vary according to the nature of the suspected disorder. The more frequently conducted tests include urine culture, arterial blood gases (ABG), electrocardiography, echocardiography, fluoroscopy, angiography, cardiac catheterization, and cardiac magnetic resonance imaging (MRI).

Defects Involving Increased Pulmonary Blood Flow

Defects involving increased pulmonary blood flow are the most common CHDs. In this type of defect, there is a communication of some type between the right and the left sides of the heart. Because of the increased pressure of the left side of the heart, some of the blood is pushed back to the right side of the heart. The increased blood on the right side of the heart then is moved to the lungs. The size of the defect and the amount of increase in blood volume determine the severity of the symptoms of heart failure.

The most common defects involving increased pulmonary blood flow are patent ductus arteriosus, atrial septal defect, and ventricular septal defect (VSD). The clinical manifestations and medical management of each are discussed in the next sections (Nursing Care Plan 32.1).

Patent Ductus Arteriosus. The ductus arteriosus is a fetal artery that connects the pulmonary artery to the aorta (see Fig. 32.1). Failure of the ductus arteriosus to close within the first weeks of life allows oxygenated blood to shunt from the high-pressure aorta to the low-pressure pulmonary artery, which causes the blood to become deoxygenated (Fig. 32.4).

Clinical Manifestations. Sometimes a small patent ductus arteriosus is asymptomatic. Children with larger defects often exhibit signs and symptoms of heart failure, including poor eating, poor growth patterns, and fatigue. Other possible clinical manifestations include a typical machine-like murmur audible at the upper left sternal border; widened pulse pressure; and bounding pulses.

Medical Management. Administration of indomethacin (a prostaglandin inhibitor) often has been effective in closing the ductus arteriosus in full-term and premature newborns. Surgical correction involves ligating the ductus arteriosus through a thoracotomy incision (surgical opening into the thoracic cavity).

Surgeons are using a new technique in some cases. Three small incisions are made on the left side of the chest, and then a thoracoscope and instruments are used to place a clip on the ductus arteriosus.

Atrial Septal Defect. An atrial septal defect is an abnormal opening in the atrial septum that enables oxygenated blood to flow from the higher pressure left atrium to the lower pressure right atrium, which causes the blood to become deoxygenated (Fig. 32.5).

Clinical Manifestations. Smaller defects (less than 5 mm in diameter) are often asymptomatic or do not produce symptoms until later in life. Larger defects produce manifestations consistent with heart failure. Additional manifestations include frequent respiratory infections and difficulty breathing. A characteristic soft systolic murmur with a split S2 may be heard during auscultation over the second intercostal space (Menillo, 2020).

Medical Management. Minor cases that are not producing symptoms often are not treated but are monitored for changes. Surgical correction consists of open heart surgery with cardiopulmonary bypass. The surgeon repairs small defects with purse-string sutures and moderate to large defects with a polyester fiber (Dacron) patch.

Nursing Care Plan 32.1 | A Child With Congenital Heart Disease

D. is a 9-month-old girl with a ventricular septal defect. She has a loud, harsh systolic murmur. She weighs 15 lb (6.8 kg); her birth weight was 7 lb (3.2 kg). The family has been told that the defect necessitates open heart surgery when she is 18–24 months of age.

PATIENT PROBLEM

Insufficient cardiac output, related to structural defect.

Patient Goals And Expected Outcomes	Nursing Interventions	Evaluation
Patient will exhibit improved cardiac output; heartbeat will be strong, regular, and within normal limits for age	Administer digoxin as ordered, and use established precautions to prevent toxicity; check dosage with another nurse for safety. Count apical pulse for 1 full min before administering drug. Withhold medication, and notify health care provider if pulse rate is less than 90–110 bpm (infants) or 75–85 bpm (older children), depending on previous pulse readings. Monitor serum potassium levels (decrease in levels enhances digoxin toxicity).	Patient's heartbeat is strong and regular.

PATIENT PROBLEM

Potential for infection, related to debilitated physical status.

Patient Goals And Expected Outcomes	Nursing Interventions	Evaluation
Patient will exhibit no evidence of infection	Use meticulous hand hygiene. Avoid contact with infected people. Monitor for signs of infection, including elevated temperature and elevated white blood cell count, which indicate possible infection. Provide frequent rest periods. Provide adequate nutrition; assess nutritional status, including daily weight. Be alert for signs of complications: • Heart failure • Digitalis toxicity • Increased respiratory effort • Hypoxemia • Cerebral thrombosis • Cardiovascular collapse	No evidence of infection is noted; temperature and white blood cell count remain within normal limits.

PATIENT PROBLEM

Potential for inability to tolerate activity, related to imbalance between oxygen supply and demand.

Patient Goals And Expected Outcomes	Nursing Interventions	Evaluation
Patient will maintain adequate energy levels	Allow for frequent rest periods. Encourage quiet, age-appropriate games and activities. Help child select activities appropriate to age, condition, and capabilities. Avoid extremes of environmental temperatures.	Patient is receiving adequate rest periods and is maintaining adequate energy levels.

PATIENT PROBLEM

Potential for atypical growth and development, related to inadequate oxygen and nutrients to tissues.

Patient Goals And Expected Outcomes	Nursing Interventions	Evaluation
Patient will achieve normal growth and development	Provide a diet high in nutrition. Provide pleasant environment for eating. Encourage patient to eat small, frequent meals. Provide snacks several times a day. Provide frequent rest periods between meals and activities. Encourage activities appropriate to the child's age and developmental level. Monitor for signs of heart failure and decreased cardiac output during activities. Arrange for continued family involvement during the child's hospitalization.	Patient is achieving normal growth and developmental milestones.

Nursing Care Plan 32.1 | **A Child With Congenital Heart Disease—cont'd**

PATIENT PROBLEMS

Potential for Injury, related to cardiac condition and therapies.
   Insufficient Knowledge, related to the disorder and methods of treatment.

Patient Goals and Expected Outcomes	Nursing Interventions	Evaluation
Family will demonstrate an understanding of the disorder and its treatments	Assess the family's understanding of the diagnosis. Reinforce the health care provider's explanation of the child's disorder and its treatments. Provide written instructions regarding medication schedules and treatment protocols. Encourage the family to verbalize questions, fears, and concerns. Allow the family to participate in the child's care when appropriate. Provide emotional support to the child and the family.	Family demonstrates understanding of child's cardiac condition as evidenced by verbal responses and therapeutic interventions.

CRITICAL THINKING QUESTIONS

1. You enter D.'s room and notice her mother sitting at her bedside crying. She states, "I don't know how I will deal with her having heart surgery." What would be an appropriate initial response to D.'s mother?
2. The mother states that D. has a very poor appetite. What two helpful suggestions may help educate the mother?
3. The mother mentions that she is concerned that D. will get an infection and become acutely ill. What are two therapeutic nursing interventions for patient teaching?

Fig. 32.4 Patent ductus arteriosus. (From James SR, Nelson KA, Ashwill JW: *Nursing care of children: Principles and practice*, ed 4, St. Louis, 2013, Saunders.)

Fig. 32.5 Atrial septal defect. (From James SR, Nelson KA, Ashwill JW: *Nursing care of children: Principles and practice*, ed 4, St. Louis, 2013, Saunders.)

Ventricular Septal Defect. A VSD is an abnormal opening in the interventricular septum, resulting in the flow of oxygenated blood from the higher pressure left ventricle to the lower pressure right ventricle, which causes the blood to become deoxygenated. The possible scope of the defect ranges from a pinhole-sized opening to absence of the entire septum (single ventricle) (Fig. 32.6).

Clinical Manifestations. Initially, such defects may be asymptomatic, but signs of heart failure eventually manifest. Other clinical manifestations include a loud, harsh systolic murmur and a palpable thrill.

Medical Management. Approximately 50% of VSDs close spontaneously; for the remainder, open heart surgery is necessary. A palliative procedure, known as *pulmonary artery banding,* can be performed in infants with symptomatic VSDs. This procedure involves impeding the flow of blood from the right ventricle to the pulmonary circulation, thus reducing pulmonary congestion. Complete surgical repair involves open heart surgery with the use of cardiopulmonary bypass. The surgeon usually repairs the defect with a polyester fiber (Dacron) patch; smaller defects sometimes necessitate only observation or sometimes necessitate surgical closure with sutures.

Fig. 32.6 Ventricular septal defect. (From James SR, Nelson KA, Ashwill JW: *Nursing care of children: Principles and practice*, ed 4, St. Louis, 2013, Saunders.)

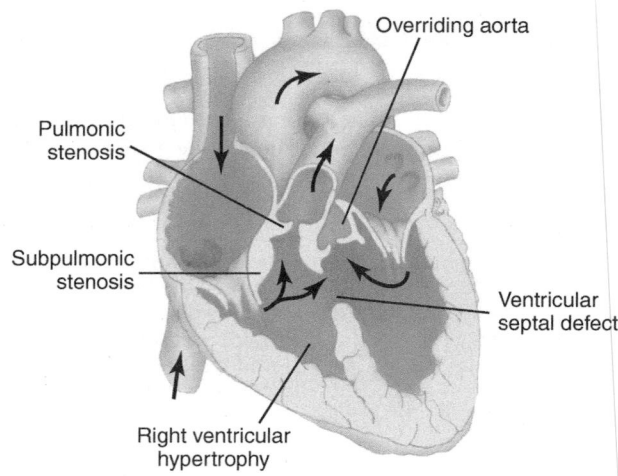

Fig. 32.7 Tetralogy of Fallot. (From James SR, Nelson KA, Ashwill JW: *Nursing care of children: Principles and practice*, ed 4, St. Louis, 2013, Saunders.)

Defects Involving Decreased Pulmonary Blood Flow

Defects involving decreased pulmonary blood flow result when there is some type of obstruction of blood flow to the lungs or if there is no connection between the right side of the heart and the lungs. Examples of defects involving decreased pulmonary blood flow include pulmonary stenosis, pulmonary atresia, and tetralogy of Fallot. The amount of obstruction or lack of connection determines the symptoms. The most common CHD resulting in decreased pulmonary blood flow is tetralogy of Fallot.

Tetralogy Of Fallot. Tetralogy of Fallot involves a combination of four defects: (1) pulmonary stenosis, (2) VSD, (3) right ventricular hypertrophy, and (4) overriding aorta (Fig. 32.7).

Clinical Manifestations. Affected infants tend to be profoundly cyanotic at birth and often experience acute episodes of severe cyanosis and hypoxia (blue spells). Older children with tetralogy of Fallot sometimes exhibit a systolic ejection murmur, clubbing of the nail beds, dyspnea, squatting, poor growth, mental slowness, syncope (fainting), and stroke.

Medical Management. In infants with profound cyanosis and hypoxia, surgeons usually perform a palliative procedure. This temporary procedure, most commonly a Blalock-Taussig shunt, creates an artificial connection between the pulmonary artery and the aorta and thus redirects blood flow back to the lungs to allow for oxygenation. Complete surgical correction involves closure of the VSD, a pulmonic valvotomy, and repair of the overriding aorta.

Mixed Defects

Mixed defects include those that do not fit into one of the other categories. These defects often include the mixing of oxygenated and unoxygenated blood in the heart or the great vessels. Symptoms are specific to the type of defects present. Examples of mixed defects include transposition of the great vessels, truncus arteriosus, and hypoplastic left heart syndrome.

Transposition Of The Great Vessels. In transposition of the great vessels, the pulmonary artery arises from the left ventricle and the aorta arises from the right ventricle. Therefore, venous blood returning to the right side of the heart exits through the aorta without being oxygenated, and oxygenated blood returning from the pulmonary system is returned via the pulmonary artery to the lungs (Fig. 32.8). Some affected infants are born with associated defects that allow for communication between the two circulations.

Clinical Manifestations. Infants born with minimal communication between the two circulations have profound cyanosis. Those who are born with an associated defect such as patent ductus arteriosus, atrial septal defect, or VSD sometimes have less cyanosis and experience manifestations of heart failure. Cardiomegaly is usually apparent on x-ray study.

Medical Management. Initially, the health care provider performs palliative procedures to provide mixing, either by enlarging an atrial septal defect that is already present or by creating one by pulling a balloon catheter through the atrial septum. Complete correction of transposition of the great vessels entails open heart surgery and involves switching the great vessels to their proper positions.

Defects Involving Obstruction to Systemic Blood Flow

Defects involving obstruction to systemic blood flow result in inability of the blood to reach the body from the heart. With this type of defect, symptoms include lack of oxygenation and decreased peripheral blood flow as a result of the obstruction, as well as symptoms of heart failure, because the blood backs up into the lungs. Defects resulting in obstruction to systemic

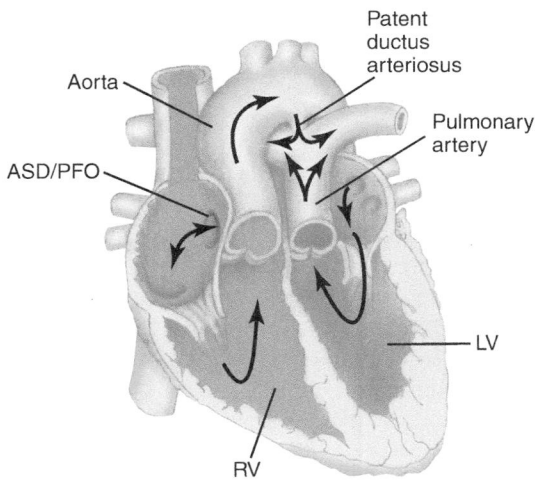

Fig. 32.8 Transposition of the great vessels. *ASD/PFO,* Atrial septal defect/patent foramen ovale; *LV,* left ventricle; *RV,* right ventricle. (From James SR, Nelson KA, Ashwill JW: *Nursing care of children: Principles and practice,* ed 4, St. Louis, 2013, Saunders.)

Fig. 32.9 Coarctation of the aorta. (From James SR, Nelson KA, Ashwill JW: *Nursing care of children: Principles and practice,* ed 4, St. Louis, 2013, Saunders.)

blood flow include aortic stenosis, pulmonary stenosis, and coarctation of the aorta.

Coarctation Of The Aorta. Coarctation of the aorta is a narrowing of the lumen of the aorta (usually at the site of the ductus arteriosus), resulting in increased pressure proximal to the defect (head and upper extremities) and decreased pressure distal to the defect (body and lower extremities) (Fig. 32.9).

Clinical Manifestations. The blood pressure in the arms is 20 mm Hg higher than that in the legs (reversal of normal pattern). Other manifestations include bounding pulses in the lower extremities, signs of heart failure, leg cramping on exertion in older affected children, and epistaxis.

Medical Management. Surgical correction involves removal of the narrowed portion of the aorta with an end-to-end anastomosis (a connection between two vessels) or graft replacement if the narrowing is extensive.

Acquired Heart Disease

Acquired heart disease refers to those disorders whose onset comes after birth. They result from a variety of reasons, including autoimmune processes, infection, familial tendencies, and environmental factors. One disease that has resurfaced and has caused concern to health care professionals is rheumatic fever.

DISORDERS OF HEMATOLOGIC FUNCTION

Childhood blood disorders encompass wide ranges of cause, severity, treatment, and prognosis. The majority of hematologic disorders occurring in infants and children stem from chronic systemic illness, nutritional deficits, and inherited blood disorders.

Anemias

Iron-Deficiency Anemia. Iron-deficiency anemia is the most prevalent blood disorder in infancy and early childhood; the incidence peaks between ages 6 and 24 months in children from lower-income backgrounds. The prevalence has decreased, probably in part because of families' participation in the Women, Infants, and Children (WIC) program, which provides iron-fortified formula for the first year of life.

Full-term, healthy infants have sufficient iron stores for the first 4 to 6 months of life. Breast-fed infants should receive adequate amounts of iron from the breast milk for the first 6 months of life. Infants who are not breast-fed should receive iron-fortified formulas for the first 9 to 12 months. Once introduction of foods begins, iron-fortified cereals and foods containing iron provide the necessary amount. The recommended daily allowance of iron for infants between the ages of 7 and 12 months is 11 mg of iron per day (USDHHS, 2021). Toddlers require 7 mg/day of iron, and to meet this requirement, a diet of iron-rich foods, such as red meat, legumes, and iron-fortified cereals, is recommended (USDHSS, 2021).

Etiology And Pathophysiology. *Anemia* is defined as a decrease in red blood cell (RBC) volume, a decrease in hemoglobin, or both. Anemia reduces the oxygen-carrying capacity of the blood and sometimes results in tissue hypoxia. Anemia is classified as either *hypoproliferative* (defective production of erythrocytes) or *hemolytic* (premature destruction of erythrocytes).

Iron-deficiency anemia develops at about 4 to 6 months of age in full-term infants and earlier in premature infants, when the maternal stores of iron become depleted and the infant becomes dependent on dietary sources of iron. Infants develop iron-deficiency anemia because milk is a poor source of iron and infants drink milk to the exclusion of solid foods. Infants who drink cow's milk have a 50% chance of increased fecal loss of blood. Anemic infants appear pale, may have poor muscle tone, and may be at increased risk for infection. Premature infants are at high risk because of a lower fetal iron supply.

Adolescents are also at risk for iron-deficiency anemia because of their rapid growth rate, combined with poor eating habits. The most common cause of anemia in adolescents is an inadequate intake of dietary iron, which is essential for hemoglobin synthesis. Other causes include acute or chronic blood loss and malabsorption of dietary iron secondary to chronic diarrhea or malabsorption syndromes.

Clinical Manifestations. The clinical signs and symptoms of mild to moderate anemia (hemoglobin values: 6 to 10 g/dL) are often vague and nonspecific. They include irritability, weakness, decreased play activity, and fatigue. When the hemoglobin value falls below 5 g/dL, the child has anorexia, skin pallor, pale mucous membranes, glossitis, concave or "spoon" fingernails, inability to concentrate, tachycardia, and systolic murmurs. Children with chronic, long-term anemia often exhibit growth retardation and developmental delays.

Diagnostic Tests. The diagnostic evaluation begins with an accurate history, including the information about the child's diet, appetite, activity, weight and rate of growth, and any recent blood loss. Initial laboratory tests include a complete blood cell count (CBC); reticulocyte count; and measurements of serum ferritin (a major iron-storage protein), serum iron concentration, and total iron-binding capacity. It is recommended that infants be screened for iron deficiency and iron deficiency anemia between the ages of 9 to 12 months of age (Mayo Clinic, 2019).

Medical Management. Therapeutic management involves iron replacement therapy, nutritional counseling, and treatment of any underlying conditions (hemorrhage or malabsorption). Health care providers usually prescribe oral iron supplementation (ferrous sulfate) until the hemoglobin level returns to normal. Citrus fruits or juices with iron supplements may be advisable because ascorbic acid enhances iron absorption. Parenteral iron may be prescribed if there is a problem with the absorption of oral iron. Packed RBCs are given only to severely anemic children. Permanent dietary changes are essential to prevent recurrence. Mothers of infants should be encouraged to breastfeed or provide iron-fortified formulas and to provide iron-rich solid foods.

Nursing Interventions. Dietary counseling is of primary importance, and the nurse's assistance to the family in choosing iron-rich foods is valuable. Advise giving oral preparations of iron three times daily between meals with citrus fruits or juices to enhance iron absorption. Parents should be informed that their child will have dark, tarry, green stools while on oral iron therapy. To avoid staining the teeth with liquid preparations of iron, teach the family to administer the medication with a syringe placed toward the back of the mouth for infants; older children can take the preparation through straws.

Patient Teaching. A primary nursing objective is to educate the family in how to prevent nutritional anemia.

For infants, discuss with parents the importance of using iron-fortified formula and the introduction of solid foods at the appropriate age. The best solid food source of iron is commercial infant cereals.

A difficulty encountered in discouraging the parents from feeding milk to the exclusion of other foods is dispelling the popular myth that milk is a perfect food. Many parents believe that milk is best for the infant and equate the weight gain with a healthy child and good parenting. They may not be concerned about providing other foods as long as the child continues to take milk. Stress that overweight is not synonymous with good health.

Diet education of teenagers is especially difficult, because teenage girls in particular are tempted to follow weight-reduction diets. Emphasizing the effects of anemia on appearance (pallor) and energy level (difficulty maintaining popular activities) is sometimes useful.

Prognosis. Serum iron levels usually return to normal within 2 months of treatment. Iron-deficiency anemia in infants and children may lead to difficulties in learning, a decrease in the attention span, and reduced alertness. In addition, iron deficiency can cause the body to absorb too much lead when exposed to the mineral.

Sickle Cell Anemia. Sickle cell anemia is one of a group of diseases collectively termed *hemoglobinopathies,* in which normal adult hemoglobin (hemoglobin A [HbA]) is replaced partially or completely by abnormal sickle hemoglobin (hemoglobin S [HbS]). Sickle cell anemia is a genetic disorder characterized by the abnormal form of hemoglobin within the erythrocyte. In the United States, the disease is most common in the African American population, with an incidence of 1 per 500 live births. Sickle cell anemia is classified as either sickle cell trait or active sickle cell disease. Sickle cell trait rarely results in clinical manifestations; however, children with sickle cell trait are carriers of sickle cell anemia. It is estimated that 1 per 13 African Americans have the sickle cell trait (Centers for Disease Control and Prevention [CDC], 2020e). The rest of this discussion focuses on active sickle cell disease, which is the most severe and potentially fatal form of the disorder.

Etiology And Pathophysiology. When oxygen is released into the tissues, the abnormal hemoglobin becomes more viscous and crystallizes, causing the erythrocyte to change from its characteristic round shape to an elongated, crescent shape (**sickled cell**). As sickled cells clump, circulation slows, resulting in obstructions with severe tissue hypoxia and necrosis. Sickling is an intermittent phenomenon; the usual precipitating factors are infection, fever, hypoxemia, dehydration, high altitudes, cold, or emotional stress.

Clinical Manifestations. Children with sickle cell disease tend to first experience pallor, irritability, fatigue, and jaundice. Growth impairment becomes apparent as the child's height and weight fall below average. Cardiomegaly and heart failure develop in response to hypoxia and decreased cardiac output. In older affected children, the joints and surrounding tissue often become edematous and painful. If sickling causes cerebral occlusion, strokes can occur, which result in sensory deficits, paralysis, or death. Persistent penile erection (priapism) sometimes occurs in response to occluded penile veins. Severe sickling leads to recurrent sickle cell crisis, an acutely painful period that occurs intermittently throughout the life of a child with sickle cell disease (Fig. 32.10). A sickle cell crisis is classified as one of three types: vasoocclusive, sequestration, or aplastic (Box 32.1).

Diagnostic Tests. Neonatal screening for sickle cell anemia is mandatory in most of the United States so that affected infants can be identified before symptoms occur. Institutions frequently use the sickle-turbidity test (SICKLEDEX) for screening purposes. It can be performed on blood from a finger stick and yields accurate results in 3 minutes. If the result is positive, the next step is to perform hemoglobin electrophoresis to determine whether the patient has sickle cell trait or sickle cell disease.

Medical Management. The treatment is primarily palliative and is outlined in Box 32.1. The only potential cure for sickle cell disease is bone marrow or stem cell transplantation.

Nursing Interventions And Patient Teaching. Nursing interventions for the child in sickle cell crisis include maintaining adequate hydration to prevent further sickling; administering analgesics as ordered; providing adequate oxygenation; and applying comfort measures such as warm baths and local heat.

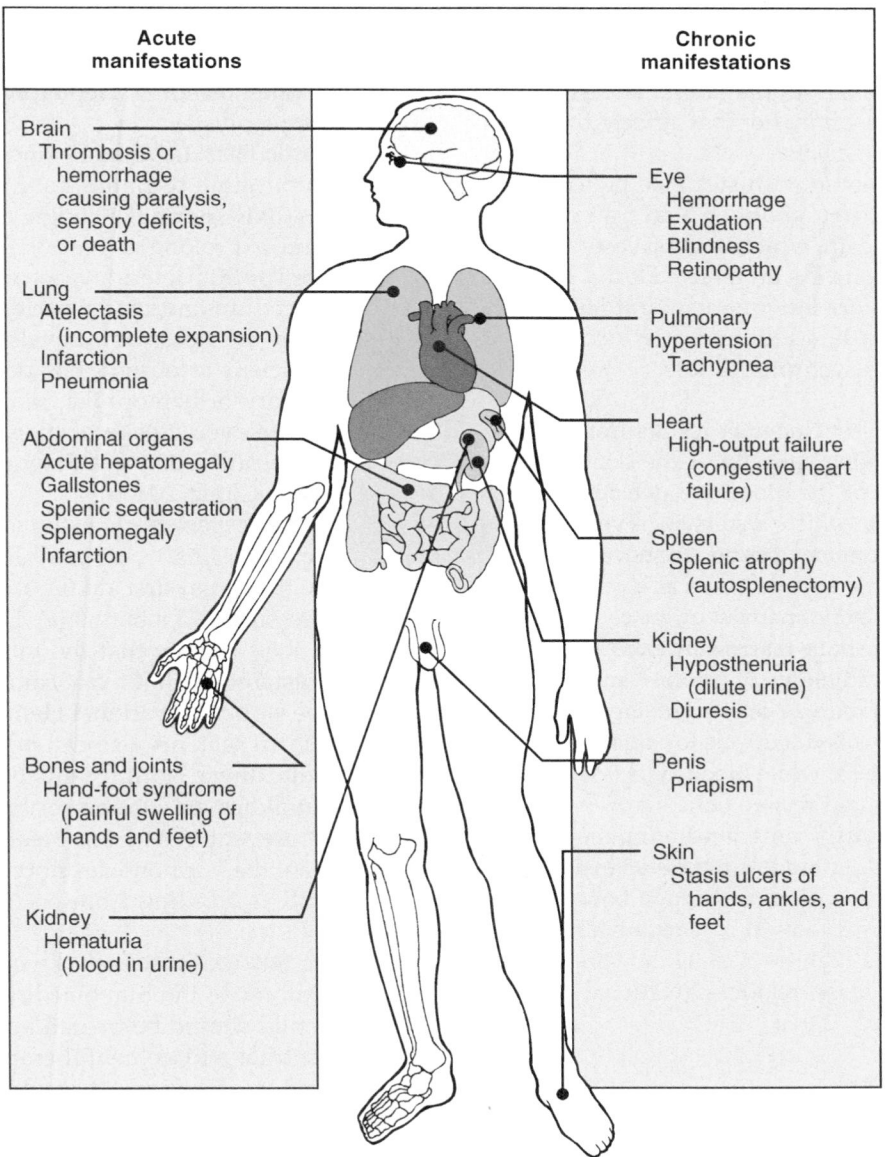

Fig. 32.10 Clinical manifestations of sickle cell disease. (From McCance KL, Huether SE: *Pathophysiology: The biologic basis for disease in adults and children*, ed 6, St. Louis, 2010, Mosby.)

Box 32.1	Types and Medical Management of Sickle Cell Crises

Vasoocclusive crisis: Obstruction of the small blood vessels of the hands and feet, resulting in edema, impaired range of motion, and pain
- Medical management: Palliative (analgesics, hydration, oxygen)

Sequestration crisis: Pooling of blood in the spleen and the liver, resulting in hepatosplenomegaly; sometimes progresses to cardiovascular collapse and death
- Medical management: Analgesics, volume expanders, transfusions; recurrent episodes treated by splenectomy

Aplastic crisis: Profound anemia, caused by premature destruction of erythrocytes
- Medical management: Transfusion of packed red blood cells

Teach families of children with sickle cell anemia to avoid situations that lead to hypoxia and sickling: infection, dehydration, emotional stress, and strenuous physical activity. Recommend that affected children wear medical alert bracelets.

Prognosis. Most people with sickle cell anemia live into adulthood. Children younger than 5 years are at the highest risk for death, which in most cases is the result of severe infections. As an affected child becomes an adolescent, crises are less frequent and less severe; however, death in early adulthood does occur. Sickle cell anemia is a serious, chronic illness.

Aplastic Anemia. Aplastic anemia results from the failure of the cell-generating capacity of the bone marrow. All formed elements of the blood are defective, underdeveloped, or absent, which results in severe anemia, leukopenia, and thrombocytopenia (pancytopenia). In some instances, aplastic anemia arises as a result of neoplastic disease of the bone marrow or, more commonly, from destruction of the bone marrow by exposure to toxic chemicals, ionizing radiation, or certain antibiotics or other medications. A failure of cell-producing capacity by aspirated bone marrow is diagnostic for aplastic anemia. In aplastic anemia, RBCs, white blood cells (WBCs), and platelets are deficient, and the red bone marrow becomes yellow and fatty. Treatment aims at restoring the function of the marrow through immunosuppressive treatment or at replacing the defective marrow through bone marrow transplantation. Survival rates at 5 years are about 70%. The rate of survival is highest in patients who received the transplant from close relatives (National Marrow Donor Program, n.d.).

Coagulation Disorders

Coagulation disorders in children characteristically involve abnormal bleeding into the skin or from internal organs, secondary to clotting factor defects, platelet dysfunction, or vascular compromise.

Hemophilia

Etiology And Pathophysiology. Hemophilia is a serious, lifelong bleeding disease inherited as an X-linked recessive disorder. Hemophilia is transmitted by female carriers and affects boys in 1 per 5000 male births. Classic hemophilia (type A) is caused by a deficiency in factor VIII, which is a necessary component of blood coagulation.

Clinical Manifestations. It is usually possible to make a diagnosis after infancy. In toddlerhood, when children typically become more active, hemophilic boys tend to have more episodes of oral bleeding and bruising. The most frequent types of internal bleeding occur within the joints (hemarthrosis) and the muscles. Pain intensifies as the bleeding continues to fill the joint cavity, limiting movement to the point where the child refuses to use the affected joint. Recurrent episodes of hemarthrosis lead to bone deformities with resulting contractures and crippling. Intracranial hemorrhage, either spontaneous or secondary to head trauma, is life threatening and accounts for more hemophilic deaths than any other bleeding. Hematomas in the spinal cord can cause paralysis.

Diagnostic Tests. Laboratory findings include normal prothrombin time (PT), normal international normalized ratio (INR), normal bleeding time, normal platelet count, and a prolonged partial thromboplastin time (PTT). For specific determination of factor deficiencies, assay procedures normally performed in specialized laboratories are necessary. Levels of factors VIII and IX are deficient or absent. For people with a known family history of hemophilia, diagnosis can be made in utero. The average age of diagnosis for children is 9 months. Nearly 100% are diagnosed by the age of 2 years (Mayo Clinic, 2020b).

Medical Management. For the most common type of hemophilia, small cuts and scrapes typically are treated with regular first aid (cleaning the cut, then applying pressure and a bandage). Deep cuts or internal bleeding may require that the missing clotting factor be administered so that a clot can form and the bleeding can be stopped (National Hemophilia Foundation, n.d.c.). Fibrin sealants also can be applied to wounds to promote direct clotting and healing of a wound. Antifibrinolytics are clot-preserving medications that can help prevent clots from breaking down. Regular infusions of the hormone desmopressin (DDAVP) help in preventing bleeding from occurring (Mayo Clinic, 2020b).

Nursing Interventions. Early recognition of the signs and symptoms of internal bleeding is very important, and the child should be treated aggressively with factor concentrate replacement therapy.

Nursing interventions focus on teaching the child and the family to avoid injury and control bleeding. The parents should be advised to give the child age-appropriate toys without rough or sharp edges, to remove throw rugs, and to place barriers at stairs.

Playtime should be supervised to minimize hazards and injuries. Physical activity, such as swimming, softball, bicycling, hiking, bowling, golf, and running, should be recommended to promote muscle development and psychological well-being. The child should be advised against contact sports, such as football, hockey, or soccer, because of their potential for injury. Early dental visits with a dentist knowledgeable about hemophilia help minimize the risk of bleeding gums. Children with hemophilia should wear medical alert bracelets. The family also should be informed about the National Hemophilia Foundation, which is a good resource for financial, medical, and psychological assistance.

Patient Teaching. Parents of children with hemophilia should be educated regarding the RICE method: *r*est, *i*ce, *c*ompression, and *e*levation. When external bleeding occurs, the affected area should be elevated while pressure and ice are applied. The child and family also should be instructed in safely administering factor products at home. Parents should seek emergency medical care if the child has signs of increased intracranial pressure, which sometimes indicates intracranial bleeding: severe headache, slurred speech, vomiting, disorientation, and loss of consciousness. The parents should be taught how to protect the child, but at the same time they should be encouraged not to be overprotective.

Prognosis. Medical advances have given children with hemophilia a normal life expectancy. Unfortunately, those who received blood transfusions before the use of the current purification techniques (before 1985) were at a high risk for exposure to the human immunodeficiency virus (HIV). During the early years of the HIV/AIDS crisis and before current purification techniques, about half of all patients with hemophilia became infected with HIV. Parents of children with hemophilia can be assured that the transfusions of factor VIII and IX are safe as there has not been any transmissions of HIV from these treatments since 1987 (National Hemophilia Foundation, n.d.a.).

Gene therapy is a major focus of research. Some promising studies are being conducted in gene therapy that include infusion of the correct version of the genes through a viral vector. Clinical trials are ongoing and a New Drug Application is expected soon (National Hemophilia Foundation, n.d.b.).

Idiopathic Thrombocytopenia Purpura

Etiology And Pathophysiology. Idiopathic (cause unknown) thrombocytopenia purpura (ITP) is characterized by a marked decrease in the number of circulating platelets with resultant bleeding beneath the skin. ITP is the most common thrombocytopenia of childhood, with onset most frequently among children aged 2 to 10 years. It occurs in either acute or chronic form. As its name implies, the cause of ITP is unknown; however, the condition is believed to be an autoimmune response to disease-related antigens. The acute form of ITP usually follows a viral infection (such as a respiratory infection, rubella, rubeola, mumps, or chickenpox; or after infection with parvovirus B19) and is self-limiting; the chronic form has periods of remission.

Clinical Manifestations. Other than bleeding, the affected child appears healthy. The platelet count drops to below $20,000/mm^3$, so clotting is impaired. Platelet counts lower than $10,000/mm^3$ are potentially life threatening. Ecchymosis and a pinpoint petechial rash are usually the first signs of ITP, and the areas most commonly involved are over bony prominences. Other manifestations include bleeding gums, bleeding lips, and epistaxis (nosebleeds). The most serious complication of ITP is intracranial hemorrhage (bleeding into the subdural, subarachnoid, or intracerebellar space), and characteristic signs are hematuria (blood in urine), hemarthrosis, melena (black, tarry stools), hematemesis (blood in vomitus), and menorrhagia (abnormally heavy menstrual periods).

Diagnostic Tests. Criteria indicating the possibility of this diagnosis are clinical manifestations. The platelet count is reduced to less than $20,000/mm^3$. Microscopic examination reveals not only a decreased number of platelets but also platelets that are large. Bleeding time and clot reaction time are prolonged, and the tourniquet test for capillary fragility, in which a blood pressure cuff is inflated to 100 mm Hg and left in place for 5 minutes, yields a positive result: the appearance of more than 15 petechiae.

Medical Management. ITP is a self-limiting illness in most cases, and about three-fourths of affected children recover without complications within 3 months. In most cases, health care providers allow ITP to run its course with supportive management. Some prescribe a short course of corticosteroids to suppress the immune attack on platelets, thereby reducing the severity of the disease. Transfusions of packed RBCs are sometimes necessary in treating severe, life-threatening hemorrhage. Use of intravenous gamma globulin (IVGG) and anti-D antibody therapy has achieved some success in treating chronic cases of ITP. Anti-D antibody therapy is a relatively new treatment that is much less expensive than IVGG. Children with symptomatic recurrent or chronic ITP that fails to respond to treatment for a year or longer usually undergo splenectomy, which eliminates the site of antiplatelet antibody production. Splenectomy removes the risk of hemorrhage, as well as the need for parents to closely monitor their child's activities. Before considering splenectomy, health care providers generally recommend waiting until the child is older than 5 years of age because of the increased risk of bacterial infection. In general, health care providers order pneumococcal and meningococcal vaccines before splenectomy. The child also receives penicillin prophylactically after splenectomy. The length of prophylactic therapy is controversial, but the usual recommendation is for a minimum of 3 years.

Nursing Interventions And Patient Teaching. Nursing interventions are largely supportive. Preventing bruising and controlling bleeding are of primary importance in managing ITP. Offer education and emotional support.

The family must be taught to protect the child while the platelet count is lower than 100,000/mm³, to restrict the child's activity, and to help the child avoid injury. It is best for children with ITP not to participate in any contact sports, bike riding, skateboarding, roller skating, gymnastics, climbing, or running. In addition, counsel the family never to depend on salicylate drugs (e.g., aspirin) for pain, because salicylates inhibit platelet function; salicylate substitutes such as acetaminophen (Tylenol) should be used instead. Instruct parents to notify their health care provider immediately if the child experiences acute head trauma and especially if the child exhibits symptoms of intracranial hemorrhage: headaches, visual disturbances, lethargy, vomiting, or disorientation.

Prognosis. For most children with ITP, the course is self-limited, with complete recovery within 6 months. For children who develop a chronic form of ITP, a splenectomy may be advised.

Neoplastic Disorders

Neoplastic disorders are the leading cause of death from disease in children past infancy. Although therapeutic advances in drug treatment (chemotherapy), radiation therapy, and surgical techniques have increased the potential for a normal lifespan, cancer remains a catastrophic, emotionally devastating diagnosis for the child and family.

Leukemia. *Leukemia* is the name given to a group of malignant diseases of the bone marrow and the lymphatic system. Leukemia is the most common malignancy of childhood and is more common in boys than in girls with an incidence peak between the ages of 2 and 6 years. It is, however, one of the forms of cancer for which survival rates have improved dramatically. Among children with acute lymphoid leukemia (ALL), the 10-year rate of survival is 90% (St. Jude Children's Research Hospital, n.d.).

Etiology And Pathophysiology. The type of leukemia that is most common in children is ALL, followed by acute nonlymphoid (myelogenous) leukemia. Although its cause is unknown, its pathologic characteristic is the uncontrollable proliferation of blast cells (immature WBCs), which accumulate in the marrow and cause crowding and depression of other healthy cells (mature WBCs, RBCs, and platelets).

Leukemia involves an overproduction of WBCs, although in the acute form of the disease, the WBC count is low. Bone marrow and peripheral blood smears show numerous, immature WBCs or blasts. Although the normal blood cells and vascular tissue are not destroyed directly by the leukemic cells, the leukemic cells infiltrate and crowd the normal cells, depriving them of the nutrients necessary for metabolism. Three

problems and effects develop as a result: (1) the decrease in RBCs causes anemia, (2) neutropenia leads to infection, and (3) the decrease in platelets causes bleeding (Hockenberry and Wilson, 2015). As nonfunctional blast cells infiltrate the lymph nodes, liver, kidneys, and spleen, they cause organ enlargement, which produces the clinical manifestations of acute leukemia.

Clinical Manifestations. Anemia, with pallor and fatigue, is often severe and often the first symptom of leukemia. Other signs are leukopenia, fever, infection, thrombocytopenia, bleeding, bruising, and petechiae. Blast cells also may invade bones, which results in bone and joint pain, limping, and edema. Bone fractures are the result of the weakening of the bone caused by the infiltration of the bone marrow by leukemic cells. Hepatosplenomegaly and enlargement of lymph nodes are often present at diagnosis. Involvement of the central nervous system (CNS) is secondary to leukemic infiltration, which sometimes causes increased intracranial pressure.

Diagnostic Tests. Diagnosis is based on review of the patient's symptoms, medical history, and results of a complete physical examination. A CBC typically indicates pancytopenia (decreased amounts of RBCs, WBCs, and platelets). Diagnostic findings in bone marrow aspirate and peripheral blood smear are immature blastic leukocyte cells. Performing a lumbar puncture is an option to determine whether the CNS has been infiltrated.

Medical Management. The health care provider institutes a highly individualized treatment protocol immediately after diagnosis. Many of the drugs used to bring about remission have the capacity to cause a serious depletion of blood elements. Therefore, the period immediately after remission is characterized by vulnerability to serious infection and hemorrhage. Supportive therapy is critical until the bone marrow recovers.

Almost immediately after confirmation of the diagnosis, induction therapy begins and lasts for 4 to 6 weeks. The principal drugs that serve for induction in ALL are corticosteroids (especially prednisone), vincristine, and L-asparaginase, with or without doxorubicin. Drug therapy for ALL includes doxorubicin or daunorubicin (or daunomycin) and cytosine arabinoside.

To prevent the development of CNS leukemia, prophylactic treatment has become a standard protocol. However, the blood-brain barrier prohibits most systemic drugs from penetrating the CNS; therefore, the intrathecal route (in which the health care provider injects the drugs directly into the cerebrospinal fluid [CSF] via lumbar puncture) is the route of choice for CNS prophylaxis. Methotrexate, the drug of choice, is given intrathecally but also may be given intravenously, along with other chemotherapeutic agents, such as triple intrathecal agent (consisting of methotrexate, cytarabine, and hydrocortisone). Once remission has occurred, the health care provider initiates maintenance therapy in an effort to maintain remission and further reduce leukemic cells. The protocol includes daily doses of 6-mercaptopurine, weekly doses of methotrexate, and monthly doses of prednisone and vincristine for 2 to 3 years.

Nursing Interventions. An important nursing intervention in dealing with children with any type of childhood cancer is to be available to the family, especially in the early phases of diagnosis and treatment.

Patient problems and interventions for a child with cancer include but are not limited to the following:

PATIENT PROBLEM	NURSING INTERVENTIONS
Potential for Infection, related to impaired immune system	Provide private room; use neutropenic precautions if necessary
	Restrict all visitors and health care providers with active infection
	Use strict hand hygiene technique
	Monitor the patient's temperature
	Use aseptic technique for all skin punctures
	Administer granulocyte colony–stimulating factor subcutaneously, as prescribed, to reduce the incidence and duration of infection in children receiving chemotherapy treatment for cancer
	In some research centers, special germ-free environments are available during complete myelosuppression from intensive chemotherapy or for bone marrow transplantation
Potential for Insufficient Nutrition, related to • Nausea • Vomiting • Anorexia	Encourage the patient to eat frequent, small meals of any food tolerated; plan to improve quality of food selections when appetite increases
	Take advantage of hungry period; serve small snacks
	Fortify foods with nutritious supplements, such as powdered milk or commercial supplements
	Allow child to be involved in food preparation and selection when appropriate
Anxiousness, related to unknown outcome	Instruct patient and family about treatments
	Promote atmosphere of open communication
	Encourage patient and family to ventilate feelings
	Recognize developmental fears associated with illness, procedures, and disturbance in self-esteem

Patient Teaching. When working with families of children with cancer, the nurse has a significant supportive role in helping them understand the therapies; preventing or managing expected side effects or toxic effects; observing for late effects of treatment; and helping the child and family live as normal a life as possible and cope with the emotional aspects of the disease. Education is a constant feature of the nursing role, especially with regard to new treatments, clinical trials, and home care. Monitor the children closely after completion of treatment to evaluate for possible recurrence or to note any long-term complications as a result of the treatment.

Prognosis. Children younger than 1 year and older than 10 years when ALL is diagnosed are considered patients at high risk. Girls appear to have a slightly more favorable prognosis than do boys. African American and Hispanic children with ALL tend to have a slightly lower cure rate than do children of other races. Of children with acute nonlymphoid (myelogenous) leukemia, those younger than 2 years tend to respond better to treatment than do older children. With both types of leukemia, children who respond quickly to treatment are more likely to have a favorable outcome (American Cancer Society [ACS], 2019).

Hodgkin Lymphoma. Childhood Hodgkin lymphoma is a malignant lymphoma distinguished by painless, progressive enlargement of lymphoid tissue, fever, night sweats, and weight loss. Although the exact cause is unknown, it is believed to develop in one specific site and to spread to nearby lymph nodes through the lymphatic vessels. Infection with the Epstein-Barr virus is a risk factor for developing the disease. Classical Hodgkin lymphoma and nodular lymphocyte-predominant Hodgkin lymphoma are the two types of childhood Hodgkin lymphoma. The most common sites for Hodgkin lymphoma to develop are in the chest, the neck, and under the arms, and groin. Lymph node biopsy helps determine the presence of Reed-Sternberg cells, an abnormal type of B lymphocyte that is the main diagnostic feature of Hodgkin lymphoma (National Cancer Institute, 2020).

Prognosis. If the diagnosis of childhood Hodgkin lymphoma is detected early and treated promptly, the prognosis is favorable for curing the disease. Factors such as the stage of the cancer, features of the cancer cells, and how well the tumor responds to treatment determine the prognosis and curability (National Cancer Institute, 2020).

DISORDERS OF IMMUNE FUNCTION

Immunodeficiency disorders result from impairment of immune function with alteration of the immune (self-defense) response. Immunodeficiency disorders are classified as primary or secondary. Primary immunodeficiency disorders result from genetic or congenital abnormalities and include X-linked agammaglobulinemia (defect in B cell development), DiGeorge syndrome (congenital absence of thymus and parathyroid glands), and severe combined immune deficiency (absence of B and T lymphocytes and of phagocytic cells). Secondary immunodeficiency disorders, the most common form of immunodeficiency, are disorders acquired in association with certain drug therapies such as corticosteroids, cancer chemotherapy, and antibiotics; radiation therapy; splenectomy; and viral infections. The common indicator in all immunodeficiency disorders is the development of unusual or recurrent, severe infections.

Human Immunodeficiency Virus And Acquired Immunodeficiency Syndrome

Etiology And Pathophysiology. AIDS is a chronic and usually fatal disease caused by an acquired dysfunction of the immune system. AIDS is caused by HIV, which has been found in blood and in varying amounts in body fluids (semen, vaginal secretions, breast milk, tears, saliva, and urine). Children may become infected with HIV by their mother while in utero, during delivery, or through breast-feeding. Additional means of infection include sexual abuse by an infected offender and participation in high-risk behaviors such as intravenous (IV) drug use and unsafe sexual activity. Children living with HIV in the United States reflect a relatively small portion of the population of children infected worldwide (UNAIDS, n.d.).

HIV targets the cells that have the CD4$^+$ molecules on their surface, especially the T helper lymphocytes. These cells are targeted because they have more CD4$^+$ receptors on their surfaces than do any other cells. Immune dysfunction occurs as a result of the destruction of T helper cells by HIV. A normal CD4$^+$ lymphocyte count is 500/μL to 1600/μL of blood. The immune system remains healthy when CD4$^+$ counts exceed 500 cells/μL. Severe immune problems occur when the CD4$^+$ count falls below 200/μL, which heightens the risk for opportunistic diseases and death from AIDS (HIV.gov, 2020).

Transmission of HIV to the infant during pregnancy, labor, and delivery has decreased to less than 10% since the 1990s. Interventions that have led to the decrease in the transmission rate include the use of antiretroviral drugs for prophylaxis, the avoidance of breast-feeding, and elective cesarean delivery (CDC, 2021c).

Clinical Manifestations. Symptoms of HIV and AIDS infection in children range from no symptoms to severe, life-threatening illnesses. Signs and symptoms common to HIV and AIDS in children include failure to thrive; weight loss; meningitis; delayed physical and developmental growth; frequent and long-lasting fevers and sweats; and frequent viral and bacterial infections (cytomegalovirus, herpes simplex virus (HSV), otitis media, sinusitis, enterocolitis, recurrent pneumonia, and septicemia).

The greatest threat to an HIV-infected infant younger than 1 year is *Pneumocystis jiroveci* (formerly *Pneumocystis carinii*) pneumonia, which is sometimes life threatening (Boston Children's Hospital, n.d.). Unique findings in the pediatric population with AIDS include lymphocytic interstitial pneumonia, oral and diaper-area candidiasis, and chronic ear infections. One of the most common causes of CNS mass lesions in HIV-infected children is malignant CNS lymphoma. In contrast to HIV-infected adults, infected children rarely contract Kaposi sarcoma. Male and female infected adolescents demonstrate more adult-oriented symptoms; girls exhibit gynecologic manifestations similar to those seen in infected women. When caring for an HIV-infected adolescent, remember that the patient is still a child and still developing cognitively, physically, and emotionally.

Diagnostic Tests. In children older than 18 months, health care providers establish the diagnosis of HIV infection by using the same serologic tests for the presence of serum HIV antibodies—enzyme-linked immunosorbent assay (ELISA) and Western blot—as in adults. The individual's blood is tested with ELISA or enzyme immunoassay (EIA), antibody tests that detect the presence of HIV antibodies. If the ELISA or EIA result is positive for HIV, then the same blood is tested a second time. If the result on the second test is positive, a more specific confirming test such as the Western blot is performed. Blood that is reactive or positive in all three steps is reported to be HIV positive. The diagnosis in a child younger than 18 months is complicated by the fact that in the seropositive mother, maternal HIV antibodies cross the placenta to the fetus. In most exposed infants up to 18 months of age, tests yield results positive for HIV antibodies, but it is unclear whose antibodies are being detected during this time.

A polymerase chain reaction (PCR) test, which tests for the presence of HIV, not for the antibody, is available to definitively diagnose HIV infection early in infants younger than 18 months. The benefits of this type of testing include early identification and treatment of the HIV-infected infant, as well as decreased anxiety and waiting time for HIV-negative parents with HIV-exposed infants.

Medical Management. There is currently no cure for HIV. Treatment is aimed at slowing the progression of the virus, prevention and treatment of opportunistic infections, maintaining normal growth and development, and maintaining quality of life.

Combinations of antiretroviral drugs help prevent reproduction of new virus particles. Antiretroviral therapy does not cure the HIV-infected patient but does assist in preventing further destruction of the immune system. The antiretroviral drugs used in HIV therapy are listed and organized by category in Box 32.2. A combination of several antiretroviral drugs is prescribed to prevent resistance to the drugs from developing. Research continues in the development of treatment for HIV-positive patients. Therapy is lifelong, which makes adherence to the regimen difficult.

Box **32.2**   Antiretroviral Drugs

NUCLEOSIDE REVERSE TRANSCRIPTASE INHIBITORS (NRTIS)
- lamivudine and zidovudine
- lamivudine, 3TC
- zidovudine, azidothymidine, AZT, ZDV
- didanosine, ddl
- abacavir sulfate, ABC

NON-NUCLEOSIDE REVERSE TRANSCRIPTASE INHIBITORS (NNRTIS)
- rilpivirine
- efavirenz, EFV
- nevirapine, NVP

PROTEASE INHIBITORS (PIS)
- tipranavir, TPV
- saquinavir mesylate, SQV
- lopinavir and ritonavir, LPV/RTV
- nelfinavir mesylate, NFV

HIV INTEGRASE STRAND TRANSFER INHIBITOR
- elvitegravir

However, if the patient's compliance with treatment results in and maintains an undetectable viral load, the HIV+ patient does not transmit the virus to others through sex and reduces the risk of perinatal transmission to less than 1% (CDC, 2021b). With proper treatment of the HIV+ mother and her newborn as well as not breast feeding, the risk of transmission is thought to be less than 1%, even with detectable viral loads (CDC, 2021cLaboratory markers ($CD4^+$ lymphocyte count, viral load) assist in monitoring disease progression and response to therapy.

It is important that HIV-infected children keep current with all childhood immunizations. The weakened immune system may not produce antibodies to vaccines. Therefore, after exposure to childhood diseases such as varicella, measles, and rubella, prophylaxis treatment may be advised.

Nursing Interventions. The nursing interventions are basically the same for the adult and pediatric populations. However, it is necessary to monitor HIV-infected children closely for signs of abnormal growth and development, which are common in this population. Complications of HIV-related infections often cause severe failure to thrive and numerous nutritional deficiencies. Because of anorexia, nausea, and diarrhea associated with recurrent illness, it is often difficult to maintain adequate nutrition. If the child exhibits weight loss and slowing of growth and development, the health care provider initiates intensive nutritional interventions (Hockenberry and Wilson, 2015). If the family is involved in the child's care, nursing interventions should be directed at emotionally supporting the family. Whenever possible, make arrangements for the intervention of social services and home health and nutritional services, such as the WIC program.

Patient problems and interventions for a child with HIV include but are not limited to the following:

PATIENT PROBLEM	NURSING INTERVENTIONS
Potential for Infection, related to • Impaired body defenses • Presence of infective organisms	Restrict contact with people who have infections, including family, other children, friends, and members of staff Practice thorough hand hygiene Place child in room with noninfectious children; restrict visitors with active illnesses Advise visitors (and hospital personnel) to practice thorough hand hygiene Promote body's remaining natural defenses (e.g., good nutrition)
Compromised Social Interaction, related to • Physical limitations • Hospitalizations • Social stigma surrounding AIDS	Administer medication as prescribed Assist child in identifying personal strengths Educate school personnel and classmates about AIDS Encourage child to participate in activities with other children
Potential for Complex Grief, related to having a child with a potentially fatal illness	Identify stage of grieving process that the family is experiencing Provide opportunities for the family to express emotions Help the parents deal with their feelings, which allows them more emotional reserve to meet the needs of their children Encourage the parents to share their moments of sorrow with their children Facilitate the family's assistance with the child's care

Patient Teaching. The adolescent population is contracting HIV infection with increasing incidence. Changing moral standards, increased sexual freedom, increased IV drug use, and misinformation about the disease in this age group render adolescents at high risk for exposure to the disease. As a patient advocate, educate adolescents directly by counseling them on matters such as avoiding casual sex and using a condom during intercourse. Promote educational messages in the media, such as radio and social media, and in places that youths frequent.

Prognosis. Infants infected in the perinatal period generally have more rapid disease progression than do children infected at older ages or adults. It has been reported that the risk of dying is higher for children in whom AIDS is diagnosed early in life and in those who develop *P. jiroveci* pneumonia. Early recognition and improved medical treatments have changed the course of HIV infection in children from a rapidly fatal illness to a chronic but still terminal disease of childhood. The ultimate prognosis for children with perinatal HIV infection depends strongly on counseling pregnant women about HIV infection, voluntary testing, and the methods currently in practice for the prevention of perinatal transmission.

Juvenile Idiopathic Arthritis

Etiology And Pathophysiology. *Juvenile idiopathic arthritis (JIA)*—also known as *juvenile rheumatoid arthritis*—is chronic arthritis occurring during childhood. JIA is the most common chronic form of joint inflammation in children, affecting girls twice as often as boys. The condition may manifest as early as 6 months of age. In most affected children, it is diagnosed by age 16 years.

JIA is characterized by chronic inflammation of the synovium with joint effusion. This inflammatory process leads to erosion, destruction, and fibrosis of the articular cartilage. The exact cause of the inflammatory process is unknown, but the supposition is that the tissue injury arises from a previous infectious process. There are several different types of JIA. The different types are classified partly on the basis of the areas of the body affected and the condition manifestations.

Clinical Manifestations. JIA may affect a single joint or numerous joints. The affected joints may be stiff and warm to the touch. Systemic manifestations may include fever and rash. The physical examination may reveal swelling in the spleen, liver, and lymph nodes. Eye involvement, such as uveitis or iritis, also may be noted. Changes in vision may include red eyes and photosensitivity, although most children with eye involvement have no symptoms, so routine eye examinations are essential to detect early clinical manifestations.

Diagnostic Tests. The diagnosis is made by the clinical presentation of the patient as well as diagnostic testing. Children who have the condition may exhibit normal findings on the traditional battery of tests performed to diagnose the disease. Initially, the history is reviewed, and other potential causes are ruled out. Laboratory tests include measurement of the erythrocyte sedimentation rate, which is elevated in the condition; CBC; measurement of C-reactive protein, to measure levels of inflammation; and search for antinuclear antibodies (ANA), which are present in the condition. Radiographic studies in early-onset JIA sometimes show the widening of joint spaces and, later, fusion and articular destruction. Regular eye examinations are indicated for a child with the condition.

Medical Management. The goals of management include the prevention of joint contractures, preservation of joint function, and relief of signs and symptoms. There is no specific cure for JIA. Nonsteroidal antiinflammatory drugs (NSAIDs), which include naproxen (Naprosyn) and ibuprofen (Motrin), are the first line of drug treatment. Stronger prescription NSAIDs may be ordered by health care providers if over-the-counter NSAIDs are not effective. In addition, corticosteroids may be ordered to control exacerbations of inflammation. Health care providers usually add slower-acting antirheumatic drugs (SAARDs) to the drug therapy when one or two of the NSAIDs no longer effectively control signs and symptoms. The SAARDs include methotrexate, sulfasalazine (Azulfidine), and hydroxychloroquine (Plaquenil).

The class of medications known as disease-modifying antirheumatic drugs (DMARDs) is used when other treatment options become ineffective. DMARDs include methotrexate (Trexall) and sulfasalazine (Azulfidine) and can be used in combination with NSAIDs. The disadvantage of this class of medications is the increased chance of infection. Tumor necrosis factor (TNF)–blocking agents such as etanercept (Enbrel) and adalimumab (Humira) are the next step of treatment when SAARDs do not control symptoms. TNF blockers help in reducing pain, morning stiffness, and joint swelling. The disadvantage of TNF blockers is the increased risk for infections, as well as the increased chance that lymphoma or another type of cancer will develop. Immune suppressants such as abatacept (Orencia) and rituximab (Rituxan) help slow the overactivity of the immune system in JIA. Symptom treatment for JIA includes physical therapy to improve joint mobility. Surgical intervention is sometimes necessary for children experiencing severe JIA that is unresponsive to therapy. Surgical procedures are performed to relieve pain or correct joint deformities. Joint replacement surgery also may be necessary.

Nursing Interventions. A key role of the nurse in care of a child with JIA begins with a thorough collection of data. Assessment of difficulties and activity intolerance should be evaluated closely. Emotional support and teaching about planned diagnostic testing are indicated. The family and child should be encouraged to express fears and concerns. The patient and parents need instruction concerning the best means to conserve strength while attempting to participate in the normal activities of daily living. Rest, exercise, and pharmacologic therapies are the cornerstones of treatment. Independence, when possible, should be stressed. Suggested physical activity for the affected child includes walking, bicycling, and swimming. Disease management strategies, such as the use of heat and cold and range-of-motion exercises, are included in the topics of education. Suggest support groups for the child and the parents that provide the necessary education and resources to cope effectively with a chronic, debilitating illness. Referrals to the Arthritis Foundation (www.arthritis.org) can provide this assistance.

Patient problems and interventions for a child with JIA include but are not limited to the following:

PATIENT PROBLEM	NURSING INTERVENTIONS
Prolonged Pain, related to joint inflammation	Provide as much relief as possible with antiinflammatory medication and other therapies to help the child tolerate the pain and cope as effectively as possible (although complete pain relief is desirable, it is probably unattainable) Apply moist heat to relieve pain and stiffness (the most efficient and practical method is tub baths)
Compromised Physical Mobility, related to joint discomfort and stiffness	Promote activities of daily living to provide satisfactory exercise and increase mobility Encourage lying in the prone position to straighten hips and knees Instruct patient and family in the purpose and correct use of any splints and appliances Instruct in use of elevated toilet seat for independent toileting

Prognosis. The course of JIA is highly variable. Children who have systemic involvement may not achieve remission and may require long-term treatment into adulthood. These children may experience joint damage and disability. Early recognition and treatment of the disease may prevent permanent joint damage, and some children will experience complete remission.

DISORDERS OF RESPIRATORY FUNCTION

Acute respiratory infections are extremely common in infants and children. The possibilities range from minor to life-threatening illnesses. Most respiratory illnesses involve viral pathogens. Bacterial infections most commonly involve groups A- and β-hemolytic streptococci (GABHS), *Staphylococcus aureus,* and *Haemophilus influenzae.*

Disorders Involving the Entire Respiratory Tract
Respiratory Distress Syndrome
Etiology And Pathophysiology. *Respiratory distress syndrome (RDS), idiopathic respiratory distress syndrome,* and *hyaline membrane disease* are synonymous terms for the severe lung disorder that is the major cause of morbidity and mortality in the neonatal period. RDS is caused by a deficiency of surfactant and occurs almost exclusively in preterm infants of low birth weight. RDS occurs more often in boys and in infants delivered by cesarean section. Other predisposing factors include maternal diabetes, asphyxia, maternal hemorrhage, and shock. Surfactant reduces the surface tension of fluids that line the alveoli, thereby enabling expansion of the lungs and alveolar inflation. Without sufficient production of surfactant, the infant is unable to keep the lungs inflated and the alveoli collapse at the end of expiration, resulting in hypoxia, atelectasis, and respiratory acidosis.

Clinical Manifestations. Respiratory signs and symptoms become apparent immediately after birth. Signs and symptoms include nasal flaring; expiratory grunting; intercostal, subcostal, or substernal retractions; dusky color involving the skin, nail beds, and mucous membranes; tachypnea (up to 80 to 120 breaths/min) initially and dyspnea; and low body temperature. Manifestations as the disease progresses include apnea, flaccidity, absence of spontaneous movement, unresponsiveness, and mottling. In severe cases, infants sometimes die within hours of the onset of signs and symptoms; those who survive gradually show improvement by the fourth day.

Diagnostic Tests. Criteria for the diagnosis of RDS consist of the clinical manifestations and the radiographic findings. Blood gas analysis indicates the degree of respiratory and metabolic acidosis.

Medical Management. The treatment of RDS is entirely supportive and aims to correct imbalances. Supportive measures include maintaining a neutral thermal environment, providing adequate oxygenation either by increasing ambient (pertaining to the surrounding area) oxygen concentration or by ventilatory assistance, and correction of respiratory and metabolic acidosis. To prevent hypoxia and the toxic effects of high concentrations of oxygen, it is necessary to evaluate oxygen therapy continually by measuring arterial oxygen. Health care providers order nutritional support through parenteral therapy during the early acute stage to prevent aspiration. Nipple and gavage feeding are contraindicated in any situation that creates a marked increase in respiratory rate because of the greater hazards of aspiration.

In infants at high risk of developing or who have developed RDS, the administration of exogenous (originating outside the body) pulmonary surfactant has reduced greatly the rates of morbidity and mortality associated with the disorder. Exogenous surfactant is administered by an endotracheal tube directly into the infant's trachea and lungs shortly after birth. Additional doses sometimes are given. In some cases, the mother is given corticosteroids such as betamethasone before delivery to increase the production of surfactant in the preterm infant.

Nursing Interventions And Patient Teaching. The primary nursing consideration in caring for an infant with RDS is to observe and assess the infant's response to therapy. Continuous monitoring and assessment are essential to adjust oxygen concentrations and ventilator settings in response to the infant's blood gas measurements and pulse oximetry readings. Perform frequent respiratory assessments, observe the infant's behavior, and observe for signs of respiratory complications and sepsis. Perform suctioning as needed, on the basis of assessment findings in the infant (auscultation, increased infant irritability, excessive moisture in the endotracheal tube). Suctioning must never be performed on a routine basis; frequent, vigorous suctioning increases the risk of bronchospasm, airway damage, infection, pneumothorax (a collection of air or gas in the pleural space that causes the lung to collapse), hypoxia, and increased intracranial pressure that can lead to intraventricular hemorrhage in the neonate. Help the infant maintain an open airway by positioning the infant on the side with the head supported in alignment. Assess the infant's skin frequently and protect the skin from impairment by frequent repositioning and the use of water mattresses or pillows and sheepskin. A water-soluble ointment is applied to reduce irritation to the nares or around the mouth, and frequent oral hygiene with water is performed to help relieve dryness caused by oxygen therapy.

Parents of such infants need emotional support. Encourage them to discuss their anxieties and concerns. Encourage parents to touch, hold, and talk to their infant and participate in the care whenever possible to promote bonding.

Prognosis. RDS is a self-limiting disease. Infants with RDS who survive the first 96 hours have a reasonable chance of recovery. Surfactant replacement therapy tends to improve the survival rate and reduce the severity of RDS.

Prevention. Prevention of premature delivery is the most effective preventive measure for RDS. Amniocentesis can determine fetal lung maturity before delivery.

Bronchopulmonary Dysplasia

Etiology And Pathophysiology. Bronchopulmonary dysplasia (BPD) is a chronic pulmonary disorder that develops in premature infants. BPD arises in association with meconium aspiration, RDS, high concentrations of oxygen, positive-pressure ventilation, and endotracheal intubation. Chronic lung changes include thickening and necrosis of alveolar walls with impairment of oxygen diffusion from the alveoli to the capillaries. Edema and inflammation of the capillary bed can cause some alveoli to collapse, some to hyperinflate, and others to rupture. Diffuse infiltrates, hyperinflation, and chronic pulmonary insufficiency characterize the disorder.

Clinical Manifestations. The clinical signs and symptoms of BPD vary. Most affected infants show evidence of respiratory distress (wheezing, retracting, nasal flaring, irritability, abundant secretions, and cyanosis when stressed). These children are vulnerable to upper respiratory infections and frequently require hospitalization because of poor respiratory status.

Diagnostic Tests. No specific signs, symptoms, or laboratory data confirm a diagnosis of BPD. Radiographic examination and ABG determinations are often helpful in making the diagnosis. Pulmonary function tests typically help determine the degree of lung dysfunction.

Medical Management. Medical management involves taking precautions to prevent RDS and to reduce requirements for ventilation and oxygen. When ventilation and oxygen are necessary, meticulous management is necessary in using the lowest concentration of oxygen and ventilatory pressures to maintain adequate gas exchange to avoid further damage of lung tissue. During weaning, bronchodilators may be used to decrease airway resistance and increase lung compliance. Management includes nutritional support, provided initially by total parenteral nutrition and later by nasogastric, gavage, or breast-feeding or formula feeding.

Nursing Interventions And Patient Teaching. Rest periods should be planned to decrease respiratory effort and conserve energy. When it is time to begin oral feedings, provide small, frequent feedings to prevent overdistention of the stomach, which can interfere with respiratory effort. You are instrumental in emotionally supporting parents and should encourage them to participate in their infant's care.

Parents also need counseling regarding ways to reduce the risk of respiratory infections. Instruct them to notify their health care provider at the first sign of a respiratory infection in their child. Teach parents cardiopulmonary resuscitation and how to manage any other possibly anticipated emergency.

Prognosis. Infants with BPD have a high mortality rate in the first year. Infants who survive are at risk for chronic lung disease. The use of exogenous surfactant in newborns with RDS has reduced the incidence of BPD greatly and its morbidity in at-risk infants.

Pneumonia

Etiology And Pathophysiology. Pneumonia is an acute inflammation of the pulmonary parenchyma (tissue), small airways, and alveoli. Pneumonia is classified according to the causative agent: bacterial, viral, mycoplasmal, or foreign body aspiration. Pneumonia is common throughout childhood, occurs more frequently in infants and young children, and usually is associated with an upper respiratory infection. Pneumonias are most common in the winter months, from November through March. Viral pneumonias are more common than bacterial pneumonias. Respiratory syncytial virus (RSV) accounts for the largest percentage of infections in infants and young children. Bacterial pneumonias most common in infants and children are caused by streptococci, staphylococci, pneumococci, and *H. influenzae.*

Box 32.3	Clinical Manifestations of Pneumonia in Children

- Abdominal pain
- Anorexia
- Chest pain
- Cough
- Fever
- Headache
- Irritability
- Lethargy
- Malaise
- Myalgia
- Nasal discharge
- Respiratory distress
- Wheeze or crackles

Clinical Manifestations. The clinical manifestations of viral and bacterial pneumonias are given in Box 32.3.

Diagnostic Tests. Radiographic examination establishes the location and the extent of infection. Peripheral blood tests sometimes reveal an elevated WBC count, which is higher with bacterial infection than viral infection. Identification of the causative organism includes culture and Gram stain of respiratory secretions and the blood, as well as diagnostic thoracentesis if fluid is suspected in the pleural cavity. In the laboratory, nasal or nasopharyngeal secretions are analyzed for RSV antigen detection. If no bacterial microorganism is identified, the pneumonia is considered viral.

Medical Management. The goal of therapy in the management of pneumonia is to improve oxygenation and prevent dehydration. Treatment includes antibiotic therapy (for bacteria-based infections), oxygen therapy, chest physiotherapy, suctioning, fluid administration, and bronchodilators. Many health care providers order antipyretics to control fever.

Premature infants, infants with CHD, and infants with chronic lung disease are considered at high risk for RSV infection. A preventive therapy for RSV, palivizumab, is recommended for these infants. Palivizumab is a genetically engineered RSV monoclonal antibiotic. At-risk infants may receive the medication monthly for a prescribed length of time, depending on their identified risk factor, to aid in prevention of RSV (Munoz et al., 2017).

Nursing Interventions And Patient Teaching. Observation of respiratory status, including skin color and respiratory effort, and monitoring of cardiovascular status are two important nursing measures. Infection control measures should be followed according to hospital protocol. Supportive nursing management includes providing adequate rest periods to conserve energy, maintaining hydration by monitoring prescribed IV fluids, administering oxygen and antibiotics as prescribed, and gentle suctioning with a bulb syringe when necessary. Oral fluids, if allowed, should be given with caution to help prevent aspiration and to decrease the possibility of aggravating a fatiguing cough.

Encourage parents to participate in their child's care, guiding them in the proper methods to feed and hold their child while in the mist tent to prevent dislodgment of IV catheters.

Prognosis. The prognosis for children with pneumococcal and streptococcal pneumonias is generally good, with rapid resolution when detection and treatment occur early. Staphylococcal pneumonias typically run a longer course, but early detection and treatment are usually effective.

Sudden Infant Death Syndrome. The sudden, unexpected, and unexplained death of an apparently healthy infant evokes a variety of familial responses ranging from hysteria and denial to stoicism (being impassive, indifferent to joy or pain). Nurses have an important role in assisting the family through the death and grieving process.

Etiology And Pathophysiology. Sudden infant death syndrome (SIDS) is the sudden, unexpected death of an apparently healthy, normal infant younger than 1 year in which a postmortem examination, investigation of the death scene, and review of the case history fail to establish a cause of death. In the United States, the rate of mortality from SIDS has declined more than 50% since 1990. Health care providers attribute the dramatic decrease to the Safe to Sleep Campaign led by the National Institute of Child Health and Human Development. SIDS always occurs during sleep and is the leading cause of death among infants aged 1 to 12 months (National Institute of Child Health and Development [NICHD], 2017). Most deaths occur between the ages of 1 to 4 months of age. Male infants have a higher incidence than female infants.

Native Americans and African Americans are most often affected, and it occurs more frequently among infants in lower socioeconomic classes. The cause of SIDS is unknown, but SIDS often is associated with premature birth and low birth weight, multiple births, and CNS and respiratory dysfunctions. There is also an association between SIDS and maternal smoking, drug addiction, and maternal age of less than 20 years. Smoking by the mother during the prenatal period and smoking in the home are linked to the incidence of SIDS. Breast-fed infants have a lower incidence of SIDS. Sleep position on the abdomen has been associated with SIDS, along with congenital abnormalities, sleep apnea, and depressed ventilator response to increased carbon dioxide or decreased oxygen blood levels. Sleeping in a prone position possibly predisposes the infant to oropharyngeal obstruction or affects ventilatory arousal. Soft, polystyrene-filled mattresses or pillows have the potential to cause suffocation in the infant sleeping in a prone position (see the Safety Alert box on preventing SIDS).

⚠ Safety Alert

Preventing Sudden Infant Death Syndrome

- Maternal smoking, prenatally and postnatally, is a possible cause of sudden infant death syndrome (SIDS) that some authorities have proposed, as are poor prenatal care and low maternal age.
- Bed sharing increases the risk of SIDS. Unlike a crib, whose design has to meet safety standards for infants, adult beds and sofas do not meet such specifications, and they carry a potential risk for accidental entrapment and suffocation.
- The infant should not be bundled too heavily. The infant should be dressed in lightweight clothing, and the room should be kept at a comfortable temperature.
- Infants always should be placed on their back for sleep until 1 year of age. Infants should be placed on a firm sleep surface. The crib or bassinet must meet current safety standards.
- Do not use soft bedding such as pillows or quilts under the infant for bedding.
- Remove items such as stuffed animals or towels from the crib while the infant is asleep to prevent possible asphyxia.
- Breast-feeding lowers the incidence of SIDS.

The use of pacifiers during sleep reduces the risk of SIDS in breastfed and bottle-fed babies. The pacifier can be used in bottle-fed newborns, but parents should wait until breastfeeding is established before introduction in breastfed babies. Do not attach the pacifier to anything and allow it to fall out during sleep.

Information from National Institute of Child Health and Human Development (NICHD): Safe sleep for your baby: Reduce the risk of sudden infant death syndrome (SIDS) and other sleep-related causes of infant death, 2019. National Institutes of Health. Modified from https://safetosleep.nichd.nih.gov/safesleepbasics/risk/reduce.

Clinical Manifestations. Death occurs during sleep, and there is no audible cry or sign of distress.

Diagnostic Tests. Confirmation of the diagnosis occurs at postmortem examination, which reveals pulmonary edema and intrathoracic hemorrhages.

Medical Management. Therapeutic management consists of emotionally assisting the family who has just lost an infant to SIDS.

Nursing Interventions. The death of an infant from SIDS propels the family into a crisis situation. The initial response is one of extreme shock and disbelief. As parents try to cope, they often experience feelings of guilt and blame.

The nurse becomes instrumental in assisting families with grief and mourning. Clean the infant, wrap the infant in a sheet or blanket, and tidy the room where the family will be able to spend time with the infant. For coming to terms with the death, ensure that the parents' last moments with their infant are quiet, peaceful, and as meaningful as possible. Offer to stay with the family or allow them private time if they wish.

Upper Respiratory Tract Infections

Acute Pharyngitis (Sore Throat)

Etiology And Pathophysiology. Acute pharyngitis is an inflammation of the pharynx. The majority of cases of acute pharyngitis are viral in origin, whereas less are diagnosed as bacterial (GABHS). Acute pharyngitis occurs frequently between the ages of 4 and 12 years, when children increasingly are exposed to infections outside the home. The infecting organism in children younger than 3 years with pharyngitis is usually *H. influenzae*. These children must be monitored for neurologic signs and symptoms that indicate possible meningitis. However, the use of the vaccine against *H. influenzae* type B (Hib vaccine) has begun to decrease the number of infections involving this organism. Acute cases of pharyngitis are more common in later winter and early spring.

Clinical Manifestations. Viral pharyngitis causes low-grade fever, malaise, anorexia, pharyngeal erythema, and throat soreness. Many affected children also complain of headache, cough, hoarseness, rhinitis, and conjunctivitis. Streptococcal pharyngitis causes high fever, throat soreness, white exudates on the posterior pharynx and tonsillar region, vomiting, and abdominal pain.

Diagnostic Tests. Although the majority of all cases of acute pharyngitis are of viral origin, a throat culture is performed to rule out GABHS.

Medical Management. Viral pharyngitis is treated symptomatically with lozenges, gargles, and acetaminophen. Streptococcal pharyngitis must be treated with a 10-day course of antimicrobial therapy to prevent complications (acute rheumatic fever and acute glomerulonephritis). Penicillin derivatives are the drugs of choice for streptococcal pharyngitis. Other medications that also treat streptococcal pharyngitis include erythromycin, azithromycin, clarithromycin, cephalosporins, and amoxicillin.

Nursing Interventions And Patient Teaching. To relieve throat discomfort in viral and bacterial infections, administer saline gargles, lozenges, warm compresses to the neck, and acetaminophen. Encourage the child to drink cool liquids (nonacid) until the throat feels better; then soft, bland foods may be introduced. Emphasize follow-up care after streptococcal pharyngitis to ensure eradication of the causative organism.

The family should be instructed in antimicrobial therapy, with emphasis on the need to finish the medication completely even though the child feels better. When a throat culture for streptococcal infection yields positive results, remind the child to discard his or her toothbrush and replace it with a new one after taking antibiotics for 24 hours.

Prognosis. The prognosis for children with acute pharyngitis is usually excellent. Inadequately treated streptococcal infections sometimes trigger a response in the heart (rheumatic fever) or kidneys (acute glomerulonephritis).

Tonsillitis

Etiology And Pathophysiology. The tonsils are masses of lymphoid tissue located in the pharyngeal cavity. They are believed to protect the respiratory and alimentary tracts from invasion by pathogenic microorganisms. They probably also play a role in antibody formation. Tonsillitis usually occurs as a result of pharyngitis and has either viral or bacterial (streptococcal) causes.

Clinical Manifestations. The signs and symptoms of viral and bacterial tonsillitis are similar and include sore throat, headache, edematous and tender cervical lymph glands, fever, hoarseness, and cough. In addition, many children with streptococcal tonsillitis exhibit vomiting, complain of muscle aches, and have difficulty swallowing or breathing.

Diagnostic Tests. The WBC count sometimes is elevated significantly. A throat culture is performed to detect streptococcal tonsillitis.

Medical Management. The treatment for bacterial and nonbacterial tonsillitis includes the comfort measures described in acute pharyngitis. In addition, treatment for bacterial tonsillitis comprises a 10-day course of penicillin (or erythromycin) to prevent complications.

Tonsillectomy is a surgical procedure that completely removes the tonsils. The primary care provider or ear, nose, and throat (ENT) specialist determines if the patient's condition warrants a tonsillectomy. Infrequent cases of pharyngitis typically do not warrant the need for a tonsillectomy. Repeated infections of the pharynx, especially streptococcal bacterial infections, may lead to a discussion regarding the pros and cons of a tonsillectomy.

Nursing Interventions. The nursing interventions for tonsillitis are the same as those described for acute pharyngitis. Before any indicated surgery, prepare the child psychologically. Assess the child for signs of infection and loose teeth and check the child's laboratory data, including findings from bleeding and clotting studies. Postoperatively, the child should be kept in a semiprone position to facilitate drainage; also, the child should be monitored frequently for excessive bleeding, which causes frequent swallowing even during sleep. Analgesics should be given as prescribed; and, after recovery from analgesia, fluids should be provided (with the exception of acidic, grape, red, or chocolate drinks so that you can distinguish fresh or old blood in emesis from ingested liquid). A soft diet follows. Postoperative hemorrhage is unusual but possible; therefore, observe the child's throat directly for evidence of bleeding, with a good source of light and, if necessary, by carefully inserting a tongue depressor. Signs of hemorrhage include increased pulse (>120 bpm), pallor, frequent clearing of the throat or swallowing by a younger child, and vomiting of bright red blood. Restlessness, an indication of hemorrhage, is sometimes difficult to differentiate from general discomfort after surgery. Decreasing blood pressure is a late sign of shock.

Patient Teaching. Appropriate discharge instructions include the following:

- Avoid foods that are irritating or highly seasoned.
- Avoid foods that are crunchy or contain seeds.
- Encourage fluid intake. Apple juice, water and grape juice are acceptable suggestions.
- Avoid the use of gargles or vigorous brushing of the teeth.
- Try to avoid coughing or clearing the throat.
- Use mild analgesics or an ice collar for pain.
- Do not use aspirin.

Hemorrhaging is possible 5 to 10 days after surgery as a result of tissue sloughing from the healing process. If parents see any signs of bleeding, they must notify the health care provider immediately.

Prognosis. The prognosis is generally excellent. Improperly treated streptococcal infections potentially result in rheumatic fever or acute glomerulonephritis.

Croup: Laryngotracheobronchitis And Acute Epiglottitis.

Croup is an acute viral disease of childhood, marked by a resonant barking cough, suffocative and difficult breathing, and laryngeal spasm.

Etiology And Pathophysiology. Laryngotracheobronchitis (LTB) is the most common form of croup. It affects children 3 months to 3 years of age and is usually viral in origin. LTB usually follows an upper respiratory infection that descends to the lower respiratory tract and has a gradual, progressive onset.

Acute epiglottitis is a severe, potentially life-threatening bacterial infection of the epiglottis in older children and usually is caused by *H. influenzae* type B. The inflamed epiglottis becomes cherry-red and edematous, which has the potential to lead to total airway obstruction. Since the advent of the Hib vaccine, the number of episodes of epiglottitis caused by *H. influenzae* type B has been decreasing.

Clinical Manifestations. Children with LTB initially demonstrate hoarseness; inspiratory stridor; tachypnea; nasal flaring; suprasternal, substernal, and intercostal retractions; and characteristic barking cough. Body temperature is usually normal or mildly elevated. A child with epiglottitis is acutely ill with high fever, muffled voice, drooling, progressive respiratory distress, anxiety, and fear.

Diagnostic Tests. Diagnostic criteria for LTB consist of a history of a preceding upper respiratory infection, CBC with differential, the clinical signs and symptoms, and physical examination.

Clinical signs and symptoms establish a tentative diagnosis of acute epiglottitis, which is considered a medical emergency. The child is taken to the operating or ambulatory surgery room, where emergency equipment is available for immediate intubation or tracheostomy in the event of further obstruction during examination of the pharynx. Health care providers sometimes obtain lateral neck radiographs in the operating room to observe for soft tissue edema and an area of obstruction. Skilled personnel with the equipment necessary to perform immediate intubation or tracheostomy never leave the child's side. The trend away from early intubation of children with LTB emphasizes the importance of nursing observation and the ability to recognize impending respiratory failure so that intubation is possible without delay. The child is put under anesthesia for visual examination of the pharynx and invasive procedures such as blood collection and insertion of IV lines. The laboratory performs culture and sensitivity testing on tracheal secretions collected at the time of intubation.

Medical Management. Management of LTB and acute epiglottitis focuses on maintaining patency of the airway. A child with LTB receives high cool-mist humidity with low-concentration (approximately 30%) oxygen by mist tent. Administration of epinephrine by aerosol helps decrease airway edema by vasoconstriction and improve oxygenation by bronchodilation. The effects of epinephrine are short lived, however, and repeated doses are needed if and when the airway edema returns a few hours after epinephrine administration. Therefore it is necessary to monitor children receiving epinephrine very closely. During the acute phase, affected children receive nothing by mouth (NPO status), because the typically rapid respirations predispose to aspiration. IV administration of fluids provides adequate hydration. The use of sedatives is contraindicated, because they mask restlessness, which is a clinical indication of hypoxia and a deteriorating condition.

Immediate treatment of a child with acute epiglottitis includes establishing an artificial airway. Respiratory care includes humidification, gentle oral suctioning, and constant observation of respiratory status. Health care providers order oxygen for moderate respiratory distress and aerosolized epinephrine to decrease airway edema by local vasoconstriction. IV antibiotics and fluids are administered as ordered. Epiglottal edema usually decreases after 24 hours of antibiotic therapy. By the third day, the epiglottis is nearly normal in size, and it is safe to extubate the child.

Nursing Interventions And Patient Teaching. LTB or acute epiglottitis tends to be a frightening experience for the child and the family. Never attempt to examine the mouth or throat in a child with LTB, because this results in epiglottal spasm and cessation of breathing. Respond quickly in a calm manner, emotionally supporting and reassuring parents that everything possible is being done for their child. Continually assess the child for signs of response to therapy or increasing obstruction. Nursing observations often provide the rationale for any treatment changes. The child is maintained in the Fowler's position, and respirations are monitored for rate, depth, retractions, and nasal flaring. Monitor the child's cardiac status because restlessness and tachycardia are signs of increasing hypoxia. Check vital signs frequently. Intubation and tracheostomy

sets are kept at the child's bedside in case of respiratory failure. Nursing interventions must be planned carefully to include frequent rest periods for the patient to conserve energy. Keep parents informed of their child's progress and encourage them to participate in care.

Prognosis. In most affected children, LTB is relatively mild. Gradual improvement to recovery occurs in 3 to 7 days. The most serious complication, and the one responsible for most deaths from croup, is laryngeal obstruction.

Without prompt diagnosis and treatment, the rapid course of epiglottitis has the potential to cause death within a few hours.

Lower Respiratory Tract Infections
Bronchitis (Tracheobronchitis)

Etiology And Pathophysiology. Bronchitis (tracheobronchitis) is an inflammation of the large airways, the trachea, and the bronchi. It usually follows an upper respiratory infection and is almost always viral in origin. The most common cause is rhinovirus, although parainfluenza, adenovirus, and RSV are other known causes. *Mycoplasma pneumoniae* is a common cause of bronchitis in children older than 6 years. Bronchitis occurs mainly in the winter months, primarily in children younger than 4 years (although it has potential to affect any age group).

Clinical Manifestations. The onset is gradual with signs and symptoms of an upper respiratory tract infection (cough, coryza, little or no fever). After 2 to 3 days, the nonproductive, hacking cough becomes productive and worsens at night.

Diagnostic Tests. For a child with severe signs and symptoms, a radiographic examination of the chest is necessary. In the majority of affected children, chest radiographs appear normal.

Medical Management. Treatment is basically palliative. If the cough interferes with resting or eating, then cough drops, lollipops, and pediatric cough preparations are usually effective. Cough suppressants are contraindicated in bronchitis unless the condition significantly affects sleep. Sometimes health care providers prescribe acetaminophen for fever. Antibiotics are not necessary in viral bronchitis. If the cough lasts beyond 10 days, a secondary bacterial infection is suspected.

Patient Teaching. Suggest the use of a cool-mist humidifier to relieve the child's cough and help liquefy secretions. Encourage consumption of fluids to decrease viscosity of secretions and prevent dehydration.

Prognosis. Acute bronchitis is self-limiting.

Respiratory Syncytial Virus And Bronchiolitis

Etiology And Pathophysiology. Bronchiolitis is an acute viral inflammation of the smaller airway passages, the bronchioles; the bronchioles become inflamed, which causes edema. The accumulation of mucus and exudate has the potential to partially or completely obstruct the lumen. RSV is the organism responsible for most cases. Bronchiolitis occurs in children younger than 2 years. The incidence peaks at 6 months of age. Cases of bronchiolitis usually begin in the fall, and the incidence peaks in the winter. The virus is transmitted through respiratory secretions. RSV can survive for hours outside a host on such items as countertops and contaminated tissues.

Clinical Manifestations. Signs and symptoms of an upper respiratory infection predominate during the first few days and worsen as respiratory distress develops. Affected infants exhibit retractions, tachypnea, nasal flaring, paroxysmal nonproductive coughing, and wheezing. Some affected infants have low-grade or very high fever; are irritable, fussy, and anxious; and have difficulty eating. Respiratory distress becomes progressively more severe during the first 72 hours. Severe disease is followed by a rise in arterial carbon dioxide tension (hypercapnia), which leads to respiratory acidosis and hypoxemia.

Diagnostic Tests. The diagnosis is based on the age of the child and the clinical signs and symptoms. Radiographic examination of the chest shows areas of atelectasis and hyperinflation. Tests providing positive identification of RSV are either ELISA or rapid immunofluorescent antibody assays of specimens obtained from direct aspiration of nasal secretions or nasopharyngeal washings.

Medical Management. There is no definitive antiviral medication suggested for use in most cases of bronchiolitis. Treatment is aimed at treating the symptoms. Hydration and oxygenation are the primary treatment modalities. High humidity, administered via mist tent, loosens secretions. If hypoxemia is present, the health care provider orders oxygen therapy with mist therapy. IV fluids are necessary if the infant is unable to tolerate oral feedings. Use of bronchodilators is sometimes an aspect of management in severe cases of bronchiolitis (Maraqa, 2021).

Nursing Interventions And Patient Teaching. Follow respiratory isolation precautions. Practice and encourage thorough hand hygiene to prevent cross-contamination, along with the use of contact precautions (gloves, gowns, masks, and goggles). Another infection control measure includes making patient assignments so that nurses assigned to children with RSV do not take care of other patients at high risk for RSV infection. Acute nursing interventions focus on promoting adequate oxygenation, frequent monitoring of respiratory status, and maintaining hydration. As with any respiratory condition, parents need reassurance and emotional support during this stressful period.

Prognosis. The disease typically lasts 7 to 10 days. With prompt treatment the prognosis is very good. Overall, the mortality in children hospitalized for bronchiolitis in different series ranges from 0.2% to 7%, depending on such factors as the stage of the infection upon diagnosis and when treatment was started (Maraqa, 2021).

Pulmonary Tuberculosis

Etiology And Pathophysiology. Pulmonary tuberculosis (TB) is a chronic bacterial lung infection caused by the bacillus *Mycobacterium tuberculosis*. TB remains a leading cause of death in many underdeveloped countries. It continues to be a public health problem in the United States primarily because of immigration, infection with HIV, and multiresistant strains of *M. tuberculosis*. The most important risk factor in the progression from TB infection to active disease is an inadequate immune response, as a result of age or an impaired immune system, as in young infants, elderly people, or people infected with HIV. Immunocompromised children and children younger than 3 years are at greatest risk for TB, but the risk increases again during the postpubertal adolescent years. The primary source of *M. tuberculosis* infection in children is exposure to an infected adult, usually a family member, babysitter, or frequent visitor.

Clinical Manifestations. When first infected, most children do not exhibit any clinical signs and symptoms. Signs and symptoms are extremely variable and develop so gradually that they often go unnoticed until the disease has progressed significantly.

Diagnostic Tests. Although not diagnostic, the tuberculin skin test, formerly known as the *Mantoux test,* is the most important screening measure in identifying infected children at risk for disease. To confirm the diagnosis, bacteriologic sputum cultures for *M. tuberculosis* must yield positive results. Infected infants and young children do not cough and expectorate sputum. Instead, they usually swallow mucus from the respiratory tract. Therefore, the best way to obtain sputum samples from infants and children is by gastric aspiration. Chest radiographs are also important in determining the presence and the extent of active lesions. The medical management and nursing interventions are basically the same as in adults with active TB.

Patient Teaching. Because the success of therapy depends on compliance with the drug regimen, it is necessary to instruct parents regarding the importance of giving medications as often and for as long as ordered. The optimal duration of therapy is unknown, but the usual course of treatment is no less than 12 months for an initial infection or 18 to 24 months for more serious forms of the disease.

Prognosis. The prognosis relies greatly on the stage of the disease at the time of diagnosis. The rate of success in treating early-onset TB is high. Complications of pulmonary TB include pneumonia, pneumothorax, and stenosis of the airways. TB of the small intestine may result in obstruction, fistula formation, and malabsorption.

Cystic Fibrosis

Etiology And Pathophysiology. Cystic fibrosis (CF) is a genetic disorder that a child inherits from both parents. This is a disorder of the exocrine (mucus-producing) glands, with the characteristic presence of excessive thick mucus that obstructs the lungs and the gastrointestinal (GI) system. CF is a multiorgan disease, but death usually is caused by pulmonary failure. The incidence of CF is greater than 30,000 people in the United States with approximately 1000 new cases diagnosed every year. More than 75% of cases are diagnosed by the age of 2 years. Fifty percent of those living with CF are over the age of 18 (Cystic Fibrosis Foundation, n.d.a.).

The abnormally thick mucus that collects in the lung airways and organ ducts causes obstruction. Bronchiolar obstruction predisposes the lung to infection, bronchiectasis, and cystic dilations. Complications include bronchial and bronchiolar obstruction, pulmonary hypertension, and cor pulmonale. Obstruction of the pancreatic ducts leads to dilation and fibrosis and a decrease in levels of pancreatic enzymes (lipase, amylase, and trypsin), which results in malabsorption. The earliest manifestation of CF is meconium ileus in the newborn, in which the small intestine is occluded with tenacious putty-like, mucilaginous meconium. Obstruction in the hepatic system leads to biliary cirrhosis, portal hypertension, and splenomegaly. Sodium chloride concentrations in the sweat and the saliva are elevated as a result of the abnormal reabsorption of chloride by epithelial cells.

Clinical Manifestations. Pancreatic insufficiency and malabsorption result in steatorrhea (bulky, foul-smelling, fatty stools), growth failure, protuberant abdomen, and thin, wasted extremities. Rectal prolapse is a common GI manifestation of CF. Appetite often is increased early in the illness in response to poor absorption. Malabsorption also has the potential to lead to a vitamin K deficiency, which results in bleeding disorders, esophageal varices, and ecchymosis. As a result of diminished subcutaneous fat, the skin appears sallow and transparent. Pulmonary complications constitute the most serious threat to life in children with CF. Many such children demonstrate respiratory symptoms before 1 year of age; others may not develop symptoms for weeks, months, or years. Pulmonary involvement is evident in chronic cough, wheezing, sputum production, and dyspnea, which results in hypoxia, clubbing of the fingers and toes, and cyanosis. Hyperinflation of the lungs sometimes causes the chest to become barrel shaped.

Diagnostic Tests. All states in the United States screen newborns for CF using a genetic test or a blood test. Diagnostic criteria for CF consist of a family history of the disorder, absence of pancreatic enzymes, chronic pulmonary involvement, and a positive result of a chloride sweat test. Typically, two sweat tests are performed to diagnose the disease. For this test, the doctor triggers sweating on a small patch of skin on an arm or leg. The provider rubs the skin with a sweat-producing chemical and then uses an electrode to provide a mild electrical current. Sweat is collected, then tested. A sweat chloride level higher than 60 mEq/L is diagnostic for CF. The normal level of sweat chloride is below

29 mmol/L in infants 6 months and younger; below 39 mmol/L for any age over 6 months (Johns Hopkins Cystic Fibrosis Center, n.d.). Chest radiographs show patchy atelectasis and evidence of obstructive emphysema. Pulmonary function tests measure ventilation and diffusion of gas across the alveolar capillary membrane and reveal evidence of pulmonary problems.

Medical Management. The goals of therapy include good nutrition, prevention and control of respiratory infections, and enabling as normal a lifestyle as possible for the child. Pulmonary therapy to ensure airway clearance is the single most important aspect of treatment. Chest physiotherapy and high-frequency chest wall oscillations have greatly improved the pulmonary status of the patient with CF. Breathing exercises are beneficial to improve aeration. Inhalation therapy with bronchodilators before chest physiotherapy facilitates secretion removal. Expectorants, mucolytic agents, and antibiotics help relieve obstruction and resolve infections. Chest physiotherapy is usually necessary twice daily (on rising and in the evening) and sometimes more frequently, especially during pulmonary infection. Positive expiratory pressure (PEP) therapy is another source of treatment. This therapy involves breathing through a device that provides resistance while exhaling. This pressure keeps the small airways of the lungs open to improve the mobility of the secretions. Digestive and nutritional therapies include pancreatic enzyme replacement, administration of fat-soluble vitamins (A, D, E, and K), and a diet high in calories, protein, and salt.

Nursing Interventions. Nursing interventions for a child with CF are highly complex and can be challenging. Management focuses on improving pulmonary function and facilitating lung clearance, preventing or managing respiratory infections, promoting normal growth and development, optimizing nutritional status, educating the patient and family about the illness and its management, planning for home care and community support, referring for counseling when needed, providing long-term emotional support and follow-up, and encouraging compliance with the medication regimen.

Improving pulmonary function involves chest physiotherapy, breathing exercises, and inhalation treatment. Chest physiotherapy performed two or more times daily helps loosen secretions in the lung with high-frequency chest wall oscillations, and postural drainage facilitates the removal of these thick secretions. To encourage breathing exercises, suggest blowing bubbles or pinwheels to help prevent tracheobronchial obstruction. The nurse or the respiratory therapist sometimes performs nebulizer treatments. Assess the child's tolerance of therapy and monitor its effectiveness. Infection control measures are instituted to prevent cross-contamination, and the family is taught to protect the child from exposure to people with respiratory infections. Strongly recommend yearly influenza immunizations. Early in the course of the illness, some children exhibit excessive appetite; as the disease progresses, the appetite decreases, and children usually experience anorexia. Before meals and snacks, administer a mix of pancreatic enzymes, needed to digest proteins, fats, and carbohydrates, together with a carbohydrate.

Children with CF have frequent hospitalizations, which are likely to interfere with normal development and impair socialization; these issues must be addressed with psychological support and appropriate activities. One of the most critical aspects in providing care to children with CF and their families is assisting them with positive coping strategies and providing emotional support. Support groups are often a source of great comfort and assistance to children with newly diagnosed disease and to their families. The Cystic Fibrosis Foundation provides education and services to families and professionals.

Patient Teaching. The family is instructed in improving the nutritional status of the child to ensure adequate growth and development. The nurse is responsible primarily for coordinating counseling, referrals to community support, and home care services, as well as for educating the child and the family in the disease process and its management. The child should receive all childhood vaccinations as recommended.

Prognosis. CF is a chronic, incurable disease. According to the Cystic Fibrosis Foundation Patient Registry, treatment of the disease has improved substantially since the 1950s. In 1955 children with CF were not expected to live long enough to attend school. The median length of survival in 2009, in contrast, was in the mid-30s. Today, 45% of the population with CF are 18 years of age or older. The life expectancy has increased for individuals with cystic fibrosis. For those born in 2019 an estimated 50% of them will live to 48 years and beyod. (Cystic Fibrosis Foundation, n.d.b.). Therapies and treatments for patients with CF are now individualized to provide the best possible outcomes, including mucus thinners, antibiotics, anti-inflammatories, and bronchodilators.

Bronchial Asthma

Etiology And Pathophysiology. Asthma is a chronic inflammatory disorder of the airways in which many cells (mast cells, eosinophils, and T lymphocytes) play a role. Bronchial asthma is a reversible obstructive respiratory disorder. Asthma accounts for the greatest number of school absences and visits to the emergency department by children. It is a leading cause of chronic disease in children with 6.2 million children affected (CDC, 2021d).

Bronchial asthma has a familial tendency and frequently occurs in association with allergic rhinitis and atopic dermatitis. A common cause of bronchial asthma is an allergic hypersensitivity to environmental factors. The common factors associated with bronchial asthma include bronchospasm, mucosal edema, and increased mucosal secretions. Bronchospasm of the bronchial smooth muscle causes bronchial edema with a decrease in the diameter of the bronchi and bronchioles; edematous mucous membranes produce thick, tenacious secretions, which cause a further narrowing of the air passages. Mucous plugs that occlude the smaller air passages cause obstruction and air trapping distal to the obstruction, which result in hypoxemia and increased respiratory effort (Fig. 32.11).

The National Heart, Lung, and Blood Institute's National Asthma Education and Prevention Program (2007) classified asthma based on symptoms that indicate the severity of the disease. The classifications are (1) mild intermittent, (2) mild persistent, (3) moderate persistent, and (4) severe persistent. These categories aid in the medical and environmental treatment of asthma.

Pulmonary function tests are useful in children after age 5 or 6 years. These tests help evaluate the presence and the degree of lung disease and responses to therapy. Health care providers often order skin testing for allergens in children with asthma to help identify and treat specific allergies.

Clinical Manifestations. Initially, many children having an asthma attack complain of a sensation of tightness in the chest, and an audible expiratory wheeze may be detected. As the attack progresses, other signs and symptoms appear: shortness of breath; inspiratory and expiratory wheezing; tachypnea; dyspnea; coarse breath sounds; prolonged expiration; restlessness; anxiety; deep, dark red color to lips; cyanosis; paroxysmal cough that progresses from dry and hacking to productive; fatigue; and diaphoresis.

Diagnostic Tests. The diagnosis is based primarily on clinical signs and symptoms; history; findings of the physical examination; results of pulmonary function tests, including spirometry and bronchoprovocation test (to assess sensitivity of airways); and serum laboratory tests such as ABG determinations and CBC. Radiographic examination of the chest and electrocardiography are standard imaging tests to rule out other disease. In general, either (1) chronic cough in the absence of infection or (2) diffuse wheezing during the expiratory phase of respiration is sufficient to establish a diagnosis.

Medical Management. Medications for treatment of asthma are divided into those given long term and those administered to manage acute exacerbations of the condition. Long-term therapies include inhaled corticosteroids, cromolyn sodium, fluticasone (Flovent Diskus, Flovent HFA), and budesonide (Pulmicort Flexhaler). These medications are administered via a nebulizer and aid in the prevention of airway inflammation. Omalizumab (anti–immunoglobulin E), which is administered by injection once or twice per month, works to prevent the body from reacting to asthma triggers. Inhaled, long-acting beta-agonists may be administered to improve control of the condition. Leukotriene modifiers such as montelukast sodium (Singulair) and zafirlukast (Accolate) reduce inflammation and work

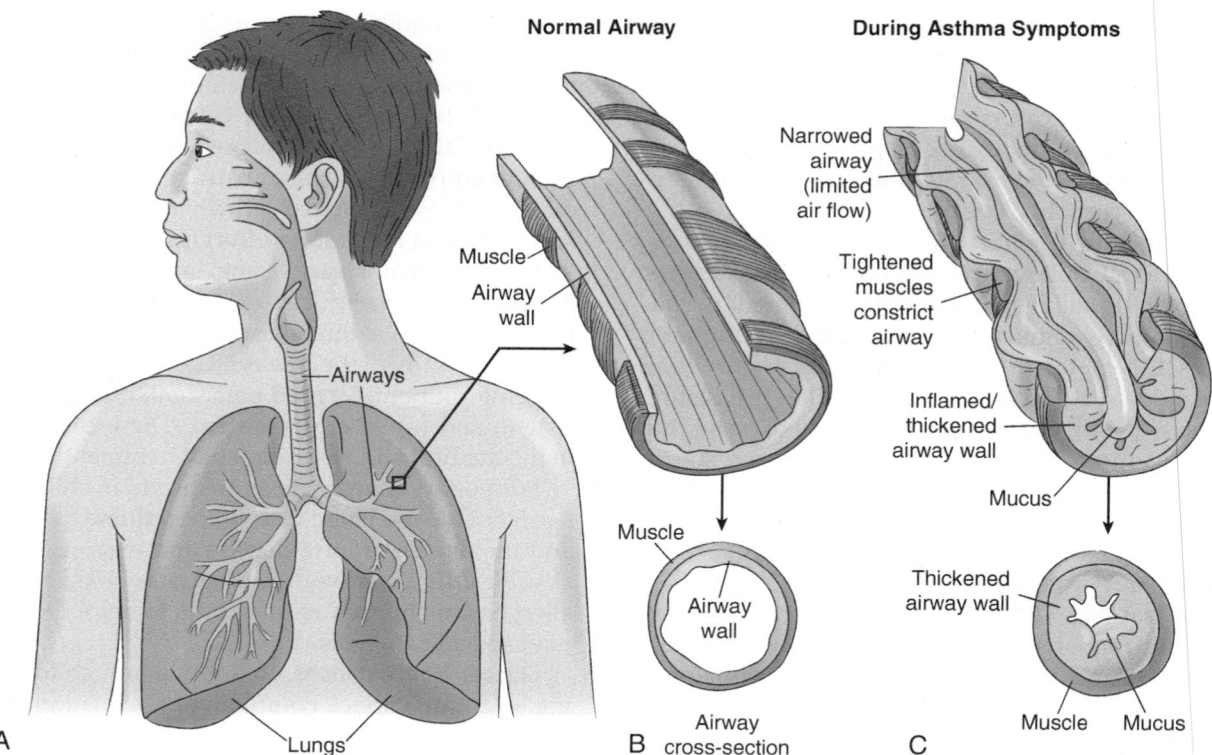

Fig. 32.11 Illustrations of lung anatomy. (A) The location of the lungs and airways in the body. (B) A cross section of a normal airway. (C) A cross section of an airway during asthma symptoms. (Redrawn from the National Heart, Lung, and Blood Institute: *What is asthma?* 2012. Available at www.nhlbi.nih.gov/health/health-topics/topics/asthma.)

to keep the airways relaxed. Long-term medications are not suitable for an acute exacerbation, because they do not work quickly enough to treat the condition.

Quick-relief (rescue) medications include short-acting beta$_2$-agonists such as albuterol (ProAir, Ventolin) and levalbuterol (Xopenex HFA). These medications act by dilating the bronchi within minutes after administration, and the effects of these medications may last for several hours. Oral and IV corticosteroids such as prednisone may be used to decrease bronchial inflammation in severe cases of asthma, but they are not used for long-term treatment because of their systemic effects on other organs. Metered-dose inhalers are used frequently to administer quick-relief and long-term medications. Health care providers typically administer nebulized medications to infants and young children who are not able to use a metered-dose inhaler. In young school-age children, the use of a spacer helps ensure that the child receives the full dose prescribed. The spacer provides a reservoir for the medication to allow the child time to inhale the full dose (Fig. 32.12). Chest physiotherapy is prescribed by some health care providers to help children with asthma strengthen their respiratory muscles and develop more efficient breathing patterns. Chest physiotherapy is not effective during an acute exacerbation of asthma.

Nursing Interventions. Nursing interventions include frequent monitoring of vital signs. Adequate hydration is maintained to replace insensible loss through

Fig. 32.12 Child using a metered-dose inhaler with spacer.

diaphoresis and hyperventilation. To facilitate optimal ventilation, the child is kept in high Fowler's position, rest periods are provided, and breathing exercises are taught. It is extremely important to provide a calm atmosphere and reassurance for the anxious child and family. Parents and children need to understand the illness and how to allay or prevent attacks at home. Allergens can be identified through skin testing, and then measures can be instituted to eliminate or avoid them.

A patient problem and interventions for a child with bronchial asthma include but are not limited to the following:

PATIENT PROBLEM	NURSING INTERVENTIONS
Inability to Maintain Adequate Breathing Pattern, related to allergenic response in bronchial tree	Teach and supervise breathing exercises and controlled breathing Teach correct use of prescribed medications Assist patient and family in selecting activities appropriate for child's capabilities and preferences Encourage regular exercise Encourage good posture Encourage physical exercise involving stop-and-start activity that does not overtax the respiratory mechanism Discourage physical inactivity

Patient Teaching. Parents need to understand the nature of the disease and, when the allergens are determined, know how to avoid or relieve asthma attacks. Teach parents and older children with asthma how to use the medications prescribed to relieve bronchospasms (see Fig. 32.12). Teach early signs and symptoms of an impending attack so that control is possible before symptoms become distressing. Older children who use a nebulizer or an aerosol device to deliver adrenergic drugs need instruction on how to use a metered-dose inhaler. The parents must be taught to avoid exposing the child to excessive cold, wind, or other extremes of weather and to smoke, sprays, or other irritants. Self-care is a hallmark of effective asthma management, and self-management programs are important in helping the child and the family cope with the disease.

Prognosis. The outlook for children with asthma varies widely. Many children lose the signs and symptoms at puberty, but no known factor predicts which children will "outgrow" their asthma. Although death from asthma is rare, the death rate has been rising steadily since 2000 despite improvements in treatment. It is important that children with asthma be assessed carefully and treated aggressively.

DISORDERS OF GASTROINTESTINAL FUNCTION

The primary function of the GI tract is the absorption and metabolism of nutrients necessary to support and promote optimal growth and development. Because the GI tract is responsible for processing nutrients for all parts of the body, an alteration in GI function has potential to affect other body systems. Failure to diagnose or treat a GI problem is likely to affect the overall health of the child. Conversely, any disease process has potential to result in manifestations of GI disturbance, even if it does not directly affect the GI tract.

Cleft Lip and Cleft Palate

Clefts of the lip and the palate are facial malformations that occur during embryologic development. A combination of cleft lip and palate is more common than an isolated occurrence of either. Approximately 2650 babies are born with a cleft palate, and 4440 babies are born with a cleft lip with or without a cleft palate.

Etiology And Pathophysiology. Cleft lip is caused by a failure of the medial nasal and maxillary processes to join (Fig. 32.13). Cleft of the palate is caused by a failure of the palatal shelves to fuse. Clefts in the palate sometimes involve only the soft palate and sometimes extend into the hard palate.

Cleft lip and palate has been linked to several environmental factors, including a folic acid deficiency in the maternal diet, maternal intake of alcohol during pregnancy, and smoking during pregnancy. Some folklore has mistakenly attempted to link the cause of cleft lip and palate to prenatal influences (see the Cultural Considerations box).

 Cultural Considerations

Cleft Lip

Beliefs in folklore and superstitions have always surrounded pregnancy and birth. Some people believe that prenatal influences affect the outcome of an unborn child, specifically with regard to birth defects. Some people believe, for example, that if a pregnant woman encounters a rabbit or hare during her pregnancy, her child will be born with a "harelip" (cleft lip).

Clinical Manifestations. Severity of cleft lip and palate may vary significantly. The cleft in the lip may be limited to a small open notch, or it may extend all the way to the base of the nose. The cleft in the palate may involve either one side or both sides of the roof of the mouth. The two clefts may combine and involve the lip and palate. Nasal shape irregularities should signal the need for further investigation. Manifestations that result from the condition may include feeding difficulties from the breast or the bottle. The extensiveness of the condition determines this ability to feed. Affected infants tend to have an ineffective suck. Saliva and intake sometimes leak into the nasal cavity, causing gagging and choking and leading to aspiration as the infant breathes.

Speech delays may develop. The most common speech-related issue is development of a hypernasal tone with poor articulation. Children with cleft palate also tend to be predisposed to recurrent otitis media or persistent otitis media with effusion as a result of eustachian tube dysfunction. Many older children with cleft lip and palate experience psychological difficulties because of the cosmetic appearance of the defect

Fig. 32.13 Variations in clefts of lip and palate at birth. (A) Notch in vermilion border, no cleft in palate. (B) Unilateral cleft lip and palate. (C) Bilateral cleft lip and palate. (D) Cleft palate alone.

and because of problems with impaired speech and faulty dentition.

Diagnostic Tests. Cleft lip and most cases of cleft palate are apparent at birth, and the facial appearance of the infant is of immediate concern to the parents. Digital examination of the mouth cavity is performed to assess the level of severity.

Medical Management. Cleft lip usually is closed within the first few months of age. Cleft palate repair occurs within the first 18 months of age. Surgical repair during this period allows for palatal changes associated with normal growth. During the period before surgical repair, the infant may be fitted with a prosthetic device that mimics the palate to improve feeding abilities. For the most positive outcome after surgical repair, interventions involve a multidisciplinary health care team that includes a pediatric plastic surgeon, an orthodontist, an otolaryngologist, a speech and language pathologist, an audiologist, nurses, and social workers (CDC, 2020c).

Nursing Interventions. Nursing interventions for a child with cleft lip and palate are focused initially on ensuring adequate nutritional support for the infant and helping the parents to deal with the diagnosis. Before surgical correction of cleft lip and palate, feeding is often a considerable problem. In addition to ensuring adequate food intake, a primary goal for nursing is to prevent aspiration. The best method for feeding is to support the infant's head in an upright position and to use care and patience during each feeding. Because infants with cleft lip and palate cannot generate the suction necessary to feed through a normal nipple or breast, the parents require assistance with learning to use special feeding devices. A variety of special "cleft-palate" nipples have had some success. However, large, soft nipples with large holes or long, soft lamb's nipples appear to offer the best means for nipple feeding (Fig. 32.14). Breast-feeding may be possible with

Fig. 32.14 Some devices used to feed an infant with a cleft lip and palate. (Courtesy Texas Children's Hospital, Houston.)

the use of a breast shield with a specially designed nipple. The ESSR feeding technique works especially well for infants with cleft lip/palate before corrective surgery. ESSR stands for the following:

*E*nlarge the nipple.
*S*timulate the suck reflex.
*S*wallow fluid appropriately.
*R*est when infant signals with facial expression.

During feedings, these infants require frequent burping because they tend to swallow large amounts of air.

Another important goal is to assist the parents in dealing with the diagnosis of cleft lip and palate and to promote bonding between the parents and the infant. To accomplish this goal, try emphasizing positive aspects of the infant's appearance and behavior. Parents may benefit greatly from viewing photographs of children who have had cleft lip and palate repairs to illustrate the positive results of surgical intervention. Postoperative nursing interventions include protecting the integrity of the suture line, promoting optimal nutrition, and continuing emotional support of the child and parents. Such infants should be positioned only on their side or back; positioning on the abdomen allows them to rub the face on the sheets. Place safety reminder devices on the child's elbows to prevent touching or rubbing of the suture line. Periodically remove the safety reminder devices to enable movement of the arms, to provide an opportunity to observe the skin underneath for signs of impairment or pressure, and to cuddle the infant.

Immediately after surgery, the infant usually is kept on NPO status until the effects of the anesthesia have disappeared. Then the infant gradually is introduced to liquids, beginning with clear liquids (water and dextrose water) and gradually progressing to formula. A soft rubber-tipped feeder is generally preferred; slip the rubber tip of the feeder into the side of the infant's mouth carefully, avoiding contact with the suture line. Breast-feeding usually is contraindicated immediately after surgery. Help the mother if she wishes to pump her breasts to promote the continued production of milk until the infant is able to feed directly from the breast. After feedings, gently cleanse the suture line with a saline-soaked cotton-tipped swab. Then place the infant in an infant seat or on the right side to promote digestion and prevent aspiration of regurgitated formula. In addition, careful aspiration of the oral and nasopharyngeal cavities is sometimes necessary to remove collections of mucus, blood, and saliva and to prevent aspiration. Analgesics should be administered as ordered.

Postoperative care after surgical repair of cleft palate is similar to that after cleft lip repair. A child with cleft palate repair should lie on the abdomen because this will facilitate drainage of mucus and serosanguineous exudate from the oral cavity. Administer analgesics as ordered. Liquid nourishments usually are provided by cup. Use of straws, pacifiers, and eating utensils is not advisable because they may injure the suture line. The child should advance gradually from a liquid diet to a blenderized diet, and parents are instructed to continue this diet after discharge until the surgeon instructs them otherwise.

Patient Teaching. Assist the family by providing them with information on agencies that provide services, information, and emotional support to families with a child who has cleft lip and palate. These agencies include the American Cleft Palate-Craniofacial Association (https://acpa-cpf.org/) and the March of Dimes (http://marchofdimes.com). Throughout the child's development, an important goal is the development of a healthy personality and self-esteem.

Prognosis. After surgery, speech impairments and middle ear infections continue to be a problem for most children with cleft lip or palate. Teach parents the signs and symptoms of upper respiratory and ear infections so that early treatment can be obtained. Early intervention is necessary in the development of normal speech patterns.

Dehydration

When the body loses more fluid than it absorbs, as in the presence of diarrhea, or when it absorbs less water than it excretes, as in the presence of vomiting, dehydration results. Dehydration occurs basically whenever the total fluid intake is less than the total fluid output. The most accurate method of assessing a child's degree of dehydration is by noting changes in the body weight. Mild, moderate, and severe dehydration correspond to fluid deficits of 5%, 10%, and 15%, respectively.

Etiology And Pathophysiology. Dehydration is the result of many possible disease processes that cause abnormal fluid losses through the skin, respiratory, renal, and (most commonly) GI systems.

Clinical Manifestations. The physical signs of dehydration are primarily the result of a deficiency in fluid volume. Because accurate record of weight before the episode of dehydration is not always available for comparison, it is easier to diagnose the degree of dehydration on the basis of its clinical manifestations (Table 32.1).

Diagnostic Tests. Health care providers diagnose dehydration on the basis of observed clinical manifestations (see Table 32.1). Laboratory tests to support diagnosis and determine severity include measurements of serum sodium, serum glucose, serum bicarbonate, and blood urea nitrogen. In general, weighing the child daily also yields useful information about the degree and severity of dehydration.

Medical Management. Refer to the discussion of medical management of diarrhea (in the section "Diarrhea and Gastroenteritis").

Nursing Interventions And Patient Teaching. Careful nursing assessment and intervention are important in the clinical detection and management of dehydration. An essential nursing function is to assess for any clinical manifestations of dehydration. This assessment begins with a general survey of the child and continues with specific observations.

Table 32.1   Clinical Manifestations of Dehydration

ASSESSMENT PARAMETER	SIGNS AND SYMPTOMS
Skin	Cold, dry, gray, loss of turgor
Mucous membranes	Dry
Eyes	Sunken
Fontanelle	Sunken
Behavior	Lethargic
Pulse	Rapid, weak
Blood pressure	Low
Respirations	Rapid

Observation includes the measurement of intake and output (I&O). This measurement accounts for oral and parenteral intake and losses from sweat, wound drainage, urine, stools, vomiting, nasogastric drainage, and fistulas. For children who are not toilet trained, wet diapers should be weighed to assess the amount of output. By subtracting the weight (in grams) of a dry diaper from the weight of the wet diaper, calculate the actual fluid content of the diaper. The volume of fluid in milliliters is equal to the weight of the fluid measured in grams. Other data that assist in the assessment of dehydration include vital signs, body weight, skin color, temperature and turgor, capillary refill, presence or absence of edema, moisture and color of mucous membranes, sensation of thirst, and, in infants, assessment of the fontanelles.

Teach the parents that infants and young children have a greater need for water than do adults and are more vulnerable to alterations in fluid and electrolyte balance. In comparison with older children and adults, infants have a greater fluid I&O relative to size. Water and electrolyte disturbances occur more frequently and more rapidly, and infants and children adjust less promptly to these alterations.

Prognosis. Shock is common with severe depletion of extracellular fluid. When medical management and nursing interventions are effective, the prognosis is favorable.

Diarrhea and Gastroenteritis

Diarrhea is one of the most common disorders affecting children; it has the capacity to quickly render the child vulnerable to fluid deficits and electrolyte imbalances. Diarrhea is a disturbance in intestinal motility, characterized by an increase in frequency, fluid content, and volume of stools. The diarrhea may be acute or chronic, and it may be either infectious or noninfectious. Diarrhea caused by an inflammatory process, such as infection, is called *gastroenteritis*.

Etiology And Pathophysiology. Although diarrhea results from a variety of causes, the most common is bacterial or viral invasion of the intestinal mucosa. The most prevalent bacterial pathogens are *Salmonella, Shigella,* and *Rotavirus* organisms. Many factors can predispose a child to diarrhea. Infants have a greater susceptibility to diarrhea, and the results are more serious because infants have a small extracellular fluid reserve. When this reserve is depleted suddenly and quickly, dehydration rapidly ensues. Children who are malnourished, debilitated, or immunocompromised are more prone to diarrhea. Poor hygiene, contaminated food or water, warm weather, and crowded and substandard living conditions also predispose children to diarrhea. Other common causes of diarrhea are the ingestion of large quantities of fruit juices, such as apple juice; food sensitivities; antibiotics; and formula intolerance.

When a pathogen invades the intestinal mucosa, the resulting enterotoxins stimulate an inflammatory reaction. As a result, water and electrolytes are secreted, and the pathogen invades and destroys the epithelial cells of the GI mucosa. Serious disturbances, such as renal failure, dehydration, metabolic acidosis, shock, and circulatory collapse, may follow.

Clinical Manifestations. In addition to the increased number of stools and the increased fluid content of stools, diarrhea has other clinical effects (Box 32.4). Assess for these, as well as for any signs of dehydration, which is a common complication of diarrhea (see Table 32.1).

Diagnostic Tests. Document the history carefully, including information regarding recent travel, exposure to infected agents, personal contact, allergies, food or formula sensitivities, living conditions, and contact with contaminated water or food. Laboratory evaluation typically includes a stool culture, examination of the stool for ova and parasites, and CBC.

Medical Management. The goals of management are to restore the fluid and electrolyte balance and to treat the underlying cause. The American Academy of Pediatrics (since 2004) no longer recommends withholding food or fluids for 24 hours after the onset of diarrhea or administering the traditional diet of bananas, rice, applesauce, and toast or tea ("BRAT" diet). It is acceptable to offer a commercially available oral rehydration solution in small amounts for the first 4 to 6 hours after the onset of diarrhea. The infant who has been breast-feeding should continue doing so as a supplement to the oral rehydration solution. Administer oral maintenance doses of the solution for the remaining first 24 hours. An older child is permitted to take clear liquids. When the number and fluid content of stools have decreased, the infant is advanced gradually to full-strength formula. In an older child, solid foods should be offered when rehydration is complete. Initially, foods that are nonirritating to the bowel should be offered. The child may resume a regular diet gradually.

In cases of severe diarrhea, hospitalization and IV therapy are required. IV administration of a saline solution containing 5% dextrose enables rehydration. This solution provides the child with fluid, sodium, and calories. Once kidney function has been verified,

| Box 32.4 | Clinical Effects of Diarrhea |

- Cool, pale skin
- Irritability progressing to lethargy
- Low blood pressure
- Malodorous stools
- Normal or elevated temperature
- Poor skin turgor
- Rapid pulse and respirations
- Sunken eyes
- Sunken fontanelles
- Vomiting
- Weight loss

it is acceptable to add potassium to the IV solution to correct any potassium depletion. IV rehydration must be continued until the diarrhea becomes less severe. Once rehydration has begun and the severe effects of the diarrhea and dehydration have abated, the focus of management shifts to determining and treating the underlying cause. This includes antimicrobial therapy as indicated.

Nursing Interventions And Patient Teaching. Nursing interventions for the infant or child with diarrhea focus on assessment, including the careful recording of I&O; promotion of rehydration; correction of electrolyte imbalances; provision of age-appropriate nutrition; prevention of the spread of the diarrhea; prevention of complications; and emotional support of the child and family.

Patient problems and interventions for a child with diarrhea and gastroenteritis include but are not limited to the following:

PATIENT PROBLEM	NURSING INTERVENTIONS
Inadequate fluid volume, related to excessive gastrointestinal losses in stool	Offer oral fluids as indicated and as tolerated Monitor intravenous fluids as prescribed Maintain strict record of intake and output (urine and stool); monitor urine specific gravity Weigh patient daily Assess vital signs, skin turgor, mucous membranes, and mental status q 4 h or as indicated
Compromised skin integrity, related to irritation caused by frequent, loose stools	Change diaper frequently Cleanse buttocks gently with bland, nonalkaline soap and water, or immerse patient in a bath for gentle cleansing Apply protective ointment (type of ointment often varies according to individual patient, and sometimes a trial period is necessary) Expose slightly erythematous intact skin to air whenever possible; apply protective ointment to very irritated or excoriated skin Observe buttocks and perineum for infection, such as Candida
Anxiousness, related to • Separation from parents • Unfamiliar environment • Distressing procedures	Provide mouth care and pacifier for infants who are on NPO status Encourage family visitation and appropriate participation in care Touch, hold, and talk to patient as much as possible Provide sensory stimulation and diversion appropriate for patient's developmental level

Parents should be instructed to avoid the use of antidiarrheals such as diphenoxylate (Lomotil) or kaolin and pectin (Kaopectate). Discuss hygiene practice and instruct the parents on hand washing after changing diapers to prevent the spread of infection. It is necessary to dispose of properly or thoroughly clean soiled diapers, bed linens, and clothes.

Prognosis. Mild or moderate diarrhea can be managed at home by simple methods. Severe diarrhea necessitates hospitalization with IV fluid therapy. When treatment is effective, the prognosis is usually excellent.

Constipation

Constipation is best defined as the passage of hardened stools, and it often occurs in association with failure to evacuate the colon completely with defecation. It is possible for constipation to manifest as a primary disorder or in association with a wide variety of GI tract or systemic disorders.

Etiology And Pathophysiology. Constipation is possible in children of any age. Newborns normally pass a first meconium stool within 24 to 36 hours after birth. Failure to do this indicates possible intestinal atresia (congenital closure of a body part usually open; in this case, any part of the intestine) or stenosis (constriction or narrowing of a passage or orifice), Hirschsprung disease, meconium ileus (ileus of the newborn caused by obstruction of the bowel with meconium), or a meconium plug. In formula-fed infants, constipation may result from a high fat or protein content or inadequate fluid in the formula. In children, constipation sometimes occurs in connection with environmental factors such as medications (e.g., iron supplements, anticonvulsant therapy, low-fiber diet, or antacids) or results from a learned repression of the urge to defecate. In children who have constipation, passage of hardened stools is painful. As a result, the child may repress the urge to defecate. Continuous repression results in dilation of the rectum, reduced sensation of the need to defecate, and decreased muscle tone in the lower rectum. This cycle results in chronic, incomplete evacuation of the colon, and the constipation becomes severe. Episodes of diarrhea or *encopresis* (leakage around the firm stool in the rectum) often lead to accidents or soiling.

Clinical Manifestations. In infancy, constipation sometimes occurs in association with hard stools or evidence of fresh blood in the stools. Accompanying symptoms may include cramping abdominal pain, anal fissures, pain on defecation, loss of appetite, and irritability.

Diagnostic Tests. Diagnosis of constipation rests largely on a thorough health history. The parents should be asked to describe the infant's or child's bowel patterns. A discussion of diet and medications is also indicated. The health care provider will perform a physical examination of the anus and rectum.

Medical Management. In the newborn, simple measures often effectively alleviate constipation. Modifying the formula with addition of more fluid or carbohydrates sometimes corrects the situation. For infants older than 5 to 6 months, adding foods with bulk (fruits and vegetables) and increasing fluid intake sometimes correct the problem. If the constipation is the result of a tightened anal sphincter or anal stenosis, the health care provider may instruct parents to dilate the sphincter manually two or three times daily until sufficient dilation is attained. The management of simple constipation in children focuses on emptying the rectum completely of stool with the use of mild laxatives or enemas and instituting dietary modifications, such as increased fluid intake and addition of high-fiber foods, to prevent further constipation. The treatment of chronic constipation in children aims at complete evacuation of the rectum and bowel retraining therapy. It is usually possible to achieve complete evacuation of the rectum through the use of enemas, manual disimpaction, and stool softeners. After complete evacuation is attained, the health care provider institutes bowel retraining therapy to sustain evacuation. This generally consists of behavioral modification, with positive reinforcement for toilet sitting and defecation, and emotional support.

Nursing Interventions And Patient Teaching. Nursing interventions begin with a careful history of bowel patterns, including stool characteristics (color, consistency, frequency, and associated pain), diet, and concomitant medications. If dietary modifications are to be instituted, educate the parents regarding these and ensure their understanding. Sometimes parents also need instruction about normal stool patterns and what constitutes constipation. Discussion of the parent's expectations and attitudes regarding toileting is helpful. Providing emotional reassurance to the parents and child is beneficial.

Instruct parents to avoid the use of raw or unpasteurized honey and corn syrup products as a home remedy for constipation in young infants. Use of these products may be associated with the development of infant botulism.

Prognosis. Simple measures ordinarily correct constipation. The underlying cause and child's age will largely affect resolution. In the more complex situations, counseling and bowel retraining are often necessary.

Gastroesophageal Reflux

Gastroesophageal reflux (GER) is the effortless regurgitation of the gastric contents into the esophagus. The passage of the gastric esophageal contents into the oropharynx is called *regurgitation*. Vomiting is the expulsion of refluxed gastric contents from the mouth. The health care provider diagnoses GER disease when gastric contents are regurgitated into the esophagus or oropharynx and produce symptoms. In affected infants, GER usually begins within 1 week of birth, and regurgitation occurs immediately after a feeding or when the infant is laid down after a feeding.

Etiology And Pathophysiology. GER results primarily from an incompetent lower esophageal (or cardiac) sphincter. As a result, gastric contents can regurgitate into the esophagus.

Clinical Manifestations. Vomiting or spitting up is the primary manifestation in the first week of life. Aspiration of the gastric contents has potential to lead to respiratory signs such as apnea, choking or gagging after feedings, and aspiration pneumonia. In affected young children, a chronic cough, wheezing, and recurrent pneumonia are common. Growth and weight gain are a problem with a majority of affected children. Continuous irritation of the esophageal lining with gastric acid can lead to esophageal ulceration and bleeding. This usually manifests as anemia, hematemesis, or blood in the stools.

Diagnostic Tests. Diagnosis begins with an evaluation of the health history and of growth and weight patterns. More invasive studies such as barium esophagography, esophageal pH, and an upper endoscopy can be performed.

Medical Management. Conservative management of GER includes feeding and positioning practices. Feeding small, frequent feedings that have been thickened with infant cereal may be implemented (Schwarz, 2019). If the infant is breast-feeding, the mother should express milk manually and mix it with cereal for feedings. The prone position improves gastric emptying and decreases GER; however, as previously discussed, to aid in preventing SIDS it is recommended to place infants to sleep on their backs. Prone positioning should be used only while the infant is awake, especially after feedings. The infant should be supervised carefully when placed in the prone position.

Pharmacologic therapies also may be prescribed. H_2-histamine receptor antagonists, such as cimetidine (Tagamet), ranitidine (Zantac), or famotidine (Pepcid), are effective in reducing the amount of acid present in gastric content and sometimes prevent esophagitis. It is also possible to give metoclopramide (Reglan) before meals and at bedtime to accelerate gastric emptying. Proton pump inhibitors such as omeprazole (Prilosec or Prevacid) and lansoprazole (Prevacid) reduce acid secretion.

Surgical management of GER sometimes is indicated in severe cases. A Nissen fundoplication, which involves wrapping the fundus of the stomach around the distal esophagus to prevent reflux of the stomach contents into the esophagus, is the most commonly performed surgical procedure.

Nursing Interventions And Patient Teaching. The nurse is often the first health care provider to whom the condition is reported. A nursing priority is to collect supportive data. The problem is distressing for children and their parents, necessitating emotional support and reassurance that the condition is physiologic in nature and not caused by emotional problems or faulty feeding patterns. Teach the plan of treatment, prescribed medications, and signs and symptoms to report.

Prognosis. In the majority of affected infants, GER is mild and normal function is achieved by 6 to 7 weeks of age. Most cases improve by about 1 year of age. Medical therapy is required in more severe cases. If GER is severe and treatment remains unsuccessful, multiple complications such as esophageal strictures and recurrent respiratory distress with aspiration pneumonia can occur.

Hypertrophic Pyloric Stenosis

Hypertrophic pyloric stenosis (HPS) is an obstructive disorder in which the gastric outlet is obstructed mechanically by a congenitally hypertrophied pyloric muscle. It is also the most common reason for an abdominal operation during the first 6 months of life. Boys are affected more often than girls. HPS most often manifests within the first 3 months of life. Genes may play a role, because children of parents who had pyloric stenosis are more likely to have this condition.

HPS occurs most often in infants younger than 6 months. It is more common in boys than in girls.

Etiology And Pathophysiology. The exact cause of HPS is not known. The incidence is higher in siblings and offspring of affected people. Other risk factors include certain antibiotics, too much acid in the first part of the small intestine (duodenum), and certain congenital diseases, such as diabetes. The circular muscle that surrounds the valve between the stomach and the duodenum becomes diffusely enlarged as the result of hypertrophy and hyperplasia (Fig. 32.15). As a result, the passage becomes narrower, and it is difficult for the stomach to empty. At approximately 4 to 6 weeks of age, infants with HPS begin to vomit almost immediately after feedings. As the condition progresses, the vomiting becomes more forceful and becomes projectile, the hallmark sign of HPS.

Clinical Manifestations. Initially, the signs begin as regurgitation that progresses to projectile vomiting 30 to 60 minutes after feeding. As the condition progresses, the affected infant exhibits lethargy, weight loss, poor skin turgor, sunken fontanelles, and loss of subcutaneous tissue as dehydration ensues (Box 32.5).

Diagnostic Tests. Examination of the abdomen is often a key assessment that assists in the diagnosis and reveals signs of HPS. Peristaltic waves that move from left to right across the epigastric region are sometimes visible, and palpation sometimes reveals an olive-shaped mass in this area to the right of the midline. If it is not possible to establish the diagnosis after history and physical examination, an ultrasonic examination usually is indicated. Ultrasonography demonstrates an elongated sausage-shaped mass with an elongated pyloric channel. If ultrasonography fails to demonstrate hypertrophy of the pylorus, health care providers order upper GI radiography to rule out other causes of vomiting.

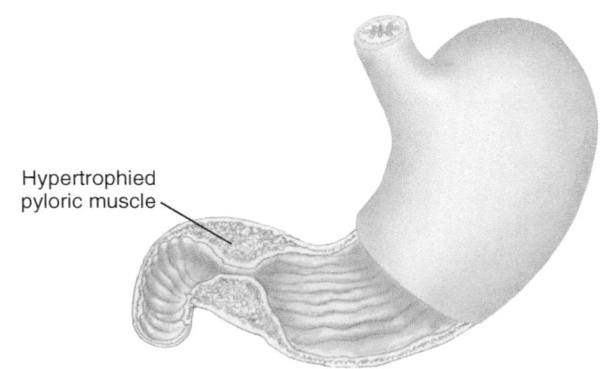

Fig. 32.15 Comparison of normal pyloric opening with evidence of pyloric stenosis. (From Ashwill JW, Droske SC: *Nursing care of children: Principles and practice,* ed 3, Philadelphia, 2007, Saunders.)

Box 32.5 **Clinical Manifestations of Hypertrophic Pyloric Stenosis**

- Projectile vomiting: vomitus is sometimes ejected 3–4 feet (0.9–1.2 m) from the child when child is in a side-lying position, 1 foot (0.3 m) or more when child is in a back-lying position:
  - Usually occurs shortly after feeding (may not occur for several hours in some cases)
  - May follow each feeding or appear intermittently
  - Nonbilious (no bile) vomitus; may be blood tinged
- Appetite: hungry, avid nurser; infant eagerly accepts a second feeding after vomiting episode
- No evidence of pain or discomfort except that of chronic hunger
- Weight loss
- Signs of dehydration
- Distended upper abdomen
- Readily palpable olive-shaped mass in the epigastrium just to the right of the umbilicus
- Gastric peristaltic waves that are visible and move from left to right across the epigastrium

---

Medical Management. Surgical relief of the pyloric obstruction as soon as establishment of the diagnosis is the standard treatment of HPS. The surgical correction of HPS consists of a pyloromyotomy, in which the pylorus muscle is surgically split down to, but not including, the submucosa; this allows for enlarging of the lumen. This procedure has a high success rate when the infant receives careful preoperative preparation to correct fluid and electrolyte imbalances.

Nursing Interventions And Patient Teaching. Nursing interventions for an infant with HPS primarily involve assisting with the establishment of a diagnosis, providing adequate nutrition, managing preoperative and postoperative care, and emotionally supporting the family. A carefully documented history, with assessment for signs and symptoms of HPS, is essential for the prompt diagnosis. Correction of any metabolic disturbances and dehydration before surgery is essential. In general, this is possible through IV administration of fluid and electrolytes. It is necessary to keep the affected infant on NPO status to eliminate vomiting. Fluid replacement needs must be assessed and are determined largely by I&O. Postoperative nursing interventions are focused on preventing complications by monitoring I&O, observing physical signs, and instituting oral feedings. Feedings of glucose water usually begin 4 to 6 hours postoperatively; then, if feedings are retained for 24 hours, full feedings are started. Encourage parents to express their concerns, visit their infant frequently, and participate in the care when appropriate. Barring complications, affected infants usually are discharged within 1 to 2 days after surgery.

Prognosis. Most infants with HPS recover completely and rapidly after pyloromyotomy. Small feedings typically are initiated within a few hours postoperatively. Postoperative complications include persistent pyloric obstruction and wound dehiscence.

Intussusception

Intussusception is the most common cause of intestinal obstruction in children between 3 months and 6 years of age. It is twice as common in male children. In general, health care providers are unable to determine the cause of intussusception.

Etiology And Pathophysiology. Intussusception is the result of the telescoping of one portion of the intestine into another (Fig. 32.16). The site most commonly affected is the ileocecal valve, at the juncture of the distal ileum and the proximal colon. As the ileum telescopes into the colon, the passage of intestinal contents distal to the defect becomes obstructed. Subsequently, as the mucosa of the intestinal walls rub against each other, blood and mucus from the mucosa leak into the intestinal lumen and form **"currant jelly" stools** (feces mixed with blood and mucus from the intestinal mucosa), a hallmark sign of intussusception. Serious complications include peritonitis, intestinal ischemia, infarction, perforation, and shock. If the condition is not treated, the child may die within 2 to 5 days.

Clinical Manifestations. In most cases, there is a sudden onset of severe abdominal pain in a previously well child.

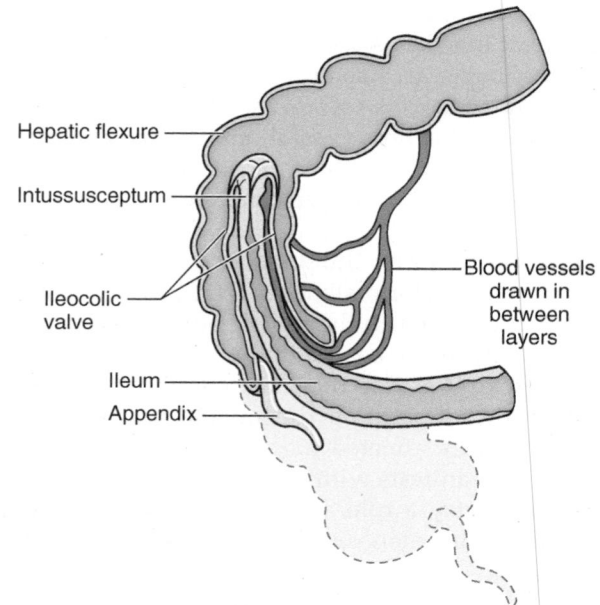

Fig. 32.16 Ileocolic intussusception.

The child assumes a fetal position in an effort to guard the abdomen. Vomiting and lethargy usually occur. Within 12 hours of the onset of abdominal pain, the child usually passes the characteristic "currant jelly" stool.

Diagnostic Tests. The signs and symptoms collected during the history and physical aid in the diagnosis of the disorder. Radiographic studies may show a perforation. Ultrasound and CT scans demonstrate intestinal obstruction caused by intussusception. Imaging of all three examinations may show a "bull's-eye," representing the intestine coiled within itself. An air or barium enema also may be used for diagnosis (Mayo Clinic, 2021).

Medical Management. In 90% of cases either of these diagnostic tests actually may correct the intussusception when the air or barium is instilled (Mayo Clinic, 2021). The force exerted by the flowing barium from the enema sometimes successfully forces the telescoped portion of the bowel into its correct position. Because the use of barium can lead to peritonitis, water-soluble contrast medium and air pressure sometimes are used instead. Surgical treatment of intussusception involves manual reduction of the invagination (the process of becoming enclosed in a sheath) and, if necessary, resection of nonviable bowel with end-to-end anastomosis.

Nursing Interventions. Nursing interventions for a child with intussusception involve documenting a thorough history from the parents and observing for physical signs that will help establish a prompt and accurate diagnosis. As soon as the health care provider establishes a diagnosis, begin to prepare the parents for the diagnostic barium enema study. Inform them that in many cases, this procedure is corrective, but if it is unsuccessful, surgery may be required. After the hydrostatic reduction, observe for the passage of barium and the return of normal bowel movements. The child is observed for at least 24 hours after the procedure to assess for the possibility of recurrence. If surgery is indicated, the child is kept on NPO status with a nasogastric tube set to intermittent low suction. Begin an IV infusion to supply adequate hydration and electrolytes. Postoperative care of the child involves measuring vital signs, monitoring the operative site, and assessing for the return of bowel sounds. When peristaltic function has returned, it is appropriate to gradually introduce oral feedings.

Prognosis. In many patients with intussusception, treatment with hydrostatic reduction is successful. Surgery is required for patients in whom the water-soluble contrast medium enema with air pressure was unsuccessful. If untreated, most patients suffer worsening or die of complications such as perforation, peritonitis, and sepsis. With early diagnosis and treatment, serious complications and death are rare.

Hirschsprung Disease

Hirschsprung disease, also known as *megacolon* (congenital aganglionic megacolon), is a functional intestinal obstruction caused by the absence of parasympathetic ganglion cells in a portion of the colon. The incidence is 1 per 5000 live births, with a predominance in boys. Hirschsprung disease is more common in children with trisomy 21 (Down syndrome) (National Organization for Rare Organization [NORD], 2017).

Etiology And Pathophysiology. In Hirschsprung disease, there is an absence of innervation to a segment of the bowel. In most cases, the lower portion of the sigmoid colon just above the anus is affected. As a result, there are no peristaltic waves in the affected portion of the colon to propel the fecal contents, which causes an intestinal obstruction and distention of the bowel proximal to the defect (Fig. 32.17).

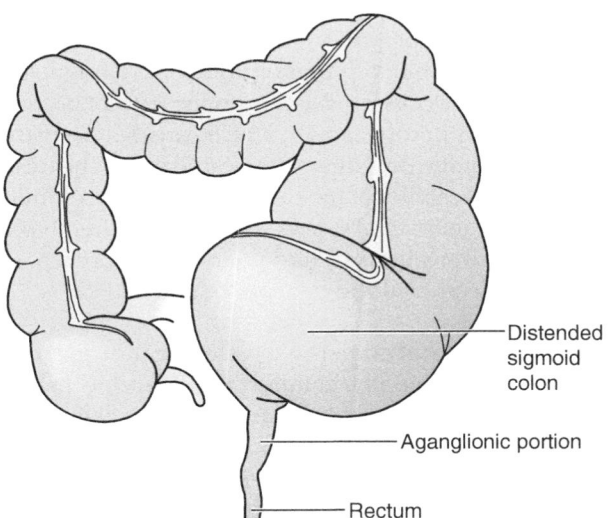

Fig. 32.17 Appearance of the affected portion of the bowel in Hirschsprung disease.

Clinical Manifestations. Clinical manifestations often vary according to age. Early observation of an affected newborn typically reveals a failure to pass meconium within 48 hours and signs of partial or complete intestinal obstruction, such as abdominal distention, vomiting, and poor feeding. Affected infants sometimes have a history of constipation or intermittent constipation and diarrhea. Dehydration, failure to thrive, abdominal distention, and fever are other possible manifestations. In affected older children, there is an association between Hirschsprung disease and chronic constipation; abdominal distention; ribbon-like, foul-smelling stools; poor weight gain; malnourishment; anemia; palpable fecal mass; and visible peristalsis.

Diagnostic Tests. A carefully obtained history, associated clinical manifestations, and a barium enema study assist in making a diagnosis of Hirschsprung disease.

Medical Management. Immediate treatment involves surgical removal of the affected portion of the bowel. The surgeon proceeds in two stages. The first stage involves placement of a temporary colostomy in the portion of normal, innervated colon just proximal to the defect. This allows for a period of rest, during which the normal bowel regains its tone. The second stage involves excising the affected segment and pulling the normal, innervated segment down through the anus, anastomosing it to the anal canal. This procedure, known as the *Soave endorectal pull-through,* usually is performed when the child reaches a weight of 20 pounds.

Nursing Interventions And Patient Teaching. The nursing interventions for the infant or child with Hirschsprung disease are focused on assisting the parents in adjusting to the diagnosis, promoting parent-infant bonding, preparing the parents for surgery, and educating them regarding colostomy care. Preoperatively, direct nursing interventions are focused on restoring the child's nutritional status with a low-fiber, high-protein, high-calorie diet or, in severe cases, total parenteral nutrition. Sometimes you must evacuate the patient's bowel with daily enemas and stool softeners. Oral antibiotics, if prescribed, are administered to decrease intestinal flora. Measure the patient's abdominal girth daily. Prepare the child, when developmentally appropriate, and the parents for the colostomy. Stress that this is a temporary procedure unless a large portion of the bowel is involved, which would necessitate a permanent ileostomy. Postoperative care includes assessing vital signs and bowel sounds, observing for the passage of flatus and stools, and monitoring the operative site. Surgeons generally place a nasogastric tube set to low intermittent suction during the surgery and order its removal as soon as peristalsis has returned, usually within 24 hours, and when a diet appropriate for age can be introduced.

Before discharge, parents need instruction regarding colostomy care; refer them as needed to a visiting nurse for assistance in caring for the colostomy.

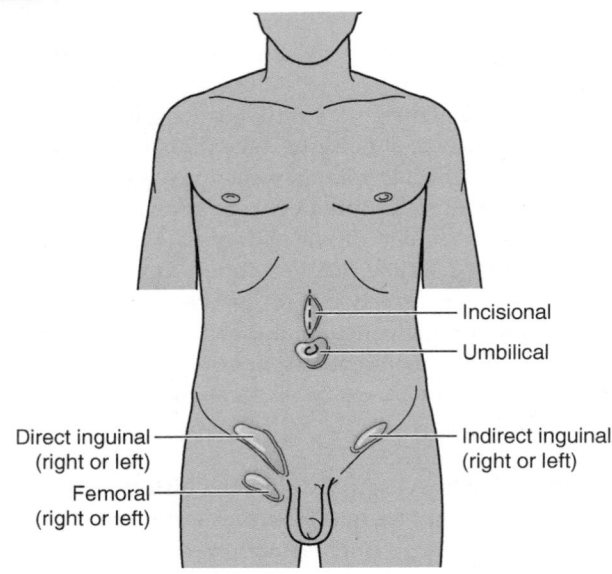

- Incisional
- Umbilical
- Direct inguinal (right or left)
- Indirect inguinal (right or left)
- Femoral (right or left)

Fig. 32.18 Locations of hernias.

Prognosis. After fluid and replacement therapy, the infant undergoes surgery, during which the surgeon creates a colostomy. One or more corrective surgeries will follow, after which time the colostomy can usually be reversed.

Hernias

A *hernia* is the protrusion of organs or portions of an organ through a structural defect or weakened muscle wall. A complication of herniation arises when the circulation to the protruding organ is impaired (known as a *strangulated hernia*) or when the pressure of protruding organs impairs the function of other organs. Incarceration of a hernia occurs when the hernia cannot be reduced manually. Fig. 32.18 and Table 32.2 illustrate and describe hernias affecting the diaphragm and the abdominal wall.

DISORDERS OF GENITOURINARY FUNCTION

Disorders of the genitourinary tract are common in children and arise from a variety of etiologic factors. The genitourinary system is responsible for maintaining fluid and electrolyte balance within the body. Disorders of the genitourinary system alter the delicate balance of fluid and electrolytes within the body and sometimes become life threatening.

Urinary Tract Infection

Urinary tract infections (UTIs) affect the upper urinary tract (kidneys and ureters), the lower urinary tract (bladder and urethra), or both. They are more prevalent in girls, uncircumcised boys, and sexually active adolescents. UTIs are caused primarily by bacteria, most frequently gram-negative organisms. Because the female urethra is short (approximately 2 cm [0.8 inch] in young girls and 4 cm [1.6 inches] in mature women), it provides an efficient access route to the bladder for organisms that are common to the perineal and perianal regions. Another factor that sometimes leads to UTIs

is urinary stasis. The urine is typically sterile, but the warm climate within the bladder provides an excellent growth medium for bacteria. Teaching parents correct perineal cleansing is imperative. In infant boys, it is necessary to retract and cleanse the foreskin with each diaper change. When older boys begin bathing themselves, it is necessary for parents to monitor this cleaning. For girls, cleansing the perineal area from front to back helps prevent UTIs from *Escherichia coli.* Some children also have a congenital anomaly such as urethral stenosis or vesicoureteral reflux (backward flow of urine from the bladder to the ureters) that can lead to urinary stasis and the development of a UTI. Signs and symptoms of UTIs are often subtle, and parents may not realize anything is wrong with the child. In affected infants, fever, weight loss, failure to thrive, feeding difficulties, vomiting, and diarrhea are common. In affected children, urinary frequency, pain during urination, foul-smelling urine, incontinence after successful toilet training, abdominal or flank pain, hematuria, and vomiting are common signs and symptoms.

Nephrotic Syndrome (Nephrosis)

Nephrotic syndrome is a clinical state characterized by proteinuria, edema, hyperlipidemia, and hypoproteinemia. Nephrotic syndrome has three forms: (1) idiopathic, or primary; (2) secondary (occurring as a result of glomerular damage caused by a known cause); and (3) congenitally acquired. In children, the idiopathic form is most common.

Etiology And Pathophysiology. For most children (90%), the cause of the syndrome is unknown. For the other 10% the most common cause is minimal change disease. Children with minimal change disease typically outgrow nephrotic syndrome by the time they reach their teen years. Minimal change disease has unknown cause, but it can be related to infections, tumors, allergic reactions, and overuse of over-the-counter medications such as ibuprofen and acetaminophen. The underlying pathologic abnormality is glomerular damage that renders the glomerulus permeable to protein (proteinuria). Loss of protein in the urine causes a decrease in the level of protein in the blood (hypoproteinemia), which causes a decrease in colloidal osmotic pressure in the capillaries. This results in hyperpermeability of the capillaries and causes fluid to leak into the interstitial spaces (edema). Children typically experience swelling around their eyes, abdomen, feet, and ankles (National Kidney Foundation, 2017).

Clinical Manifestations. The development of manifestations is subtle. Initially, children may develop periorbital edema, which is noticed primarily on awakening. Abdominal distention is sometimes apparent as fluid accumulates in the abdominal cavity (ascites). As the syndrome progresses, the edema becomes generalized and severe (anasarca) (Fig. 32.19). Vomiting, anorexia, diarrhea, and irritability are common. Increased body weight,

| Table 32.2 | Hernias Affecting the Diaphragm and the Abdominal Wall |

HERNIAS TYPE	CLINICAL MANIFESTATIONS AND DIAGNOSTIC TESTS	INTERVENTIONS
Diaphragmatic		
Protrusion of a portion of the abdominal organs through the foramen of Bochdalek (and opening in the diaphragm)	Respiratory distress within hours of birth; cyanosis, tachypnea, retractions, dyspnea, respiratory acidosis, and absence of breath sounds on the affected side (bowel sounds may be present) Abdominal pain, vomiting Diagnosis made by radiography	**Medical** Immediate surgical repair of the diaphragm with replacement of the herniation; placement of chest tubes **Nursing** *Preoperative:* Support of respiratory function; comfort measures; placement of patient in semi-Fowler's position; suctioning, oxygen administration, and monitoring of IV fluids *Postoperative:* Maintenance of routine postoperative care and monitoring; placement of patient in semi-Fowler's position; physiotherapy and positive pressure ventilation; monitoring of oxygenation; comfort measures; emotional support of parents
Hiatal		
Intermittent protrusion of the stomach through the esophageal opening in the diaphragm	Vomiting, dysphasia, dyspnea, gastroesophageal reflux, respiratory distress, bleeding Diagnosis based on history and radiography	**Medical** Surgical repair of the esophageal opening **Nursing** Routine preoperative and postoperative care, as for diaphragmatic hernia
Inguinal		
Prolapse of a loop of intestine through the inguinal ring above the scrotal sac because of muscle weakness; can be either unilateral or bilateral	Usually asymptomatic and found only in the course of routine examination; can become strangulated or incarcerated (i.e., a portion of the intestine becomes tightly caught in the hernia sac, restricting blood supply) Sometimes accompanied by hydrocele or undescended testes	**Medical** Usually possible to reduce by gentle manipulation of the trapped intestine; after surgery (herniorrhaphy), overnight hospital stay not necessary **Nursing** Applying ice to the scrotum to reduce edema; comfort measures and quieting of the patient with an incarcerated (trapped) inguinal hernia so that the surgeon can reduce the incarceration; no diapers used postoperatively, even if the child is not toilet trained; instruction of parents not to give tub baths until healing is complete
Umbilical		
Protrusion of the intestine through a weakness in the abdominal wall around the umbilicus	Inspection and palpation of abdomen High incidence in African American infants Spontaneous closure at 1–2 years of age	**Medical** Spontaneous closure by age 2 years with small defects (<2 cm); surgical closure if condition persists after age 2–5 years or for defects larger than 2 cm **Nursing** Discouraging use of home remedies (i.e., coins, belly bands, abdominal taping); reassurance of parents

decreased urine output, and marked edema are hallmark signs. Other signs include white nails, lusterless hair, and soft ear cartilage.

Diagnostic Tests. A thorough physical examination and clinical manifestations such as weight gain, edema, and lab analyses are used in the diagnosis of nephritic syndrome. Analysis of the urine reveals marked proteinuria with a high specific gravity. The urine is frequently dark and frothy. RBCs, hyaline casts, and fat bodies also may be present. Serum protein levels are reduced, and serum lipid levels are elevated. A renal biopsy may help determine the extent of glomerular damage and evaluate the response to therapy.

Medical Management. The principal goal of management of nephrotic syndrome is to reduce the edema. Steroid therapy is the primary means to accomplish this. Health care providers order adrenocortical steroids (prednisone) to reduce the proteinuria and subsequently the edema. This response usually occurs within 7 to 21 days of initiation of the therapy; administration of the

Fig. 32.19 Appearance of the genitals of a boy with nephrotic syndrome. (Courtesy Harry C. Shirkey, Fort Thomas, Kentucky.)

steroids slowly tapers over a period of several weeks and discontinues when the child has no symptoms. Bed rest is encouraged in the acute phase of the illness, with progression to ambulation as the edema subsides. The child typically is placed on a low-sodium diet during the period of severe edema. A child with nephrotic syndrome may receive diuretic therapies to reduce edema. Treatment for relapses consists of a repeated course of high-dose steroid therapy (NIDDK, n.d.).

Nursing Interventions And Patient Teaching. Nursing interventions focus on clinical observation of the child in the acute phase and monitoring the effects of therapeutic interventions. Careful monitoring of I&O, body weight, and abdominal girth is essential in assessing the status of fluid retention or excretion. Provide meticulous skin care to prevent impairment of edematous skin and secondary infections. Frequent monitoring of vital signs is necessary to detect early signs of complications, such as infection or shock. Because children with nephrotic syndrome have a poor appetite, nutrition is likely to be a challenge. It is essential that the child have a good protein intake to offset the loss of protein through the urine. Preferred foods should be offered frequently in small amounts and served in an attractive manner. Dietary restrictions include low levels of salt and fluid restrictions. Because increased susceptibility to infection is a common side effect of steroid therapy, it is necessary to keep the child free of exposure to communicable diseases and sources of infection. As the edema decreases, it is appropriate to increase the child's activity. Provide continuous emotional support to the family during the acute phase of the illness and while the child recovers.

Teach parents about testing urine for albumin, administration of medications, diet restrictions (if any), and the common effects of steroid therapy. Instruct parents about preventing contact with infected playmates, although it is permissible for the child to attend school. Parents should learn how to assess for signs of relapse; ensure they understand to seek immediate medical attention if these signs occur.

Prognosis. The chance for ultimate recovery in most cases is good. The response is more likely to be satisfactory when detection of any relapses and institution of therapy occur promptly. Remissions are longer when the prescribed treatment regimen is followed. Most affected children actually outgrow the disease during their teens or by early adulthood. Even if a child has numerous attacks, most will not develop permanent kidney damage. The children who do not outgrow it or who do not respond to treatment may become candidates for kidney transplantation (National Kidney Foundation, 2017).

Acute Glomerulonephritis

Glomerulonephritis is inflammation of the glomeruli of the kidney. Most commonly, it occurs after a pneumococcal, streptococcal, or viral infection. *Acute poststreptococcal glomerulonephritis* (APSGN) is the most common form. APSGN affects primarily children of early school age, with onset peaking at ages 6 to 7 years, and the disease occurs twice as often in boys as in girls.

Etiology And Pathophysiology. APSGN follows a streptococcal infection of the throat or skin. Immune complexes that develop as a result of infection with certain strains of group A β-hemolytic streptococci become fixed to the basement membrane of glomeruli. Most streptococcal infections do not cause APSGN. A latent period of 10 to 21 days occurs between onset of the streptococcal infection and the onset of clinical manifestations. The glomeruli become edematous and infiltrated with WBCs. As a result, the glomerular filtration rate decreases, which causes an accumulation of sodium and water in the blood, which in turn leads to circulatory congestion and edema. Inflammation and damage to the glomeruli result in increased permeability, allowing protein molecules to escape into the urine (proteinuria).

Clinical Manifestations. Manifestations of APSGN usually appear 10 to 14 days after the streptococcal infection occurs. Initial characteristics are a sudden onset of hematuria, proteinuria, and oliguria. The child's urine sometimes appears cloudy, smoky brown, or what parents describe as tea or cola colored. Edema, abdominal pain, pallor, low-grade fever, anorexia, vomiting, and headache are sometimes present. Hypertension and heart failure are possible results of hypervolemia. Fluid retention does not explain completely the hypertension associated with acute glomerulonephritis. Overproduction of renin also sometimes occurs.

Diagnostic Tests. Urinalysis reveals proteinuria, hematuria, and elevated specific gravity. Some patients have elevated levels of blood urea nitrogen and creatinine as a result of impaired glomerular filtration. Results of the urine culture are typically negative. Cultures of the throat or skin yield positive results for the streptococcal organism. The *antistreptolysin O titer* (antibodies formed against streptococci) is elevated, indicating that the patient has had a recent streptococcal infection. Renal ultrasonography, renal biopsy, electrocardiography, and chest radiography also commonly are performed to determine the extent of the disease.

Medical Management. The acute phase of glomerulonephritis generally lasts 1 to 2 weeks. During this time, health care providers usually recommend bed rest, although many children set their own limits according to their tolerance of activity. Dietary fluid, sodium, potassium, and phosphate are restricted initially. Regular measurement of vital signs, body weight, and I&O is necessary to monitor the progression of the disease and detect any complications. It is necessary to anticipate acute hypertension and identify it early. Antihypertensive medications and diuretics help control hypertension. Antibiotic therapy is indicated only for children who have a persistent streptococcal infection.

Nursing Interventions And Patient Teaching. Nursing interventions focus on promoting rest and adequate nutrition, preventing and detecting complications, and providing emotional support to the child and family. During the acute phase of the illness, some health care providers place the child on bed rest. Provide activities that require minimal energy expenditure and will keep the child's interest. Ensure that meals reflect the child's preferences and yet adhere to any dietary restrictions that have been ordered. Measurements of vital signs, body weight, and I&O provide information about the disease's progression and help detect the presence of complications.

Educate the parents about the disease and its therapy and allow them to express their feelings and concerns.

Prognosis. Most children with APSGN recover completely, with few or no complications. Specific immunity is conferred so that subsequent recurrences are uncommon. Dialysis is required if the disease is not controlled and causes acute or chronic renal failure. If acute renal failure occurs, kidney transplantation is considered.

Wilms Tumor (Nephroblastoma)

Wilms tumor (or nephroblastoma) is the most common renal and intraabdominal malignant tumor of childhood, accounting for 5% of all cancers in children. About 500 new cases of Wilms tumor are diagnosed each year in the United States. The incidence of these tumors peaks at ages 3 to 4 years. It is uncommon in children older than 6 years of age (American Cancer Society, 2020).

Etiology And Pathophysiology. Wilms tumor most commonly affects the left kidney. Both kidneys are affected in 10% of cases. Wilms tumor has hereditary and nonhereditary origins. The most common sites for metastasis are the lungs, the lymph nodes, the liver, the brain, and bone.

Clinical Manifestations. Most Wilms tumors manifest as enlarging, asymptomatic, and firm abdominal masses.

Other manifestations of the tumor include abdominal pain, hematuria, fever, hypertension, weight loss, and fatigue. If Wilms tumor has metastasized, dyspnea, cough, and chest pain may be present.

Diagnostic Tests. Parents may detect many tumors when they feel an enlarged abdominal mass while bathing, dressing, or carrying the child. In addition to a thorough history and physical examination, diagnostic studies include radiography, abdominal ultrasonography, abdominal and chest computed tomography (CT), MRI, and hematologic and chemistry studies. The definitive (final) diagnosis is based on findings of surgical biopsy. Because the tumor is encapsulated, it is important not to palpate the child's abdomen more than is necessary for diagnosis. This decreases the possibility of rupture of the capsule and spillage of the malignant cells into the abdominal cavity.

Medical Management. Treatment of Wilms tumor involves surgical resection as soon as possible after diagnosis, usually within 24 to 48 hours of admission. The surgeon performs an exploration of the abdomen to determine the extent of the disease and whether the tumor has metastasized. If one kidney is affected, the surgeon removes the tumor, the kidney, and the adrenal gland, with meticulous care during resection to avoid rupture of the capsule and spread of cancer cells throughout the abdomen. The other kidney is examined for evidence of disease. If both kidneys are involved, the surgeon removes part of the kidney on the less affected side and the entire kidney on the opposite side. Most children with Wilms tumor receive radiotherapy after surgery. Chemotherapy is indicated for all affected children. The usual course of treatment ranges from 6 to 15 months.

Nursing Interventions And Patient Teaching. Preoperative nursing interventions involve preparing the child and family for surgery. This is a challenging responsibility for the nurse because most surgeries take place within 24 hours of diagnosis. Postoperative nursing interventions are similar to those provided to children undergoing abdominal surgery with an emphasis on monitoring renal function. Be sensitive to the parents' feelings about their child's diagnosis; it is common for parents to believe that they should have identified the mass earlier.

The overall objective in discharge planning is to return the child to a normal preoperative lifestyle. Emphasize the usual needs for discipline and moderate protection from infection. Help plan treatment schedules to allow uninterrupted school attendance. Because the child is left with one kidney, certain precautions, such as avoiding contact sports, should be recommended to prevent injuring the remaining organ. Prompt detection and treatment of any genitourinary signs or symptoms are mandatory.

Prognosis. Reinforce to parents that prognosis is excellent and survival rates have improved with the development

Table 32.3   **Defects of the External Genitourinary Tract**

DEFECT	MEDICAL MANAGEMENT
Hypospadias	
Urethral opening located along the ventral (anterior) surface of the penile shaft (see Fig. 32.20)	Surgical correction involves extending the urethra to a normal position. After repair, the child is expected to have normal reproductive and urinary function.
Epispadias	
Urethral opening located along the dorsal (posterior) surface of the penile shaft	Surgical correction involves penile and urethral lengthening and possibly bladder neck reconstruction.
Phimosis	
Narrowing or stenosis of the opening of the foreskin	Mild cases are treated with manual retraction. Severe cases are treated with circumcision.
Hydrocele	
Fluid in scrotal sac	Surgical correction is indicated if spontaneous resolution has not occurred in 1 year.
Cryptorchidism	
Failure of one or both of the testes to descend into the scrotum	Medical management involves administration of human chorionic gonadotropin. Surgical correction consists of orchiopexy, which is surgical fixation of a testis. Treatment is aimed at preventing testicular damage and malignancies.
Inguinal Hernia	
Protrusion of the abdominal organs through the inguinal canal and into the scrotal sac (see Fig. 32.18)	Surgical correction involves closure of the inguinal canal.

Fig. 32.20 Hypospadias. (Courtesy H. Gil Rushton, MD, Children's National Medical Center, Washington, D.C. From Hockenberry MJ, Wilson D: *Nursing care of infants and children*, ed 9, St. Louis, 2011, Mosby.)

of new treatment protocols. Children with a localized tumor (stages I and II) have a 90% chance of cure with appropriate therapy.

Structural Defects of the Genitourinary Tract
Structural defects of the genitourinary tract have serious implications for the psychological well-being of the child. Prompt correction is necessary to avoid a negative psychological effect on the child, as well as to prevent physical complications. The major structural defects and their medical management are presented in Table 32.3 and hypospadias is depicted in Fig. 32.20.

Nursing Interventions And Patient Teaching. Nursing interventions for a child with a defect of the genitourinary tract are focused on assisting with diagnosis and preparing the child and family for procedures and corrective surgeries. Provide the child and the parents with emotional support and opportunities to express their concerns, questions, and fears.

Prognosis. Surgical repair is successful for the more common disorders and takes place or begins as early as possible.

DISORDERS OF ENDOCRINE FUNCTION
The endocrine system is responsible for the production and secretion of the major chemical regulators of the body, namely, the hormones. Disorders are caused primarily by an undersecretion or oversecretion of these hormones. Endocrine system dysfunctions affect all aspects of body function, including appearance, growth, and physical and psychological well-being.

Hypothyroidism
Hypothyroidism results from deficient production of thyroid hormone by the thyroid gland. The main function of the thyroid gland is to regulate metabolism by

Box 32.6	Clinical Manifestations of Hypothyroidism

CONGENITAL
- Cool, mottled skin
- Dyspnea
- Hypothermia
- Lethargy
- Poor appetite
- Poor sucking reflex
- Prolonged jaundice

ACQUIRED
- Constipation
- Dry skin
- Growth delay
- Lethargy
- Mental slowness
- Puffy eyes

Box 32.7	Clinical Manifestations of Hyperthyroidism

- Accelerated growth
- Advanced bone age
- Excessive appetite
- Exophthalmos (protruding eyeballs)
- Heat intolerance
- Hyperactivity
- Hypertension
- Irritability
- Nervousness
- Palpable thyroid gland
- Tachycardia
- Tachypnea
- Thyroid storm: rapid onset with severe hyperthermia, vomiting, diarrhea, severe tachycardia; may advance to delirium, coma, death
- Tremors
- Warm skin
- Weight loss

the production of thyroxine (T_4), triiodothyronine (T_3), and calcitonin. Thyroid-stimulating hormone (TSH) from the anterior pituitary controls the secretion of these hormones.

Etiology And Pathophysiology. Hypothyroidism has two forms: primary and acquired. Primary causes include (1) congenital defects and (2) defective synthesis resulting from an autoimmune process. Acquired causes of hypothyroidism include (1) insufficient stimulation of the gland by the pituitary gland or the hypothalamus and (2) systemic resistance to thyroid hormone.

Clinical Manifestations. The clinical manifestations of hypothyroidism are described in Box 32.6.

Diagnostic Tests. It is also possible to detect hypothyroidism when serum levels of thyroid hormone (T_4 and T_3) are decreased and serum TSH levels are increased (if the defect is in the thyroid) or decreased (if the defect is in the pituitary gland). A screening test for hypothyroidism is mandatory at birth. The screening is performed with a blood sample taken from the baby's heel.

Medical Management. The treatment of choice for congenital and acquired hypothyroidism is oral thyroid hormone replacement therapy. Prompt treatment is especially critical in an infant with congenital hypothyroidism to avoid permanent cognitive impairment.

Nursing Interventions And Patient Teaching. In addition to assisting in detection of the condition and implementation of thyroid hormone replacement therapy, nursing interventions focus on assisting the child and family in compliance with the medical regimen and periodic monitoring of its effects. As the child begins to mature, it is appropriate to place responsibility for treatment with the child.

Prognosis. If hypothyroidism is congenital, it is necessary to start treatment shortly after the patient's birth for

normal physical and intellectual growth to occur. The most significant factor adversely affecting eventual intelligence appears to be inadequate treatment, which in some cases is related to noncompliance with the medical regimen.

Hyperthyroidism

Hyperthyroidism is rare in young children; it affects primarily young adolescents. The most common form of childhood hyperthyroidism is Graves disease.

Etiology And Pathophysiology. Although the exact causal mechanism is unknown, the most accepted theory is an autoimmune process that results in the production of immunoglobulins that have thyroid-stimulating properties.

Clinical Manifestations. The clinical manifestations of hyperthyroidism are described in Box 32.7.

Diagnostic Tests. In addition to clinical manifestations, the diagnosis of hyperthyroidism is based on increased serum levels of T_4, T_3, and radioactive iodine uptake. An ultrasound study of the neck also may assist in determining the presence of nodules or inflammation.

Medical Management. The management of hyperthyroidism aims to decrease the rate of thyroid hormone secretion. To accomplish this, the child receives antithyroid medications, including propylthiouracil and methimazole (Tapazole); subtotal thyroidectomy; or administration of radioactive iodine (iodine-131).

Nursing Interventions And Patient Teaching. Nursing interventions for a child with hyperthyroidism are focused on intervening with the physical manifestations of the disease. Sudden episodes of crying or elation exemplify the emotional lability typical of many affected children. Promote rest and provide a quiet, nonstimulating environment in the initial phase of treatment. To alleviate heat intolerance, the child should be dressed in lightweight clothing, the room temperature should be adjusted, and lightweight blankets should be offered for sleeping comfort. Dietary modifications include increased calories and daily vitamin supplementation. If surgery is recommended, inform the child and family of the nature of the surgery, where the incision will be located, and what to expect postoperatively. Postoperative care includes strict observation of bleeding and complications. The child's neck should be kept slightly flexed and supported to prevent strain on the suture line.

On discharge, make a referral to a public health nurse, school nurse, or home health care nurse to facilitate continuity of care and increase compliance with the medical regimen.

Prognosis. In general, after drug treatment, improvements are noted within the first 2 weeks. In many affected children, complete remission of the disorder follows an initial treatment course of 1 to 2 years. Those who experience relapse sometimes benefit from a second course of medication therapy, but some of them are also candidates for surgical intervention.

Diabetes Mellitus

Diabetes mellitus is a syndrome characterized by a deficiency of insulin that results in alterations in protein, carbohydrate, and fat metabolism. Type 1 diabetes mellitus is the endocrine disorder most frequently diagnosed in children.

The terms currently used for diabetes mellitus are *type 1* and *type 2.* Type 1 was classified previously as insulin-dependent diabetes mellitus and type 2 as non–insulin-dependent diabetes mellitus. These previous classifications could be confusing because the disease name could contradict the actual treatment (some people with type 2 diabetes required insulin).

Type 1 Diabetes. Type 1 diabetes usually begins in childhood or early adulthood, but its onset can occur in adults. Each year, approximately 18,000 cases of type 1 diabetes are diagnosed in young people (American Diabetes Association, 2018). In type 1 diabetes, there is destruction of the pancreatic beta cells that produce insulin, which generally results in total insulin deficiency. In type 1 diabetes, a person with a genetic predisposition who is exposed to a precipitating event, such as a viral infection, experiences autoimmune destruction of the beta cells.

Type 2 Diabetes. In the past, type 2 diabetes was most common in people who were older than 40 years, had a family history of diabetes, and were overweight. Type 2 diabetes results from insulin resistance and the body's improper use of insulin with relative—not absolute—insulin deficiency.

There has been a substantial increase in the number of cases of type 2 diabetes diagnosed in young children. Contributing factors to the rise of type 2 diabetes in children include a low level of physical activity, exposure to diabetes in utero, and an obesity epidemic in the United States. Type 2 diabetes typically is diagnosed in children between the ages of 10 and 19 years, who are obese, who have a strong family history for diabetes, and who have insulin resistance. The rates of children with type 2 diabetes are increasing as the rates of obesity in children are increasing. In 2017, nearly 6000 children were diagnosed with type 2 diabetes (American Diabetes Association 2018).

Prediabetes

Prediabetes is diagnosed when a patient has blood glucose levels above normal but are not quite diagnostic for diabetes. Most people who have type 2 diabetes had prediabetes beforehand. The identification of a prediabetic child is an opportunity to address modifiable risk factors and prevent or delay the onset of type 2 diabetes.

Etiology And Pathophysiology. Hyperglycemia results when there is no insulin or not enough insulin is being secreted from the pancreas. This is due to the inability of glucose to enter the cells without the presence of sufficient amounts of insulin. Carbohydrates, fats, and proteins can only enter nerve cells and vascular tissue cells without the presence of insulin, resulting in damage to these tissues. When glucose levels rise above normal, the renal threshold is exceeded and glucose spills into the urine (glycosuria). When this occurs, glucose attracts water into the bladder, resulting in excessive urination (polyuria). Polyuria leads to dehydration and potential electrolyte imbalances. Dehydration causes excessive thirst (polydipsia).

When glucose does not enter the cells, the body breaks down protein to convert it to glucose in the liver (glucogenesis), again resulting in hyperglycemia. The body breaks down body fat and protein because it cannot use carbohydrates because of the insulin deficiency. The cells' lack of glucose causes excessive hunger (polyphagia). The three cardinal signs of type 1 diabetes are polyuria, polydipsia, and polyphagia.

Ketoacidosis. As discussed above, because glucose cannot be used for energy in diabetics the body breaks down fats for energy. Ketones are the product of fat metabolism and are formed by the fatty acids and glycerol that build up during this process. The ketone bodies are an alternative source of fuel; however, the rate of their use in the cells is limited. The body eliminates excess ketone bodies in the urine (ketonuria) or the lungs (acetone breath). The excessive ketone bodies in the blood (ketonemia) are toxic to the body and create strong acids (hence the term acidosis), thus resulting in ketoacidosis. As the serum pH decreases during acidosis, hyperventilation occurs to help the body eliminate carbon dioxide (acid) from the body. The characteristic Kussmaul respirations (abnormally deep and rapid respirations) are present during ketoacidosis.

Diabetic ketoacidosis is a life-threatening condition. The blood glucose level continues to rise during diabetic ketoacidosis and can reach levels that result in coma and death. The patient is treated in an acute care setting for this disorder. Diabetic ketoacidosis typically happens in type 1 diabetics because the ability to get glucose into the cells is compromised to a greater degree than the type 2 diabetic.

Diagnostic Tests. Diabetes mellitus is diagnosed on the basis of test results, including an 8-hour fasting glucose test, random blood glucose testing, and hemoglobin A_{1C}. Any of these tests may be used to diagnose diabetes. The doctor ordering the test will usually repeat the test on another day before making the diagnosis of diabetes. The normal fasting glucose level for a child is less than 100 mg/dL. A fasting glucose level of 100 to 125 mg/dL is considered prediabetes. If the doctor identifies a fasting level higher than 125 mg/dL accompanied by classic signs of diabetes, such as (1) glycosuria, polyuria, weight loss despite good appetite and (2) manifestations of metabolic acidosis with or without stupor or coma, a diagnosis of diabetes can be made. In the absence of the classic symptoms, the doctor may confirm the suspected diagnosis with a second test, such as a random blood glucose level that is higher than 200 mg/dL. The level of glycosylated hemoglobin (hemoglobin A_{1C}) is another important parameter. Nondiabetic hemoglobin A_{1C} levels are between 4% and 6.5%. A hemoglobin A_{1C} value of 6.5% or higher on two separate tests is indicative of diabetes in children. These tests can be used to identify children with type 1 and type 2 diabetes because both types are characterized by hyperglycemia. Glucosuria may be identified in both types of diabetic patients. The presence of glucose in the urine indicates excessive glucose in the blood, however the absence of glucose in the urine does not indicate a normal blood glucose. For this reason, it is not a good screening tool. If glucosuria is found unexpectedly, bloodwork to screen for diabetes is indicated.

Clinical presentation and additional labs help to differentiate between type 1 and type 2 in children. The presence of obesity is suspicious for type 2 diabetes. The presence of excessive ketones (ketoacids), metabolic acidosis (from excessive ketones in the blood), or specific antibodies points the clinician to a diagnosis of type 1 diabetes.

Medical Management. Medical management of diabetes mellitus in the child is a lifelong commitment to the prescribed regimen. A multidisciplinary approach must involve the family, the child (if appropriate), and a team of professionals that may include a pediatric endocrinologist, a diabetes nurse educator, a dietitian, and an exercise physiologist. Insulin therapy is necessary for the child. There are four types of therapeutic insulin: rapid, short acting, intermediate acting, and long acting. All insulins are prepared

in strengths of 100 U/mL. The dosage of insulin for a child varies according to levels of glucose in the blood. Blood glucose monitoring is discussed in Chapter 23.

The appropriate daily insulin dosage depends on food intake, activity level, and exercise level. Management for children involves various types of insulin and must be determined through a consideration of the child's normal activities, eating schedule, and disease process. Possible insulin regimens may include a twice-daily insulin protocol combining rapid-acting insulin, such as lispro (Humalog), or short-acting insulin, such as regular insulin (e.g., Humulin R or Novolin R), with intermediate-acting insulins, such as Humulin N or Novolin N. The child receives the injections of insulin before breakfast and before dinner. Long-acting insulin therapy may be used alone or in combination with the other categories of insulin. Long-acting insulin is given once a day, usually before bedtime; formulations include glargine (Lantus) and detemir (Levemir). It is necessary to adjust the insulin dosage during growth spurts, periods of increased exercise, illnesses, infections, and surgery.

The insulin pump, which mimics the release of the insulin hormone from the islet cells of the pancreas, is also an option for children. The insulin pump delivers predetermined amounts of insulin continuously, or the dosage can be adjusted to meet the needs for dietary intake, glucose level, or activity. Blood glucose monitoring is necessary throughout the day to ensure that the correct dosage of insulin is being delivered. Education about the pump, as well as follow-up evaluation of the correct use of the pump, is important. The insulin pump comprises a small device that houses the insulin container and that is clipped to a belt or waist of clothing. Tubing attaches the insulin container to a very small needle that is embedded in the subcutaneous tissue and covered with a transparent dressing. The needle typically is changed every 48 hours, and the site of insertion is rotated. The insulin pump often affords better glucose control because repeated injections are not required, and it is not necessary to carry the equipment for injections.

Because the management of diabetes mellitus in children also centers on nutrition and exercise, a dietitian or nutritionist is an important resource person for the child and family. The diet is essentially the same healthy diet that is encouraged for all children, with an emphasis on avoiding foods high in sugars, carbohydrates, and fats. Choosemyplate.gov (www.choosemyp late.gov) is an excellent resource for meal planning. The amount of exercise also effects the food consumption needed and the amount of insulin required to maintain a normal glucose level. Exercise should be encouraged because it helps in lowering blood glucose levels.

Nursing Interventions And Patient Teaching. Nursing interventions for a child with diabetes mellitus should focus on educating the child and the family about the disease and its treatment and possible complications, along with providing emotional support and reassurance. Because the treatment of diabetes mellitus relies on principles of self-management, it is essential that the child and the family understand the disease and its treatment. Encourage the parents and the child to express their questions, fears, and concerns about the disease and its management. Provide emotional support to the child and the family in their adjustment to the disease and provide them with concrete suggestions that will have a positive effect on their attitudes about diabetes mellitus and its management.

It is important that the child and family receive instruction about meal planning from a nutritionist and for the nurse to reinforce these instructions. The child and family need to be educated about the action of insulin, including the onset, peak, and duration of action, as well as about manifestations of hyperglycemia and hypoglycemia. They must also be aware of how to recognize manifestations of diabetic ketoacidosis. Instruct the child and the family in the proper techniques of insulin injections or use of the insulin pump. They should be taught to develop a rotation pattern if insulin injections are administered daily so that they do not give injections repeatedly in the same sites. Teach the parents and the child the principles and techniques of home glucose monitoring (see the Health Promotion box).

Prognosis. Advancements in diabetes treatment have improved the prognosis of patients living with diabetes and have decreased the risk of long-term complications. This improved outlook is highly dependent on the compliance of the patient with the prescribed long-term treatment plan. Diabetes mellitus affects the vasculature of all organs, especially those of the eyes, kidneys, and heart. Diabetic retinopathy, renal failure, and heart disease are complications of diabetes mellitus that may result but are less likely to have a major effect if diabetes is well

---

⍗ Health Promotion

Child With Diabetes Mellitus

- Blood glucose self-monitoring has improved diabetes management and is used successfully by children from the onset of their diabetes. By testing their own blood, children and parents can adjust the insulin regimen to maintain the blood glucose level. The normal range in children is 70–99 mg/dL. Diabetes management depends to a great extent on self-monitoring.
- Essentially, the nutritional needs of children with diabetes are no different from those of unaffected children. Children with diabetes require no special foods or supplements. They need sufficient calories to balance daily expenditure for energy and to satisfy the requirement for growth and development. They also need consistent intake and timing of food.
- There is no one diet for diabetes. General guidelines exist, such as to eat less fat and saturated fat and to eat more whole grains, fruits, and vegetables. Sugars and sweets, or simple sugars, do not raise blood glucose any more quickly than do starches, or "complex carbohydrates." Healthy nutrition advice is to eat sugars and sweets in moderation. It is important to base diabetes meal plans on individual needs and develop them with expert assistance from a registered dietitian.
- Exercise should be encouraged and never restricted unless other health conditions indicate the need to do so. It is part of diabetes management, and planning it around the child's interests and capabilities is important. However, in most instances, children's activities are not rigidly scheduled. Parents should compensate for the inevitable decreases in the blood glucose level by providing extra snacks before (and, if prolonged, during) the activity. Besides providing a feeling of well-being, regular exercise aids in the body's use of food and often decreases insulin requirements.
- Even a child with well-controlled diabetes typically experiences occasional mild symptoms of hypoglycemia, but if the child and caretakers recognize the signs and symptoms early and relieve them promptly with appropriate therapy, it is not usually necessary to interrupt the child's activity for more than a few minutes.
- Families need to understand the treatment method and the insulin prescribed, including the effective duration, onset, and peak action. They also need to know the characteristics of the various types of insulin and the proper mixing of insulin. The amount of time that insulin is considered acceptable to use once opened is dependent on the type of insulin and whether it is stored at room temperature or refrigerated. The manufacturer's guidelines for each type of insulin should be followed.
- Insulin must never be stored at very cold (<36°F [2.2°C]) or very hot (>86°F [30°C]) temperatures. Extreme temperatures destroy insulin.
- The site selected for insulin injection may depend on who administers the insulin. The upper arms, the thighs, the hips, and the abdomen are usual injection sites for insulin. The child can reach the thighs, the abdomen, and part of the hip and arm easily, but sometimes help is needed to inject other sites. For example, a parent can pinch a loose fold of skin on the arm while the child injects the insulin.
- Some children are candidates for continuous subcutaneous insulin infusion with a portable insulin pump. The health care provider teaches the child and the parents to operate the device, including the mechanics of the pump, battery changes, and alarm systems. They learn how to load the syringe, insert the catheter, adjust the insulin flow for routine needs and for illnesses, and connect and disconnect the catheter. Nurses should become familiar with the operation of the specific device that their facility uses and the protocol of the regimen.
- Self-management techniques that the child and the family need to master are the testing of blood, administration of insulin, and adjustment of insulin and diet with alterations in day-to-day activities and unusual occurrences.

controlled (National Institute of Diabetes and Digestive and Kidney Diseases [NIDDK], 2017).

DISORDERS OF MUSCULOSKELETAL FUNCTION

Musculoskeletal problems in childhood are common and are a result of genetics, rapid growth, or the child's natural tendency to engage in active mobility. Many musculoskeletal conditions are temporary, and normal function ultimately returns.

Developmental Dysplasia of the Hip

Etiology And Pathophysiology. Developmental dysplasia of the hip (DDH) is a developmental abnormality of the femoral head, the acetabulum, or both. The abnormality has familial tendencies and is more prominent in girls. DDH is associated with such conditions as first pregnancy, spina bifida, and breech presentation. The defining characteristic of subluxation of the hip is incorrect position, or partial dislocation, of the femoral head in the acetabulum. Subluxation is the degree of DDH most common in infants. In dislocation, the femoral head has no contact with the acetabulum.

Clinical Manifestations. In affected infants, the femur on the affected side is shortened; thigh and gluteal folds are uneven (or increased on the affected side) when the infant is placed in the prone position, and abduction of the hip on the affected side is limited (Fig. 32.21). In children who are able to stand and walk, the affected leg is shorter than the other, and they demonstrate a waddling gait or limping.

Diagnostic Tests. Early diagnosis of DDH in the newborn tends to enhance the success of treatment and minimize complications. Nursing assessment of the previously listed manifestations alerts the health care provider to the possibility of DDH. Physical assessment by the health care provider reveals an audible clunking sound when the hips are manually manipulated. In addition, radiographic examination is sometimes helpful in establishing the diagnosis.

Medical Management. Once DDH is diagnosed, treatment begins immediately. Any delay in treatment is likely to result in worsening of the deformity and a poorer prognosis. Treatment depends on the severity of the dysplasia and the age of the infant. Treatment for infants younger than 6 months consists of positioning the head of the femur within the acetabulum and maintaining the hip in abduction for 4 to 6 months with the use of a Pavlik harness (Fig. 32.22). Once this therapy achieves abduction, a hip spica cast maintains positioning for several months until the hip is stable. Treatment for a child with DDH between the ages of 6 and 24 months may require manipulation of the head of the femur into the socket while the child is under anesthesia. Surgical open reduction is necessary in some cases if soft tissue obstructs the head of the femur from entering the acetabulum. Immobilization

in a hip spica cast follows open reduction. The management of affected children older than 24 months is more extensive because adaptive changes have taken place. Open surgical reduction, osteotomy, and arthroplasty are sometimes necessary. A hip spica cast is necessary after these procedures.

Nursing Interventions And Patient Teaching. Nurses play an important role in identifying signs of DDH and other congenital defects in newborns, and the earlier the defect is identified and treated, the better is the chance for a favorable outcome. The primary goals in caring for a child in a corrective device or cast are to maintain the position of the hip joint, prevent complications, and provide the stimulation necessary for the developing infant or child. As early as possible, involve parents in caring for their baby to build confidence in their ability to provide care at home. Box 32.8 provides general guidelines for the nursing interventions for a child in a corrective device or cast.

Parents and all other caregivers need to understand that children in corrective devices need involvement in all the activities of any child in the same age group. They must not confine the child or exclude the child from family activities.

Prognosis. With early treatment, the prognosis is more favorable for the restoration of normal body function. It is essential that parents make follow-up visits to ensure that treatment is effective. These visits are necessary until the child's growth is complete.

Legg-Calvé-Perthes Disease (Coxa Plana)

Etiology And Pathophysiology. Legg-Calvé-Perthes disease (coxa plana) is a disorder caused by decreased blood supply to the femoral head, which results in epiphyseal necrosis and degeneration of the femoral head, followed by regeneration or calcification. It occurs more often in boys and affects children from 4 to 10 years of age. The cause of the disorder is unknown, and the disease process itself is self-limited. The blood supply usually is restored, and new cells replace the necrotic bone. This entire process may take 2 to 3 years.

Clinical Manifestations. Signs and symptoms are usually insidious. Affected children usually complain of pain, exhibit a limp on the affected side, and have limited range of motion (ROM). The disease in the affected hip causes the leg to be shorter than that on the unaffected side. The condition is aggravated by activity and improves with rest. Knee pain, thigh and groin pain, hip stiffness, and muscle atrophy in the thigh are also common.

Diagnostic Tests. The presence of the common signs raises the suspicion of Legg-Calvé-Perthes disease. Radiographic examination helps confirm the diagnosis. MRI is sometimes necessary if the diagnosis cannot be determined from clinical manifestations and radiographs.

Fig. 32.21 Signs of congenital dislocation of the hip. (A) Asymmetry of gluteal and thigh folds. (B) Limited hip abduction, as seen in flexion. (C) Apparent shortening of femur, as indicated by level of knees in flexion. (D) Ortolani's click (if infant is younger than 4 weeks). (E) Positive Trendelenburg sign or gait (if child is weight bearing).

Fig. 32.22 Child in Pavlik harness. (From Ashwill JW, Droske SC: *Nursing care of children: Principles and practice*, ed 3, Philadelphia, 2007, Saunders.)

Medical Management. The goal of treatment is to maintain the head of the femur within the acetabulum so that the femoral head will preserve its normal shape as it

Box 32.8	**Care of a Child in a Cast or Corrective Device**

- Perform neurovascular assessment of the five *P*s (impairments to be reported immediately): *p*ain, *p*allor or cyanosis, *p*aresthesia (numbing or tingling, decrease in sensation), *p*ulselessness, and *p*uffiness.
- Monitor skin frequently for erythema or tenderness.
- Wash and dry skin at least daily.
- Smooth or pad a sharp cast or brace edges with gauze or adhesive tape.
- Teach the family cast or brace maintenance and cleaning.
- Assess circular dressings for excessive tightness.
- Stimulate circulation with gentle massage over pressure areas.

regenerates. If this effort is successful, full ROM can be maintained. Bracing may help keep the head of the femur contained within the acetabulum. Physical therapy and ROM exercises, along with antiinflammatory medications, help prevent joint stiffness and pain. Activities such as running may be limited, and nighttime traction may be used to prevent the head of the femur from becoming displaced. Bed rest is necessary only to treat bouts of severe pain. Surgical procedures are required only if all other treatments are ineffective.

Nursing Interventions And Patient Teaching. While the child is in traction or in casts, braces, or harnesses, skin care and neurovascular assessment are essential. Box 32.8 details care of the child in a cast or corrective device. Appropriate education of the family and child includes purpose, function, application, and care of the corrective device. Correct use of the corrective device is vital for the long-term success of treatment. It is important that the child and parents understand how to use the device properly.

Prognosis. With patient compliance and early diagnosis, the prognosis is excellent. Legg-Calvé-Perthes disease is self-limiting, and early, efficient treatment and the age at onset are important factors in a positive outcome. If the diagnosis is made after the age of 6, the child is at higher risk for a hip deformity and osteoarthritis in later years.

Scoliosis

Etiology And Pathophysiology. The most common skeletal deformity of adolescence is scoliosis. The condition is a lateral curvature of the spine that causes changes in the shapes of the spine, the chest, and the hips. Severe curvature has the potential to affect cardiopulmonary and neurologic function and result in a negative self-image. Scoliosis can occur at any age but is most common in adolescent girls.

Clinical Manifestations. A child with idiopathic scoliosis has unequal hip heights and shoulder heights, scapular and rib prominence, and a posterior rib hump that is visible when the child bends forward at the waist.

Diagnostic Tests. Early identification and treatment of scoliosis are vital for a good prognosis. Routine screening of children from 10 to 15 years of age involves posterior observation of the undressed child (bending forward at the waist with arms and head hanging downward) for curvature, asymmetry, and rib hump. Radiographs confirm the diagnosis. If the health care provider suspects an underlying cause for the scoliosis, such as a tumor, he or she orders additional tests, including MRI, CT, and bone scan.

Medical Management. Curvatures of less than 20 degrees necessitate no treatment. Treatment for moderate curvatures consists of bracing, which potentially slows the progression of scoliosis until the spine is mature. Two types of braces are used to treat scoliosis: the Milwaukee brace and the thoracolumbosacral orthotic (TLSO) brace. The TLSO brace is used most commonly. It fits under the arm and is shaped to conform to the body (Fig. 32.23). The Milwaukee brace covers the entire torso and has a ring that encircles the neck with rests for the chin and the back of the head. This brace typically is used only if the TLSO brace is not effective. Surgical intervention is indicated in severe scoliosis or scoliosis that does not respond to bracing. Surgery consists of spinal fusion and the insertion of a stabilizing rod such as a Harrington rod or an L-rod.

Nursing Interventions And Patient Teaching. Many adolescents who must wear casts or braces have difficulty complying with the treatment plan. Developmentally, adolescents are trying to fit in with peers by conforming to peer norms and need plenty of reassurance to feel attractive and worthwhile during treatment. Instruction on maintaining skin integrity is essential for adolescents in a brace or cast. Box 32.8 outlines care for the child in a corrective device or cast.

Provide proper instruction to the child and the parents regarding the appliance, the anticipated results, and the desired goal.

Prognosis. Treatment for scoliosis is a lengthy process, inasmuch as it occurs during a major growth period of the child. The prognosis depends on the severity of the condition and compliance with the prescribed treatment. Information and techniques for providing emotional support of the patient are available from the National Scoliosis Foundation (www.scoliosis.org).

Talipes Equinovarus (Clubfoot)

Etiology And Pathophysiology. Talipes equinovarus is the most common congenital deformity of the foot and ankle. The incidence is 1 per 1000 live births and is twice as high among boys as among girls. The cause of talipes equinovarus is not known, but theories point to an inherited or environmental disorder. The incidence of talipes equinovarus is significantly higher in families that already have a child with the defect and in Hawaiians and Maoris (Sheth, 2021).

Clinical Manifestations. Talipes equinovarus varies in severity. It most commonly involves one foot but may involve both feet. In talipes equinovarus, the foot is pointed downward and inward (Fig. 32.24). The muscles of the affected calf and foot may be smaller and shorter than normal.

Fig. 32.23 Braces for idiopathic scoliosis. (A) Standard thoracolumbosacral orthotic (TLSO) brace. Note the color and design incorporated into the brace to make it more acceptable to children and adolescents. (B) Variation of a standard TLSO brace that fastens in the back (C) to provide needed support for the spine curvature. (From Hockenberry MJ, Wilson D: *Wong's essentials of pediatric nursing*, ed 9, St. Louis, 2013, Mosby.)

Fig. 32.24 Bilateral congenital talipes equinovarus (congenital clubfoot) in a 2-month-old infant. (From Zitelli BJ, McIntire SC, Davis HW: *Zitelli and Davis' atlas of pediatric physical diagnosis*, ed 6, St. Louis, 2012, Saunders.)

Fig. 32.25 Casting of feet for correction of bilateral congenital talipes equinovarus. (From Perry S, Hockenberry M, Lowdermilk D, et al: *Maternal-child nursing care*, ed 3, St. Louis, 2007, Mosby.)

Diagnostic Tests. Talipes equinovarus is evident at birth, and examination, manipulation, and radiographs are used to make the diagnosis.

Medical Management. Treatment of talipes equinovarus consists of manipulation and the application of a series of short leg casts (Fig. 32.25). The earlier the treatment begins, the more favorable the outcome, and serial casting typically begins shortly after birth. The health care provider gently manipulates the foot into a more normal position and then applies a cast to maintain the correction. The health care provider changes the cast weekly to allow for further manipulation and to accommodate the rapidly growing infant. The manipulation and the application of casts continues until marked overcorrection is reached. After completion of the casting series and correction of the deformity, the foot (or feet) undergo a combination of passive stretching exercises and corrective splints or shoes to prevent the deformity from recurring. The child usually must wear a brace or corrective shoes, depending on the surgeon's preference, for several years.

In severe cases, casting may not successfully correct the deformity, and surgical intervention is required. A minor surgical procedure, called a *tenotomy*, is the surgical release of the Achilles tendon. The tenotomy, followed by additional serial casting, may be all the surgery that is required. More extensive surgery involves the repositioning of the anterior tibial tendon.

Nursing Interventions And Patient Teaching. After the diagnosis of talipes equinovarus, parents need emotional support and education. Very often, parents need time to adjust to the distressing fact that their child has a deformity. Educate parents while encouraging them to express their feelings and concerns. Nursing care for an infant with casts is the same for any child in a cast (see Box 32.8). Many affected newborns receive the cast before discharge from the hospital. Keeping casts clean and dry is relatively easy with a small infant. The parents should be taught to inspect casts carefully for rough edges, which will irritate newborn skin. They should observe the toes

frequently for coldness, pain, blueness, or edema, which, if present, must be reported to the health care provider immediately. Casts are cumbersome and heavy. Assist the parents to find comfortable positions for feeding, playing, and cuddling. Sponge baths are necessary until the infant no longer needs casting. Casts also tend to hinder the infant's ability to kick, move the legs, and roll over. During this time of limited activity, suggest that parents provide audio, visual, and tactile stimulation to encourage normal development. Treatment and follow-up care usually take place on an outpatient basis.

Nursing responsibilities include the teaching of passive stretching exercises with a return demonstration by the parent, if parent participation is part of the treatment plan. Teach parents about cast care and how to handle the infant. Instruct them to perform stretching exercises several times a day; many parents find it easier to remember to perform the exercises if they do them together with another regular activity such as diaper changing or after feedings.

Prognosis. Some feet respond to treatment rapidly; some respond only to prolonged, vigorous, and sustained efforts; and the improvement in others remains disappointing even with maximal effort on the part of all concerned. Serial casting achieves the most reliable correction of talipes equinovarus. If surgical intervention is required, scar tissue can result in long-term pain and stiffness.

Duchenne Muscular Dystrophy

Etiology And Pathophysiology. Duchenne muscular dystrophy (DMD) is a sex-linked inherited disorder whose defining characteristic is gradually progressive skeletal muscle wasting and weakness. The pattern of inheritance is such that primarily only males are affected. Women, however, can be carriers of the gene. DMD is the most severe and most common form of all dystrophies. The onset of signs and symptoms typically occurs between ages 2 and 4 years.

Clinical Manifestations. Initial signs and symptoms, which are mild and progress gradually, are easy to overlook. Parents tend to be the first to notice that the child is clumsy, frequently falls, has a waddling gait, and experiences difficulty running, climbing, and riding a bicycle. The muscles of the pelvic girdle are frequently involved, and the child shows evidence of this weakness by rising from the floor in a classic manner: The child lies on the side and flexes the knees (or gets on all fours), then extends the knees and uses the hands to "walk up" the thighs (Gowers sign). As the disorder progresses, there is severe muscle wasting, which results in contractures and deformities. By 12 years of age, ambulation may no longer be possible. Respiratory tract infection usually occurs in the final stages, when the diaphragm and the accessory muscles used in respiration become affected.

Diagnostic Tests. The health care provider considers the possibility of DMD based on the clinical signs and symptoms and the family history. Electromyography, elevated levels of serum creatine kinase and aspartate aminotransferase, and muscle biopsy that reveals fibrous and fatty tissue confirm the diagnosis. Because of the frequent cardiac complications, the American Academy of Pediatrics recommends that the patient undergo a complete cardiac evaluation early in childhood and then undergo annual follow-up at the age of 10 years and on.

Medical Management. There is no effective treatment to arrest DMD. Therefore, the goals are to maintain ambulation and independence for as long as possible. Physical therapy serves to optimize ROM and to delay muscle atrophy; braces sometimes help provide additional support; and surgical intervention to release muscle contractures is another element of management.

Nursing Interventions And Patient Teaching. The most important nursing consideration in the care of a child with DMD is to assist the child and the family in developing positive coping strategies to deal with the progressively debilitating aspects of the illness. The goal is to maintain independence for as long as possible. Because of the progressive nature of the illness, assess the child's capabilities frequently. The care of a child with DMD, or any child with a chronic, debilitating terminal illness, is extremely demanding and stressful for the family. Help the family lessen their anxiety and fears through teaching and active listening. The family also needs assistance with anticipatory grieving. A referral to the Muscular Dystrophy Association of America opens the door to many supplementary services to patients and their families.

Help the family plan an exercise program to encourage muscle strength and delay the onset of some of the physical disabilities. Counsel the family about good nutrition to prevent obesity, which sometimes causes affected children to become prematurely wheelchair bound.

Prognosis. As the condition progresses, cardiomyopathy, congestive heart failure, and scoliosis are noted with increasing frequency. Affected children rarely live past age 20; death results from respiratory or cardiac complications.

Septic Arthritis (Septic Joint, Suppurative Arthritis)
Etiology And Pathophysiology. Septic arthritis (septic joint, suppurative arthritis) is an infection of a joint, which possibly arises from bacteria in the blood or as a direct extension of an existing infection such as osteomyelitis. Potential causes include ear infections, bites (human, cat, dog, rat, or tick), infected wounds, and open fractures. The infection causes joint irritation and damage to the synovial membrane; synovial fluid increases and causes distention within the joint. As the infection progresses, pus accumulates and breaks down the articulating cartilage (which does not have the capacity to regenerate) and leads to permanent damage. In infancy, the incidence of septic arthritis is equal among boys and girls; in the adolescent age group, it occurs predominantly in boys. The joints most commonly affected are the hip, knee, shoulder, wrist, and ankle. Streptococci and staphylococcus are the most common bacteria. In rare cases, fungal and viral infections may be the culprits.

Clinical Manifestations. The affected joint is erythematous, edematous, warm, and excruciatingly painful. The temperature of the joint also is elevated. ROM usually is limited. The child maintains the affected extremities in a flexed position. If the lower extremities are involved, the child often limps or refuses to walk. Except in infants, fever is usually present. The onset of septic arthritis is very rapid, and the condition is considered a medical emergency.

Diagnostic Tests. Radiographic examination may reveal joint edema. The health care provider aspirates the synovial fluid and sends purulent matter for Gram stain examination and culture. A blood culture is necessary. Serologic testing reveals leukocytosis and elevated erythrocyte sedimentation rate in children; infants do not always demonstrate these findings.

Medical Management. Joint aspiration and surgical irrigation are essential for managing the condition. Surgical drainage and irrigation ensure that the joint is decompressed, safeguard the vasculature, clear the joint of destructive purulent matter, eradicate the infection, and prevent secondary bloodborne spread of infection. The health care provider initiates broad-spectrum IV antibiotic therapy and switches it to more specific antibiotics once the laboratory has identified the organism. IV therapy continues for 10 to 14 days; once the IV response is good, the regimen can change to oral antibiotics. Oral therapy continues to complete a 4-week course. Additional pharmacologic interventions may include antipyretics and analgesics.

Nursing Interventions. Because of the lengthy pharmacologic therapies, parents need education concerning the importance of compliance with the regimen. Discuss which signs and symptoms of medication side effects to report. Range-of-motion exercises to maintain joint strength and flexibility are included in the regimen.

Prognosis. The prompt management of this condition is paramount for a successful outcome. Left untreated, the condition may result in permanent damage and destruction of the joint and adjacent structures. Involvement of the hip joint—where avascular necrosis can develop and cause deformity—may result in long-term disability.

Fractures

Although any bone can be fractured, the most common fracture sites in children are the long bones of the extremities, the clavicles, the wrists, the fingers, and the skull. Fractures vary from complete (bone and periosteum separate completely) to incomplete or greenstick (the bone splits but does not completely break). Spiral fractures affect the length rather than the width of the bone and are frequently the result of child abuse.

Clinical Manifestations. A bone fracture usually manifests with deformity, loss of normal function, and swelling. Pain and tenderness are also often present.

Diagnostic Tests. Physical assessment of the affected area helps provide an initial diagnosis. The diagnosis ultimately is confirmed with radiographic studies. Fractures that protrude through the skin (open or compound) also are evaluated with serologic testing, including a CBC and probably subsequent culture and sensitivity testing to detect the possibility of infection.

Medical Management. Upon confirmation of the fracture, the treatment includes realignment of the bones. This may be done in either a closed or open reduction. The closed reduction entails the external manipulation of the bones to return to a point of normal alignment, after which casting is performed to maintain this positioning. An open reduction requires surgical intervention to realign the bones. Pins, wires, plates, and screws are devices used to secure the bone fragments and maintain alignment to allow for healing. The open reduction may be followed by casting or traction. Pharmacologic therapies may include analgesic or antiinflammatory medications. Open fractures necessitate prophylactic antibiotic therapy.

Nursing Interventions. Evaluating a possible traumatic injury involves assessment of the injury and soft tissue damage. The affected area is assessed for pain and point of tenderness, color, sensation, motion, and pulses distal to the injury. Limitations in function also should be noted. If the child is upset, it is necessary to calm and reassure the child and the parents.

Assist in care of the child as the health care provider realigns the extremity. If the injury necessitates casting, specific nursing measures are instituted. Assess pain and administer comfort measures and analgesics as prescribed. After alignment, nursing interventions include maintaining skin integrity and monitoring

skeletal traction sites, as applicable, for infection. Observe for complications of immobility, especially circulatory compromise and muscle spasms. Patients undergoing surgical management for a fracture require routine postoperative care interventions.

Prognosis. Most fractures in children heal without incidence. Complications, although rare, include nonunion of the bones (bones do not heal together at the site of the fracture) and osteomyelitis (infection within the bone).

DISORDERS OF NEUROLOGIC FUNCTION

Disorders that affect neurologic function belong to three major categories: (1) increased intracranial pressure, (2) hypoxia, and (3) seizure activity. The residual effects of neurologic disorders often have profound effects on the child's function and future performance. It is essential to identify neurologic impairments at an early stage so that they can be diagnosed properly and interventions can be instituted.

Meningitis

Meningitis is a significant cause of illness in the pediatric age group. Meningitis is an infection of the meninges (protective covering of the brain). Most cases affect children younger than 5 years. Its importance lies primarily in the frequency with which it occurs in infancy and childhood and the unnecessarily high death rates and residual damage caused by undiagnosed and untreated or inadequately treated cases.

Etiology And Pathophysiology. Although many bacterial, viral, and fungal organisms have the capacity to cause meningitis, bacterial meningitis is the most common. The advent of antimicrobial therapy has had a marked effect on the course and prognosis of bacterial meningitis, although the use of Hib vaccine, beginning in 1990, led to the most dramatic decrease in bacterial meningitis caused by *H. influenzae*. Bacterial meningitis caused by other organisms remains a serious illness in children. Organisms generally spread to the meninges after an upper respiratory infection, by lymphatic drainage, or by direct deposit through a lumbar puncture or skull fracture. After it invades the meninges, the organism enters the CSF and travels throughout the subarachnoid space, spreading the infection. As the meninges become infected, an inflammatory process ensues, causing a thick exudate and WBC accumulation. With continued inflammation, CSF flow becomes occluded, and the brain becomes hyperemic (increased blood to a part) and edematous.

Clinical Manifestations. Meningitis manifests sometimes insidiously and sometimes suddenly, beginning with fever, vomiting, headache, irritability, photophobia, and **nuchal rigidity** (pain and stiffness in the neck when flexed) or opisthotonos (arched back); level of consciousness may decrease, and seizures may occur. Affected infants typically exhibit a bulging fontanelle and a characteristic high-pitched cry. Classic signs of meningeal irritation include a positive *Kernig sign* (resistance to knee extension in the supine position with the hips and knees flexed against the torso) and a positive *Brudzinski sign* (flexion of the knees and hips when the neck is flexed rapidly onto the chest). Meningococcal meningitis, the most readily transmissible type of meningitis, sometimes also produces petechiae and rapidly progresses to death if proper treatment is not initiated promptly.

Diagnostic Tests. The diagnosis of meningitis is based on a carefully documented history, results of a physical examination, and analysis of CSF obtained by a lumbar puncture. CSF culture and sensitivity testing that shows an elevated WBC count, elevated protein level, and decreased glucose level indicates a bacterial infection. If signs of increased intracranial pressure (papilledema, neurologic deficits, and a bulging fontanelle) are present, a lumbar puncture is contraindicated because of the risk of brainstem herniation. CT or MRI also is used to assess the level of meningeal irritation.

Medical Management. The management of bacterial meningitis involves immediate IV administration of appropriate antibiotic therapy. Therapy continues for at least 10 days or until the CSF culture result is negative. Intensive care often is employed until the antibiotic therapy has been under way for at least 24 hours.

If seizures occur, antiseizure medications are ordered. The choice of antibiotic is based on the known sensitivity of the pathogen. Appropriate hydration, antipyretics, and comfort measures are important aspects of management. Closely observe the child for complications of meningitis, including seizures, disseminated intravascular coagulation syndrome, and shock. After discharge, the health care provider monitors the child closely to assess for any sequelae of the disease, such as hearing impairments and cognitive, perceptual, language, and behavioral problems.

Nursing Interventions And Patient Teaching. Initial nursing interventions focus on rapid identification of a child with meningitis and prompt institution of appropriate antibiotic therapy. Take all necessary isolation precautions to prevent the spread of the disease.

Promote rest for the child in the initial phase of the disease and minimize environmental stimuli (especially noise and bright lights). Institute safety measures because the child may develop seizures. The child is likely to be most comfortable without a pillow and with the head of the bed elevated. Observe vital signs, level of consciousness, I&O, and neurologic signs at frequent intervals. Provide emotional support to families throughout the course of the disease; they are usually unprepared for the sudden acuteness of the disease and may feel guilty for not recognizing it earlier.

Prevention. The spread of bacterial meningitis can be avoided in the exposed siblings by administration of prophylactic rifampin. Primary prevention strategies consist of vaccine administration.

Meningococcal polysaccharide (Menomune) and quadrivalent meningococcal conjugate (Menactra) are two available vaccines in the United States to immunize children against meningitis. The choice of vaccine is based on the patient's age. The mortality rate associated with bacterial meningitis is high, but early immunization can spare families from experiencing the tragic death or disability of a child from this disease. The nurse plays a significant role in educating families regarding preventive measures.

Prognosis. Although antimicrobial therapy often has a significant effect on the course of illness, meningitis remains a potentially life-threatening disease. The age of the child, the type of causative organism, the severity of the infection, the duration of the illness before the onset of therapy, and the sensitivity of the organism to antimicrobial drugs are important factors in the prognosis. Residual deficits are possible; these include communicating hydrocephalus and possible hearing loss, blindness, seizures, learning disorders, and attention-deficit disorder.

Encephalitis

Encephalitis is defined as an inflammation of the CNS: namely the brain tissue and the spinal cord. The course of the disease closely resembles that of meningitis and the care for each is similar.

Etiology And Pathophysiology. Encephalitis is a rare condition and its cause is varied. A variety of organisms have the capacity to cause encephalitis, such as bacteria, spirochetes, fungi, protozoa, and viruses. Most cases of encephalitis occur as a result of direct invasion of the CNS by a virus or from postinfectious involvement after a viral illness, such as measles, mumps, or varicella. Other factors that may result in encephalitis include contact with infected respiratory secretions and insect bites (National Library of Medicine [NLM], 2020b).

Clinical Manifestations. An upper respiratory tract infection or GI infection may precede the onset of symptoms. The onset of encephalitis may be gradual or sudden, and manifestations may include malaise, fever, headache, dizziness, nuchal rigidity, nausea, vomiting, ataxia, tremors, seizures, and coma.

Diagnostic Tests. The diagnosis of encephalitis is based on clinical manifestations associated with the disease and, if possible, identification of the virus. Laboratory detection of the virus is possible through serologic tests or CSF cultures. MRI and CT also are performed to assess inflammation.

Medical Management. A child suspected of having encephalitis is hospitalized promptly for strict observation and supportive care. Treatment is primarily supportive, focusing on controlling fever, ensuring adequate hydration and nutrition, monitoring vital signs, and observing for complications. Pharmacologic therapies include organism-specific antibiotics or antiviral medications. Corticosteroids such as dexamethasone are prescribed to reduce brain inflammation. In addition, antiseizure and antipyretic agents may be prescribed. Analgesics are used with extreme caution because they may mask neurologic changes.

Nursing Interventions And Patient Teaching. Nursing interventions for children with encephalitis are the same as those for children with meningitis. The major focus of care is on administering medication, controlling fever, monitoring neurologic status and vital signs, and providing emotional support to the child and the family.

Follow-up care with periodic reevaluation and rehabilitation is important for survivors with residual effects of the disease. Encourage the parents to keep appointments for follow-up examinations.

Prognosis. The prognosis depends on the child's age, the type of organism, and any residual neurologic damage. Children younger than 2 years of age sometimes exhibit increased neurologic disability, including learning disabilities and seizure disorders. In severe cases, encephalitis may lead to death.

Hydrocephalus

Hydrocephalus is a condition whose defining characteristic is an excess of fluid within the cranial vault, the subarachnoid space, or both. It is caused by an imbalance between the production and the absorption of CSF within the ventricular system. Hydrocephalus can develop during infancy (as a congenital lesion) and throughout life.

Etiology And Pathophysiology. Hydrocephalus is caused by increased production of CSF, by obstruction within the ventricular system (noncommunicating hydrocephalus:

no passage of fluid between the ventricles), or by defective reabsorption of the CSF (communicating hydrocephalus: passage of CSF between the ventricles). Overproduction of CSF results most commonly from a tumor in the choroid plexus. Obstruction within the ventricular system is caused most frequently by atresia (the absence of a normal body opening, duct, or canal), most commonly along the aqueduct of Sylvius (Fig. 32.26). Other causes of obstruction include a hemorrhage, a growing tumor, or an infection. Defects in the body's reabsorptive process are sometimes caused by an extensive hemorrhage within the subarachnoid space, which obscures the absorptive surface of the membrane.

As CSF accumulates within the cranium, the brain is compressed against the skull, and the ventricular vessels become dilated, which increases intracranial pressure (see Fig. 32.26). If hydrocephalus occurs before the fusion of the cranial sutures, the skull becomes markedly enlarged.

Clinical Manifestations. In early infancy, manifestations of hydrocephalus include widening and bulging of the fontanelles, separation of the cranial sutures, dilation of scalp veins, thin and shiny scalp, and rapidly increasing head circumference. As CSF accumulation continues, frontal bossing (prominence of the forehead) becomes apparent. Other manifestations are depression of eyes with setting sun sign (sclera is seen above the iris), slow pupil response to light, irritability, high-pitched cry, difficulty in being consoled, lethargy, altered level of consciousness, and difficulty in sucking and feeding. In children, manifestations may include headache on awakening, hyperactive reflexes, strabismus, unsteady gait, irritability, papilledema (edema of the optic disk), lethargy, disorientation, and progression to stupor.

Diagnostic Tests. In infants, measurement of the head circumference is the most important diagnostic technique. It is important to measure the head circumference routinely in all infants. Any measurement that crosses one or more

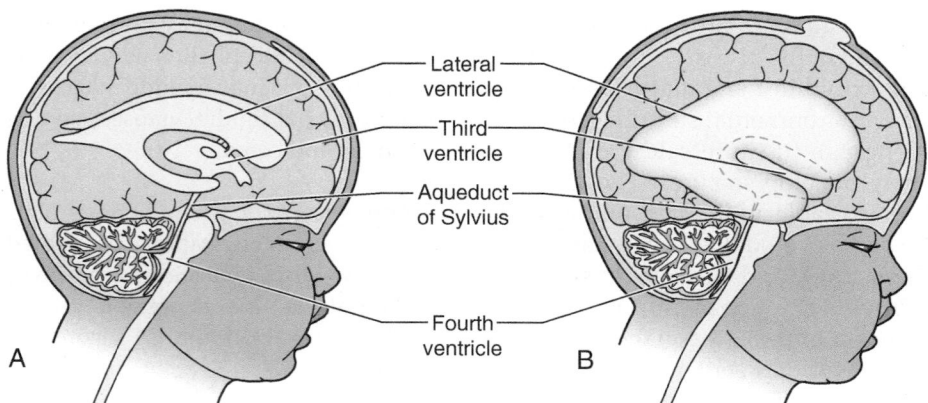

Fig. 32.26 Appearance of the brain with normal cerebrospinal fluid flow and in hydrocephalus. (A) Normal: patent cerebrospinal fluid circulation. (B) Hydrocephalus: enlargement of lateral and third ventricles, caused by obstruction of cerebral spinal fluid circulation at the aqueduct of Sylvius.

Fig. 32.27 Ventriculoperitoneal shunt placement. Catheter is threaded subcutaneously from small incisions at the sites of ventricular and peritoneal insertions.

grid lines on the growth chart within a 2- to 4-week period is suggestive of hydrocephalus. Other diagnostic assessments include observation of neurologic signs that indicate the possibility of increased intracranial pressure, CT, and MRI.

Medical Management. Treatment of hydrocephalus is aimed at relieving the pressure on the ventricles and correcting the cause of the ventriculomegaly. Complications that occur as a result of the hydrocephalus must be identified and treated. If a tumor is the cause of hydrocephalus, the surgeon removes it. If the cause of the hydrocephalus is obstruction, the treatment involves surgical diversion of excess CSF from the ventricles to the peritoneum with a ventriculoperitoneal shunt (Fig. 32.27). Revisions in the ventriculoperitoneal shunt are needed when the shunt malfunctions, becomes infected, or becomes too short as the child grows.

Nursing Interventions. Nursing interventions for a child with hydrocephalus involve assisting with prompt diagnosis, observing for complications of the disease and shunt placement, and providing emotional support and education to the family. Nutrition is likely to become an issue if intracranial pressure increases. The child should not be handled before, during, and after feedings because handling sometimes leads to vomiting. Small, frequent feedings are usually better tolerated, and it is best to place infants on their sides after feedings to avoid aspiration. After the child's surgery, observe the child for signs of increasing intracranial pressure, assess vital signs, and closely monitor I&O. Usually the child is placed on the nonoperative side to avoid putting pressure on the shunt site. Perform meticulous skin care, especially to the scalp, preoperatively and postoperatively. A sheepskin pad should be placed under the child's head, and the child's position should be changed every 2 hours. Provide emotional support to the family during the hospitalization and prepare them for discharge.

Patient problems and interventions for a child with hydrocephalus include but are not limited to the following:

PATIENT PROBLEM	NURSING INTERVENTIONS
Potential for Infection, related to presence of mechanical drainage system	Perform hand hygiene before contact with patient Limit visitors to reduce the number of organisms in patient's environment, and restrict visitation by individuals with any type of infection Encourage adequate diet to maintain optimal nutritional status Maintain asepsis for dressing changes and wound care
Impaired family processes, related to situational crisis (child with a physical defect)	Facilitate family's acceptance of infant: • Allow family's expression of feelings • Convey attitude of acceptance of infant and family Indicate by behavior that infant is a valuable human being

Patient Teaching. To prepare for the child's discharge and home care, instruct the parents in how to recognize signs that indicate shunt malfunction or infection and how to manually drain the shunt if necessary. Safe transportation is an essential issue to discuss with parents. Small infants may be restrained in a reclining position in an approved car bed. It is important to emphasize that hydrocephalus is a lifelong problem and that the child will require evaluation on a regular basis. The overall aim is to establish realistic goals and an appropriate educational program that will assist the child to achieve optimal potential.

Prognosis. The prognosis for children with treated hydrocephalus depends largely on the rate at which hydrocephalus develops, the duration of raised intracranial pressure, the frequency of complications, and the cause of hydrocephalus. With prompt diagnosis and proper shunt functioning, the survival rate for children with hydrocephalus is 80%.

Cerebral Palsy

Cerebral palsy is the most common permanent physical disability of childhood, with an average prevalence of 3.3 per 1000 live births in the United States. It occurs more often in boys than girls (CDC, 2019b). Cerebral palsy is a general term for a group of nonprogressive disorders of motoneuron impairment that result in motor dysfunction. In addition, affected children sometimes exhibit intellectual, visual, language, and neurologic impairments. The primary manifestations of cerebral palsy involve abnormal muscle tone and poor coordination.

Etiology And Pathophysiology. Many antenatal, perinatal, and postnatal factors share some of the responsibility in the development of cerebral palsy. Antenatal factors include maternal infections, maternal drug ingestion, hypoxia in utero, and blood incompatibilities. Perinatal factors include cerebral trauma and anoxia during birth. Anoxia plays the most significant role in the pathologic process of brain damage. Anesthesia or analgesia during labor and delivery, prematurity, and metabolic or electrolyte disturbances are also factors. Postnatal factors include infection, head trauma, cerebrovascular accident, and poisoning.

Clinical Manifestations. The clinical manifestations of cerebral palsy range from moderate to severe and are described in Box 32.9.

Diagnostic Tests. The diagnosis of cerebral palsy is based on history and physical examination. A thorough antenatal and birth history must be documented. A thorough neurologic examination is an essential component of the physical examination process and often aids in establishing a diagnosis of cerebral palsy. Additional tests may include CT, cranial sonography, electroencephalography, MRI, and a serum metabolic screening.

Medical Management. There is no cure for cerebral palsy. Common treatments include medicine, surgery, braces, and physical, occupational, and speech therapy. Treatment of the disorder should start as soon as the diagnosis is determined. The Individuals with Disabilities Education Act (IDEA) consists of four parts. Part C of this law ensures care for children during the first 36 months of age. Part B supplies services to children from 3 to 21 years of age. Services and supports are available based on the individual's needs. Various therapies, counseling, transportation, and assistive devices may be provided. Assistive devices include such items as braces, orthopedic devices, wheelchairs and walkers, and communication aids. These assistive devices are used to increase independence and participate more fully in everyday activities. Typically, medical treatment is provided in a hospital or similar setting. However, IDEA expands the evaluation and treatment of children into the school setting. The professionals that provide the services hold the same or similar qualifications as the ones the child would see in a hospital setting. IDEA ensures protection of the child's right to a free, appropriate public education in the least restrictive environment. The child may have a special school plan that includes modifications and accommodations that will give the opportunity to learn alongside peers in the general education setting. If a child is suspected of having a disability, the school must conduct a timely evaluation by a professional qualified to evaluate the child's condition, for example, a physical therapist, psychologist, or a speech language pathologist. These measures are to protect the child's educational rights (Saleh, n.d.).

In addition to the varied physical therapies to manage cerebral palsy pharmacological management is often indicated. The focus of the medications is geared toward reduction of the symptoms experienced. Broad categories utilized include anti-depressants, antispasmotics, anticonvulsants, antiinflammatories, and anticholinertics.

Botulinum toxin (Botox) is a drug used in the treatment of spasticity for cerebral palsy. Botox is injected into the muscle, where it acts to inhibit the release of acetylcholine into a specific muscle group, thereby preventing abnormal contractions. When administered early in the course of the disease, it often can prevent contractures, particularly in lower extremities, and eliminate the need for surgical procedures with possible adverse effects. The goal is to allow stretching of the muscle as it relaxes and permit ambulation with an ankle-foot orthosis. The major reported adverse effect of Botox injection is pain at the injection site.

Intrathecal or oral baclofen therapy is best suited for children with severe spasticity that interferes with activities of daily living and ambulation. The medication suppresses the release of excitatory neurotransmitters, thus reducing spasticity. If the medication is administered by the intrathecal route, a pump is implanted surgically. Benzodiazepines are used for seizure activity that may occur in the patient with cerebral palsy. Several other classes of drugs may be used as well to treat symptoms of cerebral palsy (CerebralPalsy.org, n.d.).

Nursing Interventions. Nursing interventions for a child with cerebral palsy focus on early recognition and prompt institution of interventions to enable optimal development. Adaptive eating utensils are used to facilitate eating. Encourage self-feeding and a high-calorie diet. It is important to encourage mobilization. Devices such as braces, wheeled scooters, and walkers are available to assist with mobility. Encourage use of protective headgear when these children are first learning to walk. Praise the children when goals are attained and encourage them to be as independent as possible within their limitations.

Patient problems and interventions for a child with cerebral palsy include but are not limited to the following:

| Box 32.9 | **Clinical Manifestations of Cerebral Palsy** |

- Arching of back
- Delayed gross motor development
- Developmental disabilities
- Difficulty swallowing and excessive drooling
- Exaggerated deep tendon reflexes
- Feeding difficulties
- Hypertonic muscles
- Involuntary movements
- Persistence of primitive reflexes
- Poor sucking
- Scissor-like gait with knees crossing
- Vision and hearing impairments

PATIENT PROBLEM	NURSING INTERVENTIONS
Compromised Physical Mobility, related to neuromuscular impairment	Encourage sitting, crawling, and walking at appropriate ages Carry out therapies that strengthen and improve control Assist the child in using appropriate leg motions when the child is learning to walk Provide incentives to promote mobility Ensure that the child has rested before attempting locomotion activities Incorporate play that encourages desired behavior Employ aids that facilitate locomotion, such as parallel bars and crutches
Inability to Bathe, Dress of Feed Self, related to physical disability	Encourage the child to assist with care as age and capabilities permit Select toys and activities that allow maximal participation by the child and that improve motor function and sensory input Assist with jaw control during feeding Adapt utensils, foods, and clothing to facilitate self-help (e.g., large-bowled spoon with padded handle; finger foods and foods that adhere to, rather than slip from, utensil; and clothing that opens in front with self-adhering closings rather than buttons) Assist parents in toilet training the child

Patient Teaching. Teach parents proper handling of their child and how to assist with activities of daily living. The family should learn to perform stretching and passive range-of-motion exercises and to select play activities that provide for maximal stimulation and participation. The parents also need education about the disorder and the resources available to them so that they can ensure optimal development for their child. Support groups are also beneficial to children and families (NINDS, n.d.).

Prognosis. Cerebral palsy is a chronic neurologic disability. There is no cure, but promotion of an optimal developmental course is vital so that affected children can realize full potential within the limits of the brain dysfunction.

Seizure Disorders

Etiology And Pathophysiology. The term *seizure* refers to a sudden, excessive, disorderly discharge of abnormal electrical impulses by the brain's neurons, causing a temporary alteration in CNS function. Some seizures are the result of such conditions as tumors, trauma, hypoxia, infections, poisons, fever, and metabolic disturbances; however, most seizures have no identifiable cause. Children are most prone to seizures during the period between birth and 2 years. More than 470,000 children between the ages of 0 to 17 years in the United States have epilepsy or recurrent seizures (CDC, 2020d). The current classification system divides seizures into two major categories: partial and generalized.

Diagnostic Testing. Data collection and review of the health history provide invaluable tools in the evaluation and diagnosis of seizure disorders. The health care provider performs a detailed neurologic examination. Electroencephalography is the most useful tool for evaluating seizure disorders. Additional diagnostic tests include CT and MRI. Single-photon emission CT gives a three-dimensional view of the brain and its vasculature. It often is used to help pinpoint the specific location of seizure activity.

Medical Management. The treatment of seizure disorders primarily involves drug therapy. Anticonvulsants that are most valuable in controlling partial or generalized seizures include carbamazepine (Tegretol), phenytoin (Dilantin), fosphenytoin (Cerebyx), and valproic acid (Depakote or Depakene). The drugs of choice for absence seizures, which belong to the class of partial seizures, are ethosuximide (Zarontin) and valproic acid. Reducing the number of drugs taken improves quality of life; therefore, experts currently recommend single-drug therapy. Additional seizure management has been achieved with gabapentin (Neurontin), lamotrigine (Lamictal), and felbamate (Felbatol). The use of felbamate is controversial because of the side effects of aplastic anemia and hepatic failure. Anticonvulsant therapy continues for a prolonged period. The health care provider modifies the dosage as the child grows. In children with a normal electroencephalogram who have been seizure free for at least 2 years, it is possible to discontinue anticonvulsant medications without increasing the risk of seizure recurrence. Discontinuing the medication gradually over 1 to 2 weeks is best. Abrupt withdrawal of anticonvulsants has the potential to result in an increase in the number and severity of seizures and sometimes even precipitates an episode of status epilepticus (continuous seizure activity).

The initial treatment of status epilepticus focuses on supporting and maintaining vital functions, including securing a patent airway, administering oxygen, establishing venous access, providing hydration, and administering lorazepam (Ativan), diazepam (Valium), or phenobarbital, as ordered. After the continuous seizure is stopped, the child will possibly receive a loading dose of phenytoin to ensure sustained control of seizures.

Nursing Interventions. Nursing interventions for a child with a seizure disorder involve assisting with the diagnosis, providing acute care during a seizure, providing for long-term management of the seizure disorder, and emotionally supporting and assisting the child and the family. To assist with the diagnosis of a seizure disorder, observe the child during a seizure and carefully document events, including any precipitating factors, if known or suspected; behavior before the seizure; time when the seizure began and ended; clinical manifestations of the seizure; and postseizure behavior and signs and symptoms. Recognize precipitating factors and prevent or minimize the child's exposure to them. Protect the child from injury during a seizure. Measures to prevent injuries during a seizure include padding the bed side rails and keeping the side rails upright; easing the child to the floor from a sitting or standing position; moving furniture out of the way; loosening restrictive clothing; and turning the child's head to the side to prevent aspiration of secretions. It is important not to force an object (e.g., tongue blade, airway) between the child's teeth during a seizure because doing so sometimes causes oral trauma. Staying with the child during and after a seizure and providing reassurance, emotional support, and explanations help minimize the child's anxiety.

A significant nursing goal is to promote a positive self-image in the child through encouragement and identification of the child's strengths and assets. Providing emotional support to the family is also essential. Encourage parents to express their fears and concerns and assist them to understand their child's condition. The family needs education regarding the nature of the disorder and possible precipitating factors, seizure precaution measures, dosage and side effects of medications, and the importance of maintaining as normal a lifestyle as possible.

Patient Teaching. The family must acknowledge the need to continue the medication regularly, without interruption, for as long as required. Help the parents plan the administration of the medication at convenient times to keep disruption of family routine to a minimum. Most neurologists prefer that patients take anticonvulsant medications in tablet or capsule form for more equal and accurate distribution of the medication. During periods of growth, medication dosage must be adjusted. Education concerning the prescribed dosages and common side effects also is needed. Teenage girls of childbearing age must be advised that selected antiseizure medications may reduce the effectiveness of hormone-based contraceptives. Individuals with seizure activity are advised to wear identification (e.g., bracelets) that highlights their seizure condition.

Prognosis. The incidence of seizures can be controlled or greatly reduced in the majority of affected children, and new studies hold the promise of progress in future treatment. Seizures do not shorten the life of the child, and the child is able to attend school, marry, and have children.

Spina Bifida (Myelomeningocele)

Spina bifida is a term that describes a variety of congenital defects of closure of the **neural tube** (the tube formed from the fusion of the neural folds and from which the brain and spinal cord arise). When the neural tube fails to close during embryonic development, a defect arises that can involve anything from a small area of the neural tube to its entire length (Fig. 32.28). Many infants with spina bifida occulta have a tuft of hair, a cleft, or a small, fatty mass over the defect. Myelomeningocele is one form of spina bifida in which portions of the spinal cord, the meninges, spinal fluid, and nerves protrude through the neural tube defect (Fig. 32.29).

Fig. 32.28 Neural tube defect: effects at each level of the defect. (From Phillips N: *Berry and Kohn's operating room technique*, ed 12, St. Louis, 2013, Mosby.)

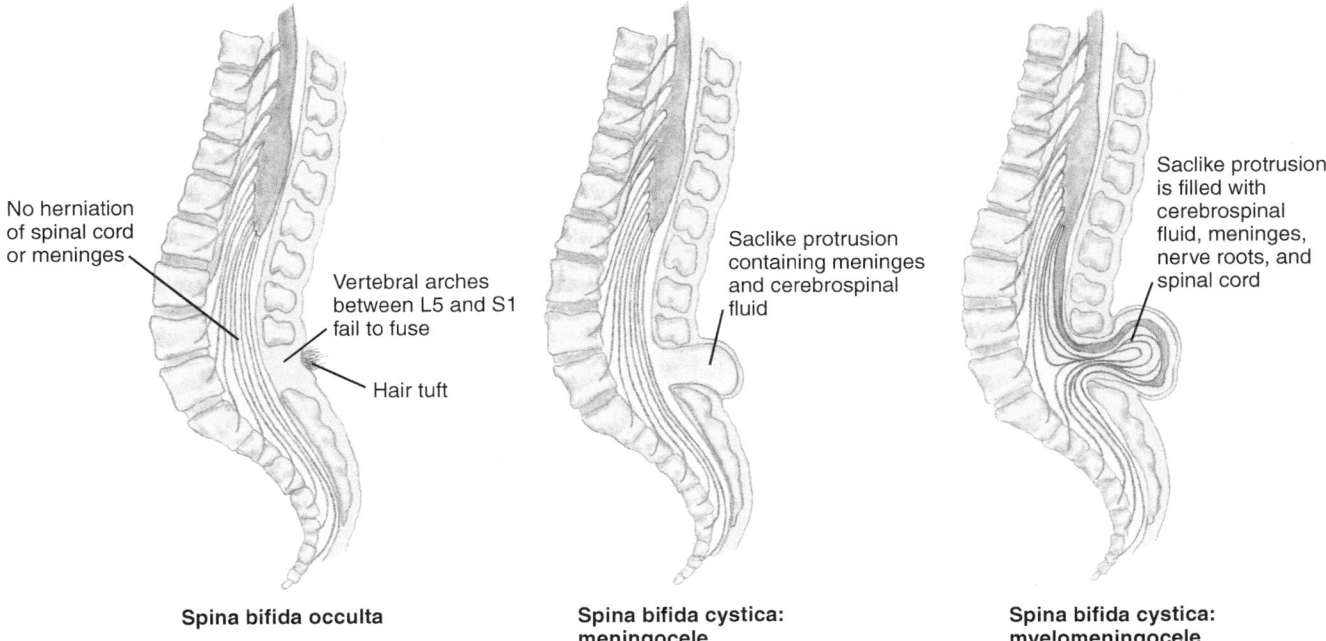

No herniation
of spinal cord
or meninges

Vertebral arches
between L5 and S1
fail to fuse

Hair tuft

Saclike protrusion
containing meninges
and cerebrospinal
fluid

Saclike protrusion
is filled with
cerebrospinal
fluid, meninges,
nerve roots, and
spinal cord

Spina bifida occulta

**Spina bifida cystica:
meningocele**

**Spina bifida cystica:
myelomeningocele**

Fig. 32.29 Three forms of spina bifida. (From James SR, Nelson KA, Ashwill JW: *Nursing care of children: Principles and practice*, ed 4, St. Louis, 2013, Saunders.)

Etiology And Pathophysiology. The cause of neural tube defects is generally unknown. Approximately 3000 children are born each year with a neural tubal defect. Poor nutrition and advanced maternal age have been implicated as contributing factors, as well as genetics, maternal antiseizure medications, and maternal obesity and diabetes. It is recommended that women of childbearing age consume 400 to 800 mcg of folic acid per day to help prevent neural tube defects. Studies show that if all women of childbearing age met these dietary requirements, 70% or more of neural tube defects could be prevented (March of Dimes, 2018).

Clinical Manifestations. In spina bifida, the spinal cord most commonly ends at the defect; therefore, all motor and sensory function below the defect is absent. Most myelomeningoceles involve the lumbar and lumbosacral areas. Depending on the level of the defect, affected infants usually have flaccid paralysis and sensory deficits of the lower extremities, bowel and bladder incontinence, talipes equinovarus defects, and a subluxated hip (a partial or incomplete dislocation of the hip). Hydrocephalus is present in the majority of affected infants.

Diagnostic Tests. It is sometimes possible to detect a neural tube defect prenatally. Uterine ultrasonography and elevated levels of maternal **alpha-fetoprotein** (antigen present in the human fetus that helps in evaluating fetal development) sometimes indicate the presence of a myelomeningocele. After birth, the health care provider makes the diagnosis on the basis of clinical manifestations. In some cases, the health care providers order a CT to assess for the presence of hydrocephalus.

Box 32.10	Nursing Interventions for a Child with Myelomeningocele

PREOPERATIVE
- Position child on abdomen.
- Cover sac with sterile, saline-soaked gauze.
- Protect sac from contact with feces and urine.

POSTOPERATIVE
- Position child on abdomen for 10–14 days (until incision is healed).
- Monitor vital signs.
- Observe for signs of bleeding and infection.

Medical Management. Treatment for myelomeningocele involves surgery to place the neural contents back within the sac to eliminate the possibility of infection. Sometimes it is necessary to insert a ventriculoperitoneal shunt to provide relief from hydrocephalus. Corrective surgeries are sometimes necessary to manage hip and lower extremity deformities. Additional measures include continuous neurologic assessments and assisting the family to deal with the diagnosis and surgery.

Nursing Interventions And Patient Teaching. Nursing interventions for a child with myelomeningocele focus on preventing infection and complications, providing postoperative care, and emotionally supporting and educating the family. Box 32.10 describes nursing interventions for children with myelomeningocele.

Parents need explanations regarding their child's condition and the surgery it necessitates. Encourage family members to express their fears and concerns and advise them of resources within their community that provide emotional support and services for families of children with spinal defects.

Because the parents will continue at home the care that began in the hospital, they need instruction on positioning, feeding, bowel training, bladder catheterization, and physical exercises.

Prognosis. The early prognosis for a child with myelomeningocele depends on the neurologic deficits present at birth, including motor ability, bladder and bowel innervation, and the presence of associated cerebral anomalies. Improved surgical techniques do not alter either the major physical disability and deformity or the chronic urinary tract and pulmonary infections and constipation that affect the quality of life for these children.

Neuroblastoma

Neuroblastoma is a malignant tumor composed principally of cells resembling neuroblasts that give rise to cells of the sympathetic nervous system. After brain tumors, neuroblastomas are the most common solid tumors in childhood, with approximately 700 new cases in children per year. The average age of diagnosis is 1 to 2 years of age with 90% diagnosed by age 5. Neuroblastoma has a high rate of dissemination, and approximately 67% of patients have metastatic disease at the time of diagnosis (ACS, 2021).

Etiology And Pathophysiology. These tumors originate from embryonic neural crest cells that normally give rise to the adrenal medulla and the sympathetic ganglia. Consequently, most tumors develop in the adrenal gland or the retroperitoneal sympathetic chain. Other sites include the head, neck, chest, and pelvis. The most common sites for metastatic disease include the liver, skin, lymph nodes, bone, and bone marrow.

Clinical Manifestations. The clinical manifestations of neuroblastoma depend on the location of the tumor. The most common location is the abdomen, and manifestations may include a palpable, firm, irregular mass that crosses the midline; anorexia; bowel and bladder alterations related to compression by the tumor; and spinal cord compression. If the tumor is located in the upper chest, manifestations include dyspnea, difficulty swallowing, and neck and facial edema. Many of the manifestations at the time of diagnosis are the result of metastatic disease. Manifestations of metastasis are hepatomegaly, splenomegaly, anemia, bone and joint pain, skin nodules (especially in infants), periorbital edema, weight loss, pallor, and weakness.

Diagnostic Tests. Initial diagnostic studies focus on locating the primary tumor site and areas of metastasis. In addition to a complete history and physical examination, studies include skeletal survey, bone scan, CT, abdominal ultrasonography, MRI, bone marrow aspiration and biopsy, and urine collection for metabolites of catecholamines

(biologically active amines, epinephrine, and norepinephrine; adrenal tumors stimulate the production of catecholamines). A biopsy of the tumor provides a definitive diagnosis and staging information.

Medical Management. The management of neuroblastoma involves a combination of surgery, radiation therapy, and chemotherapy. If the tumor is localized, the surgeon removes the tumor, and radiation therapy follows. If disease is widely disseminated, the surgeon removes as much of the tumor as possible, and the child receives follow-up chemotherapy and radiation therapy.

Nursing Interventions And Patient Teaching. Initial nursing interventions focus on preparing the child for diagnostic and operative procedures. Postoperative care is similar to that for any child undergoing abdominal surgery, including observation for any postoperative complications. Psychological support of the family is essential and involves helping them to prepare for the diagnostic and operative procedures and postoperative complications. Parents need an opportunity to express their fears and concerns. Because of the high incidence of metastasis at diagnosis, parents sometimes feel guilty that they did not seek medical attention sooner.

Parents also must be educated about any chemotherapy or radiation therapy that is needed.

Prognosis. Because this tumor is so frequently invasive, the prognosis for children with neuroblastoma is poor. In general, the younger the child is at diagnosis (especially younger than 1 year of age), the better the survival rate is. Neuroblastoma is one of the few tumors that may regress spontaneously, possibly as a result of maturity of the embryonic cell or the development of an active immune system.

Lead Poisoning

Lead poisoning is one of the most common, preventable, serious health care problems affecting children in the United States. The CDC defines lead poisoning as a blood lead level higher than 10 mg/dL. Lead levels too low to produce symptoms nonetheless can cause neurologic deficits insidiously. Lead levels as low as 10 µg/dL may cause significant health concerns in children, including long-term cognitive and behavioral problems.

Etiology And Pathophysiology. The leading cause of lead poisoning is ingestion or inhalation of environmental lead. Sources include lead-based paint, contaminated soil, and lead-contaminated pipes. The use of lead as an ingredient in household paint has been illegal in the United States since 1978. Older architectural structures still pose a threat to children's safety. Additional dangers for contamination may lurk in older painted toys and furniture. There are nearly 24 million housing units in which the children living in them are being exposed to lead because of deterioration of walls with lead paint (CDC, 2019a).

Ingested lead is excreted slowly from the body through the GI and genitourinary tracts. Any lead that is retained is stored in the bone, where it remains inactive. When the level of lead exceeds the amount that bone can absorb, lead travels through the circulatory system and causes anemia. Lead poisoning occurs more rapidly in children with iron deficiencies. Lead poisoning can damage the CNS seriously and is particularly dangerous to younger children.

Clinical Manifestations. Manifestations of lead poisoning include anemia, anorexia, abdominal pain, lethargy, aggression, impulsiveness, irritability, learning difficulties, delinquency, decreased attention span, decreased curiosity, hearing deficits, growth and developmental failure, and pica (craving to eat nonfood substances). Neurocognitive effects are possible results from lead poisoning and lead to long-term complications such as lowered IQ scores, developmental delays, speech and language problems, reading deficits, lower academic achievements, visual-spatial problems, and visual-motor problems.

Diagnostic Testing. Direct measurement of blood levels remains the primary diagnostic technique in the assessment of lead poisoning. A complete history and physical examination and an environmental assessment provide valuable information that identifies exposed children and environments at highest risk. Lead paint screening begins with blood testing. Screening is mandated for children in some states. Although blood lead levels higher than 10 mg/dL are considered diagnostic, counseling and follow-up are needed for children whose blood levels of lead exceed 2 mg/dL. CBCs, coagulation studies, and iron levels also are evaluated. Radiographic studies of the abdomen and long bones also may be performed. Lead lines (areas of increased density) near the epiphyseal lines may be identified.

Medical Management. The management of lead poisoning varies according to the blood level of lead. The primary objective of treatment is to remove lead from the body and prevent further exposure to lead. Pharmacologic treatment, such as chelation therapy (in toxicology, the use of a compound to bind to a toxic substance and render it nonactive and thus nontoxic), is a key intervention for children who have excessive lead levels. The precise course of therapy and the chelating agent depend on the preference of the health care provider and the severity of the child's condition. There is also an emphasis on ameliorating nutritional deficiencies and preventing infection.

Nursing Interventions And Patient Teaching. The challenges of lead poisoning provide a unique opportunity for pediatric nurses. The main goal of prevention strategies is to identify and deal with lead sources for the population of children at risk and the communities in which they live. To reach this goal, a thorough environmental and health questionnaire is completed at each routine health examination. The questionnaire is used to assess the child's risk for lead exposure. Provide parents with referrals to help them access resources for help with this problem.

Parent guidelines for reducing lead in the child's environment are described in Box 32.11.

Prognosis. Although most of the pathophysiologic effects of lead are reversible, the most serious consequences of high- and low-level lead exposure are the effects on the CNS. In children with lead-induced encephalopathy, permanent brain damage results in cognitive impairment,

---

Box 32.11   Parent Guidelines for Reducing Blood Lead Levels

- Make sure child does not have access to peeling paint or chewable surfaces painted with lead-based paint, especially windowsills and wells.
- If house was built before 1960 and has hard-surfaced floors, wet mop them at least once a week with a high-phosphate solution such as trisodium phosphate (available in hardware stores). Wipe other hard surfaces (such as windowsills and baseboards) with a similar solution. Do not vacuum hard-surfaced floors or windowsills or wells because this spreads dust. Use vacuum cleaners with agitators to remove dust from rugs rather than vacuum cleaners with suction only.
- Wash child's hands and face before the child eats.
- Wash toys and pacifiers frequently.
- If soil around home is likely to be contaminated with lead (e.g., if home was built before 1960 or is near a major highway), plant grass or other ground cover; plant bushes around outside of house so that child is not able to play there.
- During remodeling of older homes, be sure to follow correct procedures. Be certain children and pregnant women are not in the home, day or night, until work is completed. After deleading, thoroughly clean house with wet mopping before inhabitants return.
- In areas where lead content of water exceeds the drinking water standard, run water for at least 2 min from cold-water tap for drinking, cooking, and making formula; use first-flush water for purposes other than consumption.
- Do not store food in open cans, particularly if cans are imported.
- For food storage or service, do not use pottery or ceramic ware that was inadequately fired or is meant for decorative use.
- Avoid folk remedies that contain lead.
- Make sure that parental occupations or hobbies are not causing exposure in the home. Household members who are employed in occupations such as lead smelting should shower and change into clean clothing before leaving work.
- Make sure child eats regular meals because more lead is absorbed on an empty stomach.
- Make sure child's diet contains plenty of iron, calcium, protein, and zinc.

Modified from Centers for Disease Control and Prevention: *Preventing lead poisoning in young children,* Atlanta, 2012, Author.

behavior changes, possible paralysis, and seizures. Low-dose exposure also has the potential to cause permanent neurologic deficits. The neurologic deficits common with lead exposure include impulsivity, short attention span, distractibility, learning disabilities, and failure in school. With treatment, improvement may be seen in children with moderate lead poisoning.

Neonatal Abstinence Syndrome. Because opioids readily cross the placental membrane, women who use drugs while they are pregnant cause a passive addiction in their unborn children. Opioids commonly abused by women during pregnancy include cocaine (including "crack"), heroin, and methadone. Shortly after birth, the affected infant exhibits signs and symptoms of drug withdrawal, including irritability, disturbed sleeping and feeding patterns, tremors, seizures, hyperreflexia (increased reflex reaction), clonus (abnormal neuromuscular activity characterized by rapidly alternating involuntary contraction and relaxation of skeletal muscles), high-pitched cry, hypertonic muscles, tachypnea, frantic sucking of hands, vomiting, diarrhea, and inability to maintain body temperature. Signs and symptoms of opioid withdrawal sometimes persist for 3 to 4 months. For infants suspected of having opioid abstinence syndrome, health care providers usually order urinalysis for metabolites of the drug. It is essential to obtain a urine sample from the infant immediately after birth because the by-products of the drugs are cleared quickly from the body.

Infants who are experiencing neonatal abstinence syndrome are most comfortable in a nonstimulating environment that is free from bright lights and loud noises. They often prefer to be tightly swaddled in a blanket, with a pacifier to satisfy their vigorous sucking needs. It is essential to monitor such infants' I&O and vital signs. Nursing interventions should be organized in a manner that reduces the amount of disturbance to the infant.

On discharge, affected infants need a referral to an early intervention program, because they are at risk for neurologic problems; parent-infant bonding difficulties; and developmental, behavioral, and learning disabilities. Their mothers need referral for parental education and drug treatment programs to enable an optimal outcome for the child and family.

DISORDERS OF INTEGUMENTARY FUNCTION

Skin function is affected by genetic factors, cleanliness, hydration, and nutrition. Dermatologic disorders in children are the reason for a significant proportion of children's visits to health care provider's offices and clinics. Many of these disorders are painful for the child and distressing for the family.

Noninfectious Disorders of the Skin
Contact Dermatitis

Etiology And Pathophysiology. Contact dermatitis is an inflammatory, delayed immune response of the skin resulting from contact with environmental antigens to which a person is hypersensitive. Contact dermatitis has the highest incidence in infants and toddlers, and many patients have a family history of allergy. The most commonly affected areas include face, neck, hands, feet, and legs. The allergens that are most commonly responsible in children include soaps, detergents, bubble baths, shoe components, metals, chemicals, cosmetics, and plants such as poison ivy, oak, and sumac.

Clinical Manifestations. The contact area becomes erythematous, edematous, and pruritic. Papules (solid, red, raised areas less than 0.5 cm in diameter) and vesicles (circumscribed raised areas filled with serous fluid and less than 0.5 cm in diameter) form and can weep and ooze if broken.

Diagnostic Tests. The health care provider makes the diagnosis by observing the pattern and the location of the rash and by documenting an accurate history to identify the causative agent. Skin testing is also helpful at times in the identification of suspected plants, foods, or animals.

Medical Management. The hypersensitive reaction is usually self-limiting; therefore, in most cases, the health care provider directs treatment toward identifying and eliminating the cause and relieving signs and symptoms. Cool, wet dressings dipped in Burow's solution (solution of aluminum acetate, used as a drying agent for weeping skin lesions) or oatmeal baths help soothe the affected area. Calamine lotion may be recommended to manage pruritus without a prescription. It is acceptable to apply topical, over-the-counter steroid creams to mild contact dermatitis areas. In more severe cases, health care providers often prescribe systemic corticosteroids. Oral antihistamines such as diphenhydramine (Benadryl) are helpful in controlling pruritus.

Nursing Interventions And Patient Teaching. Advise the family to keep the child's fingernails clipped short to prevent scratching, which can result in a secondary bacterial infection. Loose, lightweight clothing during the healing phase is also comfortable and decreases irritation.

Teach parents to keep an accurate history of possible causative agents. Once it is clear what the primary irritant is, teach them to avoid it. If the skin does come in contact with the causative agent, teach parents to wash the affected area with a mild soap and water and dry it thoroughly. It is best to avoid talcum powder, overheating, and hot baths. Teach the parents to apply topical medications only as directed by a health care provider.

Prognosis. The reaction is usually self-limiting and normally resolves within 2 weeks.

Diaper Dermatitis

Etiology And Pathophysiology. Diaper dermatitis is one of the most common skin disorders in infancy and the cause of great concern for many parents. Diaper

Fig. 32.30 Diaper dermatitis. (From Habif TP: *Clinical dermatology: A color guide to diagnosis and therapy*, ed 3, St. Louis, 1996, Mosby.)

dermatitis is a form of contact dermatitis and usually caused by an external irritant (Fig. 32.30). The most common irritating agents include prolonged exposure to urine or feces; inadequate cleaning of the diaper area; soaps, detergents, or fabric softeners; excessive use of powders or ointments; and the use of plastic pants. Fair-complexioned infants tend to have more sensitive skin and are more vulnerable to diaper rash than are infants with darker complexions. The occurrence peaks at 9 to 12 months of age, and the incidence is higher in formula-fed infants than in breast-fed infants.

Clinical Manifestations. The rash appears as erythematous papular lesions (similar in appearance to a scald) on the areas that come into direct contact with the diaper: the buttocks, the labia or the scrotum, the inner thighs, and the mons pubis. Skinfolds frequently are spared. In many cases, excoriation in the perianal area is caused by frequent diarrhea. The inflammation does not take on a specific configuration; rather, a variety of patterns are possible. The moist, warm, dark environment created by the diaper also tends to promote the growth of secondary bacterial or fungal infections. An infant with diaper dermatitis is usually uncomfortable and likely to be fussy, irritable, and restless.

Diagnostic Tests. Clinical observation of the characteristics and the location of the rash and an assessment of possible irritants are diagnostic for diaper dermatitis. Bacterial or fungal cultures are sometimes necessary to investigate persistent secondary infections.

Medical Management. Keeping the diaper area clean and dry is of primary importance. Measures to promote healing and prevent diaper dermatitis from recurring include changing diapers as soon as they become soiled, thoroughly cleansing the diaper area with a mild soap and water and then gently drying at each diaper change, exposing the affected area to the air several times a day, and avoiding occlusive plastic pants. For more severe cases, a topical glucocorticoid sometimes is required.

Nursing Interventions And Patient Teaching. The prophylactic use of protective ointments such as Desitin, A+D ointment, or zinc oxide is often helpful. Keep the diaper area clean. An excessive amount of powder is contraindicated because in the presence of moisture,

Box 32.12	**Parent Guidelines for Controlling Diaper Rash**

- Keep skin dry.
- Use superabsorbent disposable diapers to reduce skin wetness. If cloth diapers are used, use only overwraps that allow air to circulate; avoid using rubber pants.
- Change diapers as soon as they are soiled, especially with stool, whenever possible and preferably once during the night.
- Expose healthy or only slightly irritated skin to air, not heat, to dry completely.
- Apply ointment, such as zinc oxide or petrolatum, to protect skin, especially if skin is very erythematous or has moist, open areas.
- When the area is soiled, wipe off top layer of ointment and reapply.
- To completely remove ointment, especially zinc oxide, use mineral oil; do not wash vigorously.
- Avoid overwashing the skin, especially with perfumed soaps or commercial wipes that are potentially irritating. It is acceptable to use a moisturizer or nonsoap cleanser, such as cold cream or Cetaphil, to wipe urine from skin. Gently wipe stool from skin with water and mild soap, such as Dove.

the powder will cake, hold the moisture, and excoriate the skin (Box 32.12).

Teach parents the basics of diaper and skin care as outlined previously. To prevent the infant's inhalation of powder dust, instruct parents to put a small amount in their hand and apply it to the infant's diaper area (see Box 32.12).

Prognosis. Quick recognition with prompt therapy leads to a good prognosis.

Atopic Dermatitis (Eczema)

Etiology And Pathophysiology. Atopic dermatitis is a pruritic, allergic response common in infancy and childhood. *Atopy* refers to an allergy for which there is a genetic or inherited predisposition. The exact cause is unknown. Many affected children have a familial history of asthma, allergic rhinitis, or dry skin. The disease also occurs in association with hypersensitivity to histamine, as well as with food allergies and abnormal skin function. Infantile atopic dermatitis can occur between 2 and 5 months of age and sometimes continues to be problematic to age 2 or 3 years, when many children seem to "outgrow" the illness. Childhood atopic dermatitis usually occurs at age 2 or 3 years and persists to 5 years of age in some cases. Adolescent atopic dermatitis usually is seen at 12 years of age and in some cases lasts indefinitely.

Clinical Manifestations. In infantile eczema, the primary lesions consist of erythema, vesicles, and papules, which typically ooze and form crusts. They appear most often on the cheeks, scalp, trunk, and extensor surfaces of the extremities. In childhood eczema, the lesions appear as erythematous, scaly patches on the trunk, elbows, knees, ankles, hands, and feet and behind the ears. The skin becomes thick and leather-like (**lichenification**). In adolescent eczema, the lesions are the same as in childhood, but the distribution involves mainly hands, feet, neck, and face. At any age, the unaffected skin is usually very dry, and the pruritus may be extremely intense. Affected children are often uncomfortable and restless. Affected infants unable to scratch often rub their faces on linens or clothing in an effort to relieve the itch. Scratching or rubbing also has the potential to lead to secondary infections, and many children with atopic dermatitis have an increased susceptibility to bacterial (*S. aureus),* viral (herpes simplex), and fungal skin infections. The signs and symptoms are better in humid climates and worse in fall and winter, when homes are heated and environmental humidity is lower.

Diagnostic Tests. The diagnosis is based on clinical observation of the type and distribution of the lesions, a positive family history of allergy, and severity of pruritus. In general, skin testing is important in severe cases to help determine specific allergens.

Medical Management. The therapeutic management includes hydration of the skin, controlling pruritus, decreasing inflammation, and preventing secondary infections. Skin hydration can be accomplished in a variety of ways. Tepid baths followed by the administration of an unscented cream or lotion help trap moisture in the skin. The application of occlusive creams or ointments helps relieve dry skin. To decrease inflammation, the health care provider orders thin applications of topical steroid creams or lotions. The strength and the type of topical steroid vary according to the degree of inflammation and the age of the child. Oral antihistamines such as diphenhydramine (Benadryl) or hydroxyzine are useful in controlling pruritus. New therapies include topical immunomodulators, which are steroid-free medications that aid in the reduction of inflammation. Tacrolimus (Protopic) and pimecrolimus (Elidel) are examples of topical immunomodulators. Dupixent (dupilumab) is an injectable monoclonal antibody that may be used in children with severe eczema. Secondary bacterial infections are managed with systemic antibiotics (Mayo Clinic, 2020a).

Nursing Interventions. The nurse's role in caring for a child with atopic dermatitis involves measures to control pruritus, promote skin integrity, and provide emotional support to the child and family. Compresses with Burow's solution (aluminum acetate) soothe itching and moisten skin. Hot baths and hot showers should be discouraged because of their drying effect on the skin. Suggest adding cornstarch to tepid bath water to provide some relief from itching, as well as to hydrate skin. Teach the child and the family to use only a mild, unscented soap such as Dove or Neutrogena, if they use any soap at all. To prevent new lesions or secondary infection, it is essential to minimize scratching. For the infant, covering the hands with mittens or socks helps reduce scratching. For the older child, gloves allow for more dexterity. At times, it may be necessary to use safety reminder devices to discourage scratching; however, it is important that the infant or child be free from these restrictions periodically.

Patient Teaching. Overheating usually intensifies itching; therefore, parents need to understand that dressing their child in lightweight, loose clothing made from cotton or cotton blends is preferable. They should wash and double-rinse clothing, linens, and blankets to ensure removal of all soap residue. It is important for parents to understand that they must apply lubricants frequently—especially after bathing, while the skin is still damp—to seal in moisture. Teach parents to keep the child's fingernails and toenails clipped short and clean to keep the risk of infection to a minimum. At any age, keeping the child's hands busy with play activities provides the distraction needed to discourage scratching. The appearance, discomfort, and irritability displayed by children with atopic dermatitis are often very upsetting for family members. Encourage parents to verbalize their feelings and provide reassurance. Teaching stress-reduction techniques is often helpful to the child and the parents because stress tends to aggravate the severity of the condition.

Prognosis. Atopic dermatitis can be controlled but not cured. Most young children with atopic dermatitis outgrow their condition before adolescence, but some continue to have symptoms throughout adulthood.

Seborrheic Dermatitis

Etiology And Pathophysiology. Seborrheic dermatitis, or cradle cap, is a chronic inflammatory reaction of the skin that is common in infancy. Although the cause of the condition is unknown, there appears to be a connection to sebaceous gland activity. Many affected infants have no family history of allergy.

Clinical Manifestations. Seborrheic dermatitis most commonly affects the scalp and appears as thick, white or yellowish, crusty or scaly patches. Mild pruritus sometimes accompanies the disorder. Other commonly affected areas include the eyebrows or eyelids (blepharitis), the postauricular area (behind the ear), the external ear (otitis externa), the nasolabial (nose and lip) folds, and the inguinal region (seborrheic diaper dermatitis).

Diagnostic Tests. Diagnosis is based on clinical observation of the characteristics and location of crusty patches. Skin biopsy of the affected area may be performed.

Medical Management. Management of seborrheic dermatitis consists of treating the signs and symptoms and simple preventive measures. The nurse and the parents can remove crusty, scaly patches by applying mineral oil to soften the affected areas (except the eyelids) and help loosen crusts, followed by shampooing with a mild, tear-free shampoo and thoroughly rinsing. Then a soft baby brush or a soft toothbrush is used to brush the hair and remove flakes from the hair. A fine-tooth comb also works well. Preventive measures include daily shampooing with an antiseborrheic shampoo. Topical corticosteroids are rarely needed.

Nursing Interventions And Patient Teaching. Soak crusts with warm water and cotton (or clean washcloth) compresses until the crusts are loosened. Then cleanse the eye area with clean cotton (or a clean washcloth) and warm water, starting at the inner canthus and continuing to the outer canthus. For each stroke, a clean piece of cotton (or clean area on the washcloth) should be used.

Patient Problems and Nursing Interventions for Children With a Disorder of Integumentary Function

PATIENT PROBLEM	NURSING INTERVENTIONS
Compromised Skin Integrity, related to irritation	Assess for signs of scratching Advise parents to keep the child's fingernails short or to cover the child's hands with mittens or socks Keep affected areas clean and dry Apply medications as directed
Potential for Infection, related to scratching and skin impairment	Assess for signs of infection Change diapers as soon as they are soiled Administer appropriate antibiotics as directed Implement standard precautions (see Chapter 7) Maintain careful hand hygiene Teach and reinforce positive habits of hygienic care
Distorted Body Image, related to perceptions of appearance	Encourage child to express feelings about personal appearance and perceived reactions of other people Hold child (remember that there is no substitute for the stimulation and comfort of human contact) Touch and caress unaffected area Teach self-care when appropriate Involve child in planning treatment schedules Emotionally support and encourage child in efforts to deal with multiple problems that sometimes occur in association with disorder, including discomfort, rejection, discouragement, and feelings of self-revulsion Encourage child to maintain usual activities

Often parents need reassurance that shampooing their infant's hair will not cause harm to the fontanelles. A demonstration on how to shampoo the hair

is sometimes necessary. If cradle cap is extensive, inform parents that several treatments may be necessary to loosen and remove all crusts. If the eyelids are involved, teach the parents how to clean these areas safely.

Prognosis. The crusts may appear shortly after birth and until old age, with periods of remissions and exacerbations.

Acne Vulgaris. Acne is an inflammatory process of the skin. It is slightly more common in boys and men. Acne most often occurs in teenagers, but it can occur at any age. Acne is a disease that involves the pilosebaceous follicles (the hair follicles and sebaceous gland complex) of the face, the neck, the shoulders, the back, and the upper chest.

Medical Management. Treatment success depends on the commitment of the adolescent. Before treatment is prescribed, it is best to determine the adolescent's level of comfort and readiness to begin treatment.

Tretinoin (Retin-A) is the only drug that effectively interrupts the abnormal follicular keratinization that produces microcomedones, the invisible precursors of the visible comedones. Tretinoin alone is usually sufficient for management of comedonal acne. The medication should not be applied for at least 20 to 30 minutes after washing, to decrease the burning sensation. It is important to emphasize the need to avoid sun and use sunscreen daily, because sun exposure has potential to result in severe sunburn. Adolescents are advised to apply the medication at night and to use a sunscreen with a sun protection factor (SPF) of at least 15 in the daytime.

Topical benzoyl peroxide is an antibacterial agent that inhibits the growth of *Propionibacterium acnes* organisms. It is effective against inflammatory and noninflammatory acne and is an effective first-line agent. This medication is available over the counter and by prescription as a cream, lotion, gel, or wash.

When inflammatory lesions accompany the comedones, some health care providers prescribe a topical antibacterial agent. These agents prevent new lesions and treat preexisting acne. Clindamycin, erythromycin, metronidazole, azelaic acid, and the combination of benzoyl peroxide with either erythromycin (Benzamycin) or glycolic acid are options for topical antibacterial therapy. The combination of 5% benzoyl peroxide and 3% erythromycin is especially beneficial. Tretinoin improves the penetration of other topical agents, and combination therapy with tretinoin and an antibacterial is helpful.

Some health care providers turn to systemic antibiotic therapy when moderate to severe acne does not respond to topical treatments. Oral antibiotics are considered safe to use to treat acne. These antibiotics include tetracycline, erythromycin, minocycline, doxycycline, clindamycin, and trimethoprim-sulfamethoxazole.

Girls and women with mild to moderate acne sometimes respond well to topical treatment and the addition of an oral contraceptive pill. These pills reduce the

Table 32.4 **Traumatic Injuries**

CLINICAL MANIFESTATION	MANAGEMENT	PREVENTION
Animal Bites (Dogs, Cats)		
Lacerations, punctures, tissue avulsion	Wound care	Supervise children during play with pets. Educate children in appropriate ways to handle pets. Teach understanding of animal behavior and respect for animals. Never leave infants alone with a pet.
Human Bites		
Lacerations	Wound care	Supervise young children at play.
Insect Bites (Fleas, Mosquitoes, Flies, Gnats)		
Hypersensitive reactions; papular urticaria; firm papules	Cool compresses, topical antihistamines, pramoxine (Caladryl) lotion	Use insect repellents (should not contain >10% N,N-diethyl-meta-toluamide [DEET]). Remove source by treating furniture, mattresses, carpets, and pets.
Insect Stings (Hornets, Wasps, Bees)		
Nonhypersensitive: local erythema, edema, tenderness, pruritus	Carefully scrape off stinger, if present; cleanse with soap and water; use cool compresses, antipruritic agents	Avoid insect breeding or nesting areas. Wear clothes that cover the extremities and feet.
Hypersensitive: systemic reactions and anaphylaxis	Intramuscular epinephrine and immediate medical attention; epinephrine kits available for home and school to prevent anaphylactic shock and death	
Sunburn		
Mild: erythema, tenderness, mild edema	Cool compresses, moisturizers	Use topical sunscreens containing para-aminobenzoic acid (PABA) and sun protection factor (SPF) 30.
Severe: severe erythema, pain, edema, vesicular formation	Immediate medical attention	Limit time spent in sun during period of maximum exposure (11 a.m. to 3 p.m.); at higher elevations, limit time on fresh snow and water, especially when sun is directly overhead.

endogenous androgen production, which may result in a decrease in acne.

Isotretinoin, or 13-*cis*-retinoic acid (Accutane), is a very potent and effective oral agent that is reserved for severe cystic acne that has not responded to other treatments. Isotretinoin is the only agent available that affects factors involved in the development of acne. However, it is essential for a dermatologist to manage any course of treatment with isotretinoin. Adolescents with multiple, active, deep dermal or subcutaneous cystic and nodular acne lesions receive treatment for 20 weeks. Multiple side effects are possible, including dry skin and mucous membranes, nasal irritation, dry eyes, decreased night vision, photosensitivity, arthralgia, headaches, mood changes, aggressive or violent behaviors, depression, and suicidal ideation. Adolescents who take this drug must be monitored for depression, depressive symptoms, and suicidal ideation. It is important to give this drug *only* at the recommended dosage for no longer than the recommended duration. The most significant side effects of this drug are teratogenic (cause developmental abnormalities in the fetus). Isotretinoin is *absolutely contraindicated* in pregnant

women. Sexually active young women must use an effective contraceptive method during treatment and for 1 month after treatment. Patients receiving isotretinoin also must be monitored for elevated cholesterol and triglyceride levels. Significant elevation sometimes necessitates discontinuation of the medication.

Nursing Interventions And Patient Teaching. An affected adolescent must be informed that benzoyl peroxide and retinoic acid are incompatible together, and thus the prescriber directs the adolescent to use them on alternate days or to use one in the morning and the other at night. The adolescent also must be informed of the side effects of topical medications, especially the erythematous skin that sometimes results from compliance with the regimen prescribed by the dermatologist. Assess the psychosocial effect of acne on the adolescent's self-image. Depression, anxiety, and low self-esteem sometimes occur during the adolescent task of developing identity. Adolescents with acne need a great deal of emotional support in dealing with feelings of self-consciousness and frustration, especially during periods of exacerbations. Teenagers should avoid oil-based cosmetics. Emphasize meticulous skin care, including removal of cosmetics at night. Involving the adolescent in developing the plan of care is sometimes the key to ensuring successful compliance with the treatment measures.

Although the disease is self-limited and not life-threatening, it is highly significant to adolescents, and it is a mistake to underestimate the effect it sometimes has on young people. See the patient problem box for patient problem statements with nursing interventions for a child with a disorder of integumentary function.

Prognosis. Acne resolves spontaneously over time, depending on the individual. Severe acne may result in scarring of the skin.

Psoriasis. Psoriasis is a chronic, proliferative skin disorder characterized by thick, scaly patches and inflammation. Psoriasis usually is not seen in children younger than 6 years of age. The disorder has characteristic remissions and exacerbations. Affected people are otherwise healthy. Humidifiers sometimes help in winter.

Traumatic Injuries

Animal, insect, and human bites in children account for a considerable number of visits to clinics and health care providers' offices. Most bites from dogs or cats are from pets belonging to the family or neighbors. Dog bites involve lacerations or tissue avulsion injuries, whereas cats inflict more puncture-like wounds. Animal bites most often occur on the child's face, scalp, and upper extremities because children tend to keep their heads close to the animal during play.

Human bites occur in young children during rough or aggressive play or when they become frustrated; bites are also possible as the result of child abuse. The most common traumatic injuries in children and their manifestations, management, and nursing interventions are outlined in Table 32.4.

Infectious Disorders of the Skin

Bacterial Infections. Impetigo, folliculitis, and cellulitis are common bacterial infections in childhood. The assessment of systemic signs and symptoms, areas involved, and appearance of lesions is helpful in establishing the type of infection. Table 32.5 lists the etiology, the clinical manifestations, the management, and the nursing interventions for these infections.

The prognosis for children with bacterial infections of the skin is favorable with proper treatment.

Herpes Simplex Virus Type 1. Herpes simplex virus type 1 (HSV-1) is a common infection. HSV-1 is transmitted by direct contact of infected body fluids with nonintact skin or mucous membranes. The children most susceptible to HSV are immunosuppressed children (those receiving steroid therapy or chemotherapy, with leukemia, or who are HIV positive), children with burns, and infants with diaper rash or eczema.

The prognosis for children with viral infections of the skin is usually good; however, the infection is sometimes fatal in children with depressed immunity. Healing occurs without scarring unless secondary infection develops.

Table 32.5	**Bacterial Infections of the Skin**	
ETIOLOGY	**CLINICAL MANIFESTATIONS**	**MANAGEMENT**
Impetigo		
Staphylococcus aureus, group A β-hemolytic streptococci, or both	Erythematous papules that progress to vesicles with exudative and honey-colored crusting stages; involves face, buttocks, and extremities; pruritus is common	Mupirocin; topical or systemic treatment with penicillin or erythromycin *Nursing interventions:* Teaching family the measures to control spread of infection; instruction in careful hand hygiene
Folliculitis		
S. aureus	Pustule with surrounding erythema of the hair follicle of the scalp or extremities; possible progression to a furuncle (a boil from the primary folliculitis), with extension into the surrounding dermis Systemic effects: malaise, if severe	Topical antibiotics and local, warm, moist compresses; in more severe cases, sometimes incision and drainage, followed by antibiotic therapy *Nursing interventions:* Teaching family the measures to control spread of infection and hygiene measures, such as careful hand hygiene
Cellulitis		
S. aureus, group A β-hemolytic streptococci, *Haemophilus influenzae* type b	Possible anywhere on the body; area is erythematous, edematous, warm, and painful; adjacent tender lymph node enlargement; sometimes progresses to abscess formation Systemic effects: fever, malaise	Antibiotic therapy, rest, and warm, moist compresses Neonates with herpes simplex virus type 1: hospitalization Children younger than 3 years of age with facial cellulitis: usually hospitalization *Nursing interventions:* Gently cleansing area with saline; observing for complications; administering antibiotics and analgesics as prescribed; instituting wound drainage precautions if drainage develops; teaching family the measures to control spread of infection, such as careful hand hygiene

Tinea Capitis, Tinea Corporis, Tinea Cruris, And Tinea Pedis (Ringworm). Tinea infections are common fungal infections of the skin in children. The infections are classified according to the area of the body that is involved. Tinea capitis is a common infection of the scalp among school-age children. Tinea corporis occurs on the trunk and on the extremities in young children; tinea cruris ("jock itch") affects the inguinal area of pubescent boys; and tinea pedis ("athlete's foot") occurs between the toes.

The prognosis for children with fungal infections of the skin, with treatment, is good.

Candidiasis (Thrush)

Etiology And Pathophysiology. The fungus *Candida albicans* causes candidiasis, or thrush. The infection is a common disorder in infants younger than 6 months and is transmitted by contaminated hands, nipples, and pacifiers. In some newborns, candidal infection results from passage through the mother's infected vagina at birth. The candidal lesion begins as a pustule on an inflammatory base. As inflammatory cells accumulate, whitish yellow or whitish gray curdlike patches appear over the infected area. The incidence of candidiasis is higher in immunocompromised children, infants of diabetic mothers, and children with oronasal malformations (cleft lip or palate).

Clinical Manifestations. The white patches of *C. albicans* frequently appear on moist tissues because the organism cannot grow on dry skin. Common areas affected include the tongue, the buccal cavity, the GI tract, and the vagina. Parents often mistake thrush for a formula coating on the tongue. In general, the condition is asymptomatic and easily treated. Severe cases sometimes result in pain, which leads to refusal to eat or drink and thus causes risk for dehydration.

Diagnostic Tests. Diagnosis is based on careful documentation of history and on clinical observation of the plaques. To distinguish thrush from formula, rinse the area with water or gently wipe the area with a wet washcloth. If the white coating remains, thrush is present. Scraping lesions is contraindicated because they bleed easily.

Medical Management. Nystatin suspension is the most common antifungal agent used to treat oral *C. albicans* infections. Nystatin suspension is administered after feedings and applied directly onto the lesions and to each side of the mouth before the child swallows. Other drugs useful in the treatment of thrush include amphotericin B, clotrimazole, fluconazole, and miconazole. Treating infections early often prevents more serious complications, such as candidal infections of the upper airway and the GI tract. When a child has oral candidiasis, it is important to also inspect the diaper area for signs of infection. Nystatin cream is prescribed for diaper candidiasis.

Nursing Interventions And Patient Teaching. Instruct parents to complete the full 7-day course of nystatin suspension, even though candidal lesions may no longer be present. Prevention of reinfection includes teaching

---

Box 32.13	**Medical Management and Nursing Interventions for Parasitic Infections**

- Treating the hair with over-the-counter medications such as pyrethrins or permethrins (be sure to follow directions closely)
- Lindane 1% lotion, cream, or shampoo (contraindicated for children younger than 2 years because of neurotoxicity) is only used as a second line treatment if other measures fail
- Simultaneous treatment of family members
- Hydroxyzine or diphenhydramine for pruritus
- Cleansing of contaminated clothing and linens on hot water setting of washer and dryer
- Dry clean or bag items for 2 weeks if they can't be washed and dried with the hot setting
- Vacuuming carpets and automobile interiors
- Discarding or treating stuffed animal or fabric toys
- Soak combs and brushes in hot water for at least 10 minutes
- Education of parents:
  - Carefully inspect the head (at the nape of the neck) of a child who scratches the head more than usual for bite marks, erythema, and nits.
  - Read directions carefully before beginning therapy.
  - Be aware of psychological effects, which can be highly stressful to children.
  - Be sure that family members do not share hats, combs, or brushes

---

parents to sterilize bottles, nipples, pacifiers, and teething objects. Emphasize proper hand hygiene. Instruct parents to report any oral discomfort that results in poor fluid intake. Review signs of dehydration with the family. If the mother is breast-feeding, advise her to wash her nipples with soap and water before and after feedings. Some health care providers also recommend the application of nystatin cream to the mother's nipples.

Prognosis. The prognosis for children with candidiasis (thrush) is good with prescribed therapy.

Parasitic Infections

Scabies And Pediculosis. Scabies is an infectious parasitic disorder caused by a mite. Scabies is most common in school-age children. The scabies mite burrows under the skin, leaving behind debris, feces, and eggs. The condition causes a linear, papular rash and intense pruritus. Transmission occurs by direct contact with an infected person, infested bed linen, or infested clothing.

Pediculosis capitis (head lice) is a scalp infection that causes intense pruritus. It is common among preschool- and school-age children. The adult louse attaches to the skin and feeds by sucking blood. On the hair shaft, the mature female louse lays her eggs (nits), which hatch in 7 to 10 days. The louse does not jump or fly and is not carried or transmitted by pets. Infestations usually occur as a result of sharing contaminated combs, brushes, hats, or clothing that comes in contact with the head. Box 32.13 outlines medical management and nursing interventions for scabies and pediculosis.

Patient teaching is as follows:

- Remove dead lice and remaining nits with a fine-tooth comb. Tweezers are necessary to remove the nits if the comb is ineffective.
- Machine wash all washable clothing, towels, and bed linens on the hot water setting of the washer and dry in a hot setting of the dryer for at least 20 minutes. Dry clean nonwashable items.
- Thoroughly vacuum carpets, car seats, pillows, stuffed animals, rugs, mattresses, and upholstered furniture.
- Seal nonwashable items in plastic bags for 14 days if they cannot be dry cleaned or vacuumed.
- Soak combs, brushes, and hair accessories in lice-killing products for 1 hour or in boiling water for 10 minutes.

The prognosis is good with treatment.

COMMUNICABLE DISEASES AND IMMUNIZATIONS

The development and use of vaccines have significantly reduced the incidence of many communicable diseases and the serious complications associated with them. However, health care providers occasionally encounter children with a preventable communicable disease. You may be the first person to observe signs of illness, such as a rash, that may be related to a communicable disease. It is important to be able to identify potentially infectious cases to institute measures to prevent exposure and transmission to others. In assessing a child with suspect signs and symptoms, determine whether the child has had any recent exposure to a known case and whether the child is experiencing any prodromal symptoms (early signs of a developing condition or disease). The immunization status of the child and a history of the illness often help rule out certain communicable diseases. The goals of nursing interventions for a child with a communicable disease are to prevent transmission of disease to other people, prevent complications, and promote supportive management. Table 32.6 describes the communicable diseases common in childhood and their medical management, specific nursing interventions, and possible complications. With accurate diagnosis, prompt treatment, and prevention of complications, the prognosis is usually good.

DISORDERS OF SENSORY ORGAN FUNCTION

Sensory impairment in young children increases the risk for serious adverse outcomes in growth and development. Prevention, early detection, and management are essential for favorable outcomes.

Hearing

Otitis Media

Etiology And Pathophysiology. Otitis media, an infection of the middle ear, is a common infection in children aged 6 months to 2 years and often follows an upper respiratory infection. A significant cause of otitis media is the accumulation of bacteria in the nasopharynx. In young children, the eustachian tube, which connects the nasopharynx and the middle ear, is shorter, more horizontal, and wider, allowing passage and trapping of nasopharyngeal flora in the middle ear. Feeding practices also have been implicated in the incidence of otitis media. It is possible that formula-fed babies have a higher incidence of otitis media than do breast-fed babies because of the more supine position assumed during bottle feeding. Always evaluate toddlers and young children for foreign bodies (pieces of toys, beads, pebbles, vegetables, and so on) in the ear canal, which have the potential to lead to hearing loss and local infection.

Clinical Manifestations. The infant or young child with acute otitis media is likely to experience otalgia (earache), fever, rhinitis, fussiness, irritability, and decreased appetite. In an affected infant, pulling, tugging, or rubbing the affected ear or rolling the head from side to side indicates possible acute otitis media. Affected older children usually complain of ear pain. On occasion, purulent discharge is present in the ear canal, which is indicative of a ruptured tympanic membrane. When this occurs, ear pain ceases suddenly.

Diagnostic Tests. Visualization of the tympanic membrane by otoscopic examination, along with clinical signs and symptoms, usually confirms the diagnosis. If drainage is in the ear canal, the material may be cultured.

Medical Management. The management of acute otitis media includes administration of antibiotics for 10 days and acetaminophen for fever and discomfort. On completion of antibiotic therapy, the health care provider examines the child to determine the effectiveness of treatment and observe for complications. An accumulation of fluid that remains in the middle ear space is often an indication for surgical insertion of tympanostomy tubes to drain the fluid and relieve the pressure. In children with chronic otitis media, some health care providers opt for tympanostomy tubes to prevent hearing loss. Tympanostomy tubes remain in the ear an average of 6 months before being ejected spontaneously.

Nursing Interventions And Patient Teaching. Children usually begin to feel better after 48 to 72 hours of antibiotic therapy. The application of heat or cold (whichever provides the greatest comfort) over the affected ear with the child lying on the affected side often also helps alleviate pain. This position also facilitates drainage of the exudate if the eardrum has ruptured or after a myringotomy. If the ear is draining, clean the external canal with sterile cotton swabs or pledgets soaked in hydrogen peroxide. If ear wicks or lightly rolled sterile gauze packs are placed in the ear after

Table 32.6 Childhood Communicable Diseases

DISEASE	CLINICAL MANIFESTATIONS	MEDICAL MANAGEMENT	NURSING INTERVENTIONS
Rubeola (Measles)			
Etiology: Paramyxovirus *Transmission:* Direct contact from respiratory tract secretions, blood, or urine of infected person *Incubation period:* 7–12 days *Communicable period:* 4 days before to 5 days after rash appears	*Prodrome:* Fever, malaise, cough, coryza, conjunctivitis; Koplik's spots (pinpoint red spots with central white speck in buccal cavity opposite lower molars) 3–4 days before rash *Acute phase:* Rash, appearing as irregular macular erythema, beginning on face and behind ears and spreading to feet, and lasting up to 7 days; possibly vomiting, diarrhea, anorexia, lymphadenopathy *Complications:* Otitis media, pneumonia, laryngotracheitis, encephalitis	*Supportive management:* Acetaminophen, fluids, and bed rest until fever subsides; dim lights or sunglasses if patient is photophobic	Institute seizure precautions (high fever is possible: 104°F [40°C]). Cleanse patient's eyes to remove crusting and decrease rubbing. Use a cool-mist humidifier for cough. Offer small, frequent meals of bland foods. Keep patient's skin clean and dry; administer tepid baths. Restrict to quiet activities until child feels better, usually by day 6 of rash. Use airborne precautions to prevent spread of infection. Teach and encourage good hand hygiene technique. Notify health care provider of ear pain, chest pain, difficulty breathing, headaches.
Rubella (German Measles)			
Etiology: Rubivirus *Transmission:* Direct contact with nasopharyngeal secretions of infected person; indirect contact with contaminated articles (fomites); transplacental transmission *Incubation period:* 14–21 days *Communicable period:* 7 days before to 5 days after rash appears	*Prodrome:* Young children—possible lymphadenopathy; adolescents and adults—low-grade fever, headache, sore throat, anorexia, clear nasal discharge, cough, lymphadenopathy for 1–5 days *Acute phase:* Pinkish red maculopapular rash beginning on face; spreads to trunk, then extremities within 3 days *Complications:* Usually none; rare complications include arthritis, encephalitis; birth defects as virus crosses placenta (teratogenic)	*Supportive management:* Acetaminophen for fever or discomfort	Provide airborne precautions to prevent spread of infection. Teach and encourage good hand hygiene technique. Institute comfort measures as needed. Isolate child from pregnant women. Reassure parents of benign nature of illness in affected child.
Roseola Infantum (Exanthema Subitum)			
Etiology: Human herpesvirus, type 6 *Transmission:* Unknown; occurs in children aged 6–24 months *Incubation period:* Unknown *Communicable period:* Unknown	Sudden-onset, persistent high fever, lasting up to 4 days; child appears well otherwise; fever rapidly falls to normal, followed by rose-pink macular or maculopapular rash on trunk and spreads to rest of body; rash lasts 1–2 days and is nonpruritic *Complications:* Febrile seizures	*Supportive management:* Acetaminophen for fever; seizure precautions if child is prone to febrile seizures; encourage child to drink fluids	Teach parents how to lower fever safely. Reassure parents as to benign nature of illness. If child is prone to seizures, discuss appropriate precautions. Follow standard precautions.

Table 32.6   **Childhood Communicable Diseases—cont'd**

DISEASE	CLINICAL MANIFESTATIONS	MEDICAL MANAGEMENT	NURSING INTERVENTIONS
Varicella (Chickenpox)			
Etiology: Varicella zoster virus (herpesvirus) *Transmission:* Direct contact with respiratory tract secretions; indirect contact with contaminated articles; airborne droplets *Incubation period:* 10–21 days (usually 13–17 days) *Communicable period:* 1 day before eruption until all lesions crusted (1 week after onset)	*Prodrome:* Low-grade fever, malaise, anorexia for 24 h *Acute phase:* Pruritic rash on trunk, face, proximal extremities, mucous membranes for 3–5 days, beginning as macules, progressing to papules and then vesicles on erythematous base; vesicles rupture, causing oozing and crusting; all three stages present in various intensities *Complications:* In children—possibly secondary bacterial skin infections; in adults—pneumonia, encephalitis, laryngeal edema, hemorrhagic varicella, thrombocytopenia	*Supportive management:* Acetaminophen for fever; systemic or topical antipruritics or systemic antihistamines; keeping skin clean and dry; antiviral treatment consisting of acyclovir ; varicella zoster immune globulin within 3 days of exposure in children at high risk (those who are immunocompromised or have leukemia; newborns)	Keep patient's nails short and smooth; give daily baths without soap; dress patient in lightweight, loose clothing; administer antipruritics or antihistamines as ordered; teach child to apply pressure on itch rather than scratching; place mittens on hands of young children. Use airborne and contact precautions in hospital. If patient is at home, instruct parents to isolate ill patient from siblings, children at high risk, and adults until lesions dry. Teach and encourage good hand hygiene technique. Administer acetaminophen as ordered. Encourage patient to drink fluids.
Erythema Infectiosum (Fifth Disease)			
Etiology: Human parvovirus B19 *Transmission:* Respiratory tract secretions and blood *Incubation period:* 4–14 days but up to 20 days *Communicable period:* Unknown; probably before signs and symptoms develop; communicability unlikely once rash develops	*Prodrome:* In children with aplastic crisis—fever, malaise, myalgia; rash usually absent *Acute phase:* Rash appears in three stages: • First stage: red rash on face, "slapped cheek" appearance (fades in 1–4 days), circumoral pallor • Second stage: maculopapular, lacelike rash on upper extremities spreading to trunk and thighs; lasts 1 week or longer • Third stage: possible for rash to recur periodically for weeks in response to heat, sunlight, cold *Complications:* Arthralgia, arthritis (infrequent in children but common in adults); encephalitis, myocarditis (rare); maternal infection (low risk for fetal hydrops)	*Supportive management:* Acetaminophen for fever; analgesic or anti-inflammatory drugs	For hospitalized child, use droplet precautions for 7 days after onset: no isolation is necessary at home. Teach and encourage good hand hygiene technique. Institute comfort measures as necessary.

Continued

Table 32.6	Childhood Communicable Diseases—cont'd

DISEASE	CLINICAL MANIFESTATIONS	MEDICAL MANAGEMENT	NURSING INTERVENTIONS
Scarlet Fever			
Etiology: Group A β-hemolytic streptococci *Transmission:* Direct contact with respiratory tract secretions of infected person *Incubation period:* 2–5 days (average, 3 days) *Communicable period:* During incubation and acute illness phases	*Prodrome:* Sudden-onset high fever, vomiting, headache, chills, malaise *Acute phase:* Tonsillitis, pharyngitis, white strawberry tongue (tongue has white coating and papillae become red and edematous) by day 1 or 2; by day 4, white coating sloughs, leaving red strawberry tongue; sandpaper-like red rash appears about 12 h after prodrome and is intense in skinfolds; cheeks are flushed and circumoral pallor is present; desquamation begins by end of first week and continues for 3 weeks or longer *Complications:* Otitis media, pneumonia, sinusitis, glomerulonephritis, carditis, peritonsillar abscess	*Antimicrobial treatment:* Full course of penicillin or, for patients allergic to penicillin, erythromycin *Supportive management:* Bed rest, analgesics, fluids	Institute respiratory precautions until completion of first 24 h of antimicrobial treatment. Teach and encourage good hand hygiene technique. Offer soft diet if child can chew; encourage drinking fluids. Restrict to quiet activities until child feels better. Offer lozenges, gargles, and cool-mist humidifier for throat. Maintain good oral hygiene. Advise parents to consult health care provider if fever persists after therapy begins. Discuss procedures for preventing spread of infection.
Diphtheria			
Etiology: Corynebacterium diphtheriae *Transmission:* Direct contact with nose, eye, throat discharges or skin lesions of infected person; in rare cases, fomite transmission or foodborne outbreaks *Incubation period:* 2–5 days *Communicable period:* Untreated person: 2 weeks to several months	Clinical manifestations vary according to diphtheritic membrane affected: • Nasal: nasal discharge—serosanguineous and mucopurulent, possible progression to epistaxis • White membrane on nasal septum • Tonsillar or pharyngeal: pharyngitis; malaise; anorexia; fever (low grade) • Membrane over tonsils, pharynx; lymphadenitis; laryngeal: cough, fever, hoarseness *Complications:* Airway obstruction, thrombocytopenia, myocarditis, vocal cord paralysis	*Antimicrobial treatment:* Penicillin or erythromycin; antitoxin, usually IV, preceded by skin testing for horse serum sensitivity; possible tracheostomy for respiratory obstruction	Institute droplet precautions. Maintain bed rest. Offer liquid or soft diet. Perform gentle suctioning, as necessary. Observe for signs of respiratory distress or obstruction: dyspnea, apprehensiveness, cyanosis; report such findings to health care provider. Keep tracheostomy set at patient's bedside. Regulate humidity for optimal liquefaction of secretions.

Table 32.6   Childhood Communicable Diseases—cont'd

DISEASE	CLINICAL MANIFESTATIONS	MEDICAL MANAGEMENT	NURSING INTERVENTIONS
Mumps (Parotitis)			
Etiology: Paramyxovirus *Transmission:* Direct contact with respiratory tract secretions of infected person *Incubation period:* 16–18 days *Communicable period:* Up to 7 days before parotid edema to 5–9 days after onset of signs and symptoms	*Prodrome:* Fever, malaise, headache *Acute phase:* Unilateral or bilateral edema and tenderness of parotid glands by day 3; chewing aggravates "earlike" pain *Complications:* Meningoencephalitis, epididymoorchitis, arthritis, sensorineural deafness, myocarditis, sterility in male patients (rare)	*Supportive management:* Acetaminophen for fever, analgesics for pain; IV fluids sometimes necessary for a child who refuses to eat or drink	Institute droplet precautions for 9 days after onset of edema or until edema has subsided. Teach and encourage good hand hygiene technique. Offer soft, bland diet; encourage child to drink fluids. Use warm or cool compresses for edema. Dress boy in tightly fitting underpants or scrotal support for orchitis.
Pertussis (Whooping Cough)			
Etiology: Bordetella pertussis *Transmission:* Direct contact or droplet spread of respiratory tract secretions of infected person *Incubation period:* 7–20 days *Communicable period:* From prodromal stage through fourth week	*Prodrome:* Upper respiratory tract infection signs and symptoms for 1–2 weeks; cough, sneezing, little or no fever, headache, anorexia *Acute phase:* Paroxysmal stage—dry, hacking cough followed by prolonged inspiration ("whoop" sound) most often at night; paroxysms usually followed by vomiting of thick, stringy mucus; lasts 4–6 weeks *Convalescent stage:* Decrease in coughing and whooping; lasts 1–2 weeks *Complications:* Pneumonia, hypoxia, atelectasis, otitis media, seizures, dehydration, weight loss, prolapsed rectum, hernia, hemorrhage (epistaxis, subconjunctival), cerebral edema, and central nervous system (CNS) disturbances	*Antimicrobial treatment:* Erythromycin or trimethoprim-sulfamethoxazole for 7–10 days *Antiseizure treatment:* For patients experiencing seizures; phenytoin; supportive management—hospitalization required for infants or children with underlying pulmonary or cardiac disease, dehydration, or severe signs and symptoms; gentle suctioning to prevent choking, high humidified oxygen therapy; IV fluids; intubation set at patient's bedside for emergency	Institute droplet precautions. Enforce strict hand hygiene. Maintain bed rest if child is febrile; offer quiet activities. Offer liquids: small amounts frequently; if child vomits, refeed. Monitor cardiac and respiratory status. Observe for signs of airway obstruction (dyspnea, restlessness, cyanosis) and report such findings to the health care provider. Provide high humidity and gentle, frequent suctioning to prevent choking. Reassure parents during paroxysms. Teach parents in the use of a cool-mist humidifier to avoid triggers of paroxysms (dust, smoke, chilling, sudden change in temperature, excitement). Teach parents how to recognize signs of respiratory distress and arrange for a public health nurse to visit after discharge from hospital.

IV, Intravenous.

surgical treatment, ensure that they are loose enough to allow accumulated drainage to flow out of the ear; otherwise the infection may migrate to the mastoid process. The wicks must be kept dry during shampoos or baths.

Emphasize the importance of taking the medication for the fully prescribed course to ensure eradication of the infection. To educate parents in the prevention of otitis media, teach them to hold their infant in an upright position when feeding. If the child has tympanostomy tubes, teach parents postoperative care. They must protect the ear during bathing, shampooing, and swimming, because bacteria from the water can be introduced into the ear.

Prognosis. The most common complication of otitis media is mild to moderate hearing loss as a result of chronic or recurrent effusion. The episodic (temporary) hearing loss that sometimes occurs during occasional bouts of otitis media is usually reversible; however, conductive hearing loss associated with chronic otitis media is in some cases permanent and has potential to interfere with language and cognitive development.

Vision

Refractive Errors (Myopia And Hyperopia). Refractive errors occur when light rays entering the lens are bent and fall in front of or behind the retina, which prevents the image from falling on a single point on the retina as it normally does. Two of the most common refractive errors in childhood are myopia (nearsightedness) and hyperopia (farsightedness), which result in loss of visual acuity. Screening tests that measure visual acuity assist in identifying refractive errors. Treatment consists of corrective lenses and periodic reevaluation. The nurse plays a vital role in ensuring vision screening, especially in the preschool years.

Strabismus. In strabismus, a lack of coordination in the extraocular musculature results in a cross-eyed appearance. Strabismus is caused by muscle imbalance, results from paralysis, or in some cases is congenitally acquired. The condition affects sometimes one and sometimes both eyes and causes the brain to receive two images (instead of one). Common clinical manifestations include squinting, closing one eye, tilting the head (to block out one image), and difficulty focusing or picking up objects. Medical management varies according to the cause of the strabismus. There is no treatment that will align the eyes perfectly. The goal is to align them as close to normal as possible. The injection of botulinum toxin (Botox) into the extraocular muscle has been effective in relaxing the muscles in strabismic patients. Often the stronger eye is patched in an attempt to strengthen the muscles of the weakened eye. Surgical intervention may be required if other measures are not effective. Nursing intervention includes adequate explanation of the treatment plan, care of corrective lenses, instruction in eye exercises, and reinforcement of occlusive patches if they become loose.

Left untreated, strabismus increases the risk for amblyopia (lazy eye; reduction or dimness of vision, especially in which there is no apparent pathologic condition of the eye), in which visual acuity is lost. This complication can be prevented if the underlying problem is corrected before the child is 6 years of age.

Periorbital Cellulitis

Etiology And Pathophysiology. Periorbital cellulitis is a serious inflammation of the eyelid and periorbital area. The condition is usually unilateral and has the potential to affect the eye and the CNS. Conjunctivitis, impetigo, insect bites, and trauma are all possible causes of periorbital cellulitis. Common causative organisms include *H. influenzae*, *S. aureus*, and group A β-hemolytic streptococci.

Clinical Manifestations. Children with periorbital cellulitis usually experience pain, tenderness, fever, erythema (of distinctive magenta color), and edema of the eyelids and periorbital area. Headache and purulent nasal discharge are also sometimes present.

Diagnostic Tests. Cultures of the eye, the nose, and the blood help identify the causative agent. Ultrasonography and CT of the orbit are sometimes useful for ruling out abscess.

Medical Management. Because of the emergency nature of the illness, the child is hospitalized for aggressive IV antibiotic administration. Analgesics and antipyretics commonly are administered for pain and fever. Warm compresses also help relieve discomfort.

Nursing Interventions And Patient Teaching. As the edema decreases, the skin around the eye becomes dry and begins to peel. Preserving skin integrity involves the application of a thin layer of petrolatum to the area.

Reassure parents that eye discoloration sometimes persists for several days and that most children recover completely without complication.

Prognosis. The edema usually subsides within 36 hours of antibiotic therapy. With appropriate treatment, the prognosis is usually excellent.

Nasal Cavity

Allergic Rhinitis

Etiology And Pathophysiology. Allergic rhinitis occurs in about 40% of the pediatric population (Asthma and Allergy Foundation of America, n.d.). Allergic rhinitis is either seasonal or perennial, and affected children have a familial predisposition to allergy. Exposure to an inhaled allergen triggers the allergic response.

Clinical Manifestations. The signs and symptoms common in the pediatric population include congestion, sniffling, mouth breathing, itchy nose, and postnasal drip. Often there is a line in the skin that is visible across the nose as a result of nasal rubbing ("allergic salute"). The medical management and nursing interventions for children with allergic rhinitis are the same as those for affected adults.

COGNITIVE DISORDERS

DISORDERS OF COGNITIVE FUNCTION

Cognitive disorders is a broad category of disorders that affect the individual's mental processes for gaining understanding, knowledge, and problem solving. Cognitive disorders include intellectual impairment, psychological disorders, learning disabilities, and developmental delays and disorders. A child's cognitive health is an integral part of the total well-being of the child. A variety of factors influence the personality and the developmental capabilities of a child, including genetic composition, environment, social support, and culture. It is appropriate to assess children for emotional as well as physical problems during all visits with a health care provider. Children in whom a cognitive impairment has been diagnosed require prompt intervention by specialists in the field of mental health, as do their families. The nurse is instrumental in providing appropriate referrals and offering emotional support to the child and the family (see the Health Promotion box).

Encouraging Healthy Behaviors for Children With a Cognitive Disorder

DOWN SYNDROME
- Provide information to parents about expected delays in milestones.
- Encourage stimulating play.
- Provide nutritionally dense foods.
- Encourage physical activity and exercise.
- Praise child for accomplishments.
- Provide consistency in matters relating to discipline.
- Ensure patients have been evaluated for atlantoaxial instability before rigorous physical activity.

ATTENTION DEFICIT/HYPERACTIVITY DISORDER
- Provide a routine for daily activities.
- Maintain a nonstressful environment, but set limits and provide rewards.
- Encourage parents to seek training in behavioral therapy to learn effective ways of dealing with their child.
- Allow child time to explain events or interactions to aid in reducing stress.
- Encourage parents to continue therapeutic regimen and to monitor for medication side effects if medications are prescribed.

DEPRESSION
- Establish a trusting family relationship.
- Review treatment plan with parents as needed.
- To discourage social isolation, provide positive reinforcement when child participates in group activities.
- Identify support groups within the community for the child and for the parents.

SUICIDE
- Alert parents to signs that include depression, social isolation, social withdrawal, changes in grades, giving away important possessions, preoccupation with death, and changes in eating and sleeping habits.
- Encourage parents and child to stay in contact with school, peers, and relatives for emotional support at this time.

Cognitive Impairment

Intellectual disability (formerly called *mental retardation*) is the most common developmental disability. It refers to significantly subaverage general intellectual functioning that exists concurrently with deficits in adaptive behavior and is manifested before the 18th birthday. Intellectual disability is identified by assessing adaptive behaviors and the intelligence quotient (IQ), an index of relative intelligence determined through the subject's answers to arbitrarily chosen questions. Usually the person with an intellectual disability has an IQ of 70 or less, but the diagnosis is not made solely on the score on the IQ test. Although the diagnostic determination is based on limitations, a thorough evaluation will include an assessment of strengths that will be used in the treatment plan (American Association on Intellectual and Developmental Disabilities [AAIDD], n.d.).

Etiology And Pathophysiology. The causes of intellectual impairment are varied and include biochemical, infectious, genetic, endocrine, and idiopathic factors. Specific causes include chromosomal abnormalities, such as Down syndrome; perinatal infections, such as cytomegalovirus, rubella, syphilis, and toxoplasmosis; perinatal anoxia; maternal drug or alcohol abuse; metabolic disorders, such as phenylketonuria; lead poisoning; hypothyroidism; and prematurity.

Clinical Manifestations. Manifestations vary according to the child's age and degree of impairment. Affected children typically fail to achieve developmental milestones at appropriate ages. In general, they tend to manifest delays in motor, social, cognitive, or language skills, or some combination of these.

Diagnostic Tests. In a child suspected of having intellectual impairment, it is important to begin assessment as soon as the parents or the health care provider realizes that the child is not developing normally. Diagnostic studies include neurologic examination, CT, serum metabolic screening, developmental screening tests (e.g., DENVER II), standardized intellectual tests (e.g., Stanford-Binet Intelligence Scale; Wechsler Intelligence Scale for Children, Revised), and chromosomal analysis and genetic screening.

Nursing Interventions. Nursing interventions for a child with an intellectual impairment focus on promoting optimal development and providing the family with emotional support, education, and referrals. The family needs support at the time of initial diagnosis, as well as encouragement to verbalize their fears and concerns. Encourage parents to enroll the child in an early intervention program that will facilitate the child's self-care abilities and assist the family with future needs. When teaching, break up each task into small, specific steps because the child cannot always understand the task as a whole. The parents are encouraged to keep their focus on the normal needs of all children—including love, social interaction, and play—regardless of children's intellectual ability (see the Safety Alert box).

Patient And Family Teaching. Provide parents with information about normal developmental milestones, stimulation techniques, safety, normal speech development, sexual development, and the role of positive self-esteem in motivating children to accomplish goals within their limitations.

Prognosis. Cognitive impairment is a chronic condition. The philosophy of care toward people with cognitive impairment has undergone major changes since the 1960s. Children with cognitive impairment are no longer automatically admitted into institutional settings; many remain at home.

Safety Alert

Children With a Cognitive Disorder

DOWN SYNDROME

- Some children with Down syndrome may have a disorder called atlantoaxial instability. This disorder is characterized by excessive movement at the junction between cervical vertebra 1 (C1) and cervical vertebra 2 (C2). Injury to the spinal cord can result, especially with physical activity. It is essential to ensure that parents are educated about this disorder and that children have been evaluated for atlantoaxial instability. Symptoms of the disorder include neck pain, weakness, and torticollis (abnormal, asymmetric head or neck position). Affected children are at risk for spinal cord compression, which places the child at risk of losing established motor skills and bladder or bowel control.
- Report immediately to a health care provider any child with the following signs of spinal cord compression:
  - Persistent neck pain
  - Loss of established motor skills and bladder or bowel control
  - Changes in sensation
- Monitor the child's airway clearance.
- Measures to decrease respiratory infections include clearing the child's nose with a bulb type of syringe, rinsing the mouth with water after feedings, increasing fluid intake, and using a cool-mist vaporizer to keep the mucous membranes moist and the secretions liquefied. Other helpful measures include changing the child's position frequently, performing postural drainage with percussion if necessary, practicing good hand hygiene, and properly disposing of soiled articles such as tissues.
- Monitor for adequate nutritional and fluid intake. The protruding tongue also interferes with feeding, especially of solid foods. Parents need to know that the tongue thrust is not an indication of refusal to feed but a physiologic response. Advise parents to use a small but long straight-handled spoon to push the food toward the back and side of the mouth. If the child thrusts the food out, the parent feeds it in again. Decreased muscle tone affects gastric motility, which predisposes the child to constipation. Dietary measures such as increased fiber and fluid intake promote evacuation. It is important to supervise dietary intake. It is sometimes necessary to scrutinize the child's eating habits to prevent obesity.

ATTENTION DEFICIT/HYPERACTIVITY DISORDER

- Keep in mind that children with attention deficit/hyperactivity disorder (ADHD) often are distracted easily by extraneous stimuli and may have difficulty following directions.
- Children with ADHD are prone to impulsive behaviors which may lead to outbursts, aggressive actions, excessive risk taking, and self-harm. These children have difficulty thinking through the consequences of such actions before acting upon their impulses
- Poor impulse control and difficulty predicting the natural consequences of actions makes parenting challenging. Parents are encouraged to prioritize the behaviors that need correction. Prioritizing the problems will increase success.
- Reward systems are effective and do not result in increased anger or aggression. Create challenging but attainable goals.
- Use pictures, demonstrations, or written lists for teaching and learning.
- Also keep in mind that such children may have difficulty switching tasks. The child generally has a difficult time planning and initiating the task then maintaining focus. The directive to move to a new task can be frustrating. The use of a visual timer can help the child with time management.

DEPRESSION

- Assess for diminished affect, fatigue with reduced motor activity, solitary play or lack of interest in play, tearfulness or crying, dependency and clinging behavior, and aggressive and disruptive behavior.
- Identification of the depressed child with suicidal tendencies and making appropriate referrals are important nursing functions.

SUICIDE

- Hospitalization is sometimes necessary for the child's self-protection.
- Provide constant monitoring to prevent self-injury.

Down Syndrome. Varying degrees of cognitive impairment and comorbidities characterize **Down syndrome,** a congenital chromosomal abnormality. It is the most common chromosomal abnormality, affecting 1 per 800 live births (CDC, 2021a).

Etiology And Pathophysiology. The incidence of Down syndrome in the United States is 1 per 800 live births. Although the risk of having a child with Down syndrome increases with maternal age, the majority of all infants with Down syndrome are born to mothers younger than 35 years old, because the majority of all babies are born to mothers in this younger age group (CDC, 2021a).

Clinical Manifestations. Children with Down syndrome have a characteristic facial appearance (Fig. 32.31). Most frequently, manifestations in the infant include a small, rounded skull with a flat occiput; upward-slanting eyes with epicanthal folds; broad, flat nose; protruding tongue; short, thick neck; hypotonic extremities; mottled skin; low-set ears; and a simian crease on the palmar side of the hand. All children with Down syndrome have some degree of intellectual impairment, ranging from low normal intelligence to severe cognitive impairment. Individual abilities vary greatly, but in general, children with Down syndrome typically display the following:

- Strengths in visual processing over auditory
- Weaknesses in grammar and language
- Delays in motor development

Children with Down syndrome are prone to upper respiratory infections and frequent otitis media, and many such children have congenital heart defects,

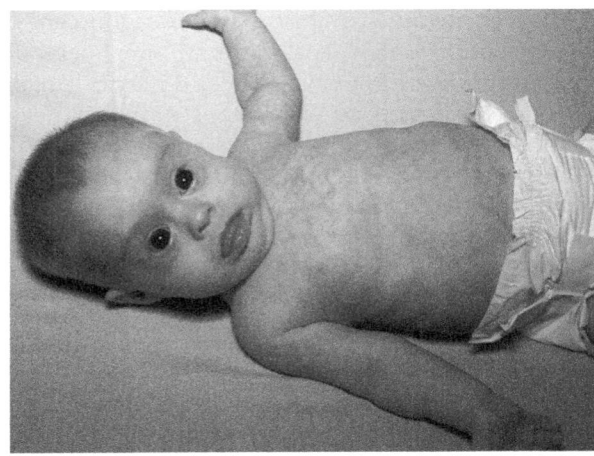

Fig. 32.31 Down syndrome in infant. Note small, square head; upward slant to the eyes; flat nasal bridge; protruding tongue; mottled skin; and hypotonia. (From Hockenberry MJ, Wilson D: *Wong's essentials of pediatric nursing*, ed 9, St. Louis, 2013, Mosby.)

which are the chief cause of death, particularly during the first year of life. Other associated health problems include increased incidence of leukemia, dysfunction of the immune system, and thyroid dysfunction, especially congenital hypothyroidism.

Diagnostic Tests. As an adjunct to the characteristic manifestations indicating the diagnosis of Down syndrome, a chromosomal analysis helps confirm the chromosomal abnormality. Individuals with Down syndrome have a higher incidence of cardiac disorders. Cardiovascular system testing, including electrocardiography and radiographic studies, may be performed to assess function and potential abnormalities.

Medical Management. In addition to routine medical care, corrective surgery is indicated in some cases for congenital heart defects. Auditory and vision screening are standard in assessing for any sensory impairments. Treatment of otitis media is necessary to prevent auditory loss, which can hamper cognitive function. Most experts also recommend thyroid function tests. If growth is delayed, it is important to carefully monitor and document nutrition, height, and weight. In an attempt to increase height, health care providers give growth hormones in some cases.

Nursing Interventions. Care for children with Down syndrome is similar to that discussed earlier for children with intellectual impairment. The child with Down syndrome is at a higher risk for other diseases and conditions. Down syndrome is a genetic disorder, not a disease, but children with Down syndrome have higher rates of certain diseases and conditions. The child may need additional screening and treatment than their typical peers. Primary nursing goals include emotionally supporting the family at the time of diagnosis and referring the child and family to agencies that provide support and services.

The language the nurse uses to discuss the disability has the capacity to enhance the therapeutic relationship between the nurse and the child and their family. As with other types of disabilities, it is important to use "person first" language when discussing the condition. Person first language states that a person "has" a condition rather than being defined by it. Children with Down syndrome have often been referred to as "Down syndrome children" rather than "children with Down syndrome." Using proper terminology shows respect for the person. It is also important to note that the terminology of "retarded" or "retardation" is often used as an insult with the intent to humiliate another person. Early terminology of "mental retardation" has been replaced by "intellectual disability" when referring to the IQ or "cognitive disability" when referring more broadly to the thought processes and problem solving as well as the intellectual impairment. The terminology of "Down's" is not preferred, as it implies ownership.

Patient And Family Teaching. The family needs education regarding their child's condition. Information regarding services available to children with Down syndrome should be conveyed to family members. The goal of treatment is to help the child reach their highest potential. Services available include speech, occupational, and physical therapy. In the United States virtually every state has early intervention programs for these children, so treatment can be initiated promptly. Children with cognitive impairments need encouragement and guidance to become self-advocates. This is especially true in children with Down syndrome because they exhibit an outward appearance that allows people to misjudge the capabilities and limitations of the individual based on appearance alone.

Prognosis. The life expectancy for people with Down syndrome has drastically improved over recent decades. In the 1960s a child born with Down syndrome would face a life expectancy of only 10 years. Over the following years, the life expectancy has made great strides. 50 years later this life expectancy has more than quadrupled (CDC, 2021a). Down syndrome is associated with earlier onset of age-related problems, such as Alzheimer disease and other types of cognitive decline. Studies support the influence of a more rapid aging process as a result of the genetic defect associated with Down syndrome (NDSS, 2017). People with Down syndrome tend to be of shorter stature and larger weight in childhood as well as adulthood. Although there is limited research on BMI in populations affected by Down syndrome, increased body mass index (BMI) is a common risk factor for comorbidities known to reduce lifespan. At this point, research into the conditions affecting people with Down syndrome is disproportionately low when compared the research into other genetic anomalies (Global Down Syndrome Foundation, 2018). As the prognosis continues to improve for these individuals, it is important to provide for their long-term health care and for their social and leisure needs.

Autism. **Autism** is a developmental disorder of brain functioning. Autism affects normal development of intelligence and behavior and results in impairments in social interactions and communications and in repetitive behaviors. *Autism spectrum disorder* refers to a broad group of developmental disabilities that vary in severity. Autism occurs in 1 in 68 children, with 1 in 42 boys and 1 in 189 girls. Autism typically is diagnosed between the ages of 2 and 3 years of age but can be diagnosed as early as 18 months of age in some cases (Autism Speaks, n.d.).

Etiology And Pathophysiology. The cause of autism remains unknown. The condition results in brain development that affects how a person perceives and socializes with others. Children and adults with autism spectrum disorder experience problems in social interaction and communication. Depending on the severity, functioning in society is often difficult.

There are several different genetic abnormalities that have been found to lead to autism spectrum disorder. Some genes are thought to affect brain development or the way that brain cells communicate. Other genetic disorders resulting in autism are related to fragile X syndrome, whereas some are related to inherited factors. Some research indicates that environmental factors also may play a role in the development of the disorder (Mayo Clinic, 2018a).

Thimerosal, a mercury-based preservative that previously was used in most childhood vaccines, was rumored to be a cause of autism. Thimerosal is no longer used in vaccinations (with the exception of some influenza vaccines). Multiple research studies have confirmed that there is no link between vaccines, vaccine schedules, or any part of vaccines and the development of autism (Mayo Clinic, 2018a; CDC, 2020f). Fears and misinformation about a connection between autism and vaccines continue. The largest autism advocacy organization, Autism Speaks, supports findings of the scientific research studies that confirm that vaccines do not cause autism. When the research studies were analyzed, over 1.2 million children had participated in the research studies that reached this conclusion (Autism Speaks, 2014).

Clinical Manifestations And Diagnostic Tests. Children with autism may demonstrate alterations in social interactions, communication, and behavior. One hallmark characteristic is the inability to maintain eye contact with another person. Parents of autistic children have noted difficulties that their infants had at a very early age with eye contact and avoidance of body contact. Children with autism also display limited functional play and sometimes interact with toys in an unusual manner.

Children with autism may display stereotypical motor activities such as rhythmic rocking of their bodies, flapping of their hands, or spinning in circles. These are referred to as *self-stimulation behaviors*. One or all the body senses may be employed in the behaviors. Some autistic children have significant GI symptoms; constipation is a common one. Social development is affected; an autistic child may be unable to understand other people's feelings. Not all children with autism have the same manifestations. Some have mild forms that necessitate minimal supervision, and some have severe forms in which self-abusive behavior is common. The majority of children with autism have some degree of cognitive disability, with scores typically in the moderate to severe range. Very low intelligence scores are more common among affected girls than among affected boys. Despite their relatively moderate to severe disability, some children with autism excel in particular areas, such as art, music, memory, mathematics, or perceptual skills, such as puzzle building.

Speech and language delays are also common in autistic children. The American Academy of Pediatrics recommends that all children be screened for developmental delays at well-child visits at the ages of 9 months, 18 months, and 24 months. It is further recommended that all children be screened for autism at 18 and 24 months of age (CDC, 2020g). Early recognition, referral, and intervention are important for improving outcomes for children with autism.

Nursing Interventions. Therapeutic intervention for a child with autism is a specialized area involving professionals with advanced training. Although there is no cure for autism, numerous therapies can be attempted. The most promising results have been achieved through highly structured and intensive behavior modification programs. In general, the objective in these programs is to promote positive reinforcement, increase social awareness of other people, teach verbal communication skills, and decrease unacceptable behavior. Providing a structured routine for the child to follow is key in managing autism.

When these children are in the hospital, the parents must be included in planning care and ideally stay with the child as much as possible. Recognize that not all children with autism have the same problems and that each one requires individual assessment and treatment. Decreasing stimulation by using a private room, avoiding extraneous auditory and visual distractions, and encouraging the parents to bring in possessions that the child is attached to usually help lessen the disruptiveness of hospitalization. Because physical contact often upsets these children, minimal holding and eye contact are sometimes necessary to prevent behavioral outbursts. Take care when performing procedures on, administering medicine to, or feeding these children, because many are fussy eaters who at times willfully starve themselves or gag to avoid eating, and many are indiscriminate gorgers, swallowing any available edible or inedible items, such as a thermometer. Eating habits of autistic children tend to be particularly problematic for families and often involve food refusal, mouthing objects, eating inedible items, and smelling and throwing food.

Children with autism need to be introduced slowly to new situations. Visits with staff caregivers should be kept short whenever possible. Because these children have difficulty organizing their behavior and redirecting their energy, they need to be told directly what to do. Communication should be at the child's developmental level, brief, and concrete.

Prognosis. Autism encompasses a broad spectrum of behaviors and levels of severity. Some children with autism ultimately achieve independence, but others may require lifelong adult supervision. Aggravation of psychiatric symptoms occurs in about half of these children during adolescence; affected girls have a tendency for continued deterioration. The earlier the diagnosis and treatment are, the better is the chance for a more positive outcome. Family involvement is needed to promote the best possible outcome. Additional information may be found at the Autism Speaks website (www.autismspeaks.org).

SCHOOL AVOIDANCE (SCHOOL PHOBIA, SCHOOL REFUSAL)

School avoidance occurs when a physically healthy child repeatedly stays home from school or is sent home from school for physical symptoms of an emotional origin. School avoidance is the most common cause of vague physical symptoms in school-age children. It affects approximately 5% of elementary school–age children and 2% of middle school students. It is possible that the incidence of school avoidance is decreasing as more mothers are in the workplace. This trend requires young children to master the conflict of separation at an earlier age.

Etiology and Pathophysiology

For some children, school avoidance is related to anxiety. Often they are worried about academic progress, peer conflicts, or marital discord in the home. Separation anxiety is also common among these children even after the normal age when this issue is mastered (3 to 4 years). These children tend to have an overprotective parent. Other children may not be anxious at all but receive secondary gains from their avoidance at school. These children stretch out an illness until they get extremely behind in their studies. Some parents of these children are too lenient, some place little value on education, and others are unconcerned about the ramifications of missing school.

Clinical Manifestations

Children who are anxious tend to have physiologic symptoms of anxiety, including headache, recurrent abdominal pain (RAP), vomiting, diarrhea, insomnia, pallor, palpitations, and hyperventilation. The child who receives secondary gains typically exaggerates or fabricates symptoms such as sore throat, leg pain, coughing tics, chest pain, and fatigue. Upon physical examination and laboratory testing, no organic cause is found. The child usually sounds very sick but appears to be well. Symptoms usually appear in the morning and decrease once the child is told he or she is not going to school.

Diagnostic Tests

Diagnostic tests are usually not indicated. Specific complaints help determine which laboratory tests, if any, may be indicated.

Medical Management and Nursing Interventions

Once the health care provider establishes the diagnosis, the nurse's primary role is to assist in convincing parents that their child is physically healthy, explain the diagnosis of school avoidance to them, and assist in returning the child to regular school attendance. Parents need to be educated that school avoidance occurs in "normal" children and that it is stress related and not a psychiatric disorder. Once parents are convinced that their child is healthy, it is necessary that the child immediately return to school. Parents are told to be firm in the morning if the child is refusing to go to school. It is important to bring any somatic complaints to the attention of the primary care provider and, if the condition is minor or without an organic cause, to then send the child to school. Reassure the child that nothing is physically wrong with him or her and that he or she is in good health. Together with the parents explain to the child that attendance at school is not negotiable. They provide emotional support and reassurance to the child who is anxious about peer or academic issues.

LEARNING DISABILITIES

It is estimated that learning disabilities affect approximately 13%, or 6.6 million, of all school-age children in the United States (National Center for Education Statistics [NCES], 2021). Learning disabilities impair a child's ability to understand, assimilate, recall, or produce information. Children with learning disabilities usually score significantly poorly on tests of academic achievement in mathematics, reading, writing, or some combination. Overall intelligence may or may not be affected. Some children display advanced ability to learn some subjects while struggling in others. The factors that underlie learning problems typically exist before school entry but often do not become apparent until academic demands are placed on the child.

Etiology and Pathophysiology

The cause of learning disabilities is multifactorial, and a specific cause often cannot be identified. Some affected children have a family history of learning disabilities. Learning problems are sometimes the result of various physiologic or environmental factors, or both, such as intrauterine exposure to alcohol, drugs, or infection; birth trauma; seizures; attention-deficit disorders; head trauma; malnutrition; and exposure to toxic substances, such as lead. Hearing or vision impairments sometimes lead to learning problems, and it is important to include the necessary screening procedures in the diagnostic assessment before the diagnosis is established. Genetic syndromes such as fragile X syndrome or Prader-Willi syndrome sometimes occur in association with learning disabilities.

Clinical Manifestations

Children with learning disabilities sometimes manifest problems with speech, behavior, or motor coordination or a combination of these; failure to master basic, grade-appropriate academic skills in one or more subject areas; and a progressive decline in school performance. Other possible manifestations include delayed acquisition of language milestones, deficient social skills, avoidance behavior in response to challenging tasks, low frustration tolerance, disorganization, and somnolence.

Diagnostic Tests

A thorough history and physical examination sometimes reveal specific indications to measure the lead level and perform electroencephalography, chromosomal studies, and hearing and vision screenings. General intelligence and achievement testing and neuropsychological testing help to identify cognitive strengths and weaknesses and in developing a comprehensive educational plan.

Medical Management and Nursing Interventions

Learning disabilities are managed primarily through appropriate educational referrals. Parents need to be educated about the special education process. Federal law requires that all schools provide a comprehensive evaluation on written request from the parents to the school principal. Therapeutic manipulation of the educational setting may include special arrangements within a regular classroom, alternative classroom placement, tutoring, and remediation assistance. Reevaluation for special education is required at least every 3 years, more frequently in certain situations, depending on age, severity of disability, and academic progression. An important referral source for parents of a child with a learning disability is the National Center for Learning Disabilities (www.ncld.org).

Prognosis

With early identification, appropriate referrals, and proper educational interventions, the negative consequences of difficulty in school can be avoided, and children with a learning disability are usually able to function optimally within their limitations.

ATTENTION DEFICIT/HYPERACTIVITY DISORDER

Attention deficit/hyperactivity disorder (ADHD) is a group of behaviors—hyperactivity, inattentiveness, and impulsivity—that appear early in a child's life, persist throughout childhood and adolescence, and sometimes extend into adulthood. ADHD is being diagnosed at an increasing rate in America. Some studies indicate that 5% of children have ADHD, whereas other studies estimate the number of children affected to be 11%. ADHD is diagnosed more frequently in boys than girls (CDC, 2020a).

Etiology and Pathophysiology

The exact cause of ADHD is unknown. The disorder does appear to have a genetic basis. Several studies have revealed a genetic link within families. Studies of twins help support the familial link. Certain environmental factors have also been linked to the disorder, such as maternal cigarette smoking and alcohol use during pregnancy. Children who are exposed to high levels of lead at young ages have a higher risk of developing ADHD. Brain injury, premature delivery, and low birth weight are additional causes linked to ADHD (CDC, 2020a).

Clinical Manifestations

Children with ADHD sometimes exhibit decreased attention span, impulsivity, failure to follow instructions, hyperactivity, poor self-regulation, noncompliance, aggression, fidgeting, immaturity during play, failure to follow rules of play in games, lack of turn-taking during play, and easy distraction by extraneous stimuli. Associated problems include poor school performance; learning disabilities; antisocial behaviors such as lying, cheating, and stealing; excessive anxiety; sleep disturbances; poor peer relationships; limited fine motor skills; and additional psychiatric diagnoses.

Diagnostic Tests

No single test is available for ADHD, and the diagnosis requires a thorough evaluation of the child over an extended period of time. Information should be obtained from the child's parents, pediatrician, teachers, as well as specialists. Vision, hearing, and other medical testing should be performed to rule out a medical cause for the child's behavior.

Medical Management

Behavioral counseling, educational intervention, and pharmacotherapy are essential components in the treatment of ADHD. Interventions aim at achieving optimal academic, emotional, social, and vocational outcomes and preserving good self-esteem. Behavior therapy is encouraged as the first line of treatment, especially with younger children.

Nursing Interventions

A critical role for the nurse is parent counseling. It is most important to allay any inappropriate feelings of guilt or responsibility that the parents may have. Educate the parents about discipline, teach them how to set limits that are appropriate and provide rewards, and encourage them to establish a strict daily routine. The parents need information about the dangers of controversial therapies (e.g., megavitamin and herbal therapies). Stress the importance of accident prevention and safety. Explain the need for increased supervision and yet foster additional responsibilities and independence. Assist in the development of the educational plan as appropriate. If the child is taking medication, explain the reasons and minimal risks of such therapy to the child's teacher and school officials as needed. Parents also need to be informed of the importance of routine follow-up of children on medication. Children should be checked for medication side effects every 6 months, and the ongoing need for medication therapy should be assessed every year or more often.

Prognosis

With intervention, ADHD can be managed successfully throughout childhood and adolescence. Symptoms may persist into adulthood. Eating healthy diets, proper exercise, and adequate sleep help in managing the disorder.

OTHER DISORDERS

Anorexia Nervosa and Bulimia Nervosa

Anorexia and bulimia are eating disorders with significant underlying psychological and emotional issues. Although these disorders affect primarily adolescents, younger children are sometimes affected. For a thorough discussion of anorexia and bulimia, refer to Chapter 35.

Substance Abuse

Substance abuse is commonly a problem of adolescence; however, it sometimes occurs in elementary school–age children. In children, substance abuse usually points to significant problems for the child, the family, or both, and professional counseling is warranted. In adolescents, the incentives are usually experimental and recreational. Drug, alcohol, and tobacco use by the adolescent tends to be symbolic of maturity or serve purposes of peer group acceptance, stress reduction, or rebellion (see Chapter 30).

Depression

Depression is defined generally as a mood disturbance with overall feelings of sadness, despair, worthlessness, or hopelessness. The prevalence of depression among young children in the United States is approximately 2%, while the prevalence for teens is approximately 8% (Anxiety and Depression Association of America, n.d.). The rate of depression is higher in girls than in boys.

Etiology And Pathophysiology. The causes of major depression have not been established. Possible risk factors are genetic or environmental. Many studies have shown that children of a parent suffering from a major affective disorder have a rate of depression three to six times higher than that in the general population. Cognitive theories attribute the development of depression to feelings of hopelessness and helplessness secondary to an actual or perceived loss. Psychosocial theories point to factors such as disturbance in family dynamics or in the parent-child relationship, a family move, the death of a loved one, divorce, or abuse or maltreatment.

Clinical Manifestations. Depressive symptoms vary with age and developmental level of the child. In infancy, separation from the primary caretaker may lead to protest (crying, panic) followed by apathy, blank staring, and sad facial expressions. School-age children with depression often demonstrate sad facial expressions, irritability, crying easily, accident proneness, social withdrawal, and eating and sleeping disturbances. Some are also likely to manifest anxiety symptoms, physical aggression, and academic underachievement. Depressed adolescents typically show signs of impulsiveness, somatization disorders (characterized by recurrent, multiple physical complaints and symptoms with no organic cause), eating disorders, drug or alcohol use, antisocial behavior, withdrawal, fatigue, and suicidal ideation.

Diagnostic Tests. Structured questionnaires or interviews (e.g., Children's Depression Inventory, Children's Depression Scale, Depression Self-Rating Scale) are useful for diagnosing depression in children and adolescents. No definitive biological tests are specific for depression.

Medical Management. Antidepressant medication, along with psychological therapies, is the mainstay of treatment of major depression. Tricyclic antidepressants or selective serotonin reuptake inhibitors such as fluoxetine (Prozac), trazodone, sertraline (Zoloft), bupropion (Wellbutrin), venlafaxine (Effexor XL), and paroxetine (Paxil) are helpful in alleviating symptoms. Parents must be aware of suicidal tendencies during the first and second weeks of therapy. In 2004 the US Food and Drug Administration ordered pharmaceutical companies to add a "black box" warning on all antidepressants to alert health care providers of an increased risk of suicidal thoughts or ideation in pediatric patients.

Psychological therapies include play therapy; art therapy; and various talk therapies, including family therapy.

Nursing Interventions. Once the mental health care provider and the primary health care provider establish the treatment plan, establish a trusting relationship with the child. In addition, provide emotional support to the child's family, using open and honest communication. Stress the importance of meeting with therapists on a regular basis when warranted.

Patient And Family Teaching. Review the treatment plan with the family and ensure that the child and the family understand the importance of following the prescribed regimen.

Prognosis. For the child and family motivated to develop better social supports and relationship skills, the prognosis is often good. Depressive episodes may recur.

Patient problems and interventions for the patient with depression include but are not limited to the following:

PATIENT PROBLEM	NURSING INTERVENTIONS
Social Seclusion, related to feelings of hopelessness	Encourage a therapeutic, trusting relationship Provide supportive reassurance as needed Provide positive reinforcement when child participates in group activities or interacts with others
Insufficient Knowledge (of child, family, or both), related to lack of information about depression and its treatment	Assess child and family's understanding of depression and its treatment Instruct child, family, and significant others about depression and its treatment Identify support groups within their community

Suicide

Suicide is defined as the deliberate act of self-injury with the intent that the injury result in death. Suicide is the third leading cause of death among 5- to 14-year-olds in the United States (NLM, 2020a). Few prepubertal children actually kill themselves, although many of them are knowledgeable about suicide. Although girls make more suicide attempts than do boys, boys more often complete the act of suicide. Girls tend to use more passive methods, such as medication ingestion or carbon monoxide poisoning, whereas boys traditionally use more violent methods, such as hanging, firearms, or wrist slashing. Drug overdose is the most common method of attempted suicide.

Etiology And Pathophysiology. Suicide is not a result of a single factor; rather, suicide is the culmination of multiple factors. These include depression (which is a common preceding factor), loss of a loved one or relationship, and social isolation. The most important individual factor is the presence of an active psychiatric disorder (e.g., depression, bipolar disorder, psychosis, substance abuse, or conduct disorder). Comorbidity of an affective disorder and substance abuse also increase the risk of suicide.

In addition, not having attained a sense of identity, a major task of adolescence, leads to self-doubt and low self-esteem.

Clinical Manifestations. Many completed suicides are the result of previous attempts. Warning signs of impending suicide include depression, preoccupation with death, perceived or actual social isolation, withdrawal, poor school performance, drug or alcohol abuse (or both), appetite and sleep disorders, and loneliness. Symptoms are usually present for at least 1 month before the attempted or completed suicide.

Diagnostic Tests. Diagnostic tests for depression (see earlier section "Depression") are useful when early recognition of depressive symptoms is part of a comprehensive effort to prevent suicidal ideation and attempts.

Medical Management. Responsibility for a suicidal patient should be shared among as many people as possible. It indicates that other people care. Individual, family, and group therapy are all helpful for adolescents. Although ordinary health care providers may be able to manage an acute depressive reaction without difficulty, the child or adolescent who has made a serious attempt or has a specific plan for suicide must receive immediate attention and competent psychiatric care.

Nursing Interventions. Mental health assessments of children and adolescents are a necessary part of every health visit. Children and adolescents are often surprisingly open in communicating their feelings with a trusted nurse in a confidential setting. If there are any concerns, ask directly whether the patient has thoughts of death or suicide, when the thoughts occurred, how long these thoughts lasted, and whether the patient has a plan. Any threat of suicide must be taken very seriously, particularly if the child has a plan, along with immediate evaluation by a mental health care provider. Help the child develop positive coping strategies in stressful situations (e.g., deep-breathing exercises, meditation, school or peer counseling) (Nursing Care Plan 32.2).

Prognosis. Prognoses vary. The children at greatest risk are those who verbalize suicidal thoughts and those who attempt suicide. It is possible for appropriate mental health care to help these children to alleviate depression and develop a more positive self-image.

Psychogenic Abdominal Pain (Recurrent Abdominal Pain)

RAP is usually multifactorial, organic, dysfunctional, or psychogenic (originating from the mind). Psychogenic RAP is most common in school-age and adolescent children and is a diagnosis that warrants consideration in children with episodes of abdominal pain that recur monthly for at least 3 consecutive months once other causes have been ruled out.

Nursing Care Plan 32.2 A Child Who Attempts Suicide

S. is a 12-year-old girl who arrives at the hospital after taking 12 of her grandmother's anti-dysrhythmia pills in an attempt to end her life. She has been despondent since her mother died of breast cancer 6 months ago. Her school performance has been declining, and she has become increasingly isolated. She is admitted to the pediatric intensive care unit and then transferred to the adolescent psychiatric unit.

PATIENT PROBLEM

Potential for injury, related to poisoning and cardiac dysfunction.

Patient Goals And Expected Outcomes	Nursing Interventions	Evaluation
Patient will exhibit improved cardiac function	Maintain open airway and air exchange. Maintain cardiac function. Monitor patient for effects of the medications. Treat any dysrhythmias.	Telemetry reveals normal sinus rhythm; no dysrhythmias noted.

PATIENT PROBLEM

Impaired Coping, related to depression.

Patient Goals And Expected Outcomes	Nursing Interventions	Evaluation
Patient will develop and use healthy coping skills	Develop a therapeutic relationship. Encourage patient to verbalize feelings and concerns. Maintain a safe environment: • Remove potentially harmful objects. • Provide direct observation monitoring as needed. • Use physical restraints as needed to prevent self-injurious behaviors. Report any changes in affect or behavior to the health care provider. Reassure child and family of the plan to protect child from suicidal attempts.	Patient is beginning to verbalize great sadness and emptiness over mother's death.

PATIENT PROBLEM

Impaired self-esteem due to current situation, related to feelings of worthlessness.

Patient Goals And Expected Outcomes	Nursing Interventions	Evaluation
Patient will express feelings of positive self-worth	Encourage expression of feelings. Approach interactions with patient in a nonjudgmental manner. Provide positive feedback for all successes and reassurance after failures. Reinforce child's and family's strengths.	Patient is making a list of her positive strengths.

PATIENT PROBLEM

Insufficient knowledge (of child, family, or both), related to no previous experience with suicide.

Patient Goals And Expected Outcomes	Nursing Interventions	Evaluation
Patient and family will verbalize understanding of signs of potential risk of suicide	Assess current level of understanding. Make appropriate referrals as needed to psychiatrist or psychologist; social worker; peer support group; hotlines. Provide information about early warning signs of ineffective coping that potentially lead to suicidal attempt or gesture: insomnia, change in weight, excessive fatigue, isolating behaviors, thoughts of death, giving away belongings, lack of interest in future, decreased social network. Encourage importance of follow-up; schedule appointments and provide phone numbers.	Patient verbalizes willingness to attend follow-up counseling sessions.

CRITICAL THINKING QUESTIONS

1. Upon entering S.'s room, the nurse notices that she is crying. She states, "I can't live without my mother; I want to be with her." What is an appropriate initial response?
2. S.'s father is concerned about taking her home after discharge. What are two therapeutic nursing interventions for patient and family teaching?
3. S. begins to express interest in others and in activities in her hospital unit. What nursing interventions would be appropriate to encourage her?

Etiology And Pathophysiology. Psychogenic RAP often is related to emotional factors in the child or family members, or both, such as poor self-esteem, anxiety, depression, school phobia, maternal depression, marital problems and divorce, or health problems in other family members. Organic causes—such as infections of the urinary tract, the GI tract, and the reproductive tract—should be assumed until proven otherwise.

Clinical Manifestations. Children with RAP are usually afebrile and sometimes have occasional vomiting and constipation. The abdominal pain is usually nonspecific, or the child complains of episodic periumbilical or epigastric pain that is unrelated to eating, defecation, or exercise.

Diagnostic Tests. For a child with RAP, it is necessary to rule out organic causes. Tests include a CBC, measurement of sedimentation rate, urinalysis and culture, serum albumin and amylase measurements, stool assessment for occult blood, and culture for bacteria and parasites.

In the adolescent girl, a pregnancy test also should be considered.

Medical Management. Once the health care provider has ruled out organic causes, it is necessary to identify and address stressors in the child's life. Consultation with a mental health care provider is often helpful. Children with psychogenic RAP sometimes must be seen as often as once every 2 or 4 weeks for pain evaluation and reassurance.

Nursing Interventions. Once the family has been advised that there is no organic cause for the abdominal pain, encourage parents to maintain a normal schedule for their child with regard to school, play, and exercise. Overprotective parents need a great deal of emotional support in helping them deemphasize their child's complaints. Also give the family instructions to call if the child's symptoms worsen.

Prognosis. Once the stressors have been addressed, the prognosis is very good.

Get Ready for the NCLEX® Examination!

Key Points

- Common skin disorders of infancy and childhood include diaper dermatitis, atopic dermatitis, and seborrheic dermatitis.
- For children with many of the musculoskeletal disorders seen in infancy, treatment initiated immediately on diagnosis often results in a better prognosis.
- Cleft lip and palate, the most common facial malformations, usually involve nutritional, dental, and speech alterations and necessitate a multidisciplinary approach to treatment.
- Congenital heart defects are classified as either acyanotic or cyanotic.
- Nursing interventions in the care of a child with heart failure are to assist in improving cardiac function, decreasing cardiac demands, reducing respiratory distress, maintaining nutritional status, promoting fluid loss, and providing emotional support to the family.
- The most common form of neoplasm in childhood is acute lymphoblastic leukemia.
- Nursing interventions for a child with hemophilia involve preventing bleeding by decreasing the risk of injury, recognizing and managing bleeding with coagulation factor replacement, preventing the crippling effects of joint degeneration, and preparing and emotionally supporting the child and the family for home care.
- For a child with iron-deficiency anemia, it is best to give oral iron preparations between meals with citrus fruits or juices to enhance absorption.

- Croup is a group of signs and symptoms of varied origin. Characteristic manifestations are obstruction or edema in the region of the larynx, which produces inspiratory stridor, hoarseness, and a cough described as "barking."
- When first infected with *Mycobacterium tuberculosis,* most children do not exhibit any clinical signs or symptoms; therefore, routine skin screening is an important measure in diagnosis.
- Characteristic signs of hypertrophic pyloric stenosis are projectile vomiting, malnutrition, dehydration, and a palpable mass in the epigastrium.
- Diabetes mellitus is a syndrome whose primary characteristic is a deficiency of insulin, resulting in alterations in protein, carbohydrate, and fat metabolism.
- Hearing, vision, and speech deficits in infants and children can be recognized early through periodic screenings and assessments.
- Although meningitis has many causes, bacterial meningitis is the most common.
- Environmental exposure through inhalation or ingestion continues to be the most important contributing factor in lead poisoning.
- Acquired immunodeficiency syndrome is associated with certain drug therapies, radiation, splenectomy, and viral infections.
- Intellectual impairment (formerly called *mental retardation*) is significantly below-average general intellectual functioning that exists concurrently with deficits in adaptive behavior and manifested before adulthood.

- The majority of cases of Down syndrome are attributable to an extra chromosome on the twenty-first pair, hence the term *trisomy 21.*
- Autism is a complex developmental disorder of brain function that occurs in the presence of a broad range and severity of intellectual and behavioral deficits.
- Learning disabilities are sometimes the result of various physiologic or environmental factors such as intrauterine exposure to alcohol, drugs, or infection; birth trauma; seizures; attention deficit disorders; head trauma; malnutrition; and exposure to toxic substances, such as lead.
- Medications, especially central nervous system stimulants such as methylphenidate (Ritalin), are highly effective in improving the behaviors of children with attention deficit/hyperactivity disorder. Positive results include increased attention span, normalization of activity level, and reduced impulsiveness.
- Suicide is the third leading cause of death among children aged 10 to 19 years in the United States.
- Psychogenic recurrent abdominal pain (RAP) often is related to emotional factors in the child or family member, such as poor self-esteem, anxiety, depression, school phobia, maternal depression, marital problems and divorce, or health problems in other family members.

Additional Learning Resources

SG Go to your Study Guide for additional learning activities to help you master this chapter content.

Be sure to visit the Evolve site at http://evolve.elsevier.com/Cooper/foundations/ for additional online resources.

Review Questions for the NCLEX® Examination

1. **The nurse is caring for a patient with nephrotic syndrome. What assessment finding does the nurse expect to find?**
   1. Gross hematuria, albuminuria, temperature of 101°F (38.3°C) to 103°F (39.4°C)
   2. Elevated blood pressure, weight loss, hematuria
   3. Albuminuria, edema, puffiness of face
   4. Edema, albuminuria, hypotension

2. **The student nurse is preparing a community presentation on urinary tract infections. What should the student include as risk factors?** *(Select all that apply.)*
   1. A short urethra in young girls
   2. Frequent emptying of the bladder
   3. Increased fluid intake
   4. Ingestion of highly acidic juices
   5. Cleaning the perineal area from back to front

3. **The nurse is answering questions from a parent whose child has acute glomerulonephritis. Which explanation of the disease is most accurate?**
   1. It is a syndrome in which there is reabsorption of bicarbonate or in which excretion of hydrogen ions is impaired.
   2. It occurs after an antecedent streptococcal infection.
   3. It is a disorder manifested by gross bacteria.
   4. It is a disorder associated with a defect in the ability to concentrate urine.

4. **A pediatric patient has received a diagnosis of Wilms tumor. Which statement regarding Wilms tumor is true?**
   1. The tumor manifests as a firm, nontender, intraabdominal mass.
   2. The tumor is sometimes difficult to distinguish from the spleen.
   3. The tumor usually crosses the midline.
   4. If the surgeon successfully removes the tumor without a tear in its capsule, no chemotherapy is needed.

5. **The nurse is assisting in preparing a care plan for a patient who has received a diagnosis of a seizure disorder. What is an important nursing intervention that should be included in caring for a child who is experiencing a seizure?**
   1. Describe and record the seizure activity observed.
   2. Restrain the child when seizures occur to prevent bodily harm.
   3. Place a tongue blade between the teeth if they become clenched.
   4. Suction the child during a seizure to prevent aspiration.

6. **In an assessment of a newborn, what findings are suggestive of hydrocephalus?**
   1. Bulging fontanelle, dilated scalp veins
   2. Depressed fontanelle, decreased blood pressure
   3. Constant low-pitched cry, restlessness
   4. Closed fontanelle, high-pitched cry

7. **A newborn was admitted to the nursery with a complete bilateral cleft lip and palate. The health care provider explained the plan of therapy and its expected good results; however, the mother refuses to see or hold her baby. What is the most therapeutic initial approach to the mother?**
   1. Restate what the health care provider has told her about plastic surgery.
   2. Encourage her to express her feelings.
   3. Emphasize the normal characteristics of her baby and the baby's need for mothering.
   4. Keep the baby and mother apart until the lip has been repaired.

8. **How is Hirschsprung disease best described?**
   1. Absence of parasympathetic ganglion cells in a segment of the colon
   2. Passage of excessive amounts of meconium by the newborn
   3. Results in excessive peristaltic movements within the GI tract
   4. Results in frequent evacuation of solids, liquids, and gas

9. **The nurse is caring for a 4-month-old patient with severe infantile diarrhea. What condition is this patient most likely to experience as a result?**
   1. Metabolic acidosis
   2. Metabolic alkalosis
   3. Respiratory acidosis
   4. Respiratory alkalosis

10. A 6-month-old patient is suspected of having cystic fibrosis. What diagnostic tests does the nurse expect to be ordered for this patient? *(Select all that apply.)*

    1. Bronchoscopy, with pulmonary washings
    2. Chest x-ray study
    3. Upper GI series
    4. Sweat test
    5. Pulmonary function tests

11. A 5-year-old patient is admitted to the pediatric unit in sickle cell crisis. Which nursing intervention will be included in the plan of care? *(Select all that apply.)*

    1. Strenuous exercise of the extremities to increase oxygen to the area
    2. Administration of IV fluids to improve circulation and hydration
    3. Administration of analgesics as ordered
    4. Administration of oxygen as ordered
    5. Applying ice packs to the affected areas

12. The nurse is caring for a child with nephrotic syndrome. The nurse is correct in questioning the health care provider's order of which class of medications? *(Select all that apply.)*

    1. Antibiotics
    2. Diuretics
    3. Vitamins
    4. Corticosteroids
    5. Antifungals

13. When interviewing parents of an infant with hypertrophic pyloric stenosis, the nurse expects the parents to report which symptom?

    1. Diarrhea
    2. Projectile vomiting
    3. Poor appetite
    4. Constipation

14. When caring for a patient who is 2½ years old and has Wilms tumor, what assessment is most likely to reveal clinical manifestations of the disease?

    1. Auscultation of lung sounds
    2. Palpation of the abdomen
    3. Assessment of skin turgor
    4. Palpation of femoral and dorsalis pedis pulses

15. The nurse is educating a new mother about infectious diseases. The mother demonstrates understanding of teaching by identifying which disorders as being contagious? *(Select all that apply.)*

    1. Impetigo
    2. *Staphylococcus aureus* infection
    3. Infantile eczema (atopic dermatitis)
    4. Pediculosis
    5. Cystic fibrosis

16. In a discussion about an 11-month-old patient's diet, which statement by her mother indicates a possible cause for iron-deficiency anemia?

    1. "Formula is so expensive. We switched to regular milk early on."
    2. "She almost never drinks water."
    3. "She doesn't really like peaches or pears, so we stick to bananas for fruit."
    4. "I give her a piece of bread now and then. She likes to chew on it."

17. When caring for a 9-month-old patient who underwent surgery to repair a cleft palate, what is the priority intervention?

    1. Referral to a parent support group
    2. Maintaining adequate nutrition
    3. Keeping an IV line open
    4. Keeping the patient sedated

18. Which statement made by a 12-year-old patient with type 1 diabetes indicates a need for more teaching?

    1. "My pancreas is sick and needs insulin until it gets better."
    2. "I will need to take my insulin every day."
    3. "I need to keep a piece of candy in my pocket in case I start to feel shaky."
    4. "My mom has to give me insulin shots twice a day."

19. The nurse is discussing possible causes of a 4-year-old child's cognitive impairment with his mother. Which causes would the nurse be correct in including in the discussion?

    1. Metabolic disorders, perinatal anoxia, hyperthyroidism
    2. Perinatal infection, metabolic disorders, and postmaturity
    3. Lead poisoning, prematurity, perinatal anoxia
    4. Iron supplementation, toxoplasmosis, maternal drug use

20. A 2-month-old infant receives a diagnosis of Down syndrome. Which clinical manifestation supports this diagnosis?

    1. Pointed nose
    2. Small, rounded skull with flat occiput; simian crease
    3. Small tongue
    4. Downward-slanting eyes

21. When a child is beginning antidepressant medications, it is important for parents to be alert for signs of _____ _____ for the first 2 weeks of treatment.

22. The parents of a 12-year-old patient are concerned about the child's recent diagnosis of school avoidance. Which response by the nurse would be the most appropriate?

    1. Emphasize that the child is sick and needs to stay home from school.
    2. Discuss the importance of the child's returning to school.
    3. Ignore any somatic complaints the child may have.
    4. Instruct them that this is a psychiatric disorder.

23. A 14-year-old patient has a positive test result for human immunodeficiency virus (HIV) and expresses a desire to kill herself. What would be the most appropriate initial response of the nurse?

    1. Tell her that they are very close to discovering a cure for HIV.
    2. Encourage her to talk to her pastor.
    3. Arrange a visit with another adolescent who is HIV positive.
    4. Immediately report the threat to a mental health care provider.

24. A 7-year-old patient has a diagnosis of recurrent abdominal pain (RAP). What nursing interventions would be most appropriate to include in the plan of care? *(Select all that apply.)*

    1. Encourage the parents to maintain a normal schedule for their child with regard to school.
    2. Support the parents in deemphasizing their child's complaints.
    3. Educate the parents to contact the health care provider if symptoms worsen.
    4. Help the parents choose appropriate exercise for the child.
    5. Discourage the parent from allowing the child to play with other children until symptoms subside.

25. A 3-year-old patient has received a diagnosis of intellectual impairment. Which intervention is most important in dealing with the patient and her family?

    1. Encourage the family to enroll the child in an early intervention program.
    2. Discourage play with "normal" children to prevent feelings of inadequacy.
    3. Instruct the family not to discuss their feelings in front of the child.
    4. Educate the family that they should treat the child in a special manner because she is "slow."

26. The mother of a child with Down syndrome expresses concerns about her child's physical health. Which response by the nurse would be the most appropriate?

    1. "Children with Down syndrome are prone to upper respiratory infections."
    2. "Congenital heart defects are uncommon in children with Down syndrome."
    3. "Your child will probably need to be institutionalized before the age of 18."
    4. "Most children with Down syndrome develop leukemia."

27. The health care provider has diagnosed depression in a 16-year-old patient. Which statement by the parents indicates that they have a proper understanding of the diagnosis?

    1. "My child will need to be placed in an inpatient mental health facility."
    2. "My child will have to take antidepressive medications for life."
    3. "The recovery process for my child is likely to be a slow, lengthy process."
    4. "Depression is nothing to worry about in a child of this age."

28. The nurse is assessing a newly admitted patient. What clinical manifestations would probably indicate that the child has autism? *(Select all that apply.)*

    1. Avoidance of body contact with other people
    2. Speech and language delays
    3. Deficits in social development
    4. Good eye contact with the nurse during the assessment
    5. Increased sensitivity to stimuli

29. A male infant, 3 months old, is brought to the ED by his parents when, after two episodes of projectile vomiting of fresh milk immediately after feeding, they both felt a firm olive-shaped mass to the right of his umbilicus when changing his diaper. They are anxious and fear he may have either a tumor or a hernia or a severe intestinal blockage. After palpation and examination, the ED physician quickly tells them she suspects possible hypertrophic pyloric stenosis without requesting an abdominal sonogram or any other diagnostic tests. The speed of this diagnosis with so little testing surprises the student nurse on ED rotation. The nurse says nothing but listens as the physician tells the parents that their son will need surgery, but that this nearly always results in complete recovery. After the physician leaves and the family is moved to pre-op, the nursing student reviews her assessment notes to determine whether her notes would also suggest hypertrophic pyloric stenosis—or something else.

Select all assessment findings that would be consistent with hypertrophic pyloric stenosis.

___ Palpable epigastric mass	___ Cool, mottled skin
___ Abdominal pain	___ Poor sucking reflex
___ Loss of appetite	___ Dehydration
___ Peristaltic left-to-right epigastric waves	___ Avid nursing at the breast after vomiting

Health Promotion and Care of the Older Adult

http://evolve.elsevier.com/Cooper/foundations/

Objectives

1. Discuss health and wellness in the aging population of the United States in relation to the aims of *Healthy People 2030.*
2. Identify some of the common myths concerning the older adult.
3. Describe biological and psychosocial theories of aging.
4. Discuss common psychosocial events that occur with the older adult.
5. Describe changes associated with aging for each of the body systems.
6. List methods of assessment used for each body system.
7. Identify patient problems appropriate to common health concerns of the older adult.
8. Describe appropriate nursing interventions for common health concerns of the older adult.
9. Discuss changes that occur with aging in intelligence, learning, and memory.
10. Discuss leading safety and security issues faced by older adults.
11. Identify ways to preserve dignity and to increase self-esteem of the older adult.
12. Discuss how finances and housing are major concerns for the older adult.
13. Compare how older adults differ from younger individuals in their response to illness, medications, and hospitalization.

Key Terms

ageism (Ā-jĭzm, p. 1085)

akinesia (ă-kĭ-NĒ-zhă, p. 1110)

aphasia (ă-FĀ-zhă, p. 1110)

ataxia (ă-TĂK-sē-ă, p. 1110)

Baby Boomers (p. 1082)

chronologic age (p. 1082)

claudication (klăw-dĭ-KĀ-shŭn, p. 1096)

dementia (dĕ-MĚN-shă, p. 1108)

dysarthria (dĭs-ĂHR-thrē-ă, p. 1110)

dysphagia (dĭs-FĀ-jă, p. 1091)

hemiplegia (hĕm-ĭ-PLĒ-jă, p. 1110)

kyphosis (kĭ-FŌ-sĭs, p. 1097)

nocturia (nŏk-TŪ-rē-ă, p. 1093)

orthostatic hypotension (ŏr-thō-STĂT-ĭk hī-pō-TĔN-shŭn, p. 1095)

presbycusis (prĕz-bē-KYŪ-sĭs, p. 1105)

presbyopia (prĕz-bē-Ō-pē-ă, p. 1104)

pruritus (prū-RĪ-tŭs, p. 1087)

respite care (p. 1086)

sandwich generation (p. 1086)

senility (p. 1108)

shearing forces (p. 1088)

HEALTH AND WELLNESS IN THE AGING ADULT

OLDER ADULTHOOD DEFINED

Older adulthood begins at about age 65 and continues until death, a possible span of 40 years or more. Older adulthood has been divided into four subgroups:

- Young-old: 65 to 74 years
- Middle-old: 75 to 84 years
- Old-old: 85 to 99 years
- Elite-old: 100 years and older

Other terms that may be used to refer to the aging population include *frail elderly,* which refers to those individuals older than 75 years of age with health concerns. *Centenarians* are those who are older than 100 years of age (Ignatavicius, 2018).

Although older adulthood is tied to chronologic age (age of an individual expressed as time elapsed since birth), chronologic age may not be an accurate predictor of health or behavior. Some individuals may be considered "old" in their 50s because of their appearance, behaviors, or health status. Today more people are living longer, active lives. Most consider maintaining activities and participating in healthy living behaviors as deflectors of typical aging perils (Fig. 33.1).

DEMOGRAPHICS

In the United States in 2019, 51 million people were 65 years of age and older, more than 16% of the population (US Census Bureau, 2020).

In the past two decades, the population of older adults (ages 65 and older) has grown twice as quickly as the rest of the population, and this increase is expected to continue. The US Census Bureau (2015)

Fig. 33.1 Exercise and activity contribute to a healthier lifestyle for older adults. (From Sorrentino SA, Remmert LA: *Mosby's textbook for nursing assistants*, ed 10, St. Louis, 2021, Mosby.)

estimates that by the year 2060 there will be 98.6 million people over the age of 65 living in the United States—more than double the number today, making them about 24% of the population. In 2018 the life expectancy in the United States was 78.5 years. This placed the United States at a ranking of 34th overall in the world (worldlifeexpectancy.com, 2018). In the past 50 years, life expectancy for Americans has increased by almost 10 years.

Health care for older people has become more complex for several reasons:
- Scientific advances in treating life-threatening conditions of the past
- Substantially increased life expectancy
- Greater focus on ethical and legal issues related to life, disease, research, and dying

Older adults are a diverse group in terms of age, life experiences, the aging process, health habits, attitudes, and response to illnesses. To best meet the challenge of delivering age-appropriate care, know the differences between normal aging versus illness or disease-related changes and be able to assess effectively older adults with delirium, dementia, and depression. To promote the patient's return to health and increase the speed of recovery, be familiar with rehabilitation care services. Older adults often are concerned about losses of function, and they need their care providers to provide respectful care that allows them to maintain their dignity.

WELLNESS, HEALTH PROMOTION, AND DISEASE PREVENTION

Wellness is more than just the absence of disease. *Wellness* is the individual operating at the optimal level of function, and even during chronic illness and dying, some level of well-being is attainable. Wellness involves a balance among the individual's emotional, spiritual, social, cultural, and physical states. Box 33.1 lists the traits of a healthy person. The role of the nurse is to assist individuals to adapt to their life situation to achieve this balance.

| Box 33.1 | Traits of a Healthy Person |

Self-responsibility: Is attuned to body messages and knowledgeable about health status and feels empowered to make healthy choices.

Nutritional awareness: Learns about healthy eating habits that reduce the risk for heart disease, high blood pressure, diabetes, osteoporosis, and cancer and that assist in achieving and maintaining a healthy body weight.

Physical fitness: Engages in regular physical activity, including aerobics, and activities that improve balance, muscle flexibility, and muscle strength.

Stress management: Identifies ways of coping with the stresses of life to be able to work productively and connect with others in the community.

Environmental sensitivity: Designs personal space to include a healthy physical and social environment with opportunities for time with friends, supportive network, giving and receiving affection, and reinforcing wellness behaviors.

From the US Department of Health and Human Services (US DHHS): National prevention strategy, 2012. Retrieved from www.healthcare.gov/prevention/nphpphc/strategy/report.html.

Health promotion takes a positive approach to health and emphasizes the strengths, resources, and abilities of an individual. Primary prevention stresses exercise to prevent cardiovascular disease, falls, and depression. Older people who quit smoking can reduce their risk of heart disease and improve lung function and circulation. A well-balanced diet without excessive sugar, fat, or alcohol is another important aspect of primary prevention. Primary prevention also includes recommended vaccinations. Immunizations recommended for older adults include an annual influenza vaccine, a tetanus/diphtheria (Td) or tetanus/diphtheria/pertussis booster every 10 years, a zoster (shingles) vaccine for those over the age of 60, and the pneumococcal vaccines (PCV13 and PPSV23) after 65 (Centers for Disease Control [CDC], 2021a). Secondary prevention in older adults focuses on early detection and treatment of disease, including screening for heart disease and hypertension (HTN), cancer, infectious disease, polypharmacy (misuse of multiple medications), nutrition, oral health, osteoporosis, falls, depression, and social isolation (Table 33.1).

HEALTHY AGING

Healthy People 2030 set forth the goals of the US Department of Health and Human Services (US DHHS) to improve health, function, and quality of life for older adults. These recommendations are in the process of being updated in *Healthy People* (Office of Disease Prevention and Health Promotion, 2021). A summary of the current 2030 goals as they relate to older adults appears in Box 33.2. The focus of these goals is on improving functional independence and the quality of life.

Table 33.1 Suggested Screening for Preventive Health for People 50 Years Old and Older

EXAMINATION OR TEST	GROUP	FREQUENCY
Complete physical, including cholesterol	Men and women	Every 1–3 years to age 75, then annually
Blood pressure	Men and women	Every 2 years for blood pressure measurements < 120/80 mm Hg; every year if systolic blood pressure measurements of 120–139 mm Hg or diastolic blood pressure measurements of 80–89 mm Hg; otherwise as directed by the health care provider
Pelvic examination, Papanicolaou (Pap) test, and breast examination	Women	Every 3–5 years
Mammogram	Women	Yearly for women ages 50–54; every 2 years for women 55 and older
Breast self-examination	Women	Monthly
Prostate examination	Men	Patients with average risk should begin discussing possible screening tests at age 50
Testicular self-examination	Men	Monthly
Stool for occult blood	Men and women	Yearly
Colonoscopy	Men and women	Baseline at age 50 until 75 years of age, every 10 years if results are normal, if abnormal as recommended by health care provider
Diabetes or prediabetes	Men and women	Starting at age 45, yearly
Depression screening	Men and women	At each visit
Fall prevention screening	Men and women	At each visit
Bone density	Men and women	Baseline at age 65 and for those who are at risk for falls, as recommended by health care provider
Lung cancer testing	Men and women	Age 55 and older with a history of smoking, as recommended by health care provider
Sexually transmitted diseases	Men and women	As recommended by health care provider
Smoking and tobacco cessation	Men and women	At each visit
Eye examination	Men and women	As recommended by the health care provider
Glaucoma test	Men and women	As recommended by the health care provider
Dental examination and cleaning	Men and women	Every 6 months for those with own teeth; every 2 years for denture wearers
Hearing test	Men and women	As recommended by the health care provider

Data from Johns Hopkins Medicine, https://www.hopkinsmedicine.org/healthlibrary/prevention/women_age,50_64; Cancer Screening Guidelines by Age, https://www.cancer.org/healthy/find-cancer-early/cancer-screening-guidelines/screening-recommendations-by-age.html; and U.S. Preventive Services Task Force, https://www.uspreventiveservicestaskforce.org/uspstf/recommendation-topics/uspstf-and-b-recommendations.

A growing number of adults are living into their 90s and beyond. A significant number of this population maintain their health and remain active up until the time of their death. The age of 65 is no longer considered old. This reality changes the circumstances of life planning, social services, employment, and social policy and the focus of health care. Keeping this population healthy, active, and moving necessitates a high standard of assessment and health promotion.

Born between 1946 and 1964, more than 70 million people are **Baby Boomers**. They make up approximately 29% of the nation's population. The older Baby Boomers are entering and approaching young-old adulthood. More than 1.5 million of them will live to 100 years of age. This group is extremely diverse and better educated, more mobile, and more aware of how to achieve and maintain good health than any previous generation. They recognize the importance of nutrition, exercise,

and a healthy environment. Many are concerned about the future in terms of available health care.

As more people take charge of their own health, many have found limitations in conventional medical approaches and have begun using alternative health strategies such as meditation, visualization, massage, magnets, aromas, and acupressure or acupuncture (see Chapter 20). Some of these therapies are effective; some are not. A method effective for one individual may not be for another. The patient must be cautioned to investigate the qualifications of the provider thoroughly, research the method under consideration, and use only one therapy at a time to allow sufficient time to identify reactions.

A holistic definition of health does not limit health to its physical and mental aspects but rather views health as a state of being, an attitude. It seems only natural to encourage people to make decisions that affect their own lives, but health care providers frequently fail to

Box 33.2   Healthy People 2030

GOAL FOR OLDER ADULTS
Improve the Health, Function, and Quality of Life

The *Healthy People 2030* objectives for older adults are designed to promote healthy outcomes for this population. Many factors affect the health, function, and quality of life of older adults. Specifically the focus is on:

- Individual behaviors that promote health, such as participation in physical activity, self-management of chronic diseases, or use of preventive health services, and can improve health outcomes;
- Social environmental factors that promote health, such as housing and transportation services that affect the ability of older adults to access care; and
- Health and social services available to older adults and their caregivers to assist them in managing chronic conditions and long-term care needs effectively.

EXAMPLES OF OBJECTIVES FOR OLDER ADULTS, AND THEIR TARGETS AND BASELINE DATA
Prevention

OA-1: Increase the proportion of older adults who use the Welcome to Medicare benefit. Target: 7%. Baseline: 6.4% of older adults used the Welcome to Medicare benefit in 2008. Target setting method: 10% improvement.

OA-2.1: Increase the proportion of males age 65 and older who are up to date on a core set of clinical preventive services. Target: 44.6%. Baseline: 40.5% of males aged 65 years and older were up to date on a core set of clinical preventive services in 2012. Target setting method: 10% improvement.

OA-2.2: Increase the proportion of females age 65 years and older who are up to date on a core set of clinical preventive services. Target: 46.8%. Baseline: 42.5% of females aged 65 years and older were up to date on a core set of clinical preventive services in 2012. Target setting method: 10% improvement.

OA-3: (Developmental) Increase the proportion of older adults with one or more chronic health conditions who report confidence in managing their conditions.

OA-4: Increase the proportion of older adults who receive Diabetes Self-Management Benefits. Target: 2.2%. Baseline: 2% of adults aged 65 and over received

Diabetes Self-Management in 2008. Target setting method: 10% improvement.

OA-5: Reduce the proportion of older adults who have moderate to severe functional limitations. Target: 26.4%. Baseline: 29.3% of older adults had moderate to severe functional limitations. Target setting method: 10% improvement.

OA-6: Increase the proportion of older adults with reduced physical or cognitive function who engage in light, moderate, or vigorous leisure-time physical activities. Target: 35.9%. Baseline: 32.6% of older adults with reduced physical or cognitive function engaged in light, moderate, or vigorous leisure-time physical activities in 2008. Target setting method: 10% improvement.

OA-7.3: Increase the proportion of registered nurses with geriatric certification. Target: 1.5%. Baseline: 1.4% of registered nurses had geriatric certification in 2004. Target setting method: 10% improvement.

Long-Term Services and Supports

OA-10: Reduce the rate of pressure ulcer-related hospitalizations among older adults. Target: 887.3 pressure ulcer–related hospitalizations per 100,000 people aged 65 years and older. Baseline: 985.8 pressure ulcer-related hospitalizations per 100,000 people aged 65 years and older occurred in 2007. Target setting method: 10% improvement.

OA-11: Reduce the rate of emergency department (ED) visits due to falls among older adults. Target: 4711.6 ED visits per 100,000 due to falls among older adults. Baseline: 5235.1 ED visits per 100,000 due to falls occurred among older adults in 2007 (age adjusted to year 2000 standard population). Target setting method: 10% improvement.

OA-12.1: Increase the number of States and the District of Columbia that collect and make publicly available information on the characteristics of victims, perpetrators, and cases of elder abuse, neglect, and exploitation. Target: 4 States and the District of Columbia. Baseline: 3 States collected and made publicly available information on the characteristics of victims, perpetrators, and cases of elder abuse, neglect, and exploitation in 2004. Target setting method: 10% improvement.

From US Department of Health and Human Services: *Older adults, 2020.* Retrieved from https://www.healthypeople.gov/2020/topics-objectives/topic/older-adults/objectives.

do so. Given sufficient information, most individuals make appropriate decisions.

Knowing the value others assign to us and being treated with respect build and sustain self-esteem (Fig. 33.2). Addressing an older individual as "Gramps" or "Grandma," "Honey," or any other similar term of familiarity is inappropriate unless the person is the caregiver's grandparent. Older adults should be called by name or by what they choose to be called; this indicates respect. Use of the person's first name is also inappropriate unless the person so specifies. Forcing changes that exceed the individual's ability to cope sometimes results in mental deterioration, physical illness, and even death. The role of the nurse includes affirmation, enhancement, and support of each person's movement through the aging process and encouragement of health and wellness.

Fig. 33.2 Self-esteem is vital for successful aging.

MYTHS AND REALITIES

Some of the myths and stereotypes of aging and older adults are presented in Box 33.3. Most myths are generalizations that focus on the negative aspects of aging. In many cases, research has proved such myths to be inaccurate.

THEORIES OF AGING

Our current knowledge about aging and the aging process is limited. In an attempt to explain aging and an individual's response to aging, experts have proposed a number of theories (Box 33.4). Biological theories attempt to explain why the body ages; psychosocial

---

Box 33.3	Common Myths Associated With Aging

Myth: Depression and loneliness are normal in older adults.

  Reality: Depression and loneliness are not a normal part of aging as the older adult has formed lasting relationships with family and friends. Most older adults have at least weekly contact with family. Many live within a 30-min drive of at least one family member. Although it is assumed that the family is the main support and source of social activity, many older people have also developed a network of friends who provide support and relationships.

Myth: Older adults need less sleep than younger adults.

  Reality: Older adults need 7–9 h of sleep a night. Adequate sleep reduces the risks of falls, improves mental well-being, and keeps the individual healthier.

Myth: Older adults cannot learn new things.

  Reality: Older adults have the ability to learn new things, create new memories, and improve a variety of skills. Engaging in activities with cognitive demands for an average of 16.5 h a week for 3 months enhanced memory function (Park et al., 2014).

Myth: It is inevitable that old people will get dementia.

  Reality: Decline is not inevitable. Creativity and intelligence do not appear to change. Memory and learning ability sometimes show slight decline because they are functions of the nervous system, which does experience some age-related changes. Serious decline in mental capabilities is generally a result of disease process, not age. In people over the age of 65 only 6%–8% have dementia. In those over the age of 85 years only one-third are affected by dementia (here are many causes of memory loss. Medications, stress, and depression are among possible culprits of forgetfulness.

Myth: Older adults should take it easy and avoid exercise, so they don't get hurt.

  Reality: Exercise and physical activity are good for mental and physical health, and can keep the individual independent during the aging process. Tai Chi and similar mind and movement balances have been shown to improve balance and stability to help prevent falls. Older adults should engage in the four types of exercise (endurance, strength, balance, and flexibility) to prevent chronic disease, maintain a healthy weight, reduce fall risk, promote sleep, lessen anxiety and stress, and improve cognitive functioning.

Myth: If a family member has Alzheimer disease, I will get it too.

  Reality: Having a family member with Alzheimer disease increases the risk. Environmental and lifestyle factors such as pollutants, diet, exercise, and smoking may affect the individual's risk. Promotion of a healthy diet, regular exercise, and smoking cessation can reduce the risk.

Myth: An older adult should give up driving.

  Reality: Approximately 42.8 million or one in five drivers are over the age of 65 (U.S. Department of Transportation Federal Highway Administration, 2016). Natural changes occur with aging that can affect the individual's ability to drive such as slower response time, diminished vision and hearing, and reduced strength and mobility. Once the individual's ability to drive safely is affected, a discussion should occur about giving up driving.

Myth: Only older women need to worry about osteoporosis.

  Reality: Osteoporosis affects both men and women. Between the ages of 65–70 both men and women lose bone mass. Risk factors could include a family history, not consuming enough calcium and vitamin D, lack of exercise, low levels of testosterone, too much alcohol, certain drugs, and smoking. Encourage the older adult to consume foods rich in calcium and vitamin D, participate in regular exercise, consume or eliminate alcohol, and quit smoking.

Myth: Older adults cannot quit smoking.

  Reality: Smoking cessation can be achieved at any age. Smoking will lower the risk of cancer, heart disease, stroke, and lung disease.

Myth: Older adults believe that once their blood pressure is lowered or returns to normal they can quit taking their medication for blood pressure.

  Reality: The reduction in blood pressure is a result of maintaining control through use of medication and lifestyle modifications. Older adults should continue to take their medications as prescribed by the primary health care provider.

Myth: Most older adults are in nursing homes or care facilities.

  Reality: About 80% of older adults own and live in their own homes.

Myth: Older adults do not have much energy and are always tired.

  Reality: Energy is largely determined by lifestyle and attitude. Sedentary individuals do not have as much energy-geared initiative.

Myth: Older adults are ill and disabled.

  Reality: Most older people have at least one chronic condition, but these conditions generally do not limit their ability to manage their household and activities of daily living. In a study of noninstitutionalized older adults, approximately 7 of 10 individuals reported their health as "good" or "excellent" as compared with that of others their own age.

National Institute on Aging. (n.d.) 10 myths on aging. Retrieved from https://www.nia.nih.gov/health/10-myths-about-aging

Park DC, Lodi-Smith J, Drew L, et al: The impact of sustained engagement on cognitive function in older adults: the synapse project, *Psychol Sci.* 25(1):103–112, 2014. doi:10.1177/0956797613499592

United States Department of Transportation Federal Highway Administration. (2016). FHWA releases new data showing nearly 20 percent of U. S. drivers are over 65. Retrieved from https://www.fhwa.dot.gov/pressroom/fhwa1652.cfm.

Box 33.4   Common Theories of Aging

BIOLOGICAL

Programmed Aging

Cells in the body can reproduce only 40–60 times. Aging takes place when more and more cells no longer have the capacity to regenerate themselves.

GENETIC FACTORS

People inherit a genetic program that determines their specific life expectancy.

IMMUNOLOGIC

The immune system becomes less effective or less able to distinguish between foreign and host cells, and aging is a result of the consequentially diminished protection from infection or disease, and the immune system destroying body cells that it misreads as defective or foreign.

FREE RADICAL

In the course of the metabolic activity of the body that produces energy, extra electrons are released that build up in the body and combine chemically, damaging cells and interfering with normal body function, resulting in aging.

WEAR AND TEAR

Cells of the body wear out from internal and external stress, including chemical damage, trauma, or dysfunction of body systems, and buildup of waste products.

PSYCHOSOCIAL

Erikson's Developmental Stages

In the last stage of life, the task is acceptance of life and one's own lifestyle, which potentially results in ego integrity. Inability to achieve a level of acceptance results in anger and despair.

Disengagement Theory

Aging is a process in which older adults and society gradually withdraw from each other to the mutual satisfaction of both.

Exchange Theory

Aging is reduced interaction between older adults and society as a result of the decreasing value that the interaction has for both.

Activity Theory

Older adults develop a positive concept of self as a result of maintaining ongoing social interactions. Well-being in later life is enhanced by substituting new roles in relation to family, recreation, and volunteer services for previous occupational roles.

Continuity Theory

Personality remains the same, and behavior becomes more predictable as people age.

theories try to give reasons for the responses and interactions older adults have with society during late adulthood (see Chapter 24).

AGEISM

Ageism is a term that describes prejudice against older adults. It reflects a negative response by younger people—a personal dread of growing old or becoming disabled, and a fear of powerlessness, uselessness, and death. Ageism systematically stereotypes and discriminates against people because they are old, just as racism and sexism stereotypes and discriminates against people on the basis of skin color and sex. To enhance the quality of life for older adults, support the patient's hope, pride, confidence, security, and integrity. All members of the health care team should work toward eliminating negative attitudes and discriminatory practices.

LEGISLATION THAT AFFECTS OLDER ADULTS

The first major legislation that attempted to provide financial security for older adults was the Social Security Act of 1935. At the time this law was passed, few people lived long enough to collect significant benefits. Over time, increasing numbers of politically active older adults sought and achieved legislation designed to benefit themselves (Table 33.2).

In 1965 the Older Americans Act (OAA) was established; it aimed to preserve the rights and dignity of the nation's older citizens. This act was updated and amended in 2006. The amendments retain provisions for low-income minorities and add emphasis on older individuals who reside in rural areas.

The increasing number of older adults also raises the issue of the needs of their caregivers. The National Family Caregiver Support Program provided a means of addressing the growing needs of caregivers (Administration of Community Living (ACL), 2021). In 2000 an additional program was added to support caregivers of American Indian elders (ACL, 2020).

The Patient Protection and Affordable Care Act (ACA) was signed into law in 2010. The results of this legislation are still developing, but the law encourages payment for preventive services to Medicare recipients and provides a drug discount for eligible seniors in the "donut hole" (USDHHS, 2021). The "donut hole" is a coverage gap that exists in most Medicare D prescription plans. The plans pay a percentage of the cost of medications up to a certain amount. When that amount is reached, Medicare recipients must pay 100% of the cost of prescriptions up to a yearly maximum out-of-pocket limit. After the maximum limit is met, the coverage gap ends and the prescription plan pays a percentage of the cost of covered drugs again. Proponents of the ACA state that the law provides new protections for seniors and cuts down on waste, fraud, and abuse. Since its inception the ACA has been met with concern over costs to those it was developed to cover and by insurers. The nation's legislators continue to propose changes in the scope, cost, and implementation of the act.

PSYCHOSOCIAL CONCERNS OF THE OLDER ADULT

STRESSES OF CAREGIVING

Older people receiving care may feel they are being a burden, be angry or frustrated about giving up their independence, or become demanding in an attempt

Table 33.2	Legislation That Has Helped Older Adults
YEAR	**LEGISLATION**
1935	Social Security Act
1965	Medicare and Medicaid established
	Administration on Aging established
1967	Age Discrimination Act passed
1972	Supplemental Security Income Program instituted
	Social Security indexed to reflect inflation, COLA (cost of living adjustments)
	Nutrition Act passed, which allows for provision of nutrition programs for older adults
1973	Council on Aging established
1978	Mandatory retirement age changed to age 70 years
1986	Mandatory retirement age eliminated for most employees
1987	Omnibus Budget Reconciliation Act (OBRA)
1988	Catastrophic health insurance established as part of Medicare
1990	Self-Determination Act: Responsibilities of care providers. Advance directives for health care provide legal clarification of an individual's wishes for limiting treatment in the event of acute illness and in dying
2004	Prescription drug plans instituted
2010	Patient Protection and Affordable Care Act (ACA) • Free Medicare preventive services • Medicare drug discount for eligible seniors who are in the "donut hole" • The health care law cracks down on waste, fraud, and abuse while providing new protections for seniors
2016	The Older Americans Act Reauthorization Act • Improved protection for vulnerable elders • Improved nutrition services

to regain control. Caregivers often feel overloaded, finding themselves pulled in many directions. There simply may not be enough time to meet all demands. Caregivers are at high risk for stress-related problems, including depression, anxiety, and increased vulnerability to physical health problems. The caregiver's coping style, how it affects caregiving, and the quality of the caregiver's support system are important to assess. Conflict is possible between family members who live near an older person and those who live at a distance because of different perspectives. It is often helpful to remind distant family members not to let apparent differences between what they see and what the local caregiver has said discredit the caregiver. Local caregivers often must compromise with the older person and accept imperfect solutions to problems.

One group of caregivers are known as the "**sandwich generation.**" These are individuals who are faced with caring for their parents while also caring for their own children. There are an estimated 44 million caregivers to the elderly in the United States. The clear majority (75%) are employed. This places stress on the "sandwiched" person. The pull of the workplace, home, and the elder can result in loss of time at work. Such situations are estimated to cost US businesses $34 billion per year.

The nursing assessment should include the needs of the caregiver. Review the demeanor and responses of the caregiver and the patient that may indicate fatigue in relation to the provision of care for the loved one. Referrals to social services and available community resources may be indicated. **Respite care** refers to the provision of care by nonfamily members with a goal of allowing the primary caregivers the opportunity for relief from the stressors and strains imposed by caring for an ill or debilitated family member.

LOSS, GRIEF, AND DEPRESSION

Significant psychosocial changes experienced by older adults typically include personal, social, and economic losses resulting from role changes, retirement, and the loss of significant others—parents, siblings, children, spouses, and friends. Physical changes often result in loss of independence and space. For some older adults, losses may occur suddenly, concurrently, or within a short period, thus increasing their impact. The ability to cope with grief and the related losses depends on many factors. Successful coping strategies to deal with grief may include avoiding isolation and self-pity, helping others, joining groups, adopting a pet, setting goals, maintaining independence, and retaining a sense of humor (see Chapter 25 for additional information).

Short-term or long-term depression may result in response to the grief from real and perceived losses. Fatigue, sadness, insomnia, anorexia, helplessness, crying, agitation, and hypochondria are frequent symptoms of depression in older adults. These symptoms are misunderstood commonly as changes that normally occur with aging. Misunderstanding and misdiagnosis too often result in many older adults failing to receive the needed treatment for depression. Depression is more common in the older adult than any other age-related group. Older people who receive psychotherapy for depression show improvement.

Patient problems and interventions for older adults with loss, grief, or depression include but are not limited to the following:

PATIENT PROBLEM	NURSING INTERVENTIONS
Complex grief, related to losses (specify)	Encourage verbalization of feelings regarding losses
	Acknowledge reality of grief
	Plan care to promote consistency and reduce stress
	Encourage participation in activities to provide distraction
	Refer to spiritual counselor or other sources of support
	Spend time with isolated individual
Helplessness, related to personal, social, and economic losses	Allow older person to make choices whenever possible
	Encourage person to do as much for self as possible
	Adapt environment to support independence
	Explain reasons for changes in plan of care

END-OF-LIFE CARE

Nurses who work with older adults assist the entire health care team to meet the physical, spiritual, and psychosocial needs of dying patients or residents. Caring for the families is an important part of this care. Knowledge about a person's culture and religious beliefs helps the team provide compassionate care.

Nurses caring for patients at the end of life need to understand the 1991 Patient Self-Determination Act (PSDA) as it relates to advance directives, living wills, durable powers of attorney, and do-not-resuscitate (DNR) orders. The health care team works closely with the patient or resident and the family to ensure that the patient's wishes are respected (see Chapter 25).

AGING BODY

Physiologic changes affect a person's biological, psychological, social, and environmental status. Physiologic changes in the aging process result in a decreased immune response, a decrease in compensatory reserve, and a loss of the body's ability to repair damaged tissue efficiently.

Numerous physiologic changes occur in all body systems during the natural aging process. There is strong evidence that inactivity is the most important contributor to declining physical mobility and function. Positive lifestyle modifications, including physical activity and proper nutrition, help optimize physical abilities and promote healthier aging. The degree and rate at which changes occur vary among individuals, systems, and organs, as does a person's ability to compensate.

In this chapter, common patient problems and nursing interventions related to each system are identified for selected age-related changes. Additional patient problem statements and nursing interventions may be appropriate to meet the individual needs of the older adult. See specific chapters for the discussion of nursing interventions that are appropriate regardless of age.

INTEGUMENTARY SYSTEM
Age-Related Changes
Aging skin is dry and thin and loses tone and elasticity. The loss of fat under the skin makes wrinkles increasingly apparent. Age spots called *lentigo* are tan or brown macules brought on by sun exposure and are more common in middle-aged and older people (Table 33.3). Hair grays and thins, and the distribution patterns often change, resulting in baldness. Nails grow slowly and often become thicker and more brittle, develop ridges, and turn yellow. Touch sensation often changes as a result of thinning skin, disease process, and responses to medication therapy. Susceptibility to infection, ecchymosis, and tearing increases with aging. Wounds tend to heal more slowly than those in a younger adult.

Assessment
- Observe skin hydration status. Pay close attention for signs of excessive dryness. Observe for skin tears or lesions. Note presence, location, and amount of exudate.
- Examine for lesions that have changed size, color, or shape. Lesions that are irregularly shaped, raised, crusted or pitting, or bleed easily should be examined by a dermatologist.
- Observe hair for excessive loss, dryness, or oiliness.
- Observe the nails for color, length, shape, symmetry, and cleanliness. Nursing interventions are indicated to manage cleanliness, excessive length, sharp edges, brittleness, increased thickening, and color changes.

Common Concerns and Nursing Interventions
Pruritus. Older people may report dryness and itching (pruritus) of the skin. This is more common in cold, dry weather because of reduced glandular secretions and moisture. Because soap tends to be drying, older adults should use soap sparingly and rinse the residue completely away. Antibacterial soap is very drying and usually is not a good option.

Skilled nursing facilities may have schedules for showering and shampooing. On nonshower days a partial bath is provided, which includes the washing of face, hands, axillary region, and perineal area.

In general, less frequent bathing is recommended for sedentary older adults because of a decrease in body oils and perspiration. Water-based or light oil-based lotions, rather than alcohol-based lotions, are best to use. Application of water-based lotions to dry areas, especially after bathing, usually increases most individuals' comfort and avoids the feeling of oil residue that some people find uncomfortable.

Moles. Most moles are benign. However, sun-related skin changes, including precancerous actinic keratosis, basal cell or squamous cell carcinoma, and malignant

Table 33.3	Integumentary Changes With Aging

PHYSIOLOGIC CHANGE	RESULTS
Decreased vascularity of dermis and decreased amount of melanin	Increased pallor in white skin
Decreased sebaceous gland function	Increased skin dryness
Decreased sweat gland function	Decreased perspiration
Decreased subcutaneous fat	Increased wrinkling
Decreased thickness of epidermis	Increased susceptibility to trauma
Increased localized pigmentation	Increased incidence of brown spots (senile lentigo)
Increased capillary fragility	Increased purple patches (senile purpura)
Decreased density of hair growth	Decreased amount and thickness of hair on head and body
Decreased melanin production in the hair bulb	Graying hair
Decreased hormone production	Decreased vaginal secretions and breast tissue mass and decreased speed of erection and the ability to maintain an erection
	Increased brittleness of nails
Decreased peripheral circulation	Increased thickening and yellowing of nails
Decreased rate of nail growth	Increased longitudinal ridges on nails
Increased androgen-to-estrogen ratio	Increased facial hair in women

melanoma, sometimes develop on sun-exposed areas. Ask a dermatologist to examine any suspicious-looking lesions.

Nail abnormalities. Bilateral clubbing of fingers indicates possible pulmonary or cardiac disease. Yellowed nails indicate possible fungal infection. Splintered nails indicate possible malnutrition, and pitting sometimes signals peripheral vascular disease (PVD), psoriasis, diabetes mellitus (DM), or syphilis. Brittle nails are often associated with fluctuations in hormones that occur during menopause.

Pressure injury. According to the Collaborative Healthcare Patient Safety Organization (CHPSO), more than 2.5 million US hospitalized patients develop pressure injury every year (CHPSO, 2017). In reviewing the literature on the rate in long-term care facilities, the numbers vary widely from a rate of 3.6% to 59% in one study to 3.4% to 32.4% in another study (Yap, 2019; Anthony, 2019). Pressure injury is a significant risk for older adults and patients with chronic disease. Thin skin and lack of subcutaneous fat predispose older adults to pressure injury development when their fragile skin is compressed between bony prominences of the body and other objects. Damage to the skin at these pressure points is best prevented by repositioning the patient at least every 2 hours. Many pressure-reducing pads and aids are available, but only those that do not restrict circulation or create pressure on surrounding areas should be used.

Fragile skin bruises and tears easily. Measures should be instituted to prevent pressure, friction, **shearing forces** (forces that can injure small blood vessels by sliding on a rough surface) (Fig. 33.3), and moisture (most commonly associated with incontinence).

Fig. 33.3 Shearing forces that result from pressure against the skin impair circulation to underlying tissues. (A) Depicts the forces occurring inside the body during shearing. (B) Depicts the forces occurring outside the body.

Friction occurs when fragile skin rubs against the bed sheets. In addition to the normal safety precautions taken to prevent injury to any patient, gentle handling during turning and transfer is necessary. Additional assistance or equipment may be needed to lift and move a resident to avoid friction burns and tearing of the skin during repositioning in bed. The use of tape on the skin of older adults should be kept to a minimum, because fragile skin can easily tear in the process of removing tape. Urine, drainage, or fecal material left in contact with the skin even for a short time potentially causes the skin to become impaired. Urine and stool tend to accelerate the formation of pressure injury at pressure points such as the coccyx or hip. Urine, drainage, and fecal material must be removed, and the skin washed, rinsed with clear water, and patted dry.

Prevention and healing of any pressure ulcer depend on good nutritional status and adequate hydration. A well-balanced diet with attention to protein, vitamins, and minerals plays an important role in maintaining skin integrity in the older adult.

Patient problems and interventions for a resident with pressure injury include but are not limited to the following:

PATIENT PROBLEM	NURSING INTERVENTIONS
Potential for Compromised Skin Integrity, related to fragile skin associated with aging	Perform daily skin inspection Reduce frequency of bathing Use mild, nonirritating soaps, and rinse thoroughly Use emollients and lotions to maintain skin moisture Turn and reposition frequently Move and transfer carefully Reduce sources of pressure Keep linens clean, dry, and free from foreign objects
Compromised Skin Integrity, related to inadequate nutritional intake	Assess nutritional intake Explain importance of nutrition Provide adequate protein, vitamins, minerals, and fluids
Potential for Infection, related to impaired skin integrity	Assess wounds daily, including size, location, and depth Obtain wound cultures if appropriate Follow strict aseptic technique when performing wound care per the health care provider's orders Use photographs to document healing or changes in pressure injury

GASTROINTESTINAL SYSTEM

A balanced diet provides fuel for the body. Good nutrition is essential to health, function, and quality of life, regardless of age. An inadequate or imbalanced diet can be tied to numerous chronic conditions, including obesity, HTN, diabetes, cancer, and cardiovascular disease. Older adults may experience a reduction in the sense of taste and smell. Medications may alter the taste of foods or result in a decrease in saliva production. Older adults living alone may report a lack of interest in preparing solo meals or may have limited financial resources to obtain nutritional foods. These occurrences contribute to undernutrition. Inactivity, boredom, and mental health concerns may result in excessive food consumption. This may result in overnutrition. Assess the patient's nutritional status. Interventions for nutritional issues can help the older adult attain higher self-esteem, improved physical well-being, and a better quality of life.

Age-Related Changes
Older adults have decreased secretion of saliva and a diminished gag response, which increases the chances of choking and aspiration. In addition, many medications taken by older adults may compound the problem by further reducing saliva production. The stomach of the older adult has decreased gastric motility as well as decreased production of bicarbonate and gastric mucus. Aging also can cause decreased production or lack of production of the intrinsic factor causing the body to become unable to use ingested vitamin B_{12}, leading to pernicious anemia.

Enzymes in the intestinal tract also are altered. The abdominal wall becomes less firm, and abdominal muscles weaken. Decreased tone of the intestine occurs, and it is common for peristalsis to become slower, leading to increased constipation (Table 33.4). The normal changes of aging often are intensified by medications commonly prescribed for other conditions, lack of fluids or dietary roughage or fiber, and lack of exercise or activity. Liver function often decreases, making drug metabolism less efficient.

Assessment
- Assess oral cavity for presence of lesions; dental caries; loose, broken, or missing teeth; dentures that do not fit well; edematous gums; and halitosis.
- Assess ability to chew and swallow.
- Assess for reports of heartburn and nausea.
- Assess dietary intake, especially of high-fiber foods, fat, and sodium. Note amount and type of food and fluid intake. Assess appetite.
- Assess weight. Compare with norms, and monitor for significant changes.
- Assess frequency, amount, odor, and consistency of bowel elimination. Assess abdomen for tenderness, distention, and active or diminished bowel sounds. Ask about intestinal cramping.
- Assess individual's ability to control defecation.
- Assess bowel elimination routines and use of laxatives.

Table 33.4 Gastrointestinal Changes With Aging

PHYSIOLOGIC CHANGE	RESULTS
Increased dental caries and tooth loss	Decreased ability to chew normally
	Decreased nutritional status
Decreased gag reflex	Increased incidence of choking and aspiration
Decreased muscle tone at sphincters	Increased incidence of pyrosis (heartburn); esophageal reflux
Decreased gastric secretions	Decreased digestion
Decreased peristalsis	Increased constipation and bowel impaction

- An annual fecal occult blood test is recommended for adults more than 50 years of age for detection of colorectal cancer, the second leading cause of cancer deaths in the United States.
- A stool DNA test may be completed for detection of colorectal cancer.

Common Concerns and Nursing Interventions

Obesity. Defined as weighing at least 20% more than ideal body weight, obesity is common in older adults. Older adults should consume less food than they did in their earlier, more physically active years. Adults 75 to 90 years of age need approximately 30 calories per kilogram of body weight (14 calories/lb), compared with 40 calories per kilogram (18 calories/lb) for people 20 to 37 years of age. This normally represents a diet of 1600 to 2400 calories daily, depending on gender and ideal weight. Along with fewer calories, older adults need to consume quality foods, such as grains, vegetables, and fruits, which contain vitamins, minerals, roughage, and fiber, to meet their daily needs without large amounts of sugar and fat. They also need foods that provide protein and are good sources of calcium.

Some foods are not as well tolerated because of changes in the digestive tract or difficulty with chewing or swallowing. Individual food preferences should be respected. A well-balanced diet is generally accepted as adequate without vitamin supplements. Vitamins A, C, and E and niacin may help slow the aging process, counteract the effects of free radicals, and extend life.

Weight loss. Gradual weight loss over time is a normal response to loss of body mass. This typically occurs with changes in body composition of fat, muscle, and fluid. Decreased nutrient intake in aging because of decreased appetite, lower metabolic rate, and diminished energy output also produces weight loss. Rapid weight loss may indicate an illness and should be reported to the health care provider. Unexplained weight loss totaling more than 5% of weight in 6 months to 1 year necessitates a medical evaluation (Mayo Clinic, 2020).

Fluids and dehydration. Fluids are necessary for the body to function and to remove the waste products of metabolism. An older person needs a minimum of 1500 mL of fluids daily. Because of arthritis or other conditions, some older adults have difficulty pouring liquids and drinking from a cup. Older adults sometimes decrease their fluid intake to control incontinence or because of an illness such as heart failure (HF).

When fluid deficit is caused by the older adult trying to control incontinence, the most appropriate interventions are to make fluids readily available and toilet facilities more easily accessible. Arranging the room so that access to the bathroom is unobstructed often helps. Sometimes the older adult needs assistance to the bathroom on a schedule, usually every 2 hours during waking hours and every 4 hours at night. If needed, a commode or urinal should be placed where the person can easily use it. Older adults who have difficulty picking up a cup or bending the neck often find that an adapted cup with a double handle (Fig. 33.4) or a cutout for the nose is a good solution. Some older adults who are disoriented likely need to be prompted to drink. Those with severe impairments often must be assisted to drink fluids on a scheduled basis.

Oral hygiene. Loss of teeth often is assumed to be normal in old age, but this is a misconception. It is *not* part of the normal aging process. Many of today's older population matured before the introduction of many modern methods of dental prophylaxis, which affects their dental health in addition to individual oral hygiene habits and the possibility of untreated periodontal disease. In the future, with good oral hygiene practices throughout life, many people will maintain their natural teeth for life.

Missing teeth make chewing difficult and tiring. Loose-fitting dentures tend to make chewing difficult and often allow food to collect under the denture, resulting in lesions. Both of these problems decrease a person's desire to eat. Oral hygiene is essential to eliminate debris that has the potential to interfere with taste or cause lesions. Recommended mouth care for older adults consists of a thorough cleansing of the entire mouth with a soft-bristled toothbrush or foam-stick applicator in the early morning and at bedtime. Mouth care is also important when an older adult has dentures. In addition to cleaning the dentures, brush the gums and the tongue, and rinse the mouth. If dentures are damaged, loose, or exert pressure on the oral mucous membranes, refer the person for dental services.

Loss of appetite. Older adults frequently experience a loss of appetite. Changes as a result of decreased saliva production and a decreased number of taste buds sometimes make food unappealing. Gastric motility slows because of the loss of smooth muscle in the stomach,

Fig. 33.4 Assistive devices for older adults.

which causes a delay in emptying time, distention, and early satiety. Anorexia and weight loss often result. In addition, many medications taken by older adults can produce side effects such as dyspepsia, nausea, vomiting, anorexia, diarrhea, and constipation, which affect the appetite.

Interventions to counteract the lack of taste buds or the lack of interest in eating may include preparing the food with color and garnishes, using attractive dishes and table settings with good lighting and bright colors, and providing foods that have more seasoning if there are no restrictions. Encourage the patient or caregiver to prepare homemade frozen dinners from extra portions of a favorite meal as an easy and effective way to provide a meal that will be enjoyed.

Individuals who have *impaired mobility* or *activity intolerance* that interferes with the ability to prepare food may benefit from community-based programs such as Meals on Wheels or home-delivered meals from a senior nutrition site. In addition, a wide variety of fresh, canned, and frozen foods in small or single servings is available in stores. Older adults should check the sodium content in canned or frozen foods to avoid consuming excessive amounts of sodium.

For most individuals, eating also is associated with a social setting. Dining alone may make eating less appealing. When an older individual has lost a spouse, or is unable to leave the house, *Despair, Grief,* and *Social Seclusion* are patient problem statements to be considered. Interventions that may assist the older adult in improving nutritional intake include community meal programs, church dinners, or senior citizen programs that provide transportation, meals, and opportunities to socialize.

Gastric reflux. Reflux occurs when the sphincter at the opening to the stomach becomes less efficient, which allows food and digestive enzymes to flow back into the esophagus. Symptoms include heartburn, sour stomach, and regurgitation of sour, bitter material. Reflux can be controlled by eating small meals, avoiding eating before bedtime, and elevating the head of the bed. Achieving and maintaining ideal body weight are also helpful.

Food intolerance. Lactose, primarily found in milk, is a common source of food intolerance. Dairy products are an important source of calcium, which is needed to prevent osteoporosis. Lactose-intolerant individuals may need to replace milk with cheese and yogurt, which is processed and easier to digest.

Dysphagia. Difficulty swallowing (dysphagia) may arise from many possible causes, including a stroke or other neurologic dysfunction, local trauma, and obstruction with a tumor. Assessment should focus on whether the dysphagia is with liquids, solids, or both and on the time frame for the progression of the symptoms. The older adult often has more difficulty swallowing fluids or foods that contain firm foods in liquid such as soup than swallowing semisolid or solid food.

Interventions for individuals who have difficulty swallowing include avoiding liquids, positioning, and verbal coaching. Thickeners can be added to liquids to improve the ability to control swallowing. The upright position, leaning slightly forward with the chin down, enlists the assistance of gravity to improve swallowing. Placing food on the unaffected side, reducing distractions in the room, and cueing the person to swallow are other ways to facilitate success.

Patient problems and interventions for the older adult with gastrointestinal (GI) system changes include but are not limited to the following:

PATIENT PROBLEM	NURSING INTERVENTIONS
Compromised Swallowing Ability, related to neurologic or vascular conditions	Refer to speech therapist for evaluation
	Assess individual's unique needs and problems
	Verify condition of teeth or fit of dentures
	Assist to sitting position with chin flexed toward chest
	Allow adequate time for meals
	Feed slowly
	Give frequent verbal cues to swallow
	Reduce distractions during meals.
	Keep suctioning equipment available in case of problems
Insufficient Nutrition, related to lack of interest in food	Assess reasons for loss of interest, such as depression or grief
	Monitor daily intake
	Weigh weekly
	Determine individual food preferences
	Provide oral hygiene before meals
	Serve meals in attractive manner; assist as needed
	Supplement meals with nutritious snacks if permitted
	Consult with dietitian
	Provide for social interaction during meals

Failure to thrive. Failure to thrive in older adults is characterized by refusal to eat, loss of weight and lean body mass, and subsequent malnutrition. This complex situation is associated with mental disorders, such as dementia and depression, and social and economic factors.

Specialized nutritional support. A patient's or resident's inability to ingest, digest, or absorb nutrients is in some cases an indication for enteral tube feedings. Feeding tubes can be placed into the stomach or the small intestine. A nasogastric or nasointestinal tube is inserted through the nose. A gastrostomy tube or percutaneous endoscopic gastrostomy (PEG) is inserted directly through the abdominal wall. Another option is a jejunostomy.

Standard enteral formulas contain whole proteins and complex carbohydrates. Other formulas contain modified protein (peptides) or amino acids. Enteral feedings sometimes are ordered short term after surgery, traumatic injury, or burns to improve nutritional intake. Transition to an oral diet occurs as soon as is feasible.

Long-term use of feeding tubes contributes to increased health risks and discomfort. The use of feeding tubes for cognitively impaired individuals is declining. Several studies suggest that the use of a tube feeding is

Fig. 33.5 Handfeeding often averts the need for feeding tubes.

not recommended for patients with advanced dementia due the possible side effects. It is suggested that careful hand feeding is the best alternative for patients with advanced dementia (Ijaopo, 2019). The use of feeding tubes has declined from 11.7% of patients with advanced dementia who had feeding tubes in 2000 to 5.7% in 2014 (Mitchell et al., 2016). Racial disparities have been noted with the use of feeding tubes. Many nursing home residents are provided with speech therapy to obtain recommendations for successful handfeeding (Fig. 33.5).

Gastrointestinal cancer. Follow-up and diagnostic testing is indicated in the presence of the following:

- Change in bowel or bladder habits
- Persistent oral lesions
- Visible or occult blood
- Indigestion or difficulty swallowing
- Unexplained weight loss
- Constipation
- Persistent bloating

Constipation has been defined broadly as an abnormally infrequent or difficult passage of hard, dry feces. Failure to relieve constipation creates the risk of a fecal impaction. Constipation can be acute or chronic. Older adults are often very attentive to their bowel function. Problems often are reported when a deviation occurs from what is perceived as normal elimination, even with relatively minor physiologic changes. Assessment relating to constipation includes dietary intake of fiber and fluids; use of medications such as opioid analgesics, antacids, iron preparations, anticholinergics, or overuse of laxatives; mechanical obstruction from fecal impaction, volvulus, adhesions, strangulated hernia, or cancer; activity and exercise patterns; and limitations such as inability to reach the toilet or a lack of privacy. Depression can be a contributing factor in some instances.

Nursing interventions include adequate fluids, exercise, and a diet that contains fiber. Bran is a good source of fiber for older adults who are unable to eat enough vegetables and fruits. Up to 10 g of bran per day may be included in the diet. This is achievable if the daily meals include two slices of whole-grain bread, two bran muffins or biscuits, and two spoonfuls of bran added to or sprinkled over other foods.

A patient problem and interventions for the older adult with constipation include but are not limited to the following:

PATIENT PROBLEM	NURSING INTERVENTIONS
Infrequent or Difficult Bowel Elimination, related to inadequate intake of fiber and fluids	Assess frequency and consistency of bowel movements Increase dietary fiber by encouraging cereals such as bran and fruits such as prunes Determine fluid preferences Keep fluids at bedside, and offer them at frequent intervals Administer stool softeners as ordered

Fecal incontinence. The most common cause of bowel incontinence in the older adult is fecal impaction associated with immobilization and inadequate fiber and fluid intake. A soft or liquid stool may ooze around the impaction, giving the appearance of diarrhea. Underlying diseases such as cancer, inflammatory bowel disease, colitis, and neurologic disease have the potential to cause fecal incontinence. A digital rectal examination by the primary health care provider may be needed to determine the nature of the problem.

Gastrointestinal bleeding. Older people have less protective mucus secretion, and therefore they are more susceptible to GI bleeding. Assess for blood in the stools in the presence of dizziness, pallor, tachycardia, or hypotension. Rectal bleeding can be a sign of hemorrhoids, rectal fissures, or cancer. In older adults, consider a guaiac-positive stool an indication of pathologic disturbance until proven otherwise. Laxatives, iron supplements, cimetidine (Tagamet), anticoagulants, aspirin and nonsteroidal antiinflammatory drugs (NSAIDs), and foods such as red meat may yield a false-positive guaiac result.

GENITOURINARY SYSTEM
Age-Related Changes
Overall kidney function decreases with age (Table 33.5). Even with a decrease of 50%, the body has adequate reserve to support normal body functions unless kidney disease is present. Bladder capacity decreases

Table 33.5 Urinary Changes With Aging

PHYSIOLOGIC CHANGE	RESULTS
Decreased number of functional nephrons	Decreased filtration rate
Decreased blood supply	Decreased removal of body wastes Increased concentration of urine
Decreased muscle tone	Increased volume of residual urine, stress incontinence, nocturia
Decreased tissue elasticity	Decreased bladder capacity
Increased size of prostate	Increased risk of infection Decreased stream of urine Increased hesitancy, frequency, nocturia

approximately 50% with age. Some bladders in older adults only hold 150 mL.

Incontinence sometimes occurs because bladder capacity decreases, urine residual increases, and bladder contractions increase. A decrease of bladder tone causes urine to remain in the bladder on emptying, which results in the sensation of a full bladder (frequency) within a brief period. Urinary tract infections also may trigger incontinence. In the older adult confusion may be the first symptom of an infection.

Urinary incontinence (UI), which affects more than 17% of women and 11% of men older than age 65 years, is embarrassing and debilitating. It is not a normal part of aging, although many believe that it is and do not seek treatment.

Changes specific to women are related to perineal changes as estrogen levels decline. Intercourse may become painful as the vaginal opening constricts and the vagina shortens, loses tone, and dries. Abnormal postmenstrual bleeding may indicate endometrial cancer and must be investigated.

Changes specific to men include enlargement of the prostate gland, which results in the occlusion of the urethra, obstructing the flow of urine; also, the scrotum becomes more pendulous. Although a man's libido does not normally decrease, erections may develop more slowly, and orgasms become less intense.

Assessment
- Assess frequency, amount, odor, color, and consistency of urine.
- Assess individual's ability to control urination.
- Assess satisfaction with sexuality and affectionate relationships.

Common Concerns and Nursing Interventions
Nocturia. At least 50% of older men and 70% of older women have to get up two or more times during the night to empty their bladders, a condition known as nocturia (urination at night). The decrease in bladder capacity may

be associated with the increase in voiding at night. This condition should be evaluated. It may also be attributed to other factors. Although nocturia does not jeopardize an individual's physical health, it is inconvenient, interferes with sleep, and tends to contribute to fatigue. Nursing interventions to decrease nocturia include limiting fluids in the evening, giving diuretic medications in the morning, and preventing fall hazards when an individual has to get up to urinate. A history of nocturia or an increase in the number of episodes necessitates medical evaluation, because it may indicate an infection and the need for medical treatment.

Urinary incontinence. Another related problem for many older individuals is incontinence. Some older adults do not leave their home for fear they will have an accident in public. The several types of incontinence include stress, urge, overflow, and functional incontinence. These types may occur in combination, causing a mixed incontinence that is common in older adults.

Stress incontinence is involuntary loss of a small amount of urine with increased abdominal pressure, such as coughing or sneezing. It is common in older women who have had multiple vaginal births or loss of muscle tone.

Urge incontinence is associated with cystitis, urethritis, tumors, stones, and central nervous system (CNS) disorders such as stroke, dementia, and Parkinson disease. Urge incontinence is characterized by involuntary urine loss after a sudden urge to void.

Overflow incontinence occurs when a chronically full bladder increases bladder pressure to a higher level than urethral resistance is able to counter, resulting in a loss of a small volume of urine. It is accompanied by a weak urine stream, difficulty starting to pass urine, interrupted voiding, or feeling of incomplete emptying. This may be the result of an atonic bladder from diabetic neuropathy, a side effect of anticholinergic medication, spinal cord injury, or mechanical obstruction (e.g., prostatic hypertrophy or a large cystocele).

Functional urinary incontinence occurs as a result of inability or unwillingness to get to the toilet because of physical limitations, depression, or confinement to bed or use of restraints. It may be related to dependence on a caregiver for assistance to the toilet.

Nursing interventions begin with an understanding that an older adult is *not* trying to get attention by requesting to go to the bathroom frequently and is not incontinent by choice. Never reprimand or humiliate an older adult for having to urinate or having accidents.

Careful evaluation of incontinence often helps identify *treatable* factors contributing to the incontinence. Treatment options include pharmacology, surgery, use of urethral inserts, and transvaginal or transrectal electrical nerve stimulation. Pharmacologic treatment possibilities include longer-acting versions of oxybutynin and tolterodine, which have fewer side effects. Behavioral therapies, such as pelvic floor–muscle

training and bladder retraining, alone or in combination with medication, have the potential to improve UI without adverse effects. Bladder retraining encourages a gradual increase in the time between voiding by designating timed intervals between voiding, rather than responding to each urge to urinate. Pelvic floor–muscle training, also known as Kegel exercises, has been effective in some cases of stress incontinence among women who performed them daily. Biofeedback techniques can be used to teach the exercises to participants by providing observable information about the location and contraction of muscles of the pelvic floor. Many other therapies are also available to assist with stress incontinence, including vaginal cone therapy, electrical stimulation devices, and a urethral plug. Be certain that an older adult has frequent and easy access to a bathroom or a urinal or commode. When other treatments are unsuccessful, many ambulatory older adults are comfortable going out in public if fitted with external collection devices, panty liners, or absorbent briefs. Never refer to an absorbent brief as a diaper when using it for an older adult.

Patient problems and interventions for the older adult with urinary system changes include but are not limited to the following:

PATIENT PROBLEM	NURSING INTERVENTIONS
Inability to Control Urination	Collect baseline bladder diaries to assess bladder habits, including frequency of urination and frequency of urinary incontinence
	Assess circumstances that precipitate incontinence (i.e., coughing, sneezing, position changes, or urgency)
	Assess awareness of dribbling and ability to control urine elimination
	Assess general health, current medications, and past medical problems, current medications, and medical, surgical, and obstetric history
	Assess use of incontinence products or other responses to incontinence
	Assess for other urinary symptoms (i.e., burning, pain, blood in the urine, difficulty getting a stream, urgency, or difficulty emptying the bladder)
	Assess physical and mental factors that may cause the patient to be unable to get to the bathroom on time
	Assess caregiver's willingness to participate in a behavioral program to treat incontinence
Inability to Control Urination, due to physical stress	Encourage the patient to use the toilet at appropriate intervals
	Teach pelvic floor exercises
	Provide toileting assistance and incontinence supplies as needed

PATIENT PROBLEM	NURSING INTERVENTIONS
Inability to Control Urination, due to urgency	Implement bladder training to increase awareness of the need to toilet Encourage the patient to use the toilet at appropriate intervals Provide information on urge inhibition Teach pelvic floor exercises Restrict caffeine intake, allowing no caffeine in the evening
Inability to Control Urination/ Urgency Due to Overflow	Allow sufficient time for voiding Teach patients the Credé method (manual expression of urine from the bladder) and encourage double voiding (urinate, relax, and repeat voiding attempt in 5 min) Notify the physician for an order for assessment of postvoid residual
Functional Inability to Control Urination	Teach caregiver to implement a prompted voiding program, increasing awareness of the need to toilet and prompting the use of the toilet at appropriate intervals Encourage fluid intake of 1500–2000 mL/day unless contraindicated Modify environment to maximize the patient's ability to get to the bathroom Obtain referral for physical or occupational therapy if indicated

CARDIOVASCULAR SYSTEM

Age-Related Changes

In general, cardiovascular changes with aging involve loss of structural elasticity (Table 33.6). Because the chambers are less elastic, the heart takes longer to contract and the chambers longer to fill. The heart valves become thicker and more rigid. A decrease in pacemaker cells occurs, and the electrical conduction is slowed or altered, which can lead to dysrhythmias. With aging, the resting heart rate tends to decrease, and the heart loses some of its capacity to increase the rate in response to exercise. Arteriosclerosis develops as the blood vessels become less elastic and are lined with deposits, resulting in increased blood pressure. In the past the definition of HTN in the older adult was less than or equal to a systolic pressure of 140 mm Hg. Some studies identify HTN in the elderly as a systolic of 150 mm Hg (Ferri et al., 2017). The patient's health care provider will determine the diagnosis of HTN in the elderly based on individualized factors.

The leading cause of death in the United States is heart disease. Two classifications are used for risk factors: nonmodifiable and modifiable. Age, gender, and family history are nonmodifiable risk factors. Modifiable risk factors include smoking, high blood pressure, a high-fat diet, obesity, physical inactivity, and stress.

Table 33.6   Cardiovascular Changes With Aging

PHYSIOLOGIC CHANGE	RESULTS
Decreased cardiac output	Increased incidence of heart failure
	Decreased peripheral circulation
Decreased elasticity of heart muscle and blood vessels	Decreased venous return
	Increased dependent edema
	Increased incidence of orthostatic hypotension
	Increased varicosities and hemorrhoids
Increased atherosclerosis	Increased blood pressure
	Increased myocardial infarction

Disparities. Although stroke death rates have been decreasing in older adults, the condition remains a growing problem for the African American community. More than 48% of women and 44% of African Americans have cardiovascular disease (The Heart Foundation, 2018). The rate of stroke in this population is twice that of whites (USDHHS, 2021). In addition, those African Americans affected are more likely to die.

Assessment

- Assess for difficulty breathing (dyspnea or orthopnea) aggravated by exertion.
- Assess cough onset and duration.
- Assess for signs of pallor, rubor, or cyanosis.
- Assess for chest pain, including onset, duration, relationship to activity, character (aching, burning, crushing), location, radiating, and severity, using a scale of 0 to 10.
- Assess apical and peripheral pulses. Compare both extremities when assessing characteristics of peripheral pulses.
- Assess capillary refill time.
- Assess for presence of vertigo, syncope, and fatigue.
- Assess blood pressure in lying, sitting, and standing positions. Note any significant change between positions (**orthostatic hypotension**).
- Assess for edema. Note location and severity.

Common Concerns and Nursing Interventions

Hypertension. HTN contributes to coronary artery disease (CAD) and stroke. It also contributes to the development of heart failure (HF), renal failure, and PVD. Pharmacologic treatment for HTN in people older than age 60 has decreased the incidence rate of coronary events significantly.

Coronary artery disease. Elevated serum cholesterol level is a major risk factor for CAD. A total cholesterol level of 130 mg/dL raises the risk for cardiac disease. Decreasing saturated fat content in the diet assists in reducing cholesterol levels. No more than 7% of calories should come from saturated fat, and no more than 200 mg of cholesterol should be consumed per day (American Heart Association [AHA], 2017). The American Heart Association recommends 20 to 30 minutes of moderate intensity exercise three to five times a week. Advise older adults to begin an exercise program with a 10- to 15-minute warm-up to achieve 75% of their maximal heart rate safely. Walking is the best aerobic exercise for older adults. They can set their own pace and choose the location. Encourage older adults with CAD to participate in cardiac rehabilitation programs to restore their physical and mental health to the highest level of function. This often involves several phases, beginning in the hospital and continuing in an outpatient setting (see the Patient Teaching box). A maintenance phase of counseling, exercise, and socialization may continue indefinitely.

Patient Teaching

Coronary Artery Disease

- Assess the knowledge and understanding of the disease process.
- Discuss the diagnosis, symptoms, and potential complications.
- Explain the purpose, dosage, side effects, and special considerations of all prescribed medications.
- Assess for modifiable cardiac risk factors and instruct the patient on the reduction of risks including:
- Diet (see Chapter 19)
  - Assess dietary intake.
  - Limit salt intake.
  - Limit intake of canned or processed foods.
- Exercise
  - As allowed by the health care provider, implement an exercise program.
  - Seniors should attempt to engage in 150 min/week (USDHHS, 2018).
- Obesity
  - Manage caloric intake to reduce BMI between 18.5 and 25.9 kg/m².
- Smoking
  - Refrain from tobacco use.
  - Avoid exposure to secondhand smoke.
- Diabetes mellitus
  - Monitor blood glucose levels daily or as recommended.
  - Maintain prescribed dietary regimens.
  - Exercise as directed.
- Avoid tobacco exposure.
- *Psychological state:* Identify sources of stress and changes that can be made to reduce these stressors.
- Implement positive sleep hygiene habits to ensure rest.

Dysrhythmias. Changes in the structure of the heart, the blood supply to the heart, and the pacemaker system sometimes make the heart more susceptible to irregular heart rhythms (dysrhythmias). Dysrhythmias cause the heart to be less effective in supplying blood to the body and have the potential to lead to heart failure. Nursing interventions for patients with dysrhythmias include

checking vital signs frequently; noting the rate, regularity, and strength of the pulse; accurately monitoring fluid intake and output (I&O); and observing and reporting an older person's response to medications. Other nursing interventions include keeping stress on the heart to a minimum by monitoring the response to activity and providing appropriate rest periods before and after activity.

Peripheral vascular disease. Vascular changes affect the arteries or veins of the older adult. Spasms or atherosclerosis allow insufficient amounts of oxygenated blood to circulate to tissues in the legs and feet. Some older adults have inadequate circulation to the muscles, which results in cold feet, numbness, and intermittent claudication (cramping pain in the calves). Inadequate supply of arterial blood to the lower extremities results in a condition called peripheral vascular disease (PVD). Another common condition is varicose veins, which involves failure of the valves to close adequately because of distention and weakening of the venous walls.

Nursing interventions include techniques to promote circulation, including walking to stimulate venous return, avoiding standing in one place for long periods, and not crossing the legs. Compression stockings provide support for varicose veins.

When inadequate circulation results in skin ulcerations and altered sensation (numbness), nursing interventions may include compression stockings, pneumatic compression pumps, Unna boots, maintenance of the cleanliness of the feet and legs, adequate shoes that give protection, and education of the older adult to be aware of situations that may cause injury, because sensation for hot and cold is decreased.

A patient problem and interventions for the older adult with PVD include but are not limited to the following:

PATIENT PROBLEM	NURSING INTERVENTIONS
Compromised Blood Flow to Tissue, related to circulatory changes with aging	Assess peripheral tissue for color, temperature sensation, movement, and the presence of pain
	Assess rate, rhythm, and volume of peripheral pulses
	Assess for the presence of edema.
	Apply antiembolism stockings as ordered
	Teach patient to avoid constrictive clothing
	Establish a walking program to slowly and steadily increase walking distance without pain
	Administer vasodilating or cardiotonic medications as ordered
	Handle gently to avoid skin tears.
	Avoid temperature extremes
	Discourage smoking

RESPIRATORY SYSTEM

Age-Related Changes

The tissues of the lungs and bronchi become less elastic and more rigid with age. The ribs become less mobile, and osteoporosis and calcification of the cartilage lead to rigidity and stiffness of the thoracic cage. Oxygen-carrying capacity (hemoglobin) often is diminished in older adults. Muscles associated with respiration sometimes weaken so that lung expansion and vital capacity are decreased. Older adults also tend to have a decrease in the number and effectiveness of cilia in the tracheobronchial tree, which results in increased difficulty in clearing secretions and increased risk of respiratory infections. This, together with less elastic alveoli, decreases vital capacity and leads to shortness of breath with activity.

Kyphosis is an abnormal curve in the upper spine sometimes called "dowager's hump." The chest wall is less able to expand because of changes in the skeletal system (Table 33.7). Overall, the older person's air exchange is reduced, and secretions and residual air remain in the lungs.

In addition, *lifestyle factors* affect lung function. Exercise has a positive effect on the respiratory and cardiovascular systems, whereas immobility has a negative effect. The lung damage that is caused by smoking and by prolonged exposure to secondhand smoke in the lungs of nonsmokers is well known. Obesity results in markedly reduced pulmonary function and increased breathlessness. Diminished cough and arousal reflexes increase the likelihood of aspiration during sleep. The increased sleep time of older adults increases the risk of aspiration and oxygen desaturation from diminished ventilatory drive and a loss of upper airway tone that predisposes to apnea or hypopnea.

Assessment

- Assess depth, rhythm, and rate of respiration at rest and with activity.
- Inspect the chest for shape and symmetry, body position, and use of accessory muscles for respiration.
- Assess breath sounds for adventitious sounds, including crackles and wheezing (inspiratory or expiratory).
- Assess the amount of activity the individual is able to tolerate. Note activities that result in increased respiratory effort.
- Ask the patient to evaluate breathlessness on a scale of 0 to 10.
- Assess for the presence of cough. Note whether cough is productive or nonproductive. Assess amount, frequency, and color of sputum production.

Common Concerns and Nursing Interventions

Chronic obstructive pulmonary disease. A common respiratory condition of older adults, chronic obstructive pulmonary disease (COPD) is not a single disease but commonly a combination of chronic bronchitis, chronic asthma, and emphysema in varying degrees as a result of

Table 33.7 Respiratory Changes With Aging	
PHYSIOLOGIC CHANGE	**RESULTS**
Decreased body fluids	Decreased ability to humidify air
Decreased number of cilia	Decreased ability to trap debris
Decreased tissue elasticity	Decreased gas exchange
	Increased pooling of secretions in lower lobes
Decreased number of capillaries	Decreased gas exchange
Increased calcification of cartilage	Increased rigidity of ribcage
	Decreased lung capacity
Possible development of kyphosis, an abnormal curve in the upper spine called "dowager's hump"	Chest wall less able to expand because of changes in the skeletal system

progressive changes that are seen as individuals become older. A smoking history increases the risk of debilitating COPD. Assessment reveals diminished breath sounds, crackles, and wheezes and a "barrel chest" characterized by an increased anteroposterior diameter. By age 90, nearly everyone has some degree of COPD.

Nursing interventions for older adults with mild to moderate COPD include pulmonary hygiene, breathing retraining, chest physiotherapy (CPT), medications, smoking cessation, and exercise programs. Pulmonary hygiene includes encouraging the patient to drink plenty of fluids to liquefy secretions and teaching deep diaphragmatic breathing and a variety of coughing techniques to remove secretions and improve airway clearance. Techniques such as pursed-lip breathing help empty the lungs of used air, which in turn promotes inhalation of adequate oxygen. CPT includes chest percussion, postural drainage, vibration, and rib shaking. Postural drainage consists of positioning the patient in a head-down position to facilitate drainage of pulmonary secretions. Medications may be given orally, via a metered-dose inhaler (MDI), or via nebulizer. Oxygen therapy also is considered a medication. The patient and the family need to learn correct oxygen liter flow, when it is to be used, and care and use of the equipment.

Patients must be taught how to adapt their lifestyles and activities of daily living (ADLs). Doing moderate intensity exercises for 20 to 30 minutes 3 to 5 days a week reduces cardiovascular disease risks, improves musculoskeletal function, helps promote weight loss, and helps prevent bone loss in older adults. In the presence of COPD, a program must be started in very small increments, such as walking for 3 to 5 minutes daily. Appropriate exercise intensity maintains a heart rate of at least 55% of the maximal rate for a patient's age, that is, a rate of 88 for a 60-year-old and 80 for a 75-year-old. Classes and exercise times usually allow for socialization with others, emotional support, and the opportunity to get out of the home.

Additional interventions include avoiding smoking and air pollution, preventing infections by avoiding crowds and people with upper respiratory infections, and receiving the flu vaccines annually. Older patients with COPD often find smoking cessation difficult, if not impossible. Success partly depends on the support of family and friends. Programs are available through the American Lung Association, the American Cancer Society, and many community hospitals.

Because respiratory function affects many other systems and the functional ability of the individual, other nursing diagnoses and interventions are likely to be appropriate for a patient with COPD.

Pneumonia. Age-related changes and decreased resistance to respiratory infections cause more older individuals to contract and die of pneumonia than younger people. Even with modern antibiotics and sophisticated medical treatment, pneumonia has the potential to be life threatening for the older adult. This is especially true if an older adult is hospitalized and has other chronic illnesses. Encourage older individuals to receive the pneumonia vaccination as recommended by the primary care provider.

Older individuals do not always exhibit the usual signs and symptoms of pneumonia, such as high fever, cough, pain, and headache. In contrast, they often show signs and symptoms only of lethargy, disorientation, anorexia, and low or mild fever. Older adults who show such signs and symptoms should consult their health care provider for diagnosis and treatment.

Interventions focus on liquefying secretions through adequate intake of fluids, taking prescribed medications, assisting removal of secretions by teaching proper coughing technique to improve airway clearance, and turning and deep breathing to improve gas exchange and prevent stasis of secretions (see the Home Care Considerations box).

🏠 Home Care Considerations

Respiratory Disorders

- Encourage fluid intake of 8–10 glasses of water a day, if not contraindicated.
- Encourage the older adult to exercise within capacity to promote thoracic muscle conditioning.
- Monitor for smoking and exposure to secondhand smoke. Encourage family members to not smoke in the presence of the older adult.
- Encourage pursed-lip breathing to control breathlessness and improve oxygenation.
- Monitor pulse oximetry to assess oxygenation.
- Encourage frequent small meals to reduce breathlessness associated with eating.
- If home oxygen is used, assess the home environment for potential safety hazards, including the possibility of the older adult tripping over oxygen tubing.
- Assess for confusion, occipital headaches, and forgetfulness. These symptoms may be indicative of carbon dioxide retention. Teach family caregivers these signs as well.

Modified from Meiner SE, Yeager JJ: *Gerontologic nursing*, ed 6, St. Louis, 2019, Mosby.

Patient problems and interventions for the older adult with respiratory changes include but are not limited to the following:

PATIENT PROBLEM	NURSING INTERVENTIONS
Inability to Clear Airway, related to excessive tenacious secretions	Assess respiratory patterns, effort, and lung sounds
	Observe for signs of cyanosis
	Teach effective breathing and coughing
	Promote adequate hydration
	Suction secretions if necessary
	Administer supplemental oxygen and nebulizer treatments as ordered
	Encourage use of spirometry as ordered
Inefficient Oxygenation, related to elevated CO2 (carbon dioxide)	Monitor oximetry readings for oxygen saturation
	Administer oxygen per protocol

Lung cancer. Lung cancer is the leading cause of cancer deaths. It is rare in people under the age of 40 but increases in incidence between ages 60 and 70. Risk factors for developing lung cancer include use of tobacco or marijuana; recurring inflammation; exposure to asbestos, talcum powder, or minerals or, less frequently, to radon; heredity; vitamin A deficiency; and air pollution. The most common form of lung cancer is small-cell lung carcinoma (SCLC), which sometimes metastasizes to the CNS, the bones, and the liver. Often no signs or symptoms are evident, or the signs are ignored or attributed to smoking or a preexisting lung disease. Nonspecific signs and symptoms may include cough, chest pain, and hemoptysis. The diagnosis of lung cancer is based on clinical history and chest x-ray studies or computed tomographic (CT) scan of the chest. Lung cancer staging provides the basis for treatment. Stage I is treatable with surgery. Treatment modalities for other stages include surgery, radiotherapy, and adjuvant chemotherapy. Stage IV treatment is palliative and includes radiotherapy, chemotherapy, and laser therapy. Nursing interventions include relief of pain, emotional support, counseling, and discussion of options and alternatives.

MUSCULOSKELETAL SYSTEM

Age-Related Changes

Some of the most obvious changes associated with aging occur in the musculoskeletal system. A gradual reduction is seen in the number and the size of active muscle fibers, and muscle tone, mass, and strength are decreased. The joints become less elastic and flexible with the loss and the calcification of cartilage. An alteration occurs in the equilibrium between bone deposition and resorption (Fig. 33.6). Falling estrogen levels in women increases bone resorption and decreases calcium deposition, resulting in bone loss and decreased bone density. The long bones and the vertebrae are

Fig. 33.6 Posture changes with aging.

Table 33.8   Musculoskeletal Changes With Aging

PHYSIOLOGIC CHANGE	RESULTS
Decreased bone calcium	Osteoporosis
	Increased curvature of the spine (kyphosis)
Decreased fluid in intervertebral disks	Decreased height
Decreased blood supply to muscles	Decreased muscle strength
Decreased joint mobility	Decreased mobility and flexibility
Decreased muscle mass	Decreased strength
	Increased risk of falls

especially vulnerable to the reduction of bone density. In the spine, narrowing of the intervertebral spaces results in a loss of 1½ to 3 inches of height. The lumbar curve of the lower back changes, which results in a shift in the center of gravity. Structural and postural changes may result in changes to the gait. The risk of fractures is increased in this population as a result of the interrelated factors (Table 33.8).

Assessment

- Assess active and passive range of motion of each joint for stiffness and limitation of movement.
- Assess joints for edema, erythema, pain, and crepitus with particular motions.
- Assess ability to perform personal care (i.e., eating, bathing, dressing, grooming, and elimination) and other activities (i.e., housework, driving, climbing stairs, caring for pets).
- Assess standing and gait, including balance, posture, base of support, size of steps, and ability to turn.
- Assess for limping, numbness or tingling, deformity, and change in skeletal contour.
- Assess for muscle weakness, paralysis, tremors, spasms, clumsiness, muscle wasting, and muscle aches.
- Assess pain using a scale of 0 to 10, location, type, onset (sudden or gradual), aggravating or alleviating factors, and position of comfort.
- Assess history of falls, traumatic injury, surgeries on joint or bone, and back problems.

Common Concerns and Nursing Interventions

Arthritis. Two forms of arthritis may occur in the older adult. Rheumatoid arthritis, a systemic inflammatory disease thought to be of immune factor origin, has the potential to affect people of any age. Osteoarthritis, or degenerative joint disease, is a noninflammatory disorder in which the cartilage in the joints deteriorates and new bone forms on the surface. This is the most common type of arthritis in older adults. Affected joints most commonly include the hands, fingers, and toes and the knees, hips, and spine.

Because the chronic nature of osteoarthritis affects an individual's functional ability and lifestyle, interventions for older individuals with arthritis involve joint protection and energy conservation through a balance between rest and exercise. Simple measures such as a warm bath or shower in the morning often reduce early morning stiffness. Recommend range-of-motion and other forms of mild exercise to maintain muscle strength and joint motion. Heat or cold therapy and gentle massage usually help to control pain and muscle spasms. Health care providers often prescribe NSAIDs and nonopioid analgesics. Injections of steroids into the joints two or three times yearly may help with chronic pain.

In more advanced situations, use of assistive devices is common (i.e., splints, walkers, adapted utensils, and clothes with Velcro fasteners). With increasing disability and severe pain, many people consider surgical options. Joint arthroplasty, a surgical replacement of the involved joint, is successful in treating arthritic pain in the shoulders, elbows, fingers, hips, and knees. Other surgical options include joint fusion, which increases function and decreases pain while eliminating some joint movement.

Hip fractures. According to the CDC (2021), one out of five falls result in serious injuries, such as broken bones or a head injury, and more than 800,000 patients are admitted each year because of head injuries or hip fractures resulting from a fall. The most frequently occurring fractures among older adults are hip, vertebral, and clavicular fractures. Fractures fall into two categories, open or closed, and vary according to location and type. The history of the patient with a fracture usually includes trauma followed by immediate local pain. Tenderness, edema, muscle spasm, deformity, bleeding, and loss of function are other manifestations common with fractures.

A fall may not be the precipitating factor in hip fractures. Commonly, weakening of the upper femur from osteoporosis causes the bone to break—and then the fall occurs (Ignatavicius, 20182018). Hip fractures are the most disabling type of fracture in older adults. A significant percentage of patients with hip fracture die within 1 year after injury. Clinicians use the locations of hip fractures to classify them. Intracapsular or subcapital fractures occur within the hip capsule. Extracapsular fractures occur below the capsule and include intertrochanteric and subtrochanteric (Fig. 33.7).

When a hip fracture occurs, the affected extremity usually is rotated externally and shortened. Tenderness and severe pain at the fracture site are often present. Immobilization of the joint is necessary. Surgical repair is the preferred treatment when the patient's condition has stabilized. Surgery depends on the location and type of fracture and often includes open reduction and internal fixation (ORIF) with pins, plates, and screws for extracapsular fractures (Fig. 33.8A) or prosthetic replacement of the femoral head for intracapsular fractures (bipolar or hemiarthroplasty; see Fig. 33.8B).

Nursing interventions after surgery require monitoring of vital signs and I&O. Frequent turning, deep breathing, coughing, and an incentive spirometer are used to prevent respiratory complications. Monitor the operative site for signs of infection and bleeding. Assess movement, circulation, and sensation of the extremity to detect impaired circulation. Monitor mental status. Postoperative delirium is possible from the anesthesia, the analgesic medications, pain, immobility, and loss of familiar surroundings. Opioid analgesics should be used cautiously. Practitioners often use lower doses of opioids to prevent changes in mental status, respiratory depression, and oversedation.

The affected extremity is kept in alignment to help keep pain to a minimum. Use pillows between the knees or an abduction splint to accomplish this. Patients who have hemiarthroplasty are at risk for dislocation, which is most likely to occur when the joint is adducted and internally rotated. Avoid movements such as crossing the legs and feet while the patient is seated and adducting the legs when the patient is lying on the unoperated side. Instruct patients to use a raised toilet seat and a shower chair, and avoid activities that have potential to cause dislocation of the hip for 6 weeks or more after surgery until the muscles that surround the joint are healed and the joint has stabilized.

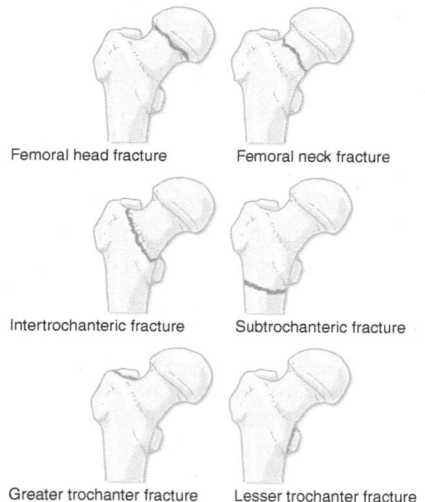

Femoral head fracture   Femoral neck fracture

Intertrochanteric fracture   Subtrochanteric fracture

Greater trochanter fracture   Lesser trochanter fracture

Fig. 33.7 Types of fractures of the hip as labeled in diagram. (From Adams JG, et al. *Emergency medicine, clinical essentials,* ed 2, Philadelphia, 2013, Elsevier.)

Fig. 33.8 ((A) and (B) Hip arthroplasty (femoral ball and socket)(B) (C) and (D) Open reduction and internal fixation (ORIF) with nails, screws, or rods.(From Cifu D, Lew HL, Oh-Park M: Chapter 3: Osteoporosis and fragility fracture. *Geriatric Rehabilitation,* ed 1, 2018, Elsevier, with permission.)

Comprehensive multidisciplinary rehabilitation focuses on the goal of returning the patient to the previous level of function. Specific areas of treatment include gait and transfer training, muscle strengthening through active assistive exercises, and teaching the use of assistive devices such as walkers and canes. During recovery, it is important to prevent depression resulting from limited independence. Consistently point out the patient's strengths, give positive feedback, and reinforce progress.

Osteoporosis. Osteoporosis, a systemic skeletal disease, is one of the most common conditions in older women. The characteristic low bone mass and deterioration of bone tissue result in a significantly increased risk of fractures. Fractures are possible in the course of routine activities such as bending, lifting, coughing, and straining at stool. Osteoporosis of the spinal vertebrae may cause a loss of height of 1½ to 3 inches or kyphosis, the development of a C shape to the cervical vertebrae, which causes a stoop that is at times severe. The visible hump on the back is also called the dowager's hump. Although osteoporosis tends to be considered a disease of old age, it actually begins in younger women. Prevention begins with children and adolescents. A diet high in calcium and vitamin D and regular weight-bearing exercise lay the foundation for later life. Bone density testing helps identify older women at risk for fractures and points the way to instituting preventive measures. Advise all women to avoid smoking and excessive alcohol and limit caffeine consumption. Additional information for osteoporosis education is available through the National Osteoporosis Foundation at www.nof.org.

For some women, osteoporosis prevention includes reducing estrogen deficiency from perimenopause with hormone replacement therapy (HRT), but its use is controversial. Although HRT has a positive effect on calcium absorption, it possibly contributes to an increased incidence of endometrial cancer, an increased risk for breast cancer, and an increase in cardiovascular disease and stroke; therefore practitioners generally do not prescribe estrogen for osteoporosis except for limited periods.

Older women need 1200 to 2000 mg of calcium daily and 600 to 800 IU of vitamin D daily (Mayo Clinic, 2020). Sixty percent of patients with hip fractures have a deficiency of vitamin D. Bisphosphonates are the most common classification of medications prescribed to treat osteoporosis. These include alendronate (Binosto, Fosamax), risedronate (Actonel, Atelvia), zoledronic acid (Reclast, Zometa), and ibandronate (Boniva). These medications improve bone density and lessen the rate of bone loss.

Patient problems and interventions for the older adult with musculoskeletal system changes include but are not limited to the following:

PATIENT PROBLEM	NURSING INTERVENTIONS
Self-care deficit, related to weakness • Bathing/hygiene • Dressing/grooming • Feeding • Toileting	Assess ability to dress, feed, bathe, and toilet self Develop plan to enhance highest level of function Allow adequate time to perform activities Provide assistive devices as indicated Consult with physical and occupational therapy Modify environment to facilitate self-care
Potential for Falling, related to age-related changes	Assess balance, gait, strength, medications that cause vertigo or drowsiness, sensory problems, and impaired mobility Maintain a regular weight-bearing exercise routine that is enjoyable Provide good lighting and assistive devices (walkers or canes) to assist balance Eliminate environmental hazards, clutter, uneven walking surfaces, and scatter rugs Encourage moving slowly from lying to standing to keep orthostatic hypotension (a sudden drop in blood pressure when standing up quickly) to a minimum

ENDOCRINE SYSTEM

Age-Related Changes
The levels of hormones secreted and the response of body tissue to hormones change with age (Table 33.9). Thyroid disturbances, especially hypothyroidism and DM, are the common endocrine disorders in the older adult.

Assessment
• Assess laboratory results and report abnormal calcium, glucose, or thyroid hormone levels.

Common Concerns and Nursing Interventions
Type 2 diabetes mellitus. There are two general types of DM: type 1 (formerly called insulin-dependent diabetes mellitus [IDDM] or juvenile diabetes), in which the body fails to produce insulin; and type 2 (formerly called non–insulin dependent [NIDDM] or adult-onset diabetes), which is characterized by the body's inability to produce and use insulin appropriately. Type 2 DM is more common than type 1 DM, and it affects 85% to 90% of adults with diabetes. Patients do not always exhibit the usual signs or symptoms of thirst, increased appetite, and large amounts of urine, as seen in type 1 DM. Repeated infections, slow healing, blurred vision, and weight gain or loss tend to be the initial signs and symptoms of DM that are more commonly seen in older adults.

Table 33.9	Endocrine Changes With Aging
PHYSIOLOGIC CHANGE	**RESULTS**
Decreased pituitary excretions of adrenocorticotropic hormone (ACTH) and steroids	Decreased muscle mass
Decreased production of thyroid-stimulating hormone	Decreased basal metabolic rate
Decreased production of parathyroid hormone (seen with osteoporosis)	Increased blood calcium levels
Decreased production and use of insulin	Increased blood glucose levels
Decreased release of testosterone, estrogen, and progesterone	Menopause in women and multiple system changes

The goal of interventions in type 2 DM is to achieve and maintain a stable metabolic state through diet management, weight control, and exercise. Diabetic education includes topics such as medication, the disease process, monitoring of blood glucose, signs and symptoms of hyperglycemia and hypoglycemia, sick-day management, foot care, eye care, and various other complications. Active involvement of the patient and family in the disease and plan of treatment promotes retention of information and compliance. Resources for patient educational handouts are available from the American Diabetes Association (ADA), and other sources.

When working with the older adult, assist in adapting a diet that meets the recommendations but also encompasses as many of the individual's personal dietary preferences as possible. This helps improve compliance. Goals should focus on achieving a BMI and weight within an acceptable range for the height and weight. A reduction in weight reduces the insulin resistance of the body's cells. Advise the person to balance intake with recommended amounts of protein, carbohydrates, fats, vitamins, and minerals. Encourage limiting refined sugar and choosing a high-fiber diet.

Older adults with DM are at a higher risk for foot problems because of changes in peripheral nerves and blood vessels. Inadequate blood flow to the feet and nerve damage contribute to the development of ulcers and infections. Hyperglycemia also plays a role because a blood glucose level of 200 mg/100 mL or higher is associated with an altered immune system leukocyte response. Although the rate of limb amputations in patients with DM has declined over the past two decades to a rate of 4 per 1000 patients, the operative loss of a limb is life altering to the patient. *Peripheral neuropathy* is the presence of abnormal sensation, numbness, and burning sensations in the extremities. This condition increases with age, particularly in people who have DM. Decreased awareness of pain, temperature changes, and diminished circulation result in risk for injury. Undetected injuries become infected easily and, if untreated, in some cases necessitate eventual amputation. Activities that promote good circulation include avoiding smoking, avoiding constricting footwear, and keeping legs uncrossed.

To prevent foot injuries, recommend daily cleansing of the feet with nondrying agents and daily inspection of the feet for blisters, cuts, or infections with a mirror. Nails are best cut or filed straight across to prevent skin injury. Recommend regular visits to a podiatrist or a health care provider who inspects the feet. Counsel individuals with neuropathy of the feet, hyperglycemia, or a history of foot infections to seek care at the first sign of a foot injury or infection.

Hypothyroidism. Aging has an impact on the thyroid gland. Over time the thyroid's function may become impaired. Neoplasms and hypothyroidism and hyperthyroidism increase in likelihood with aging. The clinical manifestations of hypo- and hyperthyroidism are more subtle. Of people older than 65 years of age 20% have thyroid problems, the most frequent of which is hypothyroidism (Touhy and Jett, 2019). Decreased thyroid function often appears in a subclinical form, and the health care provider becomes aware of it through the results of routine serum testing. Almost all cases are inconspicuous and progress slowly toward thyroid failure. Signs frequently linked to hypothyroidism in older adults include unexplained elevation in triglycerides or plasma cholesterol, nonspecific cognitive impairment, slow metabolism, chest pain or atrial fibrillation, constipation, macrocytic anemia, vague arthritic reports, cold intolerance, and depression with underlying apathy and withdrawal. The goal for interventions is stabilization of thyroid levels with medication (levothyroxine). The practitioner monitors the response to therapy through thyroid-stimulating hormone (TSH) levels. Nursing interventions center on patient and family education related to disease signs and symptoms and medication therapy. Careful management of medication therapy is essential. With treatment, patients generally experience increased energy and weight loss.

REPRODUCTIVE SYSTEM

Age-Related Changes

The major changes in the reproductive system related to aging are diminished levels of estrogen and progesterone in women and diminished levels of androgen and testosterone in men. The process of aging diminishes sexual function but does not put a halt to it. The lack of the circulating hormone testosterone in men and estrogen, progesterone, and androgen in women results in changes with arousal, orgasm, post-orgasm, and genitalia. Although it takes longer for a man to be sexually aroused and achieve erection and ejaculation, men maintain the ability for sexual function into their 80s and 90s. For women, menopause is marked by a decrease in hormones, the inability to procreate, and tissue atrophy of ovaries, fallopian tubes, cervix, and vulva. A decrease is seen in the amount of vaginal secretions, and the pH becomes more alkaline. Although age-related changes occur, they do not diminish the older woman's capacity to achieve orgasm and enjoy sexual relations (Table 33.10).

The provision of holistic care requires the introduction of subjects that may be difficult. Sexuality and any related concerns should be included in the assessment. To begin the assessment, consider making a general statement about the continuing sexual needs of older adults. After this, open-ended questions regarding the patient's sexuality are likely to be useful. For example:

"Tell me how you express your sexuality."
"What concerns do you have about fulfilling your continuing sexual needs?"
"In what ways has your sexual relationship with your partner changed as you have aged?"

The Permission, Limited Information, Specific Suggestions, and Intensive Therapy (PLISSIT) model has been used to assess and manage adults' sexuality. The model includes obtaining *p*ermission from individuals to initiate sexual discussion, providing the *l*imited *i*nformation they need to function sexually, giving *s*pecific *s*uggestions for individuals to proceed with sexual relations, and providing *i*ntensive *t*herapy regarding the issues of sexuality. The goal of assessment is to gather information that allows individuals to express sexuality safely and to feel uninhibited by normal or pathologic problems.

Nurses and nursing students commonly feel uncomfortable with assessing the sexual desires and functions of older patients. Regardless, a sexual assessment is a necessary part of the routine nursing assessment. Skill and comfort come with practice.

Assessment

- Assess past experiences or difficulties and sexually transmitted infections (STIs).
- Assess for signs of vaginal or penile ulceration, edema, or discharge.
- Assess for presence of lumps, dimpling, or drainage from the breast.

Common Concerns and Nursing Interventions

Sexual function. The misconceptions that older adults are impotent and asexual or that they are perverse if they are sexually active are common reasons for sexual dysfunction in older adults. If individuals continue to be sexually active on a regular basis, they retain the capability to respond sexually. If an older adult indicates that sexual intercourse is difficult or uncomfortable because of vaginal dryness, suggest use of estrogen creams or water-soluble lubricants to relieve the discomfort.

Table 33.10	Reproductive Changes With Aging

PHYSIOLOGIC CHANGE	RESULTS
Female	
Decreased estrogen levels	Vagina shortens, narrows, and loses some of its elasticity
	Decreased vaginal secretions
	Decreased pubic hair
	Increased vaginal tissue fragility and irritation
	Decreased size of uterus and vagina
	Increased pain with intercourse (dyspareunia)
	Decreased breast tissue mass
Increased vaginal alkalinity	Increased risk of infection
Male	
Decreased testosterone	Decreased amount of facial and pubic hair
	Lack of energy
	Erectile dysfunction
	Decrease in libido
Decreased circulation	Decreased rate of ejaculation
	Decreased force of ejaculation
	Decreased speed gaining erection

Research and information from a variety of sources indicate that aging individuals have the potential to be sexual, continue to have interest in sex, and are indeed sexual beings. For many older adults, the lack of a sexual partner is the main factor for decreased sexual activity.

Sexuality also encompasses sexual identity as a man or woman, intimacy (emotional closeness to others), and touch. Regardless of age, it is important to feel good about oneself as a male or female and to have close relationships with other people. Sexual intimacy is more than intercourse; it includes caressing, stroking, and kissing and being an emotional companion to the partner. A positive correlation exists between sexuality and physical health. This relationship makes the preservation of sexual activity and function a source of health promotion. To best assist patients and their significant others, examine your feelings about sexuality and aging and become informed about age-related changes in sexual function. The sexuality of older adults can also be supported by encouraging and helping them to look their best, complimenting them when they look nice, respecting and allowing them to have their privacy, allowing their expressions of affection for one another, and using touch to communicate acceptance. A pat on the arm or a hug is a potential way to communicate concern and caring to almost anyone.

A patient problem and interventions for the older adult with sexual dysfunction include but are not limited to the following:

PATIENT PROBLEM	NURSING INTERVENTIONS
Impaired Sexual Expression, related to lack of privacy	Allow verbalization of concerns regarding sexual needs
	Provide privacy for interaction between alert, consenting individuals
	Assist individual to maintain good physical hygiene and meet cosmetic needs
	Provide distraction and alternative activities for disoriented individuals who masturbate; if unsuccessful, provide privacy

SENSORY PERCEPTION

Age-Related Changes

The senses provide a link with the environment by receiving and interpreting various stimuli including but not limited to vision, hearing, taste, and smell (Table 33.11). Visual and hearing impairments interfere with communication, social interactions, and mobility, leading to social isolation. In the past, we recognized five senses: sight, hearing, taste, smell, and touch. Today we acknowledge additional senses and categorize all senses into two major groups: general and special. General senses include touch, pressure, pain, temperature, vibration, and proprioception. Special senses are produced by highly localized organs and sensory cells including sight, hearing, taste, smell, and balance. Sensation, or perception, is the conscious awareness and interpretation of sensory stimuli by sensory receptors.

Vision. Visual changes increase with aging. Significant changes are associated with ages over 65 years. The pupil is reduced in size. Acclimating to changes in light in the room becomes increasingly difficult. The muscles of the eyes become less effective causing changes in visual acuity. Discerning differing colors of similar hue becomes difficult. Tear production is also lessened (National Library of Medicine [NLM], 2018). Visual impairments can lead to injury because of falls. The four leading causes of visual impairment are cataracts, glaucoma, macular degeneration, and diabetic retinopathy (Bedinghaus, 2020). Undiagnosed visual disorders are increasing among older adults, especially in ethnic and cultural minorities.

Age-related changes in vision include **presbyopia** (farsightedness resulting from a loss of elasticity of the lens of the eye), or narrowing of the peripheral field of vision, decreased ability to focus on near objects, and a decrease in visual acuity as the pupil becomes smaller and less responsive to light. There is some clouding of the lens of the eye. Yellowing of the lens and changes in color perception cause older adults to have difficulty differentiating shades of some colors such as green, blue, and violet. Depth perception is distorted, and vision in dim light becomes difficult. General vision screening for individuals who wear glasses or contact

Table 33.11 Sensory Changes With Aging

PHYSIOLOGIC CHANGE	RESULTS
Vision	
Decreased number of eyelashes	Increased risk of eye injury
Decreased tear production	Increased risk of eye irritation
Increased discoloration of lens	Decreased color perception
Decreased tissue elasticity	Increased blurring
Decreased muscle tone	Decreased diameter of pupil
	Increased refractive errors
	Decreased night vision
	Increased sensitivity to glare
Hearing	
Decreased tissue elasticity	Decreased ability to distinguish high-frequency sounds
Decreased joint mobility	Decreased ability to distinguish high-frequency sounds
	Decreased hearing ability
Decreased number of hair cells in inner ear	Increased problems with balance
Taste and Smell	
Decreased number of papillae on tongue	Decreased ability to taste
Decreased number of nasal sensory receptors	Decreased ability to detect smells

lenses involves observation of reading print from a newspaper. Note the distance from the eyes the person holds the newspaper, and verify the person's ability to see print clearly (Fig. 33.9). Limited vision indicates the need for a more detailed eye examination. Although age-related changes decrease visual capability, blindness is not a normal result of aging.

Glaucoma. Glaucoma, the second leading cause of blindness in the United States, is caused by an occlusion in the drainage of the fluid in the anterior chamber of the eye, which produces an increase in intraocular pressure. Pressure transfers to the optic nerve, where damage or blindness is a possible result. Primary open-angle glaucoma, the most common type, makes up 90% of all cases of primary glaucoma. This type of glaucoma has the capacity to reduce vision so gradually and painlessly that a person is unaware of a problem until the optic nerve is badly damaged. Visual loss begins with deteriorating peripheral vision. Early diagnoses of primary open-angle glaucoma allows for control and prevention of serious visual impairment (National Eye Institute, 2020).

In contrast, acute angle-closure glaucoma occurs suddenly as a result of complete occlusion in the path of the aqueous humor. Signs and symptoms of acute

Fig. 33.9 Vision screening with use of a newspaper.

angle-closure glaucoma include severe eye pain, erythema, clouded or blurred vision, nausea and vomiting, rainbow halo surrounding lights, pupil dilation, and a steamy appearance of the cornea. Severe problems develop in acute angle-closure glaucoma when intraocular pressure rises above 50 mm Hg (normal range is 10 to 22 mm Hg). In the absence of emergency medical attention, severe vision loss occurs; blindness results in 2 days. An iridectomy is a helpful option to reduce the intraocular pressure (Ou, 2017).

Medical follow-up and eye medication are required for the rest of the person's life. Eye drops are necessary to continue even in the absence of symptoms. After administration of eye drops, pressure on the lacrimal duct for 1 minute prevents rapid systemic absorption. Use a medical-alert bracelet or card to identify glaucoma and the prescribed eye drop solution.

Cataracts. Cataracts are the most common disorder found in the aging eye. By the age of 80 an estimated 50% of people either have cataracts or have had surgery to correct them. A cataract is a clouding of the normally clear and transparent lens of the eye. Degenerative changes to the lens protein and fatty deposits (lipofuscin) in the lens are causative factors in the development of cataract. The lens focuses light on the retina to produce a sharp image. When a cataract forms, the lens sometimes becomes so opaque that the transmission of light to the retina becomes impossible. The size and the location of a cataract determine the amount of interference with sight. Cataract symptoms include dimmed, blurred, or misty vision; the need for brighter light to read; and sensitivity to glare and light.

Management and treatment of cataracts is conservative until visual impairments affect normal activities such as reading and driving. Several types of surgery exist, but the most recent technique involves the use of ultrasound to break the lens into small fragments, which allows removal from a tiny incision. A substitute lens is used to restore vision, which is a permanent, plastic intraocular lens. Cataract surgery is highly successful.

Hearing and balance. It is possible to consider the organs of hearing and balance in three parts: the external ear, the middle ear, and the inner ear. The inner ear is involved in hearing and balance. Hearing loss is not a normal part of aging and is necessary to evaluate.

The incidence of hearing impairments in older adults is frequent. Losses may be sudden in onset or occur gradually. Between the ages of 65 and 74 years about one-third of people have a hearing impairment. For those over the age of 75 years this sharply increases to almost half of this population. Aging causes rigidity of the ossicles, which results in a loss of elasticity (National Institute on Deafness and Other Communication Disorders, 2018). Atrophic changes of the auditory nerve and end organs of the inner ear affect hearing. Because of exposure to a variety of loud noises throughout life and age-related changes, older individuals often have hearing losses of different tones, which cause some sounds to be distorted and others to be absent. Older adults often deny their hearing loss and need encouragement and support to explore various methods to improve hearing.

Cerumen impaction is a reversible, often overlooked cause of conductive hearing loss. Assess for itching and a feeling of ear fullness. Removal of the blockage sometimes restores hearing acuity and relieves symptoms associated with impaction. Removal includes instillation of a softening agent. The health care provider then irrigates the ear with a syringe device on its low setting, and finishes by draining excessive fluid from the ear.

Hearing impairment falls into three categories: conductive, sensorineural, and mixed. Conductive hearing loss results from interruption of the transmission of sound through the external auditory canal and middle ear and usually is related to cerumen impaction, otitis media, and fixation of the auditory ossicles.

Sensorineural hearing loss results when the inner ear, the auditory nerve, the brainstem, or the cortical auditory pathways do not function properly so that sound waves are not interpreted correctly. Mixed hearing loss is a conductive hearing loss superimposed on a sensorineural hearing loss.

Presbycusis is a sensorineural hearing loss and the most common form of loss in older adults. Typically, the loss is bilateral, resulting in difficulty hearing high-pitched tones and conversational speech. The sounds usually lost first are *f, s, th, ch,* and *sh*. As hearing loss progresses, the sounds of *b, t, p, k,* and *s* also become difficult to distinguish. The cause is unclear. Indications of hearing loss include behaviors such as increasing the volume on the television or the radio, tilting the head toward the person speaking, cupping a hand around one ear, trouble following conversation when more than one person is speaking, watching the speaker's lips, speaking loudly, and not responding when spoken to. Diagnosis involves audiometric evaluation. Treatment options include surgical placement with a cochlear implant, hearing devices, and auditory rehabilitation to facilitate communication.

Nursing interventions to improve communication with hearing loss include providing good visual contact to allow lip reading, avoiding situations in which there is glare or shadows on the person's field of vision, reducing or eliminating background noise, and speaking at a normal rate and volume. Do not overarticulate or shout. Use short sentences and pause at the end of each sentence. Use facial expressions or gestures to give clues. Ask listeners what assists them to hear better, and be patient.

Touch. Touch involves tactile information involving pressure, vibration, and temperature. Age-related changes that affect the sense of touch and position include a decrease in the number of receptor cells throughout the skin and joints. Older adults have increasing difficulty sensing temperature and maintaining balance, which places them at risk for burns and falls. The most common disorders to affect tactile ability include stroke, PVD, and diabetic neuropathy. All these conditions involve decreased blood flow to various parts of the body. Nursing interventions should focus on prevention of accidental trauma and injury in the affected limbs.

Smell and taste. Olfactory receptors decline in number, which tends to reduce or alter a person's ability to smell. A decrease is also seen in the number of taste buds, which often influences appetite and causes the person to use more seasoning.

Assessment of the Sensory Organs
- Assess eyes for dryness, tearing, or signs of irritation.
- Assess ability of individual to see close up and at a distance. Ask about problems with or recent changes in vision.
- Assess hearing; note use of hearing aids and effectiveness.
- Assess for reported changes in taste or smell.

Common Concerns and Nursing Interventions
Decreased vision. With increasing age comes decreasing visual capability. Many interventions are possible to compensate for age-related changes in vision; be sure the patient's eyeglasses are clean and are available, increase the amount of light in the environment, reduce glare with use of shades on windows and lights, and use nightlights to avoid abrupt light-to-dark changes. The use of low-vision aids such as large print, strongly contrasting colors (black on a white background), and magnifying glasses helps compensate for the decrease in visual acuity.

Decreased hearing. The decreased ability to hear is frequently a frustration to the older adults who are affected and the individuals who are trying to talk to them. Hearing aids sometimes help in situations in which amplification has the potential to improve hearing but hearing aids do not compensate for nerve damage or effectively screen out other distracting noises. To communicate with an individual with a hearing loss, face the individual and speak at a normal or slightly slower pace without exaggerating or shouting, lower the tone of voice (because hearing loss is frequently in the higher tones), and eliminate background noise whenever possible. Another effective communication technique is using nonverbal communication such as gestures, smiles, nodding the head with the verbal message, and written communication. When communication is difficult, carefully avoid expressing annoyance or impatience to the patient who has a hearing loss.

A patient problem and interventions for the older adult with altered senses include but are not limited to the following:

PATIENT PROBLEM	NURSING INTERVENTIONS
Disturbed sensory perception (specify)	Assess for sensory changes Alert all caregivers to sensory problems of the individual Determine most effective methods of communicating with individual with sensory impairment Modify environment to remove hazards and reduce risks Verify that assistive devices such as hearing aids or glasses are clean and functional

NERVOUS SYSTEM

Age-Related Changes

Structural and functional changes of the nervous system are complex and depend on a number of variables, including the individual's genetic makeup and the specific brain regions affected. Changes associated with aging include a decline in the number of brain cells and peripheral nerve cells and fibers, and synaptic changes that affect transmission and the sensitivity of target cells to neurotransmitters. Physiologically, nerve impulse transmission in the nervous system slows, resulting in a longer reaction time for older adults. Until recently, neuron death was accepted widely as an inevitable result of normal aging. Age-related declines in neuron numbers are not a significant part of normal aging. Unless pathologic degeneration occurs, changes in neuron size and weight bring few if any negative behavioral effects. Autonomic nervous system changes include decreased efficiency in maintaining normal body temperature and in the pulse returning to normal after exercise or stress (Table 33.12).

Functional ability in older people does not consistently decline. Changes in sensorimotor and motor function, memory, cognition, sleep patterns, and proprioception occur at varying rates. Distinctive patterns of behavior, thoughts, and emotions, which constitute an individual's personality, generally remain consistent during normal aging.

Table 33.12 Neurologic Changes With Aging

PHYSIOLOGIC CHANGE	RESULTS
Decreased number of brain cells	Decreased reflexes
Decreased number of nerve fibers	Decreased coordination
Decreased number of neuroreceptors	Decreased perception of stimuli
	Decreased motor responses

Memory. Common memory concerns for older adults include forgetting names, misplacing items, and poor recall of recent events or conversations. Changes in short-term memory are common with aging. Long-term recall usually is maintained. Strategies for adapting, such as making lists or posting reminders, are useful to manage short-term memory loss (Fig. 33.10).

Cognition. The process by which information is acquired, stored, shared, and used is termed cognitive function. The elements of this process include state of consciousness, general appearance and behavior, orientation, memory, language, intelligence, perception, insight and problem-solving ability, judgment, attention span, and mood and affect. Outcomes from cognitive function are thinking, remembering, perceiving, communicating, and calculating. Many people think that cognitive abilities decline in old age. Only some older people experience some deficits, and the decline occurs at different times in their lives. Generalizations about cognitive decline in older adults are inappropriate. Intelligence and continued ability to learn is possible throughout the lifetime. Teaching strategies may need modification, and learning may require reinforcement because of the age-related changes in the senses and nervous system.

Sleep. Sleep disturbances are reported frequently by older adults. The causes for these complaints are varied. Difficulty sleeping may be related to an inability to go to sleep or interrupted sleep. Reports may include feelings that the sleep achieved is not of a good restful quality. Causes may be physiologic and relate to a disease such as Alzheimer disease, changes to the body's natural clock, or secondary to pain from another illness. The roots of sleep disorders may be psychological and linked to depression or other mental health concerns. Medications including diuretics and corticosteroids may interrupt sleep. Alcohol and drugs can alter the pattern of sleep or totally interrupt it. The intake or use of stimulants such as nicotine or caffeine will limit sleep.

Proprioception. Proprioception, the ability to maintain an upright position without falling, depends on the ability to use balance, posture, and movement. This requires a great deal of sensory input, motor output, and central integration of balance and locomotion. Aging results in slower reflexes, diminished strength of muscles for posture, and

Fig. 33.10 The older adult making a list as a memory tool.

increased postural sway. Conditions such as damage to the structures of the inner ear may affect peripheral and central control of mobility and thus affect balance. The ability to achieve proprioception declines with age.

Personality. Personality remains stable during normal aging. Consider any signs of impaired emotional control, diminished initiative, or withdrawal as indicators of other problems or an initial sign of brain dysfunction.

Assessment

- Assess level of consciousness including alertness, eye opening, verbal responses, and ability to follow simple commands.
- Assess appropriateness of behavior and responses.
- Assess mental status. Mental status examination tools vary depending on the setting. The Mental Status Questionnaire (MSQ) and Mini-Mental State Examination (MMSE) are examples. These assess orientation, immediate and recent memory, attention, calculation, and language and motor skills.
- Assess for the presence of pain. Note severity, location, quality, duration, and precipitating events.
- Assess sleep patterns. Note onset, duration, and quality of sleep and daytime napping.
- Assess laboratory results for electrolyte imbalance, anemia, liver function, thyroid function, drug levels, and vitamin B_{12}.
- Assess CT scan or magnetic resonance imaging (MRI) results if there is reason to suspect tumor, subdural hematoma, or stroke.

Common Concerns and Nursing Interventions

Insomnia. It is not unusual for older adults to report difficulty with sleep. It is commonly known that the sleep pattern changes with age. With aging, there are fewer periods of deep sleep and frequent periods of wakefulness, giving the impression of sleeplessness even though the total sleep time is the same or only slightly reduced from that of young adulthood.

Nursing interventions to help an older person sleep begin with encouraging a bedtime ritual and promoting an environment conducive to sleep. For most people, this typically includes brushing the teeth, reading a book or the paper, using a favorite pillow, and listening to the radio. Exercise and activity during the day increase the likelihood of falling asleep easily at night. Activities or dietary intake that promotes stimulation should be avoided before retiring.

To manage sleep disorders, older adults may resort to either over-the-counter preparations or medications prescribed by their health care provider. Sleep aids can be habit forming, and their use must be monitored closely. In addition, sleep aids may cause safety concerns related to falls.

Delirium. **Senility** (the state of mental and physical deterioration associated with aging) is a fear and a myth associated with aging. Delirium is a reversible condition of rapid onset. It has a fluctuating and traditionally brief course. The symptoms of delirium may manifest as behavioral changes including restlessness, agitation, or appearing withdrawn. Emotional changes may be strong, such as personality changes or mood shifts or subtler changes including apathy or depression.

Delirium is not a disease of the nervous system; it is a syndrome that results from one or more causes, including the following:
- Fever or infection
- Dehydration or malnutrition
- Electrolyte imbalances (hyponatremia or hypocalcemia)
- Sleep deprivation
- Alcohol or drug use, abuse, or withdrawal
- Pain
- Medications (analgesics, hypnotics, psychotropics)
- Physiological conditions resulting in inadequate oxygenation to the brain

When an older adult has sudden mental changes, it is important to look for a cause. Once the cause of the delirium is identified, treatment is possible. Research is focused on identifying risk factors and prevention strategies (Meiner, 2019). See Table 33.13 for a comparison of characteristics associated with delirium, dementia, and depression.

Nursing interventions to prevent delirium include education of nursing staff about the signs and symptoms of delirium, orientation and communication, mobilization, environmental modifications, education of caregivers, pain control, and management of elimination, medication management, and discharge planning.

Reality orientation. Reality orientation is a useful intervention for delirium. Guidelines for reality orientation include the following:
- Call patients by their correct names or by the name they wish to be called.
- Make eye contact.
- Converse about familiar subjects.
- Provide familiar objects in the older adult's environment.
- Explain events and procedures in concise, simple language.
- Be honest.
- Set a routine and be consistent.
- Engage the older adult in familiar and simple activities that have a purpose, such as washing the face or brushing the teeth.

Dementia and Alzheimer disease. Experts define **dementia** as a progressive impairment of intellectual (cognitive) function. The reduction in mental performance affects interpersonal relationships and other activities. It is characterized by loss of memory and at least one other disturbance of intellectual function (e.g., orientation, attention, calculation, language, motor skills). Dementia affects short-term, intermediate, and long-term memory. The individual has difficulty with abstract thinking, and it is not uncommon for those experiencing dementia or Alzheimer disease to have difficulty with identifying objects or choosing words to use in conversation. Aphasia (inability to understand words), agnosia (inability to recognize familiar objects), apraxia (problems manipulating things), and agraphia (difficulty writing and drawing) are symptoms of dementia, as well as noticeable changes in the personality.

Alzheimer disease is the most common cause of dementia. Dementia of the Alzheimer type is a progressive disorder in which the brain atrophies. Research has focused on genetic, viral, environmental, immunologic, and other causes. It usually arises in individuals older than 60 years of age and includes loss of cortical neurons, enlarged ventricles, and senile plaques and neurofibrillary tangles that appear in the cortex of the brain. Experts divide the progression of Alzheimer disease into three stages. The early stage consists of a gradual onset of memory loss and difficulty focusing attention. The middle stage involves difficulty with language, object recognition, and judgment. The terminal (final) stage is characterized by some urinary and fecal incontinence, inability to ambulate or provide self-care, and inability to communicate. There is little or no response to surroundings or recognition of family members. In late stages, the individual becomes mute and bedridden. The average duration of the illness is 8 years, but it can last as long as 20 years or more.

Multiinfarct dementia. Multiinfarct dementia (MID, vascular dementia) is the second most common cause of dementia in older adults. It results from the interruption

Table 33.13   Comparison of Characteristics Associated With Delirium, Dementia, and Depression

	DELIRIUM	DEMENTIA	DEPRESSION
Onset	Sudden	Insidious, relentless	Sudden or insidious
Duration	Hours to days	Persistent	For longer than 2 weeks
Time of day	Increases and decreases during the day	Stable or no change	Throughout the greater part of the day
Cognitive impairment	Impairment of memory, attentiveness, consciousness, numerous errors in assessment tasks	Minimal cognitive impairment initially, progresses to impaired abstract thinking, judgment, memory, thought patterns, calculations, agnosia	Impaired concentration, reduced attention span, indecisiveness, slower thought processes, impaired short-term and long-term memory
Activity	Increased or decreased; may fluctuate	Unchanged from usual behavior	Insomnia or excessive sleeping, fatigue, restlessness, anxiety, increased or decreased appetite
Speech and language	Rambling and irrelevant conversation, illogical flow of ideas, incoherent	Disordered, rambling, or incoherent; struggles to find words	Slower speech
Mood and affect	Rapid mood swings; fearful and suspicious	Depressed, apathetic, uninterested	Sad, hopeless, feels worthless, loss of interest or pleasure
Delusions or hallucinations	Misperceptions, illusions, hallucinations, and delusions	Misperceptions usually absent, delusions, no hallucinations	No delusions or hallucinations
Reversibility	Potential	No; progressive	Can be treated

From Seidel HM, Ball JW, Dains JE, et al: *Mosby's guide to physical examination*, ed 7, St. Louis, 2011, Mosby.

of blood flow to the brain. As a result, multiple strokes occur. This condition is related to vascular disorders within the brain that possibly result from stroke and severe HTN; characteristics of the condition are periods of remission (absence of symptoms), preservation of personality, and mood swings. Risk factors for development of MID include arteriosclerosis, blood dyscrasias, cardiac decompensation, HTN, atrial fibrillation, cardiac valve replacements, systemic emboli arising from other causes, DM, PVD, obesity, smoking, and vasospasms in the brain called transient ischemic attacks (TIAs). The usual progression of MID follows a stair-step decline rather than the slow, steady decline of Alzheimer disease. Symptoms depend on the location of the infarct. Abrupt-onset symptoms include confusion and problems with recent memory; wandering; getting lost in familiar places; moving with rapid shuffling steps; loss of bladder or bowel control; inappropriate display of emotions; and difficulty following instructions. Some intellectual impairment is common.

Other dementia-related diseases. Dementia may also occur in patients who have other diseases including Huntington disease, Creutzfeldt-Jakob disease, and human immunodeficiency virus (HIV) (Table 33.14).

In management of dementia-related diseases, the goals are to maintain maximum self-care abilities and prevent injury. ADLs such as dressing often must be broken down into small steps, and each step should be explained to the patient in specific and simple terms. The individual may need coaching about what to do

Table 33.14   Other Dementia-Related Diseases

DISEASE	CHARACTERISTICS
Huntington disease	Age range at diagnosis is 5–70 years; not necessarily a disease of old age. Characterized by uncontrollable writhing movements and mental deterioration that terminates in severe dementia. Begins with disturbances of gait and slurred speech. Life expectancy after diagnosis is 16 years.
Creutzfeldt-Jakob disease	Rare and rapidly progressive; associated with viral etiology, although isolation of a specific virus has not occurred. Average age of onset 50–60 years. Terminal within 6–12 months. No known treatment.
HIV-associated dementia	Characterized by forgetfulness, slowness, poor concentration, and difficulties in problem solving. Rapidly progressive.

when eating, and often it is better to give finger foods or only one item at a time. Keep the environment calm and eliminate distracting stimuli. Care of an older adult with dementia or Alzheimer disease requires patience. Routine is very important, and changes should be introduced very slowly. Remember that the individual no longer thinks logically or understands the surroundings.

When understanding and communication become impaired, nonverbal communication becomes more important. Use a calm pleasant tone of voice and gestures that correspond to the verbal message, maintain contact through touch, and use listening skills. Music has a positive influence, including improved capacity to communicate, reminisce, and recall memories. Reminiscence therapy uses the exchange of information between the affected individual and their caregivers, family, and friends. It employs the use of photographs, familiar smells and tastes, and objects that carry some autobiographical meeting for the individual. The processes may provide a link to things past, assist with conflict resolution, and provide closure in dealing with unresolved issues.

Alterations in cognition make the assessment of pain challenging. Unrelieved or chronic pain can lead to depression, social isolation, feelings of worthlessness, and a sense of a loss of personal power. Visual analog scales, word descriptor scales, and numeric scales have not been tested for accuracy of pain assessment in older adults, so using two types of assessments may yield a more accurate response.

Wandering is a behavior frequently associated with dementia. In some situations, it is an attempt to find the bathroom or familiar surroundings; for some individuals, it is their way of coping with anxiety. For individuals unable to locate the bathroom or their own rooms, easily read signs with universally accepted symbols and familiar objects are a means to help them find the way. Safety measures to prevent falls are essential.

Parkinson disease. Parkinson disease is the second most common disorder that affects the nervous system in the older adult. It is a progressive, degenerative disease whose defining characteristics are muscle rigidity, tremors, and **akinesia** (an abnormal state of motor and psychic hypoactivity). The individual has a masklike appearance, drooling, and shuffling gait and often experiences emotional instability. In most cases, stress and frustration increase signs and symptoms.

Medication therapy with levodopa, amantadine, and anticholinergics such as benztropine mesylate and trihexyphenidyl HCl sometimes helps to slow the process of the disease or in some cases temporarily improves a patient's condition, but side effects from the drugs also have potential to cause disorientation, blurred vision, delirium, and drowsiness.

Nursing interventions for an older adult with Parkinson disease include observing the response to medication therapy and maintaining mobility through exercise and activity. Range-of-motion exercises and massages help relieve muscle spasms and maintain joint mobility. Interventions for a safe environment, such as removing throw rugs and furniture from walkways and providing handrails and good lighting, are important because the patient's lack of balance and general unsteadiness typically contribute to falls and injuries. Canes, walkers, and adaptive aids for ADLs

sometimes prolong the independence of an individual with Parkinson disease.

Intellectual function is not impaired, but the tremors and involuntary movements cause difficulty in communication and much frustration for the individual and others with whom he or she is trying to communicate. Give the individual time to respond, encourage efforts to communicate, and show acceptance of the individual through actions and nonverbal communication to help alleviate some of the feelings of frustration.

Transient ischemic attacks. The changes in the vascular system in older adults include thickening of the vessel walls and the presence to some degree of atherosclerosis and arteriosclerosis. Specific medical diagnoses related to arterial conditions common in the older adult are TIAs and cerebral vascular accident (CVA), or stroke.

TIAs are small spasms or occlusions in the cerebral vessels of the brain. Signs and symptoms of TIA vary, depending on the vessel's location in the brain. The most common signs and symptoms are changes in vision, headache, disorientation, **ataxia** (impaired ability to coordinate movement), and drop attacks (falling without losing consciousness). Symptoms sometimes last for as little as 20 minutes. One in three individuals who experience a TIA has a stroke within 5 years. The patient with a TIA must have a neurologic examination and screening to determine whether there are atherosclerotic plaque-like formations in the carotid arteries or other pathologic changes in the cerebral vasculature. The occurrence of strokes can be reduced greatly by identifying high-risk or stroke-prone older adults and providing the appropriate prophylactic interventions.

Stroke. Cerebrovascular accident (stroke) is the fifth leading cause of death in the United States and increases in likelihood after 55 years of age. Many of the risk factors for a stroke also are seen with increasing age. These include heart disease, DM, and physical inactivity. Possible symptoms of a stroke include **hemiplegia** (paralysis of one side of the body), **dysarthria** (difficult, poorly articulated speech, resulting from interference in the control over the muscles of speech), *dysphagia* (difficulty in swallowing), sensory changes such as *hemianopia* (defective vision or blindness in half of the visual field), **aphasia** (an abnormal neurologic condition in which language function is defective or absent because of an injury to certain areas of the cerebral cortex), and intellectual and emotional changes.

Nursing interventions immediately after the stroke involve support of life functions. Although some of the initial neurologic involvement is likely to disappear in 3 to 6 months, most individuals have some residual dysfunction. Interventions focus on rehabilitation to accomplish ADLs and to be as independent as possible. Older adults sometimes need to learn to use the

Fig. 33.11 Hemiplegia of dominant right side necessitates learning to use nondominant hand for activities of daily living (ADLs).

PATIENT PROBLEM	NURSING INTERVENTIONS
Excessive Demand on Primary Caregiver, related to difficulty coping with cognitive losses and progressive deterioration of self-care abilities	Assess family support network and available resources Establish opportunities for respite or timeout from caregiver role Access community support groups Provide stress management strategies Assess for signs of depression
Inability to Perceive or Use One Side of the Body, related to neurologic involvement	Position bed so that people approach and provide care from the unaffected side Ensure that affected body parts are safely positioned Provide range-of-motion exercises to affected side Adapt the environment to focus on the unaffected side (placement of personal items, television, or reading materials) Keep side rails up on affected side

nondominant hand because of hemiplegia (Fig. 33.11) and often require adaptive and assistive devices for ADLs, such as special utensils, reaching devices, and pull-on or easily secured clothing. Wheelchairs and canes are sometimes necessary for weakness, loss of balance, and loss of leg control. Encourage or assist the patient to do the exercises and activities the therapist prescribes.

Communication techniques for older adults with aphasia include listening carefully, turning down or decreasing competing stimuli such as the radio or the television, using pictures and appropriate gestures, speaking slowly, using short direct statements, and not interrupting. With all interventions, be sure not to rush the older adult, and give encouragement and praise for effort and success in performing tasks. In many settings, physical therapy and occupational therapy provide a valuable role in assessment and treatment of changes related to neurologic problems.

Patient problems and interventions for the older adult with neurologic problems include but are not limited to the following:

PATIENT PROBLEM	NURSING INTERVENTIONS
Compromised Verbal Communication, related to memory loss and difficulty focusing attention	Assess communication patterns Provide calm environment with minimal distraction Use gestures to match simple verbal messages Use touch to increase attention Use familiar music to enhance recall

SAFETY AND SECURITY ISSUES FOR OLDER ADULTS

FALLS

Falls are the leading cause of accidental death in individuals older than age 65. Approximately 25% of adults older than 65 years fall each year. Falls are considered an underreported occurrence between the older adult and the health care provider. The falls are caused by a combination of an environmental factor (e.g., a wet floor, stairs) and a physiologic problem (e.g., impaired vision or cognition, gait problems) or secondary to a disease or age-related change (see the Safety Alert box). Decreased circulation to the brain; diminished coordination, space, and position perception; decreased ability to balance; decreased muscle strength; changes in gait; and slowed nervous system responses are some of the major factors. Others include limited activity, side effects of medications, disorientation, and environmental hazards such as poor lighting and objects obstructing the pathway.

Prevention *begins* with exercise that increases strength, balance, endurance, and body awareness. Exercise must be weight bearing to maintain strength of muscles and bones and must be pleasurable to be continued in the long term.

For a reduced risk of falls, an environment that is free of hazards must be maintained. Some adaptations to prevent falls include providing assistive devices such as walkers and canes to aid balance, raised toilet seats, handrails on stairs, grab bars in the bathroom, nonskid shoes, and removal of small scatter rugs. Teach older adults to sit on the side of the bed when they arise and to stand for a minute or so before walking as

Safety Alert

General Fall Prevention Guidelines

GENERAL CARE
- Assess shoes for safety.
- Avoid wearing back-less shoes or flip flops.
- Wear leather or rubber-soled shoes.
- Illuminate darkened areas.
- Avoid storing items in overhead compartments.
- Assess assistive walking devices to ensure the tips and wheels are intact and functional.
- Use caution when standing from a sitting position. Allow time for the body to acclimate to positional changes.
- Avoid the use of alcohol.
- Do not use ladders or step stools unattended.

STEPS AND FLOOR SURFACES
- Avoid the use of throw rugs.
- Assess carpets for holes or frayed areas.
- To avoid missing a step count them to ensure placement.
- Install banisters in stairways.
- Keep walk areas clear.
- On landings, use carpeting that has color contrast.

BATHROOM
- Use assistive rails in the bath and shower area.
- Use a shower stool as needed.

---

a technique to cope with orthostatic *hypotension* (sudden low blood pressure that occurs when an individual assumes the standing posture) that sometimes arises from poor vascular perfusion or medications.

POLYPHARMACY

Polypharmacy refers to the use of five or more medications. Medications may be those prescribed by a health care provider or purchased over the counter. Although medications have therapeutic benefits, each has side effects and a risk for adverse effects. With each medication added, the risk intensifies for not only adverse effects with each drug taken, but with drug-to-drug interactions. In a study of 295 individuals 65 years and older, 11.5 was the mean number of medications taken per person for this age group (Keine, 2019). Among commonly used medications are laxatives, analgesics, cardiovascular medications, vitamins and supplements, and psychoactive medications (Table 33.15).

Medication therapies are implemented initially to manage a health concern. There are some individuals who are at a higher risk for an adverse effect of their medications. This includes those who are on increasing numbers of medications; borrow medications from friends or families; do not regularly check in with their health care provider when refilling medications; or combine prescribed medications with over-the-counter medications without consultation with their providers. A review of all medications, including over-the-counter medications, is essential in assessment. Ask patients when each was prescribed, its purpose, and how it affects them. Encourage use of one pharmacy for all medications so that the pharmacist can check for dangerous interactions.

Age-related changes in body function also contribute to some adverse reactions (Fig. 33.12). Research indicates that the body's ability to absorb, transport, and eliminate medications declines with age because of impaired circulation, changes in vessel walls, and a decrease in the number and efficiency of the glomeruli in the kidneys. Metabolism of medications also is reduced as a result of decreased blood flow in the liver, fewer functioning liver cells, and a decrease in the liver enzymes that function to break down and transform medications. Because of all the changes, many medications remain in the body of an older adult longer than in a younger person. Dosages sometimes must be reduced to prevent toxicity because the normal adult dosage is typically for a 150-lb, 20-year-old individual. Many older adults also have conditions such as liver or kidney disease that further impair the body's ability to metabolize and excrete medications.

Nursing interventions begin with assessing the older person's ability to take medications properly. Most older adults are interested in learning about the medications they are taking and appreciate techniques that help them take the correct dose at the correct time, such as a chart or pill box with compartments labeled with the time and where the pills can be placed for each time they are to be taken. Also, be alert to the possibility of medication interactions and signs and symptoms of toxicities, which are easy to misinterpret as "signs of old age." Disorientation, fatigue, anorexia, falls, and vertigo are frequent indications of a medication reaction; these must be reported to the health care provider for evaluation. Nursing actions and patient teaching for homebound older adults promote safe medication practices in the home environment (see the Health Promotion box).

ELDER ABUSE AND NEGLECT

Abuse and neglect of the older adult refer to violence toward individuals older than age 65. Increasing concern has led the American Medical Association (AMA) to issue guidelines for the identification and treatment of abuse in five classifications: (1) physical or sexual abuse; (2) psychological abuse; (3) misuse of assets; (4) medical abuse (withholding necessary treatment or aids for ADLs); and (5) neglect. Common reasons for abuse and neglect include frustration and exhaustion of a caregiver; alcoholism; turbulent lifestyles; and lack of financial, emotional, family, and community resources. The National Center on Elder Abuse identifies the two most important indicators of abuse as: (1) an older person's frequent unexplained crying; and (2) an older person's unexplained fear of or suspicion of a particular person(s) in the home. Older adults are often afraid

Table **33.15**   Common Groups of Medications Used by the Older Adult

MEDICATION GROUP	NURSING INTERVENTIONS
Antacids	Observe for signs and symptoms of diarrhea, constipation.
	Teach older adult to check sodium and sugar content on the label.
	Encourage older adult to take antacid 1 hour after meals and not with other medications.
	Caution about use with a history of cardiac or renal conditions.
Antibiotics	Observe for disorientation, changes in hearing.
	Encourage fluid intake.
	Monitor weight, intake and output (I&O), specific gravity of urine.
	Observe for secondary yeast or fungal infections of mouth, vagina.
Antidepressants, antipsychotics	Observe for tremor, spasms.
	Teach techniques to use with vertigo when changing positions and methods to counteract dry mouth.
	Caution about use with glaucoma, prostate, or cardiac conditions.
	Observe for urinary retention.
Antihistamines	Observe for changes in blood pressure.
	Observe for anticholinergic effects—restlessness, delirium.
	Caution about use with glaucoma, prostate, or cardiac conditions.
Antihypertensives	Observe for depression, anxiety, disorientation.
	Monitor for bradycardia, angina, hypotension.
Antiinflammatory agents	Teach importance of taking with food.
	Explain need for avoidance with a history of peptic ulcer.
	Observe for nausea, vomiting, gastrointestinal (GI) bleeding.
	Observe for psychological disturbances and masking of infections.
Cardiovascular agents	Explain importance of keeping appointments for laboratory examinations.
	Observe for orthostatic hypotension.
	Monitor heart rate, rhythm, and blood pressure.
	Observe for adverse reactions—disorientation, depression, vertigo, lethargy.
Diuretics	Observe for orthostatic hypotension, delirium, changes in mental function.
	Explain reasons for taking in the morning.
	Observe for hypokalemia.
	Weigh daily.
	Record I&O.
Opioids	Observe for hypotension.
	Observe for adverse or idiosyncratic reactions—hallucinations, agitation, disorientation.
	Monitor respiratory function.
Oral anticoagulants	Monitor prothrombin time (PT) and international normalized ratio (INR).
	Observe for bleeding.
	Explain importance of keeping appointments for laboratory examinations.
	Explain the need to avoid aspirin-containing products.
	Institute safety measures to prevent injury.
Oral hypoglycemic agents	Observe for signs of hypoglycemia—weakness, headache, malaise.
	Monitor blood glucose levels.
Tranquilizers and sedatives	Observe for signs of oversedation—lethargy, disorientation, agitation.
	Explain the need to avoid other depressants and alcohol.
	Observe for adverse and idiosyncratic reactions—delirium, orthostatic hypotension, cardiac dysrhythmia.

to admit that they are being abused or neglected. Most states now have mandatory laws that require the reporting of older adult mistreatment. Be aware of the reporting policies within your area of practice (Box 33.5).

FINANCES

When asked what concerns them the most in their later years, older adults often answer "health" and "finances." The two are frequently related. For older

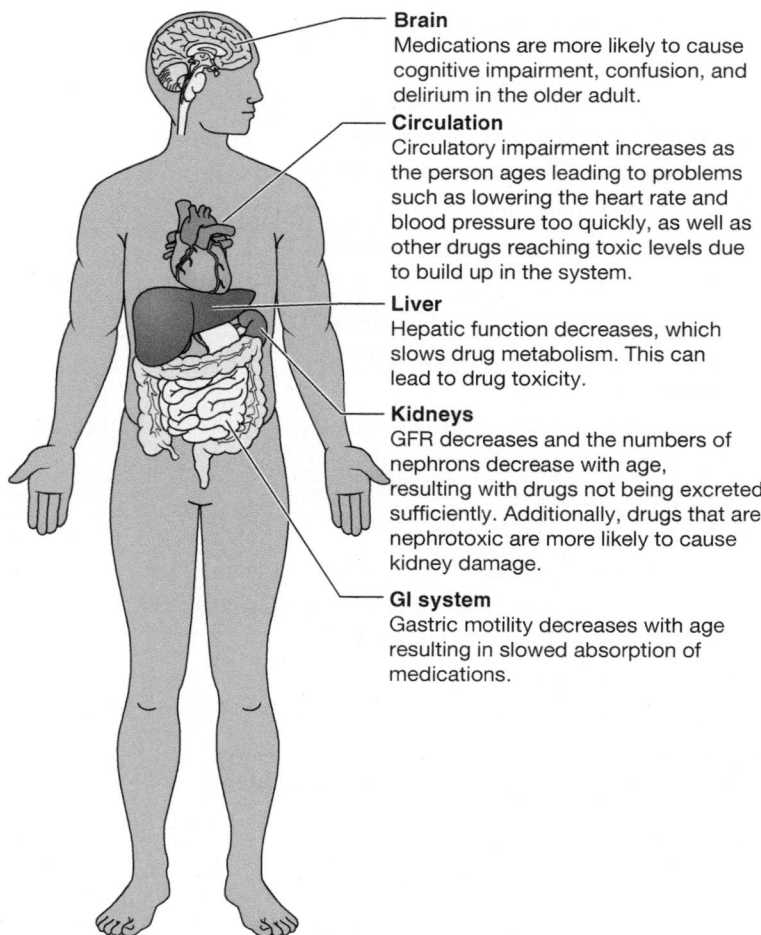

Brain
Medications are more likely to cause cognitive impairment, confusion, and delirium in the older adult.

Circulation
Circulatory impairment increases as the person ages leading to problems such as lowering the heart rate and blood pressure too quickly, as well as other drugs reaching toxic levels due to build up in the system.

Liver
Hepatic function decreases, which slows drug metabolism. This can lead to drug toxicity.

Kidneys
GFR decreases and the numbers of nephrons decrease with age, resulting with drugs not being excreted sufficiently. Additionally, drugs that are nephrotoxic are more likely to cause kidney damage.

GI system
Gastric motility decreases with age resulting in slowed absorption of medications.

Fig. 33.12 Changes in the aging body alter medication effects.

people, health care often becomes a major expense and can devastate their financial security. Because of chronic health problems in addition to acute episodes, older adults spend a greater percentage of their income on health care than younger individuals do. Older adults may be assisted financially by Medicare, Medicaid, or both. Older adults who can afford to pay the premiums for Medicare supplemental insurance have a coinsurance, which pays the 20% of expenses that Medicare does not cover. Medicare Part D prescription drug plans are also available through insurance companies and private companies approved by Medicare. Some Medicare Advantage plans also have prescription plans. Many older adults are on a fixed income from Social Security or retirement pensions and have only limited savings to pay for the rising costs of housing, food, and health care.

For individuals in lower socioeconomic groups, pensions are not always available, and low salaries and seasonal work prevent saving enough to provide basic needs later in life. Some women who never work outside the home depend entirely on their spouses

financially and become impoverished when their husbands die; others may be eligible to receive Social Security survivor benefits.

Financial problems are all too possible when people have not planned carefully for retirement. Many people assume that adequate pensions will be available if they have to retire or if their spouse dies. Another assumption is that Social Security benefits are available to everyone. Unfortunately, this is not true. Retirement planning, including financial planning, must begin early in life for men and women. Because people live longer, sometimes retirement lasts as long as 40 years. A number of agencies and senior programs in the community are available to help older adults who have limited resources. Such programs can include homemaking assistance, legal services, low-cost housing or housing improvement, heating assistance, multiservice senior programs, recreation programs, and information and referral services.

HOUSING

Housing represents a certain degree of self-concept and status. The insecurity that older adults feel when

Medication Practices for Homebound Older Adults

- During each home visit, assess the prescription and the nonprescription medications being taken by the homebound older adult.
- Document and notify the primary health care provider of the homebound older adult's medication regimen and of multiple health care provider sources for medications.
- Teach the possible complications and interactions of all over-the-counter medications to homebound older adults and their caregivers.
- Collaborate with social workers to identify community resources for financial assistance with pharmaceutical needs.
- Use laboratory parameters to monitor overuse and underuse of medications and interactive states of medications.
- Monitor urinary output status of older adults, because changes in renal excretion sometimes necessitate a decrease or increase in drug dosage.
- Teach the homebound older adult to set up a daily or weekly schedule of medications with a method or tool that fosters safe, independent administration.
- Reduce the chance of medication error by labeling or color-coding medication bottles.
- Keep an accurate record of the homebound older adult's weight, because many medication dosages are calculated by body weight.
- Teach drug safety in the home environment by instructing older adults to do the following:
- Keep drugs in original, labeled container.
- Dispose of outdated medications appropriately; never dispose of them in the trash within reach of children.
- Never "share" drugs with friends or family members.
- Always finish a prescribed medication; do not save it for a future illness.
- Read labels carefully and follow all instructions.
- Instruct older adults who have difficulty opening childproof containers to request their health care providers ask for non-childproof containers when writing prescriptions.

Modified from Meiner SE, Yeager JJ: *Gerontologic nursing*, ed 6, St. Louis, 2019, Mosby.

Box 33.5   Types of Elder Mistreatment[a]

Physical abuse: The use of physical force that has potential to result in bodily injury, physical pain, or impairment.
Sexual abuse: Nonconsensual sexual contact of any kind with an elderly person, including those individuals unable to give consent.
Emotional or psychological abuse: The infliction of anguish, pain, or distress through verbal or nonverbal acts, including intimidation or enforced social isolation.
Medical abuse: Subjecting a person to unwanted medical treatments or procedures; medical neglect occurs when a medically necessary and desired treatment is withheld.
Financial or material abuse or exploitation: The illegal or improper use of older adult's funds, property, or assets.
Neglect: The refusal or failure to fulfill any part of a person's previously agreed obligation or duties to an elder dependent on the person for care or assistance.
Abandonment: The desertion of an elder by an individual who had assumed the responsibility of providing care or assistance.

[a] Elder mistreatment implies that the recipient of the mistreatment is in a situation or condition in which the ability to protect oneself is limited in some way. Otherwise the actions are more accurately described as domestic violence, sexual assault, or fraud.
From Touhy T, Jett K: *Ebersole & Hess' Toward healthy aging: Human needs and nursing response,* ed 10, St. Louis, 2019, Mosby.

moving from one site to another in their later years is difficult for many to comprehend. In addition to the stress of relocation and the initial anxiety of adapting to a new setting, older adults typically move to more restrictive environments, sometimes against their wishes. Moving also may entail parting with possessions that have been acquired over a lifetime, making this transition more difficult. Housing is often the largest budgetary expenditure.

Relocation may be necessary as a result of physical or financial concerns. Ideally, the new setting should be as close to the old one as possible to reduce the stress of the move. Options may include downsizing to a smaller home or apartment. There are various arrangements for maintaining independent living, as long as people use some energy to develop the plan creatively. Renting may reduce the upkeep associated with home ownership. Older adults who are unable to live alone may decide to move in with their adult children.

Some older adults choose assisted living in a long-term care residence. Assisted-living facilities do not provide 24/7 skilled nursing care, but they do provide more assistance than an older adult receives in an independent-living environment. Assisted-living facilities are more expensive than completely independent settings; however, they are less costly than skilled nursing homes. Currently the average cost of an assisted living facility ranges from $2000 to $7000 per month depending upon amenities selected. This is less than a skilled nursing long-term care facility which averages ranging from monthly costs of $7,650 to $8720 (Witt, 2021).

CONTINUUM OF OLDER ADULT CARE

As the nation's population ages, nurses will care for increasing numbers of older adult patients. The increase in the aging population correlates to an increase in consumption of health care resources. An estimated 80% of older adults have a chronic illness, and half of those over the age of 65 have at least two chronic conditions.

HOSPITALIZATION, SURGERY, AND REHABILITATION

Age-related changes place the older adult at risk when faced with illness. Increased risks for the development of complications such as drug reactions, falls, infection, and delayed healing require knowledge of the specialized needs of the older adult. Although responses are individual, older adults have less reserve to cope physically and emotionally with the effects of hospitalization and surgery. They need longer postoperative recovery and convalescent periods. The normal effects of immobility on body systems, including stasis of secretions, orthostatic hypotension, and digestive and perceptual disorders, must be kept to a minimum. When adults in their 80s and 90s undergo surgery, their rehabilitation must begin as soon after surgery as their condition stabilizes.

Especially important are measures to prevent complications of immobility and techniques to support coping skills and independence. Turning, deep breathing, coughing, or other techniques for ventilation and removal of respiratory secretions are important with older adults because of the age-related changes in the respiratory tract that increase the risk of atelectasis and pneumonia. Depending on the type of surgery, older individuals are best ambulated within 8 to 24 hours to decrease the risks of stasis in the circulation, kidneys, bladder, and respiratory tract. Getting up, even to stand or take a few steps, usually helps to stimulate peristalsis, peripheral vascular circulation, and muscle activity; expand the lungs; and improve mental outlook (Fig. 33.13).

Encourage older individuals to perform self-care activities at their own level of tolerance and with rest periods. Remember that the hospitalization and the surgical intervention have the potential to increase signs and symptoms of other chronic conditions, such as arthritis, which sometimes is cause for reports of discomfort or difficulty in ADLs.

DISCHARGE PLANNING

Older adults need to have the necessary knowledge, skill, and resources to meet self-care needs at home before discharge from a health care facility. Planning begins with assessment of the biophysical, psychosocial, educational, self-care, and environmental needs. Strategies depend on physical and emotional readiness to learn, educational level, and family and community resources available. Written or visual guidelines that reinforce verbal instructions should be provided. Learning is enhanced when the older adult is actively engaged in the learning process (see the Patient Teaching box on discharge planning). Preserving as much of the older adult's autonomy as possible is a prime consideration. First consider the individual's physical strength and remaining functional abilities, not just the current disabilities, before making any modification to the home environment.

Fig. 33.13 Ambulation decreases the risks of stasis in the circulation, kidneys, bladder, and respiratory tract.

Patient Teaching

Discharge Planning for the Older Adult

- Teach when the older adult is alert and rested. Allow for several shorter sessions, watching for signs of fatigue.
- Involve the individual in discussion or activity.
- Focus on the person's strengths.
- Use approaches that adapt for the presence of pain and impaired range of joint motion, impaired reception of stimuli such as slower reaction time, muscular weakness, reduced pain and temperature perception, reduced depth perception and color discrimination, and reduced visual acuity.
- Consider need for adaptive devices, such as a syringe magnifier.
- As needed, enlist the help of the patient's significant other, or provide assistive personnel.

HOME CARE

Hospital lengths of stay are getting shorter for most illnesses. Early discharge for older adults may present unique challenges. Referrals to community-based services may be indicated to promote their independence and ability to return home.

To be eligible for the Medicare home health benefit, an individual must be homebound; have a condition that requires skilled, intermittent care; and have a referring health care provider who approves the plan of treatment in writing. The home health nurse assesses the physical, functional, emotional, socioeconomic, and environmental well-being of patients and works in collaboration with other members of the home health team, including the physical therapist, occupational therapist, speech therapist, social worker, and home health aide (HHA) or personal care attendant (PCA). Nurses initiate the plan of care and provide care that requires judgment and skill including health and self-care teaching; this teaching includes medications, medication administration, wound and decubitus care, urinary catheter care, ostomy care, postsurgical care, and care of the terminal patient. Some home health nurses provide intravenous therapy, enteral and parenteral nutrition, and chemotherapy. Once the registered nurse (RN) establishes the plan of care, licensed practical or vocational nurses (LPNs/LVNs) are permitted to provide skilled nursing and HHAs to provide personal care such as ADLs, hygiene, vital signs, and other tasks ordinarily done by the patient or family. Families often hire PCAs for cases in which only a sitter is required rather than personal or skilled care. They usually prepare meals, assist patients to the bathroom, assist with dressing and ambulation, and perform light housekeeping.

ASSISTED LIVING

Assisted living is one of the fastest growing industries in the United States. Placed between home health and the long-term care facility in the continuum of long-term care settings, assisted living offers meals, assistance with bathing and dressing, social and recreational programs, laundry and housekeeping services, transportation, emergency call system, health checks, and medication administration. Many services are purchased individually as needed by the resident.

Other options for living arrangements include retirement villages, senior housing apartments, single-family homes, group living, and sharing of a home.

LONG-TERM CARE FACILITIES

Emphasis on reducing costs in the hospital setting through earlier discharge has led to the shift of more acutely ill residents to skilled nursing facilities, traditionally referred to as nursing homes or long-term care facilities. Skilled nursing facilities may include care such as intravenous infusions, feeding tubes, ventilator care, wound vacuum-assisted closure devices, and peritoneal dialysis. Each skilled facility differs in the level of care provided and the type of patients they can accept based on the skill set of the nurses and the resources available.

Resident Characteristics

People who live in skilled or long-term care facilities are referred to as residents. The facility is their temporary or permanent home, and some residents need nursing care until death. The CDC (2021b) reports that approximately 1.3 million individuals are currently living in these facilities in the United States. Estimates project a sharp increase in this number as the older population, particularly those over 85 years of age, grows exponentially over the next 30 years. The demographic of nursing facility residents is nearly 70% female. The majority (more than 80%) are over the age of 65 years (Harris-Kojetin, 2019).

Long-term care residents usually need 24-hour care, which is not possible to provide in the home environment because of the increased scope of needs and the family's inability to provide the necessary care. The facility usually provides medical, nursing, dietary, recreational, rehabilitative, social, and spiritual care.

Care Costs

The average cost of a long-term care facility is affected by location. Amenities chosen and the type of room selected will also impact overall cost. Some Americans purchase long-term care insurance; however, individuals or state and federal Medicaid programs pay the majority of costs. Medicare will pay up to the first 100 days in each benefit period for days of skilled and rehabilitative care in most circumstances. Medicaid provides coverage for all levels of care, if the resident qualifies. Presently government officials are trying to address concerns about the abilities of the state and federal governments to continue shouldering these costs. Future legislation undoubtedly will focus on this matter.

Quality of Care

Long-term care facilities are highly regulated. The Omnibus Budget Reconciliation Act (OBRA) of 1987 and subsequent revisions aimed to improve the quality of care and have had a positive outcome. OBRA requirements include comprehensive resident assessments, increased training requirements for unlicensed assistive personnel (UAP), a greater number of nursing staff, availability of social workers, standards for nursing home administrators, and quality assurance activities.

Legislation has been passed to protect the rights of residents of nursing homes, and it is mandatory to inform the residents of these rights. Staff are required to promote and protect these rights, which are posted in the long-term care facility so that the residents are readily able to see them (Box 33.6). The Long-Term Ombudsman Program is a national effort to support the rights of the residents and the facilities. Each long-term care facility is obliged to post the name and the contact information of the ombudsman assigned to each facility.

Box 33.6	Bill of Rights for Long-Term Care Residents

- The right to voice grievances and have them remedied.
- The right to information about health conditions and treatments and to participate in one's own care to the greatest extent possible.
- The right to choose one's own health care providers and to speak privately with one's health care providers.
- The right to consent to or refuse all aspects of care and treatments.
- The right to manage one's own finances if capable or choose one's own financial advisor.
- The right to be transferred or discharged only for appropriate reasons.
- The right to be free from all forms of abuse.
- The right to be free from all forms of restraint to the extent compatible with safety.
- The right to privacy and confidentiality concerning one's person, personal information, and medical information.
- The right to be treated with dignity, consideration, and respect in keeping with one's individuality.
- The right to immediate visitation and access at any time for family, health care providers, and legal advisors; the right to reasonable visitation and access for others.

NOTE: This list of rights is a sampling of federal and several states' lists of rights of residents or participants in long-term care. Nurses should check the rules of their own state for specific rights in law for that state.
From Touhy T, Jett K: *Ebersole & Hess' Toward healthy aging: Human needs and nursing response,* ed 10, St. Louis, 2019, Mosby.

Residents' rights include the following: the right to autonomy and active participation and decision making in their care and life, including the right to self-administer medications; the right to informed consent for the use of side rails and chemical and physical restraints; and the right to withdrawal or withholding of life-sustaining treatments.

Interdisciplinary functional assessment of residents is the cornerstone of clinical practice in long-term care. The minimum data set (MDS) is a tool intended to develop a complete picture of each resident. It includes a comprehensive assessment of background information, cognition, communication, hearing, vision, physical function, mood, behavior, activity, bowel and bladder continence, disease diagnoses, nutrition and dental status, skin condition, medication use, and special treatments and procedures. This information is used to develop an individualized, comprehensive plan of care for each resident.

Get Ready for the NCLEX® Examination!

Key Points

- Although the efficiency of body systems declines with age, the body has reserves and compensatory mechanisms that normally, in the absence of disease, allow an individual to function well in late adulthood.
- Regardless of age, individuals have the same basic needs for physiologic function, safety, security, belonging, and self-esteem.
- Although older adulthood is tied to chronologic age, note that *chronologic age* may not be an accurate predictor of health or behavior.
- Wellness is based on a belief that each person has an optimal level of function and that even in chronic illness and dying some level of well-being is attainable.
- The role of a nurse includes affirmation, enhancement, and support of each person's movement through the aging process and encouragement of health and wellness.
- *Ageism* is a term that describes prejudice against older adults. All members of the health care team should work toward eliminating negative attitudes and discriminatory practices in the treatment of the elderly.

- Symptoms of depression are commonly misunderstood as changes that normally occur with aging. As a result, few older adults receive treatment for depression, although depression is common in this age group.
- Pressure injuries are a significant risk for older adults and patients with chronic disease. The best way to prevent damage to the skin is to reposition patients at least every 2 hours.
- Nutritional problems account for one-third to one-half of all health problems in older adults. Many independently living older adults have nutritional deficiencies.
- Urinary incontinence is not a normal part of aging, although many believe that it is and do not seek treatment.
- COPD is not a single disease but commonly a combination of chronic bronchitis, chronic asthma, and emphysema in varying degrees as a result of progressive changes as individuals age. By 90 years of age, nearly everyone has some degree of COPD.
- Repeated infections, slow healing, blurred vision, and weight gain or loss are often the initial signs and symptoms of diabetes mellitus in older adults.

- A common reason for sexual dysfunction in older adults is the misconception that older adults are impotent and asexual or that they are perverse if they are sexually active; however, if individuals continue to be sexually active on a regular basis, they retain the capability to respond sexually.
- About one-fifth of people older than age 70 years have visual impairments that limit activity and increase the risk of falls. Age-related changes in vision include presbyopia, a decrease in visual acuity, clouding of the lens of the eye, yellowing of the lens, and changes in color perception and depth perception.
- Cognitive decline is not a universal process of aging. Research indicates that most older people retain their intelligence and are capable of learning throughout their lives.
- Cerebrovascular attack (stroke) is the fifth leading cause of death in the United States and increases in likelihood after 55 years of age.
- Falls are the leading cause of accidental death in individuals older than the age of 65 years. Approximately one-third of people 70 years or older report falls in a single year.
- Forty percent or more of adults use alternative pharmacotherapy. Encourage older adults to avoid taking any herb, supplement, or other over-the-counter products without contacting the health care provider or a pharmacist who will review the complete drug profile.

Additional Learning Resources

SG Go to your Study Guide for additional learning activities to help you master this chapter content.

Be sure to visit the Evolve site at http://evolve.elsevier.com/Co oper/foundations/ for additional online resources.

Review Questions for the NCLEX® Examination

1. **Which statement best describes demographic changes in relation to the aging population in the United States?**
   1. The older adult population is growing twice as fast as the rest of the population.
   2. Aging is a gradual process that has a predictable pattern based on gender and race.
   3. The term *old-old* refers to those more than 100 years of age.
   4. In the past 50 years, life expectancy for older Americans has increased by almost 10 years.
   5. Of the population older than age 65 years, approximately 60% are men and 40% are women.

2. **The nursing student is discussing older adults. Which statements demonstrate an understanding of the population?** *(Select all that apply.)*
   1. "Most people become senile when they become old."
   2. "Approximately 33% of older Americans have impaired hearing."
   3. "Most older adults have at least weekly contact with family."
   4. "Approximately 25% of the older adult population resides in a long-term care facility."
   5. "Most older people have at least one chronic condition and rate their health as 'good'."

3. **According to the "disengagement theory," people who are aging:**
   1. inherit a genetic program that determines their specific life expectancy.
   2. gradually withdraw from society.
   3. have the inability to achieve a level of acceptance, which results in anger and despair.
   4. experience a change of personality and behaviors related to illness and loneliness.

4. **Which assessment finding is associated with normal aging?** *(Select all that apply.)*
   1. The integumentary system loses elasticity.
   2. There is loss of muscle tone, which increases the incidence of choking and aspiration.
   3. There is a gradual loss of weight because of loss of muscle tissue and fluid.
   4. There is increased resistance to infection from improved immune response.
   5. Personality changes are anticipated as the individual approaches age 70 years.

5. **When caring for an older adult patient who is resistant to getting light exercise, the nurse should tell the patient that which of the following are benefits of this activity?** *(Select all that apply.)*
   1. Improved circulation
   2. Decreased constipation
   3. Reduced incidence of osteoporosis
   4. Reduced incidence of gouty arthritis
   5. Enhanced hearing

6. **Which change is suggestive of osteoporosis?**
   1. Decreased muscle strength and joint mobility
   2. Increased curvature of the spine and decreased height
   3. Loss of balance and unsteady gait
   4. Nocturia and sleep pattern disturbances

7. **What description for the term dementia is most appropriate?**
   1. A sudden change in mental status that results from hypoxia, electrolyte imbalances, or some other treatable condition
   2. A state of physical and mental deterioration associated with normal aging
   3. Loss of awareness of person, place, and time
   4. A progressive impairment of intellectual function that interferes with normal activities

8. **When administering medications to older adults, it is important that the nurse keep what concepts in mind?** *(Select all that apply.)*
   1. Absorption, transport, and elimination of medications tend to decrease with age.
   2. Doses sometimes must be increased to achieve desired effects.
   3. Many older adults have conditions such as liver or kidney disease that impair the body's ability to metabolize and excrete medications.
   4. Up to 40% or more adults use alternative pharmacotherapy, such as herbal remedies, that have the potential to alter the effectiveness of certain prescribed medications.
   5. Older people use a high percentage of over-the-counter (OTC) medications, which enhance the excretion of other drugs.

9. The nurse is caring for an older adult patient who has been diagnosed with depression. The nurse correctly recognizes what characteristics about depression in the older adult as being correct?

    1. Depression is uncommon in older adults.
    2. Older people who receive psychotherapy for depression show improvement.
    3. Symptoms of depression are commonly misunderstood as normal changes of aging.
    4. Many older adults are treated for depression.
    5. Symptoms of depression in older adults may include crying, agitation, and hypochondria.

10. A patient has been experiencing visual changes from a loss of elasticity of the lens of the eye. What condition is associated with this phenomenon?

    1. Cataracts
    2. Presbyopia
    3. Glaucoma
    4. Macular degeneration

11. Older adults often have an *atypical response* to illness or infection. What is an *atypical response* in a previously active and alert older adult?

    1. Disorientation, weakness, or incontinence
    2. Fever, loss of appetite, pain
    3. Cough, shortness of breath, and fever
    4. Purulent drainage, redness, and warmth at the site of an injury

12. A patient with three school-age children cares for her mother who has Alzheimer disease. Her mother can no longer safely stay at home alone and needs continual supervision. A nursing diagnosis of *caregiver role strain* is made. Which nursing intervention is most appropriate?

    1. Provide a calm environment with minimal distraction.
    2. Access community support to provide opportunity for the caregiver to do errands and spend time with her children.
    3. Assess communication patterns between the patient and her mother.
    4. Encourage the use of gestures and touch to enhance communication.

13. Which is an appropriate nursing diagnosis for an older adult male with neurologic problems? *(Select all that apply.)*

    1. Decreased cardiac output
    2. Impaired verbal communication
    3. Impaired urinary elimination
    4. Risk for disturbed sensory perception
    5. Risk for infection

14. In data collection from an older adult, the patient discusses intimacy concerns. When developing the plan of care, the nurse correctly recognizes which of the following as the primary reason for decreased sexual activity in many older adults?

    1. Painful sexual intercourse because of vaginal dryness or pain
    2. Loss of interest as a normal part of the aging process
    3. Treatment of other conditions with medications that induce impotence
    4. Lack of a sexual partner

15. Aging often causes a decreased production of intrinsic factor from the stomach, thus interfering with the body's ability to use vitamin B_{12}. What disease develops from this deficiency?

    1. Iron-deficiency anemia
    2. Aplastic anemia
    3. Pernicious anemia
    4. Sickle cell anemia

16. In a review of the patient's medical record, the intraocular pressure is noted within normal limits. What range confirms this finding?

    1. 2 to 8 mm Hg
    2. 10 to 22 mm Hg
    3. 25 to 32 mm Hg
    4. 50 to 60 mm Hg

17. A man, 87, lives in a nursing facility for seniors where his favorite activities include a wood-working class and a chair fitness class, where he enjoys teasing the instructor. He takes the antihypertensive verapamil (480 mg/day) for his high blood pressure and rarely achieves a systolic pressure less than 159 mm Hg. Lately, he has begun to experience shortness of breath during chair fitness class, and he has chronic difficulty in clearing respiratory secretions. Despite the issue of occasional dust, he winks and persists in attending woodworking, saying, "…it's always worth a little dust to put another bird house out in the world." He is prone to frequent respiratory infections. During an outbreak within the facility, the patient develops a respiratory tract infection. He does not need hospitalization, but his physician prescribes monotherapy with the antibiotic levofloxacin, with a 500-mg initial dose, then 250 mg every 24 hours. The unit nurse advises the staff on how to monitor this patient in order to avoid or minimize adverse effects.

18. The Licensed Vocation Nurse/Licensed Practical Nurse (LVN/LPN) is doing a skin assessment on the older adult during a home visit. There are several bruises on the clients' forearms that look like fingerprint marks. Which actions are appropriate for the LVN/LPN? *(Select all that apply.)*

    1. Confront the caregiver.
    2. Say nothing as it is not your business.
    3. Use the personal cell phone to take pictures.
    4. Report the findings to the supervising registered nurse.
    5. Document the location, size, and distribution of the bruising.

Answers: 4, 5

19. A patient who sustained a head injury is being discharged to home after a recent fall. The discharge teaching should include which of the following? (Select all that apply.)

    1. Avoid the use of throw rugs.
    2. Keep walk areas clear.
    3. Place a night light in the hallway.
    4. Wear flip flops on the way to the bathroom.
    5. Use a shower stool as needed in the bathroom.

Answers: 1, 2, 3, 5

20. The Licensed Vocation Nurse/Licensed Practical Nurse (LVN/LPN) is talking with the patient about urinary incontinence. Which statement by the older adult indicates a need for further teaching?

    1. " I should make sure the pathway is clear to the bathroom."
    2. "I cannot go out in public, because I will have an accident."
    3. "I can wear an incontinent pad and change it as it becomes soiled."
    4. "I should go to the bathroom when I first feel the urge, instead of rushing at the last minute."

Answer: 2

21. The Licensed Vocation Nurse/Licensed Practical Nurse (LVN/LPN) received training for care of patients with delirium. Which statement by the LVN/LPN demonstrates reality orientation with the patient while caring for the patient?

    1. "Honey, everything is going to be alright."
    2. "Let's talk about what you did last night."
    3. Explain events and procedures in a concise, and simple language.
    4. "Yes, Sally, we will make that call to heaven so you can talk to your husband."

Answer: 3

Use an X to indicate which intervention is associated with each of this patient's medications. All should be used and can be used only once.

INTERVENTION	VERAPAMIL	LEVOFLOXACIN
Observe for sudden changes in hearing.		
Monitor for oral yeast infection.		
Observe for depression.		
Monitor for anxiety.		
Monitor for bradycardia.		
Monitor specific gravity of urine.		
Monitor for angina.		

34

Concepts of Mental Health

http://evolve.elsevier.com/Cooper/foundations/

Objectives

1. Describe the mental health continuum.
2. Identify defining characteristics of people who are mentally healthy and those who are mentally ill.
3. Describe the parts of personality.
4. Describe the factors that influence an individual's response to change.
5. Identify factors that contribute to the development of emotional problems or mental illness.
6. Identify barriers to health adaptation.
7. Identify sources of stress.
8. Identify stages of illness behavior.
9. Identify major components of a nursing assessment that focuses on mental health status.
10. Identify basic nursing interventions for those experiencing illness or crisis.

Key Terms

adaptation (ăd-ăp-TĀ-shŭn, p. 1128)

anxiety (ăng-ZĪ-ŭ-tē, p. 1127)

behavior (bē-HĀV-yŭr, p. 1122)

conflict (p. 1128)

coping responses (KŌ-pĭng rē-SPŎNS-ŭz, p. 1128)

crisis (KRĪ-sĭs, p. 1131)

defense mechanisms (dē-FĔNS MĔK-ŭn-ĭz-ŭmz, p. 1128)

deinstitutionalization (dē-ĭn-stĭ-TU-shŭn-ŭl-ĭz-Ā-shŭn, p. 1124)

frustration (p. 1128)

humoral theory (HYŪ-mōr-ăl THĔR-ē, p. 1123)

illness (ĬL-nŭs, p. 1130)

mental health (MĔN-tŭl HĔLTH, p. 1122)

mental health continuum (MĔN-tŭl HĔLTH kŏn-TĬN-yū-ŭm, p. 1125)

mental illness (MĔN-tŭl ĬL-nŭs, p. 1123)

motivation (p. 1128)

Omnibus Budget Reconciliation Act (OBRA) (ŎM-nĭ-bŭs BŬD-jĭt rĕ-kŏn-sĭl-ē-Ā-shŭn ĂKT, p. 1125)

personality (pŭr-sŭn-ĂL-ŭ-tē, p. 1126)

self (SĔLF, p. 1127)

self-concept (SĔLF KŎN-sĕpt, p. 1127)

stress (STRĔS, p. 1127)

stressor (STRĔS-ŭr, p. 1127)

A licensed practical/vocational nurse (LPN/LVN) is likely to use mental health nursing principles in a variety of health care settings. Basic mental health concepts are useful in understanding a patient's behavioral responses to disease and dysfunction. **Behavior** can be defined as the manner in which a person performs any or all of the activities of daily life. Individuals respond differently to changes in daily activities, such as the changes created by illness and hospitalization. All individuals have unique personalities and resources that affect their behavior in dealing with changing situations and the changing environment. An individual's mental health sometimes varies in accordance with the situation and the available support systems.

Mental health can be defined as a person's ability to cope with and adjust to the recurrent stresses of everyday living. Mental health is dynamic and fluctuates along a continuum. Mentally healthy individuals are able to enjoy life's activities, adapt successfully to changes, set realistic goals, solve problems, have satisfying working relationships, and maintain interpersonal relationships with family and friends (Fig. 34.1).

Factors affecting mental health include inherited characteristics, childhood nurturing, and life's circumstances. The influence of these factors on the individual's response to daily stressors in life is sometimes positive and sometimes negative. Possible positive influences include inherent adequate coping ability, mother-child bonding at birth, success in school, good physical health, and financial security. Possible negative influences include cognitive impairment, schizophrenia, extreme sibling rivalry, parental rejection, deprivation of maternal love, poor physical health, poverty, and dysfunctional relationships.

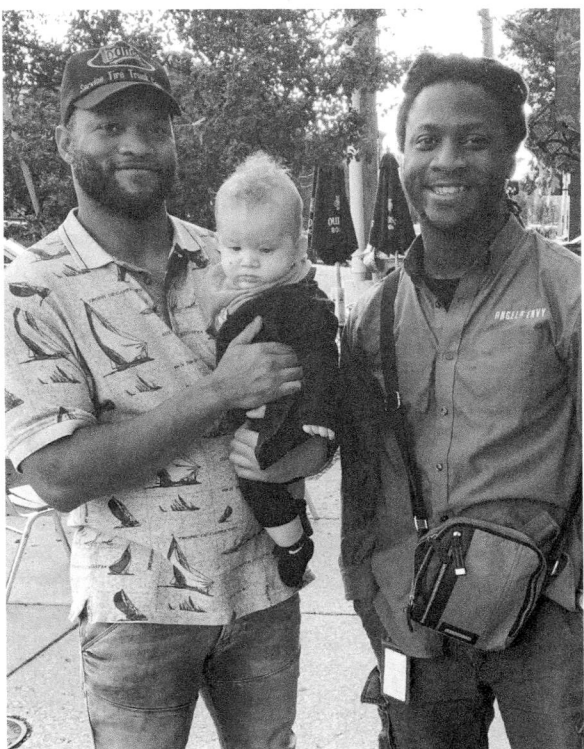

Fig. 34.1 Maintaining interpersonal relationships with family members provides a positive influence that affects mental health.

Evidence of mental illness often consists of a pattern of behaviors that are conspicuous, threatening, and disruptive of relationships or that deviate significantly from behaviors that are considered socially and culturally acceptable. Mental illness or disorder is a manifestation of dysfunction (behavioral, psychological, and biological).

Changes in society and in the economy have altered the status and situation of many individuals. According to the National Institute of Mental Health (2021), 18.1% of adults in the United States received treatment for a mental health problem in 2018. This population includes all adults who receive inpatient or outpatient care or used prescription medication for mental or emotional problems. Twice as many people actually have a mental health disorder. An astounding 60% of people in the United States will develop a mental health disorder in their lifetime. The discrepancy between individuals seeking treatment and those not treated for mental illness should serve as an alert to nurses who in their practice encounter patients and families who have mental health concerns (NAMI, 2019)). The nurse may have daily contact with battered spouses, abused children, people who are homeless as a result of mental illness, substance abusers, or patients experiencing depression, anxiety, or other mental health alterations. Regardless of the practice setting, nurses frequently encounter patients who are in need of emotional support.

Nurses can help patients by providing nursing interventions in situations involving interpersonal exchanges. Patients express their feelings in a variety of ways. The nurse is responsible for assessing and intervening while maintaining a caring relationship of trust with the patient. The emphasis of the mental health aspect of nursing is to assist the patient and family to achieve satisfying and productive ways of dealing with the positive and the negative aspects of daily living and to cope with situations that necessitate a change in lifestyle.

HISTORICAL OVERVIEW

The history of mental health care began in ancient times. During early history, people thought that a physically or mentally ill person was possessed by evil spirits. For mental illness, the shamans or medicine men focused on removing evil spirits by magical treatments such as spells, potions, noises, or sacrifices, and by physical treatments such as vomiting, bleeding, massage, and trephining (cutting holes in the skull to release evil spirits). If these tribal rites were unsuccessful, the community abandoned the affected individual to die by starvation or attack by wild animals.

Historical records show that there was an interest in mental health and illness and its treatment in the Greco-Roman era. The Greeks introduced the idea that it is possible to explain mental illness by observation of behavior. Hippocrates viewed mental illness as an imbalance of humors based on the fundamental elements of the world: air, fire, water, and earth. Each basic element corresponded to a particular fluid in the body: blood, yellow bile, phlegm, and black bile, respectively. This view of illness is called the humoral theory (pertaining to body fluids or substances contained in them). Roman physicians were interested in making their patients comfortable by providing physical care such as warm baths, massage, and music.

During medieval times, about AD 500 to 1400, society lost track of this concept of mental illness. The church became powerful and kept much knowledge locked away in the monasteries. Early Christians believed that mental illness was punishment for sins committed, evidence of possession by the devil, or an effect of witchcraft. Exorcisms, physical punishment and imprisonment, or banishment became the treatment for mental illness. Toward the end of the medieval period, Arabic influences in Europe reawakened awareness of the relation between emotions and disease and medical treatment for mental illness. The first English institution for the mentally ill was Bethlehem Royal Hospital, founded in the 16th century under Henry VI. The English word for a place of confusion and disorder, *bedlam,* originated from this hospital's nickname (Fig. 34.2). This term is still used today. To raise money

Fig. 34.2 Artist's representation of Bethlehem Royal Hospital, London, otherwise known as *Bedlam*. (From "The Rake in Bedlam," c. 1735. From the series titled *The Rake's Progress*, copyright The Trustees of the British Museum, London, England.)

to run the institution, it was common to shackle or cage the residents and display them for a price to people who were curious to see them. This practice continued for several hundred years.

During the Renaissance and the Reformation (15th and 16th centuries), little changed in the treatment of mental illness. The Reformation brought the closing of many Catholic institutions, which put the poor, the sick, and the insane back onto the streets.

The 17th and 18th centuries were a period of further growth of the sciences, literature, philosophy, and the arts, but conditions for the mentally ill were worse than ever. Common treatments included bleeding, starving, beating, purging, and confinement. During the last half of the 18th century, psychiatry became a separate branch of medicine.

Dr. Philippe Pinel, director of two Paris hospitals, changed the concept of care for the mentally ill. Pinel advocated humane care and maintenance of case history and conversation records. He classified illnesses by behaviors. In England about the same time, William Tukes, a Quaker, built an asylum similar to a Quaker household. His philosophy of care was to encourage acceptable behavior by providing a nurturing atmosphere. This concept of care became very popular.

In the United States, Dr. Benjamin Rush, a signer of the Declaration of Independence, established the Pennsylvania Hospital (1731) in Philadelphia for treatment of the mentally ill. Harsh treatment of the mentally ill still prevailed in the United States, as it did in Europe. Some newer therapies and devices (e.g., the tranquilizing chair) were used to encourage the rational mind to come forth. Dr. Rush used the newer, more humane therapies in his practice. He became known as the father of American psychiatry. The first

public psychiatric hospital in the United States, Eastern Psychiatric Hospital, opened in 1773 in Williamsburg, Virginia.

The 19th century saw the flourishing of institutions and asylums. Overcrowding and bureaucracy brought the decline of care these institutions were able to provide. Dorothea Dix, a retired schoolteacher, was appalled by the care of the mentally ill and set out to change it. She surveyed jails, almshouses, and asylums throughout the United States, Canada, and Scotland, and presented her findings to anyone who would listen: presidents, legislatures, civic groups, and concerned citizens. As a result of her efforts, millions of dollars were raised for the development of mental hospitals throughout the United States. In 1882, McLean Hospital in Waverly, Massachusetts, provided the first psychiatric training school for nurses.

The 20th century ushered in the reform of mental health care as the population became increasingly interested in social issues. Clifford Beers, a college student who had attempted suicide, spent 3 years as a patient in a mental hospital. Upon his release, he wrote *A Mind That Found Itself* (1908), in which he described the beatings, isolation, and confinement that he experienced and witnessed while he was institutionalized. As a result of Beers's work, the Committee for Mental Hygiene formed in 1909. This committee focused on prevention of mental illness and removal of the stigma of mental illness. Around this same time, Sigmund Freud, a neurophysiologist now known as the father of psychiatry, was introducing his elaborate theories and treatment for mental illnesses.

During the 1930s, mental health practitioners developed electroconvulsive therapy and insulin shock therapy and used them to treat schizophrenia. Frontal lobotomy—a surgical procedure in which the frontal lobes are severed from the thalamus—was also used to eliminate violent behaviors. By 1939, about half of all nursing schools offered psychiatric courses in their curriculum.

In the 1940s, the passage of the National Health Act and the establishment of the National Institute of Mental Health were among the most important developments in psychiatric medicine in the United States. The institute established research funding for the causes, the prevention, and the treatment of mental illnesses.

In the 1950s, psychotherapeutic drugs were introduced. This allowed psychiatric patients to be treated in regular hospital settings. These drugs also allowed individuals to control their behavior and thus spend more time in the community, which was a primary goal of mental health care. At this time, the government started the movement of **deinstitutionalization,** the release of psychiatric patients from institutions to live and receive treatment in the community setting. During the 1960s and 1970s, legislatures brought about further changes in mental health treatment at the community level. A goal of community treatment is to return the individual to the home environment as soon as possible and to provide a support system within the community to facilitate treatment and bring about functioning as near to normal as possible.

President Jimmy Carter established the President's Commission on Mental Health in 1978. This commission assessed mental health care needs of the nation and made recommendations of action for the government to take. Martha Mitchell, a nurse educator and clinical specialist in psychiatric–mental health nursing, was among those appointed to this commission. This was the first time nursing had representation in a commission of this type. From this commission's recommendations, the most comprehensive mental health care bill in US history, the Mental Health Care Systems Act, was passed in 1980.

During President Ronald Reagan's administration, the Omnibus Budget Reconciliation Act (OBRA) of 1981 was passed; it drastically reduced funding for the mental health system and put remaining funds into block grants for use and disbursement at the community level. Rapid, if not indiscriminate, deinstitutionalization was one consequence of the severe fiscal cuts. Continued declines in federal and state budgets have resulted in the loss of services to vulnerable populations). In 2018, national funding was increased to support research and services to support substance abuse services, veteran services, and in several areas, substance abuse, research, jail diversion, and re-entry. This increase in funding is a crucial step in supporting those with mental illness, but much more support is needed.

In the 21st century, health care providers put mental health concepts and principles into practice in a variety of settings, including public health and home health care agencies, outpatient settings, and acute care hospitals. Psychiatric and mental health care centers are not the only settings in which mental health care is practiced. There are patients in need of emotional support in every health care setting. The community-based mental health movement and the holistic health movement have brought awareness to the public that all individuals, sick or well, have emotional needs to be met.

BASIC CONCEPTS RELATED TO MENTAL HEALTH

Nursing is a person-oriented profession. Every interaction that a nurse has with a patient affords an opportunity for assessment of the patient's emotional state. The nurse has the power and responsibility to create an environment that allows the patient to have as positive an experience as possible. Most people have an innate ability to heal themselves that is influenced by mental attitude. The nurse can help the patient use this inner healing capacity through nursing interventions.

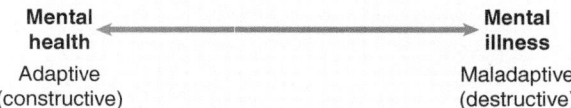

Fig. 34.3 Mental health continuum.

Box 34.1	Characteristics Identified in Mental Illness

- Poor self-concept
- Feelings of inadequacy
- Dependent behavior resulting from feelings of inadequacy
- Constant pessimism
- Poor judgment
- Inability to cope with daily events
- Irresponsibility
- Inability to accept responsibility for actions
- Avoidance of problems (no attempt to handle them)
- Inability to recognize own talents
- Inability to recognize limitations
- Inability to perceive reality
- Maladaptive behavior
- Demanding or seeking immediate gratification
- Inability to establish a meaningful relationship

MENTAL HEALTH CONTINUUM

Mental health and mental illness are the opposite ends of a mental health continuum (Fig. 34.3). Functioning is normal on the healthy end of the mental health continuum. This form of wellness includes an assertive communication style, acceptance of strengths and weaknesses, and available energy to deal with life's situations. The influences of daily stressors, although affecting the mentally healthy individual, do not normally disrupt mental health. Continued stressor exposure results in a deterioration of mental health and alterations in behaviors. The longer and the more intense the exposures are, the more likely behaviors are to become dysfunctional. Loss of contact with reality can result when an individual is at the illness end of the continuum. The midpoint on the continuum represents normal mental health. Although a person at this point probably displays some lack of insight, this midpoint level is characterized by adequate coping skills, problem-solving ability, and satisfactory responses or adjustments to life changes with some growth or possibly some mild regression. Although many individuals function in a relatively healthy manner, periods of crisis or biochemical imbalance have the potential to decrease functional capacity, moving one toward the illness end of the continuum (Box 34.1).

To determine a patient's placement on the continuum, it is necessary to assess several components of mental health. These components include a positive self-concept, awareness of responsibility for one's own behavior and its consequences, maintenance of

Fig. 34.4 Recognition and use of a support system of family and friends is one of the mental health components that determines placement on the mental health continuum. (From Varcarolis EM: *Foundations of psychiatric mental health nursing*, ed 5, Philadelphia, 2006, Saunders.)

satisfying interpersonal relationships, adaptability to change, effective communication, awareness and acceptance of emotions and their expression, effective problem solving, and recognition and use of supportive systems (Fig. 34.4).

The point at which a person is deemed to be mentally ill is determined by the behavior the person exhibits, as well as the context in which the behavior occurs. Mental illness results from an inability to cope with a situation that an individual finds overwhelming. The maladaptive behavior is often part of a response to acute anxiety (see Box 34.1).

PERSONALITY AND SELF-CONCEPT

Personality refers to the relatively consistent set of attitudes and behaviors particular to an individual. Personality consists of unique patterns of mental, emotional, and behavioral traits, woven together. Thoughts, feelings, values, and beliefs evolve into a consistent set of such traits that characterize an individual. Personality development comes under the influence of genetics and interactions with the environment. From infancy and throughout life, individuals have interactions that affect their personal security, values, personal identity, and relationships with others. Personality may be viewed as the total of internal and external patterns of adjustment to life. There are many theories about growth process and the development of personality. All are attempts to explain why people behave the way they do, as well as how each individual evolves emotionally and physically.

Erik Erikson provided a framework for understanding personality development in terms of task mastery (see Chapter 24). Erikson is one of the most widely read and influential theorists of development, and his concepts of identity and identity crisis have had major professional influence throughout the social sciences.

Box 34.2   Parts of the Personality According to Freud

ID
- Basic innate drive for survival and pleasure
- Characterized by a demand for constant gratification
- Constitutes the individual's entire personality at birth
- Is not changed by experience because it is not in contact with the external world
- Goals: to reduce tension, to increase pleasure, and to keep discomfort to a minimum

EGO
- "Reality factor"
- Helps the individual perceive conditions accurately
- Determines decisions about how to act and when to act
- Portion of the psyche that is in contact with external reality: enables reasoning and good sense (whereas the id stands for untamed passion)

SUPEREGO
- Parental or societal value system
- Characterized by striving for perfection and morality
- Develops from the ego
- Serves as a judge or censor over thoughts and activities of the ego; Freud described three functions of the superego: conscience, self-observation, and the formation of ideals

Modified from Thornton SP: Sigmund Freud (1856–1939). *Internet encyclopedia of philosophy.* Retrieved from www.iep.utm.edu/freud/#H3.

According to Erikson's framework, if a person does not master a given task, then it is possible to predict a certain set of behaviors.

Sigmund Freud described personality development as having three parts: id, ego, and superego (Box 34.2). The id functions on a primitive level; its aims are primarily experiencing pleasure and avoiding pain. The ego functions to integrate and mediate between the self and the rest of the environment. It is the ego that experiences anxiety. The superego is the moralistic censoring force. It develops from the ego in response to reward or punishment from other people. When all three substructures function in harmony, the individual experiences emotional stability; that person is considered to have a healthy self-concept. A mature, well-adjusted personality is under the leadership of the ego.

Freud delineated levels of awareness: conscious, preconscious, and unconscious. At the conscious level, experiences are within a person's awareness; an individual is aware of and able to control thoughts (Thornton, n.d.). *Preconsciousness* refers to thoughts, feelings, drives, and ideas that are outside of awareness but that can be recalled easily to consciousness. The preconscious state helps screen certain thoughts and repress unpleasant thoughts and desires. The unconscious level holds memories, feelings, and thoughts that are not available to the conscious mind. This is the most significant level because of the effect it has on behavior.

Self is a complex concept comprising four distinct parts that influence behavior: personal identity, body image, role, and self-esteem. Personal identity is the organizing principle of the self; it is the "I." A person with a strong personal identity knows who he or she is and is not in regard to such things as beliefs, values, and goals in life. Body image comprises the mental picture of and the feelings toward one's body. Body image includes feelings about the way an individual looks, the way his or her body functions, the person's gender, body size, and whether one's body helps the person realize personal gains. Manifestations of body image include stance, posture, clothing, and jewelry.

Role performance is the expected behavior of an individual in a social position. Roles are ascribed or assumed. An ascribed role—for example, being female or male—involves no personal choice. An assumed role (e.g., occupation) is selected by the individual. In a lifetime, individuals fill many overlapping roles; combining these roles to achieve an integrated pattern of functioning is necessary. Self-esteem is the assessment one makes about personal worth. Self-esteem comprises the thoughts and feelings that an individual holds about himself or herself.

Self-concept is more than the total of the four parts of self. It is the frame of reference used for all that a person knows and experiences. Self-concept includes all perceptions and values held and all behaviors and interactions performed.

Through the process of growth and development, individuals accumulate and process information that helps form a basic perception of who they are, how they look, and how others react to them. How a person sees himself or herself determines behavior and interactions with others. Disturbances in self-concept commonly arise in people with mental illness or emotional problems.

STRESS

Individuals are exposed continually to a variety of situations that produce stress, and their mental health fluctuates along with their ability to adapt to and deal with life situations or events. Any event that requires change leads to stress. It is possible for the event to be either pleasant or unpleasant. **Stress** is the nonspecific response of the body to any demand made on it. An individual's response to a stressful situation or event is often a learned or conditioned behavior.

A **stressor** is a situation, activity, or event that produces stress. Stressors can be physical, social, economic, chemical, spiritual, or developmental, or some combination of all of these. The meaning of the stress to an individual determines whether that individual feels distress. Stress is highly subjective, uniquely perceived by the person experiencing it. Stress in itself is neither good nor bad; however, it has positive and negative effects. Stress that facilitates individual growth and development and promotes change and adaptation brings positive results. Some stressors have the potential to be overwhelming, yielding the negative results characteristic of ineffective coping.

Mental health nursing focuses on behavior, particularly a person's response to stressors. Health factors affect this response. The stress of being ill greatly influences a person's emotional well-being and coping ability. How a person perceives stress determines whether the stress produces anxiety. A person's response to a stressful situation or event is often a result of learned or conditioned behavior and thus is, at least in theory, amenable to change. The nurse can serve as a resource in helping a patient develop adaptive patterns of behavior.

ANXIETY

Anxiety can be defined as a vague feeling of apprehension that results from a perceived threat to the self, although the source is often unknown. Anxiety is said to be a universal emotion and is a response to a stressful event. Anxiety is an internal process that a person experiences when there is a real or perceived threat to the physical body or self-concept. Anxiety is a major component of all mental health disturbances. In mild forms, anxiety readies the body for action and reaction to danger. Mild levels of anxiety enable the body to meet stressful demands by promoting problem solving and constructive action. Higher levels of anxiety immobilize coping skills and result in emotional chaos. In severe forms, anxiety interferes with daily activities.

Anxiety usually is described in terms of levels, and each level is associated with certain behaviors (Box 34.3). Signs of higher levels of anxiety include vocal changes; rapid speech; increased pulse, respirations, and blood pressure; tremors; restlessness; increased perspiration; nausea; decreased appetite; diarrhea; frequent urination; and occasionally, vomiting.

Anxiety arises as the result of inner conflict, and subsequent behavior stems from the anxiety. Maladaptive behavior is often a defense against anxiety. Individuals learn a variety of ways to respond to anxiety as they move through the various stages of growth and development. Behavior exhibited in response to stress and anxiety results from many factors. The degree of anxiety experienced is influenced by the following:

- How the individual views the stressor
- The number of stressors the individual is handling at one time
- Previous experience with similar situations
- The magnitude of change that the event represents for the individual
- The degree of physical and emotional health being experienced at the time of the stress

Events that have the potential to precipitate feelings of anxiety include the following:

- *Threats to physical integrity:* Decreased ability to perform activities of daily living; impending physiologic

Box 34.3   Levels of Anxiety

An individual's response in a given situation depends on the level of anxiety.

MILD
- Slight increase in vital signs measurements and an awareness of danger
- Ability to think and make connections; heightened awareness
- Readiness for action
- Increased motivation

MODERATE
- Feeling of tension
- Decreased perception
- Continuing alertness, but only to specific information
- May display a proneness to arguing, teasing, or complaining
- Appearance (often) of physical signs and symptoms: headache, diarrhea, nausea, vomiting, low back pain, and stronger vital signs

SEVERE
- Feeling of impending danger
- Significant narrowing and distortion of perceptual field
- Possible distortion of communication and difficulty in making self understood
- Feeling of fatigue
- Changes in vital signs, potentially evident on assessment

PANIC
- Extreme terror
- Possible immobilization
- Distortion of reality
- Potential further disintegration of personality
- Potential to cause harm to self and others

disability (surgery, diagnosis of a life-threatening disorder, pain, infection, trauma)
- *Threats to self-esteem and insults to the identity:* Loss of significant relationships, loss of spouse, difficulty at work, loss of job, change in jobs, relocation to a new home

Anxiety is relieved through various coping and mental mechanisms. These mechanisms are partly conscious and partly unconscious; they protect individuals from situations perceived as dangerous. Anxiety is an inevitable part of life. Part of the emotional growth process is to learn to deal with stress and anxiety in an adaptive or corrective manner.

MOTIVATION

Motivation is the gathering of personal resources or inner drive to complete a task or reach a goal. This inner drive is generated by anticipation of the reward or the punishment an individual expects when the needed task is performed. Motivation is an important aspect in treating emotional problems. The motivation to participate in care helps the patient through the stages of recovery quickly.

FRUSTRATION

Frustration is the emotional response to anything that interferes with goal-directed activity. This concept is important for understanding the individual's response to frustration. Some people are more flexible and adaptable than others. When adaptive behavior fails, anxiety increases.

CONFLICT

Conflict is a struggle, usually a mental one, either conscious or unconscious. Conflict results from the simultaneous presence of opposing or incompatible thoughts, ideas, goals, or emotional forces, such as impulses, denials, or drives. Some conflicts are resolved easily, whereas others are more complicated and lead to serious levels of anxiety. An example of conflict is the situation in which a person is ill and needs to see a physician but does not for fear of getting bad news.

ADAPTATION AND COPING

Adaptation refers to the ability to adjust to changing life situations by using various strategies. Any kind of change in routines or patterns of living causes stress in varying degrees. Illness, family problems, lack of money, and inadequate transportation may be viewed as stressful. An inability to meet basic needs or role expectations has the power to precipitate emotional upheaval. Feelings and emotions are part of a person's behavior. An individual who develops ways to deal with stress and resolve it has achieved adaptation. Adaptation, however, may be viewed as positive or negative. Growth or regression is a possible result of a stressful experience.

Coping responses are the responses used to reduce anxiety brought on by stress. Common coping responses include overeating, drinking, drug use, smoking, withdrawal, seeking out someone to talk with, yelling, exercising or other physical activity, fighting, pacing, or listening to music. People often use coping responses consciously and unconsciously to adjust to stress without changing their actual goal.

Use of defense mechanisms—unconscious, intrapsychic reactions that offer protection to the self from a stressful situation—is another way of coping with anxiety. **Defense mechanisms** are behavioral patterns that protect individuals against a real or perceived threat; they are used to block conscious awareness of threatening feelings. This type of behavior develops when an unconscious conflict or a threat to self-concept is experienced (Table 34.1).

If defense mechanisms are used inappropriately or overused to help one cope, the behavior is termed *maladaptive.*

HOW ILLNESS AFFECTS MENTAL HEALTH

There is a misconception that mental health principles are applicable only in a mental health care facility or center. In reality, all nurses address the mental health

Table 34.1 Commonly Used Defense Mechanisms

MODE	DESCRIPTION	EXAMPLE
Compensation	Making up for a "deficiency" in one area by excelling in or emphasizing another area.	A boy who is small in stature places his emphasis on academics rather than attempting sports.
Conversion	Turning emotional conflicts into a physical symptom, which provides the individual with some sort of benefit (secondary gain).	An individual who witnesses a murder then experiences sudden blindness with no organic cause.
Denial	Disregard for reality.	A patient who had a severe myocardial infarction is told that he will have to severely restrict his physical activity. The evening nurse finds him on the floor of his room, doing sit-ups and push-ups.
Displacement	Expression of emotions toward someone or something other than the actual source of the emotion. Unconsciously, the individual does not feel safe expressing the feelings directly to the actual source.	A man has an argument with his employer and comes home and yells at his family.
Dissociation	Separation and detachment of emotional significance and affect from an idea or situation.	A person who has been traumatically victimized retells her situation, while smiling and joking about it.
Identification	Incorporation of a characteristic (thought or behavior) of another individual or group. The individual does not give up personal identity.	A teenager who dresses like a favorite rock singer.
Introjection	A quality or attribute of another person is internalized and becomes part of the individual's behavior.	A child follows her parents' instructions when the parents are not present (e.g., carefully crossing the street).
Projection	Attributing problems to other characteristics that the person does not want to admit possessing; blaming personal shortcomings on someone else.	A student who does poorly on an examination states, "That test was unfair. The teacher did not present the material correctly."
Rationalization	A process of constructing plausible reasons to explain and justify one's behavior. The person denies actual thoughts and justifies actions by giving untrue, but seemingly more acceptable, reasons for the behavior.	A young boy who was instructed to make up his bed and clean his room before leaving for school chooses to play instead. In the afternoon, when he and his mother arrive home and she becomes angry at his disregard of her instructions, he states, "But Mom, Dad was in a hurry this morning and told me that if I wanted a ride to school, I'd better get in the car."
Reaction formation	Conscious behavior that reflects an emotion opposite to the emotion actually felt.	A person is excessively polite to an individual whom the person dislikes.
Regression	Exhibition of behavior, thoughts, or feelings used at an earlier stage of development.	An 8-year-old reverts to bedwetting and thumb-sucking while hospitalized.
Repression	The unconscious process of barring from conscious thought of painful, disagreeable thoughts, experiences, and/or impulses. Energy is expended in this process, so the individual has less available energy.	A patient who was incontinent after surgery suppresses the embarrassment and totally represses the event.
Sublimation	The discharge of sexual or aggressive energy and impulses in a socially acceptable way.	A teenager engages in many competitive sports.
Suppression	An intentional (conscious) exclusion of painful thoughts, experiences, or impulses. (Some authorities do not consider this a defense mechanism.)	A student fails to keep an appointment for academic counseling.

Box 34.4	Patient Problem Statements for Psychiatric-Mental Health Nursing

Anxiousness
Compromised social interaction
Compromised verbal communication
Despair
Distorted body image
Fearfulness
Grief
Impaired coping
Impaired decision-making ability
Impaired family processes
Impaired personal sense of identity
Impaired role functioning
Impaired sexual expression
Inability to sleep
Obstructive denial
Potential for impaired self-esteem due to current situation
Potential for impaired spiritual beliefs
Potential for ineffective belief system

needs of their patients. The stress of being ill greatly influences an individual's mental state and level of functioning.

Individuals like to feel in control of their lives. Illness reduces that control and sometimes creates instability of circumstances, causing anxiety. When a person is hospitalized, the familiarity of home and work is exchanged for the unfamiliar hospital setting. Upon entering the hospital setting, the patient exchanges his or her clothes for hospital wear, submits bodily fluids for testing and body parts for imaging, and endures the same questions again and again. Sometimes visitation with family and friends is limited. The patient must adapt to being one entry on someone else's scheduled daily duties: the nurse's.

Most people do not expect to become ill or have lifestyle alterations resulting from illness or accidents. Serious injury and illness have the capacity to alter dramatically a person's self-concept, body image, lifestyle, and role performance in family life, recreation, and work. Regardless of whether the situation is temporary or permanent, mental and emotional states undergo a disturbance. The nurse is able to provide effective nursing interventions only if the patient's emotional state is considered.

Meeting the psychosocial needs of the individual is a task for the health care team as a whole. Patients and their families remember the nurses who care for them, whether the nurse showed a little extra consideration or was short-tempered or judgmental. One of the steps to meeting these needs is effective patient education. It helps to build trust and encourages the patient to have faith in the care given. Patient support groups, family connections, and community involvement are important to maintain during an illness.

Box 34.4 lists psychiatric patient problem statements that nurses often use to address a patient's psychosocial needs (see the Lifespan Considerations for older adults box).

 Lifespan Considerations

Older Adults

Aging and Mental Health

- Older people experiencing significant sensory changes in hearing or vision sometimes display behavioral changes that are easy to mistake for disorientation.
- Behavioral changes in elderly patients may be related to the many medications that they may be prescribed. The absorption, distribution, and clearance may be affected by aging and potentially by the interaction between medications.
- Social isolation of older adults is frequently a result of physical or financial limitations.
- The behavioral characteristics and personalities of older people are often an exaggeration of their behavior at a younger age.
- Many losses—including loss of loved ones, home, job, and independence—occur with aging. These losses result in varying amounts of grief. The number of losses and the rapidity with which they occur have the potential to affect the coping ability of the older person and result in anxiety, fear, and depression.
- Relocation from home to hospital, or even from room to room, has potential to cause stress in the older person, which manifests as behavioral change.
- Hopelessness, helplessness, and depression are common in older adults. These feelings sometimes lead older people to lose the will to live and even progress to committing suicide.
- Reminiscence and life review are effective techniques to help older adults cope with changing life circumstances.
- Alcoholism, often hidden or denied, is common among the older population. It is possible to use alcohol as an attempted means of coping with grief, depression, loneliness, or boredom. If unrecognized, alcoholism poses the risk of exacerbating medical conditions and leading to serious drug reactions.

ILLNESS BEHAVIORS

Illness is a state of homeostatic imbalance. When an individual is ill or sick, he or she does not feel good. This is the body's way of saying, "Pay attention to my needs." The experience of being ill involves stages that are subjective and very personal. The illness experience starts with awareness of symptoms that are not healthy, and the individual takes on the sick role. The sick role allows the individual to be excused from everyday responsibilities, including social, to rest and heal. If an appropriate attempt at this stage does not cure the ailment, professional medical help is sought. The sick person receiving professional care assumes a dependent role—with the expectation of getting well. Keeping the patient informed and emotionally supported is a focus of professional care. Recovery and rehabilitation are the last stages of an illness event. The nurse assists the patient by setting attainable short-term goals to enable the patient to be aware of his or her recovery and rehabilitation.

CRISIS

A crisis can be defined as an unstable period in a person's life, characterized by the inability to adapt to a change from a precipitating event. It most often results when a person is faced with a turning point in life, accumulating stressors, or illness. Successful management of a crisis period is needed to prevent disorganization within the individual or the family unit. Difficulty or inability to manage the crisis successfully results in physical illness or emotional breakdown. The manifestations associated with an inability to navigate a crisis situation may include denial, hostility, anger, vulgarity, noncompliance, aggression, manipulation, apathy, and depression.

The sick role often produces secondary gains as well as personal attention: for example, when a mother becomes very ill every time her daughter plans a trip out of town, or when a person obtains renewal of disability benefits because the injury flares up when reevaluation is scheduled. It is possible for the sick role to become a way of life. Secondary gains are sometimes a ploy used to manipulate and cope with various emotional conflicts. It is important for the nurse to recognize this to plan appropriate interventions to meet emotional and psychological needs of the patient who uses the sick role in a destructive manner (Box 34.5).

Behavior is learned through life experiences. Interactions between a patient and the health care system are influenced largely by the patient's past. A serious illness, the breakup of a relationship, a car accident, or the death of a loved one potentially can trigger a crisis response in an individual or family. Cultural and ethnic backgrounds affect the patient's and family's behavior during illness. For example, many men received the message as boys to be stoic or ignore feelings when hurt. As adults, these men are less likely to seek medical treatment in the early stages of disease. A family may provide home remedies that generations of their forebears used to treat colds and flu. The United States is teeming with cultural diversity; thus, consider cultural influences on all patients' behavior (see Chapter 6). The nurse's responsibility is to note and to respond therapeutically to all behavior. By understanding the relationship of stressors, anxiety, and culture to behavior, nurses can facilitate healthy adaptation.

An *identity crisis* is a condition of instability that arises from an emotional or situational upheaval and results in extreme or decisive change. An identity crisis

| Box 34.5 | Behaviors Common With Illness |

DENIAL
A refusal to admit being ill. Short-term denial is often useful in mobilizing internal resources, but long-term denial usually results in maladaptive behavior patterns.

ANXIETY
Feelings of apprehension and uncertainty about the illness. Fear has the capacity to produce sympathetic nervous response (fight-or-flight response). The measurement of vital signs often helps in the assessment of level of anxiety.

SHOCK
An overwhelming emotion that paralyzes the individual's ability to process information. The individual is incapable of making decisions and unable to sort through information received.

ANGER
A response to feeling mistreated, injured, or insulted. Anger behaviors are directed inward, outward toward others, or both. Sometimes anger is an irrational response to minor events of the day and interrupts the person's social functioning.

WITHDRAWAL
Removal of self from interaction with others and the environment. Withdrawal is often a sign of depression. Family members sometimes withdraw from an ill person, or an ill person sometimes isolates herself or himself from the family.

represents potential opportunity, as well as danger. From that period of vulnerability, personal growth and strength often are developed. Nurses deal with people in identity crises nearly every day.

Phases of crisis are similar to stages in grief and dying (see Chapter 25). The initial phase consists of confusion, disbelief, and high anxiety. This progresses to a denial phase, with grasping of the conviction that everything will be all right. Once the reality of the situation becomes evident, generally anger and remorse are expressed. Sadness and crying constitute a phase of grief seen during a crisis. In this phase, the individual acknowledges and expresses the loss of what was and never will be again. The final phase of reconciliation is reached with the person's acceptance that life will continue but will be different from how it had been, and adaptation occurs.

Help the individual or family get through a crisis by providing accurate information that aids in realistic perception of the situation (see the Patient Teaching box).

Encourage expression of feelings and provide empathic gestures such as silent physical closeness, holding a hand, or giving a hug when appropriate (but not with an angry, hostile patient). These validate the individual's feelings of anger, denial, remorse, and grief as normal responses to crisis.

Patient Teaching

Improving Mental Health

Teach the patient to do the following:
- Recognize constructive aspects of mild or moderate anxiety in learning, growth, and movement toward self-actualization.
- Recognize personal characteristics that indicate presence of anxiety.
- Describe current state of anxiety.
- Analyze current expectations, goals, beliefs, and values within the context of perceptions of what is actually happening.
- Recognize the healing power of positive thinking.
- Recognize sayings that support negative thinking, and change those sayings to reflect a positive feeling.
- Develop assertive communication skills.
- Develop problem-solving and decision-making skills.
- Use progressive muscle relaxation.
- Increase repertoire of strategies to reduce anxiety, including the following: talking or being with someone; simple, concrete tasks; walking; noncompetitive sports; professional assistance; listening to soothing music; meditation or prayer; deep-breathing exercises; and relaxation exercises.

Identifying family supports and adequate coping mechanisms helps the nurse recognize family communication patterns. Dysfunction in relationships sometimes indicates a need to include other psychosocial professionals in the care of the individual or family in crisis. Active listening, restating the facts, and using other therapeutic communication techniques during family conferences are ways to help address the problem constructively. Offer as much flexibility in visiting hours as possible to reduce the frustration of separation in the individual and the family.

With or without crisis intervention, a crisis often tends to resolve over a 4- to 6-week period. The development of coping mechanisms and the redefinition of goals and roles in life often result from a crisis. The short-term active support the nurse provides in focusing on problem solving helps facilitate a positive resolution to the crisis (Box 34.6).

APPLICATION OF THE NURSING PROCESS

In every setting, nurses use the nursing process to meet the many needs of patients. An LPN/LVN participates in the nursing process by observing patient behavior and assisting in establishing patient problem statements, as well as working with the registered nurse (RN) on outlining appropriate nursing interventions. The LPN/LVN and RN implement the plan by using therapeutic communication techniques, and continue to observe and report behavior. Analysis of these observations makes it possible to adjust the plan of care appropriately.

Box 34.6   Crisis Intervention

GOALS
1. The victim's emotional stress will be decreased, and the nurse will protect the victim.
2. The nurse will assist the victim to organize and mobilize resources.
3. The victim will return to precrisis status or a higher functional level.

STEPS
1. Assess the situation and individual or individuals involved in the crisis.
2. Determine possible interventions with input from a spiritual care provider, other family members, significant others, or close friends, as well as health care providers.
3. Implement the intervention plan.

OUTCOME
The crisis resolves, and/or an anticipatory plan emerges from the solution to the problem.

Box 34.7   Assessment of Emotional Status

GENERAL APPEARANCE
Describe the patient's dress, makeup, and hygiene.

GENERAL BEHAVIOR
Describe the patient's general activity level, posture, gait, and response to examination.

SPEECH PATTERN
Describe the rate, tone, loudness, and quantity content of the patient's speech (descriptions include "response to questions too detailed"; "extreme distractibility"; "unable to complete an answer"; "uses rhyming").

CONTENT OF THOUGHT
Describe the patient's thinking: reality oriented, delusional, showing evidence of hallucinations, or showing evidence of ideas of reference or other non–reality-based thinking.

MOOD AND AFFECT
Describe the patient's overall feeling state and affect.

SENSORIAL FUNCTION
Describe the patient's orientation, memory, attention, and ability to think abstractly.

INSIGHT AND JUDGMENT
Assess whether the patient understands the current situation and what the individual is willing to do about it.

POTENTIAL FOR DANGER
Assess the patient's potential for violence or self-harm, degree of impulse control, and previous history of violence or aggression toward others.

Box 34.7 outlines basic nursing assessments of emotional status. Other possible assessments include observations for risk for violence, level of anxiety, use of defense mechanisms, and use of coping methods if the illness is severe or long lasting.

Get Ready for the NCLEX® Examination!

Key Points

- Historically, mental health care reflected fear and ignorance of mental illness, directly influencing the attitude toward mental illness that prevails today.
- Individuals have unique personalities. According to Freudian theory, the personality consists of the id, the ego, and the superego.
- All behavior has meaning. An individual's behavior is the best that person is capable of within his or her current environment.
- Corrective emotional experiences assist the individual to change. The therapeutic relationship should be directed to facilitate this change.
- *Personality* refers to the relatively consistent set of attitudes and behaviors particular to an individual. Cultural and ethnic backgrounds influence personality development.
- Self is an important part of personality; self consists of identity, body image, role, and esteem.
- Anxiety is a universal response to a real or imagined threat to self.
- Defense mechanisms are automatic behaviors used to protect the personality in times of stress.
- Coping mechanisms are usually adaptive methods used to deal with uncomfortable feelings or stressors.
- Stress is the nonspecific response of the body to demands. Stressors are factors causing stress. High or chronic stress has the potential to hamper the immune response to illness.
- It is possible to view mental health and illness as existing on a continuum.
- Physical illness affects the mental health of an individual. Behavior incorporating the sick role and dependency until recovery occurs allows the individual to cope with body image changes and keep the self intact.
- The use of therapeutic communication is a dynamic method of interaction with patients for problem solving and growth.
- Observe and evaluate behavior to determine a patient's progress and the effectiveness of the care plan.

Additional Learning Resources

SG Go to your Study Guide for additional learning activities to help you master this chapter content.

Be sure to visit the Evolve site at http://evolve.elsevier.com/Cooper/foundations/ for additional online resources.

Review Questions for the NCLEX® Examination

1. Who was the English Quaker who advocated humane care and built an asylum to reflect a household?
   1. Florence Nightingale
   2. William Tukes
   3. Sigmund Freud
   4. Benjamin Rush

2. Changes in the delivery of mental health care that resulted from the development of electroconvulsive therapy and psychotherapeutic drugs brought about which phenomenon in the 20th century?
   1. Behavioral therapy
   2. Personality disorganization
   3. Deinstitutionalization
   4. Brain surgery

3. What is the best description of personality?
   1. The level of mental health that a person attains in life
   2. The relatively consistent set of attitudes and behaviors particular to an individual
   3. The result of a positive self-concept and acceptable behavior
   4. The ability to manage stress

4. The nurse is reviewing the assessment findings for a patient hospitalized with a stress disorder. What findings support the diagnosis? *(Select all that apply.)*
   1. A vague feeling of depression
   2. An assumed role to protect the ego
   3. A main reason for all mental illnesses
   4. A distortion of reality in response to a stressor
   5. A response to any demand made upon the individual

5. The nurse is caring for a patient who is currently voicing feelings of anxiety. The nurse correctly recognizes what as the best description of the feelings that the patient is experiencing?
   1. A vague feeling of apprehension
   2. Feelings of paranoia
   3. Emotional stability
   4. Concerns about the impressions that others have of her

6. An assembly-line manager in a factory was told that he would be laid off if his line did not meet the hourly quota. He promptly went to his workers and threatened to fire anyone who was found taking even 1 minute extra on a break. What is the manager displaying?
   1. Denial
   2. Regression
   3. Displacement
   4. Identification

7. Punishment and abandonment were how mentally ill people were treated in medieval times. These practices continued until the 17th and 18th centuries. Which care practice that is still being used today did Dr. Philippe Pinel of France advocate?
   1. Electroshock therapy for melancholy
   2. Humane care with record keeping of behaviors
   3. Psychoanalysis
   4. Home care in the community

8. The student nurse is working on a presentation regarding OBRA. What was the result of this landmark legislation? *(Select all that apply.)*

   1. Deinstitutionalization
   2. Prohibition of electroshock therapy
   3. Limited access to psychotropic medications
   4. Approved surgical treatment for schizophrenia
   5. Increased construction of state facilities for residential mental health care

9. A 52-year-old patient experienced cardiac arrest from a myocardial infarction. During his acute care stay in the hospital, the patient flirts with all his female nurses. When he is asked to stop, he withdraws and later complains of chest heaviness. What is a possible explanation for the patient's behavior?

   1. Boredom from restricted activity
   2. Lack of motivation to recover
   3. Frustration from illness
   4. Threatened self-concept

10. A 14-year-old tells the school nurse that she is self-conscious about her recent breast development. She reports that the boys in her class are teasing her. What is the first step for the nurse to take?

    1. Call her parents.
    2. Ask her to describe what happened.
    3. Ask who her friends are.
    4. Provide her with a pamphlet outlining the changes associated with puberty.

11. The nurse is instructing a wife to give insulin injections to her husband. The wife is unable to sit still, frequently asks to repeat parts of the instruction for understanding, and sighs often with rapid respirations. What degree of anxiety is the wife experiencing?

    1. Mild
    2. Moderate
    3. Severe
    4. Panic

12. A 17-year-old patient was admitted to the orthopedic unit with pelvic fracture, wrist fracture, and multiple contusions and abrasions from an auto accident. She yells for the nurse every 5 minutes, refuses to use her call light, and breaks out in tears when she does not get her way. How would this behavior best be described?

    1. Regression
    2. Compensation
    3. Denial
    4. Displacement

13. A college student is brought to the emergency department by her roommate. The roommate states that when the patient returned from her date, she was crying and said she had been raped. The patient recounts the evening's events, cracking jokes about her date's trouble keeping an erection, and asking if the nurse knows where she can get a replacement for her favorite outfit, which has been torn. How is this defense mechanism best described?

    1. Displacement
    2. Compensation
    3. Denial
    4. Dissociation

14. A teenager wrecks the family car by rear-ending a truck turning left. The teenager says, "It wasn't my fault. I came over the hill and that truck was just sitting there. It was his fault for turning left." What defense mechanism is the teenager using to deal with his situation?

    1. Compensation
    2. Conversion reaction
    3. Projection
    4. Rationalization

15. After a few days of hospitalization, a patient is participating in plans to be transferred to a rehabilitation facility to continue therapies to enhance his activities of daily living. Which statement indicates the patient is beginning to adjust to his new situation and future? *(Select all that apply.)*

    1. "I know that once I can walk without assistance, I can go back to my own home."
    2. "My wife will not be able to help take care of me until I get stronger."
    3. "I'm going to show everybody that I can make it on my own; just you wait!"
    4. "I don't know why everybody is making a big deal; I was by myself before I got sick."
    5. "I am ready to get started with therapy so I can hopefully go home soon."

16. What factor is most predictive of the onset of a crisis for an individual?

    1. The individual has no support system.
    2. The individual perceives a stressor to be threatening.
    3. The individual is exposed to a precipitating stressor.
    4. The individual experiences a stressor and responds with ineffective coping efforts.

17. During crisis intervention, what is the highest priority of nursing care?

    1. Managing anxiety
    2. Identifying situational supports
    3. Patient safety
    4. Teaching specific coping skills that the patient lacks

18. The leader of a self-help group is discussing the use of defense mechanisms. What information should be included about their use? *(Select all that apply.)*

    1. Once used, they are irreversible.
    2. Defense mechanisms are pathologic.
    3. They are a means of managing conflict.
    4. Defense mechanisms are predominantly unconscious.
    5. Defense mechanisms are primarily used to blame others.

19. What interventions can the nurse use to enhance the assessment of an older adult patient? *(Select all that apply.)*

    1. Identify and accommodate physical needs first.
    2. Pledge complete confidentiality on all topics to the patient.
    3. Interpret information with consideration of the patient's spiritual or cultural background.
    4. Adhere firmly to the sequence of questions on the standardized assessment tool.
    5. Determine whether there are any sensory changes in hearing or vision before beginning the assessment.

20. The nurse manager has completed an educational program with her staff regarding patient education and improving mental illness. Which statement by a participant would indicate a need for further education? *(Select all that apply.)*

   1. "I need to teach my patients ways to recognize and describe their levels of anxiety."
   2. "My patients will not need to worry about learning relaxation skills if they don't want to."
   3. "Patients who use passive communication skills have better mental health than those who use assertive communication skills."
   4. "Learning problem-solving skills can help improve a person's overall mental health."
   5. "The power of positive thinking patterns is a topic I need to discuss with my patients."

21. A woman, age 22, is driving to the beach for a bachelorette party for her friend who's getting married the following weekend. She's running late, and the bride has texted her twice. As she is crossing a busy bridge over an inlet, she is answering a text when she almost drops the phone. Jerking slightly to catch it, she inadvertently turns the wheel and her car swerves and hits a bicyclist, who, along with his bike, is thrown over the rail into the bay and is killed. The woman makes it through the police interview, the ticketing, and the ambulance once-over (she is uninjured). An officer suggests she call someone to come drive home with her, but instead, after everyone leaves, she drives on to the beach party. Over the next few days, when she tells her story, she smiles and even makes a few self-deprecating jokes. But on the one-week anniversary of the accident, she experiences severe weakness and tremors in both hands. She is tested at a neurology clinic where results indicate that the weakness and tremors are real, but no neurological or physiological cause can be determined. She is referred to a therapist and after four cancellations, her mother goes to her apartment and finds she has taken a significant number of sleeping capsules. The mother calls an ambulance and after being treated in the ED for the overdose, the patient is admitted to the psychiatric unit and assessment begins. Her mother has already told a nurse that her daughter has a history of intermittent bouts of depression with chronic self-deprecation and low self-esteem.

   Choose the *most likely* options to complete the statement below.

   This patient's descriptions of the accident with smiling and a little self-deprecating humor are most likely indicative of _____1_____, while her new weakness and tremors suggest _____2_____. During her unit intake, the nurse recognizes that a **priority need** is to assess this patient for _____3_____.

OPTIONS FOR 1	OPTIONS FOR 2	OPTIONS FOR 3
Compensation	Compensation	Clear insight and judgment regarding current situation
Conversion	Conversion	Mood and affect including level of depression or anxiety
Denial	Denial	Content of thought, including delusion or other non–reality-based thinking
Displacement	Displacement	Potential for self-harm
Dissociation	Dissociation	Speech pattern, including extreme distractibility
Introjection	Introjection	Activity level and responsiveness
Sublimation	Sublimation	General appearance and hygiene

Care of the Patient With a Psychiatric Disorder

Objectives

1. Identify and describe the major mental disorders.
2. List five warning signs of suicide.
3. Identify basic interventions for patients experiencing various mental health problems.
4. Describe the general care and treatment methods for patients experiencing mental health problems.
5. Name two alternative therapies used for mental disorders.

Key Terms

anorexia nervosa (ăn-ō-RĔK-sē-ă nŭr-VŌ-să, p. 1151)
anxiety (ăng-ZĪ-ŭ-tē, p. 1145)
bulimia nervosa (bū-LĒ-mē-ă nŭr-VŌ-să, p. 1152)
compulsions (kŭm-PŬL-shŭnz, p. 1148)
cyclothymic disorder (sī-klō-THĪ-mĭk dĭs-ŌR-dŭr, p. 1145)
delirium (dĭ-LĬR-ē-ŭm, p. 1137)
delusion (dĭ-LŪ-zhŭn, p. 1137)
dementia (dĭ-MĔN-shŭ, p. 1137)
depression (dĭ-PRĔSH-ŭn, p. 1144)
hallucination (hă-lū-sĭ-NĀ-shŭn, p. 1143)
hypomanic episode (hī-pō-MĂN-ĭk ĔP-ĭ-sōd, p. 1144)
illusions (ĭl-LŪ-zhŭnz, p. 1149)

mania (MĀ-nē-ŭ, p. 1144)
multiaxial system (mŭl-tē-ĂK-sē-ăl SĬS-tŭm, p. 1136)
neurosis (nū-RŌ-sĭs, p. 1136)
obsessions (ŏb-SĔSH-ŭnz, p. 1148)
paraphilias (păr-ă-FĬL-ē-ŭz, p. 1150)
phobia (FŌ-bē-ŭ, p. 1148)
psychosis (sī-KŌ-sĭs, p. 1136)
schizophrenia (skĭt-sō-FRĔ-nē-ŭ, p. 1137)
serotonin syndrome (sĕr-ō-TŌ-nĭn SĬN-drōm, p. 1156)
somatic (sō-măt-ĭk, p. 1150)
sundowning syndrome (SŬN-DOUN-ĭng SĬN-drōm, p. 1137)

All nurses need to have a basic understanding of the classifications of human responses and methods of treatment for mental illness. Many patients on a medical unit have, in addition to a physiologic disorder, a history of psychiatric problems. An even more common situation is the ill patient's experience of emotional disturbance from the effects of the illness. It is important to be able to interact therapeutically with the physical and the emotional aspects of patient care.

A person's ability to handle a stressful event depends on that person's psychological state. Neurosis is a term describing ineffective coping with stress that causes mild interpersonal disorganization. People with a neurosis have insight that they have a psychiatric problem. A person with a neurosis remains oriented to reality but has some degree of distortion of reality manifested by a strong emotional response to the trigger event. The trigger event may be an everyday stressor, such as environmental stressors or family relationships. Various complaints of nervousness or emotional upset, compulsions, obsessiveness, and phobias are common with a neurosis. Many neurotic people exhibit poor self-esteem and have social relationships that are impaired by the various complaints noted. Treatment for patients with a neurosis usually is completed in an outpatient setting, if they seek treatment at all.

In contrast, a person with psychosis is out of touch with reality and has severe personality deterioration, impaired perception and judgment, hallucinations, and delusions. A psychotic person does not recognize the fact that he or she has a psychiatric illness. Treatment for psychosis often necessitates hospitalization with follow-up regularly through an outpatient setting. Some psychotic patients seek voluntary admission for treatment. Involuntary admission (commonly called *probating*) is also possible when a person is thought to be a danger to self or others. Although laws vary from state to state, a judge and either a clinical psychologist or a physician, or both, must be involved to complete an involuntary admission.

The *Diagnostic and Statistical Manual of Psychiatric Disorders*, Fifth Edition (DSM-V), published by the American Psychiatric Association (APA, 2013), includes signs and symptoms for all psychiatric illnesses. In previous editions, the *DSM* described a multiaxial system to document psychiatric illnesses. This system is not currently being used. Most hospitals and health care providers in the United States today use the

DSM-V to facilitate medical diagnosis and as a guide to clinical practice.

Mental disorders discussed in this chapter include the following:

- Organic mental disorders (e.g., delirium and dementia)
- Thought process disorders (e.g., schizophrenia)
- Affective (mood) disorders
- Anxiety disorders
- Personality disorders
- Sexual disorders
- Psychophysiologic (somatoform) disorders
- Eating disorders

A basic description of some of the major disorders and a summary of treatment, prognosis, and related nursing diagnoses are included in Table 35.1.

TYPES OF PSYCHIATRIC DISORDERS

NEUROCOGNITIVE MENTAL DISORDERS

Neurocognitive disorders differ from other mental health disorders. An identifiable brain disease or dysfunction is the basis for the behavior. These disorders affect cognitive or intellectual abilities. The effects range from mild lapses in memory to severe memory loss and behavioral changes. A predominant characteristic of the type of disorder is disorientation.

Delirium

Delirium is a change in consciousness that occurs rapidly over a short time. Occurrence of this disorder is possible at any age. Delirium is associated with reduced awareness and attention to surroundings, disorganized thinking, sensory misinterpretation, and irrelevant speech. Sleep patterns often are disturbed. Possible causes of delirium include physical illnesses, such as fever, heart failure, pneumonia, azotemia, or malnutrition; drug intoxication; and anesthesia. Treatment for delirium involves determining the cause and correcting it. If the cause is a homeostatic imbalance such as hypoxemia, electrolyte imbalance, or malnutrition, treatment is focused on the problem causing the imbalance. If the cause is chemical agents, the chemicals or drugs should be withdrawn or the dosage reduced. A person with nocturnal delirium, or sundowning syndrome, displays increased disorientation and agitation only during the evening and nighttime.

Dementia

Dementia is a term describing an altered mental state secondary to cerebral disease. Dementia is usually a slow and progressive loss of intellectual function that is often irreversible. Symptoms are often severe enough to interfere with activities of daily living. Alzheimer disease is the most common type of dementia in the United States, accounting for 60% to 80% of dementia cases. According to 2018 statistics from the Alzheimer's Association, 5.7 million people in the United States have Alzheimer disease. It is projected that 12.7 million people will have dementia related to Alzheimer's disease by the year 2050 if significant improvements in treatment are not developed (Alzheimer's Association, 2021). Using reality orientation techniques and providing a safe environment are two key aspects of nursing interventions in caring for patients with dementia (see Table 35.1).

SCHIZOPHRENIA

The main characteristic of thought process disorders is bizarre, non–reality-based thinking. Schizophrenia is one of a large group of psychotic disorders whose defining characteristics are gross distortion of reality; disturbance of language and communication; withdrawal from social interaction; and the disorganization and fragmentation of thought, perception, and emotional reaction. Schizophrenia is one of the most profoundly disabling mental illnesses that a nurse will ever encounter. The onset of schizophrenia typically occurs in young adulthood. It occurs in both sexes equally, and approximately 1% of the population will experience schizophrenia at some point in their lives. Schizophrenia is a chronic disorder with residual disability in functioning. The family of a patient with schizophrenia typically experiences emotional and financial devastation. Schizophrenia is prone to exacerbation from stresses in life.

Research findings have indicated a biological basis for the disease, dispelling the early theory of poor mother-child relationship as the cause, and researchers have noted brain tissue changes. The ventricles of the brain are larger than normal, with the left ventricle larger than the right, and the cerebral cortex is smaller than normal. This is thought to account for the disorganized thinking, hallucinations, and delusions. The neurotransmitter dopamine is present in excess amounts in the brain with schizophrenia. Pupils of the eyes differ in size, and blinking rate is sometimes faster or slower than normal. Clumsiness and difficulty in distinguishing the right and left sides of the body sometimes occur and are attributable to the enlargement of the ventricles of the brain.

Behaviors that individuals with schizophrenia display fall into different categories: positive, or excessive, and negative, or absent. The prognosis for individuals who exhibit positive behavior patterns is good; such patients have fewer structural changes in the brain and respond better to drug therapy. Positive behavior patterns include delusions, hallucinations, and disordered thinking. Negative behavior patterns include apathy, social withdrawal, and flat affect.

Positive Behavior Patterns

A delusion is a false, fixed belief that cannot be corrected by feedback and that other people in the same cultural context do not accept as true. The affected individual believes that a false premise is true. The individual fits this false premise logically into his or her interpretation of reality. Because of the strong logic supporting the false premise, it is difficult for the individual to accept what is really true. There are several types of delusions (Table 35.2).

Table 35.1 Psychiatric Disorders

CHARACTERISTICS	TREATMENT AND PROGNOSIS	ASSOCIATED PATIENT PROBLEMS	NURSING INTERVENTIONS
Neurocognitive Psychiatric Disorders			
Dementia			
Slow and progressive worsening of symptoms: impaired memory and judgment, personality changes, decreased cognitive function, impaired orientation	Treatment depends on the cause. Prognosis is poor; essential feature of this condition is the slow deteriorating rate of mental function.	Impaired Cognitive Function Fearfulness Potential for Injury Anxiousness Inability to Bathe Self Excessive Demand on Primary Caregiver	*Reality orientation techniques:* Place large clock and calendar in view; keep curtains opened and lights on during the day; and use calm, supportive approach. *Decrease sensory stimuli:* Do not expose patient to crowds; give instructions one step at a time, and keep in simple terms. *Provide for safety:* Place bed in lowest position; side rails useful to aid patient in turning. Ensure that hallway rails, chair, bed alarms, and call light are within reach; place personal articles within reach; and ensure sufficient night lighting. *Adequate nutrition:* Reduce dining distractions such as television; encourage snacks if patient is unable to eat a sufficient amount at one time; monitor weight monthly; and have family bring in patient's favorite foods.
Delirium			
Acute, rapid onset of symptoms: disorientation, incoherent thought content, impaired cognitive function, symptoms worsen at night, illusions, hallucinations	Treatment depends on the cause. Prognosis is guarded.	Potential for Injury Potential for Harming Others Impaired Cognitive Function Inability to Bathe Self	*Self-care support:* Assist as needed with ADLs and toileting; encourage mobility and other activities that use large muscle groups with activities such as "Simon says" or armchair aerobics; try to keep the daily routine the same times of each day; and, if possible, have same group of staff assist with ADLs.
Schizophrenia			
Inappropriate emotional responses, bizarre behaviors, impaired communications, delusions, illusions, hallucinations, inability to relate to other people, self-care deficit, symptoms present at least 6 months, with positive behaviors for 1 months. or more	Treatment is milieu therapy (environment), psychotherapy, antipsychotic drug therapy, and long-term social support. Prognosis is variable and depends on the extent of the symptoms and responses to treatments. Many patients with paranoid type of schizophrenia are reluctant to seek treatment.	Impaired Cognitive Function Disturbed Sensory Perception Anxiousness Inability to Bathe Self Inability to Dress Self Compromised Social Interaction Impaired Role Functioning Impaired Family Processes Ineffective Sleep Pattern Impaired Coping Impaired Personal Sense of Identity	*Establish therapeutic relationship:* Be available and listen actively; use clear, simple statements in communications; ensure that your body language is in tune with the message; and avoid hand gesturing when talking, to prevent distraction from the message. *Reality orientation techniques:* Use verbal reminding; place large clock and calendar in view; reduce stimuli to help patient focus on reality; and establish and reinforce a daily routine. *Reduce anxiety:* Avoid having patient make choices; problem solve with patient on ways to reduce anxiety; encourage socialization by invitation, not assignment; decrease sensory stimuli; and accept and support patient's feelings (empathy reduces anxiety). *Manage positive behaviors:* Ask patient directly about his or her hallucinations; watch for cues that indicate that the patient is hallucinating; focus on reality; do not argue with the patient or enter into the patient's hallucination; if the patient is having delusions, be open and honest in interactions to reduce suspicion; respond calmly and matter-of-factly to suspicions; have the patient describe who "he" or "she" is, but do not argue the logic; and if the delusion is very strong, try to help the patient find a distraction from the delusion so as not to dwell upon it. Remember that hallucinations and delusions have the potential to provoke aggressive behavior. Watch for signs of growing agitation. Provide safety. *Manage negative behaviors:* Encourage self-care, assist only as indicated; help patient recognize own feelings of the event that just occurred; and encourage social participation, but do not force it onto the patient. *Medication management:* Be alert for early recognition of serious side effects; administer medications in liquid form if you suspect the patient of hoarding pills; encourage the patient to take medications routinely, to adjust to ideas of taking them for rest of life; and provide good nutrition.

Table 35.1   Psychiatric Disorders—cont'd

CHARACTERISTICS	TREATMENT AND PROGNOSIS	ASSOCIATED PATIENT PROBLEMS	NURSING INTERVENTIONS
Affective (Mood) Disorders			
Major Depression			
Prolonged, intense unhappiness Symptoms: apathy, pessimism, multiple physical complaints, guilt feelings, anxiety, isolation, suicidal thoughts, appetite disturbance, fatigue, sleep disturbance, constipation, limited attention span, short-term memory disturbance	Treatment possibilities include antidepressant drug therapy, individual family or group psychotherapy, and electroconvulsive therapy when drug therapy is ineffective or drugs are contraindicated. An estimated 50% of all individuals have at least one additional episode of depression.	Potential for Violence Upon Self Despair Impaired Coping Inability to Bathe Self Inability to Dress Self Compromised Verbal Communication Ineffective Sleep Pattern Helplessness Potential for Insufficient Nutrition Impaired Belief System	*Establish therapeutic relationship:* Use a kind but firm manner in addressing the individual; be honest and consistent; and show compassion, composure, and patience. Remember that depressed individuals have slower-than-normal physical responses. Manic individuals are not able to stay focused. *Communications: For depression:* Encourage expression of negative feeling; point out any specific improvement; reinforce assertive behavior; recognize and point out manifestations of self-destructive thoughts or behavior to the individual; and discuss and practice alternative ways to respond to stress. *For mania:* Keep directions specific and simple; use a calm approach; present reality without arguing; be consistent and keep to the rules; attempt to provide a focus in the conversation; interrupt to slow the individual down in conversation; and phrase questions that require a brief answer. *Planned activity:* Avoid competitive activities that require the individual to continually pay attention in order to participate (e.g., volleyball). Bowling and exercise such as yoga are better choices for group activities. When providing activities for the patient, do so in patient's room to reduce distractions. Small-group activities help build self-esteem. Allow for rest periods. *Nutritional risk:* Select well-balanced meals and snacks, and include high-fiber foods in the diet to reduce constipation. Handheld foods (e.g., individual sandwiches, fresh vegetables and fruits, crackers) work well for manic patients. Avoid junk food (snacks that are high in concentrated sugar and fats). Monitor for dehydration. Weigh weekly. *Do not remove salt* from the diet while a patient is taking lithium. (Reduced salt intake can contribute to lithium toxicity.) *Drug therapy:* Monitor lithium levels. Normal loading range is 1–1.5 mEq/L; common range for maintenance is 0.6–1.2 mEq/L. In charting, note presence or absence of adverse effects of lithium. Note changes in individual's behavior and thoughts individual expresses. Document all behaviors that can be considered a suicide threat or action. Remind patient that antidepressant medications take about 2 to 4 wks. to produce any effects.
Bipolar Affective Disorder			
Mood swings with manic episodes, alternating with or without episodes of depression Symptoms of mania: grand or self-confident mood, overresponsiveness to stimuli, insomnia without fatigue, impaired judgment, irritability, psychomotor overactivity	Treatment possibilities include psychotherapy; antimanic drugs (lithium); and family and individual support, with education regarding drug use. Prognosis depends on response to medication and treatment.	Potential for Injury Inability to Tolerate Activity Potential for Violence Upon Self or Others Impaired Cognitive Function Compromised Social Interaction Potential for Insufficient Nutrition	

Continued

Table 35.1 Psychiatric Disorders—cont'd

Anxiety Disorders

Generalized Anxiety

Description	Treatment	Nursing Diagnoses	Interventions
Characterized by a steady, pervasive level of anxiety; possible at any age but commonly occurs around ages 20–30; lasts 6 months or longer. Symptoms: apprehension, irritability, insomnia, poor concentration, fear of unknown, can be either preoccupied with or neglectful of self-care, autonomic hyperactivity; conversation dominated by physical complaints	Treatment possibilities include relaxation techniques, exercise, visual imagery, massage, biofeedback imagery, and antianxiety drug therapy. Prognosis is variable; condition sometimes lasts 6 months or longer.	*Impaired Coping* *Anxiousness* *Insufficient Nutrition* *Fearfulness*	*Establish therapeutic relationship:* Encourage the patient to share thoughts and feelings. Be supportive and provide assistance. Encourage the patient to use more realistic thoughts, such as "Whatever happens, I can deal with it" or "I've been through this procedure before, and I handled it." Encourage self-care and simple decision making. Avoid reinforcing concerns over physical complaints; but do not ignore them without further assessment. *Reduce anxiety:* Decrease environmental stimuli to reduce agitation. It is sometimes a good idea to restrict visitors to decrease stimuli, but allow the patient that control. Instruct about staff routine. Teach the individual relaxation techniques such as the following: 1. Practice abdominal or deep breathing. 2. Imagery: In comfortable position, use deep breathing and focus on a pleasant image and all its details. 3. For painful procedures, have the patient imagine how a favorite hero or role model would tolerate the procedure. 4. Brisk walks, back rubs, hot showers or baths, or a heating pad also can help the patient relax. *Communications:* Include in therapeutic communications explanations of all procedures and treatments, and keep family informed about the hospital regulations (e.g., visiting hours) and the goals of the care provided (e.g., the need to reduce stimuli). Be punctual with treatments and medications. This builds trust. Anticipate needs.

Panic Disorders

Description	Treatment	Nursing Diagnoses	Interventions
Severe anxiety, intense fear; exhibiting physical manifestations suddenly without apparent reason; onset frequently in late 20s. Types of posttraumatic stress disorder: acute (occurs within 6 months of event), chronic (lasts more than 6 months.), and delayed (starts 6 months. or more after event)	Use treatments for generalized anxiety disorders. Attacks last minutes to hours and possibly recur several times a week. Debriefing techniques (as used by the military) are often helpful.	*Anxiousness* *Fearfullness* *Impaired Coping* *Physical or Sexual Assault Trauma Condition* *Impaired Family Processes*	Panic attacks are a form of Generalized Anxiety Disorder. In addition to interventions for Generalized Anxiety Disorder the nurse can help the patient reduce anxiety during a panic attack by: 1. Remaining calm during the panic attack. 2. Giving the patient space during the attack so they do not feel smothered. 3. Encouraging distractions such as physical activity, which also reduces stress.

Table 35.1	Psychiatric Disorders—cont'd		
CHARACTERISTICS	**TREATMENT AND PROGNOSIS**	**ASSOCIATED PATIENT PROBLEMS**	**NURSING INTERVENTIONS**
Phobias			
Characterized by persistent and irrational fear of a specific object, situation, or activity; leads to lifestyle of self-protective avoidance; social phobias are more common in women	With desensitization, patient learns to relax while reentering phobia-producing situation in imagination and then in real life. Anxiety and fear are kept to a minimum. Prognosis is variable and depends on response to treatment.	*Anxiousness* *Impaired Coping* *Fearfulness* *Impaired Family Processes*	Phobias are a form of Generalized Anxiety Disorder. In addition to interventions for generalized anxiety disorder the nurse can help the patient reduce anxiety experienced with a phobia by: 1. Reassuring the patient that they are safe. 2. Be accepting of the patient's fear. 3. Help the patient to identify stressors.
Obsessive-Compulsive Disorders (OCDs)			
Anxiety condition characterized by inability to stop persistent, irrational, and uncontrollable acts (compulsions) or thoughts (obsessions) contrary to person's standards or judgment; usually appears after adolescence, resulting from fear, guilt, and anticipation of punishment; person is usually orderly, meticulous, dependable, and scrupulous, although with tendency to be rigid and stubborn; mild forms are common; equally distributed between men and women; increases with stress	Treatment often consists of psychotherapy, to uncover the basic fears and to help the person distinguish objective dangers from imagined dangers. Drug therapy with clomipramine (Anafranil) has been of great value. Prognosis is more severe than with other anxiety disorders; complete recovery is rare. However, complete disability occurs only in a minority of cases.	*Impaired Coping* *Anxiousness* *Fearfulness* *Altered Thought Processes* *Ineffective Sleep Pattern* *Social Seclusion* *Impaired Role Functioning*	OCDs are a form of Generalized Anxiety Disorder. In addition to interventions for Generalized Anxiety Disorder the nurse can help the patient reduce anxiety experienced with OCD by: 1. Involving family with the treatment plan. 2. Helping the patient to recognize irrational thoughts and how best to address them. 3. Encouraging participation in support groups for those diagnosed with OCD.

Continued

Table 35.1   Psychiatric Disorders—cont'd

Personality Disorders

		Compromised Social Interaction	Establish therapeutic relationship: Maintain a therapeutic environment. Be firm and consistent.
Range of behaviors, depending on the type of disorder present	Treatment possibilities include psychotherapeutic drug therapy, group therapy, reality therapy, support groups, and family counseling.	Impaired Coping	Set limits on behaviors: Establish consequences for violating limits. Provide positive feedback for appropriate behavior; encourage ventilation of feelings.
		Impaired Family Processes	Communications: Encourage decision making and patient participation. Discuss incidents with patient. Approach in a calm, confident manner.
Common characteristics: poor impulse control (heavy drinking, overeating, substance abuse, assaultive behavior), self-destructive acts (such as self-mutilation), manipulation of or dependency on other people, inappropriate behavior for situation, disregard for rules; usually accompanied by denial of maladaptive behaviors	Prognosis is guarded; antisocial personality disorder is the more socially malignant of the disorders and appears to have the most severe consequences.	Potential for Violence Upon Self or Others	Safety and security: Know where patient is at all times. Be alert for manipulating behaviors. Assist in ADLs as necessary.
		Compromised Parenting Skills	
		Stress Response Condition	

Table 35.2   **Types of Delusions**

TYPE OF DELUSION	DEFINITION	EXAMPLE
Grandeur	Belief of being someone with great powers to control any situation	"I am God."
Ideas of reference	Belief that an event has special personal meaning	"The lady on TV is telling me to buy the soap."
Persecution	Belief that someone is out to harm him or her	"They put a transmitter in my tooth to monitor my every word."
Somatic delusions	False belief pertaining to body function or image	"I have diabetes." (in the absence of the disease)
Thought broadcasting	Belief that others know his or her ideas without action on his or her part to convey the thoughts	"You all know the thoughts I have been having today."
Thought insertion	Belief that ideas are put in his or her mind	"You put these thoughts in my head for your own pleasure."
Thought withdrawal	Belief that thoughts are being removed from his or her mind	"You have been stealing my thoughts."

A **hallucination** is a sensory experience without a stimulus trigger. Auditory hallucinations are the type that people experience most often. Visual, olfactory, and tactile hallucinations are also possible in the individual with schizophrenia.

Disordered thinking occurs when the individual is not able to interpret information being received in the brain. Loose association-making in speech sometimes makes this evident; conversation does not flow logically. *Concreteness* is sometimes a sign of disordered thinking. For example, when someone is taking a picture and the individual with schizophrenia hears "Watch the birdie!" the individual will look up into the tree for the bird instead of smiling for the camera.

Negative Behavior Patterns

Negative, or absent, behavior patterns also are associated with schizophrenia. They may manifest alone or together with positive behavior patterns. Negative behavior includes apathy (avolition), social withdrawal, alogia, blunted emotional responses, and anhedonia. *Apathy* is a lack of energy or interest. An unkempt appearance or lack of appropriate hygiene is often a reflection of apathy. *Social withdrawal* occurs in an attempt to reduce stimuli to the brain. Some individuals with schizophrenia are frightened or overwhelmed by the experience of trying to communicate with other people and find it easier to withdraw from the contact. *Alogia* is defined as reduced content of speech. Alogia sometimes occurs as part of the overload of information that occurs in conversation; the individual with schizophrenia needs time to sort out the message received. *Affect* is the outward display or expression of emotion that is felt. *Flat affect* and *anhedonia* are terms describing the lack of expressed feelings. *Flat affect* is the lack of nonverbal expression of emotions, such as by means of facial expression or tone of voice, and *anhedonia* is the inability to experience happiness or joy. Other behaviors sometimes exhibited by an individual with schizophrenia include bizarre posturing or behaviors such as laughing when receiving news about a death in the family. Adverse effects of drugs also have the potential to produce negative or absent behaviors. It is important to assess the situation surrounding the behavior.

Subtypes of Schizophrenia

Schizophrenia is a cluster of behaviors. There are five subtypes of this category of illness:

1. *Disorganized:* Flat or inappropriate affect, incoherence; prognosis is poor.
2. *Paranoid:* Delusions, auditory hallucinations; prognosis is good with treatment.
3. *Catatonic:* Stupor, negativism, rigidity, excitement, posturing; prognosis is fair.
4. *Undifferentiated:* Delusions, hallucinations, incoherence, gross disorganization (does not fit criteria of other types); prognosis is fair.
5. *Residual:* Typical signs and symptoms associated with schizophrenia without evidence of gross disorganization, incoherence, delusions, and hallucinations; prognosis is poor.

Stages of Schizophrenia

The course of schizophrenia involves four stages and features acute episodes of psychosis alternating with periods of relatively normal function. The *prodromal phase* often begins in adolescence and begins with lack of energy or motivation and withdrawal. Other symptoms common in this stage are as follows: affect becomes blunted; beliefs and ideas become odd; the person sometimes develops an excessive interest in philosophy or religion; self-care and personal hygiene decline; emotional lability is present; speech is difficult to follow; and the person often complains about multiple physical problems. Magical thinking, or believing that one's thoughts control events, is also a symptom.

Quiet, passive behavior is typical of the *prepsychotic phase.* The individual prefers to be alone. Hallucination and delusions sometimes occur in this stage. Odd, unusual, or eccentric behavior patterns are present.

Family members report that they feel the individual has changed into a stranger.

During the *acute phase,* signs and symptoms sometimes vary widely, but disturbances in thought, perception, emotion, and behavior are very apparent. Often the individual loses contact with reality and is unable to function in the most basic ways.

The *residual phase* features a group of symptoms similar to that in the prodromal phase. The residual phase follows the acute phase. Following the residual phase is a remission period, in which the individual is able to experience some relief of symptoms and to manage some basic activities in life. Prognosis for recovery is fair to poor because of the complex aspects of this disorder.

Treatment for schizophrenia involves a number of psychotherapies to allow the individual self-expression, antipsychotic drug therapy to control symptoms, and a therapeutic relationship maintained over the years to provide continuity for the individual with a lifelong illness.

MAJOR MOOD DISORDERS

Mood disorders, also known as *affective disorders,* are any of a group of psychotic disorders whose defining characteristics are severe and inappropriate emotional responses, prolonged and persistent disturbances of mood and related thought distortions, and other symptoms associated with either depressed or manic states. *Mood,* as defined by the *DSM-V* (APA, 2013), is a prolonged emotion that affects a person's psyche. Extremes in mood range from depression to mania. Hereditary factors account for 60% to 80% of cases of mood disorders. The levels of the neurotransmitters norepinephrine and serotonin are deficient in depressed individuals, and the level of norepinephrine is excessive in manic individuals. Neurotransmitter imbalances are sometimes the result of heredity and sometimes are caused by environmental factors such as prolonged stress or brain trauma. Most people experience some type of depression and maintain their life; however, the individual with a mood disorder has these extreme moods for months or years without relief.

Depression

Depression is a mood disturbance characterized by exaggerated feelings of sadness, despair, lowered self-esteem, loss of interest in former activities, and pessimistic thoughts. Depression is more than a state of mind; in any given 2-week period, almost 8% of Americans report symptoms of moderate or severe depression (Centers for Disease Control and Prevention [CDC], 2021a). Depression is found in all races, ethnic groups, age groups, and socioeconomic levels. Women are affected twice as often as men.

Depression can be so severe at times that an affected person contemplates, or actually succeeds at, committing suicide. Suicide falls in the top 10 leading causes of death in the United States; where the statistic falls

in the top 10 depends on the age group (CDC, 2021b). Many deaths supposedly caused by accidental overdoses, automobile accidents, and refusal of medical care may be viewed as hidden suicides even though they are not reported as such. Suicide attempts also are not included in the statistics. Although the highest rate of suicide is among the older population, suicide among teenagers is on the rise in this country. Children must be taught effective coping skills.

There is great controversy over the terminally ill patient's right to commit suicide. Some people believe that deliberately ending one's life is a rational decision in certain circumstances, such as terminal illness, and defend the right to commit suicide. There is growing support for right-to-die legislation, which removes the criminal stigma from suicide. Most people who commit suicide in the hospital setting have received the diagnosis of an incurable or painful illness. It is important to evaluate terminally ill individuals and treat them for depression, as well as for their physical disorders, to ease their pain and enhance their quality of life.

To help prevent suicide, recognize warning signs and learn the kinds of actions that often can avert suicide attempts (Box 35.1). Consider as warning signals verbal statements such as "I wish I were dead" or "You won't see me coming back here again" and questions about specific methods of suicide. Actions such as giving away possessions, refusing medications, or neglecting hygiene are also possible warning signals. Many people have anxiety because of a moral conflict within themselves. Many suicidal individuals manage to leave that anxiety behind by making the decision to commit suicide.

Major depression, or *persistent depressive disorder,* is defined as repeated, severe depressive episodes lasting more than 2 years (National Institute of Mental Health, 2018). Estimates are that up to 15% of people with major depressive disorder die from suicide. *Dysthymic disorder* is daily moderate depression that lasts more than 2 years. This disorder often ends up as a lifestyle in which the individual is able to function but not enjoy life.

Bipolar Disorders

Bipolar disorders, or *manic-depressive disorders,* feature shifts between emotional extremes from depression to mania. Mania is a mood disorder whose major characteristic is persistent, abnormal overactivity and a euphoric state. The early phase of a manic episode often is referred to as a hypomanic episode when symptoms are not severe. Often the manic person is engaging, outgoing, and charming, as well as achieving and successful; has excessive energy and optimism; and is possibly a very productive member of the community. Unfortunately, a manic episode has potential to accelerate.

As it intensifies, the episode of mania changes from cheerfulness into excessive feelings of euphoria, rapid speech, flight of ideas, unrealistic beliefs in abilities, no sleep, poor judgment, denial that anything could

Box 35.1 Suicide Warnings and Precautions

WARNING SIGNS OF SUICIDE
- Withdrawing from family or friends
- Talking about death, the hereafter, or suicide
- Giving away prized possessions
- Drug or alcohol abuse
- Personality changes, such as unusual anger, boredom, or apathy
- Unusual neglect of appearance; difficulty concentrating on work or school; complaints of physical problems that have no organic cause; disturbed sleeping or eating patterns; loss of self-esteem; feelings of helplessness, hopelessness, extreme anxiety, or panic
- Previously failed attempts with verbalized regrets of failure

SUICIDE PRECAUTIONS IN THE HOSPITAL ENVIRONMENT
- Remove articles that can be used for suicide: belts, straps, shoelaces, sheets, breakable items for sharp edges, razor blades, curtain cords, bed coils, and personal care items.
- Remove any furniture that can be used for self-injury, as well as doors to closets. Make sure windows are shatterproof.
- Designate a room close to the front desk of the unit or a room with a closed TV monitor.
- Check the patient approximately every 15 min on an irregular schedule around the clock.
- Instruct visitors not to leave gifts in the room until the staff examines them for anything that can be used for self-injury.
- Make sure the patient swallows all medications administered. Administer liquid forms when available. Administer injectables if the patient refuses oral forms as ordered.
- Attend the patient during meals, and keep track of eating utensils and dinnerware. Make sure used trays are not sitting where the patient has the opportunity to walk by and remove tableware.
- Make frequent therapeutic verbal contact.

possibly go wrong, increased sex drive, and obnoxious or provocative behavior such as robbing a store without the fear of being caught. If untreated, delirium may ensue, and death from exhaustion or accident is possible.

Cyclothymic disorder is a pattern that also involves repeated mood swings of hypomania and depression, although they are less intense. There are no periods of normal function with this condition. It is considered a muted version of bipolar disorder. Many individuals with cyclothymic disorder progress to bipolar disorder.

Other affective disorders are seasonal affective disorder (SAD) and postpartum depression. Both of these disorders are connected with hormonal imbalances and respond well to treatment. Practitioners treat SAD, also known as *winter depression,* with phototherapy. Postpartum depression often clears within days, but it is best to further investigate the problem if symptoms continue longer than 2 weeks.

Medical Treatment

Medical treatment for mood disorders includes antidepressants and lithium, electroconvulsive therapy (ECT), and psychotherapy. Antidepressants, such as fluoxetine (Prozac), trazodone, amitriptyline, and venlafaxine (Effexor XR), take 2 to 4 weeks to alleviate the depression. Some antidepressants such as amitriptyline work best when taken at bedtime because of a transient adverse effect of sedation; this regimen sometimes also helps normalize the sleeping pattern. Selective serotonin reuptake inhibitors (SSRIs), such as fluoxetine (Prozac) and paroxetine (Paxil), do not seem to produce as many of the anticholinergic and sedating side effects that sometimes cause patients to stop taking their medications. Some antidepressants, such as fluoxetine, work best when taken in the morning to prevent the adverse effect of insomnia. (See the later section on antidepressant medications for further discussion.)

Practitioners frequently use lithium to treat bipolar disorder. Lithium has a narrow therapeutic range, and patients who take it must be monitored closely for safety. Patients taking lithium also need to monitor the amount of sodium in their diet and fluid intake.

Other drugs in the pharmacologic toolbox to treat mental illness symptoms include duloxetine (Cymbalta), bupropion (Wellbutrin), and mirtazapine (Remeron). Bupropion is also a first-line medication for smoking cessation.

ECT is an option to consider when drug therapy is ineffective or is contraindicated (see Box 35.2 and Nursing Care Plan 35.1).

ANXIETY DISORDERS

Anxiety is a normal response to stress or threat. Anxiety is a state or feeling of apprehension, uneasiness, agitation, uncertainty, and fear resulting from the anticipation of some threat or danger. Experts describe many types of anxiety. *Signal anxiety* is a learned response to an event such as test taking. *Free-floating anxiety* is associated with feelings of dread whose source cannot be identified. *Anxiety trait* is a learned aspect of personality. Individuals with anxiety trait have anxious reactions to relatively nonstressful events. Such individuals respond more quickly and more strongly to stress and are slower than normal to calm down. (See discussion of normal anxiety response in Chapter 34).

Generalized anxiety disorders are characterized by a high degree of anxiety and/or avoidance behavior. An individual with generalized anxiety disorder tends to worry or fret over many things and finds it difficult to concentrate on the task at hand (Fig. 35.1).

Panic can be defined as an attack of acute, intense, and overwhelming anxiety accompanied by a degree of personality disorganization, such as inability to solve problems or think clearly. In a panic attack, symptoms occur abruptly and peak within 10 minutes. Panic attacks are

---

| Box 35.2 | Electroconvulsive Therapy |

Electroconvulsive therapy (ECT) is administered on either an inpatient or an outpatient basis.

PATIENT PREPARATION

1. Purpose of ECT is relief from depression. Patient signs forms of consent for treatment.
2. Common side effects include headache, confusion upon awakening, and short-term amnesia. Patient should take acetaminophen (Tylenol) for persistent headache.
3. Patient needs to be on nothing-by-mouth (NPO) status for at least 8 h before treatment.
4. Patient should wear loose-fitting clothes with access to the arm for intravenous line insertion.
5. Patient must arrange for someone to accompany him or her to and from the treatment. No treatment will take place if patient is unaccompanied.
6. Patient must avoid driving or operating machinery for at least 1 day after treatment.
7. Patient should avoid making any major decisions—about job, finances, relationships, and so forth—until the course of treatment is completed.
8. Patient should take any prescribed medications on time.

TREATMENT

1. Nurse measures baseline vital signs.
2. Nurse applies cardiac, blood pressure, and oximetry monitors to the patient.
3. Nurse establishes an intravenous line for administration of sedative and neuromuscular blockade.
4. Nurse applies electroencephalographic monitor to the patient.
5. After administration of intravenous drugs to patient, practitioner establishes an airway and delivers electrical shock for a few seconds.
6. A controlled seizure lasts 30–60 s. Neuromuscular blockade eliminates most body flexion, thereby reducing risk of spinal injury, bone fracture, or muscle tears.
7. Patient usually sleeps for about 1 h after treatment.

POSTTREATMENT CARE

1. Nurse monitors vital signs and level of consciousness.
2. It is acceptable to discharge the patient with a responsible adult when patient is alert and walking. Confusion is sometimes present, and some patients do not remember coming to the hospital for treatment and leaving afterward.

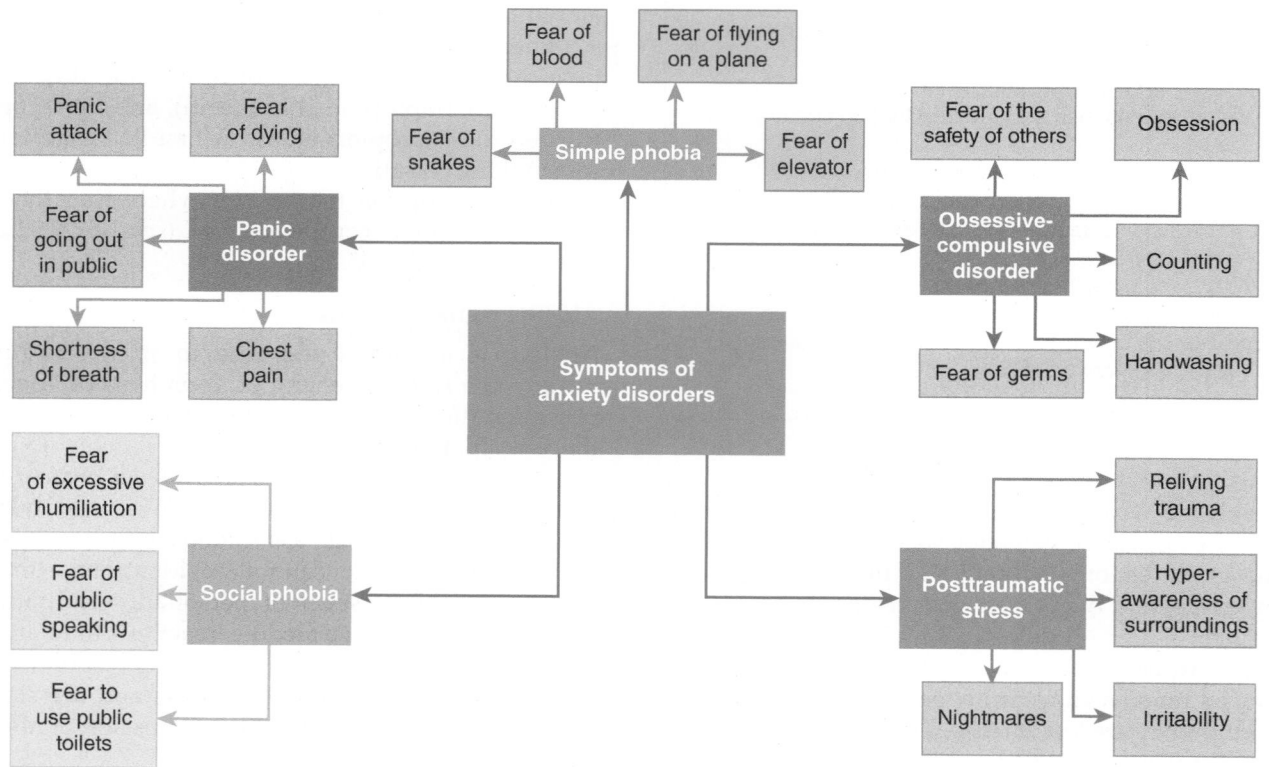

Fig. 35.1 Anxiety disorders. (Modified from Pathways Real Life Recovery, Sandy, UT.)

characterized by at least four of the following: heart palpitations or accelerated heart rate; sweating, trembling, or shaking; feelings of dyspnea or choking; chest pain; nausea or abdominal distress; feeling dizzy or faint; fear of losing control or going crazy; fear of dying; paresthesias (a sensation experienced as numbness, tingling, or "pins and needles"); and chills or hot flashes. Panic disorders are more common in women than in men.

Agoraphobia is considered a type of panic disorder. Agoraphobia is extreme anxiety brought on by situations in which a panic attack is possible. People with agoraphobia avoid people, places, or events that have the potential to trigger an attack. Fear of not receiving any help or embarrassment when an attack occurs in a public place are characteristics of agoraphobia.

Nursing Care Plan 35.1 | **The Patient With Depression**

Mr. W. is a 69-year-old widower whose wife died from cancer 9 months ago. He entered the open psychiatric unit with the diagnosis of major depression. Mr. W.'s unmarried daughter lives out of state and is a partner in a law firm. Mr. W. has severe hypertension and early-stage chronic obstructive pulmonary disease (COPD). On admission, Mr. W. states, "I just can't go on all alone like this. … I have so little energy, and I can't sleep the way I used to." Mr. W. has lost 32 pounds in the past 6 months; he weighs 145 pounds and is 5 feet 11 inches tall. Mr. W. rarely leaves his house, although friends ask him out frequently. He is tearful at times, sighs often, and has poor eye contact during the admission interview. When asked, he admits to thoughts of killing himself. He states that he attempted to do so with an overdose of his hypertension medication, but he wanted to see his daughter one last time before he dies, so he came to the emergency department.

PATIENT PROBLEM
Impaired Coping

Patient Goals and Expected Outcomes	Nursing Interventions	Evaluation
Patient will engage in reality-based interactions Patient will express feelings directly and express anger or hostility outward in a safe manner	Establish a therapeutic relationship; keep staff assignment as consistent as possible. Use a firm, kind manner; tell patient that you can see that he is sad but that he still needs to complete his personal hygiene and activities of daily living. If the patient is ruminating, convey that you will talk about reality or his feelings, but limit the attention you give to repeated expressions of rumination.	Evaluation is ongoing. Weekly care meetings of staff to discuss the patient's progress. Good daily documentation reflecting the patient's progress. Patient is beginning to verbalize to staff his feelings of loss and grief resulting from his wife's death. Patient is expressing need to interact more with his daughter.

PATIENT PROBLEM
Compromised Social Interaction

Patient Goals and Expected Outcomes	Nursing Interventions	Evaluation
Patient will communicate with others Patient will participate in activities	Initially, interact with the patient on a one-on-one basis. Progress to facilitating social interactions between patient and other patients, from small groups to larger groups. Encourage the patient to pursue personal interests, hobbies, and recreational activities. Encourage the patient to identify supportive people outside the unit and to develop these relationships.	Evaluation is ongoing. Patient is beginning to interact with other patients. Patient is beginning to become active in personal interests (e.g., attending a movie or reading a book).

PATIENT PROBLEM
Potential for Violence Upon Self

Patient Goals and Expected Outcomes	Nursing Interventions	Evaluation
Patient will avoid harming himself Patient will identify alternative ways of dealing with stress and emotional problems	Determine appropriate level of suicide precautions, and institute the precautions immediately. Convey that you care about the patient and that you believe he is a worthwhile individual. Involve the patient as much as possible in planning his treatment. Plan with the patient how he will recognize and deal with feelings and situations that have precipitated suicidal feelings in the past.	Evaluation is ongoing. Patient states that he does not intend to harm himself. Patient is verbalizing more acceptable ways of dealing with his depression with other staff members.

Continued

Nursing Care Plan 35.1 | The Patient With Depression—cont'd

PATIENT PROBLEM
Insufficient Nutrition

Patient Goals and Expected Outcomes	Nursing Interventions	Evaluation
Patient will maintain a regular, adequate eating pattern Patient will maintain normal body weight	Monitor patient's eating. Keep intake and output records. Encourage consumption of fluids (e.g., water, juices). Find out what foods the patient likes and dislikes. Try six small feedings per day. Discourage use of nonnutritional substances such as artificial sweeteners, coffee creamers, diet soda, tea, and coffee.	Evaluation is ongoing. Patient is eating 50% to 60% of each meal. Patient is beginning to demonstrate interest in sitting down and eating with a group.

PATIENT PROBLEM
Ineffective Sleep Pattern

Patient Goals and Expected Outcomes	Nursing Interventions	Evaluation
Patient will sleep 5–6 h per night before discharge Patient will verbalize ability to use relaxation techniques when awake at night	Plan for the patient to engage in physical activity while awake. Encourage only planned naps. Teach progressive relaxation exercises. Help the patient establish a consistent time to go to sleep.	Evaluation is ongoing. Patient is sleeping about 6 h per night. Patient is going to sleep at a scheduled time each night.

CRITICAL THINKING QUESTIONS
1. Mr. W. is admitted to the psychiatric unit and placed on suicide precautions. He sits stoically staring out the window and does not respond to the nurse's greeting. What safety interventions should the team incorporate into Mr. W.'s care to prevent his self-destruction?
2. Mr. W. sleeps poorly, approximately 2–3 h a night. What therapeutic interventions should be used to correct his sleep pattern disturbance?
3. Mr. W. has lost 32 pounds. What are some options for the staff to help him meet adequate nutritional requirements?

Treatment for panic disorders focuses on educating the individual about the nature of the disorder, assisting the individual to develop better coping mechanisms with anxiety, and blocking attacks pharmaceutically. Emotional support and reassurance are important nursing measures for individuals suffering with panic disorder.

Phobias

A phobia is different from normal fear. A phobia is irrational fear, in which the thoughts of the individual tend to dwell on the object of the phobia. The individual sometimes recognizes the irrationality of the fear but is still unable to control paralyzing anxiety. Characteristics of phobias vary with the culture. In some cultures, fear of hexes, magical spirits, snakes, and unseen forces have the power to trigger phobic fear reactions. Consider the patient's cultural background when assessing the phobic response.

Obsessive-Compulsive Disorder

Obsessive-compulsive disorder has two features. Obsessions are thoughts that are recurrent, intrusive, and senseless. These thoughts are anxiety producing and distressing in that they are uncontrollable. Compulsions are behaviors that are performed in response to an obsessive thought. The repetitive, ritualistic behaviors, such as checking the locks 10 times before going to bed, typically reduce the anxiety and tension produced by the obsession. Affected patients sometimes recognize the behavior as absurd but still are compelled to perform the ritual to relieve tension. Such patients tend to have difficulty expressing emotions and are often introspective. Stopping the repetitive act results in extreme anxiety. Depression is a feature that often occurs in association with this disorder. Individuals may isolate themselves or try to "make up" for actions as a way of trying to prevent anxiety. Interpersonal relationships and occupations suffer because of the time-consuming behaviors.

Experts believe that activity addictions such as compulsive gambling, sexual promiscuity, excessive Internet use, or overeating arise from obsessive-compulsive behavior disorders. See Chapter 36 for more information concerning addiction.

Posttraumatic Stress Disorder

Posttraumatic stress disorder (PTSD) describes a response to an intensely traumatic experience beyond the usual range of human experiences. These experiences—such as war, rape, a major auto accident, being tortured or observing someone being tortured, or witnessing a violent death—tend to evoke feelings of terror and helplessness. One such experience was witnessing the attack on New York City's World Trade Center on September 11, 2001. The people who escaped the World Trade Center towers before the collapse and emergency personnel who responded to the attack were the most likely to suffer from PTSD. Also at high risk are veterans returning from Iraq, Afghanistan, and other war-torn areas of the world. The experience often is relived repeatedly in dreams or flashbacks. Flashbacks often arise in response to a trigger, a stimulus that resembles the experience or perhaps the anniversary of the event. Flashbacks sometimes include illusions (false interpretation of extreme sensory stimuli, usually visual or auditory, such as a mirage in the desert or the sound of voices in the wind) and hallucinations. Avoidance behavior associated with this disorder sometimes includes emotional detachment, guilt about being a survivor, amnesia of the event, insomnia, irritability, difficulty concentrating, and wariness. Physical response to severe anxiety occurs with each relived episode. Depression and substance abuse often occur in association with PTSD.

There are three types of PTSD: acute, chronic, and delayed. In acute PTSD, symptoms occur within 6 months of the event and last about 6 months. Chronic PTSD is characterized by symptoms that last 6 months or longer. Delayed PTSD involves symptoms that start 6 months or more after the event.

Treatment for PTSD includes antidepressant or antiseizure medications; cognitive therapy, which focuses on breaking negative thought patterns; and behavioral therapy, which aims to break off a conditioned response that has become automatic. Debriefing people right after the event is one strategy that practitioners recommend to prevent PTSD.

PERSONALITY DISORDERS

Personality disorders are inflexible, maladaptive patterns of behavior or thinking that accompany significant impairment of functioning. The disorder usually surfaces during adolescence or earlier and continues through adulthood. The associated behaviors are generally more troublesome to other people than to the affected individual (Box 35.3). Personality disorders are characterized by the following:

- Lack of insight; concrete thinking; poor attention; inability to understand the consequences of behavior or learn from them
- Distorted self-perception; either hatred or idealization of self

---

Box 35.3	Personality Disorders

CLUSTER A: ODD OR ECCENTRIC BEHAVIOR
- Schizoid personality disorder
- Paranoid personality disorder
- Schizotypal personality disorder

CLUSTER B: DRAMATIC, EMOTIONAL, OR ERRATIC BEHAVIOR
- Antisocial personality disorder
- Borderline personality disorder
- Narcissistic personality disorder

CLUSTER C: ANXIOUS FEARFUL BEHAVIOR
- Avoidant personality disorder
- Dependent personality disorder
- Obsessive-compulsive personality disorder

Data from Mayo Clinic: Personality disorders, 2016. Retrieved from http://www.mayoclinic.org/diseases-conditions/personality-disorders/symptoms-causes/dxc-20247656.

- Impaired relationships; projecting own feelings onto others; poor impulse control; inability to maintain healthy interpersonal relationships
- Inflexible behavioral response patterns that do not allow the individual to handle change easily

The *DSM-V* (APA, 2013) has classified 10 distinct personality disorders. These disorders can be clustered into groups of similar behavior. Cluster A includes disorders with odd or eccentric behavior. Cluster B includes behaviors that are dramatic, emotional, or erratic. Cluster C disorders include behaviors that are anxious and fearful (see Box 35.3).

SEXUAL DISORDERS

Sex is ranked as a basic need in Maslow's hierarchy of human needs (Maslow, 1970). Human sexuality is the sum of physical and psychological attributes that express a person's gender identity and sexual behavior. Sexual disorders are of either physical or psychological origin, but often physical and psychological factors play a part in the perceived disorder.

Defining normal sexual behavior is difficult against the inescapable backdrop of cultural influences, religious institutions, and societal laws that affect an individual's beliefs regarding acceptable and unacceptable sexual behavior. Sexual behavior may be thought of on a continuum from adaptive sexual behavior to maladaptive sexual behavior. Adaptive sexual behaviors occur in private between two consenting adults, are satisfying, and are not forced on each other. Maladaptive sexual behaviors are harmful to self or others and possibly are performed publicly and sometimes without the consent of all those involved.

Sexual orientation is the preference or choice for a sex partner. *Heterosexual* is the term describing individuals who express their sexuality with members of the opposite sex. *Homosexual* is the term describing individuals who express their sexuality with members of the same sex. The *DSM-V* (APA, 2013) lists sexual and gender identity disorders in three main clusters:

(1) sexual dysfunctions, (2) paraphilias, and (3) gender dysphoria. This list does not address sexual dysfunction caused by medical problems, such as impotence secondary to diabetic neuropathy.

Sexual dysfunction is a disturbance during sexual response. *Dyspareunia* (painful intercourse), hypoactive sexual desire, and premature ejaculation are examples of sexual dysfunction that have a possible psychological component, as well as a physical component. Some medications cause sexual dysfunction by altering sexual desire or the ability to perform. Medications are now available to treat men with erectile dysfunction, if the dysfunction has physical causes.

Paraphilias are a group of sexually gratifying activities that are not common in the general public and are illegal in some countries, including the United States. The suffix *-philia* means "attraction to." Adding a descriptive prefix, such as *pedo-*, rounds out the descriptions of what the sexual attraction is to. Thus *pedophilia* means fondling or pursuing other sexual activities with a prepubescent child by an adult.

Other paraphilic disorders include *exhibitionism* ("flashing"), which means exposing one's genitals to one or more unsuspecting people to achieve sexual arousal; *voyeurism,* which means obtaining sexual gratification by observing others during intercourse or viewing another's genitals; *frotteurism,* which is sexual arousal achieved by rubbing against or touching a nonconsenting individual; and *fetishism,* which is the use of an object, usually an article of clothing, to attain sexual arousal. Masturbation usually accompanies or follows an act of fetishism. *Transvestic fetishism* involves wearing clothing of the opposite sex (cross-dressing) to obtain sexual gratification.

Other paraphilic disorders are sexual sadism and masochism. *Sadism* refers to achieving sexual arousal from inflicting pain or humiliation on another person. Possible manifestations of sexual sadism vary from mild behavior, such as spanking, to more violent behavior, such as stabbing or strangulation. *Sexual masochism* refers to sexual arousal by receiving mental or physical abuse. A diagnosis of sexual masochism is appropriate if a person finds punishment necessary to achieve sexual gratification.

Gender identity is one of the first parts of personality development established. With gender dysphoria, biological sex identity conflicts with gender perception. Many individuals with gender dysphoria truly believe that they were born with the wrong body. *Transsexualism* is a persistent desire to be the opposite sex and to have the body of the opposite sex. Transvestic fetishism is associated with this disorder. For a biological sex change to take place, psychological counseling, hormone treatments, and major surgical procedures must occur over the course of several years. The surgical procedure is not reversible, which is one of the reasons for the lengthy counseling.

Therapeutic interventions depend on the type of disorder. Treatment for most individuals takes place on an outpatient basis. Some psychosexual problems are complex, and treatment requires the skill of specially educated health care providers, nurses, or sex therapists.

Many nurses encounter medical-surgical patients who also have a sexual disorder. Nurses must be aware of their own attitudes and values about sexual behaviors. A nurse's nonverbal messages of disapproval have the capacity to hinder development of a therapeutic relationship and affect the quality of nursing judgment.

SOMATIC SYMPTOM DISORDERS

Physical signs of emotional distress are sometimes very real. Just as eating too much at the Thanksgiving table can cause nausea; so can receiving a very distressing piece of news. The term **somatic** symptom disorder refers to a physical disorder arising as a result of a psychological trigger. This term developed a negative connotation because it acquired the implication that "it's all in your head." The more recent term somatic *illness* addresses the stress-related problems that have the potential to result in physical signs and symptoms. Somatic symptom disorders are thought to have an emotional basis, manifested as a physical illness.

The body responds to continual or repeated stress by overactivating its stress response mechanism; this tends to result in many physical signs and symptoms, such as diarrhea, heart palpitations, backaches, and headaches. The gastrointestinal tract appears to suffer the most from chronic stress.

Physical disorders thought to have psychological underpinnings include ulcerative colitis, irritable bowel syndrome, hypertension, cardiac disease, asthma, arthritis, some skin disorders, irregular menstruation, and migraine headache.

The typical characteristics of somatic symptom disorders are recurrent, multiple, physical complaints and symptoms for which there is no organic cause. It is a process by which an individual's feelings, needs, and conflicts are manifested physiologically. To establish the diagnosis of somatoform disorder, all possible physical causes of dysfunctions, all drug or other toxic substance reactions, and all mental health problems that are possibly related to the symptoms must be eliminated.

EATING DISORDERS

An eating disorder is an illness that disrupts the normal eating pattern. The three most common eating disorders are anorexia nervosa, bulimia nervosa, and binge eating. These are complex psychiatric disorders related to a number of factors, including individual mental and emotional processes, family relationships, cultural values, and genetic predisposition. Eating disorders are serious, potentially life-threatening conditions affecting emotional and physical health. Eating disorders frequently appear during the teen years or young adulthood; however, younger children and older adults also develop these disorders. Statistics show that eating disorders affect mostly girls and women, but increasing numbers of boys, older women, and men are affected (Fig. 35.2). Because of the secretiveness and shame associated with eating disorders, many cases may go unreported. Early detection and treatment of eating disorders increase the likelihood of recovery. Table 35.3 lists the diagnostic criteria used to identify eating disorders.

Recognizing and treating eating disorders early offers some hope of lessening their effects. Table 35.4 lists some danger signs of these disorders. In educating patients about eating disorders, place the greatest focus on prevention and concentrate on good health rather than on thinness. Encourage individuals to respect and value their uniqueness.

Anorexia Nervosa

Anorexia nervosa is an eating disorder characterized by self-imposed starvation. It typically develops in the early to middle stages of adolescence.

Common characteristics in individuals with this disorder include an intense drive for thinness, an intense fear of gaining weight or becoming fat, and a distorted body image such that individuals view themselves as "fat" even when their weight is much less than average for their height. Some affected patients exhibit obsessive-compulsive behaviors toward food, attempting to maintain strict control over intake by counting calories meticulously, practicing unusual food behaviors and rituals, making excuses to avoid eating, and hiding food that they claim to have eaten. Some affected patients enjoy food vicariously by cooking it, serving it, or being around it without eating it. Periods of starvation, compulsive exercising, and purging after meals are among the most common behaviors. Common purging behaviors are self-induced vomiting and the misuse of diuretics, laxatives, emetics, and enemas.

Weight loss and maintenance of weight at or below 85% of goal weight are apparent physical symptoms. Other physical symptoms include cessation of menstruation in women, loss of sexual drive, cold intolerance, the growth of fine hair on the body and the face (lanugo), hypotension, and heart irregularities. Bone density is compromised, which leads in some cases to compression of vertebrae and stress fractures. The gastrointestinal tract is affected, with delayed gastric emptying, slowed peristalsis, and severe constipation. The lining of the digestive tract often deteriorates so that when the patient does eat, he or she experiences malabsorption, flatulence, and diarrhea. This further compounds the negative perception of food. Brain activity is affected, leading to altered thinking patterns, disturbed sleep, and bad dreams. There is also evidence of structural brain abnormalities (tissue loss), some of which may be irreversible. Personality and emotional changes often are pronounced. Depression and apathy are possible.

A multidisciplinary approach to treatment is best and involves nutrition therapy and individual psychological counseling along with family counseling. Nutritional goals include increasing and improving dietary intake to reverse nutrient deficiencies, achieving a healthy weight for height, and reestablishing normal eating patterns.

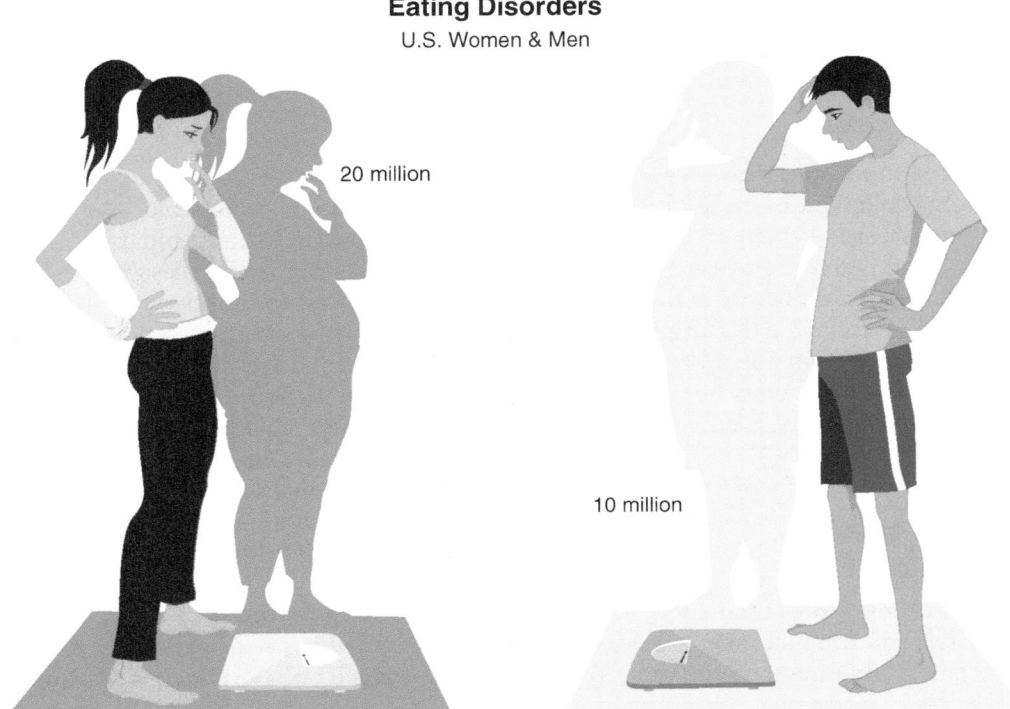

Eating Disorders

U.S. Women & Men

20 million

10 million

Fig. 35.2 Gender comparison of eating disorders in the United States.

Table 35.3 Comparison of Eating Disorder Diagnoses

CHARACTERISTIC	ANOREXIA NERVOSA	BULIMIA NERVOSA	BINGE-EATING DISORDER
Body weight and other physical indicators	Body weight at or below 85% of normal for age, sex, and height Amenorrhea (in women)	Possibly underweight, normal weight, or overweight	Usually obese
Eating behaviors	1. Restricting type: self-imposed starvation or semistarvation 2. Binge-eating or purging type: regular episodes of binge eating (eating an amount of food the patient considers to be excessive)	Recurrent episodes of binge eating: the compulsive eating of an excessive amount of food while feeling a lack of control over eating Binge eating or purging occurs at least twice per week for a period of 3 months or more	Recurrent episodes of binge eating: the compulsive eating of an excessive amount of food while feeling a lack of control over eating Episodes occur at least twice per week for a period of 6 months and are associated with at least three of the following: 1. Eating until uncomfortably full 2. Eating when not physically hungry 3. Eating rapidly 4. Eating alone because of embarrassment 5. Feeling guilt, disgust, or depression after overeating
Compensatory behaviors (purging)	1. Restricting type: may use excessive exercise 2. Binge-eating or purging type: regular episodes of self-induced vomiting or misuse of laxatives, diuretics, or enemas	1. Purging type: regular episodes of self-induced vomiting or the misuse of laxatives, emetics, diuretics, or enemas 2. Nonpurging type: use of fasting or excessive exercise	None
Psychological indicators	Distorted body image: patient perceives self as fat Intense fear of becoming fat Denial of the problem and its seriousness	Feelings of self-worth disproportionately based on body weight, shape, and size Usually awareness that there is a problem	Poor self-esteem, possible depression Awareness that there is a problem

Bulimia Nervosa

Bulimia nervosa is an eating disorder characterized by periods of binge eating followed by purging or other inappropriate compensatory behavior to prevent weight gain. Binge eating is the compulsive eating of an amount of food considered excessive in normal circumstances. Binge eating is followed by purging—self-induced vomiting and the misuse of diuretics, laxatives, emetics, and enemas—or by other compensatory behaviors such as severe caloric restriction, excessive exercising, or the use of diet pills.

People with bulimia are usually within a normal weight range and are aware that their eating patterns are abnormal. However, bulimic people may express a lack of control over the eating. They often experience fear of not being able to stop eating and experience depression, guilt, and remorse after a binge. In addition, bulimia tends to occur in combination with other psychiatric disorders such as depression, obsessive-compulsive disorder, substance abuse, and self-injurious

behavior. Clinical symptoms of bulimia include possible tooth erosion, calloused knuckles, swollen parotid (salivary) glands, broken blood vessels in the eyes or face, stomach lacerations, and esophageal and sinus infections resulting from excessive vomiting. Electrolyte imbalances lead to muscle weakness and cramps, abnormal heart rhythms, cardiac complications, and, occasionally, sudden death. Proper treatment for bulimia, like that for anorexia nervosa, is multidisciplinary. Psychological counseling and therapy are necessary. Nutritional goals include improving dietary intake to correct nutritional deficiencies and electrolyte imbalances, and cessation of binge-purge behavior with reestablishment of normal eating patterns.

Binge-Eating Disorder

Binge-eating disorder is a disorder sometimes referred to as compulsive overeating. Some authorities believe that this is the most common eating disorder, affecting millions of Americans. Binge-eating disorder is

Table 35.4	Signs and Symptom of Eating Disorders
CATEGORY	**SIGNS OR SYMPTOMS**

Emotional	1. Change in attitude or performance
	2. Inability to concentrate
	3. Body image complaints or concerns:
	  • Refers to self as fat, gross, ugly; overestimates body size; believes he or she is fat when of normal weight or thin
	  • Unable to accept compliments
	  • Constantly compares self to others; self-disparaging comments
	  • Mood affected by thoughts about appearance; seeks outside reassurance about looks
	4. Appears sad, depressed, anxious; expresses feelings of worthlessness
	5. Obsessed with maintaining low weight to enhance performance in sports, dance, acting, modeling, and the like

Physical	1. Sudden weight loss, gain, or fluctuation in a short time 2. Abdominal pain; feeling full or "bloated"; bouts of constipation or diarrhea 3. Feeling fatigue or faint, "weak," or "dizzy" 4. Dry hair or skin, dehydration, poor circulation in hands and feet 5. Cold intolerance 6. Lanugo hair (fine hair on body and face) 7. Edematous glands in the neck or beneath the jaw 8. Erosion of tooth enamel, cavities, tooth pain, changes in tooth appearance 9. Amenorrhea in women of childbearing age 10. Insomnia

Behavioral	1. Caloric restriction and preoccupation with dieting
	2. Chaotic food intake; skipping meals; exhibiting peculiar eating rituals
	3. Extreme preoccupation with food; constantly talking about food
	4. Secretive eating; binge eating
	5. Carrying own food; eating small amounts or nothing in front of others
	6. Wearing baggy clothes:
	  • To hide a very thin body
	  • To hide weight gain
	  • To hide a normal-sized body because of distorted body image
	7. Spending increasing amounts of time alone; withdrawal from family and friends
	8. Displaying compulsive or obsessive behaviors
	9. Spending frequent and increasing amounts of time in the bathroom
	10. Abusing laxatives, diuretics, enemas, or diet pills
	11. Excessive amounts of exercise

Modified from National Eating Disorders Association: Educator toolkit, n.d. Retrieved from www.nationaleatingdisorders.org/sites/default/files/Toolkits/EducatorToolkit.pdf.

characterized by frequent, recurrent episodes of binge eating; that is, eating a larger amount of food than normal during a short period of time. People with a binge-eating disorder often report a feeling of lack of control over eating during the binge episode. Unlike bulimia nervosa, binge-eating disorder is not associated with purging or inappropriate compensatory behavior.

Many people with binge-eating disorder are obese. Encourage them to consider treatment that focuses on their binge-eating behavior before they attempt to lose weight. Treatment typically includes some combination of cognitive-behavioral therapy, interpersonal psychotherapy, antidepressants, and self-help groups.

TREATMENT METHODS

COMMUNICATION AND THE THERAPEUTIC RELATIONSHIP

Therapeutic communication is an important technique that practitioners use in treatment of psychiatric disorders. Psychiatric nursing is a science and an art. Each

individual has unique value and potential for growth. Applying your own self-concept in the context of a therapeutic relationship requires self-knowledge.

The key component in psychiatric–mental health treatment is the development of a helping-trust relationship. The relationship maximizes the patient's strengths, maintains self-esteem, and assists the patient in developing and using coping skills. The helping-trust relationship is a therapeutic professional relationship; it is not social. In a therapeutic relationship, the nurse assists the patient in learning new ways of responding to people and situations.

Therapeutic communication is a dynamic process in which both participants (the nurse and the patient) share meaning and interact in the interests of problem solving and growth. To be therapeutic, communication must assist with the corrective experiences that help the patient in meeting predetermined goals. Therapeutic techniques for communication are described in Chapter 4. These techniques can be used in every nursing situation. The therapeutic dialogues in the Communication box demonstrate therapeutic nurse-patient interactions.

There are different types of relationships. Most are social; that is, the participants are involved equally in exchanging information and meeting individual needs. In a therapeutic relationship, both participants agree on goals and work toward them. The nurse assists the patient to learn new ways of interacting to function more effectively. The nurse attempts to establish rapport with the patient and obtain trust to facilitate positive interactions that will lead to corrective behavior. In day-to-day interactions with a patient, the patient is more responsive and amenable to instruction if the nurse has obtained the patient's trust and the patient sees the nurse as a competent professional.

Psychotherapy

In treating psychiatric problems, health care providers often use one or more of the following psychological techniques. *Behavior therapy* relieves anxiety through the conditioning and retraining of behavioral responses by repetition. It is often possible to resolve phobias with this technique. *Cognitive therapy* focuses on breaking negative thought patterns and developing positive feelings about memories or thoughts. These therapy types are interrelated and build upon each other. As individuals become aware of the negative actions and embrace the positive feelings, they are able to begin the process of demonstrating therapeutic behaviors (Fig. 35.3). *Group therapy* is often a useful modality in a hospital setting or day treatment

---

 Communication

Starting the Conversation

Possibilities for starting a conversation with a patient include several approaches:
- "What circumstances brought you to the hospital?"
- "Tell me a little about what has been going on with you."
- "Ms. J., I am Linda, and I'll be your nurse today."
- "Tell me how you are feeling."

THERAPEUTIC DIALOGUE 1

Ms. J. underwent a hysterectomy 1 week ago for several fibroid tumors. She is 32 years of age and has a 3-year-old child. She has been married 5 years. The nurse who admitted her after surgery enters the room and finds her crying.
Nurse: (Walks over to Ms. J., touches her arm, and stands there quietly.)
Patient: (Continues to cry but looks up at the nurse and starts to quiet.)
Nurse: You look upset; please tell me what's upsetting you. (Pulls up a chair and sits at eye level.)
Patient: My whole life is ruined.
Nurse: Your life is ruined?
Patient: I wanted other children; we were going to have a large family.
Nurse: Tell me what a large family means to you.

Many patients experiencing loss need to cry. Crying begins to release emotion; the patient needs the nurse to accept it. The nurse's close physical presence and touch communicate acceptance. Acknowledgment of feelings encourages further expression, and then it is possible to explore the patient's sense of loss.

THERAPEUTIC DIALOGUE 2

Mr. H., 65 years of age, has received a diagnosis of cancer of the lung. The day nurse is making initial patient rounds and enters the room. The nurse notices that Mr. H. looks uncomfortable.
Nurse: (Walks over to the bed.) Good morning, Mr. H. You look uncomfortable.
Patient: I'm tired; I stayed awake all night.
Nurse: You had difficulty sleeping?
Patient: I have a lot on my mind. I couldn't sleep.
Nurse: (Sits down next to the patient and pats his hand.) Tell me what has been worrying you.

Encourage patients to talk (ventilate). Be observant for nonverbal communication and for underlying meanings in the stated words. Talking reveals emotions, at which point it is possible to identify and deal with them.

You and the patient bring your physiologic, psychological, developmental, and spiritual components into the therapeutic relationship. Other elements that you bring into the relationship are previous life experiences, needs, aspirations, and frustrations. You have an opportunity to help the patient explore a life event and the meaning that it has for the patient.

THERAPEUTIC DIALOGUE 3

Ms. K., who has been pacing the halls, is now staring out the window. She is toying with a ring on her finger. You notice that Ms. K. is vigorously tapping one foot on the floor.
Nurse: (Walks over to patient and sits beside her.) Ms. K., I have noticed that you seem a little restless. Is something troubling you?
Patient: No, not really. Well, maybe I am a little upset.
Nurse: Is there something in particular that is upsetting you?
Patient: I don't know. I'm just anxious.
Nurse: Tell me how you feel.
Patient: I feel jittery and nervous.
Nurse: Is there something specific that is worrying you right now?
Patient: My husband is going to lose his job in another month, and here I am in the hospital. I just don't know how we'll pay the bills. It scares me.
Nurse: Have you and your husband discussed this situation?
Patient: (Continues to share her feelings with the nurse.)

Anxiety is an unpleasant feeling of tension and apprehension. A person experiencing anxiety is sometimes unaware of the exact source of the tension. An array of physical and psychological symptoms usually accompanies anxiety. Resolution of the anxiety begins with awareness of the anxiety's source. A person seeks ways to resolve the tension (problem solving) to be rid of the tension.

Fig. 35.3 Cognitive behavioral therapies. (Copyright © vaeenma/iStock/Thinkstock.)

programs. A group of patients with similar problems obtain insight through discussion and role playing. *Play therapy* often helps children express themselves by using toys such as puppets as their "spokesperson" of feelings.

Hypnosis helps a patient recover deeply repressed emotions and speed recovery. It also helps a patient change habits such as smoking.

Psychoanalysis was developed by Sigmund Freud. It is a long-term and intense form of therapy that enables the patient to bring unconscious thoughts to the surface. *Free association* (speaking thoughts without censorship) and dream interpretation are among the tools in psychoanalysis.

Adjunctive therapies include occupational therapy, recreational therapy, music therapy, magnetic therapy, art therapy, and hydrotherapy. These types of therapy allow expression of feelings, help increase self-esteem, and promote positive interaction and reality orientation. Such forms of adjunctive therapy can be used in a group setting or individually.

Limits of Confidentiality

Confidentiality is sometimes a dilemma when therapeutic effectiveness of care depends on the patient's willingness to talk about feelings and thoughts. It is important that the patient knows that each member of the health care team will share any information he or she receives with the others. No one member of the team keeps any secrets from the others. This practice also curtails patients' manipulating the staff or pitting one staff member or patient against another.

Just as the nurse has a duty to report child abuse, the nurse also has a duty to warn. Sometimes a patient expresses intent to kill someone when he or she is released, and the nurse is obligated to notify the appropriate authorities. Families of victims have filed—and won—lawsuits against health care workers for not warning the victim.

ELECTROCONVULSIVE THERAPY

In the late 1930s, two Italian physicians, Ugo Cerletti and Lucio Bini, introduced electroconvulsive therapy (ECT) to treat psychiatric disorders. Over the years, ECT has been refined. Muscle relaxants and anesthesia are now part of the therapy; these reduce the incidence of fracture, contusion, and sprains from the induced seizure.

ECT is a treatment for depression, mania, or schizoaffective disorders that do not respond to other treatment modalities. The course of ECT usually consists of approximately 10 treatments over several weeks. Only a very small amount of electrical current is required to trigger a tonic-clonic (grand mal) seizure; thus there is no risk of electrocution. Temporary memory loss after treatment is expected and lasts from a few hours up to a few days. Confusion right after a treatment usually dissipates in a few hours.

ECT usually is provided on an outpatient basis. There is a potential danger with the treatment, and it necessitates a great deal of care. When administered properly, for the right illness, ECT can help as much as or more than any other treatment.

Before a patient receives ECT, it is necessary to perform several tests. A thorough physical examination (which includes a blood chemistry survey, complete blood count, and urinalysis) detects any unsuspected conditions.

The practitioner completes a thorough mental examination. Electroencephalography is performed to rule out any existing electrical abnormalities. Chest and lumbosacral spine radiography rule out any skeletal abnormalities. Electrocardiography is also necessary because the treatment can put a strain on the heart.

In preparing the patient for ECT, treat the patient as a surgical candidate. In collecting data, make sure that all tests have been completed and that the health care provider has received the reports. Measure vital signs, height, and weight. If the patient has a knowledge deficit about the procedure, answer all of the patient's questions before the patient can sign a consent form. Describing the steps of the day, the room where the treatment is given, and where recovery takes place helps reduce anxiety.

Ensure that the patient is on nothing-by-mouth (NPO) status for at least 8 hours before the treatment. Just before the treatment, the patient is instructed to void. The patient must remove all watches, jewelry, glasses or contact lenses, dentures, and hairpins. If the patient is an outpatient, it is acceptable to wear loose clothing such as a sweat suit or a hospital gown.

Administer ordered pre-ECT medications, usually including a sedative. An intravenous line is established for the anesthesiologist to use during the treatment.

Post-ECT care is similar to that for any postsurgical patient in the recovery room. Once the patient is fully awake and his or her gag reflex is present, the patient should be given a light meal or snack with acetaminophen. Assisting with mobility after the patient regains consciousness is sometimes also part of the care. Sometimes the patient is confused afterward and needs supervision and reassurance. Make sure family members understand the need to attend to the patient constantly because of the temporary confusion. Do not allow the patient to drive until the confusion is gone.

Continual reassurance, support, and attentiveness before and after each treatment help the patient deal with anxiety about ECT (see Box 35.2).

PSYCHOPHARMACOLOGY

Psychotropic (psychoactive) medications in conjunction with other therapies help modify a patient's behavior. Medication helps control symptoms. Monitoring for signs of effectiveness and evidence of side effects is a very important nursing responsibility. Understanding the medications used is clearly part of the nurse's role (Table 35.5).

Antidepressants

There are many antidepressant medications. In the newest class are the SSRIs and SNRIs, which include fluoxetine (Prozac), sertraline (Zoloft), venlafaxine (Effexor XR), citalopram (Celexa), and paroxetine (Paxil). As mentioned earlier, clinicians and patients tend to prefer these drugs over the other classes because they have fewer side effects. Other classes of antidepressants are tricyclic agents; monoamine oxidase inhibitors (MAOIs); and triazolopyridines, which are similar to tricyclic agents and include trazodone (Desyrel). Bupropion (Wellbutrin) is of the aminoketone subclass of MAOIs.

These medications work in different ways in the brain to alleviate signs and symptoms of depression, such as decreased appetite or sleep pattern disturbances, prolonged sadness, and lack of concentration. None of them take effect immediately; they generally take 2 to 4 weeks to effect any improvement. Patients often describe the change that drug therapy accomplishes in depression as a "fog lifting." Antidepressant therapy must be maintained for several months to a year to prevent symptom recurrence.

Serotonin syndrome. Serotonin syndrome is a potentially life-threatening condition that occurs usually as a result of an interaction between an SSRI and another serotonergic agent. It also can occur in older adult patients taking only an SSRI. Symptoms include altered mental status, autonomic dysfunction, and neuromuscular abnormalities.

Confusion, delirium, agitation, and mutism are some of the altered mental states that practitioners sometimes fail to recognize as side effects in chronically ill older adults living in long-term care facilities, a population in which the rate of depression is sometimes as high as 50%. Autonomic dysfunction can include blood pressure fluctuation, tachycardia,

hyperthermia, marked pupil dilation (mydriasis), shivering, and diaphoresis. Possible neuromuscular symptoms include some that are similar to those produced by antipsychotic medications (see the later, more detailed, discussion of extrapyramidal symptoms): akathisia (a jittery feeling inside that causes restlessness), ataxia (incoordination), dystonia, dyskinesia, hyperreflexia, tremors, and seizures. Older adult patients are more likely to display neuromuscular side effects, which raises their risk of injury from falls. Serotonin syndrome worsens Parkinson disease. Laboratory values indicative of serotonin syndrome include an elevated level of creatine phosphokinase as a result of muscle disintegration, elevated levels of white blood cells and transaminases, and a decreased level of serum bicarbonate.

Treatment for serotonin syndrome is to decrease the dosage of the drug slowly. Sudden discontinuation has potential to cause dizziness, nausea, vomiting, muscle pain, headaches, fatigue, anxiety, crying spells, and irritability. Instruct the patient about calling for assistance in ambulating until side effects have subsided. In the home setting especially, it is a good idea for the home health care nurse to encourage the patient to take an active role in managing medications by reporting even minor side effects or concerns. Review any over-the-counter medication that the patient takes. Emphasize the importance of informing the nurse and the prescribing health care provider when the patient uses an over-the-counter medication.

When assessing the patient for efficacy of antidepressants, be familiar with the actions of each drug, possible drug interactions, and serious side effects.

Antimanic Agents

Lithium carbonate is the primary drug that health care providers use to stabilize the mood and behavior of a patient with mania. A therapeutic blood level is required and sometimes takes 7 to 10 days to achieve. During the interim, practitioners frequently prescribe antipsychotic medications to control behavior. Toxicity is a problem with lithium usage. Poor fluid intake and salt restriction in the diet increase the risk of toxicity. Be aware of the signs of toxicity: nausea, vomiting, diarrhea, drowsiness, muscle weakness, and ataxia. If the patient does not stop taking the drug, toxicity potentially leads to seizures and death. Stopping the medication abruptly can also cause increased anxiety, nausea, and significant mood changes. Patient education is an important factor in lithium administration. The therapeutic level of lithium is fairly narrow—0.4 to 1.3 mEq/L—and each patient must be evaluated individually and carefully monitored. The blood lithium level must be checked frequently to determine whether the therapeutic level has been obtained. Initially, daily level measurements may be ordered. Once a therapeutic level has been obtained, monthly measurements of the level typically are ordered.

Table 35.5   **Medications for Psychiatric-Mental Health Disorders**

GENERIC NAME	SIDE EFFECTS AND PRECAUTIONS	NURSING IMPLICATIONS
Antimanic Agents		
lithium carbonate divalproex sodium carbamazepine	Aplastic anemia, agranulocytosis, kidney damage from long-term lithium use Lithium toxicity: Serum levels >1.5 mcg/L Symptoms: Indigestion, rashes, drowsiness, nausea, vomiting, abdominal cramps, polyuria, polydipsia, ataxia, tremor, slurred speech, disorientation, and seizures	Teach patient signs and symptoms of toxicity and to maintain high fluid intake and stable salt use. Periodic blood tests to assess drug level are necessary. Risk for injury is high if patient is drowsy or ataxic. Teach patient to avoid alcohol use. Instruct patient to take medication with food if medication causes indigestion.
Antipsychotic Agents		
chlorpromazine thioridazine HCl trifluoperazine HCl fluphenazine HCl perphenazine thiothixene haloperidol	Anticholinergic effects: Dry mouth, blurred vision, constipation, urinary retention, postural hypotension Extrapyramidal side effects (EPS): Akathisia (severe restlessness—inability to stand still, foot tapping) Parkinsonian effects: Rigidity, resting tremor, shuffling gait Dystonias: Bizarre movements of the face and neck, torticollis, oculogyric crisis Other side effects: Lowered seizure threshold, tardive dyskinesia (involuntary movements of lips, tongue, jaw after medications are stopped or decreased) Rare: Neuroleptic malignant syndrome (hyperthermia, muscle rigidity, labile BP, confusion, cardiovascular collapse)	Suggest sugarless candy or gum for dry mouth. Teach patient that it is important to take the medication on time and not to stop taking the medication abruptly. Instruct patient to wear sunscreen. Establish baseline vital sign measurements and blood cell counts. May need to increase salt intake during hot weather. Explain need to rise slowly from sitting to standing. Watch for developing ataxia, clumsiness, or nervousness when dose increased. Watch for EPS, and use anticholinergic medications as ordered prn (benztropine [Cogentin], diphenhydramine [Benadryl]). Monitor for neuroleptic malignant syndrome.
Atypical Antipsychotic Agents		
Used in treating resistant forms of schizophrenia; usually more expensive but also less occurrence of adverse effects		
clozapine	Low risk of EPS and tardive dyskinesia; 1%–2% incidence of agranulocytosis; weekly serum monitoring necessary	Suggest sugarless candy or gum for dry mouth. Explain need to rise slowly from sitting to standing.
olanzapine	Significant improvement of negative behaviors; most common effects are dry mouth, dyspepsia, drowsiness, postural hypotension; no association with agranulocytosis	
risperidone	Low rate of EPS, and no association with agranulocytosis	
Antianxiety Agents		
alprazolam buspirone chlordiazepoxide HCl clorazepate dipotassium lorazepam oxazepam	Drowsiness, ataxia, muscle weakness, occasionally disinhibition, "morning hangover," transient hypotension Potentially habit forming, aggravates depression or psychosis	Monitor for increased side effects in older adults. Teach patient not to operate machines or drive if drowsiness is occurring. Teach patient to avoid alcohol use. Instruct patient not to stop taking medications abruptly. Explain need to rise slowly from sitting to standing.
Antidepressants		
Tricyclic Agents		
amitriptyline amoxapine desipramine HCl imipramine HCl nortriptyline HCl	Anticholinergic effects (see Antipsychotic Agents) Should not be administered to patients with severe liver disease or after myocardial infarction; should be administered with caution to patients with cardiac disease Sudden stoppage of medication sometimes causes sleep disturbance	Monitor BP for hypotension. Suggest sugarless candy or gum for dry mouth. Explain that appetite sometimes increases. Caution against strenuous exercise or high temperature because of reduced diaphoresis.

Continued

Table 35.5 Medications for Psychiatric-Mental Health Disorders—cont'd

GENERIC NAME	SIDE EFFECTS AND PRECAUTIONS	NURSING IMPLICATIONS
Monoamine Oxidase Inhibitors (MAOIs)		
phenelzine sulfate tranylcypromine sulfate	Orthostatic hypotension, headache, abnormal heart rate and rhythm, blurred vision, dry mouth, fatigue, nausea, vomiting, constipation, urinary hesitancy and retention Hypertensive crisis may result from eating foods containing tyramine (red wine, beer, aged cheese, chocolate, licorice, yogurt, caffeine-rich foods, liver, and broad beans)	Monitor BP; explain need to rise slowly from sitting to standing. Teach patient that tyramine-rich foods pose risk of life-threatening effects and their intake must be restricted. Teach patient to consult health care provider before taking over-the-counter cough or cold medicines. Teach patient drug interactions; consult resource when health care provider prescribes additional medications. Monitor intake and output.
Selective Serotonin Reuptake Inhibitors (SSRIs)		
fluoxetine fluvoxamine paroxetine HCl sertraline	Anticholinergic effects (see Antipsychotic Agents), appetite loss, transient fatigue, weight loss, diarrhea or constipation, diaphoresis, anxiety, tremors, insomnia, tachycardia, sexual dysfunction	Because of insomnia, take medication in the morning and early afternoon. Avoid alcohol use. Call health care provider before taking other medications. Use cautiously in patients with renal or hepatic impairment. Monitor for symptoms of serotonin syndrome.
Other Antidepressants		
venlafaxine maprotiline nefazodone bupropion trazodone mirtazapine	Same as for SSRIs	Same as for SSRIs. Instruct patient to take bupropion in three divided doses to minimize seizure risk. Suggest taking trazodone with food to decrease vertigo. Instruct patient not to take mirtazapine within 14 days of MAOI use: It has potential to cause hypertension, seizures, and death. Assess complete blood cell count and liver function periodically.

Antipsychotic Agents

Antipsychotic medications or major tranquilizers are used for acute and chronic management of (1) schizophrenia, (2) organic mental disorders with psychosis, and (3) the manic phase of bipolar mood disorder. These drugs provide symptom control but are not a cure. Responses to these drugs are highly individualized. It is best to use the lowest effective dose.

A number of dose-related side effects occur in association with antipsychotic agents. Postural hypotension and sedation are common when patients first start taking these drugs. Consider implementing safety measures to prevent falls. Photosensitivity is another side effect; patients should wear sunscreen, hats, special clothing, and sunglasses to prevent sunburn. Autonomic reactions include urinary retention, dry mouth, constipation, edema, and weight gain. Increasing fluid intake not only relieves dry mouth but also actually triggers the body to release excess fluid from the tissues.

Various abnormal neuromuscular symptoms occur in association with these drugs. The extrapyramidal symptoms include pseudoparkinsonism (e.g., tremor with rigid posture); *akathisia,* or an inability to sit still, with continuous hand, mouth, or body movements (e.g., foot tapping); *dystonias,* or aberrant posturing (e.g., hand spasms); and *dyskinesia,* or involuntary movements (e.g., lip smacking or tongue protruding). *Tardive dyskinesia* is an extrapyramidal reaction that occurs in long-term use of neuroleptic agents and it is sometimes a permanent effect. Immediate action is necessary to combat extrapyramidal effects. Options to consider include stopping the drug or reducing the dosage, administering parenteral diphenhydramine, and follow-up use of antiparkinsonian drugs such as trihexyphenidyl or benztropine.

Antianxiety Agents

Antianxiety drugs (anxiolytics) or minor tranquilizers often help individuals experiencing moderate to severe anxiety. Practitioners prescribe benzodiazepine sedatives such as lorazepam (Ativan) to relieve the tension without sacrificing motivation. Abuse of drugs in this category is common.

Ongoing maintenance for severe persistent (chronic) mental illness is often very challenging for the patient and the family. Rehospitalization, when it occurs, reminds them that a cure for the disorder is not available and that close monitoring is still necessary, even when the patient is relatively free of symptoms. The special needs of long-term mentally ill individuals must be addressed by community mental health care and support, partial hospital programs, and assisted living environments.

ALTERNATIVE THERAPIES

Use of natural or herbal medications has become tremendously popular (see Chapter 20). However, their use has been integrated very little into the current system, which is based on prescription and over-the-counter drugs. The control and manufacture of these medications does not fall under the laws of the US Food and Drug Administration; as a result, the quality and the potency vary from manufacturer to manufacturer. Claims and clinical study results are not always consistent. Nonetheless, millions of people use herbal medicine on the basis of only advertising claims. When obtaining a drug history from the patient, inquire about the use of herbs.

St. John's wort (*Hypericum perforatum*) is one of the most common weeds in the world, and studies have shown its possible effectiveness in treating mild depression with few side effects when the patient takes therapeutic doses. St. John's wort potentially interacts with MAOIs and has the capacity to trigger hypertension if taken with allergy medication that contains monoamines or phenylalanine or with amino acid supplements containing tyrosine.

Kava (*Piper methysticum*) is an herb taken by some people to treat anxiety and insomnia because of its sedative effects. Scaly rash on the backs of the hands and forearms and on the soles of the feet is a common side effect. Alcohol potentiates the sedative effect, and if kava is taken with benzodiazepines, it produces toxicity and induces coma. Other side effects are neuromuscular abnormalities similar to the side effects of antipsychotics. Another herb useful in treating anxiety is gotu kola (*Centella asiatica*), an herb that practitioners of ayurvedic medicine prescribe. The effectiveness of gotu kola is comparable to that of diazepam in reducing anxiety.

Ginkgo (*Ginkgo biloba*) and ginseng (various *Panax* spp.) are also popular herbs that some people believe improve memory and boost energy. Ginkgo provides moderate memory and cognitive improvement in treatment of early Alzheimer disease by promoting cerebral blood flow, but it sometimes potentiates the action of anticoagulant drugs such as aspirin and warfarin (Coumadin), which poses the risk of fatal hemorrhage. Ginkgo has the capacity to affect insulin secretion, and ginseng sometimes lowers blood glucose in diabetic patients.

Many foods and beverages now contain herbs. Instruct the patient to read labels and avoid drug interactions with herbal additives. Encourage the patient to seek information about herbs from the pharmacist or health care provider before any herbs are used.

Aromatherapy has gained a foothold in the American way of life; however, its effects are limited. Its use is generally to enhance or potentiate another remedy. It is used in the forms of scented oils for massage, volatile oils to sniff or inhale, and scented candles or incense. Users believe that certain odors trigger chemical activity in the brain to relieve imbalance in the body.

Citrus essences, peppermint, cedarwood, rosemary, sandalwood, chamomile, and lavender are a few essential oils that many people believe help relieve stress and anxiety. It is possible to use such oils in a variety of ways—for example, chamomile tea, a sandalwood candle, or a hot bath with lavender oil. Aromatherapy focuses on the atmosphere of the moment and uses the body's senses to try to achieve mental balance. It has a definite place in holistic care.

APPLICATION OF THE NURSING PROCESS

In the psychiatric setting, as in every setting, the nurse uses the nursing process to meet the many needs of the patient, including assessment, formulation of patient problem statements, planning, intervention, and evaluation. The licensed practical nurse/licensed vocational nurse (LPN/LVN) participates in the nursing process as a member of the mental health care team that includes nurses, therapists, and health care providers. The LPN/LVN's observations of patient behavior and therapeutic communications with the patient assist the registered nurse (RN) in collecting data to form nursing diagnoses. The LPN/LVN's contributions in developing patient problem statements with the RN ensure appropriate interventions for the patient. The LPN/LVN and the RN work together to implement the plan of care for a therapeutic nurse-patient relationship.

Health promotion interventions are focused on preventing relapse and managing symptoms by practicing a healthy lifestyle. Patient teaching is most successful when it is simple, concrete, and clear. Patients need to realize that it is possible to manage their behaviors by recognizing when these behaviors are becoming problematic and by talking with their health care provider, therapist, or both.

Evaluation of the patient will be ongoing. At intervals or when the patient's response dictates, update the care plan. Examination of the documentation and personal observations are considerations when the plan of care is evaluated.

Clearly document all phases of the nursing process. Most of the documentation methods the nurse uses are ongoing and include the assessment criteria that the health care team uses. Ensure notes are accurate and descriptive. Terms such as "appears depressed" should be avoided; instead, specify behaviors, such as "no eye contact noted during conversation." Documentation of the patient's actual conversation is very valuable.

Working with patients who have a mental disorder is always a challenge. Honesty with a caring attitude goes a long way in helping such a patient deal effectively with his or her problem.

Get Ready for the NCLEX® Examination!

Key Points

- The nurse uses the nursing process in the psychiatric context; it includes assessment, formulation of patient problem statements, planning, intervention, and evaluation. The care plan documents this process.
- To help prevent suicide, it is necessary to recognize its warning signs and learn the kinds of actions that are possible to avert it.
- Therapeutic communication is a dynamic method of interacting with patients for problem solving and growth.
- In psychiatry, medications assist patients in dealing with feelings and behaviors.
- The nurse and the health care team observe and evaluate behavior to determine a patient's progress and the effectiveness of the care plan.

Additional Learning Resources

SG Go to your Study Guide for additional learning activities to help you master this chapter content.

Be sure to visit the Evolve site at http://evolve.elsevier.com/Cooper/foundations/ for additional online resources.

Review Questions for the NCLEX® Examination

1. An 82-year-old man was admitted to the long-term care facility with moderate to severe heart failure and is unable to take care of himself at home. After dinner, the patient becomes agitated and confused. There are no significant changes in vital signs, and he has received the same medications he had been taking at home. What cause of acute confusion should the nurse consider?

   1. Alzheimer disease
   2. Sundowning syndrome
   3. Electrolyte imbalance
   4. Acute renal failure

2. A patient with Alzheimer disease continually wanders. Which snack will best meet the patient's nutritional needs? *(Select all that apply.)*

   1. Candy bars and ice cream sundaes
   2. Eggnog milk shakes and oatmeal-raisin cookies
   3. Protein bars and juice
   4. Root beer and potato chips
   5. Cheese and crackers and milk

3. The psychiatrist makes a diagnosis with the use of which system guide?

   1. The Physicians' Desk Reference
   2. The Diagnostic and Statistical Manual, Fifth Edition
   3. The hospital formulary
   4. Freud's The Ego and the Id

4. A delusional patient becomes agitated while watching television and states, "If I don't buy Crest toothpaste right now, I will have cavities." What is the nurse's best response?

   1. "The advertisement on the TV is saying its product will reduce tooth decay if you use their product regularly."
   2. "If you feel that it is absolutely necessary, we can go to the store now and purchase Crest toothpaste."
   3. "You can't believe everything you hear or see on TV."
   4. "Any toothpaste can be used to help prevent cavities; not just Crest toothpaste."

5. The nurse is assessing a patient with a diagnosis of schizophrenia for negative, or absent, behavior patterns. For which symptoms would the nurse assess? *(Select all that apply.)*

   1. Delusions
   2. Social withdrawal
   3. Hallucinations
   4. Disordered thinking
   5. Apathy

6. The nurse is assessing a patient admitted with depression. Which symptoms would the nurse expect the patient to exhibit? *(Select all that apply.)*

   1. Extreme fatigue
   2. Restlessness
   3. Flight of ideas
   4. Hallucinations
   5. Low self-esteem

7. What is the therapy of choice for bipolar, or manic-depressive, disorder?

   1. Chlorpromazine
   2. Lithium carbonate
   3. Electroconvulsive therapy
   4. Fluoxetine

8. A patient admitted to the emergency department is complaining of a panic attack. What manifestations are consistent with an anxiety attack? *(Select all that apply.)*

   1. Hypotension and bradycardia
   2. Lethargy and thready pulse
   3. Hyperventilation and tachycardia
   4. Hallucinations and apathy
   5. Inability to solve problems or think clearly

9. A 47-year-old patient is in the hospital for severe depression. She is unkempt and has lost 15 pounds in the past 2 months. Her family states that she always keeps a knife in her purse. The nurse will consider which intervention for this patient?

   1. Suicide precautions to prevent self-injury
   2. Occupational therapy to build self-esteem
   3. Art psychotherapy to help her express feelings
   4. Large-portioned meals to improve nutritional status

10. Antipsychotic medications have a number of side effects that discourage compliance by the patient. Which effect has the potential to lead to a serious permanent problem?

   1. Photosensitivity
   2. Postural hypotension
   3. Chronic constipation
   4. Tardive dyskinesia

11. A patient says the anchorwoman on the television news talks to him and told him that there was a car bombing in Israel today. What is the nurse's best response?

   1. "I don't think you understand how television projection works."
   2. "She is reporting the world news to everyone in the room. It only appears she is looking at you but she is looking in a TV camera that sends a picture to the TV."
   3. "If you look in the back of the TV console, you will see there is no person inside."
   4. "You are delusional. That is only a projected image of a person reading the news to a camera far away."

12. A 24-year-old woman was admitted for medication adjustment for bipolar disorder. The patient has not slept for 2 days and is unable to sit for more than a few minutes at a time. She has lost 11 pounds in the past week. Which factor will facilitate the best nutrition for the patient while she is in her manic phase?

   1. Have her take her meals in her room to reduce distracting stimuli.
   2. Have the kitchen double her meal portions, because she eats only half of the food served.
   3. Allow the patient to snack on candy bars between meals to gain back her lost weight.
   4. Keep sandwiches, granola bars, fruit, and noncaffeinated beverages available at the desk.

13. A patient who was sexually abused as a child recently married but finds sexual intercourse painful. She confides in her friend, who is a nurse. What is the appropriate response from her friend?

   1. "You should see your gynecologist right away in case you have torn tissues."
   2. "It is normal to have pain at first, but you will adjust to your husband over time."
   3. "You should seek counseling and make sure to get a good physical examination."
   4. "Did you report this abuse to the police?"

14. A patient is a broker on Wall Street who smokes half a pack of cigarettes a day. He avoids caffeine because he has trouble sleeping. He also often complains of an aching lower back. His physician was not able to find anything wrong physically. What is a possible cause of his back pain?

   1. Congenital anomaly
   2. Psychophysiologic origins
   3. Possible renal calculi forming
   4. Dependent personality disorder

15. A 17-year-old patient is worried about her weight. When she is out with friends, she eats junk food until she vomits and then exercises the next day for 4 hours. If she does not have a daily bowel movement, she takes a laxative. Her dentist has noticed her front teeth have signs of erosion. Her family has noticed her hair falling out, and now they have decided to take her to the family health care provider. What diagnosis do these symptoms support?

   1. Anorexia nervosa
   2. Laxative addiction
   3. Bulimia nervosa
   4. Gastroenteritis

16. A 37-year-old patient is not responding to drug therapy for depression. The health care provider has recommended ECT treatments for 1 week as an outpatient. The nurse will stress which point in the pretreatment teaching? *(Select all that apply.)*

   1. "You will need someone to take you to and from the clinic."
   2. "You may take acetaminophen after the treatment if you experience a headache."
   3. "Eat a good breakfast because you will sleep through lunch."
   4. "Scrub your forearms before coming to the clinic."
   5. "Take a laxative the night before so that you won't have an accident during the treatment."

17. The nurse is aware of the phases of schizophrenia. Arrange the following symptoms in the correct order according to the phases of schizophrenia.

   1. Odd or eccentric behavior
   2. Loss of contact with reality
   3. Lack of energy and motivation
   4. Some relief of symptoms

18. A 17-year-old boy tells his mother he is writing a paper for class on all the rock stars who have killed themselves. In the past few months, he has let his hair grow long, bathes only once a week, and stays in his room when he is at home. He is tired and irritable. His mother asks a friend who is a nurse if this is normal teenage behavior. What is the best response?

   1. "Yes; all teenagers go through a grunge stage."
   2. "Yes; he is just tired from the rapid growth spurt during adolescence."
   3. "No, and if he doesn't snap out of it, you might want to take him to a health care provider."
   4. "No; he should see a health care provider or counselor right away."

19. A 70-year-old patient is in the hospital for pneumonia and has been taking sertraline (Zoloft) for 1 year for depression. On the third day of her hospitalization, the patient has a pulse rate of 100 beats/min, demonstrates trembling in her hands, has an oral temperature of 103°F, and is diaphoretic. What is the nursing assessment?

    1. Anxiety, related to hospitalization
    2. Increased cranial pressure
    3. Impaired airway
    4. Serotonin syndrome

20. To effectively communicate with a patient demonstrating manic, elevated mood behaviors, the nurse will incorporate which technique into the plan of care?

    1. Provide detailed explanations to the patient.
    2. Joke and use puns with the patient.
    3. Be brief and concrete with the patient.
    4. Offer prn medications to the patient.

21. What is the priority nursing intervention when working with the patient with a personality disorder?

    1. Encouraging group activity participation
    2. Reassuring the patient that he or she is a "good person"
    3. Setting limits with the patient
    4. Supporting the patient's decisions consistently

22. When providing care for a depressed patient, what assessment data warrant immediate attention from the nurse?

    1. Anorexia and weight loss
    2. Lowered self-esteem
    3. Inability to care for self effectively
    4. Suicidal ideation

25. The nurse is assessing a patient diagnosed with schizophrenia and has noted several symptoms that correlate this diagnosis. Which symptoms would the nurse document as positive symptoms? *(Select all that apply.)*

    1. Auditory hallucinations
    2. Delusional belief that he is the president
    3. Avolition
    4. Apathy
    5. Tardive dyskinesia

26. A man, 58, with a comorbid history of schizophrenia and social anxiety disorder, complicated by a history of adverse reactions to antipsychotic medications (particularly akathisia), is admitted to the psychiatric unit after he walked into a busy downtown restaurant and caused disruption by shouting that the restaurant was trying to poison him. He lives in a small apartment just above the restaurant and claimed that God had warned him that the cooking scents coming up through his vents were a poisonous gas. When the restaurant staff tried to usher him out, coaxing him with a free take-away meal, he shrieked and slapped at the meal, shouting, "Get that away from me!" When a waiter tried to touch him, he hit the waiter, knocking him down. The police were called. Once settled in the unit, he continued to experience hallucinations. The treatment team will keep him for three to 7 days to stabilize his medication regimen and provide therapy. Place a check mark to indicate each potential intervention in the left column that is appropriate for this client at this time. Check all that apply.

POTENTIAL INTERVENTION	APPROPRIATE
Use hand gestures while giving clear, concise instructions.	
Decrease sensory stimuli.	
Avoid having the patient make choices.	
Provide mandatory, pre-assigned socialization opportunities.	
Ask patient directly about his hallucinations.	
Gently challenge and correct any demonstrated delusions.	

Care of the Patient With an Addictive Personality

36

Objectives

1. Name two traits that characterize an addictive personality.
2. Describe the three stages of dependence.
3. Describe one legal effort that has decreased the incidence of substance abuse.
4. Describe three disorders associated with alcoholism.
5. Explain the two phases of recovery: detoxification and rehabilitation.
6. Identify six types of drugs of abuse.
7. Describe possible steps to help the chemically impaired nurse.

Key Terms

abuse (ŭ-BŪS, p. 1163)

addiction (ŭ-DĬK-shŭn, p. 1163)

addictive personality (ŭ-DĬK-tĭv pŭr-sŭn-ĂL-ĭ-tē, p. 1164)

Alcoholics Anonymous (AA) (ăl-kŭ-HŎL-ĭks ŭ-NŎN-ĭ-mŭs, p. 1169)

alcoholism (ĂL-kŭ-hŏl-ĭz-ĭm, p. 1163)

amotivational cannabis syndrome (ā-mō-tĭ-VĀ-shŭn-ăl KĂN-ă-bĭs SĬN-drŏm, p. 1175)

cannabis (KĂN-ă-bĭs, p. 1175)

club drugs (KLŬB DRŬGZ, p. 1171)

delirium tremens (DTs) (dŭ-LĬR-ē-ŭm TRĔM-ĭnz [dē-TĒZ], p. 1166)

depressants (dĭ-PRĔS-ŭntz, p. 1171)

detoxification (dĕ-tŏk-sĭ-fĭ-KĀ-shŭn, p. 1168)

gateway drug (GĀT-wā DRŬG, p. 1166)

group therapy (GRŬP THĔR-ŭ-pē, p. 1169)

hallucinogens (hă-LŪ-sĭ-nō-jĕnz, p. 1174)

Healthcare Integrity and Protection Data Bank (HIPDB) (HĔLTH-căr ĭn-TĔG-rĭ-tē ĂND prō-TĔK-shŭn DĀ-tŭ BĂNGK, p. 1178)

huffing (HŬF-ĭng, p. 1176)

inhalants (ĭn-HĀ-lŭnts, p. 1176)

peer assistance programs (PĔR ŭ-SĬS-tŭns PRŌ-grămz, p. 1178)

psychoactive drugs (sī-kō-ĂK-tĭv DRŬGZ, p. 1164)

raves (RĀVZ, p. 1171)

street drugs (STRĔT DRŬGZ, p. 1171)

tolerance (TOL-ŭr-ŭns, p. 1165)

The treatment of patients with addictive behaviors is an important concern for nurses. Problems associated with the abuse or misuse of alcohol, tobacco, caffeine, nicotine, and other drugs consume a major proportion of current health care dollars. Many patients seeking care from acute care facilities and a variety of outpatient settings also suffer from some type of addictive behavior. Nurses often encounter problems of substance abuse and addiction in patients suffering from other medical conditions. It is not uncommon for patients to deny or hide their substance abuse problems. Substance abuse may not be addressed until withdrawal symptoms become apparent. Patients suffering from chronic pain have a high risk of developing tolerance to and addiction to opioids. Patients suffering from anxiety and depression sometimes self-medicate with alcohol, marijuana, or other substances. Investigate what the patient does to relieve stress or pain when you collect data about the patient. These data often help identify addictive behavior patterns that can impede the patient's recovery from acute illness.

ADDICTION

Addiction consists of four elements: (1) excessive use or abuse of a substance, (2) display of psychological disturbance, (3) decline of social and economic function, and (4) uncontrollable consumption of the substance, indicating dependence. Alcoholism is the addiction to alcohol. It is possible to suffer from more than one addiction at the same time. For example, an alcoholic person also may be a smoker and a compulsive gambler.

In the adult population (age 18 years and older), 89.64% report having consumed an alcoholic drink sometime in their lifetime, and 54% reported having a drink in the last 30 days. About 6% of these people have an alcohol use disorder (National Institute on Alcohol Abuse and Alcoholism, 2021). Age at the onset of drinking is strongly predictive of the development of alcohol dependence in the lifespan; of people who start drinking at the age of 14 or younger, 44% develop alcoholism. Alcohol and drug abuse are increasing in the older population. Older adults sometimes turn to alcohol, prescription and nonprescription drugs, caffeine, and nicotine to help cope with physiologic and sociologic changes associated with aging. Aging causes changes in absorption, distribution, metabolism, and excretion of drugs; thus, the risk of misuse and abuse increases with age.

Alcohol is involved in 31% of all deaths caused by motor vehicle accidents. About 95,000 deaths each year are related to alcohol consumption. Approximately 70% of these deaths are among males. These statistics make alcohol consumption the third leading cause of preventable death in the United States (National Institute on Alcohol Abuse and Alcoholism, 2021).

The use of alcohol and drugs predates recorded history. In cultures from many parts of the world, alcohol and drugs have been used as medicine, in celebrations, and as a part of worship services. In the history of the United States, legal positions on the use of alcohol have varied. The temperance movement in the 1800s stressed moderation in or total avoidance of the use of alcohol. The Eighteenth Amendment to the US Constitution, known as *Prohibition,* which forbade the production, transport, and sale of alcoholic beverages, was passed in 1919 and later repealed in 1933. There has been a decrease in alcohol use over the years that experts attribute to the education of the public and laws set forth to limit the availability of alcohol to minors.

Although there has been a long-term decline in overall alcohol use, many people still use illicit drugs. Nearly 12% of people aged 12 years and older reported having used illicit drugs in the previous month. Approximately 80% of these users admitted to using only marijuana (Centers for Disease Control and Prevention [CDC], 2021b). The goal of the Comprehensive Drug Abuse and Controlled Substance Act of 1970 (commonly referred to as the *Controlled Substance Act*) was to provide legal control over drugs that previous federal drug-related laws did not cover. The Bureau of Drug Abuse Control moved from the US Food and Drug Administration to the Department of Justice and later merged into the Drug Enforcement Agency, which today is the leading agency responsible for enforcing the 1970 act. All prescribing physicians and dispensing pharmacies register with the Drug Enforcement Agency. Smuggling and other illegal activities provide the public with illicit drugs.

Certain common traits have been identified in addicted people. These traits often have been grouped under the term **addictive personality** (exhibiting a pattern of compulsive and habitual use of a substance or practice to cope with psychic pain from conflict and anxiety). These personality traits include low tolerance for stress, dependency, negative self-image, feelings of insecurity, and depression. It is not clear whether these traits are present before the development of dependence or result from it.

STAGES OF DEPENDENCE

Psychoactive drugs, including alcohol, make the user feel good. Social use of drugs creates a relaxed atmosphere, encouraging people to socialize more openly. Movies, television commercials, and other media have suggested that individuals "need a drink" after a hard day at the office. Unfortunately, every psychoactive drug, including caffeine and nicotine, can be abused or become addicting. In the 1970s, alcoholism and drug addiction acquired recognition as diseases. Experts published diagnostic criteria and established treatment centers for addiction in the United States—a psychoactive drug-oriented society. When does substance abuse become a disease and a problem? The indicator appears to be the loss of control. The disease of dependence is a chronic, incurable, progressive one with three characteristic stages of dependence: early, middle, and late (Box 36.1).

Box 36.1   Stages of Dependence

EARLY STAGE	MIDDLE STAGE	LATE STAGE
Increased drug tolerance	Moderate impairment	Severe impairment in all areas of function
Strong denial	Withdrawal signs with abstinence	Continuous use but inability to achieve "normal" feeling
Defending drug use in response to family concerns	Using drug to feel "normal"	Worsening medical problems; organ involvement
More socializing with users	Established pattern of use	Worsening malnutrition
Increased tardiness to or time off from work/school	Further alienation from family	Poor problem solving and judgment
Possible legal problems	Drug-related behavior such as lying, stealing, mood swings	Manipulativeness; denial of problems
Good prognosis for recovery, even without a treatment program	Decline in physical health	Unemployment
	Noticeable weight loss	Often homelessness
	Blackouts	No chance of improvement without treatment
	Financial/legal problems	
	Job loss or frequent job changes	
	Low chance of recovery without treatment	

EARLY STAGES

As a person uses an increasing amount of an addicting substance and uses it more frequently to achieve the same effect, tolerance develops. The user experiences the untoward effects of insomnia, anxiety, cramps, heart palpitations, changes in sexual libido, and accidental injury. Some users decrease or stop to prove that they have control of their substance use. Family and friends probably comment about their concern for the user's overinvolvement with drugs. The user may make light of the concern or become hostile and defensive. Some users avoid family and socialize only with other users. Users are prone to legal problems, such as charges of driving while intoxicated. Users sometimes miss work or show up late for work after a weekend of use. A pattern of absenteeism emerges. If a user is a student, truancy and falling grades with an uncaring attitude are common. Mood swings, decreased self-esteem, shame, guilt, remorse, resentment, and irritability are typical, with a tendency for these feelings to focus on drug use. Financial difficulties arise in connection with greater expenditures for drug use.

The prognosis with treatment is good in this early stage, and recovery without treatment is possible.

MIDDLE STAGE

In this stage, the dependent user is moderately impaired. With difficulty, the user makes efforts to decrease or stop, but these efforts are followed by heavier use. Abstinence brings on signs and symptoms of withdrawal. The user now uses the substance just to feel "normal." The user has a pattern of use in regard to time, place, and situation. Family relationships and friendships are weakened by drug-related behavior such as arguing, lying, stealing, incest, physical abuse, and child neglect. Physical health declines. Common problems that arise during this stage include weight changes; anorexia; malnutrition; gastrointestinal problems such as nausea, diarrhea, and gastritis; suicide attempts; blackouts of short-term memory; sexual problems; sexually transmitted infection; accidental injury; infections; and overdose. Job loss is common because of absenteeism, drug use on the job, and uncooperative attitudes. Employers sometimes ask users to seek treatment. Social isolation increases, and users continue to have legal and crime-related problems. Some dependent users stay in this stage a long time; with multidrug use, however, progression into the late stage is faster.

Very few people in this stage recover without treatment.

LATE STAGE

In this stage, the dependent user displays severe impairment in all areas of function. Drug use is nearly continual in an attempt to avoid emotional and physical pain, but the user is not able to achieve a feeling of normality. Medical problems worsen. Liver disease, pancreatitis, toxic psychosis, kidney failure, sexual impotence, and stroke are possible, along with malnutrition. Users in the late stage neglect personal hygiene. Intravenous (IV) drug users are at great risk for infection with human immunodeficiency virus (HIV) or hepatitis B or C virus and for developing septicemia, abscesses, or infective endocarditis. Some users become suicidal or homicidal. Users are manipulative, are in denial of their problems, and have poor problem-solving ability and judgment. Users in this stage are usually unemployed, associate only with dealers or other users, and may be homeless.

People in this stage cannot recover without treatment.

ALCOHOL ABUSE AND ALCOHOLISM

Alcoholism is a national health problem whose prevalence is surpassed only by those of heart disease and cancer. No one theory explains the cause of alcoholism. Several factors probably contribute to the development of alcoholism. Some authorities believe that people are more likely to develop alcoholism because of some biological reason, such as an inner urge controlled by the nervous system or a dysfunction of the endocrine system. Alcoholism has genetic links. The incidence of alcoholism in members of certain families is high: the sons of alcoholic men are four times more likely to develop alcoholism over their lifetime (National Council on Alcoholism and Drug Dependence, Inc., 2015). Deficiencies in some hepatic enzymes necessary to metabolize alcohol contribute to the development of alcoholism in some people. Many Asians, Native Americans, and Inuits (indigenous people living largely in Alaska, Canada and Greenland) have deficiencies in these enzymes; alcoholism rates are higher in these ethnic groups than in the general public. Jews, Mormons, and Muslims have very low rates of alcoholism, whereas people of French descent and those of Irish descent have high rates. Bariatric weight loss surgery has been associated with an increased incidence of the development of alcoholic use disorder (AUD). Patients having the procedures have an increased incidence of AUD in the first years after the surgery.

Other theories rest on the belief that some part of the personality leads to the development of alcoholism. Some people still believe that alcoholism develops as a result of a moral fault. This theory provided the basis for much of the early treatment of alcoholic patients. Health care providers trained to provide treatment regimens that are based on this moral theory have difficulty assimilating newer biological theories into their care.

Wide cultural differences concerning drug and alcohol use have been found in US society. Most young people in the United States have their first drink at an early age. In the past, girls were typically older than boys when they took their first drink of alcohol. Currently there are conflicting studies on what age girls and boys begin drinking. In 2019 girls drank more than boys with 1.7% vs 1.5% in the age group of 12 to 13 year olds; ages 14 to 15 years saw 9.3% of girls compared to 5.9% of boys report alcohol use. In the 16 to 17 age range 20.8% of girls vs 17.8% of boys drank (NIAAA, 2021). Alcohol sometimes serves as an informal rite of passage into adulthood. Drinking beer or other alcoholic beverages is the way many Americans celebrate certain holidays (e.g., St. Patrick's Day). Experts consider drinking to be the leading health problem in the African American community. Hispanic populations and many other ethnic groups celebrate life while drinking alcohol. Alcohol often serves as a gateway drug. Many multidrug users began by abusing alcohol and progressed to abusing other substances.

Etiology and Pathophysiology

Alcohol is a central nervous system (CNS) depressant. The so-called stimulating effect occurs because the first areas affected by alcohol are the higher centers of the brain, including the frontal cortex, which governs self-control. Judgment is blocked, but the memory of pleasure is retained. As a person continues to ingest alcohol, it affects the nucleus accumbens in the limbic system (the most primitive part of the brain; it regulates hunger, thirst, and sexual desire). Repeated alcohol consumption affects the basal ganglia of the brain, where it unbalances compulsion controls, leading to obsessive-compulsive behavior. Rapid, large-quantity consumption can lead to unconsciousness, during which respiration is sometimes affected. Death from acute alcohol poisoning is possible.

The active ingredient of alcoholic beverages is ethyl alcohol or ethanol. There are similar amounts of alcohol in 12 ounces of beer, 4 ounces of wine, and 1½ ounces of hard liquor. Alcohol does not require digestion, and the body absorbs it readily in the stomach and the intestines. An empty stomach increases the rate of absorption. After ingestion, the body loses small amounts through breathing and in the urine, but 90% is metabolized by the liver.

Alcohol has a diuretic effect. The urine of a heavy drinker sometimes contains increased amounts of electrolytes, especially potassium, magnesium, and zinc. Prolonged use of alcohol has a toxic effect on the intestinal mucosa that results in decreased absorption of vitamin B_1 (thiamine), vitamin B_9 (folic acid), and vitamin B_{12} (cobalamin).

Alcohol does not undergo conversion to glycogen; it does provide the body with calories but no minerals or vitamins. One ounce of alcohol provides 200 kcal but no other nutritional value. Blood alcohol levels depend on the amount of alcohol ingested and the size of the individual. Most states designate blood alcohol serum levels of 80 mg/dL (0.08%) as the legal limit for driving a motor vehicle. Increasing blood alcohol serum levels have increasingly serious side effects (see Chapter 16, Table 16.1).

DISORDERS ASSOCIATED WITH ALCOHOLISM

Fetal Alcohol Syndrome

Fetal alcohol syndrome (FAS) is a congenital anomaly resulting from maternal use of alcohol during pregnancy. Although the condition is more common in mothers who drank heavily during pregnancy, no specific amount of alcohol has been identified as the amount that results in the syndrome. As few as two drinks per day have the potential to cause adverse effects in an infant. Experts agree that during pregnancy, it is best to avoid alcohol ingestion completely. The damage seems to be greater when alcohol is consumed during the first trimester of pregnancy. Birth defects related to alcohol use include cognitive delays; growth disorders; craniofacial abnormalities, including wide-set eyes and a flattened face; and malformed body parts. The effect on the pregnancy may include spontaneous abortion or stillbirth. Some of the effects of FAS such as cognitive delays or behavioral problems may not be evident until the toddler and preschool years or later.

Alcohol Withdrawal Syndrome

Alcohol withdrawal syndrome occurs in a person who has developed physiologic dependence and quits drinking abruptly. The risk for having alcohol withdrawal syndrome is highest in older adults, people who have previously suffered DTs, malnourished people, and people who have another acute illness. The range of possible signs and symptoms varies from mild tremor and flulike signs and symptoms to severe agitation and hallucinations. Signs and symptoms associated with the cessation of alcohol consumption include diaphoresis; tachycardia; hypertension; tremors; nausea or vomiting, or both; anorexia; restlessness; disorientation; hallucinations; and seizures.

The tremors from alcohol cessation occur 6 to 48 hours after the last drink and sometimes last for 3 to 5 days. Tremors usually occur in the hands but also may be present in the tongue, the chin, the trunk, and the feet. Seizures can occur 12 to 24 hours after alcohol cessation. Usually, these are tonic-clonic (grand mal) seizures and often are not preceded by an aura.

Delirium Tremens

Delirium tremens (DTs) is a complication of alcohol withdrawal. This acute psychotic reaction is a result of excessive alcohol consumption over a long period. The risk of death from this complication is as high as 15%, even with treatment. Signs of DTs are tremors; increase in activity, sometimes to the point of extreme agitation; disorientation; fear with an appearance of panic; hallucinations; and elevated temperature. DTs most often occur 1 to 4 days after cessation of alcohol use and usually last from 2 days to a week.

Korsakoff Psychosis and Wernicke Encephalopathy

Korsakoff psychosis and Wernicke encephalopathy are two brain disorders that sometimes occur in people with chronic alcoholism. Characteristics of Korsakoff psychosis are short-term memory loss, disorientation, muttering, delirium, insomnia, hallucinations, polyneuritis, and painful extremities, with footdrop affecting the gait. Wernicke encephalopathy occurs in association with thiamine (vitamin B_1) deficiency, causing

Table 36.1   Disorders Associated With Alcoholism

SYSTEM	DISORDERS
Gastrointestinal (GI)	Gastritis; pancreatitis; cancer of mouth, esophagus, and stomach; esophageal varices; GI bleeding; malabsorption of nutrition; ascites
Hepatic	Hepatitis, cirrhosis, fatty liver, liver failure, hepatic encephalopathy
Cardiovascular and hematologic	Hypertension, enlarged heart, high cholesterol, heart failure, portal hypertension, low blood glucose level, anemia, poor clotting ability, increased susceptibility to infection
Respiratory	Decreased cough reflex, aspiration pneumonia
Urologic/ reproductive	Prostatitis, impotence, urinary flow problems
Musculoskeletal	Myopathies, bone fractures from falls, joint damage from injury
Neurologic	Neuritis, organic brain diseases such as Wernicke encephalopathy and Korsakoff psychosis, nerve palsies, gait changes, short-term memory loss

Box 36.2   CAGE Questions

Two or more affirmations to these questions indicate probable alcoholism:
1. Have you ever felt you ought to **c**ut down on your drinking?
2. Have people **a**nnoyed you by criticizing your drinking?
3. Have you ever felt bad or **g**uilty about your drinking?
4. Have you ever had a drink first thing in the morning to steady your nerves or for your hangover (i.e., **e**ye-opener)?

brain damage in the temporal lobes of the brain. It features memory loss, aphasia, involuntary eye movement and double vision, lack of muscle coordination, and disorientation with confabulation (i.e., the patient fills in memory gaps with inappropriate words).

Because alcohol affects all tissues in the body, chronic alcohol ingestion has the potential to cause damage to all parts of the body. Table 36.1 lists other disorders arising from chronic alcohol use.

NURSING PROCESS

Assessment

It is important to collect subjective and objective data about the patient who has a substance abuse or dependence problem. *Subjective data* include the person's normal using or drinking pattern, as well as the date and time of the last drink or use of a drug. The specific substance and the quantity the person uses are important. Other complaints such as nausea, indigestion, sleep disturbance, or pain sometimes indicate the simultaneous occurrence of another disease process, in addition to the side effects of substance abuse. Assessment of normal dietary patterns, the presence of any disease that necessitates treatment with prescribed medications, and regular use of any over-the-counter drugs help complete the picture of the patient's present state of wellness. Obtain this information in as much detail as possible by asking about drug allergies or unusual responses to anesthesia, sedatives, or preoperative medications. Maintaining a concerned, nonjudgmental attitude when asking for details helps reassure the patient, as does the promise of confidentiality about this private part of his or her life.

Assess for any history of tremors, hallucinations, delusions, seizures, or DTs. Note any past periods of

abstinence. Ask about any problems with occupation, family, or legal matters. Document any family history of substance dependency. Remember that denial is strong in people with untreated substance abuse or dependence, and information from such patients is often inaccurate. It is helpful to validate the information with families or significant others if possible. Beneficial in affirming alcohol abuse is the CAGE questionnaire, whose title arises from an acronym formed from among the tool's four questions (Box 36.2).

Objective data include height, weight, vital sign measurements, and findings of physical assessment. The presence of tremor or skin conditions, especially on the forearms, should be noted. Needle tracks and small scabs on forearms, backs of hands, and insteps indicate IV use. The acne-like facial rash is possibly related to the use of 3,4-methylenedioxymethamphetamine (MDMA, or Ecstasy). Excessive gum and tooth erosion and extreme vasoconstriction may indicate methamphetamine ("meth") use.

Frequent sniffling, stuffy nose, or harsh nonproductive cough is possibly related to drug use. Assess general behavior and cognitive abilities for impairment. The presence of tachycardia, hypertension, petechiae, and neuropathies is significant. A urine or blood sample positive for drugs or alcohol or the presence of ascites alerts the nurse to the need for further investigation of the patient's history.

Diagnostic Tests

Blood and urine tests help screen for toxins. Certain foods sometimes cause a false-positive reading in a urine screen. If a person ate a poppy seed roll and later gave urine for a drug screen, the result may appear positive for heroin. Abnormalities in routine blood tests are sometimes directly related to alcoholism. Elevated levels of liver enzymes, hypoglycemia, and abnormal blood protein levels occur with alcoholism. Magnesium levels are decreased in some cases. Anemia and other evidence of poor nutrition are common in addicted patients. Some practitioners also order testing for hepatitis and HIV.

Patient Problem

Patient problems and interventions for the patient with an addiction cover emotional needs and physical needs (Box 36.3).

| Box 36.3 | Possible Patient Problems for Addiction |

PHYSICAL CONDITIONS	EMOTIONAL CONDITIONS	EDUCATIONAL CONDITIONS
Acute confusion	Defensive coping	Deficient knowledge
Functional urinary incontinence	Disturbed personality identity	Ineffective family therapeutic regimen
Impaired physical mobility	Dysfunctional family processes	management
Insomnia	Impaired individual resilience	Readiness for enhanced family
Risk for electrolyte imbalance	Ineffective impulse control	processes
Risk for imbalanced fluid volume	Risk for compromised human dignity	Readiness for enhanced self-concept
Risk for impaired liver function	Social isolation	Risk-prone health behavior
Risk for poisoning	Spiritual distress	
Sleep deprivation	Stress overload	

From Ralph S, Taylor C: *Nursing diagnosis reference manual*, ed 9, Philadelphia, 2014, Wolters-Lippincott.

Nursing Interventions

Care for the addicted patient starts with **detoxification**, the removal of the poisonous effects of a substance. A controlled setting in which the patient can be observed closely and treated for any complications is important during this acute phase of recovery.

Safety of the patient is a primary concern. If the patient is intoxicated, a patent airway must be maintained. The side-lying position and oral suctioning should be considered if oral secretions can be aspirated or if vomiting could occur. If swallowing is intact, the head of the bed should be elevated at least 30 degrees to encourage better air exchange. IV fluids may be administered to correct the patient's fluid and electrolyte imbalance. The IV site must be monitored often, especially if the patient is restless. The facility's seizure precautions—such as padded side rails, floor pads, and moving the patient to a room close to the nurse's station—should be instituted.

Practitioners usually treat tremors, nervousness, and restlessness with drugs such as chlordiazepoxide (Librium) or lorazepam (Ativan). Scheduled doses must be given on time. Environmental stimuli should be reduced. The patient should be allowed to ambulate or perform other benign activities that help ease nervousness, but the patient must refrain from overexertion. The patient should be attended while ambulating if he or she is unsteady from coordination disturbance or the lack of conditioning. As weakness subsides, a regular exercise regimen should be included in the care plan (Nursing Care Plan 36.1.)

Cardiorespiratory distress is a possible result of stimulant abuse. Health care providers sometimes prescribe beta-adrenergic agents such as propranolol (Inderal) and calcium channel blockers such as nifedipine (Procardia) and oxygen. Continuous cardiac monitoring and frequent checks on vital signs with respiratory assessment help the nurse detect any adverse changes early before they have the chance to become life threatening.

Keep explanations to the patient simple. Speak in a calm voice, planning time for the patient's verbalizations. Therapeutic conversation techniques are used to assist the patient in understanding himself or herself (self-realization). Reinforce teaching about the disease concept of addiction. Denial is confronted in a nonjudgmental manner. The family is encouraged to participate in planning for sobriety. Counselors sometimes initiate individual therapy to assist the patient in the rehabilitation phase of recovery.

For patients who are extremely restless, health care providers sometimes order magnesium sulfate to raise the seizure threshold or another anticonvulsant medication such as phenytoin (Dilantin). High doses of chlordiazepoxide (Librium) have the potential to cause urinary retention. Intake and output measurements are appropriate in some cases.

Disorientation is possible, especially at night. Nightlights in the room and frequent visits by nurses tend to help. If a patient is not able to sleep at night, he or she should sit up and have a snack; then give the patient a back rub and encourage him or her to rest. If the patient appears fearful or panicky and unable to reacquire orientation to reality, notify the supervising nurse. Check vital signs (including temperature) before the health care provider is notified. Physical restraints have the potential to escalate aggressive behavior but are sometimes necessary if the patient poses a risk for harm to self or others.

Many addicted patients are malnourished and suffer from loss of appetite. Incorporating nutritious foods and inquiring about food preferences help meet nutritional deficits. Providing between-meal snacks is also helpful. Administration of multivitamins and thiamine as ordered helps the patient improve his or her nutritional state.

Rehabilitation

After detoxification, the acute phase of recovery, it is time to start rehabilitation. The object of rehabilitation is to help the patient abstain from substance abuse. Because there is no cure for addiction, abstinence is the practical equivalent to the control of the disease. Administration of disulfiram (Antabuse) is sometimes a way to encourage abstinence. It causes facial flushing, nausea, tachycardia, dyspnea, dizziness, and confusion when the patient consumes alcohol. The purpose is to

Nursing Care Plan 36.1   **The Patient Who Abuses Alcohol**

Mr. J., 56 years of age, was a corporate executive. His employer confronted him about his increasing tendency to call in sick, last-minute rescheduling of meetings, and excessive alcohol use during luncheon meetings. Later, after the confrontation, the police cited him for driving while intoxicated for the third time and jailed him. Sentencing included the requirement to complete a treatment program for alcoholism.

PATIENT PROBLEM

Obstructive denial, related to the inability to admit being alcoholic

Patient Goals and Expected Outcomes	Nursing Interventions	Rationale
Patient will participate in program Patient will identify negative effects of drinking on other people Patient will abstain from alcohol use Patient will express acceptance of alcoholism as a disease Patient will express acceptance of responsibility for own behavior Patient will maintain abstinence after discharge	Confront the patient's denial by relating incidents and problems to its use. Reinforce teaching about the disease of alcoholism. Encourage the patient to identify behaviors that have caused problems in his or her life. Do not allow the patient to rationalize or to blame others.	It is necessary to address the problem of alcoholism first. Providing knowledge about the disease and having the patient identify the relationship between alcohol and his or her problems will help the patient overcome denial. Blaming others is an excuse to continue drinking behavior.

PATIENT PROBLEM

Impaired coping, related to abnormal use of alcohol

Patient Goals and Expected Outcomes	Nursing Interventions	Rationale
Patient will express feelings directly and express anger or hostility outward in a safe manner Patient will practice using nonchemical alternatives to deal with stress or difficult situations Patient will verbalize increased self-esteem	Encourage the patient to explore alternative ways of dealing with a stressful situation. Involve the patient in a group to provide confrontation, positive feedback, and sharing of feelings. Avoid discussion of unanswerable questions, such as why he drinks.	Patient perhaps has minimal experience of dealing with stress without alcohol. Groups of peers are honest and supportive. Asking why when there is no answer is dwelling on the negative and in the past. Focus on positive and the future, for which change has the power to make a difference.

CRITICAL THINKING QUESTIONS

1. During Mr. J.'s assessment, the nurse notes that he has tremors, is agitated, and verbalizes visual hallucinations. What therapeutic interventions are appropriate to perform to prevent injury to the patient?
2. As Mr. J.'s physical condition improves, he discloses his hopelessness and lack of desire to continue living. What is an appropriate response by the nurse?
3. During group therapy, Mr. J. states, "Now that I am physically better, I know I will be able to stop drinking. I don't need any help. There really isn't anything wrong with me." What is the appropriate staff intervention at this time?

reduce alcohol consumption by aversion conditioning. Treatment programs often include family members in part of the treatment plan. Some of these programs are inpatient, and some are outpatient or day-treatment programs.

Group therapy. Group therapy is an effective treatment modality. Group therapy provides a caring, emotionally supportive atmosphere in which the patient is able to acknowledge the relationship of substance abuse with negative consequences in his or her life. The group tends to point out negative defense mechanisms such as denial or displacement and to offer possible solutions to its members. Families should be encouraged to attend support groups to help the patient and family to grow together, not apart. Group therapy sometimes continues after the completion of an inpatient program. Group therapy is an important part of all recovery programs.

Alcoholics Anonymous. Alcoholics Anonymous (AA) is an international nonprofit organization that began in 1935 as a way for abstinent alcoholic people to help other alcoholic people become and stay sober through group

Box 36.4	Twelve Steps of Alcoholics Anonymous

1. We admitted we were powerless over alcohol—that our lives had become unmanageable.
2. Came to believe that a Power greater than ourselves could restore us to sanity.
3. Made a decision to turn our will and our lives over to the care of God *as we understood Him.*
4. Made a searching and fearless moral inventory of ourselves.
5. Admitted to God, to ourselves, and to another human being the exact nature of our wrongs.
6. Were entirely ready to have God remove all these defects of character.
7. Humbly asked Him to remove our shortcomings.
8. Made a list of all people we had harmed and became willing to make amends to them all.
9. Made direct amends to such people wherever possible, except when to do so would injure them or others.
10. Continued to take personal inventory and when we were wrong promptly admitted it.
11. Sought through prayer and meditation to improve our conscious contact with God *as we understood Him,* praying only for knowledge of His will for us and the power to carry that out.
12. Having had a spiritual awakening as a result of these Steps, we tried to carry this message to alcoholics and to practice these principles in all our affairs.

The Twelve Steps are reprinted with permission of Alcoholics Anonymous World Services, Inc. ("AAWS"). Permission to reprint the Twelve Steps does not mean that AAWS has reviewed or approved the contents of this publication, or that AAWS necessarily agrees with the views expressed herein. AA is a program of recovery from alcoholism only—use of the Twelve Steps in connection with programs and activities which are patterned after AA, but which address other problems, or in any other non-AA context, does not imply otherwise.
From Alcoholics Anonymous: The twelve steps of Alcoholics Anonymous, 2016. Retrieved from http://www.aa.org/assets/en_US/smf-121_en.pdf.

Box 36.5	Addiction Issues to Consider

The medical community has overcome its fear of addiction and focuses on providing adequate pain management for acute and chronic pain conditions.

- Postoperative care with the use of opioids in patient-controlled administration devices has shown that opioid need and the severity of pain decrease. Many patients are using nonopioid medications for pain control by the third postoperative day. No development of tolerance or addiction occurs. However, the patient sometimes suffers undue fears of addiction when told that opioids will be used to control postoperative pain. Explanation of the pain management regimen usually helps allay the patient's fears of addiction. The patient's use of the self-medication before activities helps the patient heal more quickly.
- Chronic pain management involves more than just a pill to relieve pain. It is very important to use imagery, physical therapy, and other methods to help the patient relieve pain without chemical intervention. Side effects of high doses of NSAIDs are not tolerated by some patients; in such cases, it is possible to use narcotics to control pain. Although opioid addiction is always a possibility, health care providers sometimes consider opioids to be cheaper and more effective than treating the serious side effects of high-dose NSAID therapy. If the patient is dying, addiction to opioid agents is not an issue, but close monitoring is necessary to avoid acute overdose.
- Acute pain management for addicted patients presents a challenge to the health care team. Accidents and surgery are usually the cause of the acute pain. Circumstances of an injury sometimes trigger withdrawal symptoms within 24 h of admission to an acute care facility. Most often, health care providers order medications to relieve pain and suppress withdrawal symptoms. Cross-tolerance and multidrug abuse necessitate careful consideration of minor changes in the patient's condition. In the plan of care, discuss referral for rehabilitation; the initial steps of rehabilitation will, in some cases, be part of the patient's acute phase of recovery.

support, shared experiences, and faith in a power greater than themselves. There are regular meetings in most communities. Listings for local AA chapters may be found in the telephone book, in the newspaper, or on the Internet. The foundation of AA is a 12-step program that assists the dependent person in admitting powerlessness over alcohol (Box 36.4). Other groups have followed up on the success of AA, usually using similar models for rehabilitation; these groups include Overeaters Anonymous, Al-Anon (for friends and family of alcoholic people), and Narcotics Anonymous.

Treatment centers. Residential treatment centers provide the opportunity for detoxification. There is no direct medical intervention; instead, trained nurses provide close physical monitoring with the assistance of counselors and recovered peers. After detoxification, the patient enters a drug- and alcohol-free residence. A primary goal of this type of treatment is the rebuilding of social skills that do not involve drug use as the primary method of interaction. The length of the stay in a treatment center ranges from 1 to 6 months; most centers operate on an ability-to-pay basis, with some governmental funding.

Pain management. Pain management sometimes involves the use of addicting substances, which sometimes complicates pain management for an addicted person. The medical community has improved greatly the regimen options for effective pain management with combinations of nonopioid, opioid, and antianxiety agents, along with nonchemical interventions. Nursing interventions require not only careful assessment of pain but also observation for developing patterns of drug-seeking behavior that indicate the patient's tolerance or addiction to the drug. Encouraging the patient to practice and use nonchemical interventions to ease pain will reduce the risk of chemical dependency for relief (Box 36.5).

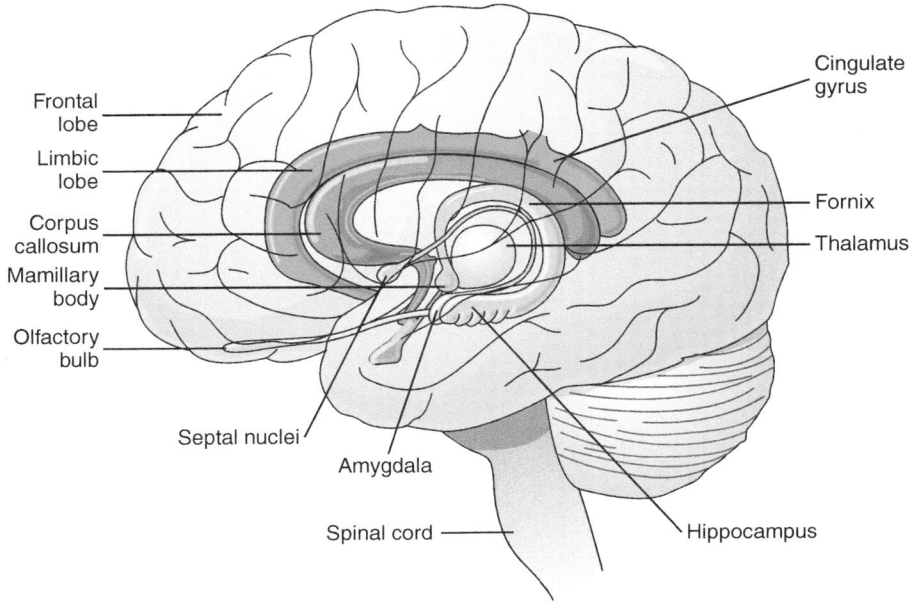

Fig. 36.1 Limbic system. The limbic system is considered to be the emotional center of the brain. An emotional response to an incoming stimulus is produced and then stored in memory. (From Copstead-Kirkhorn LE, Banasik J: *Pathophysiology*, ed 5, St. Louis, 2013, Mosby.)

DRUG ABUSE

Although alcohol abuse is present most frequently in patients fighting addiction or in patients who are being treated for other health problems, drug abuse is also a growing problem in the health care setting. Many people think only of illegal drugs when drug abuse is mentioned, but abuse of prescription and over-the-counter drugs is common. More than 46 people die every day because of a prescription drug overdose (CDC, 2021a). Prescription drugs are sometimes traded or shared. Drug abusers may seek excessive prescriptions from their health care providers, purchase them on the streets, or divert them from the supplies of friends or family members. Rationalizations such as "If it worked for me, it will work for my friend" and "If one pill works, two pills will work better" often deny or justify misuse or abuse of many prescription and over-the-counter drugs.

When a person takes drugs for reasons other than medical issues or in a dose higher than recommended, the term *misuse* or *abuse* applies. Club drugs refer to substances that people frequently take for euphoric effect at parties, concerts, dance clubs, or all-night raves (also called trance parties: dance parties with extremely loud music). Club drugs are often street drugs. Street drugs are substances that users buy from illegal drug dealers. These drugs come from illegal manufacturers without strict controls, are illegally obtained prescription drugs, or are not approved for use in the United States. Chronic abuse has the potential to lead to psychological or physical dependence, or both. Many commonly abused drugs act on the limbic system of the brain and

potentially cause permanent damage to that area (Fig. 36.1 and Box 36.6). Commonly abused drugs discussed in this chapter are depressants, opioids, stimulants, hallucinogens, cannabis, and inhalants (Box 36.7).

DEPRESSANTS

CNS depressants include alcohol, sedative-hypnotic medications, and opioid analgesics. The sedative-hypnotic medications most often abused include barbiturates and benzodiazepines (minor tranquilizers). People usually take them orally in tablet or capsule form. Box 36.8 lists the effects of depressants.

Barbiturates entered into medical use in the beginning of the 20th century; they are useful in the clinical context for their sedative, hypnotic, anesthetic, and anticonvulsant effects. Problematic side effects include respiratory depression, rapid tolerance, and dependency; untoward effects (e.g., seizures or status epilepticus) accompany sudden withdrawal. In the 1960s, benzodiazepines became popular as a safer alternative

---

Box 36.6   Limbic System of the Brain

The structures of the limbic system, which are sometimes referred to as the *limbic lobe*, are involved in feeding, defense, reproduction, emotional responses, and the consolidation and retention of memory. The limbic lobe is not a separate structure; rather, it comprises border areas of the frontal, parietal, and temporal lobes with inner brain structures around the ventricles. Structures included are basal ganglia, amygdala, hippocampus, thalamus, hypothalamus, nucleus accumbens, cerebral cortex, olfactory cortex, and connecting nerve tracts.

Box 36.7	Commonly Abused Drugs and Their Street Names

Amphetamines: Speed, truck drivers, copilots, black beauties, crank, go
Barbiturates: Reds, blues, yellow jackets, rainbows, bluies
Benzodiazepines: Downers, chill pill, vitamin V
Chloral hydrate: Mickey Finn, mickey
Cocaine: Snow, crack, blow, coke, nose candy, toot, white dust, toot sweet
Gamma-hydroxybutyrate (GHB): Soap, easy lay, Georgia homeboy, liquid Ecstasy
Heroin: H, smack, scag, junk, caca
Ketamine: Special K, vitamin K
Lysergic acid diethylamide (LSD): Acid, windowpane, gelcap, microdots, blotter, purple haze
Marijuana: Pot, reefer, grass, dope, weed, green, cannabis, Jamaican, Acapulco gold
Methamphetamine: Speed, crystal, ice
3,4-methylenedioxymethamphetamine (MDMA): Ecstasy, E, XTC, hug, love bug, beans, Adam, Molly
Nitrous oxide: Nitrous, whippets
Phencyclidine (PCP): Angel dust, rocket fuel, wack, ozone
Psilocybin: Shroom, magic mushroom
Rohypnol: Roofies, rough, rope, roach

Box 36.8	Signs and Symptoms Produced by Central Nervous System Depressants

- Ataxic gait (staggering)
- Decreased respirations
- Memory loss
- Nausea and vomiting
- Passiveness, listlessness
- Pinpoint pupils (opioid effect)
- Reduced hunger or thirst
- Reduced sexual drive
- Slurred speech
- Sense of heaviness in extremities

to barbiturates. Flurazepam (Dalmane) and chlordiazepoxide (Librium) were the first benzodiazepines, and diazepam (Valium) became available shortly after.

Valium soon became the most frequently prescribed antianxiety agent. The effects of addiction and overdose with benzodiazepines were not apparent at first, but by 1981, Valium dropped to the sixth most prescribed drug in the United States. In the 1990s, alprazolam (Xanax) was the most frequently prescribed benzodiazepine for the treatment of acute anxiety (American Society of Addiction Medicine, n.d.). Xanax is prescribed for anxiety and also is used as a drug of abuse.

Another benzodiazepine that gained notoriety in the 1990s was flunitrazepam (Rohypnol). Perpetrators of sexual assault frequently have administered this drug to victims, and people thus sometimes refer to it as a "date-rape drug." It is easy to mix it secretly into an alcoholic drink so that the victim consumes it unknowingly. Its effects include muscle relaxation and amnesia. Alcohol increases these effects; the two together are sometimes a lethal combination. Flunitrazepam is not legal for use in the United States. Klonopin (clonazepam) is a common benzodiazepine drug that is now prescribed for anxiety and recently has been seen as a drug of abuse.

Some people in the United States have abused gamma-hydroxybutyrate (GHB) for its euphoric, sedative, and body-building (anabolic) effects. Its abuse as a synthetic steroid is common at fitness centers and gyms. As with flunitrazepam, GHB has been associated with club drug use and sexual assault. Flunitrazepam and GHB are odorless, tasteless, and colorless. They are easy to mix with drinks and quickly cause unconsciousness. These drugs also rapidly cause relaxation of voluntary muscles and potentially cause the victim to have long-term amnesia for events occurring while the victim is under the influence of the drug.

OPIOID ANALGESICS

Opioid analgesics are drugs made from the opium poppy. Hippocrates praised the poppy's pain-relieving properties. During the 16th century, laudanum, an opium compound, was the most popular medication in Europe. Heroin is a widely abused drug in the United States. In 2016, about 948,000 Americans reported using heroin in the past year, with 626,000 being heroin users dependent on the drug (National Institute on Drug Abuse, 2021). Heroin is a schedule I drug that has no medical use. People take heroin by snorting, smoking, or injecting it into a vein. Morphine and its synthetic derivatives are schedule II drugs. They can be taken orally or injected. Opioids replace natural endorphins in the CNS, which makes these drugs highly addictive. Besides being excellent pain suppressants, opioids act as cough suppressants, slow peristalsis in the gastrointestinal system, and mildly contract the bladder. Tolerance develops rapidly, but abstinence reverses tolerance. Cross-tolerance with other opioids is possible. Three general types of opioid abusers are (1) street abusers who get opioids illegally, (2) abusers of opioids from medical sources (prescription opioids), and (3) methadone abusers. Nurses often deal with people in the second group, who are predominantly middle-class older adults, health care professionals, women, and patients with chronic pain syndrome.

Symptoms of acute opioid overdose include severe respiratory depression, pinpoint pupils, and stupor or coma. Aspiration is possible. Treatment involves supporting ventilation and administering naloxone (Narcan) as prescribed. Health care providers sometimes prescribe clonidine (Catapres) to help reduce withdrawal symptoms. It is important to continue monitoring for recurrent symptoms of toxicity when naloxone is discontinued.

In addicted people who consume huge amounts of morphine and heroin, predictable withdrawal signs

Box 36.9	Signs and Symptoms Produced by Central Nervous System Stimulants

- Anorexia
- Anxiety and paranoia
- Bronchodilation
- Bruxism (grinding of teeth)
- Delirium and hallucinations
- Diarrhea
- Dilated pupils
- Drug-induced psychosis
- Elation
- Euphoria
- Hostility and anger
- Hyperreflexia
- Hypertension
- Increased concentration
- Insomnia
- Mental alertness
- Nausea
- Peripheral vasoconstriction
- Tachycardia
- Twitching and tremors

and symptoms typically begin approximately 6 hours after the last dose. Withdrawal symptoms include flu-like signs and symptoms and body aches, watery eyes and runny nose, dilated pupils, vomiting, cramps and diarrhea, diaphoresis, tachycardia, hypertension, and chills and fever. The term "cold turkey" comes from the gooseflesh that is common during withdrawal. The intensity of signs and symptoms usually peaks in 2 to 3 days. Signs and symptoms subside within 5 to 10 days.

Methadone (Dolophine) is a synthetic opioid that helps suppress withdrawal symptoms in the morphine or heroin addict. Once the patient's condition stabilizes, the methadone dosage decreases daily until the addict is methadone-free. Methadone is sometimes a drug of abuse for people formerly addicted to heroin. The success of any cessation program depends on the motivation of the user.

STIMULANTS

CNS stimulants include a wide variety of substances. The category ranges from caffeine (the most widely consumed substance in the world) to cocaine and amphetamines. Box 36.9 lists the effects of stimulants.

Caffeine

Caffeine is present in foods such as coffee, tea, chocolate, and soft drinks and in over-the-counter medications such as cold and sinus medications and appetite suppressants. It is chemically related to theophylline, which is useful in the treatment of chronic obstructive pulmonary disease. Stimulant effects of caffeine are usually mild and typically last 5 to 7 hours after consumption. Abrupt cessation of habitual use of five to seven cups of caffeinated beverages per day can cause withdrawal symptoms of headache, fatigue, and irritability. Caffeine potentially can aggravate anxiety disorders and schizophrenia, as well as heart conditions.

Nicotine

Nicotine is a drug present in tobacco. Tobacco use is a legally sanctioned form of substance abuse. The number of Americans who smoke is declining, but the number of female smokers and underage smokers is rising. The effects of nicotine include increased alertness and concentration, appetite suppression, and vasoconstriction. People who smoke heavily or persistently quickly develop tolerance and dependence. Smokers sometimes switch to smokeless, oral forms of tobacco (snuff or chew) to reduce hazards from smoke. People who smoke heavily and stop suddenly experience withdrawal symptoms that include craving, irritability, restlessness, impatience, hostility, anxiety, confusion, difficulty in concentration, disturbed sleep, increased appetite, and decreased heart rate. Treatment for nicotine dependence includes the use of agents that deliver decreasing doses of nicotine. These agents include nicotine gum, transdermal patches, and nasal spray; agents that block the reinforcing effect of smoking; an antidepressant, bupropion; and combinations thereof. Behavioral therapy is also often beneficial in remaining smoke free. As many as 70% of people who quit smoking experience relapse within 1 year.

Cocaine

Cocaine is a white powder that is used as a topical, local, and regional anesthetic and as a vasoconstrictor for some types of surgery of the eye, ear, nose, and throat. Crack cocaine is an inexpensive form of cocaine mixed with baking soda. Freebasing is a method of smoking a drug, such as cocaine. To use powder cocaine, it is arranged into lines on a flat surface and snorted. Cocaine also can be taken intravenously. The rush occurs within 30 seconds, but the effect is very short lived. The "crash" that follows the rush consists of intense craving, agitation, and moderate to severe depression. Crack cocaine addiction occurs rapidly. The cravings have the potential to persist months into abstinence, which makes treatment difficult. The use of powder and crack cocaine became epidemic in the 1980s and 1990s.

Cocaine is a strong CNS stimulant. Chronic abuse by snorting erodes the nasal septum and often causes sinusitis and rhinitis. Smoking cocaine poses the risk of bodily injury from burns, and the caustic chemicals that people use to make it sometimes cause hemoptysis and pneumonitis. Overdose potentially produces cardiorespiratory distress and seizures. It is best to hospitalize the user to stabilize heart abnormalities and protect him or her from suicide if profound depression occurs.

Health care providers have used dopaminergic drugs such as amantadine and bromocriptine (Parlodel), which assist treatment of Parkinson's disease, to reduce the craving. If psychotic symptoms do not resolve in 3 days, it is appropriate to start conventional treatment. Neonates of addicted mothers need close monitoring for complications. Swaddling or wrapping such babies snugly is often comforting; stimuli such as bright lights, loud noises, and excessive handling should be minimized.

Amphetamines

Amphetamines and their analogs (e.g., methylphenidate) gained popularity as club drugs in the 1990s. Amphetamine is a powder that is snorted, smoked, or injected. People often mix it with other drugs such as heroin or marijuana. Methamphetamine is a potent, addictive amphetamine that causes a powerful release of the neurotransmitter dopamine. Over time, dopamine depletion in the brain results in parkinsonian-like symptoms. Brain cell damage is sometimes permanent. CNS stimulation is so strong that hallucinations and paranoia are possible. Weight loss and malnutrition from the anorexia effect are sometimes severe. Overstimulation of the heart sometimes raises blood pressure, which potentially causes damage to blood vessels, leading to heart attack or stroke. Brain damage at the cellular level and sudden death have occurred with amphetamine use. Treatment for withdrawal corresponds to the severity of the symptoms. People who suffer from chronic abuse typically exhibit flat affect, forgetfulness, and difficulty in concentration as a result of irreversible brain damage after they complete detoxification.

HALLUCINOGENS

Hallucinogens, either natural or synthetic, affect several areas of the brain. These drugs alter perception and thinking, and some of their effects sometimes last 6 to 12 hours. Deaths have occurred as a result of altered perceptions that have the potential to trigger the fight-or-flight response, which then leads to possible cardiac arrest or dangerously altered thinking, such as the user's notion that he or she has the ability to fly.

Drugs in this group are phencyclidine (PCP); lysergic acid diethylamide (LSD); 3,4-methylenedioxymethamphetamine (MDMA), known as Ecstasy, and its parent drug, methylenedioxyamphetamine (MDA); ketamine; mescaline; and psilocybin.

Phencyclidine

PCP entered the street scene in the 1960s and quickly gained a reputation for causing adverse drug reactions. PCP is a powder that easily dissolves in water or alcohol; users often sprinkle it in other drugs such as marijuana. Some people take it without knowing, unaware that PCP is mixed into another street drug. Experts consider it addictive with regular use. In low to moderate doses, symptoms of generalized numbness and poor coordination occur. Flushing and sweating occur with a rise in blood pressure and pulse. Some users report feelings of increased strength and power. Overdosage of PCP sometimes becomes apparent through symptoms of schizophrenia-like psychosis with extreme violence or attempted suicide. Seizures and coma are possible. At high doses, a drop in respirations, pulse, and blood pressure accompanies the loss of balance, blurred vision, nausea, and vomiting.

Lysergic Acid Diethylamide

LSD also entered the street scene in the 1960s. It is one of the most potent hallucinogenic drugs. Because its effects potentially last more than 12 hours, an LSD experience is referred to as a "trip." Dilation of pupils, sweating, loss of appetite, dry mouth, sleeplessness, and tremors occur. Crossover of sensory perception such as "hearing colors" and "seeing sounds" occurs. Altered perceptions such as melting walls and fear of insanity and death sometimes trigger panic attacks. Flashback of symptoms is possible, occurring suddenly within a few days or more than a year after LSD use. These flashbacks usually occur in chronic users. Risks of LSD use include flashbacks, bad "trips," lingering mental disorders such as severe depression and schizophrenia, and general impairment of mental function. LSD does not produce compulsive drug-seeking behavior, and experts consider it nonaddictive.

3,4-Methylenedioxymethamphetamine

MDMA, also known as Ecstasy or Molly, has been a popular club drug since the 1980s. MDMA use is estimated to reach approximately 3% among high school seniors, and 11.5% among the 18- to 25-year-old age group in 2013 (National Institute on Drug Abuse, 2020). It is considered a hallucinogenic stimulant that is neurotoxic, causing the release of the neurotransmitter serotonin until it is depleted in the brain cells (Fig. 36.2). Because serotonin is involved with regulating mood, aggression, sex drive, sleep, and pain perception, there are many risks of lingering problems. Normal growth and development are altered in adolescents who use MDMA.

MDMA produces physical symptoms of muscle tension, bruxism (grinding of the teeth), nausea, blurred vision, chilling or sweating, and faintness. In high doses, it can trigger malignant hyperthermia, which leads to kidney and heart failure. MDMA gives the user a feeling of euphoria, like being in love. Many people with MDMA addiction use baby pacifiers to ease the teeth-grinding effect. Heat exhaustion results from physical exertion (movement eases muscle tension) and excess fluid loss. Drug effects potentially last 6 hours or longer. Users report drug cravings and lasting psychological difficulties such as confusion, sleep disturbance, poor concentration, and anxiety.

MDMA's parent drug, MDA, has properties similar to those of MDMA and is related to the amphetamine

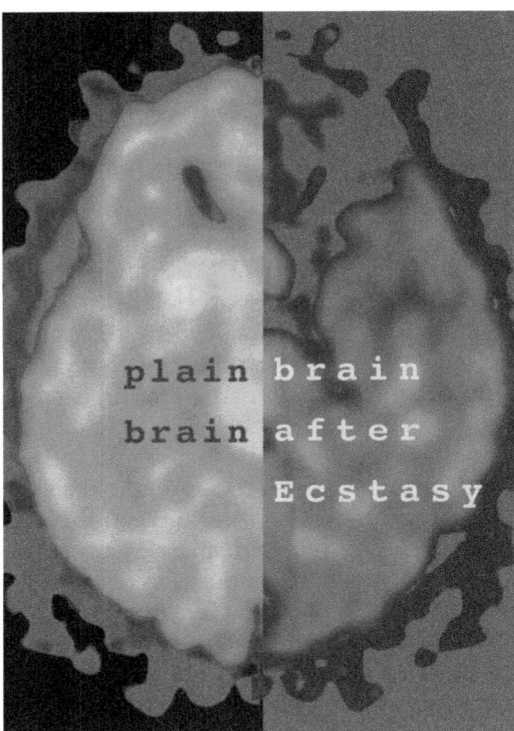

Fig. 36.2 Differences in human brain function with regard to drugs. *Left,* Scan of the brain of an individual who never used drugs; *right,* scan from an individual who had used the club drug 3,4-methylenedioxyamphetamine (MDMA or Ecstasy) many times but had not used any drugs for at least 3 weeks before having the scan. The left, bright-reddish half shows active serotonin sites in the brain. The dark sections in the right half represent serotonin sites that are not present even after 3 weeks without any drugs. In addition to these changes in serotonin sites, Ecstasy injures serotonin neurons. Although these have the capacity to regrow, they do not grow back normally, or sometimes they grow back but in the wrong location. (From National Institute on Drug Abuse, Bethesda, MD, 1999, National Institutes of Health.)

group. Lingering parkinsonian-like tremor has been reported with regular use of this drug.

Ketamine

Ketamine is an anesthetic drug that the US Food and Drug Administration has approved for human and veterinary use. Most ketamine that people sell legally in the United States is intended for veterinary use. Ketamine users either snort or inject it. It produces a dreamlike state with hallucinations. At higher doses, amnesia, impaired motor function, and delirium are possible. Sometimes it is used as a date-rape drug. Fatal respiratory problems have occurred.

Mescaline and Psilocybin

Mescaline and psilocybin are naturally occurring hallucinogens. Mescaline is derived from the peyote cactus. When dried, the round cactus looks like a button. Descendants of the Apache Native American tribe won the legal right to continue peyote use in their religious ceremonies. Psilocybin comes from a mushroom. Both produce the same types of hallucinations and side

effects of LSD, but their effects are not as long-lasting as those of LSD. Because of the general lack of availability, the abuse potentials of these drugs are low.

CANNABIS

People have used cannabis or marijuana for thousands of years. Its first descriptions are in Chinese writings of 2700 BC. No other drug has evoked so much controversy over the appropriateness of legalization and use for medical purposes. Marijuana remains a schedule I drug because of its high abuse and addiction potential in the absence of proven medical use. Evaluation of its therapeutic use as an analgesic, an antiemetic for chemotherapy, a tranquilizer, glaucoma medication, and an antispasmodic for multiple sclerosis has shown only fair results. Medicinal and recreational use of marijuana is legal in some states.

Marijuana and hemp are common names for the herb *Cannabis sativa.* Hashish is the concentrated resin from the plant. Delta-9-tetrahydrocannabinol (THC) is the main active ingredient present in marijuana. Users usually smoke marijuana in a cigarette (or "joint" or "nail") or in a pipe (or "bong"). Marijuana eaten in foods such as brownies produces a longer-lasting effect. Physical effects are short lived, but THC potentially does accumulate in the body because of its fat solubility. THC sometimes remains in the body up to a month or longer after last use; thus, tests for this illegal drug may yield positive results for a long time.

Effects of marijuana include distorted perception; difficulty in problem solving, memory, and learning; euphoria; uncontrolled laughter; increased appetite; dreamy or sleepy affect (being "stoned"); anxiety and panic attacks; dry mouth and dry eyes; increased sexual interest; loss of coordination; and increased heart rate.

Chronic abuse sometimes has long-lasting effects. Some physical effects include a stuffy nose, bronchitis and asthma, lung cancer, abnormal sleeping and eating patterns, decreased testosterone and sperm count, and decreased immune function. Accidents occur because of altered perception and judgment. Some observers report craving and drug-seeking behavior. Psychological effects include panic reactions, hallucinations, and delusions from acute toxicity; organic brain syndrome; and amotivational cannabis syndrome.

Characteristics of amotivational cannabis syndrome are decreased goal-directed activities, abrupt mood swings, abnormal irritability and hostility, apathy, and decline of personal grooming. Depression, paranoia, and suicidal thoughts or attempts are possible. Abstinence reverses this syndrome.

Research on marijuana use among people 18 years of age and younger has shown a trend of lower achievement than in nonusers, more acceptance of deviant and delinquent behavior, poorer relationships with parents, and greater rebelliousness. Marijuana use had remained constant for several years. Sadly, its use has increased and is being combined with the use of vaping devices. More than 40% of 12th-grade students report having vaped marijuana (National Institute on Drug Abuse, 2019). Many of those teenagers who use marijuana as seniors continue to use marijuana into adulthood. It remains the most commonly used illicit drug in the United States.

Some experts consider marijuana a gateway drug similar to alcohol. Many people who abuse other drugs have reported starting with marijuana. Each year, more people enter treatment centers for their primary addiction to marijuana. Some people report withdrawal symptoms, which suggests that physical dependence as well as psychological dependence is possible.

INHALANTS

Inhalants are volatile chemicals that have the capacity to alter thinking and emotions when people inhale them. This group includes solvents, glues, aerosols, refrigerants, and anesthetic gases. The use of inhalants during religious rites and healing ceremonies dates back to ancient Egypt. Today, inhalants are favorite drugs of abuse among young people between the ages of 14 and 17. Inhalants serve, in some cases, as gateway drugs to more dangerous drug abuse.

In the 1960s, the number of reports about abuse of model airplane glue, lighter fluid, and cleaning fluids grew rapidly. The federal government banned the use of carbon tetrachloride after reports attributed a number of deaths to it and benzene. Rates of use are higher among people from minority groups, such as Mexican Americans and Native Americans. Men are more likely to abuse inhalants than are women. Users in a group setting sometimes put solvents onto a cloth or into a paper or plastic bag and pass it around; inhaling in this way is sometimes called huffing. Effects are short lived and include a euphoric or intoxicated feeling, auditory hallucinations, feeling weightless or floating on air, ataxia, slurred speech, wheezing, cough, photophobia, irregular heartbeat, anorexia, and nausea. High doses pose the risk of respiratory arrest and irreversible damage to the brain, kidneys, or other organs. Most fatalities have occurred with butane, adhesive solvents, and cleaning fluid solvents containing toluene and other halogenated hydrocarbons.

Some people used anesthetic gases, chloroform, and ether as anesthetics and parlor entertainment until less-flammable gases gained notoriety. Nitrous oxide (laughing gas), which dentists use today, is available as a street drug and in balloons at outdoor festival activities. After inhalation, its effects last only a few minutes. "Whippets" are nitrous oxide cartridges for commercial use. Amyl nitrate and butyl nitrate ("poppers"), whose proper use is to treat heart disease, are cloth-covered ampules that a user has to break and inhale.

Most inhalants are not detected in a routine drug screen, but people who use them chronically sometimes develop organic brain disorders, general myalgia and neuritis, mood disorders, and cognitive impairment. Liver and kidney failure are possible results of chronic exposure to inhalants (Table 36.2).

CHEMICALLY IMPAIRED NURSES

An estimated 10% of nurses in the United States have a drug dependency problem. The high-stress work environment, potential for work-related injuries, and accessibility to drugs are believed to be contributing factors. In 1982, the American Nurses Association adopted a policy that recommends offering treatment to chemically impaired nurses before taking disciplinary action. Today, most states have programs that offer chemically impaired nurses the option to receive treatment and rehabilitation in order to keep their license. Nurses who are referred for monitoring programs will be expected to enter into a recovery agreement. Failure to remain compliant or complete the programming may result in licensure sanction.

Nurses are as vulnerable as the general public to substance abuse and addiction. Denial by the abuser as well as by colleagues may be intense. Many of the same indicators of substance abuse that are evident in patients appear in addicted nurses. Family history, a chronic medical condition necessitating opioid analgesics, physical signs and symptoms of use, memory loss, mood swings, and changes in work performance and work relationships sometimes point to substance abuse.

Some nurses who abuse drugs request to work the night shift or assignments that facilitate access to drugs. Behaviors indicating possible use on the job include frequent trips to the bathroom, with behavioral changes noted afterward, and sudden absence from the unit. Impaired nurses become illogical and careless in performing documentation responsibilities and duties. Discrepancies in narcotics counts, patients who feel less pain relief when a particular nurse is on duty, and unusual variation in the quantity of medications dispensed to the patients on the unit are indications of drug diversion by an impaired nurse.

As addiction progresses, an impaired nurse sometimes signs out medications and reports spillage. Some impaired nurses steal drugs from patients' bedsides after the supply count for the shift is done. Some nurses have stolen entire deliveries with the sign-out sheets and then claimed that it was an accounting error (Box 36.10).

Impaired nurses put their patients at risk for injury, medication error, and slower recovery. It is important for nursing colleagues to report suspect behavior. It is the duty of every nurse to uphold the standards of the profession. Most state boards of nursing accept anonymous tips. These reports do require verification. The nursing boards have the resources to initiate an investigation into the complaint. Although it is easy to ignore or cover up the problem, reporting suspicious behavior anonymously or to the supervisor will begin

Table 36.2   Acute Intoxication and Withdrawal of Psychoactive Substances

SIGNS AND SYMPTOMS	TREATMENT	WITHDRAWAL SYMPTOMS
Alcohol		
Behavior dependent on blood serum levels: slurred speech; ataxia; blurred vision; decreased level of consciousness; possible nausea, vomiting, and diarrhea; loss of consciousness and respiratory depression with a high blood level	Maintain ventilation. Position unconscious patient lying on the side. Monitor vital signs every 30–60 min until they are stable. Check emesis and stool for occult blood. Offer fluids and small amounts of bland foods when swallowing ability is intact. Allow the patient to get up as tolerated, but prevent overexertion. Give thiamine as ordered; possible to give IM or IV initially, then PO daily. Give sedative as ordered for tremor and restlessness; watch for urine retention with a high dosage of chlordiazepoxide (Librium); some health care providers order naltrexone or lorazepam (Ativan). Seizure medications such as phenytoin (Dilantin) or magnesium sulfate may be given if indicated. Provide teaching of health risks. Encourage patients to seek a recovery program such as AA.	Mild to severe tremors of the hands, jaw, torso Restlessness, pacing Illogical thinking Demanding, drug craving Manipulating Diaphoresis Chain smoking Visual and auditory hallucinations Confusion If the patient is unable to reorient, appears panicked, and temperature is elevated, suspect DTs.
CNS Depressants (Including Barbiturates, Benzodiazepines, Narcotics)		
Range of relaxation to sleepiness to coma; depressed vital signs; pinpoint pupils; respiratory depression	Lavage if ingestion was recent. Maintain ventilation. Position unconscious patient lying on the side. Monitor vital signs every 15–30 min until stable. Administer drugs as ordered for cardiac dysrhythmias. Barbiturate dosages must be tapered down to reduce the risk of status epilepticus. Maintenance therapy can start with methadone or LAAM. Clonidine may be given for opioid withdrawal, as may naltrexone (ReVia). Provide teaching concerning health risks. Encourage the patient to seek a recovery program.	Opioids: restlessness, yawning, lacrimation, diaphoresis, rhinorrhea, anorexia, abdominal cramping, body ache, tremors, gooseflesh, insomnia, drug craving, possible seizures with barbiturates, symptoms such as DTs.
CNS Stimulants (Including Cocaine, Amphetamines, MDMA)		
Elevated vital sign values, cardiac dysrhythmias, flushing or pallor, agitation, paranoia, fever, convulsions, cardiac arrest	Monitor vital signs. Provide a quiet environment. Reorient patient to reality. Encourage consumption of fluids and nutrition. Give cardiac drugs as ordered; beta blockers (Inderal) and calcium channel blockers (Procardia) can be administered for dysrhythmias. Amantadine (Symmetrel) and other antiparkinsonian drugs may be given to reduce cocaine craving. Provide teaching concerning health risks. Encourage the patient to seek a recovery program.	Mild withdrawal: apathy, somnolence, fatigue, irritability, depression Severe withdrawal: drug craving, "crashing," depression, paranoia, suicidal ideation, tachycardia, heart failure, malnutrition.
Hallucinogens (Including LSD, PCP, Ketamine, MDMA)		
Strong psychological effects; emotional lability (laughing or crying); acute panic attacks; acute psychosis from a bad "trip"; flashback episodes	Provide a quiet supportive environment. Remind the patient that experience from the drug will subside when the drug is out of the body. Monitor vital signs routinely. Some health care providers order an antianxiety drug for severe anxiety or agitation. Encourage consumption of fluids. Provide teaching concerning the health risks and possible permanent damage.	No evidence of withdrawal symptoms.

Continued

Table 36.2	Acute Intoxication and Withdrawal of Psychoactive Substances—cont'd		
SIGNS AND SYMPTOMS	**TREATMENT**		**WITHDRAWAL SYMPTOMS**
Cannabis			
Mild anxiety to panic attacks, emotional lability, increased appetite, dilated pupils, dry mouth, dry eyes, drowsiness	Provide supportive environment. Give antianxiety medication as ordered for agitation. Provide teaching concerning health risks and amotivational cannabis syndrome.		Mild withdrawal symptoms: drug craving, irritability, anorexia, insomnia.
Inhalants			
Usually short-acting effects: euphoria, intoxication	Usually, chronic use impairs cardiopulmonary function and causes hepatic and renal failure. Provide teaching concerning health risks (e.g., plastic bags lead to possible suffocation death).		No withdrawal symptoms; drug craving by chronic users noted.

AA, Alcoholics Anonymous; *CNS,* central nervous system; *DTs,* delirium tremens; *IM,* intramuscular (route); *IV,* intravenous (route); *LAAM,* levo-alpha-acetylmethadol; *LSD,* lysergic acid diethylamide; *MDMA,* 3,4-methylenedioxymethamphetamine; *PCP,* phencyclidine.

Box 36.10	**Warning Signs of Nurse Impairment**

When observing a nurse who is suspected of impairment observations of appearance, behaviors and dispensing of controlled substances may be impacted.
Changes in job performance:
- Absences from the unit for extended periods
- Frequent trips to the bathroom
- Arriving late or leaving early
- Making an excessive number of mistakes, including medication errors.

Behavioral changes can be physical:
- Subtle alterations in appearance that escalate overtime
- Increasing isolation from colleagues
- Inappropriate verbal or emotional responses
- Diminished alertness, confusion, or memory lapses.
- **When nurses are abusing drugs and are unable to obtain them from a treating health care provider, they may turn to the workplace for access, often causing narcotics discrepancies.** Incorrect controlled substance counts
- Large amounts of controlled substance wastage
- Numerous corrections of medication records
- Frequent reports of ineffective pain relief from patients
- Offers to medicate coworkers' patients for pain
- Altered verbal or phone medication orders

Variations in controlled substance discrepancies among shifts or days of the week.
From National Council State Boards of Nursing. A Nurse Manager's Guide to Substance Abuse Disorder in Nursing. https://www.ncsbn.org/Mgr_SUDiN_Brochure_2014.pdf

the healing process for an impaired nurse. Other nurses should report observations objectively and keep a diary in case it becomes necessary to recall an event. When action is necessary, the supervisor or the state board of nursing contacts the peer assistance program. Sometimes investigation reveals that mental illness, rather than drug abuse, is responsible for the behavioral manifestations. Either way, people in authority will approach the nurse and ask him or her to seek treatment.

Peer assistance programs (called *diversion programs* in some states) are usually under the jurisdiction of the state board of nursing. These programs administer contract agreements requiring that the nurse undergo treatment and monitoring for a period of several years to keep his or her license in good standing. Many programs have requirements of continued attendance at Alcoholics Anonymous or Narcotics Anonymous, with random drug screening as part of the monitoring during return to work. Nurses having permission to continue employment will have worksite monitoring. The worksite monitor submits reports of the nurse's performance and any identified areas of concern. Some job modification is necessary in some cases to reduce stress and decrease the opportunity for relapse. These programs maintain confidentiality as much as possible, but it is necessary for a nurse to notify employers if he or she is in the program. It is not permitted in most states to subpoena any records the program keeps.

In 1999, the US Department of Health and Human Services established a national data bank, **Healthcare Integrity and Protection Data Bank (HIPDB).** It requires federal and state government agencies (including nursing boards and health agencies) to report all final adverse actions taken against a health care provider, supplier, or practitioner since August 1996. This provides an incentive for impaired nurses to enter treatment and avoid any final action that must be reported to the HIPDB.

Finally, nurses who are suffering from addiction or another health problem that affects performance on the job must be truthful and seek help. Being proactive results in benefits to his or her own personal life and career, to the welfare of patients, and to the overall functioning of the health care setting.

Get Ready for the NCLEX® Examination!

Key Points

- Many patients who enter acute care facilities with other diagnoses also have problems with drug and alcohol abuse.
- *Substance abuse* and *drug dependency* are terms often used interchangeably in reference to addiction.
- Alcoholism is a chronic, incurable, progressive disease.
- Common traits of an addictive personality include low tolerance for stress; dependency; negative self-image; depression; and feelings of insecurity.
- The three distinct stages of dependence disease are early, middle, and late.
- Morality-based theories about alcoholism are falling in favor because of biological findings. Changes in brain activity, hepatic enzyme deficiencies, and genetic links prove the existence of a disease process.
- Alcohol and drug use weaves its way into the multicultural society of the United States through family traditions, peer pressure, and mass media advertising.
- Chronic alcohol abuse is toxic to multiple organs and results in the development of physical disorders.
- Denial and delusions are coping mechanisms common among untreated substance abusers.
- Maintaining a professional, nonjudgmental attitude when communicating about use sometimes allows the user to be honest about use.
- The goal of detoxification is to keep the patient free from complications while ridding the body of the substance.
- Safety is of primary concern during detoxification.
- Malnourishment occurs in many people who chronically abuse alcohol or drugs.
- Like illegal drugs, over-the-counter drugs and prescription drugs are abused.
- Street drugs pose a risk of severe side effects and sometimes permanent damage because there are no controls in the manufacturing of these drugs.
- Peer assistance programs are available for helping impaired nurses into recovery without taking away the privilege to practice nursing.

Additional Learning Resources

SG Go to your Study Guide for additional learning activities to help you master this chapter content.

Be sure to visit the Evolve site at http://evolve.elsevier.com/Cooper/foundations/ for additional online resources.

Review Questions for the NCLEX® Examination

1. An early age at the onset of drinking alcohol is a strong risk factor for developing which disorder?
   1. Alzheimer's disease
   2. Alcohol or substance abuse
   3. Resistance to chemical dependency
   4. Immunity to alcohol

2. In all deaths related to motor vehicles and fatal intentional injuries, alcohol is involved in what percentage of them?
   1. 7%
   2. 10%
   3. 17%
   4. 38%

3. Two days after surgery, a patient is agitated and asking to be discharged home because he cannot get any rest in the hospital. Slight tremors in his hands are noted. The admission records indicate that the patient states he does not use alcohol or drugs. Which coping mechanism is this patient probably using?
   1. Denial
   2. Regression
   3. Guilt
   4. Hostility

4. A patient was found unconscious in his apartment with four empty bottles of whiskey and was brought to the hospital by his family. Upon admission, he moans out loud and is having dry heaves and diarrhea. What is the best way to maintain his airway?
   1. Elevate the head of the bed to ease breathing, and place an emesis basin on the patient's lap.
   2. Place the patient in the side-lying position until the swallowing reflex is intact.
   3. Adjust the bed to the reverse Trendelenburg position until the patient regains consciousness.
   4. Tape an oral suction catheter in place to avoid aspiration.

5. What area of the brain is affected most often by psychoactive substances and has the potential to sustain permanent damage?
   1. Brainstem
   2. Limbic system
   3. Cerebellum
   4. Corpus callosum

6. A patient with a history of alcoholism nervousness has escalated, and this evening he keeps looking over his shoulder. He shouts out, "There's a fire!" Upon entering his room, the nurse finds the patient huddled in a corner, diaphoretic and with a fearful expression. The nurse reassures him that there is no fire and assesses him, finding the following: blood pressure of 160/95, pulse rate of 132, respiration rate of 30, and temperature of 100°F. Which of these manifestations is consistent with delirium tremens? *(Select all that apply.)*
   1. Fever
   2. Abdominal cramping
   3. Nervousness
   4. Fear
   5. Disorientation

7. A 25-year-old patient entered the hospital with diagnoses of septicemia and infective endocarditis. He admits to using IV heroin regularly. For what withdrawal symptoms should the nurse monitor?

   1. Red rash similar to that of chickenpox
   2. Head cold and flulike signs and symptoms
   3. Intractable singultus
   4. Severe joint pain and back pain

8. The nurse is caring for a patient who is in the emergency department after a suspected "date rape." What benzodiazepine drug is most likely to be suspect?

   1. Diazepam (Valium)
   2. Flunitrazepam (Rohypnol)
   3. PCP
   4. LSD

9. The nurse is caring for a patient who has been using MDMA (Ecstasy). Why is this substance considered to be neurotoxic?

   1. Serotonin is depleted in the brain, which damages brain cells.
   2. Dehydration causes neurologic damage.
   3. Heart damage results from malignant hyperthermia.
   4. Inner ear damage leads to deafness.

10. Amotivational cannabis syndrome is suspected in a patient. What findings would support this diagnosis? *(Select all that apply.)*

    1. Periods of euphoria
    2. Obsession with personal hygiene
    3. Apathy
    4. Sharp increases in appetite, commonly referred to as the "munchies"
    5. Irritability

11. A nurse with a history of drug-related charges has action taken against her practitioner's license. Where is this reported?

    1. National Health and Welfare Records Department
    2. Healthcare Management Organization of the United States
    3. Federal Drug Enforcement Agency
    4. Healthcare Integrity and Protection Data Bank

12. A patient is scheduled for abdominal surgery. He tells the nurse that his uncle became addicted to narcotics after his surgery; fearing that he too could become addicted, he does not want to receive any narcotics. What is the nurse's most appropriate response?

    1. "Don't worry. You can refuse to take them."
    2. "Usually narcotics are given in the first few days after surgery; then you will be given a milder pain reliever for your pain. You will not be given narcotics long enough to become addicted."
    3. "Your fear of addiction is unfounded, but I will tell your health care provider about your concern."
    4. "I've never heard of anyone getting hooked on narcotics after surgery."

13. The nurse is ready to give the end-of-shift report to the nurse in charge of the unit for the next shift. When the oncoming nurse arrives 15 minutes late, she does not make eye contact, she smells of mints, her hands are trembling, her uniform is disheveled, and her shoes are untied. She asks no questions regarding any patients and leaves the room when the report is completed. What should the first nurse do?

    1. Go home because the shift is completed.
    2. Call the supervisor and report observations.
    3. Stay on the unit until she is sure the oncoming nurse has no questions regarding the patients.
    4. Call the state board of nursing and report the oncoming nurse's behavior.

14. A patient has begun a substance abuse outpatient treatment program and is allowed to return to work with supervision. Which statement by the patient indicates that she is recovering from her substance abuse problem?

    1. "I wish I knew who turned me in to administration; I would like to give that nosy witch a piece of my mind!"
    2. "Just because I had a glass of wine with a meal before I came to work once or twice, I'm going to be watched like a hawk. What a pain!"
    3. "I realize that I'm going to have to regain the trust of my coworkers and administrators, but I can do that, one day at a time."
    4. "If other people took their jobs as seriously as I take mine, they wouldn't have time to rat on other people."

15. The nurse is performing a physical assessment on a patient who has a history of long-term cocaine use. Which finding is indicative of long-term cocaine use?

    1. Constricted pupils
    2. Red, irritated nostrils
    3. Conjunctival redness
    4. Muscle aches

16. A person addicted to heroin is likely to exhibit which symptoms of withdrawal? *(Select all that apply.)*

    1. Nausea and vomiting, diarrhea, and diaphoresis
    2. Tremors, insomnia, and hypotension
    3. Incoordination and unsteady gait
    4. Decreased heart rate and flushing
    5. Chills and fever

17. A patient has begun attending AA meetings. Which statement reflects the patient's understanding of the purpose of this organization?

    1. "I will attend meetings and have a support person to help me stay sober. I must not drink any alcohol again."
    2. "I'll dry out in AA, and then I can have a social drink once in a while."
    3. "AA is only for people who have reached the bottom."
    4. "If I lose my job, AA will help me find another."

18. The nurse is caring for a patient who is in the acute care unit for elective surgery. What findings during the patient's hospitalization would be consistent with alcohol withdrawal? *(Select all that apply.)*

    1. Euphoria and hyperactivity
    2. Depression and hypersomnia
    3. Diaphoresis and nausea
    4. Below normal temperature and bradycardia
    5. Vomiting and tremors

19. The nurse has completed an educational program on impaired nurses. Which statements by a participant indicated the teaching was successful? *(Select all that apply.)*

    1. "Impaired nurses tend to work day shift so their patients are awake and will request more pain medication."
    2. "Frequent bathroom breaks with varied behavior may be an indication of an impaired nurse."
    3. "Impaired nurses commit all medication errors."
    4. "Patients being cared for by impaired nurses may complain of inadequate pain control."
    5. "Nurses who are impaired cannot work as a nurse until they complete a recovery program."

20. The nurse is reviewing a patient's chart admitted with substance abuse. The nurse notes that the previous nurse charted that the patient has developed tolerance. Which statement by the patient would support this?

    1. "When I wake up in the morning, my hands shake until I take my first drink."
    2. "I used to drink 4 to 5 drinks every night but now I drink 10 to 12 drinks to feel the same way."
    3. "My wife won't quit nagging me to quit drinking. I work hard and deserve the chance to relax."
    4. "I think I've hit rock bottom. I need help to quit drinking."

21. A nurse, 47, has been working at the same nursing home with an excellent performance record for the past 7 years. Then, a few months ago, she began crying at work, shouting into her cell phone while moving from room to room, and losing her temper with both patients and staff. She was given a warning by the nurse leader, who learned that the nurse was going through a painful and messy divorce. She was given a week off with pay but then needed to get back to work. When she returned on the night shift, at first things seemed back to normal, except that she was making frequent trips to the bathroom and staff noticed more mood swings and apparent memory loss. She also began to seem a little reckless with detailed tasks like documentation and now a new problem has arisen. Three patients on Klonopin (clonazepam) have begun experiencing increased pain during the nights, while documentation shows they have received their meds. A closer inspection, however, showed an unusual discrepancy in the quantity of medications apparently dispensed to other patients. A diversion of these drugs is suspected. A meeting between the two floor leaders raises suspicions that this same nurse may be stealing clonazepam for her own use. Still, they would need more specific signs before making such an accusation. Which of these additional behaviors would support possible theft and misuse of Klonopin?

Use an X to indicate which behavior is associated with each drug's effects of overuse. All should be used and can be used only once.

ASSESSMENT FINDINGS	CNS DEPRESSANT EFFECTS	CNS STIMULANT EFFECTS
Pinpoint pupils		
Dilated pupils		
Euphoria		
Anxiety and paranoia		
Bruxism		
Ataxic gait		
Slurred speech		
Listlessness		

CNS, Central nervous system.

37

Home Health Nursing

Objectives

1. List at least three types of home health (HH) agencies.
2. Summarize governmental financing possibilities for HH nursing.
3. Discuss new developments that are occurring in HH care, including remote electronic monitoring.
4. Relate seven steps to breaking through cultural barriers to communication.
5. List at least four services possible to provide with HH care.
6. Define skilled nursing services.
7. Describe the role of the licensed practical/vocational nurse (LPN/LVN) in the delivery of skilled nursing care.
8. Relate the nursing process to HH care practice.
9. List two sources of reimbursement for home care services.

Key Terms

accreditation (ă-crĕd-ĭ-TĀ-shŭn, p. 1184)
certification (sŭr-tĭ-fĭ-KĀ-shŭn, p. 1184)
diagnosis-related groups (DRGs) (p. 1183)
home health care (p. 1182)

Medicaid (p. 1192)
Medicare (p. 1192)
telehealth services (p. 1186)

Recently, a shift to community-based care has led to an increased number of acutely ill home care patients, which changes demands on health care providers. Home health care services enable individuals of all ages to remain in the comfort and security of their homes while receiving health care. Family support, familiar surroundings, and participation in the care process contribute to feelings of worth and dignity. Possible services include skilled nursing, physical therapy, psychiatric therapy, pain education and management, speech and language therapy, occupational therapy, social services, intravenous (IV) therapy, nutritional support, respiratory therapy, acquisition of medical supplies and equipment, home health (HH) aide, homemaker, pet care assistance, and companion care.

Patients most often receive referrals for HH services on discharge from the hospital. However, the patient, the family, or the health care provider can request HH care at other times.

For qualified coverage by Medicare, a health maintenance organization (HMO), or various types of insurance, the patient must be "homebound," meaning unable to leave the home or needing a great deal of effort to travel for appointments to see the health care provider. The health care provider will create a plan of care for the patient with regular reviews. In addition, the patient plan of care certifies that the patient is in need of intermittent skilled services, nursing, or therapy (Medicare.gov, n.d.a.).

In 2018, patients older than 65 years account for more than 88.6% of all HH patients, with 33% 85 years and older. Patients of all ages with various diagnoses account for the rest(Centers for Medicare and Medicaid Services [CMS], 2020). On discharge from a hospital or a rehabilitation center, patients who have had a stroke, chronic obstructive pulmonary disease, fractured hips with or without surgical interventions, and joint replacement procedures often are referred to HH agencies. HH care includes wound care, ostomy assistance, setting up of oral medications, prefilling of insulin syringes, administration of injections, IV administration, nutrition therapy, postoperative assistance for patients who have undergone total hip and total knee replacements, and monitoring of patients with heart failure, diabetes, and hypertension Medicare.gov, n.d.b.). The frequency and length of HH visits vary depending on the services needed. The visits occur sometimes as often as twice daily and as seldom as monthly.

Health care providers are referring patients to home care more today than ever before. Advancing technology has enabled more care to be delivered in the home. Americans are living longer and thus have more health concerns that necessitate care. The length of hospital stays continues to shrink, resulting in an increasing number of patients who need nursing care on discharge from the facility.

The best approach to patient care is one of teamwork and blending of disciplines. The licensed practical/vocational nurse (LPN/LVN) is a valuable member of this important health care team. Registered nurses (RNs) are involved primarily in case management, the administration and management of agencies, and the supervision of nursing interventions. Although home care traditionally has been a part of public and community health services, its focus is now much narrower.

HOME HEALTH CARE DEFINED

HH care preserves individual independence and integrity and keeps families together. The following are definitions of HH care as viewed from four different perspectives:

- *Official:* A component of comprehensive health care in which individuals and their families receive services in their place of residence for the purpose of promoting, maintaining, or restoring health, or of minimizing the effects of illness and disability.
- *Patient:* Skilled and compassionate care provided on a one-to-one basis in the comforting and familiar surroundings of the home. Providers base care on individual needs and personalized schedules and do so over a given period to enable adjustment, change, and learning to take place effectively.
- *Family:* A means to keep the family together as a functioning, integrated unit. The goals are learning to adapt to change, preventing dysfunctional patterns from setting in, and attaining family wellness within the scope of an individual member's illness or disability. It provides needed emotional support and linkage with the larger community support systems.
- *Provider:* Challenges all disciplines involved to provide excellent care in often less-than-excellent conditions and surroundings. Independence, creativity, communication, and excellent clinical skills are integral aspects of daily practice. It is an opportunity for nurses to demonstrate the best of their profession and themselves in cooperation with the health care team to patients and families with physical and psychological needs.

HISTORICAL OVERVIEW

A series of legislative events have facilitated the growth and expansion of HH care. In 1965, Title XVIII (known as Medicare) and Title XIX (known as Medicaid) amendments to the Social Security Act were passed, which directly affected HH care. Medicare provided direct federal funds for the health care of all citizens 65 years and older (or disabled), regardless of socioeconomic status. The companion Medicaid bill covered the care needs of the poor and indigent of all ages. When Medicare became effective in 1966, it revolutionized home care by (1) changing it to a medical rather than nursing model of practice; (2) defining and limiting the services it reimbursed; and (3) changing the payment source and even changing the reason for providing home care (see the Lifespan Considerations for older adults box).

Lifespan Considerations
Older Adults

Home Care Services

- The growing number of older adults has resulted in an increased need for HH care services.
- Early discharge policies have resulted in very ill older adults leaving the hospital. This increases the importance of patient teaching, early discharge planning, and appropriate referral to HH agencies by hospital staff nurses.
- Many older adults do not need total care but do need a limited amount of assistance. Home care reduces disruption of lifestyle and is more cost effective than institutional placement.
- Transfer to a hospital or nursing home even on a temporary basis increases the stress level of older people. Stress is decreased if they receive care in a familiar environment.
- Caregivers must learn the importance of preserving the older adult's autonomy and make any modifications to the home environment with consideration of the older adult's physical strengths and remaining functional abilities, not just the patient's disabilities.
- Many agencies assist older adults in their communities. The services offered by some of these agencies include Meals on Wheels, HH aides, homemakers, and home-based physical therapy services. Be familiar with HH services available in your area of service.

The next major influence on home care occurred in 1983. Congress enacted the prospective payment system (PPS) as a part of the Tax Equity and Fiscal Responsibility Act for hospitals receiving Medicare reimbursement. This system, based on major diagnostic categories and diagnosis-related groups (DRGs), pays a set rate (according to diagnosis) for the hospitalized patient's care rather than the "cost," or charges an institution traditionally bills according to its own schedule of fees. The net effect of the change was a major shift of patients out of hospitals and into their homes, extended-care facilities, or skilled nursing facilities. Discharge for such patients occurred earlier in their convalescence; thus, the patient needed more nursing care. This created a challenge to home care in terms of the volume of patients seen, the need to provide more skilled nursing care over more intensive periods, and the evolution of highly technical procedures in the home. Existing agencies expanded, and new ones developed to meet the demand.

In an effort to control HH expenditures, Congress imposed new limits on HH payments through a provision of the Balanced Budget Act of 1997 (BBA) called the interim payment system (IPS). Until BBA, there were no limits on payment for covered HH services provided to qualifying patients as long as visit costs were within "reasonable" cost limits. To reduce the growth in HH, the IPS imposed lower per-visit limits and imposed a new agency-specific, aggregate per-beneficiary limit based on agencies' federal fiscal year spending in 1994 (CMS, 2021).

The effects of IPS were more far reaching than either Congress or the Health Care Financing Administration (HCFA) intended, producing a reduction in beneficiaries served and a reduction in overall expenditures, leading to a reduction to use of HH care services in some instances. The effect on individual agencies that were unable to maintain costs within per-visit and per-beneficiary limits was devastating. Once the current PPS was put into place in the year 2000, HH care use saw a rise again. According to 2018 statistics, 11,170 Medicare-certified HH agencies were in operation throughout the United States. The number of beneficiaries receiving HH care services was 3,365,951, and 103,969,027 home visits were made (CMS, 2020).

BBA provided the authority for the development of a PPS for HH, which went into effect in 2000. With HH PPS, Medicare pays providers of HH services at fixed predetermined rates for services and supplies to cover an episode of care during a specific 60-day period. The goal of PPS is to produce incentives for the HH provider to be more efficient in the delivery of HH services and still remain financially viable. The goal is for HH care agencies to be more cognizant of limiting excess expenditures, thus saving money paid out by Medicare. This is especially important given the concerns that have arisen over the last several years about the amount of funds available through Medicare. In 2016, the Home Health Value-Based Purchasing Model was implemented to provide incentives to Medicare-certified HH agencies with the goal of achieving higher quality and more efficient care (CMS, 2019).

Home care visits and Medicare expenditures for home care quadrupled between 1980 and 1991. This was attributed directly to shorter hospitalizations, more seriously ill patients being discharged to home, and increased acceptance of the delivery of higher technological care in the home. HH care grew five times faster than the average of other health care industries between 1990 and 1997 and accounted for more than 6% of health service jobs. The annual growth rate for HH care had been 1.7% in 2010, a 20% increase from 2002 with a slight decrease in costs. (Morse, 2017). The industry continues to grow today.

TYPES OF HOME CARE AGENCIES

In the broadest terms, delivery of home care services is possible by any individual, service group, organization, or agency with the desire to provide services to the older adult, disabled, or ill of any age. The type and qualifications of personnel used, the quality of services delivered, and the standards of care can vary widely, and these often depend on funding sources. The agency typically has to comply with federal, state, and local laws and regulations via the following:

- *Licensure by the state.* This gives legal permission to operate within that state only. Regulations vary widely. Not all states have such laws.
- *Certification by the state certifying body that the federal government designates.* The federal government sets the rules that govern **certification** (a process in which the government evaluates and recognizes an individual, institution, or educational program as meeting certain predetermined standards). Only certified agencies are permitted to receive Medicare payments. Many states piggyback Medicaid reimbursement to certification, as do some insurers.
- *Certificate of need.* Some states grant this according to rules and formulas that state regulators devise. Cost of starting and running the agency, availability of personnel, and need for their services generally are considered in this process.
- Accreditation by an outside agency that evaluates and judges how well the agency meets certain standards that the accrediting organization sets. An agency sometimes obtains this **accreditation** (a process whereby a professional association or nongovernmental agency grants recognition to a school or institution for demonstrated ability in a special area of practice or training) from organizations such as the National League for Nursing Community Health Accreditation Program, The Joint Commission, or the Community Health Accreditation Partner (CHAP). Other groups sometimes grant accreditation to special programs or specialized agencies. Some of these national accrediting agencies are seeking "deemed status" from federal regulators, which allows their accreditation also to serve as the required certification. This eliminates the need for separate surveys for some agencies.

Before Medicare, the provision of HH care was primarily the task of visiting nurse associations, nursing divisions of state or local health departments, and hospitals. Now agencies are classified according to (1) *tax status,* for profit or not for profit; (2) *location,* freestanding or institution-based; and (3) *governance,* private or public. Table 37.1 summarizes the six generally accepted types of HH agencies. The structure of some of these agencies is subject to change and variation. For example, some visiting nurse associations have reorganized and placed their HH agencies into private, nonprofit structures to ensure reimbursement that covers the cost of providing services.

Growth in the number of agencies has mirrored the growth of home care. Although the late 1980s saw a decrease in agencies, the numbers rebounded, largely

Table **37.1**   **Home Health Agencies**

STATUS	GOVERNANCE	SOURCE OF SUPPORT	SERVICES OFFERED	NATURE OF STAFF	TIME OF SERVICE	EXAMPLE
Voluntary						
Public; nonprofit; freestanding	Community-based board of directors	Tax-deductible contributions; grants; fees from all sources	Community health; public health; home health	RN; LPN/LVN; aide; homemaker; social worker; therapists	Generally 30min to 8h	Visiting nurse association
Official						
Public; nonprofit; freestanding	State, county, city, or other local unit of government and volunteer board representatives of the area	State, local, or county revenues; grants; fees from limited sources; charitable contributions	Community health; public health; home health	RN; LPN/LVN; aide; homemaker; social worker; therapists	Generally 30min to 4h	State health departments; county health departments; city health departments
Combination						
Public; nonprofit; freestanding	Jointly operated by the two types of agencies previously mentioned under a combined board of directors	State, local, or county revenues; grants; fees from limited sources; charitable contributions	Community health; public health; home health	RN; LPN/LVN; aide; homemaker; social worker; therapists	Generally 30min to 4h	County-based visiting nurse association
Hospital						
Private; nonprofit or for profit; institution-based; hospital	Hospital board of directors	Fees from all sources	Home health; community health (limited)	RN; LPN/LVN; aide; social worker; therapists	Generally 30min to 4h	XYZ hospital home health agency
Proprietary						
Private; for profit; freestanding	Governed and owned by individual, corporation, or other organization; many paid boards of directors appointed by the owner	Fees from most sources; some do and some do not participate in Medicare-Medicaid	Some offer limited home health; private duty; homemaker	RN; LPN/LVN; aide	1–24h	Home health care of XYZ
Private Not for Profit						
Private; not for profit; freestanding	Governed and owned by individual, corporation, or other organizational structure; board appointed by the owner	Fees from most sources; some do and some do not participate in Medicare-Medicaid	Some offer limited home health services; private duty; homemaker	RN; LPN/LVN; aide	30min to 24h	ABC home health agency
Other						
Private; for profit or nonprofit; institution-based	Based within a formalized institution; governed by that board or designated board	Fees from all sources	Home health services; limited homemaker	RN; LPN/LVN; aide; therapists; may have homemaker; social worker	30min to 8h	ABC nursing home—home health agency; ABC rehabilitation facility; home care

LPN/LVN, Licensed practical/vocational nurse; *RN*, registered nurse.

Fig. 37.1 Telehealth care. (Courtesy Philips Healthcare. Used with permission.)

because of increases in hospital-based agencies and specialized agencies that provide highly technical types of care, including IV therapies, peripherally inserted central catheter (PICC) line care, and ventilator-dependent care services. A newer method of care delivery is telehealth services. This innovative approach to the provision of care allows for patient and care provider interaction and monitoring through the use of telephones, computers, televisions, and two-way monitors. The use of technology allows patient care to take place outside of the traditional inpatient setting. A computerized system can call a patient on the telephone at home and ask recorded questions such as, "What is your blood pressure?" The patient is able to respond by using the phone's keypad. In this way, the nurse is able to review the patient's progress efficiently without making a home visit. Over the past several years, advances in technology and forward-thinking HH agencies have helped spur a jump in the adoption of telemonitoring for HH patients. Advantages include a return of the patient to the family unit, conservation of financial resources, family participation in care delivery, and increased care delivery options in rural settings or settings at a distance from the health care provider (Nelson & Staggers, 2017) (Fig. 37.1). For example, a patient with recently diagnosed diabetes can receive telehealth monitoring with the use of a glucometer to read blood sugar, which may be transmitted electronically to a health care provider, who then may evaluate the results for the need of additional intervention without having to visit the patient.

CHANGES IN HOME HEALTH CARE

Some recent changes have occurred in HH care, including the establishment of ethics committees to handle ethical issues that arise in the home. Another includes Medicare reimbursing psychiatric nurse clinicians for home visits. Psychiatric patients are required to be under the care of a psychiatrist and have a psychiatric diagnosis. The psychiatric nurse clinician provides therapy and education and counsels family members.

Social workers have been taking a more active role in HH care. Social workers provide assistance with a patient's emotional, financial, and household problems, thus allowing the nurse more time to perform nursing interventions.

More HH agencies are employing nurse pain specialists to assess and manage pain control in the home. They can provide education to patients and staff and provide greater benefits in the relief of pain and reduce the cost of ineffective pain management.

Most agencies are obtaining a separate Medicare certification to provide hospice care. Medicare-certified hospices receive per diem payments rather than a fee for the visit. This method of payment is more economical for insurers and taxpayers.

Pet care programs are a new inclusion in some areas to reduce stress for HH patients who are too ill to care for their pets. A "durable power of attorney for pet care" allows patients to make arrangements for pet care if they become hospitalized or die. Some HH agencies provide special pet services, such as the transportation of pets to veterinarian appointments or in-home pet care.

One of the most rapidly growing segments in HH is home infusion therapy; an increasing number of HH agencies are offering home infusion services in an effort to compete for patient referrals. Health care facilities are eager to have HH agencies provide this service because home IV therapy complements their cost-cutting strategies. Until the 1980s, patients needing infusion therapies were managed by admission to hospitals or long-term care facilities, resulting in elevated costs to patients and insurers. Antibiotics, hydration, and total parenteral nutrition (TPN) are three of the most common forms of home IV therapy, and the practitioner may order them for patients at home without prior hospital admission. The list of medications for home IV therapies has grown and includes analgesics, chemotherapeutic agents, hormones, and antiemetic agents.

SERVICE COMPONENTS

Most HH agencies follow the basic Medicare model of services they offer. State licensing boards and professional organizations dictate functions and scopes of practice. Primary services include the following:
- Skilled nursing
- Physical therapy
- Speech-language therapy
- Occupational therapy
- Medical social services
- Homemaker-HH aide

Other therapy services (e.g., respiratory) or professional services (e.g., nutritional counseling, pharmacy, podiatry, dentistry, and psychiatric or mental health) are sometimes offered. Provision of support services (e.g., homemaker, companion, and respite) is common but not directly reimbursable by Medicare. The service mix depends on patient diagnosis, patient and family needs, and availability of resources. The agency commonly provides medical supplies, including durable medical equipment (DME). Home medical equipment ranging from the traditional hospital bed to highly sophisticated items such as respirators and apnea monitors is possible to buy or lease from companies that specialize in equipment provision (see the Health Promotion box).

🏃 Health Promotion

Home Care

- Common diagnoses for home care patients are diabetes mellitus, hypertension, heart and circulatory diseases, osteoarthritis, stroke, acute and chronic wounds, chronic obstructive pulmonary disease, cancer, and endocrine disorders.
- Commonly performed treatments in the home include administration of infusion therapy (i.e., antibiotic administration), patient-controlled analgesia for pain management, enteral feedings, parenteral nutrition, chemotherapy, hydration therapy, and psychiatric counseling and education.
- The nurse and a rehabilitation team member sometimes also provide medical equipment in the home to facilitate medical treatment and safety, such as electrical beds, wheelchairs, commodes, walkers, and other assistive devices.

Medicare and Medicaid home care services are based on the medical model of treatment and depend on the physician for entry into the formalized system. Medicare requires a plan of treatment signed by the physician that outlines all disciplines, treatment, frequency, and duration. The physician or a designated medical provider (nurse practitioner or physician assistant), working in conjunction with the physician, must provide a face-to-face visit with the patient. If the patient is to receive home care benefits beyond the original 60-day period, a recertification must be completed for each subsequent 60-day period. This recertification requires a face-to-face encounter and the medical provider and each of the primary disciplines involved to sign the plan of treatment (CMS, 2015). Third-party payers sometimes do and sometimes do not have similar requirements. This chapter explains only the primary services.

SKILLED NURSING

Currently licensed RNs provide and direct skilled nursing services. Some agencies require that nurses have a bachelor's degree in nursing, whereas others employ nurses from differing educational levels (e.g., LPN) of all types of RN programs and teach them agency policies and specific procedures. Not all nurses have the ability to be effective HH nurses. The LPN/LVN provides nursing care under the direction of the RN whose responsibility is the development of the plan of care.

Service Goals

Skilled nursing services revolve around four major goals:

1. *Restorative:* Returning to a previous level of functioning as appropriate and realistic.
   Restorative goals may include: Patient able to feed self without signs of choking.
2. *Improvement:* Achieving better health and a higher level of functioning than at admission.
   Improvement goals may include: Patient verbalizes understanding of signs of impending heart attack or brain attack and when to call emergency assistance.
3. *Maintenance:* Preserving functional capacities and independence by maintaining the current level of health.
   Maintenance goals may include: Patient demonstrates compliance with a daily exercise routine to maintain strength and prevent further decline.
4. *Promotion:* Teaching healthy lifestyles that keep the effect of illness or disability to a minimum and prevent the recurrence of illness.
   EXAMPLE: The patient who just had a stroke
   Promotion goals may include: Patient demonstrates compliance in a low-fat, low-cholesterol, low-sodium diet.

Provider Attributes

Nurses who practice in the home setting are caregivers, teachers, counselors, case managers, and advocates. Attributes of an effective HH nurse are technical proficiency and self-motivation, good organizational skills, innovation, independence in decision making, and response to problems promptly. The home care patient must be able to depend on the honesty and reliability of the assigned nurse. Positive communication skills and rapport with the patient are essential. Ongoing assessment and reinforcement of the teaching plan are crucial in caring for patients in their homes. When services are provided in the patient's home, the nurse needs to feel comfortable with the unknown and accept differences in ethnic cultures and value systems. Nurses who prefer the structure of the institutional setting and benefit from immediate direction and frequent peer support find the independence of home care practice difficult.

Those working in the home care setting must remember that they are walking into the home of the patient and family. In doing so, remember, as a guest in this home, to respect the cultural values and beliefs. At times, this may include the use of alternative or complementary medicine. Always remember to include the use of herbal remedies and alternative treatments in the assessment and to incorporate these in the plan of care if not contraindicated and if approved by the medical provider signing the plan of care.

Strong communication skills are essential for teaching, counseling, interviewing, and listening. A high energy level, cheerfulness, and a positive attitude are valuable attributes because nurses often are called on to work with patients and families who are under stress. Respect for the patient's dignity, privacy, and need for autonomy is an integral part of providing effective nursing services. Commitment to professional standards of practice, ongoing continuing education, and skills updates are important.

ROLE OF THE LPN/LVN

RNs have been the primary providers of skilled service by tradition and regulation. However, skilled service has become a growing field of practice for the LPN/LVN as agencies cope with increased staffing needs, nursing shortages, and recognition of the many contributions the LPN/LVN makes to home care.

An RN has to supervise LPN/LVNs. Although LPN/LVNs are not empowered to make detailed patient assessments or clinical judgments, their observations, reporting, documentation, teaching, and technical care capabilities are important to home care.

Provider Attributes

Personal and professional attributes described for RNs also apply to the LPN/LVN. Independent practice is not allowed, but self-direction, motivation, creativity, clinical proficiency, flexibility, compassion, empathy, and patience are essential attributes. Good communication skills—written and spoken—are necessary. The ability to work alone, follow directions, recognize important changes in condition, and assist in patient teaching is needed. Evaluation of care interventions and recommendations for alteration of the plan of care constitute a part of the role. It is important to understand and practice the concept of teamwork.

Functions

Depending on the agency, agency policies, and state practice acts, the LPN/LVN may provide the following services in the home as directed by the plan of care established:

- Bowel and bladder training
- Catheter care and teaching
- Emotional support
- Enemas for special conditions
- Finger sticks for blood glucose readings
- Injection administration
- Insertion of urinary catheter, irrigation, and observation for infections
- Monitoring of physical status (such as lung sounds, bowel sounds, pulses, edema, and weight)
- Nutrition; assessment of nutrition and hydration status; teaching about prescribed diet; administration of nasogastric, gastrostomy, and jejunostomy tube feedings, and teaching families about tube feedings
- Ostomy care and teaching

Fig. 37.2 Educating the patient in the home setting.

- Pain management
- Patient and family teaching (Fig. 37.2)
- Prefilling of insulin syringes
- Preventive health measures
- Respiratory care, management of oxygen therapy, mechanical ventilation, and physiotherapy
- Specimen collection
- Teaching, monitoring, or setting up medications
- Therapeutic diet teaching or reinforcement
- Tracheostomy care, including suctioning
- Vital signs
- Wound care and sterile dressing changes

⚠ Safety Alert

Home Oxygen Use

MASK OR CANNULA
- Ensure that the straps are not too tight.
- Remove the straps two or three times a day to wash, dry, and stimulate skin.
- Pad any pressure points.
- Observe the tops of the ears for skin impairment from pressure points.

ORAL AND NASAL MUCOUS MEMBRANES
- Assess oral and nasal mucous membranes two or three times a day.
- Use water-based gel on lips and nasal mucosa.
- Provide frequent oral hygiene.
- Provide humidification via humidifier or nebulizing device.

DECREASING RISK FOR INFECTION
- Remove mask or collar and cleanse with water two or three times a day.
- Cleanse skin carefully at this time and observe for cuts, scratches, and ecchymosis.
- Change disposable equipment frequently.
- Remove secretions that are expectorated.

DECREASING RISK OF FIRE INJURIES
- Post "No Smoking" warning signs in home where they are clearly visible.
- Do not allow open flames, wool blankets, or mineral oils in the area where oxygen is in use.
- Do not allow smoking in the home.

Assistance with highly technical procedures, such as IV therapies, home dialysis, and respirator management, is occurring in HH care.

HH care offers a new and challenging area of practice for the LPN/LVN who enjoys practicing nursing in a less restrictive environment. LPN/LVNs employed in HH agencies cite satisfaction in terms of flexibility, pay, and one-on-one relationships with patients. The need for this level of nursing practice will continue to grow. Commitment to quality of care is a common thread through skilled nursing services; the LPN/LVN has the responsibility also to pursue frequent in-service updates and continuing education to ensure current practice.

PHYSICAL THERAPY

A qualified and licensed physical therapist is required to provide services. A physical therapy assistant under the supervision of a licensed therapist is permitted to deliver limited services. The goals of treatment have to be restorative for Medicare reimbursement but in some cases are for maintenance or prevention for other payer sources. The therapist completes a detailed assessment of the patient and then determines treatment, education, and assistive devices needed for rehabilitation. These are included as a part of the physician-approved plan of treatment. Treatments range from muscle strengthening to transcutaneous nerve stimulation and ultrasound treatments, which also may aid in pain management. Patients who have orthopedic conditions, such as repair of a fractured hip or a total hip or total knee replacement, frequently receive physical therapy services in the home care setting. Other common reasons for HH physical therapy include wound care, heart failure complications, and diabetes medication teaching. The therapist actively teaches the patient and the family the rehabilitation plan to promote self-care and independence. Communication with the physician and the RN is mandatory and promotes continuity of care.

SPEECH-LANGUAGE THERAPY

For Medicare reimbursement, a master's-prepared clinician who has been certified by the American Speech and Hearing Association is required to provide speech services. Other insurers sometimes accept a practitioner prepared at the bachelor's level. Therapy goals include reducing to a minimum communication disorders and their physical, emotional, and social impact. Independent functioning and maximum rehabilitation of speech and language abilities are primary treatment goals. Often, the provision of services occurs after stroke or surgery. Possible therapies range from language relearning to working with eating or swallowing disorders or teaching lip-reading to those with hearing disorders. Pathologists work closely with the patient and family for rehabilitation or adjustment to a new disability.

OCCUPATIONAL THERAPY

Occupational therapy services deal with life's practical tasks. Therapists have the opportunity to earn the occupational therapist, registered (OTR) designation if they meet the registration requirements of the National Occupational Therapy Association. The certified occupational therapy assistant is permitted to provide some services under the supervision of the OTR. On the basis of a complete evaluation of functional level, the therapist chooses and teaches therapeutic activities designed to restore functional levels. Services include the following:
1. Techniques to increase independence
2. Analysis of activities as they relate to patients' skin, their environment, their families, and their routines
3. Expanding the disease management approach into a lifestyle management approach
4. Design, fabrication, and fitting of orthotic or self-help devices
5. Assessment for vocational training

Occupational therapists assist patients to improve in their performance of activities of daily living (ADLs) and their sensory-motor, cognitive, and neuromuscular functioning. Patient-centered education is an integral part of attaining independence in self-care (Bureau of Labor Statistics, 2021).

MEDICAL SOCIAL SERVICES

Social workers prepared at the master's level provide medical social services. Workers with bachelor's degrees are permitted to provide services under the supervision of a social worker with a master's degree (Master of Social Work, MSW). Their focus is on the emotional and social aspects of illness. The patient, family, or other support systems undergo evaluation for social, emotional, and environmental factors. The care plan includes education, counseling, payment source identification, and referrals. Coping with stress and crisis intervention are also part of social worker services. Social services in HH are generally short term.

HOMEMAKER-HOME HEALTH AIDE

Medicare refers to the homemaker-home health aide (HM-HHA) as an HHA. These workers are an integral part of the HH care team. They provide the basic support services that sometimes enable an elderly individual, disabled adult, or dependent child to remain at home. Medicare requires that a primary skilled or therapy service (speech or physical) be provided before HHA services are arranged. Medicaid and some insurers have less stringent requirements. Many insurers do not reimburse this care. Family members and individuals are often willing to pay privately to prevent institutionalization.

Most aide services fall into one of three categories: (1) *personal care*, or assistance with bathing, oral hygiene, eating, dressing, and toileting (see the Coordinated Care box); (2) *physical assistance* with transfers, medications, and ambulation; or (3) *household chores,* or cooking, light housekeeping, shopping, and laundry. Medicare does not cover visits made solely for the third reason.

Coordinated Care

Delegation

Patient Bathing

Skills of bathing are often acceptable to delegate to unlicensed assistive personnel (UAP); however, skin and range-of-motion (ROM) assessments require critical thinking and knowledge application unique to the nurse. As a nurse, do the following:

- Instruct the care provider as to which type of bath (complete, partial assist, tub, shower) is appropriate to the patient's diagnosis, needs, and ability.
- Remind the care provider to notify you of any skin integrity problems so that you can be sure to inspect areas of impairment or potential impairment.
- Remind the care provider to use an organized approach and reassuring tone of voice so that the patient feels safe and comfortable during bathing.
- Instruct the care provider to encourage the patient to report any concerns or discomfort during the bath.
- Instruct the care provider to encourage as much independence in the patient's self-care skills as appropriate and to provide positive feedback.

Although training of aides has long been required by Medicare, rules governing type, length, and content of preparation have been nonexistent; hence, skills and standards were not uniform. Part of the Omnibus Budget Reconciliation Act of 1987 involved the formulation of new standards for training and competency evaluation that are now in effect.

Medicare and Medicaid require on-site supervision of the aide every 2 weeks, principally by the RN. Supervision by a licensed physical therapist is acceptable if skilled nursing is not involved (US Government Publishing Office, 2020). Private payers, however, often do not have such requirements. Aide services sometimes are provided in blocks of time ranging from 1 to 2 hours for Medicare to 8 to 24 hours for private or other payment sources.

TYPICAL HOME HEALTH PROCESS

REFERRAL

The entry point to the HH care system is by referral. This comes from the patient, the family, a social service agency, the hospital, the physician, or another agency. Agencies have a variety of methods of intake for referrals, ranging from a formalized hospital discharge planning process with a central agency intake coordinator to a direct call from the patient's physician to the agency staff.

ADMISSION

The RN makes the initial evaluation and admission visit within 24 to 48 hours of the referral. In some

instances, if nursing is not necessary at the start of care, the physical therapist may be the one completing this admission process. The physician often gives general orders before this visit, but agencies sometimes make an evaluation visit without orders if agency policy permits. The evaluation and admission process generally includes at least the following:

1. Complete patient evaluation, including physical and psychosocial factors
2. Environmental assessment relating specifically to safety and ability to provide services effectively in the home
3. Identification of primary functional impairments
4. Identification of the impact of the disease or disability on the patient and the family
5. Assessment of the support system of the family or the significant other
6. Determination of knowledge and adherence to treatments and medications
7. Determination of desire for care and services
8. Involvement of the patient and the family in the development of the plan of care and goals
9. Notification of the patient of rights as a patient, along with information on costs, payment sources, and billing practices
10. Explanation of the patient's right to self-determination, including information and implementation policies for advanced directives
11. Provision of initial nursing interventions (obtain an initial set of orders from the health care provider and proceed with providing the specific interventions ordered)

The admission process typically takes a minimum of 1 hour. It takes longer if the patient is disoriented or in need of nursing interventions. Some hospital-based agencies initiate an abbreviated evaluation visit while the patient is still in the hospital.

CARE PLAN

If the agency is to admit the patient, the physician must be contacted for specific orders before the delivery of care. Agency staff drafts a treatment plan cooperatively with the physician. This plan describes the current physical status of the patient, medications, treatments, the disciplines needed to provide care, the frequency and the duration of services, the goals and outcomes, and the time frame for implementation. The physician is required to sign the plan of treatment, which serves as the traditional physician orders. The treatment plan is possible to alter at any time (based on patient needs) through additional written, signed orders, and it is obligatory to review and renew it on a regular schedule for Medicare and Medicaid patients. Separate care plans that are discipline specific, such as nursing and physical therapy, are possible. A separate, detailed HH aide care plan always is required.

VISITS

Skilled visits for interventions by the disciplines are conducted according to the orders in the plan of treatment and serve to meet the patient-centered goals and make progress toward identified outcomes. Skilled nursing interventions typically take 30 to 45 minutes, but the duration potentially increases to several hours for complex procedures. Therapy visits range from 30 minutes to 1 hour. With increasing federal pressure to decrease home care and hospice costs, and with the current Medicare PPS, clinical efficiency is critically necessary within the industry. The current method of developing individual care plans, that is, having a home care nurse visit a patient for a predetermined number of visits per week during each episode of care, is no longer tenable. Patients who use telemonitoring are "seen" daily, thereby allowing agencies to plan home visits, not for regular patient assessment (such as vital signs), but to provide hands-on intervention or face-to-face teaching when necessary. The purpose of telehealth is not to replace nurses but to generate data that professional caregivers need to make critically important clinical decisions, allowing them to use their time and talents more effectively and efficiently (HealthIT.gov, 2020). Aide visits average 1 to 2 hours but sometimes are longer depending on needs and payment source. Patients receive visits as infrequently as once a month for diabetic monitoring to several times a day over a short period to provide complex care. Some patients receive only skilled nursing services, and others receive assistance from all disciplines. Greater and more frequent use of LPN/LVNs is occurring when clinically appropriate. Patients sometimes remain on the caseload for a week or years, depending on the needs of the patients.

DOCUMENTATION

Throughout the care process, concise and complete documentation is essential. This documentation may be handwritten. With increasing frequency, agencies are moving toward computerization. These systems are beneficial on many fronts. They provide the following benefits (HealthIT.gov, 2018):

- Provide extended periods of health information
- Allow medical documentation to be accessible by varying members of the health care team
- Monitor patient compliance and care needs
- Promote quality of care

Many agencies are beginning to use various problem classification schemes linked with patient problems (Box 37.1), specific interventions, and defined patient outcomes. Documentation that follows the nursing process model provides an accurate picture of the type and the quality of care. It reflects the effectiveness of the plan of care and progress toward goals and outcomes, or it reflects the nature of and the reasons for lack of progress or deterioration and includes alternative interventions. Communications with the home

---

Box 37.1   Selected Patient Problems for Home Health Care

Inability to bathe self, related to:
- Decreased endurance
- Musculoskeletal impairment
- Neurologic impairment
- Pain

Excessive demand on primary caregiver, related to:
- Inability to manage the care needs of the family member
- Inability to participate in activities away from the home

Insufficient knowledge, related to:
- Cognition limitation
- Lack of experience

Insufficient nutrition, related to:
- Economic deprivation
- Inability to absorb nutrients
- Inability to ingest or digest food

Compromised skin integrity, related to:
- Impaired circulation (pressure)
- Inadequate nutrition
- Physical immobility
- Radiation

Impaired family processes, related to:
- Changes in family resources
- Illness-necessitated role changes

Discomfort, related to:
- Chronic illness (e.g., rheumatoid arthritis)
- Terminal cancer

Potential for infection, related to:
- Inadequate acquired immunity
- Inadequate primary or secondary defenses
- Malnutrition

Social seclusion, related to:
- Feelings of being homebound with ill family member
- Limited contact with family and friends

---

care team and referral sources are also necessary to document.

Other factors also influence documentation. Staff members must recognize the record as a legal document subject to close scrutiny at any time. Professional standards, accountability, and quality of care are linked closely to legal implications and to internal evaluation purposes. Reimbursement sources have a major influence on documentation requirements by setting forth specific forms and formats that are necessary to follow. Medicare requires extensive paperwork. Private insurer requirements are generally less cumbersome.

DISCHARGE PLANNING

Discharge planning for home care, as in hospitals, begins with admission. When patient goals or other specific criteria are met, the discharge occurs. Agencies encourage patient and family participation in discharge planning. The agency consults the physician regarding the discharge, and the physician issues the final order. Many agencies follow up on a postdischarge basis to track patient progress and elicit patient satisfaction information. The purpose of discharge planning is to promote continuity of care in the patient's home.

QUALITY ASSURANCE, ASSESSMENT, AND IMPROVEMENT

Quality assessment programs provide documentation for outside organizations and for internal measures for improvements and refinements of policies and procedures. Assessment of quality involves evaluation of all aspects of the agency operation. Quality management is the guidelines and techniques used to meet the needs of the home care clients and continuously improve (continuous quality improvement) the quality of care provided. Three major elements are included:

1. *Structural criteria:* The agency's overall organization, philosophy, policies, procedures, bylaws, personnel practices, supervision, orientation, contracts, and physical facilities.
2. *Process criteria:* Evaluation of care delivery. Authorities scrutinize the activities of the health professionals and paraprofessionals and support in the management of patient care, documentation, and patient care conferences.
3. *Outcome criteria:* Measurement of change in patient behavior, the results of patient care in terms of changes, health indicators, and satisfaction. Care standards and expected outcomes are integral parts of this area.

Those responsible for quality assessment develop specific criteria and measures in each area and evaluate them for compliance and effectiveness. Evaluation is possible to accomplish in some areas by management, and in others by a multidisciplinary committee or by groups of outside professionals and consumers.

In the past, measures of quality of the agency, the care delivered, and the staff were subjective, with little standardization and agreement. Quality assessment plans now reflect standards, objectives, and measurable outcomes and include plans for remediation or improvement as an integral part of the process. There is a move by a national accreditation body (The Joint Commission) and many businesses to redefine quality assessment activities in terms of quality improvement. The following major principles are involved:

- Quality of patient care and desired outcomes are possible to improve by assessing and improving governance, management, and clinical and support processes that affect patient outcomes.
- Processes are carried out by individuals (managers, clinicians, support) and jointly by these groups.
- Coordination and integration of processes are necessary.
- Employees of an organization are motivated and competent to carry out processes. It is appropriate to give them opportunities to improve continuously through continuing education and certification.

This move will have a direct effect on all staff members and provide a different emphasis on how many agencies will operate.

REIMBURSEMENT SOURCES

Reimbursement for HH services comes from a variety of sources, and covered services and disciplines vary. Medicare and Medicaid are primary sources of income for the majority of agencies, but reliance on these sources for reimbursement has decreased in recent years.

MEDICARE

Medicare is a federal program that requires agencies to be certified as meeting the federal conditions of participation, which set forth specific requirements for organization, staffing, training, types of services covered, and agency evaluation. Regulations further mandate eligibility requirements. Beneficiaries of services are required to be 65 years or older or disabled or have end-stage renal disease. In addition, they have to be under the care of a licensed physician. In 2011, it was mandated through the Affordable Care Act that beneficiaries of services must be seen in a face-to-face visit with a physician or nurse practitioner up to 90 days before or 30 days after the beginning of HH care for payment to occur. This face-to-face visit may be an office visit or a telehealth visit (Center for Medicare Advocacy, 2016). Home care recipients also must be homebound and in need of skilled nursing or therapy services on an intermittent basis. Types of services covered and length of coverage are delineated further in guidelines developed by the HCFA. Ten regional fiscal intermediaries, who act on behalf of the HCFA, receive claims for payment, process reimbursement, and determine coverage.

MEDICAID

The Medicaid program pays for home care services to indigent and low-income people of all ages. The state administers it, but state and federal funding subsidize it. Many states require Medicare certification for participation in the Medicaid program. Services covered vary from state to state, but most include the basic services covered by Medicare plus expansion of aide and personal care services.

THIRD PARTY

Third-party insurers pay for limited home care services. Coverage, requirements, and payment rates vary. Reimbursement often is tied to posthospitalization recoveries. A few progressive companies are paying for nursing and aide services for new mothers who return home within 24 hours of delivery.

There is a wide practice of case management by or on behalf of insurance companies and worker compensation plans. A case manager (commonly a nurse or social worker) determines and arranges for a mix of home care, therapy services, counseling, supplies, and equipment for a patient. The availability of these combined, paid-for services often allows earlier discharges and provides a planned approach to rehabilitation.

A similar approach to case management for the older adult is commonly the goal of area Agencies on Aging, social service departments, community or public health agencies, independent case managers, or contracts with groups or companies that provide such services. Costs sometimes are fully paid depending on how the service is provided.

PRIVATE PAY

Individuals sometimes also pay directly for HH services. Possible charges range from the standard full charge to scaled-down rates based on the ability of the patient to pay.

OTHER SOURCES

HMOs and preferred provider organizations (PPOs) have negotiated contracts with HH agencies to provide services to their patients. Both organizations are prepaid health plans operated independently or through employer groups. Again, requirements and coverage differ.

CULTURAL CONSIDERATIONS

Nurses encounter great diversity in a variety of cultural interactions. This factor must be considered when providing nursing interventions in the hospital, nursing home, or community. Culture is present in the lives of patients, families, and health care providers and is especially apparent in the home environment. Frustration occurs when values conflict, thus increasing the complexity involved in nursing interventions. As a nurse, you need to anticipate potential cultural problems and identify your own and other's values. Cultural health practices are acceptable to incorporate with traditional medical care in the home environment provided it does not conflict with the prescribed treatment.

Apply all of the strategies you use to communicate with patients in general and to patients from different cultures. In addition, several other steps should be taken to ensure clear and effective communication with patients from other cultures (see the Cultural Considerations box; see Chapter 6).

🌐 Cultural Considerations

Breaking Through Cultural Barriers to Communication

STEP 1: ASSESS PERSONAL BELIEFS OF PERSONS FROM DIFFERENT CULTURES
- Review your personal beliefs and past experiences.
- Set aside any attitudes, values, and biases that are judgmental.

STEP 2: ASSESS COMMUNICATIONS VARIABLES FROM A CULTURAL PERSPECTIVE
- Learn as much as possible about the patient's cultural customs and beliefs.
- Encourage the patient to reveal the cultural interpretation of health, illness, and health care.
- Be sensitive to the uniqueness of the patient.
- Identify sources of discrepancy between the patient's and your own conceptions of health and illness.
- Communicate at the patient's level of functioning.
- Assess cultural factors that have the potential to affect your relationship with the patient and respond appropriately.

STEP 3
- Be attentive to signs of fear, anxiety, and confusion in the patient. Be alert for feedback that the patient does not understand the communication taking place.
- Respond in a reassuring manner in keeping with the patient's cultural orientation.
- Be alert to words the patient seems to understand and use them frequently.
- Keep messages simple and repeat them frequently.
- Avoid using medical terms and abbreviations that the patient perhaps does not understand.
- Be aware that in some cultural groups discussion with others concerning the patient possibly will cause offense and impede nursing practices.

- Use an appropriate language dictionary or chart.
- Use appropriate language translation service according to agency policy.

STEP 4: RESPECT PATIENTS AND THEIR COMMUNICATED NEEDS
- Use a kind and attentive approach to convey respect.
- Learn how people signal that they are listening in the patient's culture; then use appropriate active listening techniques.
- Adopt an attitude of flexibility, respect, and interest to help bridge barriers imposed by culture.
- Be considerate of reluctance to talk when the subject involves sexual matters; be aware that in some cultures, people do not discuss sexual matters freely with members of the opposite sex.

STEP 5: COMMUNICATE IN A NONTHREATENING MANNER
- Use a caring tone of voice and facial expression to help alleviate the patient's fears.
- Speak slowly and distinctly but not loudly.
- Conduct the interview in an unhurried manner.
- Follow acceptable social and cultural amenities.
- Ask general questions during the information-gathering stage.
- Be patient when the respondent gives information that seems unrelated to the patient's health problem.
- Develop a trusting relationship by listening carefully, allowing time, and giving the patient your full attention.
- Use gestures and pictures to help the patient understand.
- Repeat the message in different ways if necessary.

STEP 6: USE INTERPRETERS TO IMPROVE COMMUNICATION
- Ask the interpreter to translate the message, not just the individual words.
- Obtain feedback to confirm understanding.
- Use an interpreter who is culturally sensitive.
- Speak to the patient, not to the interpreter.

Modified from Giger JN, Haddad LG: *Transcultural nursing: Assessment and intervention*, ed8, St. Louis, 2021, Mosby.

Fig. 37.3 In the home, the nurse encourages the patient to use imagery to relax and relieve pain.

❖ NURSING PROCESS FOR HOME HEALTH CARE

The role of the licensed practical/vocational nurse (LPN/LVN) in the nursing process as stated is that the LPN/LVN will:

- Participate in planning care for patients based on patient needs
- Review patient's plan of care and recommend revisions as needed
- Review and follow defined prioritization for patient care
- Use clinical pathways, care maps, or care plans to guide and review patient care

HH nursing uses the basic nursing process to assess the needs, establish a patient-centered plan of care, implement nursing actions, evaluate the effectiveness of actions, and plan for the modification or resolution of identified problems. Possible interventions range from wound care to IV chemotherapy. Teaching sometimes involves diabetes mellitus instruction or perhaps the management of complex support equipment in the home. Teaching is always patient centered, with the primary goals being self-care and independent functioning within the confines of the illness or disability (Fig. 37.3). In the counseling role, the nurse sometimes provides emotional support to the dying patient and the family or provides skilled psychiatric interventions (if properly qualified). Case management possibly includes only supervision of the HH aide or involves the coordination of complex care plans with services, supplies, and equipment provided by many different disciplines.

◆ ASSESSMENT

Begin assessment by considering the patient and the family members and the patient's attitude toward the family. Also, assess functions of the patient and the family. These include the ability of the family to provide emotional support for the patient, the ability to cope with the current health problem or situation, ways that goals are set, and progress everyone makes toward the achievement of goals. Work within the structure of the family when providing care.

◆ PATIENT PROBLEM

The patient problem often focuses on the family's ability to cope with the illness of the family member. During times of acute illness, the family in some cases becomes extremely distressed and possibly focuses solely on the patient, neglecting the needs of other members. While caring for a patient, sometimes you will learn of such difficulties and have the opportunity to help or refer the family to other resources. Maintain a family nursing perspective. Possible patient problems related to the HH patient and family are included in Box 37.1.

◆ EXPECTED OUTCOMES AND PLANNING

When planning nursing interventions for the patient, work with the patient and the family in setting goals. The patient and the family must understand and agree on the goals as you set them together. Also, consider ways that the older adult affects family structure. The following is an example of a family-oriented goal and outcome:

Goal: The patient and family voice understanding and demonstrate effective coping with the health problems of its member.

Outcome: The patient and family are able to meet the needs of all members.

◆ IMPLEMENTATION

After goal setting has taken place, assist the patient and family to learn health promotion practices. Providing accurate health information about the diagnosis and the prognosis helps the patient and the family members to understand the patient's experience and the best ways to be effective caregivers.

◆ EVALUATION

Be prepared to revise a plan of care depending on the findings of the evaluation. Determine whether expected outcomes have been met. An example of a goal and evaluative measure related to the family follows:

Goal: The family voices understanding and demonstrates effective coping with the health problems of its members.

Evaluative measure: The family members are able to perform care measures correctly.

CONCLUSION

Current trends support the growth of home care as an economic, compassionate, preferred health delivery system for many types of care. Advances in medical knowledge, coupled with high-technology health care, have increased the number of individuals surviving birth traumas, prematurity, infectious diseases, acute illnesses, accidents, and other maladies that were formerly fatal.

Medical management and control rather than cure are the standard of care for many illnesses. This has increased the number of potentially debilitating chronic illnesses. Dependency and disability are more prevalent in all age groups. Home care provides the assessment and evaluation of chronic illnesses necessary to prevent acute episodes. Aides and homemakers have the capacity to provide necessary support in ADLs to enable the patient to remain in the home.

The birth rate has declined, resulting in an aging population. In the 1900s, only 2% of the US population was 65 years or older. That figure was 13% (40 million people) in 2010 and is projected to reach 20% by 2030. Nearly 20% of this group falls into the categories of the poor or the near-poor. Some 80% of this group is estimated to have at least one chronic disability. The age group of older than 85 years is the fastest-growing group today, with a projection of growing from 5.5 million in 2010 to possibly 19 million by 2050. About 40% of those 85 years and older need help with physical activities (Federal Interagency Forum on Aging-Related Statistics, 2020). Assistance in daily living is essential to this group. Skilled nursing and therapy offer rehabilitation and prevention of deterioration and methods to cope with physical changes.

Federal and private insurers are trying to cap the rapidly rising cost of health care by shortening hospital stays and controlling admissions. Home care agencies are filling the gap for patients who are released early but still need complex care or rehabilitation. In many cases, home care services offer the means to prevent hospitalization by providing enteral, parenteral, IV, and blood transfusion services.

The movement toward deinstitutionalization of technology-dependent children and adults now is becoming feasible as Medicaid and third-party payers change reimbursement criteria. Home care support makes "family life" a reality for people who once thought of hospital personnel as parents because of their dependency on various machines for sustaining life.

HH providers support an emphasis on healthy living and illness prevention as part of the plan of care. This one-on-one education teaches specific techniques to prevent recurrences of illness or deterioration of condition. Individuals want to be at home as long as possible. Care provided by HH agencies and support from social service agencies and others are now making this possible throughout the lifespan.

Get Ready for the NCLEX® Examination!

Key Points

- Home health care allows individuals to maintain personal control and to participate in the direction of their own care.
- Families are an important part of the success of home care services as health care workers provide care, supervision, assistance, and support in attaining the care plan goals.
- Home health care is not a new concept; however, legislative, regulatory, and current health care trends have changed the way it is provided.
- A number of different professional and paraprofessional disciplines provide home care services based on a coordinated plan of care approved by a physician. Teamwork is an essential component of the concept.
- Home health agencies are organized groups that employ or contract with professionals and paraprofessionals to provide services. Different types of agencies usually are subject to varying federal, state, and local laws and regulations.
- Skilled nursing care is the most frequently provided service. RNs and LPN/LVNs under the supervision of RNs provide direct care of different levels of complexity.
- Providers of care in the home must possess special qualities to practice effectively in this nontraditional environment.
- Home health care agencies strive to provide the highest quality of services economically. Success is evaluated through quality assurance plans.
- Home health services are reimbursed by federal, state, local, group, and private sources.
- Congress imposed new limits on home health payments through a provision of the BBA called the Interim Payment System (IPS), which later became the PPS.

- Quality assessment of safe and effective care in the home is significant.
- Although some aspects of nursing interventions in the home are the same as those practiced in other health care settings, home health care nurses pay particular attention to interaction and cooperation among family members, the patient, and other members of the health care team.
- The acuity levels of patients who need care in their homes continue to rise, and the technological aspects of care, including use of mechanical equipment and invasive procedures such as IV therapies, are increasing in home care. These factors, when combined with shorter hospital stays, require extensive discharge planning to prepare patients and family for home health care.

Additional Learning Resources

SG Go to your Study Guide for additional learning activities to help you master this chapter content.

Be sure to visit the Evolve site at http://evolve.elsevier.com/Cooper/foundations/ for additional online resources.

Review Questions for the NCLEX® Examination

1. A 79-year-old patient recently fractured her hip and had a hemiarthroplasty (bipolar) hip repair. Her daughter works during the day but provides care in the evening. Which service agency is most appropriate to provide for this patient's daily care?

   1. Private duty agency
   2. Home health care agency
   3. Nursing home facility
   4. Outpatient rehabilitation agency

2. A student nurse asks her nurse educator why there is an increased demand for home health care. Which response is the most accurate for the nurse educator?

   1. More family members want to care for their ill members at home.
   2. There is a shortage of nurses who want to work in acute hospital care settings.
   3. There is an increase in the number of older patients with chronic illnesses.
   4. There is increased technology in hospitals, which provokes anxiety in many patients.

3. The nurse is assigned to home health care for an 83-year-old patient with a stroke who has right-sided hemiplegia, difficulty swallowing, and speech impairment. He is receiving care in his home from his wife and daughter. Which should the home care nurse provide?

   1. Strict regimen and care plan
   2. Holistic, nonjudgmental philosophy
   3. Teaching plan for all family members
   4. Means of transporting the patient to his physician

4. Which is an example of an evolving future health care trend?

   1. Increased reimbursement for home health care services
   2. Keeping patients in the hospital longer because of the severity of their illnesses
   3. Increased use of telehealth
   4. Slowed growth in the number of agencies involved in home care

5. A 68-year-old patient is recovering from an abdominoperineal resection with a permanent colostomy. Her physician has ordered home health care nursing on her discharge. What is the primary patient goal?

   1. The patient will be able to return to previous lifestyle.
   2. The patient will avoid dependency on medication therapy.
   3. The patient will establish self-care and independence.
   4. The patient will maintain a friendly relationship with family members.

6. The home health nurse has been assigned to provide care for a patient with cultural values that differ from the nurse's. What is the best action for the nurse to take? (Select all that apply.)

   1. Ask for an assignment change to allow a colleague who has cultural values more in line with those of the patient to be assigned.
   2. Accept the assignment and provide the patient with information on the values of the nurse to facilitate communication.
   3. Take time to consider the differences between the values held and those of the assigned patient.
   4. Research the culture of the assigned patient.
   5. Review past experiences with cultural dilemmas.

7. When arranging home care for a patient, from whom should the home health care nurse collect data? (Select all that apply.)

   1. Home care agency
   2. Patient
   3. Primary care provider
   4. Community volunteer agencies
   5. Family members as per patient wishes

8. The nurse is reviewing a patient's eligibility for home services reimbursed by Medicare. What criteria are needed to be eligible? (Select all that apply.)

   1. Age 60 years or older
   2. Under the care of a nurse practitioner
   3. Homebound
   4. In need of intermittent skilled nursing services
   5. In acute renal failure

9. A group of nursing students is preparing a presentation on the major diagnostic categories and diagnosis-related groups. What is the correct name for this system?

   1. Prospective payment system (PPS)
   2. Medicaid
   3. Medicare
   4. Older American Act

10. Which 1997 congressional act imposed new limits on home health payments?

    1. Social Security Administration
    2. National Institutes of Health (NIH)
    3. Balanced Budget Act (BBA)
    4. Human and Health Services (HHS)

11. What was instituted by the Health Care Financing Administration (HCFA) in 2000?

    1. A new payment system for home health agencies
    2. Medicare-certified agencies
    3. The Joint Commission
    4. Rules governing certification of home health agencies

12. What are the major nursing considerations crucial for patients in their homes and in structured facilities? (Select all that apply.)

    1. Immediate medical direction
    2. Nursing assessment
    3. Frequent peer support
    4. Reinforced patient teaching
    5. Individualized care

13. A patient is discussing the need for home health care services with the primary care provider. Which statement by the patient indicates the need for reinforced teaching? (Select all that apply.)

    1. "My Medicaid will pay for a nurse to stay at my house for up to 60 days."
    2. "Having home health care will let my doctor make house calls."
    3. "My home health nurse can help set up my daily medications."
    4. "I will be able to receive my IV medications at home instead of coming in to the hospital."
    5. "The federal government pays for all of the Medicaid bills."

14. Over the past several years, technology advances have helped increase the adoption of _____ to monitor the patient's vital signs, oxygen saturation, and weight in the home by the home health agency.

15. The nurse is beginning orientation for a position in a medical practice that employs telehealth. What statement by the nurse indicates an understanding of telehealth?

    1. "The patient must have a computer in the home to utilize the services."
    2. "Blood glucose monitoring may be performed with telehealth services."
    3. "Telehealth is more expensive than traditional health care services."
    4. "Insurance rarely covers telehealth-related expenses."

16. A young woman, 18, was born with cystic fibrosis and has spent a quarter of her life in the hospital and now she and her siblings have a new plan: for her to spend the rest of whatever might remain of her life at home with them. Her older brother and his wife have set up a room just for her with a private bath, right off the living room and kitchen (with a deck overlooking the yard) so that she can participate as fully as possible with family yet still retain the comfort and privacy of her own space. Unfortunately, both her brother and his wife work full time. Her mother, who is 69, had her daughter late in life and is now fairly debilitated herself with severe rheumatoid arthritis. However, she wants to help her children's plan succeed and begins to stay with her daughter during the day. Unfortunately, the patient is reaching the end stage of her disease and after a failed lung transplant, she is bedridden and begins to have increasing struggles with mucus blocking her airways frequently. As digestion becomes difficult, her condition becomes a lot for her family members to handle, especially as she is now entering late-stage pancreatic and respiratory failure. They feel both grief and panic, fearful of letting her down. Her physician suggests they call a home health agency. Choose the *most likely* options to complete the statement below. This client *most likely* qualifies for _____1_____–oriented skilled nursing services, with an LPN providing _____2_____, while the HHA provides ___3_____.

OPTIONS FOR 1	OPTIONS FOR 2	OPTIONS FOR 3
Restorative	Assessment	Assessment
Improvement	Nursing diagnoses	Nursing care plans
Maintenance	Clinical decisions	Personal care
Promotion	Technical and skilled care	Technical and skilled care

Objectives

1. Describe settings of long-term care services.
2. Identify patients of long-term care services.
3. Discuss federal and state regulations related to long-term care.
4. Identify the sources of reimbursement for long-term care services.
5. Define chronic and acute health services.
6. Describe the goals of long-term care health services.
7. Describe long-term care nursing services.
8. Describe services available from each type of agency: home health agency, hospice agency, adult daycare, assisted living facility, continuing care community, and long-term care facility.
9. Identify 2017 Nursing Care Center Safety Goals and strategies to meet these goals.

Key Terms

activities of daily living (ADLs) (p. 1200)
adult daycare (p. 1201)
age in place (p. 1200)
assisted living (p. 1202)
continuing care retirement community (CCRC) (p. 1203)
functional assessment (p. 1207)
hospice (HŎS-pĭs, p. 1201)
instrumental activities of daily living (IADLs) (p. 1202)
long-term care (p. 1198)
Medicaid (p. 1206)

Medicare (p. 1206)
minimum data set (MDS) (p. 1207)
palliative care (p. 1207)
quality of life (p. 1198)
resident assessment instrument (RAI) (p. 1207)
residential care (p. 1202)
restorative nursing care (p. 1205)
skilled nursing care (p. 1203)
subacute unit (p. 1203)

Long-term care is defined by the US Centers for Medicare and Medicaid Services as an array of services an individual may find necessary to help in meeting various personal care needs (Medicare.gov, n.d.). Rather than medical care, most long-term care residents only require assistance with meeting their activities of daily needs. The goal of all long-term care is to keep people as independent as possible. The need for long-term care arises when an individual is not capable of meeting daily needs independently, perhaps because of physical or psychological impairment. The term *long-term care* often makes people think of older adults in a nursing home setting, but patients of all age groups may need long-term care at any given time in various types of facilities. Long-term care encompasses a range of services, including health maintenance and care, rehabilitation, treatment of disease processes, and assistance with activities of daily living (ADLs). The need for these services may follow an acute illness such as a traumatic injury or may be for the effects of a chronic illness such as diabetes or schizophrenia.

There are various settings for and a broad spectrum of long-term care services. The types of settings and services necessary depend on the individual and unique needs of each patient. Care is aimed at providing patient-centered care and maintaining quality of life. The term **quality of life** is an individualized concept, but it generally refers to an individual's overall well-being and feeling of physical, social, and spiritual happiness. Quality of life is important in maintaining self-esteem and a sense of well-being and in experiencing the pleasures of life (Fig. 38.1). *Healthy People 2020* includes the initiative health-related quality of life. HRQoL addresses the need for physical, mental, emotional, and social well-being and the impact a person's health status has on the quality of life (CDC, 2018).

Culture is a system of values, beliefs, and practices that guides a person's behavior. Culture plays a large role in shaping patients' beliefs about health and illness and therefore greatly influences health behaviors. Religion is one of the universal components of culture (see the Cultural Considerations box on religion among older adult populations). Ethnicity is a person's identification with a certain ethnic group based on shared traditions, national origin, physical characteristics, and other markers such as language, religion, food, and dress. The composition of the older adult population is changing—racial and ethnic diversity

Fig. 38.1 Family is important in helping to maintain quality of life for the older adult.

is increasing (see the Cultural Considerations box on diversity in the long-term care setting). In 2017, there were 48.2 million Americans aged 65 and over and 6.4 million aged 85 and over living in the United States. By the next year, this total increased to 52 million over the age of 65. As the nation's population continues to age, the segment of the population that will be composed of seniors will also increase. By 2050, an estimated 22% of the population will be composed of seniors 65 years and older (Statista, 2021). The demographic make-up of the population represented by populations other than Caucasian will also increase. Knowledge of cultural and ethnic groups is important to the ability to provide comprehensive nursing interventions.

 Cultural Considerations

Religion Among Older Adult Populations

- In the long-term care facility, one goal of the interdisciplinary team is to provide opportunities for residents to participate in worship services that support their religious beliefs. Worship services to meet spiritual needs are important; visitation and support from the clergy of any denomination also are encouraged.
- Nursing, social services, and the dietary department provide support through an interdisciplinary team approach.
- Dietary services take into consideration any food preferences or foods to avoid based on the resident's culture and religion.
- The long-term care facility consistently provides opportunities to practice one's religious faith.

Historically, providers of long-term care have managed these services based on a medical model that includes expert nursing services and medical management. Patient safety in any setting has been and always will be a priority. As the patient population changes, health care in the long-term care industry will evolve to meet the needs of older adults with functional impairments related to normal changes of aging, in addition to any health disorders they experience.

Cultural Considerations

Diversity in Long-Term Care Facilities

Although residents of long-term care facilities are currently predominantly white women, residents are becoming older and ethnically more diverse. The population in the United States is expected to grow from 310 million in 2010 to 439 million in the year 2050. By 2042, the ethnicity that now makes up the minority of the population is expected to become the majority. By 2030, one in five residents in the United States will be 65 years of age and older. By 2050, 42% of the population will be of older age. Between 2010 and 2050, the white elderly population is projected to decrease from 87% to 77%. The Asian elderly population will increase from 3% to 9% by 2050, and the African American elderly population will increase from 9% to 12%. By 2050, the elderly population of the American Indian and Alaskan Native will increase from 235,000 to 918,000 and the Hawaiian and other Pacific Islander elderly population will grow from 39,000 to 219,000. The largest growth of cultural diversity in this age group will be in those who are of two or more races, with an increase from 278,000 in 2010 to 1.3 million in 2050.

Data from the US Census Bureau: The next four decades: The older population in the United States: 2010 to 2050, 2010. Retrieved from: https://www.census.gov/content/dam/Census/library/publications/2010/demo/p25-1138.pdf

SETTINGS FOR LONG-TERM CARE

As the population of older adults continues to grow, so will the need for long-term care. Statistically, the majority (52%) of people will require long-term care at some point in their lives (LTC Consulting Services, 2018). Many changes are occurring in the long-term care system in regard to types of settings, criteria for admission, services offered, and reimbursement. In 2018, an estimated 14 million people needed the services provided by long-term care. Of those, 56% were over the age of 65 years (Hado, 2019). The setting for the care delivery will vary based upon the level of care needed in response to the degree of impairment. The greatest number of individuals receive care in their homes. Most of these individuals will be cared for in the home setting, which leaves approximately 40% who need admission to a nursing home facility. Of those admitted to the nursing home, about 10% will remain in the facility for 5 years or longer (Medicare.gov, n.d.b). Long-term care will continue to evolve over the coming years. At present, there are numerous settings for long-term care, including the home, community, and specialized facilities (Fig. 38.2).

Ethnicity differences are seen in the residential nursing home demographics. The overwhelming majority of residents are white, non-Hispanic (77.9%). Black, non-Hispanics at 14.2%. and Hispanics at 5.36% (Statista, 2016). Women being the majority of elderly living at home is not surprising since the age expectancy of women is higher than for men.

Least restrictive

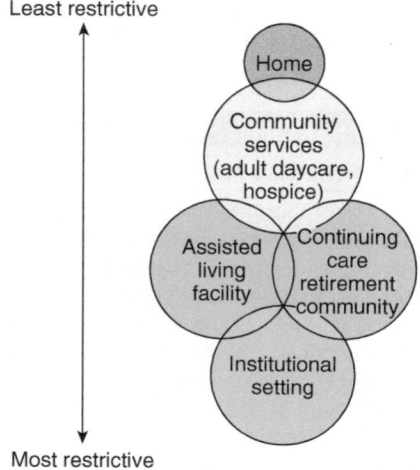

Fig. 38.2 Available settings that provide long-term care services.

Fig. 38.3 Caring for aging parents is one of the tasks of middle adulthood.

HOME

Most older adults live in a home setting, with only a small percentage of those age 65 and older residing in an institutional setting. There are an estimated 47 million seniors in the United States. Approximately 3% are in long-term care facilities. The remaining 45 million reside in home settings. Many seniors hope to **age in place.** This refers to remaining in their desired home setting as they age. The goal is to remain in that environment until they are unable to do so. There are benefits to aging in place. Remaining in the home location promotes independence. It is less expensive. Staying at home is also familiar and thus comfortable (Witt, 2021). Choosing to age in place successfully requires planning.

| Box 38.1 | Services to Support Home Care Providers for Older Adults |

- *Respite care:* Scheduled stays for the older adult who needs care at a long-term care facility to give the caregiver a break from the responsibility of providing care.
- *Daycare:* A setting that provides structured age-appropriate activities during the day; frequently used by family members and caregivers who work during the day.
- *Home health care:* Includes homemakers, shoppers, respite care workers, personal care attendants, home health aides, and nursing care staff.
- *Nutrition programs:* Community programs, such as senior centers, or home delivery of one hot meal per day (Meals on Wheels); some programs are funded by the community, and others charge a small fee for services.
- *Senior centers:* Government or community-funded centers that provide recreational activities, lunch, health screening, exercise classes, educational classes, and transportation to and from the site if needed.
- *Transportation services:* Community- or government-funded service to grocery shopping or medical appointments. Some of these services may charge a fee.

Data from the National Institute on Aging: Long-term care: Facility-based services, n.d. Retrieved from https://www.nia.nih.gov/.

The individual will need to approach their health with a proactive attitude seeking to promote health and wellness. Resources needed to remain in the home require planning and evaluation. Even if a senior opts to age in place, supportive services may be indicated.

Care of the older adult at home sometimes involves a great deal of participation from loved ones. Caregivers also may be caring for a spouse, children, grandchildren, and even great-grandchildren in a multigenerational household (Fig. 38.3). Without the support of families, there undoubtedly would be even more admissions to long-term care facilities. The cost savings to society cannot be ignored. Care for an older adult at home costs approximately half as much as care in a long-term care facility, unless the older adult has a great degree of physical impairment. Many of those who care for older adults at home rely on valuable community services to assist them (Box 38.1).

One of these services, the home health agency, strives to fulfill the needs of homebound patients for as long as possible (see Chapter 37). The increased rate of growth of the over-65 population and the increased cost of institutional long-term care continue to be driving forces in the continued progression of home health care. The needs of the home health care patient range from complex skills such as central line intravenous care or mechanical ventilation to more simple needs such as help with **activities of daily living (ADLs).** ADLs are daily routines of hygiene, dressing and grooming, toileting, eating, and ambulating each person carries out independently throughout life.

Home health agencies provide services that focus on rehabilitation with physical therapy, occupational therapy, speech therapy, respiratory therapy, access to social services, nutritional support by a registered dietitian, the rental or purchase of durable medical equipment, and nursing services. Home health agencies offer nursing services from shoppers, respite care workers, personal care attendants, certified nursing assistants (CNAs), home health aides (HHAs), licensed practical/vocational nurses (LPN/LVNs), as well as registered nurses (RNs) to provide the more complex care and education.

Medicare and Medicaid offer a program called the Program of All-Inclusive Care for the Elderly (PACE), which helps people remain in their homes while still receiving necessary care. Services are offered by an interdisciplinary team in the home, community, and PACE centers. To qualify for PACE, a person must be 55 years or older, live in a service area that has a PACE organization, qualify for nursing home–level care, and be deemed safe to live at home with the help of PACE services. Payment is dependent on the patient's financial state. Some of the services include dentistry, home care, meals, adult day care, physical therapy, and medications (Medicare.gov, n.d.c).

Role of the Licensed Practical Nurse/Licensed Vocational Nurse and the Registered Nurse in the Home Care Setting

Often, the role of the LPN/LVN in the home health care setting involves private duty or shift work. Responsibilities sometimes include home visits to gather data to evaluate care provided by the personal care attendants, CNAs, and HHAs. The LPN/LVN also provides a valuable human resource as staffing coordinator, intake coordinator, or medical chart auditor or reviewer. The staffing coordinator receives information from the intake coordinator describing the requested home care for the patient. The staffing coordinator, on the basis of established protocols, schedules the appropriate care provider to meet the needs of the patient and verifies financial coverage for the care. A medical chart auditor or reviewer uses knowledge of health care to fulfill the quality assurance documentation guidelines (see the Coordinated Care box).

 Coordinated Care

Delegation

Licensed Practical/Vocational Nurse as Staff Coordinator

An important example of delegation of care by the LPN/LVN is the role of staffing coordinator. As with any delegation, the LPN/LVN must consider the scope of practice and the individual abilities of the caregiver when scheduling and assigning care. In some states, LPN/LVNs are not authorized to delegate; only RNs have the power to delegate, by regulation.

In home health care, the RN provides intermittent visits for holistic care, supervisory home visits, comprehensive assessments, referrals, nursing interventions, health care education, health maintenance, and home management. Within the home health care agency, the RN also functions as a manager and administrator.

HOSPICE

Hospice agencies provide services to patients and families as the end of life approaches. These services are available to any age group, not just older adults. Medical certification is required for terminal care. Hospices care for terminally ill cancer patients and a growing number of patients with other chronic, life-threatening illnesses, such as end-stage heart and lung disease, and amyotrophic lateral sclerosis (ALS) (see Chapter 40).

The philosophy of the overriding value of maintaining comfort as death approaches is central to hospice care. Palliative care extends the principles of hospice care to a broader population that has the possibility to benefit from comfort care earlier in an illness or disease process. This agency provides nursing interventions to meet basic needs, ADLs, pain and symptom management, and spiritual and psychosocial support for the patient, the family, and significant others. Care providers include CNAs, HHAs, LPN/LVNs, and RNs for case management. Volunteers provide respite relief for caregivers and socialization and companionship for the patient. If the patient belongs to a religious community, parish nurses sometimes serve as an adjunct to hospice care to assist the patient and family with psychosocial concerns and bereavement issues. Hospice or terminal care is possible to provide in the home setting; in an inpatient hospice unit located in an institutional setting, such as a long-term care facility; and in stand-alone hospice facilities. Patients enter an inpatient hospice unit generally for one of the following reasons: pain or symptom management, respite for the family, or terminal care. If hospice care is given in the home setting, family members or loved ones are the primary caregivers with hospice staff making regular visits while available 24 hours a day (see Chapter 40).

COMMUNITY RESOURCES

Adult Daycare

Adult daycare services are community-based programs designed to meet the needs of functionally or cognitively impaired adults through supervised health care and social and recreational activities. These structured, comprehensive programs provide a variety of services, including physical care, mental stimulation, socialization, assistance with health maintenance, and health referrals, during any part of the day but for less than 24 hours a day (Box 38.2). These centers generally operate during regular business hours, with the patient returning home to family or caregivers at night, although some offer services during evening and weekend hours.

Adult daycare centers are designed to serve adults who need supervision, social opportunities, or assistance because of physical or cognitive impairment. The typical adult who attends daycare is disabled and 75 years of age. Many need assistance with one to three ADLs.

Box 38.2	**Typical Services Offered by Adult Daycare Centers**

- Transportation
- Social services
- Assistance taking medications
- Mental stimulation
- Health monitoring (vital signs)
- Meals
- Limited nursing care
- Personal care
- Counseling
- Therapeutic activities
- Rehabilitation therapies
- Crafts
- Recreational activities

Family Care America, Inc: What is adult day care?, 2019. National Caregivers Library. Retrieved from: http://www.caregiverslibrary.org/Caregivers-Resources/GRP-Caring-For-Yourself/HSGRP-Support-Systems/What-Is-Adult-Day-Care-Article.

Fig. 38.4 Social interaction and acceptance are important aspects of care for the older adult.

Adult mental health centers and senior centers are additional places where families are able to turn for adult daycare services. These centers sometimes are located in churches or public-use areas within the community. Their staff includes a director, an activities coordinator, and a personal care attendant. The director of an adult daycare center is usually either a social worker or an RN. The activities coordinator has specialized training and education in activities to promote the maintenance of functional abilities and independence in the environment (Fig. 38.4). The personal care attendant assists with ADLs. The CNA or personal care attendant has to meet state requirements of training in assistance with ADLs and basic observation skills.

Transportation Services

Transportation services are offered in many communities to older or disabled people. These services may be funded by the community or may be operated privately and charge a fee. Transportation is provided to and from health care–related appointments, shopping centers, grocery stores, and other community agencies.

Respite Care

Respite care is care provided to give family members or caregivers a "break" from the responsibility of care to patients who are unable to care for themselves. Respite care is available in varying time options from a single hour or several days. The service is available in various settings, including the person's home, long-term care facilities, and respite care facilities. Respite care is reimbursed by some private and some government-sponsored insurance.

RESIDENTIAL CARE SETTINGS

Residential care settings serve the older adult population and the mentally or physically disabled person and offer a wide variety of services. Among the most popular types of residential care facilities are assisted living facilities, congregate care facilities, and continuing care retirement communities. In the following section, two of the more popular types of settings, assisted living and continuing care retirement communities, are discussed.

Assisted Living

Assisted living is a type of residential care setting in which the adult patient rents a small one-bedroom or studio-type apartment and has the option of receiving several personal care services such as bathing, dressing, and administration of medications. Assisted living services are possible to provide in freestanding residences, near or integrated with skilled nursing homes or hospitals, as components of continuing care retirement communities, or at independent housing complexes. Virtually unheard of before 1990, in 2014, there were nearly 28,000 residential care communities that represent nearly 1 million beds in the United States according to the CDC (2020). Approximately 60% of these residents will live in these facilities for an average of 22 months before moving to a skilled nursing facility (American Health Care Association [AHCA], 2020).

Personal care services included in assisted living environments include housekeeping and laundry. The patient receives encouragement to partake in communal dining and various social activities. Some facilities offer transportation for organized recreational activity or personal business (Fig. 38.5). Nursing care varies from minimal care for patients with impairments in ADLs or instrumental activities of daily living (IADLs) to more complex daily tasks such as shopping and using the telephone and assistance with medications, to more complex care such as tube feeding and oxygen therapy. Some facilities even contract for outside hospice care. Key features of assisted living are listed in Box 38.3.

Staffing requirements for caregivers in assisted living facilities vary from state to state, as do regulations for the facilities. Many states have age and skill requirements for caregivers (e.g., first aid, cardiopulmonary

Fig. 38.5 A bulletin board at a senior center shows times when legal help is available.

- Services and supervision available 24 h/day
- Services to meet scheduled and unscheduled needs
- Care and services provided or arranged to promote independence
- Emphasis on resident's dignity, autonomy, and choice
- Emphasis on privacy and a homelike environment

resuscitation [CPR]), and some require special credentialing such as CNA or HHA. Administrators are sometimes RNs or LPN/LVNs, and others are licensed long-term care administrators.

Continuing Care Retirement Communities

A continuing care retirement community (CCRC) offers a complete range of housing and health care accommodations from independent living to 24-hour skilled nursing care. Usually, older adults enter a CCRC when they are in relatively good health and capable of living independently or with little assistance. In most cases, signing a contract to enter a CCRC is a lifetime commitment. CCRCs offer residents this complete range of housing and care for the rest of their lives, enabling older adults the opportunity to experience a gradual transition from independent living to continuous skilled nursing care (if needed) while remaining at the same location. For an older couple, the knowledge that they will be able to stay together is comforting, even though one of them may come to need long-term care (AARP, 2019).

CCRCs offer apartments, townhomes, or detached dwellings, or a combination of these; they sometimes accommodate several hundred residents, although they sometimes also provide much smaller settings. Facilities range from luxurious settings with tennis courts, swimming pools, and hotel-style dining rooms to more modest facilities with similar but less plush amenities. Many CCRCs have long waiting lists for admission.

Nursing interventions for a resident in a CCRC depend on the functional abilities of the older adult. With more independent residents, a personal care attendant, CNA, or HHA can provide assistance with ADLs or IADLs. Nursing interventions are possible for residents who need skilled nursing interventions by LPN/LVNs or RNs. Some CCRCs contract with outside agencies to provide needed services, such as hospice care. Some CCRCs contract with nursing registries to provide personnel for long-term care in a resident's apartment. The reward of nursing in this setting is, again, the opportunity to care for a patient over a longer time frame.

INSTITUTIONAL SETTINGS

Subacute Unit

The subacute unit is a type of institutional setting that has become extremely popular since the late 1980s, when the advantage became clear of a less expensive alternative to acute care for patients with high-acuity medical and nursing intervention needs. The subacute unit is possible to view as a bridge between acute care and long-term care. Most subacute units are located in long-term care facilities, which provide skilled nursing care; others are former hospital units that have been reclassified to provide subacute care. Subacute units have a stronger rehabilitative focus and shorter length of stay than a long-term care facility. The level of care that subacute units provide is at nearly the same acuity as in the hospital. In fact, the typical older adult in a subacute unit today corresponds to some medical-surgical patients.

Subacute care has become necessary because of our increased lifespan as well as changes in hospital reimbursement. Modern medicine now saves lives that, before technological advances, were unable to be saved. This has led to a ripple effect. The intensive care unit (ICU) cares for patients whose condition is so critical that they formerly would not have survived. Patients whose condition is so serious that they formerly would have been cared for in the ICU are now on the medical-surgical unit. Patients who would have been on the medical-surgical units are now discharged out of the hospital, but often their conditions are too complicated for home care, hence the evolution of the subacute unit.

In the acute care setting, strict rules about length of stay and limitations in cost reimbursement limit the amount of time an adult can be hospitalized. The reimbursement rules for acute care are different from those that apply to subacute care provided in a skilled nursing facility setting. The cost savings of the subacute setting has been one of the reasons for its growth.

Patients with numerous disorders make up much of the population in a subacute facility. Patients are able to receive a variety of therapies, including intravenous medication administration via peripheral or central venous catheters, complex dressing changes, peritoneal dialysis, and even mechanical ventilation. Physical rehabilitation, stroke rehabilitation, wound care, and recovery from hip fracture are among the most common care needs in the subacute setting. The nurse employed in a subacute unit needs to have a variety of assessment, rehabilitative, medical-surgical, and leadership skills. The assessment and technical skills of a medical-surgical nurse are required, along with the knowledge about reimbursement and interdisciplinary team skills of a long-term care nurse.

Long-Term Care Facility

Commonly known as a nursing home or extended-care facility, this institutional setting mostly provides services to adults, primarily older adults (older than age 65), although a person of any age can be cared for in a long-term care setting. Long-term care facilities provide 24-hour care to individuals who do not need expensive inpatient hospital services but who do not have options for care at home or by other community agencies or services. Because the long-term care facility becomes a home for the adult, on either a long-term or a short-term basis, the adult is referred to as a resident rather than a patient. As of 2019, approximately 54.1 million people age 65 and older lived in the United States (ACL, 2020). In 2015, the number of residents of the age of 65 and older in long-term care was 1.3 million (CDC, 2019). With the projected increase in the elderly population, these numbers are expected to grow.

Most residents of long-term care facilities have more than one health disorder when they are admitted. The most common disorders on admission include cardiovascular disease, hypertension, depression, dementia, and type 2 diabetes.

It is a common misconception that most older adults live in long-term care facilities. As noted in the previously mentioned statistics, the vast number of the population over the age of 65 do not live in long-term care facilities.

Although cardiovascular disorders are the most common diagnoses on admission, they are not necessarily the main reasons why an older adult enters into long-term care. Cognitive impairment, incontinence, inability to perform ADLs, and the state of being single or widowed and unable to care for oneself are also important factors that determine placement into a long-term care facility. Patients with cognitive disorders, such as Alzheimer's disease, pose a challenge to manage at home or in other less restrictive care environments because of the patient's short-term memory loss, confusion, disorientation, restlessness, wandering, and hallucinations. A major safety event, such as forgetting to turn off the stove, is often the precipitating event in long-term care facility placement. As patients with Alzheimer's disease advance in age, their ability to participate in their ADLs declines, eventually becoming totally dependent on others for care. In the final stages of the disorder, they often have impaired mobility.

Two categories of residents generally are found in a long-term care facility. The first category is the short-term resident, sometimes called the short-stay resident. These residents have often been transferred from an acute care facility to which they had been admitted for an acute illness or the worsening of a chronic illness. The residents are admitted principally for rehabilitation and are expected to be discharged within 6 months. These residents and the residents of a subacute unit have many similarities. The second category is the traditional type of resident who lives in the facility on a long-term basis. Such residents usually stay in the facility until they die or are transferred to an acute care facility. These residents require numerous nursing intervention needs and may be cognitively impaired. Most residents in the typical long-term care facility are of the traditional category, although the trend is toward admitting more short-term residents. As a result, the overall nursing interventions of long-term care residents have become increasingly complex.

The long-term care facility industry is large and will continue to grow as the population ages, although it is changing. Fewer, but larger, long-term care facilities are found today. The greatest population growth is occurring in the older adult group, the oldest-old or frail elderly, those older than age 85. The philosophy in a long-term care facility is to maintain and restore health and functional abilities to the resident's highest level and to provide a homelike atmosphere, promoting dignity, independence, restoration, maintenance, and assistance in ADLs, and skilled nursing interventions (Box 38.4).

Long-term interdisciplinary care team. The long-term care facility is an interdisciplinary setting. In this setting, health care professionals work together as an interdisciplinary team to meet the needs of the resident. Members of the team possibly include the resident, nursing personnel (gerontologic clinical nurse specialists, RNs, LPN/

Box 38.4 **Selection of a Nursing Home**

CONSIDERATIONS WHEN CHOOSING A NURSING HOME
- Five-star quality rating based on health inspections, staffing, and quality measures
- Health inspections from regulatory agencies. Evaluation includes management of medications, protection of residents from physical or mental abuse, general care of the residents, environment of the facility, and storage and preparation of food
- Staffing ratios of licensed and nonlicensed personnel to residents
- Fire safety standards
- Medicare published quality measures, which include whether residents are receiving flu vaccines, weight loss statistics, and pain control measures

Data from Medicare.gov: Compare nursing home quality, n.d.a. Retrieved from: https://www.medicare.gov/what-medicare-covers/what-part-a-covers/compare-nursing-home-quality.

LVNs, CNAs), the primary or facility health care provider, social worker, pharmacist, dietitian, activities director, and rehabilitation specialists (from the areas of physical therapy, occupational therapy, and speech therapy), and a podiatrist, psychiatrist, audiologist, and dentist. As mentioned, the long-term care industry is now challenged to provide a homelike environment and an individualized approach to residents with more complex care needs than this setting used to accommodate. The interdisciplinary care planning meetings (often called ICPs) are mandated by the *Omnibus Budget Reconciliation Act (OBRA)* to occur on a regular basis. The team meets regularly to review a resident's care plan, with each team member offering a unique perspective.

The goal is to have a plan of care that accurately reflects the resident's needs and goals and, as much as possible, retains life as it was at home. The care plan sometimes has many components and properly includes input from the direct care providers, CNAs, and nurses. In some states, the resident's family members or significant others, or health care power of attorney, are required to receive an invitation to attend these interdisciplinary team meetings. If CNAs are not part of the official meeting, it is up to the LPN/LVN to communicate closely with them. LPN/LVNs must make sure their viewpoints are represented, because they are usually the ones who work most closely with the older adults, performing the majority of physical care in the long-term care setting. Involvement of all categories is crucial to successful implementation of the interventions developed at the meeting.

The long-term care facility is managed by an administrator and a director of nursing (DON). The facility has nursing services, social services, dietary services, activities or recreation, rehabilitation or physical therapy, building maintenance, and housekeeping departments. These departments and the provision of care are highly regulated by state and federal agencies to ensure quality services are supplied to a potentially vulnerable population, the frail older adult.

Nursing services is the largest department, as it is in most health care facilities. The DON is an RN. Depending on the size of the facility or the number of beds, the facility sometimes has an assistant director of nursing (ADON), a staffing coordinator, and RNs as managers of nursing units and shift charge nurses. In many facilities, LPN/LVNs function in these management roles and provide direct nursing care. LPN/LVNs are sometimes facility supervisors, medical record technicians, staff development assistants, and admission coordinators because of their nursing assessment and data collection abilities. Within the nursing department, CNAs provide the largest percentage of nursing care. The CNA receives educational preparation to encourage the patient's independence within the environment, offer restorative nursing interventions, and assist with ADLs.

This group of nursing care providers also learns basic observation, reporting, and recording skills to support nursing care.

A unique member of the caregiving team in the long-term care facility setting in some states is the certified medication aide or certified medication technician (CMA/CMT). This caregiver is first required to be a CNA and then has the option to complete an educational course in the administration of medications. In the long-term care facility, medication administration is permitted by the RN, LPN/LVN, and CMA/CMT. The CMA/CMT works under the guidance of the licensed nurse and is prohibited from administering certain types of medications. In regard to medication administration, the difference between long-term care and acute care is the vast number of patients to whom the medication administration person sometimes administers medications. In some states, this ratio is as high as one medication administration person to 60 residents; in long-term care, there is a 2-hour window for legal administration of medications (1 hour before the scheduled time to 1 hour after), although the individual facility's policy is important to check. Restorative nursing assistants are CNAs who have completed an educational program that focuses on restorative nursing care, or basic concepts of physical therapy for maintenance of functional mobility and physical activity.

Legal, Ethical, and Financial Issues

Legal and ethical issues among long-term care agencies are similar, but subtle differences exist depending on the provider setting. Most providers are subject to regulation by federal and state guidelines or use them as minimal standards for health care services, reimbursement, or quality indicators. The OBRA of 1987, also known as the nursing home reform legislation, was a landmark law that affected long-term care facilities. OBRA defines requirements for the quality of care given to residents and covers many aspects of institutional life, including nutrition, staffing, qualifications required of personnel, and many others.

Some of the positive outcomes of OBRA include empowerment of residents, focus on residents' rights, reduction or elimination of physical restraint use, and improved staffing, although many nurses believe that staffing continues to need greater improvement in many facilities. The enactment of OBRA led to the requirement for long-term care facilities to use greater numbers of licensed nursing staff, which led to greater opportunities for employment for the LPN/LVN. Other aspects of the OBRA law helped expand the role of the LPN/LVN to include areas such as intravenous therapy and team leading.

The Centers for Medicare and Medicaid Services (CMS) administers and monitors the OBRA guidelines through institutional surveys. Surveyors are required by law to visit the long-term care facility unannounced (on an annual basis and as needed) to assess the quality of life for the residents by assessing each department and its services, the physical layout of the facility, and records. The HCFA makes available the information it obtains about the quality of long-term care facilities to beneficiaries, providers, researchers, and state surveyors. The Patient Protection and Affordable Care Act is the newest legislation implemented for the protection of the elderly population. It was passed in 2013 (Box 38.5).

The long-term care facility is able to receive Medicare (a federally funded national health insurance program in the United States for people older than age 65) funding by adhering to the HCFA guidelines for reimbursement. Medicaid (a federally funded, state-operated program of medical assistance to people with low incomes), financial assistance provided to anyone who qualifies, is a large source of revenue for the long-term

care facility. An increasing number of individuals have invested in long-term care insurance in anticipation of the possibility of needing these services as they age. Private pay is another method of payment for care in a long-term care facility. Unfortunately, private pay often results in older adults spending all of their assets in a short time. The resident sometimes then qualifies for Medicaid to cover the continued costs of living in a long-term care facility.

Long-term care facilities, like all other health care providers, come under the regulation of the Occupational Safety and Health Administration (OSHA). The inclusion of long-term care facilities in the OSHA guidelines significantly increases the cost of care in this setting but ensures a safe environment for the personnel, which is mandatory today.

Resident rights are a universal priority in all long-term care settings (Box 38.6). Residents and staff of each agency receive communications about setting-specific

---

Box 38.5 Patient Protection and Affordable Care Act

The Patient Protection and Affordable Care Act (PPACA) is the first comprehensive law in a generation to improve the care and safety of the elderly and people with disabilities in nursing homes and other long-term care settings. A protective addition to the PPACA is the Elder Justice Act. This legislation seeks to provide increased protection of seniors from abuses. It seeks to prevent, identify, act upon and prosecute elder abuses. Updates in 2020 entitled "Emergency Support for Nursing Homes and Elder Justice Reform Act of 2020" were implemented (US Senate Committee on Finance, 2020). A large portion of the updates were to aid long-term care agencies in manage the Covid-19 pandemic. Provisions included:

- Financial support for personal protective equipment for long-term care facilities.
- Promote transparency about Covid-19 related cases and fatalities and staffing levels in nursing homes.
- Establishing strike teams—These teams will be established statewide or regionally to respond to the needs of the nursing homes in relation to Covid-19.
- Promoting identification and reporting of abuse and neglect in long-term care facilities.
- Promoting quality of life of long-term care facility residents through televisitation.
- Upgrading nursing home compare and the Five-Star rating system.
- Enhancing federal oversight of nursing homes participating in Medicare and Medicaid.
- Continuing funding for Elder Justice Act of 2010 programs.
- Increasing resources to investigate abuse and neglect and extend services to victims.
- Protecting Americans with dementia.
- Reducing racial and ethnic disparities in long-term care facilities.
- Achieving savings in health care programs.
- Information to guide families in one of the most difficult decisions they ever make: the choice of a nursing home

to care for a loved one. The PPACA expands information about the quality of individual nursing homes on the Medicare website, Nursing Home Compare; helps consumers avoid homes that provide poor care; and creates incentives for Medicare and Medicaid providers to improve staffing, services, and safety in their facilities.

- Public disclosure of nursing home owners and operators that allows government regulators and consumers to identify who is responsible for care in facilities.
- More accountability in individual facilities and better oversight of corporations that operate nursing homes in multiple states.
- A stronger consumer complaint system.
- Disincentives for nursing homes to delay compliance by filing meritless appeals.
- Adequate notification and appropriate relocation of residents when facilities decide to close.
- Training of nursing assistants in the care of people with dementia and in the prevention of abuse.
- Better training for long-term care ombudsmen and state inspectors.
- A program to support national criminal background checks on people who work with vulnerable adults who receive long-term care in institutions or in their own homes.
- Mandatory reporting of the abuse, neglect, or exploitation of anyone in a long-term care facility that receives federal funds.
- Better coordination among agencies that prevent, investigate, and prosecute neglect, exploitation, and abuse of the elderly.

Box **38.6**	Other Ethical Issues Related to Long-Term Care

- Adherence to a patient's bill of rights
- Advance directives
- Do-not-resuscitate (DNR) orders
- Guardianship
- Power of attorney
- Responsible party designation

interpretations as a part of orientation for the personnel and orientation to the services for the recipient of health care services. Advance directives are imperative and valuable in the long-term care facility. Do-not-resuscitate (DNR) orders from the physician are always the result of discussion with the resident, family, and significant others, and documentation by the physician is required. These directions help promote dignity in the last stages of life.

Power of attorney, guardianship, and responsible party designation are all varying degrees of decision-making mechanisms for the resident. The legal system is the route to establish the power of attorney and guardianship, and documentation (legal papers) in the resident's chart is necessary. A responsible party is a person the patient designates, not necessarily with legal formality, to take care of financial and business affairs.

Functional assessment and documentation. Several different types of nursing are present in the long-term care setting: team nursing, functional nursing, total resident care, or a combination of these. The goal remains the same—that is, to provide nursing interventions to a special population over a long period, based on individual assessment and fulfillment of the resident's wishes and needs at this time in life.

The interdisciplinary functional assessment of the resident is the cornerstone of clinical practice in this setting. OBRA prescribed the method of resident assessment and care plan development in an instrument known as the resident assessment instrument (RAI). The LPN/LVN is permitted to complete this assessment tool under the direction of the RN, but it must be signed by the RN. The RAI consists of three parts: the minimum data set (MDS), the resident assessment protocols (RAPs), and the utilization guidelines. The MDS provides a system for assessment of each resident's functional, medical, mental, and psychosocial status on admission to a facility and at regular intervals thereafter. It is an assessment instrument that consists of more than 400 items that usually help identify a resident's problems, strengths, needs, and preferences so that a resident's function can be maintained or enhanced.

After the nurse completes the MDS on a resident, responses to specific items trigger further assessment with the RAPs. RAPs are assessment guides that address common clinical problems, such as delirium, falls, and urinary incontinence. RAPs have accompanying utilization guidelines, the third component. These contain a wealth of clinical information to assist in assessment and care planning. The functional status of the resident is the ability to perform normal, expected, or required activities. In reference to the older adult, it is the capacity to perform self-care activities (ADLs) and the more complex personal, household, and social activities (IADLs) necessary for independent living. The MDS incorporates many of the same assessment factors as a functional assessment tool and requires input from nursing and social services within a specified time frame. The comprehensive assessment provided by the RAI is intended to lead to improved care planning and provision of care for long-term care facility residents.

In this setting, documentation of the resident's condition is different from that in the acute care setting. A summary, including vital signs and weights, is required only monthly. The exception to this charting is a condition change, acute illness, or incident reporting, which is necessary to document at or soon after the time of occurrence.

SAFETY ISSUES IN THE LONG-TERM CARE SETTING

To aid in meeting the safety needs of residents in the long-term care setting, The Joint Commission has established national patient safety goals (TJC, 2021). In addition, The Joint Commission has also provided suggestions on strategies to meet these goals. The five major patient safety goals are:
- Identify residents correctly
- Use medicine safely
- Prevent infection
- Prevent residents from falling
- Prevent pressure injuries

Strategies to meet each of these goals can be found in Box 38.7. Chapter 10 addresses all other safety concerns of patients and residents in health care facilities, including the long-term care setting.

❖ NURSING PROCESS

The role of the LPN/LVN in the nursing process as stated is that the LPN/LVN will:
- Participate in planning care for patients based on patient needs
- Review patient's plan of care and recommend revisions as needed
- Review and follow defined prioritization for patient care
- Use clinical pathways, care maps, or care plans to guide and review patient care

The nursing process is used in long-term care on admission to the facility and is an ongoing process.

Box 38.7 **2017 TJC Nursing Care Center National Patient Safety Goals**

SAFETY GOAL	STRATEGY TO MEET GOAL
Identify residents correctly	Use a minimum of two identifiers for patients or residents. Suggestions are name and date of birth.
Use medicines safely	Use caution with patients or residents on anticoagulants. Upon admission ensure a current medication list is obtained. Follow policy to confirm correct medications are administered. Provide resident with written instructions regarding their medications.
Prevent infection	Use good hand hygiene at all times to prevent the spread of infection among patients or residents.
Prevent residents from falling	Determine which patients or residents are at risk for falls. Institute fall protocol for these patients or residents according to facility policy.
Prevent skin breakdown	• Skin inspection, skin cleansing, care for dry skin, use of moisture barriers, and massage • Nutritional support based on an individualized nutritional needs assessment • Avoidance of skin injury from friction or shear forces through the use of positioning, transferring, and turning techniques • A plan to maintain and, when appropriate, to increase mobility and activity level • Improvement in positioning, repositioning, transferring, and turning techniques to reduce skin injury caused by friction and shear force • Use of repositioning devices and mechanical loading and support surfaces to reduce skin injury caused by friction or shear force • Staff educational programs on the assessment, prevention, and treatment protocols.

Data from The Joint Commission (TJC): Nursing care center: 2021 national patient safety goals, 2021. Retrieved from: https://www.jointcommission.org/standards/national-patient-safety-goals/nursing-care-center-national-patient-safety-goals/.Data from

---

◆ **ASSESSMENT**

The assessment of a long-term care resident occurs on admission and is an ongoing process for the collection of data and information to meet a resident's needs. Communication with the resident, significant other, or family member is essential for complete data collection. The nursing assessment includes a health history, medication history (including herbal products and nutritional supplements) and current medication usage, a functional assessment related to ADLs, personal preferences (e.g., routines, likes and dislikes, hobbies), a physical assessment to document baseline information, and a mental status assessment. The MDS and nursing admission forms document a great deal of this information. In long-term care, the interdisciplinary team reviews the resident's plan of care every 90 days for resolution of problems or revision of goals and interventions.

 Safety Alert

Herbal Products and Nutritional Supplements

When eliciting a medication history and current medication usage patterns, ask about the use of herbs and nutritional supplements. These products, which are marketed as "safe" and "natural," are unregulated by the US Food and Drug Administration (FDA) and potentially have actions and side effects similar to medications. They also have the potential to interact with medications the health care provider prescribes for the resident and in some cases affect medical conditions (either beneficially or detrimentally). Take a complete history of vitamin and mineral usage (and look at the label on the bottle if available); some multivitamin and multimineral products actually contain multiple herbs as well. Residents sometimes are unaware that they are consuming herbal products.

◆ **PATIENT PROBLEM**

The nurse and the team identify patient problems from the assessment. Prioritize risk patient problems for the long-term care resident according to that individual's needs. Possible selections are available in the following list of patient problems (which is not all inclusive):
- *Anxiousness, related to financial difficulties*
- *Complex Grief, related to multiple losses*
- *Compromised Physical Mobility, related to abnormal gait*
- *Functional Ability to Control Urination, related to decreased bladder capacity*
- *Impaired Cognitive Thinking, related to cognitive impairment*
- *Inability to Bathe Self, related to musculoskeletal weakness*
- *Inability to Clear Airway, related to chronic respiratory conditions and musculoskeletal weakness*
- *Inefficient Oxygenation, related to chronic respiratory conditions*
- *Insufficient Cardiac Output, related to cardiovascular disease*
- *Insufficient Nutrition, related to decreased appetite and cognitive impairment*
- *Potential for Aspiration Into Airway, related to impaired swallowing, ill-fitting dentures, musculoskeletal weakness, and medical conditions such as stroke*
- *Potential for Compromised Skin Integrity, related to malnutrition*
- *Potential for Inadequate Fluid Volume, related to the altered thirst mechanism*
- *Potential for Injury, related to forgetfulness, impaired balance*

- *Prolonged Confusion, related to cognitive impairment*
- *Prolonged Low Self-Esteem, related to physical impairment*
- *Social Seclusion, related to homebound status*

◆ EXPECTED OUTCOMES AND PLANNING

The planning process must be patient-centered and individualized to meet the needs of the patient. Priorities begin with the consideration of meeting basic physiologic needs (airway, breathing, and circulation) and go on to consider the patient's multiple conditions or needs. Emotional and psychosocial needs of the patient are also necessary to consider and include in the plan of care.

Properly formulated, the expected outcomes reflect the input of the patient, significant others, and the interdisciplinary team. Expected outcomes have to be measurable, be specific to the patient's problem, and include a time element. Examples are as follows:

Expected outcome 1: Patient will have respirations of 16 to 20 breaths/min during the next 90 days.

Expected outcome 2: Patient will have a pulse rate between 60 and 100 beats/min during the next 90 days.

Expected outcome 3: Patient will verbalize two positive attributes about his or her appearance within 2 days.

◆ IMPLEMENTATION

Nursing interventions basic to long-term care include making rounds and monitoring for resident safety *every* 2 hours. The interpretation of this includes seeing the resident, changing the resident's position, assessing for incontinence, providing skin care, and offering fluids. For example, the LPN/LVN or RN has the responsibility of assessing and intervening to support progress toward the first patient-centered expected outcome in the previous section with the following interventions. Assess the resident for the following:

- Respiratory rate, noisy respirations, signs of suprasternal or intercostal retractions, or nasal flaring
- Color of skin, lips, mucous membranes, and nail beds; cyanosis
- Adventitious lung sounds: describe character and phase of the respiratory cycle (inspiration or expiration) when they occur
- Oxygen administration: note the method of oxygen delivery (nasal cannula versus mask); verify flow rate with physician order; post a "No Smoking" sign on room door; secure the tank for safety; assess tubing or mask for proper fit on resident's face; assess skin for impairment; maintain tubing off the floor
- Offer a sip of water cautiously to assess the resident's ability to swallow fluids

- Assess for cough, sputum characteristics, and ability to expectorate
- Elevate the head of the bed to 30 degrees or greater
- Offer periods of rest between activities
- Alternate foods and fluid when assessing with meals

◆ EVALUATION

Although the RN is officially responsible for the evaluation and modification of the plan of care for the patient, the LPN/LVN's contribution is crucial. The data gathered, along with observation of changes in the patient, make the difference in whether the plan of care is successful.

Nursing evaluation must be aimed directly at patient outcomes. The outcomes identified earlier in the chapter are straightforward and objective, and they require nursing assessment and data gathering to evaluate progress. Evaluation of other outcomes possibly requires additional investigation, such as consulting various sources of information (including reading the progress notes, discussing the plan with the resident, speaking with family and significant others, listening to the nursing report, and investigating laboratory data). In addition, the nursing evaluation also has to take into consideration individual interventions used and which ones were effective and which ones were less useful. This written evaluation is helpful for all nurses implementing the care plan.

The evaluation of care is based on questions such as the following: Was the expected outcome reached for and with the resident? Is the outcome what the resident wishes to accomplish? Are significant others and family members supportive of the outcomes developed by the interdisciplinary team with the resident? After consideration and analysis of the evaluative measures, with use of the nurse's knowledge base, the team makes a decision to continue the current regimen or to implement a change in the nursing interventions to better achieve the patient-centered expected outcome and offer a better quality of life the resident desires. For example:

Expected outcome 1: Patient will have respirations of 16 to 20 breaths/min.

Evaluative measure: Is the resident experiencing shortness of breath during activity or rest? Is there a color change of lips during activity? What is the resident's respiratory rate before, during, and after activity?

The nursing services in long-term care center on functional assessment. Nursing interventions also must be provided based on the following prioritized list of nursing needs: airway, breathing, circulation, nutrition, fluids, elimination, sexuality, safety and security, belonging, self-esteem, and self-actualization.

Get Ready for the NCLEX® Examination!

Key Points

- The need for long-term care services arises after the acute stage of an illness has resolved, when the patient continues to need services to maintain the current and changing physical and psychosocial status and functional abilities.
- Settings that provide long-term care include the home, residential care settings, and institutional settings.
- Services that assist those caring for older adults in the home include adult daycare, hospice, home health agencies, and other community agencies and services.
- Residential care settings offer a wide variety of services to the older adult; two of the more popular types are assisted living facilities and continuing care retirement communities.
- Institutional facilities include subacute units and long-term care facilities.
- Most long-term health care providers are under regulation by federal and state guidelines or use them as minimal standards for health care services, reimbursement, and quality indicators.
- Ethical issues related to long-term care services include adherence to a patient's bill of rights, advance directives, DNR orders, power of attorney, guardianship, and responsible party designation.
- In the long-term care facility, the resident's plan of care is reviewed every 90 days for resolution of problems or revision of expected outcomes and interventions by the team.
- Identification of safety concerns, goals, and ways to meet safety goals are important aspects of care in the long-term care setting.

Additional Learning Resources

SG Go to your Study Guide for additional learning activities to help you master this chapter content.

Be sure to visit the Evolve site at http://evolve.elsevier.com/Co oper/foundations/ for additional online resources.

Review Questions for the NCLEX® Examination

1. **The student nurse is researching long-term care. What does the student identify as being the overall goal for residents in long-term care?**

    1. The resident will remain free of disease.
    2. The resident will return home as soon as possible.
    3. The resident will enjoy their long-term care experience.
    4. The resident will remain as independent as possible in the long-term care setting.

2. **Which person would benefit most from long-term care services?**

    1. A 98-year-old widow who lives at home independently and can perform ADLs but needs a ride to church every Sunday
    2. A 65-year-old widower who is recovering from a stroke and is unable to move his left side
    3. A 75-year-old woman who lives with her husband and has arthritis and osteoporosis with reports of mild to moderate stiffness every morning
    4. A 70-year-old man who lives alone and has a history of coronary artery disease and hypertension

3. **The nurse identifies which patient as having the highest priority need for hospice care?**

    1. A 65-year-old woman who has metastatic lung cancer and receives home health services
    2. A 77-year-old man who has end-stage prostate cancer and lives in a long-term care facility
    3. A 44-year-old woman who has AIDS and lives in a continuing care retirement community
    4. A 70-year-old woman who recently was diagnosed with ovarian cancer

4. **A patient is receiving hospice care for his end-stage cardiac disease. Which statement by his wife alerts the nurse for the need for further education regarding hospice care?** *(Select all that apply.)*

    1. "What are the side effects of my husband's pain medication?"
    2. "Are there support groups to help with the grieving process?"
    3. "My husband finally slept for more than 2 hours last night."
    4. "How will I know when it is time to call 9-1-1?"
    5. "We will only need hospice care until my husband gets better."

5. **What institutional setting is a bridge between acute care and long-term care?**

    1. Subacute care
    2. Nursing home care
    3. Residential care
    4. Adult daycare

6. **Which scenario best illustrates the effect OBRA has had on the professional practice of LPN/LVNs in the long-term care setting?** *(Select all that apply.)*

    1. The LPN/LVN may be responsible for administering intravenous therapy.
    2. The LPN/LVN provides direct bedside resident care.
    3. The LPN/LVN performs dressing changes.
    4. The LPN/LVN functions as medication nurse.
    5. The LPN/LVN has the responsibility of being a team leader.

7. **Which is the best example of an interdisciplinary team?**

    1. Director of nurses, charge nurse, staff nurse, CNA, resident
    2. Resident, nurses, physician, social worker, pharmacist, dietitian, activities director, rehabilitation specialists, podiatrist, psychiatrist, audiologist, dentist
    3. Attending physician, resident physician, intern, medical student, CNA, CMA/CMT, physical therapist
    4. Gerontologic clinical nurse specialist, physician, pharmacist, social worker, clergy, resident

8. The new nurse has questions about palliative care. Which response by the nurse best describes this type of care?

 1. "Palliative care is usually provided in acute care facilities."
 2. "Palliative care is typically recommended for individuals with less than 6 months' life expectancy."
 3. "Palliative care is usually affiliated with a church and provided by parish nurses."
 4. "Palliative care extends the principles of hospice care to a broader population that has the possibility to benefit from comfort care earlier in the disease process."

9. Which statement by the student nurse is most accurate in regard to the elderly population?

 1. Most live in a long-term care facility.
 2. Most attend an adult daycare facility.
 3. Most live in a home setting.
 4. Most live in an assisted living setting.

10. The nurse working in an outpatient clinic refers which patient to PACE based on the nurse's assessment?

 1. A 52-year-old who is being treated for hypertension and lives alone
 2. A 70-year-old who has no support system and has chronic venous ulcers requiring treatment at the local wound center
 3. A 90-year-old who has type 2 diabetes controlled by oral diabetic agents and lives with family
 4. A 49-year-old who is disabled because of a chronic debilitating neuromuscular disease and requires physical therapy services three times per week

11. In accordance with National Patient Safety Goals for Nursing Care Centers, which action by the nurse demonstrates an understanding of these goals? *(Select all that apply.)*

 1. The nurse asks the patient to state his or her name and hospital ID number before administering them their medication.
 2. The nurse provides indwelling catheter care to a patient by following facility policy and procedures.
 3. The nurse performs a thorough skin assessment of a new resident upon admission to the health care facility.
 4. The nurse performs a sterile dressing change to the central line of a resident as directed by facility policy.
 5. The nurse asks the resident's family to bring in all home medications to ensure the list given by the patient upon admission to the facility is accurate.

12. An LPN has just begun his first job in his new profession at a long-term care facility for seniors, and he's looking forward to it. "I lived with grandparents as part of an extended household growing up," he says, "and I really gained a lot from it. I wouldn't trade that experience for the world and I feel like I'm a natural fit for working in elder care. This was my absolute first choice!" But on his first day, he finds himself a bit overwhelmed by the assessment instruments under OBRA's resident assessment instrument (RAI). "It's a little overwhelming," he says, "trying to understand the difference in function between the minimum data set (MDS) and the resident assessment protocols (RAPs)."

Use an X to indicate whether each function belongs to either the minimum data set (MDS) and the resident assessment protocols (RAPs). All should be used and can be used only once.

FUNCTION	MINIMUM DATA SET (MDS)	RESIDENT ASSESSMENT PROTOCOLS (RAPS)
Assesses each resident's overall status *on admission* to a facility		
Expands on specifics for key assessment items		
Offers assessment guidelines that address common clinical problems		
Assesses each resident's overall status at regular intervals *after* admission		
Responses to items trigger further investigation		
Provide utilization guidelines to assist in care planning		
Consists of more than 400 items to identify problems, strengths, needs, and preferences		

Objectives

1. Define the philosophy of rehabilitation nursing.
2. Identify patients who would benefit from rehabilitation services.
3. Discuss the goals of rehabilitation therapies.
4. Describe the interdisciplinary rehabilitation team concept and the function of each team member.
5. Discuss the role of the nurse in the specialized practice of rehabilitation.
6. Recognize the importance and significance of family-centered care in rehabilitation.
7. Discuss two major disabling conditions.
8. Recognize polytrauma as a difficult challenge for rehabilitation.
9. Recognize how important it is for the nurse on the rehabilitation team to be knowledgeable about posttraumatic stress disorder (PTSD) and assess for its presence.
10. Describe the goals of pediatric and gerontologic rehabilitation nursing.

Key Terms

chronic illness (KRŎN-ĭk ĬL-nĭs, p. 1213)
Commission on Accreditation of Rehabilitation Facilities (kŭ-MĬSH-ŭn ŎN ŭ-krĕd-ĭ-TĀ-shŭn ŬV rē-ŭ-bĭl-ĭ-TĀ-shŭn fŭ-SĬL-ŭ-tēz, p. 1214)
comprehensive rehabilitation plan (kŏm-prē-HĔN-sĭv rē-ŭ-bĭl-ĭ-TĀ-shŭn PLĂN, p. 1214)
disability (dĭs-ŭ-BĬL-ŭ-tē, p. 1213)
exacerbation (p. 1213)
family-centered care (FĂM-ŭ-lē SĔN-tŭrd KĀR, p. 1217)
functional limitation (FŬNG-shŭn-ŭl lĭm-ĭ-TĀ-shŭn, p. 1213)
gerontologic rehabilitation nursing (jĕr-ŏn-tŭ-LŎJ-ĭk rē-ŭ-bĭl-ĭ-TĀ-shŭn NŬR-sĭng, p. 1224)
impairment (ĭm-PĀR-mĭnt, p. 1213)

interdisciplinary rehabilitation team (ĭn-tŭr-DĬS-ŭ-plĭn-ăr-ē rē-ŭ-bĭl-ĭ-TĀ-shŭn TĒM, p. 1215)
multidisciplinary rehabilitation team (mŭl-tē-DĬS-ŭ-plĭn-ăr-ē rē-ŭ-bĭl-ĭ-TĀ-shŭn TĒM, p. 1215)
pediatric rehabilitation nursing (pē-dē-ĂT-rĭk rē-ŭ-bĭl-ĭ-TĀ-shŭn NŬR-sĭng, p. 1224)
physiatrist (fĭz-ē-ĂT-rĭst, p. 1215)
posttraumatic stress disorder (PTSD) (pōst-trăw-MĂT-ĭk STRĔS dĭs-ŎR-dŭr, p. 1219)
spinal cord injury (SCI) (SPĪ-nŭl CŌRD ĬN-jŭr-ē, p. 1220)
transdisciplinary rehabilitation team (trănz-DĬS-ŭ-plĭn-ăr-ē rē-ŭ-bĭl-ĭ-TĀ-shŭn TĒM, p. 1216)
traumatic brain injury (TBI) (trăw-MĂT-ĭk BRĀN ĬN-jŭr-ē, p. 1223)

The focus of rehabilitation nursing is to support patients in the restoration of a health state or in the adaptation of changes that have resulted from chronic illness, disability, or injury. Rehabilitation nursing is holistic. The patient's physical, mental, emotional, and social needs are assessed and incorporated into the plan of care. The participation of the family is encouraged. In rehabilitation nursing, these concepts are used throughout the continuum of care and across the lifespan of the patient.

It is possible to define rehabilitation in a variety of ways. This chapter will focus on rehabilitation from a medical aspect. Mental health–focused rehabilitation is addressed in Chapters 34 through 36. Rehabilitation is a process of outcome-focused patient care delivered by an interdisciplinary team (such as

nurses, physical and occupational therapists, speech therapists, and mental health professionals) with the goal of restoring the patient to the fullest physical, mental, social, vocational, and economic capacity of which he or she is capable. Rehabilitation helps an individual regain function or adjust to a new set of needs by finding new ways to do the things previously done. The underlying philosophy of rehabilitation is to focus on abilities rather than disabilities, to continually make the most of the abilities that remain intact. The individual, the family, and the support system are the focus of all rehabilitation efforts. Quality rehabilitation results in the person continually striving to reach his or her highest potential. The setting for rehabilitative activities may be inpatient or outpatient.

NEED FOR REHABILITATION

Rehabilitation is required and valuable in a variety of circumstances. What precipitates the need for rehabilitation may include one or more of the following:

- **Impairment:** Any loss or abnormality of psychological, physical, or anatomic structure or function.
- **Disability:** The loss of ability to participate in one or more major life activities as a result of mental, emotional, or physical impairments. This includes activities such as school, employment, home, community, or social events (ADA National Network, 2021). The impairment may limit participation in a manner within a range of ability that is considered normal.
- **Functional limitation:** Any loss of ability to perform tasks or activities of daily living (ADLs).
  Chronic illness: A chronic illness generally refers to a condition or state that lasts for 3 months or longer. A chronic illness can have periods of remission and **exacerbation.**

It is important to recognize the differences between these terms and the uniqueness of each term. In rehabilitation nursing, the individual is recognized to have a disability, and the focus is on the individual rather than on the disability. Thus, rehabilitation nurses work with people who have disabilities, rather than "the disabled."

CHRONIC ILLNESS AND DISABILITY

Although managing chronic illness and disability is one of the biggest health care problems facing developed countries, the US health care system is not yet positioned to provide optimal care for the individuals who need it. The emphasis on acute care persists, even though the largest group of health care consumers consists of people with chronic illnesses: 113 million Americans have a chronic illness. This accounts for 40% of the population. The risk of chronic illness intensifies with age: An estimated 80% of individuals aged 65 and older are living with a chronic disease (National Rehabilitation Information Center [NARIC], 2016). Aging causes an accumulation of lifelong risk factors and behaviors that may not have been health promotional. Children are not exempt from this plight. In the population aged 5 to 17 years, 8% experience loss of functionality related to a chronic condition. Medical costs for chronic conditions such as mental health disorders represent about 90% of these health care expenditures (CDC, 2021). Healthy People is a systematic approach for promoting improved health and wellness for the nation. The government initiative by the US Department of Health and Human Services (DHHS) spans each decade. Many of the initiatives relate to access to care and the management of chronic illness (Box 39.1). A concerned public as well as committed and knowledgeable professionals are necessary to accomplish these goals.

Box 39.1	*Healthy People 2030* Focus Areas Related to Chronic Illness and Disability

- Increase access to comprehensive, high-quality health care services
- Arthritis, osteoporosis, and chronic back conditions
- Cancer
- Chronic kidney disease
- Chronic Pain
- Dementias
- Diabetes
- Disability and health
- Hearing and other sensory or communication disorders
- Heart disease and stroke
- Infectious Disease
- Mental health and mental disorders
- Overweight and obesity
- Respiratory disease
- Sensory or Communication Disorders

From US Department of Health and Human Services: Office of Disease Prevention and Health Promotion: *Healthy People 2030*, n.d. Retrieved from: https://health.gov/healthypeople/objectives-and-data/browse-objectives#health-conditions

Health care providers must learn to recognize the special needs of the person with a chronic illness or disability and to organize, plan, and provide care to meet these needs. To appreciate the need for a specific, unique approach to planning and providing care for individuals with chronic illnesses and disabling conditions, providers first need to understand the concepts of chronicity and disability.

CHRONICITY

Unlike acute illnesses, which are usually abrupt in onset and self-limiting (the illness is either resolved or death ensues), chronic illnesses have the potential to be either abrupt or insidious in onset and, by definition, persist for an extended and indefinite period. Affected patients are still able to function, but often with some limitation because of the chronic illness.

SCOPE OF INDIVIDUALS REQUIRING REHABILITATION

Rehabilitation is a bridge for the patient, spanning the gap between uselessness and usefulness, between hopelessness and hopefulness, between despair and happiness. The scope of conditions that necessitate rehabilitation is broad and spans the life continuum. Living longer in the United States presents an interesting paradox between retiring and enjoying the so-called golden years and a strong probability of acquiring one or more chronic, disabling conditions. Chronic illness and physiologic changes of aging increase the likelihood of physical limitations and disability disproportionately for older people in comparison with younger adults. Although many families continue to care for older people with disabling conditions in their homes, many also live in nursing homes. Whether an older patient is in the acute stage of an illness or injury, rehabilitation services are built around maintaining functional abilities, ensuring safety, promoting effective coping, preventing complications, and modifying the environment for maximal independence.

A disability has a number of potential effects on the patient and the family, including behavioral and emotional changes, as well as changes in roles, body image, self-concept, and family dynamics.

GOALS OF REHABILITATION

Rehabilitation is a goal-oriented (outcome-oriented) process. These goals are personal, and the rehabilitation team individualizes them to meet the holistic needs of each patient served. To determine goals, a collaborative goal-setting process includes the members of the rehabilitation team, with the patient and the family at the center of the process.

It is appropriate to include the following criteria in all rehabilitation goals:

- The goals maximize the quality of life of the patient.
- The goals address the patient's specific needs.
- The goals assist the patient with adjusting to an altered lifestyle.
- The goals are directed toward promoting wellness and minimizing complications.
- The goals assist the patient in attaining the highest degree of function and self-sufficiency possible.
- The goals assist the patient with home and community reentry.

All rehabilitation efforts must be outcome-focused, comprehensive, and must constitute an educational process.

CORNERSTONES OF REHABILITATION

Rehabilitation involves several important aspects of care in helping the patient meet agreed-upon goals. The following are important factors to keep in mind in helping the patient to reach these goals:

- *Focus on the individual:* All efforts of rehabilitation are centered on the patient's goals and objectives. When the patient sets or holds goals that are not realistic, the team works with the patient in reshaping expectations.
- *Community reentry:* Rehabilitation is considered successful if the patient is able to reenter the community through participation in social, vocational, and recreational activities.
- *Independence:* The goals of rehabilitation focus on promoting and maintaining the patient's physical and emotional independence.
- *Functional ability:* Progress in rehabilitation is measured in terms of functional outcomes.
- *Team approach:* Rehabilitation goals are achieved through the work of the rehabilitation team members, including the patient and the family.

- *Quality of life:* Goals focus on improving the quality of life, rather than increasing the quantity of life.
- *Prevention and wellness:* Because many problems that necessitate rehabilitation are long-standing, rehabilitation goals focus on preventing complications and maximizing function.
- *Change process:* Patients who experience a disabling condition or chronic illness experience the change process, as do their families. The rehabilitation team is responsible for directing the change in as positive a manner as possible.
- *Adaptation:* Although patients with disabilities do not always accept their disability, learning to adapt to the circumstances created by the limits of their abilities is a positive method of coping.
- *Patient and family education:* Knowledge and skills are essential components of the rehabilitation program. Patients with substantial disability have the potential to obtain a degree of independence through patient education, which enables them to direct their own care.

COMPREHENSIVE REHABILITATION PLAN

The more comprehensive the rehabilitation program is, the better are the chances for higher functional outcomes of the people served. According to the **Commission on Accreditation of Rehabilitation Facilities** (a nonprofit, private, international standard-setting and accreditation body whose mission is to promote and advocate the delivery of quality rehabilitation), it is necessary to initiate an overall individualized **comprehensive rehabilitation plan** of care within 24 hours of the patient's hospital admission and have it ready for review and revision by the rehabilitation team within 3 days of the admission. The results of the interdisciplinary admission assessment provide the basis for developing the plan. Underlying it are individual goals incorporating the unique strengths, needs, abilities, and preferences of the patient. This plan reflects the environment where the patient will go upon hospital discharge. The goals must be measurable, must be described in functional or behavioral terms, and must have associated time frames for achievement. The responsible team member or members must be listed, as well.

All clinicians treating the patient use this comprehensive plan of care. Evaluation conferences and family conferences take place on a regular basis. The active participation of the patient and family is an integral part of planning and implementing the discharge process.

REHABILITATION TEAM

Because a single discipline does not offer the knowledge and expertise necessary to provide all the components of the rehabilitation program, the rehabilitation team is composed of people from multiple

Table **39.1**   Rehabilitation Team

MEMBER	ROLE	ACTIONS
Patient	Key member	Participates in goal setting Takes control of own life
Physiatrist	Rehabilitation physician	Is team leader and coordinator of program
Rehabilitation RN	Coordinator, educator	Provides support Educates patient and family concerning rehabilitation process Promotes independence
Rehabilitation LPN/LVN	Care provider; patient's advocate	Provides support Reinforces education to the patient and family concerning the rehabilitation process Assists in treatment plan and implementation
Physical therapist	Designing exercise program	Provides therapy Assesses patient's needs Provides training
Occupational therapist	Assessing independent living needs	Recommends equipment modifications Adapts equipment
Speech-language pathologist	Performing assessment of communication and swallowing abilities Designing rehabilitation communication program	Helps patient regain communication skills Teaches patient
Therapeutic recreation therapist	Recreation planner	Plans leisure activities Promotes patient's interest in activities
Clinical psychologist	Emotional evaluator	Assesses patient's position on the mental health continuum Promotes patient's independence by maximizing active participation Assists patient in developing realistic positive attitudes
Chaplain	Spiritual consultant	Provides spiritual support and guidance
Vocational rehabilitation counselor	Vocational planner	Helps patient obtain training for new or current employment

LPN/LVN, Licensed practical nurse or licensed vocational nurse; *RN,* registered nurse.

disciplines. The patient's specific illness and needs ultimately determine the team's composition. Members of the interdisciplinary team may include a physician, a nurse practitioner, a physiatrist (physicians specializing in physical medicine or rehabilitation), a physical/occupational/speech therapist, a recreational therapist, a nutritionist, a psychologist, a spiritual adviser, and a social worker. It always includes the patient, too. The team coordinates the comprehensive rehabilitation program for each patient in an individualized manner (Table 39.1 and Fig. 39.1).

MODELS OF TEAM FUNCTIONING

There are three primary models of rehabilitation team functioning. One model, primarily of service in the past, is the multidisciplinary rehabilitation team. Characteristic of this model are discipline-specific goals, clear boundaries between disciplines, and outcomes that are the sum of each discipline's efforts. Effective communication is the key to success for this type of team.

The type of team most commonly used today in rehabilitation hospitals is the interdisciplinary rehabilitation

Fig. 39.1 Members of the rehabilitation team helping a patient with ambulation.

team. This type of team collaborates to identify individual's goals and features a combination of expanded problem solving beyond the boundaries of the individual disciplines, together with discipline-specific work toward goal attainment.

A third type of team is the transdisciplinary rehabilitation team. What characterizes this model is the blurring of boundaries between disciplines, as well as cross-training and flexibility to minimize any duplication of effort toward individual goal attainment.

Major strengths of the team methods of care delivery are that they are well established, promote good communication and collaboration among disciplines, address comprehensive aspects of care, energize staff, and view the patient holistically. These models provide a structure for rehabilitation. It is still necessary to integrate services to ensure a comprehensive, appropriate experience.

REHABILITATION NURSE

The rehabilitation nurse with diverse expertise, roles, and work settings plays a vital, unique role on this team. Rehabilitation nurses are with the patient on a 24-hour basis. Because of this constant exposure, nurses can notice small, often imperceptible changes. It is necessary for rehabilitation nurses to have broad knowledge of the pathophysiology of a wide range of medical-surgical conditions and highly specialized knowledge and skills regarding rehabilitation (Box 39.2).

In addition to a set of specialized knowledge and skills, rehabilitation nursing is an attitude. In rehabilitation, the work is predicated on the belief that

---

Box 39.2   Roles of the Rehabilitation Nurse

- Educator
  - Reinforces the teaching delivered by other members of the health care team
  - Discusses wellness and health promotion activities
  - Provides information about the disease process and the plan of care
- Provider of care
  - Performs holistic patient assessments
  - Provides or oversees physical care of the patient
  - Plans nursing care
- Collaborator
  - Works to streamline the interactions of the health care team
  - Develops realistic, patient-focused goals
- Patient advocate
  - Actively listens to the needs and wishes of the patient
  - Seeks to incorporate the requests of the patient in the plan of care

The above copyrighted information was reprinted with permission from the Association of Rehabilitation Nurses, 8735 W. Higgins Road, Suite 300, Chicago, IL 60031; © 2015. Information may not be reprinted or altered without written permission from the Association of Rehabilitation Nurses.

---

individuals with functional disabilities or chronic illnesses have an intrinsic worth that transcends the disability or illness. William Barclay put it this way (197:

"One of the highest of human duties is the duty of encouragement… It is easy to laugh at men's ideals; it is easy to pour cold water on their enthusiasm; it is easy to discourage others. The world is full of discouragers… We have a duty to encourage one another. Many a time a word of praise or thanks has kept a man on his feet. Blessed is the man who speaks such a word."

Rehabilitation nurses are obliged to offer encouragement on a regular basis. The role of a rehabilitation nurse is to put the individual in charge of his or her own care rather than taking charge.

The Association of Rehabilitation Nurses (2021) gives the following definition:

Rehabilitation nursing is a specialty practice area within the scope of professional nursing. It involves the diagnosis and treatment of human responses of individuals and groups to actual or potential health problems resulting from altered functional ability and altered lifestyle.

The goal of rehabilitation nursing is to assist individuals with disabilities and chronic illness in the restoration, maintenance, and promotion of optimal health. The rehabilitation nurse is skilled at treating alterations in functional ability and lifestyle resulting from injury, disability, and chronic illness.

Rehabilitation nurses provide comfort, therapy, and education; promote health-conducive adjustments; support adaptive capabilities; and promote achievable independence. Rehabilitation nurses provide holistic, comprehensive, and compassionate end-of-life care, including promotion of comfort and relief of pain.

Specialized training is necessary to become an effective team member. Although each team member contributes to the rehabilitation process, it is the rehabilitation nurse who reinforces teaching and training completed by the other disciplines on a 24-hours-a-day, 7-days-a-week basis. Efficacious rehabilitation nursing is essential for a successful rehabilitation outcome.

Rehabilitation nursing is practiced in a variety of settings across the continuum of care: primary care clinics, home health agencies, outpatient services, hospitals and rehabilitation facilities, skilled nursing facilities, subacute or transitional care facilities, residential facilities, daycare agencies, insurance companies, and private companies. The rehabilitation nurse is a vital member of the interdisciplinary rehabilitation team and is responsible for taking on many roles: educator, caregiver, counselor, care coordinator, case manager, patient advocate, consultant, researcher, administrator or manager, and expert witness.

The focus in rehabilitation is on enabling the patient to move from a totally dependent state to a level of independence. In the optimal scenario, each patient receives individual treatment from specific nurses and therapists so that bonds of trust and friendship can develop through the difficult rehabilitation process. Extensive family and patient education, modern adaptive equipment, numerous community integration activities, specialized programs, and professional, effective team therapies combine to help patients learn to make the most of their lives.

Basic rehabilitation can be used whether the patient is suffering from arthritis, multiple sclerosis, mental illness, brain attack or stroke, spinal cord injury, burn, or traumatic brain injury. The nurse's responsibility is to apply appropriate concepts and techniques throughout the continuum of care. All basic nursing measures are essential—these include position changes and maintaining body alignment, which prevent skeletal and muscular deformities (contractures) and pressure ulcers.

Rehabilitation nursing is a challenge that requires knowledge, teamwork, coordination, planning, and patience. To care for people with disabilities, it is important for rehabilitation professionals to learn and stay abreast of current knowledge and techniques.

The phenomenon of change as it relates to the human experience is a central concept in nursing. This is especially true for rehabilitation nurses, who regularly interact with people experiencing great change. The focus of this chapter is on the individual patient, who is the central member of the rehabilitation team. Understanding and promoting the change process is therefore an integral part of the role of a rehabilitation nurse.

Nursing Assessment

The nurse begins to develop a plan of care for the patient by assessing the ability of the patient to perform ADLs in a safe manner, and this assessment helps the nurse determine the patient's level of independence. This assessment is performed best through observation of the patient completing different basic tasks, such as ambulation and bathing. Observation of the abilities or disabilities of the patient provides information on which to base the plan of care. Additional areas to observe include ability of the patient to dress himself or herself, including fastening clothing, and self-feeding ability, including holding utensils and chewing and swallowing food and liquids.

Patient Problem

The major patient problem for a patient receiving rehabilitation services is related to performing ADLs. Based on assessment findings, any of the following patient problem statements could be used in relation to inability to perform ADLs:

* *Inability to bathe self*
* *Inability to dress self*
* *Inability to feed self*
* *Inability to toilet self*

Additional patient problems for consideration in the rehabilitation setting include the following:

* *Compromised maintenance of health*

* *Excessive demand on primary caregiver*
* *Helplessness*
* *Insufficient knowledge*
* *Interrupted family processes*
* *Potential for inability to tolerate activity*

NURSING INTERVENTIONS

Nursing interventions are geared to support and reinforce activities included in the interdisciplinary plan of care. Additional nursing interventions may include the following:

* Assisting the patient with repetition and practice of exercises
* Minimizing distractions that would prevent patient participation in therapy
* Providing cues and reminders as needed

The following five-step approach is an option to guide this process:

1. Assess the patient's and the family's needs, abilities, and concerns.
2. Plan interventions on the basis of these needs, abilities, and concerns.
3. Implement the educational plan.
4. Document the educational process.
5. Evaluate and revise the educational plan.

FAMILY AND FAMILY-CENTERED CARE

Family-centered care is a philosophy that recognizes the pivotal role of the family in the lives of children with disabilities or other chronic conditions. It is a philosophy by which health care providers strive to support families in their natural caregiving roles by building on the parents' unique strengths as individuals. This perspective promotes normal patterns of living at home and in the community, and families and professionals are viewed as equals in a partnership committed to excellence at all levels of health care. The ability and willingness of nurses and health care providers to share knowledge and control of health resources with families, empowering family members to act as advocates for themselves and their children, is an integral part of family-centered care.

The key elements of family-centered care are as follows:

* Incorporating into policy and practice the recognition that the family is the constant in a child's life, whereas the service systems and support personnel within those systems are transitional
* Facilitating family-professional collaboration at all levels of hospital, home, and community care
* Exchanging complete and unbiased information between families and professionals in a supportive manner at all times
* Encouraging and facilitating family-to-family support and networking
* Appreciating the unique characteristics of families and children with a recognition of the wide range

of strengths, concerns, emotions, and aspirations beyond their need for specialized health and developmental services and support (Bamm, 2008)

Collaboration between family and the professional is essential for providing appropriate and optimal care.

Family-centered care is an evolving concept. It is a process that differs according to variations in situations, families, cultures, health care settings, and providers. Family-centered care requires learning new ways of relating to and working with families, in rehabilitation and throughout the continuum of care.

CROSS-CULTURAL REHABILITATION

Society is in a state of transformation. Demographic shifts, in combination with an increasingly wide range of ethnic identification, religions, material reality, beliefs, and behaviors, lead to rich diversity and cultural complexity. At the same time, health professionals, including rehabilitation teams, are becoming much more aware of the need to become culturally knowledgeable to be effective in their interaction with patients.

The relationship between the rehabilitation team, the patient, and family members is often extended. To be successful, the collaboration must be genuine. The quality of this relationship will impact the outcome. Disability exists in all societies, but the definition and significance of disability in an individual culture depends on that culture's values. Attitudes also vary toward individuals with a disability; toward concepts of rehabilitation; toward the sociocultural, biological, and economic implications of disability; and toward policy affecting individuals with a disability. (See Chapter 6 for a detailed discussion of culture and ethnic considerations.)

Cultural competence requires the acknowledgment and awareness of one's own cultural norms. Then, it involves the awareness and acceptance of those cultural values and behaviors of another. The incorporation of cultural competence into the assessment, planning, and delivery of care enables the patient to receive holistic care.

The following describes a culturally competent practitioner:

- Has the capacity for cultural self-assessment
- Provides health care that is sensitive to the culture and values of the patient and is linguistically appropriate
- Is conscious of the dynamics of difference
- Disseminates cultural knowledge
- Adapts to diversity in race, color, ethnicity, national origin, immigration status, religion, age, gender, sexual orientation, political beliefs, social and economic status, education, occupation, spirituality, and any other differences

In summary, what characterizes cultural competence is acceptance and respect for difference, continuing self-assessment regarding culture, vigilance toward the dynamics of difference, ongoing expansion of cultural knowledge and resources, and adaptability of services.

People develop *cultural proficiency* when they hold culture in high regard. The culturally proficient professional recognizes the need to conduct research, disseminates the results, and develops new approaches that promise to increase culturally competent practice. Rehabilitation professionals have an ethical responsibility to strive for cultural competence and cultural proficiency.

ISSUES IN REHABILITATION

In rehabilitation, several forces drive the rendering of care. The issues involved include, but are not limited to, the following:

- *Quality of life versus quantity of life*: Rehabilitation focuses on continually improving the quality of the person's life, not merely maintaining life itself.
- *Care versus cure*: Because of the suddenness and catastrophic effect of many conditions that necessitate rehabilitation, it is necessary to consider the care of the individual in relation to the cure of the condition. Many conditions are irreversible, making the focus of care on the adaptation to a condition rather than its resolution.

High cost of interdisciplinary care versus long-term care: Rehabilitation is expensive. The care team involves a number of highly trained professionals. Planning for rehabilitation should ideally begin in the first days of the initial illness. Early entry into rehabilitation is beneficial. Benefits include cost savings due to a reduced length of stay in both ICU and acute care facilities. In addition, early rehabilitation efforts will lessen physical or mental declines. In some cases, the success of rehabilitation is viewed as a person's return to productive employment. In other cases, a disability means that two people become unemployed—the individual with the disability and the caregiver. Rehabilitation in this scenario can be successful, and the savings still considerable, if the individual with the disability becomes independent enough to not require a caregiver even though he or she remains unable to return to work.

CHRONIC CONDITIONS NECESSITATING REHABILITATION THERAPY

CARDIAC REHABILITATION

An insult to the cardiovascular system, such as a myocardial infarction or cardiac surgery, may require the patient to participate in rehabilitation to improve function and facilitate a return to normal activities. A cardiac rehabilitation program is designed to meet the needs of the patient through exercise, education about heart healthy living, and counseling in stress reduction in an effort to reduce modifiable risk factors associated with cardiac disease and to prevent future hospitalizations (American Heart Association [AHA], 2016).

The rehabilitation team evaluates baseline levels of physical fitness and develops an individualized program. The focus is also on improving the patient's emotional adaptation to the cardiac condition and related limitations.

PULMONARY REHABILITATION

Patients with chronic breathing problems, such as chronic obstructive pulmonary disease, and those who require or who have just recently undergone lung surgery may benefit from pulmonary rehabilitation. This type of rehabilitation includes an exercise program; counseling regarding diet and nutrition; education regarding the lung disease process; and management, energy conservation techniques, and breathing strategies (American Lung Association, 2016). The program may be located in the hospital or offered on an outpatient basis in the community. Home-based services are common. Health care team members involved in pulmonary rehabilitation include primary care providers, nurses, respiratory therapists, physical and occupational therapists, dietitians, and nutritionists. Social services also may be represented.

POLYTRAUMA AND REHABILITATION NURSING

Soldiers wounded in conflicts abroad in locales such as Iraq and Afghanistan have brought about challenges to today's health care system. These soldiers experience multiple traumas with variable patterns—a phenomenon known as polytrauma/blast-related injury (PT/BRI)—as a result of explosions (US Department of Veterans Affairs, 2021a). Rehabilitative nurses in the military and in the Veterans Administration have responded to these challenges (Fig. 39.2).

Blast-related injuries are categorized as primary, secondary, tertiary, or quaternary (miscellaneous) (Pennardt, 2016). Air-filled cavities in the body (ears, lungs, and gastrointestinal tract) and organs enveloped

Fig. 39.2 Wounded army veteran receiving rehabilitative nursing care. (US Army photo by Spc. Cody Barber/Released.)

by fluid (brain and spinal cord) are most susceptible to compression damage from high-explosive blasts. These injuries are considered primary blast-related injuries. Injuries from airborne debris, bomb fragments, and shrapnel embedded in any body part are considered secondary blast-related injuries. Any injury sustained from being thrown as the result of an explosive shock wave or dynamic overpressure is a tertiary blast-related injury. Examples include broken bones and traumatic head and spinal cord injuries. Inhalation of and exposure to toxic chemicals, traumatic amputations of limbs, and burns are examples of quaternary injuries (Tan, 2021).

In an effort to deal more effectively with PT/BRI, the plans for treatment and rehabilitation will include medical, mental health, and surgical needs. A primary goal will be the reduction of disabilities associated with these injuries. The rehabilitation teams for soldiers who have experienced PT/BRI gear their care toward discovering and treating additional injuries that were not detected during the post-acute phase, as well as treating those originally identified injuries. Early onset for the rehabilitation plans will aid in a reduction of costs for the total period of treatment.

It is important to understand, identify, and treat PT/BRIs to avoid focusing care solely on the more visible injuries. Identification of this newly identified group of injuries allows successful treatment of a variety of conditions, ranging from concussions that cause cognitive and vestibular deficits to posttraumatic stress disorder (Rosenfeld, 2010).

POSTTRAUMATIC STRESS DISORDER

Posttraumatic stress disorder (PTSD) is defined as a mental health condition related to the experience or witnessing of a traumatic event (Mayo Clinic, 2018). These events may be those imposed on one personally, such as a rape or serious accident, or may be linked to a national crisis/disaster. PTSD has been tied to the terrorist attacks of September 11, 2001, the California forest fires, and hurricanes. For the majority of those experiencing PTSD, the symptoms begin within a few months of the event, although some may not experience them for several years. Instead of getting better over time, the symptoms get worse. The person may repeatedly experience the traumatic event through flashbacks or nightmares, causing difficulty in sleeping and concentrating. A person experiencing PTSD tries to avoid people, places, and activities that serve to remind him or her of the traumatic event (Anxiety & Depression Association of America [ADAA], 2017).

The American Psychiatric Association first identified PTSD in 1980. Before 1980, the field described soldiers who experienced the symptoms now known as PTSD as suffering from "shell shock" or "war neurosis" (Glass, 1969), and many people believed that affected soldiers were making up the symptoms to avoid being involved in further combat (Clark, 1997). After the Vietnam War, PTSD received acceptance as a psychiatric diagnosis, and other forms of trauma, such as rape and natural disasters, were also identified as causes of PTSD (American Psychiatric Association, 1980).

The veracity of the disorder still raises doubt among some family members and health care providers. PTSD diagnosis is considered if the symptoms do not improve, or worsen, after at least 1 month and are dependent on the identification of a traumatic event—either personally experienced or witnessed—and/or the reliving of the traumatic events, either through dreams or reoccurring vivid memories or flashbacks, which interferes with normal life functions (Mayo Clinic, 2018).

Without proper identification and treatment, PTSD has been known to lead to other mental health problems such as depression, anxiety, alcohol or drug use, and even suicidal thoughts or actions. Effective treatments for PTSD have included psychotherapy and pharmacotherapy. Studies have shown that a combination of cognitive and prolonged-exposure therapy is the most effective in treating the disorder, sometimes with the aid of medications such as selective serotonin reuptake inhibitors (US Department of Veterans Affairs, 2021b).

For the nurse on the rehabilitation team, it is important to be aware that other psychological conditions often accompany PTSD. The nurse plays a critical supportive role during rehabilitation in assisting the patient to adapt to or regain control over the symptoms of PTSD. Through early assessment of PTSD symptoms and the use of therapeutic communication, nurses are able to assist patients in achieving the goal of treatment. Therapeutic communication techniques include listening, reframing, normalizing responses, and working to develop trust in the nurse-patient relationship. Nurses also need to be aware of their own reactions, emotions, and communication skills when caring for trauma victims. Nurses who are feeling overwhelmed sometimes need to consult with a mental health care provider.

DISABILITY

The Americans with Disabilities Act became law in 1990. This landmark legislation provides protection against discrimination of people with disabilities. Universally accepted, the Americans with Disabilities Act defines an individual as disabled if he or she has a physical or mental impairment that substantially limits one or more major life activities, has a record of such an impairment, or is regarded as having such an impairment.

As is the case with chronic illness, it is important to recognize that having a disability is just one of many variants of the normal human experience. One way to look at it is to assert that all individuals are only temporarily able-bodied and that at some point in life, everyone experiences some form of disability. It is essential to develop this level of awareness to avoid labeling groups of people in ways that risk disenfranchising them.

People with disabilities are not defined by their illness or their disability. They are complex individuals with unique combinations of skills, and identifying them as such is obligatory. The basis for planning care that promotes health and positively affects the quality of life is a holistic, person-first approach in which the shared experience of being human, along with the uniqueness of the individual, is honored and the strengths, as well as impairments, are recognized.

Providers are called on to offer interventions that address the needs of people with chronic illnesses or disabilities to develop personally within the context of that illness or disability.

The following sections concern two of the major conditions for which dedicated rehabilitation efforts are necessary.

SPINAL CORD INJURIES

A **spinal cord injury (SCI)** is any injury in which the spinal cord undergoes compression by fracture or displacement of vertebrae, by bleeding, or by edema. Injury at each level has its unique characteristics, but in general, the higher the injury point, the greater the loss of function. The body parts and the functions located above the injury point continue to operate as they should. Injury to the spinal cord is irreversible in that the cord is unable to repair itself. Spinal function is sometimes present below the level of the lesion. In general, however, the effects of an injured spinal cord include paralysis, loss of normal bowel and bladder function, and loss of sensation (Fig. 39.3). Terminology associated with SCI includes, but is not limited to, the following:

- *Complete injury:* No motor or sensory function below the level of injury
- *Incomplete injury:* Some or all motor or sensory function below the level of injury
- *Quadriplegia:* Damage to the cervical spine or the neck that involves weakness or paralysis in all four extremities
- *Paraplegia:* Damage below the cervical area that involves weakness or paralysis in the trunk and lower extremities
- *Paresis:* A slight paralysis, incomplete loss of muscular power, or weakness of a limb
- SCIs are categorized as follows:
  - *Cervical cord injury:* Level of injury is at the cervical spine (C2 to C7) and involves paralysis of all extremities and trunk, respiratory failure, bladder and bowel disturbance, bradycardia, perspiration, elevated temperature, and headache.
  - *Thoracic cord injury:* Level of injury is at the thoracic spine (T1 to T12) and involves paralysis of lower extremities. Initially after the injury, muscles are flaccid (weak, soft, flabby, lacking normal muscle tone) and later become spastic (having spasms or other uncontrolled contractions of the skeletal muscles). Other potential symptoms are paralysis of bladder, bowel, and sphincters; pain in chest or back; abdominal distention; and loss of sexual function.

C
1
2
3
4
5
6
7
8

QUAD. C1 to C4   Usually requires respiratory
assist (respirator) and usually requires skilled care.

QUAD. C5 to C8   In general, each level is more
independent as progression from C1 to C8 occurs.
  1. Nonambulatory
  2. Transfer with assistance
     a) C4-5 complete dependent transfer
     b) C5-6-7 assistive transfer
  3. ADL needs assist
  4. C5-6-7 drive with assist
  5. Intellectual work or avocation

T
1
2
3
4
5

T1 to T5
  1. Nonambulatory (may have
     exercise ambulation with braces)
  2. ADL independent
  3. Bladder independent care. Bowel may need
     help.
  4. Driving with hand controls
  5. Intellectual work or bench or sedentary
     work

6
7
8
9

T6 to T9
  1. Limited ambulation with braces
  2. ADL independence
  3. Bladder independent care; may need
     help with bowel
  4. Driving with hand controls
  5. Vocation most likely at desk or bench

10
11
12

T10 to T12
  1. Functional ambulation
  2. Complete ADL independence
  3. Bowel and bladder independent care
  4. Driving
  5. Appropriate work

L
1
2
3

L1 to L3
  1. Functional ambulation
  2. Complete ADL independence
  3. Bowel and bladder independent care
  4. Driving
  5. Appropriate work

4
5

L4 and Below
  1. Full ambulation
  2. Complete ADL independence
  3. Bowel and bladder control
  4. Driving
  5. Appropriate work

S
1
2
3
4
5

C4 injury

Cervical

C6 injury

Thoracic

Spinal
cord

T6 injury

L1 injury

Lumbar

Sacral

Fig. 39.3 Levels and loss of function by location of spinal cord injury. *ADL*, Activities of daily living.

• *Lumbar cord injury:* Level of injury is at the lumbar spine (L1 to L2), with paralysis of lower extremities, bladder, and rectum, as well as loss of sexual function (see Fig. 39.3).

SCIs occur mainly as a result of traumatic accidents, and the individuals paralyzed are primarily young men. Because of improved emergency and medical care techniques, typical patients are more likely to survive the injury. Most of these patients are young enough that they have vocational potential. Injury level and the extent of damage to the spinal cord largely determine functional disabilities. Functional limitations occur in nearly every aspect of an individual's life after an SCI.

The effect of SCI on the individual remains one of the most compelling challenges in the field of rehabilitation. Patients with SCI often require considerable motivation and reeducation to regain a satisfying quality of life and to ensure community reintegration. Crucial for rehabilitation is the communal effort of an interdisciplinary team whose members work together to meet the specific needs of the patient and the family.

Common medical complications experienced by patients with SCI include, but are not limited to, postural hypotension, autonomic dysreflexia, heterotopic ossification, and deep vein thrombosis. Patient problems for a patient with SCI include, but are not limited to, those listed in Nursing Care Plan 39.1.

Nursing Care Plan 39.1 | **The Patient With a Spinal Cord Injury**

T., a 26-year-old man, was admitted to the acute rehabilitation unit with T1 paraplegia, secondary to a motor vehicle accident 10 days earlier. Initially, he was in spinal shock, and during his acute care phase, he had periods of despondency and signs of depression. Before the accident, T. was scheduled to be married in 2 weeks. His future wife and his family were attentive and supportive but apprehensive about their future. The young couple was in the process of purchasing a house and moving out of state, where T. was scheduled to begin employment as a mechanical engineer.

PATIENT PROBLEM
Grief

Patient Goals and Expected Outcomes	Nursing Interventions	Evaluation
Patient will acknowledge disability	Offer guidance and support through early stage of grieving.	
Patient will verbalize sense of loss from enforced changes	Encourage expression of feelings regarding disability and enforced lifestyle changes.	Patient is able to verbalize his distress with his altered lifestyle.
	Assist patient in using current abilities in the performance of self-care skills, leisure activities, and family and community socialization.	
Patient and family will reorganize life incorporating the patient's current strengths and abilities	Guide realistic goal setting and planning to meet goals.	Patient and fiancée set alternative wedding date.
Patient will refocus energies to promote positive changes	Reinforce active planning and implementation of future vocational options.	Patient is exploring alternative employment options.
Patient will participate in social interaction	Provide contacts for appropriate group support.	
Patient will participate in leisure activities or verbalize plan to incorporate leisure activities		
Patient will identify value in altered lifestyle		

PATIENT PROBLEM
Compromised Physical Mobility

Patient Goals and Expected Outcomes	Nursing Interventions	Evaluation
Patient will be able to perform independent bed mobility skills, transfers, and wheelchair mobility	Instruct and assist the patient in maximizing his ability to move around in the environment (e.g., locomotion by wheelchair).	Patient will achieve optimal independence in transfers from one surface to another. Patient will achieve independence in wheelchair mobility.
Patient will demonstrate the ability to direct others to assist him to achieve optimal mobility	Instruct and assist the patient in maximizing his ability to transfer from one surface to another (e.g., bed to chair).	Patient will learn to use adaptive equipment to achieve his optimal level of independence in performing activities of daily living.
	Instruct and assist the patient in the use of adaptive or assistive equipment.	
	Instruct and assist the patient in methods that help increase mobility in bed.	
	Instruct and assist the patient in methods that help maximize energy and maintain safety during movement.	
	Instruct and assist the patient in maintaining optimal body alignment to promote skin integrity and prevent contracture.	Patient will maintain intact skin integrity. Patient will be free of contractures.

CRITICAL THINKING QUESTIONS
1. Describe the stimuli or precipitating factors associated with bowel functioning or management that have potential to cause autonomic dysreflexia. What are the appropriate interventions if it does occur?
2. The patient has T1 quadriplegia. How is it possible to lessen the patient's potential for developing orthostatic hypotension?
3. When explaining orthostatic hypotension to a new nursing assistant, what commonly occurring signs and symptoms should the nurse describe, and what instructions should be given to the nursing assistant?

Postural Hypotension

Some patients with SCIs have a marked drop in blood pressure while sitting in a wheelchair. It is common for many quadriplegic patients to have a blood pressure of 90/60 mm Hg (or lower) when sitting as a result of the pooling of the blood in the lower extremities and in the abdominal area. Returning the patient to the horizontal position usually stops dizziness. To lessen hypotension, raise the head of the bed 15 to 20 minutes before moving the patient to the wheelchair. Elastic stockings (thromboembolic disease [TED] hose) and abdominal binders may also be used.

Autonomic Dysreflexia

Patients with spinal cord lesions above T5 sometimes experience sudden and extreme elevations in blood pressure, caused by a reflex action of the autonomic nervous system. It is the result of some stimulation of the body below the level of the injury, usually bladder distention from a blocked catheter. Any stimulation has potential to produce the syndrome, including constipation, diarrhea, sexual activity, pressure ulcers, position changes (from lying to sitting), and wrinkles in clothing or bed sheets. In addition to high blood pressure, possible symptoms include diaphoresis, shivering or goose bumps, flushing of the skin, and a severe, pounding headache.

Treatment for autonomic dysreflexia is to find and remove the source of irritation. Once the irritation is gone, the blood pressure returns to normal within a few minutes. The patient should be raised into a sitting position immediately. This helps reduce the elevated blood pressure before damage occurs.

Heterotopic Ossification

Heterotopic ossification is the abnormal formation of bone cells in joints. It commonly arises in people with SCIs and occurs below the level of the lesion. The formation of extra bone in these joints usually results in limited range of motion. The most commonly affected joints are the hips and sometimes the knees. It occurs most frequently 1 to 4 months after the injury and rarely occurs more than 1 year afterward. Symptoms include localized edema around the area—after several days, a firm mass can be palpated in underlying tissue. After several weeks, range of motion is diminished. Treatment options involve aggressive range-of-motion exercises, medications, and occasionally surgery.

Deep Vein Thrombosis

Patients with spinal injuries have the potential to develop deep vein thrombosis in the lower extremities. Deep vein thrombosis is a clotting of blood within vessels of the legs caused by slowing of the circulation or an alteration in the blood vessel walls. Clinical signs include localized swelling, redness, and heat in the involved area. If these signs are present, aggressive movement to that leg is unwise because it has the potential to detach the blood clot, which in turn has the potential to lodge in the lung (as an embolus). Anticoagulants (blood thinners) prevent deep vein thrombosis. Passive and active range-of-motion exercises are other possible preventive measures.

TRAUMATIC BRAIN INJURIES

Every year, nearly 3 million Americans suffer from traumatic brain injury (TBI). The injuries range from mild concussion to the more devastating type that renders injured people comatose for the remainder of their lives. The age groups impacted most often are those aged 75 years and older, children under the age of 4 years, and youths ages 15 to 24 years. An estimated 5.3 million people are living the aftereffects of a TBI. Although some people are fortunate enough to return to their previous functioning level shortly after receiving their injury, more than 50,000 people will die from their TBI annually. While this may appear bleak, there have been slight declines in TBI-related deaths. This is largely attributed to an increasing public awareness and use of safety items such as helmets. Of individuals who do survive, 500,000 receive injuries severe enough to necessitate hospitalization, and 90,000 of those injuries result in severe and permanent disability. Most brain-related disabilities, including physical, cognitive, and psychosocial difficulties, necessitate at least 5 to 10 years of difficult and painful rehabilitation; many affected patients require lifelong treatment and attention. When these statistics expand to include families of individuals with brain injuries, the number of people whose lives are forever altered by TBI rises to staggering proportions.

The primary goal of the rehabilitation professional treating the survivor of brain injury is to restore the patient to the highest possible level of independent functioning.

Head injuries are classified as either penetrating or closed-head injuries. In penetrating injuries, an object lacerates the scalp, fractures the skull, and injures the soft tissue in its path, thus destroying nerve cells. In a closed-head injury, some application of force causes the brain to collide with an inner surface of the skull. There is often violent twisting action, which causes the upper section of the brain to rotate while the lower end remains securely anchored in a stationary position. This results in widespread damage called *shearing* (when the brain mass is rotated in the cranial vault). Brain injuries are also possible as a result of other traumas (e.g., electrocution, drug overdose).

Brain injuries are classified as *mild, moderate, severe,* or *catastrophic.* Brief or no loss of consciousness characterizes mild brain injury, which is the majority of head injuries. Neurologic examination findings are often normal. Post-concussive syndrome sometimes persists for months, years, or indefinitely. Signs and symptoms include fatigue, headache, vertigo, lethargy, irritability, personality changes, cognitive deficits, decreased information processing speed, and difficulties with memory, understanding, learning, and perception. These symptoms can lead to feelings of incompetence, guilt, and frustration. Family members may also become impatient and frustrated at times.

Moderate brain injuries are characterized by a period of unconsciousness ranging from 1 to 24 hours. Cognitive skills—including planning, sequencing, judgment, reasoning, and computation skills—are usually impaired. In general, some psychosocial problems also occur, such as self-centeredness, denial, mood swings, agitation, depression, lethargy, sexual dysfunction, emotional lability, low tolerance for frustration, poor judgment, and behavioral outbursts.

Patients with severe brain injuries experience unconsciousness or posttrauma amnesia for longer than 8 days. Cognitive, psychosocial, and behavioral disabilities result.

In catastrophic brain injury, a defining characteristic is a coma lasting several months or longer. Affected individuals sometimes appear to be awake. However, they generally never regain significant, meaningful communication with their environment.

The nurse performing a rehabilitative assessment of the patient with TBI commonly observes inconsistent performance, anger, and frustration. However, ineffective problem-solving strategies can be modified (unless the injury is neurogenic). Cognitive barriers to rehabilitative recovery include problems in thinking and reasoning (impaired memory), impaired concentration and attention, and impaired informational processing speed. Psychosocially, the patient appears to lack initiative. However, this is a normal consequence of a head injury. Egocentric (self-centered) behavior often is noted in brain-injured individuals, as is depression. In general, the more the memory improves, the more the patient becomes depressed. Abstinence from alcohol is a primary injunction for any patient with a brain injury, because alcohol increases the chance of abnormal electrical impulses and seizure activity.

Continuous and honest involvement of the family, as a victim of the injury and an equal participant in the rehabilitation process, is crucial for successfully rehabilitating a patient with TBI. Rehabilitation professionals must be available and honest when reporting to families. Equal communication with all family members is important, as is encouraging the family to become involved in counseling and education. Family members should be reminded to be aware of each other's needs and interests. Help them become involved in a support group and inform them of available community resources.

Regardless of personality types, any disability, particularly a TBI, is a crisis that threatens many aspects of the patient's and family's life: job income, pleasures, family, community ties, health, and life. The fears are valid.

Patient problems for a patient with TBI include, but are not limited to, those in Nursing Care Plan 39.2.

PEDIATRIC REHABILITATION NURSING

Pediatric rehabilitation nursing is a specialty practice area that also continues to expand within the field of rehabilitation. The field of pediatric rehabilitation has undergone marked development since the early 1900s. The number of children with chronic disabling conditions has increased as a result of improved rates of survival from illnesses and injuries that once were fatal.

Since the 1990s, the field has evolved from a mere combination of pediatrics and rehabilitation into a true specialty committed to the care of children with disabilities or other chronic conditions and their families. Nurses in this field, in a collaborative relationship with the interdisciplinary team, provide a continuum of care so that affected children can become contributing members of society and function at their maximal potential. Infants, children, and adolescents with a variety of disabling conditions receive specialized care from hospital to home, from clinic to school. Physical, emotional, social, cultural, educational, developmental, and spiritual dimensions are subjects of consideration in a holistic approach to care. The goal is to cherish and foster the unique qualities of each child.

When rehabilitation is needed for children, there is one key fundamental difference from an adult client. The developmental age and related capabilities of the child must be incorporated in the plan of care. Children and adolescents can receive an injury resulting in disability at any age, with very different consequences for the patient's future, depending on the age and developmental level at which the trauma occurred. In some cases, the child may regress to an earlier, less mature developmental status as a result of the injury or illness. Children who are born with genetic disorders, who are premature, or whose fetal development is affected by maternal disease, injury, or substance abuse require services focused on habilitation rather than rehabilitation. Whereas *rehabilitation* refers to the relearning of skills or behaviors lost as a result of disease or injury, *habilitation* refers to the process of acquiring skills and behaviors by an individual whose development has been affected by disease or other disabling conditions since birth or very early childhood.

In summary, as leader, advocate, and educator, the pediatric rehabilitation nurse has the power to have a very positive influence on the lives of children with disabilities and chronic conditions, as well as on their families. By facilitating transition from hospital to home and community, as well as by offering counseling and support to families, the nurse provides assistance in meeting identified needs. By designing an individualized plan of care that incorporates the values and beliefs supported in rehabilitation, the nurse has the opportunity to affect the quality of the child's life for the better and to facilitate the child's interactions with family and friends within the community.

GERONTOLOGIC REHABILITATION NURSING

Gerontologic rehabilitation nursing is a specialty practice that focuses on the unique requirements of older adult rehabilitation patients. Because the needs of

Nursing Care Plan 39.2   **The Patient With Traumatic Brain Injury**

J. is a 33-year-old man employed as a chemist for a large pharmaceutical company. He lives alone in a second-floor apartment. After not reporting to work for 2 days, he was found unconscious on the floor of his bathroom. He was taken to the hospital, where he remained in a deep coma for 5 days as a result of an electrical injury that caused anoxic encephalopathy. After 4 weeks, J. was transferred to an acute rehabilitation unit. He was experiencing disorientation, short-term memory loss, and reduced cognition.

PATIENT PROBLEM

- Impaired Neurovascular Function

Patient Goals and Expected Outcomes	Nursing Interventions	Evaluation
Patient will provide accurate responses to orientation testing	Provide reality orientation and testing. Provide orientation cues such as clocks and calendars.	Patient is able to consistently respond accurately when reality testing is done.
Patient will have increased attention span	Implement memory training program. Implement visual and auditory cues. Control environmental stimuli when working with patient to reduce distractions.	Patient is able to follow a three-step command consistently. Patient is able to recall names and activities completed during the previous 3 days. Patient is able to complete a task once it is begun.
Patient will demonstrate appropriate behavior that is based on reality	Provide appropriate level of interactions with a gradual increase in socially appropriate interactions.	Patient is able to demonstrate good judgment in abstract problem-solving situations given to him.
Patient will demonstrate improved accuracy in problem solving	Cue patient on the focus of task before he starts, and reorient him as required. Implement sensory stimulation program.	Patient is able to use information to reach appropriate conclusions.

PATIENT PROBLEM

- Potential for Harm or Damage to the Body

Patient Goals and Expected Outcomes	Nursing Interventions	Evaluation
Patient will demonstrate an awareness of potential safety hazards	Initiate appropriate safety precautions to protect patient from injury.	Periodically evaluate and document patient's progress toward prevention of injury.
Patient will demonstrate safety in activities of daily living (ADLs) and mobility activities	Establish behavior modification program for isolated safety activities.	Consult with other health care professionals on methods to prevent patient from sustaining injury.
Patient will demonstrate knowledge and use of safety devices	Use verbal cueing to prevent injury in all activities.	
Patient will obtain assistance for activities appropriately to ensure safety	Reinforce use of appropriate measures to compensate for the patient's physical or cognitive deficits.	
Patient will remain injury free	Explain side effects of medications that have potential to affect the patient's safety. Anticipate the patient's needs (e.g., toileting, eating, and drinking) to minimize impulsive movement. Use calm, controlled, and consistent manner. Use short-term, goal-directed techniques. Assume nothing: review, review, review.	

CRITICAL THINKING QUESTIONS

1. Deficits with socialization, motivation, and sexual behaviors that occur after brain injury result from damage to which portion of the brain? Discuss appropriate nursing interventions for a patient with this type of injury.
2. A patient recovering from a traumatic brain injury has problems telling the difference between objects that have a similar shape. What is this type of deficit, and what nursing interventions are appropriate for a patient with this deficit?
3. What interventions are most appropriate to begin establishing communication with a patient who is just emerging from coma after a brain injury?

From Centers for Disease Control and Prevention: Explosion and blast injuries: A primer for clinicians, n.d. Retrieved from https://www.cdc.gov/masstrauma/preparedness/primer.pdf.

older adults differ from those of the rest of the population, the knowledge and skills needed to provide quality patient care warrant special attention. Gerontologic rehabilitation nurses are knowledgeable about techniques of caring for the aged, as well as rehabilitation concepts and principles. This unique type of nursing combines knowledge of the aging process and rehabilitation practice in the specialized task of caring for older adults with a disability or long-term health problem.

A primary goal in gerontologic rehabilitation nursing is the assistance of older adult patients in achieving their personal optimal level of health and well-being through holistic care in a therapeutic environment. This aim is similar to that of general rehabilitation nursing but with a special focus on the geriatric population, considering their special needs, roles, and social relationships, and the potential physical limitations that are possible as a result of the aging process.

Gerontologic rehabilitation nurses strive not only to provide rehabilitative care, but also to include preventative health teaching. The gerontologic rehabilitation nurse has an opportunity to function within primary, secondary, and tertiary levels of care, with the universal goal of helping older adult patients to achieve optimal wellness and self-care.

CONCLUSION

Rehabilitation nursing is a career with several key requirements and rewards. This type of responsibility should be taken seriously because it can significantly affect the future of patients with disabilities. Rehabilitation nurses facilitate the change from resistance to openness, turning inertia into action. The focus must be maintained on the assets and the successes of people who have disabilities.

Ralph Waldo Emerson (1803 to 1882) summed it up succinctly when he wrote, "It is one of the most beautiful compensations of this life that no man can sincerely try to help another without helping himself."

Get Ready for the NCLEX® Examination!

Key Points

- Rehabilitation is the process of maximizing an individual's capabilities or resources to foster optimal independent functioning.
- The patient is the most important team member and must be involved in planning the programs and learning in detail about the disabilities, the ways of accomplishing the goals, and the options available.
- Rehabilitation nursing aims toward preventing complications of disease or trauma and toward maintaining or restoring function.
- Basic rehabilitation is possible regardless of the cause of disability. The rehabilitation team individualizes care by developing a goal-directed, comprehensive care plan for each patient.
- A disability has a number of potential effects on both the patient and the family, including behavioral and emotional changes and changes in roles, body image, self-concept, and family dynamics.
- Holistic nursing interventions are used to assist the patient in attaining an optimal level of functioning and well-being.
- A comprehensive rehabilitation plan is multifaceted and properly involves a functional assessment, an evaluation conference, and a family conference.
- The focus of all rehabilitation is on the patient's abilities, not on his or her disabilities.

Additional Learning Resources

SG Go to your Study Guide for additional learning activities to help you master this chapter content.

Be sure to visit the Evolve site at http://evolve.elsevier.com/Cooper/foundations/ for additional online resources.

Review Questions for the NCLEX® Examination

1. When setting goals for an elderly patient, the nurse should consider what primary goal of rehabilitation?
   1. Enabling patient's return to work
   2. Teaching safe mobility
   3. Improving quality of life
   4. Reducing cellular destruction

2. When working on the multidisciplinary rehabilitation team, it is imperative to have clear set _____ and _____ for each discipline.

3. An 11-year-old boy had a head injury from being struck in the skull by a baseball bat. When he awakens in the hospital 3 weeks later, how would his head injury be classified?
   1. Mild brain injury
   2. Moderate brain injury
   3. Severe brain injury
   4. Catastrophic brain injury

4. A patient has been in the intensive care unit for several days after a head injury. His condition is stable, but today he has shown no signs of improvement. Over the past shift, the patient's father has seemed increasingly upset over small concerns. Toward the end of the shift, he yells at the nurse when the intravenous (IV) alarm goes off. What would be the most appropriate response by the nurse?
   1. "You sound upset."
   2. "I am going to get my supervisor for you."
   3. "You need a break."
   4. "Maybe you had better speak to the physician."

5. What term is the student nurse referring to that describes a disadvantage for a person that results from an impairment or a disability and limits that person's fulfillment of his or her normal roles?

   1. Disability
   2. Impairment
   3. Handicap
   4. Inconvenience

6. The nurse is considering a position on a rehabilitation care unit that uses the concept of a transdisciplinary rehabilitation team. The nurse must be aware that this type of care will require what characteristics? *(Select all that apply.)*

   1. The ability to work with all members of the rehabilitation team
   2. Organized approaches to care
   3. Skills in all therapies that are provided
   4. Willingness to cross-train with other disciplines
   5. Developing expertise in a limited number of skills

7. Which are barriers to cultural competence? *(Select all that apply.)*

   1. Respect for the beliefs of others
   2. Knowing all members of a cultural group are not necessarily alike
   3. Believing that one's own culture is better than others
   4. Treating one group better than another on the basis of culture or race
   5. Performing self-assessment of awareness of various cultural beliefs
   6. An inability to fluently speak the patient's native language
   7. Recognition that one's personal religious beliefs differ from their assigned patient
   8. Being assigned to care for others who have different cultural beliefs than those personally held
   9. Speaking up when feeling overwhelmed about cultural clashes.
   10. Asking to be transferred to another assignment when faced with a cultural diversity

8. As part of the rehabilitation treatment team, why is the nurse often the first professional to detect symptoms of posttraumatic stress disorder (PTSD)?

   1. Nurses are more intuitive than other members of the team.
   2. The rehabilitation team has no need to address this issue.
   3. Nurses are the only members of the team knowledgeable about PTSD.
   4. Nurses are in the unique position of having extended time to talk with patients and hear their concerns, feelings, and needs.

9. The nurse is caring for a veteran who has shrapnel embedded in his eye as a result of a polytrauma/blast-related injury (PT/BRI). How should the nurse classify this injury?

   1. Primary
   2. Secondary
   3. Tertiary
   4. Quaternary

10. When caring for a patient with PTSD, what should the nurse's initial action with the patient be?

    1. The nurse should first communicate the planned routine for the rehabilitation unit.
    2. The nurse should first work with the patient to establish goals for the plan of care.
    3. The nurse should first determine the family's level of involvement with care.
    4. The nurse should establish a therapeutic nurse-patient relationship.

11. Which nurse is demonstrating a desired quality of a rehabilitation nurse? *(Select all that apply.)*

    1. The nurse is focusing on helping the patient work toward a cure for his condition.
    2. The nurse includes the patient's family in the plan of care.
    3. The nurse helps the patient achieve the goal of reentry into the home or community.
    4. The nurse uses therapeutic communication skills with the patient and family.
    5. The nurse encourages the patient to delay rehabilitation until his strength increases.

12. When dealing with the patient, what must the rehab nurse remember?

    1. The nurse is frequently interacting with people experiencing change.
    2. The nurse must ensure change is occurring with each patient.
    3. The nurse is always changing.
    4. The nurse is the center of change.

13. Family-centered care recognizes that, when caring for a child with disabilities, which of the following is true?

    1. The family needs assistance.
    2. The family and professional are equals in a partnership.
    3. The family is in charge.
    4. The family must understand they must change.

14. Reasons a patient may be admitted for rehabilitation include which of the following? *(Select all that apply.)*

    1. Post coronary bypass
    2. Cardiopulmonary disease
    3. Diabetic ketoacidosis
    4. Urinary tract infection
    5. Cardiovascular accident

15. A 10-year-old patient keeps crying and saying, "No, no," moving as if uncomfortable, then returns to sleep every few hours throughout the night. Her mother is not sure why this is happening. What should the nurse suspect?

    1. The patient is not comfortable in her bed and should be awakened to assess comfort level.
    2. The patient may have experienced a traumatic event, which may need further investigation.
    3. The mother is upsetting the patient by staying in the room.
    4. The patient is acting out because of staying in a strange place.

16. A group of nurses are working on the transdisciplinary rehabilitation team. When working on goals, the nurses are aware that boundaries are _____ between _____.

Objectives

1. Discuss the philosophy of hospice care.
2. Differentiate between palliative care and curative care.
3. Discuss four criteria for admission to hospice care.
4. Name the members of the interdisciplinary team, and explain their roles.
5. Develop a care plan with patient goals related to the common symptoms of terminal illness.
6. Discuss the usefulness of pain assessments and when it is best to complete them.
7. Discuss the role of hospice in families' bereavement period.
8. Discuss two ethical issues in hospice care.

Key Terms

adjuvant (ĂJ-ŭ-vănt, p. 1236)
bereavement (bĭ-RĒV-mĭnt, p. 1234)
cachexia (kă-KĔK-sē-ŭ, p. 1239)
curative treatment (KYŬR-ŭ-tĭv TRĔT-mĭnt, p. 1230)
holistic (hō-LĬS-tĭk, p. 1231)
hospices (HŎS-pĭs-ĕz, p. 1229)
interdisciplinary team (ĭn-tŭr-DĬS-ŭ-plĭn-ăr-ē TĔM, p. 1231)

pain assessment (PĀN ŭs-SĔS-mĭnt, p. 1235)
palliative care (PĂL-ē-ă-tĭv KĂR, p. 1229)
primary caregiver (PRĪ-măr-ē KĂR-gĭv-ŭr, p. 1231)
psychosocial (sī-kō-SŌ-shŭl, p. 1233)
respite care (RĔS-pĭt KĂR, p. 1233)
terminal illness (TŬR-mĭn-ŭl ĬL-nŭs, p. 1228)
titrated (TĪ-trāt-ĭd, p. 1236)

The philosophy of hospice is to provide care and support to patients with a **terminal illness** (a disease in an advanced stage with no known cure and poor prognosis) and their families. An interdisciplinary team promotes comfort, care, and support through compassion, interest, and genuine concern (Box 40.1) to promote quality of life as the end approaches. With hospice support, the patient and the family recognize that dying is a natural part of life. The goals are to maximize the quality of life and keep the patient as comfortable as possible in the home or setting that he or she chooses. Studies have shown that patients cared for in a hospice setting experience an improved quality of life with less pain and more mobility, and live longer than those terminally ill patients not in this type of setting (SSM Health, 2018).

HISTORICAL OVERVIEW

"Hospice" is from the Latin word *hospitium,* meaning "hospitality" and "lodging." The concept originated in Europe, where hospices were resting places for travelers. Monks and nuns believed that service to one's neighbor was a sign of love and dedication to God. Typical medieval hospices run by monks and nuns were a combination guesthouse and infirmary. They were places of refuge for the poor, the sick, and travelers on religious journeys. They provided food, shelter, and care to ill guests until the guests were strong enough to continue their journey or died. As centuries passed and hospices developed into hospitals, the emphasis on physical care increased, and spiritual care became less important.

The idea of hospice was renewed in the 1960s in London, when Dame Cicely Saunders, a nurse and physician, realized that terminally ill patients needed a different kind of care. She had a patient who was dying of a terminal illness, and she found that quality of life was not the main emphasis of his care. She then devoted her life to improving pain management and symptom control for people who were dying. She believed it is important for each patient to know his or her own contribution to life and that his or her life had meaning. She began her work at St. Joseph's Hospice, operated by the Irish Sisters of Charity. In 1968 St. Christopher's Hospice of London was opened, and this hospice continues to serve as a national and international education, training, and research center for professionals involved in the hospice approach to care of terminally ill patients.

The philosophy of hospice migrated to the United States in the early 1970s; the first hospice program opened in Connecticut in 1971. Since then, health care providers, nurses, clergy, social workers, and many nonprofessional volunteers have worked together to

Frequently I am asked whether it is depressing to work with terminally ill patients and death every day. Frankly, I cannot think of doing anything else. Death is as much a part of life as is birth, and through hospice, I am challenged to find very individualized and innovative ways to give back the control that dying patients have lost while being treated for various kinds of terminal illnesses.

As a hospice nurse, I am guided by a dedicated interdisciplinary team to achieve symptom control so that quality of life can again be realized. Many hopes and dreams can become reality once a patient is comfortable. Frequently, comfort enables our patients to take one more family trip, attend a great family reunion, and go to a special wedding, graduation, or anniversary. What could be more rewarding than playing a part in that and seeing the joy it brings? Together we rejoice in the celebration of life, see families reunited, see peace made with God, review each triumph, and weep over each disappointment and loss. Families are enabled to say all the things they could not find words for before: "Thank you"; "I'm sorry"; "Forgive me"; "I love you"; and finally the good-byes.

Of course there is sadness, but there are also reconciliation, peace, and beauty, for this is a part of life and these are the important things in life. Daily, I feel so personally grateful for every person I have known and loved and lost, for I know that I have learned far more about living from them than I could ever teach them about dying. Through it all, I have become closer to God, more compassionate, more open to people, and more sensitive to the needs of others. Hospice nursing has given me direction and hope.

Kathleen Carsten, CRNH
Hospice Nurse

develop more than 4300 hospice programs serving between 1.6 and 1.7 million patients throughout the United States. Despite the rates of hospice use there are some consistent myths. These include the following (Morrow, 2020a):

Myth 1: Hospice means giving up hope.

Myth 2: Hospice means I must sign a do-not-resuscitate (DNR) order.

Myth 3: Hospice is only for cancer patients.

Myth 4: Hospice is only for patients actively dying or close to death.

Hospices serve patients with various primary disease processes, the most common being cancer, which accounts for 30.1% of the patient population. Dementia-related disease processes account for 15.6% of the client population, and cardiac and lung diseases account for almost 28.6% of the primary diagnoses of the patients served by hospice (National Hospice and Palliative Care Organization [NHPCO], 2020).

Hospices vary in structure and organization. Inpatient facilities and residences may be hospital-based or free standing. The freestanding hospices have an atmosphere that is more like that of a friendly dormitory than that of a hospital. The patients usually wear their own clothes, move about the hospice

as they choose, and socialize with each other and with the staff. The kitchen is always open for individually prepared food, as well as for conversation. Some hospices are operated by a home health agency or community-based organization in which care usually is provided in the patient's home, wherever that home may be. Hospice care also may be given in a long-term care setting. On occasion, a hospice patient goes into the hospital and receives hospice services for control of acute pain or for 5-day respite care for the family or care provider on an occasional basis. Hospice care can be delivered intermittently or continuously. Skilled team members, including health care providers, nurses, hospice aides, social workers, spiritual leaders, bereavement coordinators, and volunteers, make visits to the home or wherever the patient most often resides. The team provides comfort measures, as well as medications and therapy. The team members also educate the patient and the caregiver with regard to disease processes, medication administration, and how to provide daily care. Expert help and support is available to the patient and the caregiver 24 hours a day, either by phone or in person.

The Medicare Hospice Benefit came into effect in 1983, and today hospice services are reimbursable through Medicare, Medicaid, and most private insurance companies. Medicare certification or state licensure ensures quality hospice services (see the Lifespan Considerations for older adults box).

 Lifespan Considerations

Older Adults

Hospice Care

The Hospice Medicare Benefit covers all expenses for palliative care related to the terminal illness, including professional staff visits, medication, equipment, occasional short periods of respite for caregivers, and acute care when needed for the control of symptoms.

Hospice often provides dying older adults with a higher level of control and dignity than do other types of health care.

The primary caregiver is often a member of the immediate family, such as the spouse or adult child.

The Hospice Medicare Benefit provides for bereavement follow-up care for up to 1 year after the patient's death.

From Centers for Medicare & Medicaid Services: Coverage of hospice services under hospital insurance. Medicare benefit policy manual (Publication No. 100-02, Rev. 10437), 2020. Retrieved from https://www.cms.gov/Regulations-and-Guidance/Guidance/Manuals/Downloads/bp102c09.pdf.

PALLIATIVE VERSUS CURATIVE CARE

Palliative care, as defined by the World Health Organization (2020), is an approach that improves the quality of life of patients and their families facing the problems associated with life-threatening illness, through the prevention and relief of suffering by means of early identification and impeccable assessment and treatment of pain and other problems, physical,

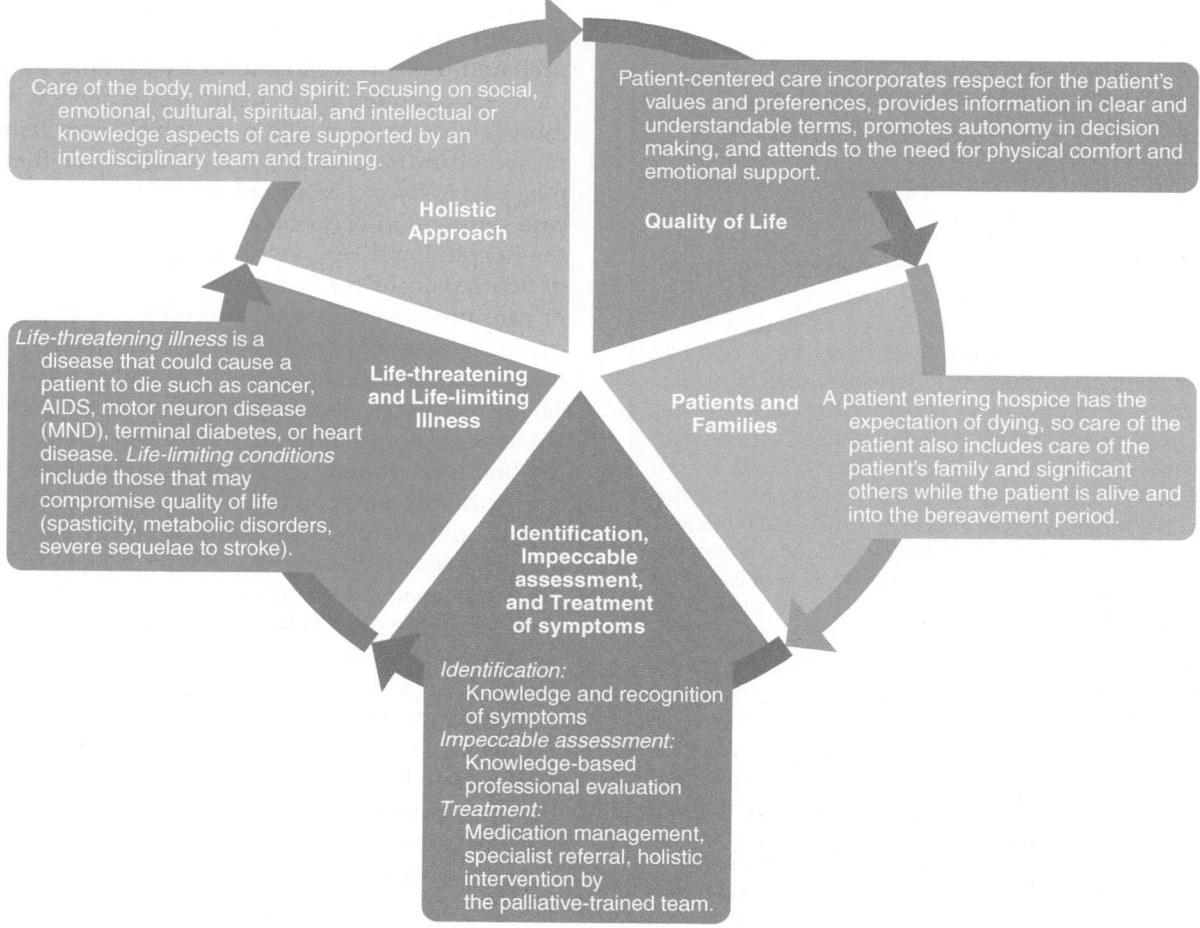

Holistic Approach

Care of the body, mind, and spirit: Focusing on social, emotional, cultural, spiritual, and intellectual or knowledge aspects of care supported by an interdisciplinary team and training.

Quality of Life

Patient-centered care incorporates respect for the patient's values and preferences, provides information in clear and understandable terms, promotes autonomy in decision making, and attends to the need for physical comfort and emotional support.

Life-threatening and Life-limiting Illness

Life-threatening illness is a disease that could cause a patient to die such as cancer, AIDS, motor neuron disease (MND), terminal diabetes, or heart disease. *Life-limiting conditions* include those that may compromise quality of life (spasticity, metabolic disorders, severe sequelae to stroke).

Patients and Families

A patient entering hospice has the expectation of dying, so care of the patient also includes care of the patient's family and significant others while the patient is alive and into the bereavement period.

Identification, Impeccable assessment, and Treatment of symptoms

Identification: Knowledge and recognition of symptoms
Impeccable assessment: Knowledge-based professional evaluation
Treatment: Medication management, specialist referral, holistic intervention by the palliative-trained team.

Fig. 40.1 Components of palliative care. (From Abernethy AP, Wheeler JL, Bull J: Development of a health information technology–based data system in community-based hospice and palliative care. *Am J Preventive Med*, 40[5 Suppl 2]:S217–S224, 2011.)

psychosocial, and spiritual (Fig. 40.1). **Curative treatment** is aggressive care in which the goal and intent are to cure the disease and prolong life at all costs. When a patient with a life-threatening illness has undergone all reasonable treatment and the disease has not been arrested or cured, it is necessary for the patient to decide whether continued active therapy is feasible or beneficial. By that time, the patient may already have experienced many debilitating physical and emotional symptoms as a result of the treatments or the progression of the disease. This situation leads the patient and family to decide whether to continue with curative treatments or to transition to palliative measures. Palliative care is not curative but aims to relieve pain and distress and to control symptoms of disease. It is important to give the patient and caregiver honest and accurate information so that they are able to make appropriate decisions.

CRITERIA FOR ADMISSION TO HOSPICE

The patient is required to meet certain criteria to be admitted into hospice:

The health care provider must certify that the patient's illness is terminal and that the patient has a prognosis of 6 months or less to live. The health care provider must have a doctorate of medicine or osteopathy to make the prognosis determination.

For the patient to qualify for Medicare or Medicaid assistance, two health care providers are required to verify that the patient is dying and has less than 6 months to live. This must be documented by the medical provider in a narrative that supports the reason for the limited life expectancy. The hospice patient who continues to live beyond the estimated time period still qualifies for Medicare if hospice criteria are still met (Medicare.gov, n.d.).

It is mandatory that the patient desires the services. The patient and caregiver must understand that all treatment will be palliative and that no further curative treatment will be rendered.

The patient and caregiver are required to understand and agree that hospice staff will plan the care according to comfort and that they will not necessarily perform life-support measures.

The patient and caregiver—or, if the patient is unable to participate, the caregiver—are required to understand the prognosis and be willing to participate in the planning of care.

Many hospices in the United States request that the patient have a **primary caregiver** (a person who assumes ongoing responsibility for health maintenance and therapy for the illness). The caregiver is sometimes an immediate family member and sometimes a significant other, a friend, or a hired caregiver. Caregivers' services become vital when patients are no longer able to care for themselves safely. If a patient resides in a freestanding hospice residence, a long-term care facility, or a residential home, the nursing staff is designated as the primary caregiver.

Once the criteria are met and a patient is admitted to hospice, the staff performs complete physical, psychosocial, and spiritual assessments, and those involved discuss the care openly. The patient and caregiver receive a complete explanation of the hospice program and the philosophy of hospice, along with the interdisciplinary team concept.

GOALS OF HOSPICE

To provide effective hospice care, an understanding of the philosophy and its relationship with the patient's responses and points of view is beneficial. The basic goals of hospice address the following:

Controlling or alleviating the patient's symptoms;

Allowing the patient and caregiver to be involved in the decisions regarding the plan of care;

Encouraging the patient and caregiver to live life to the fullest;

Providing continuous support to maintain patient and family confidence;

Educating and supporting the primary caregiver in the home setting that the patient chooses.

INTERDISCIPLINARY TEAM

In this approach of hospice, defined as **holistic** (pertaining to the total patient care in which the physical, emotional, social, economic, and spiritual needs of the patient are considered), an interdisciplinary team manages the problems (Fig. 40.2). The **interdisciplinary team** (a multiprofessional health team whose members work together in caring for a terminally ill patient) develops and supervises the plan of care in conjunction with all those involved with the care. The core interdisciplinary team members are the medical director, the nurse coordinator, the social worker, and the spiritual coordinator. To provide support to the dying patient and the caregiver, the interdisciplinary team considers all aspects of the family unit. They include the family in all decisions and care planning because families also experience the stresses of the terminal illness and death of the patient (Fig. 40.3). These stresses also extend into the bereavement period after the patient dies.

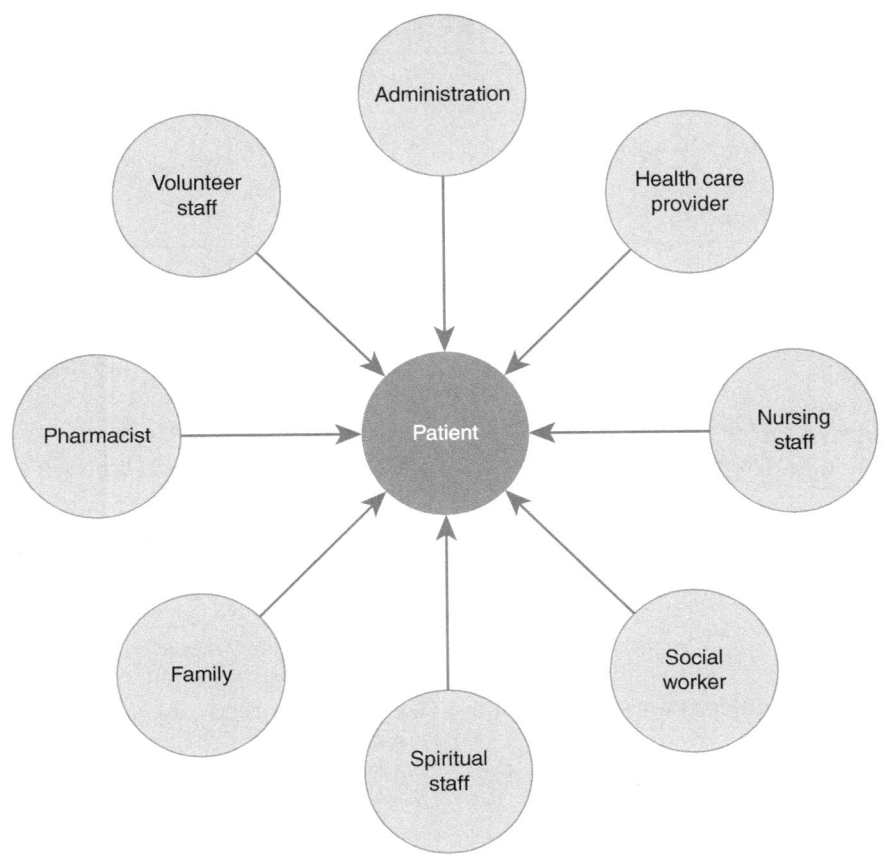

Fig. 40.2 The relationship between the hospice team members and the patient.

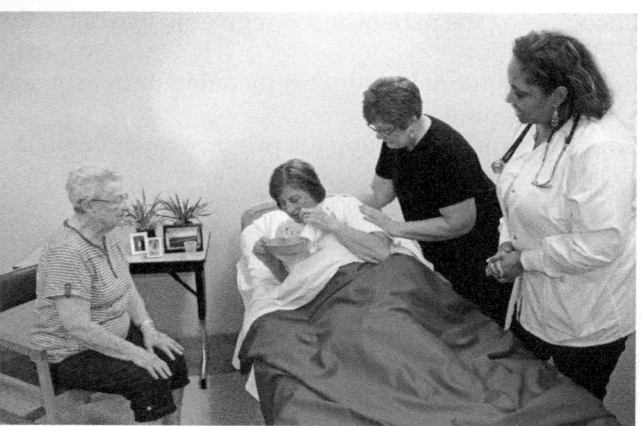

Fig. 40.3 Family member participation with the hospice care team.

Each hospice patient is assigned a primary team that consists of the patient's own health care provider, the primary hospice nurse, the social worker, a primary hospice aide, a primary volunteer, and a spiritual leader. This group of professionals, along with the interdisciplinary team, develops and is responsible for carrying out the plan of care. Regular and frequent team meetings are held to discuss the patient's physical, mental, and spiritual conditions; the plan of care is revised as needed. The effectiveness of the plan of care is also discussed. The team meeting is the forum for bringing together all members' observations and thoughts respectfully, and the team strives to function as a cohesive unit to use all expertise and resources in the interest of providing quality patient care (see Tables 40.1 and 40.2).

Table 40.1   Core Interdisciplinary Hospice Team

TEAM MEMBER	BACKGROUND	FUNCTION OR RESPONSIBILITY
Medical director	Licensed physician	Mediates between the hospice team and attending medical provider Provides consultation relative to the medical aspect of care
Nurse coordinator	Licensed registered nurse	Manages the patient's care Explains the service, admits the patients, assigns the primary team
Social worker	Bachelor's degree in social work	Evaluates the patient's psychosocial needs Serves as resource for potential community services Assists with counseling in grief issues
Spiritual coordinator	Seminary degree	Serves as liaison between the patient and the spiritual community Coordinates spiritual support

Table 40.2   Primary Hospice Team

TEAM MEMBER	BACKGROUND	FUNCTION OR RESPONSIBILITY
Volunteer coordinator	Experience in volunteer work	Recruits and trains the volunteers Coordinates assignments of volunteers
Bereavement coordinator	Professional with grief experience	Assesses and supports the bereaved survivor Facilitates support groups
Hospice pharmacist	Licensed registered pharmacist	Provides drug consultation
Primary health care provider	Licensed physician	Responsible for the medical aspect of symptom control for the patient
Primary nurse	Licensed registered nurse	Serves as liaison between (1) patient and (2) caregiver, health care provider, and interdisciplinary team Evaluates patient's response to treatment Educates the patient and family in disease process and care Assesses symptom management Provides emotional support to patient and caregiver
Primary spiritual leader	As required by religious group	Supports patient and caregiver in coping with fears and uncertainty about spiritual issues
Hospice volunteer	Completion of volunteer training	Provides companionship for patient and caregiver Available for short periods of respite care
Hospice aide	Certified as a home health aide	Administers personal care and assistance with bathing

MEDICAL DIRECTOR

The medical director has a doctorate of medicine or osteopathy and assumes overall responsibility for the medical component of the hospice patient's care program. The medical director does not take the place of the patient's health care provider but acts as a consultant for the health care provider. The medical director, with consultation from the interdisciplinary team, medically certifies the patient's eligibility for hospice care. The medical director is a mediator between the interdisciplinary team and the health care provider. He or she oversees the plan of care, ensuring that the care being provided and ordered is palliative in nature.

NURSE COORDINATOR AND HOSPICE NURSES

The nurse coordinator is a registered nurse who coordinates the implementation of the plan of care for each patient. The nurse coordinator often performs the initial assessment, admits the patient to the hospice program, and develops the plan of care along with the interdisciplinary team. The nurse coordinator also ensures that the plan of care is being followed, coordinates assignments of the hospice nurses and aides, facilitates meetings, and determines methods of payment.

Hospice nurses coordinate services of the hospice team, which includes hospice health care providers, pharmacists, dietitians, physical therapists, social workers, clergy, certified nursing assistants, and hospice volunteers. Hospice nurses must possess compassion, excellent teaching skills, and the ability to adapt therapeutically to the hospice patients' many needs. It is also necessary for a hospice nurse to be especially adept in pain and symptom control.

SOCIAL WORKER

The social worker evaluates and assesses the **psychosocial** (a combination of psychological and social factors) needs of the patient. The social worker assists with accessing community resources and filing insurance papers, supports the patient and caregiver with emotional and grief issues, and, in some cases when communication difficulties are present, also assists with counseling. The social worker provides these services under the direction of the health care provider and in accordance with the plan of care.

SPIRITUAL COORDINATOR

The spiritual coordinator, who may be affiliated with any religion, is the liaison between the spiritual community and the interdisciplinary team. The spiritual coordinator assists with the spiritual assessment of the patient and, in keeping with patients' and families' beliefs, develops the plan of care with regard to spiritual matters. If the patient desires spiritual assistance and does not have a spiritual home, the spiritual coordinator assists in finding the spiritual support desired. The spiritual coordinator is vital in assisting the patient and caregiver to cope with fears and uncertainty. Possible support includes dealing with unfinished business and regrets and providing opportunities for reconciliation, prayer, and spiritual healing. Funeral planning and performing funeral services also are included in this role, as is continued support for the family throughout the bereavement period. In addition, the spiritual coordinator is one resource to assist with cultural differences (see the Cultural Considerations box).

 Cultural Considerations

DEATH AND DYING

The United States is becoming increasingly multicultural, and hospice care is challenged to meet the needs of people from other cultures.

Compassionate and empathic care bridges cultures, but it is necessary to learn as much as possible about a patient's culture to provide appropriate assistance. Each person has a different reaction and tradition regarding death and dying, but all people experience grief.

A cultural assessment of the patient and the family must include factors such as the following:

Religious beliefs

Primary decision-making person and process

Dietary preferences

Preferred language and the need for translation services as needed, as well as written information provided in the language of preference for the patient and the family

Support measure preferences such as alternative medicine, as well as who is allowed to support the patient

The patient's perspective of death, dying, and burial

The family's grief processes, burial practices, and perspective of death.

The team may need to be prepared for a change in expectations regarding the death of the patient because of differences in belief systems between the patient and the surviving family members.

Changes regarding the plan of care must not be made without discussing them with all family members.

The following sections describe additional members of the team whose services are needed to provide adequate care for the patient.

VOLUNTEER COORDINATOR

The volunteer coordinator must have experience in volunteer work. The volunteer coordinator assesses the needs of the patient and caregiver for volunteer services. When families are responsible for the total care of the patient in the home, caregiver "burnout" becomes a concern. This is when the services of volunteers become vital. They provide companionship, caregiver relief through **respite care** (a period of relief from responsibilities of caring for a patient), and emotional support. Appropriate services for the volunteer to provide are what are considered typical of a good neighbor: perhaps grocery shopping, yard work, reading to the patient, or keeping the patient company while the caregiver leaves the home for short periods.

The volunteer coordinator ensures that the volunteer is adequately trained and prepared for working with the dying patient. Responsibilities also include assigning the proper volunteer to the appropriate patient. Hospice volunteers are an instrumental part of the hospice experience. To retain funding, agencies that receive Medicare and Medicaid funding are required to demonstrate that at least 5% of the work being completed is done by volunteers. Training is needed to ensure the volunteers have an understanding of the role and clear expectations relating to what they will encounter as a hospice volunteer. Training programs vary and normally last about 30 hours (Morrow, 2020b).

BEREAVEMENT COORDINATOR

Bereavement is a period of mourning or an expression of grief in reaction to the death of someone close. The bereavement coordinator is a professional who has experience in dealing with grief issues. The bereavement coordinator assesses the patient and the caregiver at admission to the hospice program and identifies potential risk factors that may arise after the death of the patient. The bereavement coordinator follows the plan of care for the bereaved caregiver for at least a year after the death. The bereavement coordinator facilitates support groups and assigns bereavement volunteers to visit the caregiver.

The bereavement coordinator sometimes also provides counseling but has the option to refer the family to other counseling if the issues are too extensive. The goals of bereavement counseling for loved ones during the patient's illness and after the death are (1) to provide support and (2) to assist survivors in the transition to a life without the deceased person. It is appropriate to incorporate grief support into the plan of care.

HOSPICE PHARMACIST

The hospice pharmacist must be a licensed pharmacist and available for consultation about the drugs the hospice patient may be taking. The pharmacist evaluates for drug-drug or drug- food interactions, appropriate drug doses, and correct administration times and routes. The pharmacist typically gives information and advice about common drugs used, administration time, and doses (Table 40.3).

NUTRITION CONSULTANT

Licensed medical nutritional therapists (LMNTs) or licensed dietitians are available for hospice consultations and for diet counseling. The hospice nurse performs the nutritional assessment at the patient's admission. If the nurse notes nutritional problems, a referral may be made to the LMNT or dietitian for assistance with diet counseling and meal planning. The LMNT or dietitian also assists with educating the caregiver about nutritional issues in end-stage diseases.

HOSPICE AIDE

The hospice aide is a certified nurse's aide who works under the supervision of the hospice nurse. The hospice aide follows the plan of care that the interdisciplinary team develops and assists the patient with bathing and hygiene, including hair, nail, oral, and skin care. The hospice aide sometimes also assists the patient or

Table 40.3 Medications Commonly Used in Hospice Care			
GENERIC NAME (BRAND NAME)	**INDICATIONS**	**SIDE EFFECTS**	**NURSING INTERVENTIONS**
morphine sulfate: immediate-release	Acute and severe pain	Constipation, nausea and vomiting, sedation	Assess pain control by using pain assessment; instruct about administration routinely.
morphine sulfate: controlled-release (MS Contin)	Moderate and severe pain	Constipation, nausea and vomiting, sedation	Assess pain control and medication effectiveness.
fentanyl transdermal system (Duragesic patch; an opioid)	Moderate and severe pain	Confusion, hypoventilation, nausea and vomiting, constipation	Instruct caregiver to clean patient's skin with water only and dry before application.
droperidol (Inapsine)	Emesis	Hypotension and tachycardia, drowsiness, dizziness	Ensure that caregiver is administering the antiemetic appropriately and routinely.
prochlorperazine	Emesis	Extrapyramidal symptoms, dry mouth, depression	Assess control of nausea and ensure that caregiver is administering the antiemetic appropriately and routinely.
senna (Senokot)	Constipation	Nausea and vomiting, diarrhea, abdominal cramping	Encourage patient to drink fluids; assess gastrointestinal status and administer the laxative routinely if patient is taking pain medication.
lorazepam (Ativan)	Anxiety	Dizziness, drowsiness, orthostatic hypotension, tachycardia	Administer routinely; instruct patient in safety issues regarding rising slowly and not driving.
Acetaminophen	Fever, headache	Nausea, Stomach pain	Carefully monitor dosages to prevent overdosage and potential liver damage

the caregiver with light housekeeping services. The patient and the hospice aide often develop a close relationship, and in some cases, the patient shares feelings with the aide more easily than with any other member of the team.

OTHER SERVICES

Other services, if needed, are available from a physical therapist, a speech-language pathologist, and an occupational therapist. These services are available not for rehabilitative purposes but to assist with improving the quality of life and care for the patient and the caregiver. The physical therapist assists with teaching the caregiver transferring skills, exercises that are sometimes useful to relieve muscle cramps, and wheelchair fittings. The speech-language pathologist helps with difficulties in communication or swallowing. The occupational therapist helps with positioning for comfort, providing adaptive equipment for the patient, or other assistance for comfort and for activities of daily living.

PALLIATIVE CARE/HOSPICE

The goal and emphasis of hospice is symptom management and palliative care. The team of caregivers routinely assesses, reassesses, and documents the severity, the treatment, and the control of symptoms of the illness.

When the patient is admitted and with each subsequent visit, the nurse and the team must assess the comfort level of the patient. One assessment tool that often is used is the Edmonton Symptom Assessment System (National Palliative Care Research Center, n.d.). This tool addresses the areas of pain, tiredness (lack of energy), drowsiness, nausea, appetite, shortness of breath, depression (feeling sad), anxiety or nervousness, and overall feeling of well-being. The patient is asked to rate each of these areas on a scale of 0 to 10. Having the patient participate in this way allows the patient to say where he or she has the most discomfort or area of greatest concern .

PAIN

Of all the symptoms that a dying patient experiences, pain is the most dreaded and feared; therefore, pain management is a priority in hospice. Pain disrupts activities as well as the quality and enjoyment of life. To a healthy person, pain is usually temporary and tolerable, but to a terminally ill patient, it can be excruciating, constant, and terrifying. Pain takes many forms such as physical, psychosocial, and spiritual, and addressing and alleviating it is correct and proper. It is all too easy for the caregiver caring for people experiencing pain to become frustrated and feel helpless as he or she tries to control the discomfort, which may lead to feelings of guilt and inadequacy.

Initially, the health care provider may order diagnostic tests to determine the exact cause of the pain.

Findings may reveal the pain to be related to tumor invasion, compression of organs or nerves, erosion of tissue, or other pathologic factors. Removing the cause is not always possible in some cases; therefore, controlling the symptoms becomes central to the successful management of pain for terminally ill patients. Initial and routine assessments are vital for managing pain, and the patient is the primary source of information. The patient's self-report of intensity, quality, and management of pain provides the most significant data. The **pain assessment** (evaluation of the factors that alleviate or exacerbate a patient's pain) should include information about the severity and the history of the pain and what brings relief to the patient. Pain assessment begins with the patient's self-report, and the patient rates the pain on a scale of 0 (no pain at all) to 10 (the worst imaginable pain). Any pain the patient rates at 5 or higher on the pain scale has a great effect on the quality of life.

Clinicians use many different pain assessments, such as OLD CARTS, which stands for *o*nset, *l*ocation, *d*uration, *c*haracter of pain, *a*ggravating factors, *r*elieving factors, *t*reatments, and *s*everity. Use the pain assessment tool available at your practicing institution. Assessment of pain is ongoing; any change in the intensity or type of pain necessitates changes to the plan of care (Box 40.2).

Box 40.2   Pain Assessment Questionnaire

1. Throughout our lives, most of us have had pain from time to time such as minor headaches, sprains, and toothaches. Have you had pain other than everyday kinds of pain today?
2. Where is the pain? (The use of a body chart often helps the patient to identify the location.)
3. Using the scale of 0–10, with 0 being no pain and 10 being the worst pain imaginable, rate the pain at its worst in the past 24 hours.
4. Using the same scale of 0–10, rate the pain at its lowest point in the past 24 h.
5. Using the same scale of 0–10, rate the pain on the average.
6. Describe your pain. (The words the patient uses to describe the pain help you to understand the type of pain for treatment purposes.)
7. What treatments or medications are you using to control the pain?
8. Using the scale of 0–10, with 0 being no relief and 10 being complete relief, rate the amount of relief received from the treatment.
9. What causes or increases the pain?
10. Does the pain interfere with any of the following?:
    General activity
    Mood
    Walking ability
    Normal work
    Relations with other people
    Sleep
    Appetite
    Enjoyment of life

Box 40.3	Pain Control

It is never right for a patient to suffer pain.

Ask the question, "Are you experiencing any pain?" If the answer is yes, ask the patient to describe the pain using the pain assessment questionnaire.

Pain is treated with medications such as morphine singularly or in combination with other medications to provide maximal relief while at the same time avoiding maximal side effects.

Proper pain relief is provided on a regular around-the-clock basis.

Medications should be available to manage episodes of breakthrough pain.

Nonpharmacologic interventions should be included in the plan of care.

The need for palliative care worldwide is enormous and will continue to increase. Symptom management and adequate pain control must be the prime objectives for the hospice nurse; at the same time, the nurse must always strive to maintain the patient's dignity and capacity to contribute to society as a full human being (Gordon, 2001).

The answers to the questions in Box 40.2 help the hospice team determine the appropriate mode of therapy that will be effective in managing the patient's pain. The goal of therapy is to prescribe a dose of effective drug sufficient to alleviate pain and allow the patient to remain alert enough to participate in activities of daily living (Box 40.3).

To effectively treat pain, it is important to determine which of the three main types of pain the patient is experiencing. *Somatic pain* arises from the musculoskeletal system and is described as aching, stabbing, or throbbing. Nonsteroidal antiinflammatory drugs, nonopioid drugs, and opioid drugs are often effective in treating somatic pain.

Pain that originates from the internal organs is called *visceral pain*. The words people commonly use to describe this are "cramping," "pressure," "dull pain," or "squeezing pain." Health care providers typically prescribe an anticholinergic medication alone or as an **adjuvant** (additional drug or treatment that is added to assist in the action of the primary pain treatment) to nonopioids or opioids.

Neuropathic pain arises from the nerves and the nervous system. Tingling, burning, or shooting pains often have neuropathic causes. Health care providers sometimes order anticonvulsants to be administered as an adjuvant to assist with pain control.

Lifestyle considerations are important in determining the route and the type of medication to administer for pain control. Oral medications may be preferable because they help the patient and the caregiver manage the scheduling and administration more easily. After the severity of pain and the type of medication to be used are determined, the dosage of the medication must be **titrated** (slowly increased to the level at which the drug is therapeutic). Mild to moderate pain sometimes can be managed with nonsteroidal antiinflammatory drugs; as the pain increases in severity with progression of the patient's condition, the health care provider often switches the analgesic regimen to an opioid drug, with or without adjuvant drugs. Nonsteroidal drugs can be administered along with the opioid to enhance the medication's effectiveness. Oral administration of analgesics is not always feasible because of nausea and vomiting, obstruction, or inability to swallow, and other routes (sublingual, subcutaneous, parenteral, rectal, or topical) may be considered. Morphine derivatives are often the drugs of choice in caring for hospice patients, because they can be delivered by all routes and the dosage can be titrated to control the pain. Breakthrough pain management is a primary need of hospice patients. Analgesics should be administered as needed.

Long-acting medications such as morphine sulfate (MS Contin), oxycodone (OxyContin), or fentanyl (Duragesic) patches often provide better pain control and are more convenient for the patient and the caregiver. As the pain increases, it is important to monitor the amount and frequency of medications administered. Increases in dosages may be needed to manage breakthrough pain.

As the patient's condition deteriorates and pain increases, the expert knowledge and skill of the hospice personnel in titrating and managing the pain are invaluable.

Ineffective pain management usually is associated with undermedication as a result of common myths and fears. The myths and fears are addiction, tolerance, and respiratory depression. With careful and expert monitoring by the hospice team, along with reassurance and support, these fears can be relieved.

An individualized approach is needed to manage pain successfully. Various alternative pharmacologic and nonpharmacologic options are available. Radiation therapy, nerve blocks, and psychological or physical methods can be tried in appropriate circumstances. Hot or cold packs at the site of discomfort, repositioning the patient, music therapy, relaxation techniques, acupuncture, and even transcutaneous electric nerve stimulation (TENS) are sometimes good alternatives (Box 40.4).

Nursing Interventions and Patient Teaching

The nurse's role is to focus on the effectiveness of the care plan: that is, to ensure that the plan achieves good control of the symptoms (Nursing Care Plan 40.1). It is necessary to assess and reassess constantly the pain and the symptoms to ensure that their management is adequate. The patient and the caregiver must be educated in the appropriate administration, scheduling, and effects of the medication to help them become aware of signs and symptoms of increasing pain. The patient and the caregiver must understand that it is possible to control pain and that using large doses of opioids is

Box 40.4   Nursing Care Plan The Hospice Patient With Metastatic Prostate Cancer

Mr. B. is a 74-year-old who has prostate cancer with bone metastasis. He complains of severe pain in his right leg and in his ribs, which he rates as a 7–8 on a scale of 0–10. Mr. B. also has shortness of breath. He is on a regimen of morphine sulfate; MS Contin, 20 mg every 12 h, and Roxanol, 20 mg every 4 h.

PATIENT PROBLEM

Pain, related to the cancer that has metastasized to the bone, manifested by complaints of pain, rating 7–8 on a scale of 0–10.

PATIENT GOALS AND EXPECTED OUTCOMES	NURSING INTERVENTIONS	EVALUATION
Pain will be controlled at a rating of 2 or less on a scale of 0–10	Assess pain control and pain level by using the pain assessment scale of 0–10 every visit. Assess patient's and caregiver's understanding of medication administration. Assess for compliance with medication schedule. Assess for side effects of the medications, and educate patient and caregiver accordingly. Notify the interdisciplinary team of any uncontrolled pain. Educate patient and caregiver of other pain control methods such as transcutaneous electric nerve stimulation (TENS), repositioning methods, and heat and cold treatments. Have the patient and caregiver keep a pain diary.	Patient rates pain at 7 or 8 on the pain scale of 0–10.

PATIENT PROBLEM

Inability to maintain adequate breathing pattern, related to disease process manifested by shortness of breath.

PATIENT GOALS AND EXPECTED OUTCOMES	NURSING INTERVENTIONS	EVALUATION
Patient will not complain of shortness of breath	Assess respiratory status and effort at every visit. Ask patient to rate respiratory effort on the scale of 0–10 at every visit. Assess need for oxygen use by measuring oximetry level as ordered. Administer oxygen per nasal cannula as needed. Notify the interdisciplinary team of any complaints of respiratory distress. Educate patient and caregiver about methods that ease respiratory distress (e.g., relaxation techniques, diaphragmatic breathing, medication usage, positioning). Provide emotional support to patient and caregiver at each visit.	Patient rates respiratory distress at 6 on a scale of 0–10. Oxygen is administered at 3 L/min by nasal cannula.

CRITICAL THINKING QUESTIONS

1. Mr. B.'s wife complains to the hospice nurse that her husband has not had a bowel movement in 3 days. What will be included in an appropriate nursing intervention that would provide relief for Mr. B.?
2. The nurse notes that Mr. B. is restless and demonstrates dyspnea. She performs an oximetry check on Mr. B. and notes that oxygen saturation is 83%. List three nursing interventions to improve his respiratory distress.

common and necessary to achieve that control. Assist the caregiver in setting a schedule for administering the medications and then monitoring the patient's response to and compliance with the established plan. This should be documented by the caregiver and monitored by the nurse at each visit to ensure compliance and to help in determining when a change in the plan of care is necessary. Encourage the use of alternative treatment such as music therapy and relaxation methods to aid in pain control. It is important to give encouragement and positive reinforcement to the patient and the family in their efforts at following the plan.

NAUSEA AND VOMITING

Nausea and vomiting tend to be very upsetting to the patient and the caregiver. Many patients consider nausea to be worse than vomiting, because sometimes it is noticeable only to the patient and therefore is overlooked by caregivers and health care professionals. It is important to assess the cause of nausea and vomiting, and to remove the cause if at all possible. Nausea is a possible side effect of chemotherapy and can result from obstruction, tumor, uncontrolled pain, constipation, and even food smells. At times, the treatment of the nausea is as simple as bringing in food already prepared so that the cooking smells do not bother the patient. Sometimes the drugs used for pain control cause nausea; antiemetics may be administered with the opioid analgesic. Nausea is a common side effect with the initiation of opioid treatment. This side effect usually subsides after a time, and the best response is to use an antiemetic rather than discontinue the opioid. Anxiety also has been known to cause nausea, which then leads to vomiting. Patients who vomit are typically anxious about why they are vomiting, which often worsens the symptoms.

Nursing Interventions and Patient Teaching

Educate the patient and the caregiver regarding the cause or the prevention of nausea and vomiting. Managing nausea and vomiting will include close monitoring of labs to ensure electrolyte imbalances are corrected, rehydration, and the administration of antiemetic medications. In the acute phases of nausea and vomiting, intravenous administration is needed. Then, oral medications can be used. Determining an effective pharmacologic regimen may be challenging. No single medication will work for each patient. Combinations of medications may be needed. Serotonin (5-HT3) antagonist medications such as ondansetron (Zofran) and dolasetron (Anzemet), and phenothiazine medications such as prochlorperazine and promethazine are frequently prescribed.

Eating slowly and in a pleasant atmosphere, with relaxation and rest periods after eating, is a good way to control the nausea. If vomiting occurs, discourage eating for a short time until peristalsis stabilizes. When the nausea and vomiting have subsided, the patient may begin drinking liquids to avoid dehydration or start eating soft, bland foods. Small, light, bland meals should be served, and sweet, greasy, spicy, or strong-smelling foods should be avoided. If anxiety and fear are causing nausea and vomiting, verbalizing the fears is often helpful. Under no circumstances is it ever acceptable to force the patient to eat food or drink fluids if he or she has no desire to eat because this also has potential to compromise dignity and be detrimental to the patient's well-being.

Patients may achieve relief from dehydration with the use of hypodermoclysis. Hypodermoclysis involves the administration of fluids subcutaneously through a butterfly needle; 0.9% sodium chloride is administered by gravity infusion. The individual state nurse practice act may allow this intervention to be performed by the LPN/LVN (Vidal et al., 2016).

CONSTIPATION

One of the most common problems of terminally ill patients is constipation. Constipation has many possible causes, and assessment as to the cause is fundamental for treating it adequately. Sometimes this problem causes more anxiety and discomfort than pain itself. Because constipation has the capacity to cause other symptoms, such as abdominal pain, nausea, or vomiting, prevention of the problem is important. Factors that contribute to constipation are poor dietary intake, poor fluid intake, hypercalcemia, hyponatremia, tumor compression of the bowel, use of opioids for pain control, and decrease in physical activity. Opioid administration can be followed by administration of a stool softener and a stimulant as well. Some opioids are more likely to cause constipation than are others; in such cases, a different opioid may be helpful. Changing the rate of administration sometimes also provides some relief. As with other drugs, if inability to swallow or nausea and vomiting are also a problem, other routes, such as suppositories or enemas, should be considered. A rectal examination may be necessary to check for an impaction, along with manual removal of stool. A small volume enema helps soften and dissolve a hard impaction whose removal is otherwise a painful procedure. Premedicating the patient with an anxiolytic and an analgesic before the removal of an impaction may help the patient better tolerate the procedure.

Nursing Interventions and Patient Teaching

Supporting and educating the patient and the caregiver are the nurse's primary concerns. The following points should be covered with the patient and the caregiver:

A decrease in oral intake will also decrease the amount of stool expelled.

Even if a patient does not have oral intake, bowel movements can still occur in some cases.

Opioids pose a risk of constipation, so patients who receive opioids should also take laxatives.

Comfort is the all-important factor. If the patient has not had a bowel movement, discomfort, bowel sounds, and firmness of the abdomen must be assessed before any active treatment.

ANOREXIA AND MALNUTRITION

Anorexia and malnutrition are major anxiety-producing symptoms of terminal illness. Poor appetite potentially arises from nausea, vomiting, constipation, dysphagia, stomatitis, tumor invasion, general deterioration of the body, depression, or infections. These complications lead to difficulty in eating, which in turn causes loss of appetite. Odors of food cooking, inability to tolerate sweet foods, or a bitter taste in the mouth also contribute to the problem. This makes food less enjoyable, so the patient does not eat.

Disease processes change the body's metabolism and appetite; these changes sometimes lead to cachexia (malnutrition marked by weakness and emaciation), usually in association with a serious disease such as cancer, resulting in muscle weakness and weight loss. If poor oral intake of either food or fluids is affecting the quality of life, it is necessary to make adjustments to the plan of care.

Nursing Interventions and Patient Teaching

Complete nutritional assessments routinely and apply the findings to the hospice plan of care as appropriate. Assess and treat causes of manifestations such as nausea, vomiting, and constipation. For depression or infection, treatment options should be discussed with the medical provider and interdisciplinary team. If anorexia is related to stomatitis or infections, good oral hygiene is important. A technique to alleviate discomfort of the mouth is to use sponge-tipped oral swabs soaked in mouthwash. Patients who have oral ulcerations may experience discomfort with mouthwash; therefore, water-soaked swabs may be a better option. Small frequent drinks, crushed ice, or artificial saliva are often useful in relieving a dry mouth. If the odor of food causes anorexia, the patient should not be in the kitchen during meal preparation, or family, friends, or volunteers may bring in meals. The meals should be made as attractive as possible, consisting of foods the patient chooses. High-protein supplements are helpful when eating is difficult. Avoid weighing the patient because sometimes the patient becomes depressed and discouraged by attention to weight loss.

Often the caregiver needs additional support when a patient is not eating; many caregivers think that a reduced diet will hasten death, and therefore, if they manage to get the patient to eat, the food will prolong life. Nurses often must reassure the patient and the caregiver that anorexia is part of the end-of-dying process and that forcing the patient to eat may be harmful. If the cause of the anorexia is untreatable, as in the case of tumor invasion, the patient and the caregiver may need additional emotional support. Rarely do artificial hydration, total parenteral nutrition, and tube feedings come into consideration. These may slow the overall cachexic effect, but they have the potential to do more harm than good, and the long-term result and quality of life will not change.

DYSPNEA AND AIR HUNGER

Dyspnea is a symptom that arises from a variety of possible conditions, such as heart failure, dysrhythmias, infection, ascites, or tumor growth. Breathing effectively is difficult for many patients, especially during the final stage of the illness. An estimated 55% to 70% of patients in the later stages of life experience difficulty breathing. Air hunger is sometimes caused by tumor pressure, fluid and electrolyte imbalance, or anemia (Morrow, 2020c). Anxiety resulting from fear or panic may accompany this problem. Some respiratory distress is relieved by oxygen, morphine, or bronchodilators. Oxygen may not actually relieve the dyspnea, but it often eases the anxiety of the patient and the caregiver. Sublingual morphine helps relax the patient's respiratory effort, thus enabling greater respiratory efficiency. Bronchodilators sometimes ease respiratory obstructions and ease the respiratory distress. In many cases, around 24 to 48 hours before death, the patient exhibits the "death rattle," which is the result of an accumulation of mucus and fluids in the posterior area of the pharynx. The sound that air makes as it passes through the mucus is coarse and loud and can upset the caregiver. Anticholinergic drugs, such as transdermal scopolamine or atropine given sublingually, are sometimes helpful in preventing excess secretions.

Nursing Interventions and Patient Teaching

The main nursing focus is in relieving the anxiety and supporting the patient and caregiver. Education on positioning, use of a fan to circulate air, use of morphine to decrease the work of respiration, use of anxiolytics to ease anxiety, and maintaining good oral hygiene help the patient and ease the caregiver's anxiety. Suctioning should be minimized, because it actually increases mucus production and is very uncomfortable for the patient. Suctioning should be performed only if the patient is choking and unable to recover.

PSYCHOSOCIAL AND SPIRITUAL ISSUES

Spiritual unrest and issues are often interrelated with psychosocial problems and have the potential to surface, especially when symptoms are uncontrolled. It is always necessary to respect any religious or spiritual concerns and meet the patient's wishes if at all possible. Spiritual assessments are meant to gather information regarding the patient's feelings and needs. When confronted with a terminal illness, some patients question their faiths and beliefs, and some search for the spiritual support that they have never had. Many symptoms such as depression, the need to suffer, bitterness, anger, hallucinations, or dreams of fire are, in some cases, indicative of unmet spiritual needs.

Nursing Interventions and Patient Teaching

Spiritual issues should be referred to the spiritual coordinator and not used as an opening to share personal feelings and beliefs unless the patient specifically asks for that perspective. The hospice organization determines whether the nurse or the spiritual coordinator performs the spiritual assessment. It is essential for the assessor to be nonjudgmental and accepting of the patient's and the caregiver's spiritual beliefs. The social worker also may assist with the relationship between the patient and the caregiver and provide counseling to resolve conflict. The social worker does not "fix" the conflicts but assists in problem solving. The development of trust between the patient and the interdisciplinary team is critical and is invaluable in dealing with these issues.

OTHER COMMON SIGNS AND SYMPTOMS

Weight loss and dehydration sometimes lead to a decrease in soft tissue, especially on the bony areas of knees, hips, elbows, and buttocks, which can lead to skin impairment.

Increased weakness is also notable in the last stages of a terminal illness; it often leads to activity intolerance and causes the patient to spend most of the time reclining. This leads to a risk for skin impairment and the formation of pressure ulcers. Poor nutrition, decreased circulation, and decreased mobility contribute to an increased risk for skin impairment. Education provided frequently to the family and the patient is necessary to promote integrity of the skin. The caregiver should observe the patient's skin and report any erythema or impairment. Instruct the caregiver to reposition the patient for comfort, use alternating air or egg-crate mattresses, and to perform good hygiene to prevent skin impairment.

Weakness is accompanied by safety issues of instability and falling. Patients often exhibit signs of depression and may make comments regarding suicide. Comments regarding suicide do not always come from the actual desire to kill oneself but are, in some cases, rather a statement of a desire for independence. Sleeplessness and insomnia sometimes occur as a result of an accumulation of signs and symptoms, and exhaustion has the potential to cause an exacerbation of all other signs and symptoms.

Nursing Interventions and Patient Teaching

It is important at this time to teach the patient and the caregiver the basics of good skin care. Cleanliness promoted by bathing is often refreshing, as well as therapeutic in promoting comfort and the feeling of self-worth. The skin should be inspected frequently and kept as dry and clean as possible. Stress the need to avoid harsh soaps, strong detergents, and irritation by buttons, snaps, or food crumbs. An egg-crate mattress, sheepskin, or an air-flotation mattress, as well as heel and elbow protectors, help cushion the bony areas. The hospice aide is often very helpful to the patient in assisting with personal care, hygiene, and bathing. If pressure ulcers occur, cleaning with normal saline, drying well, and applying a skin protector are helpful measures. Caregivers must be able to prevent

falls and injuries; provide information regarding home safety. Listening and providing emotional support are important nursing interventions for the patient with depression and suicidal thoughts. The social worker is influential in these situations.

The hospice interdisciplinary team realizes that a terminal illness is potentially the most difficult time in a person's life. The team takes as honest and straightforward an approach as possible in all matters affecting the patient and caregiver. It is thought that the fear of the unknown is always greater than the fear of the known. Because of this, education is an important part of the care that the team provides to the patient. Educating the caregiver about symptom management, hands-on care of the patient, caring for body functions, and the signs and symptoms of approaching death is important to help relieve fears (Table 40.4).

PATIENT AND CAREGIVER TEACHING

BEREAVEMENT PERIOD

Hospice care does not conclude once the patient dies. Loss and grief are individualized emotions. The need for support is provided by the hospice for an extended period after the death. The family, especially the primary caregiver, continues to need support after the patient dies. Even though the family feels they have prepared for the death, facing the future without the person who died is difficult. Many people believe that four full seasons must pass before bereaved persons are able to think of the deceased without feeling intense emotional pain, but this period is different for everyone. The death of a loved one is a devastating agony that takes time to heal and subside. Depending on the size of the program, special bereavement teams with counselors may be available for the caregiver and family. Some teams facilitate a bereavement support group that meets on a regular basis, providing these families the opportunities to communicate and share their feelings. Volunteers and pastors keep in touch by visits, phone calls, cards, and remembering the bereaved person on holidays and anniversaries.

The hospice staff also goes through a grieving period for each patient who dies. It is a good idea to encourage the team members to attend funeral services, attend memorials, or visit the caregivers as appropriate after the death to help ease their grief. Each hospice provides support to its staff with support meetings and time to vent their feelings and heal.

ETHICAL ISSUES IN HOSPICE CARE

Ethical issues that sometimes arise when dealing with hospice patients include withholding or withdrawing nutritional support, the right to refuse treatment, allowing a natural death, and DNR orders. Families find it difficult to discontinue nourishment, even when death is clearly approaching. If the patient is unconscious,

Table 40.4 **Signs and Symptoms of Approaching Death**

SIGNS AND SYMPTOMS	NURSING INTERVENTIONS
The arms and legs of the body sometimes become cool to the touch, and the underside of the body sometimes becomes darker.	Keep warm blankets on the patient to prevent feeling of coldness.
The patient may spend more and more time sleeping during the day and at times is difficult to arouse.	Assist caregiver in planning time to be with the patient when the patient is most alert.
The patient may become increasingly confused about time, place, and identity of close and familiar people.	Reorient the patient as appropriate to the time of day and who is present. Do not upset the patient.
Incontinence of urine and bowel movements often happens when death is imminent. Sometimes there is a significant decrease in urine output.	Educate the caregiver in keeping the patient clean and dry. Provide pads or adult diapers as needed.
Oral secretions sometimes become more profuse and collect in the back of the throat. This produces the sound often referred to as the "death rattle."	Provide a cool-mist humidifier to increase the humidity in the room when oral secretions build up. Elevate the head of the bed with pillows or obtain a hospital bed to make breathing easier.
Clarity of hearing and vision decrease slightly.	Keep lights on in the room when vision decreases and never assume that the patient is not able to hear you.
Restlessness, pulling at the bed linen, and having visions of people or things that do not exist sometimes occur.	Talk calmly and assuredly with the confused patient so as not to startle or frighten him or her further.
The patient's need for food and drink decreases.	Inform the caregiver that the patient will not starve to death or die of dehydration. Much reassurance is needed in this area.
Breathing patterns change to an irregular pace; there are sometimes 10- to 30-second periods of no breathing (apnea).	Elevating the head of the bed often relieves the patient who has irregular breathing patterns. Oxygen sometimes is and sometimes is not beneficial.
Changes in vital signs occur, with decreased blood pressure and elevated pulse.	Inform the family that these changes are normal and expected and are not uncomfortable for the patient.

decision-making regarding these issues sometimes falls on one family member, which has the potential to create guilt feelings if other family members disagree. There are no simple answers to any of these concerns. It is helpful when the patient makes his or her wishes known in advance, as in a living will or an advance directive, or assigns a durable power of attorney.

An advance directive is a document prepared while an individual is alive and competent. It provides guidance to the family and the health care team in the event that the individual is no longer capable of making decisions. The directive states the individual's preferences concerning life-support measures and organ donations and sometimes gives authority to another person to make decisions for the individual, who at that point may be in a coma.

Physician Orders for Life-Sustaining Treatment (POLST) is a form completed by the medical provider and the patient to inform health care providers of the patient's wishes. This form may be referred to by other names in different states. It is a shorter form than the advance directive with a few simple questions that can be filled out in a few minutes. This may be used in addition to or instead of the advance directive; it has proven to be more effective in preventing medical errors that arise from not following patients' wishes. Completion of this form is encouraged for all nursing

home patients and for patients entering a hospital or hospice; 29 states have adopted or are considering or working on adoption of the National POLST (National POLST, n.d.). The other 21 states are using POLST forms developed by the individual state.

Nurses must be aware of their organization's ethics policies and procedures so that they and their colleagues are able to address any questions and concerns appropriately and correctly. No discrimination is ever tolerable for patients in hospice, regardless of sex, race, age, religion, and diagnosis. It is never acceptable for hospices to exclude or refuse patients who need high-cost care; their mandate is to serve everyone regardless of ability to pay. Services are to be available 7 days a week, 24 hours a day.

A hospice patient may have suffered many losses throughout the illness: health, job, independence, self-esteem, family, and financial security. Hospice attempts to assist the patient in maintaining dignity and control. Hospice places the emphasis on living and not dying. It is important for the hospice team to be sensitive to the patient's and the caregiver's needs and to maintain honesty at all times. The team must make sure to include the patient and the caregiver in all aspects of care and decision- making. Provide opportunities for expressing concerns and fears because this will make the process less fearful and threatening. Allowing the patient and the caregiver to live fully, comfortably, and with dignity until death occurs naturally is the main goal of hospice care.

FUTURE OF HOSPICE CARE

Trends indicate that as more patients and families are educated about its many benefits, hospice is increasingly attractive as an alternative to facing death in a clinical setting. Nevertheless, only a fraction of people who have the option of hospice care choose to participate in it. Health care providers, patients, and family members may be unwilling to begin hospice care for several reasons. The patient or family sometimes believe that availing themselves of the services of hospice denotes giving up hope, and some health care providers are hesitant to prescribe hospice care if they perceive the patient's worsening condition a personal failure on their part. The average length of service is 76.4 days, with seven days or less for 27.8% of the population receiving services. This statistic highlights the need for increased attention and education to the benefits of hospice to patients, families, and members of the health care team (NHPCO, 2019).

Get Ready for the NCLEX® Examination!

Key Points

- Hospice is a philosophy of care about providing support to patients with a terminal illness and to their families.
- "Hospice" comes from the Latin word hospitium, meaning "hospitality" and "lodging."
- Hospice care is appropriate when active treatment is no longer effective and supportive measures are necessary to assist a terminally ill patient through the dying process.
- The Hospice Medicare Benefit covers all expenses for palliative care related to the terminal illness, including professional staff visits, medication, equipment, respite care, and acute care.
- Hospice care emphasizes quality, not quantity, of life.
- Palliative care is appropriate when a cure is not possible but care is still necessary.
- The goal of palliative care is to control pain and other symptoms for the prevention of distress.
- Palliative care is the treatment used to relieve or reduce discomfort of disease processes and may be used at any point during treatment, but is used most often when curative therapy has failed.
- Entering a hospice program is the decision of a patient and family.
- An important criterion for the patient to be admitted into hospice is certification by the attending health care provider and a second health care provider that the patient has a prognosis of 6 months or less to live.
- Hospice care consists of a blending of professionals and nonprofessionals to meet the total needs of the patient and family.
- Hospice care is delivered by an interdisciplinary team because no individual or individual profession is able to meet all the needs of terminally ill patients and families all the time.
- Hospice care accounts for all aspects of the lives of patients and their families. Stresses and concerns have the potential to arise in many ways when families are faced with a terminal illness.
- In a hospice care program, the patient and family are considered together as the unit of care because families experience much stress and pain during the terminal illness of one of their members.
- Family participation in caregiving is an important part of palliative care.
- Hospice care is available 24 hours a day, 7 days a week, because needs may arise at any time.
- Hospice care entails respect for all patient and family belief systems, wherein resources to meet the physical, psychosocial, and spiritual needs of the family unit are sought.
- Hospice care for the family continues into the bereavement period. Needs of the family continue after the patient dies.

Additional Learning Resources

SG Go to your Study Guide for additional learning activities to help you master this chapter content.

Be sure to visit the Evolve site at http://evolve.elsevier.com/Cooper/foundations/ for additional online resources.

Review Questions for the NCLEX® Examination

1. The health care provider is explaining to a 74-year-old patient that his prostate cancer is progressing and that curative treatment is no longer feasible. The health care provider has recommended hospice to the patient and his wife. What information may be included with a recommendation to hospice?
   1. "We can provide support and control your symptoms and discomfort so that you have good quality days."
   2. "With hospice, we would continue with aggressive curative care."
   3. "There is no hope left for you, and you should just go home and wait to die."
   4. "We can no longer guarantee controlled symptoms or a dignified life, but we can still provide sympathy."

2. The patient's wife calls the hospice nurse and reports that her husband is complaining of pain in his leg and is not able to get comfortable. What action by the hospice nurse may be implemented?

   1. Explain to the wife that pain will increase because of the progression of the disease and there is nothing to be done.
   2. Ask the wife how the patient rates his pain and whether he has taken any medication for breakthrough pain.
   3. Advise the wife that her husband must be a complainer.
   4. Advise the wife to wait until morning and call the health care provider.

3. When the nurse makes a home visit, the patient is experiencing shortness of breath and has increased anxiety. Place the hospice nurse's interventions in order.

   1. Assess the respiratory status.
   2. Increase morphine dosage to the higher end of the prescribed scale.
   3. Check pulse oximetry.
   4. Contact the primary care provider for a possible order for oxygen.

4. The patient is experiencing a decreased appetite and voices concerns about his weight loss. What action by the hospice nurse is most appropriate?

   1. Encourage the patient's wife to cook all of his favorite foods, and maybe he will eat.
   2. Tell the patient to force himself to eat.
   3. Explain to the patient that decreased appetite is normal.
   4. Contact the primary care provider for an order for an appetite stimulant.

5. The patient's wife is exhausted and expresses a need to get away for a short time. How can the volunteer coordinator help in this situation?

   1. Advise the wife that a volunteer will not help the situation at all.
   2. Instruct the wife that it is best for her to just stay with her husband because he might die while she is away.
   3. Assign a volunteer to sit with the patient for a couple of hours two or three times a week so that the wife is able to either take a nap or to leave for a short time to do errands.
   4. Assign a volunteer to do errands so that the patient's wife does not have to leave.

6. As a part of the hospice program, the patient has a core interdisciplinary team that manages his care. What members make up the core interdisciplinary team? (Select all that apply.)

   1. Spiritual coordinator
   2. Physical therapist
   3. Nurse coordinator
   4. Social worker
   5. Medical director

7. The patient's wife tells the hospice aide that she is having problems meeting their financial obligations. What action by the hospice aide is most appropriate?

   1. Tell no one because this is confidential information.
   2. Ask her for permission to report this to the interdisciplinary team, and have the social worker make a visit to see whether it is possible to provide assistance.
   3. Report this to the patient's church to see whether there is some financial assistance available.
   4. Encourage the patient's wife to consider government assistance during this difficult time.

8. The patient is complaining of constipation. He has had very little food intake the past 4 days. What action by the nurse is most appropriate?

   1. Advise his wife to stop all food and water.
   2. Assess for bowel sounds, abdominal distention, and possible impaction.
   3. Explain that reduced intake will result in reduced stool output.
   4. Instruct him to bear down to assist in elimination of his stool.

9. The patient is complaining of pain at a level of 5 on a pain scale of 0 to 10. What action by the nurse is indicated?

   1. Assume that because the pain is rated a 5, no further treatment is necessary or no changes are appropriate.
   2. Ask the patient what he wants his pain goal to be; if it is below 5, then you will have to notify the health care provider.
   3. Explain that the patient needs to try to tolerate a pain rating 5 or less.
   4. Automatically give the patient an additional analgesic.

10. The _____ is the mediator between the hospice team and the attending health care provider.

11. The nurse is discussing hospice with the spouse of a patient who has been diagnosed with dementia. During the session, which statement by the patient's spouse indicates the need for further discussion?

   1. "My wife will be happier that we can keep her at home during her hospice care."
   2. "My wife does not meet the criteria for using hospice."
   3. "The hospice care team is available around the clock."
   4. "I am glad to know that my family does not have to sign any documents allowing her to be without resuscitation should the time come."

12. The patient is nearing death. His wife, who is the primary caregiver, asks the nurse if it is still appropriate to turn the patient every 2 hours even as it creates discomfort and causes him to become restless. What would be the nurse's best response?

    1. "You should always reposition the patient every 2 hours no matter what."
    2. "Yes, you do not want the patient to develop pressure ulcers."
    3. "Position changes at this stage can be limited and performed only when he appears to be uncomfortable."
    4. "Position changes should be avoided from this point on."

13. The patient has never attended church and on hospice admission requested no spiritual support. Now he is within days of death and voiced some spiritual concerns to the nurse. What action by the nurse is indicated?

    1. Share personal spiritual beliefs with him.
    2. Advise him that it is too late and no church would accept him.
    3. Contact the interdisciplinary team to ask that the spiritual coordinator make a home visit.
    4. Communicate this information to the social worker.

14. The patient died peacefully and with dignity, but his wife is still having problems dealing with the death. What services by the hospice team can be anticipated?

    1. Continued bereavement support for her for the next year.
    2. Dismiss the wife from all hospice services.
    3. Encourage her to begin to explore activities outside of the home.
    4. Have the hospice aide continue with her visits to the home.

15. For the patient to qualify for assistance from Medicare or Medicaid for hospice care, which criteria are necessary? (Select all that apply.)

    1. The health care provider's statement that the patient has less than 6 months to live
    2. The fact that the patient is receiving chemotherapy or radiation
    3. Two health care providers' verification that the patient is dying
    4. The patient's prognosis of less than 1 year to live
    5. The patient's or caregiver's understanding of the plan of care

16. The bereavement coordinator on the hospice team follows a plan of care for the bereaved caregiver for what length of time after the death of the patient?

    1. 3 to 4 months
    2. 9 to 10 months
    3. Up to 13 months
    4. Up to 3 years

17. What elements are included in the definition of palliative care according to the World Health Organization? (Select all that apply.)

    1. Focusing on controlling pain and other symptoms, as well as reducing psychological, social, and spiritual distress for the patient and the family
    2. The active total care of patients whose disease is not responsive to curative treatment
    3. The framework for hospice care
    4. The active total care of patients by providing treatments to assist in improving patient prognosis
    5. The care in this setting initiated at the final stages of the dying process

18. A female patient, 48, is in hospice end-of-life care at home for Type III ECL-cell carcinoid abdominal cancer, Stage IV. Her key symptoms have been those of carcinoid syndrome: flushing, abdominal pain, constriction of the bronchial tubes in the lungs, and heart valve dysfunction. She was having diarrhea for a while, but that symptom has disappeared as she now rarely eats more than a cup of broth, Jello, or tea. Over the last 36 hours she has had half a cup of tea; for the last 24, she has been semi-conscious, accepting only ice chips when awake. Up to this point, she has preferred to rely on ibuprofen for pain control so that she can be present with her family for as long as possible. Tonight, the patient is experiencing dyspnea, which is making her and her family panic, and the family is alarmed by strange gurgling noises at the back of the patient's throat as she breathes.

Place a checkmark next to appropriate actions to take for this patient:

___ Administer sublingual morphine	___ Move patient into Trendelenburg position
___ Administer oxygen	___ Move patient into Sims position
___ Warm steam humidifier	___ Administer sublingual atropine
___ Turn off any fans	___ Suction frequently to reduce secretions

Professional Roles and Leadership

Objectives

1. Discuss the processes used to look for and secure employment.
2. Describe the traditional work shifts of a licensed nurse.
3. Discuss confidentiality.
4. List the advantages of membership in professional organizations.
5. Discuss certification programs and programs that further educational goals.
6. Discuss the computerized adaptive testing (CAT) in the National Council Licensure Examination (NCLEX) for the licensed practical nurse or licensed vocational nurse (LPN/LVN) candidate (NCLEX-PN examination).
7. Discuss Nurse Practice Acts.
8. Identify three important functions of a state board of nursing.
9. Discuss mentoring.
10. Discuss career opportunities for the LPN/LVN.
11. Discuss the guidelines and duties for being an effective leader in nursing.
12. Discuss styles of leadership for nurses.
13. Discuss delegating nursing tasks.
14. Discuss nursing informatics.
15. List the three types of health care provider's orders and discuss the legal aspects of each.
16. List three ways to ensure accuracy in transcribing health care providers' orders.
17. List the pertinent data necessary to compile an effective change-of-shift report.
18. Discuss the importance of malpractice insurance.
19. Identify strategies for burnout prevention.
20. Discuss the chemically impaired nurse.

Key Terms

advancement (ăd-VĂNS-mŭnt, p. 1250)
articulate (ăr-TĬK-yū-lāt, p. 1246)
as necessary (prn) (ĂS NĔS-ŭ-sĕr-ē, p. 1250)
burnout (BŬRN-out, p. 1267)
certification (sŭr-tĭf-ĭ-KĀ-shŭn, p. 1252)
contract (KŎN-trăkt, p. 1247)
endorsement (ĕn-DŌRS-mŭnt, p. 1255)
interview (ĬN-tŭr-vyū, p. 1246)

negligence (NĔG-lĭ-jĕns, p. 1257)
Nurse Practice Act (NŬRS PRĂK-tĭs, ĂKT, p. 1248)
per diem (PŬR DĒ-ŭm, p. 1250)
preceptor (prē-SĔP-tŭr, p. 1252)
reciprocity (rĕs-ĭ-PRŎS-ĭ-tē, p. 1255)
resignation (rĕz-ĭg-NĂ-shŭn, p. 1250)
résumé (REZ-ū-mā, p. 1246)
transcribes (trăn-SKRĪBZ, p. 1264)

FUNCTIONING AS A GRADUATE

There are ample options for employment in today's health care system for a licensed practical/vocational nurse (LPN/LVN). It is important for the newly licensed LPN/LVN to consider career plans and options that best fit his or her strengths, skills, and areas of interest. The role of a graduate nurse is exciting and challenging, and a career-planning tool or career planning resource (e.g., http://nalpn.org) helps the recent graduate navigate the road toward gainful employment. This chapter provides some guidelines for being a conscientious nurse while assuming this new role as well as methods to assist in securing a job, including a cover letter, a résumé, and the interview process. In addition, most colleges and universities offer career placement services to graduates. Box 41.1 provides an eight-step tool for helping the new nurse in career planning.

FINDING AND SECURING A JOB

Cover Letters

Cover letters are a means of introducing a job applicant to a potential employer. Key components of the cover letter include identification of interest in employment, a brief statement of qualifications, and availability for the position being sought. It is important to personalize the cover letter and to emphasize strengths and desired qualities applicable to the position. When writing the cover letter, consider the fit of the prospective

1. *Take stock:* the most important step of the career-planning process
   a. Read, listen, watch, learn; find out as much as possible about the trends in health care.
   b. Assess your professional strengths and weaknesses honestly and objectively.
   c. Ask yourself whether you hold certain beliefs that have any potential to undermine your attitude; such beliefs—myths, even—sometimes interfere with job performance and satisfaction.
2. Explore the options.
   a. Consider what kind of nursing positions are likely to enhance your strengths.
   b. Discuss your options with a mentor.
3. Gather more information.
   a. Attend health care job fairs.
   b. Research different nursing positions.
   c. Visit with colleagues who are doing the kinds of work you are interested in doing.
   d. Call nurse recruiters.
   e. Read professional journals and newspapers.
4. Narrow your focus.
   a. Consider the education and skills required for each position.
   b. Evaluate the responsibilities involved in each position.
   c. Consider salary range, days and hours, travel time, and availability of that job in your area.
5. *Make a decision:* List the pros and cons of each position and narrow the field to two or three possibilities.
6. *Get specific:* Learn as much as you can about other candidates for a nursing position.
   a. Obtain additional training if needed.
   b. Investigate the possibility of tuition reimbursement.
   c. Find out if on-the-job training is available.
7. Map your strategy.
   a. Record each step of your strategy.
   b. Develop a résumé.
   c. Develop interviewing skills.
   d. Practice interviewing by role-playing with a mentor or friend.
8. *Manage your career:* Periodically review where you are in your career and your life; choose a special date each year (e.g., your birthday) to make your reassessment.

Remember that successful careers do not happen accidentally. You make choices and changes along the way.

position for your personal skills and strengths. This aids in the development of a document that identifies you more clearly to the interview team. The cover letter should not exceed a single page. It also should contain contact information and a signature line. Cover letters (Fig. 41.1) may be mailed to the employer or uploaded as an attachment if the applicant is completing an online application.

Résumé

The **résumé** is a one- or two-page summary of educational and professional experiences, activities and honors, and concrete skills and interests. A concise, comprehensive, well-prepared résumé will impress future employers. It should be well organized, neat, and accurate. The applicant should be certain to use a variety of descriptive terms (e.g., "highly motivated," "exceptional ability," or "outstanding skills") when preparing the résumé. The résumé is the tool used by the employer to preview job candidates and select candidates to interview.

The three primary types of résumés are the chronologic, functional, and combination. In the chronologic résumé, the applicant's job history is listed in reverse chronologic order, with the most recent job listed first. The chronologic résumé often is considered the easiest to prepare because it requires a recall of work and education-related activities. Critics of the chronologic résumé report it does little to highlight a candidate's skillset. It also can emphasize gaps or a lack of experience. The functional résumé promotes the applicant's skills and experiences. It does not reference dates of the experiences listed. The combination type of résumé blends the two types. It allows a systematic, easily followed recall of work history and focuses on skills and experiences. The applicant should choose the résumé style that best demonstrates his or her strengths and abilities. The employer is seeking the employee with the most potential for the job, and the résumé is likely to be one of the first means by which the employer obtains an impression of the applicant (Fig. 41.2).

Personal Interview

The **interview** is a face-to-face meeting, an online meeting via a webcam or Skype, or a telephone call during which the employer assesses the potential candidate's qualifications and personality. The interview is a vital part of the application process. It is important for the applicant to be prepared for the interview process (Box 41.2). First impressions have a lasting effect, so it is imperative to make the most of the initial contact with a potential employer (Box 41.3). Applicants should **articulate** (speak clearly, distinctly, and to the point) and present themselves with clarity and effectiveness to make a good first impression.

Processes used for interviews vary by organization. The interview may be conducted by a single person or a panel. Members of the interviewing team may include the department's management team as well as representation from the work unit. The interview process may consist of a single meeting or a multistep series of contacts. In some settings, an initial screening may be performed by a member of the human resources staff or a nurse recruiter. The initial screening is often by telephone. The next stage of the interview process consists of meetings between the applicant and the nursing division.

For a good working relationship, it is best if the applicant's skills and nursing care values are in harmony with the objectives of the job description (Boxes 41.4 and 41.5).

July 1, 2021

Ms. Kelly Borrell
Nurse Recruiter
Kell-Russell Health and Rehabilitation Center
1650 East Health Valley Lane
Brazil, IN 47805

Dear Ms. Borrell,

In the next few weeks I will be completing my course work and graduating from the Practical Nursing program at Indiana College of Health and Nursing. I plan to sit for my licensure examination shortly after. During my nursing education, I was assigned clinical rotations at your facility. The experience provided me with a close view of the quality of care and the collegiality displayed by the health care team. As I begin my career these are qualities I will value in my nursing practice and I would like to have in my employer.

I have noted your website indicates there are open positions for licensed practical nurses on the memory care unit and I would like to meet with members of your team to discuss opportunities for employment. I will contact you next week to discuss this matter.

Sincerely,

Kim Dennis
3917 Marquette Ave
Brazil, IN 47805
Kimdennis555@qualitynurse.com
(811) 555-0011

Fig. 41.1 Sample cover letter.

Box 41.2   Preparing for a Successful Interview

1. *Build contacts.* Employers fill a majority of positions through personal contacts.
2. *Know the institution.* Learn everything possible about the institution to which you are applying.
3. *Take your personal inventory.* Record your strengths.
4. *Write or review your résumé.* Prepare or update your work history and professional accomplishments.
5. *Rehearse questions and answers.* Some standard interview questions are as follows:
   a. "Would you tell me about yourself?"
   b. "What are your major strengths and weaknesses?"
   c. "How do you think you will fit into this position?"
   d. "Give an example of when you have shown leadership skills or initiative."
6. *Make a good impression.* You have only a very short time to make a good impression.
7. *Understand the goal.* Interviewers need to determine four things about a job applicant: qualifications, attitude, adaptability, and affordability.
8. *Market yourself.* Think of a job interview as a sales pitch; you are assertively promoting yourself and your skills.
9. *Answer effectively.* How you answer a question is often more important than what you say.
10. *Practice role-playing.* Have different friends practice interviewing with you; video-record these role-plays and review the recording.

Job Shadowing

The entry into practice can be a frightening transition. School-based clinical experiences provide an introduction to the nursing care environment but do not often give a full picture of the culture of some nursing units. New graduates may have apprehension about the clinical environment and work expectations. There may be concerns about which units would best meet their needs and goals. Job shadowing provides a means for the individual to follow a nurse during a normal shift. This gives a snapshot of the unit culture, types of patients cared for, and expectations of the licensed caregiver. In addition, the opportunity provides an invaluable contact for the individual's professional network. Shadowing may begin before graduation. Multiple shadow opportunities provide experiences for comparison. Shadow experiences normally are coordinated by the human resources department.

CONTRACTS AND STARTING OUT

A **contract** is a promise or a set of promises between two or more people that creates a legal relationship with legal obligation between them. The usual contract that LPN/LVNs encounter is the employment contract. Today, the contract between the employee and employer is often verbal and implied. Under the employment contract, it is the nurse's obligation to perform nursing functions with the skill and knowledge that

<table>
<tr><td align="center">

Kim Dennis
3917 Marquette road
Brazil, IN 47805
(811) 555-0011

Kimdennis555@qualitynurse.com

Career objective

Hard-working practical nursing major (2.67 GPA) currently attending allied College of nursing and health science, with work experience in healthcare is seeking an entry licensed practical nursing position to increase skills and gain experience. Frequently praised as focused and dedicated by my peers, I can be relied upon to work as a team member in the quest for the delivery of quality patient care.

Experience
Kell-memorial health and rehabililtation center, Indianapolis, IN
Certified nursing assistant, july 2017 – present
- ❖ Change linens and make beds
- ❖ Assist with patient nutritional needs
- ❖ Measure and record input, output and reporting of changes to charge nurse
- ❖ Provide physical support to assist patients to perform daily living activities, such as getting out of bed, bathing, dressing, toileting, standing, walking, or exercising

Whitfield family pharmacy, terre, haute, IN
Cashier, jan 2015 – june 2017
- ❖ Receive payments by cash, check, or credit hard
- ❖ Issue receipts, refunds, credits
- ❖ Greet customers entering establishment

Education
Allied college of nursing and health science
Indianapolis, IN
Technical certificate practical nursing (anticipated completion may 2022)
- ❖ **GPA:** 3.52
- ❖ **Extracurricular activities:** Student nursing club, student government association (SGA)

Horrall institute
Brazil, IN
Certified nursing assistant, december 2016 – june 2017

</td></tr>
</table>

Fig. 41.2 Sample résumé.

is in accordance with the standards of the profession under that state's Nurse Practice Act. The employer is responsible for providing a safe working environment, sufficient and competent fellow workers, and safe equipment. Failure on the part of the nurse or the employer to perform these duties is a breach of contract. It is possible for breach of contract to result in a lawsuit, in which the court may order the breaching party to perform the obligations of the contract or to pay money to the party who suffered damage because of the breach. Because the contract is one for personal services, a nurse usually is not forced to work for the employer. Rather, the nurse may be liable for money damages to an employer for breach of contract.

The employment contract properly specifies the length of the contract period; hours that the nurse is to work; salary; vacation; sick leave pay; medical, maternal, disability, and liability insurance coverage; educational benefits; and any other benefits or working conditions to which the nurse and employer agree. The employment contract can be terminated legally, without a breach, by completion of all obligations under the terms of the contract or by consent of all parties to the termination.

New employees usually find that facilities provide orientation programs, which vary in length, depending on the facility policy. Many facilities also require newly graduated nurses to take examinations or tests to assess competencies in medication and math skills.

Recent graduates also are often required to serve a probationary period before acquiring the status of a benefit-earning member of the staff. Internships or residency programs sometimes are offered by employers to nurses who have graduated recently. An internship helps with the transition to professional nursing. Some facilities provide a mentor or preceptor (person who supports a new or transferred employee through clinical orientation) to assist the new graduate during this internship period. Probationary policies such as internships or orientations should be discussed during the interview process.

Encountering Problems

Despite the best intentions, problems may arise during employment. It is important to follow the chain of command. Be aware of the organizational chart of your

Box **41.3**   Steps to a Successful Interview

1. Be well groomed. Dress conservatively and appropriately. Try on the planned clothing to ensure you are comfortable prior to the day of the interview.
2. Arrive at the interview 10 min earlier than the appointment; if a receptionist or secretary greets you, identify yourself, and give the name of the person you are to see.
3. Be cheerful and polite.
4. Be knowledgeable about the position for which you are applying.
5. Be patient while waiting for an interview.
6. Smile and give your name distinctly when greeting the interviewer.
7. Use a firm handshake.
8. Address interviewer by last name, using "Mr.," "Mrs.," or "Ms."
9. Have at least three extra copies of your résumé and reference list and a neatly typed list of references.
10. Do not slouch or fidget; sit upright and be attentive. Do not chew gum.
11. Maintain eye contact with the interviewer.
12. Allow the interviewer to take the initiative; be an attentive listener.
13. Put purses or portfolios on the floor beside you, not in your lap. Avoid looking at your watch.
14. Answer questions concisely. Try to make the interview interesting and informative. Use the time effectively.
15. Be prepared to be interviewed by a group or committee or to have the interview recorded. Look at each member of the interview team. Shake hands with each one, using his or her name.
16. Articulate your speech.
17. Be factual.
18. Avoid being critical.
19. Convey genuine interest and enthusiasm.
20. Avoid discussing personal problems unless they are applicable to the job.
21. Be prepared to relate qualifications and experiences.
22. Inquire about job description, work schedule, and benefits.
23. If you are asked, state desired salary; if salary offered is unacceptable, do not mislead the interviewer.
24. Inquire about starting salary, pay increases, and maximum salary allowed.
25. If you are asked, indicate your preference of positions (if more than one position is open or if the interviewer invites you to "dream a little").
26. Look for clues when the interview is over. Usually an employer asks, "Do you have any more questions?" Hold any questions not covered until this time. If you do not have questions, this is probably a good time to say, "No, thank you, but I enjoyed our interview and hope that you will consider me for the position with your company."
27. Express appreciation for the interview.
28. Suggest when and where you may be contacted, if necessary.
29. Send additional information promptly on request.
30. Be aware that most beginning nursing positions require rotating shifts, even night shifts and working every other weekend. Many facilities require that you have medical-surgical experience before they will assign you to a specialty area such as obstetrics or pediatrics.
31. Follow up the interview with a thank-you letter or an email to the interviewer within 48 h.

Box **41.4**   Common Interview Questions

1. Tell me about yourself.
2. What are your top strengths and weaknesses?
3. Tell me about your last position.
4. Do you prefer working with others or independently?
5. What are your travel or relocation limitations?
6. How would you prefer people to criticize you, and how do you criticize others?
7. How many hours per week do you think someone should spend on the job?
8. What do you know about our facility?
9. Why do you want to work for us?
10. What important trends do you see in our industry?
11. What are your three most important accomplishments thus far in your career?
12. Give an example of your creativity.
13. How do you define success?
14. Is your current (or past) income commensurate (in proportion to or adequate) with your abilities?

Box **41.5**   What an Interviewer Can and Cannot Ask

CAN ASK	CANNOT ASK
• Criminal history	• Financial or credit status
• Hobbies	• Sexual preferences
• Community or social activities	• Marital status
• Future professional goals	• Age
• Education	• Color
• Work experience	• Religious beliefs
• Strengths and weaknesses	• Race
• Reason(s) for leaving previous job	• Creed
• Reason(s) why applicant thinks he or she is qualified	• Nationality
• Reason(s) for applying for this job	• Political affiliation
	• Level of financial debt

facility, as well as the grievance process for circumstances that cannot be resolved easily or if treatment is perceived to be unfair. Open communication is the best way to resolve most disagreements.

Work Schedule

Flexible scheduling is offered in most health care facilities. Common options include part-time and full-time schedules, straight evenings or straight nights, weekends only, shared jobs, **per diem** shifts or as needed or **as necessary (prn)** shifts, 12-hour shifts, 10-hour shifts, and 8-hour shifts. Eight-hour shifts are common in clinics, health care providers' offices, and care environments such as rehabilitation and long-term care facilities in which continuity of care is key to the health and stability of the patient population.

Many employers offer sign-on incentives or bonuses, as well as tuition reimbursement for nurses who choose to further their education. Nurses working flex time sometimes are allowed to set their own hours, which enables them to fit their work schedule around personal or family responsibilities. Nurses working the 12-hour shift may work three 12-hour shifts per week; some employers consider this a full-time schedule. Twelve-hour shifts are traditionally from 7 a.m. to 7 p.m. or 7 p.m. to 7 a.m. Care units such as the emergency department or surgery may have a variety of other shifts designed to provide increased coverage during peak activity times. Patient care is not limited to weekdays. Most care units require some type of weekend rotation by employees. Some nurses find satisfaction working a "weekend only" shift option. Mandatory overtime is sometimes a concern. If no nurses are available for the oncoming shift, those who worked the preceding shift are obliged to remain on duty. Some hospitals have been forced to turn away patients because they did not have adequate staffing. In an effort to provide an adequate number of care providers, facilities may opt to require a "call schedule." Call schedules require nurses to remain available to the unit on days or shifts for which they are scheduled off. Another tool that may be used to provide staffing are the development of short term contracts in which a nurse agrees to increase their weekly hours for a prescribed period of time. The nurse in the contracted arrangement traditionally agrees to a bonus payment or a substantial increase in their base salary rate. The amount of call shifts or hours required of a nurse varies by agency policy. Nurses continue to express their concerns and negotiate to improve patient care and working conditions.

Frequently, newly hired nurses in acute and long-term care facilities find themselves working the night shift, to which it may be difficult for some nurses to adapt. For nurses required to work the night shift, some suggestions on how to best adapt to working this shift are listed in Box 41.6.

Box 41.6 **How to Cope With the Night Shift**

STAYING ALERT AT WORK
- Remain hydrated.
- Eat before your shift
- Determine when and how many caffeinated beverages work for you.
- Eat light, balanced meals.

GETTING TO SLEEP
- Attempt to get 7–9 h of sleep per day.
- Make your sleeping area cool, comfortable, quiet, and dark, with blackout shades or blinds, a sleep mask, earplugs, or a white noise machine. Unplug the phone and turn down the doorbell volume.
- Limit caffeinated beverages and foods a few hours before attempting sleep. Stop drinking.
- Do not use alcohol or a sedative to get to sleep.
- Avoid smoking prior to retiring. Nicotine is a stimulant and may impact sleep.
- Develop a routine for the hours after work. Retire at the same time each day.
- Avoid exercise just prior to retiring.
- Wear sunglasses on the drive home to reduce the melatonin-inhibiting effect of sunlight.

BALANCING YOUR LIFE
- Eat right, exercise regularly, and get some fresh air and sunlight.
- Take short naps as needed, especially before driving home from work if necessary.
- Engage family and friends to help with sleep and work schedules.

ADVANCEMENT

Advancement (a rise in rank or importance; a promotion; progress; improvement) is a possible result of additional preparation or additional experience. A nurse may achieve advancement by learning the position more thoroughly and by assuming new and greater responsibilities. Advancements, together with the difficulties and obstacles that they bring, stimulate interest and enthusiasm. They usually are based on a person's qualifications, behavior, performance, and preparation. Facilities may employ a career ladder. Career ladders allow nurses who seek increasing responsibility and committee involvement to receive recognition for their contributions. Agency policies govern the application process and advancement. Nurses who seek to advance along the ladder may find financial compensation or other benefits provided for their participation.

TERMINATING EMPLOYMENT

Resigning from a position properly is another skill with which the LPN/LVN should be familiar. Employers sometimes raise questions about a résumé that reflects frequent job changes. Remaining at the first place of employment for at least 1 year is recommended. If this is impossible, follow the proper procedure for **resignation** (the act of resigning to give up a position of employment).

A verbal statement and a written resignation, providing at least a 2-week notice, is considered professional courtesy and maintains a good relationship with the employer. The letter should be kept brief, with concise terms stating the reason for leaving the position and providing the last planned date of employment. Some organizations may request an exit interview with the individual who is leaving. This traditionally is conducted by a representative from human resources. The exit interview may include returning any items that have been assigned to you, such as an identification badge or cell phone, discussing areas of improvement suggested for the organization, and reviewing benefits available after termination such as insurance. Failing to provide adequate notice may harm your reputation or leave the employer with an inadequate amount of time to find a replacement for the position. Positive references may be difficult to obtain from employers who feel they were abandoned or where the nurse did not act in a professional manner.

TRANSITION FROM STUDENT TO GRADUATE

KNOW YOUR ROLE

Sometimes it is difficult to gain a clear understanding of the exact responsibilities of each health team member. The LPN/LVN is responsible to a registered nurse (RN) or to the health care provider. The role of the LPN/LVN, like the roles of other health care professionals, is changing constantly. As the services of health care facilities attempt to meet the increasing demand of the population, the role of the LPN/LVN does not remain static. Many technical and scientific changes in the health care system have resulted in a multiplicity and complexity of responsibilities placed in nurses' job descriptions. In view of these developments, the LPN/LVN must continue to keep the patient as the focus of care. Patients quickly recognize a nurse's genuine concern for their individual needs.

CONFIDENTIALITY

All patient information must remain confidential. Patient information should be exchanged only with other members of the health care team responsible for the care of the patient. Release of information to anyone other than the health care team without the consent of the patient is a violation of the right to privacy. Refer to Chapter 2 for additional information regarding confidentiality (Box 41.7).

ROLE OF THE LICENSED PRACTICAL/ VOCATIONAL NURSE IN THE COMMUNITY

The LPN/LVN participates in activities that promote the community's positive attitude toward health care. The LPN/LVN uses community resources to promote a better understanding of the health services available to the general public and promotes and participates in community health projects and other health-oriented activities such as maternal and child health clinics,

---

Box **41.7**	Confidentiality Reminders

1. Discuss patient information only in conferences or reports. Be mindful of conversations in the cafeteria and at the nurses' station.
2. Keep confidential all information gathered from medical records, reports, or conferences.
3. Be nonjudgmental in observations of patients, hospital staff, family members, and other personnel.
4. Do not store patient statistics on any retrievable or permanent computer system unless authorized.
5. Do not keep or copy any patient information except when necessary for required report. All notes should be shredded after use.
6. Never copy any original medical records for any reason unless following the policies of the healthcare facility.
7. Do not leave a patient chart or electronic health record where unauthorized people are able to access it.
8. When using computers, always completely log off the system when stepping away from the device.
9. It is generally not the nurse's responsibility to release patient information to the police, media, relatives, or visitors.
10. Familiarize yourself with how patient information is to be handled within the facility.
11. You are obligated ethically to treat information about your patient as confidential.
12. Be aware of the actions of unlicensed personnel with whom you work. If necessary, teach others the importance of safeguarding a patient's privacy.

disabled children clinics, mental health clinics, blood pressure clinics, and community health fairs.

PROFESSIONAL ORGANIZATIONS

To have a voice in one's profession, join a professional organization. No organization has the power to be any more active or effective than its members. Some professional health care organizations provide opportunities for continuing education to their members and associated allied health staff.

Two national organizations exist to support and meet the needs of the LPN/LVN: the National Association for Practical Nurse Education and Service (NAPNES) and the National Federation of Licensed Practical Nurses (NFLPN).

Founded in 1941, the purpose of NAPNES is to promote an understanding of practical nursing schools and continuing education for LPN/LVNs. The organization also developed a position on the education of the practical nurse, defines ethical conduct, and publishes standards of practical and vocational nursing practice. The *Journal of Practical Nursing* is its official publication, and *NAPNES Forum* is the newsletter that informs members of activities. Membership is open to students, graduates, faculty, and other people who are interested in practical or vocational nursing. NFLPN, founded in 1949, serves the interests specifically of LPN/LVNs. It restricts membership to only LPN/LVN students and graduates. It informs members of the most current issues of interest and makes available to its members insurance coverage for malpractice, personal liability, health, and accident. The NFLPN also lobbies on the state and national levels for issues that are of interest and concern to its members. *Licensed Practical Nurse* is its official publication. For further information about NAPNES, visit its website (www.napnes.org). For further information about NFLPN, visit its website (www.nflpn.org). Members of these two organizations share the common goals of the LPN/LVN.

CONTINUING EDUCATION

The health care system is changing constantly as a result of rapidly developing technology and research, and keeping current with nursing trends and issues is crucial. There are abundant avenues by which to gain additional nursing skills and knowledge. Facilities frequently offer employees continuing education through seminars, conferences, or workshops (Box 41.8). Continuing education credit is also available through some nursing journals.

To renew nursing licenses, some states require a given number of hours per year in continuing education units (CEUs). These requirements are intended to improve the quality of patient care by educating nurses about the most recent trends in nursing interventions. Not all continuing education opportunities are accepted by all state boards of nursing for renewal of licensure. The LPN/LVN is responsible for acquiring the required number of CEUs and for ensuring that the credits are attained from approved providers.

CERTIFICATION OPPORTUNITIES

Certification is a process by which the nurse is granted recognition for competency in a specific area of nursing. Various certification opportunities are available to LPN/LVNs through seminars or self-guided study courses and successful completion of examinations. Knowledge is the basis for improved nursing skills and safety in patient care. Presently, certification through NAPNES is available for the LPN/LVN in pharmacology, long-term care, rehabilitation, and intravenous (IV) therapy. To be eligible, nurses must be licensed in their state. In many states or agencies, certification is also the basis for salary increases and advancement.

Certification in Managed Care

The American Board of Managed Care Nursing offers curriculum and testing that certifies the nurse in delivery of care that is patient centered. The nurse certified in managed care develops and puts into practice wellness and disease prevention/management programs, as well as quality management programs. The certification examination is a national examination, and recertification is required every 3 years.

Box 41.8 Continuing Education

ORIENTATION TO THE FACILITY

Provides an opportunity to learn about variations in routine and a review of selected previously learned information and skills. Orientations vary in length, depending on the type of facility; orientation periods may last from days to weeks. The new employee may be assigned a **preceptor** to work with during the orientation period.

IN-SERVICE EDUCATION

Information chosen to meet specific needs within a facility. Attendance at some in-service programs, such as a yearly update on bloodborne pathogens, is required. Usually, a specified amount of time is required for in-service programs, such as 1 h a month or three times a year, according to the agency policy. Depending on the credentials of the instructor, continuing education credits or units may be earned.

WORKSHOPS

Forum in which information is presented, discussed, and practiced. Workshops provide excellent opportunities to learn new skills. The length varies according to the content. Some agencies pay the workshop fee or expenses if the topic is specific to and enhances the employee's nursing skills. Workshops are also a major source of continuing education credits or units required by many states as a part of relicensure.

CONTINUING EDUCATION CLASSES

There are often classes on complex nursing skills such as intravenous therapy, physical assessment, LPN/LVN charge nurse responsibilities, mental health concepts, nursing process for LPN/LVNs, and so on. Some vocational schools and community colleges provide courses that a nurse is interested in if the nurse requests them and if there are enough potential students to make up the required minimum enrollment. Many of these classes provide continuing education credits, as opposed to course credit. A certificate is awarded when course work is completed satisfactorily.

SHARING INFORMATION

One of the most valuable benefits of continuing education classes is the opportunity to meet with other working LPN/LVNs. Networking allows for the exchange of ideas and practices among nurses. Keep a personal record of all in-service programs, seminars, and workshops offered, including dates, credits, and topics, for future reference. Ensure that the employer includes these records in personnel files at your place of employment.

LPN/LVN, Licensed practical nurse or licensed vocational nurse.

Certification in Pharmacology

NAPNES pharmacology certification addresses principles of pharmacology and medication administration, including dosage calculation. The LPN/LVN has the option of taking the challenge examination without benefit of a course. Courses are available, however, and some sponsoring agencies mandate the course as an initial step. Recertification is required every 3 years.

Certification in Long-Term Care

NAPNES offers certification in long-term care that addresses issues across the lifespan for individuals faced with chronic illness and for elderly patients. Once the examination is successfully completed, the certification allows the nurse the extended title of certified in long-term care (CLTC).

Certification in Intravenous Therapy

For nurses who desire to enhance their practice skills in IV therapy and phlebotomy, NAPNES offers IV therapy certification. This certification is offered through an examination as well as course work if desired. Nurses must consider the limits of their state's Nurse Practice Act when seeking IV therapy certification.

LPN/LVN Refresher Course

For LPN/LVNs who seek to enhance their knowledge and skills, NAPNES offers an online self-study and self-paced refresher course. LPN/LVNs who have been inactive in their profession, are seeking reactivation of their license, or are seeking to update their knowledge and skills may benefit from this course. Information for the LPN/LVN refresher course can be found on the NAPNES website (www.napnes.org).

Further Education: LPN/LVN-to-RN Programs

Many community colleges, private schools, and universities have programs that offer a specialized curriculum that leads to obtaining an RN license for LPN/LVNs who wish to further their education or career. There are *degree* programs such as the associate of science in nursing (ASN) and baccalaureate of science in nursing (BSN). Further degree outcomes for the LPN/LVN offer opportunities of completion for Master of Science in nursing (MSN). Some programs offer an accelerated pace for completion of the degree and may offer an online curriculum or a combination of classroom and online courses. These programs build on the education obtained in the LPN/LVN program. The state board of nursing is an excellent source of information about programs in each area. Colleges vary in their admission requirements and offer differing credits for previous education. Program length is variable.

LICENSURE EXAMINATION

REGISTRATION FOR THE EXAMINATION

Completion of the nursing program's course of study results in the conferment of a degree or certificate. The type varies by institution. Graduation from the program of nursing does not provide licensure. Licensure is granted by the state. Completion of the nursing program does not automatically provide eligibility to sit for the licensure examination. Most state boards require a criminal background check and fingerprinting before permission is granted for a candidate to take the NCLEX-PN. If there is a question about the candidate's work history or criminal background, the state's board of nursing may require the applicant come in for a personal appearance. This hearing is a means to provide more information about the areas of concern. The applicant may choose to appear alone or be represented by legal counsel. A person who is knowledgeable about the candidate sometimes writes a recommendation regarding the candidate's moral character. The state board has the authority to accept or reject a candidate's request to take the licensure examination. The board may feel the candidate should be licensed but may have lingering concerns about the applicant, The board of nursing may place restrictions upon passage of the NCLEX-PN such as probation, work site limitations, or the requirement of a work site monitor. The monitor would be charged with providing updates on the nurse's work activities.

Each state enforces its own Nurse Practice Act that addresses various issues, including licensure. The board of nursing in the jurisdiction where the candidate will take the NCLEX-PN approves the candidate's application. The state board of nursing has the authority to refuse any candidate the right to take the examination.

The scope of practice and titles of the graduate prior to licensure will rest with the state board of nursing. When seeking employment prior to licensure, it is imperative that the individual have an understanding of expectations and limitations that will be faced until passing of the licensure exam.

TEST PREPARATION

Some nursing programs administer an exit examination before graduation that will provide the graduate with an estimated likelihood of passing the National Council Licensure Examination for Practical Nurses (NCLEX-PN) Examination. The score on an exit examination is a good indicator of how much preparation the graduate will need for success on the NCLEX-PN.

Review courses are available to assist the graduate nurse in preparing for the NCLEX-PN. Before registering for a review course, the graduate should evaluate which course will be most beneficial. In considering a review course, the graduate must remember that the objective is not primary learning but review. Some review courses focus on content and others on test taking skills. Faculty members from the graduate's program may be able to provide recommendations for a reputable review course. Review material also may be found at the learning extension website of the National Council of State Boards of Nursing (NCSBN; www.learningext.com).

The graduate should take the following steps:
- Plan ahead and make an intelligent decision regarding a review course.
- Carefully evaluate the need for a review course.
- Look for a course that uses faculty from outside the nursing program.

- Investigate the course modality. Some are taught in a classroom setting and others online.
- Consider the cost; review courses may range from $250 to $500.
- Know the following: how long the course will last, where the course is held, the size of the class, and when the course is offered.
- Find out what guarantees the review vendor places on the review with regard to NCLEX success on the initial attempt.
- Determine if the review will provide a probability score tied to the likelihood of exam success.

Review books, online sources, and smartphone applications are available to aid the new graduate in preparing for the NCLEX-PN. It is important to select a review resource that meets individual study needs. Review resources undergo revision approximately every 3 years. Students should be sure to use current review resources because they follow the current NCLEX test plan. Nursing faculty frequently can offer suggestions for quality review resources.

Testing centers are available in each state as well as outside of the United States. After submitting an application to the state board of nursing, the candidate—if approved—registers with Pearson VUE to receive an authorization to test (ATT). The candidate also receives information that describes the test, the protocol for making an appointment for the examination, and a list of available centers and their contact information. Once the ATT is received, the testing location, date, and time are reserved.

TAKING THE TEST

The NCSBN adopted computerized adaptive testing (CAT) for the NCLEX in 1994. The maximum time length for administration of the NCLEX-PN is 5 hours. Some candidates are able to complete the examination in less time.

CAT test centers are quiet and comfortable, with specially designed workstations to enhance security while providing a personal testing environment. Upon entry, candidates are required to provide identification and have their fingerprints and photograph taken. The candidate sits at an individual computer terminal and answers questions that appear on the screen. Test staff maintain security by directly observing the testing session in addition to continuous monitoring. The proctor is able to observe all candidates simultaneously and continuously during testing without entering the room, which eliminates the noise and distraction of people moving about the room.

In April 2005, test administrators revised the test format by introducing *alternate format items*. An alternate-item format is an examination item that takes advantage of new technology through the use of a format to assess candidate ability that differs from the standard one of four multiple-choice options with one correct response. Possible alternate-item formats include

questions with multiple correct responses, fill-in-the-blank questions (including calculation and ordered-response item types), and "hot-spot" items, for which a candidate is to identify an area, picture, or graphic. All NCLEX-PN item formats, including current standard multiple-choice items, sometimes include charts, tables, or graphic images; the intent of alternate-item formats is to assess each candidate's ability to critically think in a way that is more flexible than with standard multiple-choice items.

Each test unfolds in an interactive way as the candidate proceeds through the material, but each one covers the same subject content (each test is based on the test plan). The goal of CAT is to determine competence on the basis of the difficulty of questions, not on how many questions are answered correctly. The interactive computerized format makes it possible to match the test questions posed to each candidate's demonstrated competence level. This makes for greater efficiency in the testing process: The program poses only questions that offer the best measurement of the candidate's competence, rather than a one-size-fits-all set that includes questions not relevant to a given candidate's situation.

Testing experts have ascertained the difficulty level of each of the thousands of questions in the computer's item bank by trying them out on thousands of candidates and then statistically analyzing the results. In the actual testing situation, the program uses a candidate's answers to calculate a competence estimate based on the known level of difficulty. It then scans through the test item bank, classified by test plan area and level of difficulty, and determines the question that will measure the candidate in the next test plan area most precisely and appropriately. It presents this selection on the computer screen as the successive test question to the candidate. This process continues, creating as it goes an examination tailored to the individual candidate's knowledge and skills and at the same time fulfilling all NCLEX-PN plan requirements.

Questions are ranked by the level of difficulty from easiest to hardest. If asked the easiest questions, most candidates answer most of them correctly. If asked only the hardest, they probably answer most incorrectly. As the examination questions progress from easy to hard, there comes a point at which an individual candidate is answering 50% of the questions correctly. Questions further along the difficulty continuum are likely to receive wrong answers (i.e., although some answers will be right, more will be wrong), and easier questions are likely to elicit correct answers. The goal of CAT is to find that point, which is different for everyone. That point is the competence level.

The minimum number of questions for the NCLEX-PN is 85 (60 "real" questions and 25 pilot, or "try-out," questions). The scores on the try-out questions are not counted toward the competence level of the candidate. If a candidate is able to answer the difficult questions correctly, there is no point wasting the candidate's time with a lot of easy questions. Likewise, if a candidate is not able to answer the easy ones correctly, there is no point in continuing with the difficult ones because the candidate is unlikely to be able to answer them. In fact, the system often has enough data to make a decision after less than the minimum of 60 questions, but a minimum of 60 scored questions is necessary to ensure coverage of the test plan. It is important that the candidates get the opportunity to answer several questions in each of the test plan content areas.

After the candidate has answered 85 questions, the system compares the competence level with the passing standard and determines (1) whether the candidate is clearly above the passing standard (the candidate passes), (2) whether the candidate is clearly below the passing standard (the candidate fails), or (3) whether the competence level is not clear. If it is not clear whether the candidate has passed, the system continues to ask questions. The system stops asking questions when the competence level is clearly above or clearly below the passing standard, when the maximum number of questions has been answered (265 for the NCLEX-RN and 205 for the NCLEX-PN), or when the candidate runs out of time (5 hours).

There is no random selection of which candidates get a long examination. The length of the NCLEX-PN is based on the performance of the individual candidate.

Candidates who are accustomed to knowing most of the answers on tests sometimes find a CAT test difficult because they know the answers to only about half the questions. However, it is in fact possible that these candidates are doing well: Because they are answering the most difficult questions in the item bank, even 50% correct scores reflect a high competence level.

Applicants having documented disabilities may request accommodations for testing. These requests are approved by the individual state boards for the location of what will be the "home state." The most frequent requests involve additional time to complete the examination, increased computer magnification, an exam reader, and an isolated testing space. Additional requests vary.

In response to the Covid-19 pandemic, NCSBN made changes to the testing environment and to the exam's requirements in 2020. Social distancing and other requirements were implemented in the testing centers. This significantly reduced the number of people who could test at any one time. NCSBN statisticians modified the exam to a minimum of 60 questions with a maximum of 130 questions. Testing time was reduced to 4 hours.

NEXT GENERATION NCLEX

Studies have shown that more than 65% of nursing errors are the result of a failure of clinical decision making (Flores-Harris, 2019). Next generation NCLEX (NGN) was developed in effort to evaluate clinical decision making and critical thinking. Case studies that feature scenarios with interrelated factors that will require evaluation to ensure the actions taken are clinically sound. Proposed items for NGN are evaluated as they are administered to testers. The questions do not "count for or against" the test taker. NCSBN reports NGN will not begin until 2023 or after.

The most current and complete information about the NCSBN and the NCLEX-PN is available from its website (www.ncsbn.org).

AFTER THE TEST

To ensure accuracy each exam is scored twice. The computer at the testing site will score the exam. The test scores are pass or fail. Test administrators print score reports and send them to the board of nursing in each jurisdiction within 24 hours. Each board of nursing schedules its own notification timetable and process. Most test results are received by candidates in 1 week or less.

Candidates who have failed their licensure examination in most states are allowed to retake the test after waiting 45 days. Additional guidelines from the state board of nursing include (1) the number of times a candidate is allowed to retake the test before being required to seek reeducation and (2) the amount of time allowed between graduation from nursing school and taking the licensure examination. Those failing exams will be provided a report from NCSBN concerning their performance in meeting each of the client need categories.

On successful completion of the examination, the candidate has the right to practice as an LPN/LVN. The licensed LPN/LVN is responsible for license renewal and keeping the state board informed of any changes of address, name, and employment (i.e., active or inactive) status. The LPN/LVN is not allowed to practice without a license. Licensure permits nurses to offer special skills to the public, but it also provides legal guidelines for protection of the public.

ENDORSEMENT AND RECIPROCITY

The NCLEX-PN makes it possible to practice nursing in states other than the one in which the nurse first qualifies (see Chapter 2). If the nurse moves after successfully passing the examination and fulfilling the educational requirements, it is necessary to apply for a license or temporary practice permit before practicing nursing. Licensure that transfers this way from one state to another is called endorsement (a statement of recognition of the license of a health practitioner in one state by another state; the applicant needs to meet the current state's licensing requirements). Some states called this licensure reciprocity; this is a mutual agreement to exchange privileges, dependence, or relationships, such as an agreement between two governing bodies to accept the credentials of caregivers licensed in each other's state. True reciprocity means that an individual licensed in one state automatically can receive licensure in the other, even if the licensing requirements of the states differ. In either case, the nurse must have a license that is unencumbered. Some states also offer temporary licensure to individuals seeking endorsement in that state. This allows the applicant endorsement to work while the application for licensure is being reviewed.

Nurse Licensing Compact and Mutual Recognition

To date, 25 states have adopted mutual recognition licensure or an interstate compact. Those states (known as *compact states*) are listed in the NCSBN's website (https://www.ncsbn.org/nurse-licensure-compact.htm).

Because mutual recognition licensure is based on the primary state of residence, every nurse is required to declare his or her primary state of residence. The primary state of residence is defined as a declared, fixed, permanent, and principal home for legal purposes (domicile). Indicators of a domicile include, but are not limited to, where real property is located and where the nurse pays state taxes, votes, and is licensed to operate a motor vehicle.

For example, if the LPN/LVN's primary state of residence is Missouri and the LPN/LVN's nursing practice is confined totally to the state of Missouri—that is, the LPN/LVN does not physically leave the state to care for patients and the LPN/LVN does not use technology (telephone, computer interface, interactive closed circuit television) to assess or provide advice to patients living outside of Missouri—this does not affect how the LPN/LVN is licensed.

If an LPN/LVN travels with a patient from one state to the other or to Canada, the LPN/LVN's license is valid for the length of the stay in the other state or Canada.

If the LPN/LVN's primary state of residence is Missouri and the state (or states) in which the LPN/LVN practices is on the list of compact states, the LPN/LVN's license entitles him or her to practice in that state after Missouri's effective date and the other compact state's effective date have passed. The LPN/LVN must be sure to maintain the Missouri license on active status. After Missouri and the other compact state's effective dates have passed, the LPN/LVN no longer needs to maintain a license in the other compact state.

If the LPN/LVN's primary state of residence is Missouri but the state in which he or she practices is not on the list of compact states, the LPN/LVN needs to maintain a license in the other state. If the LPN/LVN's primary state of residence is Missouri but the LPN/LVN practices in one or more states that are on the compact state list and one or more states that are not on the compact state list, the LPN/LVN is permitted to practice in the compact states because of the Missouri license, but the LPN/LVN must maintain a separate license in any states that are not on the list.

Also, the LPN/LVN should consider maintaining the Missouri license in anticipation of other states' adopting mutual recognition licensure.

Nurses who are on active duty in the armed forces or employed by the US Public Health Service, the US Department of Veterans Affairs, or any other federal institution must meet the licensure requirements of those federal institutions. The nurse licensure compact does not replace the federal requirements and thus does not necessarily affect licensure status. However, the LPN/LVN still is required to declare his or her primary state of residence. If the LPN/LVN is a federal employee and holds a second (civilian) job in nursing, the compact does not apply to the civilian position, and the LPN/LVN must obtain licensing by the usual route of applying to the state board of nursing. Some states that do not accept mutual recognition still require endorsement or reciprocity.

State boards of nursing differ, so contact the board of nursing in the state where licensure is being sought for the specific requirements of that state.

NURSE PRACTICE ACTS

The Nurse Practice Act is a statute enacted by the legislature of any of the states or by appropriate officers of the districts or possessions.

A **Nurse Practice Act** is the licensing law. It defines the title and the regulations governing the practice of nursing. The act delineates the legal scope of the practice of nursing within the geographic boundaries. Its provisions assist the nurse in staying within the legal scope of nursing practice in each state. Some states have separate governing boards for professional and practical or vocational nursing. The Nurse Practice Act defines the regulations for practical nursing and includes requirements for an approved school of nursing. It also states the requirements for licensure and conditions under which a license may be revoked or suspended (see Chapter 2).

STATE BOARD OF NURSING

Each state has a board of nursing. The composition of the boards is determined by individual state statute. The majority of state boards are composed of LPN/LVNs and RNs. A few states have separate boards for the different practices. Boards are appointed by the state's governor or designee. The duties of the state boards have a focus on the promotion of public safety and the oversight of nursing licenses and educational programs. The duties may vary but generally include the following:

- Interpretation and enforcement of the state Nurse Practice Act
- Administration and development of nurse licensure policies
- Discipline as determined of nurse licenses

- Development of nurse practice standards
- Accreditation and monitoring activities for nursing education programs

The purpose of the board is to protect the public by administering the Nurse Practice Act. The board is responsible for approving schools of nursing and for renewing and issuing licenses. The board also has the authority to suspend or revoke a license. Some of the conditions under which a nurse's license is suspended or revoked include inability to perform competently as a result of drug addiction, alcohol abuse, and lack of mental or physical well-being. A nursing license may also be revoked for negligence in patient care (the commission of an act that a prudent person would not have committed or the omission of a duty that a prudent person would have fulfilled, resulting in injury or harm to another person; proof is necessary that other prudent members of the same profession would ordinarily have acted differently under the same circumstances), for endangering a patient's life, or for failing to comply with the standard and requirements of the Nurse Practice Act of the state in which the nurse is practicing (see Chapter 2). Sanctions also may be taken in response to criminal actions that are outside of the realm of nursing practice.

MENTORING AND NETWORKING

A mentor is a nurse with more experience and knowledge who is willing to help a novice nurse learn the skills of the profession through counseling, role modeling, and teaching. Nurses need to demonstrate caring behaviors for themselves, each other, and patients. Much attention has been given to the benefits of mentoring in nursing. Retention rates for new graduates—and for nurses in general—have been found to increase for agencies that have a mentoring program in place (Cottingham et al., 2011; Ketola, 2009). The loss of a nurse from a position results in significant cost to the employer. Cost estimates vary but can add up to thousands of dollars. The loss is not limited to the care that would have been administered by the nurse but extends to include the cost of sharing the message of the open position, interviewing, loss of productivity, and impact of morale of the remaining members of the health care team (Box 41.9).

If a facility does not have a mentoring or preceptor program, the new graduate (mentee) should locate a nurse (mentor) who demonstrates similar clinical interests and displays actions and behavior that are desirable. The mentee should evaluate how receptive to questions the potential mentor seems and whether he or she seems likely to take time to explain and clarify information.

If the new graduate is unable to identify a mentor or the facility does not have a mentoring program, there are some ways to self-mentor. Suggestions include the following:

| Box **41.9** | Cost of Nursing Turnover |

- Human Resource costs for advertisements, interviews, and background checks
- Coverage needed to replace the nurse until a replacement is able to assume responsibilities (this may involve overtime, travel or agency nurses)
- Orientation and training
- Decreased productivity until the replacement employee is ready to assume all duties
- Potential patient errors, compromised quality of care related to reduced staffing levels
- Potential declines in unit morale
- Loss of organizational knowledge
- Additional turnover

- Interact with nurses. Ask questions, listen, and clarify what you know with other nurses to enhance your understanding.
- Discover and use references. Read books and journal articles.
- Observe other nurses who are knowledgeable and insightful.
- Enroll in educational programs, especially those that include skill practices.
- Determine solutions for yourself, reflect on them, and work through them on your own.

Another strategy is networking, which is an effective method for interacting with and gaining support from other people employed in the same setting. Information and suggestions are shared when a nurse is networking with others in the same field. In addition to networking within a facility, there are various Internet resources through which nurses network with each other.

CAREER OPPORTUNITIES

Never before has nursing been so exciting. Today, the new graduate has an unprecedented variety of job opportunities available. Making the correct career decision requires considerable thought for the graduate. The job opportunities for the LPN/LVN extend beyond those in the long-term care facility and the hospital. When entering the field of nursing, the new graduate should be aware of the average wage, number of jobs available, and the job outlook for the LPN/LVN. This demographic information better prepares the new graduate for employment opportunities (Box 41.10).

Some nurses believe that it is better for the LPN/LVN to seek employment first in a hospital or long-term care facility with a subacute unit. This provides the opportunity to sharpen clinical skills and solidify the LPN/LVN's knowledge base, providing a strong foundation. This decision depends on the individual's goals and personal situation. For example, if the LPN/LVN knows that he or she can work only days and needs weekends off, a health care provider's office or clinic may be a preferable first job.

| Box 41.10 | **LPN/LVN Demographics in the United States in 2017** |

1. Median pay: $47,480 per year ($22.83 per hour)
2. Number of jobs: 721,700
3. Job outlook from 2019 to 2029: 9% increase (faster than average occupations)
4. Projected employment change in number of jobs from 2019 to 2029 +65,700 Places of employment:
   Nursing and residential care facilities : 38%
   Hospitals; 15% Physician offices: 13%
   Home health care services: 13%
   Government: 6%
5. Work schedules: The majority of LPN/LVNs worked full time in their place of employment; the remainder worked part time.

LPN/LVN, Licensed practical nurse/licensed vocational nurse.
Modified from US Department of Labor, Bureau of Labor Statistics: Occupational outlook handbook: Licensed practical and licensed vocational nurses, 20182021. Retrieved from: https://www.bls.gov/ooh/healthcare/licensed-practical-and-licensed-vocational-nurses.htm.

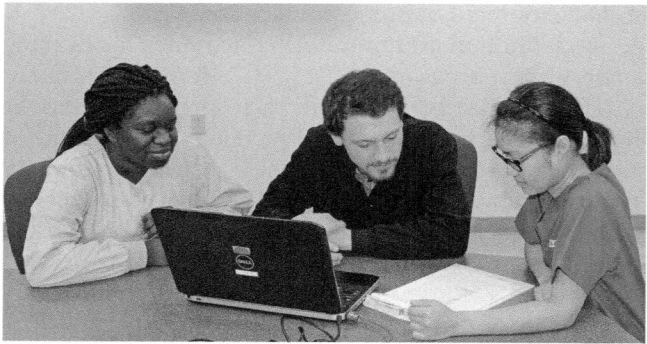

Fig. 41.3 Various positions on the health care team are available in the long-term care setting.

HOSPITALS

Because of health care economics, hospitals are responsible for providing quality care as economically as possible. Under the supervision of an RN, the LPN/LVN is legally able to provide most bedside care to patients in the hospital setting. Because the LPN/LVN salary is lower than that of the RN, it makes economic sense to employ a number of LPN/LVNs. It also makes sense because the LPN/LVN is prepared to give excellent bedside care.

The LPN/LVN has opportunities in various departments throughout the hospital, including coronary care, intensive care, emergency department, surgery scrub, outpatient surgery, and pediatrics. Policies vary by facility and locality. In the hospital setting, the LPN/LVN has responsibility for supervising nursing assistants, whereas overall management of a unit is the responsibility of an RN.

Salaries in a hospital setting may include shift differential and extra pay for holidays and perhaps weekends. Benefits tend to be good in hospitals, and some provide for 12-hour shifts and special schedule plans such as a 3-day weekend work schedule. Other opportunities in the hospital setting include work in infection control and employee health, as well as serving on various committees.

When seeking employment, the LPN/LVN should consider a number of different types of hospitals. Some have a wide range of services, and some are more specialized. Common specialized hospitals include pediatric facilities, orthopedic facilities, and rehabilitation facilities. Some hospitals operate in conjunction with a university and are the site of a great deal of teaching and research.

LONG-TERM CARE FACILITIES

LPN/LVN work is the backbone of long-term care facilities (previously called *nursing homes*). LPN/LVNs

in this setting frequently advance to charge nurse and supervisory capacity with RN supervision. The LPN/LVN in the long-term care setting often is involved in staff development and recruitment and serves on various committees. Management and leadership skills have ample opportunity for development in the long-term care setting (Fig. 41.3).

Salaries for LPN/LVNs vary by clinical environment and regional location. The LPN/LVN earns the most amount of money in governmental agencies. Slightly lower earnings were reported in ambulatory settings such as physician practices. In 2017, the median salary was $45,030. In long-term care facilities, salaries are currently similar to those in the hospital setting (Bureau of Labor Statistics, 2021). Shift differential pay and scheduling alternatives may be available. Benefit packages also tend to be good in the long-term care setting.

Many positive changes have occurred in the facilities. The long-term care facility is just that: a facility for patients who require long-term care. Hospitals no longer are an option for patients after the period of acute illness. Alternatives include rehabilitation hospitals if patients meet the qualifications, home health care, or a long-term care facility. Residents are of any age, and the level of care depends on the unit. Subacute units provide care that in years past was possible only in the hospital setting. Physical, speech, occupational, and other therapies are available. Many patients receive therapy and are able to return home.

HOME HEALTH

The degree to which home health care opportunities are available to LPN/LVNs varies in different parts of the United States. The LPN/LVN is capable of providing much of the care required, but RN supervision must be available. The advantages of home health care include patient preference, nurse autonomy, and the lower cost of care in comparison with hospital stays. Home health care also allows for continuity of care since the nurse often is assigned a caseload that he or she follows during the entire time the patient is receiving home health care.

HEALTH CARE PROVIDER'S OFFICE OR CLINIC

Health care providers' offices and clinics are a common place of employment for LPN/LVNs. It is important for the LPN/LVN to be aware that certain skills may be required in these settings that were not included in his or her educational program, such as phlebotomy and electrocardiography. In some cases, the health care provider teaches these skills, or certification classes may be available. The LPN/LVN should check his or her state's Nurse Practice Act to ensure that any additional skills are within the scope of practice. Computer skills are essential in virtually every health care setting, and insurance coding skills may be necessary in smaller offices.

Salary in offices tends to be lower than that in hospitals and long-term care facilities. Often, the benefits package is not as complete as in the other settings. The schedule of primarily days with minimal weekend work is a definite advantage. There is an opportunity to focus on prevention in these settings, as well as opportunities for patient teaching.

INSURANCE COMPANIES

Insurance companies may employ LPN/LVNs in their preadmission and claims departments. These positions are office positions with few requirements involving manual dexterity. Companies usually require prior experience in medical-surgical nursing. The nurse's role may include performing basic physical examinations for potential policyholders or consultation for current policyholders. Practice environments largely determine the earning potential of the LPN/LVN in this field. Regional variables also determine earning capabilities.

TEMPORARY AGENCIES

There are opportunities to work for staffing agencies. These agencies provide nurses to meet the staffing needs in a variety of health care facilities. The salary is usually very good, but sometimes the benefits package is limited. The LPN/LVN must be very flexible to adjust to various work settings when working for a temporary agency.

Advantages of employment with a temporary agency are the right to refuse an assignment and the variety of assignments available. When employed by a temporary agency, the LPN/LVN has the right to say no on a given day when called upon to work, which provides flexibility in one's personal schedule. The nursing experiences are more varied than when working every day at the same facility on the same unit.

A disadvantage is the uncertainty that work is available. If the number of patients is low in a facility, temporary employees are not called to work, so it is important for the new LPN/LVN to budget appropriately in the event of no work. Another disadvantage is that it may be difficult to create friendships or obtain the feeling of being the part of a team.

TRAVEL OPPORTUNITIES

Experienced nurses may explore opportunities to travel and work for specified periods in areas in need of nurses through a type of temporary agency with an expanded area of service. These agencies match employers' needs with nurses' experience and interest in living in that area for a time. Lodging usually is provided in addition to salary. This affords nurses who have the flexibility to travel the chance to visit an area and work there for a period of time.

PHARMACEUTICAL SALES

Pharmaceutical sales companies sometimes employ nurses as sales representatives. These companies usually require experience in specific areas and an expertise in science and pharmacology. Salary usually is based on sales. There is no direct patient care. Sales representatives contact health care providers, pharmacists, and nurses in various clinical settings to present the advantages of products and to teach about side effects and precautions.

OTHER MEDICAL SALES

Opportunities are also available for nurses with companies selling medical supplies. Responsibilities and compensation are similar to those in pharmaceutical sales. Sometimes nurses in this line of work hold inservice programs at facilities to demonstrate product use. Products vary widely, from such items as incontinence products to surgical equipment.

MILITARY

Opportunities are available for the LPN/LVN in military service. Active duty and the reserves are options. Local recruiters can provide information regarding a military career. Benefits of serving in the military as a nurse include the opportunity to serve one's country and educational opportunities. Various programs assist with tuition if the LPN/LVN chooses to further his or her education.

ADULT DAY SERVICES

Some communities may provide adult day services that require nursing supervision. These facilities are designed for individuals who require medical supervision while their family members work or take a break from the responsibility of care. The pace is relaxed, and the schedule is excellent. Many nurses find it to be a rewarding experience to work in a facility providing this kind of service to the adults and their family members who need it.

SCHOOLS

Opportunities are available in some communities to work as a school nurse. Health screening, emergency care, and health teaching are the major responsibilities. The nurse may work in one school or travel to different schools. Working only during the school year and during school hours is an advantage for nurses who themselves have children.

PUBLIC/COMMUNITY HEALTH

There are sometimes opportunities for LPN/LVNs with the public health department. Responsibilities usually include working in clinics and home visits. The nurse sometimes also participates in health inspections. Teaching is a major area of responsibility. The focus is on prevention. Day schedules are usually available. Salaries tend to be lower than in hospitals and long-term care facilities. In addition, community health opportunities include employment in areas such as weight-loss clinics, Head Start programs, and camp programs.

OUTPATIENT SURGERY

Work is available in a large number of outpatient facilities, especially for outpatient surgery. The LPN/LVN is sometimes employed to prepare patients for surgery, as a scrub nurse, or to work in the recovery room under the supervision of an RN. This is typically a Monday through Friday position. Some facilities are freestanding, and others are part of a hospital complex.

PRIVATE DUTY

The private duty nurse gives total care to one patient. The setting for the private duty nurse changes from patient to patient, but the job description is basically the same. This type of nursing is totally independent nursing care service when the nurse self-contracts. Private duty nursing takes place in the hospital, the home, or other facility and during travel abroad or in the United States. When performing private duty nursing, the LPN/LVN cares not only for the patient but also for the family. The nurse is paid directly by the patient or responsible person. When the setting for private duty nursing is in a health care facility, the nurse is expected to follow the policies and procedures of that facility.

In private duty nursing, the nurse is legally responsible for his or her own actions. If the nurse ever has any doubt about an order or procedure, he or she must obtain clarification from the health care provider before carrying out the order or procedure. It is important to keep charts carefully. In the home, the nurse can set up a type of record in which to list necessary items, such as medications given, vital sign measurements, and the conditions of the patient. This home record is sometimes requested by and released to the health care provider. The nurse returns any narcotics not used to the health care provider before leaving the assignment.

The major disadvantages of private duty nursing are the irregularity of assignments and the economic aspects. In private duty nursing, there is no certainty of work or payment. Also, the private duty nurse must keep accurate records for tax and Social Security purposes.

An advantage of private duty nursing is the option of working as many days as desired and the opportunity to accept an assignment for as long a period as desired. There are also more freedom and fewer restrictions in the workday.

GOVERNMENT (CIVIL SERVICE)

Some LPN/LVNs work in a Veterans Administration (VA) hospital or other government hospitals. Advantages are competitive salary, benefits, retirement plans, and tuition reimbursement programs. In addition, many VA nurses feel rewarded by caring for veterans who have served their country in the military (US Department of Veterans Affairs, n.d.).

OCCUPATIONAL HEALTH

The focus in occupational health nursing is on promoting wellness and preventing accidents. The emphasis is on safety and administering first aid care. Job responsibilities include physical assessment, health surveys, insurance form preparation, and health education as well as nursing intervention for patients injured in industrial accidents. The LPN/LVN works under the supervision of an RN or a health care provider. Depending on the size of the industrial or facility site, this type of nursing sometimes offers shifts and benefits different from those of other career opportunities.

REHABILITATION

This field requires responsibility for guiding the patient toward health and independence. The role of the rehabilitation nurse includes assisting patients to meet maximum functioning capabilities, caring for patients with disabilities or chronic disease, and working closely with not only the patient but also the patient's family. An important aspect of rehabilitation nursing is collaboration with the rehabilitation team (Association of Rehabilitation Nurses, 2012).

MENTAL HEALTH–PSYCHIATRIC NURSING

Mental health–psychiatric facilities employ LPN/LVNs in a variety of settings. Venues for this type of nursing vary from inpatient units in a general hospital to outpatient clinics, mental health agencies, and psychiatric hospitals. Residential rehabilitation facilities are another site in which the LPN/LVN works with patients experiencing mental health or psychiatric issues.

HOSPICE

Hospice nursing offers the opportunity to care for terminally ill patients in either an institution or a home setting. The qualifications for hospice nurses are to have a clear understanding of their own feelings concerning death and to understand the philosophy of the hospice setting. The nurse closely supports the patient and family without interfering with family interpersonal relationships. Advantages of hospice nursing are steady employment, an environment that is less formal, and opportunities to provide good bedside care that is concerned with pain relief and comfort measures.

Disadvantages are the fact that the nurse cares only for dying patients and the possibility of having to travel to more than one home each shift (see Chapter 40).

CORRECTIONAL FACILITY NURSING

Employment in correctional facilities is a growing field for nursing. Nurses work in county and city jails, as well as state and federal prisons. Duties vary from basic first aid care to extensive nursing care. Some larger state and federal prisons are finding it more beneficial and economical to house all medical services within the facility rather than transporting inmates to surrounding hospitals and clinics. This trend will increase the number of correctional nurses needed to adequately staff such units. Certifications in correctional nursing are available for nurses and nurse managers.

LEADERSHIP AND MANAGEMENT

Leadership is the art of getting other people to want to do something that the leader believes must be done. One root of the word *lead* means "to go." Leaders typically have a vision of where to go: a direction in which they influence other people to follow. Leaders are the ones who show the way and envision the "big picture."

Management is closely related. The word *management* comes from a word meaning "hand." Managers handle the day-to-day operations to achieve a desired outcome. Successful organizations require leadership and management (see the Coordinated Care box for responsibilities of the nurse manager).

When determining rules of supervision, team members typically supervise other team members who have a lesser scope of practice. Understandably, an LPN/LVN would not supervise the RN but could be responsible for other LPN/LVNs. Other members of the health team who would be managed by the LPN/LVN would include medical assistants, certified medical assistants, orderlies or transport workers, clerks, and technicians. The majority (38%) of LPN/LVNs are employed in long-term or assistive care facilities (US Bureau of Labor Statistics, 2021). In these settings, nurses may work in a position of leadership or management. In addition, some states may view LPN/LVNs as supervisors or they may have waivers that allow them to have increased supervisory responsibilities (Chron, 2020).

Leadership is an important factor in determining the effectiveness of any undertaking. Management style is the approach or manner that a leader uses to influence the behavior of other people in various situations. Leadership styles relate to the amount of control or freedom the manager allows the group. Such styles range from total control by the manager to extreme permissiveness. The most common styles are autocratic, democratic, and laissez-faire.

 Coordinated Care

Supervision

Responsibilities of the Nurse Manager

- Assist staff in establishing annual goals for the unit and determining the systems needed to accomplish goals.
- Monitor professional nursing standards of practice on the unit.
- Develop an ongoing staff development plan, including one for new employees.
- Recruit new employees (interview and hire).
- Conduct routine staff evaluations.
- Establish yourself as a role model for positive customer service (customers include patients, families, and other members of the health care team).
- Submit staffing schedules for the unit.
- Conduct regular patient rounds and help resolve patient or family complaints.
- Establish and implement a quality improvement plan for the unit.
- Review and recommend new equipment needs for the unit.
- Conduct regular staff meetings.
- Conduct rounds with health care providers.
- Establish and support necessary staff and interdisciplinary committees.

AUTOCRATIC STYLE

The autocratic leader retains all authority and responsibility and is concerned primarily with tasks and goal accomplishment. This type of leader assigns clearly defined tasks and establishes one-way communication with the group. The input of other team members is not sought or considered. The autocratic leader is firm, insistent, and dominating. Such a leader stresses prompt, orderly performance and uses power to intimidate or pressure employees who fail to adhere to expectations. This leader displays little trust or confidence in employees and therefore makes all the decisions. Because employees generally fear this type of manager, there tends to be some stifling of individual initiative and creativity.

The autocratic style of leadership is appropriate in certain situations. In situations in which immediate action is required and there is no time for group decisions, the autocratic leader is able to take quick action. Autocratic leaders excel in times of crisis (e.g., code situations) and in environments where staff turnover is rapid. This environment doesn't allow for development of leadership skills in employees so the autocratic leader makes the decisions. (RN.org, 2019).

DEMOCRATIC STYLE

The democratic style is a people-centered approach that allows employees more control and individual participation in the decision-making process. The emphasis is on team building and on collaboration through the joint effort of all team members. Democratic leaders function to facilitate goal accomplishment while stressing the self-worth of each individual. These leaders treat each staff member as an adult and expect the same in return. Criticism focuses on behaviors, not on personality, and its purpose is to promote growth and development of the staff.

The democratic style works best with mature employees who work well together in a group. This style sometimes does not work as well with ancillary staff, who in many cases need more direction. The group decision-making process sometimes seems slow and frustrating to those who expect prompt action on an issue. Disagreements are more likely and sometimes require more time to resolve. This style tends to demand more of the leader, but many employees value it for the sake of the professional growth and development of the staff that it facilitates. The results of the democratic leadership style in health care settings are evident in shared governance (an organized, systematic approach to decision making that enables nurses at all levels to participate), self-directed work teams, and staff committees concerned with quality improvement.

LAISSEZ-FAIRE STYLE

This leadership style often is referred to as the "free-run style" or "permissive leadership." This type of leader relinquishes control completely and chooses to avoid responsibility by delegating all decision making to the group. Laissez-faire leaders want everyone to feel free to "do their own thing," and as a result, there is no sense of direction unless provided by the group or an informal leader. This style sometimes works well with highly motivated professional groups (e.g., a research staff), but it seldom works well in health care settings because of the complexity of the work environment.

SITUATIONAL LEADERSHIP

Situational leadership is a comprehensive approach to the issue of management that takes into account the style of the leader, the group being managed, and the situation at hand. Supporters of situational leadership contend that no single leadership style is best but rather that the best style for the manager to use is contingent on the situation at hand.

The basis of situational leadership theory is the flexibility of the manager in adapting to the needs of the individual or the work group. In a typical work setting, the manager may be directive in dealing with staff who are in orientation and simultaneously act as a coach for those on another shift who are more experienced but still need some guidance. For seasoned staff nurses, the manager is more of a support person. The situational leadership style enables professional growth for manager and staff (Hill and Howlett, 2013).

TEAM LEADING

Sometimes, an LPN/LVN is assigned the role of team leader. This role entails assisting and guiding the nursing team in providing care for a select group of patients. The team leader assigns patients to each team member and takes responsibility for the delivery of care to patients, as well as for supervision of all members of the team, including nursing assistants. Duties of a team leader include the following:

- Receiving reports on assigned patients
- Making assignments for team members
- Making rounds and assessing all assigned patients
- Giving team members reports about assigned patients
- Assisting in administering medications and treatments
- Providing time in the early part of the shift to have a conference with team members on priority patients (those with the most urgent needs) to keep everyone informed of progress in patient care, provide continuity of care, and allow the team member to answer questions and resolve problems

An advantage of team nursing is the collaborative style that encourages each member of the team to help others.

DELEGATION

Delegation of tasks is an important aspect of patient care. Delegation of care refers to the act of making another individual responsible for a specific task. One of the benefits of delegation is that licensed personnel are allowed more time to focus on higher level tasks.

Delegation mandates clear communication of all aspects of the delegated care to the person completing the task. Consider the job description, the legal responsibility, the educational level, the ability, and the licensure of the person to whom you are delegating complete care. The staff member performing the care must be able to perform tasks independently and have the ability and knowledge to complete the task (see the Coordinated Care box on the five rights of delegation). Do not assign care to an unqualified staff member. For example, the LPN/LVN may delegate ambulation of a patient to a certified nursing assistant, but the LPN/LVN is responsible for determining the degree of assistance necessary for the patient.

TIME MANAGEMENT

Time management is an aspect that is sometimes difficult for the new LPN/LVN. For a new nurse, the patient load is often heavier than that during nursing school and there are added responsibilities as a licensed professional. It is important for the new LPN/LVN to evaluate his or her time management skills to determine whether time is being used effectively. Suggestions for time management are listed in the Coordinated Care box on prioritization and time management.

Coordinated Care
Delegation

The Five Rights of Delegation

RIGHT TASK

The right task refers to delegating care for a specific patient and ensuring that the task delegated is within the health care professional's scope of practice. If a task is delegated to unlicensed assistive personnel, the task should be a skill that is repetitive, requires little supervision, is relatively noninvasive, has predictable results, and poses minimal risk to the patient.

Right Circumstances

Consider the appropriate patient setting, available resources, and other relevant factors. In an acute care setting, patients' conditions often change quickly. Good clinical decision making is necessary to determine what to delegate.

Right Person

The right person is delegating the right tasks to the right employee for performance on the right patient.

Right Direction and Communication

Give a clear, concise description of the task, including its objective, limits, and expectations. It is essential for communication to be ongoing between the registered nurse (RN) and assistive personnel during a shift of care.

Right Supervision and Evaluation

Provide appropriate monitoring, evaluation, intervention as needed, and feedback. Assistive personnel must feel comfortable asking questions and seeking assistance.

Be aware that accountability remains with the delegating nurse in many situations. A major advantage of delegation is that tasks are completed in a more timely manner when all staff are working together to reach the common goal for the patient (Fig. 41.4).

Data from American Nurses Association: Joint statement on delegation: American Nurses Association (ANA) and National Council of State Boards of Nursing (NCSBN), n.d. Available at *https://www.ncsbn.org/Delegation_joint_statement_NCSBN-ANA.pdf*.

Coordinated Care
Prioritization

Principles of Time Management

GOAL SETTING

Review the patient's goals of care for the day and your goals for activities, such as completing documentation, attending a patient care conference, giving the staff report on time, or preparing medications for administration.

Time Analysis

Reflect on how you use your time. While you work in a clinical area, keep track of how you use your time in different activities. Such tracking often provides valuable information and reveals how well organized you really are.

Priority Setting

Schedule the priorities that you have established for patients within set time frames. Determine the best time for activities such as conducting teaching sessions, planning ambulation, and providing times for rest.

Interruption Control

Everyone needs time to socialize or to discuss issues with colleagues. However, do not let this interrupt important patient care activities. Use time during reports, meal breaks, or team meetings to the best advantage. Also, plan time to assist colleagues so that it complements your patient care schedule.

Evaluation

At the end of each day, take time to think about how effectively you used your time. If you are having difficulties, discuss them with a more experienced colleague.

Employer/Nurse Leader Responsibilities
- Identify a nurse leader
- Determine nursing responsibilities that can be delegated, to whom, and in what circumstances
- Develop delegation policies and procedures
- Periodically evaluate delegation process
- Promote positive culture/work environment

Communicate information about delegation process and delegatee competence level

Training and Education

Public Protection

Licensed Nurse Responsibilities
- Determine patient needs and when to delegate
- Ensure availability to delegatee
- Evaluate outcomes of and maintain accountability for delegated responsibility

Two-way Communication

Delegatee Responsibilities
- Accept activities based on own competence level
- Maintain competence for delegated responsibility
- Maintain accountability for delegated activity

Fig. 41.4 Delegation model. (From National Council of State Boards of Nursing: National guidelines for nursing education, *J Nurs Reg* 7:5–14, 2016.)

NURSING INFORMATICS

Nursing informatics has become a well-recognized term since it first was introduced. The American Nurses Association (2008) recognized nursing informatics as a specialty that "integrates nursing science, computer science, and information science to manage and communicate data, information, knowledge, and wisdom in nursing practice." Numerous computer systems are available in the health care setting, so nurses are trained on the particular system used at their place of employment. Nurses incorporate nursing informatics into the daily routine in various ways, including entering health care information into the patient's *electronic medical record (EMR)*, documenting medication administration, and researching medical information from online sources. Both certifications and graduate degrees in nursing informatics are available.

TRANSCRIBING HEALTH CARE PROVIDERS' ORDERS

Health care providers convey orders for patient care through writing, telephoning, or verbalizing the orders to the nurse. The health care providers' order may be handwritten in the patient's records by the health care provider. In an attempt to prevent errors in transcription, many facilities are now requiring the health care provider to submit orders directly into the computer system of the facility. Some acute care facilities employ ward clerks, ward secretaries, or unit secretaries to transcribe the health care providers' orders. Conversely, in most long-term care facilities, there are no unit secretaries. In facilities that do employ unit secretaries, the secretaries usually do not work at night. In many facilities, an expectation of the nurse is to transcribe the order from the patients' record if it was not submitted electronically. Some orders are difficult to read. If in doubt, clarify the order with the health care provider. Review the orders while the health care provider is on the unit so that clarification can be obtained in person immediately rather than later over the phone (Fig. 41.5). Also, if the written order seems unusual or does not seem congruous with the patient's condition, clarify the order with the health care provider. It is imperative to understand each order before carrying it out.

The health care provider is in charge of directing the patient care, and nurses carry out these orders for care unless the nurse believes that the orders are in error or will be harmful to the patient. In this case, contact the health care provider to confirm or clarify the orders. If you still believe the orders to be inappropriate, immediately contact the nursing supervisor and put in writing the reason the orders are not being carried out. A nurse who carries out an erroneous or inappropriate order is at risk of being held liable for harm experienced by the patient. Nurses are responsible for their actions regardless of who told them to perform those actions.

Fig. 41.5 Clarifying the health care provider's order. (Copyright 1999–2012 Thinkstock. All rights reserved.)

The policies for verbal or telephone orders vary in different facilities. Check the facility's policy for accepting verbal or telephone orders. Orders given by telephone or verbal communication are more subject to error. If you are responsible for accepting this type of order, be certain of its accuracy. Clarify the order by repeating it to the person giving it and document that this was done. This gives both people a chance to hear the order. A telephone or verbal order always must be written down immediately. If the order is given too rapidly, ask the giver to repeat it more slowly. When the correct spelling of a medication is questionable, refer to a list of commonly ordered medications or to the *Physicians' Desk Reference*. Be cautious about medications whose spellings look alike or similar and those that sound alike. Several medications sound alike but have very different actions (e.g., Xanax [alprazolam] and Zantac [ranitidine]; Xanax is an antianxiety agent, and Zantac is a histamine antagonist for the treatment of ulcers).

When the nurse transcribes (writes or types a copy of) health care providers' orders, a number of precautions must be used to prevent errors (see the Medication Safety Alert box on precautions for transcribing orders).

Orders requiring transcription are those concerning diet, preoperative and postoperative instructions, all medical treatments, activity, procedures, medications, diagnostic imaging and other diagnostic studies, and laboratory tests. When a patient undergoes surgery, all preoperative orders are canceled automatically. The health care provider must rewrite the orders postoperatively if continuation of the orders is desired. Many health care providers have routine postoperative orders, which have been prepared beforehand. There is a protocol for each order according to the facility's policy. When transcribing any order, follow through all

! Medication Safety Alert

Precautions for Transcribing Orders

The following information applies to all health care providers' orders:

1. Check that written/computer entry orders correspond correctly to the intended chart.
2. If there is more than one order, read through all orders before beginning to transcribe them.
3. Process stat orders first. (A stat order is for a single dose of medication to be administered immediately and only once.)
4. If there is some confusion during a telephone order, have another nurse listen for clarification.
5. When you take telephone or verbal orders, write the order on the order sheet, read the order back to the person giving it, and document that you read the order back.

The following items are basic guidelines and sometimes vary from one facility to another. The LPN/LVN should refer to agency policy.

6. Order the medication needed from the pharmacy per facility policy; include date, patient's name and identification number, date of birth, room number, time of administration, medication, route of administration, dosage, and frequency.
7. Record the orders in the required areas, such as the medication administration record (MAR), unless the orders are computer generated. Be certain to include the date.
8. Make very certain that all orders have been carried out and recorded in the proper record. (The new graduate should have a second nurse verify for accuracy until experience is obtained.)
9. Check off each order on the health care providers' order sheet if it is handwritten; otherwise follow the policy of the facility for computerized systems. Most facilities require the nurse's signature or initials to verify that orders have been transcribed.
10. Make sure to notify the nurses responsible for administering medications of any new order.
11. Follow the facility policy for identifying new orders for the staff.
12. When there is an order to discontinue or change a medication, take the steps in the Medication Safety Alert box on the procedure for discontinuing or changing a medication (this procedure varies in different facilities).

! Medication Safety Alert

Procedure for Discontinuing or Changing a Medication

1. If the medication administration record (MAR) is not on the computer, the discontinued medication should be marked off on the MAR by crossing through with a highlighter and documenting the discontinue date on the MAR. If the order is being changed, a new order should be written. If the MAR is a computerized system, follow the policy of the program or facility.
2. Notify the nurse responsible for carrying out new orders about discontinued and newly ordered medications.
3. On the health care provider's order sheet, verify that the order has been carried out.

Fig. 41.6 The MedStation, a computerized system for narcotics distribution. A variety of medications are housed in individual compartments that the nurse can access. (Courtesy CareFusion Corporation.)

steps completely as described previously with medication orders.

Some drugs may be distributed as floor stock. Floor stock are medications distributed to the nursing unit in bulk (either individually wrapped or in bottles). In general, medications appropriate for floor stock are those that health care providers tend to prescribe routinely on an as-needed (prn) basis. Medication dispensing systems, such as computer-assisted or electronic devices, are variations of unit-dose and floor stock systems. For example, the Pyxis MedStation (Care Fusion Products) (Fig. 41.6) has the capacity to carry a variety of medications, housed in individual compartments, that the nurse can access after requesting the medication from a computerized screen. The MedStation often houses medications that are used frequently, such as floor stock and narcotics, as well as individual patient medication bins. All medications that nurses retrieve from the MedStation must be recorded in the system's computer. (See Chapter 17 for more detailed discussion of medication administration.)

CHANGE-OF-SHIFT REPORT

The purpose of the change-of-shift report is to provide the staff on the next shift with pertinent information about the patient (AHRQ, n.d.). The quality of nursing care that the patient receives is contingent on how well the staff on each shift communicate with the staff on other shifts. The LPN/LVN's work environment may require participation in the reporting activities.

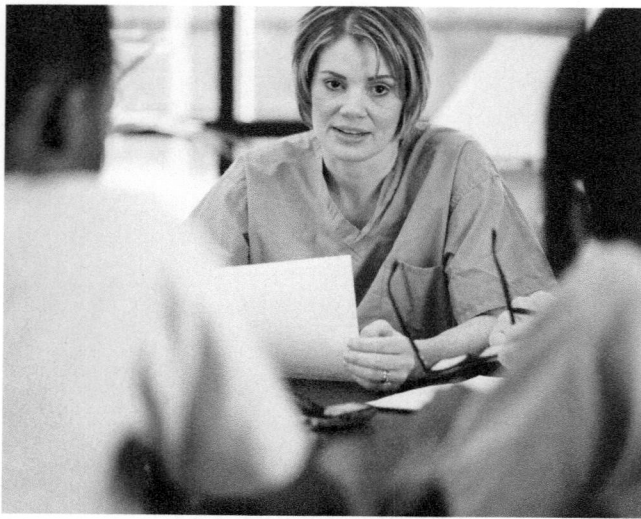

Fig. 41.7 Giving a change-of-shift report. (Copyright 1999–2012 Thinkstock. All rights reserved.)

The change-of-shift report may be given in person or documented on a recording device, or the report may be given by making rounds from patient to patient (Fig. 41.7). Oral reports are given in a conference room with nurses from both shifts participating. When a recording device is used, the report is recorded before the end of the shift. This allows the nurses who are preparing to leave to finish last-minute tasks while the oncoming staff listens to the report. Allow time for clarification or updates before nurses leave the unit. Giving reports in person or on rounds allows immediate feedback. Research supports bedside reports. It engages the patient in the exchange of information.

Before beginning the report, consider what information regarding the patient is important to communicate, and avoid reporting unnecessary information.

Typically, information that is considered important includes vital sign measurements (if abnormal), type of IV fluids (including rate of infusion, amount left to infuse, and IV site), intake, and output of feces, urine, and gastric secretions. The following should be reported using accepted medical and nursing terminology (Boxes 41.11 and 41.12):

- Output from all drainage tubes and appearance of drainage
- Any prn medications, including the time of administration and the effect, as well as the presence and amount of patient-controlled analgesia used
- Assessment data that are pertinent to the patient
- Dressing changes, amount and color of exudate, and the condition of any incisions or wounds
- Any abnormal signs and symptoms, such as dyspnea, tachycardia, or abnormal mental status or level of consciousness
- Neurologic deficits

Box 41.11 **Information for Change-of-Shift Report**

1. State patient's room and bed number, name, age, health care provider, all diagnoses, and date of surgery if patient is in a postoperative period.
2. Summarize patient's day (or evening or night).
3. Report all pertinent nursing care.
4. Describe change in patient's condition. Usually, most facilities report only abnormal vital sign measurements except for first postoperative day, when the last set of vital signs is measured.
5. Report special medications, intravenous (IV) solutions, infusion rate, amount of fluid remaining, and IV site. State time, method, and dosage of analgesics given and the effect.
6. Report all intake and output.
7. Report status of lungs and bowel sounds.
8. Report patient's mental status and level of consciousness.
9. Report circulatory checks, pedal pulses, and skin abnormalities in turgor or color.
10. State diagnostic procedures, such as computed tomography scans, x-ray studies, magnetic resonance imaging, endoscopy, proctoscopy, thoracentesis, and surgery. Report diet changes, special permits, preoperative procedures, daily weights, activity status, blood glucose measurements, blood in stools, clean-catch urine for analysis or culture and sensitivity (C&S), sputum specimen for C&S, respiratory therapy, and physical therapy orders. Report all nursing interventions, such as dressings, ostomy care, and oxygen.
11. Discuss patient and family education.
12. Note other services, such as social services, pastoral care, and discharge planning.
13. State any pertinent information helpful in patient care.
14. Report "no code" or do-not-resuscitate (DNR) status.
15. Present the report in an unbiased, nonjudgmental manner.

MALPRACTICE INSURANCE

Malpractice insurance for nurses is becoming increasingly important in a society that has become litigious. Paying for the defense of a lawsuit and any possible judgment is beyond the financial means of most people. To protect their employees and themselves against any legal and financial consequences that have potential to arise from provision of services, institutional employers carry malpractice liability insurance. Because individuals are responsible for their own actions, it is still possible for an employee to be sued personally. This is true even in states in which charitable immunity—the protection of nonprofit hospitals from legal liability—applies.

Some nurses choose to obtain a personal professional liability (malpractice) insurance policy separate from the employer's policy. The decision about whether to carry malpractice insurance is a personal choice. When making this decision, consider your state's malpractice

Box **41.12**	Sample of a Change-of-Shift Report

Room 348A Mabel L., age 87, patient of Dr. B., in with heart failure and stasis ulcer of the right leg. She is alert and cheerful, has had a comfortable day. Edema in her ankles bilaterally has decreased from +2 to +1 after she received an additional 40 mg of Lasix orally at 1000 [10 a.m.]; weight is 165 lb [75 kg], down 10 lb [4.5 kg] since admission 2 days ago. Vital signs unremarkable except BP 168/100 mm Hg. Has an IV infusion of D_5W with 20 mEq of KCl infusing at 60 mL/h with 600 mL remaining. IV site in right forearm is without edema or erythema. Patient has been up about 1 h today. Appetite has been good; ate 75% of breakfast and lunch. Received Vicodin [hydrocodone] tablets two at 1400 [2 p.m.] for pain in right leg. Intake 480 mL IV, 350 mL oral; voided 650 mL of clear, amber urine. Lung sounds clear except for fine crackles in base of right lung. She is expectorating a small amount of clear mucus. No dyspnea noted. Bowel sounds present; abdomen soft. Had moderate amount soft brown stool. Pedal pulses 2+ in strength bilaterally. Has a 2- to 3-cm stasis ulcer of right leg, treated with whirlpool and Hydrogel dressing. The dressing is to be changed every 24 h; antiembolic hose are on. There is an order for Hematest of stools ×3, midstream urine for C&S, and a chest x-ray. She is to be NPO after midnight for surgery at 0900 [9 a.m.] for debridement of the ulcer of her right leg. A preoperative consent form is needed. Social services will be seeing the patient and her daughter Ann Z. for discharge planning a few days after surgery.

BP, Blood pressure; *C&S,* culture and sensitivity (testing); *D_5W,* dextrose 5% in water solution; *IV,* intravenous; *KCl,* potassium chloride; *NPO,* nothing-by-mouth status.

compensation law, as well as the amount and type of malpractice insurance that your facility carries. Enlist the help of a knowledgeable expert to determine what, if any, additional amounts (dollar value) and type (occurrence or claims-based) of personal coverage is necessary or desired. (See Chapter 2 for further discussion of liability and professional liability insurance.)

BURNOUT

The term *burnout* has been used frequently over the years in health care. Maslach and Jackson (1986) identified burnout as a state of emotional exhaustion, depersonalization (responding in an impersonal manner toward patients/clients), and reduced sense of personal accomplishment in one's work, seen among human service, education, business, and government professions. The symptoms of burnout may include physical, psychological, and behavioral changes. The responsibilities of providing safe patient care are daunting. When combined with increasing acuity levels in facilities, less available support staff, and the nursing shortage, the risk of burnout is heightened. Burnout may lead to more job turnover and patients' dissatisfaction with care being received from nurses. There is also an impact on patient safety. Eleven percent of nurses reported having made an error due to

Box **41.13**	Symptoms of Burnout

PHYSICAL
- Fatigue
- Changes in sleeping, eating
- Lack of energy
- Loss of interest in sex

PSYCHOLOGICAL
- Irritability
- Hypersensitivity
- Frustration
- Negative outlook
- Forgetting

SPIRITUAL
- Loss of commitment
- Loss of meaning
- Loss of integrity

fatigue. In one study, more than 60% of nurses reported job related burnout (NSI Nursing Solutions, 2021). . The significance of burnout on the health care workplace can be underscored by the reports that the greatest challenge for health care administrative teams is the need to uplift the morale of the care team. This was prioritized above the recruitment and compensation of workers.

Signs and Symptoms of Burnout

Be aware of your feelings and emotional state to be alert to signs of burnout.

Box 41.13 identifies physical, psychological, and spiritual symptoms of burnout. Burnout is characterized by constant exhaustion, depression, irritability, insomnia, negative feelings toward one's job, difficulty focusing, becoming emotionally detached, and believing that one's actions do not make a difference to other people.

For the nurse experiencing burnout, it becomes increasingly difficult to delegate responsibility because of the fear that others may not perform a task as well. There seems to be less and less time available, and the nurse finds little time for replenishing the self. Time for other people (e.g., family or friends) is limited, and every demand on the nurse's time seems like an intrusion. The nurse is always tired and preoccupied with work and rarely experiences emotional pleasure.

Self-needs become buried by rationalizations, such as "As soon as I get the unit staffed…" or "As soon as I get my degree…" Despite working harder and enjoying it less, the nurse feels alone and isolated, misunderstood, and unappreciated. Repressed self-needs find maladaptive expression in overeating, overspending, addictions, snapping at family, or avoiding friends. Insomnia during the week, preoccupation with tasks, and utter exhaustion on the weekend or days off suggest a serious imbalance in lifestyle.

Strategies for Burnout Prevention

Awareness. The first step in burnout prevention is awareness. Deliberately reflecting on the stress in one's life immediately puts it in perspective. If in doubt, ask colleagues as well as family and friends if they perceive any signs or symptoms of burnout. Solutions become possible once the problem is identified.

Balance. Another important step in dealing with or preventing burnout is restoring balance to one's life. A *healthy balance* among work, family, leisure, and lifelong learning enhances personal judgments, satisfaction, and productivity. Actively scheduling time for each of these activities is the best way to ensure that time will be made for them.

Choice. People experiencing burnout usually do not think they have any choice other than to keep doing what they have been doing, but life is a series of choices and negotiations. Nurses are especially fortunate in that there are a number of career paths in nursing. Transfers within facilities are usually available for the nurse who experiences burnout while working on a particular unit or department in a facility. Another option is employment in a totally different field of nursing by leaving the current place of employment for another. Choosing not to delegate tasks is another cause of burnout, so it is important for the nurse to learn to delegate appropriately.

Compartmentalizing. Being able to compartmentalize responsibilities helps the nurse complete as much of a job at hand as possible. Focusing on a job or project to the best of one's ability and then, at the end of the day or the time designated to the project, dropping it completely helps prevent burnout. Saying to oneself that something is "sufficient for the day" is a stress management strategy that puts boundaries on life tasks.

Altruistic egoism. Potential burnout victims generally put everyone and everything ahead of themselves. They ignore their own needs or minimize their importance. *Altruistic egoism* simply means paying as much attention to your own personal needs as you do to the needs of others. Although this seems obvious, many nurses consider paying attention to their own needs as being selfish. Nothing is further from the truth. In the long run, a balance between self-needs and the needs of others enhances the quality of care that the nurse is able to give to patients.

Focus. People who are focused are often able to achieve their goals more easily than other people. Focusing full energy on one thing at a time and finishing one project before starting another has several benefits: It is more likely that a person will enjoy each activity more and being able to give full attention will make for a better product. A powerful contributor to the development of burnout is having several unfinished projects all demanding similar amounts of one's attention.

Goals. This step is closely aligned with focus, with an emphasis on outcome. An excellent burnout prevention strategy is identifying goals that are realistic, achievable, and in line with one's personal values. Being able to identify goals and the path to achieve goals enhances the chance for success.

Hope. People who feel burned out experience helplessness and hopelessness about changing their situation. The despair that accompanies emptiness and futility can be reversed by simply seeking out connections with other people who are empathetic. Their advice and caring support, even in one encounter, is a considerable antidote to inner emptiness. However, be sure to seek support from people who will help in developing solutions and not merely sympathize with how horrible the situation is. A solution-focused—rather than problem-oriented—approach is essential in the development of hope.

Integrity. Restoring personal integrity is important in the process of combating burnout. It is easy for the nurse experiencing burnout to lose sight of personal values. The nurse forgets what is important to him or her and instead tries to conform to others' expectations. Recognizing and reversing this process can go a long way in reversing burnout.

CHEMICALLY IMPAIRED NURSES

Chemical impairment is a concern for the nursing profession. At any given time, an estimated 10% to 15% of nurses are impaired or in a recovery program. The number of nurses who illegally use drugs and abuse alcohol will continue to increase as addiction to drugs and alcohol increases in the general population. Some of the excuses that nurses give for resorting to using drugs, alcohol, or both include job-related stress, inability to cope with changes in the workplace, overwhelming personal responsibilities, a feeling of frustration and helplessness in their personal and professional lives, and easy access to drugs. Addiction may begin as a workplace injury, requiring medications to manage, which eventually spiral out of control. The work environment of nurses allows a unique level of access to addictive medications. Emergency room nurses have a higher level of addiction.

Addiction is a chronic disease much like diabetes or hypertension. It requires the same care and ongoing attention and management. Nurses should receive the same care and support as other people with an addiction. With proper treatment, nurses can remain employed in their field and be able to provide quality care to their patients.

Each state's board of nursing has implemented nurse assistance programs to meet the needs of chemically impaired nurses. The makeup and monitoring of each state's program varies by statute. Many programs are abstinence based. This means that upon entry to the program, full compliance requires that all addicting substances be discontinued. This can be a challenge because a nurse may have a chronic condition that is managed by a prescription medication that is not allowed for a nurse in monitoring. In this case, efforts are made using a team approach between the nurse's physician and the nurse assistance program. Monitoring of the nurse in recovery includes counseling; random, unannounced urine drug screenings; worksite monitor reports; and participation in group activities such as Alcoholics Anonymous. There is often a change to the status of the nurse's license to practice nursing. If the addiction is deemed to be out of control and the nurse a danger to him- or herself, the license may be suspended. Probation commonly is imposed to allow the nurse the opportunity to work while providing oversight safeguards.

It is the nurse's responsibility to himself or herself and to the patients being cared for to avoid the abuse of prescription or nonprescription medications. If a nurse or a coworker does become addicted to drugs or alcohol, the only option is to seek immediate assistance. Referring oneself or someone else to the state board of nursing for voluntary treatment and a rehabilitation program may not only save a career but also save a life. See Chapter 36 for further discussion of chemical dependency.

Get Ready for the NCLEX® Examination!

Key Points

- Today's health care system is complex with a highly competitive job market.
- A well-prepared résumé broadens interview opportunities.
- An interview is important; every effort should be made to guarantee a successful one.
- Learning does not cease after graduation; it is a continuous process. The LPN/LVN must stay current with new concepts and technologies.
- Various job opportunities are available to new graduates. Each option requires considerable thought.
- A mentor is a nurse with more experience and knowledge who is able and willing to assist a novice nurse to learn the skills of the profession.
- Nursing care continues 24 hours a day in facilities to ensure continuity of care for all patients.
- LPN/LVNs are legally liable for their actions; therefore, they need to understand the legal framework within which they are practicing.
- Endorsement or reciprocity enables the nurse to practice in another state without retaking the NCLEX-PN.
- The National Council of State Boards of Nursing has adopted computerized adaptive testing for the NCLEX-PN.
- The Nurse Practice Act is the licensing law.
- It is a good idea for the LPN/LVN to take advantage of the knowledge available from certification seminars or self-guided study courses.
- The main function of a state board of nursing is to ensure safety for consumers of nursing services.
- Licensure permits people to offer special skills to the public, but it also provides legal guidelines for protection of the public.
- Leadership skills are an important aspect of nursing today.
- Although no single leadership style is always best, the overall approach of a leader has to foster the professional growth of other people and facilitate their professional development so that they become less dependent on the leader.
- The more that nurse managers adapt their leadership styles to work situations and the needs and abilities of staff, the more effective they are as managers.
- Effective problem-solving skills are key for providing quality nursing care.
- Nursing informatics continues to influence the delivery of nursing care.
- Correct procedure and facility policy should be followed in transcribing health care providers' orders.
- The health care provider oversees directing the patient's care, and nurses carry out the health care provider's orders, unless they believe that the orders are in error or will be harmful to the patient.
- The purpose of the change-of-shift report is to communicate pertinent patient information accurately from staff of one shift to staff of another.
- Burnout occurs more often in people who have excessive expectations of themselves and who believe that they need to do everything correctly. Nurses are especially prone to this characteristic.
- Malpractice insurance is available to nurses.

Additional Learning Resources

SG Go to your Study Guide for additional learning activities to help you master this chapter content.

Be sure to visit the Evolve site at http://evolve.elsevier.com/Cooper/foundations/ for additional online resources.

Review Questions for the NCLEX® Examination

1. **Which are functions of the state board of nursing?** *(Select all that apply.)*
    1. Assisting health care facilities in the training of nursing staff
    2. Imposing discipline on a nursing license
    3. Monitoring the schools of nursing within the state
    4. Approving the students admitted to nursing programs in the state
    5. Enforcement of the state's Nurse Practice Act

2. **Which organizations are totally committed to practical and vocational nursing and its continuing education?** *(Select all that apply.)*
    1. APNES

2. ANA
3. NFLPN
4. NCSBN

3. The LPN/LVN has been hired at a long-term care facility. The nurse questions if the role will include supervision of other staff members. What response is most correct? *(Select all that apply.)*

1. "You will be expected to organize and delegate as needed the care of patients on the unit of care."
2. "You will be expected to supervise any nurse on your assigned wing who has less seniority."
3. "The limit of charge or supervisory roles expected of the LPN/LVN is low."
4. "In the long-term care setting you may find you are in a leadership role."
5. "It is expected that you would supervise those staff members having less scope of practice than the LPN/LVN."

4. What is the main purpose of state requirements that nurses be licensed to practice nursing?

1. To protect the LPN/LVN employer and the nurse
2. To provide legal guidelines to protect the public
3. To protect the patient and employer
4. To protect the LPN/LVN from malpractice lawsuits

5. The style of leadership that takes into account the style of the leader, the maturity of the groups, and the circumstances at hand is which type of leadership style?

1. Autocratic
2. Situational
3. Democratic
4. Laissez-faire

6. When transcribing orders, the LPN/LVN knows that which health care provider order takes priority?

1. prn orders
2. One-time-only orders
3. Routine orders
4. Stat orders

7. Which act of the state legislature delineates the legal scope of the practice of nursing within the geographic boundaries of the jurisdiction?

1. NLN Act
2. Nurse Practice Act
3. NCLEX Act
4. JCOAH Act

8. In the change-of-shift report, which information should the outgoing nurse pass on to the receiving nurse? *(Select all that apply.)*

1. The number of visitors that the patient has had during the shift
2. The amount of time the patient has been able to nap during the shift
3. The list of patient problem statements found in the care plan
4. The patient's blood glucose levels for the shift
5. The patient's total intake and output for the shift

9. Which statement best reflects the autocratic style of leadership?

1. "Everyone knows their work assignment, so let's not meet together unless we have an unexpected crisis."
2. "Let's discuss this case study thoroughly and decide on a plan of action as a group."
3. "I'll consider each of your requests and then give you the guidelines for establishing new acuity ratings for our patients."
4. "I'll try to pair you in comparable work teams, and we'll evaluate the success of this approach in 2 weeks."

10. Which actions demonstrate effective time management skills for the nurse? *(Select all that apply.)*

1. Meeting all of the patient's major needs in the early morning hours
2. Anticipating possible interruptions in the plan of care for the day
3. Doing each of the patient's assessments and treatments individually at separate times
4. Leaving each day unplanned to allow for adaptations in treatments
5. Planning care based on prioritizing the needs of the patient

11. To settle a conflict between two staff members, the nurse manager should focus on which strategy?

1. Developing a compromise solution to solve the conflict
2. Investigating what the conflict parties want to achieve as an outcome
3. Identifying the real issues and assisting in solving them
4. Limiting the number of possible solutions to the conflict

12. Why is it beneficial to become certified in other areas after becoming an LPN/LVN?

1. The certifications are designed to increase nursing knowledge and skill.
2. The nurse will gradually be able to assume the work of an RN without becoming an RN.
3. Use of the extended title(s) will improve the nurse's status among other employees and peers.
4. Unless the state board of nursing acknowledges the certification, it serves no purpose.

13. Which is a primary function of the LPN/LVN?

1. Teaching professional and practical nursing students
2. Providing direct patient care
3. Being in charge in various health care settings
4. Directing nurses and other personnel who are employed in the hospital setting

14. The student nurse demonstrates understanding of the NCLEX-PN with which statement?

1. "The NCLEX-PN measures the LPN/LVN student's ability to compete in the job market."
2. "The NCLEX-PN measures the LPN/LVN student's entry-level competencies."
3. "The NCLEX-PN measures the LPN/LVN student's proficiency-level competencies."
4. "The NCLEX-PN measures success of the nursing program."

15. **What will a new graduate include on a résumé?** *(Select all that apply.)*

    1. Person to notify in an emergency
    2. Review of professional experience
    3. Grade transcripts from nursing schools
    4. Education history
    5. Only current work
    6. References from at least 5 former employers
    7. Personal history, including number of children
    8. Desired benefits package
    9. Name of spouse if married
    10. Nursing license number

16. **What is a quality of an effective mentor?**

    1. Inconsistent
    2. Unaccountable
    3. Inaccessible
    4. Informative

17. **What will the nurse wish to consider when obtaining malpractice insurance?**

    1. Malpractice insurance is becoming less important for the nurse in today's health care environment.
    2. If the employer has a claims-based policy in force, a personal policy is not necessary.
    3. Most employers carry insurance for the employee, which will more than cover any expenses that will be incurred.
    4. A separate personal malpractice insurance policy in addition to the employer's policy is a personal choice.

18. **The nurse coworker of an LPN/LVN confides in the LPN/LVN that he is abusing alcohol. What is the best initial action for the LPN/LVN to take?**

    1. Talk to the coworker about the state's nurses assistance program for chemically impaired nurses.
    2. Immediately report this information to the nurse manager.
    3. Encourage the coworker to take a leave of absence from his current position.
    4. Report the coworker to the state board of nursing.

Abbreviations

Common Abbreviations

ABBREVIATION	MEANING	ABBREVIATION	MEANING
°C	degrees Centigrade	CT	computed tomography
°F	degrees Fahrenheit	dL	deciliter
@	at	DNR	do not resuscitate
≥	greater than	DTR	deep tendon reflex
≤	less than	Dx, dx	diagnosis
↑	increase	ECG, EKG	electrocardiogram
↓	decrease	EEG	electroencephalogram
1°	primary	elix	elixir
2°	secondary	ER/ED	emergency room/department
Δ	change	ESR	erythrocyte sedimentation rate
ABGs	arterial blood gases	ETOH	ethyl alcohol
ac	before meals	FUO	fever of unknown origin
ad lib	freely as desired	Fx, fx	fracture
ADL	activities of daily living	g/G	gram
AED	automated external defibrillator	GI	gastrointestinal
AIDS	acquired immunodeficiency syndrome	gr	grain
ama, AMA	against medical advice	gtt	drop; drops
BE	barium enema	GTT	glucose tolerance test
bid, BID	two times a day	h, hr	hour
BM	bowel movement	H&P	history and physical examination
BMI	body mass index	HCT, Hct	hematocrit
B/P, BP	blood pressure	Hgb	hemoglobin
BRP	bathroom privileges	HIV	human immunodeficiency virus
BSA	body surface area	hs	at bedtime, hour of sleep
BUN	blood urea nitrogen	I&O	intake and output
C&S	culture and sensitivity	IM	intramuscular
c̄	with	IV	intravenous
cap	capsule	IVP	intravenous pyelogram
CBC	complete blood count	K+	potassium
		kg	kilogram
CDC	Centers for Disease Control and Prevention	KUB	kidney, ureters, and bladder (radiograph)
		KVO	keep vein open
cm	centimeter	L	liter
c/o	complains of	LLL	left lower lobe
CO	carbon monoxide	LLQ	left lower quadrant
CO_2	carbon dioxide	LMP	last menstrual period
CPR	cardiopulmonary resuscitation	LOC	level of consciousness

Common Abbreviations—cont'd

ABBREVIATION	MEANING	ABBREVIATION	MEANING
LUL	left upper lobe	prn	as often as necessary, when needed
LUQ	left upper quadrant	q	every
M	meter	qid, QID	four times a day
mcg	microgram	RLL	right lower lobe
mg	milligram	RLQ	right lower quadrant
mL	milliliter	ROM	range of motion
mm	millimeter	RUL	right upper lobe
mm Hg	millimeters of mercury	RUQ	right upper quadrant
MRI	magnetic resonance imaging	Rx	medication, prescription
NG	nasogastric	$\bar{s}$	without
NKA	no known allergies	Sub-Q, subcut	subcutaneous
NPO	nothing per os, nothing by mouth	$\dot{s}\dot{s}$	half
O_2	oxygen	SSE	soapsuds enema
OD	optical density; overdose	stat	immediately
oz	ounce	tid, TID	three times a day
pc	after meals	TKO	to keep open
PERRLA	pupils equal, round, and reactive to light and accommodation	TPN	total parenteral nutrition
		TPR	temperature, pulse, and respirations
pH	hydrogen ion concentration (acidity and alkalinity)	TX, tx, Tx	treatment
PO, po	orally, per os, by mouth	WBC	white blood cell

The Joint Commission "Do Not Use" Abbreviation List[a]

DO NOT USE	POTENTIAL PROBLEM	USE INSTEAD
U, u (unit)	Mistaken for "0" (zero), the number "4" (four), or "cc"	Write "unit"
IU (International Unit)	Mistaken for IV (intravenous) or the number 10 (ten)	Write "International Unit"
Q.D., QD, q.d., qd (daily)	Mistaken for each other	Write "daily"
Q.O.D., QOD, q.o.d., qod (every other day)	Period after the Q mistaken for "I" and the "O" mistaken for "I"	Write "every other day"
Trailing zero (X.0 mg)[b]	Decimal point is missed	Write X mg
Lack of leading zero (.X mg)	Decimal point is missed	Write 0.X mg
MS	Can mean morphine sulfate or magnesium sulfate	Write "morphine sulfate"
MSO_4 and $MgSO_4$	Confused for one another	Write "magnesium sulfate"

[a]Applies to all orders and all medication-related documentation that is handwritten (including free-text computer entry) or on preprinted forms.
[b]EXCEPTION: A "trailing zero" may be used only where required to demonstrate the level of precision of the value being reported, such as for laboratory results, imaging studies that report size of lesions, or catheter/tube sizes. It may not be used in medication orders or other medication-related documentation.
© The Joint Commission, Facts about the official "Do Not Use" list of abbreviations, 2019. Reprinted with permission.

Laboratory Reference Values

http://evolve.elsevier.com/Cooper/foundations/

Reference Intervals for Hematology

TEST	CONVENTIONAL UNITS	SI UNITS
Acid hemolysis (Ham test)	No hemolysis	No hemolysis
Alkaline phosphatase, leukocyte	Total score, 14–100	Total score, 14–100
Cell counts		
Erythrocytes		
Males	4.6–6.2 million/mm^3	4.6–6.2 × 10^{12}/L
Females	4.2–5.4 million/mm^3	4.2–5.4 × 10^{12}/L
Children (varies with age)	4.5–5.1 million/mm^3	4.5–5.1 × 10^{12}/L
Leukocytes, total	5000–10,000/mm^3	4.5–11.0 × 10^9/L
Leukocytes, differential counts[a]		
Myelocytes	0%	0/L
Band neutrophils	3%–5%	150–400 × 10^6/L
Segmented neutrophils	54%–62%	3000–5800 × 10^6/L
Lymphocytes	20%–40%	1000–4000 × 10^6/L
Monocytes	3%–6%	100–600 × 10^6/L
Eosinophils	1%–4%	50–250 × 10^6/L
Basophils	0.5%–1%	15–50 × 10^6/L
Platelets	150,000–400,000/mm^3	150–400 × 10^9/L
Reticulocytes	25,000–75,000/mm^3	25–75 × 10^9/L
Coagulation tests	(0.5%–1.5% of erythrocytes)	
Bleeding time (template)	2.75–8.0 min	2.75–8.0 min
Coagulation time (glass tube)	5–15 min	5–15 min
D-Dimer	<0.5 mcg/mL	<0.5 mg/L
Factor VIII and other coagulation factors	50%–150% of normal	0.5–1.5 of normal
Fibrin split products (Thrombo-Welco test)	<10 mcg/mL	<10 mg/L
Fibrinogen	200–400 mg/dL	2.0–4.0 g/L
Partial thromboplastin time, activated (aPTT)	20–25 s	20–35 s
Prothrombin time (PT, Pro-time)	12.0–14.0 s	12.0–14.0 s
International normalized ratio (INR)	0.8–1.1	
Coombs' test		
Direct	Negative	Negative
Indirect	Negative	Negative
Corpuscular values of erythrocytes		
Mean corpuscular hemoglobin (MCH)	26–34 pg/cell	26–34 pg/cell
Mean corpuscular volume (MCV)	80–96 mm^3	80–96 fL
Mean corpuscular hemoglobin concentration (MCHC)	32–36 g/dL	320–360 g/L

Reference Intervals for Hematology—cont'd

TEST	CONVENTIONAL UNITS	SI UNITS
Haptoglobin	20–165 mg/dL	0.20–1.65 g/L
Hematocrit		
Males	40–54 mL/dL	0.40–0.54
Females	35–47 mL/dL	0.37–0.47
Newborns	49–54 mL/dL	0.49–0.54
Children (varies with age)	35–49 mL/dL	0.35–0.49
Hemoglobin		
Males	13.0–18.0 g/dL	8.1–11.2 mmol/L
Females	12.0–16.0 g/dL	7.4–9.9 mmol/L
Newborns	16.5–19.5 g/dL	10.2–12.1 mmol/L
Children (varies with age)	11.2–16.5 g/dL	7.0–10.2 mmol/L
Hemoglobin, fetal	<1.0% of total	<0.01 of total
Hemoglobin A_{1C}	3%–5% of total	0.03–0.05 of total
Hemoglobin A_2	1.5%–3.0% of total	0.015–0.03 of total
Hemoglobin, plasma	0.0–5.0 mg/dL	0.0–3.2 μmol/L
Methemoglobin	30–130 mg/dL	19–80 μmol/L
Erythrocyte sedimentation rate (ESR)		
Wintrobe		
Males	0–5 mm/h	0–5 mm/h
Females	0–15 mm/h	0–15 mm/h
Westergren		
Males	0–15 mm/h	0–15 mm/h
Females	0–20 mm/h	0–20 mm/h

aConventional units are percentages; SI units are absolute cell counts.
SI, International System of Units.

Reference Intervalsa for Clinical Chemistry (Blood, Serum, and Plasma)

ANALYTE	CONVENTIONAL UNITS	SI UNITS
Acetoacetate plus acetone		
Qualitative	Negative	Negative
Quantitative	0.3–2.0 mg/dL	30–200 μmol/L
Acid phosphatase, serum (thymolphthalein monophosphate substrate)	0.1–0.6 units/L	0.1–0.6 units/L
Adrenocorticotropic hormone (ACTH), plasma, 8 AM	10–80 pg/mL	2–18 pmol/L
Alanine aminotransferase (ALT), Serum glutamic pyruvic transaminase (SGPT)	1–45 units/L	1–45 units/L
Albumin, serum	3.3–5.2 g/dL	33–52 g/L
Aldolase, serum	0.0–7.0 units/L	0.0–7.0 units/L
Aldosterone, plasma		
Standing	5–30 ng/dL	140–830 pmol/L
Recumbent	3–10 ng/dL	80–275 pmol/L
Alkaline, phosphatase (ALP), serum		
Adult	35–150 units/L	35–150 units/L
Adolescent	100–500 units/L	100–500 units/L
Child	100–350 units/L	100–350 units/L
Ammonia nitrogen, plasma	10–50 mmol/L	10–50 μmol/L
Amylase, serum	25–125 units/L	25–125 units/L

Reference Intervals[a] for Clinical Chemistry (Blood, Serum, and Plasma)—cont'd

ANALYTE	CONVENTIONAL UNITS	SI UNITS
Anion gap, serum calculated	8–16 mEq/L	8–16 mmol/L
Ascorbic acid, blood	0.4–1.5 mg/dL	23–85 µmol/L
Aspartate aminotransferase (AST), Serum glutamic-oxaloacetic transaminase (SGOT)	1–36 units/L	1–36 units/L
Base excess, arterial blood, calculated	0 ± 2 mEq/L	0 ± 2 mmol/L
Bicarbonate		
Venous plasma	23–29 mEq/L	23–29 mmol/L
Arterial blood	21–27 mEq/L	21–27 mmol/L
Bile acids, serum	0.3–3.0 mg/dL	0.8–7.6 µmol/L
Bilirubin, serum		
Conjugated	0.1–0.4 mg/dL	1.7–6.8 µmol/L
Total	0.3–1.1 mg/dL	5.1–19.0 µmol/L
Calcium, serum	8.4–10.6 mg/dL	2.10–2.65 mmol/L
Calcium, ionized, serum	4.25–5.25 mg/dL	1.05–1.30 mmol/L
Carbon dioxide, total, serum or plasma	24–31 mEq/L	24–31 mmol/L
Carbon dioxide tension (PCO_2), blood	35–45 mm Hg	35–45 mm Hg
β-Carotene, serum	60–260 mcg/dL	1.1–8.6 µmol/L
Ceruloplasmin, serum	23–44 mg/dL	230–440 mg/L
Chloride, serum or plasma	96–106 mEq/L	96–106 mmol/L
Cholesterol, serum or EDTA plasma		
Desirable range	<200 mg/dL	5.20 mmol/L
Low-density lipoprotein (LDL) cholesterol	60–180 mg/dL	1.55–4.65 mmol/L
High-density lipoprotein (HDL) cholesterol	30–80 mg/dL	0.80–2.05 mmol/L
Copper	70–140 mcg/dL	11–22 µmol/L
Cortisol, plasma		
8:00 AM	6–23 mcg/dL	170–630 nmol/L
4:00 PM	3–15 mcg/dL	80–410 nmol/L
10:00 PM	<50% of 8:00 AM value	<50% of 8:00 AM value
Creatine, serum		
Males	0.2–0.5 mg/dL	15–40 µmol/L
Females	0.3–0.9 mg/dL	25–70 µmol/L
Creatine kinase (CK), serum		
Males	55–170 units/L	55–170 units/L
Females	30–135 units/L	30–135 units/L
Creatinine kinase MB isoenzyme, serum	<5% of total CK activity	<5% of total CK activity
	<5% of ng/mL by immunoassay	<5% of ng/mL by immunoassay
Creatinine, serum	0.6–1.2 mg/dL	50–110 µmol/L
Erythrocytes	145–540 ng/mL	330–120 nmol/L
Estradiol-17β, adult		
Males	10–65 pg/mL	35–240 pmol/L
Females		
Follicular	30–100 pg/mL	110–370 pmol/L
Ovulatory	200–400 pg/mL	730–1470 pmol/L
Luteal	50–140 pg/mL	180–510 pmol/L
Ferritin, serum	20–200 ng/mL	20–200 mcg/L
Fibrinogen, plasma	200–400 mg/dL	2.0–4.0 g/L

Reference Intervals[a] for Clinical Chemistry (Blood, Serum, and Plasma)—cont'd

ANALYTE	CONVENTIONAL UNITS	SI UNITS
Folate, serum	3–18 ng/mL	6.8–4.1 nmol/L
Follicle-stimulating hormone (FSH), plasma		
Males	4–25 mU/mL	4–25 units/L
Females, premenopausal	4–30 mU/mL	4–30 units/L
Females, postmenopausal	40–250 mU/mL	40–250 units/L
Gastrin, fasting, serum	0–100 pg/mL	0–100 mg/L
Glucose, fasting, plasma or serum	70–115 mg/dL	3.9–6.4 nmol/L
γ-Glutamyltransferase (GGT), serum	5–40 units/L	5–40 units/L
Growth hormone (hGH), plasma, adult, fasting	0–6 ng/mL	0–6 mcg/L
Haptoglobin, serum	20–165 mg/dL	0.20–1.65 g/L
Immunoglobulins, serum (see table of Reference Intervals for Tests of Immunologic Function)		
Iron, serum	75–175 mcg/dL	13–31 mmol/L
Iron-binding capacity, serum		
Total	250–410 mcg/dL	45–73 mmol/L
Saturation	20%–55%	0.20–0.55
Lactate		
Venous whole blood	5.0–20.0 mg/dL	0.6–2.2 mmol/L
Arterial whole blood	5.0–15.0 mg/dL	0.6–1.7 mmol/L
Lactate dehydrogenase (LD), serum	110–220 units/L	110–220 units/L
Lipase, serum	10–140 units/L	10–140 units/L
Lutropin (LH), serum		
Males	1–9 units/L	1–9 units/L
Females		
Follicular phase	2–10 units/L	2–10 units/L
Midcycle peak	15–65 units/L	15–65 units/L
Luteal phase	1–12 units/L	1–12 units/L
Postmenopausal	12–65 units/L	12–65 units/L
Magnesium, serum	1.3–2.1 mg/dL	0.65–1.05 mmol/L
Osmolality	275–295 mOsm/kg water	275–295 mOsm/kg water
Oxygen, blood, arterial, room air		
Partial pressure (PaO$_2$)	80–100 mm Hg	80–100 mm Hg
Saturation (SaO$_2$)	95%–100%	95%–100%
pH, arterial blood	7.35–7.45	7.35–7.45
Phosphate, inorganic, serum		
Adult	3.0–4.5 mg/dL	1.0–1.5 mmol/L
Child	4.0–7.0 mg/dL	1.3–2.3 mmol/L
Potassium		
Serum	3.5–5.0 mEq/L	3.5–5.0 mmol/L
Plasma	3.5–4.5 mEq/L	3.5–4.5 mmol/L
Progesterone, serum, adult		
Males	0.0–0.4 ng/mL	0.0–1.3 mmol/L
Females		
Follicular phase	0.1–1.5 ng/mL	0.3–4.8 mmol/L
Luteal phase	2.5–28.0 ng/mL	8.0–89.0 mmol/L
Prolactin, serum		
Males	1.0–15.0 ng/mL	1.0–15.0 mcg/L

Continued

Reference Intervals[a] for Clinical Chemistry (Blood, Serum, and Plasma)—cont'd

ANALYTE	CONVENTIONAL UNITS	SI UNITS
Females	1.0–20.0 ng/mL	1.0–20.0 mcg/L
Protein, serum, electrophoresis		
Total	6.0–8.0 g/dL	60–80 g/L
Albumin	3.5–5.5 g/dL	35–55 g/L
Globulins		
α_1	0.2–0.4 g/dL	2.0–4.0 g/L
α_2	0.5–0.9 g/dL	5.0–9.0 g/L
β	0.6–1.1 g/dL	6.0–11.0 g/L
γ	0.7–1.7 g/dL	7.0–17.0 g/L
Pyruvate, blood	0.3–0.9 mg/dL	0.03–0.10 mmol/L
Rheumatoid factor	0.0–30.0 IU/mL	0.0–30.0 kIU/L
Sodium, serum or plasma	135–145 mEq/L	135–145 mmol/L
Testosterone, plasma		
Males, adult	300–1200 ng/dL	10.4–41.6 nmol/L
Females, adult	20–75 ng/dL	0.7–2.6 nmol/L
Pregnant females	40–200 ng/dL	1.4–6.9 nmol/L
Thyroglobulin	3–42 ng/mL	3–42 mcg/L
Thyrotropin (hTSH), serum	0.4–4.8 mIU/mL	0.4–4.8 mIU/L
Thyrotropin-releasing hormone (TRH)	5–60 pg/mL	5–60 ng/L
Thyroxine (FT_4), free, serum	0.9–2.1 ng/dL	12–27 pmol/L
Thyroxine (T_4), serum	4.5–12.0 mcg/mL	58–154 nmol/L
Thyroxine-binding globulin (TBG)	15.0–34.0 mcg/mL	15.0–34.0 mg/L
Transferrin	250–430 mg/dL	2.5–4.3 g/L
Triglycerides, serum, after 12-h fast	40–150 mg/dL	0.4–1.5 g/L
Triiodothyronine (T_3), serum	70–190 ng/dL	1.1–2.9 nmol/L
Triiodothyronine uptake, resin (T_3RU)	25%–38%	0.25–0.38
Troponin I	0.05–0.50 ng/mL	0.05–0.5 ng/mL
Urate		
Males	2.5–8.0 mg/dL	150–480 µmol/L
Females	2.2–7.0 mg/dL	130–420 µmol/L
Urea, serum or plasma	24–49 mg/dL	4.0–8.2 nmol/L
Urea, nitrogen, serum or plasma	11–23 mg/dL	8.0–16.4 nmol/L
Viscosity, serum	1.1–1.8 × water	1.1–1.8 × water
Vitamin A, serum	20–80 mcg/dL	0.70–2.80 mcmol/L
Vitamin B$_{12}$, serum	180–900 pg/mL	133–664 pmol/L

[a]Reference values may vary depending on the method and sample source used.
EDTA, Ethylenediaminetetraacetic acid; *SI,* International System of Units.

Reference Intervals for Therapeutic Drug Monitoring (Serum or Plasma)[a]

ANALYTE	THERAPEUTIC RANGE	TOXIC CONCENTRATIONS	PROPRIETARY NAME(S)
Analgesics			
acetaminophen	10–40 mcg/mL	>150 mcg/mL	Tylenol, Datril
salicylate	100–250 mcg/mL	>300 mcg/mL	Aspirin, Bufferin
Antibiotics			
amikacin	20–30 mcg/mL	*Peak* >35 mcg/mL *Trough* >10 mcg/mL	Amkin
gentamicin	5–10 mcg/mL	*Peak* >10 mcg/mL *Trough* >2 mcg/mL	Garamycin
tobramycin	5–10 mcg/mL	*Peak* >10 mcg/mL *Trough* >2 mcg/mL	Nebcin
vancomycin	5–35 mcg/mL	*Peak* >40 mcg/mL *Trough* >10 mcg/mL	Vancocin
Anticonvulsants			
carbamazepine	5–12 mcg/mL	>15 mcg/mL	Tegretol
ethosuximide	40–100 mcg/mL	>250 mcg/mL	Zarontin
phenobarbital	15–40 mcg/mL	40–100 ng/mL (varies widely)	Luminal
phenytoin	10–20 mcg/mL	>20 mcg/mL	Dilantin
primidone	5–12 mcg/mL	>15 mcg/mL	Mysoline
valproic acid	50–100 mcg/mL	>100 mcg/mL	Depakene
Antineoplastics and Immunosuppressives			
cyclosporine A	150–350 ng/mL	>400 ng/mL	Sandimmune
methotrexate, high-dose, 48 h	Variable	>1 μmol/L, 48 h after dose	
sirolimus (within 1 h of 2-mg dose)	4.5–14 ng/mL	Variable	Rapamune
sirolimus (within 1 h of 5-mg dose)	10–28 ng/mL	Variable	Rapamune
tacrolimus (FK-506), whole blood	3–20 mcg/L	>15 mcg/L	Prograf
Bronchodilators and Respiratory Stimulants			
caffeine	3–15 ng/mL	>30 mcg/mL	Elixophyllin
theophylline (aminophylline)	10–20 mcg/mL	>30 mcg/mL	Quibron
Cardiovascular Drugs			
amiodarone (obtain specimen more than 8 h after last dose)	1.0–2.0 mcg/mL	>2.0 mcg/mL	Cordarone
digoxin (obtain specimen more than 6 h after last dose)	0.8–2.0 mcg/mL	>2.4 ng/mL	Lanoxin
disopyramide	2–5 mcg/mL	>7 mcg/mL	Norpace
flecainide	0.2–1.0 mcg/mL	>0.1 mcg/mL	Tambocor
lidocaine	1.5–5.0 mcg/mL	>6 mcg/mL	Xylocaine
mexiletine	0.7–2.0 mcg/mL	>2 mcg/mL	Mexitil
procainamide	4–10 mcg/mL	>12 mcg/mL	Pronestyl
procainamide plus NAPA (*N*-acetyl procainamide)	8–30 mcg/mL	>30 mcg/mL	
propranolol	50–100 ng/mL	Variable	Inderal
quinidine	2–5 mcg/mL	>6 mcg/mL	Cardioquin, Quinaglute
tocainide	4–10 ng/mL	>10 ng/mL	Tonocard

Continued

Reference Intervals for Therapeutic Drug Monitoring (Serum or Plasma)[a]—cont'd

ANALYTE	THERAPEUTIC RANGE	TOXIC CONCENTRATIONS	PROPRIETARY NAME(S)
Psychopharmacological Drugs			
amitriptyline	120–150 ng/mL	>500 ng/mL	Elavil, Triavil
bupropion	25–100 ng/mL	Not applicable	Wellbutrin
desipramine	150–300 ng/mL	>500 ng/mL	Norpramin
imipramine	125–250 ng/mL	>400 ng/mL	Tofranil
lithium (obtain specimen 12 h after last dose)	0.6–1.5 mEq/L	>1.5 mEq/L	Lithobid
nortriptyline	50–150 ng/mL	>500 ng/mL	Aventyl, Pamelor

[a]Values may vary depending on the method and sample collection device used. Always consult the reference values provided by the laboratory performing the analysis.

Reference Intervals[a] for Clinical Chemistry (Urine)

ANALYTE	CONVENTIONAL UNITS	SI UNITS
Acetone and acetoacetate, qualitative	Negative	Negative
Albumin		
Qualitative	Negative	Negative
Quantitative	10–100 mg/24 h	0.15–1.5 µmol/day
Aldosterone	3–20 mcg/24 h	8.3–55 nmol/day
D-Aminolevulinic acid (d-ALA)	1.3–7.0 mg/24 h	10–53 µmol/day
Amylase	<17 units/h	<17 units/h
Amylase-to-creatinine clearance ratio	0.01–0.04	0.01–0.04
Bilirubin, qualitative	Negative	Negative
Calcium (regular diet)	<250 mg/24 h	<6.3 nmol/day
Catecholamines		
Epinephrine	<10 mcg/24 h	<55 nmol/day
Norepinephrine	<100 mcg/24 h	<590 nmol/day
Total free catecholamines	4–126 mcg/24 h	24–745 nmol/day
Total metanephrines	0.1–1.6 mg/24 h	0.5–8.1 µmol/day
Chloride (varies with intake)	110–250 mEq/24 h	110–250 mmol/day
Copper	0–50 mcg/24 h	0.0–0.80 µmol/day
Cortisol, free	10–100 mcg/24 h	27.6–276 nmol/day
Creatine		
Males	0–40 mg/24 h	0.0–0.30 mmol/day
Females	0–80 mg/24 h	0.0–0.60 mmol/day
Creatinine	15–25 mg/kg/24 h	0.13–0.22 mmol/kg/day
Creatinine clearance (endogenous)		
Males	110–150 mL/min/1.73 m^2	110–150 mL/min/1.73 m^2
Females	105–132 mL/min/1.73 m^2	105–132 mL/min/1.73 m^2
Cystine or cysteine	Negative	Negative
Dehydroepiandrosterone		
Males	0.2–2.0 mg/24 h	0.7–6.9 µmol/day
Females	0.2–1.8 mg/24 h	0.7–6.2 µmol/day
Estrogens, total		
Males	4–25 mcg/24 h	14–90 nmol/day
Females	5–100 mcg/24 h	18–360 nmol/day
Glucose (as reducing substance)	<250 mg/24 h	<250 mg/day

Reference Intervals[a] for Clinical Chemistry (Urine)—cont'd

ANALYTE	CONVENTIONAL UNITS	SI UNITS
Hemoglobin and myoglobin, qualitative	Negative	Negative
Hemogentisic acid, qualitative	Negative	Negative
17-Hydroxycorticosteroids		
Males	3–9 mg/24 h	8.3–25 µmol/day
Females	2–8 mg/24 h	5.5–22 µmol/day
5-Hydroxyindoleacetic acid		
Qualitative	Negative	Negative
Quantitative	2–6 mg/24 h	10–31 µmol/day
17-Ketogenic steroids		
Males	5–23 mg/24 h	17–80 µmol/day
Females	3–15 mg/24 h	10–52 µmol/day
17-Ketosteroids		
Males	8–22 mg/24 h	28–76 µmol/day
Females	6–15 mg/24 h	21–52 µmol/day
Magnesium	6–10 mEq/24 h	3–5 mmol/day
Metanephrines	0.05–1.2 ng/mg creatinine	0.03–0.70 mmol/mmol creatinine
Osmolality	38–1400 mOsm/kg water	38–1400 mOsm/kg water
pH	4.6–8.0	4.6–8.0
Phenylpyruvic acid, qualitative	Negative	Negative
Phosphate	0.4–1.3 g/24 h	13–42 mmol/day
Porphobilinogen		
Qualitative	Negative	Negative
Quantitative	<2 mg/24 h	<9 µmol/day
Porphyrins		
Coproporphyrin	50–250 mcg/24 h	77–380 nmol/day
Uroporphyrin	10–30 mcg/24 h	12–36 nmol/day
Potassium	25–125 mEq/24 h	25–125 mmol/day
Pregnanediol		
Males	0.0–1.9 mg/24 h	0.0–6.0 µmol/day
Females		
Proliferative phase	0.0–2.6 mg/24 h	0.0–8.0 µmol/day
Luteal phase	2.6–10.6 mg/24 h	8–33 µmol/day
Postmenopausal	0.2–1.0 mg/24 h	0.6–3.1 µmol/day
Pregnanetriol	0.0–2.5 mg/24 h	0.0–7.4 µmol/day
Protein, total		
Qualitative	Negative	Negative
Quantitative	10–150 mg/24 h	10–150 mg/day
Protein-to-creatinine ratio	<0.2	<0.2
Sodium (regular diet)	60–260 mEq/24 h	60–260 mmol/day
Specific gravity		
Random specimen	1.003–1.030	1.003–1.030
24-h collection	1.015–1.025	1.015–1.025
Urate (regular diet)	250–750 mg/24 h	1.5–4.4 mmol/day
Urobilinogen	0.5–4.0 mg/24 h	0.6–6.8 µmol/day
Vanillylmandelic acid (VMA)	1.0–8.0 mg/24 h	5–40 µmol/day

[a]Values may vary depending on the method used.
SI, International System of Units.

Reference Intervals for Toxic Substances

ANALYTE	CONVENTIONAL UNITS	SI UNITS
Arsenic, urine	<130 mcg/24 h	<1.7 μmol/day
Bromides, serum, inorganic	<100 mg/dL	<10 mmol/L
Toxic symptoms	140–1000 mg/dL	14–100 mmol/L
Carboxyhemoglobin, blood	Saturation, percent	
Urban environment	<5%	<0.05
Smokers	<12%	<0.12
Symptoms		
Headache	>15%	>0.15
Nausea and vomiting	>25%	>0.25
Potentially lethal	>50%	>0.50
Ethanol, blood	<0.05 mg/dL, 0.005%	<1.0 mmol/L
Intoxication	>100 mg/dL, 0.1%	>22 mmol/L
Marked intoxication	300–400 mg/dL, 0.3%–0.4%	65–87 mmol/L
Alcoholic stupor	400–500 mg/dL, 0.4%–0.5%	87–109 mmol/L
Coma	>500 mg/dL, 0.5%	>109 mmol/L
Lead, blood		
Adults	<20 mcg/dL	<1.0 μmol/L
Children	<10 mcg/dL	<0.5 μmol/L
Lead, urine	<80 mcg/24 h	<0.4 μmol/day
Mercury, urine	<10 mcg/24 h	<150 nmol/day

SI, International System of Units.

Reference Intervals for Tests Performed on Cerebrospinal Fluid

TEST	CONVENTIONAL UNITS	SI UNITS
Cells	<5 mm³; all mononuclear	$<5 \times 10^6$/L; all mononuclear
Protein electrophoresis	Albumin predominant	Albumin predominant
Glucose	50–75 mg/dL (20 mg/dL less than in serum)	2.8–4.2 mmol/L (1.1 mmol/L less than in serum)
IgG		
Children, <14 years	<8% of total protein	<0.08 of total protein
Adults	<14% of total protein	<0.14 of total protein
IgG index	0.3–0.6	0.3–0.6
Oligoclonal banding on electrophoresis	Absent	Absent
Pressure, opening	70–180 mm H_2O	70–180 mm H_2O
Protein, total	<15–45 mg/dL	150–450 mg/L

SI, International System of Units.

Reference Intervals for Tests of Gastrointestinal Function

TEST	CONVENTIONAL UNITS
Bentiromide	6-h urinary arylamine excretion. 57% excludes pancreatic insufficiency
β-Carotene, serum	60–250 ng/dL
Fecal fat estimation	
Qualitative	No fat globules seen by high-power microscope
Quantitative	<6 g/24 h (>95% coefficient of fat absorption)
Gastric acid output	
Basal	
Males	0.0–10.5 mmol/h
Females	0.0–5.6 mmol/h
Maximum (after histamine or pentagastrin)	
Males	9.0–48.0 mmol/h
Females	6.0–31.0 mmol/h
Ratio: basal/maximum	
Males	0.0–0.31
Females	0.0–0.29
Secretion test, pancreatic fluid	
Volume	>1.8 mL/kg/h
Bicarbonate	>80 mEq/L
D-Xylose absorption test, urine	>20% of ingested dose excreted in 5 h

Reference Intervals for Tests of Immunologic Function

TEST	CONVENTIONAL UNITS	SI UNITS
Autoantibodies, Serum, Adult		
Anti-CCP antibody	0–19 units	
Anti-dsDNA antibody	0–40 IU	0–40 IU
Antinuclear antibody	<1:40	
Rheumatoid factor (total IgG, IgA, IgM)	0–30 mg/dL	
Complement, Serum		
C3	85–175 mg/dL	0.85–1.75 g/L
C4	15–45 mg/dL	150–450 mg/L
Total hemolytic (CH_{50})	150–250 units/mL	150–250 units/mL
Immunoglobulins, Serum, Adult		
IgA	70–310 mg/dL	0.70–3.1 g/L
IgD	0.0–6.0 mg/dL	0.0–60 g/L
IgE	0.0–430 mg/dL	0.0–430 mg/L
IgG	640–1350 ng/dL	6.4–13.5 mcg/L
IgM	90–350 mg/dL	0.90–3.5 g/L

Anti-CCP, Anticyclic citrullinated peptide; *dsDNA,* double-stranded DNA; *Ig,* immunoglobulin; *SI,* International System of Units.

Reference Intervals for Lymphocytes Subsets, Whole Blood, Heparinized

ANTIGEN(S) EXPRESSED	CELL TYPE	PERCENTAGE	ABSOLUTE CELL COUNT
CD2	E rosette T cells	73–87	860–1880
CD3	Total T cells	56–77	140–370
CD3 and CD4	Helper-inducer cells	32–54	550–1190
CD3 and CD8	Suppressor-cytotoxic cells	24–37	430–1060
CD3 and DR	Activated T cells	5–14	70–310
CD16 and CD56	Natural killer (NK) cells	8–22	130–500
CD 19	Total B cells	7–17	140–370

Helper-to-suppressor ratio: 0.8–1.8.

Reference Values for Semen Analysis

TEST	CONVENTIONAL UNITS	SI UNITS
Volume	2–5 mL	2–5 mL
Liquefaction	Complete in 15 min	Complete in 15 min
pH	7.2–8.0	7.2–8.0
Leukocytes	Occasional or absent	Occasional or absent
Spermatozoa		
Count	$60–150 \times 10^6$ mL	$60–150 \times 10^6$ mL
Motility	>80% motile	>0.80 motile
Morphology	80%–90% normal forms	>0.80–0.90 normal
Fructose	>150 mg/dL	>8.33 mmol/L

SI, International System of Units.

References

CHAPTER 1

American Association of Colleges of Nursing: Enhancing diversity in the workforce, 2019. Retrieved from: https://www.aacnnursing.org/News-Information/Fact-Sheets/Enhancing-Diversity.

American Hospital Association (AHA): The patient care partnership: understanding expectations, rights and responsibilities, Atlanta, 2003, Author.

Bureau of Labor Statistics (BLS): Occupational employment and wages, May 2020: 29-2061 licensed practical and licensed vocational nurses, 2020. Retrieved from: https://www.bls.gov/oes/current/oes292061.htm

Bureau of Labor Statistics (BLS): *Occupational Outlook Handbook, Licensed* Practical and Licensed Vocational Nurses, 2021. Retrieved from: https://www.bls.gov/ooh/healthcare/licensed-practical-and-licensed-vocational-nurses.htm

Centers for Disease Control and Prevention (CDC): Healthy People, 2020. Retrieved from: https://www.cdc.gov/women/healthypeople2020/index.htm.

Centers for Disease Control and Prevention (CDC): National Center for Health Statistics: health expenditure, 2019. Retrieved from: https://www.cdc.gov/nchs/fastats/health-expenditures.htm

Centers for Medicare and Medicaid Services: National health expenditure data: historical, 2020. Retrieved from: https://www.cms.gov/Research-Statistics-Data-and-Systems/Statistics-Trends-and-Reports/NationalHealthExpendData/NationalHealthAccountsHistorical

Centers for Medicare and Medicaid Services: Resident rights, n.d. Retrieved from: https://www.medicare.gov/what-medicare-covers/what-part-a-covers/rights-protections-in-a-nursing-home.

Commonwealth Fund, The: U.S. health care from a global perspective, 2015. Retrieved from: http://www.commonwealthfund.org/publications/issue-briefs/2015/oct/us-health-care-from-a-global-perspective.

Early J: The Nurse Pinning Tradition, 2015. Retrieved from: http://www.nursinghistory.org/pinning-tradition/.

Ellis H: Florence Nightingale: creator of modern nursing and public health pioneer, *J Perioper Pract* 18(9):404–406, 2008.

The Henry J. Kaiser Family Foundation (KFF): Total number of professionally active nurses, 2017. Retrieved from: http://kff.org/other/state-indicator/total-registered-nurses/?currentTimeframe=0&selectedDistributions=licensed-practical-nurse-lpn.

Hill SS, Howlett HA: In *Success in practical/vocational nursing: from student to leader*, ed 7, St. Louis, 2013, Saunders.

McCarthy N: How U.S. healthcare spending compares with other countries, Forbes, August 8, 2019. Retrieved from: https://www.forbes.com/sites/niallmccarthy/2019/08/08/how-us-healthcare-spending-per-capita-compares-with-other-countries-infographic/?sh=350c9f55575d

Medscape Today News: Celebrating nurses: What happened to the cap? Part 2: Losing our tradition. slideshow. n.d. Retrieved from: www.medscape.com/features/slideshow/nurse-caps-pt2.

National Association for Practical Nurse Education and Service (NAPNES): Standards of practice and educational competencies of graduates of practical/vocational nursing programs, 2007. Retrieved from: http://napnes.org/drupal-7.4/sites/default/files/pdf/standards/standards_read_only.pdf.

National Council State Boards of Nursing (NCSBN): National Nursing Workforce Study, 2017. Retrieved from: https://www.ncsbn.org/workforce.htm

National League for Nursing Education (NLNE): History of the National League of Nursing (1893-2018), n.d. Retrieve from: http://www.nln.org/docs/default-source/about/nln-timeline9c00c85c78366c709642ff00005f0421.pdf?sfvrsn=4.

National League for Nursing (NLN): Nurse Educator Demographics, 2017. Retrieved from: http://www.nln.org/newsroom/nursing-education-statistics/nurse-educator-demographics

NLN Board of Governors: NLN Vision Series. A Vision for Recognition of the Role of Licensed Practical/Vocational Nurses in Advancing the Nation's Health. A Living Document from the National League for Nursing, 2014. Retrieved from: http://www.nln.org/docs/default-source/about/nln-vision-series-(position-statements)/nlnvision_7.pdf.

Payne C: More men entering nursing profession, USA Today, 2013. Retrieved from: http://www.usatoday.com/story/news/nation/2013/02/25/men-nursing-occupatins/1947243.

Smith T: A policy perspective on the entry into practice issue, Online J Issues Nurs 15(1):2009. Retrieved from: www.nursingworld.org/MainMenuCategories/ANAMarketplace/ANAPeriodicals/OJIN/TableofContents/Vol152010/No1Jan2010/Articles-Previous-Topic/Policy-and-Entry-into-Practice.html.

Society for Women's Health Research: Women's Health Research, 2020. Retrieved from: https://swhr.org/about/womens-health-research/

Stringer H: IOM Future of Nursing report care: Progress after 10 years. nurse.com, 2019. Retrieved from: https://www.nurse.com/blog/2019/07/01/iom-future-of-nursing-report-card-progress-after-10-years/

US Army Heritage Center Foundation: Soldier stories, n.d. Retrieved from: https://www.armyheritage.org/programs/soldier-stories/.

US Census Bureau: Health insurance coverage in the United States: 2018, 2019. Retrieved from https://www.census.gov/library/publications/2019/demo/p60-267.html.

US Census Bureau: Income, poverty, and health insurance coverage: 2011 Highlights, 2011. United States Department of Commerce, 2011. Retrieved from: www.census.gov/hhes/www/hlthins/data/incpovhlth/2011/highlights.html.

CHAPTER 2

American Nurses Association (ANA) and National Council of State Boards of Nursing (NCSBN): ANA and NCSBN unite to provide guidelines on social media and networking for nurses, 2011. Retrieved from:

Cornell University Law School: Cruzan v. Director, Missouri Department of Health, (88-1503), 497 U.S. 261 (1990), 1990. Retrieved from: https://www.law.cornell.edu/supct/html/88-1503.ZO.html.

Levin SM: H.R.4449–Patient Self-Determination Act of 1990, 1990. Retrieved from: https://www.congress.gov/bill/101 st-congress/house-bill/4449.

Miller and Zois Attorneys at Law 2020. Retrieved from: https://www.millerandzois.com/nurse-malpractice-statistics.html.

Missouri Department of Health & Senior Services: Negligence and malpractice, n.d. Retrieved from: http://health.mo.gov/living/lpha/phnursing/negligence.php.

Motacki K, Burke K: In *Nursing delegation and management of patient care*, ed 2, St. Louis, 2017, Elsevier.

National Council of State Boards of Nursing (NCSBN): Filing a complaint, n.d. Retrieved from: https://www.ncsbn.org/filing-a-complaint.htm.

Stokowski LA: Social media and nurses: promising or perilous? 2011. Retrieved from: https://www.medscape.com/viewarticle/753317_3.

CHAPTER 3

American Hospital Association: Patient Care and Information, n.d. Retrieved from: https://www.aha.org/ahia/promoting-healthy-communities/patient-care-and-information.

Centers for Medicare and Medicaid Services (CMS): Home Health Agency Center, n.d. Retrieved from: https://www.cms.gov/Center/Provider-Type/Home-Health-Agency-HHA-Center.html.

The Joint Commission: Inadequate hand-off communication. Sentinel Event Alert, issue 58, September 12, 2017. Retrieved from: https://www.jointcommission.org/-/media/tjc/documents/resources/patient-safety-topics/sentinel-event/sea_58_hand_off_comms_9_6_17_final_(1).pdf

The Joint Commission: National Patient Safety Goals, 2020. Retrieved from: https://www.jointcommission.org/standards_information/npsgs.aspx

Mayo Clinic Staff: Personal health records and patient portals, 2020. Retrieved from: https://www.mayoclinic.org/healthy-lifestyle/consumer-health/in-depth/personal-health-record/art-20047273

The Office of the National Coordinator for Health Information Technology: EMR vs. EHR. What's the difference?, 2011. Retrieved from: https://www.healthit.gov/buzz-blog/electronic-health-and-medical-records/emr-vs-ehr-difference/

CHAPTER 4

Ackley BJ, Ladwig GB: *Nursing diagnosis handbook: an evidence-based guide to planning care*, ed 12, St. Louis, 2020, Mosby.

Arnold E, Bogg KJ: *Interpersonal relationships: professional communication skills for nurses*, ed 7, Philadelphia, 2016, Saunders.

Balzer Riley J: *Communication in nursing*, ed 9, St. Louis, 2021, Elsevier.

Krauss Whitbourne S: Polish off your personal space. PsychologyToday, 2012. Retrieved from: www.psychologytoday.com/blog/fulfillment-any-age/201211/polish-your-personal-space.

Maier-Lorentz MM: Transcultural nursing: its importance in nursing practice, *J Cultural Divers* 15(1):37–43, 2008.

Old N, Kai T: Survival of the funniest: using therapeutic humour in nursing, *Nurs N Zealand* 18(8):17–19, 2012.

Potter PA, Perry AG: *Fundamentals of nursing*, ed 10, St. Louis, 2021, Mosby.

Yoshikawa Y, Ohmaki E, Kawahata H, et al.: Beneficial effect of laughter therapy on physiological and psychological function in elders, *Nurs Open* 6(1):93–99, 2019.

CHAPTER 5

American Nurses Association (ANA): *Nursing: scope and standards of practice*, Silver Spring, Md, 2015, Author.

American Nurses Association (ANA): What is nursing? n.d.a. Retrieved from: http://nursingworld.org/EspeciallyForYou/What-is-Nursing.

American Nurses Association (ANA): The nursing process, n.d.b. Retrieved from: https://www.nursingworld.org/practice-policy/workforce/what-is-nursing/the-nursing-process/.

Butcher HK, Bulechek GM, McCloskey JM, et al.: *Nursing interventions classification (NIC)*, ed 7, St. Louis, 2019, Mosby.

Carpenito LJ: *Nursing diagnosis*, ed 16, Burlington, MA, 2021, Jones & Bartlett Learning.

Moorhead S, Johnson M, Maas M, et al.: *Nursing outcomes classification (NOC)*, ed 6, St. Louis, 2018, Mosby.

North American Nursing Diagnosis Association–International (NANDA-I): Nursing diagnoses: glossary of terms, n.d. Retrieved from: https://nanda.org/publications-resources/resources/glossary-of-terms/.

Papathanasiou IV, Kleisiaris CF, Fradelos EC, et al.: Critical thinking: the development of an essential skill for nursing students, *Acta Inform Med*(4)283–286, 2014, https://doi.org/10.5455/aim.2014.22.283-286.

CHAPTER 6

Beauregard JL, Hamner HC, Chen J, Avila-Rodriguez W, Elam-Evans LD, Perrine CG: Racial disparities in breastfeeding initiation and duration among U.S. infants born in 2015, *Weekly* 68(34):745–748, 2019. Retrieved from https://www.cdc.gov/mmwr/volumes/68/wr/mm6834a3.htm.

Centers for Disease Control and Promotion (CDC): Disability and Health Overview, 2020. Retrieved from https://www.cdc.gov/ncbddd/disabilityandhealth/disability.html

Chamorro-Premuzic T: Science explains why unconscious bias training won't reduce workplace racism. Here's what will. Fast Company, 2020. Retrieved from: https://www.fastcompany.com/90515678/science-explains-why-unconscious-bias-training-wont-reduce-workplace-racism-heres-what-will

Giger JN: *Transcultural nursing: assessment and intervention*, ed 7, St. Louis, 2017, Elsevier.

Healthy People 2020: Lesbian, gay, bisexual, and transgender health, Office of Disease Prevention and Promotion, 2020. Retrieved from https://www.healthypeople.gov/2020/topics-objectives/topic/lesbian-gay-bisexual-and-transgender-health

Marcelin JR, Siraj DS, Victor R, et al.: The impact of unconscious bias in healthcare: how to recognize and mitigate it, *J Infect Dis* 220(2):S62–S73, 2019.

Medicinal Medicinal remedies from Appalachia, 2012. Retrieved from: https://blindpigandtheacorn.com/medicinal-remedies-from-appalachia/

United Cerebral Palsy: Disability etiquette, 2018. Retrieved from: https://ucp.org/resource-guide/disability-etiquette

US Census Bureau: Census data 2010, 2010. Retrieved from: www.census.gov/2010census/data.

US Census Bureau: Most children younger than age 1 are minorities, 2012. Retrieved from: https://www.census.gov/newsroom/releases/archives/population/cb12-90.html.

CHAPTER 7

Agency for Healthcare Research and Quality (AHRQ): Universal ICU Decolonization: An Enhanced Protocol, 2013, Retrieved from: https://www.ahrq.gov/hai/universal-icu-decolonization/universal-icu-ape3.html

Association of periOperative Registered Nurses (AORN): *Perioperative standards and recommended practices*, Denver, 2019, Author.

Boyce JM, Pittet D: HICPAC/SHEA/APIC/IDSA Hand Hygiene Task Force, CDC Healthcare Control Practices Advisory Committee: Guideline for hand hygiene in health-care settings, *Am J Infect Control* 30(8), 2002.

Centers for Disease Control and Prevention (CDC): Anthrax as a Bioterrorism Weapon, 2020. Retrieved from: www.cdc.gov/anthrax/bioterrorism/index.html

Centers for Disease Control and Prevention (CDC): Current HAI Progress Report: 2019. https://www.cdc.gov/hai/data/portal/progress-report.html

Centers for Disease Control and Prevention (CDC): Updated U.S. Public Health Service guidelines for the management of occupational exposure to HIV and recommendations for postexposure prophylaxis, Washington, D.C., 2013, Author. Retrieved from: http://stacks.cdc.gov/view/cdc/20711/cdc_20711_DS1.pdf

Centers for Disease Control and Prevention (CDC): Precautions to prevent transmission of infectious diseases, 2019. Retrieved from: https://www.cdc.gov/infectioncontrol/guidelines/isolation/precautions.html#:~:text=There%20are%20two%20tiers%20of,Precautions%20and%20Transmission%2DBased%20Precautions.rganisms%20in%20health%20care%20settings,%202006.%20Retrieved%20from:%20www.cdc.gov/ncidod/dhqp/pdf/ar/mdroGuide%20line2006.pdf

Centers for Disease Control and Prevention (CDC): Preventing Healthcare-Associated Infections, 2015. Retrieved from: https://www.cdc.gov/hai/prevent/prevention.html

Centers for Disease Control and Prevention (CDC): Isolation precautions, 2019. Retrieved from: https://www.cdc.gov/infectioncontrol/guidelines/isolation/index.html

Centers for Disease Control and Prevention (CDC): Handwashing: clean hands save lives: show me the science—how to wash your hands, 2020. Retrieved from: https://www.cdc.gov/handwashing/show-me-the-science-handwashing.html.

Centers for Disease Control and Prevention: Healthcare providers, 2021. Retrieved from: https://www.cdc.gov/handhygiene/providers/index.html

Centers for Disease Control and Prevention (CDC): Anthrax as a Bioterrorism Weapon, 2020. Retrieved from: https://www.cdc.gov/anthrax/bioterrorism/index.html.

Centers for Disease Control and Prevention (CDC): Four steps to food safety: clean, separate, cook, chill, 2020. Retrieved from: http://www.cdc.gov/foodsafety/groups/consumers.html.

Centers for Disease Control and Prevention (CDC): HAI data, 2018a. Retrieved from: https://www.cdc.gov/hai/surveillance/index.html.

Centers for Disease Control and Prevention (CDC): Healthcare-associated infections: HAI Data, 2020 Retrieved from: https://www.cdc.gov/hai/data/portal/index.html

Centers for Disease Control and Prevention (CDC): New ICD-10-CM code for the 2019 Novel Coronavirus (COVID-19), 2020. Retrieved from: https://www.cdc.gov/nchs/data/icd/Announcement-New-ICD-code-for-coronavirus-3-18-2020.pdf#:~:text=On%20March%2011%2C%202020,COVID%2D19%20Outbreak.

Centers for Disease Control and Prevention (CDC): Strategies to prevent *clostridioides difficile* infection in acute care facilities, 2016. Retrieved from: https://www.cdc.gov/hai/prevent/cdi-prevention-strategies.html

Centers for Disease Control and Prevention (CDC): Transmission-Based Precautions, 2016. Retrieved from: https://www.cdc.gov/infectioncontrol/basics/transmission-based-precautions.html

Centers for Disease Control and Prevention (CDC): Travel-Related Infectious Diseases, 2019. Retrieved from: https://wwwnc.cdc.gov/travel/yellowbook/2020/travel-related-infectious-diseases/tuberculosis

Johns Hopkins Medicine: CHG bathing to prevent healthcare associated infections. Retrieved from: https://www.hopkinsmedicine.org/health/treatment-tests-and-therapies/chg-bathing-to-prevent-healthcareassociated-infections.

The Joint Commission: National Patient Safety Goals, 2017. Retrieved from: https://www.jointcommission.org/assets/1/6/NPSG_Chapter_NCC_Jan2017.pdf.

Mayo Clinic: Drugs and supplements: anthrax vaccine (intramuscular route, subcutaneous route), 2021. Retrieved from: https://www.mayoclinic.org/drugs-supplements/anthrax-vaccine-intramuscular-route-subcutaneous-route/description/drg-20074564.

Mayo Clinic: Handwashing: do's and don'ts, 2020. Retrieved from: https://www.mayoclinic.org/healthy-lifestyle/adult-health/in-depth/hand-washing/art-20046253.

National Capital Poison Center, 2019. Retrieved from: https://www.poison.org/poison-statistics-national

Nuclear Regulatory Commission (NRC), 2020. Retrieved from: https://www.nrc.gov/waste.html

Potter PA, Perry AG, Stockert P: *Essentials for nursing practice*, ed 9, St. Louis, 2019, Elsevier.

Siegel JD, Rhinehart E, Jackson M, et al; Healthcare Infection Control Practices Advisory Committee: Guideline for isolation precautions: Preventing transmission of infectious agents in healthcare settings, 2007. Retrieved from: https://www.ajicjournal.org/article/S0196-6553(07)00740-7/fulltext

US Food and Drug Administration: Safety alerts for human medical products, 2016. Retrieved from: http://wayback.archive-it.org/7993/20170110235327/http://www.fda.gov/Safety/MedWatch/SafetyInformation/default.htm.

US Food and Drug Administration: Anthrax, 2018. Retrieved from: https://www.fda.gov/vaccines-blood-biologics/vaccines/anthrax

US Food and Drug Administration: Doxycycline and Penicillin G Procaine for Inhalational Anthrax (Post-Exposure) 2017. Retrieved from https://www.fda.gov/drugs/bioterrorism-and-drug-preparedness/doxycycline-and-penicillin-g-procaine-inhalational-anthrax-post-exposure

US Food and Drug Administration: Emergency preparedness (drugs), 2019. Retrieved from: https://www.fda.gov/drugs/emergencypreparedness/default.htm.

US Food and Drug Administration: What you should know about flu antiviral drugs, 2021. Retrieved from: https://www.cdc.gov/flu/treatment/whatyoushould.htm#antiviral-drugs

World Health Association: Glove use information leaflet, 2009. Retrieved from:https://www.who.int/gpsc/5may/Glove_Use_Information_Leaflet.pdf?ua=1

CHAPTER 8

Ackley BJ, Ladwig GB: *Nursing diagnosis handbook*, ed 12, St. Louis, 2020, Mosby.

Borojeny LA, Albateneh AN, Dehkordi AH, Gheshlagh RG: *The incidence of pressure ulcers and its associations in different wards of the hospital: a systematic review and meta-analysis*. Retrieved from: https://www.ncbi.nlm.nih.gov/pmc/articles/PMC7716611/, 2020.

Centers for Disease Control and Prevention (CDC), National Institute for Occupational Safety and Health (NIOSH): Safe patient handling and mobility (SPHM), 2017. Retrieved from: https://www.cdc.gov/niosh/topics/safepatient/default.html.

National Library of Medicine (NLM): Compartment syndrome, 2014. Retrieved from: https://medlineplus.gov/ency/article/001224.htm.

Potter PA, Perry AG, Stockert PA, et al.: *Fundamentals of nursing: concepts, process, and practice*, St. Louis, 2017, Mosby.

Rasul, Jr, AT: Acute Compartment Syndrome, 2020. Retrieved from https://emedicine.medscape.com/article/307668-overview#a8.

CHAPTER 9

Agency for Healthcare Research and Quality (AHRQ): Preventing pressure ulcers in hospitals: a toolkit for improving quality of care, 2014. Retrieved from: www.ahrq.gov/professionals/systems/hospital/pressureulcertoolkit/index.html.

Medscape: A closer look at pressure ulcers: "Reasonably preventable," 2008. Retrieved from: www.medscape.org/viewarticle/574206_2.

National Pressure Ulcer Advisory Panel (NPUAP): National Pressure Ulcer advisory panel NPUAP announces a change in terminology from pressure ulcer to pressure injury and updates the stages of pressure injury, 2016. Retrieved from: https://www.woundsource.com/blog/national-pressure-ulcer-advisory-panel-npuap-announces-change-in-terminology-pressure-ulcer

CHAPTER 10

Asthma and Allergy Foundation of America: Latex allergy. Retrieved from https://www.aafa.org/latex-allergy/

Campbell R: Fires in health care facilities, 2017. Retrieved from: http://www.nfpa.org/news-and-research/fire-statistics-and-reports/fire-statistics/fires-by-property-type/health-care-facilities/fires-in-health-care-facilities.

Centers for Disease Control and Prevention (CDC), National Occupational Research Agenda (NORA): Sharps injuries, 2019. Retrieved from: https://www.cdc.gov/nora/councils/hcsa/stopsticks/sharpsinjuries.html

Centers for Disease Control and Prevention (CDC), National Occupational Research Agenda (NORA): Sharps injuries: Bloodborne pathogens, 2019. Retrieved from: https://www.cdc.gov/nora/councils/hcsa/stopsticks/bloodborne.html .

Centers for Disease Control and Prevention (CDC): Bioterrorism agents/diseases. Retrieved from http://emergency.cdc.gov/agent/agentlist.asp#.

Centers for Disease Control and Prevention (CDC): Home and recreational safety: Poisoning, 2015. Retrieved from: https://www.cdc.gov/homeandrecreationalsafety/poisoning/.

Centers for Disease Control and Prevention (CDC): Vaccine information for adults: healthcare workers, n.d. Retrieved from: https://www.cdc.gov/vaccines/adults/rec-vac/hcw.html.

Environmental Protection Agency (EPA): Radionuclides in drinking water, 2015. Retrieved from: https://cfpub.epa.gov/safewater/radionuclides/radionuclides.cfm?action=Rad_Disposal%20Options.

The Joint Commission (TJC): Sentinel event, n.d. Retrieved from: www.jointcommission.org/sentinel_event.aspx.

The Joint Commission (TJC): Active shooter planning and response, 2017. Retrieved from: https://www.jointcommission.org/-/media/tjc/documents/resources/workplace-violence/2017_active_shooter_planning_response_healthcare_settingpdf.pdf.

King KC, Strony R: Needlestick. StatPearls [Internet]. Treasure Island (FL), 2021 StatPearls Publishing. Retrieved from: https://www.ncbi.nlm.nih.gov/books/NBK493147/.

National Capital Poison Center: Poison statistics: national data 2019, 2019. Retrieved from: http://www.poison.org/poison-statistics-national.

Occupational Safety and Health Administration (OSHA): Decontamination, n.d. Retrieved from: https://www.osha.gov/SLTC/hazardouswaste/training/decon.html.

Rossen LM, Bastian B, Warner M, Khan D, Chong Y: *Drug poisoning mortality: United States, 1999–2018*, National Center for Health Statistics, 2020.

Stobart-Gallagher MA: Needle-stick guideline, 2019. Retrieved from: http://emedicine.medscape.com/article/784812-overview#a6.

US Bureau of Labor Statistics (BLS): Fact Sheet: workplace violence in healthcare, 2018, 2020. Retrieved from https://www.bls.gov/iif/oshwc/cfoi/workplace-violence-healthcare-2018.htm.

US Department of Homeland Security: Active shooter: how to respond, 2008. Retrieved from: https://www.dhs.gov/xlibrary/assets/active_shooter_booklet.pdf.

US Department of Labor, Occupational Safety and Health Administration: Workplace violence, n.d. Retrieved from: https://www.osha.gov/SLTC/healthcarefacilities/violence.html.

CHAPTER 11

The Joint Commission (TJC): Standards FAQ details: Nursing assessments—Licensed practical nurse, n.d. Retrieved from: https://www.jointcommission.org/standards/standard-faqs/critical-access-hospital/provision-of-care-treatment-and-services-pc/000001666/.

Kind AJH, Smith MA: Documentation of mandated discharge summary components in transitions from acute to subacute care, n.d. Retrieved from: https://www.ahrq.gov/downloads/pub/advances2/vol2/Advances-Kind_31.pdf.

Maslow A: *Motivation and personality*, ed 2, New York, 1970, Harper & Row.

CHAPTER 12

American Heart Association: Heart-health screenings, 2019. Retrieved from: http://www.heart.org/HEARTORG/Conditions/Heart-Health-Screenings_UCM_428687_Article.jsp#.WI1OvvIsOSo.

Goldman LR, Shannon MW: Committee on Environmental Health: Technical report: mercury in the environment: implications for pediatricians, *Pediatrics* 108(1), 2001.

National Library of Medicine (NLM): Body temperature norms. n.d. Retrieved from: https://medlineplus.gov/ency/article/001982.htm.

CHAPTER 13

Center for Disease Control and Prevention (CDC): Clinical guidance for carbon monoxide poisoning after a disaster, 2020. Retrieved from: https://www.cdc.gov/disasters/co_guidance.html

Centers for Disease Control and Prevention (CDC): Standard precautions for all patient care, 2016. Retrieved from: https://www.cdc.gov/infectioncontrol/basics/standard-precautions.html.

Jarvis C: In *Physical examination and health assessment*, ed 8, St. Louis, 2020, Elsevier.

The Joint Commission: Patient safety. Retrieved from https://www.jointcommission.org/resources/patient-safety-topics/patient-safety/.

CHAPTER 16

Aboubakr M, Alameda G: Brain Death Criteria. [Updated 2021 May 29]. In: StatPearls [Internet]. Treasure Island (FL): StatPearls Publishing; 2021 Jan-. Retrieved from: https://www.ncbi.nlm.nih.gov/books/NBK545144/.

American Burn Association: Burn Incidence Fact Sheet, 2016. Retrieved from: https://ameriburn.org/who-we-are/media/burn-incidence-fact-sheet/.

American Heart Association (AHA): Hands-Only CPR Factsheet, n.d. Retrieved from: https://ahainstructornetwork.americanheart.org/idc/groups/ahaecc-public/@wcm/@ecc/documents/downloadable/ucm_504171.pdf.

American Heart Association (AHA): CPR and ECC Guidelines, 2020. Retrieved from: https://cpr.heart.org/en/resuscitation-science/cpr-and-ecc-guidelines.

Centers for Disease Control and Prevention: Rabies: Postexposure prophylaxis, 2019. Retrieved from: https://www.cdc.gov/rabies/medical_care/index.html.

Harrison L: Should POLICE replace RICE as the ankle therapy of choice? 2014. Retrieved from: http://www.medscape.com/viewarticle/823217_2.

Immunization Action Coalition: Rabies: Questions and answers: information about the disease and vaccines, n.d. Retrieved from: www.immunize.org/catg.d/p4216.pdf.

Jiang L, Zhang JS: Mechanical cardiopulmonary resuscitation for patients with cardiac arrest, *World J Emerg Med* 2(3):165–168, 2011, https://doi.org/10.5847/wjem.j.1920-8642.2011.03.001.

Johns Hopkins Medicine: Snake bites, n.d. Retrieved from: https://www.hopkinsmedicine.org/health/conditions-and-diseases/snake-bites.

Keany JE, McKeever D: Femoral shaft fracture in emergency medicine clinical presentation, 2019. Retrieved from: https://emedicine.medscape.com/article/824856-clinical.

Mayo Clinic: Hypothermia, 2020. Retrieved from: https://www.mayoclinic.org/diseases-conditions/hypothermia/symptoms-causes/syc-20352682.

Proehl JA: *Emergency nursing procedures*, ed 4, St. Louis, 2009, Saunders.

Rumsfeld JS, Brooks S, Aufderheide TP, et al: Use of mobile devices, social media, and crowdsourcing as digital strategies to improve emergency cardiovascular care: A scientific statement from the American Heart Association. Circulation 134:e87-e108, 2016. Retrieved from: https://www.ahajournals.org/doi/10.1161/CIR.0000000000000428.

Tactical Emergency Casualty Care (TECC): *Guidelines for BLS/ALS medical providers*. Retrieved from: http://www.c-tecc.org/images/4-2019_TECC_ALS_BLS_Guidelines_.pdf, 2019.

Vyas KS, Wong LK: Oral rehydration solutions for burn management in the field and underdeveloped regions: a review, *Int J Burns Trauma* 3(3):130–136, 2013.

Wheeless CR, editor: *Wheeless' textbook of orthopaedics*, 2016, Duke Orthopaedics and Data Trace Internet Publishing. Retrieved from: www.wheelessonline.com.

Zonnoor B: Frostbite treatment and management, 2020. Retrieved from: https://emedicine.medscape.com/article/926249-treatment.

CHAPTER 17

American Nurses Association (ANA): Safe needles save lives, n.d. Retrieved from: https://www.nursingworld.org/practice-policy/work-environment/health-safety/safe-needles/safe-needles-law/.

Belle DJ, Singh H: Genetic factors in drug metabolism, *Am Fam Physician* 77(11):1553–1560, 2008.

Bollinger MB: How do patients determine that their metered dose inhaler is empty? *Pediatrics* 116(Suppl 2):2005. Retrieved from: http://pediatrics.aappublications.org/content/116/Supplement_2/563.1.

Brewster LM, Seedat YK: Why do hypertensive patients of African ancestry respond better to calcium blockers and diuretics than to ACE inhibitors and β-adrenergic blockers? A systematic review, *BMC Med* 11:141, 2013.

Kee JL, Hayes ER: *Pharmacology: a nursing process approach*, ed 7, St. Louis, 2012, Elsevier.

National Library of Medicine (NLM): Furosemide, 2017. Retrieved from: https://medlineplus.gov/druginfo/meds/a682858.html.

Ortega VE, Meyers DA: Pharmacogenetics: Implications of race and ethnicity on defining genetic profiles for personalized medicine, *J Allergy Clin Immol* 133(1):16–26, 2014.

The Joint Commission: Official "do not use" list, 2018. Retrieved from: https://www.jointcommission.org/assets/1/18/dnu_list.pdf.

US Food and Drug Administration (FDA): What are generic drugs? 2009. Retrieved from: www.fda.gov/Drugs/ResourcesForYou/Consumers/BuyingUsingMedicineSafely/UnderstandingGenericDrugs/ucm144456.htm.

CHAPTER 18

Brinkman JE, Sharma S. Respiratory Alkalosis. [Updated 2020 Jul 26]. In: StatPearls [Internet]. Treasure Island (FL): StatPearls Publishing; 2021 Jan. Retrieved from: https://www.ncbi.nlm.nih.gov/books/NBK482117/.

Infusion Nurses Society: Infusion nursing standards of practice, *J Intraven Nurs* 34(1S):S65, 2011.

Ray-Barruel G, Polit DF, Murfield JE, Rickard CM: Infusion phlebitis assessment measures: a systematic review, *J Eval Clin Pract* 20(2):191–202, 2014.

CHAPTER 19

American Diabetes Association: Diabetes basics: Facts about type 2, n.d.a. Retrieved from: www.diabetes.org/diabetes-basics/type-2/facts-about-type-2.html.

American Diabetes Association: Diabetes basics: Type 1 diabetes, n.d.b. Retrieved from: www.diabetes.org/diabetes-basics/type-1.

American Heart Association: Trans fat, 2017. Retrieved from: https://www.heart.org/en/healthy-living/healthy-eating/eat-smart/fats/trans-fat .

Centers for Disease Control and Prevention (CDC): Adult obesity facts, 2021. Retrieved from: https://www.cdc.gov/obesity/data/adult.html

Centers for Disease Control and Prevention (CDC): Hip fractures among older adults, 2013. Retrieved from: www.cdc.gov/homeandrecreationalsafety/falls/adulthipfx.html.

The Food and Drug Administration (FDA): The new nutrition facts label, n.d. Retrieved from: https://www.fda.gov/food/nutrition-education-resources-materials/new-nutrition-facts-label

March of Dimes: Caffeine in pregnancy, 2020. Retrieved from: https://www.marchofdimes.org/pregnancy/caffeine-in-pregnancy.aspx.

The National Academies of Sciences, Engineering, Medicine: Dietary reference intakes (DRIs): recommended dietary allowances and adequate intakes, Elements, n.d. Retrieved from: http://nationalacademies.org/hmd/activities/nutrition/summarydris/dri-tables.aspx?_ga=2.139664307.1693095242.1531251493-1603260316.1531251493.

US Department of Health and Human Services (USDHHS), National Institutes of Health (NIH), National Heart, Lung and Blood Institute (NHLBI): Calculate your body mass index, n.d.a. Retrieved from: https://www.nhlbi.nih.gov/health/educational/lose_wt/BMI/bmicalc.htm?source=quickfitnesssolutions.

US Department of Health and Human Services (USDHHS), National Institutes of Health (NIH), National Heart, Lung and Blood Institute (NHLBI): DASH eating plan, n.d.b. Retrieved from: https://www.nhlbi.nih.gov/health-topics/dash-eating-plan.

US Department of Health and Human Services (USDHHS), National Institutes of Health (NIH), National Heart, Lung, and Blood Institute (NHLBI): Your guide to lowering cholesterol with TLC, 2005. Retrieved from: https://www.nhlbi.nih.gov/files/docs/public/heart/chol_tlc.pdf.

US Department of Health and Human Services (USDHHS), National Institutes of Health (NIH), National Institute of Diabetes and Digestive and Kidney Diseases (NIDDK): Bariatric surgery, n.d.a. Retrieved from: https://www.niddk.nih.gov/health-information/weight-management/bariatric-surgery#SurgAdult.

US Department of Health and Human Services (USDHHS), National Institutes of Health (NIH), National Institute of Diabetes and Digestive and Kidney Diseases (NIDDK):

Lactose intolerance, n.d.b. Retrieved from: http://digestive.niddk.nih.gov/ddiseases/pubs/lactoseintolerance.

US Department of Health and Human Services (USDHHS), National Institutes of Health (NIH), Office of Dietary Supplements: Calcium Fact Sheet for Health Professionals, 2017. Retrieved from: https://ods.od.nih.gov/factsheets/Calcium-HealthProfessional/.

US Department of Health and Human Services (USDHHS), National Institutes of Health (NIH), Office of Dietary Supplements: Chromium Fact Sheet for Health Professionals, 2018a. Retrieved from: http://ods.od.nih.gov/factsheets/Chromium-HealthProfessional.

US Department of Health and Human Services (USDHHS), National Institutes of Health (NIH), Office of Dietary Supplements: Folate Fact Sheet for Health Professionals, 2018b. Retrieved from: http://ods.od.nih.gov/factsheets/Folate-HealthProfessional.

US Department of Health and Human Services (USDHHS), National Institutes of Health (NIH), Office of Dietary Supplements: Iron: Fact Sheet for Health Professionals, 2018. Retrieved from: https://ods.od.nih.gov/factsheets/Iron-HealthProfessional/.

US Department of Health and Human Services (USDHHS), National Institutes of Health (NIH), Office of Dietary Supplements: Potassium Fact Sheet for Health Professionals, 2018d. Retrieved from: https://ods.od.nih.gov/factsheets/Potassium-HealthProfessional/.

US Department of Health and Human Services (USDHHS), National Institute of Health (NIH), Office of Dietary Supplements: Vitamin E Fact Sheet for Health Professionals. 2018e. Retrieved from: https://ods.od.nih.gov/factsheets/VitaminE-HealthProfessional.

US Department of Health and Human Services (USDHHS), National Institutes of Health (NIH), Office of Dietary Supplements: Vitamin B12 Fact Sheet for Health Professionals, 2018f. Retrieved from: https://ods.od.nih.gov/factsheets/VitaminB12-HealthProfessional/.

US Department of Health and Human Services (USDHHS), National Institutes of Health (NIH), Office of Dietary Supplements: Vitamin C Fact Sheet for Health Professionals, 2018g. Retrieved from: https://ods.od.nih.gov/factsheets/VitaminC-HealthProfessional/.

US Department of Health and Human Services (USDHHS), National Institutes of Health (NIH), Office of Dietary Supplements: Vitamin D Fact Sheet for Health Professionals, 2018h. Retrieved from: https://ods.od.nih.gov/factsheets/VitaminD-HealthProfessional/.

US Department of Health and Human Services (USDHHS), National Institutes of Health (NIH), Office of Dietary Supplements: Vitamin K Fact Sheet for Health Professionals, 2018i. Retrieved from: https://ods.od.nih.gov/factsheets/VitaminK-HealthProfessional/.

US Department of Health and Human Services (USDHHS) and US Department of Agriculture (USDA): 2015–2020 Dietary Guidelines for Americans, 8th Edition. December 2015. Available at: https://health.gov/our-work/food-nutrition/previous-dietary-guidelines/2015

US Department of Health and Human Services (USDHHS) and US Department of Agriculture (USDA): UDSA-HHS Development of the Dietary Guidelines, n.d. Available at: https://www.dietaryguidelines.gov/usda-hhs-development-dietary-guidelines

CHAPTER 20

American Cannabis Nurses Association (ACNA). n.d. Retrieved from: https://cannabisnurses.org.

American Optometric Association: Head-down yoga poses increase eye pressure in glaucoma patients, 2016. Retrieved from: http://www.aoa.org/news/clinical-eye-care/head-down-yoga-poses-increase-eye-pressure-in-glaucoma-patients?sso=y.

Clark TC, Black LI, Stussman BJ, et al.: Trends in the use of complementary health approaches among adults: United States, 2002-2012, *Natl Health Stat Report* 79, 2015.

Glaucoma Research Foundation: Doing yoga with glaucoma: modify your yoga routine to avoid increased IOP, 2017. Retrieved from: https://www.glaucoma.org/news/blog/doing-yoga-with-glaucoma-how-to-modify-your-yoga-routine-to-avoid-increased-iop.php.

Harvard Health Publishing, Harvard Medical School: The health benefits of tai chi, 2019. Retrieved from https://www.health.harvard.edu/staying-healthy/the-health-benefits-of-tai-chi

King BA, Jones CM, Baldwin GT, Briss PA: The EVALI and youth vaping epidemics — implications for public health, *N Engl J Med* 382:689–691, 2020, https://doi.org/10.1056/NEJMp1916171. 2020. Retrieved from.

Mayo Clinic: Pet therapy: Animals as healers, 2020. Retrieved from: https://www.mayoclinic.org/healthy-lifestyle/consumer-health/in-depth/pet-therapy/art-20046342.

Mayo Clinic: Biofeedback, 2021. Retrieved from: https://www.mayoclinic.org/tests-procedures/biofeedback/about/pac-20384664.

The Medical Cannabis Institute (TMCI): About TMCI Global (TMCI), n.d. Retrieved from: https://themedicalcannabisinstitute.org/about/.

National Academies of Sciences, Engineering, and Medicine: The Health Effects of Cannabis and Cannabinoids: The Current State of Evidence and Recommendations for Research, 2017. Washington, DC: The National Academies Press. Retrieved from: https://doi.org/10.17226/24625

National Center for Complementary and Integrative Health (NCCIH): Accuracy in the media, n.d.a. Retrieved from: https://www.nccih.nih.gov/health/know-science/facts-health-news-stories/page-7.

National Center for Complementary and Integrative Health (NCCIH): Main page, n.d. Retrieved from https://www.nccih.nih.gov/.

National Center for Complementary and Integrative Health (NCCIH): Magnets for pain, 2013. Retrieved from: https://nccih.nih.gov/health/magnet/magnetsforpain.htm.

National Conference of State Legislatures (NCSL): State medical marijuana laws, 2021. Retrieved from: https://www.ncsl.org/research/health/state-medical-marijuana-laws.aspx#2.

National Institute on Drug Abuse (NIDA): What is the scope of marijuana use in the United States?, 2020. Retrieved from: https://www.drugabuse.gov/publications/research-reports/marijuana/what-scope-marijuana-use-in-united-states.

Pa Patients Out of Time, n.d. Retrieved from: http://patientsoutoftime.org/.

Russo EB: Synthetic and natural cannabinoids: the cardiovascular risk, *British J Cardiol* 22(1):7–9, 2015. Retrieved from: https://www.researchgate.net/publication/273203570_Synthetic_and_natural_cannabinoids_The_cardiovascular_risk.

Russo EB: Cannabis therapeutics and the future of neurology. *Front Integr Neurosci* 12:51, 2018. Retrieved from: https://www.frontiersin.org/articles/10.3389/fnint.2018.00051/full.

Russo EB: Cannabis and pain, *Pain Medicine* 20(11):2083-2085, November 2019. https://doi.org/10.1093/pm/pnz227.

U.S. Food and Drug Administration (FDA): FDA approves first drug compromised of an active ingredient derived from marijuana to treat rare, severe forms of epilepsy, 2018. Retrieved from: https://www.fda.gov/news-events/press-announcements/fda-approves-first-drug-comprised-active-ingredient-derived-marijuana-treat-rare-severe-forms

University of Michigan Health System: Guided imagery, 2020. Retrieved from: http://www.uofmhealth.org/health-library/aa84044spec.

Yang, J-M: What is Taijiquan?, 2013. Retrieved from: https://ymaa.com/articles/2013/05/what-is-taijiquan

CHAPTER 21

McCaffery M: Your patient is in pain. Here's how you respond, *Nursing* 32(10):35–2002, 2002.

McCaffery M, Pasero C: In *Pain: clinical management*, ed 3, St. Louis, 2003, Mosby.

Meinhart NT, McCaffery M: *Pain: a nursing approach to assessment and analysis*, New York, 1983, Appleton-Century-Crofts.

Racine M: Chronic pain and suicide risk: A comprehensive review. *Prog Neuropsychopharmacol Biol Psychiatry*. 20;87(Pt B): 269-280, 2018 December. doi: 10.1016/j.pnpbp.2017.08.020. Epub 2017 Aug 26. PMID: 28847525.

The Joint Commission (TJC): Pain management standards for accredited organizations, n.d. Retrieved from: https://www.jointcommission.org/resources/patient-safety-topics/pain-management-standards-for-accredited-organizations./.

U.S. Federal Drug Administration (FDA): Abuse-deterrent opioid analgesics, 2021. Retrieved from: https://www.fda.gov/drugs/postmarket-drug-safety-information-patients-and-providers/abuse-deterrent-opioid-analgesics

CHAPTER 22

Carvalho RLR, Campos CC, Franco LMC, Rocha AM, Ercole FF: Incidence and risk factors for surgical site infection in general surgeries. *Rev Lat Am Enfermagem*. 2017;25:e2848. Published 2017 Dec 4. doi:10.1590/1518-8345.1502.2848.

National Healthcare Safety Network (NHSN): Surgical site infection event (SSI), 2020. Centers for Disease Control and Prevention (CDC). Retrieved from: https://www.cdc.gov/nhsn/pdfs/pscmanual/9pscssicurrent.pdf.

Xue M, Jackson CJ: Extracellular *Matrix Reorganization During Wound Healing and Its Impact on Abnormal Scarring, Adv Wound Care (New Rochelle)* 4(3):119–136, 2015, https://doi.org/10.1089/wound.2013.0485.

CHAPTER 23

Infusion Nurses Society: Infusion nursing standards of practice, *J Infus Nurs* 39(suppl 1), 2016.

Occupational Safety and Health Administration (OSHA): Bloodborne pathogens and needlestick prevention, n.d. Retrieved from: https://www.osha.gov/bloodborne-pathogens.

CHAPTER 24

American Academy of Child & Adolescent Psychiatry (AACAP): TV violence and children, 2014. Fast Facts for Families®, no 13. Retrieved from: http://www.aacap.org/AACAP/Families_and_Youth/Facts_for_Families/FFF-Guide/Children-And-TV-Violence-013.aspx.

American Academy of Child & Adolescent Psychiatry (AACAP): Screen Time and Children, 2020. Fast Facts for Families®, no. 54. Retrieved from: https://www.aacap.org/AACAP/Families_and_Youth/Facts_for_Families/FFF-Guide/Children-And-Watching-TV-054.

American Academy of Pediatric Dentistry: Frequently asked questions, n.d. Retrieved from: http://www.aapd.org/resources/frequently_asked_questions/.

American Academy of Pediatrics (AAP): AAP clinical report highlights early introduction of peanut-based foods to prevent allergies, n.d.a. Retrieved from: https://www.healthychildren.org/English/news/Pages/Early-Introduction-of-Peanut-based-Foods-to-Prevent-Allergies.aspx.

American Academy of Pediatrics (AAP): Infant food and feeding. n.d.b. Retrieved from: https://www.aap.org/en-us/advocacy-and-policy/aap-health-initiatives/HALF-Implementation-Guide/Age-Specific-Content/Pages/Infant-Food-and-Feeding.aspx/.

American Cancer Society (ACS): American Cancer Society recommendations for prostate cancer early detection, 2021a. Retrieved from: https://www.cancer.org/cancer/prostate-cancer/detection-diagnosis-staging/acs-recommendations.html.

American Cancer Society (ACS): American Cancer Society recommendations for the early detection of breast cancer, 2021b. Retrieved from: : https://www.cancer.org/cancer/breast-cancer/screening-tests-and-early-detection/american-cancer-society-recommendations-for-the-early-detection-of-breast-cancer.html.

Centers for Disease Control and Prevention (CDC): Violence prevention: bullying, 2020. Retrieved from: https://www.cdc.gov/violenceprevention/youthviolence/bullyingresearch/fastfact.html.

Centers for Disease Control and Prevention (CDC): Defining childhood overweight & obesity: BMI for children and teens, 2021a. Retrieved from: www.cdc.gov/obesity/childhood/defining.html.

Child Welfare Information Gateway: Foster care statistics 2019, 2021. Number and Trends, Children's Bureau, Administration for Children and Families. U.S. Department of Health and Human Services. Retrieved from: https://www.childwelfare.gov/pubs/factsheets/foster/.

Family Equality Council: LGBTQ family fact sheet, 2017. Retrieved from: https://www2.census.gov/cac/nac/meetings/2017-11/LGBTQ-families-factsheet.pdf.

Fleming S: US life expectancy is falling – here's why, 2020. World Economic Forum. Retrieved from: https://www.weforum.org/agenda/2020/01/us-life-expectancy-decline/.

Generations United: African American grandfamilies: helping children thrive through connection to family and culture, n.d.a. Retrieved from: https://www.gu.org/resources/african-american-grandfamilies-helping-children-thrive-through-connection-to-family-and-culture/.

Generations United: Grandfamilies, n.d.b. Retrieved from: https://www.gu.org/explore-our-topics/grandfamilies/2020/.

Mather M, Jacobsen L, Pollard K: Aging in the United States, *Popul Bull* 70(2):2015. Population Reference Bureau. Retrieved from: https://www.prb.org/wp-content/uploads/2016/01/aging-us-population-bulletin-1.pdf.

Murman DL. The impact of age on cognition. *Semin Hear*. Aug; 36(3):111–121, 2015. Retrieved from: https://www.ncbi.nlm.nih.gov/pmc/articles/PMC4906299/

National Children's Alliance: National statistics on child abuse, n.d. Retrieved from: https://www.nationalchildrensalliance.org/media-room/national-statistics-on-child-abuse/.

Ortaliza J, Ramirez G, Satheeskumar V, Twitter K: *How does U.S. life expectancy compare to other countries? Chart Collections Health & Wellbeing.* 2021. Retrieved from: https://www.healthsystemtracker.org/chart-collection/u-s-life-expectancy-compare-countries/#item-start

Stibich M: What is the genetic theory of aging? How genes affect aging and how you may "alter your genes", 2020. Retrieved from: https://www.verywellhealth.com/the-genetic-theory-of-aging-2224222http://www.acf.hhs.gov/sites/default/files/cb/data_brief_foster_care_trends1.pdf.

US Department of Health and Human Services, Office of Disease Prevention and Health Promotion: Healthy People 2020,

2014. Retrieved from: https://www.healthypeople.gov/2020/About-Healthy-People.

Wang W: The majority of U.S. children still live in two-parent families, 2018. Institute for Family Studies. Retrieved from: https://ifstudies.org/blog/the-majority-of-us-children-still-live-in-two-parent-families.

Zill N: The adoptive difference: new evidence on how adopted children perform in school, 2018. Institute for Family Studies. Retrieved from: https://ifstudies.org/blog/the-adoptive-difference-new-evidence-on-how-adopted-children-perform-in-school.

CHAPTER 25

Aging With Dignity: Five Wishes, n.. Retrieved from: https://agingwithdignity.org/programs/five-wishes/.

Centers for Disease Control and Prevention (CDC): Suicide and self-inflicted injury, 2021. Retrieved from: https://www.cdc.gov/nchs/fastats/suicide.htm.

Death With Dignity: Death with dignity acts, n.d. Retrieved from: https://www.deathwithdignity.org/learn/death-with-dignity-acts/.

Eskanazi Health: No One Dies Alone, 2016. Retrieved from: https://www.eskenazihealth.edu/programs/noda.

Kapel S: Dying boy's letter pleads for empathy, Kansas City, March 8, 1974, *Kansas City Times*.

National Consensus Project for Quality Palliative Care: Clinical Practice Guidelines for Quality Palliative Care, ed 4. Richmond, VA: National Coalition for Hospice and Palliative Care; 2018. Retrieved from: https://www.nationalcoalitionhpc.org/ncp. National Organ Transplantation Act, Public Law 98-507, 10-14, 1984. Retrieved from: https://history.nih.gov/research/downloads/PL98-507.pdf.

NICU Helping Hands, The Angel Gown® Program, n.d. Retrieved from: https://nicuhelpinghands.org/programs/angel-gown-program/.

Now I Lay Me Down to Sleep: Our mission, vision, and reach, n.d. Retrieved from: https://www.nowilaymedowntosleep.org/about-us/our-mission-vision-reach/mission/reach/.

The Oregon Death With Dignity Act, 1997. Retrieved from: http://public.health.oregon.gov/ProviderPartnerResources/EvaluationResearch/DeathwithDignityAct/Documents/statute.pdf.

procin ProCon.org: Opinion Polls/Surveys, 2011. Retrieved from: http://euthanasia.procon.org/view.resource.php?resourceID=000134.

Worden JW: *Grief counseling and grief therapy: a handbook for the mental health practitioner*, ed 4, New York, 2009, Springer.

World Health Organization: Palliative care, n.d. Retrieved from: https://www.who.int/health-topics/palliative-care.

CHAPTER 26

American College of Obstetricians and Gynecologists (ACOG), n.d. Prenatal genetic testing chart. Retrieved from: https://www.acog.org/en/Womens%20Health/Infographics/Prenatal%20Genetic%20Testing%20Chart.

American College of Obstetricians and Gynecologists' Committee on Obstetric Practice, et al: *Methods for estimating the due date*, Committee Opinion, Number 700, 2017.

Davidson M, London M, Ladewig P: *Olds' maternal-newborn nursing and women's health across the lifespan*, ed 9, Upper Saddle River, NJ, 2010, Pearson.

Edgren AR: Hyperemesis gravidarum. In *Gale encyclopedia of medicine*, The Gale Group, Inc, 2008.

Harman CR: Assessment of fetal health. In Creasy RK, Resnik R, Iams JD, editors: *Maternal-fetal medicine: principles principles and practice*, ed 6, Philadelphia, 2008, Saunders.

Hockenberry MJ, Lowdermilk DL, et al.: *Wong's maternal-child nursing care*, ed 8, St. Louis, 2007, Mosby.

Lowdermilk DL, Perry SE, Cashion K, et al.: *Maternal and women's health care*, ed 10, St. Louis, 2012, Mosby.

May KA: Three phases of father involvement in pregnancy, *Nurs Res* 31(6):337–342, 1982.

National Library of Medicine (NLM): Nuchal translucency test, 2020a. Medline Plus. Retrieved from: https://medlineplus.gov/ency/article/007561.htm.

Moldenhauer JS: Postpartum Care, 2020. Merck Manual: Professional edition. Retrieved from: https://www.merckmanuals.com/professional/gynecology-and-obstetrics/postpartum-care-and-associated-disorders/postpartum-care.

National Library of Medicine (NLM): Pica, 2020b. Medline Plus. Retrieved from: https://medlineplus.gov/ency/article/001538.htm.

Perinatology.com: Reference values during pregnancy, 2010. Retrieved from: http://www.perinatology.com/Reference/Reference%20Ranges/Reference%20for%20Serum.htm.

Perry S, Hockenberry M, Lowdermilk D, et al: *Maternal-child nursing care*, ed 5, St. Louis, 2014, Mosby.

CHAPTER 27

Centers for Disease Control and Prevention (CDC): National vital statistics reports: Birth: Final data for 2013. National Vital Stat Rep 64 (1), 2015. Retrieved from: https://www.cdc.gov/nchs/data/nvsr/nvsr64/nvsr64_01.pdf.

DONA International: Benefits of a doula, n.d. Retrieved from: https://www.dona.org/what-is-a-doula/benefits-of-a-doula/.

Lowdermilk DL, Perry SE: In *Maternity and women's health care*, ed 9, St. Louis, 2007, Mosby.

CHAPTER 28

American Academy of Pediatrics (AAP), Task Force on Circumcision: Circumcision policy Statement, 2012. Retrieved from:http://pediatrics.aappublications.org/content/130/3/585.

American Academy of Pediatrics: Swaddling: Is it safe?, 2020. Retrieved from: https://www.healthychildren.org/English/ages-stages/baby/diapers-clothing/Pages/Swaddling-Is-it-Safe.aspx.

Centers for Disease Control and Prevention (CDC): Sudden unexpected infant death and sudden infant death syndrome, 2020. Retrieved from: https://www.cdc.gov/sids/parents-caregivers.htm.

Ferguson H: Planning letter-perfect postpartum care, *Nursing* 17(5):50, 1987.

Gagandeep, Sagar Nidhi, Mamta, Kaur Jasbir: Efficacy of cabbage leaves in relief of breast engorgement among postnatal mothers, 2013, *Int J Nurs Educ* 5(2):76–79, 2013.

Governors Highway Safety Association: Child passenger safety laws, n.d. Retrieved from: http://www.ghsa.org/state-laws/issues/child%20passenger%20safetywww.ghsa.org/html/stateinfo/laws/childsafety_laws.html.

CHAPTER 29

American Cancer Society (ACS): Gestational trophoblastic disease causes, risk faster, and prevention, 2017. Retrieved from: https://www.cancer.org/content/dam/CRC/PDF/Public/8645.00.pdf.

Centers for Disease Control and Prevention (CDC): Infant mortality, 2021. Retrieved from: https://www.cdc.gov/reproductivehealth/maternalinfanthealth/infantmortality.htm

Centers for Disease Control and Prevention (CDC): Reproductive health: Maternal mortality, 2020. Retrieved from: https://www.cdc.gov/reproductivehealth/maternal-mortality/index.html.

Centers for Disease Control and Prevention (CDC): National Center for Health Care Statistics: Multiple births, 2021. Retrieved from: https://www.cdc.gov/nchs/fastats/multiple.htm.

Davidson MC, London ML, Ladewig PW: In *Olds' maternal-newborn nursing & women's health across the lifespan*, ed 9, Upper Saddle River, NJ, 2012, Pearson Prentice Hall.

Johns Hopkins Medicine: Gestational trophoblastic disease, n.d. Retrieved from: https://www.hopkinsmedicine.org/health/conditions-and-diseases/gestational-trophoblastic-disease.

Jones F: Equal access to maternal, prenatal care crucial for mothers, 2020. *Capitol Weekly*. Retrieved from: https://capitolweekly.net/equal-access-to-maternal-prenatal-care-crucial-for-mothers/.

Kamal R, Hudman J, McDermott D: What do we know about infant mortality in the U.S. and comparable countries?, 2019. Peterson-KFF Health System Tracker. Retrieved from: https://www.healthsystemtracker.org/chart-collection/infant-mortality-u-s-compare-countries/#item-start.

Langdon K: Postpartum blues, n.d. Postpartumdepression.org. Retrieved from: https://www.postpartumdepression.org/postpartum-depression/types/blues/.

Lowdermilk DL, Perry SE: In *Maternity and women's health care*, ed 9, St. Louis, 2007, Mosby.

Moore LE: Hydatidiform mole, 2016. Retrieved from: http://emedicine.medscape.com/article/254657-overview#a6.

Office of Minority Health (OMH): Infant mortality and African americans, 2021. U.S. Department of Health and Human Services, Retrieved from: https://www.minorityhealth.hhs.gov/omh/browse.aspx?lvl=4&lvlid=23.

National Library of Medicine (NLM): Choriocarcinoma, 2020. Medline Plus. Retrieved from: https://medlineplus.gov/ency/article/001496.htm.

Osterman MJK, Martin JA: Timing and adequacy of prenatal care in the United State, *National Vital Stat Rep* 67(3):2018, 2016.

Stremick JK, Couperus K, Ashworth SW: Ruptured tubal ectopic pregnancy at fifteen weeks gestational age. *Clin Pract Cases Emerg Med*, 3 (1), 2019. Retrieved from: https://westjem.com/case-report/ruptured-tubal-ectopic-pregnancy-at-fifteen-weeks-gestational-age.html.

CHAPTER 30

American Academy of Child & Adolescent Psychiatry (AACAP): Video games and children: playing with violence, 2015. Fast Facts for Families®, no 91. Retrieved from: https://www.aacap.org/AACAP/Families_and_Youth/Facts_for_Families/FFF-Guide/Children-and-Video-Games-Playing-with-Violence-091.aspx.

Anderson CA, Bushman BJ, Bartholow BD, et al.: Screen violence and youth behavior. *Pediatrics*, 2017. Retrieved from: https://pediatrics.aappublications.org/content/140/Supplement_2/S142

Ballard J: Teens use these social media platforms the most. October 25, 2019. YouGovAmerica. Retrieved from: https://today.yougov.com/topics/lifestyle/articles-reports/2019/10/25/teens-social-media-use-online-survey-poll-youth .

Berchick ER, Mykyta L: Children's public health insurance lower than in 2017, 2019. United States Census Bureau. Retrieved from: https://www.census.gov/library/stories/2019/09/uninsured-rate-for-children-in-2018.html.

Casselbury K: Children with poor nutrition, 2018. SFGate. Retrieved from: https://healthyeating.sfgate.com/children-poor-nutrition-6555.html.

Centers for Disease Control and Prevention (CDC): Childhood overweight and obesity, 2017a. Retrieved from: https://www.cdc.gov/obesity/childhood/index.html.

Centers for Disease Control and Prevention (CDC): National Center for Health Statistics (NCHS): Over half of U.S. teens have had sexual intercourse by age 18, new report shows, 2017b. Retrieved from: https://www.cdc.gov/nchs/pressroom/nchs_press_releases/2017/201706_NSFG.htm

Centers for Disease Control and Prevention (CDC): National Center for Health Statistics (NCHS): Health, United States, 2018 – Data Finder, 2019. Retrieved from: https://www.cdc.gov/nchs/hus/contents2018.htm?search=Vaccination.

Centers for Disease Control and Prevention (CDC): Smoking & tobacco use: electronic cigarettes, 2020a. Retrieved from: https://www.cdc.gov/tobacco/basic_information/e-cigarettes/index.htm .

Centers for Disease Control and Prevention (CDC): Smoking & tobacco use: smokeless tobaccos: health effects, 2020b. Retrieved from: https://www.cdc.gov/tobacco/data_statistics/fact_sheets/smokeless/health_effects/index.htm

Centers for Disease Control and Prevention (CDC): Smoking & tobacco use: youth and tobacco use, 2020c. Retrieved from: https://www.cdc.gov/tobacco/data_statistics/fact_sheets/youth_data/tobacco_use/index.htm

Centers for Disease Control and Prevention (CDC): Prevalence of childhood obesity in the United States, 2021a.Retrieved from: https://www.cdc.gov/obesity/data/childhood.html

Centers for Disease Control and Prevention (CDC): Physical activity: children, 2021b. Retrieved from: https://www.cdc.gov/physicalactivity/basics/children/index.htm.

Centers for Disease Control and Prevention (CDC): Smoking & tobacco use: hookahs, 2020c. Retrieved from: https://www.cdc.gov/tobacco/data_statistics/fact_sheets/tobacco_industry/hookahs/index.htm.

Centers for Disease Control and Prevention (CDC): Vaccines and preventable diseases: HPV vaccine recommendations, 2020d. Retrieved from: https://www.cdc.gov/vaccines/vpd/hpv/hcp/recommendations.html.

Engeln R: Does social media use really cause depression in teens? May 21, 2019. *Psychology Today*. Retrieved from: https://www.psychologytoday.com/us/blog/beauty-sick/201905/does-social-media-use-really-cause-depression-in-teens.

Guttmacher Institute: Adolescent sexual and reproductive health in the United States, 2019. Retrieved from: https://www.guttmacher.org/fact-sheet/american-teens-sexual-and-reproductive-health.

Halbrook YJ, O' Donnell AT: When and how video games can be good: a review of the positive effects of video games on well-being, 2019. Retrieved from: https://journals.sagepub.com/doi/abs/10.1177/1745691619863807

Harvard T.H. Chan School of Public Health: Television watching and sit time, n.d. Retrieved from: https://www.hsph.harvard.edu/obesity-prevention-source/obesity-causes/television-and-sedentary-behavior-and-obesity/.

Herold B: Teen social medica use is skyrocketing. But don't panic, new research says. September 10, 2018. EducationWeek. Retrieved from: https://www.edweek.org/technology/teen-social-media-use-is-skyrocketing-but-dont-panic-new-research-says/2018/09.

Jacobo J: Teens spend more than 7 hours on screens for entertainment a day: report, Oct 29 2019. *ABC News*. Retrieved from: https://abcnews.go.com/US/teens-spend-hours-screens-entertainment-day-report/story?id=66607555/

Juergens J: Health effects of teen substance abuse, 2021. Addiction Center. Retrieved from: https://www.addictioncenter.com/teenage-drug-abuse/health-effects-teen-substance-abuse/.

Let's Move: America's move to raise a healthier generation of kids. Retrieved from: https://letsmove.obamawhitehouse.archives.gov/.

MaineHealth: Let's Go!, n.d. Retrieved from: https://mainehealth.org/lets-go.

News Medical Life Sciences: AAP report addresses new phenomenon, "Facebook depression", 2012. Retrieved from: https://www.news-medical.net/news/20120131/AAP-report-addresses-new-phenomenon-Facebook-Depression.aspx.

Paresky PB: Teen overall drug use is down, but marijuana use is up, December 23, 2017. *Psychology Today*. Retrieved from: https://www.psychologytoday.com/us/blog/happine

ss-and-the-pursuit-leadership/201712/teen-overall-drug-use-is-down-marijuana-use-is.

Riley LK, Rupert J, Boucher O: Nutrition in toddlers, *Am Fam Physician* 98(4):227–233, 2018.

Schaeffer K: Most U.S. teens who use cellphones do it to pass time, connect with others, learn new things, August 23, 2019. Pew Research Center. Retrieved from: https://www.pewresearch.org/fact-tank/2019/08/23/most-u-s-teens-who-use-cellphones-do-it-to-pass-time-connect-with-others-learn-new-things/.

Stopbullying.gov: Facts about bullying, n.d. Retrieved from: https://www.stopbullying.gov/media/facts/index.html#stats.

Unite for Sight: Module 2: Unique barriers to health care for children and adolescents, n.d. Retrieved from: http://www.uniteforsight.org/women-children-course/barriers-children.

U.S. Department of Health and Human Services. Physical Activity Guidelines for Americans, ed 2. Department of Health and Human Services, 2018. Retrieved from: https://health.gov/our-work/physical-activity/current-guidelines.

US Department of Health and Human Services (USDHHS), Office of Disease Prevention and Health Promotion (ODPHP): Healthy People 2030, 2021. Retrieved from: https://health.gov/healthypeople.

US Department of Health and Human Services (USDHHS) and U.S. Department of Agriculture (USDA). 2015–2020 Dietary Guidelines for Americans, ed 8. December 2015. Retrieved from: http://health.gov/dietaryguidelines/2015/guidelines/.

US Food and Drug Administration (FDA): Cervarix, 2019a. Retrieved from: https://www.fda.gov/vaccines-blood-biologics/vaccines/cervarix.

US Food and Drug Administration (FDA): Gardasil, 2019b. Retrieved from: https://www.fda.gov/vaccines-blood-biologics/vaccines/gardasil.

Vaughn E: More LOLs, fewer zzzs: teens may be losing sleep over social media, October 22, 2019. *NPR*. Retrieved from: https://www.npr.org/sections/health-shots/2019/10/22/772415313/more-lols-fewer-zzzs-teens-may-be-losing-sleep-over-social-media.

CHAPTER 31

American Academy of Pediatrics (AAP): Breastfeeding and the use of human milk, *Pediatrics* 129(3):e827–e841, 2012. Retrieved from: http://pediatrics.aappublications.org/content/129/3/e827.full.pdf+html.

American Academy of Pediatric Dentists (AAPD), n.d. Retrieved from: https://www.aapd.org/globalassets/media/policy-center/year1visit.pdf.

American Academy of Pediatrics (AAP): Reduce the risk of SIDS and suffocation, 2017. Retrieved from: https://www.healthychildren.org/English/ages-stages/baby/sleep/Pages/Preventing-SIDS.aspx.

American Nurses Association (ANA): Scope of practice, n.d. Retrieved from: https://www.nursingworld.org/practice-policy/scope-of-practice/.

American Nurses Association (ANA): Nursing's social policy statement, MD, 2003, Silver Springs. Nursesbooks.org.

Centers for Disease Control and Prevention (CDC): Achievements in public health 1990-1999: healthier mothers and babies, *MMWR Morb Mortal Wkly Rep* 48(38):849–858, 1999. Retrieved from: https://www.cdc.gov/mmwr/preview/mmwrhtml/mm4838a2.htm.

Centers for Disease Control and Prevention (CDC): Community water fluoridation, 2020. Retrieved from: https://www.cdc.gov/fluoridation/index.html.

Forum on Child and Family Statistics: America's children at a glance, 2019. Retrieved from: http://childstats.gov/americaschildren/glance.asp.

Healthychildren.org: Cholesterol levels in children and adolescents, 2020. Retrieved from: https://www.healthychildren.org/English/healthy-living/nutrition/Pages/Cholesterol-Levels-in-Children-and-Adolescents.aspx

Hockenberry MJ, Wilson D: In *Wong's nursing care of infants and children*, ed 10, St. Louis, 2015, Mosby.

Leifer G: In *Introduction to maternity and pediatric nursing*, ed 8, St. Louis, 2019, Saunders.

National Institute of Child Health and Human Development (NICHD): What are the recommendations for breastfeeding? n.d. Retrieved from: https://www.nichd.nih.gov/health/topics/breastfeeding/conditioninfo/recommendations.

Office of Population Affairs: Adolescent health, n.d. U.S. Department of Health & Human Services (USDHHS). Retrieved from: https://opa.hhs.gov/adolescent-health?adolescent-development/reproductive-health-and-teen-pregnancy/teen-pregnancy-and-childbearing/trends/index.html.

Robertson J, Robertson J: Separation and the very young, London, 1990, Free Association Books.

Spitz RA: Hospitalism—an inquiry into the genesis of psychiatric conditions in early childhood, *Psychoanal Study Child* 1:53–74, 1945.

Spitz RA: Hospitalism; a follow-up report on investigation described in volume I, 1945, *Psychoanal Study Child* 2:113–117, 1946.

U.S. Department of Health & Human Services (DHHS): *Administration for Children and Families, Administration on Children, Youth and Families*, Children's Bureau, 2020.

Child Maltreatment 2018. Retrieved from: https://www.acf.hhs.gov/cb/research-data-technology/statistics-research/child-maltreatment.

CHAPTER 32

American Association on Intellectual and Developmental Disabilities (AAIDD): Definition of intellectual disability, n.d. Retrieved from: https://www.aaidd.org/intellectual-disability/definition.

American Cancer Society [ACS]: Prognostic factors in childhood leukemia (ALL or AML), 2019. Retrieved from: https://www.cancer.org/cancer/leukemia-in-children/detection-diagnosis-staging/prognostic-factors.html.

American Cancer Society: What are the key statistics about Wilms tumor?, 2020. Retrieved from: https://www.cancer.org/cancer/wilms-tumor/about/key-statistics.html.

American Cancer Society: Key statistics about neuroblastoma, 2021. Retrieved from: https://www.cancer.org/cancer/neuroblastoma/about/key-statistics.html.

American Diabetes Association: Statistics about diabetes, 2018. Retrieved from: https://www.diabetes.org/resources/statistics/statistics-about-diabetes.

Anxiety and Depression Association of America (ADAA): Depression, n.d. Retrieved from: https://adaa.org/understanding-anxiety/depression.

Asthma and Allergy Foundation of America (AAFA): Allergy facts and figures, n.d. Retrieved from: http://www.aafa.org/page/allergy-facts.aspx.

Autism Speaks: What is autism?, n.d. Retrieved from: https://www.autismspeaks.org/what-autism.

Autism Speaks: New meta-analysis confirms: No association between autism and vaccines, 2014. Retrieved from: https://www.autismspeaks.org/science-news/new-meta-analysis-confirms-no-association-between-autism-and-vaccines.

Boston Children's Hospital: Congenital HIV symptoms and causes, n.d. Retrieved from: http://www.childrenshospital.org/conditions-and-treatments/conditions/c/congenital-hiv/symptoms-and-causes.

Centers for Disease Control and Prevention (CDC): Childhood lead poisoning prevention: Children, 2019a. Retrieved from: https://www.cdc.gov/nceh/lead/prevention/children.htm.

Centers for Disease Control and Prevention (CDC): Disease or condition of the week: Cerebral palsy, 2019b. Retrieved from: https://www.cdc.gov/dotw/cerebral-palsy/index.html.

Centers for Disease Control and Prevention (CDC): Attention-deficit/hyperactivity disorder (ADHD): Data and statistics, 2020a. Retrieved from: https://www.cdc.gov/ncbddd/adhd/data.html

Centers for Disease Control and Prevention (CDC): Autism spectrum disorder (ASD): Screening & diagnosis, 2020b. Retrieved from: https://www.cdc.gov/ncbddd/autism/screening.html

Centers for Disease Control and Prevention (CDC): Birth defects: cleft lip/cleft palate, 2020c. Retrieved from: https://www.cdc.gov/ncbddd/birthdefects/cleftlip.html

Centers for Disease Control and Prevention (CDC): Epilepsy: Data and statistics, 2020d. Retrieved from: https://www.cdc.gov/epilepsy/data/index.html.

Centers for Disease Control and Prevention (CDC): Sickle cell disease (SCD): Data and statistics on sickle cell disease, 2020e. Retrieved from: https://www.cdc.gov/ncbddd/sicklecell/data.html.

Centers for Disease Control and Prevention (CDC): Vaccine safety: Autism, 2020f. Retrieved from: https://www.cdc.gov/vaccinesafety/concerns/autism.html.

Centers for Disease Control and Prevention (CDC): Autism Spectrum Disorders, 2020g. Autism Spectrum Disorders. Retrieved from: https://www.cdc.gov/ncbddd/autism/hcp-recommendations.html.

Centers for Disease Control and Prevention (CDC): Birth defects: Down syndrome, 2021a. Retrieved from: https://www.cdc.gov/ncbddd/birthdefects/downsyndrome.html.

Centers for Disease Control and Prevention (CDC): HIV: HIV treatment as prevention, 2021b. Retrieved from: https://www.cdc.gov/hiv/risk/art/index.html.

Centers for Disease Control and Prevention (CDC): HIV: Pregnant women, infants and children, 2021c. Retrieved from: https://www.cdc.gov/hiv/group/gender/pregnantwomen/.

Centers for Disease Control and Prevention (CDC): National Center for Health Statistics: Asthma, 2021d. Retrieved from: https://www.cdc.gov/nchs/fastats/asthma.htm.

CerebralPalsy.org: Treatment for cerebral palsy, n.d. Retrieved from: https://www.cerebralpalsy.org/about-cerebral-palsy/treatment.

Cystic Fibrosis Foundation: About cystis fibrosis, n.d.a. Retrieved from: https://www.cff.org/What-is-CF/About-Cystic-Fibrosis/.

Cystic Fibrosis Foundation: Understanding changes in life expectancy, n.d.b. Retrieved from: https://www.cff.org/Research/Researcher-Resources/Patient-Registry/Understanding-Changes-in-Life-Expectancy/.

Global Down Syndrome Foundation: Fact and FAQs about Down syndrome, 2018. Retrieved from: https://www.globaldownsyndrome.org/about-down-syndrome/facts-about-down-syndrome/.

HIV.gov: What are HIV and AIDS?, 2020. US Department of Health and Human Services (USDHHS). Retrieved from: https://www.hiv.gov/hiv-basics/overview/about-hiv-and-aids/what-are-hiv-and-aids.

Hockenberry MJ, Wilson D: In Wong's nursing care of infants and children, ed 10, St. Louis, 2015, Mosby.

Johns Hopkins Cystic Fibrosis Center: Diagnostic testing, n.d. Retrieved from: https://hopkinscf.wpengine.com/knowledge/diagnostic-testing/#section3.

Maraqa NF: Bronchiolitis, 2021. Medscape. Retrieved from: http://emedicine.medscape.com/article/961963.

March of Dimes: Neural tube defects, 2018. Retrieved from: https://www.marchofdimes.org/complications/neural-tube-defects.aspx.

Marshall BC: Survival trending upward, but what does this really mean? Cystic Fibrosis Foundation, 2017. Retrieved from: https://www.cff.org/CF-Community-Blog/Posts/2017/Survival-Trending-Upward-but-What-Does-This-Really-Mean/.

Mayo Clinic: Autism spectrum disorder, 2018a. Retrieved from: https://www.mayoclinic.org/diseases-conditions/autism-spectrum-disorder/symptoms-causes/syc-20352928.

Mayo Clinic: Congenital heart defects in children, 2018b. Retrieved from: https://www.mayoclinic.org/diseases-conditions/congenital-heart-defects-children/symptoms-causes/syc-20350074.

Mayo Clinic: Iron deficiency in children: prevention tips for parents, 2019. Retrieved from: http://www.mayoclinic.org/healthy-lifestyle/childrens-health/in-depth/iron-deficiency/art-20045634.

Mayo Clinic: Atopic dermatitis (eczema), 2020a. Retrieved from: https://www.mayoclinic.org/diseases-conditions/atopic-dermatitis-eczema/diagnosis-treatment/drc-20353279.

Mayo Clinic: Hemophilia, 2020b. Retrieved from: http://www.mayoclinic.org/diseases-conditions/hemophilia/basics/tests-diagnosis/con-20029824.

Mayo Clinic: Intussusception, 2021. Retrieved from: http://www.mayoclinic.org/diseases-conditions/intussusception/diagnosis-treatment/diagnosis/dxc-20166997.

Medscape: Cerebral palsy medication, 2016. Retrieved from: http://emedicine.medscape.com/article/1179555-medication#2-#4.

Menillo AM, Lee LS, Pearson-Shaver AL. Atrial Septal Defect. [Updated 2020 Nov 25]. In: StatPearls [Internet]. Treasure Island (FL): StatPearls Publishing; 2021 Jan-. Retrieved from: https://www.ncbi.nlm.nih.gov/books/NBK535440/

Munoz FM, Ralston SL, Meissner HC: RSV recommendations unchanged after review of new data, AAP News, October 19, 2017. Retrieved from: http://www.aappublications.org/news/2017/10/19/RSV101917.

My Child Without Limits (MCWL): Down syndrome prognosis, 2018. Retrieved from: http://www.mychildwithoutlimits.org/understand/down-syndrome/down-syndrome-prognosis.

National Asthma Education and Prevention Program, Third Expert Panel on the Diagnosis and Management of Asthma. Expert Panel Report 3: Guidelines for the Diagnosis and Management of Asthma. Bethesda (MD): National Heart, Lung, and Blood Institute (US); 2007 Aug. Retrieved from: https://www.ncbi.nlm.nih.gov/books/NBK7232/.

National Cancer Institute: Childhood Hodgkin lymphoma treatment (PDQ®) – patient version, 2020. National Institutes of Health. Retrieved from: https://www.cancer.gov/types/lymphoma/patient/child-hodgkin-treatment-pdq.

National Center for Education Statistics (NCES): Children and youth with disabilities, 2021. Institute of Education Sciences. Retrieved from: https://nces.ed.gov/programs/coe/indicator/cgg.

National Down Syndrome Society (NDSS): Aging and Down Syndrome, 2017. Retrieved from: https://www.ndss.org/wp-content/uploads/2017/11/Aging-and-Down-Syndrome.pdf.

National Hemophilia Foundation: Blood and blood product safety, n.d.a. Retrieved from: https://www.hemophilia.org/advocacy/federal-priorities/blood-and-blood-product-safety.

National Hemophilia Foundation: Frequently asked questions, n.d.b. Retrieved from: https://www.hemophilia.org/bleeding-disorders-a-z/treatment/future-therapies/frequently-asked-questions.

National Hemophilia Foundation: Hemophilia A , n.d.c. Retrieved from: https://www.hemophilia.org/bleeding-disorders-a-z/types/hemophilia-a.

National Institute of Child Health and Development (NICD): Fast facts about SIDS, 2017. National Institutes of Health. Retrieved from: https://www.nichd.nih.gov/sts/about/SIDS/Pages/fastfacts.aspx.

National Institute of Diabetes and Digestive and Kidney Diseases (NIDDK): Childhood Nephrotic Syndrome. n.d. Retrieved from: https://www.niddk.nih.gov/health-information/kidney-disease/children/childhood-nephrotic-syndrome.

National Institute of Diabetes and Digestive and Kidney Diseases (NIDDK): Type 1 diabetes, n.d. National Institutes of Health. Retrieved from: https://www.niddk.nih.gov/health-information/diabetes/overview/what-is-diabetes/type-1-diabetes.

National Institute of Mental Health: Major depressive disorder in children, n.d. Retrieved from: www.nimh.nih.gov/statistics/1MDD_CHILD.shtml.

National Institute of Neurological Disorders and Stroke (NINDS). Cerebral Palsy: Hope through research. Retrieved from: https://www.ninds.nih.gov/Disorders/Patient-Caregiver-Education/Hope-Through-Research/Cerebral-Palsy-Hope-Through-Research#3104_17.

National Kidney Foundation: Childhood nephrotic syndrome, 2017. Retrieved from: https://www.kidney.org/atoz/content/childns.

National Library of Medicine (NLM): Death among children and adolescents, 2020a. Medline Plus. Retrieved from: https://medlineplus.gov/ency/article/001915.htm.

National Library of Medicine (NLM): Encephalitis, 2020b. Medline Plus. Retrieved from: https://medlineplus.gov/ency/article/001415.htm.

National Marrow Donor Program: Severe aplastic anemia, n.d. Retrieved from: https://bethematch.org/patients-and-families/about-transplant/blood-cancers-and-diseases-treated-by-transplant/severe-aplastic-anemia--saa-/.

National Organization for Rare Disorders (NORD): Hirschsprung disease, 2017. Retrieved from: https://rarediseases.org/rare-diseases/hirschsprungs-disease/.

Saleh M: Your child's rights: 6 principles of IDEA, n.d. Retrieved from: https://www.smartkidswithld.org/getting-help/know-your-childs-rights/your-childs-rights-6-principles-of-idea/.

Schwarz SM: Pediatric gastroesophageal treatment & management, 2019. Medscape. Retrieved from: http://emedicine.medscape.com/article/930029-treatment.

Sheth U, Shirley E, Kay R: Clubfoot (congenital talipes equinovarus), 2021. *Ortho Bullets*. Retrieved from: https://www.orthobullets.com/pediatrics/4062/clubfoot-congenital-talipes-equinovarus.

St. Jude Children's Research Hospital: Acute lymphoblastic leukemia (ALL), n.d. Retrieved from: https://www.stjude.org/disease/acute-lymphoblastic-leukemia-all.html.

UNAIDS: Global HIV & AIDS statistics —fact sheet, n.d. Retrieved from: http://www.unaids.org/en/resources/fact-sheet.

US Department of Health and Human Services (USDHHS), National Institutes of Health (NIH), Office of Dietary Supplements: Iron: Fact sheet for health professionals, 2021. Retrieved from: https://ods.od.nih.gov/factsheets/Iron-HealthProfessional/.

CHAPTER 33

Administration for Community Living (ACL): Services for Native Americans (OAA Title VI), 2020. US Department of Health and Human Services (USDHHS). Retrieved from: https://www.acl.gov/programs/services-native-americans-oaa-title-vi.

Administration for Community Living (ACL): National family caregiver support program, 2021. US Department of Health and Human Services (USDHHS). Retrieved from: https://www.acl.gov/node/314.

American Heart Association: The skinny on fats, 2020. Retrieved from: https://www.heart.org/en/health-topics/cholesterol/prevention-and-treatment-of-high-cholesterol-hyperlipidemia/the-skinny-on-fats

Anthony D, Alosoumi D, Safari R: Prevalence of pressure ulcers in long-term care: A global review, *J Wound Care* 28(11):702, 2019. 209.

Bedinghaus T: An overview of glaucoma, 2020. Retrieved from: https://www.verywellhealth.com/glaucoma-overview-3421722.

Centers for Disease Control and Prevention (CDC): Facts about falls, 2021. Retrieved from: https://www.cdc.gov/falls/facts.html.

Centers for Disease Control and Prevention (CDC): Immunization schedules: Adult immunization schedule, 2021a. Retrieved from: https://www.cdc.gov/vaccines/schedules/hcp/imz/adult.html.

Centers for Disease Control and Prevention (CDC): National Center for Health Statistics: Nursing home case, 2021b. Retrieved from: https://www.cdc.gov/nchs/fastats/nursing-home-care.htm

Collaborative Healthcare Patient Safety Organization (CHPSO): By the numbers: CHPSO pressure injury data, 2017. Retrieved from: https://www.chpso.org/post/numbers-chpso-pressure-injury-data.

Harris-Kojetin L, Sengupta M, Lendon JP, Rome V, Valverde R, Caffrey C. Long-term care providers and services users in the United States, 2015–2016, 2019. National Center for Health Statistics. *Vital Health Stat* 3(43).

Ignatavicius DD, Workman ML, Rebar CR: In *Medical-surgical nursing: concepts for interprofessional collaborative care*, ed 9, St. Louis, 2018, Elsevier.

Ijaopo EO, Ijaopo RO: Tube feeding in individuals with advanced dementia: a review of its burdens and perceived benefits, 2019. *J Aging Res*, 2019, 7272067. Retrieved from: https://www.hindawi.com/journals/jar/2019/7272067/

Keine D, Zelek M, Walker JQ, Sabbagh MN: Polypharmacy in an elderly population: Enhancing medication management through the use of clinical decision support software platforms, *Neurol Ther* 8(1):79–94, 2019.

Mayo Clinic: Calcium and calcium supplements: Achieving the right balance, 2020. Retrieved from: https://www.mayoclinic.org/healthy-lifestyle/nutrition-and-healthy-eating/in-depth/calcium-supplements/art-20047097.

Mayo Clinic: Unexplained weight loss, 2021. Retrieved from: https://www.mayoclinic.org/symptoms/unexplained-weight-loss/basics/definition/sym-20050700.

Meiner SE, Yeager JJ: In *Gerontologic nursing*, ed 6, St. Louis, 2019, Mosby.

Mitchell SL, Mor V, et al: Tube feeding in U.S. nursing home residents with advanced dementia, 2000-2014, *JAMA* 316(7):769–770, 2016. Retrieved from: https://www.ncbi.nlm.nih.gov/pmc/articles/PMC4991625/.

National Eye Institute: Glaucoma, 2020. National Institutes of Health. Retrieved from: https://www.nei.nih.gov/learn-about-eye-health/eye-conditions-and-diseases/glaucoma.

National Institute on Deafness and Other Communication Disorders: Hearing loss and older adults, 2018. National Institutes of Health. Retrieved from: https://www.nidcd.nih.gov/health/hearing-loss-older-adults.

National Library of Medicine (NLM): Aging changes in the senses, 2020. Medline Plus. Retrieved from: https://medlineplus.gov/ency/article/004013.htm .

Office of Disease Prevention and Health Promotion: Development of the National Health Promotion and Disease

Prevention Objectives for 2030, 2021. US Department of Health and Human Services (USDHHS). Retrieved from: https://www.healthypeople.gov/2020/About-Healthy-People/Development-Healthy-People-2030.

Marak C: Assisted living costs: Review the average costs of assisted living by state, n.d. SeniorCare.com. Retrieved from: https://www.seniorcare.com/assisted-living/resources/assisted-living-costs/.

Tan S: Myths of aging, 2011. *Psychology Today*. Retrieved from: https://www.psychologytoday.com/us/blog/wise/201101/myths-aging.

The Heart Foundation: African Americans and heart disease, 2018. Retrieved from: https://theheartfoundation.org/2018/09/07/african-americans-and-heart-disease/.

Touhy T, Jett K: *Ebersole & Hess' toward healthy aging: human needs and nursing response*, ed 10, St. Louis, 2019, Mosby.

US Census Bureau: 65 and older population grows rapidly as baby boomers age, 2020. Retrieved from: https://www.census.gov/newsroom/press-releases/2020/65-older-population-grows.html.

US Department of Health and Human Services (USDHHS): Physical Activity Guidelines for Americans, ed 2, 2018. Retrieved from: https://health.gov/sites/default/files/2019-09/Physical_Activity_Guidelines_2nd_edition.pdf

US Department of Health and Human Services (USDHHS): About the Affordable Care Act, 2021. Retrieved from: www.healthcare.gov/law/timeline/full.html#top

US Department of Health and Human Services (USDHHS) Office of Minority Health: Stroke and African Americans, 2021. Retrieved from: https://www.minorityhealth.hhs.gov/omh/browse.aspx?lvl=4&lvlid=28.

Worldlifeexpectancy.com: United States: Life expectancy, 2018. Retrieved from: https://www.worldlifeexpectancy.com/united-states-life-expectancy.

Witt S, Hoyt J: How much does assisted living and home care cost in the US?, 2021. Retrieved from: https://www.seniorliving.org/assisted-living/costs/

Yap TL, Kennerly SM, Ly K: Pressure injury prevention: Outcomes and challenges to use of resident monitoring technology in a nursing home, 2019. *J Wound Ostomy Continence Nurs*, 46(3), 207-213.

CHAPTER 34

Beers CW: *A mind that found itself*, New York, 1908, Longmans, Green & Co.

National Alliance on Mental Illness (NAMI): Mental health by the numbers, 2019. Retrieved from: https://nami.org/mhstats.

National Alliance on Mental Illness (NAMI): Mental health investment by states slowed in 2014, 2014. Retrieved from: https://www.nami.org/Blogs/NAMI-Blog/December-2014/Mental-Health-Investment-By-States-Slowed-in-2014.

National Institute of Mental Health (NIMH): Mental illness, 2021. Retrieved from: https://www.nimh.nih.gov/health/statistics/mental-illness.

Thornton SP: Sigmund Freud (1856–1939). Internet Encyclopedia of Philosophy, n.d. Retrieved from: www.iep.utm.edu/freud/#H3.

CHAPTER 35

Alzheimer's Association: 2021 Alzheimer's disease facts and figures, 2021. Retrieved from: https://www.alz.org/alzheimers-dementia/facts-figures.

American Psychiatric Association: In *Diagnostic and statistical manual of mental disorders*, ed 5, Arlington, VA, 2013, American Psychiatric Publishing.

Centers for Disease Control and Prevention (CDC): Mental health conditions: depression and anxiety, 2021a. Retrieved from: https://cdc.gov/tobacco/campaign/tips/diseases/depression-anxiety.html.

Centers for Disease Control and Prevention (CDC): National Centers for Health Statistics: Leading causes of death, 2021b. Retrieved from: https://www.cdc.gov/nchs/fastats/leading-causes-of-death.htm.

Maslow AH: *Motivation and personality*, New York, 1970, Harper & Row.

National Eating Disorders Association: Educator toolkit, n.d. Retrieved from: www.nationaleatingdisorders.org/sites/default/files/Toolkits/EducatorToolkit.pdf.

National Institute of Mental Health: Depression, 2018. Retrieved from: https://www.nimh.nih.gov/health/topics/depression/index.shtml.

CHAPTER 36

Centers for Disease Control and Prevention (CDC): Drug overdose: Prescription opioids, 2021a. Retrieved from: https://www.cdc.gov/drugoverdose/deaths/prescription/index.html

Centers for Disease Control and Prevention (CDC): National Center for Health Statistics: Illicit drug use, 2021b. Retrieved from: https://www.cdc.gov/nchs/fastats/drug-use-illicit.htm

National Council on Alcoholism and Drug Dependence, Inc. (NCADD): Facts about alcohol, 2015. Retrieved from: https://www.ncadd.org/about-addiction/alcohol/facts-about-alcohol.

National Institute on Alcohol Abuse and Alcoholism: Alcohol facts and statistics, 2021. Retrieved from: https://www.niaaa.nih.gov/alcohol-health/overview-alcohol-consumption/alcohol-facts-and-statistics.

National Institute of Alcohol Abuse and Alcoholism: Underage drinking, 2021. Retrieved from: https://www.niaaa.nih.gov/publications/brochures-and-fact-sheets/underage-drinking

National Institute on Drug Abuse: Vaping of marijuana on the rise among teens, 2019. Retrieved from: https://www.drugabuse.gov/news-events/news-releases/2019/12/vaping-of-marijuana-on-the-rise-among-teens.

National Institute on Drug Abuse: MDMA (ecstasy/molly) trends & statistics, 2020. Retrieved from: https://www.drugabuse.gov/drug-topics/mdma-ecstasymolly/mdma-ecstasymolly-trends-statistics.

National Institute on Drug Abuse: What is the scope of heroin use in the United States?, 2021. Retrieved from: https://www.drugabuse.gov/publications/research-reports/heroin/scope-heroin-use-in-united-states

Robinson L, Smith M: Underage drinking and teen alcohol use, 2021. Retrieved from: https://www.helpguide.org/articles/addictions/underage-drinking.htm.

CHAPTER 37

Center for Medicare Advocacy: Medicare home health benefit's face-to-face encounter requirement, 2016. Retrieved from: http://www.medicareadvocacy.org/medicare-home-health-benefits-face-to-face-encounter-requirement/

Centers for Medicare & Medicaid Services (CMS): CMS manual system Department of Health & Human Services (DHHS), Pub 100-01, Medicare general information, eligibility, and entitlement, 2015. Retrieved from: www.cms.gov/Regulations-and-Guidance/Guidance/Transmittals/downloads/R68GI.pdf

Centers for Medicare and Medicaid Services (CMS): The home health value-based purchasing (HHVBP) model, 2019. Retrieved from: https://www.cms.gov/Medicare/Quali

ty-Initiatives-Patient-Assessment-Instruments/Value-Based-Programs/Other-VBPs/HHVBP.

Centers for Medicare and Medicaid Services (CMS): MDCR HHA 2. Medicare Home Health Agencies: Persons with Utilization, Total Service Visits, Total Episodes, and Total Program Payments for Original Medicare Beneficiaries, by Demographic Characteristics and Medicare-Medicaid Enrollment Status, Calendar Year 2018, 2020. Retrieved from: https://www.cms.gov/files/document/2018-mdcr-hha-2.pdf.

Centers for Medicare & Medicaid Services (CMS): Home health PPS, 2021. Retrieved from: https://www.cms.gov/medicare/medicare-fee-for-service-payment/homehealthpps.

Federal Interagency Forum on Aging-Related Statistics: Older Americans 2020: key indicators of well-being, 2020. Washington, D.C., United States Government Printing Office. Retrieved from: https://www.agingstats.gov/docs/LatestReport/OA20_508_10142020.pdf.

HealthIT.gov: Health IT and health information exchange basics, 2018. Retrieved from: https://www.healthit.gov/topic/health-it-and-health-information-exchange-basics/health-it-and-health-information-exchange.

HealthIT.gov: Telemedicine and telehealth, 2020. Retrieved from: https://www.healthit.gov/topic/health-it-health-care-settings/telemedicine-and-telehealth.

Medicare.gov: Home health services, n.d.a. Centers for Medicare and Medicaid Services. Retrieved from: https://www.medicare.gov/coverage/home-health-services.html.

Medicare.gov: What's home health care?, n.d.b. Centers for Medicare and Medicaid Services. Retrieved from: https://www.medicare.gov/what-medicare-covers/whats-home-health-care.

Morse, S: Medicare proposed changes would cut home health reimbursement, 2017. *HIMSS Media*. Retrieved from: https://www.healthcarefinancenews.com/news/home-health-agencies-concerned-about-cuts-proposed-medicare-payments.

Nelson R, Staggers N: In *Health informatics: an interprofessional approach*, ed 2., St. Louis, 2017, Mosby.

US Bureau of Labor Statistics: Occupational outlook handbook: occupational therapists, 2021. Retrieved from: https://www.bls.gov/ooh/healthcare/occupational-therapists.htm.

US Government Publishing Office: State Operations Manual Appendix B - Guidance to Surveyors: Home Health Agencies, 2020. Retrieved from: https://www.cms.gov/Regulations-and-Guidance/Guidance/Manuals/downloads/som107ap_b_hha.pdf.

CHAPTER 38

AARP: How continuing care retirement communities work, 2019. Retrieved from: https://www.aarp.org/caregiving/basics/info-2017/continuing-care-retirement-communities.html.

Administration for Community Living: Aging and disability in America, 2020. Retrieved from: https://acl.gov/sites/default/files/Aging%20and%20Disability%20in%20America/2020ProfileOlderAmericans.Final_.pdf.

American Health Care Association (AHCA): Facts & figures, 2020. Retrieved from: https://www.ahcancal.org/Assisted-Living/Facts-and-Figures/Pages/default.aspx.

Centers for Disease Control and Prevention (CDC): Health-related quality of life (HRQOL): HRQOL concepts, 2018. Retrieved from: https://www.cdc.gov/hrqol/concept.htm.\

Centers for Disease Control and Prevention (CDC): National Center for Health Statistics: Residential care communities, 2020. Retrieved from: https://www.cdc.gov/nchs/fastats/residential-care-communities.htm

Centers for Disease Control and Prevention (CDC): National Center for Health Statistics: Nursing home care, 2019. Retrieved from: https://www.cdc.gov/nchs/fastats/nursing-home-care.htm.

Hado E, Komisar H: Long-term services and supports: Fact sheet 648, 2019. AARP Public Policy Institute. Retrieved from: https://www.aarp.org/content/dam/aarp/ppi/2019/08/long-term-services-and-supports.doi.10.26419-2Fppi.00079.001.pdf.

The Joint Commission (TJC): Nursing care center: 2021 national patient safety goals, 2021. Retrieved from: https://www.jointcommission.org/standards/national-patient-safety-goals/nursing-care-center-national-patient-safety-goals/.

LTC Consulting Services: Long-term care statistics you need to know in 2018. Retrieved from: https://www.ltccs.com/blog/long-term-care-statistics-2018/.

Medicare.gov: Compare nursing home quality, n.d.a. Retrieved from: https://www.medicare.gov/what-medicare-covers/what-part-a-covers/compare-nursing-home-quality.

Medicare.gov: Long-term care, n.d.b. Retrieved from: https://www.medicare.gov/coverage/long-term-care.html.

Medicare.gov: PACE, n.d.c. Retrieved from: https://www.medicare.gov/your-medicare-costs/get-help-paying-costs/pace.

Statista: Share of nursing home residents U.S. 2014, by ethnicity, 2016. Retrieved from: https://www.statista.com/statistics/717618/percent-of-nursing-home-residents-in-us-by-ethnicity/.

Statista: U.S. – seniors as a percentage of the population 1950-2050, 2021. Retrieved from: https://www.statista.com/statistics/457822/share-of-old-age-population-in-the-total-us-population/.

US Census Bureau: Quick facts, 2017. Retrieved from: https://www.census.gov/quickfacts/fact/table/US/PST045217.

US Senate Committee on Finance: Emergency support for nursing homes and Elder Justice Reform Act of 2020, Retrieved from: https://www.finance.senate.gov/imo/media/doc/2020-07-01%20Emergency%20Support%20for%20Nursing%20Homes%20and%20Elder%20Justice%20Reform%20Act%20Section-by-Section%20Summary2.pdf.

Witt S, Hoyt J: Aging in place – What does aging in place really mean?, 2021. Retrieved from: https://www.seniorliving.org/aging-in-place/.

CHAPTER 39

ADA National Network: What is the definition of disability under the ADA?, 2021. Retrieved from: https://adata.org/faq/what-definition-disability-under-ada.

American Association of Physiatrists: About the AAP, 2013. Retrieved from: www.physiatry.org.

American Heart Association (AHA): What is cardiac rehabilitation?, 2016. Retrieved from: https://www.heart.org/en/health-topics/cardiac-rehab/what-is-cardiac-rehabilitation.

American Lung Association: How pulmonary rehab helps you breathe, 2016. Retrieved from: http://www.lung.org/about-us/blog/2016/03/pulmonary-rehab-helps-breathe.html.

American Psychiatric Association (APA): *Diagnostic and statistical manual of mental disorders*, ed 3, Washington, D.C., 1980, American Psychiatric Press.

Anxiety & Depression Association of America (ADAA): How to prevent trauma from becoming PTSD, 2017. Retrieved from: https://adaa.org/learn-from-us/from-the-experts/blog-posts/consumer/how-prevent-trauma-becoming-ptsd.

Association of Rehabilitation Nurses: Certified rehabilitation registered nurse: Examination candidate handbook, 2021. Retrieved at: https://rehabnurse.org/uploads/certification/2021_CRRN_Handbook_March_-_ONLINE.pdf

Bamm EL, Rosenbaum P: Family-centered theory: origins, development, barriers, and supports to implementation in rehabilitation medicine, *Arch Phys Med Rehab* 89(8):1618–1624, 2008.

Barclay W: *Letters to the hebrews (the new daily study bible)*, London, 1976, Westminster John Knox Press.

Centers for Disease Control and Prevention (CDC): Explosion and blast injuries: a primer for clinicians, n.d. Retrieved from: https://www.cdc.gov/masstrauma/preparedness/primer.pdf.

Centers for Disease Control and Prevention (CDC): Health and economic costs of chronic disease, 2018. Retrieved from: https://www.cdc.gov/chronicdisease/about/costs/index.htm

Centers for Disease Control and Prevention (CDC): National Center for Chronic Disease Prevention and Health Promotion (NCCDPHP), 2021. Retrieved from: https://www.cdc.gov/chronicdisease/index.htm

Clark CC: Posttraumatic stress disorder: how to support healing, *Am J Nurs* 97(8):27–33, 1997.

Glass AJ: Introduction. In Bourne PG, editor: *The psychology and physiology of stress*, New York, 1969, Academic Press.

Mayo Clinic: Post-traumatic stress disorder (PTSD), 2018. Retrieved from: https://www.mayoclinic.org/diseases-conditions/post-traumatic-stress-disorder/symptoms-causes/syc-20355967.

National Rehabilitation Information Center (NARIC): Can a chronic disease diagnosis motivate healthy lifestyle changes? 2016. Retrieved from: http://www.naric.com/?q=en/rif/can-chronic-disease-diagnosis-motivate-healthy-lifestyle-changes.

Pennardt A: Blast injuries, 2016. Medscape Retrieved from: http://emedicine.medscape.com/article/822587-overview.

Rosenfeld JV, Ford NL. Bomb blast, mild traumatic brain injury and psychiatric morbidity: a review. *Injury*. 2010 May;41(5):437-443. doi: 10.1016/j.injury.2009.11.018. Epub 2010 Feb 26. PMID: 20189170.

Tan DK: Blast injuries: 4 types EMS providers need to know, 2021. EMS1. Retrieved from: https://www.ems1.com/ems-training/articles/blast-injuries-4-types-ems-providers-need-to-know-kZROn8iPonrbJBYn/.

US Department of Health and Human Services: Office of Disease Prevention and Health Promotion: Healthy People 2030, n.d. Retrieved from: https://health.gov/healthypeople/objectives-and-data/browse-objectives#health-conditionsUS Department of Veterans

Affairs: Polytrauma/TBI system of care, 2021a. Retrieved from: https://www.polytrauma.va.gov/index.asp.

US Department of Veterans Affairs: PTSD: National Center for PTSD, 2021b. Retrieved from: https://www.ptsd.va.gov/.

CHAPTER 40

Gordon A: End of life issues, *Caring* 20(21):6, 2001.

Medicare.gov: Your Medicare coverage: hospice and respite care, n.d. Retrieved from: https://www.medicare.gov/coverage/hospice-and-respite-care.html.

Morrow A: The 4 common myths about hospice, 2020a. Retrieved from: https://www.verywellhealth.com/hospice-myths-1132617.

Morrow A: How to become a hospice volunteer, 2020b. Retrieved from: https://www.verywellhealth.com/lend-a-caring-hand-1132290.

Morrow A: How to manage dyspnea in dying patients, 2020c. Retrieved from: https://www.verywellhealth.com/dyspnea-in-the-dying-1132408.

National Hospice and Palliative Care Organization (NHPCO): Facts and figures: Hospice care in America, 2020. Retrieved from: https://www.nhpco.org/wp-content/uploads/NHPCO-Facts-Figures-2020-edition.pdf.

National Palliative Care Research Center: Guidelines for using the Edmonton Symptom Control Assessment (ESAS), n.d. Retrieved from: http://www.npcrc.org/files/news/edmonton_symptom_assessment_scale.pdf.

National POLST: National POLST maps, n.d. Retrieved from: http://polst.org/programs-in-your-state/.

SSM Health: Early admission to hospice can improve quality of life, 2018. Retrieved from: https://www.ssmhealth.com/blogs/ssm-health-matters/july-2018/early-admission-to-hospice-can-improve-quality.

Vidal M, Hui D, Williams J, Bruera E: A perspective study of hypodermoclysis performed by caregivers in the home setting, *J Pain Symptom Manage*, 2016;October 4.

World Health Organization (WHO): Palliative care, 2020. Retrieved from: https://www.who.int/news-room/fact-sheets/detail/palliative-care.

CHAPTER 41

Agency for Healthcare Research and Quality (AHRQ): Nurse bedside shift report training, n.d. Retrieved from: https://www.ahrq.gov/sites/default/files/wysiwyg/professionals/systems/hospital/engagingfamilies/strategy3/Strat3_Tool_3_Pres_video_508.pdf.

American Nurses Association (ANA): *Nursing informatics: Scope and standards of practice*, Silver Springs, Md, 2008, Author.

American Nurses Association (ANA) and National Council on State Boards of Nursing (NCSBN): Joint statement on delegation, n.d. Retrieved from: https://www.ncsbn.org/Delegation_joint_statement_NCSBN-ANA.pdf.

Association of Rehabilitation Nurses: History of rehabilitation nursing, n.d. Retrieved from: https://rehabnurse.org/about/history.

Chron: Can an LPN be a nurse manager?, 2020. Retrieved from: http://work.chron.com/can-lpn-nurse-manager-13874.html.

Cottingham S, Dibartolo MC, Battistoni S, et al.: Partners in nursing: a mentoring initiative to enhance nurse retention, *Nurs Educ Perspect* 32(4):250–255, 2011.

Flores-Harris, M: A radical change in the nursing board exams, 2019. Medscape. Retrieved from: https://www.medscape.com/viewarticle/917116.

Hill S, Howlett H: In *Success in practical/vocational nursing*, ed 7, St. Louis, 2013, Mosby.

Ketola J: An analysis of a mentoring program for baccalaureate nursing students: does the past still influence the present? *Nurs Forum* 44(4):245–255, 2009.

Maslach C, Jackson SE: In *Burnout inventory manual*, ed 2, Palo Alto, CA, 1986, Consulting Psychologists Press.

NSI Nursing Solutions: 2021 NSI national health care retention and RN staffing report, 2021. Retrieved from: https://www.nsinursingsolutions.com/Documents/Library/NSI_National_Health_Care_Retention_Report.pdf.

Rehab Center: Nurses and addiction: A quiet epidemic, 2019. Retrieved from: https://www.rehabcenter.net/nurses-and-addiction/.

RN.org: Clinical supervision: Leadership styles, 2019. Retrieved from: https://www.rn.org/courses/coursematerial-252.pdf.

US Bureau of Labor Statistics: Occupational outlook handbook: Licensed practical and licensed vocational nurses, 2021. Retrieved from: https://www.bls.gov/ooh/healthcare/licensed-practical-and-licensed-vocational-nurses.htm#tab-3.

US Department of Veterans Affairs: Nursing, n.d. Retrieved from: https://www.vacareers.va.gov/Careers/Nursing.

Glossary

A

abduction Movement of an extremity away from the midline of the body.

ableism Discrimination and prejudice toward people with disabilities where the person is defined by their disabilities and preference is giving to people without disabilities.

abortion Loss of a pregnancy before 20 weeks' gestation.

abuse Misuse, as of an addictive substance such as alcohol, tobacco, nicotine, and so forth.

abuse deterrent Medications have properties that allow the management of pain but also have properties limit their use for abusive purposes.

accountability Being answerable for one's own actions.

accreditation Process whereby a professional association or nongovernmental agency grants recognition to an institution or agency for demonstrated ability in a special area of practice.

acid-base balance Homeostasis of the hydrogen ion (H^+) concentration in the body fluids.

acquired heart disorder Abnormality occurring after birth that compromises heart function.

acquired immunodeficiency syndrome (AIDS) Acquired condition that impairs the body's ability to fight infection; the end stage of the continuum of HIV infection, in which the infected person has a CD_4^+ (lymphocyte) count of ≤200 cells/ mm^3.

acrocyanosis Peripheral cyanosis; the blue discoloration of the hands and feet in most infants at birth that sometimes persists for 7 to 10 days.

active listening Giving full attention and a concerted effort to understand the message being sent.

active transport The movement of materials across the cell membrane by means of chemical activity (the energy of metabolism), which allows the cell to admit molecules larger than would otherwise be able to enter.

activities of daily living (ADLs) Those activities of daily life, such as toileting, bathing, dressing, and grooming, that promote maintenance of functional abilities and independence in the environment.

actual nursing diagnosis Statement of a health problem that a nurse is licensed and competent to treat.

acupressure Complementary and alternative therapy that uses gentle pressure at points on the body; used primarily to prevent and relieve symptoms of muscle tension.

acupuncture Complementary and alternative therapy that stimulates certain points on the body by the insertion of special needles to modify the perception of pain, normalize physiologic functions, and to treat or prevent disease.

acute Having a short and relatively severe course; a disease process characterized by a relatively short duration of signs and symptoms that are usually severe and begin abruptly.

acute pain Intense, unpleasant sensation of short duration, lasting less than 6 months.

adaptation Adjustment to changing life situations by using various strategies.

adaptive immunity Protection that provides a specific reaction to each invading antigen and has the unique ability to remember the antigen that caused the attack.

addiction Excessive use or abuse of a substance or practice, displayed by psychological disturbance, decline of social and economic function, and uncontrollable consumption, indicating dependence.

addictive personality One who exhibits a pattern of compulsive and habitual use of a substance or practice to cope with psychological pain from conflict and anxiety.

adduction Movement of an extremity toward the axis of the body.

adenosine triphosphate A substance produced in the mitochondria from nutrients and capable of releasing energy that in turn enables the cell to work.

adjuvant Additional, as in additional drug or treatment.

admission Entry of a patient into a health care facility.

adoptive family Family unit with adoptive children who are chosen and taken into the family by legal process and raised as the family's own.

adult daycare A community-based program designed to meet the needs of functionally or cognitively impaired adults through an individualized plan of care.

advance directives Signed and witnessed documents providing specific instructions for health care treatment in the event that the individual is unable to make those decisions personally at the time they are needed.

advancement Rise in rank or importance; a promotion, progress, improvement.

adverse drug reaction A harmful, unintended reaction to a drug administered at a normal dosage.

advocate A person who acts on behalf of another person.

affect External manifestation of inner feeling or emotions, often reflected by facial expression.

against medical advice (AMA) Charting notation when a patient leaves a health care facility without a physician's order for discharge.

age in place Seniors remaining in their desired home setting as they age.

ageism Process of systematic stereotyping of and discriminating against people because of their advanced age.

aggressive communication Interacting with another in an overpowering and forceful manner to meet one's own needs at the expense of others.

agonist Drug that produces a predictable response at the intended site of action.

agoraphobia An anxiety disorder characterized by a fear of being in an open, crowded, or public place such as a field, tunnel, bridge, congested streets, or busy stores, where escape may be difficult or help unavailable if anxiety incapacitates the person. If untreated, the individual often refuses to leave the home.

air embolism A blockage or obstruction in a vessel caused by a bubble of air.

akinesia Abnormal state of motor and psychic hypoactivity.

Alcoholics Anonymous (AA) Nonprofit organization founded in 1935, consisting of abstinent alcoholics helping other alcoholics to become and stay sober through group support.

alcoholism Addiction to alcohol.

alignment Relationship of various body parts to one another.

allergen A substance that can produce a hypersensitive reaction in the body but is not necessarily inherently harmful.

allopathic medicine Traditional or conventional Western medicine.

allow natural death *See* do-not-resuscitate.

alopecia Loss of hair resulting from destruction of hair follicles.

alpha-fetoprotein (AFP) Antigen present in the human fetus; can be used to evaluate fetal development.

altered cognition A decrease or lack of cognitive ability to receive, process, and send information.

alternative therapies Nontraditional therapies that may include the same interventions as complementary therapies but that often become the primary treatment modalities that replace allopathic (traditional) medicine. Examples are exercise, massage, acupuncture, and herbalism.

Alzheimer's disease A presenile dementia characterized by confusion, memory failure, disorientation, restlessness, agnosia, speech disturbances, inability to carry out purposeful movements, and hallucinosis. Also called *senile dementia— Alzheimer's type (SDAT)*.

amblyopia Lazy eye; reduction or dimness of vision, especially when there is no apparent pathologic condition of the eye.

amino acids Building blocks out of which proteins are constructed; the end products of protein digestion.

amniocentesis Obstetric procedure in which a small amount of amniotic fluid is removed for laboratory analysis; usually performed between the 16th and 20th weeks of gestation to aid in the diagnosis of fetal abnormalities.

amniotomy Artificial rupture of the fetal membranes (AROM).

amotivational cannabis syndrome Follows the use of cannabis and is characterized by decreased goal-directed activities, abrupt mood swings, abnormal irritability, etc.

anabolism The building aspect on which the energy released from catabolism allows the cells to build more complex, usable forms of nutrients; the building and repairing phase of metabolism; opposite of catabolism.

anaphylactic shock Severe, life-threatening hypersensitivity reaction to a previously encountered antigen.

anasarca Severe, generalized edema.

anion Negatively charged ion that, when in solution, is attracted to the positive electrode.

anorexia nervosa A psychoneurotic disorder characterized by a prolonged refusal to eat; self-imposed starvation.

antagonist Drug that will block the action of another drug.

antepartal First stage of the maternity cycle. Also called the *prenatal* or *antenatal* period.

anterior fontanelle A diamond-shaped space covered by tough membranes between the bones of an infant's cranium. The posterior fontanelle is triangular.

anticipatory grief Expectation of or preparation for the loss of one or more valued or significant others; accomplishment of part of the grief work before the actual loss occurs.

anticipatory guidance Psychological preparation of a patient for an event expected to be stressful, such as preparing a child for surgery by explaining what will happen and what it will feel like. It is also used to prepare parents for normal growth and development of their children.

antigen A substance recognized by the body as foreign that can trigger an immune response.

antioxidant Chemical or other agent that delays or prevents the breakdown of a substance by oxygen.

antiseptic A substance that tends to inhibit the growth and reproduction of microorganisms; may be used on humans.

anxiety Condition in which an individual experiences a vague feeling of apprehension resulting from a real or perceived threat to the self.

aphasia Abnormal neurologic condition in which language function is defective or absent because of an injury to certain areas of the cerebral cortex.

apical pulse Heartbeat as measured with the bell or disk of the stethoscope placed over the apex of the heart; represents the actual beating of the heart. Most authentic of all pulses.

apnea The absence of breathing.

approved program Program that meets minimum standards established by the state agency responsible for overseeing education programs.

aromatherapy An alternative therapy that uses essential oils produced from plants to provide health benefits.

articulate Speaking clearly, distinctly, and to the point; presenting yourself with clarity and effectiveness.

as necessary (prn) The completion of activities as the condition demands; as needed.

ascites An accumulation of fluid and albumin in the peritoneal cavity.

asepsis Free of pathogenic microorganisms.

assertive communication Interaction that takes into account the feelings and needs of the receiver.

assessment Evaluation or appraisal of a condition; includes observing, gathering, verifying, and communicating pertinent data, usually information about the patient.

assisted living Residential care whereby the adult patient rents a small one-bedroom or studio apartment and can receive personal care services such as assistance with bathing, dressing, eating, etc.

asterixis Hand-flapping tremor usually induced by extending the arm and dorsiflexing the wrist; frequently seen in patients who are in a hepatic coma.

ataxia Abnormal condition characterized by impaired ability to coordinate movement.

atelectasis Collapse of lung tissues, preventing the respiratory exchange of carbon dioxide and oxygen.

atony Lack of normal tone or strength.

attention deficit/hyperactivity disorder (ADHD) A group of behaviors—hyperactivity, inattentiveness, and impulsivity— that appear early in a child's life, persist throughout childhood and adolescence, and may extend into adulthood.

attenuation The process of weakening the degree of virulence of a disease organism.

attitude In obstetrics, the relationship of fetal body parts to one another.

auditors People appointed to examine patient charts and health records to assess the quality of care.

auscultate/auscultation To listen for sounds within the body to evaluate the condition of the heart, lungs, pleura, intestines, or other organs or to detect fetal heart sounds.

autism A complex developmental disorder of brain function accompanied by a broad range of severity of intellectual and behavioral deficits that impairs the child's ability for appropriate social interaction, communication skills, and behavior.

autocratic family pattern Family unit with unequal relationships; parents attempt to control with strict, rigid rules and expectations.

autoimmune/autoimmunity Immune response (autoantibodies or cellular immune response) to one's own tissues.

autologous Something that has its origin within an individual, especially a factor present in tissues or fluids.

autolysis Self-dissolution or self-digestion in tissues or cells by enzymes in the cells.

autopsy Examination performed after a person's death to confirm or determine the cause of death.

axilla Underarm area or armpit.

B

baby boomers The segment of the population who were born between 1945 and 1964.

ballottement Technique of palpating an organ or floating structure by bouncing it gently and feeling it rebound. Ballottement of a fetus within the uterus is a probable objective sign of pregnancy.

bandage A strip or roll of cloth or other material that may be wound around part of the body in a variety of ways for multiple purposes.

basal metabolic rate (BMR) Amount of energy used by the body at rest to maintain vital functions such as respiration, circulation, temperature, peristalsis, and muscle tone.

base of support Area on which an object rests; a stance with feet slightly apart.

basic life support (BLS) The role of cardiopulmonary resuscitation (CPR) and emergency cardiac care (ECC) to preserve circulatory or respiratory function or both in the emergency treatment of a victim of cardiac or respiratory arrest.

bedpan Device for receiving feces or urine from a patient who is confined to bed; may be used for specimen collection.

behavior Manner in which a person acts or performs. Any or all of the activities of a person, including physical actions, that are observed directly, and mental activity that is inferred and interpreted. Kinds of behavior include abnormal, automatic, invariable, and variable.

benign Not recurrent or progressive; opposite of malignant.

bereavement Common depressed reaction to the death of a loved one.

bereavement overload The individual's experience of an initial loss compounded with an additional loss before resolution of the initial loss.

bicarbonate A main anion of the extracellular fluid.

binder Bandage made of large pieces of material to fit a specific body part (e.g., abdominal or breast binder).

biofeedback A technique that is nonpharmacological and noninvasive used to control body responses.

biographic data The facts and events of a person's life.

biologic death Results from permanent cellular damage caused by a lack of oxygen.

biomedical health belief system A belief that health and illness are controlled by a series of physical and biochemical processes that can be analyzed and manipulated by humans. Primary health belief in the United States.

biopsy The removal of a small piece of living tissue from an organ or another part of the body for microscopic examination to confirm or establish a diagnosis, estimate a prognosis, or follow the course of a disease.

bioterrorism Use of biologic agents to create fear and threat in a terrorist act.

birth defect (congenital anomaly) Any abnormality present at birth, particularly a structural one that may be inherited genetically, acquired during gestation, or inflicted during parturition (process of giving birth).

bladder training Development of the use of the muscles of the perineum to improve voluntary control over voiding.

blastocyst Embryonic form that is a spherical mass of cells having a central fluid-filled cavity (blastocele) surrounded by two layers of cells; the outer layer forms the placenta, and the inner layer later forms the embryo.

blended (reconstituted) family Family unit formed by parents who bring unrelated children from prior marriages into a new joint living situation. Also called a *stepfamily.*

blood buffers Compounds that work to enable the body to maintain homeostasis in the body's pH. These compounds include carbon dioxide, carbonic acid, and bicarbonate acid.

blood pressure Pressure exerted by the circulating volume of blood on the arterial walls, veins, and chambers of the heart.

body mass index (BMI) An estimate used to determine if a person may be at health risk because of excessive weight.

body mechanics Physiologic study of the muscular actions and the functions of muscles in maintaining the posture of the body.

body surface area (BSA) Total area exposed to the outside environment.

bonding *See* parent-child attachment. Emotional attachment between parent and child.

borborygmi Loud, gurgling sounds that accompany increased motility of the bowel.

botulism An often fatal food poisoning that results from ingestion of the toxin produced by the bacillus *Clostridium botulinum.*

bradycardia Slow cardiac rhythm characterized by a pulse rate of fewer than 60 beats per minute.

bradypnea A slow respiratory rate of fewer than 12 breaths per minute.

brain death Irreversible form of unconsciousness characterized by a complete loss of brain function while the heart continues to beat. The legal definition of this condition varies from state to state.

Braxton Hicks contractions Irregular tightening of the pregnant uterus that begins in the first trimester and increases in frequency, duration, and intensity as pregnancy progresses. Near term, strong Braxton Hicks contractions are often difficult to distinguish from real labor.

brown fat Source of heat unique to the neonate; it is capable of greater thermogenic (heat-producing) activity than ordinary fat. Deposits are formed around the adrenal glands, kidneys, and neck; between scapulas; and behind the sternum, and they remain for several weeks after birth.

bruit Abnormal swishing sound heard over organs, glands, and arteries.

bruxism Teeth grinding.

buccal In or directed toward the cheek.

buffer Chemical compound that neutralizes excess acids or bases by contributing or accepting hydrogen ions to form a weaker acid or base; can be considered chemical sponges.

bulimia nervosa An eating disorder involving an insatiable craving for food, often resulting in continual eating followed by periods of depression, self-deprivation, and/or purging. Also called *bulimia.*

burnout Physical, emotional, and spiritual exhaustion among caregivers.

burping Belching or eructation.

C

CABs Mnemonic for assessing status of an emergency patient: Circulation, Airway, Breathing; used in one- or two-rescuer CPR.

cachexia General ill health and malnutrition marked by weakness and emaciation; usually associated with a serious disease such as cancer.

calcium Silvery yellow metal; the most abundant mineral in the body; a positively charged ion, called a cation.

cannabidiol A cannabis compound purported to have anti-inflammatory effects.

cannabinoid Compounds found in marijuana. There are more than 60 of these compounds. It is responsible for the feelings of being "high" that are associated with the use of marijuana.

cannabis Marijuana.

canthus Angle at the medial and lateral margins of the eyelid (inner and outer corners of the eye).

carcinogen Substance known to increase the risk for the development of cancer.

carcinoma The term used for a malignant tumor composed of epithelial cells; it displays a tendency to metastasize.

cardiac arrest Sudden cessation of functional circulation.

cardinal movements of labor Seven movements in sequence that the fetus undergoes in the process of labor, delivery and birth. These movements include engagement, descent, flexion, internal rotation, extension, externa rotation and expulsion.

cardiopulmonary resuscitation (CPR) Basic emergency procedure for life support, consisting of artificial respiration and manual external cardiac massage.

career A profession for which one trains and is undertaken as a permanent calling.

carrier Person or animal who harbors and spreads an organism, causing disease in others but does not itself become ill.

case management The assignment of a health care provider to oversee the case of an individual patient.

catabolism Breakdown or destructive phase of metabolism. Catabolism occurs when complex body substances are broken down to simpler ones; opposite of anabolism.

catheterization Introduction of a rubber or plastic tube through the urethra and into the bladder.

cation Positively charged ion that, when in solution, is attracted to the negatively charged electrode.

cellular immunity Acquired immunity characterized by the dominant role of small T lymphocytes. Also called *cell-mediated immunity.*

Centers for Disease Control and Prevention (CDC) Federal agency that provides facilities and services for investigation, identification, prevention, and control of disease; headquartered in Atlanta, Georgia.

cephalocaudal Growth and development that proceeds from the head toward the feet. The infant's head is large compared with the rest of the body.

cephalopelvic disproportion The head of the fetus is larger than the pelvic outlet. Also called *pelvic disproportion.*

cerclage Technique that uses suture material to constrict the internal os of the cervix. Aids in preserving the pregnancy.

certification Process in which an individual or institution, agency, or educational program is evaluated and recognized as meeting certain predetermined standards.

cerumen Yellowish or brownish waxy secretion produced by vestigial apocrine sweat glands in the external ear canal; earwax.

chart (health care record) Legal record that is used to meet many demands of the health accreditation, medical insurance, and legal systems.

charting Process of recording information on a patient's chart.

charting by exception Recording only new data or changes in patient status or care; charting the exceptions to the previously recorded data.

charting, documenting, or recording Process of noting data in a patient record, usually at prescribed intervals.

chelation therapy In toxicology, use of a compound to group a toxic substance and make it inactive and thus nontoxic. Chelating agents are used in the treatment of metal poisoning.

chevron A method of applying tape to secure an intravenous line; a narrow piece (0.5-inch wide) of sterile tape is placed under the hub of the catheter with adhesive side up and then crisscrossed over the hub to form an inverted V. This method is no longer frequently used.

Cheyne-Stokes respiration An abnormal pattern of respiration characterized by alternating periods of apnea and deep, rapid breathing.

child maltreatment Physical and emotional neglect, and physical, emotional, and sexual abuse of children.

children with special needs Infants and children with congenital abnormalities, malignancies, gastrointestinal diseases, and central nervous system anomalies.

chiropractic therapy Nontraditional therapy that includes manipulation of the musculoskeletal system.

chloride Negatively charged extracellular anion; a salt of hydrochloric acid.

cholesterol Fat-soluble sterol found in animal fats and oils, organ meats, and egg yolk.

chorionic villi Tiny vascular protrusions of the chorionic surface that project into the maternal blood sinuses of the uterus and help form the placenta. This occurs when conception has occurred.

chorionic villus sampling Aspiration of a small amount of tissue from the placenta to test for genetic disorders of the fetus.

chromosomes Threadlike structures in the nucleus of a cell that function in the transmission of genetic information.

chronic Developing slowly and persisting for a long period, often for the remainder of an individual's life.

chronic illness An irreversible presence, accumulation, or latency of disease states or impairments that involve the total human environment for supportive care, function, and prevention of further disability.

chronic pain Pain lasting longer than 6 months; can be as intense as acute pain; can be continuous or intermittent.

chronologic age Age of an individual expressed as time elapsed since birth.

Chux Waterproof, disposable underpad.

circumcision Surgical procedure in which a part of the foreskin is removed, leaving the glans penis uncovered.

circumorbital Around an orbit; often referring to the eye.

clarifying Restating the patient's message in a manner that asks the patient to verify that the message received is accurate.

claudication Weakness of the legs accompanied by cramp-like pain in the calves caused by poor circulation of the blood to the leg muscles.

clinical death Occurs when heartbeat and respiration have ceased.

clinical pathway Multidisciplinary plan that schedules clinical interventions over an anticipated time frame for a high-risk, high-volume, high-cost type of case.

closed posture A formal, distant body position, generally with the arms and possibly the legs tightly crossed.

closed question Focused question that seeks a particular answer (e.g., yes or no).

club drugs Drugs taken for euphoric effect at parties, concerts, dance clubs, and raves.

code System of notification that allows information to be transmitted rapidly.

cognitive impairment Significantly subaverage general intellectual functioning; existing concurrently with deficits in adaptive behavior and manifested during developmental period (formerly referred to as mental retardation).

cohabitation *See* social contract family.

collaborative problem Actual or potential health problem (complication) that focuses on the pathophysiologic response of the body for which nurses are responsible and accountable for identification and treatment in collaboration with the physician.

collagen Fibrous, insoluble protein found in connective tissue, including skin, bone, and ligaments.

colostomy A procedure in which the large intestine is brought through the abdominal wall for evacuation of stool.

colostrum Breast fluid that may be excreted from the second trimester of pregnancy onward but is most evident in the first 2 or 3 days after birth and before the onset of true lactation. This thin, yellowish fluid is rich in proteins and calories in addition to antibodies and lymphocytes.

Commission on Accreditation of Rehabilitation Facilities (CARF) A not-for-profit, private, international standards–setting and accreditation body. Its mission is to promote and advocate delivery of quality rehabilitation. It is governed by a board of trustees who are responsible for accreditation decisions. Surveyors are peers involved in administrative or professional positions within an organization that is eligible for CARF accreditation.

communication Use of words and behaviors to construct, send, and interpret messages.

compartment syndrome Pathologic condition caused by progressive development of arterial compression and reduced blood supply to an extremity. Increased pressure from external devices (casts, bulky dressings) causes decreased blood flow, resulting in ischemic tissue necrosis; most often occurs in the extremities.

compatibility Quality or state of existing together in harmony.

complementary therapies/complementary and alternative therapies Therapies that are used in addition or as a complement to nontraditional therapies. Examples are exercise, massage, reflexology, acupuncture, and herbalism.

complicated grieving *See* dysfunctional grieving.

comprehensive rehabilitation plan An overall individualized plan of care that is initiated within 24 hours of admission and ready for review and revision by the team within 3 days of admission for each individual; a planned, orderly sequence of services for a disabled individual designed to help the patient realize maximum potential.

compress A soft pad, usually made of cloth, used to apply heat, cold, or medication to the surface of a body area, or over a wound to help control bleeding.

compulsion Irresistible, repetitive, irrational impulse to perform an act that is usually contrary to one's ordinary judgments or standards yet results in overt anxiety if not completed.

computer on wheels, or COWs Point-of-care systems housed on wheeled carts.

conception (fertilization) Beginning of pregnancy.

concrete operational phase Phase of Piaget's theory in which thoughts become increasingly logical and coherent so that the child is able to classify, sort, and organize facts while still being incapable of generalizing or dealing with abstractions; occurs between 7 and 10 years of age.

conflict Mental struggle, either conscious or subconscious, resulting from the simultaneous presence of opposing or incompatible thoughts, ideas, goals, or emotional forces, such as impulses, desires, or drives.

congenital heart disease (CHD) An abnormality or anomaly of the heart, present at birth.

connotative meaning Reflects the individual's perception or interpretation of a given word.

contamination Condition of being soiled, stained, touched, or otherwise exposed to harmful agents by the entry of infectious or toxic material into a previously clean or sterile environment; making an object potentially unsafe for use as intended.

continuing care retirement community Offers complete range of housing and health care accommodations from independent to 24-hour skilled nursing care.

continuity of care Continuing of established patient care from one setting to another.

contract Promise or a set of promises between two or more people that creates a legal relationship between them and a legal obligation that one or more of them must fulfill.

contracture Abnormal, usually permanent condition of a joint characterized by flexion and fixation and caused by atrophy and shortening of muscle fibers.

contusion An injury that does not break the skin, is caused by a blow, and is characterized by edema, discoloration, and pain.

coping responses Voluntary patterns of behavior used to relieve stress or anxiety.

cotyledon One of the 15 to 28 visible segments of the placenta on the maternal surface, each made up of fetal vessels, chorionic villi, and intervillous space.

crackle(s) Short, discrete, interrupted crackling or bubbling adventitious breath sounds heard on auscultation of the chest, most commonly upon inspiration. They are produced by passage of air through the bronchi that contain secretions of exudate or are constricted by spasms or thickening; usually heard during inspiration; formerly called rales.

crepitus Sound that resembles the crackling noise heard when rubbing hair between the fingers or throwing salt on an open fire. It is associated with gas gangrene, the rubbing of bone fragments, or the crackles of a consolidated area of the lung in pneumonia.

crime Breaking of any law; an offense to society that is punishable.

crisis Time of change or turning point in life when patterns of living must be modified to prevent disorganization of the person or family.

crown-rump length The measurement from the top of the fetal head to the buttocks.

cryptorchidism Failure of testes to descend into the scrotum.

cue Word, phrase, or symptom that indicates the nature of something perceived. Cues are grouped to assist the nurse in interpretation of data, as in formulating the patient's plan of care.

cultural bias The beliefs and practices of their particular culture are best.

cultural competence Awareness by the nurse of his or her own cultural belief practices and an understanding of the limitations that these beliefs put on the nurse when dealing with those from other cultures. This understanding should give the nurse the ability to react to others with openness to and understanding and acceptance of cultural differences between them.

cultural healing beliefs Beliefs that reflect a specific culture's concept of health and illness.

culture (1) A set of learned values, beliefs, customs, and practices that are shared by a group and passed from one generation to another. (2) A laboratory test involving cultivation of microorganisms or cells in a special growth medium.

cumulative A drug that builds up in the body; can lead to a toxic or even lethal (deadly) effect.

curative treatment Aggressive care with the goal and intent of curing the disease and prolonging life at all costs.

"currant jelly" stools Feces mixed with blood and mucus from the intestinal mucosa.

customs Habitual practices; the usual way of acting under given circumstances.

cyanosis Slightly bluish, gray, slatelike, or dark purple discoloration of the skin resulting from the presence of abnormally reduced amounts of oxygenated hemoglobin in the blood.

cyclothymic disorder A pattern that involves repeated mood swings of hypomania and depression that are less intense than with bipolar disorder. There are no periods of "normal function" with this condition. It is thought to be a muted version of bipolar disorder.

cytology/cytologic evaluation Study of cells and their formation, origin, structure, biochemical activities, and pathology.

D

database Large store or bank of information, as in forming the patient's nursing diagnosis.

deaf culture A set of beliefs that are influenced by beliefs centered around an inability to hear

death Cessation of life.

deciduous teeth Set of 20 teeth that normally appear during infancy.

defecation Elimination of bowel waste.

defense mechanisms Unconscious, intrapsychic reactions that offer protection to the self from stressful situations.

defining characteristics Clinical signs and symptoms that a problem exists.

dehiscence Partial or complete separation of a surgical incision or rupture of a wound closure.

deinstitutionalization Release of institutional psychiatric patients to be treated in the community setting.

delirium An acute, organic mental disorder characterized by confusion, disorientation, clouding of consciousness, incoherence, fear, anxiety, excitement, and often illusions and hallucinations. Symptoms are of short duration and reversible with treatment of the underlying cause, such as fever or electrolyte imbalance.

delirium tremens (DTs) An acute psychotic reaction that is a complication of alcohol withdrawal.

delusion A persistent, aberrant belief or perception held inviolable by a person despite evidence to the contrary.

dementia A slowly progressive, organic mental disorder characterized by chronic personality disintegration, deterioration of intellectual capacity and function, and memory loss that leads to confusion, disorientation, and stupor. An example is Alzheimer's disease.

democratic family pattern Family style in which the adult members are considered equal and children are treated with respect and recognized as individuals.

denominator Bottom number of a fraction.

denotative meaning The commonly accepted definition of a particular word.

dentures Artificial teeth not permanently fixed or implanted.

deposition Out-of-court, under-oath statement of a witness.

depressant A drug that depresses the central nervous system, such as alcohol, sedative-hypnotic medications, and opioid analgesics.

depression An emotional disorder brought on by an imbalance of the neurotransmitter serotonin in the brain, which brings about exaggerated feelings of sadness, melancholy, emptiness, worthlessness, and frustration. Fatigue, inability to concentrate, short-term memory loss, and sleep pattern disturbance, as well as slowed body functions, can be seen with this disorder.

descent In obstetrics, the downward progress of the presenting part belonging to the fetus. The amount of progress measured by comparing the lowest point of the presenting part with the ischial spines of the mother.

detoxification Removal of poisonous effects of a substance from a patient.

development Gradual process or change and differentiation from a simple to a more advanced level of complexity.

diagnose To identify a disease or condition by a scientific evaluation of physical signs, symptoms, history, laboratory tests, and procedures.

diagnosis-related group (DRG) System that classifies patients by age, diagnoses, and surgical categories; used to predict the use of hospital resources, including the length of stay.

diaphoresis The secretion of sweat, especially the profuse secretion of sweat.

diastole The period of time between contractions of the atria or the ventricles, during which blood enters the relaxed chambers from the systemic circulation and the lungs.

diastolic pressure The second number recorded in the blood pressure reading; represents the minimum level of blood pressure measured between the contractions of the heart.

dietary fiber Generic term for nondigestible chemical substances in plants.

differentiation Process of cellular development in which unspecialized cells or tissues are systematically modified to achieve specific and characteristic physical forms, physiologic functions, and chemical properties.

diffusion A process in which solid particles in a fluid move from an area of higher concentration to an area of lower concentration.

dilemma Situation requiring a choice between two equally desirable or undesirable alternatives.

dimensional analysis A method of dosage calculation that employs the use of three factors, which include the drug label factor, conversion factor, and drug order factor.

direct Coombs' test Laboratory blood test to detect foreign antibodies that have adhered to red blood cells, which can cause cellular damage. These antibodies result in hemolytic anemia. Normal findings: negative, no agglutination.

disability Any restriction or lack (resulting from an impairment) of an ability to perform an activity in the manner or within the range considered normal for a human being.

disaster manual Written agency instructions specifying departmental responsibilities, chain of command, callback procedures for the receipt and management of casualties, and policies related to the overall management of supplies and equipment.

disaster situation Uncontrollable, unexpected, psychologically shocking event.

discharge Release of a patient from a health care facility.

discharge planning Schedule of events often planned by a multidisciplinary team leading to the return of a patient from hospital confinement to life at home or another health care setting.

disease Any disturbance of a structure or function of the body; a pathologic condition of the body.

disengagement stage Period of family life when the grown children depart from the home. In some family units this stage is brief because the adult children return to live in the family home.

disinfectant A chemical that can be applied to objects to destroy microorganisms.

disinfection Process by which pathogens, but not necessarily their spores, are destroyed.

disorientation Mental confusion characterized by inadequate or incorrect perceptions of place, time, and identity.

disoriented Having lost awareness or perception of space, time, or personal identity and relationships.

disuse syndrome A condition that results from an extended period of physical activity. The resulting condition impacts both the physical and mental capabilities of the individual.

diuresis Secretion and passage of large amounts of urine.

dizygotic Of or pertaining to twins from two fertilized ova.

do-not-resuscitate (DNR) A note written in a patient's record and signed by a qualified attending physician instructing the staff of the institution not to attempt to resuscitate the patient in the event of cardiac or respiratory failure. Also called *no code.*

documenting Process of adding information to the chart, usually at prescribed intervals.

doctrine of informed consent The requirements on a physician to provide information to the patient about a procedure that will include both the risks and benefits of the intervention planned.

dominant group Group of people exercising authority or influence; ruling or prevailing group.

Dorothea Dix A retired teacher who was appalled by the care of the mentally ill. In 1841, she began her crusade for placing individuals with mental illnesses in specially built hospitals. Her efforts brought millions of dollars toward developing mental hospitals in the United States.

dorsal Toward the back.

dorsal (supine) Lying horizontally on the back.

dorsal recumbent Supine position with patient lying on the back, with head, shoulders, and extremities moderately flexed and legs extended.

dorsiflexion Bending or flexing backward, as in upward bending of the fingers, wrist, foot, or toes.

double bagging Infection control practice of placing a bag of contaminated items into another bag that is clean and held outside the isolation room by a second staff member.

Down syndrome A congenital condition usually resulting from having three copies of chromosome 21 and characterized by varying degrees of cognitive disability and multiple physical defects.

drainage Free flow or withdrawal of fluids from a wound or cavity by some sort of system such as a urinary catheter or T-tube.

DRG *See* diagnosis-related group.

drip factor A method that is used to deliver measured amounts of intravenous solutions at specific flow rates based on the size of drops of the solution.

drug interaction Modification of the effect of a drug when administered with another drug.

dullness Low-pitched thudlike sound upon percussion of the body.

dumping syndrome Combination of profuse perspiration, nausea, vertigo, and weakness experienced by patients who have had a subtotal gastrectomy; symptoms are felt soon after eating, when the contents of the stomach empty too rapidly into the duodenum.

durable powers of attorney A signed and notarized document that appoints another person to make decisions in the event of the patient's incompetence. Usually completed by the patient while still able to function.

dysarthria Difficult, poorly articulated speech resulting from interference in the control over the muscles of speech.

dysfunctional grieving Unresolved grief or complicated mourning.

dysphagia Difficulty swallowing.

dyspnea Shortness of breath or difficulty in breathing; may be caused by disturbances in the lungs, certain heart conditions, and hemoglobin deficiency.

dysrhythmia Any disturbance or abnormality in a normal rhythmic pattern, specifically irregularity in the normal rhythm of the heart. Also called *arrhythmia*.

E

ecchymosis Discoloration of an area of the skin or mucous membrane caused by the extravasation of blood into the subcutaneous tissues. Also called a *bruise*.

eclampsia Most severe form of pregnancy-induced hypertension, characterized by toxic and grand mal convulsions, coma, hypertension, albuminuria, and edema. Also called *gestational hypertension (GH)*.

ectoderm Outer layer of embryonic tissue that gives rise to skin, nails, and hair.

ectopic pregnancy Implantation of the fertilized ovum outside the uterine cavity, such as in the abdomen, fallopian tubes, or ovary.

edema Abnormal accumulation of fluids in interstitial spaces of tissue; a combining form meaning swelling.

effacement Thinning and shortening of the cervix as it is stretched and dilated by the fetus. This occurs during late pregnancy, labor, or both.

efficacy The effectiveness of the therapy to produce the intended effect.

electrocardiogram (ECG) Graphic representation of electrical impulses generated by the heart during a cardiac cycle.

electrolyte Substance that is sometimes called a mineral or salt; it develops tiny electrical charges when dissolved in water and breaks up into particles known as ions.

electronic health record An electronic patient record designed for health information exchange between facilities.

electronic medical record An electronic patient record designed for health information exchange only within a facility.

elopement Leaving the care agency/provider by a patient without medical approval and support. The action may be intentional or unintentional.

embolism An abnormal circulatory condition in which an embolus (e.g., a foreign substance, blood clot, fat, air, or amniotic fluid) travels through the bloodstream and becomes lodged in a blood vessel.

emergency medical services (EMS) National network of services coordinated to provide aid and medical assistance from primary response to definitive care, involving personnel trained in the rescue, stabilization, transportation, and advanced treatment of traumatic or medical emergencies.

empathy Ability to recognize and, to some extent, share the emotions and states of mind of another and to understand the meaning and significance of that person's behavior.

endemic A characteristic or condition that is associated with a group.

en face position Position in which the adult's face and the infant's face are approximately 8 inches apart, as when the mother holds the infant up in front of her face or when she nurses the infant.

endoderm Innermost cell layer; from the endoderm arises the lining of cavities and passages of the body and covering for most internal organs.

endogenous Growing within the body; originating from within the body, or produced from internal causes, such as a disease caused by the structural or functional failure of an organ or system.

endorphin Any one of the neuropeptides composed of many amino acids, elaborated by the pituitary gland and acting on the central and peripheral nervous systems to reduce pain.

endorsement Statement of recognition of the license of a health practitioner in one state by another.

endotracheal tube The placement of a tube through the mouth or nose into the trachea. The purpose is to maintain a patent airway.

enema The instillation of a solution into the rectum of the sigmoid colon for the purpose of evacuating the bowel or introducing a medication.

engagement Fixation of the presenting part of the fetus in the maternal pelvis. The lowest part of the presenting part is at or below the level of the ischial spines.

engagement or commitment stage Period when the couple prepares for marriage and becomes free of parental domination.

engorgement Swelling of the breast tissue brought about by an increase in blood and lymph supply to the breast; occurs about 48 hours postpartum and usually reaches a peak between the third and fifth days after delivery.

enteral Within, or by way of, the intestine.

enteral nutrition Administration of nutrients into the gastrointestinal tract; usually referred to as *tube feeding*.

enteric-coated Encasement of a tablet in a candylike shell to prevent medications from being absorbed in the stomach; absorption takes place in the intestine.

enzyme-linked immunosorbent assay (ELISA) Antibody test that uses a rapid enzyme immunochemical assay method to detect HIV antibodies.

epidemic A large, unchecked spread of an infectious condition through a population.

episiotomy Surgical incision of the perineum at the end of the second stage of labor to facilitate delivery and avoid laceration of the perineum.

epistaxis Hemorrhage from the nose; nosebleed.

epistaxis digitorum Self-inflicted local digital trauma (i.e., from nose-picking).

ergonomics Processes geared toward the movements in a manner that takes into consideration ways to avoid injury and undue fatigue.

erythema Redness or inflammation of the skin or mucous membranes resulting from dilation and congestion of superficial capillaries. Examples are mild sunburn, nervous blushes, injury resulting from trauma or infection.

erythematous Pertaining to erythema (redness).

erythroblastosis fetalis Hemolytic anemia in newborns resulting from maternal-fetal blood group incompatibility, especially involving the Rh factor and ABO blood groups.

esophageal varices A complex of longitudinal, twisted veins at the lower end of the esophagus.

essential nutrient Carbohydrates, proteins, fats, minerals, vitamins, and water necessary for growth, normal function, and body maintenance. These substances must be supplied by food; they are not synthesized by the body in the quantities required for normal health.

establishment stage Period in a couple's life between their wedding and the birth of their first child.

ethical dilemma Situation that does not have a clear correct or incorrect answer.

ethics The way one should behave; how a person ought to act.

ethnic stereotype A fixed concept of how all members of an ethnic group act or think.

ethnicity A shared common social and cultural heritage based on traditions, national origin, and physical and biologic characteristics. It often includes social practices such as language, religion, dress, music, and food.

ethnocentrism A perception that the practices and beliefs of one's own culture are superior to those of other cultures.

etiology The study of all factors that may be involved in the development of a disease; the cause of disease.

euthanasia Deliberately bringing about the death of an individual suffering from an incurable disease or condition; can be done actively or passively.

evaluation The determination made about the extent to which the established outcomes have been achieved in the nursing care plan.

evisceration Protrusion of an internal organ through a disrupted wound or surgical incision.

exacerbation An increase in the seriousness of a disease or disorder; marked by greater intensity in the signs or symptoms of the patient being treated.

exogenous Outside the body; originating outside the body or produced from external causes, such as a disease caused by a bacterial or viral agent foreign to the body.

expectant stage The period of family life that begins when conception occurs and continues through the pregnancy.

expectorate To eject mucus, sputum, or fluids from the trachea and lungs by coughing or spitting.

expressive aphasia A physiologic condition in which an individual is unable to communicate a desired message.

expulsion Having the tendency to drive out or expel.

extended family A family group consisting of the parents, their children, the grandparents, and other family members.

extension Movement allowed by certain joints of the skeleton that increases the angle between two adjoining bones.

external rotation Occurs as the head and body move through the birth canal, using the same maneuvers as the head. The shoulders are delivered similarly to the fetal head, with the anterior shoulder pressing under the symphysis pubis, which again acts as a leverage point and assists in delivery of the posterior shoulder.

extracellular Fluid outside the cells of the body.

extremes Outer terms of the proportion. Very severe or drastic.

exudate Fluid, cells, or other substances that have been slowly exuded or discharged from body cells or blood vessels through small pores or breaks in cell membrane.

F

failure to thrive The abnormal retardation of growth and development of the infant resulting from conditions that interfere with normal metabolism, appetite, and activity.

family-centered care Philosophy of care that recognizes the family as the constant in the child's life and holds that systems and personnel must support, respect, encourage, and enhance the strengths and competence of the family.

febrile Body temperature above normal.

fecal impaction The presence of stool that is obstructive and not passed without intervention to relieve it.

feces Waste from the intestine; bowel movement (BM).

fetal lie Relationship existing between the long axis of the fetus and the long axis of the mother.

fetal position The relationship of the occiput, sacrum, chin, or scapula on the presenting part of the fetus to its location in the front, back, or sides of the maternal pelvis.

fetal presentation The part of the fetus that enters the pelvis first and lies over the inlet; head, face, feet, or shoulders.

fetopelvic disproportion The head of the fetus is larger than the pelvic outlet. Also called *cephalopelvic disproportion.*

filtration The transfer of water and dissolved substances from an area of higher pressure to an area of lower pressure.

fixative Any substance used to preserve gross or histologic specimens of tissue for examination.

flagellation Whiplike movement.

flail chest Two or more ribs fractured in two or more places resulting in instability in part of the chest wall with associated hemothorax, pneumothorax, and pulmonary contusion.

flatness Soft, high-pitched, flat sound produced by performing percussion over tissue such as muscle tissue.

flatulence Excess formation of gases in the stomach or intestine.

flatus Air or gas in the intestine that is passed through the rectum.

flexion Movement of certain joints that decreases the angle between two adjoining bones.

flow meter A device to measure the outflow of a gas, such as oxygen.

focus charting Expansion of the data and need columns in nurses' notes to include topics concerning the whole patient, such as behavior or treatment and response. The charting format is data, action, response (DAR).

focused assessment Concentration of attention on the part of the body where signs and symptoms are localized or most active in order to determine their significance.

focusing A communication technique used when more specific information is needed to accurately understand the patient's message.

folk health belief system Belief that health and illness are controlled by supernatural forces. May use native healers, plants, religious rituals, and prayers.

folk medicine The traditional healing practices that are passed down within a culture.

fomite Nonliving material, such as bed linens, stethoscope, needles, and many other objects that may host and transfer pathogenic microorganisms.

fontanelle Broad area or soft spot consisting of a strong bond of connective tissue between an infant's cranial bones.

formal operational thought phase Piaget's phase that begins during adolescence, permitting abstract reasoning and systematic scientific problem solving.

foster family Family unit that cares for, supervises, and nurtures children whose parents are unable to care for them.

Fowler's Known as the standard patient position. The patient is lying with legs straight or bent at the knees and the head of the bed is elevated between 30 and 90 degrees.

fraction of inspired oxygen (FiO_2) The percentage of oxygen being breathed in.

frustration Emotional response to anything that interferes with a goal-directed activity.

functional assessment The assessment of the functional status of the patient, which is the ability of an individual to perform normal, expected, or required activities of daily living.

functional disease May be manifested as an organic disease, but careful examination fails to reveal evidence of structural or physiologic abnormalities.

functional limitation Any loss or ability to perform tasks and obligations of usual roles and normal daily life.

fundus Top part of uterus.

G

gate control theory Suggests that pain impulses can be regulated or even blocked by gating mechanisms located along the central nervous system.

gateway drug A drug, for example, alcohol, that is the first drug of abuse, later followed by other drugs.

gauge A standard or scale of measurement.

genupectoral Patient kneels so weight of body is supported by knees and chest.

gerontologic rehabilitation nursing Specialty practice that focuses on the unique requirements of elderly rehabilitation patients.

gestational diabetes mellitus (GDM) Disorder characterized by an impaired ability to metabolize carbohydrates, usually caused by a deficiency of insulin; occurs in pregnancy and disappears after delivery but in some cases returns years later.

gestational hypertension (GH) *See* pregnancy-induced hypertension.

gestures Movements used to emphasize the idea being communicated.

glomerular filtration rate A measure of kidney function that captures the rate of blood passing through the glomeruli each minute.

glomerulonephritis Inflammation of the glomeruli of the kidney.

glycogen Polysaccharide that is the major carbohydrate stored in animal cells.

glycosylated hemoglobin This test produces an accurate long-term index of the patient's average blood glucose level by measuring the patient's glycohemoglobin (GHB). Glycohemoglobin is a minor hemoglobin that makes up 4% to 8% of the total hemoglobin. It is a combination of hemoglobin and blood glucose. This test can have a blood sample drawn at any time because it is not affected by short-term variations. This test reflects the average blood sugar level for the 100- to 120-day period before the test.

goal The purpose to which an effort is directed.

Good Samaritan law Legal stipulation for protection of those who give first aid in an emergency situation.

Goodell's sign Softening of the uterine cervix; a probable sign of pregnancy.

Gowers' sign Classic sign of Duchenne's muscular dystrophy; the child positions on all fours and uses the hands to walk up the thighs.

graduated Container that has interval markings of measurement.

grandfamilies Families with children under the age of 18 years who live with or in the custody of grandparents.

granulation Soft, pink, fleshy projection consisting of capillaries surrounded by fibrous collagen that slowly fills the incision during the process of healing.

gravida A pregnant woman.

grief A pattern of physical and emotional responses to bereavement, separation, or loss; a natural response to loss.

grief therapy Mental treatment aimed at helping an individual deal with the pain of loss; a program in assisting the bereaved to cope with their loss.

grief work Adaptation process of mourning a loss.

group therapy Provides a caring, emotionally supportive atmosphere for a patient in a recovery program.

growth Increase in the size of an organism or any of its parts.

gynecomastia Development of abnormally large mammary glands in a male that sometimes may secrete milk. When observed in the newborn, it is in response to maternal hormones; may be noted in either sex of the newborn.

H

hallucination A sensory experience without a stimulus trigger that occurs in the waking state. It can occur in any of the senses.

hallucinogen A drug that alters perception and thinking.

harlequin sign Rare color change of no pathologic significance occurring between the longitudinal halves of the newborn's body; when the infant is placed on one side, the dependent half is noticeably pinker than the superior half.

Hazard Communication Act Requires hospitals to inform employees about the presence of or potential for harmful exposures and how to reduce the risk of exposures.

health A condition of physical, mental, and social well-being and the absence of disease or other abnormal conditions.

health care facility Agency or institution that provides health care.

health care system The complete network of agencies, facilities, and all providers of health care in a specific geographic area.

health disparities Preventable, negative health outcomes that disproportionately affect socially and economically disadvantaged populations.

Healthcare Integrity and Protection Data Bank (HIPDB) National data bank created in 1999 to which federal and state agencies report all final adverse actions taken against a health care provider.

Hëgar's sign Softening of the isthmus of the uterine cervix early in gestation; a probable sign of pregnancy.

Heimlich maneuver An emergency procedure for dislodging a bolus of food or other obstruction from the trachea to prevent asphyxiation.

hemarthrosis Bleeding into a joint space, a hallmark of severe disease usually occurring in the knees, ankles, and elbow.

hematemesis Vomiting blood.

hematuria Blood in the urine.

hemiplegia Paralysis of one side of the body.

Hemoccult test Detects occult (hidden) blood in the feces.

hemoptysis Expectorating blood from the respiratory tract.

hemothorax Collection of blood into the pleural space.

herbal therapy An alternative therapy that uses herbs to provide health benefits.

high-risk pregnancy Condition in which the life or health of the mother or infant is jeopardized by a disorder coincidental with or unique to pregnancy.

HIPAA The federal law governing patient privacy is the Health Insurance Portability and Accountability Act (HIPAA) of 1996, which went into effect on April 14, 2003. It mandates national standards for protecting all verbal or documented health information from improper alteration, access, or loss. The goal is to ensure the security and privacy of this data.

HIV disease Symptomatic human immunodeficiency virus (HIV) infection that is not severe enough for a diagnosis of acquired immunodeficiency syndrome (AIDS); symptoms of HIV disease are persistent unexplained fever, night sweats, diarrhea, weight loss, and fatigue.

HIV infection State in which HIV enters the body and, under favorable conditions, multiplies and produces injurious effects to the body.

holistic Pertaining to the total patient care that considers the physical, emotional, social, economic, and spiritual needs of the person.

holistic health belief system Belief that forces of nature must be kept in natural balance or harmony.

holistic health care A system of comprehensive or total patient care that considers the physical, emotional, social, economic, and spiritual needs of the person; the response to the illness and the effect of the illness on the person's ability to meet self-care needs.

holistic nursing The practice of nursing that focuses on the entire person.

Homans' sign Early sign of thrombophlebitis of the deep veins of the calf in which there are complaints of pain when the leg is in extension and the foot is dorsiflexed.

home health agency An organization that provides health care in the home.

home health care Services that enable individuals of all ages to remain in the comfort and security of their homes while receiving health care.

homeostasis A relative constancy in the internal environment of the body, naturally maintained by adaptive responses that promote healthy survival.

homosexual family Family group made up of same-sex adults who share bonds of emotional commitment and roles of childrearing.

hospice From the Latin word *hospitum,* meaning hospitality; a resting place for travelers on a difficult journey; philosophy of care that provides support to terminally ill people and their families.

host A person or group who, because of risk factors, may be susceptible to disease or illness; an organism in which another, usually parasitic, organism is nourished and harbored.

huffing Typically in a group setting, breathing in solvents from a cloth, paper, or plastic bag.

humoral immunity One of the two forms of immunity that respond to antigens such as bacteria and foreign tissue. It is mediated by B cells.

humoral theory A theory dating back to Hippocrates. He viewed mental illness as an imbalance of humors (the fundamental elements of the world: air, fire, water, and earth). Each basic element was represented in the body by certain fluids: blood, yellow bile, black bile, and phlegm.

hydramnios Abnormal condition of pregnancy characterized by an excess of amniotic fluid.

hydrogenation Process in which hydrogen is added to vegetable oil to make it more solid and stable to rancidity.

hydrostatic pressure The outward force exerted on a vessel wall.

hygiene The science of health and its maintenance; system of principles for preserving health and preventing disease.

hyperbilirubinemia An excess of bilirubin in the blood of the newborn.

hyperextension Position of maximum extension; extreme or abnormal stretching.

hypersensitivity An abnormal condition characterized by an excessive reaction to a particular stimulus.

hypertension Occurs when the elevated blood pressure is above normal.

hyperthermia Condition of abnormally high body temperature.

hypertonic A solution of higher osmotic pressure.

hypomanic episode The early phase of a manic episode when symptoms are not severe.

hypotension Occurs when the blood pressure is below normal.

hypothermia Condition of abnormally low body temperature.

hypotonic A solution of lower osmotic pressure.

hypoxia An inadequate, reduced tension of cellular oxygen.

I

idiopathic Cause unknown.

idiosyncratic An individual's unique hypersensitivity to a particular drug.

ileostomy The placement of the end of the small intestine through an opening in the abdominal wall and creating a stoma.

illness An abnormal process in which aspects of the social, emotional, or intellectual condition and function of a person are diminished or impaired.

illusion A false interpretation of an external sensory stimulus, usually visual or auditory, such as a mirage in the desert or voices on the wind.

imagery Visualization techniques to create mental images to evoke physical changes in the body, improve perceived well-being, and enhance self-awareness.

immobility Inability to move around freely, caused by any condition in which movement is impaired or therapeutically restricted.

immunity The quality of being unsusceptible to or unaffected by a particular disease condition.

immunization A process by which resistance to an infectious disease is induced or increased.

immunocompetence/immunocompetent The ability of an immune system to mobilize and deploy its antibodies and other responses to stimulation by an antigen.

immunodeficiency An abnormal condition of the immune system in which cellular or humoral immunity is inadequate and resistance to infection is decreased.

immunogen Any agent or substance capable of provoking an immune response or producing immunity.

immunology Study of the immune system; the reaction of tissues of the immune system of the body to antigenic stimulation.

immunosuppression/immunosuppressive Administration of agents that significantly interfere with the ability of the immune system to respond to antigenic stimulation by inhibiting cellular and humoral immunity.

immunosurveillance The immune system's recognition and destruction of newly developed abnormal cells.

immunotherapy A special treatment of allergic responses; involves the administration of increasingly larger doses of the offending allergens to gradually develop immunity.

impaction Condition of being tightly wedged into a part, such as eruption of a tooth blocked by other teeth; the presence of a large or hard fecal mass in the rectum or colon which the patient is unable to pass.

impairment Any loss or abnormality of psychological, physical, or anatomic structure or function.

implantation Embedding of the fertilized ovum in the uterine mucosa.

implementation The phase of the nursing process that includes ongoing activities of data collection, prioritization, and performance of nursing intervention and documentation.

incision Surgical cut produced by a sharp instrument to create an opening into an organ or space in the body.

incompetent cervix Passive and painless dilation of the cervix during the second trimester of pregnancy; it is variable and exists as a continuum that is determined in part by cervical length.

incontinence The inability to control urination or defecation.

indirect Coombs' test Laboratory blood test that detects circulating antibodies against red blood cells (RBC). The test can detect Rh antibodies in maternal blood and is used to anticipate hemolytic disease of the newborn.

induration Hardening of a tissue, particularly the skin, because of edema, inflammation, or infiltration by neoplasm. May be seen with an IV infiltrate.

infant mortality The death of a child who is under 1 year of age.

infant mortality rate The number of deaths of children who are under 1 year of age. It is measured per 1000 children born.

infection Caused by an invasion of microorganisms such as bacteria, viruses, fungi, or parasites that produce tissue damage.

infection control The policies and procedures of a hospital or other health care facility to minimize the risk of nosocomial or community-acquired infection spreading to patients or other members of the staff.

infection prevention and control Activities geared toward stopping and limiting the transmission of infection.

infectious process Condition caused by the invasion of the body by pathogenic microorganisms.

infiltration The process whereby a fluid passes into the tissues.

inflammation Protective response of body tissues to irritation, injury, or invasion by disease-producing organisms. The cardinal signs include erythema, edema, heat, and loss of function.

inflammatory response A tissue reaction to injury.

informatics The process of retrieving, storing, and transmitting data.

informed consent doctrine A legal doctrine that requires the patient to fully understand any proposed treatment and consent to it; this document gives the competent adult the choice to accept or reject any treatment modalities.

inhalant A volatile chemical that can alter thinking and feeling when inhaled.

innate immunity The body's first line of defense; provides physical and chemical barriers to invading pathogens and protects the body against the external environment.

inquest A legal inquiry into the cause or manner of a death.

inspection Visual examination of the external surface of the body and of its movements and posture, including observation of moods and all responses and nonverbal behaviors.

instrumental activities of daily living (IADLs) Daily tasks that are more complex than ADLs, such as shopping or using the telephone.

intelligence quotient (IQ) Index of relative intelligence determined through the subject's answers to arbitrarily chosen questions.

Integrative care Care is the assimilation of complementary therapies into conventional medical care.

interdisciplinary When health care professionals work together as a team to meet the needs of a patient.

interdisciplinary hospice team Multiple-professional health team, such as physicians, nurses, social workers, and pastors, working together in caring for the terminally ill patient.

interdisciplinary rehabilitation team Team that collaborates to identify an individual's goals and is characterized by a combination of expanded problem solving beyond discipline boundaries and discipline-specific work toward goal attainment.

interdisciplinary team A diverse team of professionals from several disciplines who collaborate to optimize care and decrease fragmentation services.

intermittent venous access device An intravenous infusion device with a male adapter covered by a rubber diaphragm for intermittent intravenous therapy. Also called *heparin* or *saline lock.*

internal rotation In obstetrics, when the largest diameter of the fetal head aligns with the largest diameter of the pelvis. This allows the fetal head to progress through the maternal pelvis.

interstitial Fluid between the cells or in the tissues of the body.

interview Meeting people for an evaluation or for questioning a job applicant.

intracellular Fluid inside the cells of the body.

intrapartal Period that begins with the onset of labor and ends with the delivery of the placenta. Also called *perinatal.*

intravascular Fluid or plasma within the vessels of the body.

intravenous (IV) Pertaining to the inside of a vein, as of a thrombus, or an injection, infusion, or catheter.

introitus An entrance to a cavity (e.g., the vaginal introitus).

involution Reduction in size of the uterus after delivery and return to its normal size.

ion Electronically charged particle resulting from the breakdown of an electrolyte; negatively or positively charged.

irrigation A gentle washing of an area with a stream of solution delivered through an irrigating syringe.

isolation precautions Practices of infection control to reduce or eliminate the transmission of pathogens; precautions include wearing protective apparel such as gowns, gloves, and masks and following the procedure for double bagging.

isotonic Having equal tension of a salt solution. Having the same osmotic pressure as blood.

J

jargon Commonplace language or terminology unique to people in a particular work setting.

jaundice Yellowish discoloration of the skin, mucous membranes, and sclera of the eyes caused by greater than normal amounts of bilirubin in the blood.

joint Any one of the connections between bones.

K

Kaposi's sarcoma (KS) Rare cancer of the skin or mucous membranes; characterized by blue, red, or purple raised lesions and seen mainly in middle-aged Mediterranean men and those with HIV disease.

Kardex/Rand A card system used to consolidate patient orders and care needs in a centralized, concise way.

kernicterus Abnormal toxic accumulation of bilirubin in central nervous system tissue caused by hyperbilirubinemia (an excess of bilirubin in the blood of the newborn).

kick count Daily counting of fetal movements felt in 1 hour while the mother is resting.

kilocalorie Unit that denotes the heat expenditure of an organism and the fuel or energy value of food; often abbreviated kcalorie or kcal.

Korotkoff sounds Sounds heard while measuring blood pressure when using a sphygmomanometer and stethoscope.

kyphosis An abnormal condition of the vertebral column; characterized by increased convexity in the curvature of the thoracic spine.

L

labia majora Two large folds of tissue extending from the mons pubis to the perineal floor; lip.

labia minora Smaller fold of tissue covered by the labia majora; lip.

labile Liable to change; unstable. As in unstable blood pressure.

lactation Function of secreting milk from the breasts for the nourishment of an infant or breastfeeding child.

lanugo Downy, fine hair characteristic of the fetus between 20 weeks of gestation and birth; most noticeable over the shoulders, forehead, and cheeks, but found on nearly all parts of the body except for the palms of the hands and the soles of the feet.

latch-on The process by which the baby attaches to the nipple for the purpose of breastfeeding.

law The reference of a rule, principle, or regulation established and made known by a government to protect or restrict the people affected.

Legg-Calvé-Perthes disease A disorder caused by decreased blood supply to the femoral head that results in epiphyseal necrosis or degeneration of the femoral head followed by regeneration or calcification.

leukopenia An abnormal decrease in the number of white blood cells to fewer than 5000 cells/mm³ due to depression of the bone marrow.

liability A legal concept that holds a person legally responsible for harm caused to another person or property.

licensure The granting of permission by a competent authority (usually government agency) to an organization or individual to engage in a practice or activity that would otherwise be illegal.

lichenification Hypertrophy of the epidermis, resulting in rough, thickened, leathery skin.

life expectancy Average number of years an individual will probably live.

lightening Sensation of decreased abdominal distention produced by uterine descent into the pelvic cavity as the fetal presenting part settles into the pelvis. It usually occurs 2 weeks before the onset of labor in nulliparas.

Linda Richards Practiced in the 1880s and has been credited as the first psychiatric nurse.

lipids Group name for organic substances of a fatty nature, including fats, oils, sterols (such as cholesterol), phospholipids, waxes, and related compounds.

lipoprotein A protein-and-lipid molecule that facilitates transport of lipids in the bloodstream.

lithotomy position Position assumed by the patient lying supine with the hips and knees flexed and the thighs abducted and rotated externally.

lithotomy Incision of a duct or organ, especially the bladder, for removal of a stone.

living will A legal document drawn up by a person who is not yet near death detailing how much medical care he or she wants to receive if terminally ill.

LOC Level of consciousness.

lochia Vaginal discharge during the puerperium consisting of blood, tissue, and mucus; following childbirth.

long-term care The range of services—physical, psychosocial, spiritual, social, and economic—needed to help people attain, maintain, and regain their optimum level of functioning.

loss When any aspect of self is no longer available to a person, that person suffers loss.

lumen Space within an artery, vein, intestine, or tube such as a needle or catheter.

lymphocytes White blood cells that occur in two forms—B cells and T cells.

lymphokine One of the chemical factors produced and released by T lymphocytes that attract macrophages to the site of infection or inflammation and prepare them for attack.

M

magnesium The second most abundant cation in the intracellular fluid of the body.

malignant Growing worse, resisting treatment; said of cancerous growths. Also tending or threatening to produce death; harmful.

malpractice (in law) Professional misconduct; behavior that fails to meet the standard of care.

mammogram X-ray examination of the breast; use of radiography of the breast to diagnose breast cancer.

managed care A health care system that involves administrative control over primary health care services in a medical group practice. Redundant facilities and services are eliminated, and costs are reduced. Health education and preventive medicine are emphasized.

mania A state characterized by an expansive emotional state, extreme excitement, excessive elation, hyperactivity, flight of ideas, increased psychomotor activity, and sometimes violent, destructive, and self-destructive behavior.

Martha Mitchell Nurse educator and clinical specialist in psychiatric mental health nursing, appointed to the President's Commission on Mental Health, established in 1978.

matriarchal family pattern A style in which the female assumes primary dominance in areas of child care and homemaking. Also called *matrilocal.*

maturational loss A loss from normal life transitions.

means Inner terms of the proportion; halfway between extremes.

meconium First stools of the infant; viscid, dark greenish brown, almost black; sterile; odorless.

Medicaid A federally funded, state-operated program of medical assistance to people with low income; authorized by Title XIX of the Social Security Act.

medical asepsis A group of techniques that inhibit the growth and spread of pathogenic microorganisms. Sometimes referred to as clean technique.

medical diagnosis The identification of a disease or condition by scientific evaluation of physical signs, symptoms, history, laboratory tests, and procedures.

medical nutrition therapy The use of specific nutrition services to treat an illness, injury, or condition.

Medicare A federally funded national health insurance for certain people older than 65 years of age.

medicine The art and science of the diagnosis, treatment, and prevention of disease and the maintenance of good health.

melena Abnormal, black, tarry stool containing digested blood.

meniscus Curved upper surface of a column of liquid as in a mercury column.

mental health One's ability to cope with and adjust to the recurrent stresses of everyday living.

mental health continuum Range of behaviors from adaptive (constructive) to maladaptive (destructive).

mental illness May be evidenced by behavior that is conspicuous, threatening, and disruptive of relationships or that deviates significantly from behavior that is considered socially acceptable. It is a manifestation of dysfunction (behavioral, psychological, and biologic).

meridians Channels of energy.

mesoderm Embryonic middle layer of germ cells giving rise to all types of muscles, connective tissue, bone marrow, blood lymphoid tissue, and all epithelial tissue.

metabolite Substance produced by metabolic action.

metastasis The process by which tumor cells spread to distant parts of the body.

microorganism Any tiny (usually microscopic) entity capable of carrying on living processes; kinds of microorganisms include bacteria, fungi, protozoa, and viruses; seen only by a microscope.

midstream urine specimen Urine collected after voiding is initiated and terminated before voiding is complete.

milliequivalent (mEq) Number of grams of soluble substance dissolved in 1 mL of normal solution.

mind-body link Connection between the physiologic and the mental as applied to healing.

minimal encouragement A subtle communication technique that communicates to the patient that the nurse is interested and wants to hear more.

minimum data set (MDS) A part of the patient assessment instrument (PAI) that incorporates many of the same assessment factors as a functional assessment tool and requires input from nursing and social services within a specific time frame.

minority group A racial, religious, ethnic, or political group smaller than and differing from the larger, controlling group in a community or nation.

mobility A person's ability to move around freely in his or her environment.

monozygotic Originating or coming from a single fertilized ovum, such as identical twins.

morbidity An illness or an abnormal condition or quality; the rate at which an illness occurs in a particular area of a population.

mores Accepted traditional customs, moral attitudes, or manners of a particular social group.

mortality The condition of being subject to death; number of deaths in a specific population, usually expressed as deaths per 1000, 10,000, or 100,000.

mortician Person trained in the care of the dead.

morula Development stage of the fertilized ovum in which there is a solid mass of cells resembling a mulberry.

motivation Inner drive to complete a task or reach a goal.

mourning Reaction activated by a person to assist in overcoming a great personal loss.

multiaxial system A system that classifies mental disorders; used by most hospitals and health care professionals in the United States. Various disorders and descriptive references are outlined.

multidisciplinary rehabilitation team Team characterized by discipline-specific goals, clear boundaries between disciplines, and outcomes that are the sum of each discipline's efforts.

multidisciplinary setting A group of health care workers who are members of different disciplines, each one providing specific services to the patient.

mummification Mortification producing a dry, hard mass.

musculoskeletal disorders (MSDs) Conditions that impact the muscles, bones, and connective tissue.

N

NANDA-I North American Nursing Diagnosis Association–International.

narrative charting Traditional system of charting in which the nurse documents in story form all pertinent patient observations, care, and responses in the nurse's notes section of the patient's records.

nasal cannula A device for delivery of oxygen by way of two small tubes that are inserted into the nares.

nasogastric tube A pliable tube that is inserted through the patient's nasopharynx and into the stomach.

negligence Failure to act as a responsible, prudent person would act in the given situation; applies to professionals and laypeople.

neoplastic Any abnormal growth of new tissue, benign or malignant.

neural tube Tube formed from the fusion of the neural folds from which the brain and spinal cord arise.

neurosis A term describing difficulty with stress that causes mild interpersonal disorganization. There is no loss of reality perception; the individual has insight that he or she has a problem.

neurotoxic Toxic or damaging to the brain.

Nissen fundoplication A surgical procedure to wrap the fundus of the stomach around the distal esophagus to prevent reflux of the stomach contents to the esophagus.

nitrogen balance Difference between intake and output of nitrogen in the body. If intake is greater, a positive nitrogen balance exists and anabolism occurs. If output is greater, a negative nitrogen balance exists and catabolism occurs. When nitrogen intake equals output, the body is in zero nitrogen balance.

nocturia Excessive urination at night.

nomenclature The process of assigning names.

nonmaleficence Ethical principle meaning "to do no harm."

non–rapid eye movement (NREM) One of two highly individualized sleeping states divided into four stages through which a sleeper progresses during a typical sleeping cycle; represents three-fourths of a period of typical sleep.

non-rebreather mask A device used to deliver oxygen to the patient. The patient can breath on his or her own. The mask is used to deliver precise concentrations of oxygen.

nontherapeutic communication Communication techniques, both verbal and nonverbal, that hinder the nurse-patient relationship.

nonverbal communication The transmission of messages without the use of words.

nosocomial infection An infection acquired in a hospital or any other health care facility; an infection acquired at least 72 hours after admission.

noxious A stimulation of the sensory nerve endings that is harmful, injurious, or detrimental to physical health.

nuchal rigidity Pain and stiffness of the neck when flexed.

nuchal translucency screening Ultrasound screening to measure fetal nuchal folds to assess for potential Down syndrome.

nuclear family A family unit consisting of the parents and their offspring.

numerator Top number of a fraction.

nurse practice act A statute enacted by the legislature of any of the states or by the appropriate officers of the district's possessions. The act delineates the legal scope of the practice of nursing within the geographic boundaries of jurisdiction.

nursing bottle caries Tooth decay caused by bottle feeding during sleep.

nursing care plan Plan of care based on a nursing assessment and a nursing diagnosis; lists nursing actions necessary to meet a patient's needs.

nursing diagnosis A clinical judgment about individual, family, or community responses to actual or high-risk (potential) health problems or life processes.

nursing health history Data collected about the patient's level of wellness, changes in life patterns, sociocultural role, and mental and emotional reactions to illness.

nursing intervention Activity performed by nurses that should promote the achievement of the desired patient outcome.

nursing notes The form on the patient's chart on which nurses record their observations, care given, and the patient's responses.

nursing physical assessment Identification by a nurse of the needs, preferences, and abilities of a patient. Assessment provides the scientific basis for a complete nursing care plan.

nursing process Systematic method by which nurses plan and provide care for patients.

nursing-sensitive outcomes The results or outcomes of nursing interventions. These outcomes or indicators are influenced by nursing and can be used to judge effectiveness of care and determine best practices.

nutrient A dietary element that is used to nourish the body.

nutrient-dense foods Foods providing a high quantity of one or more nutrients in a small number of calories are nutrient dense.

nutrient density Nutrients relative to calories.

O

obesity Abnormal increase in the proportion of fat cells, mainly in the viscera and subcutaneous tissues of the body; grossly overweight.

objective data Of or pertaining to a clinical finding that is observed, palpated, or auscultated. Laboratory findings, as well as radiologic and other studies, are included; observable and measurable signs.

obsessions Persistent thoughts and ideas that are recurrent, intrusive, and suggest an irrational act. The mind is continually and involuntarily preoccupied. These thoughts are anxiety producing and distressing in that they are uncontrollable.

occlusion An obstruction or closing off in a canal, vessel, or passage of the body.

occult Hidden.

Occupational Safety and Health Administration (OSHA) Federal agency responsible for monitoring safety and health standards in the workplace.

oligohydramnios Abnormally small amount or absence of amniotic fluid; often indicative of fetal urinary tract defect.

oliguria A diminished capacity to form and pass urine (less than 500 mL in 24 hours); result is that the end products of metabolism cannot be excreted efficiently.

Omnibus Budget Reconciliation Act (OBRA) Federal legislation that mandates specific standards governing the care of older adults in U.S. nursing facilities and prohibits routine use of safety reminder devices (SRDs; restraints) in nursing homes.

oncology The sum of knowledge regarding tumors; the branch of medicine that deals with study of tumors.

one-way communication A structured form of communication in which the sender is in control.

open-ended question A question that does not require a specific response and allows the individual to elaborate freely on a subject.

open posture A relaxed stance with uncrossed arms and legs while facing another individual.

opportunistic Disease characteristic caused by a normally nonpathogenic organism in a host whose resistance has been decreased by a disorder such as AIDS.

oral hygiene Care of the oral cavity (mouth).

organic disease Results in a structural change in an organ that interferes with its functioning.

orthopneic Pertaining to the posture assumed by the patient sitting up in bed at a 90-degree angle; patient may also lean forward supported by a pillow or over a bed table.

orthostatic hypotension A drop of 25 mm Hg in systolic pressure and a drop of 10 mm Hg in diastolic pressure when moving from a lying to sitting position.

osmosis Passage of water across a selectively permeable membrane; the water moves from a less concentrated solution to a more concentrated solution.

ostomy A surgical opening in the body. Some ostomies are created to allow the body to eliminate wastes.

outcome Description of the specific measurable behavior (outcome criteria) that the patient will be able to exhibit after the nursing interventions.

oxygen saturation Measurement of how much oxygen has combined with hemoglobin in the red blood cell.

oxytocin Hormone produced in the hypothalamus and stored in the posterior pituitary gland; when needed, promotes the release of breast milk and stimulates uterine contractions during labor.

P

pain assessment An evaluation of the factors that alleviate or exacerbate a patient's pain.

palliative Designed to relieve pain and distress and to control the signs and symptoms of disease; not designed to produce a cure.

palliative care Preventing, relieving, reducing, or soothing symptoms of disease or disorders without effecting a cure. Extends the principles of hospice care to a broader population that could benefit from comfort care earlier in their illness or disease process.

palpation A technique used in physical examination in which the examiner feels the texture, size, consistency, and location of certain parts of the body with the hands.

panic disorder An anxiety disorder that exhibits a sudden onset of acute, extreme anxiety. Feelings of terror and intense apprehension are accompanied with physical manifestations such as dyspnea, palpitations, sweating, trembling, and dizziness. An attack may last for several minutes and may be triggered again in certain situations.

Papanicolaou test (Pap smear) A simple smear method of examining stained exfoliative cells; used most commonly to detect cancers of the cervix.

para- A combining form meaning "similar, beside." Also a combining form meaning a woman who has given birth after 20 weeks' gestation (e.g., nonpara, unipara, bipara).

paracentesis A procedure in which fluid is withdrawn from the abdominal cavity.

paraphilia Sexual perversion or deviation. One of three main clusters of sexual and gender identity disorders.

paraphrasing A communication technique that involves restating the patient's message in the nurse's own words to verify that the nurse's interpretation of the message is correct.

parenchyma Tissue of an organ as distinguished from supporting or connective tissue.

parent-child attachment (bonding) Initial phase in a relationship characterized by strong attraction and a desire to interact.

parenteral nutrition Administering nutrients by a route other than the alimentary canal, such as intravenously.

parenteral Pertaining to treatment other than through the digestive system.

parenteral nutrition The administration of nutrients intravenously.

parenthood stage Begins at the birth or adoption of the first child.

partial rebreather mask A device used for oxygen delivery of 50-70%. The devise includes a collection bag for exhaled air.

PASS A mnemonic used to outline the steps needed to use a fire extinguisher. (*P*ull the pin, *A*im low, *S*queeze handle, *S*weep the unit).

passive listening Receiving a message without any response or indication of understanding.

passive transport The movement of small molecules across the membrane of a cell by diffusion; no cellular energy is required.

passivity The acceptance of the actions of others with no active response or resistance.

patency A condition of being opened and unblocked.

pathogenic Capable of causing disease.

patient A recipient of a health care service, usually thought of as a recipient who is ill or hospitalized.

patient assessment instrument (PAI) A method of patient assessment and care plan development prescribed by OBRA in 1987.

patient-controlled analgesia (PCA) A drug delivery system that dispenses a preset intravenous dose of an opioid analgesic into a patient's vein when the patient pushes a switch on an electric cord.

patriarchal family pattern A family style in which the male assumes the dominant role.

pediatric rehabilitation nursing Specialty practice that focuses on the care of children with disabilities or other chronic conditions and their families.

peer assistance program Administers contract agreements requiring a nurse to undergo treatment and monitoring to keep his or her license in good standing.

peer review An appraisal by professional co-workers (of equal status) of the way an individual nurse conducts practice, education, or research.

per diem An agreed upon daily rate of payment for a service.

percent Hundredths; symbolized as %.

percussion Using fingertips to tap the body's surface to produce vibration and sound.

percutaneous Through the skin or mucous membrane.

perinatal Period during pregnancy that begins with the onset of labor and ends with delivery of the placenta; sometimes called intrapartal.

perineal care Care given to the genitalia.

peripheral Pertaining to the outside, surface, or surrounding area of an organ, other structure or field of vision.

pernicious anemia A progressive megaloblastic, macrocytic anemia that results from a lack of intrinsic factor essential for the absorption of vitamin B_{12}.

personal health record An electronic record in which patients are allowed to input and update their own health information.

personal hygiene Self-care measures that people use to maintain their health.

personality Refers to the relatively consistent set of attitudes and behaviors particular to an individual; it consists of a pattern of mental, emotional, and behavioral tracts of a person.

pesthouse A home or hospital used to house and care for patients with infections.

phagocytes White blood cells that are able to surround, engulf, and digest microorganisms and cellular debris.

pharmaceuticals Drugs, or drug-based products or preparations.

pharmacology Study of drugs and their actions on the living body.

phobia An anxiety disorder characterized by obsessive, irrational, and intense fear of a specific object or activity.

phosphorus Chiefly, an intracellular anion in fluid of the body.

phototherapy Treatment for hyperbilirubinemia and jaundice in the newborn that involves the exposure of light; accelerates the excretion of bilirubin in the skin, decomposing it by photooxidation.

physiologic jaundice Jaundice usually occurring 48 hours or later after birth, gradually disappearing by the 7th to 10th day; caused by the normal reduction in the number of red blood cells. The infant is otherwise well.

pica Craving to eat nonfood substances.

placebo effect Positive response to treatment that has no known medical effect.

placental barrier Obstruction, boundary, or separation provided by the placental tissue between the fetal and maternal circulation; substances of small size, excluding blood cells, may cross this barrier.

planning In the five-step nursing process, a category of nursing behavior in which a strategy is designed for the achievement of the goals of care for an individual patient, as established in assessing and analyzing. Planning includes developing and modifying a care plan for the patient, cooperating with other personnel, and recording relevant information.

pleural space The potential space between the visceral and parietal layers of the pleurae.

pneumothorax A collection of air or gas in the pleural space, causing the lung to collapse.

point-of-care (POC) Computer electronic health record systems that are located at the patient's bedside.

poison A substance that is toxic.

poisoning The condition or physical state produced by the ingestion, injection, inhalation, or exposure of a poisonous (toxic) substance.

polydactyly More digits (finger or toes) than normal.

POMR *See* problem-oriented medical record.

portfolio A file of items accumulated that highlight an individual's educational and professional accolades.

postmortem care Care of the body after death.

postpartal The final stage of the maternity cycle; from Latin *post*, "after."

posture The position of the body. It may refer to the position when standing, sitting or lying.

potassium The dominant intracellular cation.

potentiation When one drug increases the action or effect of another drug.

preceptor Person assigned to support a new or transferred employee through clinical orientation.

preeclampsia An abnormal condition of pregnancy characterized by the onset of acute hypertension after the 24th week of gestation.

pregnancy-induced hypertension (PIH) A disease encountered during pregnancy or early in the puerperium, characterized by increasing hypertension, albuminuria, and generalized edema. Also called *gestational hypertension (GH)*.

prenatal Before birth; occurring or existing before birth; referring to both the care of the woman during pregnancy and the growth and development of the fetus.

preoperational thought stage Piaget's phase of child development during the period of 2 to 7 years of age, when the child focuses on the use of language as a tool. The child has the emerging ability to reason.

presbycusis A normal loss of hearing acuity, speech intelligibility, auditory threshold, and pitch associated with aging.

presbyopia Defect in vision in advancing age involving loss of accommodation or recession of near vision; due to loss of elasticity of crystalline lens.

priapism Persistent penile erection.

primary caregiver One who assumes ongoing responsibility for health maintenance and therapy for the ill.

primary (deciduous) teeth Baby teeth that normally appear during infancy.

primary intention A wound that has been made surgically and has little tissue loss; skin edges are close together and minimal scarring results.

problem Any health care condition that requires diagnostic, therapeutic, or educational action.

problem list Prioritized master list of the patient's active, inactive, temporary, and at-risk medical or other problems; serves as an index to the rest of the record.

problem-oriented medical record (POMR) Method of recording data about the health status of a patient in a problem-solving system. Parts included are the database, problem list, initial plan, and progress notes.

prodromal Early sign of a developing condition or disease.

prolactin A hormone secreted from the anterior pituitary gland that is responsible for stimulating milk production in the mammary alveolar cells.

pronation Palm of the hand turned down.

prone Lying face down on the abdomen.

proning Turning the patient to a prone position for better posterior lung field ventilation and clearing of secretions.

proportion Shows that the relationship between two ratios has equal value.

proximodistal Growth and development that moves from the center toward the outside. The infant gains control of the shoulders before developing control of the hands and fingers.

pruritus The symptoms of itching; an uncomfortable sensation leading to the urge to scratch; scratching often leads to secondary infection. Some causes of pruritus are allergy, infection, elevated serum urea, jaundice, and skin irritation.

pseudomenstruation Discharge of blood-tinged mucus from the vagina of the newborn, which occurs in response to maternal hormones.

psychoactive drugs Drugs that make the user feel good but have the potential to be abused or addicting.

psychogenic Relating to causes that are emotional, psychological, or nonorganic in origin.

psychosis Any major disorder characterized by gross impairment in reality testing; the affected person exhibits moderate to severe personality disintegration.

psychosocial A combination of psychological and social factors.

puerperium Period of time after the third stage of labor and lasting until involution of the uterus takes place, usually about 3 to 6 weeks.

pulse A rhythmic beating or vibrating movement; regular recurrent expansion and contraction of an artery produced by waves of pressure caused by the ejection of blood from the left ventricle of the heart as it contracts.

pulse deficit A condition that exists when the radial pulse rate is less than the ventricular rate as auscultated at the apex of the heart.

pulse oximeter Device used to measure the oxygen saturation.

pulse pressure Difference between the systolic and diastolic blood pressures, usually 30 to 40 mm Hg.

pulverized Crushed to a powder.

puncture A perforation that my be the result of an accidental or intentional action.

purulent Producing or containing pus.

Q

Qi Life force.

quality assurance/assessment/improvement In health care, any evaluation of services provided and the results achieved as compared with accepted standards.

quality of life A measure of the optimum energy that endows a person with the power to cope successfully with the full range of challenges encountered in the real world.

R

RACE A formula to enable nurses to be prepared when safety is threatened by fire; *R*escue the patient, sound the *A*larm, *C*onfine the fire, *E*xtinguish or *E*vacuate.

race A group of people who share biologic and physical characteristics.

racism Any ethnocentric activity—cultural, individual, or institutional, deliberate or not—that is based on a belief in the superiority of one racial group over other racial groups; the oppression of, thus maintaining control over, these groups.

range of motion (ROM) Normal movement that any given joint is capable of making. Any body action involving the muscles, joints, and natural directional movements.

rapid eye movement (REM) One of the two highly individualized sleeping states that follows NREM state. May last from a few minutes to a half an hour and alternate with NREM periods; dreaming occurs during this time.

ratio Relationship of one number or quantity to another number or quantity.

raves All-night parties or "trances"; often the scene of club drug use.

receiver The individual or individuals to whom a message is conveyed.

receptive aphasia A physiological condition in which an individual cannot recognize or interpret the message being received.

receptivity Willingness to take in and accept new experiences.

receptors Molecules that recognize or respond to specific invaders.

reciprocity Mutual agreement to exchange privilege, dependence, or relationships as an agreement between two governing bodies to accept the credit of caregivers licensed in each state. True reciprocity means that individuals licensed in one state can automatically receive licensure in the next, even if the licensure requirements of the states differ.

recording Process of adding written information to the chart, usually at prescribed intervals.

Reed-Sternberg cells Atypical histiocytes; large, abnormal, multinucleated cells in the lymphatic system, found in Hodgkin's lymphoma.

referred pain Pain that is felt at a site other than in the injured or diseased organ or part of the body.

reflecting A communication technique that assists the patient to "reflect" on inner feelings and thoughts rather than seeking answers or advice from someone else.

reflexology A form of complementary and alternative medicine based on the premise that zones and reflexes in different parts of the body correspond to all parts, glands, and organs of the entire body. In reflexology it is thought that the entire body can be reached by applying pressure to specific areas on the feet.

Reiki A form of alternative health treatment that originated in Japan. It is focused on the promotion of health and wellness through relaxation techniques.

relaxation The state of generalized decreased cognitive, physiologic, or behavioral arousal.

relaxin Ovarian hormone that softens and relaxes joints and ligaments to facilitate labor and delivery.

reservoir Any natural habitat of a microorganism that promotes growth and reproduction.

resident assessment instrument (RAI) A comprehensive tool that includes the minimum data set, resident assessment protocols, and guidelines for functional assessment of the resident.

residential care A care setting for older adults, providing a wide range of services, such as assisted living and continuing care.

residual urine Urine remaining in the urinary tract after voiding.

residue Bulk in the colon that includes undigested food, fiber, bacteria, body secretions, and cells.

resignation Act of resigning; giving up a position of employment.

respirations The taking in of oxygen, its use in the tissues, and the giving off of carbon dioxide; the act of breathing (i.e., inhaling and exhaling).

respite care Period of relief from responsibilities for the care of a patient.

restating A communication technique that involves the nurse repeating to the patient what the nurse believes to be the main point that the patient is trying to convey.

restitution In obstetrics, the turning of the fetal head to the left or right after it has completely emerged from the introitus of the vagina as it assumes a normal alignment with the infant's shoulders.

restorative nursing care Basic concepts of physical therapy for maintenance of functional mobility and physical activity.

résumé A summary of educational and professional experiences, including activities and honors, to be used in seeking employment for biologic citations on professional meeting programs or related purposes; curriculum vitae.

retrovirus Lentivirus that contains reverse transcriptase, which is essential for reverse transcription (the production of a deoxyribonucleic acid [DNA] molecule from a ribonucleic acid [RNA] model).

risk nursing diagnosis A clinical judgment that an individual, family, or community is more vulnerable to develop the problem than others in same or similar situation.

role A socially expected behavior pattern associated with an individual's function in various social groups.

S

safety reminder device (SRD) Any one of numerous devices used to immobilize a patient; formerly referred to as a restraint.

saline infusion ultrasound Facilitates visualization of the uterus by infusing saline through a small catheter.

sandwich generation A group of people who find themselves captured between caring for their own children and their aging parents.

sanguineous Pertaining to blood.

sarcoma Malignant tumor of connective tissues such as muscle or bone; usually presents as a painless swelling.

satiety Feeling of fullness and satisfaction from food.

savants Children with autism who excel in particular areas such as art, music, memory, mathematics, or perceptual skills such as puzzle building.

sex trafficking A type of maltreatment that refers to the recruitment, harboring, transportation, provision, or obtaining of a person for the purpose of a commercial sex act.

schema Innate knowledge structure that allows a child to organize his or her mind.

schizophrenia Any one of a large group of psychotic disorders characterized by gross distortion of reality, disturbances of language and communication, and disorganized and fragmented thought, perception, and emotional reaction.

school avoidance Repeated absence from school of a child who is physically healthy.

school violence Anything that physically or psychologically injures schoolchildren or damages school property.

secondary intention Healing that occurs when skin edges of the wound are not close together or when pus is formed.

self A complex concept comprising four distinct parts: personal identity, body image, role performance, and self-esteem.

self-concept How an individual views the self; pertains to personal identity, body image, role, and self-esteem.

semi-Fowler's position The position a patient assumes while lying in bed; the head of the bed is raised to about 30 degrees, and the foot of the bed is raised slightly.

sender The person conveying a message.

senescence stage The last stage of the life cycle that requires the older adult to cope with a long range of changes.

senile The state of physical and mental deterioration associated with aging.

senility Pertaining to or characteristic of old age or the process of aging.

sensitivity A laboratory method of determining the effectiveness of antibiotics. A report of resistance means that the antibiotic is not effective in inhibiting the growth of a pathogen, whereas use of an effective antibiotic results in a sensitive report.

sensorimotor stage The developmental phase of childhood encompassing the period from birth to 2 years of age, according to Piaget's psychology. In this stage, an infant's knowledge of the world comes about primarily through sensory impressions and motor activities.

sensory deprivation An involuntary loss of physical awareness caused by detachment from external sensory stimuli.

sentinel event Any unexpected occurrence involving death or serious physical or psychological injury, or the risk thereof.

separation anxiety Fear and apprehension caused by separation from familiar surroundings and significant people.

sequestrum A fragment of necrotic bone that is partially or entirely detached from the surrounding or adjacent healthy bone.

seroconversion The development of detectable levels of antibodies; a change in serologic tests (e.g., ELISA and Western blot) from negative to positive as antibodies develop in reaction to an infection.

seronegative Negative result on serologic examination. The state of lacking HIV antibodies; confirmed by blood tests.

serosanguineous Thin, red exudate composed of serum and blood.

serotonin syndrome A potentially life-threatening condition that can occur as a result of an interaction between a selective serotonin reuptake inhibitor (SSRI) and another serotonergic agent.

serous Thin, watery exudate composing the serum portion of blood.

severe preeclampsia An elevation in blood pressure of 160/100 or higher accompanied by severe proteinuria in a pregnant woman that results after 20 weeks' gestation. The elevated blood pressure readings must be on at least two occasions 6 hour apart.

shearing forces Applied forces or pressure exerted against the surface and layers of the skin as tissue slides in opposite but parallel planes.

shock Abnormal condition of inadequate blood flow to peripheral tissues, with life-threatening cellular dysfunction, hypotension, and oliguria.

sickled cell Erythrocyte whose characteristic round shape has altered to an elongated crescent shape.

sign An objective finding as perceived by the examiner; a sign can be seen, heard, measured, or felt by the examiner.

simple face mask A device used to administer oxygen at a rate of 5 to 8 L/min.

Sims' position Lying on the left side with the right knee and thigh drawn upward toward the chest; the chest and abdomen are allowed to fall forward.

single-parent family Family group that occurs when one parent leaves the nuclear family because of divorce, separation, desertion, or death. May also be the result of an unwed parent living alone or the decision of a single person to adopt a child.

SBAR (Situation, Background, Assessment, Recommendation) A common communication tool used in health care between the care team. It focuses on identifying pertinent issues related to the situation, background, assessment, and recommendation.

situational loss Loss occurring suddenly in response to a specific external event.

skilled nursing care The provision of care by a team of trained and/or licensed heath care providers.

skilled nursing facility Houses a subacute unit with a stronger rehabilitative focus and shorter length of stay than a long-term facility.

SOAPE Charting format used in POMR. Components include subjective data (S) reported by the patient; objective data (O) acquired by inspection, percussion, auscultation, and palpation and by tests, usually measurable findings; assessment (A) of the problem; plan (P) of care; and evaluation (E) of the patient's response to the treatment plan.

SOAPIER Same as SOAPE charting except that intervention (I) and revision (R) are added. Interventions are specific actions carried out, and revisions are the changes to be made to the original plan.

social contract family/cohabitation Unmarried couple living together and sharing roles and responsibilities similar to those of the nuclear family structure.

society A nation, community, or broad group of people who establish particular aims, beliefs, or standards of living and conduct.

sodium The most abundant electrolyte in the body; the major extracellular electrolyte; it is a cation.

somatization A disorder characterized by recurrent, multiple, physical complaints and symptoms for which there is no organic cause.

souffle cup Ungraduated, disposable paper cup.

specimen A small sample of something, intended to show the nature of the whole, such as a urine specimen.

sphygmomanometer Device for measuring arterial blood pressure.

spinal cord injury (SCI) An injury in which the spinal cord is compressed by fractures or displaced vertebrae, bleeding, or edema.

spore The reproductive cell of some microorganisms such as fungi or protozoa. These cells are highly resistant to heat and chemicals. Under proper environmental conditions they may revert to an actively multiplying form of bacterium (e.g., gas gangrene or tetanus).

stages of dependence The three characteristic stages of dependence, which are chronic, incurable, and progressive.

standard precautions A set of guidelines set forth by the CDC to reduce the risk of transmission of bloodborne pathogens and pathogens for moist body substances. These precautions promote handwashing and use of gloves, masks, eye protection, and gowns when appropriate for patient contact. These precautions are designed to reduce the risk of transmission of microorganisms from both recognized and unrecognized sources of infection.

standardized languages A structured vocabulary that provides nurses with a common means of communication.

standards of care Those acts that are permitted to be performed or prohibited from being performed by a prudent person working within the limits of the training, licensing, experience, and conditions existing at the time of the duty to give care.

stapedectomy The removal of the stapes of the middle ear and insertion of a graft and prosthesis.

steatorrhea Excessive fat in the feces.

stereotype A generalization about a form of behavior, an individual, or a group.

sterilization A process by which all microorganisms, including their spores, are destroyed.

stethoscope Instrument placed against patient's body to hear heart, lung, or bowel sounds.

stimulants Drugs that affect the central nervous system.

stomatitis Inflammation of the mouth due to destruction of normal cells of the oral cavity that may result from infection by bacteria, viruses, or fungi from exposure to certain chemicals or drugs, vitamin deficiency, or systemic inflammatory disease.

street drugs Substances (drugs) sold to users illegally by drug dealers and that are manufactured without strict controls, illegally obtained prescription drugs, or drugs not approved for use in the United States.

stress The nonspecific response of the body to any demand made on it.

stressor A situation, activity, or event that produces stress.

stridor Harsh sound made during respirations; high pitched and resembling the blowing of wind; due to obstruction of air passages.

subacute unit Institutional setting that provides a less expensive alternative to acute care; a bridge between acute care and long-term care.

subculture A group that shares many characteristics with the primary culture but has characteristic patterns of behavior and ideals that distinguish it from the rest of a cultural group.

subjective data Symptoms; verbal statements provided by the patient. That which arises from within or is perceived by the individual and related to the examiner.

sublingual Under the tongue.

subluxation Partial dislocation.

sundowning syndrome Sometimes referred to as nocturnal delirium. Manifested by increased disorientation and agitation only during the evening and nighttime. Seen more often in older adults.

supination Kind of rotation that allows the palm of the hand to turn up.

supine Being in the horizontal position, lying face upward.

surfactant Lipoprotein necessary for normal respiratory function that prevents alveolar collapse (atelectasis); may be necessary for preterm infants.

surgical asepsis A group of techniques that destroy all microorganisms and their spores (sterile technique).

surrogacy The agreement a woman makes to be artificially inseminated, voluntarily or for a fee, to bear a child and then relinquish parental rights to the baby's natural father or another couple.

surveillance Exercise of continuous scrutiny of and watchfulness over the distribution and spread of infections and factors related thereto, of sufficient accuracy and completeness to be effective control.

symptom Subjective indication of a disease or a change in condition as perceived by the patient.

syncope A transient loss of consciousness due to inadequate blood flow to the brain (fainting).

syndactyly Malformation of digits, commonly seen as a fusion of two or more toes to form one structure.

syndrome nursing diagnosis Used when a cluster of actual or risk nursing diagnoses are predicted to be present in certain circumstances.

synergistic Action of two or more substances or organs to achieve an effect of which each is capable.

systolic The number or reading that represents ventricles contracting, forcing blood into the aorta and pulmonary arteries. In blood pressure readings, it is the higher of the two readings.

T

T-tube A tube inserted through the skin to provide drainage from a wound or cavity.

tachycardia An abnormal condition in which the myocardium contracts regularly but at a rate greater than 100 beats per minute.

tachypnea An abnormally rapid rate of breathing.

T'ai chi/Taiji Martial arts practice that emphasizes relaxing the body and focusing the mind; Tai chi movement is performed slowly, accentuating the intention, mechanics, accuracy, and precision of motion.

temperature Relative measure of sensible heat or cold.

teratogen Any substance, agent, or process that interferes with normal prenatal development, causing the formation of one or more developmental abnormalities in the fetus.

teratogenic agent *See* teratogen.

terminal illness An advanced stage of disease with no known cure and poor prognosis.

terrorism Use or threats of violence by individuals or organized groups using biological, chemical, or nuclear weapons against society or government for political gain.

tertiary intention Healing that occurs by primary intention with delayed suturing of a wound in which two layers of granulation tissue are sutured together.

tetanus toxoid Active agent prepared from detoxified tetanus toxin that produces an antigenic response in the body, conferring permanent immunity to tetanus infection.

tetrahydrocannabinol A compound of marijuana.

thanatologist One who studies dying and death.

thanatology The study of dying and death.

therapeutic Beneficial.

therapeutic communication A form of communication that facilitates the formation of a positive nurse-patient relationship.

therapeutic diet A diet used as a medical treatment.

therapeutic massage The manipulation of the soft tissues of the body to assist with healing.

third-party payers Entities (persons or elements) other than the giver or receiver of service responsible for payment (e.g., Medicare or an insurance company).

thrill Fine vibration sensation along the artery, which is palpated by the examiner.

thrombocytopenia An abnormal hematologic condition in which the number of platelets is reduced to fewer than $100,000/mm^3$.

titrate Slowly increasing the amount of drug to find the therapeutic dose.

tolerance A state that develops as the amount and frequency of use of an addicting substance increases to achieve the same effect.

topical application Applied to the skin.

TORCH (*Toxoplasmosis, Other, Rubella virus, Cytomegalovirus,* and *Herpes* simplex viruses) Group of agents that can infect the fetus or the newborn infant, causing a constellation of morbid effects called TORCH syndrome.

total parenteral nutrition (TPN) The administration of a hypertonic solution into a large central vein, usually the superior vena cava, via a catheter threaded through either the subclavian or internal jugular vein.

tourniquet Constricting device applied to control bleeding.

toxicity The level of exposure to a substance that the body will experience detriment.

toxicologic analysis Scientific study of poisons, their detection, and their effects.

tracheostomy A surgical opening into the trachea through which an indwelling tube may be inserted; created by a tracheotomy.

traditional (block) chart Conventional patient chart broken down into sections or blocks; included are admission data, physicians' orders, history and physical examination, nursing care plan, nurses' notes and graphics, progress notes, and test data.

transcribe To write or type a copy.

transcultural nursing An integration of the nurse's understanding of culture into all aspects of nursing care.

transcutaneous electrical nerve stimulation (TENS) A type of pain control that is managed with a pocket-sized, battery-operated device that provides a continuous, mild electrical current to the skin via electrodes.

transdisciplinary rehabilitation team Team characterized by the blurring of boundaries between discipline and by cross-training and flexibility to minimize duplication of effort toward individual goal attainment.

transfer Moving a patient from one unit to another (intra-agency transfer) or moving a patient from one health care facility to another (interagency transfer).

transgender family A family unit that is composed of one or both of the parents who have undergone gender reassignment or who are nonconforming to their gender as identified at birth.

traumatic brain injury Head injury classified as either penetrating or closed; may also be classified as mild, moderate, severe, or catastrophic.

Trendelenburg's position A position in which the patient is lying supine with the head lower than the body with body and legs elevated and on an incline.

triage Process of classifying a group of patients as to the severity of injury and need of care.

trimester One of the three periods of approximately 3 months into which pregnancy is divided.

tube feeding Administration of nutritionally balanced liquefied food or formula through a tube inserted into the stomach, duodenum, or jejunum by way of nasoenteric or a feeding ostomy.

turgor The normal resiliency of the skin caused by the outward pressure of the cells and interstitial fluid; may be assessed as increased or decreased skin turgor.

two-way communication A form of communication that requires that both the sender and the receiver participate equally in the interaction.

tympanic Membranous eardrum.

tympany A high-pitched drumlike sound produced by performing percussion over a hollow organ such as the stomach.

U

ultrasonography The process of imaging deep structures of the body by measuring and recording the reflection of pulsed or continuous high-frequency sound waves. Also called *sonography*.

umbilicus Point on the abdomen at which the umbilical cord joined the fetus. In most adults it is marked by a depression.

unassertive communication A style of communication in which the sender sacrifices legitimate personal rights to meet the needs of the receiver, often resulting in feelings of resentment.

unconscious bias An inherent decision-making shortcut that nearly all people possess as a part of brain efficiency

unresolved grief A disturbance in the normal progression toward resolution.

urinal A device for receiving urine; may be used with male or female; may be used for specimen collection.

urinary catheter A hollow, flexible tube that can be inserted into the bladder through the meatus and urethra to withdraw urine or instill medication or an irrigant.

urinary retention The inability to empty the bladder completely.

urostomy An opening through the skin created to provide an outlet for urinary elimination.

uterine inertia Absence or weakness of uterine contractions during labor.

V

Vacutainer Container used in blood collection.

vacuum-assisted closure An intervention used to provide wound healing and closure by withdrawing fluids from the cavity and pulling the wound closed by use of negative pressure.

value clarification A process of self-inspection to identify one's own beliefs, morals, and values.

values Individual's intrinsic (or personal) beliefs about the importance of a particular idea, object, or custom that will influence behavior.

vapotherm Non-invasive, mask-free high flow oxygen delivery device delivering up to 40L/min.

variance The unexpected event that occurs during the use of a clinical pathway; can be positive or negative.

vasoconstriction When the lumen of the blood vessel narrows, thus hindering blood flow and resulting in less edema.

vasodilation When the lumen of the blood vessel widens, thus increasing the blood flow.

vastus lateralis muscle Located on the anterior (front) of thigh, this site is preferred for injections in children.

vector A living carrier for transmission of microorganisms.

vegan Vegetarian whose diet excludes all foods of animal origin.

vehicle The means by which organisms are carried about.

venipuncture Most common method of drawing a blood sample, involving inserting a hollow-bore needle into the lumen of a large vein.

venturi mask An oxygen delivery device used to administer a precise concentration of oxygen to a patient.

verbal communication A form of communication that involves the use of spoken or written words or symbols.

verdict Decision rendered based on the facts of a case, evidence and testimony presented, credibility of witnesses, and laws pertaining to the case.

vernix caseosa Protective, gray-white fatty substance of cheesy consistency covering the fetal skin at birth.

vertigo The sensation that the outer world is revolving about oneself or that one is moving in space.

villi Short vascular processes or protrusions clustered over the entire mucous surface of the small intestine.

virulent Having the power to produce disease; of or pertaining to a very pathogenic or rapidly progressive condition.

visual analog scale An objective means of assessing pain severity; it consists of a straight line, representing a continuum of intensity, and has visual descriptors at each end.

vital signs Measurement of temperature, pulse, respiration, and blood pressure.

W

weaning Gradually eliminating breastfeeding or bottle feedings, replaced by cup and table feeding.

wellness A dynamic state of health in which an individual progresses toward a higher level of functioning, achieving an optimum balance between internal and external environments.

wellness nursing diagnosis A clinical judgment about an individual, group, or community in transition from a specific level of wellness to a higher level of wellness.

Western blot A laboratory blood test to detect the presence of antibodies to a specific antigen; used in diagnosing HIV.

Wharton's jelly Gelatinous tissue that remains when the embryonic body stalk blends with the yolk sac within the umbilical cord.

wheeze Adventitious breath sounds that have a whistling or sighing sound resulting from narrowing of the lumen of a respiratory passageway. May be heard both on inspiration and expiration. Wheezes characteristically clear on coughing.

wound An injury to body tissue. The injury may be intentional or accidental.

Y

yoga Holistic system of mind-body connection that includes control of the body through correct posture and breathing, control of the emotions and mind, and meditation and contemplation.

Z

zygote Cell formed by the union of two reproductive cells; the fertilized ovum resulting from the union of a sperm and ovum from the time it is fertilized until, as a blastocyst, it is implanted in the uterus.

Index